WATSON'S
Medical–Surgical Nursing and Related Physiology

WATSON'S
Medical–Surgical Nursing and Related Physiology

FOURTH EDITION

EDITED BY

Joan A. Royle RN, MScN

Associate Professor, School of Nursing,
Faculty of Health Sciences, McMaster University;

Clinical Nurse Specialist, St Joseph's Hospital,
Hamilton, Ontario, Canada

AND

Mike Walsh BA, RGN, PGCE, DipN

Course Coordinator, BA Nursing Studies,
St Martin's College, Lancaster, UK

Baillière Tindall

LONDON PHILADELPHIA TORONTO
SYDNEY TOKYO

This book is printed on acid free paper.

Baillière Tindall 24–28 Oval Road
W.B. Saunders   London NW1 7DX

The Curtis Center
Independence Square West
Philadelphia, PA 19106–3399, USA

55 Horner Avenue
Toronto, Ontario M8Z 4X6, Canada

Harcourt Brace Jovanovich Group (Australia) Pty Ltd,
30–52 Smidmore St
Marrickville, NSW 2204, Australia

Harcourt Brace Jovanovich Japan Inc.
Ichibancho Central Building, 22–1 Ichibancho
Chiyoda-ku, Tokyo 102, Japan

First edition published 1972 by W.B. Saunders Company as
Medical–Surgical Nursing and Related Physiology, by Jeannette E.
Watson.
Second edition published 1979 by W.B. Saunders Company
Third edition published 1987 by Baillière Tindall as _Watson's
Medical–Surgical Nursing and Related Physiology_, by Jeannette E.
Watson and Joan Royle
Fourth edition published 1992 by Baillière Tindall as _Watson's
Medical–Surgical Nursing and Related Physiology_, by Joan A. Royle
and Mike Walsh

Typeset by Columns Design and Production Services, Reading
Printed in Great Britain by Butler and Tanner Ltd, Frome, Somerset

A catalogue record for this book is available from the British
Library

ISBN 0–7020–1515–6

Contents

UK Contributors

This Edition has been extensively revised and adapted for UK usage by experts in clinical nursing and nurse education:

June Andrews, MA, RMN, RGN
Assistant Director, DMPP, Royal College of Nursing, London, UK (Chapter 4)

Patricia A. Cooksley, RGN, CMBI, DipN (Lond.)
Clinical Nurse Specialist, Department of Neurology, Derriford District General Hospital, Plymouth, Devon, UK (Chapter 21)

Susan Day, BSc, RGN, Cert Ed
Senior Lecturer in Nursing, Bristol Polytechnic, Bristol, UK (Chapters 18, 19)

Sylvia Denton, RGN, RHV, ONC CERT, FRCN
Commissioning Nurse/Clinical Nurse Manager, Mid Kent Oncology Unit, Maidstone, Kent, UK; formerly Group Senior Nurse, Breast Unit, Royal Marsden Hospital, London, UK (Chapter 23)

Nancy Hallett, SRN, DipN, DipNEd
Senior Nurse, Cancer Services, Directorate, St Bartholomew's Hospital, London, UK (Chapter 9)

Cathryn P. Havard, BA (Hons), DipN (Lond.), RGN, Oncology Nursing Certificate
Senior Lecturer in Nursing, Bristol Polytechnic, Bristol, UK (Chapter 10)

Damaris Jones, RGN, BA (Hons)
Clinical Nurse Manager (Operating Theatres), Bristol Royal Infirmary, Bristol, UK (Chapter 11)

Maggie Judd, BA, RGN, Cert Ed, RNT
Nurse Teacher, Avon College of Health, Glenside Hospital, Bristol, Avon, UK (Chapters 24, 25)

John Perry, RGN, OND, RNT
Director of Nursing Services, Manchester Royal Eye Hospital, Manchester, UK (Chapter 28)

Miriam K. Rowswell, MSc, BSc (Hons), RGN, DipN (London)
Lecturer in Nursing, Department of Nursing Studies, King's College London, London, UK (Chapter 13)

David R. Thompson, BSc, PhD, RGN, RMN, ONC
Clinical Nurse Specialist, Coronary Care Unit, Leicester General Hospital, Leicester, UK (Chapter 14)

Anne E. Topping, RGN, BSc (Hons), Cert Ed (FE)
Senior Lecturer in Nursing/Health Studies, School of Human & Health Studies, The Polytechnic, Huddersfield, UK (Chapters 16, 17, 20)

Mike Walsh, BA, RGN, PGCE, DipN
Course Coordinator, BA Nursing Studies, St Martin's College, Lancaster, UK (Chapters 1, 2, 3, 5, 6, 7, 8, 12, 15,26)

Barbara A. Walters, RGN, RM, PDN Cert, RCT DipN (Lond.), DNE (Lond.) RNT
Nurse Tutor, St Bartholomew's College of Nursing & Midwifery, London, UK (Chapter 22)

Janet Whelan, BSc, SRN, MSc
Macmillan Lecturer in Cancer Nursing, Royal Marsden Hospital, London, UK (Chapter 27)

North American Contributors

M. Leslea Anderson, RN, MS
Clinical Nurse Specialist,
Hamilton Psychiatric Hospital

Associate Clinical Professor,
McMaster University,
Hamilton, Ontario, Canada
(Chapter 24)

Andrea Baumann, RN, PhD
Associate Dean Health Sciences (Nursing)
McMaster University,
Hamilton, Ontario, Canada
(Chapter 21)

Margaret Black, RN, MScN
Assistant Professor,
McMaster University

Clinical Nurse Consultant (Gerontology)
Hamilton-Wentworth Regional Department of Public Health
Services,
Hamilton, Ontario, Canada
(Chapter 4)

Lee Ann Bourdon, RN, BScN, BA
Head Nurse, Acute Care Unit,
St Joseph's Hospital,
Hamilton, Ontario, Canada
(Chapter 12)

Donna Ciliska, RN, PhD
Associate Professor,
McMaster University

Clinical Nurse Consultant,
Hamilton-Wentworth Regional Department of Public Health
Services, Hamilton,
Ontario, Canada
(Chapters 2, 18)

Geoff Coates, MB, BS, MSc, FRCP
Professor Radiology and Nuclear Medicine,
McMaster University,
Director Research, Associate Chairman,
Department of Radiology,
Chedoke-McMaster Hospitals,
Hamilton, Ontario, Canada
(Sections on Nuclear Medicine)

Michael D. Coughlin, PhD
Ethics Consultant,
St Joseph's Hospital

Associate Professor,
Biomedical Sciences, McMaster University,
Hamilton, Ontario, Canada
(Sections on Ethics)

Mary Fawcett, RN, BScN, MHSc
Associate Professor,
McMaster University

Clinical Nurse Specialist,
Hamilton General Hospital,
Hamilton, Ontario, Canada
(Chapter 21)

Ingrid Fell, RN, BScN, MSc (Teaching)
Nursing Supervisor,
St Elizabeth Visiting Nurses Association,
Hamilton, Ontario, Canada
(Chaper 7)

Cheryl Forchuk, RN, PhD (candidate)
Clinical Nurse Specialist,
Hamilton Psychiatric Hospital

Associate Clinical Professor,
McMaster University,
Hamilton, Ontario, Canada
(Sections in Chapter 5)

Jo Ann E.T. Fox Threlkeld, RN, BN, MSc, PhD
Professor, McMaster University,
Hamilton, Ontario, Canada
(Sections on Gastrointestinal Physiology)

Esther Green, RN, BScN, MSc (Teaching)
Director of Nursing, Education and Practice
The Ontario Cancer Institute, Incorporating the Princess
Margaret Hospital, Toronto

Clinical Lecturer, McMaster University,
Hamilton, Ontario, Canada
(Chapter 3)

Tracy Hildebrandt, RN, MN
Clinical Nurse Specialist,
St Boniface General Hospital,
Winnipeg, Manitoba, Canada
(Sections on HIV infection)

Diane Isaac
Coordinator, Volunteer Services,
Village Clinic Inc.
Winnipeg, Manitoba, Canada
(Sections on HIV infection)

Colina Jones, MB, ChB, DPH, FRCP(C), DTM&H
Professor of Pathology,
McMaster University

Head of Service, Microbiology,
St Joseph's Hospital,
Hamilton, Ontario, Canada
(Chapter 6)

Janet W. Kenney, RN, PhD
Associate Professor, College of Nursing,
Arizona State University,
Tempe, AZ, USA
(Chapter 1)

Judy Knighton, RN, MScN
  Clinical Nurse Specialist,
  Wellesley Hospital,
  Toronto, Ontario, Canada
  (Chapter 26)

Deborah C. Marcellus, BSc(OT), MD, FRCP(C), MSc
  Terry Fox Fellow with the National Cancer Institute of
  Canada,
  McMaster University,
  Hamilton, Ontario, Canada
  (Consulted on Chapter 13)

Margaret MacLean-Wade, RN, MSN
  Clinical Nurse Specialist (Oncology),
  St Joseph's Health Center,
  Toronto, Ontario, Canada
  (Section on Breast Cancer)

Alba Mitchell, RN, MSc, PhD (candidate)
  Associate Professor,
  McMaster University,
  Hamilton, Ontario, Canada
  (Sections on Inflammatory Bowel Disease)

Sandy Mitchell, RN, MScN
  Clinical Nurse Specialist,
  The Ontario Cancer Institute
  incorporating the Princess Margaret Hospital,
  Toronto, Ontario, Canada
  (Chapter 10)

Jane Stephens Mosley, RN, MScN
  Clinical Nurse Specialist (Cardiology),
  St Joseph's Health Center

  Clinical Associate, University of Toronto,
  Toronto, Ontario, Canada
  (Chapter 14)

Betty Oka, RN, MN
  Ryerson Polytechnical Institute,
  Toronto, Ontario, Canada
  (Chapter 8)

Patricia A. Porterfield, RN, MScN
  Clinical Nurse Specialist,
  Vancouver General Hospital,
  Vancouver, British Columbia, Canada
  (Chapter 9)

Marietta Pupo, RN, MHSc
  Clinical Nurse Specialist,
  St Joseph's Hospital

  Assistant Clinical Professor,
  McMaster University,
  Hamilton, Ontario, Canada
  (Sections on Tracheotomy)

John Rawlinson, MA, FRCS, FRCR
  Fellow in Radiology,
  McMaster University Medical Center,
  Hamilton, Ontario, Canada
  (Sections on Radiology)

Elizabeth Rideout, RN, BN, MHSC, MSc
  Associate Professor,
  McMaster University, health problems,
  Hamilton, Ontario, Canada
  (Chapters 5, 25)

Carolyn Sara Roberts, RN, PhD
  Associate Professor,
  College of Nursing,
  Arizona State University, Tempe, AZ, USA
  (Chapter 1)

Lee Robinson, RN, BN, MSc
  Clinical Nurse Specialist,
  Health Sciences Center,
  Winnipeg, Manitoba, Canada
  (Consulted on Chapter 15)

Joan A. Royle, RN, MScN
  Associate Professor, School of Nursing,
  Faculty of Health Sciences, McMaster University

  Clinical Nurse Specialist, St Joseph's Hospital,
  Hamilton, Ontario, Canada
  (Chapters *6, *7, *8, 13, 15, 16, 17, *18, 19, *20, 23, 26 *Co-
  authored chapters)

Charlene Sandilands, RN, BScN
  Program Manager, Emergency Department,
  St Joseph's Community Health Center,
  Hamilton, Ontario, Canada
  (Chapter 12)

Donna Shields-Pöe, RN, MSc
  Clinical Nurse Specialist
  Mt Sinai Hospital

  Clinical Associate
  University of Toronto
  Toronto, Ontario, Canada
  (Chapter 22)

Lori Schindel Martin, RN, MS (Community Health Nursing)
  Clinical Nurse Specialist,
  St Peter's Hospital,
  Hamilton, Ontario, Canada
  (Chapter 20)

Leslie Vincent, RN, BScN, MScA
  Associate Program Director,
  Nursing and Clinical Nurse Specialist,
  Mount Sinai Hospital

  Clinical Associate, Faculty of Nursing,
  University of Toronto,
  Toronto, Ontario, Canada
  (Chapter 10)

Jan Westwell, RN, MScN
  Clinical Nurse Specialist,
  Hamilton Psychiatric Hospital

  Assistant Clinical Professor,
  McMaster University,
  Hamilton, Ontario, Canada
  (Sections in Chapter 5)

Betty Wong, BScPhm
  Coordinator Clinical Services,
  Pharmacy Department,
  St Joseph's Hospital,
  Hamilton, Ontario, Canada
  (Sections on Pharmacology)

Preface

The Fourth Edition of this major textbook has been prepared with the rapidly changing environment of health care in the early 1990s in mind. Higher standards in nursing education, such as the development of undergraduate courses and the Project 2000 reforms, have occurred at the same time as the emphasis has started to shift from illness to health and from hospital to community care. Nursing is now emerging as a profession in its own right, complementary to medicine but distinct, with its own expanding, research based, discrete body of knowledge. In addition, the threats to health continue to change as the effects of unhealthy lifestyles, poverty and an increasingly aged population take their toll, alongside disease processes such as AIDS.

The student nurse in the 1990s is therefore learning in a different environment to that experienced by his or her counterpart of only a few years ago. It is in response to these changes that the Fourth UK Edition of this well known and respected text has been extensively adapted by a team of UK nursing experts working with Canadian colleagues. The aim has been to make the text as up to date as possible and both clinically and educationally relevant to the needs of the nursing student in the UK.

One of the key foundations of nursing care remains a sound understanding of the physiology of the various systems of the body together with the disease processes which may affect them. This approach, which has long been a feature of this text, has been retained and strengthened for this Edition. However, the roles of psychological and social processes which have often been neglected in the past (and sadly still are in the traditional medical model) are also recognized and incorporated into the caring model which this book offers as good nursing practice. The authors firmly believe that a synthesis of the psychosocial and physiological approaches to care is a fundamental requirement of professional nursing. It is only through this process that the patient is placed where he or she belongs, centre stage as a real person with a whole range of problems needing care and support from the nurse.

The editors would like to acknowledge the following people: Jeannette Watson, teacher, mentor and friend, who personally wrote the first two editions of this text. Her contributions to the nursing literature have influenced the development of several generations of nursing students in many countries. The Canadian authors of chapters in previous editions of this text whose work provided a sound basis for the current revisions: Patricia M. Kearns, RN, MScN, Director of Education and Professional Standards, St Joseph's Health Center, Toronto and Rose Kinash, RN, MScN, Associate Professor, College of Nursing, University of Saskatchewan, Saskatoon.

We also thank the health professionals who shared their clinical knowledge and expertise for this current revision: Phyllis Allen, RN, Enterostomal Therapist, St Joseph's Hospital, Hamilton; Denise Bryant Lukosius, RN, BScN, Nurse Clinician, Haematology/Oncology, Henderson General Hospital, Hamilton; W. Peter Cockshott, MD, Professor, Department of Radiology, McMaster University, Hamilton; Barbara Ferraro, FN, BScN, Head Nurse and Susan Gudelis, RN, BScN, Primary Care Nurse, St Joseph's Hospital, Hamilton; Maureen Montemuro, RN, BScN, MHSc, Clinical Nurse Specialist, St Joseph's Hospital and Assistant Clinical Professor, McMaster University, Hamilton; Diane Ollinger, RN, BA, BScN, Nurse Manager, Nephrology, Vancouver General Hospital, Vancouver; Kathy Parker, RN, BScN, Diabetes Nurse Educator, St Joseph's Hospital, Hamilton; Jennifer Skelly, RN, MHSc, MSc, Clinical Nurse Specialist, St Joseph's Hospital and Assistant Clinical Professor, McMaster University, Hamilton, Ontario, Canada.

Aileen Hewer and Ann Fusic of McMaster University School of Nursing for not only the secretarial support they provided but also the many extra tasks and responsibilities they assumed to facilitate communication and maintain schedules.

Finally, we would like to thank all the UK contributors for their hard work in meeting deadlines and getting the job done to such a high standard as well as the publishing and editorial staff without whom I do not know how this would all have been completed!

Joan A. Royle
Mike Walsh

Publisher's Acknowledgements

The publisher would like to thank the following for their kind permission to reproduce material in this book:

Table 1.1 & Table 1.2: Christensen PJ & Kenney JW (eds) (1990) *The Nursing Process: Application of Models*. 3rd edn, St Louis: Mosby.

Table 1.4: Curtin L & Flaherty MJ (1982) *Nursing Ethics: Theories and Pragmatics*. Bowie MD, Brady pp. 59–63.

Table 2.1 & Figure 2.2: Pender N (1987) *Health Promotion & Nursing Practice*. Norwalk, CT: Appleton and Lange.

Figure 2.1: adapted from *Community Health Nursing in Canada* by Miriam Stewart, et al., Chapter 27 "Health Promotion Strategies by Jean Innes and Donna Ciliska. Copyright © Gage Educational Publishing Company. All rights reserved.

Table 3.1: *Safer Sex Guidelines: A Resource Document for Educators and Counsellors*, a report from the Canadian AIDS Society Consultation on Safer Sex (March 1988) Ottawa: Canadian AIDS Society.

Table 3.2: Adams R, Fliegelman E. & Grieco A (1987) *Medical Aspects of Human Sexuality*. **21**: 74–75 New York: Cahners Publishing Company.

Table 3.3: Lewis HR & Lewis ME (1987) What you and your patient need to know about safer sex. *RN* **50(9)**: 53–58. Montvale, NJ: Medical Economics Publishing.

Figure 4.1: Life expectancy at birth, at age 45 and at age 65, England and Wales. Department of Health, UK.

Figure 4.2: UK population and projections (index 1948 = 100) *Annual Abstracts of Statistics*. Newport: Central Statistical Office.

Figure 4.3: Elderly people in residential accommodation in the UK. *Social Trends* © Crown copyright. Newport: Central Statistical Office.

Table 4.1: Gioella EC & Bevil CW (1985) *Nursing Care of the Aging Client: Promoting Healthy Adaptation*. Norwalk CT: Appleton and Lange.
Taylor C, Lillis C & Lemone P (1989) *The Fundamentals of Nursing: The Art and Science of Nursing Care*. Hagerstown, MD: JB Lippincott.

Table 4.2: Whitman et al (1986) *Teaching in Nursing Practice: A Professional Approach*. Norwalk CT, Appleton and Lange.

Figure 5.1: Thornbury KM (1981) Coping: implications for health practitioners *Patient Counselling in Health Education*. Vol. 4, No. 1, p. 6 Shannon: Elsevier Scientific Publishers Ireland Ltd.

Figure 6.1: Burton GRW (1988) *Microbiology for the Health Sciences*. 3rd edn, Hagerstown, MD: JB Lippincott.

Figure 6.4: Dalgleish, AG, Malkovsky & Habeshaw J (1990) in RD Cohen et al (eds) *The Metabolic and Molecular Basis of Acquired Disease*. London: Baillière Tindall. Vol. 2, p.2063.

Table 6.1: Centers for Disease Control (1986) *Morbidity and Mortality Weekly Report*. **37**: 229–234.

Table 6.2: Gauthier DK & Turner JG (1988) The antibody test for AIDS. *AAOHN Journal*. **36**: 266–273. Atlanta, GA: American Association of Occupational Health Nurses.

Table 6.3: Gauthier DK & Turner JG (1989) *American Journal of Infection Control*. **17**: 213–225. St Louis, MO: Mosby-Year-Book Inc.

Table 6.4 & Table 6.5: Beaufoy A, Goldstone I & Riddell R (1988) Aids: what nurses need to know. *The Canadian Nurse/L'infirmière Canadienne*. **84(7)**: 16–27.

Table 6.6: Wittenberg J & Lazenby A (1989) Aids in infancy: diagnostic therapeutic and ethical problems *Canadian Journal of Psychiatry*. **34**: 576–580.

Table 6.7: Centers for Disease Control (1988) *Morbidity and Mortality Weekly Report*. **37**: 377–388.

Table 7.4: Kim et al (1984) *Pocket Guide to Nursing Diagnosis*. St Louis, MO: Mosby Year-Book Inc. Carpenito IJ (1989) *Nursing Diagnosis: Application to Clinical Practice*. 3rd edn, Hagerstown, MD: JB Lippincott.

Table 7.6: Rice V (1984) Shock Management. Part I: Fluid Volume replacement. *Crit. Care Nurs*. **Nov/Dec** pp. 71–73.

Figure 8.1 & Figure 12.1 & Figure 19.3: Vander AJ, Sherman JH & Luciano DS (1990) *Human Physiology: The Mechanisms of Body Function*. New York: McGraw-Hill, p. 595.

Table 9.1 & Table 9.2: McCaffrey M & Beebe A (1989) *Pain: Clinical Manual for Nursing Practice*. St Louis, MO: Mosby Year-Book Inc.

Table 9.4: Narcotics: Approximate Analgesic Equivalences. *MS Contin Product Monograph*. Pickering, Ontario: Purdue Frederick Drug Company.

Figure 9.2: Raiman J *London Hospital Pain Chart*. London Hospital Medical College.

Figure 10.1: Ten most common cancers per new case registered in the UK in 1985. Cancer statistics – Registrations 1985. HMSO 1990.

Figure 10.2 & 10.3: Ten most common causes of cancer deaths registered in the UK in 1989. Five year relative survival % England and Wales 1981. London: Cancer Research Campaign.

Table 10.2: Glasel M (1985) Cancer prevention: the role of the nurse in primary and secondary cancer prevention *Cancer Nursing*. 8 (i) supplement 5–12. New York: Raven Press Ltd.

Table 13.2: Hoffbrand AV & Pettit JE (1984) *Essential Haematology*. Oxford: Blackwell Scientific Publications Ltd.

Table 13.4: Smith LH & Thier SO (1981) *Pathophysiology*. 2nd edn. Philadelphia: WB Saunders.

Figure 13.5: Hirsh J & Brain EA (1983) *Haemostasis and Thrombosis A Conceptual Approach*. 2nd edn. New York: Churchill Livingstone.

Table 13.10: Selfcare management of long term central venous catheters. St Joseph's Hospital, Hamilton, Ontario.

Figure 14.2: Wyper S & Walsh E (1989) The patient with cardiovascular problems. In Lang B & Phillips J. *Medical-Surgical Nursing*. 2nd edn. St Louis: Mosby-Year Book Inc.

Figure 14.7 & Figure 20.4: Guyton AC (1986) *Textbook of Medical Physiology*. 6th edn. Philadelphia: WB Saunders.

Figure 14.8: Vacek J, Smith W & Philips J (1984) Cardiac Electrophysiology. An Overview. *Practical Cardiology*. 10(4) 83–97.

Table 14.3 & Table 14.5: Holloway N (1988) *Nursing the Critically Ill Adult*. 3rd edn. California: Addison Wesley.

Table 14.4: Range of normal resting haemodynamic values. Grossman W & Barry W (1988) In E Braunwald (ed) *Heart Disease*. 3rd edn. Philadelphia: WB Saunders.

Figure 15.18: Secor (1969) *Patient Care in Respiratory Problems*. Philadelphia: WB Saunders, (Courtesy of Harris Calorific Co. Cleveland Ohio).

Table 15.8: Robinson LA & Pugsley SO (1981) Dealing with chronic airflow obstruction. In Anderson SVD and Bauwens EE (eds) *Chronic Health Problems*. St. Louis: Mosby-Year Book Inc.

Figure 16.3: Sleisenger MH & Fordtran JS (eds) (1978) *Gastrointestinal Disease*. 2nd edn. Philadelphia: WB Saunders.

Figure 16.4 & Figure 21.33: Luckman & Sovenson T (1980) *Medical-Surgical Nursing: A Psychophysiologic Approach*. 2nd edn. Philadelphia: WB Saunders, pp. 1415 & 530.

Figure 16.9: Rolsted BS (1987) Innovative surgical procedures and stoma care in the future *Nursing Clinics of North America* 22(2): p. 353.

Figure 16.11: Erickson BJ (1987) Ostomies: the art of pouching *Nursing Clinics of North America*. **22**: 316–317.

Table 16.1 & Table 13.4: Genong WF (1989) *Review of Medical Physiology*. 14th edn. Norwalk CT: Appleton & Lange.

Table 16.5: Metheny N (1988) *Nursing Research*. **37(6)**: 324–329.

Table 16.13: Shipes E (1987) *Nursing Clinics of North America*. **22(2)**: 305.

Table 17.3: Patton F (1981) Hepatitis: Current Concepts. *Crit. Care Nurs*. Vol. 1, no. 3, p. 24. Critical Care Nursing Association.

Figure 17.4: Mount Sinai Hospital, Toronto, Canada.

Table 18.3: Janes EMH (1986) Changing our eating habits *Nursing*. **3(7)**: 269. London: Mark Allen Publishing Ltd.

Figure 19.7: Notkins AL (1979) The causes of diabetes. *Sci. Am*. Vol. 241, no. 5, pp. 62–73.

Figure 20.5: Smith K (1980) *Fluids and Electrolytes: a Conceptual Approach*. Edinburgh: Churchill Livingstone.

Figure 20.8: Lewis SM (1981) Pathophysiology of Chronic renal failure. *Nursing Clinics of North America* Vol. 16, no. 3, p. 504.

Figure 20.15: Turpie ID & Skelly J (1989) *Geriatrics*. **44(9)**: 32–36. Cleveland, OH: Edgell Communications.

Figure 20.16: Sabiston DC Jr (eds) (1981) *David-Christopher Textbook of Surgery*. Philadelphia: WB Saunders.

Table 20.7: McFarland G & MacFarlane EA (1989) *Nursing Diagnosis & Intervention: Planning for Patient Care*. St Louis: CV Mosby-Year Book Inc. pp. 282–283.

Figure 21.6: Penfield W & Rasmussen T (1950) *The Cerebral Cortex of Man*. New York: Macmillan Publishing Company.

Figure 21.7: Guyton AC (1984) *Physiology of the Human Body*. 6th edn. Philadelphia: WB Saunders.

Table 21.2: Guyton AC (1981) *Human Physiology and Mechanisms of Disease*. 3rd edn. Philadelphia: WB Saunders.

Figure 22.2: Hensle TW (1987) In Gillenwater et al (eds) *Adult and Paediatric Urology*. Chicago: Yearbook Medical Publishers p. 1918.

Figure 22.12: Jacob SW, Francome CA & Lossow WJ (1982) *Structure and Function in Man*. 5th edn. Philadelphia: WB Saunders.

Figure 22.13: Speroff L, Glass RH & Kase N (1983) *Clinical Gynaecologic Endocrinology and Infertility*. 3rd edn. Baltimore MD: Williams & Wilkins, p. 81.

Figure 22.14: Matsumoto S et al (1968) Environmental anovulatory cycles. *Int. J. Fertility*. **13(1)**: pp. 15–23.

Figure 22.16: Masters WH & Johnson VE (1966) *Human Sexual Response*. Boston MA: Little Brown, p. 183.

Figure 22.17 & Figure 22.18: Cavanagh D (1969) The vaginal examination. *Hosp. Med*. 5 pp. 35–51.

Table 22.2 & Table 22.3: Katchadourian HA & Lunde J (1987) *Fundamentals of Human Sexuality* 3rd edn. New York: Holt Rinehart & Winston.

Table 22.7: Andrist L (1988) *Nursing Clinics of North America*. **23(4)**: 959–973.

Table 22.9: Toole K & Vigilante P (1990) *American Journal of Maternal–Child Nursing*. **15**: 170–175.

Figure 23.1: Soterakos M (1981) Nursing Care of the patient with breast cancer. In Bouchard-Kurtz & Speese-Owens, *Nursing Care of the Cancer Patient*. 4th edn. St. Louis: CV Mosby, p. 160.

Figure 23.2: de Graaf KM (1984) *Human Anatomy*. Iowa: Wm C Brown, p. 649.

Figure 23.3: 'Be Breast Aware.' NHS Breast Screening Program. Oxford: Cancer Research Campaign.

Figure 23.5: Breast Care and Mastectomy Association of Great Britain.

Table 23.1: Morton PG (1985) *Health assessment in Nursing* Springhouse PA, Springhouse.

Figure 24.6 & Figure 24.17: Gartland JJ (1974) *Fundamentals of Orthopaedics* 2nd edn. Philadelphia: WB Saunders, pp. 349–350.

Figure 24.7 AB: Stewart & Hallet (1986) *Traction and Orthopaedic Appliances*. Edinburgh: Churchill Livingstone.

Figure 24.7C: Steer-Nicholson (1984) The Belfast Fixator. *Nurs Times*. Feb 22nd.

Figure 25.3: *Rheumatic Disease Occupational Therapy and Rehabilitation* (1977) Philadelphia: FA Davis.

Table 25.3: Meenan RF et al (1988) *Arthritis and Rheumatism*. **23(2)**: 146–152. Hagerstown, MD: JB Lippincott.

Table 26.1: Norton D, McLaren R & Exton-Smith AN (1975) *An Investigation of Geriatric Nursing Problems in Hospital*. Edinburgh: Churchill Livingstone.

Table 26.5: Feller I & Archambeault-Janes SC (1973) *Procedures for Nursing in the Burns Patient*. Ann Arbour MI, The National Institute for Burn Medicine.

Figure 27.7: Shah N. *Glue Ear*, Royal National ENT Hospital, Grays Inn Road, London.

Figures 28.5, 28.6, & 28.7: Nave CC & Nave BC (1980) *Physics for Health Sciences*. 2nd edn. Philadelphia: WB Saunders, pp. 283, 287 & 285.

Figure 28.9: Smith and Nephew Ltd, Hessle Road, Hull (Booklet *Understanding Cataract*).

Figures 14.3, 14.6, 15.2, 15.3, 21.9, 21.12, 21.13, 21.16, 22.5, 24.2, 26.1: Hinchliff S & Montague S (1989) *Physiology for Nursing Practice*. London: Baillière Tindall.

Publisher's Notes

Dosages Every effort has been made to ensure any dosage recommendations are precise and in agreement with standards officially accepted at the time of publication. However it is urged that you check the manufacturer's recommendations for dosage.

Clinical Situations Throughout this book various *Clinical Situations* are described which aim to enhance aspects of the text by providing realistic clinical scenarios. Please note that the identity of each person described in these *Clinical Situations* is fictitious, and that any resemblance to known individuals, alive or dead, is thus entirely coincidental.

The Nature of Nursing

OBJECTIVES

This chapter provides the reader with the opportunity to:

- Identify three trends in the delivery of health care that influence the practice of general nursing
- Identify changes of emphasis in the focus of nursing practice in the recent past
- Discuss the concepts central to nursing
- Discuss the relationships between models of nursing, theories from other disciplines and the nursing process
- Use a series of theoretical concepts central to nursing to guide nursing practice
- Specify the characteristics of the nurse–patient relationship
- Use the nursing process to provide nursing care
- Discuss the ethical basis of nursing
- Apply an ethical analysis model to the resolution of ethical dilemmas

What is nursing? This simple question has exercised the minds of many nurses over the years, yet it is only in the relatively recent past that nursing has been seen as an independent profession. The evolution of nursing is in an exciting and constantly changing state, drawing upon the biological and behavioural sciences and areas such as ethics and social policy. This is occurring at the same time as major changes within society affecting the delivery of health care. It is the relationship between these themes that will form the basis of this chapter.

HEALTH CARE SERVICES

Changes in the delivery of health care services have been in response to three major social trends in the second half of the 20th century: the explosion in scientific knowledge, the escalating costs of health services and the changing needs of the health care consumer population. These trends give rise to complex issues which involve economic, political, social, cultural, educational and ethical considerations.

Scientific discoveries in medicine, notably advanced medical technology, have influenced the delivery of health care services and nursing practice. Advances in medical technology permit intense monitoring of and interventions into human biological processes on a scale hitherto unimagined. Life and death decisions may be made on the basis of nurses' interpretations of information from high technology equipment. These advances have led to increasing specialization within nursing, in both hospital and community settings.

Advances in computer technology, as part of the explosion in scientific knowledge, have influenced the delivery of health care. Computers have automated and consolidated information and increased the speed and efficiency of information processing. Nurses in a variety of health care settings are using computers to enter, store and retrieve patient information, check nursing and medical orders, and request services for their patients from other sectors of the health care system as diverse as pharmaceutical and social services.

A second trend, the rising cost of restoration to health through acute care hospitalization, in competition with other public needs and wants and in the face of finite resources, has evoked a search for alternative health care delivery strategies and sites. Health promotion and health maintenance through public education and community based programmes have become widespread. Nurses have played a significant role in providing these alternatives. In addition, increased attention has been given to threats to human health emanating from personal life-styles, pollution of the environment and poor socioeconomic circumstances.

A third trend, the changing needs of the health care consumer population, stems from changing patterns of mortality and morbidity, coupled with consumers' increased participation in their own health care decisions. The proportion of the population who are elderly is increasing, as is the incidence of chronic illness. Many patients are less willing to be passive recipients of care.

Longitudinal studies show a pattern of decreasing mortality and increasing incidence of morbidity (illness) for middle-aged and older people. Previously, acute infectious diseases were the greatest threat to health; today, chronic disabling diseases, from infancy to old age, represent our major health problems. These disabling diseases are attributed to detrimental social, environmental and life-style factors, which are much more difficult to control than infections. Chronic illness represents a broad spectrum of diseases. Some are life threatening, such as heart disease, cancer, acquired immune deficiency syndrome (AIDS) and stroke, while

Table 1.1 Major concepts of six nurse theorists.

Theorist	Nursing	Patient	Health	Environment
King's theory of goal attainment	An interaction process between patient and nurse, whereby during perceiving, setting goals and acting on them, transactions occur and goals are achieved	An individual (personal system) or group (interpersonal system) unable to cope with an event or a health problem while interacting with the environment	An ability to perform the activities of daily living in one's usual social roles; a dynamic life experience of continuous adjustment to environmental stressors through optimum use of resources	Any social system in society; social systems are dynamic forces that influence social behaviour integration, perception and health, such as hospitals, clinics, community agencies, schools and industry
Leininger's transcultural nursing model	A humanistic and scientific mode of helping a patient, through specific cultural caring processes (cultural values, beliefs and practices) to improve or maintain a health condition	An individual, family, group, society or community with possible physical, psychological, or social needs, within the context of their culture, who is a recipient of nursing care	Defined by specific culture and the local people's viewpoint; technology-dependent cultures view health and health care differently from non-technology-dependent societies	Any culture or society worldwide where ethnocaring is practised by nurses assisting patients
Neuman's health care systems model	Assisting patients to reduce stress factors and adverse conditions that affect optimum functioning	Individual, family or group with an identified or suspected stressor that may disrupt harmony and balance	Level of wellness in which all needs are met and more energy is built and stored than is expended	Internal and external forces surrounding the patient at the time; nurse–patient settings are not described
Orem's self-care model	A service of deliberately selected and performed actions to assist individuals or groups to maintain self-care, including structural integrity, functioning and development	Individual or group unable to continuously maintain self-care in sustaining life and health, in recovering from disease or injury, or in coping with their effects	Individual or group's ability to meet self-care demands that contribute to maintenance and promotion of structural integrity, functioning and development	Any setting in which a patient has unmet self-care needs/requisites and in which a nurse's presence is implied, but not specified
Peplau's interpersonal model	Goal-directed interpersonal process to promote patients' forward movement of their personality and personal living	Any individual who feels or recognizes unmet needs	Ability to accomplish interpersonal activities and developmental tasks within a productive level of anxiety	Any health related setting is implied, but not defined
Roger's science of unitary human beings	Science and art to facilitate and promote symphonic patterning of human beings and their environment	Any human being and his or her environment; energy field	Expression of the life process, characterized by behaviours emerging from mutual, simultaneous interaction between human beings and their environment	Four dimensional negentropic energy field identified by pattern and organization and encompassing all that is outside any given human field; any setting worldwide where nurse and patient meet

Table 1.1 *continued*.

Theorist	Nursing	Patient	Health	Environment
Roy's adaptation model	Promotion of the patient's adaptation in the four modes to enhance health using the nursing process	Person, family, group, or community with unusual stresses or ineffective coping mechanisms; adaptive being	State and process of being and becoming an integrated whole person	All conditions, circumstances, and influences surrounding and affecting the development and behaviour of persons and groups; focal, contextual and residual stimuli

Modified from Christensen and Kenney (1990).

others are more physically or cognitively debilitating, such as diabetes or Alzheimer's disease.

Illness does not affect members of society equally. For example, the death rate amongst men between 15 and 64 years of age is almost twice as high as that for women, but women visit their general practitioners more than men (Townsend, 1988). Social class also exerts a major influence over both mortality and morbidity, with the mortality rate for social class V (unskilled labourers) being 2.5 times that for class I (professionals). This difference is found in both chronic illness and trauma, in children and in adults. Work by Whitehead (1988) has updated these findings and confirmed their persistence well into the 1980s, showing that major variations exist between different areas of the UK and, to a lesser extent, within areas. Poverty and wealth, education and class are all factors that influence the incidence of health and illness.

The immigrant community in the UK shows health trends that also reflect the importance of society. Marmot et al (1984) found that immigrants live longer than average for their country of birth, with the notable exception of the Irish, although there is disturbing evidence that stillbirths and perinatal mortality rates are higher for women born in Pakistan, Bangladesh and India compared with those born in the UK, while infant mortality rates in the Pakistani community are nearly twice as high as the UK average.

Consumers' involvement in their own health care has changed considerably in the latter half of the twentieth century. In the 1970s, the women's movement and other activist groups began to assert their rights in health care. Today, consumers are much more knowledgeable about health problems and interventions. Many consumers want to participate actively in their health care; they seek information to make informed decisions. The formerly dependent, acquiescent patient may now prefer to be an active partner with the health care team members.

Nurses have responded to the changing needs of patients by focusing less on the medical emphasis of disease cure and more on the holism of patient health promotion, maintenance and restoration. Thus, the role of the nurse incorporates that of adviser, counsellor and collaborator. Nurses work in partnership with patients. Many nurses serve as patient advocates by providing information which patients seek, assisting them to examine their own values, beliefs and goals, and helping them to evaluate and choose from available courses of action (Gadow, 1983).

THE FOCUS OF NURSING

Nursing is recognized as an emerging profession with a unique perspective on people, environment and health. It is the application of nursing knowledge to the promotion, maintenance and restoration of health for the individual and family through stressful events, which may include death and bereavement. In recent years, nursing has derived its focus not from the medical model, with its emphasis on the treatment and cure of pathological problems, but from the relationships between people, the environment and health outlined in nursing models. Specifically, the focus of nursing is derived from the interrelationships of people seeking health within their environment as they interact with nursing.

Many nurse scholars have defined the focus of nursing over the years. Henderson's definition remains the best known; she describes the nurses' unique function as 'assisting the individual, sick or well, in the performance of those activities contributing to health or its recovery (or to a peaceful death) that he would perform unaided if he had the necessary strength, will, or knowledge' (Henderson, 1966). Table 1.1 summarizes some current understandings of the focus of nursing.

It is noteworthy that, from the time of Nightingale, nursing has described as its focus the health of human beings. What has changed over time are the skills, scope and settings of nursing practice.

THE PROFESSION OF NURSING

The profession of nursing is derived from the perspective which nursing brings to knowledge from the physical, biological, behavioural, social and medical sciences, for the promotion, maintenance and restoration of health. It is the body of knowledge which defines nursing and provides the rationale for nursing education, practice and research.

Does the profession of nursing have a sound theoretical basis for practice? The purpose of theory is to describe, explain, predict and control the phenomenon of interest. Disciplines construct theories, frameworks and models to organize the knowledge and information of interest to the discipline. Theory provides us with ways of viewing the portion of the world of interest. It orders our thinking. The functional components of theories are the major concepts and their definitions. Writers such as Pearson and Vaughan (1986), Kershaw and Salvage (1986) Aggleton and Chalmers (1986) and Walsh (1991) have provided introductions to some of the more common nursing models and examples of how they may be used to plan care. An analysis of models by Aggleton and Chalmers (1987) suggested three distinct approaches may be discerned:

1. Systems models which emphasize a balance between physiological or social systems (e.g. Roy, Orem, Henderson, Roper).
2. Interactionist models which concentrate on the individual's perceptions of the world and how the individual relates to other people (e.g. Riehl, King).
3. Developmental models which concentrate on the growth and development of the individual and the nurse–patient relationship (e.g. Peplau).

These are not rigid categories, however, as different models draw upon various sources for their views of nursing: thus Orem's model has a strong developmental component, while King's model also relies upon systems theory.

The various conceptual frameworks that outline philosophies of care have been the subject of much debate. Walsh (1991) has summarized the arguments by suggesting that while these nursing models do not achieve the status of theories, as encountered in the physical sciences, they are still of value in that they help to define nursing by giving a coherent philosophy and approach to care.

Nurses need to use models in a flexible way if care is to meet the wide range of needs that characterize patients. A clinical unit should be prepared to use several models, reflecting the different individual needs of patients. There is no one single model that is right while all others are wrong; humans and their holistic health environment are too complex for such a simplistic approach.

The immature state of nursing theory, coupled with the complexity of that which we are trying to understand, i.e. human beings and health, suggests that it is premature to talk of nursing theories in the same way as theories in the physical sciences. The expression 'nursing model' is therefore commonly used, suggesting a looser framework of ideas, a philosophy of care, or a hypothesis in need of developing and testing.

The four major concepts of all existing nursing models are patient, environment, health and nursing. Nursing models differ in their definitions of these concepts and in the relationships among the concepts; each describes the concepts and their relationships in a unique way (Table 1.1). However, these differences in perspective are complementary rather than competitive in their organization of nursing knowledge.

CONCEPTS CENTRAL TO NURSING

The Patient

The patient is the recipient of nursing care and may be conceptualized as an individual, family, group, community or society by different nurse theorists. However, all nurse theorists include in the concept the notion of patient as person. An understanding of the patient as person is basic to nursing. The patient is viewed in the context of being both a human being and being unique, with a particular make-up, experiences and responses. The person has a distinct identity, in addition to being a member of a family and community, and is in constant interaction with the environment. Interactions and responses are influenced by sociocultural background, life-style, set of values, capabilities, interests, past experiences and the patterns of behaviour laid down as a result of those experiences. These factors contribute to the uniqueness of the person, who should be regarded as having worth, dignity and the right to pursue health, happiness, love, security, purpose and freedom. The nurse considers the individual holistically by focusing the nurse–patient encounter on the total person and not merely the component parts.

There is consensus among nursing theorists that the recipient of care should be informed about his/her health status, make informed decisions compatible with personal beliefs and values, and actively participate (as far as possible) in the care process. All people have essential basic human needs; nursing intervention may be indicated when the individual cannot independently satisfy these needs. Basic biological needs include the intake of oxygen, fluids and food, the elimination of wastes, rest, sleep, activity, and maintenance of body temperature within a definite range. Significant psychosocial needs of each person include: a sense of security, the maintenance of an identity as an individual, acceptance, a sense of being wanted and belonging, the opportunity for socializing, independence (and at times dependence and interdependence), freedom to make decisions, and opportunities to develop and use innate potential. He or she should have interests and goals and the opportunity to feel self-respect, in addition to feeling useful and having a sense of achievement.

Environment

The relationship between the individual and the environment is dynamic and influences both health and life-style. Some nurse theorists understand the environment to be external to the person, while others conceptualize internal and external environments. When considering the internal and external environments within the context of nursing, the internal environment comprises everything within the skin and mucous membranes of the body. It encompasses all structural and physiological aspects of the human body and may be modified by assimilated psychological and sociocultural experiences. The external environment includes physical surroundings, patterns of relationships and interactions with family and society, outside resources, and the ways in which the individual has contact with a health-care delivery system.

Nursing is directed towards managing the way in which the patient interacts with the environment, promoting health, preventing disease and delivering care in illness. Specific strategies and actions enabling the nurse to direct or manage the patient–environment interaction vary according to the individual, the environment and the health problem.

Health

Nurse theorists differ in their conceptualization of health. Some see health as a state, others as a process. Most recognize health as a goal to be attained and maintained. How health is perceived by the individual is influenced by cultural and educational background and past experiences. An individual's health is measured against some yardstick or set of standards. The standard used may be absolute; for example, it may be the presence or absence of disease, or the ability or inability to function as a contributing, independent member of society. Other measurements may be relative and give greater consideration to subjective components such as the sense of well-being and quality of life (see Chapter 2).

Besides the physiological and functional aspects of health, nursing is also concerned with subjective factors contributing to the quality of life and the opportunity the individual has to realize potential. Effects of the internal environment on functioning, well-being and life-style are readily apparent. The effects of un-favourable external environmental factors significant to health, such as polluted air, water, noise and adverse living conditions, are complex and more difficult to identify and change. Other factors related to life-style, such as the amount of physical exercise a person takes, dietary and smoking habits, levels of stress and the relationships one has with others, can also affect health and perception of health. These issues are considered in more detail in Chapter 2.

Nursing

Theorists agree that nursing takes place within the context of the nurse–patient relationship, which is characterized as a professional or therapeutic relationship. This differs from a social relationship in that it is collaborative and is directed towards meeting the patient's goals. It may be time-limited and take place within a structured and designated setting, such as a hospital. People often have preconceived ideas about the nurse as well as about how they themselves should behave as patients. Clarification of these perceptions may be necessary before an effective rapport can develop. The professional purpose of the relationship gives direction to the role assumed by the nurse and to

the way in which the nurse applies nursing knowledge and skills. The nurse brings to the relationship respect for the person's uniqueness and integrity and an appreciation of the patient's right to participate in or receive care. The patient, as an active participant, brings certain abilities and values, as well as a background of culture, education, experiences and needs, with the right to demonstrate and apply these in decisions and in the care process. Mutual acceptance is fundamental to the effectiveness of the nurse–patient relationship.

As the nurse develops empathy with the patient and strives to earn trust and confidence, the patient should develop trust and confidence in the nurse. With each encounter, the nurse's role is mutually agreed upon by the nurse and patient. A sincere interest and willingness to help may be demonstrated by the nurse being non-judgemental, accepting the patient, demonstrating thoughtfulness, anticipating needs, showing concern and, most importantly, by being ready to listen and answer questions. Recognition of identity by addressing the patient by name, respect for personal preferences and the demonstration of flexibility contribute to a satisfactory relationship. Appreciation of the family's concerns and each member's need for an interpretation of what is happening fosters trust and confidence. Expressing and sharing information with the family may prove therapeutic for them as well as the patient.

During the total nurse–patient relationship, the nurse's responsibilities include that of being the advocate. When acting on behalf of the patient, attempts are made to assess the situation carefully from the patient's point of view, rather than simply deciding what is 'good for' the patient on the basis of past nursing experience. As advocate, the nurse should provide information to assist the patient and/or the family to make informed decisions about the individual's health care (e.g. about a procedure, a form of therapy or a change in circumstances). Confidentiality must be respected; it is an important factor in establishing and maintaining good nurse–patient relationships. When information must be shared with other members of the health care team, the patient should be advised of the reasons and the advantages of communicating it to others.

While the nurse is under an obligation to attend anyone, regardless of race, nationality, politics or creed, there may be practical situations where the patient's choice is in conflict with the nurse's personal values and beliefs. The resolution of such ethical dilemmas is, however, very difficult. The United Kingdom Central Council (UKCC) does provide guidelines in its code of professional conduct and recognizes that the patient has the right to make decisions and choices.

The development of the nurse–patient relationship occurs in three distinct phases: (1) initial phase, (2) working phase, and (3) termination phase (Peplau 1978). The length and scope of each phase is determined by its purpose and the situation in which it occurs. In a brief encounter with a critically ill patient in an accident and emergency department, the relationship is based on efforts directed towards meeting life-threatening needs and is usually terminated in a short time. In long-term or community health settings, when the patient presents with multiple and complex problems, the interaction may extend over several weeks, months or years. The patient and family may need help in adjusting to chronic disability or preparing for impending death.

The *initial phase* includes introduction to the patient, the creation of an atmosphere conducive to interventions and the establishment of a mutual contract for nursing activity. The initial interview is structured by the nurse to establish a rapport with the patient, obtain pertinent clinical data and make plans for care. During this phase, initial roles are defined and the patient's expectations of health care are explored.

The *working phase* involves providing information and nursing actions that are directed towards assisting the patient to alleviate problems, make informed choices, set goals and participate in care. The nurse provides direct intervention when the patient is unable to undertake self-care. Goals are reviewed frequently and are redefined as the patient's situation and condition change.

The *termination phase* requires planning and is built into the relationship from the beginning. It is directed by the purpose and goals of the relationship. The nurse supports the patient in assuming independence, makes referrals and identifies resources to assist in the move towards self-management. The ease or difficulty with which this is accomplished depends on the effectiveness of the nurse–patient relationship throughout the three phases. The patient and nurse evaluate the outcomes in relation to how well defined goals have been achieved.

NURSING MODELS APPLIED TO PRACTICE

Models Related to Theories of Other Disciplines

Nursing models, which describe the relationships between patient, environment, health and nursing, provide a perspective through which to view theories from other disciplines. Within different nurse–patient relationships, the nurse may find theories from other disciplines very useful in describing, explaining, making predictions about, or controlling the events which occasion the relationship. For example, the nurse may derive insights from knowledge of the psychological and physiological changes associated with ageing to assist the elderly patient; alternatively, learning theory may assist the nurse in patient teaching. Depending upon the context, theories from other disciplines have considerable relevance to nursing as descriptions, explanations and/or predictors of the relationships between patient, environment and health and as the basis for rational nursing actions. It is, however, nursing's unique perspective which directs us to select from among the theories of other disciplines those which are useful in each nurse–patient relationship.

Models Related to the Practice of Nursing

The major concepts of nursing models provide a perspective to guide the practice of nursing, and these views can be applied to each component of the nursing process, which is a logical way of organizing and delivering planned, individualized nursing care. Models of nursing attempt to influence and determine the broad strategy of that care and their use makes the use of the nursing process essential, otherwise the individualized care that is the goal of any nursing model cannot be delivered. A model guides the nurse in patient assessment and helps in the formulation of patient problems and goals. Nursing care and interventions will also be influenced by a model, although there is also a large component of practical nursing that is common to any model. It is important that nurses have rationales for their actions (although intuition also has a place) and models help provide a basis for understanding and planning care. Doing something because we have always done it or because 'Sister likes it that way' is not a sufficient foundation for professional practice and leads to ritualistic, unthinking nursing that may be positively harmful to the patient (Walsh and Ford, 1989).

THE NURSING PROCESS

The purpose of the nursing process is to provide a systematic framework for nursing practice. The nursing process unifies, and directs nursing practice in a consistent, logical manner. As the core of nursing practice, the nursing process provides the structure for nursing care. The nursing process involves a certain amount of time spent writing out care plans but this time may yield a rich dividend in terms of the benefits that flow from planned care. Only in this way can care be individualized and made relevant to each patient's needs. Communication involving nurses and other staff, such as social workers, should be greatly improved by the keeping of written records, which will also permit careful evaluation of care to assess it's effectiveness. A logical care planning system also permits the full involvement of the patient in planning care and setting goals.

Kenney (1990a) has identified seven major characteristics of the nursing process which enhance its use in practice:

1. It is purposeful as a goal-directed tool to provide quality patient-centred health care.
2. It is systematic and provides an organized, logical approach to nursing care.
3. It is dynamic by virtue of being an ongoing process focused on the changing responses of the patient.
4. It is applicable to individuals, families and community groups at any point on the health–illness continuum.
5. It is adaptable to any practice setting or specialization, and the components may be used sequentially or concurrently.

6. It is interpersonal and based on the nurse–patient relationship.

7. It may be used with any type of nursing model.

Use of the nursing process enables the nurse to plan care, based upon a sound assessment of the patient's needs, that will be individualized and directed towards patient-centred goals. Consistency of care and communication can be greatly improved if a 'primary nursing system' is also implemented. MacGuire (1988) has described this as a system whereby each nurse retains overall responsibility for the care of a group of patients, even when not on duty. This 'primary' nurse is held responsible for the patients' care, which is delegated to other 'associate' nurses when the primary nurse is off duty. If no one nurse is responsible for a care plan, in practice it either falls into disuse and becomes out of date and irrelevant to the patient's needs or confusion reigns as different nurses write different and sometimes contradictory statements in the plan. Primary nursing therefore goes hand in glove with the nursing process as a means of delivering patient care. Five interacting components, with various steps, comprise the nursing process as outlined in Table 1.2.

Assessment

Assessment is a continuous process of collecting data about the patient's responses, health status, strengths and concerns. The data are comprehensive and multifocal, reflecting both historical and current data about biological, psychological and social functioning, as well as environmental and life-style factors which may affect health. The patient is the primary source of data, but a variety of data sources should be used, such as the family, health records and other health professionals. Assessment techniques include the interview, direct observation and measurement. Validation of data and any assumptions made are essential to ensure that messages conveyed by the patient are being received and accurately interpreted by the nurse.

Data may be categorized as subjective or objective. Subjective data are obtained from the patient, family or friends regarding the patient's feelings or perceptions about health concerns, e.g. fear, anxiety or pain. Objective data are obtained through observation and measurements, including the physical examination and laboratory tests. Height and weight are examples of objective data.

Problem Identification

Problem identification must have the patient as a focus; a correctly stated patient problem is the starting point for effective, individualized nursing care. Data obtained in the assessment need to be sorted into categories and compared with accepted norms, as defined by sciences such as anatomy, physiology or psychology, in order that actual or potential health problems may be discovered. It is also essential to seek the patient's point of view, as the patient may not agree with the nurse that a behaviour constitutes a problem, for example the

Table 1.2 The nursing process.

Components	Definitions	Activities
Assessment	An ongoing process of data collection to determine the patient's strengths and health concerns	Data Collection 　Interview 　History 　Examination 　Records review
Problem identification	The analysis/synthesis of data to identify patterns and compare with norms and models resulting in a clear, concise statement of health problems appropriate for nursing interventions	Data Analysis and Synthesis 　Identify gaps 　Categorize 　Recognize patterns 　Compare to norms and models
Goal setting	The setting of realistic, measurable and mutually agreed long- or short-term goals with the patient	Discuss with patient 　Establishment of priorities 　Consider how goals may be measured
Implementation	The patient and nurse carry out the plan	Write care plan 　Carry out care plan with patient 　Update/revise care plan 　Record progress made
Evaluation	A systematic, continuous process of comparing the patient's response with written goals/ outcome criteria	Compare responses to goals/outcome criteria 　Determine progress 　Revise plan of care

Modified from Kenney (1990b).

patient may see smoking as beneficial because it is perceived as reducing stress.

Models of nursing have the advantage of offering a structure or series of categories for the process of problem identification; for example, Roy's adaptation model requires the nurse to look at physiology (broken into subcategories such as oxygenation and circulation, fluid balance, etc.), self concept, role function and interdependence in order that a holistic view of the patient may be obtained. The model also offers a nursing perspective of a norm, in Roy's case the ability to adapt to outside and inside stimuli. Failure of adaptation is seen as a patient problem; thus the patient may develop pressure sores in response to prolonged immobility as the skin and subcutaneous tissue is not able to adapt to the stimulus of prolonged pressure. Whatever nursing model is used, it is essential to try and include the cause when making a problem statement as this gives guidance towards the nursing interventions required.

Goal Setting

Goal setting (planning) occurs when the patient and nurse identify activities to prevent, reduce or correct the patient's problems. The steps in planning are to:

1. Set priorities among the identified problems
2. Establish patient goals and outcome criteria
3. Identify intervention strategies
4. Weigh alternative actions and predict outcomes
5. Determine nursing interventions
6. Write the nursing care plan.

Once patient problems (actual and potential) have been identified, priorities are set to provide direction for nursing interventions. Knowledge, experience and, in some critical situations, intuition are applied in setting priorities. If the situation is life threatening, airway, breathing and circulation (ABC) assume priority. In many situations, priority setting involves patient and family participation to prevent conflicts arising and to enhance active co-operation in care activities.

There is no one tool or framework available that assists in making decisions on priorities of care in all situations. Emergency and life-threatening circumstances readily dictate priorities for intervention; other situations may require different considerations. Maslow's framework, which presents an ordered classification of human needs, may be used to rank patient problems (Maslow, 1970). It is based on motivation theory and implies that the patient contributes to the decision. Physiological needs (for oxygen, water, food) are ranked as the most immediate priorities, followed by safety and security, love and belonging, self-esteem and self-actualization. Communicating the reasons for priorities helps in establishing mutual goals; failure to consider what is important to the patient may create conflict and delay in achieving health goals.

Goals and objectives describe the patient's expected behavioural outcomes. Each goal is derived from the identification of patient problems and the goals are directed towards the promotion, maintenance and restoration of health, the alleviation of suffering and the giving of support to the dying. Goals may be either short-term or long-term statements reflective of realistic resolution of the identified problem and within the patient's capabilities and limitations. Short-term goals may be discrete short-term steps leading to achievement of a specific long-term goal and should always reflect mutual planning with the patient. An important feature of a patient goal is that it must be measurable, otherwise how will we know if the patient has achieved it? A 'fluid intake of 3 litres per day' represents a measurable goal which also contains a statement of the time limit on goal achievement, whereas a statement such as 'increase fluid intake' is too vague to be measurable as a goal and has no concept of time attached to it. Goals should therefore be stated in terms of observable behaviour and should also be realistic. Goals that are unrealistic will only discourage both patient and nurse and are a waste of time.

Nursing intervention strategies are selected with the patient from alternatives. They are considered in light of anticipated effectiveness in achieving outcomes, the benefits and risks involved, and the availability of resources, including people, equipment, time, finances and facilities.

The nursing care plan should contain written statements describing the nursing interventions required to help the patient achieve the various goals outlined in the plan. They should be stated in concise, specific terms, and in the sequence in which they are to occur. They may include strategies for the promotion, maintenance or restoration of health, or for peaceful dying. The nursing interventions support the medical regimen of care and should be kept current, revised, and describe alternate plans, as necessary. The scientific rationale for the nursing orders may be stated to explain the basis for the plan of nursing care. If so, the reason for each nursing intervention is clearly identified. Rationale may include principles, theory, research findings and current literature.

When problems are identified by the nurse that are outside the realm of nursing, a referral may be made to the appropriate member of the health care team. Similarly, when problems are identified that are beyond the expertise of one particular nurse, referrals may be made to other qualified nursing colleages. These may be clinical nurse specialists, nurses practising in a special care area or speciality, or community nurses. Collaboration, cooperation and sharing of knowledge and skills provide quality and continuity of care. Medical orders and the plans developed by other health care workers should be integrated with the planned nursing actions to develop an overall schedule for patient care.

Implementation

Implementation is the performance of nursing interventions described in the nursing care plan. The scope of nursing actions include:

- Supportive measures that are designed to assist with activities the patient is unable to perform and to reinforce adaptive coping mechanisms.
- Therapeutic measures.
- Continuous data collection and monitoring of the patient's health status.
- Health promotion and health maintenance activities such as teaching.
- Co-ordination of care by other members of the health care team.
- Reporting, recording and consultation.

Evaluation

Evaluation encompasses comparing the patient's health status with the goals and objectives of health care, and determining progress toward goal achievement. Evaluation is a continuous process which occurs during ongoing assessment and implementation of nursing care. When behaviour indicates that goals have been achieved, the nurse and patient either move to the next level of expectation or the relationship is terminated. If the goals were not achieved, the nurse may explore the reasons for this by questioning. For example: Were the goals realistic? Were they stated in measurable terms? Were the actions inappropriate, or did the patient's situation alter? Goals are then re-examined, modified if

necessary, and priorities are re-established in relation to the patient's level of achievement and/or change in health status.

DOCUMENTATION

The patient's health record can be used as a legal document. The nurse is accountable for ensuring that information recorded in the notes is accurate, clear, concise, factual and complete. Data collection, identification of patient problems, plan of care, interventions and results of the interventions, and evaluation of the outcome criteria are recorded.

All members of the health care team should share the patient's record. It thus becomes a means of providing information about the patient's condition and the health professionals' care plans, and contributes to continuity of care. Accurate and comprehensive written documentation facilitates collaboration and co-operation among members of the various health care professions to ensure optimum use of resources on the patient's behalf. The record is a confidential document; it is only available to those participating in the care by permission of the health authority. Table 1.3 describes the steps involved in giving planned nursing care.

Table 1.3 Steps involved in carrying out planned, individualized nursing care.

---

1. *Assessment*
Collection of data about the patient's physical, psychological and social status. Data should be both objective (measurable) and subjective (e.g. patient's feelings) and should also be relevant to the present situation. The patient, family, significant others and already existing records provide the sources for data, which should be collected and recorded in an orderly and systematic way

2. *Problem identification*
Data are categorized and each category compared with others to see if patterns and relationships appear. Observations are compared with norms and standards and the patient's views of the health problems are considered. A holistic view of the patient's health status should be attained in order that both actual and potential problems may be identified, together with possible causes. Statements should be patient centred

3. *Goal setting*
Goals must be prioritized in order that the most urgent problems are dealt with first. The patient should be involved in goal setting and prioritization, with nurse–patient negotiations aiming to resolve differences of opinion. Goals should be patient-centred, realistic and measurable. Statements should be phrased in such a way that a time scale is set for goal achievement, together with a means of measuring goal attainment (outcome criteria)

4. *Intervention*
The steps required for nursing care should be agreeable to the patient, relevant to the patient's goal and clearly written in the care plan in a form that is readily understood by other staff. They should have sound rationales which justify the action planned. Written statements of planned care should be dated and signed by the nurse responsible and should be revised as appropriate. The care carried out should reflect the written plan and be with the patient's consent at all times. Care given should be accurately documented and signed for. As a test of the adequacy of a written care plan, a nurse new to the patient should be able to come on duty and, working from the plan, immediately give high quality nursing care relevant to the patient's needs. If a care plan does not permit such action it is inadequate and needs rewriting

5. *Evaluation*
Continual monitoring of patient progress is essential, particularly with reference to patient goal statements. The plan of care should be modified as appropriate if goals are not achieved or new patient problems are identified

---

Table 1.4 Critical ethical analysis model.

1. *Data base*
What is the information relevant to the situation? Who is involved? What information is available (scientific, cultural, sociological, psychological, physiological)? Information is ordered and ranked according to its direct relevance for the decision at hand to more precisely determine the problem.

2. *Identification and clarification of ethical components*
What type of ethical problem is at hand? Not all problems are ethical. What moral principles are involved? What is the source of moral conflict? Is there more than one conflict?

3. *Individuals involved in decision making*
All persons involved in the decision must be identified. The rights, duties, authority and capabilities of the decision makers is clarified. What is the basis of their respective rights and duties? Conflicts are identified and ranked. Consider how free each person is to make a choice. Is the patient in pain? Is the family stressed? Is the professional facing a conflict of duties? Determine whose decision it is, and why.

4. *Options, possible courses of action and projected outcomes*
Explore all options, courses of actions and projected outcomes for all involved. Identify the good and harm that can result from each action for all involved.

5. *Reconciling facts and values: holding multiple values in tension*
The facts of the situation are reconciled with the principles. Principles, values and facts are held in creative tension simultaneously to arrive at a decision. Actions which produce more harm than good, and actions which debase the human being are to be avoided. Different rankings of the rights and duties of those involved result in different weightings of the facts and principles which, in turn, result in different decisions in different situations. The reasons for the decision must be rationally given and defended.

6. *Resolution*
The choices are difficult. There are times when the resolution is influenced by the law or social expectations. These may or may not coincide with what is right conduct.

Adapted from Curtin L and Flaherty MJ (1982) *Nursing Ethics: Theories and Pragmatics*. Bowie MD: Brady. pp. 59–63.

NURSING ETHICS

Recent authors in nursing, Gadow, Watson and Fry, have argued that the moral premise of nursing practice is founded in the nurse–patient encounter, embodied in the concept of caring. Gadow (1987) concerned for the protection and enhancement of the human dignity of patients, views caring as the nursing actions of truth-telling and touch. Through truth-telling, the nurse empowers patients to make choices for themselves, and through touch, affirms their personhood. Watson (1985) suggests that the moral premise of caring needs to be extended beyond acts, to a philosophy of caring from which caring acts are derived. Fry (1989) believes that a theory of nursing ethics will be derived from a philosophical view founded on caring as the moral basis for both the social role of nursing as a profession, and for nursing actions. At this writing, caring, as the moral premise for nursing, either as acts or as a philosophical view, is just beginning to be developed.

Nursing ethics is currently based on the approach to biomedical ethics derived from analytical philosophy. This ethic is governed by an appeal to principles of moral conduct. These principles of moral conduct, sometimes expressed as moral duties, include:

- *Autonomy:* the obligation to respect the personal choices another person makes

- *Beneficence:* the obligation to do good
- *Fidelity:* the obligation to keep one's word
- *Justice:* the equitable distribution of risks and benefits among people
- *Non-maleficence:* the obligation to do no harm
- *Veracity:* the obligation to tell the truth.

The principles of moral conduct have been derived from several different world views of human relationships. The world views articulate rights and obligations in human encounters through principles of moral conduct. One world view, teleology, argues that the goodness of an act is determined by its consequences. It further argues that the collective good takes precedence over the good of the individual: the greatest good and least harm to the greatest numbers. In contrast, a second world view, deontology, argues that the goodness of an act is independent of its consequences and is determined by its conformity to obligations that arise from the fact of being human. It further argues that the good of the individual takes precedence over the collective good, based on the premise that no one be treated as a means to the ends of another.

Conduct based upon any one of the principles, and not in conflict with any other principles, is morally right conduct. However, when two or more moral courses of conduct come into conflict, we have an ethical dilemma.

Nursing ethics wrestles with problems which arise when alternating courses of conduct, each moral in itself, come into conflict in a particular situation. An example in nursing practice of conflicts between alternative courses of moral conduct is the conflict between beneficence and autonomy. For example, consider the person who refuses nursing care which would greatly benefit his or her health. If the nurse respects the person's autonomy, the health status may be harmed. If the nurse coerces the individual into receiving nursing care, or fails to elicit consent for nursing care, the nurse violates the autonomy of the person, and possibly the law, as such an act may be construed as common assault, for which a patient may sue to obtain damages. The nurse may have to choose one over the other as a basis for the course of action.

An alternative ethical dilemma often occurs over the issue of how much information to give a patient. Webb (1987) has rightly stressed the role of the nurse as patient advocate and how this involves giving information in order that a patient may make informed decisions about treatment and care. The UKCC code of practice requires nurses to be truthful with patients. The doctor, however, is responsible for medical decisions and may decide to withhold information about a patient's true diagnosis, typically in cases of malignant disease, or even the range of treatments that are available (e.g. in breast cancer). The nurse may therefore be placed in the position of having to choose between lying to the patient when asked 'What is wrong with me?' or telling the truth and contradicting the doctor in the process.

The legal position of the nurse and the balance of power in the nurse–doctor relationship have been discussed by writers such as Dimond (1987), Darbyshire (1987) and Walsh and Ford (1989). There are no easy answers, except to say that nurses must be able to support their actions with sound rationales (such as the UKCC code of conduct), and in cases of difficulty would also derive great benefit from membership of a professional organization.

The need to choose between moral courses of action is known as an ethical dilemma. Several dilemma resolution models are available in the literature. The model presented here (Table 1.4) was selected because it recognizes that an ethical resolution of a dilemma is independent of both social expectations and legal requirements of conduct.

SUMMARY

The practice of nursing is dynamic and evolving, shaping and being shaped by the contexts within which nursing practice takes place. This chapter has briefly explored five of these contexts.

The first context discussed is changes in the health care delivery system in response to the knowledge explosion, changing health care priorities and changing needs of health care consumers. These changes influence the scope, skills and settings for the practice of nursing.

Nursing also has to be seen in the context of a movement away from the medical model focus on pathology and cure. Rather, the emerging focus of nursing is on people seeking health within their environments as they interact with nursing.

The third context for the practice of nursing is the emergence of a theoretical body of nursing knowledge, based upon understandings of the relationships between people, environments, health and nursing practice. Nurse theorists have provided perspectives unique to nursing that emphasize the knowledge, research, ethics and practice of the profession. These perspectives provide a framework for applying theories from other disciplines to the practice of nursing, delineating the nurse–patient relationship and using the nursing process to deliver high quality nursing care.

The nursing process provides the next context against which nursing must be seen; it is the core of nursing practice, a systematic framework which provides the structure for nursing care. The nursing process is the vehicle through which theoretical knowledge is applied to actual or potential patient health problems.

A final context is the ethical practice of nursing. Nursing ethics is premised upon principles of moral conduct which include autonomy, beneficence, fidelity, justice, non-maleficience and veracity. The United Kingdom Central Council provides guidelines for the ethical practice of nursing in its code of professional conduct.

The following chapters in this text provide the reader with the knowledge, rationale and nursing perspective for the practice of nursing. However, excellence depends upon the nurse applying the knowledge gleaned from these chapters within the contexts of nursing practice discussed in this chapter. These contexts render each nurse–patient encounter unique.

REFERENCES AND FURTHER READING

Aggleton P & Chalmers H (1986) *Nursing Models and the Nursing Process*. Basingstoke: Macmillan.

Aggleton P & Chalmers H (1987) Models of nursing; nursing practice and nursing education. *Journal of Advanced Nursing* **12**: 573–581.

Christensen PJ & Kenney JW (eds) (1990) *The Nursing Process: Application of Models* 3rd edn, pp. 26–27. St Louis: Mosby.

Darbyshire P (1987) The burden of history. *Nursing Times* **83(4)**: 32–34.

Dimond B (1987) Your disobedient servant. *Nursing Times* **83(4)**: 28–31.

Fry ST (1989) Toward a theory of nursing ethics. *Advances in Nursing Science* **11(4)**: 9–22.

Gadow S (1983) Basis for nursing ethics: paternalism consumerism or advocacy? *Hospital Progress* **64(8)**: 62–78.

Gadow S (1987) Nurse and patient: the caring relationship. In Bishop AH & Scudder JR (eds) *Caring, Curing, Coping: Nurse, Physician, Patient Relationships*. Birmingham, AL: University of Alabama Press.

Henderson V (1966) *The Nature of Nursing*. New York: Macmillan, p. 15.

Kenney JW (1990a) Theory based nursing practice. In Christensen PJ & Kenney JW (eds) *The Nursing Process: Application of Models*. St Louis: Mosby.

Kenney JW (1990b) Components, definitions and activities in the nursing process. In Christensen PJ & Kenney JW (eds) *The Nursing Process: Application of Models* 3rd edn, chap. 3. St Louis: Mosby.

Kenney JW (1991) The evolution of nursing science and practice. In Deloughery N (ed) *Theories and Trends in Nursing*, chap 3. St Louis: Mosby.

Kershaw B & Salvage J (1986) *Models for Nursing*. London: Wiley.

MacGuire J (1988) I'm your nurse. *Nursing Times* **83(30):** 32–36.

Marmot M, Adelstein A & Bulusu L (1984) Immigrant Mortality in England and Wales 1978–79. OPCS Studies on Medical and Population Subjects No. 47. London: HMSO.

Maslow A (1970) *Motivation and Personality*. New York: Harper & Row.

Peplau HE (1978) *Interpersonal Relations in Nursing*. London: Macmillan.

Pearson A & Vaughan B (1986) *Nursing Models in Practice*. Oxford: Heinemann.

Townsend P (1988) (ed.) *Inequalities in Health*. London: Penguin.

Walsh M (1991) *Models in Clinical Nursing: The Way Forward*. London: Baillière Tindall.

Walsh M & Ford P (1989) *Nursing Rituals, Research and Rational Action*. Oxford: Heinemann.

Watson J (1985) *Nursing: Human Science and Human Care*. New York: Appleton Century Crofts.

Webb C (1987) Professionalism revisited. *Nursing Times* **83(35):** 39–41.

Whitehead M (1988) *The Health Divide*. London: Penguin.

Wright S (1989) *My Patient – My Nurse*. Lancaster: Gazelle.

Health Promotion

OBJECTIVES

On completion of this chapter, the reader will be able to:
- Recognize that there are many different definitions of health promotion
- Differentiate between health promotion as life-style change and as a sociopolitical process
- Identify the role of the nurse in health promotion
- Be able to assess an individual's life-style and make suggestions for strategies to change behaviour
- Recognize the unresolved ethical dilemmas associated with health promotion

Definitions

In order to comprehend the content of this chapter, some words, particularly *health* and *health promotion*, must be defined. Many different definitions of each are found in the literature. It is important to realize that there is not one 'right' definition, but the definitions chosen will give the reader a basis for understanding the other concepts presented. Some historical perspectives will also be discussed.

HEALTH

It is important in thinking of health not just to see it in biological terms for, as Aggleton (1990) has explained, there is also a significant social component and, in the main, modern theories of health differ principally on how much weight they attach to these two components. Alternatives to the biomedical model of health include social-positivist theories which, according to Aggleton, apply the methods of the natural sciences to social enquiry in order to try and identify the causes of health and illness, while interactionist explanations concentrate on the meanings that people give to the experiences of health and illness. Finally, there is the structuralist approach, which sees health in terms of how power and authority are distributed in the broader context of society; the effects of capitalism, class structure and the power of men over women are examples of how this view seeks to explain health.

Whichever view of health is chosen, every nursing model defines health in relation to the overall model and requires distinct approaches to the patient. Thus, there are several different acceptable definitions. However, a commonly cited definition is that of the World Health Organization (WHO, 1958): 'health is a state of complete physical, mental, and social well-being, not merely the absence of disease and infirmity.' This definition was an acknowledgement that health is more than non-disease, but it has been criticized for proposing an ideal, rather than a measurable goal for which strategies for achievement can be devised. It has since been altered from health as a 'state' to reflect health as a 'resource' (WHO, 1986):

'Health is the extent to which an individual or group is able, on the one hand, to realize aspirations and satisfy needs and on the other hand to change or cope with the environment. Health is seen as a resource for everyday life, not the objective of living, it is a positive concept emphasizing social and personal resources as well as physical capacities.'

However, this definition has not increased its measurability.

Pender (1987) provides an excellent overview of the historical development and evolving nature of the definition of health as it relates to individuals, family and community, then goes on to identify her definition:

'Health is the actualization of inherent and acquired human potential through goal-directed behaviour, competent self-care, and satisfying relationships with others while adjustments are made as needed to maintain structural integrity and harmony with the environment.'

In contrast to the WHO, Pender has proposed criteria for evaluating health to reflect her definition. For this reason, Pender's definition will be used for this chapter. The criteria are presented in Table 2.1. From this definition health can be seen as more than preserving a status quo, it also involves a dynamic process of change as the individual strives to achieve a high level of wellness in order to get the most out of life physically, mentally and socially. It is interesting to see how Hartweg (1990) has analysed these views of health and shown that the Orem self-care model of nursing is very appropriate for nurses to use as a vehicle for health promotion. As Pender has described, the definition is a combination of actualizing and stabilizing tendencies, and reflects the process of development characterized by experiences of challenge, achievement and satisfaction.

PREVENTION

Early public health strategies were related to the eradication of illness and prevention of communicable disease. Prevention is commonly described in three levels:

1. *Primary:* activities to decrease the probability of illness and to protect against illness. It includes both risk avoidance and risk reduction.

2. *Secondary:* activities for early diagnosis and early intervention to reduce the duration and severity of illness.

3. *Tertiary:* rehabilitation, coping with disability or chronic disease.

Prevention and health protection are still important activities, but emphasis has shifted to allow inclusion of health promotion activities, with a 'wellness' focus of optimizing functioning as opposed to an 'illness' focus of preventing disease. Both are important and complementary activities.

HEALTH PROMOTION

Early definitions of health promotion were related to changing life-style behaviours which could be damaging to health, or to changing behaviours which would lead to maximizing health and functioning. The importance of life-style choices first gained credence with the publication of the Alameda County study (Belloc and Breslow, 1972). This large population longitudinal study found that there were seven critical health practices which, if followed, resulted in longer life. The seven practices were:

- Eating breakfast daily
- Using alcohol not at all or in moderation
- Being physically active for 20 minutes three times per week
- Eating three meals per day at regular times
- Maintaining weight at that desirable for height
- Getting 6–8 hours of sleep per night
- Not smoking

Men of 45 years of age reporting between six and seven of the above practices had a life expectancy 11 years longer than those reporting four practices. Women of the same age reporting 6–7 practices had a life expectancy of seven years more than those reporting four.

About the same time, a Canadian report was published which became a model for many countries (Lalonde, 1974). In this report, leading causes of mortality and morbidity were related to life-style choices, and a model was presented, the Health Field Concept, which made life-style as important a determinant of health as the health care services. Health promotion became a reaction to consumers' disillusionment with traditional medicine, as well as an excuse for governments to reduce funding for tertiary care in response to pressures to contain high health care costs. Both the social and political climates were emphasizing self-help, individual control over health and personal responsibility for health. A wave of programmes and media messages admonished people to start exercising, stop smoking, reduce their weight, cut down on their fat intake, and, in many other ways, gave the directive to change behaviour in order to maximize health. Health promotion was the 'buzz' word in health and social service agencies for the next decade.

Table 2.1 Proposed criteria for evaluating health.

1. Exhibits personal growth and positive change over time
2. Identifies long-term and short-term goals that guide behaviour
3. Prioritizes identified goals
4. Exhibits awareness of alternative behavioural options to accomplish goals
5. Perceives optimum health as a primary life purpose
6. Engages in interpersonal relationships that are satisfying and fulfilling
7. Actively seeks new experiences that expand knowledge or increase competencies for personal care
8. Displays a high tolerance for new and unusual situations or experiences
9. Derives satisfaction from the experience of daily living
10. Expends more energy in acting on the environment than in reacting to it
11. Recognizes barriers to growth and deals constructively in removing or ameliorating them
12. Uses self-monitoring and feedback from others to determine personal and social effectiveness
13. Maintains conditions of internal stability compatible with continuing existence
14. Anticipates internal and external threats to stability and takes preventive actions

From Pender (1987) with permission.

However, a backlash also occurred. How many options (for joining exercise groups or getting support from friends to stop smoking) exist for the socially disadvantaged female, single head of the household, on social security, with three children? Health promotion interventions are based on the assumptions that an individual has a great deal of control over personal decisions and actions regarding life-style behaviours, and that changes in these behaviours can significantly affect health outcomes. The work of Townsend (1988) and Whitehead (1988) referred to in the previous chapter showed the great inequalities that exist in health in the UK. Social factors such as wealth, education, culture and class play a major role in determining health. The simplistic approach to health promotion described above ignored the effects that the social and physical environment, coupled with lack of resources, have on health behaviour. There is now an acknowledgement of the social inequities that exist in morbidity, mortality, health behaviours and well-being, and a sensitivity to the possibility of 'victim-blaming'. Victim-blaming was first labelled by Ryan (1971). He argued that society places a double burden on the sick: it creates the conditions that lead to illness, then establishes a model of health care which makes the individual responsible for the sickness, and even stigmatized for it.

Naidoo (1986) has argued that there are three main criticisms of concentrating on the individual alone in health promotion: firstly, such an approach denies that health is a social product; secondly, it assumes free choice exists; and finally, it simply does not work. The case for health being strongly influenced by society is overwhelming, while the notion of free choice is severely limited for, as Tones (1990) has argued, factors such as lack of knowledge, low self-esteem, addictions, and the various structural barriers that exist in society mitigate against free choice. There is also the dilemma of one person's freedom of choice adversely affecting another person's health; passive smoking is a typical example. Naidoo critically examines various individually-structured health campaigns (such as the Great British Fun Run of 1985) to show their failings in support of her third point, i.e. individualistic health promotion campaigns often do not work.

There is a marked difference in approach between the USA and Europe in the field of health promotion. This has been analysed by Salmon (1989), who concludes that in the USA the focus is very much on the individual, with profit acting as a major motive for health promotion, while in Europe a much broader approach, involving the social and physical environment, is distinguishable. Efforts concentrated in the field of public policy and social change will, according to Salmon, be more beneficial than concentrating simply on trying to make individuals behave more responsibly.

Support for this view comes from writers such as Mitchell (1989), who considers that politicians overstate the case for individual responsibility in order to mask the inadequacies of the available services and the inequalities in health that exist and for which they, as members of Government, are ultimately responsible.

This reaction to the individualistic, life-style modification approach to health promotion has led to a socioecological model of health promotion being widely adopted, and this has been supported by the WHO. Their Ottawa charter (WHO, 1986) defines health promotion as 'the process of enabling people to increase control over and improve their health'. It argues that there are basic prerequisites for health: peace, shelter, education, food, income, stable ecosystem, sustainable resources, social justice and equity. Further, it states that the principal means of attaining these prerequisites are political: advocacy (making sure health appears on the political agenda), enablement (allow people to achieve fullest health potential), and mediation of different societal interest. The WHO suggests that the key strategies are: to build healthy public policy, create supportive environments, strengthen community action, develop personal skills and reorient health services. The WHO is trying to implement the socioecological model through its motto and plans of *Health for All by the Year 2000* (WHO, 1979), which includes the 'Healthy Cities' and 'Healthy Communities' projects around the world. These projects are using local community-level coalitions to alter problems at the same level, whether they be environmental, housing, access to health services, provision of food, or many other issues.

Progress being made in the Healthy Cities campaign in the UK has been reviewed by Adams (1989) and, amongst the problems identified, institutional racism has been recognized as a major cause for concern, denying ethnic minority populations their rightful place in society. Pearson (1986) has offered an interesting analysis of how health promoters, by focusing specifically on health problems seen as unique to ethnic groups, are behaving in a racist manner by falling into the trap of stereotyping and victim-blaming. It is clear that only a multiracial health promotion team of equals can be truly effective in getting rid of racial stereotypes and acting in the best interests of *all* members of society.

The Healthy Cities campaign can be made to work by making health a matter of civic pride. First, however, a health profile of a city is needed to show the extent of the problem. Binyish (1989) has discussed how this approach has been used in Coventry to stimulate greater activity by both the local authority and by local people acting on their own initiatives to improve health. A different perspective on this problem is offered by Farrant and Taft (1988), who presented a case study of the problems in Paddington and North Kensington, most of which, according to the authors, lie outside the traditional remit of health workers, e.g. poverty, homelessness, unemployment, etc. This wide range of social problems which are adversely affecting health are strongly related to national and local government policy. There is therefore a need to confront political issues in the interests of health promotion.

HEALTH PROMOTION AS A ROLE FOR NURSES

In the UK, health promotion was originally seen as a role for health visitors, with the emphasis very much on child health, although the health promotion needs of the elderly have become increasingly important. Current government initiatives to reform the NHS are radically changing the role of the general practitioner and the way community staff will work in the future, so much so that the specialist health visitor role is now under threat, together with that of the community nurse. The future may well bring a generic community health nurse working under the direction of the general practitioner; even so, it is apparent that health promotion should be a key ingredient of any such future developments.

This approach shifts the centre of gravity of health promotion activity away from the individual into the community, a view strongly supported by Green and Raeburn (1988) in their discussion of the meaning of health promotion and its future. They argue strongly that the primary concern of health promotion should be the people whose health is at stake, rather than competing ideologies, and they stress the need for an enabling approach. This involves giving people power over resources and health, a strategy that may run into conflict with Governments and health care professionals. It is striking that, despite widespread opposition from the public and health professions alike, the UK Government refused to allow ballots during 1989–1990 on the subject of the health reforms which were to lead to the setting up of 'opted out' hospital trusts.

Health promotion can, however, be integrated into all settings where nurses work. Innes and Ciliska (1985) developed a model for defining areas of nursing

Figure 2.1 Model for the integration of health promotion into nursing practice. Modified from Innes and Ciliska (1985) with permission.

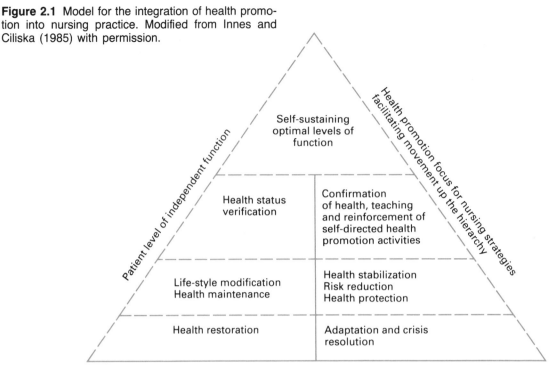

Note: Hierarchical progression of subgoals toward self-sustaining optimal levels of function and focus for health promotion strategies.

practice relative to health promotion with individuals or families (Figure 2.1). In their model, health promotion is defined as 'activity that is deliberately planned and purposefully directed toward increasing a person's ability to function and facilitating a maximal state of physical, mental and social well-being'. It is not directed solely to the 'well', who want to be at a higher level, but to people who need their health restored from an illness, and all stages in between. The ultimate goal of health promotion activity by nurses is for the patient to achieve self-sustaining optimal levels of function and well-being. At this level, people do not need nursing or other professional health care. They have achieved a healthy and harmonious life-style, and they are able to manage their self-care. After a thorough assessment, it may be discovered that the person is already at this level, or the level may be reached by nursing interventions to assist the patient in achievement of three hierarchically-arranged subgoals (Figure 2.1):

1. *Health restoration:* adaptation and crisis resolution for people experiencing some health threat or health deficit.
2. *Health maintenance and life-style modification:* health stabilization for people with chronic conditions, risk reduction and health protection for people without identified illness.
3. *Health status verification:* confirmation of health through periodic assessments, and teaching and reinforcement of self-directed health promotion activities.

Using this model, it is easy to see that health promotion may occur in any setting; although the nurse

must always consider the social factors which affect the patient's health, these may not be so apparent in hospital. Hospitalized patients, even in critical care, may benefit from a health promotion intervention. For example, the nurse could support a middle-aged male and help his family adapt to the crisis of a myocardial infarction. The second level of the hierarchy involves stabilization (which may also occur in a tertiary setting), and risk reduction (which may be in hospital or the community). Health status verification often occurs in occupational health and community settings.

A change has occurred in interpersonal relations between nurses and patients, away from the view of the health professional as the expert who always knows what is best for the patient. Nurses, together with others on the health care team, are affected by the consumer movement in health care, in which the public is asking to be more informed about choices for treatment, side-effects of drugs, and the reasons for and against various treatments. The expectation is that the nurse is a partner, as is the patient, on the health care team. This new partnership requires a shift in terminology away from words or phrases which imply dependency and powerlessness in the relationship such as 'compliance with treatment', to terms which imply co-operation such as 'negotiation'.

Health Assessment

A comprehensive health assessment includes a history of the presenting complaint, family history, psychosocial history, a life-style evaluation, assessment of beliefs and attitudes towards health behaviours and susceptibility to disease, physical examination and mental health status examination. Life-style evaluation will be addressed here, followed by a model to determine likelihood of behaviour change.

Several assessment tools are available to assess life-style: risk appraisals and less formal self-report measures. In interpreting such tools, the social context in which the patient's life-style is located must always be considered.

HEALTH RISK APPRAISAL

Health risk appraisal (HRA) tools, computerized or self-scoring, compute a risk score for mortality and morbidity. Health Risk Appraisal (also called Health Hazard Appraisal) has been found to elicit reliable information from people in the areas of family history, cigarette smoking and relative weight, but self-reported scores of blood pressure, cholesterol, diet, physical activity and stress are far less reliable. The implication for health promotion programmes is that if people do not perceive themselves at risk, they are less likely to adopt new behaviours. Risk estimates are targeted to the 'perceived benefits' area of the health promotion model (presented below); a behaviour is more likely to be pursued if the individual believes the change will be of benefit.

SUBJECTIVE TOOLS

In this case the score does not reflect a computation of risk, but is simply an awareness of the various components involved in life-style over which the individual may potentially have some control. These tools usually include items such as smoking, alcohol, drug use, nutritional intake, anxiety, depression, quality of relationships with family and friends, and purpose in life.

Conceptual Models for Directing Assessment and Intervention

Two models have been chosen to help understand factors important in health promotion behaviours. They illustrate factors to consider in assessment. In addition, they identify appropriate areas of intervention, reflecting the range of strategies for health promotion programming. The models are Pender's Health Promotion Model and the Ecological Model of Health Promotion (McLeroy et al, 1988).

PENDER'S HEALTH PROMOTION MODEL

Pender's Health Promotion model (Figure 2.2) was derived from social learning theory, which emphasizes cognitive processes in determining health behaviours. Its purpose is to determine or help predict health promoting behaviour of individuals and it offers some guide-lines for areas of intervention to increase the likelihood that a patient will engage in positive behaviours.

The categories of factors chosen for the model were based on a literature review. The categories are summarized here. The *cognitive-perceptual* factors are the main reasons that are thought to lead people to acquiring and maintaining health promoting actions. Valuing health is related to finding out about health topics; perceiving that the individual has control over health should lead to positive health practices such as weight loss (conversely, having a strong desire for control but little perceived control may result in helplessness, frustration and inhibition of desired behaviours). It is expected that people with positive perceptions of their skills, i.e. they think they can achieve their goals, will be most likely to initiate the behaviour and maintain it. Personal definition of health would result in different behaviours if one defined health as an absence of disease, as opposed to self-actualization, or simply 'getting the most out of life'. Perceptions of good health are associated with higher levels of exercise and life satisfaction. Perceived barriers (such as inconvenience, difficulty, lack of availability or access) reduce the likelihood of health-promoting behaviours occurring, regardless of whether or not the barriers are real.

Modifying factors consist of demographic characteristics, biological characteristics, interpersonal influences, situational and behavioural factors. These factors exert their influence over the cognitive-perceptual factors discussed above. Characteristics such as age, sex, ethnicity, education and socioeconomic level all influence positive health behaviours. Biological factors such as weight or physical disabilities have a modifying influence on life-style behaviours such as exercise. Interpersonal influences are highly influential and are dealt with in this chapter under social support. Situational factors are primarily issues of availability of choices and actions, for example the types of food available in a works cafeteria. Behavioural factors refer to previous experience with actions, which tends to make it more likely that a positive health behaviour will occur.

Cues to action is the last part of the Health Promotion Model and consists of activating cues or triggers that spark off health promotion activity, such as mass media campaigns or conversations with friends.

Although this is essentially an individualistic view of health promotion, it still contains useful insights into how a person may be helped, providing the nurse considers at all times the wider social and physical factors in the environment which affect the patient.

THE ECOLOGICAL MODEL OF HEALTH PROMOTION

The Ecological Model of Health Promotion is a broader model than Pender's, and is applicable to individuals, groups, communities or countries. It blends the two potentially conflicting views of health promotion, i.e. the individual 'life-style' health behaviour idea and the concept of sociopolitical influences affecting health and disease. In it, behaviour is viewed as being determined by:

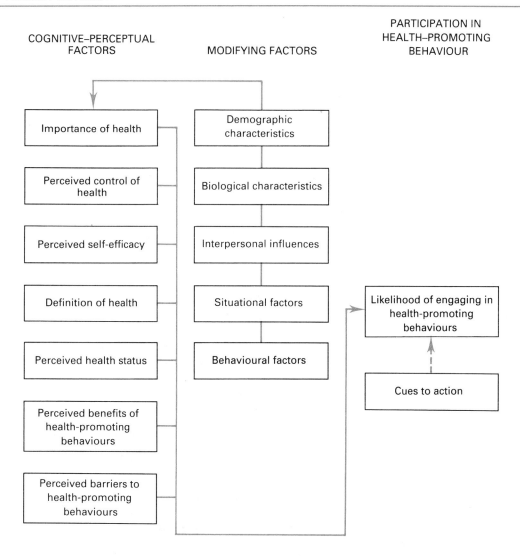

COGNITIVE–PERCEPTUAL FACTORS

MODIFYING FACTORS

PARTICIPATION IN HEALTH–PROMOTING BEHAVIOUR

Importance of health

Perceived control of health

Perceived self-efficacy

Definition of health

Perceived health status

Perceived benefits of health-promoting behaviours

Perceived barriers to health-promoting behaviours

Demographic characteristics

Biological characteristics

Interpersonal influences

Situational factors

Behavioural factors

Likelihood of engaging in health-promoting behaviours

Cues to action

Figure 2.2 Health promotion model. Modified from Pender (1987) with permission.

1. *Intrapersonal factors*—characteristics of the individual such as knowledge, attitudes, behaviour, self-concept, skills, etc. This includes the developmental history of the individual.
2. *Interpersonal processes* and primary groups—formal and informal social network and social support systems, including the family, work groups, and friendship networks.
3. *Institutional factors*—social institutions with organizational characteristics, and formal (and informal) rules and regulations for operation.
4. *Community factors*—relationships among organizations, institutions, and informal networks within defined boundaries.
5. *Public policy*—local, state, and national laws and policies.

The Ecological Model clearly overlaps, and is consistent with Pender's Health Promotion Model in the interpersonal and intrapersonal factors. The additions of interest beyond Pender's model are the notions of institutional and community factors and public policy (although these may well be 'situational factors' in Pender's model, the Ecological Model has made' these factors more explicit).

As with Pender's model, the Ecological Model can be used as an assessment guide and for directing intervention. Interventions at the intrapersonal level involve educational programmes, peer support and mass media campaigns targeted to the individual's knowledge, skills, attitudes or intention to change behaviour. Those at the interpersonal level are developed to change the nature of existing social influences and norms, such as adolescent drug use or sexual practices. Organizational factors are needed to support long-term behavioural changes by changing the culture to support health issues such as smoking cessation or physical activity.

The ecological approach requires collective action. Ewles and Simnett (1985) give a good introductory account to this concept, stressing the importance of planning and getting to know the community before working to bring people together and forming a campaign organization with clear goals and priorities. These concepts are explored further by Kickbush (1989), who emphasizes the need to see health education as much more than an individual process. Public policy can have a tremendous impact on health behaviours by restrictions such as no smoking policies, by incentives (positive or negative) such as taxes on alcohol and cigarettes, and by implementing policies which allocate support to programmes. The authors of this model emphasize that ecological strategies must minimize the possibility of coercion and paternalism through active involvement of the target population in all phases by the process of consensus building.

For a good overview of various health education techniques and how they may be deployed in various fields, such as smoking and diet, the reader is referred to the work of Ewles and Simnett (1985); Smith and Jacobson (1988) provide a good source-book of UK health information, with some clear policy suggestions for the rest of this century.

Interventions

The following discussion deals with strategies which can be used with an individual, family or small group. It is recognized that behaviour change involves at least a two-step process of acquiring knowledge and skills for initiating the change, then a different set of skills for maintaining the change. Often, programmes use a variety of strategies combined to try to increase the power of the intervention. Strategies are categorized here under cognitive, behavioural and supportive interventions. Community strategies are also discussed.

COGNITIVE STRATEGIES

Cognitive strategies attempt to alter thinking, problem-solving, reasoning and coping. The most common cognitive strategy is instruction for education. Education involves both information giving and skill development. Information is aimed at increasing awareness, sensitivity, possibly attitude change and motivation to change. Educational strategies will be further explored below. In addition, modelling will be described as a strategy for skill acquisition.

Education is done in a variety of ways. Pamphlets, mass media campaigns, one-to-one or group instruction, books, audiotape and videotape instruction are used for a variety of health promotion activities. It is important that the information is appropriate to the target group in the way in which it is delivered. The audience needs to feel that it has the knowledge and the skill to carry out the behaviour change in order for the message to have

an effect. Principles of adult education should be applied to any instruction given. Learning will be more effective if learners are active participants, if they set goals and monitor their progress, and if they get support from others in the process (see Chapter 3).

Modelling is a cognitive strategy to learn new skills or methods of coping. The strategy is based on social learning theory and is often employed in media campaigns to model positive behaviours such as teenagers saying 'No' to drugs, alcohol or smoking. Through modelling, people can learn skills, strengthen or weaken an existing behaviour, and provide prompts for behaviour which has already been learned. To be most effective, the model must be perceived to be like the observer and the outcomes of the behaviour must be clear. Nurses should always remember their own very powerful role as a model for healthy behaviour, as Melvin (1987) rightly points out.

BEHAVIOURAL STRATEGIES

The behavioural approach is based on the assumption that behaviour is determined by stimuli and is more likely to recur if positive reinforcement is given. Behavioural strategies include self-monitoring, stimulus control and contracting.

Self-monitoring is a tool to increase self-awareness. It involves diary-keeping to observe and record one's behaviour and its relationship to the antecedents (or stimuli) and the consequences (or reinforcers). It is considered an essential preparatory phase because of baseline data which is collected, and the resulting increased self-awareness. It is useful in documenting almost any behaviour including tobacco, alcohol and drug use, food intake, exercise and sleep patterns.

Self-monitoring allows for the analysis of stimuli for 'stimulus control'. A behaviour change plan may involve cue restriction (staying away from places or people with whom one associates smoking while one is trying to reduce cigarette consumption) or cue expansion (having the kitchen stocked with several varities of fresh fruits, vegetables and whole grain products when trying to reduce consumption of refined carbohydrates). Stimulus control may also involve analysis of barriers which tend to block the new behaviour. This analysis allows for increased awareness and planning for overcoming barriers in the environment.

Contracting consists of an agreement on paper with oneself, or between two or more people (Figure 2.3). It is a way to individualize interventions, and it also helps to build commitment through two mechanisms: (1) by making a public announcement, and (2) by keeping a written record of the plan. Contracts have been used for a variety of self-behaviour changes, such as stopping smoking, use of birth control, exercise, nutrition and procrastination. One of the most difficult areas of the contract to develop is that of rewards. Help the patient by 'brainstorming' possible internal and external rewards. Internal rewards may be the positive feelings of control, efficacy or increased self-esteem which result from completing new behaviour. External rewards should be something that the patient finds desirable, but would not otherwise obtain unless new behaviour is achieved. The

CONTRACT

GOAL: _____

OBJECTIVES: _____

_____

_____

PLAN:

Over the next week I will (be as specific as possible about time, place and people involved):

_____

_____

_____

_____

_____

_____

I will enlist the SUPPORT of: _____

_____

Their role: _____

_____

REWARDS: _____

_____

TIME contract will be evaluated and renegotiated:

_____

SIGNATURES: _____   _____

           Helper   Contract owner

Figure 2.3 A contract.

external rewards should be inexpensive enough for the patient to be able to afford to get the reward, or else a point system could be developed so that after a certain number of points are collected, they may be 'cashed in' on the desired item.

Use of fear in health promotion messages, punishment after unwanted behaviour or other aversive techniques are generally not effective and are not supported in the literature.

SUPPORTIVE STRATEGIES

One of the most potentially powerful strategies for making and maintaining behaviour change is to enlist the support of others. Certainly the nature of the nurse–patient relationship builds upon the inherent support of the nurse, but the nurse and patient can actively enlist family, neighbours and co-workers to provide support.

Social support has been conceptualized to encompass emotional (psychological support when one has a problem), informational (knowledge about resources and action), instrumental (assistance in performing behaviour) and appraisal support (how one is doing in terms of competence or importance). The literature relates lower morbidity and mortality and faster recovery from illness to stronger social ties with spouse, family, friends and formal and informal group associations. It is not known whether the mechanism for this protective effect is (1) a health-promoting effect at all times, perhaps by increasing resistance, or (2) a protective effect in times of high stress.

Self-help groups are another means of finding support for patients. Also called 'mutual aid' groups, they are usually small groups of people with similar problems or handicaps who come together to share experiences, provide mutual support, share treatments, and offer coping strategies to bring about personal and/or social change. They are usually informal, care-giving networks which can protect and improve peoples' health by acting as a buffer to stress and increasing resistance to disease; however, some have been sufficiently organized to become formal, with paid staff. They may serve as a lobby group to bring about changes in health care provision and societal attitudes. The processes rather than the activities are thought to be important, but there is little research regarding different groups or how they actually enhance coping.

COMMUNITY STRATEGIES

Community strategies for health promotion are derived from the socioecological framework presented earlier in this chapter. Education may be carried out community wide but other interventions are usually required to deal with social and political issues which relate to health. These issues usually require a high degree of community participation and a community development focus. The nurse working in community health needs skills in community assessment, community organization, and consultation. Community development projects are often neighbourhood based, where a community development officer meets with the residents to identify their health needs and interests (very broadly defined) and to help them to organize themselves to meet these needs. Community development projects are often directed to the inequalities in health or unequal access to health care services. The WHO Healthy Cities project emphasizes the words 'enabling' and 'empowerment' to signify that resources (knowledge, skills, power and money) for health matters should be distributed to people in the community, who should be involved in setting priorities.

ETHICAL ISSUES

What are appropriate target outcomes of health promotion programmes? For example, in weight loss repeated attempts at losing weight may be more harmful than an overweight person staying at a stable but higher weight (see Chapter 18 for supporting argument). What rights do people have not to be 'intervened upon'? What rights do people have to practice self-destructive behaviour (indeed, drug and alcohol abuse or risk-taking behaviour may lead to a positive feeling of well-being)? Other sources of potential conflict have been identified by the WHO (1988):

1. Health promotion will be viewed as the ultimate goal incorporating all life (sometimes called 'healthism') and could lead to others prescribing what individuals should do for themselves, how to behave.
2. Health promotion programmes may be inappropriately directed at individuals at the expense of tackling economic and social problems, as in the 'blame the victim' circumstance.
3. Resources, including information, may not be useful to people, that is not presented in ways which are sensitive to their expectations, beliefs, preferences and skills, thereby increasing social inequalities. Information is not enough; it may raise awareness without the likelihood of change, thereby increasing anxiety and powerlessless.
4. There is a danger that health promotion will become the job of one professional group or subgroup and become specialized to the exclusion of other professionals and community citizens.

The WHO has identified these ethical issues and potential conflicts in health promotion but have so far offered few, if any, solutions. They argue that the participation of communities in decisions that affect them will help prevent/resolve these ethical problems (WHO, 1988). Given the resources committed to health promotion, it must be asked whether there is any valid way of measuring progress, for if health promotion efforts produce no measurably beneficial results, there must be pressure to switch scarce resources elsewhere in the health field. The ethical dilemma of resource allocation arises: the money spent on one health campaign, which might benefit many people, could also finance a series of hip replacement operations which would relieve pain and immobility, but for fewer people.

The issue of developing health promotion indicators has been tackled by Dean (1988), who points out that they are very different from health indicators such as morbidity and mortality rates. There are vast quantities of data available, but Dean reminds us that this data must be analysed with care in order that that which is both meaningful, relevant and valid in health promotion is extracted. Dean is particularly critical of overemphasizing statistics collected on individual areas such as smoking and alcohol consumption, for if they are not interpreted in their complex social context, they can be very misleading. Energy might be better expended on developing indicators of the cultural, structural and situational processes that influence health, as these more accurately reflect the complexity of health and health promotion.

CONCLUSIONS

The effectiveness of programmes for life-style intervention are hampered by high drop-out rates. they produce inconsistent results in behaviour change, even when attitudes and beliefs have changed. People tend to fall back to old habits when the programme is finished. Innovations geared to improving these issues have included booster sessions or reminder calls or letters to help maintenance of behaviour change, the development of support groups for reinforcement, and the enlistment of spouse, family and friends in building supportive environments. Community development projects take much more time than most funding agencies are willing or able to allow. It is true to say that why people behave the way they do in matters of health is at best only partly understood, while the process of changing behaviour is fraught with difficulties. However, progress is being made and the potential benefits are so great as to make it more than worth the effort. It is a sobering thought that at present the best means of dealing with AIDS is through health promotion aimed at changing the population's beliefs about human immunodeficiency virus (HIV), and changing high-risk behaviours such as having unprotected sexual intercourse and sharing intravenous injection equipment. In this and other situations health promotion saves lives where nothing else can. Life-style has been closely linked with a range of health promotion opportunities but concentration on the individual alone ignores the social origins of health and the restraints on freedom of choice that the individual has to cope with. A broader approach to health promotion, involving the social and physical environment, is therefore required.

LEARNING ACTIVITIES

1. Use Pender's Health Promotion Model (see Figure 2.2) to look at one area of your own life where your life-style behaviour could be more positive. What aspect of your own thoughts, interpersonal relationships or environment are keeping you from displaying more positive behaviour? What could be altered that would make the behaviour easier, or more likely to occur?
2. Self-behaviour change exercise: use a self-contract to begin your own life-style change. Experiencing the pleasures and pitfalls will help you to be more effective in developing contracts with patients. (Figure 2.3 provides a useful format for this exercise.)

REFERENCES AND FURTHER READING

Adams L (1989) Healthy cities, healthy participation. *Health Education Journal* **48**: 4.

Aggleton P (1990) *Health*. London: Routledge.

Belloc NB & Breslow L (1972) Relationship of physical health status and health practices. *Preventive Medicine* 409–412.

Binyish K (1989) The health of Coventry. *Health Education Journal* **48(2)**: 94–96.

Black D *et al* (1982) *Inequalities in Health*. London: Penguin.

Blair SN (1989) Physical fitness and all cause mortality: a prospective study of healthy men and women. *Journal of the American Medical Association* **262(17)**: 2395–2401.

Dean K (1988) Issues in the development of health promotion indicators. *Health Promotion* **3(1)**: 13–20.

Ewles L & Simnett I (1985) *Promoting Health*. Chichester: Wiley.

Farrant W & Taft A (1988) Building healthy public policy in an unhealthy political climate: a case study from Paddington and North Kensington. *Health Promotion* **3(3)**: 287–297.

Hartweg D (1990) Health promotion self care with Orem's general theory of nursing. *Journal of Advanced Nursing* **15**: 35–41.

Innes J & Ciliska D (1985) Health promotion strategies. In Stewart M, Innes J, Searl S & Smillie C (eds) *Community Health Nursing in Canada*. Toronto: Gage.

Kickbush I (1989) Approaches to an ecological base for public health. *Health Promotion* **4(4)**: 265–268.

Lalonde M (1974) *A New Perspective on the Health of Canadians*. Ottawa: Government of Canada.

McLeroy KR, Bibeau D, Steckler A & Glanz K (1988) An ecological perspective on health promotion programmes. *Health Education Quarterly* **15(4)**: 351–377.

Melvin B (1987) Promoting health by example. *Nursing Times* **83(17)**: 42–43.

Mitchell L (1989) Whose health for all? *Nursing Times* **85(34)**: 48–50.

Naidoo J (1986) Limits to individualism. In Rodmell S & Watt A (eds) *The Politics of Health Education*. London: Routledge.

Pearson M (1986) Racist notions of ethnicity and culture in health education. In Rodmell S & Watt A (eds) *The Politics of Health Education*. London: Routledge.

Pender N (1987) *Health Promotion and Nursing Practice*. Norwalk, CT: Appleton & Lange.

Ryan W (1971) *Blaming the Victim*. New York: Vintage Books.

Salmon W (1989) Dilemmas in studying social change versus individual change; considerations from political economy. *Health Promotion* **4(1)**: 43–49.

Smith A & Jacobson B (1988) *The Nation's Health*. London: King's Fund.

Tones K (1990) Why theorise? Ideology in health education. *Health Eduction Journal* **49(1)**: 2–6.

Townsend P (1988) (ed.) *Inequalities in Health*. London: Penguin.

Whitehead M (1988) *The Health Divide*. London: Penguin.

WHO (1958) *The First 10 Years of the WHO*, Geneva: WHO, p. 459.

WHO (1979) *Formulating Strategies for Health for All by the Year 2000*. Geneva: WHO.

WHO (1986) *Ottawa Charter for Health Promotion*. Ottawa: WHO.

WHO (1988) *Research Policies for Health for All*. Copenhagen: WHO.

Health Education and Patient Teaching

OBJECTIVES

As a result of reading this chapter, the reader should be able to:

- Develop a conceptual framework for patient education
- Identify the responsibilities of the nurse and the patient
- Explore the implications that compliance/noncompliance has on learning
- Outline the process of patient education as a clinical skill
- Describe how cultural values influence learning
- Formulate nursing strategies for facilitating learning

This chapter presents an overview of patient education. The philosophical basis of patient education outlined here is that the patient must be an active participant if learning and application of knowledge are to occur. The nurse's role is to act as a facilitator to help the patient learn and solve problems independently. The goal of patient education is to help individuals incorporate knowledge and skills into healthy behaviours in order to improve health outcomes. Patient education involves exchange between the patient and nurse; it is not something done *to* the patient but rather done *with* the patient.

It is important to understand that there is a difference between health promotion, as discussed in the last chapter, and health education, as applied to individual patients in this chapter. The former represents a broad objective; health education is one specific way to help achieve that objective. Patient education is one of the tactics by which the strategy of health promotion may be achieved.

Health promotion, according to French (1990), encompasses health education, disease prevention, health politics and disease management. He sees health education as ensuring that health information is available in an understandable form to every individual (patient education) but that it should also involve educating the policy makers in society and placing health on their agenda. This leads to a view that health education should empower communities to take health initatives and that all workers in the field should use social action methods to affect the way political, environmental and economic systems function in relation to health. Social action involves communities using the political process and, if necessary, confrontational methods to effect change. Health education is therefore a very powerful weapon in the armoury of health promotion.

In this chapter the emphasis will be upon the patient education dimension of health education; the reader who wishes to explore this area further should start with the work of Freire (1972).

BELIEFS ABOUT PATIENT EDUCATION

Patient education is an important function of nursing practice. Henderson (1966) suggested that it is part of the nurses' role to improve the patient's level of understanding and, by doing so, to improve the patient's health. Education is recognized as an integral part of health care and Lask (1989) has shown how it may be incorporated into basic nursing education. It is an important factor in disease prevention, e.g. safe sex to prevent AIDS, and in compensatory care, e.g. in adapting to loss of function following amputation of a limb or in adapting to changes in technology which affect conditions managed by the patient at home, such as asthma or diabetes.

Health eduation has been described simply by Tones (1990) as any planned activity which promotes learning about illness or health so that there is some relatively permanent change in a person's knowledge and ideas. Ewles and Simnett (1985) fill in some detail by stressing that this process involves the whole person throughout their entire life, regardless of how ill or well that person may be at any one time. They see health education as helping people to help themselves, either individually, in families or in larger communities, by using a wide range of teaching techniques to achieve goals which often involve changing behaviours, attitudes and social circumstances. In the past, nurses have tended to teach patients within a disease-oriented framework rather than from a health perspective. Focussing only on the disease is a narrow and blinkered approach that ignores a wide range of social and psychological factors and is also very limited in its goals. As Seedhouse (1986) reminds us, a major theme in health education tends to be the prevention of illness rather than the creation of wellness. In his view, health is the foundation for all human achievement; this gives a much deeper significance and meaning to health education.

Wilson-Barnett and Osborne (1983) viewed patient

Table 3.1 Degree of risk for specific sexual practices.

No possibility of transmission of HIV: no theoretical risk and no evidence of transmission
  Solo masturbation
  Mutual masturbation
  Dry kissing
  Body-to-body rubbing
  Erotic talk
  Massage/touch/caresses
  Erotic bathing or showering
  Nipple stimulation (without drawing blood)
  Nibbling/biting (without blood)
  Receptive cunnilingus with barrier
  Receptive anilingus with barrier
  Insertive anilingus with barrier

Minimal possibility of HIV transmission: theoretical risk without evidence of transmission
  Wet kissing
  Anilingus without a barrier
  Insertive fellatio without a condom
  Insertive fellatio with a condom
  Receptive fellatio without a condom
  Receptive fellatio without a condom, no ejaculation
  Receptive fellatio without a condom, ejaculation without swallowing
  Insertive cunnilingus without a barrier outside menstruation
  Insertive cunnilingus with a barrier
  Receptive cunnilingus with a barrier
  Receptive cunnilingus without a barrier

Low possibility of HIV transmission: theoretical risk with small evidence of transmission
  Insertive cunnilingus without a barrier during menstruation
  Receptive fellatio without a condom and with swallowing of ejaculate
  Insertive penile–vaginal intercourse with a condom
  Receptive penile–vaginal intercourse with a condom
  Insertive penile–rectal intercourse with a condom
  Receptive penile–rectal intercourse with a condom

Very high possibility of HIV transmission: high theoretical risk and high evidence of transmission
  Receptive penile–rectal intercourse without a condom
  Receptive penile–vaginal intercourse without a condom
  Insertive penile–rectal intercourse without a condom
  Insertive penile–vaginal intercourse without a condom
  Coitus interruptus (intercourse with withdrawal before ejaculation) without a condom

From *Safer Sex Guidelines: A Resource Document For Educators And Counsellors*, a report from the Canadian AIDS Society Consultation on Safer Sex, March 1988, published by the Canadian AIDS Society in Ottawa, 1988, pp. 11–15.

Hospitals and other health care agencies have also created organizational barriers that prevent the patient from having the freedom to make decisions about health.

If we accept that health education is a patient-centred activity, what are it's goals? To say 'education about health' is very trite and not very helpful. Ewles and Simnett (1985) list a series of goals that should be the aim of the nurse and patient/family working together. These range from broad objectives, such as raising health consciousness so that the patient is aware of issues in the field of health, through to a goal of changing social circumstances which makes it easier for the patient to make healthy choices in life. Other goals relate to knowledge, attitude change, self-awareness, decision making and behaviour changes.

Taking a philosopher's view of health, Seedhouse (1986) commented that the meaning of health cannot be understood from a dictionary, nor is it enough to say that health is desirable and then leave the issue at that; action is needed. In his view, health education has two main, broad aims: (1) to ensure that people have a good standard of general education; (2) to develop people's powers of intellectual conception so that they can maximize the information with which they are presented. This is very much an enabling point of view, giving people the tools with which to tackle their own health problems; health education is definitely not about indoctrination and propaganda.

Every patient has the right to seek information and participate in the educational plan. Simply providing information about health matters is a waste of time. The purpose of education is to encourage patients to use knowledge to modify behaviour and perform activities that will result in improved health status. The role of the nurse, therefore, is to plan learning experiences with the patient, as a component of total care, so that adults share responsibility for health. Ideally, the outcome of learning is that the patient is able to make rational decisions with respect to health, participate effectively in self-care and adjust to the realities of the life-style changes that are required. However, as the discussion on p. 14 shows, various environmental factors can seriously hinder the patient's ability to change life-style.

education as an interactive process whereby learning, which may subsequently be used to influence behaviour, takes place. This is a more humanistic view of patient education in which the nurse and patient share responsibility for learning.

Fahrenfort (1987) supports the belief that in patient-centred education, autonomy is the key. In education that is medically centred, notions of compliance and a paternalistic viewpoint tend to dominate. Fahrenfort embraces Paulo Freire's concept that real education must entail emancipation; that is, liberating people to make their own decisions on their own terms. Historically, however, nurses and other professionals have hesitated to allow patients the control that they need to make their own choices and decisions. At times this reluctance has stemmed from our maternalistic/paternalistic view of patients, our need to 'do' for others.

PRACTISING HEALTH EDUCATION: AN EXAMPLE

A prime example of the importance of health education is provided by AIDS where, in the absence of any known cure or immunization programme, the main defence against the disease is education. Nurses are one of the key groups who can carry out the educational function in a wide range of situations and, in view of the importance of the issue of health education and AIDS, it is worth exploring in some detail.

There are critical goals in the global management of HIV infection. First and foremost, intervention needs to be focused on the prevention of transmission of the virus into healthy individuals. Information about HIV infection can be integrated into the nurse's interaction with all patients. School health, well-baby clinics and patients admitted for elective surgery all present the nurse with opportunities to discuss HIV infection and ways to prevent its transmission. Prevention of HIV infection also needs to focus on decreasing sexually transmitted disease in general, as mucosal integrity may be a factor in susceptibility to HIV. Second, intervention must be focused on appropriate and humane care of individuals affected by the virus. Self-care for the person is critically important.

Prevention of HIV infection is everyone's responsibility. Abstaining from or minimizing the degree of risky behaviours is an important deterrent in decreasing transmission of the virus. It is crucial that information be provided in a culturally acceptable manner and in a language that is easily understood. Previously, the weight of responsibility has fallen on individuals infected with HIV to practise safer sexual practices or to inform sexual partners of their HIV status. However, self-protection is

equally the responsibility of a non-infected partner. Sexual relationships require individual responsibility. For individuals to be motivated to adopt a new behaviour they must perceive a certain degree of risk or vulnerability. One of the problems of preventive education is that repression and denial are often used to minimize the degree of threat to the person. Therefore, individuals do not adopt safer behaviours because they deny they are at risk (Archer, 1989).

The nurse can inform people of the importance of using safer sexual practices (Table 3.1); however, it is often difficult to motivate individuals to change practice. It is usually more effective to focus teaching around both partners. An atmosphere that feels safe needs to be created so that individuals will feel comfortable discussing intimate behaviours. Safer sexual practices need to be incorporated so they are pleasurable and in keeping with the individual's cultural and moral values. The individual needs to understand that safer sex is used because the person wants to stay healthy, not because their partner is suspect. Attention needs to be given not only to the mechanics of sexual behaviour but also to

Table 3.2 Information on condoms and lubricants.

When used correctly and consistently during sexual intercourse, good quality latex condoms can create a protective barrier against all sexually transmitted diseases, including HIV infection. Latex dental dams are useful for mouth-to-vaginal or mouth-to-anal contact. Latex dams can be made by carefully cutting the tip off a latex condom and cutting it lengthwise to make a square.

ALWAYS BE PREPARED
- Condoms should be made of latex not animal skin
- Condoms should have a reservoir tip
- Condoms should be checked for the expiry date
- Condoms should be stored in a cool place not in a trouser pocket or glove compartment as heat can damage them
- Condoms need to be applied correctly:
  —be sure it is put on after the penis is erect and before either partner is extremely aroused
  —be careful not to tear it with your fingernail
  —unroll the condom to the base of the penis
  —leave 0.5–1 cm extra space at the tip of the condom to catch the ejaculate
  —remove the condom before the penis is completely relaxed
  —never use a condom more than once
- Lubrication is essential to avoid condom breakage
- Lubricants:
  —should be used in addition to condoms, not as a substitute
  —should be water-soluble, avoid petroleum jelly or vegetable oil as they can damage condoms
  —may contain nonoxynol-9, a chemical barrier against sexually transmitted diseases (should not be used for anal intercourse as it can damage the rectal mucosa)
  —should be applied over the condom after it has been put on
  —should *not* be used on the shaft of the penis as the condom will likely fall off during intercourse

Modified from Adams *et al* (1987).

Table 3.3 How to talk about condoms.

If your partner says	You can reply
I know I'm disease-free. I haven't had sex with anyone in months.	As far as I know I'm clean too. But either of us could have an infection and not know it.
I can't feel anything when I wear a condom. It's like shaking hands with a rubber glove.	I know there's some loss of feeling. Why don't we try putting a bit of lubricant in the tip of the condom. It'll be fun.
Condoms are messy and smell funny.	With a condom we'll be safe. Let's try some of the scented ones. This could be a whole new experience.
I think I'll lose the mood if I use a condom.	Let's try building it in as part of foreplay. We may feel a bit awkward at first but it will pass and its fun to try new things together.
I'll lose my erection if I stop to put on a condom.	I'll help you put it on. That will help you keep it.
I love you, I wouldn't give you anything.	I love you too, and because I love you I want to protect our relationship. Many people don't know they're infected.
I just don't feel ready to use a condom.	Maybe it's better if we wait for awhile until we can work this out, or maybe we can try things other than intercourse.

After Lewis and Lewis (1987).

areas of maintaining intimacy and closeness. The loss of or alteration in sexual freedom for an individual may manifest in typical grieving responses. In addition to information on safer sexual practices, the nurse also needs to provide information on the use of condoms and lubricants (Table 3.2). Obstacles to incorporating behaviour change may include knowledge deficits, fear, lack of skill, lack of social support or inadequate resources to purchase products such as condoms. The nurse can be of vital importance in helping individuals learn how to negotiate a sexual relationship. In particular, it may be difficult to get a sexual partner to use condoms. Many individuals are unsure as to how to initiate this discussion. Among men, a variety of reasons have been cited for the underutilization of condoms, including lack of ready access, failure to plan for sexual intercourse, the use of alcohol and drugs prior to sex, beliefs that condoms impair sexual pleasure, and the belief that condoms are unnatural or immoral (Valdiserri et al, 1989). These same questions have not been asked of women. It may be useful to role-play prospective situations to try and minimize these barriers (Table 3.3). When people are empowered with information and negotiating skill, they are less likely to place themselves in risky situations.

EXPECTATIONS FOR PATIENT EDUCATION

Patients are becoming better consumers of health care. They are better informed and they want to know more. Because of the consumer movement and greater media attention to health care issues, patients are aware of their rights and are more demanding about receiving information on their condition and treatment. Many want to be involved in decision-making regarding their care and treatment.

Patient education is now viewed as an integral part of high quality health care. Quality assurance is increasingly being recognized as an essential component of health care, particularly in light of recent NHS reforms. It is the process of setting standards for care, monitoring the achievement of those standards and taking corrective action when standards are not met. The health care system should have a focus on quality.

Patient education has become part of total, comprehensive patient care. In order to provide quality care, all the patient's needs must be addressed, including the need to know about health education, disease prevention and health promotion.

Cook's meta-analysis of 100 research studies revealed substantial evidence of the impact of patient education on patients undergoing surgery (Cook, 1984). Patient education was shown to reduce anxiety, encourage postoperative self-care and reduce complications. This analysis confirms that patient education can have an impact on the length of hospital stay and can positively affect the quality of care.

Wilson-Barnett and Osborne (1983) also reviewed several studies evaluating the effectiveness of patient teaching. They found that patients gained from and appreciated having more information; that patient anxiety was reduced; that patients participated in the teaching process; and that they felt an increased sense of control over their lives.

Other factors influence the need for more education. Shorter hospital stays, reduced convalescent facilities and higher incidence of chronic illness mean that more patients are being cared for at home by family carers. Family carers cannot be expected to care for ailing relatives without learning the necessary skills.

Some writers feel that nurses should play a major role in patient education and that teaching patients is an essential component of patient care (Benbow Plewes, 1984; Smith, 1984). There is a view that nurses should be responsible for teaching patients to cope with health and illness. Tones (1983) suggested that one of the principles in deciding who should take responsibility for health education is that it should be done by those who have close contact with an individual. The nurse appears to have more opportunity for patient teaching than any other member of the health care team, since the nurse spends more time with the patient and is in a better position to determine learning needs and readiness to learn.

On the other hand, doctors also perceive the importance of their role in patient teaching, believing that the doctor is in a unique position of responsibility and opportunity to understand, detect and improve compliance because of the relationship established with the patient. It is interesting to look at the work of Williams et al (1989). They investigated the attitudes of 424 general practitioners towards health education and found that overall there was strong agreement that they had a role to play in this area. However, there was apprehension amongst general practitioners about how to respond to patients who reacted negatively to health advice; this apprehension might indicate a deficiency in traditional medical training. The research also demonstrated that older general practitioners were more reluctant to become involved in health education work although a small number of the younger ones also had negative views about its value. Wood et al (1989) have confirmed the findings of Williams and colleagues, noting that the one area that general practitioners thought it inappropriate to explore with patients was the effect of poverty. In the previous chapter we saw that social factors such as poverty were thought of as crucial to any understanding of health and health promotion, yet this appeared to be a 'blank spot' in this sample of doctors. The patients who were identified as being most in need of health education were high-risk smokers, pregnant women and drug abusers. Overall, female general practitioners rated health education as more important than did their male colleagues.

Some nursing authors question whether nurses should be responsible for patient education. In a literature review, Close (1988) examined the role of nurses as patient teachers. She found that, while there was general agreement that patient education was part of the nurse's role, in reality nurses do little teaching. She found that there were many reasons for this, not the least of which was inadequate knowledge and skill development for such a role. Nursing realities, such as staffing shortages, time pressures and the needs of patients who are acutely ill, often force nurses to put teaching low on their list of priorities.

While teaching is a stated goal of nursing and nurses do value the concept, the actual practice of patient teaching often falls short of the goal. Runions (1988) surveyed staff nurses and administrators about their beliefs about patient teaching and their perceptions of the impediments to its practice in a hospital setting. While the nurses confirmed their belief that patient teaching is part of the nurse's role, nevertheless the impediments outweighed that belief. Impediments to patient teaching identified by the nurses included lack of knowledge, time limitations, role ambiguity, lack of continuity, lack of teaching competence and limitations in interpersonal skills.

Tilley et al (1987) studied the level of agreement between the perceptions of patients and nurses in relation to the nurse's role in patient education. They found that, while the patients identified a general teaching function for nurses, they most frequently preferred that a doctor teach them specific information related to their condition. These authors suggested that nurses need to develop a clear definition of their role in patient education, to validate patients' desires for teaching and to examine the organizational factors influencing performance in the patient-teaching role.

In summary, it is clear that there are expectations placed on nurses to teach. Quality assurance standards, professional standards and a focus on risk management emphasize the nurse's role in patient education. Nurses perceive that patient education is an important component of total patient care, yet are faced with external constraints that limit their ability to teach effectively. These constraints include time restrictions, unrealistic expectations of managers, patients who are too acutely ill to learn, and workload factors. With greater expectations on the part of patients who want to learn and demand to know, the challenge is for nurses realistically to meet these expectations.

The emphasis so far has been on hospital situations; what evidence is there that nurses can make a contribution to health in the community? The role of the health visitor stands out as a clear example, but what of the future? Government reforms could weaken that role and we have already seen a dramatic increase in practice-based nurses. The potential benefits that might flow from nurses working in this way have been shown by Robson et al (1989), who looked at how nurses might work in a disease prevention role. In this study a health promotion nurse, after appropriate training, was employed in a large, inner city general practice. The study looked at the recording of preventative activities carried out on patients seen by doctors alone, and those where the doctor and nurse worked together. The results were startling. A substantially higher (and statistically significant) proportion of patients in the nurse–doctor group had such screening procedures as blood pressure monitoring and cervical screening carried out, together with the recording of risk factors, such as smoking or a family history of ischaemic heart disease. The research concluded that, after 2 years, employing a nurse with a health promotion role made an important contribution to the recording of risk factors and the follow-up of patients with known risks.

This study shows how nurses can make contributions to health in the community, not only by screening, as in this case, but also by increasingly taking on a health education role. Health education is not the sole prerogative of health visitors; all community nursing staff must become involved. Stuttle and Pears (1988) have described an innovative example of community-based health education in which they put together a 'continence' roadshow that travelled around five different non-medical venues in their health authority area. The multidisciplinary team helped 80 people in 5 days and were still receiving enquiries weeks later. Health education has to be made available to people; nurses should be prepared to venture outside hospitals and health centres if they are to communicate effectively with those who most need health education.

Health education in the community must focus on the elderly as well as the younger section of the population. It is a myth that old people are too set in their ways to learn. Minkler and Checksway (1988) have argued for the empowerment of elderly people and their families by stressing the strengths of the elderly and the need to give them the information they require to improve their health. The family and informal care givers should not be forgotten in such a community-based programme of health education.

IS PATIENT EDUCATION EFFECTIVE?

Before adopting a framework for patient education, nurses need to know whether patient education works. What do we know about the effectiveness of the education process? What can be learned from research studies conducted to evaluate patient education programmes, interventions and strategies?

One of the most frequently quoted authors on educational effectiveness is Steven Mazzuca. Mazzuca (1982) completed a meta-analysis on 30 research studies focusing on educational interventions in chronic disease. He concluded that patient education programmes, conceived and designed to help patients cope with their unique self-management plan, are more likely to improve the course of their chronic disease than are standard presentations of medical facts and rules. Behaviourally-oriented programmes which encouraged and supported patients to care for themselves were consistently more successful in improving the patient's condition and course of illness.

Hathaway (1986) also completed a meta-analysis of experimental studies focusing on preoperative instruction. In the review of 68 studies, she confirmed that preoperative instruction did have positive effects on postoperative outcomes. Maximum patient learning occurs when the teaching process accommodates patient differences.

Brown et al (1987) measured knowledge about medication, side-effects and compliance in a before-and-after design. They found that written and verbal instruction were more effective in influencing knowledge than was verbal instruction alone.

Lindeman (1988), on the basis of an extensive review of studies spanning a 20-year period, concluded that patient education worked regardless of the strategies employed. Programmed instruction, booklets, lectures, modelling and other techniques appear to be equally effective in their ability to influence knowledge and skills. Results of these findings are summarized in Table 3.4.

COMPLIANCE

Much time, effort and expense is devoted to patient education by health professionals. As a result, there are expectations for and interest in the benefits that education can provide. Patient education, if viewed as a total process, can be a key component in enabling patients to act on the recommendations of the health professionals. However, patients cannot carry out a treatment or recommendation that they do not understand or *do not accept*. The degree to which patients follow recommendations is usually called *compliance* or *patient adherence*.

Compliance should not be viewed as coercive obedience but as a negotiated agreement. In this sense, compliance is part of the helping relationship between the health professionals and patient; it is the outcome of nurse–patient communication and interaction. It may be defined as the 'Extent to which an individual chooses behaviours that coincide with a clinical prescription . . . achieved through negotiations between the health professional and the patient' (Dracup and Meleis, 1982).

Increased attention to the area of compliance has been generated because of the impact of compliance or non-compliance on health outcomes. It appears that a high percentage of patients do not follow the recommendations of health professionals. On average, only one of three individuals will comply with the treatment plan (Becker, 1985). Non-compliance is therefore costly; it wastes medical and human resources and may have serious consequences for the patients and their families or significant others.

Non-compliance can take many forms: failure to keep scheduled appointments, to take medications as directed, to follow recommended dietary or life-style change or to follow recommended preventive health practices. Factors which may contribute to non-compliance include financial problems (inability to pay for expensive prescriptions), inconvenience (such as taking medications during working hours), denial of illness, lack of family or other support, feelings of fear or shame, feelings of helplessness or lack of control. All of these factors can impact on the patient's decision not to follow suggestions or recommendations regarding health.

Consider what patients are asked to do! Diabetics for example, must change every aspect of their life-style: eating, drinking, working and enjoying life. Then there are the additional stressors of taking daily injections and testing blood glucose levels. When we ask patients to follow directions, we must be sensitive to the impact

Table 3.4 Results of patient education research findings.

Psychological factors are not strong predicators of patient teaching outcomes.

Patient education materials tend to be written at reading levels beyond the capabilities of most patients.

Patient education outcomes are not influenced by the timing of teaching.

Instruction of the family benefits the patient.

Patient education does influence learning.

Most teaching strategies are effective.

Group teaching is effective and may be preferred by patients.

All patient groups respond to patient education.

Adapted from: Lindeman CA (1988). Patient education. *Annual Review of Nursing Research*. **6**: 29–60.

that these will have on their lives. It is difficult, and even stressful, to change patterns which have been a part of one's life for a long time. Therefore, the nurse *must appreciate* and *understand* the implications of the changes that are required to adapt to an illness or modify life-style.

The Health Belief Model is useful in determining why some patients comply and others do not. The Health Belief Model theorizes that the likelihood of patient compliance varies with:

1. The patient's perception of susceptibility to the disease.
2. The prediction of the impact of the illness on the patient's life.
3. The patient's perception of barriers to taking recommended action.
4. The patient's perception of the benefits of taking the action.

It is important for nurses to understand that all individuals are influenced by their beliefs and values (attitudes) about their health or illness. Nurses are also influenced by their own beliefs and values. At times, the individual's values and the nurse's beliefs may be very different. For effective teaching to occur, the nurse has to base the educational plan on the individual's perception of what is important and achievable because beliefs are strong motivators of human behaviour.

Locus of control is a concept which is linked with beliefs and compliance. Individuals who perceive that they control their own actions have an internal locus of control. Those who seek influence from others, such as family or friends, or luck, have an external locus of control. The individual with an internal locus of control will ask for information on which to make decisions and will accept responsibility for health behaviour.

Yet another factor influencing control is the rapport and relationship established between the nurse and patient.

Listening to the patient and checking understanding of what has been said will greatly enhance learning. The active participation of patients is a preferred goal.

Finally, Green (1987) made several recommendations to health professionals about working with patients who need to adhere to medication regimens:

1. Instructions should be *specific* in teaching a simple short-term regimen.
2. When teaching long-term regimens, multiple strategies are necessary.
3. Providing *cues* is an effective strategy to increase compliance.
4. Rewards may help to sustain behaviour change.
5. Counselling, group sessions, support and self-monitoring are successful strategies to increase compliance.

Contracting with patients has been shown to be effective in achieving compliance. The purpose of a contract is to promote the patient's active participation in health care by assisting the patient to identify and accomplish specific goals. Contracting helps to facilitate the patient's self-esteem, as well as promoting a trusting relationship.

Contracting promotes the patient's autonomy, involvement and responsibility for health. The patient exercises the right to self-determination and ability to solve problems. Furthermore, when a nurse uses contracting as a strategy, he or she is demonstrating belief in the dignity and worth of the patient.

Steps in developing a contract include:

1. Identification of the priority health concerns or needs of the patient.
2. The setting of *mutual* goals.
3. Writing the contract.
4. Implementation of the tasks or activities agreed upon.
5. Evaluation of the outcomes of the contract.

An example of a format that may be used for a written contract is shown in Figure 2.3. This example illustrates the main points of setting the goals and objectives and clearly outlining the tasks, and the importance of the patient and nurse signing the agreement.

When helping patients to adjust to major life-style changes, the nurse can use contracting as a method to achieve compliance. Contracting breaks down what might be overwhelming change into small incremental steps. The patient, who feels in control of what can be accomplished, will be more likely to achieve the desired objective.

INFLUENCE OF CULTURE ON PATIENT EDUCATION

Culture determines many of the beliefs and values held by individuals; it therefore has a strong influence on health behaviour. Conflicts can arise when the nurse and patient hold different beliefs and values about what constitutes appropriate health behaviour.

Assessment of the beliefs, values and practices of the patient is vital to tailoring educational interventions. The

Table 3.5   Assessment of patients' educational needs.

Patient characteristics
   Attitudes to health and customs
   Past experience with illness
   Physical condition
   Emotional state
   Intellectual level
   Support systems
   Preferred methods of learning.

Other factors influencing learning
   Patient/family perceptions of learning needs
   Patient goals
   Factors facilitating learning
   Barriers to learning
   Learning needs identified by health professionals
      and validated by patient/family

patient should be assessed as an individual, so that cultural preferences come out naturally, rather than being forced into a preconceived ethnic stereotype.

For example, to teach about therapeutic changes in diet, the nurse must determine the patient's preferred and current diet and the meaning of food in the patient's life.

The nurse needs to elicit the patient's views on the illness experience. For example, in some cultures it may be undesirable for a man to be bathed by a woman and to put the patient in this situation would jeopardize his self-esteem. Conflicts in perspectives should be acknowledged openly and clarified. The nurse cannot enforce a teaching plan that contradicts the patient's beliefs. The patient's plan may not be the nurse's first choice but it may be more acceptable than the patient rejecting all interventions.

When English is the patient's second language, it is important for the nurse to speak slowly, use simple sentence structure, avoid medical/technical jargon, provide sequential steps in teaching, and not assume that the patient understands. Even if English is the first language, jargon and abbreviations should be avoided. The nurse should also consider the educational level of the patient and, without being patronizing, speak in terms that are appropriate and readily understood by the individual.

THE PROCESS OF PATIENT EDUCATION

The process of patient education parallels the steps of the nursing process and includes: data collection and analysis to identify learning needs; goal setting and planning; implementation; and evaluation. The discussion of each step of the process involves collaboration between the nurse and the patient. Documentation is an essential component of each step. Table 3.5 outlines a framework for collection of the data that are relevant to the patient's educational needs.

Assessment

Assessment begins with identifying those patient characteristics that influence learning. Biographical data, results of diagnostic studies and the medical plan of care can be obtained from the patient's health record. Much information about the individual can be gathered during any physical examination in history taking and when giving care. Factors which influence patient education processes and which therefore need to be included in the assessment process are given below.

Attitudes to health and customs. The patient's attitudes towards health, and the degree of belief that it is possible to be in control of one's health, will influence learning. Religious and cultural beliefs influence eating habits, life-style and receptiveness to health care and prescribed therapy. This information is also useful to the nurse who is helping the patient make decisions about care.

Past experience with illness. Information about past health history should be collected, including how the person coped with illness and what changes in health habits and life-style resulted.

Physical condition. The patient's general feeling of well-being or illness influences the capacity and readiness to learn. The ability to carry out activities of daily living and to manage tasks and procedures necessary for self-care should be assessed. Vision, hearing, touch, manual dexterity and mobility all need assessment because they are important to physical functioning.

Emotional state. Emotions affect an individual's readiness to learn and to respond to teaching. In illness, and when there is a permanent loss of function, patients may progress through stages of adaptation or grieving. These stages include denial, anger and resentment, recognition and acknowledgement of the problem. When recognition and acknowledgement occur the patient begins to participate in decision making.

Intellectual ability. As well as willingness and desire to learn, the patient's ability to understand the condition and solve related problems will contribute to effective learning. The length of the individual's attention span, basic knowledge and fluency in the language being used should be kept in mind when considering comprehension and learning.

Support system. The response of family and friends to the situation can play an important part in the patient's education. If supportive, it facilitates learning and provides reinforcement for positive changes in behaviour.

Barriers to learning. Individual deterrents to learning include sensory deficits, decreased ability to comprehend, lack of orientation to time, place and person, decreased manual dexterity and loss of physical mobility. Learning is also inhibited by lack of motivation.

Severe anxiety can interfere with learning, so that worries about lack of social and financial support and resources may inhibit effective patient education. If the language or form of words used by those teaching is unfamiliar or too technical (or perhaps too patronizing), that can also act as a barrier to understanding.

Identification of Learning Needs

A learning need is the educational gap between the present and the desired or required level of competence. It is mutually identified by the nurse and the patient from the analyses of the data collected and the needs expressed by the patient. The identification of learning needs should include a description of what the patient should know or be able to do and the factors influencing this.

When patients are in hospital, nursing staff tend to take over all responsibility for giving medication, yet upon discharge patients are expected to manage their own drugs. If a patient does not understand facts, such as the effects and side-effects of medication, dosage and timing, it should not be surprising that after discharge there is a strong possibility that the medication regimen will not be followed, which might contribute to the patient's readmission. Patients need to fully understand their medication before discharge, which suggests that teaching programmes are essential, including, where appropriate, self-medication while still in hospital. The concept of the traditional 'drug round' is in need of review.

The patient may not perceive the needs that are identified by health care personnel as priority needs, or may not wish to acquire the knowledge and skills required. It is therefore necessary that the learning needs identified by professionals are discussed with the patient and family and an explanation given as to why these needs are relevant to the patient's health.

The family should receive teaching on how they can best assist with the daily activities that the patient cannot carry out alone and on what resources and environmental changes can be provided to promote patient self-care.

The patient's preferred method of learning. Certain methods of teaching and learning work better than others with different patients. Past educational experience will influence the effectiveness of various teaching methods and learning styles. It is useful to identify whether the patient learns best by reading, viewing an audiovisual programme or carrying out a learning activity, and whether there is a preference for one-to-one or group teaching or, indeed, a combination of several methods.

Patient/family perceptions. Identifying educational needs and setting priorities requires assessing the patient's and family's present knowledge, how they see the patient's present level of functioning and what the desired level of competence may be. It is important to know if they are able to look at the long-term implications or are only able to focus on what is happening today. This sort of assessment must be a continuous process, as changes occur once the patient has achieved the initial goals, coped with the impact of illness and begun to accept the changes in life-style.

Patient goals. The patient's goals and priorities for present and future functioning should be determined. Motivation and readiness to assume responsibility for health care require assessment as this may reveal that the patient's goals differ from those of the health professionals and of relatives, resulting in conflicts and confusion which hinder learning.

Planning

SETTING GOALS

Once learning needs have been identified, the nurse works with the patient to establish goals for learning, to determine priorities for teaching content and to select methods of teaching. Learning goals are usually divided into *short-term goals*, for immediate learning needs and *long-term objectives* for defining the eventual expected outcomes. The knowledge or skill to be achieved is defined, and the expected level or degree to which it will be met is stated. The final component of objective-setting is defining the time in which the desired change is expected to occur. Behavioural objectives are worded in simple, basic terms that are clear to the patient and to all members of the health care team. Action verbs such as 'state', 'describe', 'demonstrate' and 'perform safely' identify what is expected of the patient and give direction for designing the content and process of the learning experiences. Objectives may include all three categories of learning:

1. Cognitive (knowledge)
2. Psychomotor skills
3. Attitudes.

Objectives break learning tasks into small, sequential steps that can be achieved independently before the total goal is mastered. The patient knows what is expected of him at each point, as well as what the overall goal is.

The teaching plan must be written and placed in the patient's record. Without a written plan, other members of the health care team cannot actively participate in the teaching process. The plan must also be shared with the patient so that he or she can actively work towards achieving results.

Using a patient with diabetes as an example, be-havioural objectives for the patient might be to:

- *State* the action of insulin.
- *Demonstrate* the technique of drawing up the

prescribed amount of insulin into a syringe.
- *Verbalize* feelings related to self-injection with in-sulin.

PRIORITY SETTING

Priority is given to what the patient perceives as important and is ready to learn. If conflicts arise between what the nurse perceives as important and what the patient needs to know, negotiation and compromise become necessary to facilitate learning and compliance. The nurse can influence the patient's receptiveness to teaching by providing the information the patient requires to make a decision. The first priority is the learning of survival skills so that the patient can provide safe self-care. For example, the patient learns about diabetes, diet and how to self-administer insulin. Following this, priority is given to other details of the therapeutic regimen (e.g. dietary exchanges, activity, etc.). Lastly, information from pamphlets, books and sources such as self-help groups should be given, if this information is perceived by the nurse and the patient to be useful.

SELECTION OF METHODS OF PRESENTATION

Planning teaching requires the selection of appropriate approaches and methods for presenting information to the patient. Teaching strategies are selected to meet the unique characteristics of the patient and to involve as many senses as possible. If the family is supportive, members are included as active participants in the plan. If the patient has a physical and/or sensory defect, a teaching method is planned that will compensate for it. For example, auditory resource material may be used with the blind.

The teaching content in patient education may relate to a patient's present illness, the general health habits of the patient and/or family, or to a specific health problem of a family member. Teaching content must be accurate, expressed in terms and language understandable to the patient and family, and adapted to age, cognitive ability, education and culture. The amount of time necessary and opportunities for questions, correction and repeti-tion should be given consideration when planning teaching programmes.

Uninterrupted periods for instruction should be planned for times when the patient is most likely to be comfortable and rested. Periods of teaching should be relatively short, as offering too much information at one time may defeat the purpose and leave the patient feeling confused and discouraged.

Practical procedures should be broken down into a logical sequence of steps. First, the procedure should be demonstrated as a whole so that the patient is provided with an overview; then each step should be shown slowly and in detail. Time and opportunity should be allowed for practising the technique as soon as possible after the demonstration. The nurse should be aware that, in teaching any body of information, the first and last parts are recalled best, therefore the most important points should come first and last. Repetition and receptiveness to questions reinforces learning.

Implementation

The actual carrying out of the teaching plan follows the guidelines developed during the planning phase and incorporates principles of learning. Many learning activities can be incorporated into patient care. For example, the nurse can provide information about drugs when they are being given; then later, can ask the patient to state what has been understood about the action of each drug. An explanation may be given each time a procedure is performed, as the patient gradually takes increasing responsibility for the task until able to complete the whole procedure, e.g. changing a stoma bag. Some learning activities require rescheduling to involve family members or a group of patients. Having learning resources (e.g. pamphlets, books, insulin syringe and needle) available for use by the patient is very helpful and frequently leads to questions being asked and problems being addressed.

Evaluation

Evaluation of the teaching programme and the patient's learning should be continuous. Revisions are made as indicated and in some instances are made on the spot if the patient is not responding positively to the planned strategy. Outcomes of teaching are assessed: what effect the teaching has had, whether the objectives have been met, and whether the patient has acquired the knowledge and skills needed. Role-playing or simulation may be used to assess changes in the patient's behavioural responses and in the ability to apply knowledge to real-life situations. The patient must also be an active participant in the ongoing and final evaluation of the educational plan. Observation and feedback are the primary ways in which the nurse determines if (behavioural) change has occurred.

DOCUMENTATION OF PATIENT EDUCATION

Communication between members of the health team is essential to achieve a co-ordinated, consistent approach to patient education. Documentation needs to include:

- Assessment data and action taken
- The teaching plan
- What has been taught
- The patient's level of understanding
- What further teaching or reinforcement of information may be needed
- Instances when the patient was not ready to learn
- When teaching was not completed prior to discharge and what referral or action was taken

To be useful, documentation need not be elaborate, nor does it need to take an inordinate amount of time. To facilitate the documentation of complex information or the teaching given to patients with similar conditions, such as diabetic patients, a flow sheet can be developed.

A documentation flow sheet for teaching might include:

- Preprinted objectives related to expected outcomes
- Space to indicate that the outcome was achieved
- Space for time, date and signature
- A section for narrative comments.

Documentation is an important component in the process of patient education. It helps make patient education effective by providing a means of communicating how much teaching has or has not been accomplished.

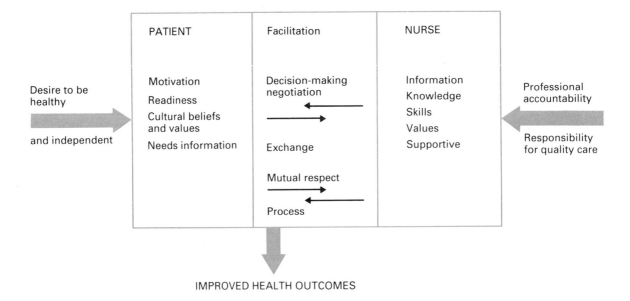

Figure 3.1 A proposed framework for patient education.

FRAMEWORK FOR PATIENT EDUCATION

An outline of the factors influencing patient education has been presented in this chapter. Beliefs and values about patient education were explored, as well as the process of patient education. From the outline presented, a schematic framework for patient education is suggested (Figure 3.1). The overall goal for patient education depicted in this diagram is the incorporation of information into health behaviours in order to improve health outcomes. Patient teaching is an interactive process wherein the role of the nurse is to support and encourage the patient to be an equal partner in decision making. The values and beliefs of the nurse and the patient influence patient education. The nurse has information, knowledge and skills to share. The patient has a desire to learn and wants information which can be used to modify health. The nurse is influenced in his or her teaching by the goals of nursing, professional accountability and responsibility for providing quality care.

LEARNING ACTIVITIES

1. *Experiencing change in life-style*
   As outlined in the chapter, patients are required to make significant changes in their life-style to accommodate illness or to prevent illness. Examples include patients with diabetes mellitus or patients with high cholesterol levels at risk of cardiovascular illness. To appreciate the impact of life-style changes and thus understand how teaching may influence the patient, try to make a significant change in your lifestyle. Try to eliminate all fats from your diet for one week and record what you experienced in doing so. Keep a log of your reactions and review this periodically as you work with patients.

2. *Measuring teaching effectiveness*
   List ways that you could use to evaluate whether your patient teaching has been effective. For example, one measurement would be to ask the patient for feedback on how the process went. What other measures could you implement?

3. *Patient medication*
   Consider the following types of drugs: β-blockers, antibiotics, non-narcotic analgesics, diuretics, bronchodilators and non-steroidal anti-inflammatory agents. Pick one example of each and write out a patient education document that would be suitable for a 70-year-old patient being discharged home on such a drug, explaining dosage, effects and side-effects, etc.

REFERENCES AND FURTHER READING

Adams R, Fliegelman E & Grieco A (1987) Patient guide: how to use a condom. *Medical Aspects of Human Sexuality* **21**: 74–75.

Archer VE (1989) Psychological defenses and control of AIDS. *American Journal of Public Health* **79**: 876–878.

Becker MH (1985) Patient adherence to prescribed therapies. *Medical Care* **23**: 539–555.

Benbow Plewes C (1984) Helping nurses become better patient educators. *Canadian Nurse* **80**: 41–42.

Brown CS, Wright RC & Christensen DB (1987) Association between type of medication instruction and patient's knowledge, side effects and compliance. *Hospital & Community Pharmacy* **38(1)**: 55–60.

Close A (1988) Patient education: a literature review. *Journal of Advanced Nursing* **13(7)**: 203–213.

Cook T (1984) Major research analysis provides proof: patient education does make a difference. *Promoting Health* **Nov.–Dec.**: 4–9.

Dracup K & Meleis AI (1982) Compliance: an interactionist approach. *Nursing Research* **31(1)**: 31–36.

Ewles L & Simnett I (1985) *Promoting Health*. Chichester: Wiley.

Fahrenhoft M (1987) Patient emancipation by health education: an impossible goal? *Patient Education and Counselling* **10**: 25–37.

French J (1990) Boundaries and horizons, the role of health education within health promotion. *Health Education Journal* **49(1)**: 7–10.

Friere P (1972) *Cultural Action for Freedom*. Harmondsworth: Penguin.

Green C (1987) What can patient health education coordinators learn from 10 years of compliance research? *Patient Education and Counselling* **10**: 167–174.

Hathaway D (1986) Effect of preoperative instruction on postoperative outcomes. *Nursing Research* **35(5)**: 269–275.

Hellenbrand D (1983) An analysis of compliance behaviour: a response to powerlessness. In Miller JF (ed.) *Coping with Chronic Illness; Overcoming Powerlessness*. Philadelphia: Davis.

Henderson V (1966) *The Nature of Nursing*. New York: Macmillan.

Lask S (1989) Teaching health education. *Nursing Times* **85(50)**: 43–44.

Lewis HR & Lewis ME (1987) What you and your patients need

to know about safer sex. *RN* **50(9):** 53–58.

Lindeman CA (1988) Patient education. *Annual Review of Nursing Research* **6:** 29–60.

Mazzuca S (1982) Does patient education in chronic disease have therapeutic value? *Journal of Chronic Disease* **35:** 521–529.

Minkler M & Checksway B (1988) Ten principles for geriatric health promotion. *Health Promotion* **3(3):** 277–285.

Robson, J, Boomla K, Fitzpatrick S, Jewell A, Taylor J, Self J, Colyer M (1989) Using nurses for preventive activities with computer assisted follow-up: a randomised controlled trial. *British Medical Journal* **298:** 433–435.

Runions J (1988) Impediments to the practice of patient teaching. *Canadian Journal of Nursing Administration* **June:** 12–15.

Seedhouse D (1986) Health: the foundations for achievement. London: Wiley.

Smith JP (1984) Prevention by example. *Nursing Mirror* **159(3):** 17–18.

Stuttle B & Pears N (1988) Continence promotion roadshow. *Nursing Times* **84(14):** 75–76.

Tilley J, Gregor FM & Thiessen V (1987) The nurse's role in patient education: incongruent perceptions among nurses and patients. *Journal of Advanced Nursing* **12:** 291–301.

Tones K (1983) Getting across the facts of life. *Health and Social Services Journal* **Feb.10:** 170–173.

Tones K (1990) Why theorise? Ideology in health education. *Health Education Journal* **49(1):** 2–6.

Valdiserri RO, Arena VC, Proctor D & Bonati FA (1989) The relationship between women's attitudes about condoms and their use: implications for condom promotions programs. *American Journal of Public Health* **79:** 499–501.

Village Clinic Inc. (1988) *Love Life. Enjoy Safer Sex.* Winnipeg: Village Clinic Inc.

Williams A, Bucks R , Whitfield M (1989) *Health Promotion* **48(1):** 30–32.

Wilson-Barnett J & Osborne J (1983) Studies in evaluating patient teaching: implications for practice. *International Journal of Nursing Studies* **20(1):** 33–44.

Wood N, Whitfield M & Bailey D (1989) *Health Promotion* **48(3):** 145–149.

Ageing and Health

4

OBJECTIVES

After studying this chapter, the reader will be able to:
- Identify the demographics of an ageing population
- Discuss the influence of myths and attitudes on behaviour towards older adults
- Describe normal ageing changes related to physiological, cognitive and psychosocial development
- Identify the principles of health promotion for older adults
- Discuss ethical issues related to the care of the elderly
- Describe a framework for the nursing care of the elderly

'Good health and affluence go together, and differences in fortune which exist throughout the life span are still there in striking form in old age.'

In ancient times, in Rome and Egypt, some people survived for over 100 years. In the UK today a few people survive to a hundred, and the event is celebrated with a telegram from Buckingham Palace because it is such an unusual achievement. The rest of the population die long before then, although the average length of life has gradually increased in this century (Figure 4.1). In many parts of the world the life span of a human is much less. The difference is largely connected to sanitary conditions and the fact that a number of childhood diseases that used to be fatal can now be treated with antibiotics or prevented by immunization, and childbirth is much safer for women (and babies). Yet, even within UK society today, a healthy old age depends on a number of social factors.

Numerous publications are available giving details of the ageing UK population. Any textbook is soon out of date but the latest figures are always available from other sources. Publications such as *Social Trends*, the *General Household Survey* and the *Family Expenditure Survey* give information on the elderly. The number of people over the age of 65 is increasing at a faster rate than the number of people under that age (Figure 4.2). Even within the group of people over 65 there are differences. Because of the casualties in the Second World War, and the people who emigrated after it, there will be a fall in the number of 'younger' old people between now and the first decade of the twentieth century.

The increasing number of elderly patients has been seen as a threat to society and is regarded as a problem rather than a logical conclusion of a healthier society. The elderly are, however, heavy consumers of health care. Thirty-five per cent of health and personal social expenditure is devoted to people aged 65 and over, and 20% to those over 75 (Phillipson, 1982), but this is not the result of inevitable decline in old age. The financial problems of elderly people contribute significantly to their health problems, for example by creating stress that may lead to mental illness. Social isolation may also lead to depression (Abrams, 1980). Those who have been affluent in earlier life are far less likely to suffer from illness in old age. Most elderly people are, however, capable of independent living, of identifying their own health needs and of making appropriate decisions regarding their health. However, Figure 4.3 shows the steady increase in the numbers of elderly people in residential homes who are no longer able to live independently.

ATTITUDES AND MYTHS

Attitude refers to a person's favourable or unfavourable evaluation of an object (Yurick, 1988). The attitudes of care-givers toward the elderly have been considered by gerontologists to have had a major influence on the kind of care provided and on the self-image of older persons. However, definition and measuring problems have created a contradictory and confusing picture. Research findings on *behaviours* of others with the elderly are now thought better to explain the care provided. Behaviour is defined as overt action taken by an individual that is studied in its own right (Yurick, 1988). The relationship between attitudes and behaviours is not clear and may only be meaningful if attitudes relate to specific nursing behaviours.

Studies have revealed that younger people respond negatively to some older adult attributes such as physical age cues, type of dress, proximity to death, passivity/dependency, slowed reactions and disruptive behaviours (Lawrence, 1974; Salter and Templer, 1979; Elliot and Hybertson, 1982; Kahana and Keyak, 1984).

Myths and stereotypes are many. 'Old biddy', 'young

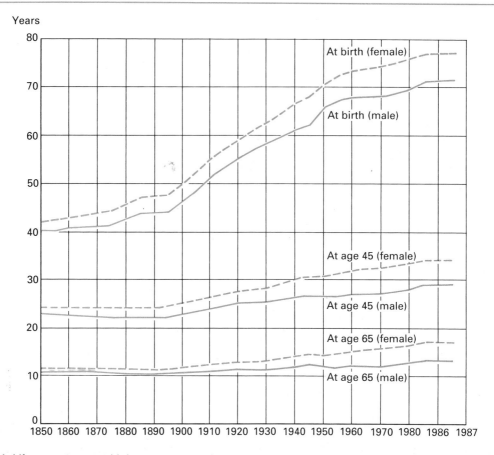

Years

Figure 4.1 Life expectancy at birth, at age 45 and at age 65, England and Wales.

for her age', 'dirty old man' are common phrases which imply an expected behaviour or appearance in old age. The belief that changes experienced by an older person must be caused by physical decline is widely accepted. However, this is often not true. For example, mental slowness could result from decreased social contact/ stimuli rather than from the effects of dementia. Older adults may be disadvantaged both by persons who overemphasize a positive view of ageing and by those who are pessimistic and emphasize a negative view.

Nurses can combat the impact of prevailing attitudes and myths through a thorough exploration of the history of older persons in order to appreciate their unique past and present coping resources. The feelings that individuals have depend on a number of factors, including previous experience and the things that are learnt through study. It is interesting to note that the attitude of student nurses towards the elderly often gets more negative during the experience of socializing (Fielding, 1986). Their positive feelings, based on human experience, seem to get overlaid with profes-sional prejudice.

Some nurses feel that future careers are not to be made in what may be perceived as the 'back-breaking, backward looking' wards where the elderly are cared for. What happens to the positive feelings that student

nurses have at the start? How do nurses develop their opinions? Where do they get these ideas from? Interestingly, the research that has been done shows that highly educated nurses, for example nurses with degrees, are attracted towards posts where there is scope for a large amount of autonomy and influence, and they are therefore attracted to the care of the elderly. Some of the most recent advances in nursing have been pioneered in care-of-the-elderly settings (Wright, 1986) and the King's Fund nursing develop-ment units have included a large proportion of care-of-the-elderly units. Nevertheless, the exposure of student nurses to the care of the elderly in the past has sometimes been a disappointing experience.

'Ageism' is the word that is used to describe the negative attitudes towards the elderly in society. Ageism does not exist in isolation. Ageing women face more discrimination than ageing men. Being affluent not only hides some of the signs of ageing, but also prevents some of the symptoms. Older women who live alone are much more likely to be poor, and therefore seen as a nuisance and a drain on society. The myth of the older person is acted out in the media images of the old. The news may be read by a mature man with grey hair, but his female companion is most likely to be young and beautiful. An elderly person with sexual desires is

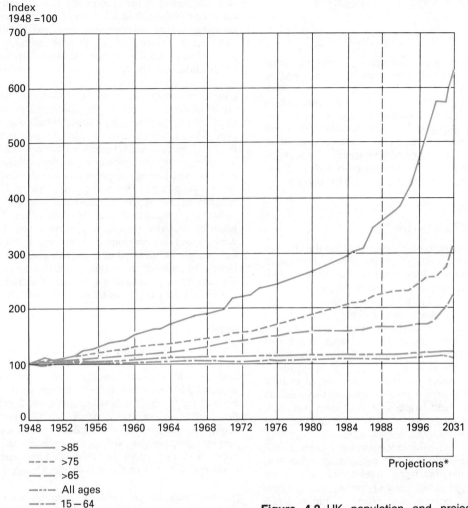

Figure 4.2 UK population and projections (index 1948 = 100).

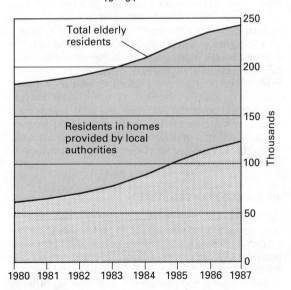

Figure 4.3 Elderly people in residential accommodation in the UK.

represented as either dirty or ridiculous. Women outnumber men by over 50% in the over-60 age group, but there is a tendency to marginalize them and ignore the issues that face them as a group.

Nurses can help to minimize the effect of stereotyping by treating and talking to each person as an individual. Listening to an elderly person who comes into your care, you will find out what makes them unique and whether or not they suffer from any of the disabilities that some people associate with old age. By finding out who they are and what their background is, you can come to respect them. The elderly woman in your care may have lived through two world wars, loved and lost husbands, brothers and children. She may be daring and outrageous and adventurous, or she may be more conservative and quiet. If you learn how to listen to elderly people with respect, you will be able to help them build on their strengths and overcome any problems that have beset them as a result of illness or poverty.

GROWTH AND DEVELOPMENT

PHYSIOLOGICAL THEORIES OF AGEING

There are many theories to explain why and how ageing occurs. These major theories can be categorized as molecular, cellular and physiological (Yurick, 1988). Physiological theories examine the interrelationships between organ systems during ageing. In particular, immunological ageing and neuroendocrine control are two mechanisms which have been studied. Some or all of these internal processes may be found to determine the ageing process, while external factors such as drugs, nutrition and the environment also likely contribute to the process.

PHYSIOLOGICAL STATUS

While it is important to distinguish between the changes in an older adult resulting from the expected course of ageing and those resulting from disease or injury, we lack precise information on normal ageing processes. Much of the research has been cross-sectional (comparing average results of a group of older persons with a younger group), so that the differences found in these studies between age groups may have been due, not to age, but to the effects of environment, diet or activities interacting with the groups at different points in time.

The accepted theory that there is a universal gradual loss in all body organs from about age 30 may need to be reassessed. New studies which have followed individuals over long periods reveal no change in renal function for those free of disease (Lindeman et al, 1985). In some instances, performance actually increases with age. It has been found that such things as exercise, diet, non-smoking and practising intelligence tests have produced changes in the level of fitness, heart reserve, blood pressure, memory and reaction time of some older adults (Fries, 1989). The existing knowledge related to changes with age can serve as general guidelines for care which is aimed at preserving and prolonging function. However, we need to recognize that new knowledge may alter these conceptions of old age.

Most older adults function well at rest but their functional capacity may be altered under conditions of stress. Such stressors as illness, surgery, trauma, physical exercise and emotional stress may exceed the body's threshold of physiological reserves, resulting in an inability to maintain homeostasis. Furthermore, the older person is more likely to develop complications from health insults and may take longer to recover than younger individuals.

Physiological changes can begin for some in adulthood or may not occur until well after 70 years of age. The older adult may continue to engage in all the activities of middle age but may modify the pace of life and take more frequent rests. Table 4.1 displays physical and functional changes that occur with ageing. Key nursing implications are noted as well.

Assessment. There are three methods of assessment: interview, observation and examination. Basic to discus-sing assessment is the recognition that the patient has the right to refuse all or any parts of the assessment. The *interview* with an older person takes time due to slower functioning, reduced energy, possible memory deficits and a longer history. It may be necessary to collect information over several episodes. Privacy, awareness of possible sensory or cognitive losses, language and education barriers must all be considered. When the nurse *observes*, all senses including vision are used. Smell is used to detect any unusual breath, excretory or skin odours. Touch can be used to assess strength, flexibility, texture and temperature. Sounds can be used to detect quality of speech or respirations. *Examination* is conducted through inspection and palpation, as with other age groups. The nurse organizes and records findings in the approved manner, taking note of the richness of the qualitative data often found in the histories of older people which can reveal both the worries and the wisdom of many years. Nurses will increasingly be involved in the health assessment of the elderly because of the requirement that general practitioners are responsible for regular health checks on elderly patients as part of their contracts.

SKIN

Ageing skin is generally characterized by diminishing function and reserve capacity. The epidermis 'thins', and decreases in elasticity, strength and vascularity. The superficial blood vessels are less efficient in dilating and contracting to regulate body temperature. Local sensation of heat, pressure and painful stimuli may be less acute. Wound healing is retarded; trauma can have serious consequences. Nail growth declines; hair follicle production and colour are influenced by genetic and endocrine factors. Patterns of body hair change with age.

Nursing Implications. Elderly patients need to be encouraged to report any lesion that bleeds, fails to heal or changes size. The older person should avoid exposure to strong sun and heat, but in the UK there is an even greater danger of death from hypothermia in the cold winter months and the nurse should be aware of the benefit of good warm clothing, and be aware that many older people cannot afford to heat their homes adequately. Careful attention to maintaining integrity and lubrication of the skin, hair and nails is important. Because of increased risk of pressure sores, frequent position changes and personal hygiene require attention. The use of a chiropodist for foot care may be necessary.

MUSCULOSKELETAL SYSTEM

Adult bone loss (osteoporosis) begins to take place in both sexes around the age of 40 and is thought to be related to diet, physical activity, hormonal changes and possibly RNA activity. The bones become weaker and compression of the vertebrae leads to a reduction in height. There is approximately a 15% slowing of nerve conduction time, which contributes to a decrease in speed, strength, reaction time, resistance to fatigue and co-ordination. However, a wide variability exists. If the

Table 4.1 Physical and functional changes related to ageing.

Changes	Nursing implications
Skin	
• Decreased elasticity • Dryness, scaling of skin • Wound healing retarded; increased vascular fragility • Nails thicken, become brittle and yellow • Thinning of hair, loss of pigmentation • Sweat glands atrophy	• Attention to skin care, nail care, position changes, and hygiene • Insulatory effect of clothing • Avoiding exposure to sun and heat
Musculoskeletal	
• Decreased subcutaneous tissue, muscle mass and strength • Bone demineralization • Joints stiffen, lose flexibility	• Accident prevention and rest • Exercise programme • Weight control • Aids to movement • Diet high in calcium, vitamin D, and protein
Neurological	
• Slowed reaction, especially to multiple stimuli (neurone loss) • Decreased temperature regulation and pain perception • Increased time for problem solving • Decreased overall sleep time and REM sleep • Sense of balance declines	• Slower pacing of activities • Monitor trauma or illness carefully • Assess sudden confusional states • 5–7 hours of night sleep may be sufficient
Special senses	
• Diminished visual activity (presbyopia); increased sensitivity to glare and difficulty adjusting to darkness • Decreased depth perception • Diminished hearing activity (presbycusis) • Diminished colour perception (especially blue and green) • Decreased sense of taste and smell	• Regular vision and hearing tests • Avoid night driving, glare • Home safety (lighting, furniture) • Communication techniques (auditory, visual and tactile) • Use of yellows, oranges against contrasting backgrounds • Use of spices/herbs and low calorie foods • Smoke detectors
Cardiopulmonary	
• Less able to increase heart rate and cardiac output with activity • Blood vessels less elastic • Venous return less efficient • Peripheral oedema and pooling may occur, especially with immobility • Pulmonary elasticity and ciliary action decrease leading to less efficient gas exchange and slowed cough reflex	• Regular blood pressure readings • Posture, breathing, and walking exercise • Avoid prolonged immobility; early ambulation • Avoid irritants • Limit salt intake • Pacing activities • Attention to prolonged infections • Vaccinations (pneumococcal and influenza)
Gastrointestinal (including dentition)	
• Diminished saliva, digestive juices, and decreased nutrient absorption • Delayed oesophageal and gastric emptying • Reduced muscle tone and decreased peristalsis • Decreased blood flow to liver lessens drug detoxication • Decreased taste buds • Teeth more brittle, some reabsorption of gum tissue	• Regular diet low in fat and calories, high in fibre and fluids • Small, frequent servings more readily digested • Discourage long-term laxative and other non-prescription drugs • Accessible toilet facilities • Community resources for help with meals • Dental and oral hygiene • Regular dental examinations
Genitourinary (including reproductive)	
• Decreased blood flow to kidneys • Bladder capacity diminishes; reduced glomerular filtration • Decrease in bladder size and sphincter control may result in incomplete emptying	• Encourage hydration • Minimum daily 1500–2000 ml of fluid • Accessible toilet and hygiene facilities • Avoid constipation

Table 4.1 *continued*

Changes	Nursing implications
• Enlarged prostate, reduced testosterone, slowed erection • Atrophy and decreased lubrication of female genital tract; reduced oestrogen	• Recognize drug toxicity • Incontinence aids • Adaptation of sexual practices
Endocrine • Decreased testosterone • Glucose tolerance deteriorates • Temperature regulation less efficient	• Maintain normal weight • Limit use of fat and sugar

Modified from Gioiella et al (1985) and Taylor et al (1989).

person remains active, the muscle tissue shows some atrophy but remains relatively strong. Disuse of the muscles leads to fatty infiltration and marked weakness. The key issue is the degree to which these changes affect function.

Nursing Implications. The older person can benefit by pacing activities, maintaining a suitable exercise programme, compensating for dysfunction through the use of aids, and eating adequate nutrients such as protein, potassium, calcium and Vitamin D. Physical and financial limitations may however limit the person's ability to consume an ideal diet. Accident prevention should be emphasized both in the home and in hospital. Weight reduction can minimize the degenerative changes in the joints and promote mobility and function.

NEUROLOGICAL SYSTEM

Simple reaction time is decreased with age due to vision impairment, decreased axons in the nerves and synapse changes resulting in slow nerve conduction. This may result in slowed reflexes, decreased pain sensation, and an increased time required for problem solving.

Nursing Implications. The elderly person needs more time to make decisions. Loss of sensation increases the potential for skin lesions to form, e.g. due to pressure localized over any particular area. Sudden confusion is not age related and needs immediate assessment as there may be a physical cause such as an hypoxia related to a chest infection. The older person requires less sleep, between 5 and 7 hours could be sufficient, and may well be used to early rising as a matter of habit. The sense of balance may deteriorate in old age (see below).

SPECIAL SENSES

Loss of acuity of the senses occurs with ageing. The change in visual acuity or blurred vision is probably caused by changes in the lens and the vitreous humour. *Presbyopia* (far-sightedness) in which the eye cannot focus on near objects as clearly begins about the age of forty. Other visual changes are poorer adaptation to dark, decreased depth perception, increased susceptibility to glare, increased need for lumination due to

decreased pupil size, and changes in colour discrimination (mostly in blues and greens). Nursing assessment considers the age-related changes, the person's methods of adapting to these changes, and the visual assets that the person does possess.

Hearing ability declines with ageing for some individuals but this is not universal. The extent of the decline is difficult to measure because other factors such as the person's concentration, attentiveness and caution may influence responses. Generally, there is difficulty hearing high frequency sounds (*presbycusis*) and consonants (S, T, Z, G, F) may not be discriminated. It is important to assess the ability of the person to hear a conversation in a setting where there are other voices, music and background noise. Because hearing loss develops slowly, the person may be able to adapt to the change, but when excess energy is required to discriminate speech the person may withdraw or become suspicious.

Communication involves the use of symbols and motor articulation or speech. With ageing, simple reaction time is decreased and learning occurs at a less rapid rate, but normal ageing alone does not account for speech difficulties. Such things as teeth alignment, breath control, atrophy of vocal cords affecting pitch may alter speech, but generally it remains functional.

There is a decreased sense of taste and smell with ageing for some individuals.

Nursing Implications. Many of the effects of visual changes can be minimized through environmental modifications. The level of illumination can be increased; glare and night driving can be avoided; and colours which enhance the visibility of objects can be introduced. Landmarks can be used to orientate the visually impaired person. Low vision aids or corrective lenses can often help but require correct assessment and training. Assessment of hearing changes should include the person's reaction to the loss. What kind of adaptation has taken place, if any? There are many tips for improving communication with the hearing impaired person, such as slowing the rate of speech, adequately lighting the face of the speaker, placing the speaker 3–6 feet from the elderly person. The use of touch, hearing aids, auditory training, speech reading, speech training and environmental aids such as telephone amplifiers are some of the many ways to improve hearing. Changes in diet through the addition of herbs to enhance flavour can compensate for potential taste changes. Safety features for those whose sense of smell is impaired (smoke alarms) can be considered, as well as diet changes to encourage healthy eating.

CARDIOPULMONARY SYSTEM

Cardiac output drops due to fibrosis and sclerosis in the endocardium, left ventricular wall thickening and increased fat infiltration in the right atrium and ventricle. The heart rate slows with age, ranging anywhere from 44 to 108 beats per minute. Cardiovascular stress response is less efficient in the older adult. Body water decreases from 80% of total body composition at birth to 50% of total for those 70 years of age. A decrease in fluids affects the removal of dust and mucous through coughing and sneezing from the tracheobronchial tree and predisposes the person to bronchopneumonia. Pulmonary elasticity and ciliary action decrease, which leads to less efficiency and contributes to bacterial growth.

Nursing Implications. Pacing activities and allowing time for rest is important. Immobility and prolonged bed rest are avoided. Regular blood pressure screenings, the moderation of sodium intake, sufficient fluid intake, smoking cessation, appropriate exercise and relaxation are all helpful. The older adult should seek attention for any respiratory infection that lasts more than 2–3 days and be encouraged to receive the influenza vaccination annually and the pneumococcal vaccine (once only), particularly if the person also has chronic respiratory or cardiac disease.

GASTROINTESTINAL SYSTEM (INCLUDING DENTITION)

The gastrointestinal system has such a large reserve capacity that decreases in normal function can occur with little effect on physiological processes. Teeth enamel is thinner and teeth may become brittle. Periodontal disease becomes the major cause of tooth loss. There is less salivary activity and a drying of the mucous membranes. The gag reflex is weaker and the cardiac sphincter is more relaxed, predisposing the older adult to aspiration problems. Decreased amounts of gastric acids and weaker musculature leads to more difficulties with large amounts of food. Decreased blood flow to the liver lessens drug detoxification. Decreased intestinal peristalsis and duller nerve sensations can cause a missed signal for defecation.

Nursing Implications. Maintaining teeth in good condition (flossing, brushing teeth, palate and tongue, regular check-ups) can enhance appetite and permit adequate chewing of food. Avoidance of high fat foods and taking small regular meals, a high fluid intake and adequate fibre can help minimize digestive problems. A healthy, well-balanced diet in the elderly is at least as important as in younger age groups. Avoidance of laxatives, responding promptly to the urge to defecate,

ensuring adequate toilet facilities and easily-removable clothing are all important factors.

GENITOURINARY SYSTEM

Degeneration of the renal system for some older adults leads to a slowing of filtration functions. Bladder capacity decreases from about 500 to about 250 ml, causing frequency and nocturia. Bladder emptying is more difficult due to a weakening of muscles, which may lead to urine retention. Tissue changes associated with oestrogen deficiency in women result in relaxed pelvic floor muscles. In men, prostrate enlargement and atrophy of periurethral structures can occur. These changes may lead to uninhibited bladder contractions (stress incontinence and dribbling).

Nursing Implications. Older adults should be encouraged to drink 2–3 litres of fluids daily as they may seek to cope with continence problems by seriously reducing their fluid intake to the point where dehydration has become an actual problem. Accessible toilet facilities, appropriate clothing and regular toileting which is tailored to the older adult's usual pattern can help to prevent urine remaining in the bladder for long periods and decrease the risk of infection, calculi and overflow. Toxic signs from drugs are important to recognize, especially for those drugs excreted by the kidneys.

REPRODUCTIVE SYSTEM

Reduced testosterone, hypertrophy of the prostate, slow erection, low-intensity ejaculation and thinner pubic hair are some age-related changes in men. Women experience cessation in ovulation and oestrogen production; the vulva, cervix and fallopian tubes become atrophied; and the vagina is less vascular and moist but is more alkaline. This can lead to painful intercourse (dysparuenia). These age-related changes do not prevent sexual function nor alter the libido and pleasure derived from sexual activity.

Nursing Implications. The older adult needs to understand that more time may be required for the male to become fully erect and greater attention should be paid to the female's more fragile vagina. A water-soluble lubricant can reduce dryness. More sensitive foreplay activities can enhance the pleasure. Other forms of intimacy can be explored (touching, hugging). Sexual dysfunction can have many causes and these need to be explored. Disease (diabetes), drugs, abstinence, overeating, fatigue, mental health problems, lack of privacy and concern over others' opinions can all contribute to dysfunction. It is important that the older women should continue to do monthly breast self-examinations and to report any vaginal bleeding as these actions can lead to the early detection of malignant changes.

Cognitive Status

Cognition refers to cerebral functioning (e.g. thinking

and reasoning) and the ability to perceive and understand one's world (Taylor et al, 1989). A loss of mental function is not a normal process of ageing. However, there is a decreased capacity for adaptation, especially in stressful or unfamiliar settings and if the person has impaired senses. Older persons experience a decreased ability to respond to multiple or complex stimuli so they tend to respond to stimuli of the greatest intensity. If all stimuli are of low intensity, the older person may become disinterested.

The older adult continues to learn and to problem solve. Intellectual performance is stable but response time declines, so that the older person takes more time to absorb, process and respond to information and environmental cues. Memory is generally stable unless reorganization is required, or distractions or time pressure are present. Mild short-term memory loss

occurs commonly, while long-term memory remains good (Siegler, 1980).

Nursing Implications. The former loss can be minimized through the use of lists, schedules and calendars which incorporate information meaningful to the daily functioning of the individual. Pacing the amount of information given and providing reinforcement and an environment conducive to learning can improve the older adult's ability to receive, retain and retrieve information. For example, in teaching an elderly person how to use a new hearing aid it may be necessary to demonstrate the hearing aid on more than one occasion. A list of the instructions would be helpful and teaching should be provided not in a busy clinic with other people walking past but somewhere quiet where the older person can concentrate on what is being

Table 4.2 Health education and the elderly.

Key developmental factors	Implications for health teaching
Physical maturation	
• Sensory changes:	• Distinct, large configurations in visual aids; glasses clean, accessible; good lighting
Decreased acuity and accommodation of vision	
Loss of perception of high tone sounds and some discrimination	• Speak clearly, at a normal rate, close to learner. Increase loudness as needed.
	• Use audiovisual aids carefully: the very elderly are not as comfortable with these resources, particularly if they move so quickly that auditory and visual cues are missed
Cognitive development	
• Affected by motivation, interest, sensory alteration	• Replace spectator learning with involvement (process) learning
	• Encourage new and unconventional approaches: use role play, singing, games, exercise; anything which proves helpful and fun
• Decreased speed of response	• Present content at a slow pace or foster self-pacing
	• Allow adequate response time
• Less efficient short-term memory	• Provide repetition, opportunities for recall
• Simultaneous activities disruptive	• Short learning sessions
	• Environment should eliminate distracting sights and sounds
	• Establish reachable short-term goals
Psychosocial development	
• Ego integrity versus despair (Erikson). Well-developed life-style habits	• Encourage participation in decision making and planning for learning
	• Integrate new behaviours with previously established ones
	• Encourage self-reward as well as praise from others
	• Identify barriers to learning (environment, values, beliefs)
• Changes in body image due to effects of ageing	• Be sure that all reminders of the dependent child-learner are gone: straight rows of chairs, attendance, rules and regulations, formal testing, comparison with other learners, censure, sarcasm and teacher domination
	• Family members could participate and serve as sources of support
• Changes in roles occur through retirement, loss of spouse (others) through death	

From Whitman et al (1986).

taught. Even better, with early detection of hearing loss, the instructions can be given to the patient at a younger age while there is still some hearing. The more highly motivated, younger patient can readily learn to use the hearing aid and hopefully continue to use it in later life. The older person with long-standing deafness may not understand, may get fed up and throw the hearing aid into a drawer. Table 4.2 summarizes conditions specific to the older learner and suggests teaching strategies which can be used.

COGNITIVE IMPAIRMENT

The incidence of mental health problems increases with age (Blazer, 1980) and can be devastating to the older adult and family. *Dementias* are a variety of organically caused disorders that progressively affect cognitive functioning. Among these disorders, the most common is Alzheimer's disease, a serious and ultimately fatal disease with no effective medical treatment. However, good nursing care can enhance the quality of life for the demented person for a long time.

Other disorders such as paranoia, schizophrenia, anxiety, brain tumours and depression may be incorrectly identified as a dementia or may coexist with a dementing illness. Once identified, some of these conditions can be treated and, if coexisting with dementia, treatment may improve the individual's overall functioning (Clarfield, 1988).

Acute confusion is a common non-specific presenting symptom of illness in old age (Hamdy 1984). It is a frequent direct cause of hospital admission of elderly patients. Unlike dementia, acute confusion can be treated and it is important to identify the underlying cause(s). Factors such as drug reactions, infections, metabolic disturbances, heart disease or surgery can all lead to a confusional state.

In acute confusion, the old person has a sudden deterioration in level of consciousness and a disturbed thought process. The older person is disorientated firstly in time and then in place. Attention and memory are poor. The patient is restless, especially at night and sleep is frequently disturbed. Speech may be affected. It has been compared to being in a fog, seeing patches of building, a tree or motor car without being able to relate them to each other (Brocklehurst, 1982).

Nursing Implications. It is important that the nurse recognizes changes in attention span, perception, thinking, memory, psychomotor behaviour, and the sleep–waking cycle of the older adult that could signal the onset of confusion. The nurse can use reminiscence therapy and reality orientation to stimulate the senses. It is also very important to help the patient and family to deal with the role changes and cope with the behaviour alterations and safety requirements that follow the onset of dementia particularly.

Reality orientation is a technique employed to rehabilitate those suffering from disorientation. Basically it consists of recalling the patient to reality repeatedly and frequently by the use of painted signs and calendars and variable prompts. Frequently drawing attention to those details which are relevant to daily life, such as the time of day and the location, can help the patient control what is happening.

Reminiscence therapy is a way of stimulating elderly people with memorabilia, films and songs meaningful to their generation. It can be used in conjunction with or in preparation for reality orientation therapy (Weller, 1989).

Psychosocial Development

There are several psychological or social theories of ageing. There is not sufficient evidence to support one particular theory (Murray, 1980).

PSYCHOLOGICAL THEORIES OF AGEING

Developmental theories seek to explain the diverse growth processes that occur with ageing. Erik Erikson's Epigenetic Theory of Development or 'eight stages of life' is probably the most well-known example (Erikson, 1964). It states that each stage of life is a psychosexual crisis that must be accomplished and lays the foundation for the next stage. Erikson proposed that the older adult searches for emotional integration and an acceptance of the past and present. He believed that it was necessary to accept physical decline without fear of death (integrity versus despair). The concept of 'life review' first described by Robert Butler came from Erikson's beliefs that the effort to relive and restructure life experiences is a way of achieving integrity.

Some view this theory as inflexible. Supporters believe that the theory can be revised so that crisis resolution would incorporate differences in the individual's culture and environment. Other critics believe that the theory sets unrealistic standards, while others call for a clearer definition and more research.

SOCIOLOGICAL THEORIES

The Disengagement Theory, originally described by Cumming and Henry (1961), contends that older adults inevitably and universally withdraw. The theory states that this process prepares one for death and is mutually beneficial for society and the elderly. This concept refutes the view of developmental theorists who regard personality as a key dimension. Some research studies have shown that persons with an active life-style are more likely to express life satisfaction. These findings have resulted in a decreased support for this theory. The degree of agreement between the individual's actual and desired participation rates seems to be the important factor.

The Activity Theory proposed by Havighurst (Havighurst, 1963) and others asserts a positive relationship between levels of participation in social activities and life satisfaction. The older person may substitute activities but does not slow down or disengage from society. Critics argue that this theory has a middle-class bias and that it assumes that one has the luxury of changing roles and developing new ones. It does not deal with the impact of health problems, reduced income or preparation for death. Research has shown partial support for this theory.

The Continuity Theory (Atchley, 1980) proposes that adaptation to ageing can proceed in several directions, depending on the person's past life. Personality and adjustment to stress remain stable over the life span. This theory has gained support as it accounts for factors in other theories and considers individual variation.

More recent theoretical approaches such as age stratification (Riley et al, 1972) and symbolic interaction view ageing as a process that encompasses the entire life-cycle and are broader based. The former considers intergenerational role strain and social class differences. The latter, symbolic interaction, emphasizes the understanding of different points of view and sees role changes as opportunities for older adults (Burggraf and Stanley, 1989).

Nursing Implications. These psychosocial theories suggest certain approaches based on how relationships between the elderly and society are viewed. These theories can form a conceptual framework or philosophy which can influence how the nurse approaches the older person. A nurse who accepts that the older adult withdraws or gives up certain activities would tend to discourage the elderly from making decisions, would aid withdrawal and tend to minimize the need to do assessments or encourage preventive activities.

A nurse who adopts a continuity approach would encourage patient control, would view the environment and the person as equally important and would highly individualize nursing care. Primary health care and prevention would be emphasized with this view.

The other more recent approaches mentioned would encourage the nurse to explore the impact of role changes on the older adult, to be aware of the danger of negative labelling and to understand that the care of older adults can be influenced by conflicts over scarce resources in the broader health and social system.

Psychosocial Status

Age-related psychosocial changes can be associated with internal stressors, such as changes in memory, sleep patterns, hearing and vision, and gastrointestinal metabolism. These and other factors may lead the older adult to feel isolated, frustrated, bored or apathetic. External stressors such as retirement, death of a spouse or friends and diminished resources can contribute to a loss of self-worth and independent functioning. Depression, severe enough to require treatment, is thought to affect 15–20% of the elderly (Shamoian, 1985), and the prevalence of undetected serious depression among hospitalized elderly patients is high (Warshaw et al, 1982). Treatment can improve the outcome for most, especially with careful assessment and early intervention. Caution should be directed at some classes of medication which can aggravate depression, such as antihypertensives, sedatives, narcotics, antihistamines and psychotropic drugs (Salzman, 1985).

Nursing Implications. Nursing care can be directed at strategies to improve self-esteem, such as increasing positive social support, encouraging life review or relaxation and reinforcing the value of appropriate treatment.

Functional Status Assessment

The domains of functional status assessment usually include physical, mental, emotional and social function. Physical function is comprised of two elements: (1) basic self-care activities such as hygiene and mobility; and (2) the more complex independent life tasks such as shopping, transport use and food preparation. With increasing age, the older adult may delegate tasks to others in order to continue independent functioning.

The assessment of function complements other diagnostic and clinical tests because loss of function frequently signals the onset of an acute illness, the progression of a chronic illness or the combined effect of concurrent ill-health and treatment interactions (Johnson and Mezey, 1989). Functional impairments in key areas combined with impaired cognitive functioning frequently lead to the need for institutional care.

The ability to detect functional changes early may enable interventions that can prevent or delay entry into an institution. The Barthel Index is an example of an established self-care assessment instrument which is sensitive to changes in function (Mahoney and Barthel, 1965). This 11-item index was designed for use in rehabilitation settings for patients with neuromuscular and musculoskeletal problems. Using direct observation, it determines the defined aspects of function which a patient can perform independently or with assistance. Functioning in feeding, bathing, dressing, walking and arising from the toilet are some of the areas measured. A numerical score (maximum = 100) is assigned to each area based on the time, amount of physical assistance and special environmental changes the patient needs. Its language is suitable for use in home assessments. Applegate and others have reviewed the use of structured instruments in the assessment of physical, cognitive and emotional function in a recent publication (Applegate et al, 1990).

Information on functional status should be gathered from a wide variety of sources including the older adult, family, doctors, visiting nurses, social workers, friends, day care centre workers and physiotherapists.

Nursing Implications. The maintenance of independence is a highly valued cultural belief among older adults (Boyle and Counts, 1988). The nurse and other members of the health care team can assist the older adult to continue in regular activities while allowing time for rest and the productive use of energy. The nurse can encourage the older adult to make decisions and to choose among health care options which are congruent with the person's beliefs and values, while also supporting self-care. The growth in the number of aids which are available to minimize disabilities in hearing, walking, speech, bathing, dressing, cooking, speak of the efforts that are being made to improve the quality of the older adult's daily life.

HEALTH PROMOTION AND WELLNESS

Some writers suggest that older adults are more likely to be interested in following favourable health practices than are other age groups, despite the fact that older adults generally have lower incomes and less education than the general population (Prohaska et al, 1985; *Prevention Index*, 1987). They are more likely to engage in health activities aimed at reducing stress and controlling emotions. However, older adults may under-report or underestimate symptoms of ill health, believing them to be due to age alone. They tend to accept these conditions as inevitable and simply a part of life (Keller et al, 1989). Still other older adults may be overly sensitive to the symptoms they experience and vigorously seek attention. It is therefore important when discussing health matters to explore the meaning that the older person places on his or her symptoms.

It has been suggested that healthy life-styles for older adults should encompass 'self-responsibility for health, nutrition, exercise, stress management, interpersonal relationships/support, spiritual growth and self-actualization, accident or injury prevention, safe/moderate use of medications and alcohol, smoking avoidance or cessation, self-care regimens for chronic illnesses and accessing preventive health services' (Walker, 1989). Balanced against this view however is the reality of poor housing, low income and an extensive range of social difficulties that many elderly people face.

A number of preventive practices have been found to yield important benefits for older adults and are summarized well by Gambert and Gupta (1989):

1. Smoking cessation, regardless of age, is beneficial to lung performance and can aid in lowering heart rate and blood pressure within a matter of days (US Department of Health, Education and Welfare, 1981).
2. Avoidance of high frequency noises, toxins (such as dyes, gases) and excessive sunlight is recommended.
3. Accurate assessment of nutrient requirements for older adults demands a knowledge of numerous factors such as genetic, physiological, environmental, pathological, pharmacological factors and food selection preferences (Roe, 1989). However, a diet rich in complex carbohydrates and low in fats (emphasizing polyunsaturated fats) is important; modest increases in soluble fibre, a daily calcium intake of at least 1000–1500 mg and adequate intakes of vitamins A and C are advocated.
4. Regular exercise that meets individual interests and health limitations (Howze et al, 1989) is encouraged.
5. Adult immunization for influenza, pneumococcus and tetanus is recommended.
6. Effective management of stress and emotional problems is beneficial.

Health education programmes are shifting from a focus on disease-specific conditions and individual responsibility to developing comprehensive health promotion programmes. These programmes are aimed at the prevention of illness/injury and the understanding of the determinants of health, such as socioenvironmental factors. Older adults and professionals recognize the need for structural changes in the underlying conditions that keep some older adults disadvantaged. This recognition has led to the development of some health promotion programmes that advocate changes by policy makers, manufacturers and mass media (Minkler and Pesick, 1986). More research studies, particularly longitudinal studies, which evaluate the effectiveness of these programmes are required.

ETHICAL ISSUES RELATED TO THE ELDERLY

Increase in age brings with it the likelihood that changes in health and economic status may threaten the older adult's autonomy and independence and erode their quality of life. In years gone by the high death rates of children and young adults in the lower socioeconomic groups reflected enormous inequalities in society. The inequalities continue to exist. People in social class 5 for example, are two and a half times more likely to die before retirement than those in social class 1. Two-thirds of pensioners are women and while married couples are more likely to live above the poverty line, the greater life expectancy of women leads to many widows living below the level of supplementary benefit. Single pensioners are more likely to be poorer than a married couple; the very old are far more likely to be poor than the recently retired. Women, particularly the very elderly, single or widowed, are most likely to be poor. Indeed poverty in this country is, for the most part, the poverty of women (Hewitt, 1974).

A common view is that old people are trapped in deteriorating bodies with deteriorating mental powers and they are viewed socially as a burden consuming disproportional amounts of health care.

It is difficult to separate the ethical issues related to the care of elderly people from the economic issues, especially when so many apparently 'ethical' problems in health care are actually problems of distribution of limited resources. It is a common 'ethical' problem when decisions are made to restrict the use of resources for elderly people because of their poor life expectancy or because their quality of life is judged to be poor. Examples of care decisions that have this kind of ethical analysis include:

- Whether to initiate or continue active treatment for a terminally ill patient
- Whether to withhold tube feeding in a severely demented patient
- Whether to transplant a kidney to an elderly individual.

The ethical principles that are often used to guide decisions in health care are discussed on p. 10. These principles can lead to conflict in nursing situations; for example, the principle of justice may conflict with the principle of beneficence.

An example of the difficulties which may be caused by

the distribution of goods and services is the situation where there is only one hospital bed but two patients requiring admission. In deciding to admit one patient rather than the other, the health care worker is taking an action which will possibly harm the second patient.

Members of the health care team must be sensitive to their own values and beliefs as they affect the team's actions and decisions. The nurse must communicate fully with the older patient and negotiate the care goals clearly. Nurses make these decisions under pressure. For example, in preparing for discharge the nurse should take the patient's wishes fully into consideration when making decisions. It may take considerable time to fully inform older patients of possible outcomes and to allow patients to decide what is in their best interest. Unfortunately, discharge from hospital is often done in a hurry and the older patient may wish to return to a situation which the family, social services and members of the health care team do not consider safe or suitable.

Careful assessment of the older person's competence to make firm decisions can be extremely important. Phillipson (1982) points out an example of a suffocating and probably unethical method of persuading old people to follow a particular course of action: 'The approach to agitated old people is very similar to that of a loving and imaginative mother to an overwrought child. She patiently presents pleasing and soothing alternatives to activities which she cannot condone' (Gray and Isaacs, 1979). An old person is not a child, a fact the nurse should never forget.

Public attention has been focused on ethical and legal issues closely related to competence by the movement for 'living wills'. The living will is an advance directive which outlines an individual's choice for care should specific conditions arise. For example, a person may state in a living will that, if ever suffering from dementia, he or she does not wish to be treated with antibiotics for any further illness. These directives can be seen as another way of increasing the older adult's choice for care. The will would be written while the individual was well and fully competent and before a crisis. Such a document has no legal standing in the UK at the moment, although it has some value and is an indication of what patient's wishes would be if he or she were competent to say so. The legislative support for this kind of action in some countries has certainly been influenced by the increasing cost of health care for all age groups.

Policy makers have been asked to rationalize decisions about who receives a particular medical care. There may be an unwritten age limit for particular kinds of surgery or for admission to intensive care. The prevailing belief that as one ages one loses value or purpose and makes way for the next generation continues to be acted out in policies and daily interactions.

It has been indicated that it is inaccurate to regard the depreciation of the elderly as a recent affair. The elderly have always suffered from changes which made their experiences outmoded. In the past some older people did retain authority; this was more because of the resources at their disposal than any particular esteem attached to old age.

Apart from access to treatment there is the question of quality of life experienced by long-term residents in institutions. There has been a long history, well documented, of depersonalization affecting female patients in geriatric wards. Norman (1980) described the authoritarianism in regimes within institutions and the lack of choice in or control of key areas of life such as diet, times of sleeping, personal clothing, etc. Phillipson (1982) suggests that the fact that women far outnumber men in old people's homes may, in itself, to some extent explain the low standards of care and privacy. Degradation reflects external beliefs about the elderly in general, and elderly women in particular.

SUMMARY

Ageing is a process of continued development, maturation and adaptation. It is now recognized that those who survive beyond the age of 65 are a highly diversified group, most of whom remain well and function independently until only a short time before death. Throughout society stereotypes about ageing still persist and frequently lead to efforts to prevent older adults from reaching their potential physically, socially, mentally and emotionally. Fortunately there is a growing body of knowledge about ageing which has begun to reach both the health professions and the public at large. This increased societal awareness and the increasing participation by the elderly themselves in the political process has helped to improve equity and access to services for the aged.

Public policy still reinforces many injustices and will require the efforts of many individuals as well as multiagency co-operation to improve the opportunities for older persons. Nurses working with elderly people will continue to require complex skills and knowledge to meet the demands of caring for the older adult, especially as care of the elderly is shifting to the community. Those older adults who are cared for in acute and long-term institutional settings will continue to have complex needs that require the nurse to have a sound theoretical and clinical base, combined with a strong background in growth and development, excellent communications skills and a philosophy which stresses mutual goal setting with the client or patient.

LEARNING ACTIVITIES

1. When do you think a person is old?
2. Imagine yourself at this stage of being old.
   (a) Draw and/or describe your physical appearance.
   (b) Describe your activities/life-style for a typical 24-hour period.
3. At this imaginary state of being old you are admitted to hospital with a fractured hip.
   (a) What characteristics would you wish to find in the nurses caring for you?
   (b) What characteristics would you expect to be the least helpful to you?
4. Find an older person who will talk with you: a neighbour, relative or perhaps someone at a local day centre who would be willing to meet you. Ask this older adult whether they plan to make any changes in their life-style to improve their health. If so, what are they? Have they experienced any barriers in the past that prevented them from making any changes? What resources are available in the community to help promote the health of older adults?
5. A 75-year-old Polish widower living alone in a cold, dirty council flat has been forgetting to pay his bills, leaving the oven on and has been eating only tinned soup and biscuits. He is brought into the hospital with the diagnosis of pneumonia secondary to malnutrition. He refuses home help and meals on wheels and insists that he wants to go home alone as soon as he is stronger. Using Table 1.4 Critical Ethical Analysis Model as a guide, explore the ethical dilemma presented.
   (a) What information is relevant to this situation?
   (b) What are the ethical components of this situation?
   (c) Who are the individuals involved in the decision making?
   (d) Explore all possible options/courses of action.
   (e) Reconcile the facts and values with the principles.
   (f) Resolution: describe the course of action you would recommend and give your rationale.
6. What kinds of assessments would it be important to make in the situation described above? Who in the health care team might contribute to the collection of information?

REFERENCES AND FURTHER READING

Abrams M (1980) *Beyond Three Score Year and Ten; a Second Report of a Survey on the Elderly.* London: Age Concern.

Alderson R (1988) Demographic and health trends in the elderly. In Wells N & Frears C (eds) *The Ageing Population; Burden or Challenge?* London: Macmillan.

Applegate WB, Blass JP & Williams TF (1990) Instruments for the functional assessment of older patients. *New England Journal of Medicine* **322(17):** 1207–1214.

Atchley R (1980) *Social Forces in Later Life.* Belmont, CA: Wadsworth.

Blazer DG (1980) The epidemiology of mental illness in late life. In Busse EW & Blazer DG (eds) *Handbook of Geriatric Psychiatry*, pp. 249–271. New York: Van Nostrand Reinhold.

Boyle JS & Counts MM (1988) Toward healthy aging: a theory for community health nursing. *Public Health Nursing* **5(1):** 45–51.

Brocklehurst JC (1982) Mental confusion as a presenting symptom. *Geriatric Medicine* **12(6):** 50.

Burggraf V & Stanley M (eds) 1989) *Nursing the Elderly: A Care Plan Approach.* Philadelphia: Lippincott.

Clarfield AM (1988) The reversible dementias: do they reverse? *Annals of Internal Medicine* **109:** 476–486.

Cumming E & Henry WH (1961) *Growing Old.* New York: Basic Books.

Elliot B & Hybertson D (1982) What is it about the elderly that

elicits a negative response? *Journal of Geriatric Nursing* **8(10):** 568–571.

Erikson E (1964) *Child and Society.* New York: Norton.

Fielding P (1986) *Attitudes revisited; an examination of student nurses attitudes towards healing old people in hospital.* London: RCN.

Fries JF (1989) *Aging Well: A Guide for Successful Seniors.* Reading, MA: Addison-Wesley.

Gambert SR & Gupta KL (1989) Preventive care: what it's worth in geriatrics. *Geriatrics* **44(8):** 61–71.

Gioiella EC & Bevil CW (1985) *Nursing Care of the Aging Client: Promoting Healthy Adaptation.* Norwalk, CT: Appleton Century Crofts.

Gray B & Isaacs B (1979) *Care of the Elderly Mentally Infirm.* London: Tavistock.

Hamdy RC (1984) *Geriatric Medicine; a Problem Orientated Approach.* London: Baillière Tindall.

Havighurst RJ (1963) Successful aging. In Williams RH, Tibbitt C & Donahue C (eds) *Process of Aging*, p. 299. New York: Lieber-Atherton.

Hewitt P (1974) London: Age Concern.

Howze EH, Smith M & DiGlio DA (1989) Factors affecting the adoption of exercise behaviour among sedentary older adults. *Health Education Research* **4(2):** 173–180.

Johnson JC & Mezey MD (1989) Functional status assessment:

an approach to tertiary prevention. In Lavisso-Mourey R, Daly S, Diserens D & Grisso JA (eds) *Practising Prevention for the Elderly*, pp. 141–152. Philadelphia: Hanley & Belfus.

Kahana EF & Keyak HA (1984) Attitudes and behaviours of staff in facilities for the aged. *Research on Aging* **6(3)**: 395–415.

Keller ML, Leventhal H, Prohaska TR & Leventhal EA (1989) Beliefs about aging and illness in a community sample. *Research in Nursing and Health* **12**: 247–255.

Lawrence JH (1974) The effect of perceived age on initial impressions and normative role expectations. *International Journal of Aging and Human Development* **5(4)**: 369–391.

Lindeman RD, Tobin J & Shock NW (1985) Longitudinal studies on the rate of decline in renal function with age. *Journal of the American Geriatric Society* **33**: 278–285.

Mahoney FI & Barthel DW (1965) Functional evaluation: the Barthel Index. *Maryland State Medical Journal* **14(2)**: 61.

Minkler M & Pesick R (1986) Health promotion and the elderly: a critical perspective on the past and future. In Dychtwald K (ed.) *Wellness and Health Promotion for the Elderly*, pp. 39–54. Baltimore, MD: Aspen.

Murray RB, Huelskoetter MM & O'Driscoll DL (1980) *The Nursing Process in Later Maturity*. Englewood Cliffs, NJ: Prentice-Hall.

Norman AJ (1980) *Rights and Risk*. London: Centre for Policy on Ageing.

Phillipson C (1982) *Capitalism and the Construction of Old Age*. Macmillan: London.

Prevention Index '87: A Report Card on the Nation's Health (1987) Summary Report Consumer's Survey by Louis Harris & Associates, Nov 1986. Emmaus, PA: Rodale Press.

Prohaska TR, Leventhal EA, Leventhal H & Keller ML (1985) Health practices and illness cognition in young, middle aged and elderly adults. *Journal of Gerontology* **40(5)**: 569–578.

Riley MW, Johnson M & Foner A (1972) *Aging and Society: A Sociology of Age Stratification*, vol. 3. New York: Russell Sage Foundation.

Roe D (1989) Nutritional needs of the elderly: Issues, guidelines and responsibilities. *Family and Community Health* **12(1)**: 59–65.

Salter CA & Templer DI (1979) Death anxiety as related to helping behaviour and vocational interests. *Essence* **3(1)**: 3–8.

Salzman C (1985) Geriatric psychopharmacology. *Annual Review of Medicine* **36**: 217–228.

Shamoian C (1985) Assessing depression in elderly patients. *Hospital and Community Psychiatry* **36(4)**: 338–339.

Siegler IC (1980) The psychology of adult development and aging. In Busse EW & Blazer DG (eds) *Handbook of Geriatric Psychiatry*, pp. 169–221. New York: Van Nostrand Reinhold.

Taylor C, Lillis C & Lemone P (1989) *The Fundamentals of Nursing: The Art and Science of Nursing Care*. Philadelphia: Lippincott.

US Department of Health, Education and Welfare (1981) Health Consequences of Smoking: The Changing Cigarette. *A Report of the Surgeon General*, DPPD(PHS) 81–50186, pp. 225–227. Washington DC: US Department of Health, Education and Welfare, Public Service Office, Office on Smoking & Health.

Walker SN (1989) Health promotion for older adults: directions for research. *American Journal of Health Promotion* **3(4)**: pp. 47–52.

Warshaw GA, Moore JT, Friedman SE et al (1982) Functional disability in the hospitalized elderly. *Journal of the American Medical Association* **248**: 847–850.

Weller BF (ed.) (1989) *Baillières Encyclopaedic Dictionary of Nursing and Health Care*. London: Baillière Tindall.

Whitman M, Graham BA, Gleit CJ & Boyd MD (1986) *Teaching in Nursing Practice: A Professional Model*. Norwalk, CT: Appleton Century Crofts.

Wright SG (1986) *Building and Using a Model of Nursing*. London: Arnold.

Yurick AG, Spier BE, Robb SS & Ebert NJ (1988) *The Aged Person and the Nursing Process* 3rd edn. Norwalk, CT: Appleton & Lange.

Psychological Effects of a Health Disorder

OBJECTIVES

On completion of this chapter, the reader will be able to:

- Describe the illness-related, personal and environmental factors that influence the patient's emotional response to disease and injury
- Demonstrate an assessment of the illness-related, personal and environmental factors in a patient experiencing disease or injury
- Assess the patient's emotional response to disease or injury
- Describe nursing interventions designed to modify factors that contribute to symptoms of anxiety, denial, anger and depression

FACTORS INFLUENCING PSYCHOLOGICAL RESPONSES TO HEALTH PROBLEMS

In this chapter we will explore some of the psychological responses to illness that the nurse may encounter. It is important, however, to try and take the knowledge gained in these pages and see it as a series of themes running through the rest of the book as we discuss the wide range of health problems that patients and their families may meet. The student should also be trying to relate these ideas to practical experience gained with patients.

Health problems are often sources of stress for patients and families, whether the problem is acute (e.g. myocardial infarction) or chronic (e.g. rheumatoid arthritis). People exposed to similar problems have different psychological, social and physical responses. Some individuals exhibit considerable distress, expressed as symptoms such as depression, anxiety or anger that interfere with daily living, while others maintain a sense of psychological well-being and participate actively in the management of their health problem as they adapt to the demands made upon them.

Each person's response is unique and is influenced by a number of factors that fall into three major categories: *illness related factors*, *personal characteristics of the individual* and *factors in the patient's environment* (see Figure 5.1) (Moos, 1977). Since it is these factors that affect the psychological response of the patient, the nurse must assess each of these areas when preparing to care for the patient.

Illness-related Factors

Moos has identified a number of adaptive tasks or stressors associated with physical illness or injury. A stressor is defined as any discrete life event or ongoing source of stress that requires adjustments in one's life pattern (Cronkite and Moos, 1984). One major task involves dealing with the symptoms, such as pain, fatigue, breathlessness or decreased mobility, that may be encountered. A whole model of nursing may be built around the aim of helping the patient adapt to stressors, be they physical or psychosocial. Callista Roy's nursing model is based on this aim (Pearson and Vaughan, 1986). It is important that the nurse fully assesses the patient in order that the various signs and symptoms being experienced are known and documented. This is a necessary step towards exploring the patient's psychological status. This must include the patient's interpretation of a sign or symptom which may be very different to that of a nurse. A patient may see obesity as a sign of good health as it is associated with eating a great deal, while the presence of a cough may be interpreted as healthy as it 'keeps the chest clear'. A patient may therefore become distressed about something that is not particularly significant, but remain unperturbed by a serious health problem.

A second task involves dealing with the hospital environment and special treatment procedures. Many demands are placed on patients: learning the breathing and leg exercises used to prevent postoperative complications; attending physiotherapy sessions to relearn how to walk following a stroke; changing colostomy and ileostomy devices; and receiving chemotherapy and radiotherapy for cancer. These are examples of expectations of patients within the hospital setting. The hospital environment itself is a potential stressor, with its strangeness and lack of privacy and the particular routines that are imposed on patients. The nurse must be aware of these sources of stress and ensure that the patient is well informed and supported. If the patient is denied the information needed to make sense of the strange hospital environment and all that is happening, this will only lead to feelings of anxiety and frustration. As Hyland and Donaldson (1989) point out, the need for information is an essential part of the need for self-

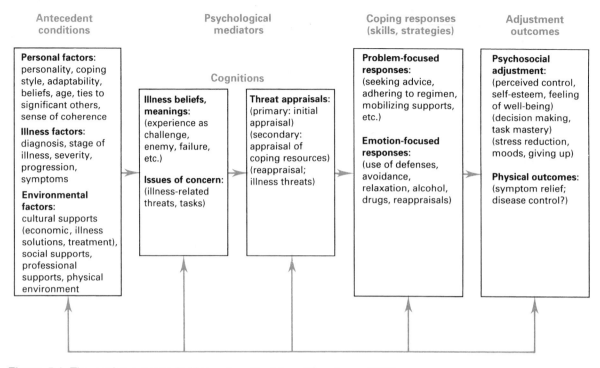

Figure 5.1 The coping process in illness (modified from Thornbury, 1981).

determination, an ability which is a fundamental human right. These authors also point out the importance of information to self-care by the patient and compliance with treatment. If unaware of what is being done and why, the patient cannot co-operate with treatment.

A third task for the patient involves establishing and maintaining adequate relationships with professional staff. Patients are often in awe of the doctor, who usually comes from a very different background, and feel much more able to communicate with nurses who they see 24 hours a day. However, asking for pain relief, for instance, may be seen as a sign of weakness by some patients, while asking for a bedpan may be just too embarrassing for others. Imagine the feelings of a patient who has been incontinent of faeces in the bed and has to ask for help. For an adult who is normally in control of all aspects of life to be reduced by disease and the effects of treatment to a state where it is necessary to ask for assistance in performing even the most basic personal tasks is a major source of stress. It is often true that the patient is old enough to be the nurse's grandparent; this too affects relationships. Fears that professional staff are withholding information from the patient and not telling the full truth about the diagnosis or treatment will also place relationships under great stress. Nurses need to work hard at establishing good channels of communication with patients to avoid embarrassment and build trust.

Maintaining relationships with family and friends is another task that is a potential source of distress for patients. The possibility that family and friends will reduce their support is a common worry, especially for patients experiencing health problems that are long term and/or disabling. The patient's role within the family may need to be changed as a result of disease or injury. For example, the wife who stayed home with children may need to seek employment when the husband is unable to work following a disabling injury.

In considering the family, the nurse should be aware that family strains may have contributed to the illness. At one extreme a woman may be admitted as a result of assault by her husband or may have taken a drug overdose as a response to severe relationship difficulties, while on a more subtle level an individual's diet, smoking and alcohol intake, for example, are strongly influenced by the family environment.

In response to a major illness event, many families do come together and rally round but, as Gillis (1988) points out, they may also split apart, cleaving along lines of weakness that have been contained within the family for many years. Recriminations, bitterness and guilt may surface and it is possible for such feelings to become displaced upon nurses and other members of staff, leading to a string of complaints and very difficult behaviour that at first light is hard to understand. In situations such as these staff should avoid being drawn into a family quarrel and only work for the patient's benefit.

Any individual who is hospitalized is subject to some loss of control. This may be devastatingly sudden in the case of acute illness or injury, or equally difficult for the patient if it is a chronic illness with little hope of improvement, e.g. multiple sclerosis. Issues of control and self-concept are further potential stressors. The nurse should be aware of these sources of distress and encourage maximum independence. Encouraging patient choices in areas such as diet, sleeping times, the time for bath and dressing changes, and teaching symptom management to the patient with a chronic disease are examples of nursing interventions that foster a sense of control for the patient. Involving patients in their care is one of the central ideas found in King's model of nursing. She considers that mutual goal setting is fundamental to nursing care (Aggleton and Chalmers, 1990).

Another task involves dealing with the uncertainty that is a part of most disease experience. Common questions asked by patients include 'Will I be able to walk again? How long will I live? Will my death be reasonably painless? Uncertainty about the future and the expected course of the health problem is cited as a particular stressor, since uncertainty reinforces lack of control and precludes any planning for the future.

Nursing interventions include helping the patient express fears and sharing information with the patient. Some or all of these stressors are associated with the experience of disease or injury. How they are experienced and responded to by the patient is influenced by personal and environmental factors.

To appreciate how a patient may respond to any clinical situation it is important to understand something of the fundamental theory of emotion. Modern thinking stems from the early experimental work of Schachter (Schachter and Singer, 1962). In his experiments Schachter was able to demonstrate that the emotional response of subjects to various situations was largely determined by previous experience and by the cues given off by other participants in the scene (Atkinson et al, 1987). Emotion seems to consist of some arousing event which produces a similar physiological response, whatever the nature of that event (characterized by sympathetic stimulation). However, the emotion that is produced can vary a great deal, despite being associated with identical physiological changes; this is where the effects of experience and other participants colours or influences the nature of the emotional response. In nursing, therefore, an event such as pain or being told bad news acts as the stimulus; what determines the emotional outcome for the patient is previous experience of similar events and the behaviour of the nurses or doctor involved. The nurse must consider the cues being given the patient; are they warm and sympathetic, calming and reassuring or anxious and uncertain, indifferent or downright hostile? Whatever is the nature of the nursing staff's emotional input will be reflected in the patient's emotional response to the various stressful situations encountered in hospital or at home.

Although much work has been done to refine and develop Schachter's ideas about emotion, they still form a sound basis for nursing practice. Other factors, such as the personality traits of the individual and environmental factors, should be considered.

Personal Characteristics of the Individual

Personal characteristics which might affect emotional response include philosophical and religious beliefs,

psychological resources such as self-esteem and a sense of personal control, previous experience with the same or similar problems and socioeconomic status.

One such personal trait is locus of control, the degree to which people feel in control of their lives (p. 28). Individuals who feel environmental events are controllable by their own actions are less likely to be adversely affected by stressful life events like disease and injury. In the instance of chronic illness, patients who seek to control the symptoms while accepting that the course of the disease is uncontrollable seem to adjust most effectively. For example, the patient with rheumatoid arthritis who learns to balance rest and activity, while understanding the incurable nature of the disease, is exerting symptom control; these individuals exhibit more positive adjustment to their disease. Assessing the patient's sense of control and reinforcing and supporting efforts to exert control are effective nursing activities.

Another personal characteristic found to influence adjustment is the appraisal made of the disease or injury. Lazarus and Folkman describe the appraisal modes of harm, threat and challenge and suggest that the way the event is appraised will influence emotional response. Appraisal is influenced by such factors as past experience, quality and quantity of available information and perceptions of how and why the disease or injury occurred. Patients who feel challenged by the disease or injury are more inclined to take action to deal effectively with it, while those who are threatened and see no immediate action are less likely to become active participants in dealing with the illness-related tasks outlined in the previous section.

The nurse should assess the patient's appraisal of the situation, using such questions as: 'What is happening to you now? Why do you think your disease/injury occurred? What do you expect to happen in the future?' The nurse must be aware of the meaning of the event to the individual in order to intervene effectively.

The individual's coping strategies and the opportunity to use them also influence emotional response. Coping strategies have been broadly categorized as problem focused and emotion focused. Neither approach is inherently adaptive or maladaptive; each has a role to play in emotional adjustment. The problem-focused approach consists of seeking relevant information, and developing and discussing possible solutions to identified problems. As Moos states, 'People who are feeling helpless and useless may find that information seeking gives them (purpose) and restores a sense of having some control.' Emotion-focused coping involves requesting reassurance and support from family, friends and health professionals. This approach is particularly important when the patient receives 'bad news'. Understanding the usefulness of this approach and providing opportunities for expression of feelings and fears are important nursing activities.

One of the most difficult coping situations is dealing with the death of a loved one. The process of grief and bereavement is a long and difficult one and it is not surprising that there are many investigations which show that the general health status of the bereaved shows a marked decline in the year after bereavement;

for example, widowers are estimated to be 40% more likely to die than a comparable control group of men of the same age (Swann, 1988).

It is interesting to see how Gass and Chang (1989) applied the ideas of Lazarus and Folkman to a study of coping mechanisms among 100 older widows and 59 older widowers. In their detailed study they found that lower threat appraisal, more problem-focused and less emotion-focused coping, greater resource strength and younger age had direct and positive effects on reducing psychosocial health dysfunction. Emotion-focused coping strategies often prevent the person from confronting the real situation and allow denial to be used as a means of coping, whereas problem-focused coping is about facing the reality of the situation and getting on with trying to solve problems.

The implication for nursing of these ideas about coping is that the nurse should be assessing how well the patient recovers from the initial shock and denial phases of bereavement, for a failure to do so, and the continued use of denial and escapist thinking, seems to be an indicator of an increased risk of physical and psychological morbidity. Encouraging a practical, problem-solving approach to bereavement, rather than not talking about it, is also likely to help the person. Great tact and gentleness should be used at all times when talking to the bereaved.

The importance of nurses understanding the processes involved in bereavement cannot be overemphasized. The nurse is involved with the family before death occurs, at the moment of death and in the aftermath. The bereaved themselves become patients in their turn, and with 3 200 000 widows and 750 000 widowers in the UK (Swann 1988) this represents a substantial proportion of the demand for nursing services.

Morris (1988) has written of how nurses shy away from death because it reminds us of our own mortality; we cannot be busy doing things before the eyes of the dying, but rather must acknowledge the dying with silent attention. Morris argues that we cannot shy away, hide or become embarrassed by a dying patient but must offer care and comfort, thus exposing ourselves to the stresses of witnessing death. It is part of the job; it is part of being human.

Maguire (1988) has pointed out that it is easier for a patient to cope with a life-threatening illness if the patient feels there is something he or she can do to fight it. This requires an understanding of what is happening, which will also help the patient cope with the stresses of the illness as it allows the use of a problem-focused coping mechanism. It also opens the door for a question to the patient, such as 'What do you think you can do to help fight this illness?'

How patients feel about their illnesses can exert a strong influence on the way they set about coping with it. The notion of an external locus of control (p. 28) may lead to bitterness directed against some external target, which impedes attempts at helping patients help themselves. If a patient sees the cause of the illness as self-inflicted, great anger and frustration may accompany anxiety and fear. AIDS or lung cancer are possible examples where a patient may think in this way.

The issue of AIDS raises the problem of stigma, which may make the whole process of death and bereavement even more difficult. In the final section of this chapter, these issues will be explored further as an illustration of the complex interplay of psychological and social factors which occurs in terminal illness.

Facing up to one's own impending death and also the process of grieving for others seems to follow a definite path with distinct phases. Kubler-Ross (1973) has described a person who is dying as passing through five stages. The first three denial, anger and bargaining occur as the person struggles with the process of coming to terms with the facts of dying. A depressive phase follows as the fact of impending death is realized. Finally there is the stage of acceptance of death. Rees and Lutkins (1967) described similar phases in the bereaved as they came to terms with death, starting again with a shocked, numbed, denial of death. This is followed by a developing awareness of death at which the person starts to react emotionally. This may vary from profound distress through to anger. Gradually emotional control returns as there is an acceptance of the loss but there still needs to be resolution, as the person adapts and adjusts the pattern of their daily life to deal with the loss. Finally the deceased is idealized as the bereaved remembers the good and positive things about their loved one.

Simpson (1989) has looked at various other models of grieving and points out that whatever model is used it is important to realize that the stages involved do not follow automatically. People may regress backwards or just get stuck at one stage, leading to significant psychological morbidity. These stages should not be thought of as a mechanistic process that all people pass through in the same way at the same rate. Each person is an individual and we all face death and dying in an individual, unique way. The work of Kubler Ross (1969, 1973) is rather a general sketch, the details may vary a great deal from person to person. Whatever model of bereavement is used, it must be agreed that in the end a great deal of emotional release is involved. Burnard (1988) has strongly argued that nurses must learn how to handle these emotional situations by methods other than walking away and being busy elsewhere. How right he is.

Tact and sensitivity, based on an awareness of the grief process, are essential in dealing with the family of the deceased. Where the dying is a slow process, anticipatory grief may be encountered. It seems as though people can start the grief work before death itself, which, if the death is greatly prolonged, may lead to perceived inappropriate responses from the family. It is not that they do not care, they have grieved in advance of the death.

Truth and honesty are essential parts of all nursing care, and never more so than in the care of the dying where a conspiracy of silence may exist to deny the patient knowledge of their condition. Nurses should not lie, even when doctors appear to withhold the truth from patients. This is a potential source of conflict between doctors and nurses. Good communication about exactly who has been told what and by whom can go a long way to reducing this problem. Problems can still remain, however, and the nurse should remember that deliberately lying to a patient about his or her health contradicts the UKCC code of professional conduct.

Attempts to justify doing something that a person knew was wrong, on the grounds that the person was 'following orders', have met with little success in courts of law. The Nuremberg war crimes trials after World War II are the most celebrated case in point. The nurse who is instructed to break the code of professional conduct by a doctor is placed in an unenviable position and should consult with senior nursing colleagues and a body such as the Royal College of Nursing before deciding on a course of action.

Factors in the Patient's Environment

The nature, type and extent of social support available to the patient comprised the most significant environmental factor affecting emotional response to disease and injury. Social support is defined as 'interpersonal transactions involving such characteristics as the provision of aid, affect and affirmation' (Antonucci and Israel, 1986). The perceived availability and adequacy of support is a core variable influencing adjustment. The relationship between support and psychosocial adjustment is supported by studies using different diseases and different measures of support (Turner and Noh, 1988; Johnson and Morse, 1990).

An assessment of the social support available to an individual should include the type of support given, the source of support and, most important, whether it is perceived as sufficient by the patient. Patients who feel they do not have sufficient support to meet their needs tend to feel isolated and abandoned and hence susceptible to feelings of depression and anxiety. The nurse can also make alternative sources of support available to patients. For example, meeting with other persons experiencing similar problems is often helpful. Referral to community agencies, including self-help groups, is also useful.

PSYCHOLOGICAL RESPONSES TO ILLNESS

In this section we will look at some of the more specific psychological responses to illness that patients may display.

Anxiety

Anxiety is a common response to illness and results from any perceived and/or actual threat to the person's self-perceptions or sense of self. Peplau (1963, 1989) describes four levels of anxiety: *mild, moderate, severe* and *panic*. Mild anxiety heightens the person's awareness and the person's ability to focus on relevant material. This anxiety can be very helpful. For example, mild anxiety might be felt by a patient learning to walk

again after a leg amputation. Moderate anxiety results in narrowing of the person's perceptual field and the focusing of attention to less relevant material. Anxiety experienced preoperatively may frequently be at the moderate level. The physiological effects of stress and anxiety are discussed in Chapter 21, under the Autonomic and Sympathetic Nervous Systems.

Severe anxiety prevents the individual from being able to focus on the presenting situation, even with assistance. An example might be the mother in the A & E department who talks only about the child's ruined dress though her child has multiple internal injuries due to a road traffic accident (RTA). During panic, the person experiences overwhelming dread, horror or terror. Behaviour such as extreme confusion, violence or hysteria may also be demonstrated.

Anxiety may serve a useful purpose, for example, anxiety about contracting a disease motivates people to take preventative measures, but as it becomes more severe it can become disabling. An alternative way of looking at anxiety is to say that it can be classed as normal (i.e. it is appropriate in a certain situation to be anxious) or neurotic, when the anxiety is seen as an inappropriate reaction (Atkinson et al, 1987). Anxiety neurosis can be generalized and free floating or specific to certain situations, when it is known as a phobia, or it may lead to compulsive behaviour patterns. In all these manifestations, anxiety can disrupt and seriously handicap a person's life. In these situations the person's anxiety has become a psychiatric problem and Moores (1987) has described how anxiety management groups led by psychiatric nurses can help people deal with such problems.

Anxiety can affect patients in a wide range of situations. The following are some typical examples. Termination of pregnancy is a very stressful event for a woman and might be expected to provoke severe anxiety. Llewelyn and Pitcher (1988) investigated this problem in a sample of 21 women, half of whom had supportive partners and half who did not. Their conclusion was that the presence of a partner reduced the postoperative anxiety felt by the woman and that this should be considered an important factor in post-termination counselling.

Surgery is another very stressful event and Biley (1989) has pointed out that there is a substantial amount of literature indicating that nurses frequently fail to recognize the true levels of fear and anxiety experienced by patients. When she surveyed a sample of preoperative patients and nursing staff she found that, while both groups rated the items in her questionnaire in broadly the same order of anxiety, nursing staff consistently assessed patients as worrying more than they actually did. This is a surprising finding, and whether these patients would still rate their anxiety lower than nurses would postoperatively is open to speculation. Different types of surgery might also produce a different outcome in terms of patient anxiety.

Thompson (1989) investigated anxiety levels in male patients who had suffered a first myocardial infarction and assessed whether a programme of supportive education and counselling would reduce anxiety and depression. He found that after 5 days in hospital those patients receiving such a programme from a nurse showed statistically significant lower levels of anxiety and depression when compared with a control group who had not received the benefit of the programme.

These three studies reinforce the importance of family support and information-giving in reducing anxiety, while reminding us that nurses frequently fail to estimate correctly the degree of anxiety that patients experience.

Although anxiety results from a perceived threat to the person's sense of self, it may not be the obvious observable emotion to either the nurse or patient. The perceived threat may be experienced as an emotion such as anger, sadness, helplessness or emptiness, and may be accompanied by obvious physical signs of anxiety such as restlessness, 'clammy' or perspiring skin, etc. Chapter 21 discusses the physiological effects of stress in more detail. Sometimes the person may not be aware of any feelings or the sense of threat. Nursing interventions with the person experiencing higher levels of anxiety need to be congruent with the narrowing field of attention. For example, the nurse must use short simple sentences.

Anxiety is a contagious emotion. It is therefore important for the nurse to monitor personal anxiety when nursing an anxious patient. Self-observations could demonstrate: increasing pace of activities, a sense of lack of control or disorganization and feelings of being pressured. When the nurse notices some of these behaviours in himself or herself, it may be useful to try to identify the sources of the anxiety to put the situation in perspective. It should be remembered that the nurse has his or her own emotional state which can significantly affect the patient's emotions. With higher levels of anxiety, self-exploration will be increasingly difficult. The nurse may then use techniques such as physically relaxing muscles, taking slow deep breaths or use silent positive self-statements such as 'I can handle this'.

Fear

Fear is sometimes seen as almost synonymous with anxiety (Beck and Emery, 1985). Both emotions are common responses to perceived threats. When distinctions are made, fear is described as being attributable to a clearly identified real threat, whereas the sources of threat for the anxious individual may be more diffuse. Burton (1979) suggests that fear is perhaps the most powerful of all emotions, sometimes inducing behavioural patterns over which fearful individuals have limited or no control. Degrees of fear, and the way fear is manifested in individuals, can also vary. What could be classed as mild fear is a common experience for the majority of people facing a hospital visit, particularly if they are unsure of what the visit will entail. Moderate to severe levels of fear can arise when individuals perceive, either consciously or subconsciously, that a hospital visit will be more threatening. A patient receiving chemotherapy on a regular outpatient basis, for example, will

often be very fearful beforehand knowing that the injection will trigger off extremely unpleasant side-effects. Indeed, many such patients suffer the symptoms of nausea and vomiting as they begin their journey to the hospital, or in response to seeing the syringe being drawn up. Some individuals, on the other hand, may enter a hospital with no conscious anxieties or fears of what the visit may entail, and yet the experience provokes a subconscious memory of, for example, a childhood period of hospitalization thus inducing a very real sensation of fear.

Whatever the causes or physical manifestations, it is vital for the nurse to recognize that anxiety and fear are real sensations for many people in hospital or community health settings, although they may not always be openly or visibly expressed. By being aware of this, and by providing such individuals with an opportunity to express and explore their feelings, the nurse can often lessen or alleviate anxiety through emphatic communication tailored to individual needs and circumstances. The supportive presence of family members or friends can also offer great comfort and reassurance. It is important to recognize, however, that in some instances family and friends may worsen anxiety by their presence, particularly if they are anxious or fearful for their relative's wellbeing.

Denial

Denial is a response to illness that may arise in some individuals in response to anxiety, or to protect the person from experiencing anxiety or fear. It could thus be said that denial is a subconscious attempt temporarily to 'cushion' the effects of unpleasant reality. As a subconscious entity, it is not within an individual's conscious awareness, yet to observers it often appears to be conscious. When a patient denies feeling anxious or afraid, for example, and yet shows physical signs that suggest otherwise, immediate action is required by the nurse in the form of listening and empathy; denial can never be taken literally in such circumstances.

Denial thus serves as a buffer, but can also act as a barrier. It serves as a buffer when it allows the person time and space to deal with an uncomfortable reality. For example, a recently diagnosed terminally ill cancer patient may initially deny the diagnosis and discuss long-term plans. This denial can be a buffer when the information is too overwhelming. It becomes a barrier if it prevents the person from ever dealing with the impending death or if it prevents a patient from seeking medical help in the early stages of illness. Patients still present, for example, with advanced fungating cancers of the breast; denial must have been at work for many months. Denial is a normal, initial response to death, dying and grief (Kubler-Ross, 1969). At times, all people use denial as a defensive or coping strategy.

Nursing interventions with the person using denial can be difficult. It is important for the nurse to recognize the unconscious nature of denial and to remember that it serves a protective function, since it protects the person from the extreme pain and anxiety of accepting the situation. Understanding this process allows the nurse to avoid directly challenging or contradicting the person's view. *No intervention is frequently the intervention of choice.* Dealing directly with denial almost always forces the person to increase the use of denial and compromises the nurse–patient relationship.

The 'back door approach' proposed by Forchuk and Westwell (1990) suggests that the nurse explore with the patient a less threatening aspect of the situation. For example, in the situation of the patient with terminal cancer making long range plans, the nurse might ask broad questions such as, 'How is your family reacting to your illness?'

The nurse does not reinforce the denial by directly agreeing with the use of denial. The nurse can use the strategy '*agreeing with truth*', by agreeing only with content the nurse believes is accurate and not responding to content that, in the nurse's perception, is unrealistic. An example of a response the nurse might make to a person suffering from alcoholism who states 'My drinking isn't hurting anyone' is 'It sounds as if you believe your drinking does not hurt anyone'. This would not be said in an provocative or challenging manner.

Anger

Some patients use anger as a response to illness. Anger develops out of anxiety and, like anxiety, can be a contagious emotion. It is important for the person experiencing anger to have the opportunity to express this feeling in a direct manner without fear of retaliation. The person who is experiencing anger may often find it impossible to discuss the situation calmly. It is important for the nurse not to take the person's anger as directed personally as this interferes with the ability to listen to the person's concerns. To do this, the nurse needs to understand his or her own attitudes and beliefs about experiencing and communicating anger.

Anger may be expressed in abusive language or even by acts of destruction. The nurse must not react externally, even though internally there may be a whole range of emotions from righteous indigation ('How dare this patient say that to me!') through to fear of attack. The nurse is the person standing there when the patient vents their feelings, just as the tree on the cliff top is standing there when a westerly gale blows in off the sea. It is not a personal attack on that tree, it just happens to be there when the wind blows. So it is with nurses and, like the tree, the nurse needs to sway with the wind and let the patient express the anger. Any attempt at confrontation or disagreement runs a grave risk of provoking further anger and even physical violence. It also helps to try and see things from the patient's point of view; anger may be more understandable when viewed from a different perspective.

Listening is an important role for the nurse in this situation. Listening requires allowing the patient to express feelings to the nurse, without the nurse responding in a defensive or advice-giving manner. For example the patient may say, 'You don't care! Nobody cares!' It is natural for the nurse to become defensive and want to reply that this is not the case. This would be denying the patient's perception and could force the discussion into premature closure, where the conversation is closed before the patient has been able to resolve feelings through verbal expression. A more helpful response would be a reflective statement, for example, 'It feels to you like no one cares.'

Anger can be dissipated in different ways, depending on the person's cultural and personal beliefs and values. Examples include: *verbally* (talking or writing out feelings), *physically* (using exercise or running) or *spiritually* (using prayer or absolution). It is also useful to determine the methods the patient has found helpful in the past to deal with feelings such as anger. In this situation the nurse should be prepared to discuss possible acts of violence that have occurred in the past and be aware of the possibility of such behaviour recurring.

Depression

Depression is a common response to illness or loss. At less serious levels depression is experienced as sadness or 'the blues'. Behaviours such as withdrawal, tearfulness, apathy, lack of interest in usual activities, alterations in eating patterns (e.g. loss of appetite) and sleep disturbances may all be indicators of depression. If depression is suspected it is important to allow the patient ample opportunity to express feelings of sadness. Again, listening is a key role for the nurse. It is also important to identify the person's previous means of dealing with feelings.

Depression becomes increasingly common in elderly people although, as Kimmel (1980) points out, it is usually mild and the majority of elderly people are not depressed. The association of depression with loss explains this observation, as elderly people are more likely to have experienced bereavement, will have retired from work, experienced a decrease in fitness and independence and a greater incidence of ill health. A useful insight into depression and the elderly came from Jiminez et al (1989) who, in a sample of 207 citizens aged over 65, demonstrated a correlation between depression and appetite, exercise and sleep. The greater the appetite, the more exercise taken and the greater the amount of sleep, the less the depression rating obtained by questionnaire. These findings are consistent with the discussion in the preceding paragraph, although it should be remembered that, as this study was conducted in Spain, cultural differences must be considered.

Depression may become more profound than the understandable feeling of sadness after an adverse life event, such as illness or loss. It may not even be associated with any such obvious event, and instead just gradually develops for no apparent reason, leading to the withdrawal of the person from everyday life. The effects may be debilitating and possibly life threatening, as self-neglect develops and possibly suicidal thoughts start to occur. In situations such as these the person needs psychiatric help and a variety of strategies, ranging from drug therapy to cognitive behavioural therapy, may be employed by psychiatrists and mental health nurses trying to help. Dodd (1988) has described how nursing staff may use this approach to try and help depressed patients overcome their negative beliefs about themselves and to help them to think more positively.

In the UK the suicide rate has remained at around 4000–5000 deaths per year for much of the twentieth century (Northcott, 1987). The last 25 years has, however, witnessed a dramatic increase in acts of deliberate self-harm, such as drug overdose, and Northcott estimates the current level of such cases at around 200 000 cases per year. This is the same order of magnitude as other workers such as Walsh (1990) have found. A strong association exists between lower social class and self-harm rates; females are more likely than males to exhibit such behaviour and there is a strong bias towards the younger age groups (16–30 years).

It is likely that the large majority of patients who deliberately inflict self-harm have no suicidal intent, rather it is a coping mechanism for dealing with stressful life events and relationship difficulties. Nurses must beware being judgemental and expressing negative feelings towards patients who have inflicted deliberate self-harm; they are not 'time wasters' but rather people with real problems who have adopted an inappropriate way of dealing with those problems. However, nurses should also be aware that some patients with a history of deliberate self-harm may, in fact, be suicidal and may carry out a successful suicide attempt while on the ward. Gaze (1989) and Blank (1989) have discussed the devastating effects this can have on nurses and also the lack of support available for staff in coming to terms with such a tragedy.

With depression there is potential for suicide. Indicators of possible suicidal risk include: a family history of suicide; a personal history of suicidal attempts; speaking of wanting to end one's life; statements that death is preferable to life; giving away possessions; tying up business (for example, wills or financial arrangements); a sudden improvement in mood after a depression; plans of methods for suicide; and access to a means of committing suicide. Use of alcohol or other disinhibiting drugs can increase the potential for suicidal behaviour. Socially isolated people are also at greater risk than those with good support networks. Since depression and suicidal ideation are potentially fatal, it is imperative for the nurse to be alert to symptoms of either. A psychiatric or mental health consultation is often helpful in determining risk and planning appropriate interventions. A key nursing intervention would be to have the individual under close or even continuous supervision when suicidal risk is present (Ashton, 1986).

The devastating impact of a fatal disease on an individual and family can be seen from considering one example, that of AIDS, and we will therefore conclude this chapter by considering this example in some depth.

PSYCHOSOCIAL IMPLICATIONS OF HIV INFECTION

Living with a chronic, life-threatening illness necessitates a constant, dynamic process of assessment and adjustment; a process of coping with the changes and demands of progressive illness. The impact of this process on the individual's psychological and social well-being, the psychosocial impact, is significant and must be considered and addressed along with physical symptoms.

This *routine of adaptation* involves the individual in an ongoing series of coping tasks:

- Maintaining a sense of normality.
- Modifying daily routines and adjusting life-style to include therapy and symptom control.
- Obtaining knowledge and skill for continuing self-care.
- Maintaining a positive concept of self.
- Adjusting to altered social relationships.
- Grieving over losses of function, ability, status, income, etc.
- Dealing with dramatic role changes within the family, social network and workplace.
- Dealing with illness-induced and treatment-induced discomfort.
- Complying with an illness-based regimen.
- Maintaining a feeling of being in control.
- Confronting the inevitability of one's own death.
- Maintaining hope in spite of uncertain or deteriorating physical condition (Miller, 1983).

People living with HIV infection face all these coping tasks. There are, however, psychosocial issues unique to it. To understand their impact, it is important to examine their origins in the deeply entrenched societal attitudes towards sexuality, sexual practice or behaviour, and sexual orientation.

Unlike the chronic conditions (e.g. heart and kidney disease) and cancers that are the most common causes of death in the western world, HIV infection is communicable and its primary means of transmission is sexual. In the West, those initially infected with HIV were homosexual men. AIDS was referred to as the 'gay plague'. Suddenly a society that for the most part rejected or ignored homosexuality and its life-style had the reality of both, together with the reality of the AIDS epidemic, thrust upon its consciousness. Homosexuality and HIV infection became synonymous, and the fear of both became inextricably linked.

Not only has homosexuality become equated with AIDS but all our social and moral values about homosexuality, sex with more than one partner or 'promiscuity' (a word loaded with negative connotations) and injection drug use have also become associated with AIDS.

Since homosexuality, promiscuity and drug use are held to be in violation of conventional morality, many in our society have come to accept AIDS as appropriate punishment for what has been defined as immoral behaviour. People with HIV infection who can not be categorized as moral transgressors (haemophiliacs, anyone transfused with contaminated blood, infants contracting the virus in utero) have often been seen as innocent victims, the implication being that others, particularly homosexual men, are guilty victims, and deserve AIDS. This judgement and blame add to the already considerable physical and psychosocial burden of AIDS. The signal that social attitudes have changed and that judgement is no longer being pronounced will occur when method of transmission is irrelevant and no one asks how one became infected with HIV.

Even though patterns of infection are changing and the percentage of diagnosed cases of AIDS among homosexual men is dropping, and the percentage of cases diagnosed among heterosexuals is rising, this association persists, making it impossible to separate the response to the disease and all its sufferers (particularly homosexual men) from the negative response to homosexuality (homophobia). While increasing numbers of people are testing positive for HIV antibodies as a result of sharing needles and heterosexual contact, the majority of people diagnosed with AIDS are still, and will continue to be for some time, homosexual men.

The importance of providing judgement-free care to patients with AIDS must be emphasized in the realization that attitudes and fears of care-givers are most certainly communicated to them. It is essential that the nurse does not contribute to the stress of living with AIDS. As a result, the first challenge for the care-giver helping the AIDS patient deal with the psychosocial implications of AIDS becomes an examination of personally held stereotypes that may well form the basis of fear of AIDS.

Having discussed some of the underlying social constructions of attitudes towards AIDS, it is important to identify the specific psychosocial issues created for people with AIDS, homosexual men in particular, their families and professional care-givers.

STIGMATIZATION

There is ample evidence for the stigma attached to AIDS. Many still advocate quarantine for everyone infected with the virus. Despite medical and scientific evidence that casual transmission does not occur, the debate still rages over whether HIV-infected children should be allowed to attend regular classes in schools; whether HIV-infected adults should be allowed to teach, work in restaurants, offices, for airlines, in hospitals; the list is long. Surveys show that many in the health care field are refusing or are reluctant to treat people with HIV infection.

AIDS is sometimes compared with leprosy, and people with AIDS with lepers. People with HIV infection are not seen solely as carrying a virus or being ill, but as tainted. The label of AIDS marginalizes those with the syndrome, most of whom (homosexual men, injection drug users) are already marginalized within society. The impact of the stigma of AIDS can be devastating.

People with AIDS are often faced with the reality of there being very few 'safe' people in their environment. They have to deal not only with the fear of the physical consequences of their illness, but of the fear of rejection and discrimination by family, friends and professional helpers. A significant part of caring for clients with AIDS becomes the creation of a safe and accepting environment.

SECRECY AND FEAR OF DISCLOSURE

Not surprisingly, people with AIDS often feel the need to maintain absolute secrecy about the nature of their condition. Because of socially entrenched homophobia, many men also wish to keep the fact of their being homosexual a secret. For them, disclosure of a diagnosis of AIDS necessitates disclosing that they are homosexual. This double disclosure is obviously traumatic and fear laden, and may fall as a double blow for family and friends. The patient may have to deal with family members coming to terms with his diagnosis while at the same time struggling with the revelation that he is homosexual. Again, non-judgement, an attitude of acceptance and caring on the part of the nurse is essential so that the patient and family can adjust to the realities of disclosure.

The nurse is also frequently required to help keep the 'secret', sometimes even when it appears to the nurse as a care-giver that disclosure is desirable. It is essential to remember that the reality for the patient is vastly different from that of an observer, and that the patient, in light of the reality of wide-spread homophobia and AIDS phobia, may face loss of family, social network and livelihood if secrecy is not maintained. The importance of allowing the patient to decide whether to disclose cannot be overstated.

Injection drug users frequently have a strong need for secrecy. In addition to their vulnerability to AIDS phobia, they may, as a result of their drug use, fear additional social censure and legal repercussions. Such fears are exacerbated by concerns over imprisonment and the treatment of HIV-positive people in jails and prisons.

The heterosexual, non-drug-using person with AIDS also feels it necessary to keep a diagnosis of AIDS secret. Again, even though the energy required to maintain such secrets is immense and may seem counterproductive and wasted, the consequences of breaking the secrecy are real and potentially severe.

REJECTION AND ABANDONMENT

Sometimes family and friends are unable to accept that the patient has AIDS, is homosexual or uses injection drugs. Those who contract HIV heterosexually are often seen as 'bad' and sinning, and are condemned and rejected on the basis of their behaviour. While there are many wonderful and inspiring examples of people rallying to support someone with AIDS, it is not uncommon for people with AIDS to be rejected and abandoned by most people in their family and social network. In these instances, care-givers become the main or only supports for the patient and it is helpful for the nurse or hospital to be aware of community-based AIDS organizations, many of which are able to augment or replace diminished networks.

ISOLATION

The need for secrecy and the stigmatization, rejection and abandonment experienced by people with AIDS frequently leads to profoundly painful isolation. Homosexual communities were the first to organize in response to the AIDS epidemic, and most urban centres have excellent community-based support and information programmes to help combat that isolation. Self-help and HIV support groups exist in almost all major cities. Because the majority of infected people are homosexual men, the majority of people attending these groups are homosexual men. While all people with AIDS have common concerns, women and heterosexual men have concerns particular to their situations, gender and sexual orientation and do not always feel comfortable or adequately served in groups comprised mainly of homosexual men. The isolation for women is more severe because of their smaller numbers and because the vast body of information about AIDS addresses male physiological responses to HIV.

DISCRIMINATION BY HEALTH CARE PROVIDERS

People with AIDS often fear discrimination by the health care professionals on whom they must rely. Patients with AIDS often test and retest the reliability of care providers to determine if they are sympathetic and safe. In view of the discrimination against people with AIDS that does exist, such testing is not surprising, and is necessary for the patient to establish a sense of security in what often feels like a hostile environment. The nurse should expect to be tested and accept that it may not be reflective of his or her care or caring, but is prompted by general and prevailing social attitudes. Such testing can also identify behaviours that do reflect negativity on the part of the nurse and can be used as an opportunity to re-examine personal attitudes and their impact on the patient.

ABANDONMENT BY THE CHURCH

There is considerable evidence of compassionate and caring individuals, functioning within the framework of organized religion, who have been supportive to people with AIDS. Unfortunately, in large part, our churches have failed to serve people with AIDS, condemning them on the grounds of immoral behaviour based on either homosexuality, promiscuity, sex outside of conventional marriage, drug abuse, etc. As a result, many people with AIDS have found themselves denied or afraid to seek spiritual counsel at a time in their lives when spiritual issues are of paramount importance.

The Family

An expanded definition of family must be established to facilitate understanding of the impact of AIDS on the families of those with the syndrome. For the purposes of this discussion, 'family' includes family of origin (parents, siblings), extended family, children, relationship partner (heterosexual or homosexual), and 'chosen' family (friends who function in place of absent members of family of origin or extended family).

In the case of homosexual men, institutionalized homophobia creates situations that are the source of considerable anxiety and concern. Since there is no recognition of homosexual relationships, same-sex partners have no legal or social status. This absence of official sanction for the position of a partner can cause ambiguity and conflict over who should be consulted for treatment decisions. Members of family of origin have challenged the right of same-sex partners to be involved, even in situations where the patient has made it known that the partner should be considered next-of-kin. Failure to respect the patient's wishes in this regard is the cause of considerable pain and anxiety for both patient and partner.

Conventional assumptions about relationships and the identity of important people to patients with AIDS may be incorrect. Sensitivity to that possibility and willingness to enquire about and respect the patient's significant relationships will go a long way toward easing much of the anxiety around this issue.

Regardless of how family is defined, anyone supporting a person with AIDS, by association, shares the stigmatization, isolation, rejection, discrimination and need for secrecy. Health care providers are often the only people with whom friends and family feel safe expressing their feelings, fears and anticipatory grief. The intensity of these feelings is increased by the isolation which they are experiencing.

Since HIV is sexually transmitted, it is possible that the spouse or partner of the patient may also be infected, raising additional concerns:

- Care partner neglecting self-care to concentrate on the care and support of partner who is more acutely ill.
- Asymptomatic care partner constantly reminded of more acute stages of HIV infection.
- Guilt or anger over source of infection.

Non-infected sexual partners of HIV positive people may feel guilt over being free of the virus in the face of their partner's seropositivity.

As much of a family's coping with their loved-one's illness is accomplished in isolation, so often is their grieving over that person's death. Care-givers who knew the individual may be among a very small number of people with whom the family can share the truth about that person's death and the full range and depth of their feelings. The secrecy frequently prolongs the grieving process and places an additional burden on family and care-giver.

Homosexual men whose partners die of AIDS must deal with psychosocial issues unique to 'gay grief':

- They do not readily fit into traditional grief support groups, the members of which are usually heterosexual women over the age of 50.
- Surviving partners of people who have died of AIDS are often themselves stigmatized and shunned.
- Low self-esteem and guilt is often exacerbated by homophobic attitudes.
- The deceased may have been the survivor's only real family.
- There is no societal approval for homosexual relationships and therefore there are no formal, ritualized mourning practices; for example, there is not even a formal title like 'widow' or 'widower' to

identify the surviving partner.

- Homophobia may have prompted the couple to keep their sexual orientation, and therefore the true nature of their relationship, secret. This makes it impossible to acknowledge the true nature of the grief in the workplace to avoid arousing questions about such a strong response to the death of a 'friend'.
- Financial benefits are not guaranteed to surviving same-sex partners. This absence of any legal protection for the survivor can result in the loss of joint assets.
- Surviving partners are sometimes excluded from planning and even attending the funeral of their partners (Klein and Fletcher, 1986).

The first two points also apply to surviving partners in heterosexual relationships.

The Care-giver

The stigma and fear that so profoundly affect people with AIDS, and their families, also touches the professionals who care for them. Nurses must often deal with their own families' fears and concerns about AIDS. Sometimes nurses' families disapprove of their caring for people with AIDS, and conflicts between professional and family responsibilities arise.

The secrecy demanded by patients requires special effort on the part of nursing staff, bringing a new dimension and complexity to medical confidentiality.

Dying is the aspect of AIDS that has the most obvious effect on care-givers. Most people who die from AIDS are young, often younger than their nurses. It is not expected that so many young people will die from chronic illness. Each death marks the beginning of a process of grief for the care-provider. The psychosocial issues that affect people with AIDS and their families also extend to grieving care-givers. The hostile response to AIDS and its sufferers often forces nurses to grieve in isolation from their family and friends. Secret grief is often prolonged or truncated, to the detriment of the mourner (Feinblum, 1986).

Self-care for nurses is essential to maintaining personal and professional effectiveness. Care-giver support groups can afford an opportunity to deal with issues arising from caring for HIV infected individuals, thus reducing the negative impact of AIDS care and minimizing the likelihood of care-givers themselves becoming marginalized.

It is clear that those psychosocial issues unique to AIDS are less the direct result of adjustment to the physical changes caused by diminished immune function, but more the result of beliefs widely held within our society. They are not associated with the disease process, but with stereotypes and attitudes towards those who suffer from the disease and the behaviour that led to infection. These social tenets are generally accepted to be truth rather than perception and are therefore rarely questioned, yet for patients to neutralize their impact and for care-givers to provide judgement-free care and treatment, the potentially painful process of challenging beliefs must be followed.

SUMMARY

Although emotional responses to illness are highly individualized, the nurse caring for ill adults can expect to frequently encounter patients and family members experiencing anxiety, denial, anger and/or depression. Recognizing these emotional responses, and giving the patient and family opportunity to express their feelings are important nursing interventions. Expression of feelings does not need to happen separately from the physical care given by the nurse. For example, the physical closeness and time required for a bed bath often provides an opportunity for the patient to express worries and concerns. The nurse needs to be aware of his or her comfort and limitations with emotional responses and to seek consultation when necessary. Comprehensive nursing assessments will consider emotional as well as physiological responses to illness.

LEARNING ACTIVITIES

1a. Identify the factors in the hospital environment that are potential sources of stress for patients.
  b. Develop an assessment guide for use in exploring a patient's responses to the hospital environment.
2. Develop an interview protocol to be used in determining a patient's appraisal of disease or injury.
3. Identify possible sources of social support for patients experiencing any disease or injury.
4. Role play with a colleague an interaction with a patient expressing denial. One student should role play the patient experiencing chest pain who is denying the presence of the pain. The second student should role play the nurse performing a pain assessment. The students should critique the nursing approach that was demonstrated.

REFERENCES AND FURTHER READING

Aggleton P & Chalmers H (1990) King's nursing model. *Nursing Times* **86(1):** 38–39.

Antonucci TD & Israel B (1986) Veridicality of social support: a comparison of principal and network member's response. *Journal of Consulting and Clinical Psychology* **54:** 432–437.

Ashton J (1986) Preventing suicide in hospital. *Nursing Times* **Dec. 31:** 36–7.

Atkinson R, Atkinson L, Smith E & Hilgard E (1990) *Introduction to Psychology.* 10th edn. London: Harcourt Brace Jovanovich.

Beck AT & Emery G (1985) *Anxiety Disorders and Phobias: A Cognitive Perspective.* New York: Basic Books.

Biley FC (1989) Nurse's perceptions of stress in preoperative surgical patients. *Journal of Advanced Nursing* **14:** 575–581.

Blank M (1989) The other victims. *Nursing Times* **85(26):** 28–30.

Burnard P (1988) No need to hide. *Nursing Times* **84(24):** 36–38.

Burton G (1979) *Interpersonal Relations, A Guide for Nurses.* London: Tavistock.

Cronkite RC & Moos RH (1984) The role of predisposing and moderating factors in the stress-illness relationship. *Journal of Health and Social Behaviour* **25:** 372–393.

Dodd H (1988) Realistic thinking. *Nursing Times* **84(32):** 55–57.

Feinblum S (1986) Pinning down the psychosocial dimensions of AIDS. *Nursing and Health Care* **7:** 255–257.

Forchuk & Westwell J (1990) Denial. In Baumann A, Johnston NE & Antai-Otong D (eds) *Psychiatric and Psychosocial Nursing,* pp. 194–195. Toronto: Decker.

Gass K & Chang A (1989) Appraisal of bereavement: coping, resources and psychosocial health dysfunction in widows and widowers. *Nursing Research* **38(1):** 31–36.

Gaze H (1989) How do we cope? *Nursing Times* **85(26):** 34–35.

Gillis L (1988) *Human Behaviour in Illness.* London: Faber & Faber.

Guttman HA (1983) Psychosocial factors on physical illness. *Medical Clinics of North America* **35:** 3324–3326.

Hyland M & Donaldson M (1989) *Psychological Care in Nursing Practice.* London: Scutari.

Jimenez JC et al (1989) Behavioural habits and affective disorders in old people. *Journal of Advanced Nursing* **14:** 356–364.

Johnson JL & Morse JM (1990) Regaining control: the process of adjustment after myocardial infarction. *Heart Lung* **19:** 126–135.

Kimmel DC (1980) *Adulthood and Aging.* New York: Wiley.

Klein SJ & Fletcher W (1986) Gay grief: an examination of its uniqueness brought to light by the AIDS crisis. *Journal of Psychosocial Oncology* **4:** 25.

Kubler-Ross E (1969) *On Death and Dying.* New York: Macmillan.

Kubler-Ross E (1973) *On Death and Dying.* London: Routledge.

Llewellyn S & Pytcher R (1988) An investigation of anxiety following termination of pregnancy. *Journal of Advanced Nursing* **13:** 468–471.

Maguire P (1988) The stress of communicating with seriously ill patients. *Nursing* **3(32):** 25–27.

Mechanic D (1986) The concept of illness behaviour: culture, situation and personal predisposition. *Psychological Medicine* **16:** 1–7.

Miller JF (1983) Coping with chronic illness. In Miller JF (ed.) *Coping with Chronic Illness: Overcoming Powerlessness,* pp. 15–36. Philadelphia: Davis.

Moores A (1987) Facing the fear. *Nursing Times* **83(27):** 44–46.

Moos RH (ed) (1977) *Coping with Physical Illness,* chap. 1. New York: Plenum.

Morris E (1988) A pain of separation. *Nursing Times* **84(42):** 54–56.

Northcott N (1987) Reflections on suicide. *Nursing* **3(20):** 6–7.

Pearson A & Vaughan B (1986) *Nursing Models for Practice.* Oxford: Heinemann.

Peplau HE (1963) A working definition of anxiety. In Burd S & Marshall M (eds) *Some Clinical Approaches to Psychiatric Nursing.* New York: Macmillan.

Peplau HE (1989) Theoretical constructs: anxiety, self, and hallucinations. In O'Toole AW & Welt SR (eds) *Interpersonal Theory in Nursing Practice,* pp. 270–326. New York: Springer.

Rudy TE, Kerns RD & Turk DC (1988) Chronic pain and depression: toward a cognitive-behavioral mediation model. *Pain* **35:** 129–140.

Schachter S & Singer JE (1962) Cognitive, social and physiological determinants of emotional state. *Psychological Review* **69:** 379–399.

Simpson K (1989) Understanding mourning. *Nursing Times* **85(4):** 43–45.

Stuart GW & Sundeen SJ (1983) The nurse as helper. In Stuart GW & Sundeen SJ (eds) *Principles and Practice of Psychiatric Nursing,* pp. 63–69. St Louis: Mosby.

Swann A (1988) Men and bereavement. *Nursing* **3(26):** 966–968.

Thompson P (1989) Randomized controlled trial of in-hospital nursing support for first time myocardial infarction patients and their partners; effects on anxiety and depression. *Journal of Advanced Nursing* **14:** 291–297.

Thornbury KM (1981) Coping: implications for health practitioners. *Patient Counselling and Health Education* **4:** 3–9.

Tschudin V (1991) *Counselling Skills for Nurses* 3rd edn. London: Baillière Tindall.

Turner RJ & Noh S (1988) Physical disability and depression: a longitudinal analysis. *Journal of Health and Social Behaviour* **29:** 23–37.

Westwell J & Forchuk C (1989) Denial; buffer and barrier. *Canadian Nurse* **85(9):** 16–18.

Infection and Disease

6

OBJECTIVES

On completion of this chapter, the reader will be able to:

- List the groups of infectious agents that interact with humans
- Describe the microbial and host factors which determine the nature and outcome of their interactions
- Describe the course of infectious disease
- List diagnostic tests used in infections
- Discuss measures relevant to the collection of specimens
- Assess local and systemic responses to infection
- Plan, implement and evaluate nursing intervention for the person with an infection
- Discuss factors influencing the occurrence of infections in populations
- Describe measures to control nosocomial infections
- Describe measures to prevent and control infection in the community
- Describe the pathophysiology of HIV infection and contrast the virus effect on healthy immune functioning
- Describe the modes of transmission of the human immunodeficiency virus
- Compare and contrast the clinical presentation of HIV in males, females and children
- Apply the principles of universal precautions in clinical practice.
- Describe common clinical manifestations of HIV infection and apply appropriate nursing interventions

Humans and animals are host to populations of micro-organisms which live on the skin and mucous membranes. The normal human fetus lives in a sterile environment until birth, when the infant soon gains a complex flora with bacteria derived from maternal flora and surroundings. Certain species of bacteria regularly inhabit different parts of the body where they constitute the normal flora of the area. Such organisms are termed *commensal*. They do not harm the normal host but achieve a balance with the host that ensures their survival and growth.

Micro-organisms that are capable of causing disease are termed *pathogens* or *infectious agents. Infection* is the multiplication of an infectious agent within the body tissues. The outcome is determined by the ability of the micro-organism to adhere, invade and damage the host (virulence) versus the host's defence mechanisms. Infection affecting specific body systems is discussed in the later chapters. This chapter concerns infection in general.

INFECTIOUS AGENTS

Groups of micro-organisms that interact with human beings and cause infections include bacteria, viruses, fungi, protozoa and parasitic worms.

Bacteria are extremely diverse, microscopic organisms and are usually 1–2 μm in length and diameter. They differ from other cells in having a unique polymer peptidoglycan in their cell wall, which can be damaged by antibiotics. They are prokaryotic organisms, i.e. they lack a nucleus, which makes them distinct from all other living cells. They are divided into two main groups by their appearance after Gram staining. Those that stain purple are called Gram-positive and those that do not, Gram-negative. Several distinct shapes are known: rod (bacillus), sphere (coccus), curve (vibrio), spiral (spirillum), and corkscrew (spirochaete).

Some bacteria form spores which are very resistant to heat and cannot be killed by boiling; this has to be considered in sterilization procedures. Spore-forming bacteria are commonly found in the soil. Many bacteria possess a gel (called a capsule) outside the cell wall, which allows them to adhere to surfaces and also confers resistance to ingestion by the host's phagocytes (cells whose function is to destroy invading micro-organisms). Others possess filaments, called flagella, that confer motility on the organism.

Bacteria multiply by binary fission (dividing into two), many of them multiply rapidly so that under suitable conditions a single cell can give rise to more than a million cells after 6 hours: a consideration when handling specimens obtained from cases of infectious disease. Bacteria are present in soil, air and water and are major constituents of the commensal flora. Most bacteria do not cause disease, they are non-pathogenic; for example, the skin is a normal habitat of staphylococci, coliform bacilli are always present in the intestine, and lactobacilli inhabit the vagina. Commensal organisms may play an essential role in the body; for instance, vitamin K, which is necessary for blood clotting, is produced by bacterial action in the intestine. The bacterial flora may be potentially pathogenic if they gain access to other areas of the body.

Viruses are small infectious agents ranging in size from 0.02 to 0.3 μm. They differ from other living cells in that they are obligate intracellular parasites of living cells, plants, animals and even bacteria. They are composed of either DNA or RNA surrounded by a protein coat, and some have a lipid envelope. They produce disease by entering the host cells, where they may cause proliferation, degeneration or destruction of the cells. Once inside the cell, they direct the host's metabolic machinery to reproduce themselves; some viruses may become integrated with the host cell genome and become established indefinitely. The initial clinical effect of the invasion may disappear and the virus remains dormant, only to reactivate later and produce symptoms, as in herpes simplex infection. When the entrance of a virus into tissue cells stimulates cell reproduction (proliferation), the new cells contain the virus. The many varieties or strains of virus and their intracellular location within the host has made effective therapy and control more difficult. Examples of viral diseases are the common cold, influenza, measles, mumps and AIDS. There is also accumulating evidence that viruses are associated with the development of some malignant diseases.

Fungi are multicellular, mould-like organisms which produce interlacing filaments or chains. A disease caused by a fungus is called a *mycosis*, or it may be indicated by the suffix -osis, preceded by the name of the causative fungus. Thrush, ringworm and histoplasmosis are examples of mycotic disease.

Protozoa are single-celled organisms that belong to the animal kingdom and are more complex in structure and activity than bacteria. Diseases that are caused by protozoa include malaria, giardiasis, amoebic dysentery and trichomoniasis.

Infection may be caused by parasitic worms, which are referred to as *helminths*. The helminthic infections most commonly seen are those caused by the roundworm, pinworm, tapeworm and *Trichinella spiralis*. The latter causes trichiniasis. The filarial worm, which causes filariasis or elephantiasis, and the hookworm are more prevalent in tropical areas.

INTERACTION BETWEEN HOST AND INFECTIOUS AGENTS

The outcome of the interaction between microorganisms and the host depends on the balance between the factors that promote establishment of the infectious agents and the host defence mechanisms. If host tissues are damaged, infectious disease occurs. The ability of a micro-organism to invade and injure host tissue is termed *virulence*.

Virulence

Determinants of virulence vary for different species and include the ability to attach to and invade host cells. Some agents display a specific attraction for certain cells and organs, e.g. *Neisseria meningitidis* attacks the meninges of the central nervous system, while *Neisseria gonorrhoeae* and *Chlamydia trachomatis* invade cervical epithelial cells. The mumps virus has a predilection for the parotid glands. Many bacteria are able to evade phagocytosis (see p. 63) by means of surface capsules or by proteins in the cell wall. *Streptococcus pyogenes*, the cause of pharyngitis, has an M protein, and *Streptococcus pneumoniae* has a thick capsule that are antiphagocytic.

Other virulence factors are the production of destructive enzymes and harmful toxins. Tissue-degrading enzymes such as collagenase, which breaks down collagen, and hyaluronidase, which hydrolyses hyaluronic acid (the ground substance of connective tissue), facilitate the spread of bacteria through tissues. Haemolysins and leucocidins destroy erythrocytes and leucocytes respectively.

Some bacteria are capable of intracellular growth within phagocytic cells. *Mycobacterium tuberculosis* and *Salmonella typhi* are examples of bacteria which multiply within macrophages (see p. 63) and are transported to other parts of the body. Some viruses are able to evade the host defences and persist in host cells for long periods of time (e.g. herpes simplex virus persists in sensory ganglial cells and produces latent infections).

Toxins are chemical substances which cause damage to the host. Endotoxins are the lipid A part of a lipopolysaccharide in the cell wall of Gram-negative bacteria. They are released when bacteria are killed and are responsible for the syndrome of septic shock (fever, leucopenia, hypotension). Exotoxins are excreted by many bacteria, both Gram-positive and Gram-negative. Some bacteria remain localized at the point of entry and produce characteristic disease by toxin production; for example, *Clostridium tetani* produces a toxin which acts on the nervous system to produce the muscular spasms characteristic of tetanus; *Staphylococcus aureus* in the vagina releases a toxin that causes toxic shock syndrome. The enterotoxins produced by certain strains of *Escherichia coli* and *Vibrio cholerae* interfere with salt and water absorption in the gut and cause diarrhoea.

Host Defences

The invasion of the body by microbes represents a major challenge to host resistance. Non-specific or innate resistance comprises defences against any injurious agent, including micro-organisms. The immune response is a specific response to specific antigens located on or produced by the micro-organisms. The term *antigen* describes a molecule which generates an immune response and which reacts with antibodies or primed T cells.

NON-SPECIFIC DEFENCES

BARRIERS

The intact skin is a protective barrier which is impermeable to most infectious agents. The damaged or broken skin, as in burns or invasion by intravascular catheters, allows invasion of bacteria. Mucous membranes are more vulnerable to attack by infectious agents. *Neisseria meningitidis* and *Neisseria gonorrhoeae* can penetrate the mucous membranes, and many viruses, e.g. the influenza virus, invade mucosal cells.

BACTERICIDAL SUBSTANCES IN BODY FLUIDS

Skin secretions contain fatty acids which inhibit and prevent the survival of many pathogens. However, *Klebsiella* may survive for many hours, which may explain its importance in nosocomial infections transmitted by hands between patients. *Staphylococcus aureus* is highly resistant to acidity and frequently resides on the skin and may infect hair follicles, causing boils. Mucous membranes secrete an external layer of mucus which traps infectious agents, preventing their adhesion to the epithelial cells. The mucus is propelled by ciliary movement (mucociliary flushing) and coughing and sneezing to the exterior.

Most body fluids have bactericidal activity. Lysozyme is present in all tissues and all body secretions except urine. It is present in high concentration in tears. It is an enzyme capable of damaging the peptidoglycan cell wall of bacteria, causing lysis and death.

Gastric juice, highly acid at pH 2.0, is lethal for nearly all bacteria except *Mycobacterium tuberculosis*, which is resistant. Ingested organisms may be protected by the bulk of food eaten. Breast milk and saliva contain lactoperoxidase, which inhibits multiplication of some bacteria. It also contains an antiviral agent (distinct from antibodies) which protects the mucosa against rotavirus infections. Prostatic secretions contain an antibacterial agent that enters the bladder at the end of micturition.

NORMAL BODY FLORA

The commensals that form the normal body flora are characteristic for a particular site. They prevent colonization and infection by pathogens. Their removal by antibiotic therapy often results in overgrowth of antibiotic-resistant organisms, which may cause an infection such as the pseudomembranous colitis caused by *Clostridium difficile*.

PHAGOCYTOSIS

Phagocytosis is the engulfment, killing and digestion of micro-organisms by polymorphonuclear leucocytes, monocytes and the macrophages, which originate from stem cells in the bone marrow.

Polymorphonuclear leucocytes are highly mobile amoeboid cells present in the blood. They contain granules filled with potent chemicals that enable them to kill and digest micro-organisms. These chemicals contribute to the acute inflammatory response. Every minute of the day the bone marrow produces 80 million of these cells.

Monocytes circulate in the blood and then migrate into tissues, where they develop into magrophages (big eaters). They are found in connective tissues in the lungs, liver, spleen, brain and lymph nodes.

Macrophages play an important role in both the non-specific and specific defence mechanisms of the body. Non-specifically, they rid the body of cell debris (micro-organisms and other worn out cells). Some bacteria, notably the mycobacteria, are capable of surviving intracellularly and migration of macrophages may be instrumental in the spread of infection to different parts of the body. The vital role of macrophages to the regulation of the immune responses and the development of inflammation will be discussed later.

COMPLEMENT

The complement system is made up of a series of about 25 proteins that work to complement the activity of antibodies in destroying bacteria, either by facilitating phagocytosis or by puncturing bacterial cell membranes. It also aids in the elimination of antigen–antibody complexes from the body. Carrying out these tasks, it induces an inflammatory response.

Complement proteins circulate in the blood in an inactive form. When the first of the series is triggered, it sets in motion a cascade effect. As each component is activated, it in turn acts on the next in a precise sequence that ends in the formation of a hole in the target cell which rapidly swells and bursts.

In addition, various fragments flung off by this cascade produce other consequences: the production of vaso-active substances by degranulation of mast cells and basophils, cause redness and swelling; the attraction of polymorphs to the area (chemotaxis); and the rendering of target cells attractive to phagocytes (opsonization).

THE INFLAMMATORY RESPONSE

The events orchestrated by phagocytic cells and complement and the tissue damage caused by the invading micro-organisms lead to the process of inflammation. The release of histamine by mast cells and basophils causes dilatation of capillaries and an increase in vascular permeability. Polymorphonuclear leucocytes migrate to the area to phagocytose the infectious agent. In so doing, they die themselves. Macrophages appear later to mop up the debris, which consists of dead leucocytes, bacteria and necrotic tissue. If the infection is severe enough, pus may be formed. The clinical events that mirror this process are local swelling, redness, heat and pain.

HOST RESISTANCE TO VIRUSES

Interferon is an important component in the defence mechanism against viruses. When certain body cells, leucocytes, fibroblasts and T lymphocytes, are infected by some viruses, they respond by producing interferon, a group of small proteins which inhibit virus multiplication within the cells. These proteins will only work in the species that produced them. Interleukins are types of interferons that aid in stimulating the antibody response (play a role in the specific immune response).

NATURAL KILLER CELLS

These non-specific lymphocytes rid the body of what they perceive as foreign or non-self cells without having to recognize a specific antigen. They migrate from the lymphoid tissue to the site of inflammation or tumour growth where they destroy the pathogens, tumour cells or virus-infected cells.

FEVER

Fever is the most common manifestation of the inflammatory response and a signal response in infectious disease. Various products of inflammation are capable of inducing fever. Among them are the endotoxins of Gram-negative bacteria and various cytokines derived from monocytes and macrophages. Most important of the cytokines is interleukin-1, also called endogenous pyrogen, which acts on the thermoregulatory centre in the hypothalamus where physiological responses result in fever.

A raised body temperature is thought to be of some host defence value but no adverse effects have been noted by the suppression of fever to make the patient comfortable. Antibody formation and T-cell proliferation are more efficient at higher body temperatures.

Interleukin-1 has a whole range of effects in addition to inducing fever. It promotes granulocyte release from the bone marrow, activation of macrophages, and proliferation of B and T lymphocytes to produce antibodies and promote cell-mediated immunity, respectively.

SPECIFIC DEFENCES

ANATOMY OF THE IMMUNE SYSTEM

The immune system consists of specialized cells and organs that are distributed throughout the body. This network of cells is able to distinguish self from non-self by recognition of foreign molecules. Nearly all body cells possess an identifiable marker. The central organs of the system are the bone marrow and the thymus, while the peripheral organs include the lymph nodes, spleen, tonsils, adenoids, appendix and the Peyer's patches of the intestine. Immune cells originate from the lymphoid stem cells of the bone marrow (Figure 6.1). About half of these cells migrate very early in life to the thymus gland, where they are processed into T lymphocytes, which are involved in *cell-mediated immune responses* and participate in the control of antibody production (Burton, 1988).

Other cells differentiate in the bone marrow to become B lymphocytes. B cells migrate to the lymphoid tissues throughout the body and are responsible for the production of antibodies or immunoglobulins. This is referred to as the *humoral response*.

The T and B lymphocytes are transported by the blood and lymph vessels. The lymph nodes, scattered throughout the lymphatic system, filter the lymph drained from the tissues, separating out antigens and exposing them to the cells of the immune system. The spleen, like the lymph nodes, contains both T and B cell areas and is particularly effective in filtering out particulate antigens such as micro-organisms. Removal of the spleen is a loss of a significant defence mechanism.

CELL-MEDIATED RESPONSE

When bacteria enter the body they are first processed by macrophages. The bacterial antigen appears on the surface of the macrophage where it is recognized by a matched T cell which binds with the antigen–macrophage complex. The macrophage produces interleukin-1 which activates the T cell. The T cell multiplies, forming three subsets of lymphocytes:

- *Effector cells* which provide the actual protective actions. Cytotoxic T cells disrupt the membranes of the invading cells and destroy them by lysis. Delayed hypersensitivity lymphocytes release lymphokines, which enhance the activities of the non-specific defence mechanisms, especially phagocytosis.
- *Regulator cells* which function to control the immune responses and to facilitate interaction between T-cell and B-cell activities. Helper T cells interact with the plasma B cells to initiate antibody production. Suppressor T cells interact with B cells to decrease or control the production of antibodies.
- *Memory cells* which are stored after the offending antigen has disappeared. They retain their sensitivity to the specific antigen, enabling them to be quickly reactivated when reinfection with the identical antigen occurs.

HUMORAL RESPONSE

Antibody secretion by the B cells, with co-operation from helper and suppressor T cells, occurs in response to a specific antigen. The production of antibodies depends on the nature of the antigen, the site of antigen stimulus, the amount of antigen present and the frequency of previous exposure to the antigen. B cells bind only with the antigen that fits their receptors. They then mulitply, producing identical clones, which differentiate into plasma cells that produce large quantities of antigen-specific antibodies for several days until they die. The antibodies are released into the circulation where they interlock with matching antigens to form antigen–antibody complexes. These bind with toxins or viruses to neutralize them, increase phagocytic activity or activate complement to destroy the bacterial cell.

The number of antigens decreases as the infection is overcome and antibody production declines as the plasma cells die and the suppressor T cells exert their control. Some activated B cells that did not become plasma cells become *memory* cells which are stored and respond later when stimulated by exposure to the same antigen.

Antibodies are immunoglobulin molecules which are composed of four interlinked polypeptide chains (two long or heavy chains and two shorter, light chains),

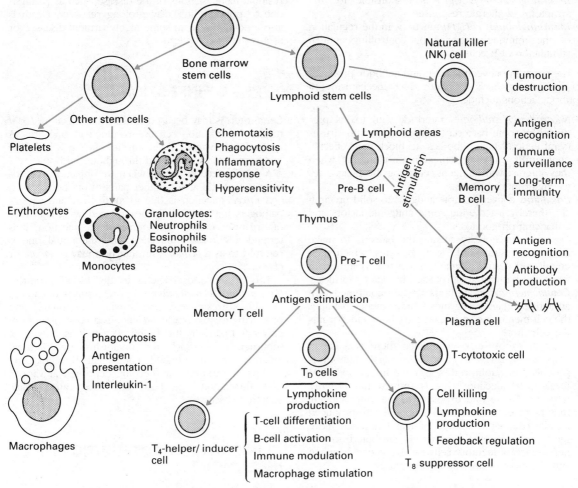

Figure 6.1 Differentiation of blood and lymph cells from bone marrow cells: development of cell-mediated immunity and antibody production. Modified from Burton (1988) with permission.

shaped to form a Y (Figure 6.2). The sections at the tips of the Y, arms called the *variable* regions, are the specific antigen combining sites. The stem of the Y, called the *constant* region, links the antibody to other molecules of the defence process, e.g. complement. The major classes of immunoglobulins (Ig) or antibodies are labelled A, D, E, G and M, preceded by the symbol Ig (i.e. IgA, IgD, IgE, IgG and IgM). There are two identified types of IgA and four of IgG.

- *Immunoglobulin G (IgG)* is the most common antibody in the blood and is able to enter tissue spaces. It crosses the placenta and provides protection against infection to the fetus and newborn.
- *Immunoglobulin M (IgM)* is large and tends to remain in the bloodstream where it produces an early line of attack against bacteria. It does not cross the placenta.
- *Immunoglobulin A (IgA)* is found in saliva, tears, respiratory and gastrointestinal secretions and colostrum, as well as the bloodstream. It serves to protect the external body openings against invasion.

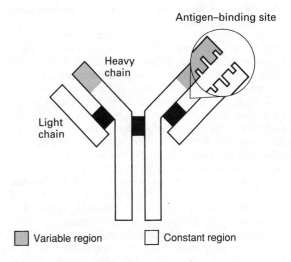

Figure 6.2 Structure of an antibody.

- *Immunoglobulin E (IgE)* is responsible for the symptoms of allergic responses.
- *Immunoglobulin D (IgD)* functions in the regulation of the immune response by controlling antigen stimulation of B cells.

The reaction between antigen and antibody produces an *antigen–antibody complex*. The mechanisms of antibody actions include:

- *Neutralizing antibodies* interlock with toxins produced by some bacteria (antitoxins) or with viruses (viral neutralizing antibodies) to block their effects.
- *Agglutinins* cause agglutination or clumping when they interact with antigens, enabling the phagocytes to engulf more bacteria.
- *Precipitins* convert soluble antigens to solid precipitate, thereby inactivating some antigenic factors and enhancing phagocytosis.
- *Opsonins* function by coating the bacteria to make them more susceptible to phagocytes, which then engulf and destroy them. This reaction is important when the bacteria are protected by outer capsules.
- *Complement-fixing* antibodies, when combined with an antigen, release enzymes (complement) that alter the cell membrane so it leaks cytoplasm and disrupts the cell (lysis).
- On first exposure to an antigen there is a lag in response of a few days or weeks. IgM antibody is produced first, followed by IgG and IgA or both. IgM levels soon decline. This is termed the *primary response*. On second exposure to the same antigen, months or even years later, antibodies are produced rapidly (the same amount of IgM but much more IgG). The prompt response is attributed to the persistence of memory cells for that specific antigen and is called the *secondary response*.

COURSE OF THE INFECTIOUS DISEASE

The course of most infectious diseases extends over the following phases.

The *incubation period* is the interval between the time the organism enters the body and the initial clinical manifestations of an infection. During this stage the organisms multiply and the host defences are mounted to counter the infection. The patient is asymptomatic but may shed the infectious agent. If the host defences overcome the causative organisms, there may be no signs or symptoms. Such inapparent or subclinical infections are detected by laboratory methods. Persons who shed infectious agents but do not have symptoms of the disease are said to be *carriers*.

The *acute illness* is the stage in which the disease reaches its full intensity. The length of the period of acute illness varies from a few hours to weeks. It is generally predictable for the specific disease.

Convalescence is the stage during which the clinical manifestations subside. Many infectious diseases are self-limiting and recovery takes place over a short, defined period of time. The development of complications or of residual manifestations of the disease, such as paralysis due to poliomyelitis, may prolong recovery. Death is also a possibility from some highly virulent diseases, or as a result of complications.

TYPES OF INFECTION

Certain terms may be used to describe infection. *Local* means the infection remains confined to one area. A *generalized systemic* infection is one in which the organisms are disseminated throughout the body.

A *focal* infection occurs when the infection spreads from a confined area to other parts of the body.

A *mixed* infection is due to more than one type of pathogen. If a person becomes infected by another type of organism during the course of an infection, it is termed a *secondary* infection, and the initial one is referred to as a *primary*. An infection may be *acute* or *chronic*.

The presence of bacteria in the blood produces *bacteraemia*. *Septicaemia* means organisms have entered the bloodstream and are actively multiplying and producing toxins. *Toxaemia* implies a concentration of bacterial toxins in the blood. *Pyaemia* is a type of septicaemia in which the organisms are clumped together or incorporated into small thrombi. The clumps or thrombi may become deposited at various sites throughout the body and may cause small, scattered abscesses.

CLINICAL CHARACTERISTICS OF INFECTION

During the incubation period, symptoms of infection are usually general and include headache and malaise. Manifestations common to many infections during the acute stage include the following systemic and local symptoms: fever, which may be preceded by chills; an increase in the pulse and respiratory rates; anorexia; nausea and vomiting; headache; apathy and fatigue; joint and muscle pain; and general malaise. The patient may appear hot and flushed, and the tongue is frequently furred and dry. There may be enlargement and tenderness of the lymph nodes that receive the lymph from the site of infection.

If the infection is local, the classic symptoms are that the area becomes red (rubric) and hot (hyperthermic) due to vasodilatation, swollen (oedema) due to increased vascular permeability, and painful (dolor) as a result of the release of chemical mediators and pressure from increased tissue fluid. These symptoms are also seen in inflammatory responses. Inflammation is always present with infection unless the patient's immune system is severely impaired. Infection, on the other hand, is not always present with inflammation as inflammation may be caused by heat, radiation or trauma, as well as by micro-organisms.

In addition to the common signs and symptoms described above, certain features characteristic of a specific infection may be present and may play an important role in the diagnosis. For example, certain infections cause a rash, while others may give rise to a marked increase in a particular type of leucocyte.

DIAGNOSTIC PROCEDURES USED IN INFECTION

LEUCOCYTE COUNT AND DIFFERENTIAL

Some infections cause an increase in the number of white blood cells well above the normal, while in others there may be a decrease below the normal. An increase in a particular type of leucocyte is recognized as being characteristic of certain infections.

ERYTHROCYTE SEDIMENTATION RATE

This is a non-specific test sometimes requested as part of the diagnostic work-up. The rate at which the red blood cells settle in a specimen of blood is increased in infection and inflammation.

IDENTIFICATION OF THE CAUSATIVE ORGANISM

Identification of the causative agent involves the isolation of the organism from the body tissue or secretion in which it is located. This is done by the following methods:

- Direct examination which involves a specimen of sputum, blood, spinal fluid, urine, faeces, discharge or of the scrapings from a lesion being stained and examined under the microscope for organisms. Appearance, shape and certain staining characteristics assist in identifying different organisms.
- Cultural growth which involves the sterile collection of suspect material from the patient and introduction of this material to nutrient culture media, chick embryo or tissue culture media. The media are observed for a period of time for the growth of organisms. The material to be cultured may be sputum, nasal or throat secretions, blood, urine, faeces, wound discharge or spinal fluid.

A pure growth of the causative organism that is isolated is tested for susceptibility to appropriate antimicrobial drugs. The results of these tests form the basis for the selection of the most appropriate, effective drug to destroy the organisms.

ANTIBODY TESTS

A specimen of blood may be examined to determine the concentration of antibodies present; this is referred to as an antibody titre. Micro-organisms act as antigens, stimulating the production of specific antibodies, and antibody titres rise as the disease progresses. Two specimens, one taken in the early stage and the other in the later or convalescent stages, are required to demonstrate an increase in the antibody titre. Tests may also be done to detect the presence of certain antigens or antibodies; a known antibody may be used to determine the presence of an antigen, or a known antigen may be used to detect antibodies.

SKIN TESTS

Two skin tests are the tuberculin and Schick tests. In the tuberculin test, a small dose of old tuberculin or purified protein derivative of tuberculin is injected intradermally on the flexor surface of the forearm. A positive reaction is indicated by swelling and oedema at the site of injection and a surrounding redness within 2–3 days; this result means the individual has or has had an infection by tubercle bacilli, acquired either naturally or following a BCG vaccine. The test is considered negative if there is no reaction. If the first test is negative, the test may be repeated with a larger dose of tuberculin.

The Schick test, which is less frequently used, determines susceptibility to diphtheria. A small dose of diphtheria toxin standard dilution (0.1 ml) is administered intradermally into a forearm, and a dose of inactivated toxin is given intradermally in the opposite arm. The latter is used as the comparative control. In a positive reaction, the site of the active toxin injection manifests redness in 48 hours; this persists for 1–2 weeks. The control shows no reaction. A positive reaction indicates that the recipient of the toxin does not have antibodies to neutralize the toxin and is considered susceptible. A negative Schick test shows no reaction on either arm and indicates the person has sufficient protective antitoxin antibodies.

Collection of Specimens

The laboratory examination of specimens is an important item in the diagnosis and therapeutic management of the patient with infection. It is particularly important for accurate diagnosis that the sample represents the conditions that prevailed at the time of collection, the quality of the specimen must therefore be preserved at all times. Controversy surrounding delivery of specimens to the laboratory frequently results in improper handling and deterioration of specimens. Each nursing unit should have guidelines for the collection and handling of specimens. When collecting specimens, these general procedures should be followed (from Burton, 1988):

1. All specimens must be collected in a sterile, leak-proof container, which must be properly labelled with the patient's name and the source of the specimen, and submitted with a requisition giving relevant clinical information, the date, time of collection, doctor's name and laboratory tests required.
2. The sample should be obtained from the site of infection and care must be taken to avoid contamination by normal body flora. The amount should be adequate for the number of tests required.
3. Specimens should be collected before the administration of antibiotics. If this is not possible,

indicate on the requisition those antibiotics given.

4. Specimen collection should be performed with care and tact to avoid harming the patient, causing discomfort or causing undue embarrassment. Patients should be given clear instructions regarding specimen collection.

5. Specimens should be protected from heat and cold, and be promptly delivered to the laboratory so the analysis will yield the organisms present at the time of collection. If delivery is delayed, some delicate pathogens will die. Anaerobes (organisms which grow in the absence of molecular oxygen) will die when exposed to air. In addition, the normal flora of the patient may overgrow the pathogens and inhibit or kill them.

6. Specimens are usually placed in a sealed plastic bag to prevent contamination of the ward messenger.

NURSING MANAGEMENT OF THE PERSON WITH INFECTION

Assessment

Health history. Specific factors from the patient's health history that are relevant to infections include: age; immunization history, including dates and type of immunization received; childhood communicable diseases; history of metabolic and chronic diseases; medication history, particularly in relation to immunosuppressive drug therapy and corticosteroids; general nutritional status; exposure to radiation; occupational and home environments and history of recent travel; and information about recent changes in life-style (marriage, deaths, new sexual partner, etc.), as well as subjective symptoms of infectious diseases (headache, chills, anorexia, nausea, apathy, fatigue, joint and muscle pain and general malaise).

Physical examination. Assessment of the patient for objective signs of infection includes: the recording of vital signs (temperature, and pulse and respiratory rates) and observing overall appearance (e.g. flushing of the skin and perspiration, general posture and body positioning). The patient should be observed for a tendency to splint, guard or failure to use certain body parts, indicating pain and discomfort. The skin is examined for rash, lesions, warmth and moisture.

Patient Health Problems

Analysis of the data collected from the patient's history, by physical examination and specific diagnostic tests will lead to the identification of potential patient problems (for the patient with an increased risk of infection) or to actual patient problems (for the patient with an actual infection).

Increased potential for infection may be related to breakdown in any link of the infectious chain resulting in the individual being exposed to the infectious agent or to factors in the individual which increase susceptibility to infection once the organism has been transmitted. These factors include inadequate acquired or innate immunity, poor nutritional status, age, metabolic disturbances or other diseases and immunosuppression, e.g. due to steroid therapy or the effects of HIV (see page 75).

The following patient health problems relate to most individuals with infectious diseases:

- Physical and social isolation associated with limitations imposed by the potential for transmission of infectious agents and the resulting infection control measures.
- Inadequate nutrition to meet the increased metabolic demands of infection.
- Alteration in comfort; pain associated with the inflammatory process.
- Alteration in certain body functions related to the manifestations of specific infectious diseases (e.g. altered bowel function with diarrhoea, or ineffective airway clearance related to increased respiratory secretions).
- Alteration in self-management related to functional loss resulting from sequelae or complications of the infection.

Planning

Nursing care may be summarized as aiming to:

- Provide a safe environment.
- Control the sources of infection.
- Prevent transmission of infectious agents.
- Protect the patient with an increased susceptibility to infection.
- Support the functioning of the individual with an infection.

Goals for the patient with an infection are to:

- Minimize the impact of physical and social isolation.
- Maintain adequate fluid and nutritional status.
- Prevent and/or alleviate discomfort.
- Maintain functioning of other body systems.
- Adapt to the psychological stress of the illness.

The person will show that these goals have been achieved by being able to:

- State the reasons for protective measures
- Demonstrate the recommended infection control measures
- Verbalize feelings and concerns about restrictions imposed by illness and isolation
- Demonstrate absence of infection: body temperature decreased to normal range; white blood count within normal range; urine output and bowel elimination normal for the person; and normal skin turgor
- State absence of pain or discomfort
- State the signs and symptoms of recurrence of the infection
- Describe plans for follow-up care.

Nursing Intervention

Five potential problems are relevant to most patients with infections. A care plan developed for an individual patient would be more specific and comprehensive by including additional problems relevant to the patient's situation.

1. PHYSICAL AND SOCIAL ISOLATION

Infection control measures are implemented to isolate the organisms, not the patient (see page 74). The nurse should assess how the patient perceives the situation in order to provide meaningful support and to decrease concerns and anxiety. Isolation may have negative and frightening connotations for the patient and family. Feelings of rejection or guilt or of being punished are not uncommon. Explanations should be given to the patient and family as to the reasons for the protective measures. Specific details as to what these measures involve for the patient, visitors and hospital personnel and the expected length of the period of isolation are outlined. The nurse should not assume that explanations made on admission will be fully comprehended, because at that time the individual was probably very anxious. Repetition of explanations and assessment of the patient's perceptions and understanding should be ongoing.

The patient, family and nurse should take time to explore feelings and to develop plans to compensate for the physical and social isolation that the patient in isolation may experience. Interests and leisure activities can be elicited which may help the patient to make plans that are realistic for the situation and meaningful to him. Books, radios, television sets, telephones, family pictures and craft articles may be made available or brought in by the family if appropriate to the patient's interest and current condition. Sedentary activities are usually preferable because of the patient's need for rest. Visitors are encouraged within the isolation limitations. The patient and family are expected to participate in the planning and carrying out of care within the limits of their interest and abilities.

When the patient is being cared for at home, the nurse helps the family to plan patient care so that there will be minimal disruption of family routine and to enable the patient to participate in decisions and important family activities.

2. ALTERED NUTRITION

Fluids. Fluids promote the dilution and excretion of toxins and are also necessary because they prevent the dehydration which can occur because of diaphoresis.

Patient assessment involves monitoring of body temperature, the presence of chills and signs of dehydration. Chills occur when the body attempts to raise its temperature. Body temperature should be measured following each episode of chills. Signs of dehydration include: loss of skin turgor, as determined by gently raising and pinching a fold of skin and observing the time it takes to return to its original shape; a decrease in urinary output (fluid intake and

output should be accurately monitored); change of shape of eyeballs, which appear sunken; depression of the fontanelles in young children when palpated; and subjective sensations of thirst and dryness.

The patient's fluid intake should be increased to a minimum of 2500–3000 ml, unless contraindicated by cardiovascular or renal impairment.

Nutrition. A high caloric, high protein and high vitamin diet (especially vitamin C, which is important in wound healing due to its effect in promoting collagen formation), is important for the patient with an infection. The metabolic rate increases as the body temperature rises, resulting in increased energy expenditure. Extra calories should be given to prevent the breakdown of body tissue and to meet the increased energy demands. Proteins and vitamins play important roles in the formation of antibodies and tissue repair. Anorexia may be a problem; frequent small amounts of foods may be necessary.

Increased rest should be planned for the patient in order to conserve energy and decrease the caloric demands of the body. Treatments and care activities are planned so that uninterrupted periods are possible. For example, when the patient must be disturbed for the administration of medication, other therapeutic and supportive measures are carried out at that time if at all possible.

3. ALTERATION IN COMFORT

Various nursing measures may be necessary to provide symptomatic relief. In the early stages of the infection, the patient may complain of chilliness; extra bedcovers and warmth should be provided. When the patient develops a fever, tepid sponges may be used to reduce the temperature, the bedcovers are reduced to a minimum, and efforts are made to maintain a cool environment.

The dry mouth and coated tongue that frequently accompany infectious disease and fever are a source of discomfort. Regular cleaning of the teeth, frequent mouth rinses and the application of a cream or oil to the lips, as well as increased fluid intake, are used to promote comfort.

Skin care is important for the patient with a rash, dry itching skin or who is sweating excessively. The skin should be bathed with warm water, using a soft cloth, and patted dry. Soaps and perfumed skin preparations should be avoided as they tend to dry and irritate the skin. If soap is required, a superfatted soap preparation should be used.

The patient may experience pain in the infected area; a bed-cradle over the area to take the weight of the bedding may help. Analgesics for the relief of pain are administered as prescribed.

An important nursing measure that contributes to the patient's comfort is the relief of the anxiety and apprehension that are common in any illness. The patient and family are kept informed of progress, treatment and anticipated results. They are encouraged to participate in planning and in implementing care activities. The nurse assesses the patient's responses to illness and treatment and provides opportunity for the patient to discuss perceptions and concerns, to ask questions and express feelings.

4. MAINTAIN FUNCTIONING OF OTHER BODY SYSTEMS

Assessment of physiological responses to infection is continuous and directed by the expected manifestations of the disease and potential complications. Bowel function is carefully monitored when the patient has an infection of the gastrointestinal tract and in children who frequently manifest gastrointestinal symptoms with a fever. Urine output is monitored in the elderly, and in patients with cardiovascular or renal disorders, due to the possibility of urinary retention or renal failure. Respiratory status is assessed for all patients with respiratory infections or who have restricted mobility which may lead to the development of a respiratory infection. Ear infections, meningitis and encephalitis are complications that can develop with measles. Changes in pain or discomfort, neurological and mental status should be observed and reported promptly. Vital signs are recorded at frequent intervals and the patient should be observed closely and examined for changes that might indicate spread of the infection or complications. For example, if there is infection in a foot, the complete limb should be examined for redness, tenderness, and swelling and the lymph nodes in the groin checked for tenderness and swelling.

Administration of anti-infective agents. Anti-infective agents are prescribed to destroy or control the causative organisms and thus limit the disease process and decrease the incidence of complications.

Prior to the administration of an anti-infective agent, the patient is questioned about any known allergies or drug reactions. The nurse must be familiar with the possible side-effects of the drug being used and must be alert for very early signs of untoward reactions. Side-effects vary with the specific drug but generally include skin rashes, nausea, vomiting and diarrhoea.

When administering antimicrobial drugs it is important to provide adequate constant serum and tissue levels of the antimicrobial agent. To achieve this, the nurse must administer the medications on time and, if given intravenously, administer in the prescribed time interval (e.g. 20 min). Aminoglycoside preparations pose the greatest potential for such problems. If they are given too early, the blood levels become excessive and toxicity develops. If administered late, prolonged periods with subtherapeutic levels decrease their effectiveness. The administration of intravenous aminoglycosides is usually planned over a 30–60 min period to provide optimum levels. Similar precautions should be taken with other antibiotics. The nurse must also be alert to the fact that penicillin has the potential to inactivate aminoglycosides. It is important to space the administration of different antimicrobial agents so that a constant serum level of the specific drug is maintained and so that incompatible drugs are not mixed together. Different intravenous lines are used or the drugs are given by different routes.

When the patient is taking antimicrobial drugs at home or is being discharged from hospital with a prescription for these agents, it is important that the nurse instruct the patient to complete the full course of the prescribed medication and give specific instructions as to when drugs are to be taken. Times are determined by assessing the patient's daily life-style. The nurse should explain that antimicrobial therapy should not be stopped when the patient feels better, as this may lead to the development of resistant strains, and that medications prescribed for a previous illness should not be substituted.

5. ALTERATION IN SELF-MANAGEMENT

The incidence of major communicable diseases has been greatly reduced as a result of improved socio-economic and environmental conditions, worldwide immunization programmes and advances in microbiology and epidemiology. Medical advances have contributed to improved management of the patient with an infectious disease and a decrease in the incidence and severity of residual effects and complications from the disease. The elderly, very young and those with debilitating diseases whose body defences are decreased, show a greater incidence of sequelae.

Specific nursing interventions for the patient with functional loss or other complications of infectious diseases will depend on the nature and severity of the impairment.

The patient and family can be helped to cope with functional loss or impending death by first identifying how they are perceiving the situation. Knowledge of the home situation, family and community resources as well as the socioeconomic status helps the patient, family and nurse to develop realistic plans for follow-up care and rehabilitation. Patient and family instruction includes knowledge of the disease, its signs and symptoms and the possibility of recurrence, as with infections such as tuberculosis and malaria. Manifestations of recurrence and the action to take are stressed. Self-care skills are taught and community resources outlined. Necessary referrals are made if continuity of care and supervision are needed. Plans for rehabilitation are made to promote optimal return of activity and independence. The family and patient should be told of the anticipated outcomes and helped to recognize and deal with the consequences of any permanent impairment. They may require considerable support and counselling to help them accept an impairment and its implications, and to make realistic plans to deal with the temporary or permanent impairment or with death.

Evaluation

Evaluation of the outcomes of nursing intervention for the person with an infection is based on the patient goals, which are to: (1) minimize the physical and emotional impact of the isolation precautions; (2) maintain fluid and nutritional status; (3) control pain and discomfort; and (4) prevent complications. The patient and family should be aware of the microbial and host factors contributing to the development of the infection. They should be able to describe measures to prevent the transmission of the infection to others and be familiar with the treatment plan and plans for follow-up care.

Evaluation of measures to prevent the transmission of infection to others may be determined by identifying the incidence of the infection in family members and associated others in the home, workplace or community, as well as from an analysis of hospital infection control reports and statistics.

OCCURRENCE OF INFECTIOUS DISEASE IN POPULATIONS

Epidemiology is the study of the occurrence and distribution of a disease within populations. An *endemic* disease is constantly present in a given population and its prevalence varies little over time. An *epidemic* is the occurrence of cases of a disease or an outbreak clearly in excess of expectancy. A *pandemic* is a worldwide epidemic.

The Chain of Infection

Infections develop as a result of a chain of events which link the *reservoir* of infectious agents with the *suscep-*

tible host. These are a mode of escape from the reservoir, a means or route of transmission, and a mode of entry into the susceptible host. All three links in the chain must be present for infections to occur. Intervention at any point in the chain can prevent the development of infection. Figure 6.3 illustrates the links that must be present for infection to occur and the factors which influence the process.

RESERVOIR OF INFECTIOUS AGENTS

Any site in which an infectious agent lives and multiplies, and from which it can be transmitted, is called a reservoir. Micro-organisms may come from sources external to the human body or may be normal inhabitants of the body. The normal flora of the body may cause disease when the host's resistance is lowered, or when the organisms are transferred to another area of the body where they are not normally found.

External reservoirs of infectious agents may be other humans, animals, insects or inanimate objects. These sources provide reservoirs where the organisms can live and propagate and from which they are transferred to the host. The most common reservoir is a human, who may be in the incubation period, acute stage or convalescence of the disease, or who may be a carrier. The carriers may appear healthy but harbour pathogenic organisms which can be transmitted to others.

Tuberculosis and brucellosis (undulant fever) are examples of infections (zoonoses) that may be contracted from cows. Animals infested with parasites may be a source of disease if their flesh is eaten raw, e.g.

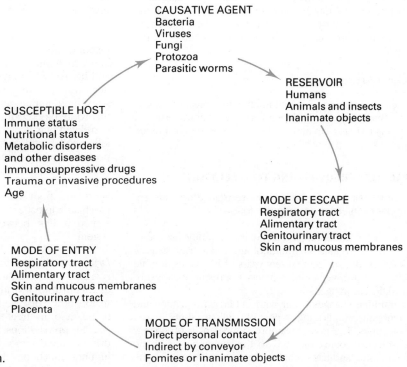

Figure 6.3 The chain of infection.

toxoplasmosis. Rabies is acquired from rabid dogs, cats or other infected animals.

The most common inanimate reservoirs are soil and decaying animal and vegetable matter. Tetanus usually develops as a result of soil contamination of a wound. Soil may also be a source of some pathogenic fungi.

MODE OF ESCAPE

Infectious agents require a means of escaping from the reservoir. Exit from human reservoirs may be by the respiratory, alimentary or genitourinary tracts, or from open lesions on the skin or mucous membranes.

MODE OF TRANSMISSION

Pathogenic agents may be transmitted from their source by direct or indirect contact. In direct spread, the infecting agent is transferred directly from the reservoir to the person. Indirect transmission implies an inter-mediate contaminated conveyor or object. Conveyors frequently support the life and growth of the organisms. Transmission of the disease-producing organism by indirect contact occurs in airborne infections (e.g. respiratory disease) and water and food infections (e.g. food poisoning, typhoid fever). *Fomites* is a term applied to inanimate objects that spread infection; examples are bedding, towels, dishes, instruments and furniture.

MODE OF ENTRY

The infecting agents may enter the host through the respiratory tract, the alimentary tract, a break in the skin or the genitourinary tract. A fetus may become infected by transplacental transmission. Normally the placenta is an effective barrier but certain organisms, such as the spirochaete that causes syphilis and viruses if present in the mother, are likely to cross the placenta and enter the fetus.

SUSCEPTIBLE HOST

The development of infection after the infectious agent has entered the body depends on the characteristics of the micro-organism and on the nature of the local tissue and systemic defences of the host.

FACTORS PREDISPOSING TO INFECTION

Factors that influence the host's resistance and suscep-tibility to infection include the following.

Age.   Both humoral and cellular immunity are com-promised in infants. Immunological maturity steadily develops during the first few years of life. Considerable variations are seen among infants as a result of exposure to different antigens.

Immune changes occur with puberty, pregnancy and menopause, indicating a possible link to shifts in sex hormones. The immunosuppression seen in pregnancy is selective, being directed to the maintenance of the fetal tissue, and has minimal clinical significance for the

woman. There is evidence of a diminished resistance to viral infections during pregnancy.

The incidence of autoimmune disease and cancer increase with ageing. The elderly are more susceptible to and have a diminished capacity to combat infection. The thymus gland begins to atrophy at about 45 years of age resulting in a decreased production of its hormones which play a role in the differentiation of lymphocytes. There is an increase in autoantibodies in the elderly which is believed to contribute to the pathological changes that occur with ageing. The response to foreign antigens decreases and the elderly are not able to sustain resistance against infection.

Occupation.   Certain occupations provide increased exposure to infecting agents or may reduce the efficiency of one's protective mechanisms.

Exposure to cold.   A lowering of the body temperature below normal is thought to decrease the ciliary movement in the respiratory tract, reduce the blood supply to superficial tissues and suppress antibody formation, all of which are natural defence mechanisms.

Nutritional imbalances.   Lymphoid tissue is vulnerable to excesses and deficiencies of many nutrients because of its rapid rate of proliferation. Protein and caloric undernutrition is a prevalent cause of impaired cell-mediated immunity. Humoral immunity and phagocytosis are less affected. Inadequate dietary intake of vitamins A, B and folic acid and of minerals such as zinc and iron affect the components of the immune system. Without the required nutrients and energy the production of antibodies, lymphocytes and the chemical mediators of the immune response is impaired. Excessive dietary intake of cholesterol and fats leads to a decrease in immunocompetence.

Stress.   Psychoneuroendocrine immunology is a de-veloping field of study that looks at the interactions between immune function, neuroendocrine responses and life stresses. Carrieri et al reviewed six studies that demonstrated the relationship between life-change stress and immunocompetence. The results indicated that white blood cell counts and lymphocyte cytotoxicity correlated negatively with life-change stress, that natural killer (NK) and cytotoxic T cell activity correlated positively with coping ability, and antibody response with ego strength (Halliburton, 1986). Naturally occur-ring, persistent stress accompanied by poor coping alters the body's immunocompetence. Studies using psychiatric in-patients and medical students have demon-strated a link between loneliness and the immune system.

Drugs and therapeutic interventions.   Immunosuppres-sive agents are used to treat autoimmune disorders such as rheumatoid arthritis, glomerulonephritis and inflam-matory bowel disease, to prevent rejection of transplanted tissue, and to treat cancers. Agents include cortico-steroid preparations, cyclophosphamide and azathio-prine. Some commonly used antibiotics may also impair immune function. All drugs are capable of initiating a hypersensitivity reaction.

Ionizing radiation reduces resistance to infection while surgical intervention, anaesthesia and all forms of shock have also been shown to alter immunocompetence. Some infections decrease the person's resistance to a secondary infection. The HIV virus depresses cell-mediated immune function and leaves the individual vulnerable to many opportunistic disorders, including *Pneumocystis carinii* pneumonia and Kaposi's sarcoma.

Smoking is a life-style factor that impairs the regulation of T cells.

Infectious Disease in Hospital Populations

NOSOCOMIAL INFECTION

Hospital-acquired or *nosocomial* infections are infections that were not present, or incubating, in hospitalized patients at the time of admission. The infection may result from endogenous organisms carried by the patient or originate from the animate or inanimate environment of the hospital. The latter is a potentially preventable infection. Hand-washing is the simplest and most effective preventive measure yet McFarlane (1990) has shown that in one study 89% of staff failed to fully wash both hands, while Phillips (1989) urges the need for washing to last 30 seconds, a quick splash under the tap is not enough! Nosocomial infections result in prolonged hospitalization, increasing the cost of treatment as well as causing discomfort and inconvenience for the patient. Such infections are determined by factors which stem from the hospital environment and its population. The reservoirs of infectious agents are the patients with infectious disease, and carriers among both these patients and hospital care personnel. These bacterial agents tend to be resistant to multiple antibiotics because the use of wide-spectrum antimicrobial drugs makes for the selection and survival of more resistant micro-organisms in the hospital environment.

The principal types of acquired infection involve surgical wounds, urinary and respiratory infections; according to Cadwaller (1989) the UK rate is 9.2% of all admissions. In studying a 600-bed district general hospital, she found not a single ward correctly practised hand-washing technique, the simplest of all preventive measures.

Infection may be endogenous as commensal organisms become opportunists, with the capacity to invade the body when host defences are impaired (e.g. *Staphylococcus epidermidis*, a common skin commensal, is a frequent cause of i.v. cannulae-related bacteraemia). The environment may be the source of infection. Organisms from environmental sources, e.g. *Pseudomonas aeruginosa* in tap water and *Legionella pneumophila* growing in hot water tanks may contaminate the atmosphere and cause disease.

If an intravenous (i.v.) infusion is used to rehydrate the patient, it should be remembered that this carries a significant infection risk in itself. Goodinson (1990) reviewed the literature, finding a range of from 7.8 to 28.4% of i.v. infusions becoming infected. She urges the use of strict aseptic techniques, a limited period of use for each site, anticoagulation and careful selection of i.v. cannulae to help reduce infection rates.

The possibility of hospital food causing a serious, life-threatening illness must not be forgotten. Ward (1988) points out that, in one study, 59% of hospital kitchens did not comply with UK food regulations and 13% were bad enough to warrant prosecution.

The transmission routes of infection are as previously described; however, hands of hospital personnel are an important vehicle of transfer of resistant bacteria, like *Klebsiella*, from one patient to the other. It has been shown that some Gram-negative organisms can survive on skin for long periods.

In addition to the general factors affecting susceptibility that have been discussed above, the patient population is also compromised by virtue of underlying disease, impairment of host defences by immunosuppressive agents, broad-spectrum antibiotics which kill the commensal flora, invasive techniques such as urethral and vascular catheterization, surgery and by implantation of prosthetic devices which may become a focus for bacterial growth.

CONTROL OF NOSOCOMIAL INFECTIONS

The nurse has a responsibility in any situation where infection is known to exist, or where there is the possibility of infection, to practise and promote measures that will confine the organisms and prevent their spread to other persons. Measures to prevent hospital-acquired infections include:

- Recognition of the possible risk of infection among hospitalized patients.
- Questioning the use of invasive procedures and implementing these procedures only when necessary.
- Following strict surgical aseptic techniques when carrying out invasive procedures (e.g. urinary catheterization, intravenous infusion).
- Instruction of patients and visitors in measures to prevent spread of organisms (e.g. hand washing, covering nose and mouth with tissues when coughing, not sharing personal objects and not visiting if an infection is suspected.)
- Prompt identification and treatment of infections in hospital personnel.
- Implementation of isolation procedures for certain infected patients.
- The practice of hand washing under running water with soap and friction before and after provision of care for a patient and/or following the handling of patient articles.
- Efficient domestic cleaning of wards, isolation rooms and other areas of the hospital (e.g. damp mopping to decrease dust, and the use of approved hospital disinfectants).

Hospitals should have in place infection control policies for the prevention of transmission of infection. The Infection Control Committee, with members representing all sections of the hospital, formulates these policies. Infection control may however become a ritualized routine of little value unless rationales are presented for actions. Walsh and Ford (1989) have argued that much nursing practice in this field is outmoded ritual and back up their arguments in convincing detail.

Isolation precautions

Patient isolation precautions are designed to protect health care providers from exposure to infectious agents and to prevent cross-infection among patients. Various approaches to infection control have been implemented over the years. *Quarantine* in the home literally segregated persons with infections from society.

Category-specific isolation, introduced in hospitals in 1970, uses seven general categories of isolation or precautions based on the suspected infectious agent, the mode of transmission of the suspected pathogen and the site and extent of the infection. The use of protective attire (gloves, gowns and masks) is dependent on the likelihood of the care-giver coming in contact with items contaminated with the agent (Streed and Wenzel, 1990).

Disease-specific isolation, introduced in 1983, considers the characteristics of each agent and infection site. It recommends the use of only those precautions needed to interrupt the transmission of the given agent. This system promotes more efficient use of care-giver time and of supplies by individualizing the precautions to be implemented but it is also dependent on knowledge of each agent and identification of the causative organism with consequent delay in its implementation.

Universal precautions were developed to provide a more generalized approach and to address growing concerns regarding the transmission of viral agents, specifically HIV and hepatitis B virus (HBV), found in blood and body fluids. Universal precautions are used for all patients. They are described in more detail in relation to HIV infections later in the chapter (page 81).

Ward (1988) cautions against the rigid enforcement of blanket isolation procedures, stressing the great psychological damage that can be inflicted on the patient – she urges a more flexible, individualized approach to isolation and feels there is a tendency to over isolate patients.

Although universal and body substance precautions are recommended for use with all patients and do not require previous knowledge of the infectious potential of the patient, the nurse and other health care providers need to be aware of the risks involved in carrying out various patient care procedures. The literature strongly supports the fact that needlestick injuries are the main source of infection transmission to hospital workers. On the basis of aggregated results from six prospective studies of the risk of HIV seroconversion among hospital workers after needlestick injury involving patients known to have AIDS, Stock and colleagues found the risk to be 0.36%; the risk was found to be 0% after skin and mucous membrane exposure to blood or other body fluids (Stock et al, 1990). The impact of universal precautions on preventing the transmission of hepatitis B has not been determined. The administration

of hepatitis B vaccine to health workers at risk is probably more effective and less expensive than universal precautions (Hart 1990). With 1000 new hepatitis B cases a year in the UK, staff must avoid complacency; as Hart points out, health service staff develop an average of 35 cases of hepatitis B per year, with death a possible outcome. Further measures to prevent needlestick injuries need to be evaluated and implemented. *Used needles should not be recapped* and the design and accessibility of puncture-resistant containers for needles and other sharp objects need to be examined. The use of needles should be avoided whenever possible.

Community Prevention and Control of Infection

COMMUNITY MEASURES

Environmental control measures in the community for the control of infectious disease are directed at various links in the chain of infection. Adequate sewage disposal and the provision of a safe water supply destroy one of the major links in the chain by removing major reservoirs for micro-organisms. These are major factors to consider in underdeveloped areas in Europe and the rest of the world. Control of diseases, such as typhoid fever and many gastrointestinal infections in children, is dependent on these two factors. The control of insects is one method of decreasing the likelihood of transmission of infectious agents, as are isolation measures to control the transfer of organisms from infected individuals. Immunization programmes are directed at increasing the immunity of susceptible people. Various types of immunity are recognized.

Active immunity results in antibody production in the individual as a result of a natural infection or is artificially induced following immunization with a specific antigenic agent.

Passive immunity results from the administration of antibodies to the individual. Natural passive immunity results with the transfer of IgG antibodies across the placenta and IgA in breast milk from the mother to the infant. Artificial passive immunity is induced through the injection of presynthesized antibodies in the form of antitoxins (e.g. tetanus antitoxin), or immune serum globulin. They are given to provide rapid, short-term protection to individuals at risk of exposure, or following exposure to specific agents.

IMMUNIZATION

The administration of an immunizing agent (antigen) induces an immune response in the individual and the production of sensitized cells that can respond later when the person is exposed to the specific agent.

Immunization schedules and practices vary in different countries and in different areas. This service is generally available through local health authorities or agencies and therefore is accessible to most individuals without concern for cost.

Routine immunization is generally provided for

diphtheria toxoid, pertussis (whooping cough), tetanus, rubella (German measles), mumps, measles and poliomyelitis. Smallpox vaccine is no longer used in routine immunization programmes.

Artificially induced immunity becomes weaker over a period of months to years; it varies in relation to the different diseases. As a result, reinforcing doses of some immunizing agents are necessary. Records of immunization received and the date it was obtained should be kept by each individual for future reference.

For individuals who have been exposed to certain pathogenic organisms, prophylactic measures include: the administration of booster or recall doses of toxoid (e.g. diphtheria toxoid, tetanus toxoid) to enhance existing immunity; human immune serum globulins and antitoxins to provide passive immunity; or antibiotics to augment body defences in combating the organisms.

Many measures to control infectious disease in the community are controlled by legislation and are monitored by international, European Community (EC), national and environmental health departments or local government authorities. The World Health Organization (WHO), an agency of the United Nations, monitors outbreaks of infectious disease throughout the world and institutes appropriate preventive and control measures.

HUMAN IMMUNODEFICIENCY VIRUS (HIV) INFECTION

A consideration of the development of AIDS illustrates some of the points which have been made in this chapter.

A disease or illness is shaped not only by its biological qualities but also by the cultural milieu into which it comes. HIV infection, primarily associated as a sexually transmitted disease, carries with it connotations and metaphors of 'sin' and 'evil'. The myths and misconceptions surrounding HIV/acquired immunodeficiency syndrome (AIDS) are rampant in the general public and amongst health care professionals. Gallagher (1990) has shown that even after an education programme, nurses still held irrational fears of contracting AIDS. The ramifications of AIDS are so great that Dimond (1990) has argued that there needs to be a special UK Bill of Rights for AIDS patients to protect their position within the law.

HIV infection presents as a spectrum of disease, with the most severe form being AIDS. HIV infection is a serious health problem in which there is impaired functioning of the body's immune system. As with other chronic illnesses, the individual with HIV infection strives to maintain a sense of normality by keeping the signs and symptoms of illness under control and by avoiding allowing the disability or illness to become all-consuming. Chronic illness requires both the patient and the health care professional to redefine their goals from 'cure' to 'wellness'.

Pathophysiology

HIV is a member of a family of RNA-containing viruses

called retroviruses. Most organisms are capable of using DNA to produce complementary molecules of RNA. Retroviruses, however, through an enzyme process known as reverse transcription, are able to synthesize DNA by using RNA as the pattern (Beaufoy et al, 1988; Gauthier and Turner, 1989). HIV has particular affinity for T_4 or T helper cells, a subset of T lymphocytes, which initiate the immune response. Once HIV invades the T_4 cell, reverse transcription occurs and viral DNA is integrated in the host cell chromosomes, where it may remain for a lifetime (Figure 6.4). After integration of viral DNA the infection may become latent. When the T_4 cell is stimulated, viral replication will occur. HIV particles are assembled in the cytoplasm of the cell and escape from the cell by budding through the cell membrane, killing the T_4 cell in the process (Gauthier and Turner, 1989). HIV is also capable of invading monocytes, macrophages and certain cells of the nervous system. As increasing numbers of T_4 cells are destroyed, the body's immune system becomes weakened, making the individual prone to a variety of opportunistic infections, malignant diseases and neuro-psychiatric complications.

Transmission

Although HIV has been isolated in body fluids such as tears, urine and saliva, the concentration is extremely low and there is no documented evidence that HIV can be transmitted by these secretions. Transmission of HIV has occurred through blood, semen, vaginal fluids and occasionally breast milk.

HIV is primarily transmitted by engaging in intimate sexual contact, by exposure to infected blood, and perinatally from an infected mother to her child. HIV cannot be transmitted through casual contact such as hugging, holding hands, crying, shared toilet seats, etc.

High-risk Behaviours

HIV was once thought to be isolated to high-risk groups such as homosexuals or individuals who used intravenous drugs. However, it is certain behaviours that place individuals at risk rather than the groups to which they belong. Specific sexual practices carry varying degrees of risk (see Table 3.1). The presence of heterosexual transmission is clearly documented. In certain African countries, for instance, transmission occurs as frequently in the heterosexual as in the homosexual population, supporting the notion that it is certain behaviours that place people at risk and not membership of a specific group.

HIV can be transmitted by infected blood or blood products. Sharing needles or drug paraphernalia with someone who is infected is risky because small amounts of infected blood are transmitted in the drug equipment. The use of drugs or alcohol does not specifically put a person at risk, although the individual is less likely to be thinking clearly when under the influence of mood-altering substances. Individuals who suffer from clotting disorders, who require multiple infusions of

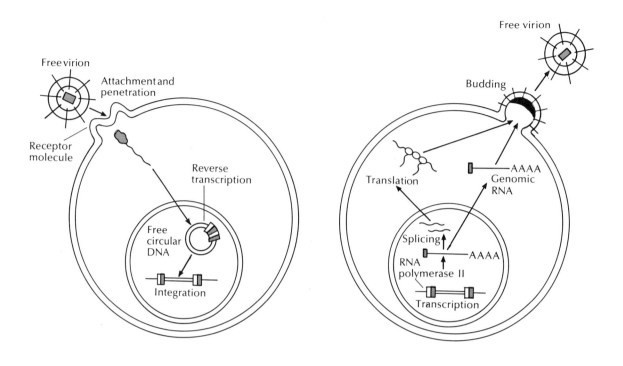

Figure 6.4 The life cycle of a retrovirus.

clotting factor concentrates manufactured from the pooled plasma of thousands of donors, were also at risk of HIV infection (Beaufoy et al, 1988). Routine HIV antibody screening (available since November 1985) and heat treatment which inactivates HIV (available since 1986) have greatly reduced this threat of transmission.

In a small number of cases health care workers have become HIV seropositive after being exposed, through percutaneous or mucous membrane contact, to the blood or body fluids of individuals who are infected. Based on health care worker surveillance data of needlestick and mucous membrane exposures, the risk of seroconversion for the health care worker is less than 1%, with percutaneous exposure carrying greater risk (McCray, 1986; McEvoy et al, 1987; Centers for Disease Control, 1988a; Losos et al, 1988; Marcus, 1988; Stock et al, 1990). Recapping of needles is the single most important action responsible for needlestick injuries. There have been recent reports of transmission from an HIV positive health care worker to some of his patients. This raises the issue of whether health care workers should inform their patients of their HIV status if it is positive.

HIV can also be transmitted from an infected mother to her child in utero or during the birthing process. Estimates of perinatal transmission rates in the literature range from 20 to 60%, with increased rates for subsequent pregnancies (Ippolito and Gibes, 1988; Stear

and Elinger, 1988). In addition to cross-placental transmission and vaginal secretion exposure at birth and breast milk may also be a source of transmission (Landesman, 1989).

Progression of HIV Infection

Persons infected with HIV may have a variety of clinical manifestations, ranging from asymptomatic infection to life-threatening cancers and opportunistic infections. The Centers for Disease Control (CDC) have attempted to summarize the spectrum of infection presented by HIV (Table 6.1).

Acute infection with HIV has been described as a mononucleosis-like syndrome, which is associated with laboratory evidence of HIV seroconversion. Symptoms of infection usually appear within 2–6 weeks after exposure and are characterized by fever, myalgia, arthralgia, headache, diarrhoea, sore throat, lymphadeno-pathy and maculopapular rash (Bryant-Armstrong, 1988; Lifson et al, 1988). After the initial manifestation of infection, which lasts approximately 2 weeks, the individual is likely to return to the premorbid state with the only evidence of infection being a seropositive result.

After acquisition of infection, persistent antibodies to HIV usually develop within 3 months, although in some

Table 6.1   CDC classification of HIV.

Group I: acute infection
Group II: asymptomatic infection
Group III: persistent generalized lymphadenopathy
Group IV: other disease

Subgroup   A: constitutional disease
Subgroup   B: neurological disease
Subgroup   C: secondary infectious diseases
    C–1: specified secondary infectious diseases listed in CDC surveillance definition for AIDS (e.g. pneumocystic pneumonia, candidiasis, cytomegalovirus, MAI, cryptococcosis, toxoplasmosis)
    C–2: other specified secondary infectious diseases (e.g. oral hairy leucoplakia, herpes zoster, tuberculosis, oral candidiasis)

Subgroup   D: secondary cancers (e.g. Kaposi's sarcoma, non-Hodgkin's lymphoma, primary lymphoma of the brain)

Subgroup   E: other conditions

From Centers for Disease Control (1986).
MAI: mycobacterium avium intercellularis.

cases it may take 6 months or longer (Ranki et al, 1987). The presence of infection is confirmed using a test called the enzyme-linked immunosorbent assay (ELISA) and the more specific western blot test. Both of these tests detect antibodies to HIV in the serum. With the ELISA no attempt is made to separate or identify antibodies to specific HIV antigens, whereas with the Western blot, antibodies that react with specific antigens can be detected (Gauthier and Turner, 1989). There are a few cases in the literature which suggest that some individuals do not produce antibodies to HIV that are detectable by current screening methods or that some individuals have transient antibody production but remain capable of transmitting the virus to others (Burger et al, 1985; Ranki et al, 1987). To guard against these concerns most blood banks around the world have instituted donor history or life-style questionnaires which exclude donors who may have factors that place them at high-risk for HIV infection.

Being tested for HIV is often an extremely sensitive time for the individual. The knowledge that the person may develop a disease with a high mortality rate places the individual under considerable stress. The stress may be compounded by the added threat of disclosure of personal behaviour which the individual may have chosen not to make public. Inadequately assessed and counselled individuals may become extremely distressed, with manifestations of acute anxiety, severe depression, drug or alcohol use, sexual hyperactivity and suicide. It is therefore crucial the person receive pretest counselling. The pretest counselling session is an opportunity to: (1) provide information about HIV infection; (2) explore with the individual the risks and benefits of being tested (Table 6.2); (3) help the person

Table 6.2   Potential benefits and risks of HIV testing.

A. POTENTIAL BENEFITS
For the individual
• Decreases anxiety in a worried, non-infected person with a low-risk life-style
• Confirms the diagnosis of AIDS in a person with other manifestations of the disease
• Provides information for making decisions regarding pregnancy or breast-feeding
• Testing of high-risk infant provides information for making decisions regarding immunization with a live virus vaccine
• Early detection of HIV infection may allow a change in life-style that may prevent other infections
• Detection of HIV infection in an asymptomatic person will allow periodic assessment of health status indicators (such as T_4 count) with possible institution of drug therapy to prevent or delay the occurrence of opportunistic infection

For others
• Reduces the risk of transmission of HIV via blood or blood products
• Reduces the risk of transmission of HIV via artificial insemination or organ transplantation
• Knowledge of HIV infection may motivate a person to modify high-risk behaviours and thus protect others
• Contributes to knowledge about the natural history of the disease, its transmission, and its prevalence in different segments of the population
• Use of test data by researchers contributes to the development of mechanisms for prevention or control of AIDS

B. POTENTIAL RISKS
For the individual
• Harmful psychological reactions to a positive test result, including depression, anxiety, suicide, desire for revenge
• Stress on relationships with family members, significant others, or friends
• Worry about the development of AIDS, leading to excess anxiety over minor symptoms that may not be related to HIV infection
• Self-imposed withdrawal from usual social contacts
• Ostracism by others who are misinformed about the modes of transmission of the virus
• Discrimination in employment, insurance, housing
• False sense of security from a negative test result, leading to a sense of invincibility and the continuation of high-risk behaviours
• Sense of survivor guilt in non-infected persons

Other risks or problems
• The probability of anti-HIV antibody testing at hospitals and clinics may prevent persons with other medical problems from seeking medical attention at these sites
• Testing must be repeated at intervals on a seronegative person whose high-risk behaviour continues
• If tests are done anonymously, there is no dependable mechanism to notify either the client or his or her partner(s) of a positive result

From Gauthier and Turner (1989).

Table 6.3 Facts about antibody tests.

The antibody to the AIDS virus is a protein the body produces in response to an infection by the AIDS virus. The AIDS virus (usually called HIV) may cause serious disease resulting in the body's inability to fight infection.

A positive test indicates that the antibody to the AIDS virus has been found in your blood. The test is not always accurate. A small percentage of persons tested may be told they have the antibody when in fact they do not. A small percentage of persons with negative test results have in fact been infected with the AIDS virus.

What a positive antibody test result means:

- Your blood sample has been tested more than once and the tests indicate that antibodies to the AIDS virus are present
- You have been infected with the AIDS virus and your body has produced antibodies
- You should assume that you are infectious and capable of passing the virus to others

What a positive test does *not* mean:

- That you have AIDS or an AIDS-related condition (ARC)
- That you will get AIDS or ARC
- That you are immune to AIDS

What a negative antibody test result means:

- No antibodies to the AIDS virus have been found at this time. There are three possible explanations for this:
  1. You have not been in contact with the virus, OR
  2. You have come in contact with the virus, but have not become infected. Repeated high-risk exposure to the virus greatly increases the likelihood of your becoming infected
  3. You have been infected with the virus but have not produced antibodies yet. It may take from weeks to months to produce antibodies. A small number of persons who become infected never produce antibodies

What a negative antibody test does *not* mean:

- That you are immune to the virus
- That you have not yet been infected with the virus (you may have been infected and have not yet produced antibodies)
- That you should stop worrying about being infected by the AIDS virus if you participate in high-risk behaviours

Modified from Gauthier and Turner (1989).

understand the meanings of the test (Table 6.3); and (4) develop a plan to maximize benefits and minimize risks. It also provides the nurse with an opportunity to assess the individual's support system and to do some preventive education in relation to safer sexual practices and drug use.

Many individuals will go on to develop clinical signs of HIV infection which may include persistent fatigue, unexplained weight loss, diarrhoea, lymphadenopathy, night sweats or fevers, and recurrent candida infections. The average length of time for symptoms to develop is 18 months, although some individuals will develop symptoms earlier and some much later (Bryant-Armstrong, 1988). Before the onset of symptoms, laboratory tests generally show a lymphocyte deficit, a decrease in T_4 cells, an abnormal $T_4:T_8$ ratio, and a deficit in platelets. The type and extent of symptoms with which the individual presents will depend on the degree of immunodeficiency as well as the causative organism. Although studies vary, it has been estimated that the average time from infection with HIV to the development of AIDS is approximately 8–11 years (Lifson et al, 1988). A diagnosis of AIDS is made when the individual presents with an opportunistic infection or neoplasm, as outlined in the CDC surveillance definition. It is not known if all individuals who are HIV infected will at some time develop full-blown AIDS. The most common opportunistic infection in individuals with AIDS is *Pneumocystis carinii* pneumonia. The most common neoplasm is Kaposi's sarcoma. Tables 6.4 and 6.5 outline the common opportunistic infections and neoplasms in people with AIDS.

HIV Infection in Women and Children

It is clear that the clinical model for HIV infection is based on homosexual male illness. HIV infection appears differently in women, with many of the symptoms being focused on gynaecological problems such as persistent and virulent yeast infections, irregular menstrual periods and hormonal imbalances. Women and their physicians have often learned to ignore these symptoms as 'women's problems', missing early opportunities for intervention and assistance. Women generally have had limited access to drug trials because of the potential effect on child bearing. In fact, some early drug trials in the USA went as far as to sterilize women before participation in trials was allowed. Therefore, little is known about the effect of experimental drugs on the female population. Women often do not have the information they require to make informed decisions about safer sex, intimacy, child care and reproductive rights. Because women have traditionally been care providers in society they may neglect their own health because the needs of family and significant others appear more important.

HIV infection is primarily transmitted to women through the sharing of infected drug equipment or through heterosexual contact with infected partners. Factors which have the potential to increase infectivity include a past history of sexually transmitted disease, trauma during sexual relations, the presence of genital ulcers, and the presence of vaginal infection (Society of Obstetricians and Gynaecologists of Canada, 1988).

Pregnancy complicates issues surrounding HIV infection for women as it affects the immune system in three important ways: (1) suppression of cell-mediated immunity; (2) increased susceptibility to some infections; and (3) a decreased T helper to T suppressor ratio, which is lowest in the third trimester and returns to

Table 6.4 Common opportunistic infections in AIDS patients.

Cause	Usual site	Symptoms	Common diagnostic tests	Therapy
Protozoa				
1. *Pneumocystis carinii*	Lungs	Dry, non-productive cough, shortness of breath, fever, night sweats	Chest X-ray, gallium scan, bronchoscopy	Dapsone Trimethoprim Pentamidine Co-trimoxazole
2. *Toxoplasma gondii*	Brain	Headache, seizures, neurological deficits, behaviour changes, may lead to dementia	CT scan (head) MRI scanning	Sulphadiazine Pyrimethamine
3. *Cryptosporidium*	GI tract	Profuse, watery diarrhoea, dehydration, debility	Stool cultures	Spiramycin Antidiarrhoeals, Antiparasitics Antiperistaltics
Fungi				
4. *Candida albicans*	Mouth (thrush) Oesophagus	Dysphagia Dysphagia (oral candida may not be present)	Visible lesions scraped and cultured Endoscopy with biopsy and culture of tissue	Nystatin, clotrimazole Ketoconazole
5. *Cryptococcus neoformans*	Brain Lungs	Headache, fever, confusion, beahviour changes Non-specific cough or fever, dyspnoea	Lumbar puncture, bone marrow aspiration Chest X-ray, sputum for culture, bronchoscopy with culture	Amphotericin B Flucytosine
Viruses				
6. Cytomegalovirus	Eyes Lungs GI tract Spinal cord	Retinitis, loss of vision Cough, dyspnoea, fever Abdominal pain, ulcer, GI bleeding Paraparesis, quadraparesis	Serology testing Bronchoscopy with biopsy and culture Endoscopy, colonoscopy Analysis of spinal fluid	DHPG Foscamet
7. Herpes simplex	Skin Spinal cord	Painful cold sore clusters at mouth and perianal area Paraparesis, quadraparesis	Histology and culture Analysis of spinal fluid	Acyclovir
Bacteria				
8. *Mycobacterium avium-intracellulare*	Disseminated, many organs affected: liver, spleen, lungs, lymph nodes, bone marrow, GI tract	Fever, profuse sweating, productive cough, lymphadenopathy, diarrhoea, weight loss	Blood cultures, bone marrow aspiration, stool for acid-fast bacilli, endoscopy, colonoscopy with culture of biopsy tissue	Isoniazid Rifampin Ethambutol Streptomycin Amikacin Biofazimine

From Beaufoy et al (1988).

normal approximately 3 months post partum (Stear and Elinger, 1988). It is not clear whether a woman who is HIV infected and pregnant will progress more rapidly to AIDS than a woman who is not pregnant. Approximately 20–60% of women who are HIV seropositive transmit the virus to their unborn child. There is no difference in rates of prematurity or low birth weight in babies delivered by women based on their HIV sero-status. Women who are addicted to intravenous drugs, however, commonly have premature and low birth weight babies.

Children who are born to mothers who are HIV infected are likely to carry passively-acquired maternal antibodies to HIV, making an accurate diagnosis of infection difficult until the child is approximately 15 months old. Maternal antibody in the infant is usually lost at between 6 to 9 months but may persist until 15 months (Stear and Elinger, 1988). Symptoms of HIV infection usually appear when the child is 6 months to 2 years of age (Cruz, 1988).

A child with HIV infection will live approximately 2 years from the time of diagnosis. Problems associated with infection are characterized by failure to thrive and developmental delays. The average age of onset of clinical signs indicating an immunodeficiency is approximately 4–6 months, with the mean age at diagnosis of AIDS being 12 months. The child is particularly prone to recurrent bacterial infections, recurrent oral thrush

Table 6.5   Secondary cancers common in AIDS patients.

Type	Site	Signs/symptoms	Diagnostic tests	Therapy
Kaposi's sar-coma	Skin	Multiple pink/purple/brown vascular lesions	Skin biopsy	Chemotherapy
	GI tract Lungs	Usually asymptomatic Symptoms often same as pneumocystic pneumonia, unless pleural thickening or effusion present	Endoscopy visualization of lesion Chest X-ray, bronchoscopy (no biopsy usually necessary)	Radiation
Lymphomas	Brain Systemic	Neurological deficits According to site	CT scan Selective brain biopsy according to site	Radiation Chemotherapy, radiation

From Beaufoy et al (1988).

and chronic diarrhoea (Table 6.6). Chronic parotid swelling and pulmonary lymphoid interstitial pneumonitis, thought to be linked to the Epstein–Barr virus, are found frequently in paediatric AIDS (Cruz, 1988). The major cause of morbidity in these children is lung disease. Children do not acquire as many opportunistic infections as do adults, with the exception of *Pneumocystis carinii* pneumonia. Opportunistic infections presenting in the first year of life are associated with a higher mortality. Kaposi's sarcoma is seldom found in children. Children also present with neurological abnormalities such as acquired microcephaly, brisk tendon reflexes, and abnormal electrophysiological findings. Developmental delays in motor, language and cognitive skills are also common. Some studies suggest the presence of HIV-induced embryopathy, while other studies conclude that there is not a consistently documented syndrome associated with HIV. Children with HIV infection should never be given live-virus vaccines, such as measles, mumps and rubella, as they may cause active infection.

Table 6.6   Major symptoms of AIDS in infancy.

Failure to thrive
Developmental delays and regressions
Persistent or recurrent fevers, bacterial or yeast infections, or diarrhoea
Chronic interstitial lymphoid pneumonitis
Chronic lymphadenopathy
Hepatosplenomegaly

Modified from Wittenberg and Lazenby (1989).

Intravenous Drug Use

The incidence of HIV infection amongst people who use intravenous drugs is on the rise. Infection in this population is complicated by poverty and social factors.

Traditionally, individuals from some subcultures are distrustful of medical and government establishments, making the building of a therapeutic relationship, and thus intervention, extremely difficult. Intravenous drug users are also not as likely to belong to formal organizations, diminishing the power of influence available through collective action. Behavioural change is made difficult by barriers such as low mean education levels, alienation from sources of accurate information and the presence of a folklore belief system that minimizes the disruption of intravenous drug use activities and values (e.g. risk taking is highly prized) (Friedman et al, 1987).

Intervention to stop transmission of HIV through sharing of needles ideally involves reaching individuals through drug treatment centres. In reality this often cannot be accomplished. The goal becomes that of getting dirty needles out of circulation. In some centres this is being done through needle-exchange programmes, where intravenous drug users will get clean needles when they turn their dirty ones in. At the very least, nurses need to be involved in teaching people how to clean their 'works'. Drug 'works' involve not only the needles and syringes that people use but also the bowls and mixing items with which drugs are prepared. Some outreach programmes distribute household bleach and directions for cleaning. As with condoms, bleach needs to be readily available if people are to use it. Bleach can be diluted with water in a 1:10 solution and the drug equipment soaked for 30 minutes, or a quicker method can be used where the needle and syringe are rinsed twice with full strength bleach and then rinsed with water. Interventions such as boiling or soaking drug equipment for long periods of time are not likely to be successful as they require too much time and forethought.

Precautionary Measures for Health Care Workers

Since a medical history and physical examination will not reliably identify individuals infected with HIV or other blood borne pathogens, in 1987 the Centers for

Disease Control recommended the use of universal blood and body fluid precautions for all individuals. Universal precautions advocate caution in the handling of blood and certain body fluids of *all* individuals regardless of their HIV or hepatitis B status. Universal precautions are intended to supplement routine infection control practices such as hand washing. To clarify misconceptions regarding universal blood and body fluid precautions, in 1988 the CDC specified the body fluids in which universal precautions applied and those to which they did not (Table 6.7).

Table 6.7   Universal precautions.

Body fluids to which universal precautions *apply*

Blood	Synovial fluid
Body fluids containing visible blood	Pleural fluid
Semen	Peritoneal fluid
Vaginal secretions	Pericardial fluid
Tissues	Amniotic fluid
Breast milk	Cerebrospinal fluid

Body fluids to which universal precautions *do not apply*

Faeces	Vomitus
Urine	Sweat
Saliva	Tears
Sputum	
Nasal secretions	

Revised from Centers for Disease Control (1988b).

Transmission of blood-borne agents in the health care setting occurs by three types of contact: (1) parenteral, (2) percutaneous, and (3) permucosal. HIV is not easily transmitted in the health care setting. Risk of exposure can be greatly minimized by using appropriate barrier techniques. The risk of exposure for each health care worker may be influenced by the degree of skill of the worker, the type of working environment and the co-operation of the patient. Therefore, health care workers must assess their personal degree of risk when caring for an individual. The following guidelines may be useful.

1. *Hand washing.* Hand washing is the single most important means of preventing transmission of infection. Hand washing should be routinely performed immediately before and after any direct patient contact. It is essential that hands and any other contaminated skin or mucosal surface be washed promptly and thoroughly if contaminated with blood or body fluids.
2. *Gloves.* Gloves should be worn:
   - For touching blood and body fluids containing visible blood, mucous membranes or non-intact skin of all clients.
   - For handling items or surfaces soiled with blood or body fluids containing visible blood.
   - For performing venepuncture and other vascular access procedures if contamination with blood is anticipated.
   - If the health care worker has open cuts or lesions on the hands.
3. *Gowns.* Gowns are not recommended for routine care but may be used if clothing is likely to be contaminated. Gowns or plastic aprons should be worn during procedures that are likely to generate splashes of blood or other body fluids containing visible blood, such as surgical interventions or other invasive procedures.
4. *Masks.* Masks are not recommended for routine care. Masks should be worn during procedures that are likely to generate droplets of blood or body fluids containing visible blood, such as surgical interventions and invasive procedures.
5. *Protective eye wear.* Protective eye wear is not recommended for routine care. Protective eye wear should be worn for procedures that commonly result in the generation of droplets, splashing of blood or other body fluids containing visible blood or the generation of bone chips during operative procedures, endoscopies and autopsies.
6. *Resuscitation devices.* Although saliva has not been implicated in the transmission of HIV, to minimize the need for emergency mouth-to-mouth resuscitation, mouthpieces, resuscitation bags or other ventilation devices should be available for use.
7. *Needles, syringes and sharps.* Extraordinary care must be taken to prevent injuries caused by needles, scalpels and other sharp instruments during procedures; when cleaning used instruments; during disposal of used needles; and when handling sharp instruments after use. To prevent needlestick injuries, needles should *not* be recapped, purposely bent or broken by hand, removed from disposable syringes, or otherwise manipulated by hand. Disposable syringes and needles should be placed in puncture-resistant containers for disposal. When immediate disposal of used needles is not possible, safe recapping may be the safest approach.
8. *Linen.* Double bagging of linen with an inner water-soluble bag and an outer cloth bag is not necessary for any patient. Soiled linen should be routinely placed in a single standard cloth bag. If linen is saturated with blood and/or body fluids it may leak through a single bag. It should be double bagged in another cloth bag to prevent environmental contamination.
9. *Dishes.* No special precautions are routinely necessary for dishes. They can be washed in hot water using household detergent.
10. *Blood and body fluid spills.* Spills should be wiped up immediately wearing gloves and using paper towels. After the visible material has been removed, the contaminated area should be disinfected using one part household bleach to ten parts water.
11. *Patient equipment.* Standard sterilization and disinfection procedures for patient care equipment are adequate to inactivate blood-borne pathogens. Family members should refrain from sharing personal hygiene items such as razors and toothbrushes.
12. *Housekeeping.* Environmental surfaces such as walls, floors and other surfaces are not associated

with transmission of infections to patients or health care workers. Extraordinary attempts to disinfect these environments are not necessary. Routine cleaning of the patient's bedside environment, bathroom and all diagnostic areas should be done on a daily basis.

13. *Waste disposal.* All bulk blood, suctioned fluids, excretions and secretions may be flushed down the toilet. Soiled dressings should be first disposed of in a sealed plastic bag then placed in the regular garbage receptacle.

14. *Specimens.* All blood and body fluid specimens should be considered potentially infectious and handled with appropriate caution. All specimens should be put in well-constructed containers with secure lids to prevent leaking, then placed in a sealed plastic bag for transportation. 'Blood and Body Fluid Precaution' stickers should not be used routinely (St Boniface General Hospital, 1988).

In the event that a health care worker is accidentally exposed to blood or body fluids, the area should immediately be cleansed and the health care worker should report the incident to the occupational health department. An assessment of risk and possible testing of the patient should ensue. The health care worker, after receiving appropriate counselling, should be given the option of being tested for HIV antibodies. A baseline assessment of the health care worker is critical for workers' compensation benefits. The health care worker should be placed on a surveillance protocol where retesting would occur at 3, 6, and 12 months post exposure.

Antiviral Therapy

Antiviral drugs can work at several points in the life-cycle of the virus. Some may work by preventing HIV from entering a cell by changing the cell membrane, others may inhibit viral proteins such as reverse transcriptase, thus stopping the production and integration of viral DNA into an infected cell, and others may block viral DNA from forming new viruses or stop the new viruses from budding from infected cells.

Azidothymidine (AZT; zidovudine, Retrovir) is the most widely-used antiviral drug. It works by altering viral proteins. Although a fairly good drug, it does not eradicate the virus altogether. AZT can be toxic and may be associated with side-effects such as sleep disturbances, headaches, and haematological disorders such as anaemia and granulocytopenia. Dideoxyinosine (DDI) is another frequently used antiviral drug, which has similar but not such severe side-effects as AZT.

New drugs or techniques such as Compound Q or passive immunotherapy are being constantly developed and tested. Access to drug trials is a controversial issue for patients. Many of them feel the drug regulations are too stringent. In response, many drugs are available through underground drug markets. Dangers are present for patients when drugs are not properly monitored. The underground drug market is also prone to fraud.

The development of a vaccine to prevent HIV infection remains to be achieved. Retroviruses are tricky entities which are difficult to understand. Clearly the strongest weapon available against the virus is education.

SUMMARY

This chapter presents an overview of the development and control of infections. The development of infection is dependent on the nature of the interaction between the host and microbial agent. Host and microbial factors which determine the outcomes of these interactions are discussed, followed by a description of the course of infectious disease. Principles relevant to the collection of laboratory specimens are described. The collection of patient data through the health history and physical examination of persons with infection are presented, together with nursing measures common to persons with infection. Discussion also includes factors which contribute to the development of infection in populations in hospitals and the community and measures to prevent and control infections in populations.

Much progress in recent decades has resulted in a marked decrease in the incidence of many infectious diseases (e.g. measles, mumps, diphtheria, typhoid fever, small pox and poliomyelitis). Knowledge of factors influencing the interaction between host and microbial agent has led to more effective preventive and control measures. Continued progress in the control and eradication of infectious diseases requires ongoing and effective health education programmes at local, national and international levels.

In the past few years, HIV infection has become known as the most serious communicable disease of our time. Its presentation is complicated not only by the seriousness of the illness but also by the social, spiritual and ethical challenges it provides. The first response to individuals with HIV infection has traditionally been fear, not only of a virus which had deadly consequences but also of people assumed to be 'different'.

Complications of HIV infection are many and varied. Individuals with HIV infection may be asymptomatic and healthy or be very ill as the immune system becomes increasingly compromised. HIV is primarily transmitted by intimate sexual contact, by exposure to contaminated blood, and from a mother to an unborn infant. Care of the individual focuses not only on the clinical manifestations of the illness but also on the psychosocial implications of infection. If the nurse is to provide competent care, there must be a willingness to explore feelings about homosexuality and intravenous drug use. As the development of a vaccine to HIV infection is far in the future, the only reliable mode of intervention is education. To be effective education must break down barriers of fear and denial. Behaviour change will only occur if individuals feel vulnerable to the effects of the virus.

Ultimately, the AIDS epidemic has the potential to unite us as a society in a sense of community. How we respond to this situation will shape history and the views of humanity.

LEARNING ACTIVITIES

1. Who is responsible for infection control in hospitals?
2. Visit a unit in your hospital and explore the measures instituted for the prevention of nosocomial infections.
3. Consider what it would be like to take an HIV antibody test yourself. How would your life change if you were told the test was positive? Who could you tell? What would be the response of your family or significant others? What effect would this have on your goals and dreams?
4. Examine your own sense of mortality. Take some time to plan your own funeral and write your Will.

REFERENCES AND FURTHER READING

Beaufoy A, Goldstone I & Riddell R (1988). AIDS: what nurses need to know. *Canadian Nurse* **84:** 16–27.

Bryant–Armstrong TB (1988) The pathophysiology of human immunodeficiency virus infections. *Journal of Advanced Medical/Surgical Nursing* **1:** 9–20.

Burger H, Weiser B, Robinson WS et al (1985) Transient antibody to lymphadenopathy-associated virus/human T-lymphotropic virus type III and T-lymphocyte abnormalities in the wife of a man who developed the acquired immunodeficiency syndrome. *Annals of Internal Medicine* **103:** 545–547.

Burton GRW (1988) *Microbiology for the Health Sciences* 3rd edn. Philadelphia: Lippincott.

Cadwaller H (1989) Setting the seal on standards. *Nursing Times* **85(37):** 70–71.

Centers for Disease Control (1986) Classification system for human T-lymphotropic virus type III/lymphadenopathy-associated virus infections. *Morbidity and Mortality Weekly Report* **35:** 334–9.

Centers for Disease Control (1987) Recommendations for prevention of HIV transmission in health-care settings. *Morbidity and Mortality Weekly Report* **36:** 38–128.

Centers for Disease Control (1988a) Update: acquired immunodeficiency syndrome and human immunodeficiency virus infection among health care workers. *Morbidity and Mortality Weekly Report* **37:** 229–234.

Centers for Disease Control (1988b) Update: universal precautions for prevention of transmission of human immunodeficiency virus, hepatitis B virus, and other bloodborne pathogens in health-care settings. *Morbidity and Mortality Weekly Report* **37:** 377–388.

Centres for Disease Control (1989) Guidelines for prevention of transmission of human immunodeficiency virus and hepatitis B virus to health-care and public-safety workers. *Laboratory Medicine* **20:** 783–797.

Cruz LD (1988) Children with AIDS. *American Operating Room Nursing* **48:** 893–910.

Dimond B (1990) AIDS and the law. *Nursing Standard* **4(17):** 52–54.

Flaskerud JH (1987) AIDS: neuropsychiatric complications. *Journal of Psychosocial Nursing* **25:** 17–20.

Friedman SR, Des Jarlais DC, Sotheran JL et al (1987) AIDS and self-organization among intravenous drug users. *International Journal of the Addictions* **22:** 201–219.

Gallagher R (1990) AIDS: the fear of contagion. *Nursing Standard* **4(19):** 30–32.

Gauthier DK & Turner JG (1988) The antibody test for AIDS. *AAOHN Journal* **36:** 266–273.

Gauthier DK & Turner JG (1989) Anti-HIV antibody testing: procedures and precautions. *American Journal of Infection Control* **17:** 213–225.

Goodinson S (1990) Risks of IV therapy. *Professional Nurse* **5(5):** 235–238.

Gurevich I (1985) Symposium on infection in the compromised host: the competent internal immune system. *Nursing Clinics of North America* **20:** 151–161.

Gurevich I & Tafuro P (1985) Nursing measures for the prevention of infection in the compromised host. *Nursing Clinics of North America* **20:** 257–260.

Halliburton P (1986) Impaired immunocompetence. In Carrieri VK, Lindsey AM & West CM (eds) *Pathophysiological Phenomena in Nursing: Human Responses to Illness.* Philadelphia: Saunders, pp. 315–342.

Hart S (1990) Hepatitis B: guidelines for infection control. *Nursing Standard* **4(45):** 24–27.

Hopkins CC (1989) AIDS: implementation of universal blood and body fluid precautions. *Infectious Diseases Clinics of North America* **3:** 747–761.

Hotter AN (1990) Wound healing and immunocompromise. *Nursing Clinics of North America* **25:** 193–203.

Ippolito C & Gibes RM (1988) AIDS and the newborn. *Journal of Perinatal and Neonatal Nursing* **1:** 78–86.

Jones PL & Millman A (1990) Wound healing and the aged patient. *Nursing Clinics of North America* **25:** 263–277.

Landesman SH (1989) Human immunodeficiency virus infection in women: an overview. *Seminars in Perinatology* **13:** 2–6.

Lewis H & Lewis M (1987) What you and your clients need to know about safer sex. *RN* **Sept.:** 53–58.

Lifson AR (1988) Do alternate modes of transmission of human immunodeficiency virus exist? A review. *Journal of the American Medical Association* **259:** 1353–1356.

Lifson AR, Rutherford GW & Jaffe HW (1988) The natural history of human immunodeficiency virus infection. *Journal of Infectious Diseases* **158:** 1360–1367.

Lindsey AM & West CM (eds) *Pathophysiological Phenomena in Nursing: Human Responses to Illness.* Philadelphia: Saunders, pp. 315–342.

Losos J, Well G, Elmslie K et al (1988) Acquired immune deficiency syndrome in Canada: the first 5 years of surveillance. *Canadian Medical Association journal* **139:** 383–388.

McCray E (1986) Occupational risk of the acquired immunodeficiency syndrome among health care workers. *New England Journal of Medicine* **319:** 1127–1132.

McEvoy M, Porter K & Mortimer P et al (1987) Prospective study of clinical, laboratory, and ancillary staff with accidental exposure to blood or body fluids from patients infected with HIV. *British Medical Journal* **294:** 1595–1597.

McFarlane A (1990) Why do we forget handwashing? *Professional Nurse* **5(5):** 235–238.

McKane L & Kandel J (1985) *Microbiology: Essentials and Applications*, New York: McGraw Hill.

Marcus R (1988) Surveillance of health care workers exposed to blood from patients infected with the human immunodeficiency virus. *New England Journal of Medicine* **319:** 1118–1123.

Miller JF (1983) Coping with chronic illness. In Miller JF (ed.) *Coping with Chronic Illness: Overcoming Powerlessness*, pp. 15–36. Philadelphia: Davis.

National Academy of Sciences (1986) *Mobilizing Against AIDS: The Unfinished Story of a Virus*. Boston: National Academy of Sciences.

Nily G (1988) AIDS: opportunistic diseases and their physical assessment. *Journal of Advanced Medical/Surgical Nursing* **1:** 27–36.

Phillips C (1989) Hand hygiene. *Nursing Times* **85(37):** 76–79.

Ranki A, Valle SL, Krohn M et al (1987) Long latency precedes overt seroconversion in sexually transmitted human immunodeficiency virus infection. *Lancet* **ii:** 589–93.

St Boniface General Hospital (1988) *Guidelines for Universal Blood and Body Fluid Precautions*, pp. 1–7. Winnipeg: St Boniface General Hospital.

Salmond SW (1987) Health care needs of the chronically ill. *Orthopedic Nursing* **6:** 39–45.

Society of Obstetricians and Gynaecologists of Canada (1988) Impact of AIDS in obstetrics and gynaecology. *SOGC Bulletin* **10:** 19–21.

Stear LA & Elinger SS (1988) Understanding acquired immunodeficiency syndrome: implications for pregnancy. *Journal of Perinatal and Neonatal Nursing* **1:** pp. 33–46.

Streed SA & Wenzel RP (1990) Isolation. In Mandell G et al (eds) *Principles of Infectious Disease* 3rd edn, pp. 2180–2182.

Stock SR, Gafni A & Bloch RJ (1990) Universal precautions to prevent HIV transmission to health care workers: an economic analysis. *Canadian Medical Association Journal* **142:** 937–946.

US Department of Health and Human Services (1988) *Understanding the Immune System*, NIH 88529. Washington DC: National Institutes of Health.

Village Clinic Inc. (1988) *Love Life. Enjoy Safer Sex.* Winnipeg: Village Clinic Inc.

Walsh M & Ford P (1989) *Nursing Rituals: Research and Rational Action.* Oxford: Heinemann.

Ward (1988) The role of the infection control nurse. *Nursing* **3:** 5–8.

Williams AB, D'Aquila RT & Williams AE (1987) HIV infection in intravenous drug abusers. *IMAGE: Journal of Nursing Scholarship* **19:** 179–183.

Wittenberg J & Lazenby A (1989) AIDS in infancy: diagnostic, therapeutic and ethical problems. *Canadian Journal of Psychiatry* **34:** 576–580.

Fluid Balance and Homeostasis

OBJECTIVES

On completion of this chapter, the reader will be able to:

- Describe the mechanisms for fluid volume regulation
- Describe the mechanisms for maintaining electrolyte and acid–base balance
- Identify the risk factors for and clinical characteristics of disturbances in fluid, electrolyte and acid–base balance
- Understand the importance of preventing fluid, electrolyte and acid–base imbalance
- Plan, implement and evaluate interventions to restore fluid, electrolyte and acid–base balance

FLUID AND ELECTROLYTE BALANCE

Normal body functioning demands a relatively constant volume of water and definite concentrations of certain chemical substances known as electrolytes. The distribution of certain proportions of total body water and certain electrolytes in the various fluid compartments is also important.

The body fluid and electrolytes are balanced when water and the various electrolytes are present in normal amounts in the major fluid compartments of the body. The relative constancy or balance is maintained by a number of regulatory processes that involve the cardiovascular and urinary systems.

Body Water

Water is essential for all body processes; it transports substances to and from the cells, promotes necessary chemical activities, and maintains a physicochemical constancy that is important in normal cellular functions.

Approximately 60–65% of the total body weight of an average adult is water, and represents about 40–45 litres in a man weighing 70 kg. The proportion of body weight that is water varies with age, sex and the amount of fatty tissue. In the newborn infant, water comprises about 75% of the body weight but progressively decreases with age to adult levels. After 3–5 years of age the percentages of extracellular fluid are the same as for adults. This level is maintained until early old age, when a gradual decrease again begins. Since fatty tissue is practically free of water, the proportion of water to body weight is less in an obese individual and in females, who have more body fat than males.

DISTRIBUTION OF BODY WATER

Body water is contained within two major physiological reservoirs: the intracellular and extracellular compartments. Intracellular fluid comprises about 40% of body weight. The extracellular fluid, which is about 20% of the total body weight, is subdivided into the intravascular and interstitial fluids (Figure 7.1). The intravascular fluid is that contained within the blood vessels and refers to the plasma component of the blood. The interstitial fluid is that contained in the tissue spaces between the blood vessels and the cells and includes that found within the lymph vessels. The interstitial fluid provides an internal environment for all cells, as well as an exchange medium between the blood and the cells. These major fluid compartments are separated by semipermeable membranes.

Another compartment of fluid is the transcellular fluid. This represents a much smaller proportion of total body water and is of less clinical significance in assessing the patient's hydration status and maintaining the normal fluid balance. The transcellular fluid includes gastrointestinal secretions, cerebrospinal fluid, intraocular fluid, and pleural, peritoneal and synovial secretions.

Normally, body water is in a dynamic state; there is constant loss and replacement, and changes in location and volume. Water enters the body through the intestinal tract via the mouth and leaves the body through the skin, lungs, intestines and kidneys.

Intracellular fluid	Extracellular fluid	
	Interstitial fluid	Plasma
25 litres	15 litres	5 litres
40% Body weight	20% Body weight	

Figure 7.1 Distribution of body water in adults.

SOLUTES IN BODY WATER

Solutes are minute particles dissolved in the body fluid and may be molecules or fragments of molecules. They include inorganic and organic substances which are important for their impact on the electrochemical and osmotic activity within each fluid compartment. When the inorganic solutes dissolve in water they dissociate into separate electrically charged atoms or radicals called ions. These charged particles are called electrolytes and act as conductors of electrical current in the solution. For example: sodium chloride (NaCl) in solution forms sodium ions (Na^+) and chloride ions (Cl^-); sodium bicarbonate ($NaHCO_3$) breaks up into sodium ions (Na^+) and hydrogen carbonate ions (HCO_3^-); and calcium chloride ($CaCl_2$) yields a calcium ion (Ca^{2+}) and two chloride ions (Cl^-) for each calcium ion, because calcium is a bivalent ion. The ions that have given up an electron are positively charged and are called cations and those that have gained an electron are negatively charged and called anions.

The organic solutes are of both large and small molecular size. The smaller organic solutes (e.g. amino acids, urea) diffuse across semipermeable membranes and are less important in the distribution of water, but if present in excessive amounts they may promote the retention of water. The large molecular organic substances are the blood proteins (albumin, globulin, fibrinogen), which have a major influence on the movement of fluid between the intravascular and interstitial compartments. The size of the molecules inhibits free diffusion of the blood proteins across the capillary membrane.

ELECTROLYTE COMPOSITION OF THE FLUIDS

Although the extracellular and intracellular fluids are separated by the cellular semipermeable membrane, marked differences exist between the electrolyte concentrations in the two compartments. The difference is maintained by the cells, which actively reject certain electrolytes and retain others. For example, sodium is in much higher concentration in the extracellular fluid; the difference is maintained by cellular action, referred to as the sodium pump, which ejects sodium from the cells.

A significant difference between the intravascular and interstitial fluids is the greater quantity of large molecular protein in the intravascular fluid. The other electrolytes diffuse readily between the two compartments, but the large particles of protein are unable to pass through the capillary membrane. The electrolytic composition of body fluids is shown in Table 7.1.

MEASUREMENT OF ELECTROLYTE CONCENTRATION AND OSMOTIC ACTIVITY

Electrolyte concentration

The presence of certain electrolytes in relatively definite concentrations in each fluid compartment of the body is necessary to maintain the volume and location of body fluid; therefore it is clinically important to be able to measure these. Since cellular and interstitial fluid are

Table 7.1 Electrolytes in body fluids.

Intracellular	Extracellular
Potassium (K^-)	Sodium (Na^+)
Phosphate (HPO_4^{2-})	Chloride (Cl^-)
Magnesium (Mg^{2+})	Bicarbonate (HCO_3^-)
Protein (Pr^-)	Protein (Pr^-)*
Sodium (Na^-)*	Calcium (Ca^{2+})*
Bicarbonate (HCO_3^-)*	Potassium (K^+)*
Sulphate (SO_4^{2-})*	Phosphate (HPO_4^{2-})*
Chloride (Cl^-)*	Magnesium (Mg^{2+})*
Calcium (Ca^{2+})*	Sulphate (SO_4^{2-})*

* Occur in much smaller amounts.

not readily accessible for examination clinically, measurements are made of the plasma. The concentration of plasma electrolytes may be measured in *millimoles per litre (mmol/l)*. A *mole* refers to the molecular weight of a substance expressed in grams. Substances in biological systems frequently are fractions of moles (mol) and are expressed, for example, as *millimoles* (mmol) or *micromoles* (μmol) (1 mmol is one thousandth or 10^{-3} of a mole; 1 μmol is one millionth or 10^{-6} of a mole).

Table 7.2 lists the normal range of electrolyte concentrations in plasma.

Table 7.2 Concentration of electrolytes in serum.

Electrolyte	mmol/l
Hydrogen carbonate (HCO_3^-)	24–28
Calcium (Ca^{2+})	2.2–2.6
Chlorine (Cl^-)	100–106
Magnesium (Mg^{2+})	0.8–1.3
Phosphate (HPO_4^{2-})	0.8–1.5
Potassium (K^+)	3.5–5.5
Sodium (Na^+)	135–145

Osmotic activity

When two solutions of differing concentrations are separated by a semipermeable membrane, the solvent (fluid) passes from the least concentrated solution to the greatest, in order to equalize the solute (solid) concentration on both sides of the membrane. This process is referred to as *osmosis*. The direction and degree of osmotic activity is proportional to the number of solute particles and is not influenced by the molecular weight of the particles. As the concentrations of solute in the two solutions approach equalization, pressure develops which decreases the flow of solvent across the membrane. This pressure is referred to as *osmotic pressure*. The *osmole* (osmol) is the unit of measurement of osmotic pressure. One milliosmole (mosmol) is one thousandth of an osmole. The osmotic activity of solutions is influenced by the extent to which the solutes ionize. An increase in the number of particles from ionization of the molecules of solute increases the osmotic pressure. A solute that does not ionize, such as glucose, produces less osmotic pressure. One mole of a substance that does not dissociate into ions is equal to 1 osmol. One mole of sodium chloride, which dissociates almost completely into sodium ions and chloride ions, equals 2 osmols. For example, 1 litre of a solution with 60 mmol of sodium chloride dissolved in it, contains 120 mosmol per litre of the solution.

Osmole concentration of the body fluids plays an important role in the distribution and exchange between compartments of water and dissolved substances. The osmotic activity is a result of the combined osmotic pressure of several solutes. *Osmolality* is the osmole concentration per unit of solvent. *Osmolarity* refers to the concentration of active particles per unit of solution. Since a litre of plasma contains about 90% water and 10% solids, such as proteins, lipids, urea and glucose, the osmolality of the solution is the more accurate measurement. The osmolality refers to the number of active particles in the volume of water, while the osmolarity measures the number of active particles in the total litre of plasma. The term *tonicity* refers to the effective osmolality of a solution. Isotonic solutions have an osmolality of 285 mosmol, which is the same as for body fluids. A hypotonic or hypo-osmolar solution has an osmolality of less than 285 mosmol per litre and a hypertonic or hyperosmolar solution has an effective osmolality greater than 285 mosmol.

EXCHANGES BETWEEN COMPARTMENTS

MOVEMENT OF WATER BETWEEN FLUID COMPARTMENTS

A continuous exchange of water takes place between the intravascular and interstitial fluids and between the cellular and interstitial fluids. Water diffuses readily through the semipermeable membranes which separate the compartments but the net exchange of water is dependent on two principal forces: the osmotic pressure created by the electrolytes and the blood proteins, and the hydrostatic pressure of the blood. When the osmotic pressure changes in one compartment, water moves across the semipermeable membrane from the area of lesser osmotic pressure to that of the greater until an equilibrium is established. The hydrostatic pressure created by the volume of blood flowing through the vessels is the driving force that causes filtration of fluid through the semipermeable membranes of the capillaries.

Exchange between intravascular and interstitial compartments

The total volume of fluid that moves across the capillary membranes is enormous because of the vast number of capillaries, but the net exchange between the intravascular and interstitial compartments is very small. Fluid moves out at the arterial end of the capillary and moves back in at the venous end.

Two opposing forces exist within the vascular compartment: the hydrostatic pressure of the blood, which forces fluid out through the semipermeable membrane, and the osmotic pressure of the blood proteins, which is a holding or pulling force opposing the flow of fluid across the vascular membrane. The volume and direction of movement of fluid depends on the difference between these two opposing forces. When the blood enters the arterial end of the capillaries the hydrostatic pressure is greater than the protein osmotic pressure, and fluid filters out of the vessels, taking with it diffusible solutes. The movement of fluid out of vessels is also facilitated by the negative hydrostatic pressure and the osmotic pressure in the interstitial spaces. As a result, the force which promotes the movement of fluid through the capillary membrane is the sum of the positive outward pressure from within the capillaries and the negative hydrostatic pressure and osmotic pressure in the interstitial spaces. The hydrostatic pressure within the interstitial spaces remains negative due to the continuous lymphatic drainage. The blood hydrostatic pressure is reduced as the blood flows through the capillaries and becomes less than the plasma osmotic pressure. As a result, fluid is drawn into the vascular compartment from the interstitial spaces at the venous end of the capillaries.

The effective forces operating in fluid movement through the capillary membrane are also outlined in Figure 7.2.

Exchange between extracellular and intracellular compartments

The net exchange of water between the cellular and interstitial fluids is governed by differences in the osmotic pressure in the two compartments (Figure 7.3). In the extracellular fluid, the principal osmotic forces are exerted by the sodium and chloride ions. Potassium, magnesium and phosphate are mainly responsible for the osmotic pressure within the cells. Normal electrolyte concentrations maintain equal osmotic pressures in both compartments, and water diffuses freely between the compartments without net gain or loss in either. A decrease in the volume of extracellular water causes an

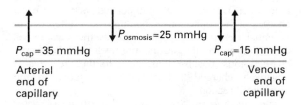

Figure 7.2 Exchange of water between intravascular and interstitial compartments. At the arterial end of the capillary the net pressure is +10 mmHg outwards, i.e. $35 - 25 = +10$. At the venous end of the capillary the net pressure is -10 mmHg inwards, i.e. $15 - 25 = -10$. Fluid therefore tends to leave the arterial end of the capillary but enter from the surrounding tissues at the venous end. Modified from Hinchliffe and Montague (1988).

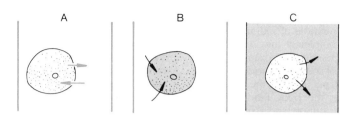

Figure 7.3 Exchange of water between intracellular and extracellular compartments. A, Osmotic pressure of extracellular fluid is equal to that within the cell. Water passes freely between the compartments without net gain or loss. B, Osmotic pressure of extracellular fluid is less than that within the cell. Water passes into the cell. C, Osmotic pressure of extracellular fluid is greater than that within the cell. Water passes out of the cell.

increase in the concentration of ions and a corresponding increase in the osmotic pressure. This results in the movement of water from the cellular compartment into the interstitial space to establish an equilibrium. Conversely, if the osmotic pressure within the cells exceeds that of the interstitial fluid, water moves into the cells.

MOVEMENT OF SOLUTES BETWEEN FLUID COMPARTMENTS

The principal mechanisms responsible for the movement of solute particles across the semipermeable membranes are diffusion, filtration, solvent drag and active transport by cell membranes.

Only small molecular solutes *diffuse* through the membranes. Although their continuous random movement results in their transfer in both directions, the net movement tends to be to the compartment having the lower solute concentration. The diffusion of solutes through the membranes occurs at a much slower rate than water. Diffusion is also influenced by the electrical charges of the solute ions. When there is a difference in potential between two compartments the ions move, attempting to equilibrate the positively and negatively charged ions; positive ions move to the area that is negatively charged and negative ions move in the opposite direction.

The *filtration* process involves the forcing of water and small molecular solutes through the semipermeable membranes. The force is created by a difference in hydrostatic pressure on the two sides of a membrane. Filtration operates across the capillary walls, promoting the movement of water and small molecular solutes in the plasma into the interstitial compartment.

The cell actively engages in the transport of sodium out to maintain a low sodium concentration in the intracellular compartment. At the same time it actively transports potassium into the cell and retains it to maintain a high potassium concentration within. Both sodium and potassium ions diffuse readily through the semipermeable membranes but are prevented from establishing equal concentrations within the intracellular and extracellular compartments by the sodium–potassium pump within the cells.

Active transport in the form of pinocytosis and phagocytosis also occurs. These processes take substances into the cell and are important in the movement of larger, non-diffusible molecules. Conversely, many substances, such as wastes and hormones, must be moved out of cells. This process may be referred to as exocytosis, or reverse pinocytosis.

Fluid Balance

A minimum daily intake equal to certain obligatory fluid losses is necessary to maintain the optimum volume and distribution of body fluid. The daily obligatory losses total approximately 1300 ml, which include the water evaporated from the skin and lungs and the minimum volume required by the kidneys to excrete solid metabolic wastes. Approximately 900 ml are lost in sweat and respiration, and 400 ml is considered the minimum quantity required by normal kidneys to eliminate the metabolic wastes (Table 7.3).

Sources of body fluid are the ingested fluid and foods and the cellular oxidation processes. The average fluid and food intake by healthy persons usually provides a volume well in excess of the obligatory losses.

A balance is maintained between the intake and output by certain mechanisms in order to preserve a constancy in fluid volume. The mechanisms involved are the sensation of thirst, neural and hormonal mechanisms and renal activity. When the intake is reduced or if there is an excessive loss, as in vomiting or diarrhoea, the urinary output is decreased and one is prompted to increase the intake by the sensation of thirst that usually develops. Conversely, if there is an increase in the intake, a corresponding increase in the urinary output occurs.

Table 7.3 An average daily water intake and output.

Intake (ml)		Output (ml)	
Fluid ingested	1300	Urine	1500
Water content of ingested food	1000	Faeces	150
Water of oxidation	250	Via lungs and skin	900
Total intake	2550	Total output	2550

When the intake volume does not equal that of the obligatory loss, body fluid is drawn upon, and the normal volume is reduced. One then develops a *negative fluid balance (dehydration)* which may seriously affect body functioning if not corrected promptly. If electrolyte concentrations and osmotic pressures are altered, abnormal fluid shifts between compartments occur. Diminished excretion with a continued intake may result in an excessive volume in the fluid compartments, producing a *positive fluid balance*. Electrolyte concentrations are changed, a harmful fluid excess develops and wastes are retained.

Thirst

This is a sensation which is interpreted as a need for fluid. The fluid may be needed to cover a loss or to reduce an elevated osmotic pressure of the extracellular fluid, which may be due to an excessive sodium or protein intake.

The thirst centre in the hypothalamus is sensitive to an increase in the osmotic pressure, a decrease in perfusion pressure of the extracellular fluid, and to angiotensin II. When osmolality rises and the intravascular volume decreases, as in haemorrhage, the cells of the hypothalamus are stimulated and the person experiences the sensation of thirst and seeks water. When osmolality falls, thirst is inhibited. Dryness of the oral and pharyngeal mucous membrane also initiates the thirst sensation.

Adjustment of kidney output

The kidneys perform the most important role in regulating the volume and chemical composition of body fluids. Certain factors from outside the kidneys influence them in the amount of fluid and electrolytes they should reabsorb or eliminate in the urine to preserve homeostasis.

A large amount of water and solutes is filtered out of the blood into the renal tubules. The production of the filtrate depends upon the hydrostatic pressure of the blood; if there is a fall in blood pressure, there is a corresponding decrease in the volume of filtrate. A prolonged period of hypotension may well provoke acute renal failure. About 80% of the filtrate is quickly reabsorbed in the proximal portion of the renal tubules. Absorption of water and salts in the distal portion of the tubules is adjusted to the amount necessary to maintain normal volume and osmotic pressure of the body fluids.

The amount of water reabsorbed by the tubules is governed by antidiuretic hormone (ADH). This hormone is secreted by the hypothalamus and is delivered to the posterior lobe of the pituitary gland (neurohypophysis) where it is stored and released as required. Within the hypothalamus are cells (osmoreceptors) that are sensitive to variations in the osmotic pressure of the extracellular fluid. An increase in the osmolality of the extracellular fluid results in impulses being delivered to the posterior pituitary lobe, which bring about the release of ADH. The increased osmotic pressure may be due to a water deficit, an increased intake of sodium chloride or an excessive amount of glucose. The hormone stimulates the wall of the collecting ducts of the renal tubules, making them permeable to water. Water is thus removed from the collecting ducts, causing an increase in the volume and a decrease in the osmolality of the extracellular fluid; this results in a decrease in the volume and an increase in the concentration of urine (Figure 7.4). Conversely, a fluid intake that lowers the osmotic pressure results in ADH being withheld and the kidneys then allow a greater loss of water.

A second hormone that indirectly influences water balance is aldosterone, which is secreted by the adrenal cortex. It stimulates the renal cortical collecting ducts and distal tubules to reabsorb sodium and excrete potassium and hydrogen. Sodium is chiefly responsible

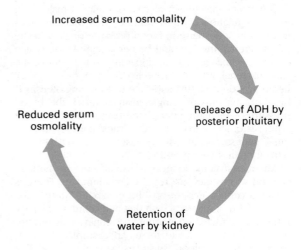

Figure 7.4 Volume regulation: ADH.

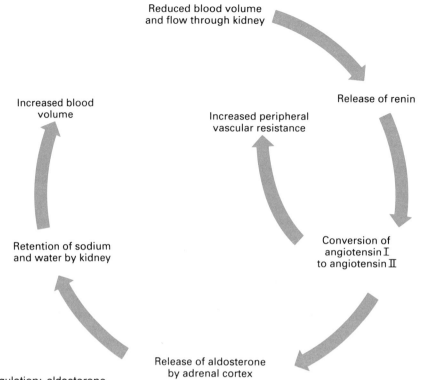

Figure 7.5 Fluid volume regulation: aldosterone.

for the osmotic pressure of the extracellular fluid; an increased absorption brings about the release of ADH and a resulting decrease in the water loss.

Aldosterone is the primary regulator of sodium reabsorption in the renal distal tubules (Figure 7.5). A less significant action of the hormone is on sodium transport in the colon and sweat glands. The secretion of aldosterone is influenced by the concentration of sodium and potassium in the extracellular fluid, angiotensin II and adrenocorticotrophic hormone (ACTH) (see p. 622).

The renin–angiotensin mechanism plays a major role in the regulation of fluid volume. This mechanism is initiated by a decrease in blood pressure or flow in the afferent renal arteriole and by nerve stimulation which causes the juxtaglomerular apparatus in the wall of the afferent renal arteriole to release renin (see p. 622). Renin acts on a plasma substrate to form angiotensin II by a plasma enzyme. Angiotensin II raises the blood pressure by increasing peripheral resistance, stimulating synthesis of aldosterone by the adrenal cortex, inducing thirst and stimulating the release of the ADH by the pituitary gland (see p. 568).

Water loss via the kidneys is also affected by the load of solid wastes they are required to eliminate. There is always a certain amount of solid metabolic waste to be excreted, but it may vary with diet and cellular activities. If there is an increased amount, the kidneys may require more water to eliminate them. An example of this is seen when the blood sugar exceeds the normal; a greater volume of water is excreted in order to eliminate the excess sugar. This accounts for the

increased urinary output and excessive thirst which are characteristic of diabetes mellitus.

The Person with Altered Fluid Balance

FLUID VOLUME DEFICIT (DEHYDRATION)

A fluid deficit is a negative fluid balance; the fluid loss exceeds the intake and there is a reduction in the normal volume of body fluid. The reduction may be due to an actual loss of fluids, failure of regulatory mechanisms or a decreased intake of fluid. A negative water balance not only implies changes in the water volume, but involves changes in electrolyte concentrations.

Extracellular fluid is depleted first and is followed by changes in the intracellular fluid volume. The osmolality of the extracellular compartment is increased (hyperosmolar state); the fluid becomes hypertonic and causes water to move out of the cells. Cellular dehydration alters cellular concentrations and eventually disrupts normal cellular activities. The movement of water from the intracellular compartment helps to maintain intravascular fluid within near normal limits, and blood pressure, pulse volume and the haematocrit may remain within normal range for a period of time. If the fluid deficit is not corrected, the intravascular fluid is eventually depleted and this is reflected in a fall in blood pressure, progressive weakening of the pulse and a rise in the haematocrit. Blood flow through the kidneys is reduced and the urinary output falls below the obligatory output. This leads to the retention of metabolic wastes and acidosis.

A deficit of water is usually accompanied by a loss of potassium ions, mainly from the cells. They are excreted by the kidneys or retained in the extracellular fluid in higher than normal concentration. The loss of potassium from the cells lowers the osmotic pressure of the intracellular fluid. As a result more cellular water is lost to the extracellular fluid.

In order to offset the fluid deficit, there is an increase in the secretion of ADH as a result of the hyperosmolality and decreased volume of the extracellular fluid. The increased reabsorption of water by the renal tubules minimizes the loss of body water.

In diabetes inspidus, with a deficit in ADH production and/or renal insensitivity to ADH, excessive amounts of dilute urine are excreted. The patient ingests large quantities of water and continues to excrete fluid in excess of intake. The hypotonic fluid loss results in a *hyperosmolar state*.

Water and solutes may be lost in equal proportions, as seen in haemorrhage, severe diarrhoea, burns and shifts of large volumes of fluid with intestinal obstructions or paralytic ileus. The loss from the extracellular volume is followed by a compensatory loss from the intracellular volume. The osmolality in both compartments is in equilibrium. This type of fluid loss may be referred to as an *isotonic fluid loss*. The decreased extracellular fluid volume stimulates the renin–angiotensin–aldosterone mechanisms resulting in retention of sodium and water by the kidneys. With continued loss of extracellular fluids the homeostatic mechanisms to replace volume will exceed the body's ability to replace solutes and a hypo-osmolar state will develop as the concentration of sodium decreases in proportion to the water replacement.

A hypo-osmolar state results when the solute loss exceeds the water excretion and the urine output is excessively hypertonic. Causes of fluid output with excessive electrolyte loss include the overuse of diuretics and loss of gastrointestinal secretions. Serum sodium and serum osmolarity are decreased. Water moves from the extracellular compartment into the area of higher osmolality in the intracellular compartment. Normal cell structure and function may be altered with serious effects. For example, intracranial pressure increases with cellular 'swelling', affecting many activities. The reduction in the extracellular fluid as it moves into the cells results in an increase in the serum haematocrit and the blood urea concentration; there is a decrease in kidney perfusion, which stimulates the release of aldosterone to bring about a retention of sodium and water in an attempt to restore normal fluid volumes and electrolyte concentrations. (The *haematocrit* represents the volume percentage of erythrocytes in whole blood. The normal range for women is 37–47%, for men 40–50%.) This compensatory mechanism will not function if the initial cause is related to renal disease or ADH insufficiency.

ASSESSMENT OF THE PERSON WITH FLUID VOLUME DEFICIT

The effects of dehydration depend on the volume of the fluid deficit, the type of fluid lost and the rate at which the loss develops. Effects are more acute when it develops rapidly, when the patient is an infant, a young child or an elderly person, and if the patient is debilitated.

Measurement of fluid volumes. In certain circumstances measurements of the extracellular fluid volume and plasma volume can be useful. These are measured with radioisotope techniques.

Table 7.4 outlines the causes of fluid deficits and common presenting conditions (clinical characteristics). A list of associated patient health problems has been

Table 7.4 Patient problem: fluid volume deficit.

Cause*	Clinical characteristics†	Associated health problems
• Excessive losses through normal routes: urinary, gastrointestinal • Excessive losses through abnormal routes: wounds, indwelling tubes • Failure of regulatory mechanisms • Increased fluid needs: fever, hyper-metabolic states • Factors affecting access to, intake of, or absorption of fluids • Medications: diuretics, laxatives • Knowledge deficit related to fluid volume	• Output greater than intake • Dry skin/mucous membranes • Increased serum sodium • Increased pulse rate • Decreased blood pressure • Decreased or excessive urine output • Concentrated urine or urinary frequency • Decreased fluid intake • Decreased skin turgor, crackles • Weight loss • Thirst/nausea/anorexia • Weakness, lethargy • Decreased level of consciousness	• Dehydration (actual or potential) • Risk of pressure sore formation due to impairment of skin integrity • Knowledge deficit related to fluid balance • Alteration in thought processes due to electrolyte/fluid imbalance • Potential for injury due to confusion • Potential alteration in individual or family coping

* Modified from Kim et al (1984).
† Modified from Carpenito (1989).

Table 7.5 The person with fluid volume deficit.

Interventions	Goals
• Prevent fluid deficit • Replenish fluid volume and electrolytes • Promote comfort and prevent further complications • Prevent mechanical injury which may occur as a result of confusion, disorientation and incoordination • Minimize the impact of undesirable physiological, psychological and environmental changes	• Patient's weight increases to normal • Fluid intake and output balance is normal • Muscle tone and strength are normal for particular patient • Skin and mucous membranes are moist and warm • Blood pressure returns to normal • Pulse is normal in rate and volume • Laboratory reports indicate that the levels of serum electrolytes, haematocrit and osmolality are within normal ranges • Specific gravity of the urine and electrolyte concentrations are within normal ranges • Coordination, concentration and thought processes return to normal

included. The characteristics of dehydration form the basis for assessment of the patient's fluid balance status. A history of fluid intake and fluid loss should be obtained, together with observations of the physical signs listed in Table 7.4. It is also important to obtain qualitative data about a patient's preferences for fluid intake if individualized care is to be practised, e.g. does the patient prefer tea or coffee, with or without sugar/milk. Alcohol intake might also be usefully assessed as significant alcohol intake may be associated with health problems.

Problems and goals (Table 7.5). If the problem of dehydration is recognized, the patient goal should be stated in both measurable and realistic terms such as 'fluid intake 2.5 litres/day' rather than vague statements such as 'increase fluid intake'.

NURSING INTERVENTION

Principles and rationale for nursing intervention to prevent dehydration

• The identification of risk factors.
• Assurance that an adequate supply of acceptable fluids is available and within reach of the patient. Patients with a potential for dehydration should be reminded to drink fluids and assistance with drinking should be provided when needed.
• Identification of factors influencing a patient's ability to meet fluid needs, and the development of a schedule with the patient and family to meet fluid needs on a daily basis, both in hospital and at home.
• The evaluation of the patient's and family's understanding of the actions and recognizable side-effects of medications and the prescribed therapeutic regimen.
• Instruction as to the purpose, action, side-effects and prescribed administration schedule of medications.
• Referring the patient to community services for continuous supervision and further teaching as needed.

Fluid and electrolyte replacement

The necessity to restore normal hydration and electrolyte concentrations is urgent in order to restore normal metabolism, circulation and renal function. The method used for the administration of replacement fluids will depend on the patient's condition. Intravenous infusion is used to re-establish a satisfactory balance quickly. When ordering the quantity and type of solution to be given the doctor considers the cause, source and volume of the losses and excesses as well as the general condition of the patient. Blood chemistry studies are done to determine possible electrolyte and acid–base imbalances. The choice of solution is an individual matter based on each patient's needs (Table 7.6). The site of the infusion should be chosen with care so that there is as little interference as possible with the patient's activities of living.

When the fluid loss is isotonic, both fluid and electrolytes are administered. Isotonic normal saline or 5% glucose solutions are usually the solutions of choice. Whole blood, plasma and plasma expanders are administered to correct vascular volume deficits.

Before the intravenous infusion is started, the nurse should explain the purpose and expectations of the procedure to the patient. It may be necessary to splint the limb that is used or provide some form of support in order to prevent dislocation of the needle and maintain the flow of solution into the vein. Displacement of the needle by withdrawal from the vein or secondary puncture results in solution running into the interstitial spaces. This causes swelling and discomfort at the site of infusion.

Once the intravenous infusion is started, the nurse is responsible for maintaining the desired rate of flow, detecting any difficulties and noting the patient's reactions. If the patient is an infant, young child, an elderly person or a patient with a cardiac or pulmonary condition, the rate of flow must be carefully controlled. Too rapid infusion may overload the circulatory system and lead to pulmonary oedema and possible cardiac failure.

Table 7.6 Guide to parenteral fluids.

Type	Description	Composition	Uses/indications	Advantages	Disadvantages	Special considerations
A. Blood and blood products						
Whole blood	500 ml unit of complete blood	Red blood cells Leucocytes Plasma Platelets Clotting factors*	To replace blood volume and maintain haemoglobin (Hb) at 120–140 g/l	Provides intravascular volume Increases the oxygen carrying capacity of the blood	Possibility of limited supply Potential associated risks of hepatitis and allergic reactions Delayed administration because of necessary typing and crossmatching Possibility of type and crossmatch errors	Whole blood should be stored at 0–10°C but warmed at least 20–30 minutes before administration (never infuse cold blood) Use *fresh* whole blood whenever possible to avoid adverse metabolic changes related to stored blood

* The concentration and state of preservation of clotting factors in whole blood depends on the duration of storage and other variables.

Type	Description	Composition	Uses/indications	Advantages	Disadvantages	Special considerations
Red blood cells (packed concentrate) Fresh	300 ml unit of whole blood minus 80% of plasma (haematocrit 70%)	Red blood cells 0.30 plasma Some leucocytes and platelets	To increase the haematocrit to a minimum level of 30% To correct red blood cell deficiency and improve the oxygen carrying capacity of the blood	Concentrate form increases the oxygen carrying capacity with less volume loading Associated with fewer risks of metabolic complications when compared to stored whole blood (decreased amount of transfused antibodies, electrolytes, etc.) Provides economic use of blood as a resource; frees other blood components, such as platelets and clotting factors, to be concentrated and stored	Slow infusion rate because of increased viscosity Decreased content of plasma proteins and coagulation factors when compared with whole blood Inadequate (alone) for volume replacement and correction of hypovolaemia Altered blood clotting with administration of more than 20 units: for every four units of red blood cells over 20, one unit of fresh frozen plasma should be administered to replenish clotting factors	Administer via Y-connector tubing with normal saline to increase infusion flow rate Washed red blood cells (resuspended in saline) can be given in shock to decrease red cell adhesiveness (washing decreases the cell's fibrinogen coating)
Human plasma (fresh, frozen, or dried)	200 ml unit of uncoagulated, unconcentrated plasma (separated from one unit of whole blood)	Plasma All plasma proteins, including albumin Clotting factors (no red cells, leucocytes or platelets)	To restore plasma volume in hypovolaemic shock without increasing the haematocrit To restore clotting factors (except platelets)	Effective for rapid volume replacement Contains clotting factors	Expensive Deficient of red blood cells	Administer fresh frozen plasma promptly after thawing to prevent deterioration of clotting factors V and VIII
Platelets	Platelet sediment from platelet-rich plasma, resuspended in 30–50 ml of plasma	Platelets Lymphocytes Some plasma	To control bleeding due to thrombocytopenia To maintain normal blood coagulability		Deficient of other coagulation factors	
Plasma protein fraction	250 ml and 500 ml units of a solution of human plasma proteins in normal saline	Albumin 44 g/l α and β Globulins 6 g/l Sodium 130–160 mmol/l Potassium 2 mmol/l Osmolality 290 mosmol/l pH 6.7–7.3	To expand plasma volume in hypovolaemic shock (while crossmatching is being completed) To increase the serum colloid osmotic pressure	Can be used interchangeably with 5% human serum albumin Osmotically equivalent to plasma Associated with low risk of hepatitis	Expensive Deficient of clotting factors Associated with larger number of side-effects such as hypotension, and hypersensitivity, than those reported with 5% albumin (due to presence of globulins) Hypotension induced by rapid intravenous administration (greater than 10 ml/min)	Plasma protein fraction as prepared from pooled plasma heated to 60°C for 10 hours. (This procedure reduces the risk of transmission of hepatitis viruses) Rapid administration of large dosages can alter blood coagulation This solution should be used cautiously in patients with congestive heart failure (due to added fluid and rapid plasma

Table 7.6—*continued*

Type	Description	Composition	Uses/indications	Advantages	Disadvantages	Special considerations
						volume expansion) and in patients with renal failure (due to added proteins)
Albumin	Aqueous fraction of pooled plasma prepared from whole blood in buffered normal saline		To increase the plasma colloid osmotic pressure To rapidly expand the plasma volume	Rare allergic reactions (less than 0.011% in all albumin solutions combined)	Potential leakage from capillaries in states associated with increased capillary permeability Possible precipitation of congestive heart failure following rapid infusion in patients with circulatory overload and compromised cardiovascular function	Albumin does not contain preservatives; therefore each opened bottle should be used at once The rate of administration of 5% albumin should not exceed 4 ml/min The rate of administration of 25% albumin should not exceed 1 ml/min 25% Albumin is reserved for use in patients with pulmonary or peripheral oedema and hypoproteinaemia. Administer with a diuretic to ensure diuresis
5%	250 and 500 ml units	Albumin 50 g/l Sodium 130–160 mmol/l Potassium 1 mmol/l Osmolality 300 mosmol/l Colloid osmotic pressure 20 mmHg pH 6.4–7.4				
25% (salt-poor)*	25 ml, 50 ml and 100 ml units	Albumin 240 g/l Globulins 10 g/l Sodium 130–160 mmol/l Osmolality 1500 mosmol/l pH 6.4–7.4				

* The term salt-poor designates the 25% albumin concentration and is a carry-over from the days when acetyltryptophan replaced a 1.8% salt solution to increase the thermal stability of the product. The term salt-poor is erroneous because both concentrations of albumin contain sodium carbonate or sodium bicarbonate to adjust the pH and sodium caprylate and sodium acetyltryptophan as stabilizers.

B. Pharmaceutical plasma expanders

Type	Description	Composition	Uses/indications	Advantages	Disadvantages	Special considerations
Dextran	Biosynthesized, water-soluble, large polysaccharide polymer of glucose		To rapidly expand plasma volume	All dextrans—associated with low incidence of anaphylactic reactions (<0.01%) less expensive than protein solutions LMWD—associated with fewer allergic reactions than HMWD LMWD—facilitates blood flow by decreasing red blood cell adhesiveness HMWD—leaks from the capillaries less readily than LMWD; can effectively increase plasma volume for up to 24 hours	LMWD—70% excreted unchanged in the urine, so the urine osmolality and specific gravity are altered LMWD—potential osmotic-nephrosis and renal tubular shut-down LMWD—possible bleeding from raw surfaces due to decreased platelet adhesiveness: side-effects include decreased haemoglobin haematocrit, fibrinogen, and clotting factors, V, VIII, and IX HMWD—50% excreted unchanged in the urine, so the urine osmolality and specific gravity are altered HMWD—higher incidence of allergic reactions when compared to LMWD HMWD—increases blood viscosity and platelet adhesiveness	Avoid the use of dextran in patients with active haemorrhage, haemorrhagic shock, coagulation disorders, and thrombocytopenia Bleeding times can be prolonged when the correct dose of dextran 70 (1.2 g/kg/ day) or dextran 40 (2 g/kg/day) are exceeded Administer dextran in dextrose solutions to patients with sodium restriction Dextran administration can interfere with typing and crossmatching of blood when the older (outdated) enzyme method is used
Low molecular weight dextran (LMWD) (dextran 40) (Rheomacrodex)	500 ml unit of solution which contains 10% dextran in either normal saline or 5% dextrose in water	Glucose polysaccharides with average molecular weight of 40 000				
High molecular weight dextran (HMWD) (Dextran 70) (Macrodex)	500 ml unit of solution which contains 6% dextran in either normal saline or 5% dextrose in water	Glucose polysaccharides with average molecular weight of 70 000				
Haemaccel	500 ml unit of a 6% solution containing a polymer of gelatin	Sodium 14.5 mmol/l Chloride 14.5 mmol/l Potassium 5.1 mmol/l	To expand plasma volume	Non-antigenic No danger of transmission or HIV or	Potential dilution of plasma proteins and decreased plasma	Use with caution if patient has pulmonary oedema or congestive

Table 7.6—*continued*

Type	Description	Composition	Uses/indications	Advantages	Disadvantages	Special considerations
	derived polypeptides	Calcium 6.25 mmol/l Gelatin-derived polypeptides crosslinked with di-isocyanate		hepatitis virus 1.5 l blood loss can be replaced with haemaccel	colloid osmotic pressure Potential dilution of clotting factors with resultant coagulation changes Potential circulatory overload in patients with severe congestive heart failure and compromised renal function	heart failure
Mannitol	Solution of mannitol in water or normal saline	Mannitol (inert form of sugar mannose)	To raise intravascular volume To reduce interstitial and intracellular oedema To promote osmotic diuresis	Reduces intracellular swelling Increases urinary output	Potential circulatory overload in patients with congestive heart failure, pulmonary congestion, and renal dysfunction	
C. Crystalloid solutions (isotonic)						
Normal saline	0.9% Sodium chloride in water	Sodium 154 mmol/l Chloride 154 mmol/l Osmolality 308 mmol/l	To raise plasma volume when red blood cell mass is adequate To replace body fluid	Considered by some to be the single most important salt for maintaining and replacing extracellular fluid Increases plasma volume without altering normal sodium concentration or serum osmolality	Potential fluid retention and circulatory overload due to sodium content	
Lactated Ringer's solution (Hartman's solution)	0.9% Sodium chloride in water with added electrolytes and buffers	Sodium 130 mmol/l Potassium 4 mmol/l Calcium 1.5 mmol/l Chloride 109 mmol/l Lactate 28 mmol/l pH 6.5	To replace body fluid To buffer acidosis	Lactate is converted to bicarbonate (in the liver) which buffers acidosis Lactate replaces bicarbonate, preventing precipitation of calcium bicarbonate and calcium carbonate Lactate is more stable than bicarbonate and more compatible with ions present in the solution	Increased lactic acidosis in shock due to lactate Fluid retention and circulatory overload due to sodium content	Lactate conversion requires aerobic metabolism; therefore, it should be used cautiously in shock and other hypoperfusion states
Ringer's solution	0.9% Sodium chloride in water with added potassium and calcium	Sodium 147 mmol/l Potassium 4 mmol/l Calcium 2.5 mmol/l Chloride 156 mmol/l	To replace body fluid To provide additional potassium and calcium	Does not contain lactate, so can be given to patients with hypoperfusion	Potential hyperchloraemic metabolic acidosis due to high chloride concentration Potential fluid retention and circulatory overload due to sodium content	
5% Dextrose	5% Dextrose in water		To raise total fluid volume	Distributed evenly in every body compartment (acts like free water) Reverses dehydration Prevents hyperosmolar state Maintains adequate renal tubular flow (facilitates water secretion)	Dilution of plasma proteins and electrolytes due to rapid metabolism of glucose and resultant free water	

Table 7.6—*continued*

Type	Description	Composition	Uses/indications	Advantages	Disadvantages	Special considerations
D. Crystalloid solutions (hypotonic) ½ Normal saline	0.45% Sodium chloride in water	Sodium 77 mmol/l Chloride 77 mmol/l	To raise total fluid volume		Potential interstitial and intracellular oedema due to rapid movement of this fluid from the vascular space Dilution of plasma proteins and electrolytes	

Phlebitis, or inflammation of the vein, is a widely recognized complication of intravenous infusion (Francombe, 1988). The presence of particulate matter and the chemistry of the intravenous solution are the most likely causes of phlebitis. Hecker (1988), in an excellent review of intravenous therapy, points out that this inflammation may lead to narrowing of the vein and reduction in flow rate some 24 hours later. Squeezing the intravenous giving set will do little to help and may lead to a tear in the vein wall at the site of cannulation, rendering the vein incompetent and causing leakage into the tissues.

The doctor who orders the intravenous infusion indicates the duration of time over which a given volume of fluid should be infused. Because the size of the drop delivered may vary with different makes of giving set, the instructions should be checked to determine the number of drops that will deliver a millilitre. The flow is monitored frequently, since the rate may change with changes in patient position, such as flexing the arm in which the infusion is sited, or if the needle is partially or totally blocked. A continual rate of infusion may be obtained by the use of an infusion pump. Leggett (1990a, 1990b) and Luken and Middleton (1990) have extensively reviewed the advantages of these devices but point out there are also disadvantages associated with their use.

The site of infusion and the vein pathway are examined for possible interstitial infusion and irritation of the vein by the solution. The patient's pulse and respirations are also assessed frequently if there is a risk of circulatory overload; dyspnoea and unfavourable changes in the pulse should be reported promptly. The usual procedure when untoward reactions are suspected is to slow the rate of flow and consult the doctor immediately (Miller, 1989).

An intravenous infusion need not interfere with the care of the patient if the intravenous cannula and distal portion of the tube are anchored securely with a sterile occlusive dressing. The patient may be turned at regular intervals or encouraged to move about if able.

Re-evaluation of the serum electrolytes and reassessment of the individual's hydrational status are necessary.

Volume and electrolyte composition of the solution are adjusted according to the results.

If the patient is permitted oral fluids, some persuasion and resourcefulness may be necessary on the part of the nurse. The patient's cooperation is sought by advising him of the importance and role of fluids in his recovery and in health. Small amounts are given at frequent intervals. Preferences for certain fluids should be ascertained and respected if possible, and the necessary assistance in taking a drink should be provided. The patient may be too sick or too weak to reach out and take the fluid himself; holding the glass and elevating his head will prove more effective than simply placing the fluid at the bedside and instructing the patient to take it.

The patient's daily fluid intake and output should be monitored and recorded. The volume, type and method of administration of the fluid intake are noted as well as the amount, type and source of fluid loss. Urine, emesis, suction drainage, wound drainage, blood loss, sweat and stools are all sources of fluid loss. Accurate measurements should be made and recorded when possible, but only where the patient's clinical condition indicates the need, otherwise this becomes a time-wasting ritual (Walsh and Ford, 1989). Estimates are made for losses by sweating and respiratory evaporation which cannot be accurately measured. The patient is weighed daily, as losses or gains help the nurse assess the deficit as well as providing a guide for fluid replacement. The individual should be weighed at the same time each day, on the same scale with an empty bladder and with the same weight of clothing.

Poor fluid intake leads to low urinary output, and stasis of urine in the bladder predispose to urinary tract infection. Support for this view comes from Pitt (1989) who demonstrated that fluid intake levels in a group of patients in the community with urinary tract infections were low when compared with a similar group of people not being treated for urinary tract infections.

Promotion of comfort. To promote patient comfort the nurse should be aware of the following and give care as necessary:

• Mouth care. The mouth requires frequent cleansing

and rinsing. Oil, petroleum jelly or cold cream may be applied to the lips to relieve dryness and prevent cracking.

- Skin care. Frequent bathing or sponging with tepid water may help to reduce pyrexia as well as provide comfort for the patient. The amount of bedding should be adjusted to the patient's temperature as far as possible.

  Observation of the skin for dryness and decrease in turgor provides information about the patient's hydrational status. Changes in turgor are best assessed over a bony prominence such as the forehead or back of the hand. Skin turgor may be difficult to assess in the elderly because of the loss of skin elasticity with age.
- Headache. A quiet environment with subdued lighting may relieve the patient's headache to some extent. Analgesia should be given according to the patient's prescription.
- Rest. The patient is encouraged to rest as much as possible in order to lessen the demand on cellular activities. Nursing care is planned so that the patient will be disturbed as little as possible.

Prevention of injury. Close observation is necessary to protect the patient if there are indications of confusion and disorientation. The patient's call-bell and any personal requirements should be left where they can be readily reached by the patient.

Dehydration and electrolyte imbalance are one cause of patient confusion. Repeated explanations of the treatments and situation are necessary to reassure the patient and increase confidence and orientation. Family members should also be reassured as to the cause of the patient's behaviour change, what is being done to correct it and that it is usually a temporary state. Relatives are encouraged to remain with the patient as much as possible. The presence of familiar objects and family beside the patient's bed may be helpful in promoting orientation and decreasing confusion.

FLUID VOLUME EXCESS

An increased volume of body fluid can result from excessive water intake, retention of fluid with normal or isotonic proportions of water and electrolytes, or from an excessive ingestion of sodium or other solutes such as protein and glucose.

Water intoxication

Excessive water intake results in a hypo-osmolar state with an increase in the volume of body fluid and a decrease in the concentration of solutes. When extreme, this state is referred to as water intoxication. The osmotic pressure of the extracellular fluid is less than that of the intracellular fluid. As a result, water leaves the interstitial spaces and enters the cells, disturbing their normal concentrations and activities. The amount of water cells will hold is limited, so an excess may also remain in the interstitial spaces.

The cause of water intoxication is a decreased urinary output with a continuing intake of water, or an excessive intake of water without salt. This may occur, for example, in renal failure.

Adaptive physiological mechanisms to restore fluid balance include the inhibition of ADH secretion, which promotes water excretion by the kidneys. The decrease in serum sodium concentration in the extracellular fluid stimulates aldosterone release and conservation of sodium by the kidneys. When the cause is related to renal disease or excessive ADH secretion, these mechanisms may fail to respond.

Isotonic fluid excess

Where the net gain in fluid is accompanied by electrolyte gains in isotonic proportions, expansion of volume in both the extracellular and intracellular compartments occurs. Causative factors include: congestive heart failure, acute renal failure, cirrhosis of the liver, nephrotic syndrome, hyperaldosteronism, steroid therapy and excessive intravenous infusions of isotonic solutions.

Regulatory responses include (1) the suppression of ADH release in response to the increased extracellular volume, which results in increased water excretion by the kidneys, and (2) increased renal perfusion as a result of the increased blood volume and thus inhibition of the renin–angiotensin–aldosterone mechanisms. In the presence of renal failure, these mechanisms fail to function. Congestive heart failure and cirrhosis of the liver also interfere with the adaptive mechanisms; in the former condition, the decreased cardiac output will result in decreased renal perfusion.

Hyperosmolar volume excess

Hyperosmolar volume excess results in an extracellular volume excess and an intracellular fluid deficit. Sodium or other solutes such as protein and glucose are present in greater proportion than normal. The increased hyperosmolality of the extracellular fluid draws water out of the cells. The causes include excessive sodium or protein intake without sufficient water (frequently seen in patients receiving nasogastric feeds) and hyperglycaemic states. The physiological response is increased renal excretion of sodium and water.

Development of oedema

Oedema may be defined as an accumulation of interstitial fluid volume in excess of the normal. It may be local or generalized and may be associated with either an increase or a decrease in intravascular volume. Table 7.7 lists the physiological factors and associated disturbances which may lead to increased interstitial fluid volume.

When the intravascular volume expands, the net outward force is increased. More fluid moves from the intravascular compartment, resulting in excess interstitial fluid. The decreased plasma volume results in reduced renal perfusion and stimulates the release of

Table 7.7   Factors influencing oedema formation.

Physiological factors	Associated disturbances
Increased hydrostatic pressure in the capillary network increasing shift of fluid out of capillaries	Venous obstruction Lymphatic obstruction Congestive heart failure Constrictive pericarditis Sodium intake in excess of renal capacity for excretion Cirrhosis of liver
Reduced osmotic pressure failing to pull fluid into the capillaries	Nephrosis Decreased albumin synthesis Increased albumin loss with burns Nutritional protein deficiency Interstitial fluid loss
Increased capillary permeability permitting excess movement of fluid out of capillaries	Local trauma Inflammation Severe hypersensitivity reactions Burns

Table 7.8   Fluid volume excess.

Cause	Clinical characteristics	Associated health problems
• Excess fluid intake • Excess sodium intake • Failure of regulatory mechanisms	• Weight gain • Oedema • Increased heart rate • Increased blood pressure • Venous distention • Decreased haemoglobin, haematocrit • Increased respiratory rate • Dyspnoea, orthopnoea • Abnormal breath sounds—crackles • Frothy sputum • Alteration in urinary output • Alteration in electrolyte concentration • Anorexia • Muscular twitching • Confusion, fatigue • Restlessness, anxiety	• Difficulty in breathing due to pulmonary oedema • Fluid volume excess, actual or potential • Risk of impairment in skin integrity due to oedema • Knowledge deficit • Alteration in thought processes • Potential for injury due to confusion • Potential alteration in individual or family coping

The patient goals in situations of fluid volume excess involve re-establishing a fluid balance and avoiding the associated health problems listed above. With regard to the former, a goal might be set that the patient will void 2 l of urine in the next 12 hours for example in acute cases, or that the patient will lose 2 kg in weight over 24 hours.

renin, angiotensin and aldosterone by the kidneys. This leads to the reabsorption of sodium and water by the kidneys. The resulting increase in the volume of body water and sodium concentration exacerbates oedema.

Normally, intravascular osmotic pressure promotes the movement of fluid into the vascular compartment at the venous ends of the capillaries. When this osmotic pressure is reduced, the normal amount of fluid does not pass from the interstitial spaces back into the vascular compartment. This reduces plasma volume and renal perfusion; the regulatory mechanisms lead to the retention of sodium and water in an effort to compensate.

Increased capillary permeability leads to local oedema. Local trauma and inflammation result in a shift of fluid into the interstitial space and a loss of vascular volume.

Oedema may be associated with any one of the three physiological circumstances already described or from any combination of these circumstances. In generalized oedema, the interstitial fluid volume and the amount of total body sodium are increased.

The interstitial fluid volume does not increase as long as the interstitial fluid pressure remains negative (normal, -5.3 mmHg). When interstitial fluid pressure exceeds 0 mmHg the interstitial fluid volume increases precipitously.

Increased lymph flow assists in preventing oedema during the initial phase when the interstitial fluid pressure is still within the negative range. The increased flow also 'washes out' most of the proteins from the interstitial spaces and decreases the interstitial osmotic pressure by about 5 mmHg. The removal of fluid and the decrease in osmotic pressure function to retain the interstitial free fluid pressure within the negative range. Once positive pressure is reached, the interstitial fluid volume expands rapidly, the tissue spaces stretch and oedema results.

ASSESSMENT OF THE PERSON WITH FLUID VOLUME EXCESS

The effects of fluid volume excess depend on the volume of the fluid retained and the rate at which the excess develops. Effects are more acute when it develops rapidly, when the patient is an infant, a young child or an elderly individual, and if the person is debilitated. Table 7.8 outlines the causative factors of fluid volume excess and common presenting conditions (clinical characteristics). A list of associated patient health problems has been included.

Table 7.9 lists the patient goals for nursing intervention for the person with fluid volume excess.

NURSING INTERVENTION

Principles and rationale for nursing intervention to prevent fluid volume overload

The prevention of fluid volume overload involves the following:

- Close monitoring of intravenous infusions and the use of automatic drip counting and regulating devices.
- Identification of the patient's and family's understanding of dietary restrictions and medication routine.
- Instruction as to the prescribed diet and medications.
- Patient teaching about the signs and symptoms of excessive fluid accumulation.
- Assisting the patient to utilize health care resources for the diagnosis, treatment and continuous management of associated diseases.

Decreasing fluid overload

The following are important in decreasing fluid overload and achieving fluid balance.

- An accurate record is made of the fluid intake and loss. The patient should be weighed daily or every other day if possible. This should be done at the same time each day, following emptying of the bladder, with the patient wearing the same amount of clothing, and on the same weighing scale each time.
- Specific orders should be received from the doctor as to the patient's fluid and salt intake. Salt is usually restricted except in localized oedema. Fluid restrictions are governed by the patient's circulatory status and urinary output. Fluids may be restricted in renal failure to as little as 500 ml a day.
- Diuretics inhibit reabsorption of water and electrolytes within the renal tubules. Serum electrolyte levels are determined, as an excessive loss may be incurred with the diuresis. The nurse should be familiar with the method of administration and peak action time of the diuretic to ensure that patient activities are planned to promote maximum rest and privacy. Diuretics administered prior to social activities may be disturbing or embarrassing to the patient. Evening administration should occur sufficiently in advance of the patient's bedtime so as not to interfere with sleep.

  If a diuretic is ordered, an accurate record should be made of the volume of urine excreted. If ambulant, the patient should be close to a toilet. Frequent use of a urinal or commode will be

Table 7.9 Patient problem: the person with fluid volume excess.

Interventions	Goals
- Prevent volume overload - Decrease fluid overload and achieve fluid balance - Maintain skin integrity - Maintain normal pulmonary function - Minimize stress caused by physiological, psychological and environmental changes	- Patient's weight decreases - Fluid intake and output are balanced and are within normal ranges - Skin is warm, dry and intact - Blood pressure is normal for the particular patient - Pulse is normal in rate and volume - Respiratory rate and sounds are normal and lungs are clear of fluid - Specific gravity of the urine and electrolyte concentrations are within the normal range - Coordination, concentration and thought processes return to normal

necessary for the bed patient, who should not be kept waiting for a urinal or commode or receive an impression that demands are excessive. The frequent voiding can be exhausting for the patient; necessary assistance in getting on and off the commode and allowing the patient to rest undisturbed between voidings help to conserve energy.

Maintenance of skin integrity

The skin requires special attention, since oedematous tissue is poorly nourished and susceptible to breakdown. The patient's position should be changed frequently and vulnerable pressure areas examined. A ripple mattress or a sheepskin may be used to protect the skin by decreasing pressure and friction respectively. The patient should be handled gently to prevent mechanical injury. Excesses of heat and cold should be avoided as sensitivity to temperature changes may be decreased.

Maintaining pulmonary function

The patient's respiratory status may be severely impaired due to pulmonary oedema, therefore it should be monitored frequently. Wheezing, dyspnoea and the use of accessory muscles in respiration are noted.

In the case of pulmonary oedema, the patient is usually placed in the semirecumbent position. This helps to decrease the venous return to the heart and lungs and may reduce the pulmonary oedema.

Patient and family coping

Changes in intracellular fluid volume lead to anxiety, apprehension, irritability and confusion. Repeated explanations should be given to the patient and family about the reasons for the behavioural changes and what is being done to correct the situation. Family members are encouraged to stay with the patient. Safety precautions such as the use of cot-sides may be necessary. The patient is observed frequently and is reminded each time of the nurse's presence and availability.

Specific Electrolytes and Imbalances

SODIUM (Na$^+$)

Sodium is the major cation found in the extracellular fluids. Its concentration is maintained relatively constant within a narrow range (135–145 mmol/l), although the amount ingested varies greatly from day to day, and between individuals.

FUNCTIONS

Sodium plays an important role in fluid balance by maintaining the normal osmolality of the extracellular fluids. The osmotic pressure created by sodium is the principal factor in the movement and volume of body water. A normal concentration of sodium in the interstitial and intravascular fluids prevents excessive fluid retention or fluid loss.

Sodium contributes to normal muscular irritability or excitability. It is essential in the transmission of electrochemical impulses along nerve and muscle cell membranes.

Cell permeability is affected by the sodium concentration; it is considered essential in the movement of some substances across the cell membrane.

Sodium ions are also important in conjunction with chloride ions and hydrogen carbonate in acid–base regulation.

REQUIREMENT, SOURCES, METABOLISM

The average diet contains sodium well in excess of the suggested body requirement of 2 g (5 g of sodium chloride). Sodium occurs naturally in unprocessed foods, and much is added in the form of sodium chloride in the preparation and preservation of foods.

Of the sodium removed from the body, 95% is excreted in the urine, with the remainder leaving the body in sweat and faeces. The adrenocortical secretions, especially aldosterone, influence the metabolism of sodium. The steroid secretions promote reabsorption of sodium by the renal tubules. A deficiency of the cortical secretions (Addison's disease) causes an increase in sodium excretion in the urine and a lower serum sodium level.

Since sodium plays a major role in the regulation of the extracellular fluid volume, changes in the concentration of sodium result in changes in fluid volume.

THE PERSON WITH SODIUM IMBALANCE

HYPONATRAEMIA (SODIUM DEPLETION)

Since normal kidneys are very efficient in conserving sodium when the intake is reduced, an adequate concentration for normal body functioning is usually maintained. Depletion of sodium ions in the extracellular fluid most often results from an excessive loss rather than a deficient intake. A low serum sodium level may also occur because of fluid retention; excessive fluid volume causes dilution of the sodium. This is referred to as dilutional hyponatraemia.

Normally, a lowered concentration of extracellular sodium initiates a decrease in the release of ADH and an ensuing increase in the volume of water excreted in the urine. This response is made in an effort to restore normal osmolality of the extracellular compartments, but it sacrifices fluid volume. Some extracellular fluid also moves into the cells; the cells become swollen, normal cellular electrolyte concentrations are altered and cell activities may be impaired. If the sodium deficit is severe, depletion of the extracellular fluid results in the development of dehydration and its manifestations.

The movement of water into cells and the excessive loss of water are considered responsible for the symptoms of sodium deficit outlined in Table 7.10. If the sodium deficiency persists, complicated by a marked reduction in total extracellular fluid, the individual lapses into unconsciousness and manifests circulatory failure and shock. Table 7.10 lists the clinical characteristics and associated health problems experienced by the person with hyponatraemia.

Table 7.10   The person with sodium imbalance.

Sodium imbalance	Cause	Clinical characteristics	Associated health problems

Sodium deficiency (hyponatraemia)	• Sodium restricted diet
	• Sodium loss by:
	  —diaphoresis in fever or high environmental temperature
	  —loss of gastrointestinal fluids with vomiting, suction, diarrhoea or fistula
	  —a deficiency of adreno-cortical secretions
	  —renal disease
	  —intracellular shift with potassium deficiency
	• Water gain through:
	  —ingestion of large volumes of water
	  —increase in ADH
	  —no excretion without corresponding fluid loss
	  —intravenous infusion of non-electrolyte solution
		• Serum sodium < 135 mmol/l
		• Apprehension
		• Lethargy
		• Headache
		• Muscular and abdominal cramps and weakness
		• Nausea and vomiting
		• Diarrhoea
		• Decreased urinary output followed by oliguria
		• Twitching, convulsions
		• Loss of consciousness
		• Hypotension
			• Knowledge deficit related to dietary and fluid regimens
			• Alteration in nutrition: less than body requirements related to inadequate sodium intake
			• Alteration in thought processes
			• Alteration in bowel elimination: diarrhoea
			• Fluid volume deficit associated with fluid and sodium losses

Sodium excess (hypernatraemia)	• Excessive sodium intake • Inadequate water intake • Loss of water and sodium • ADH deficiency • Adrenal hyperactivity • Corticosteroid therapy • Renal disease • Intravenous administration of excessive sodium bicarbonate	• Serum sodium > 145 mmol/l • Mucous membranes dry and sticky • Tongue dry and rough • Thirst • Decreased reflexes • Restlessness • Hypertension • Lethargy • Confusion • Loss of consciousness	• Knowledge deficit related to dietary restrictions of sodium and of fluid requirements • Alteration in nutrition more than body requirements related to excessive sodium intake • Fluid volume deficit associated with inadequate fluid intake • Alteration in thought processes • Alteration in patterns of urinary elimination related to renal failure, ADH deficiency, corticosteroid treatment

Nursing intervention and treatment

Nursing interventions related to the patient health problems identified for each electrolyte imbalance are discussed in detail in subsequent chapters.

Nursing intervention and treatment of hyponatraemia consists of the administration of a salt-containing solution or, if necessary, an intravenous infusion of an isotonic sodium chloride solution (0.9%). The volume and additional electrolytes that may be needed are determined by the presenting symptoms, pulse rate and volume, blood pressure, urinary output, and laboratory reports of serum electrolytes. While receiving the intravenous infusion of sodium chloride, the patient should be observed closely for the disappearance of the symptoms manifested and the appearance of other changes. The rate of administration of the infusion is usually reduced after the first litre has been given. A rapid increase in extracellular sodium and osmolality may induce the movement of an excessive amount of water from within the cells to the interstitial compartment. If the low serum sodium level is due to dilution, the intake of water is restricted and diuresis may be initiated by the administration of a diuretic, such as frusemide (Lasix).

The individual at risk of developing hyponatraemia is taught to replace body fluid losses with electrolytes as well as water. Saline solutions or sodium chloride tablets may be taken when fluid loss is excessive.

HYPERNATRAEMIA (EXCESS SODIUM)

An excess of sodium in extracellular fluid and consequent hyperosmolality may develop as a result of an excessive ingestion of sodium chloride, an inadequate water intake, water loss without a corresponding excretion of sodium or decreased renal excretion of sodium.

Normally, the responses to an increase in the osmolality of the extracellular fluids above normal include an increased release of ADH, thirst, decrease in sweating and movement of water out of the cells.

The clinical characteristics and associated health problems of an elevated serum sodium are listed in Table 7.10.

Nursing intervention and treatment

The disorder is treated by giving water orally and/or by the administration of dextrose 5% in water by intravenous infusion. The underlying cause must also be investigated and treated. A low sodium diet is prescribed; depending on the cause of the hypernatraemia, the restriction may vary from 'No added salt' (2–3 g) to the more severe restriction of being permitted only 500 mg per day.

The patient is taught to prevent hypernatraemia by following prescribed dietary restrictions of sodium and maintaining an adequate fluid intake.

POTASSIUM (K⁺)

Potassium is the major cation found in the intracellular fluids and, to maintain homeostasis, the amount in the body is kept relatively constant within a range of 3.5–5.5 mmol/l of blood serum. The amount of total body potassium is about twice that of sodium. It is present only in small amounts in the extracellular fluids but is especially abundant and active within the cells.

FUNCTIONS

Within the cells, potassium plays a significant rôle in creating the osmotic pressure that is important in preserving normal cellular fluid content. Normal volume of water, in turn, contributes to the maintenance of normal electrolyte concentrations. Potassium also influences the acid–base balance.

Potassium ions in the extracellular fluids are essential for the normal functioning of all muscle tissue, and are especially important in cardiac muscle activity. In conjunction with sodium and calcium, potassium regulates neuromuscular excitability and stimulation and is necessary for the transmission of the nerve impulses that prompt contraction of muscle fibres.

Potassium is also active in carbohydrate metabolism. It is required in the conversion of glucose to glycogen and in its subsequent storage. This element is also used in fairly large amounts in the synthesis of muscle protein.

REQUIREMENT, SOURCES, METABOLISM

Potassium is widely distributed in foods; a deficiency is unlikely if there is an adequate intake of food, since the average daily diet contains 2–4 g. Meats, whole grains, bananas, oranges, apricots, prunes, tomatoes, legumes and broccoli have a high potassium content. Potassium is readily absorbed from the small intestine. The digestive secretions contain potassium but this portion, as well as much of that found in digested foods, is normally reabsorbed.

Kidney activity is the chief regulatory mechanism for potassium; reabsorption, secretion and excretion of potassium ions by the tubular cells operate to maintain an optimum serum concentration. The kidneys can readily increase the excretion of potassium if the intake is high. The excretion of the ions is influenced by changes in the acid–base balance; the serum potassium level is higher in acidosis and lower in alkalosis. The serum level may also be influenced by the adrenocortical secretion, aldosterone. The latter promotes renal excretion of potassium ions and the conservation of sodium.

THE PERSON WITH POTASSIUM IMBALANCE

Even small variations outside the narrow normal range should receive prompt attention because of possible serious effects on cardiac activity. Slight variations in extracellular fluids are readily reflected in electrocardiographic changes.

HYPOKALAEMIA (POTASSIUM DEPLETION)

When the potassium concentration of the extracellular fluid is depleted, potassium tends to move out of the cells, creating an intracellular deficit. The cells retain more sodium and hydrogen ions in an effort to establish an ionic balance. These ionic shifts seriously affect normal cell functioning, and the normal alkalinity of the extracellular fluid is altered because of its loss of hydrogen and sodium ions.

Nursing intervention and treatment

Hypokalaemia may be prevented in patients known to be predisposed to it because of their receiving diuretic or steroid therapy by increasing foods high in potassium in their diet, and by taking a supplementary preparation. Patients receiving digitalis should be followed up closely and observed for early symptoms of potassium depletion. Even a slightly below normal serum level may precipitate digitalis toxicity, manifested by bradycardia (slow pulse), irregular pulse, anorexia, vomiting and/or diarrhoea and yellow vision. Patients are taught to include foods high in potassium, such as citrus fruits, yeast extract and bananas, in their diets. Instruction should be given on the actions of prescribed diuretics and the relationship between digitalis toxicity and a potassium deficit. The patient is taught to observe for signs and symptoms of potassium deficiency and of digitalis toxicity.

Medical treatment of hypokalaemia involves the administration of potassium orally or by intravenous infusion. If the patient's condition permits, oral administration is preferred because the low normal concentration can readily be exceeded and the problem may become one of hyperkalaemia. Potassium-rich foods are given, and potassium chloride may be prescribed in liquid or tablet form. Potassium supplements should be given with food to avoid gastric distress. Liquid preparations must be diluted prior to administration.

Considerable caution is necessary if the patient is

Table 7.11 The person with potassium imbalance.

Potassium imbalance	Cause	Clinical characteristics	Associated health problems
Potassium deficiency (hypokalaemia)	• Inadequate potassium intake • Excessive urinary loss; renal tubular diease, uncontrolled diabetes mellitus, increased adrenocortical secretion, steroid therapy • Gastrointestinal loss; diarrhoea, intestinal fistula, vomiting, nasogastric aspiration • Intracellular shift; alkalosis, intravenous administration of glucose or insulin • Side-effect of diuretics	• Serum potassium < 3.5 mmol/l • Alkalosis • Muscle weakness and decreased tone • Numbness • Decreased reflexes • Cardiac dysrhythmias • ECG changes • Cardiac/respiratory arrest • Hypotension • Muscular paralysis • Abdominal distension • Nausea and vomiting • Decreased or absent bowel sounds • Increased urine output	• Knowledge deficit related to dietary measures and actions of diuretics and digitalis • Alteration in nutrition less than body requirements related to potassium intake • Alteration in patterns of urinary elimination • Alteration in bowel elimination: constipation • Alteration in tissue perfusion • Activity intolerance • Ineffective breathing pattern
Potassium excess (hyperkalaemia)	• Decreased renal excretion: renal failure, oliguria caused by dehydration or adreno-cortical insufficiency • Extracellular shift; tissue destruction from crush injuries or burns and metabolic acidoses • Excessive intake with rapid intravenous administration	• Serum potassium > 5.5 mmol/l • Muscle weakness • Paralysis • Decreased reflexes • Lethargy • Confusion • ECG changes • Cardiac dysrhythmias • Cardiac arrest • Abdominal cramps • Diarrhoea	• Knowledge deficit related to dietary restrictions for patients with renal failure • Alteration in patterns of urinary elimination • Alteration in bowel elimination: diarrhoea • Activity intolerance • Ineffective breathing pattern

receiving potassium by intravenous infusion. It is necessary to note what the patient's urinary output has been and to keep a close record of it during and following the infusion. Potassium is not usually prescribed if the patient has oliguria or if there is any question about the adequacy of renal function, since it is the major channel by which excess is eliminated. The rate of administration of a solution with potassium is generally kept within the range of 8–10 mmol/l depending upon the severity of the deficit, and is usually given in normal saline rather than dextrose 5% since the latter may result in still further decrease in the serum level. Glucose promotes movement of potassium into the cells, thereby decreasing serum levels. Adequate dilution of potassium is essential to decrease irritation and prevent thrombophlebitis.

HYPERKALAEMIA (EXCESS SERUM POTASSIUM)

An excessive concentration of serum potassium may be the result of decreased renal excretion, increased catabolism or the administration of excessive amounts (Table 7.11). In practice, renal failure is the most common cause of high serum potassium levels. The destruction of tissue causes the release of intracellular potassium into the extracellular fluid. Metabolic acidosis

also causes hyperkalaemia as potassium shifts from the cells. The disorder rarely occurs as a result of an excessive intake if renal function is normal.

Manifestations of high serum potassium levels resemble those of low levels in many respects (Table 7.11).

Nursing intervention and treatment

It is important to recognize the possibility of hyperkalaemia developing in patients with impaired kidney function and oliguria. The serum level should be checked, the intake controlled and observations made of early indications of increased extracellular potassium. As myocardial contraction and the conduction of cardiac impulses are impaired in hyperkalaemia, the electrocardiogram (ECG) should be monitored. The ECG shows tall, peaked T waves and a prolonged P–R interval. Impaired cardiac function may progress to ventricular fibrillation (rapid, irregular, weak and ineffective contractions) and cardiac arrest.

Treatment of hyperkalaemia involves measures to restrict the intake of potassium, antagonize the effects of the high concentration of potassium, move potassium into the cells and increase the excretion of potassium.

Medication containing potassium and foods high in potassium are restricted. Intravenous therapy should not include any potassium-containing solution.

A slow intravenous injection of a calcium solution (calcium gluconate or chloride) may be given by the doctor to counteract the effects of the potassium on the heart.

Glucose and regular insulin may be given intravenously to promote the movement of potassium ions into the cells. If there is no oedema or cardiovascular overload, a solution of sodium bicarbonate may be added to the glucose or administered separately intravenously to enhance the shift of potassium into the cells, especially if the ECG reflects serious cardiac disturbance.

Potassium ions may be removed from the body by giving a cation-exchange resin such as calcium resonium. It may be prescribed to be given orally (20–50 g) or by rectum (50 g dissolved in 200 ml of water and given as a retention enema). When oliguria is present, haemodialysis or peritoneal dialysis (see pp. 638–644) may be used to reduce extracellular potassium ions.

CALCIUM (Ca^{2+})

Calcium is present in the body in a greater amount than any other mineral. It comprises about 2% of the body weight and most of it (approximately 99%) is in the bones and teeth in the form of calcium phosphate. A relatively small amount is present and essential in the body fluids. Normal total serum calcium is within the range of 2.2–2.6 mmol/l. About half of this calcium is in the form of free diffusible calcium ions (1.1–1.3 mmol/l and the remainder is bound with plasma proteins or occurs as part of other compounds. The degree of protein building decreases with acidosis and increases with alkalosis.

FUNCTIONS

In addition to being the major inorganic constituent of bone tissue, calcium has an essential role in the blood clotting process, normal muscle contraction and relaxation, and nerve impulse transmission. It influences cellular permeability and is necessary for the activation of some enzymes; for example, it activates adenosine triphosphatase in the release of energy for muscle fibre contraction.

REQUIREMENT, SOURCES, METABOLISM

The minimum daily requirement of an adult is estimated to be 600–800 mg; the latter is equivalent to about three 224-ml glasses of milk. Demands are greater during the growth period and during pregnancy and lactation. It is currently being recommended that adult women have a daily calcium intake of 1200–1500 mg. Calcium absorption is reduced with decreased oestrogen production in the menopause and renal calcium reabsorption is less efficient.

Dairy products are the richest source of calcium. Other sources, although they contribute much less, include egg yolks, fish, nuts, green leafy vegetables, legumes and whole grains.

Absorption of calcium from the intestine is largely dependent upon the presence of vitamin D. It is also influenced by the contents of the diet; a high phosphate concentration tends to reduce absorption, and free fatty acids may cause the formation of insoluble, non-absorbable calcium salts. An increased pH (increased alkalinity) of intestinal fluid reduces absorption. Serum calcium ion concentration also affects calcium absorption; even a slight decrease promotes increased absorption.

The principal regulator of calcium concentration in the body fluids is the parathyroid hormone (parathormone, PTH), which is secreted by the parathyroid glands. A decrease in serum ionized calcium stimulates the secretion of parathyroid hormone, which in the presence of vitamin D causes a withdrawal from the stores of calcium within bone tissue, decreased excretion by the kidneys and probably increased reabsorption of the mineral from the intestine (Figure 7.6). When the serum level of calcium is increased above normal, parathyroid hormone is not released, less calcium is added to the body fluids and more is excreted by the kidneys. Calcitonin, secreted by the parathyroid glands, functions to decrease blood calcium ion concentration. Its effect on plasma calcium is transient, but it produces a prolonged effect by decreasing the rate of bone remodelling and increasing the amount of calcium salts deposited in bone. Urinary excretion is the principal mechanism by which excess serum calcium is eliminated from the body. A small amount is also excreted with the intestinal digestive secretions, especially bile. Unabsorbed dietary calcium is excreted by the intestinal tract.

A reciprocal relationship exists between phosphorus and calcium levels in the extracellular fluids. An elevation in one accompanies a decrease in the other, but their functions are not comparable.

THE PERSON WITH CALCIUM IMBALANCE

HYPOCALCAEMIA (CALCIUM DEFICIT)

Calcium is the mineral most likely to be deficient in the human diet because of its relatively limited sources. Decreased intestinal absorption may result from a deficiency of vitamin D, increased alkaline or fatty acid intestinal content, or disease of the intestine. Absorption may also be reduced if the content is hurried through the small intestine and eliminated, as in diarrhoea, or if it is lost in the drainage of an intestinal fistula.

A decrease in parathyroid hormone secretion produces an abnormally low concentration of calcium. This may occur as a result of a new growth in the parathyroid glands or of trauma during a surgical procedure, such as thyroidectomy.

Calcium depletion may also develop in chronic renal disease because of impaired reabsorption of the ions from the filtrate or because abnormal amounts of phosphate are being retained, resulting in a compensatory decrease in calcium.

Table 7.12 lists the causes and clinical characteristics of calcium imbalance.

Figure 7.6 Regulation of serum calcium concentration.

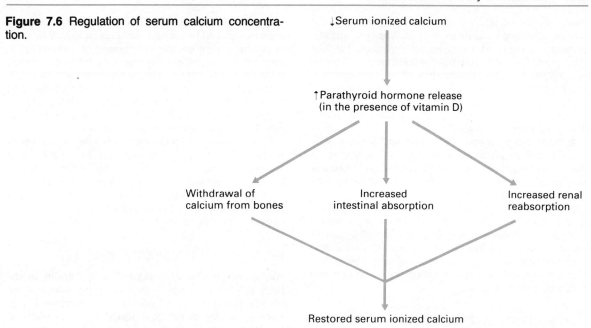

Table 7.12 The person with calcium imbalance.

Calcium imbalance	Cause	Clinical characteristics	Associated health problems
Calcium deficiency (hypocalcaemia)	● Inadequate calcium intake ● Decreased intestinal absorption ● Hypoparathyroidism ● Impaired renal function	● Serum calcium < 2.2 mmol/l ● Muscular irritability ● Tetany ● Numbness and 'pins and needles' in extremities ● Twitching of facial muscles ● Painful muscular spasms ● Convulsions ● Diplopia ● Abdominal cramps ● Urinary frequency ● Increased tendency to bleed	● Knowledge deficit related to calcium requirements and dietary sources and absorption of calcium ● Alteration in comfort: muscle spasm and cramps ● Alteration in bowel elimination: diarrhoea ● Alteration in patterns of urinary elimination ● Increased potential for injury (bleeding)
Calcium excess (hypercalcaemia)	● Excessive vitamin D intake ● Excessive intake of calcium ● Hyperparathyroidism ● Thyrotoxicosis ● Prolonged immobility ● Malignant disease ● Impaired renal function	● Serum calcium > 2.6 mmol/l ● Anorexia ● Nausea and vomiting ● Loss of muscle tone ● Weakness ● Constipation ● Increased urinary output ● Thirst ● Dehydration ● Mental dullness ● Confusion ● Coma ● Bone pain	● Alteration in comfort: bone pain ● Alteration in bowel elimination: constipation ● Alteration in patterns of urinary elimination ● Alteration in thought processes ● Activity intolerance ● Increased potential for injury (fractures)

Nursing intervention and treatment

Treatment depends on the cause of the deficiency. Acute hypocalcaemia may be rapidly corrected by the intravenous administration of a calcium solution (e.g. calcium gluconate 10% or calcium chloride 5%).

Following the initial administration of 10–30 ml a continuous infusion of a weaker solution may be given to maintain a satisfactory calcium concentration. Laboratory assessment of the serum level is made at intervals and the individual observed for positive changes or increasing severity of symptoms. Oral calcium supplements should be given if the condition permits. If the patient is allowed foods, those with high phosphorus content are omitted to promote maximum calcium absorption. Vitamin D, 100 000–200 000 units (2.5–5.0 mg) per day for 3–4 days, may be prescribed if the deficit is severe; the dosage is reduced in 2–3 days since the drug is accumulative. Calcitrol, an activated form of vitamin D, may be substituted in persons with renal or liver failure. The usual dose is 0.25 µg per day.

If the cause if hypoparathyroidism and is not readily corrected by intravenous calcium, parathyroid extract in doses of 100–200 units may be prescribed. Environmental stimuli should be minimized to decrease the likelihood and effects of seizures.

Patients should be instructed as to the recommended daily requirements for calcium. Calcium supplements may be recommended for older women. The patient should also be informed that caffeine in coffee and cigarette smoking interfere with calcium absorption. Calcium absorption is best if tablets are taken between meals or in the evening.

HYPERCALCAEMIA (EXCESS SERUM CALCIUM)

The major cause of hypercalcaemia is hyperparathyroidism. The increased PTH secretion increases calcium uptake from the bones into the blood and enhances phosphorus excretion by the kidney. Some malignant tumours secrete PTH-like substances that function in a similar manner. Excessive intake of vitamin D leads to increased intestinal absorption of calcium. Prolonged immobility may lead to increased bone remodelling and release of calcium into the blood.

Nursing intervention and treatment

Medical treatment is directed to the primary cause, and to prompt lowering of the serum calcium level because of the serious, adverse effects on neuromuscular functions. Since renal sodium excretion is accompanied by calcium excretion, an intravenous infusion of saline is given. A diuretic such as frusemide (Lasix) may also be prescribed to promote sodium excretion. Serum levels of the electrolytes sodium, potassium and calcium are determined at intervals to ascertain progress and to determine whether serum sodium and potassium are being depleted by the diuresis.

If the hypercalcaemia is secondary to sarcoidosis (a collagen disease) or new growth, a corticosteroid preparation such as prednisone may be given, which is thought to decrease intestinal absorption and renal tubular reabsorption from the glomerular filtrate. The level of serum sodium is monitored in case hypernatraemia develops.

If the increased serum calcium is the result of malignant neoplasm in bone tissue, mithramycin, a cytotoxic chemotherapeutic agent, is occasionally administered intravenously because of its side-effect of hypocalcaemia. If given, the nurse should observe the patient for other possible side-effects, which include bleeding as a result of a decrease in thrombocytes and impaired renal function.

If hypercalcaemia is associated with immobility, a regimen of full passive and active physiotherapy exercises should be carried out; a tilt table may be used to permit weight on the long bones; or ambulation is promoted to decrease calcium loss from the bones. Fluid intake should be increased to 3000–4000 ml daily if the patient's cardiovascular system will tolerate that volume. The increased fluids serve to minimize the precipitation of the calcium in the renal tubules which may lead to the formation of kidney stones.

Dietary intake of foods with high calcium content is restricted. Care of the patient involves precautions against falls and heavy lifting because of the weakened bone structure and the predisposition to fractures.

Other disorders associated with calcium metabolism include osteoporosis, osteomalacia and rickets, discussed further in Chapter 24.

PHOSPHORUS (PHOSPHATE; HPO_4^{2-})

Phosphorus is closely associated with calcium in the body and occurs mainly in the form of phosphate. About 80–85% of the total phosphorus is combined with calcium in the bones and teeth. The remainder is combined with protein, lipid and carbohydrate compounds, and with enzymes and other substances throughout all body cells. The normal serum level is 0.8–1.5 mmol/l.

FUNCTIONS

Phosphate functions as a component in the structure of bone tissue and teeth. It is essential in the metabolism of almost all cells and is especially important in the absorption process of glucose and glycerol in the intestine, and in the formation of many enzymes essential to the intracellular oxidation process and production of energy. As part of the buffer system, it is active in maintaining acid–base balance. Through its combination with fatty acids and the formation of phospholipids it prevents an excess of free fatty acids. Monohydrogen phosphate (HPO_4^{2-}) acts as a urinary buffer by taking up hydrogen ions and is then excreted as dihydrogen phosphate (HPO_4^-) in the urine.

REQUIREMENT, SOURCES, METABOLISM

The requirement is comparable to that of calcium (800 mg daily) and, since phosphorus is present in nearly all foods, a dietary deficiency is not likely to occur. Dairy products and lean meats have a high phosphate content.

The metabolism is closely associated with that of calcium, as mentioned in the previous discussion. Vitamin D facilitates the absorption of phosphorus from the intestine but it not actually essential for its transfer. The kidneys regulate the serum phosphorus level by their tubular excretion and reabsorption mechanisms. This regulation is influenced by the parathyroid hormone. With an increase above normal in the serum phosphate level, the parathyroid hormone is released to block renal tubular reabsorption of phosphorus from the glomerular filtrate, with an ensuing increase in the amount excreted in the urine. Conversely, a decrease

Table 7.13 The person with phosphorus imbalance.

Phosphorus imbalance	Cause	Clinical characteristics	Associated health problems
Phosphate deficiency (hypophosphataemia)	• Malabsorption disorders (coeliac disease, sprue) • Hyperparathyroidism • Osteomalacia • Excessive use of phosphate binding gels, e.g. aluminium hydroxide (Aludrox) • Alcoholism	• Serum phosphate < 0.8 mmol/l • Lethargy • Muscle weakness and wasting • Anorexia • Hypoxia	• Activity intolerance • Knowledge deficit related to adverse effects of phosphate binders • Alteration in nutrition: less than body requirements
Phosphate excess (hyperphosphataemia)	• Renal failure • Hypoparathyroidism • Hypomagnesaemia	• Serum phosphate > 1.5 mmol/l • Metastatic calcifications • Signs of hypocalcaemia (cramps, tetany, convulsions), usually asymptomatic	• Alteration in nutrition: more than body requirements

below the normal serum level results in increased reabsorption in the renal tubules.

THE PERSON WITH PHOSPHORUS IMBALANCE

HYPOPHOSPHATAEMIA (PHOSPHATE DEFICIT)

Phosphorus may be depleted as a result of impaired intestinal absorption, hyperparathyroidism and osteomalacia, in which there is an imbalance of calcium and phosphorus (Table 7.13).

Management

The primary disease that leads to the phosphorus deficit is treated. Foods high in phosphorus, such as milk, cheeses, whole grain cereals and nuts, are increased in the diet. The person should also be instructed to avoid excessive use of phosphate-binding medications such as aluminium hydroxide gels.

HYPERPHOSPHATAEMIA (EXCESS PHOSPHATE)

A serum phosphate level above normal may occur because of renal failure or hypoparathyrodism. Serum calcium falls and the patient may manifest the effects of hypocalcaemia.

Management

Correction of the hyperphosphataemia is aimed at the primary causative condition. Phosphate-binding medications (aluminium hydroxide gels) are administered. Constipation is a side-effect of this medication. Calcium supplements and vitamin D are administered to lower the serum phosphate level.

MAGNESIUM (Mg^{2+})

The adult body contains about 20–21 g of magnesium; 50–60% is insoluble and in combination with calcium and phosphorus in bone tissue. The remainder is found in soft tissue and in body fluids. The normal serum level of magnesium is within the range of 0.8–1.3 mmol/l.

FUNCTIONS

Magnesium is essential in the function of many enzyme systems, especially those involved with carbohydrate metabolism and protein synthesis. It also influences neuromuscular activity, the maintenance of normal ionic balance, osmotic pressure and bone metabolism.

REQUIREMENT, SOURCES, METABOLISM

The suggested daily requirement for an adult is 300–350 mg. The main food sources are whole grains, legumes, seafood, soy beans, cocoa and milk. The metabolism of magnesium is similar to that of calcium.

THE PERSON WITH MAGNESIUM IMBALANCE

HYPOMAGNESAEMIA (MAGNESIUM DEFICIT)

Hypomagnesaemia is usually caused by reduced dietary intake or decreased intestinal absorption. Excessive urinary or gastric loss may also result in a magnesium deficit. Magnesium deficits are often compounded by other electrolyte deficiencies.

Nursing intervention and treatment

The serum level is determined and the deficit corrected by increased intake of foods high in magnesium, such as green vegetables, meat, milk and fruits or by in-

Table 7.14 The person with magnesium imbalance.

Magnesium imbalance	Cause	Clinical characteristics	Associated health problems
Magnesium deficiency (hypomagnesaemia)	• Gastric loss through vomiting, diarrhoea, suctioning • Starvation • Hypoparathyroidism • Alcoholism • Prolonged intravenous therapy without magnesium supplementation • Malabsorption disorders	• Serum magnesium < 0.8 mmol/l • Muscular weakness • Muscular twitching and tremors • Convulsions • Nystagmus • Restlessness • Confusion • Hypertension • Cardiac arrhythmias	• Altered nutrition less than body requirements • Activity intolerance • Alteration in thought processes
Magnesium excess (hypermagnesaemia)	• Renal insufficiency	• Serum magnesium > 1.3 mmol/l • Bradycardia • Decreased reflexes • Drowsiness • Weakness • Coma • Respiratory and cardiac arrest	• Activity intolerance • Alteration in thought processes • Alteration in tissue perfusion • Breathing pattern ineffective • Knowledge deficit related to side-effects of antacids with magnesium

travenous administration of a magnesium sulphate or chloride preparation (e.g. 50 mmol of $MgSO_4$ in glucose 5% or in normal saline). The solution is given very slowly over 12–24 hours because it is a strong central nervous system depressant. This may be repeated daily until the serum concentration returns to nearly normal levels.

HYPERMAGNESAEMIA (EXCESS SERUM MAGNESIUM)

An excessive concentration of serum magnesium is usually associated with renal insufficiency. Clinical characteristics of magnesium excess are listed in Table 7.14.

Nursing intervention and treatment

Treatment is directed toward promoting urinary output and magnesium excretion. Haemodialysis or peritoneal dialysis may be used to reduce the blood level of magnesium rapidly. Magnesium-rich foods should be decreased in the diet. Antacids with magnesium, such as magnesium hydroxide gels, are avoided.

CHLORINE (Cl⁻)

Chlorine is a vital electrolyte for the maintenance of homeostasis, and occurs in the body as the chloride ion. It is found in greatest concentration in extracellular fluids; it is the major anion in the extracellular compartment.

FUNCTIONS

Chloride ions, along with sodium, help to maintain normal extracellular osmotic pressure and regulate water balance. Chloride is important in the chloride shifts that occurs between red blood cells and plasma. In this latter function it contributes to acid–base equilibrium. Chloride ions are also essential for the production of hydrochloric acid by gastric mucosal cells to provide the necessary acid medium for normal gastric digestion.

REQUIREMENT, SOURCES, METABOLISM

No actual requirement for chlorine has been established. The intake is satisfactory if the sodium intake is adequate. Both intake and output are inseparable from those of sodium. Chloride is almost completely absorbed from the intestine; only an insignificant amount is lost in faeces. It is excreted by the kidneys according to the need to maintain acid–base balance. The reabsorption of chloride ions, as with sodium, is promoted by adrenocorticoid secretion, especially aldosterone.

Disorders of chloride metabolism are generally associated with disorders of sodium; excessive sodium losses, as in Addison's disease (adrenocortical insufficiency), diaphoresis and diarrhoea, are accompanied by chloride depletion.

A loss of chloride ions in excess of sodium may occur with the loss of gastric secretions incurred by prolonged vomiting, prolonged gastric aspiration or suction, or pyloric or duodenal obstruction, causing hypochloraemia. As a result of the chloride deficit there is an increase in bicarbonate ions, and alkalosis develops.

ACID–BASE BALANCE

The acidity or alkalinity of a solution depends upon the concentration of hydrogen ions (H^+). When these are in excess of those contained in a neutral solution, the chemical reaction is *acid*; if fewer, it is *alkaline*. Normally body fluids are slightly alkaline; slight deviations in hydrogen ion concentration result in an imbalance that is disturbing and threatening to body metabolism.

Acids are substances which contain hydrogen ions that can be freed or donated by chemical reaction to other substances. Conversely, *bases* are chemical substances that can combine with hydrogen ions in a chemical reaction. A compound that completely dissociates its hydrogen ions is referred to as a strong acid; for example, hydrochloric acid, which completely dissociates when placed in water, is a strong acid ($HCl \rightarrow H^+ + Cl^-$). One that only partially frees its hydrogen ions is referred to as a weak acid; for example, a molecule of carbonic acid dissociates into one hydrogen ion and a hydrogen carbonate ion ($H_2CO_3 \rightarrow H^+ + HCO_3^-$), and therefore is termed a weak acid.

Hydrogen ion concentration ($[H^+]$) is measured in nanomoles per litre; the normal concentration in extracellular fluid is 40 nmol/l. An increase in the hydrogen ion concentration above 40 nmol/l indicates acidity, while a decrease in the concentration of hydrogen ions indicates alkalinity.

Traditionally, hydrogen ion concentration has been measured by the pH scale. The symbol pH is used to express the hydrogen ion concentration, or the degree to which a solution is acidic or alkaline. It represents the negative logarithm of the hydrogen ion concentration. For example, a neutral solution, such as water, with a pH of 7 contains 10^{-7} hydrogen ions per litre. A solution with a pH of 6 contains 10^{-6} hydrogen ions per litre; it contains 10 times as many hydrogen ions as a solution with a pH of 7. Since a solution of pH 7 is neutral, as the pH decreases below 7 the hydrogen ion concentration increases, and the solution becomes acidic. Conversely, as the pH increases above 7 and the hydrogen ion concentration decreases, the solution becomes alkaline. In other words, a pH of 7 denotes neutrality. A pH of less than 7 indicates acidity, and the smaller the figure, the greater the degree of acidity; a pH greater than 7 denotes alkalinity, and the greater the figure, the greater the degree of alkalinity.

Acid–Base Regulation

Cellular chemical processes produce relatively large amounts of acids, but the body is equipped with control mechanisms that maintain the pH or hydrogen ion concentration within a very limited range. Blood normally has a hydrogen ion concentration of 35–45 nmol/l or a pH of 7.35–7.45. An arterial blood hydrogen ion concentration below 20 nmol/l or over 120 nmol/l (or a pH below 6.8 or over 7.8) is considered incompatible with normal cellular activity and life.

The chief acid resulting from metabolism is carbonic acid, which is formed by the chemical combination of water and carbon dioxide ($H_2O + CO_2 \rightarrow H_2CO_3$). The combination is promoted by the enzyme carbonic anhydrase within the cells. In addition to carbonic acid, cellular activity produces a substantial quantity of stronger acids such as sulphuric, phosphoric, lactic, uric, acetoacetic, β-hydroxybutyric and hydrochloric acid. The acids must be rapidly neutralized or weakened by chemical reactions and, since their production is continuous, there must be a constant elimination of them from the body.

CONTROL MECHANISMS

The optimum pH of body fluids is maintained by acid–base buffer systems in the body fluids, respiratory excretion of carbon dioxide, and selective excretion of hydrogen ions or bases by the kidneys.

BUFFER SYSTEMS

Buffers are substances which tend to stabilize or maintain the constancy of the pH of a solution when an acid or a base is added to it. They do this by rapidly converting a strong acid or base to a weaker one which does not dissociate as rapidly.

A buffer system consists of two substances: a weak acid and a salt of that acid. The buffer systems of body fluids include the following pairs:

carbonic acid	H_2CO_3
sodium (or potassium) bicarbonate bicarbonate	$NaHCO_3$ (or $KHCO_3$)
acid phosphate	NaH_2PO_4
alkaline phosphate	Na_2HPO_4
acid plasma protein	HPr
proteinate	Na proteinate
haemoglobin	Hb
potassium haemoglobinate	KHb
oxyhaemoglobin	$H \cdot HbO_2$
potassium oxyhaemoglobinate	$KHbO_2$

Bicarbonate buffer system

The principal buffer pair of the plasma is the carbonic acid–sodium bicarbonate system. Maintenance of a normal pH is greatly dependent upon the ratio of carbonic acid concentration to that of sodium bicarbonate, which normally occurs as 1:20. *As long as there are 20 hydrogen carbonate ions to one carbonic acid molecule, the pH will remain within the normal range, regardless of the actual amounts of the two substances.*

When a strong acid is added to a fluid that contains the carbonic acid–sodium bicarbonate system, it combines with the hydrogen carbonate ion to form carbonic acid. Thus, the strong acid which dissociates readily to yield many hydrogen ions is replaced by a weaker acid which frees fewer hydrogen ions.

Phosphate buffer system

When an acid is added to a solution with the acid phosphate–alkaline phosphate system, it combines with the alkaline phosphate to form acid phosphate, a weaker acid. The phosphate system is especially active in the kidneys where the acid phosphate that has been formed is eliminated. It is also important in the intracellular fluids which have higher concentrations of phosphate than those found in the extracellular fluids.

Haemoglobin

Oxyhaemoglobin and reduced haemoglobin act as the acids of buffer pairs in the erythrocytes, and the potassium salt of the haemoglobin forms the other part of the system. When carbon dioxide diffuses into the red blood cells it combines with water to form carbonic acid:

$$CO_2 + H_2O \xrightarrow{\text{carbonic anhydrase}} H_2CO_3$$

The carbonic acid is buffered by potassium haemoglobinate to form the weak acid haemoglobin and potassium bicarbonate ($H_2CO_3 + KHb \rightarrow HHb + KHCO_3$.

When the acid haemoglobin is oxygenated to oxyhaemoglobin in the lungs it becomes a stronger acid and is rapidly buffered by potassium bicarbonate to form potassium oxyhaemoglobinate and carbonic acid ($HHbO_2 + KHCO_3 \rightarrow KHbO_2 + H_2CO_3$).

Carbonic anhydrase reverses its action and the carbonic acid is broken down into carbon dioxide and water; the carbon dioxide diffuses out of the cells into the blood and into the alveoli of the lungs.

Protein buffer system

The protein buffer system is the most abundant buffer in the body cells and plasma. Plasma proteins have the capacity to buffer either hydrogen ions (H^+) or excess hydroxide ions (OH^-), forming water. Thus proteins act as both acidic and basic buffers.

Intracellular buffering affects the movement of other ions, notably chloride, sodium and potassium. When hydrogen carbonate and hydrogen ions are formed from carbonic acid, some of the hydrogen carbonate diffuses out of the red blood cells into the plasma in exchange for another negatively charged ion, chloride. This movement is called the chloride shift. The remainder of the hydrogen carbonate remains in the red cells where it attaches to the intracellular potassium.

When hydrogen ion concentration is decreased extracellularly, some of the hydrogen ions released from the carbonic acid, move to the extracellular fluid in exchange for either potassium or sodium ions from the extracellular fluid. Conversely, if the extracellular hydrogen ion concentration is high, hydrogen ions will move into the cells in exchange for intracellular potassium or sodium.

Although the function of each buffer system has been discussed separately, within the body they work together in complementary and interchangeable reactions. Any condition that changes the balance of any one of the buffer systems also changes the balance of all the others, for the buffer systems also buffer each other.

RESPIRATORY REGULATION

A second important factor in the maintenance of the normal pH of body fluids is the elimination of carbon dioxide in respiration. Carbon dioxide is constantly produced in cellular metabolism and diffuses from the cells into the blood and erythrocytes. As a result, carbon dioxide is in greater concentration in the blood when it enters the pulmonary capillaries than in the air in the alveoli of the lungs. The pressure gradient results in some carbon dioxide diffusing from the blood into the alveoli from which it is exhaled. This reduces the amount available to form carbonic acid in the body fluids.

The neurones of the respiratory control centre in the medulla are extremely sensitive to the concentration of carbon dioxide and hydrogen ions in body fluids. An increase in either stimulates the centre to increase the rate and volume of respirations so more carbon dioxide may be eliminated. Conversely, a decrease in the concentration of carbon dioxide or hydrogen ions below the normal results in slower shallow respirations so that carbon dioxide is retained to form carbonic acid.

Obviously any condition that impairs the capacity of the lungs to eliminate carbon dioxide from the body predisposes to an increase in the carbonic acid level and a decrease in the pH of body fluids; on the other hand, increased pulmonary ventilation may increase the pH of the body fluids by the excessive loss of carbon dioxide.

KIDNEY REGULATION

The kidneys play an important role in maintaining the acid–base balance by excreting hydrogen ions and forming hydrogen carbonate in amounts as indicated by the pH of the blood. The cells of the distal portion of the renal tubules are sensitive to changes in the pH; when there is a decrease below the normal, hydrogen ions are excreted and hydrogen carbonate is formed and retained. Conversely, when there is an increased alkalinity above the normal, hydrogen ions are conserved and base-forming ions are excreted. In other words, the kidneys may excrete many or few hydrogen ions and form more or less hydrogen carbonate according to the need.

Renal regulation of hydrogen ion secretion involves three major processes: the reabsorption of hydrogen carbonate, the titration of urinary buffers, and the excretion of ammonium ions.

In summary, to preserve the normal pH, the kidneys reabsorb hydrogen carbonate and sodium ions in exchange for hydrogen ions. The phosphate and ammonia buffer systems result in increased sodium bicarbonate concentrations in the extracellular fluid. Hydrogen ions are secreted in the form of water, acid and as ammonium.

The Person with Alteration in Acid–Base Balance

Normally the hydrogen ion concentration (pH) of blood is maintained within the narrow range of (pH) 7.35–7.45. Acidosis or acidaemia is present when the pH is less than 7.35. Alkalosis or alkalaemia exist when the pH is greater than 7.45.

TESTS FOR ACID–BASE IMBALANCE

Blood gases

An estimation is made of the carbon dioxide and oxygen concentrations of the blood (see p. 369).

Arterial blood values for blood gases are used clinically more often than venous estimations. The collection of arterial blood samples for the evaluation of blood gases involves certain measures to prevent exposure of the specimen to the air. True values cannot be obtained if air contacts the blood sample.

A readily accessible artery, such as the radial or femoral, is used. The site is cleansed with an antiseptic. A solution of heparin is drawn up into the syringe to be used to rinse the inner surface, and is then discarded. All air must be excluded from the syringe and needle.

When the needle is passed through the arterial wall, the patient is likely to experience deep sharp pain; the patient is advised of this during the preparation for the procedure and asked not to move the limb. Anticipating this possibility, the assisting nurse provides the necessary support. If arterial blood gases are to be taken frequently, an arterial line may be inserted.

When the needle is withdrawn it is quickly inserted into the rubber stopper or capped to prevent the entry of air. The syringe is placed in an insulated container or a container of crushed ice, labelled and, with the requisition, is delivered immediately to the laboratory. If the analysis is delayed, true values are altered.

Pressure should be applied to the arterial puncture site for at least 8 minutes. When the nurse is assured that there is no bleeding, a sterile dressing is applied. The area and the area directly beneath it are checked at 15-minute and then half-hourly intervals for 2–3 hours for possible bleeding.

ACIDOSIS

When the hydrogen ion concentration is increased in body fluids, the three control mechanisms (buffer systems, respiration and kidney activity) endeavour to re-establish a normal pH. If the carbonic acid:bicarbonate ratio can be kept normal by increased respiratory elimination of carbon dioxide and by increased kidney elmination of hydrogen ions and formation of sodium bicarbonate, the pH (and hydrogen ion concentration) is kept within normal range. The condition is then said to be *compensated acidosis*. If the mechanisms cannot compensate adequately, a decrease in the carbonic acid:bicarbonate ratio develops, the pH falls below normal (i.e. the hydrogen ion concentration rises), and a state of uncompensated acidosis exists.

Acidosis may be classified according to the cause as respiratory or metabolic.

RESPIRATORY ACIDOSIS

This condition develops as a result of hypoventilation; the elimination of carbon dioxide does not keep pace with its production. The $Paco_2$ level is elevated and the condition may be referred to as hypercapnia. The level of serum carbonic acid rises above normal and the pH of body fluids decreases. Impaired carbon dioxide excretion by the lungs is usually accompanied by reduced Pao_2 (hypoxia) because of the decreased alveolar gas exchange. Since respiratory impairment is the cause of the acidosis, the primary adaptive response is increased renal excretion of acid.

The kidneys respond to the increased level of carbon dioxide by secreting an excess of hydrogen ions, resulting in an increase in sodium bicarbonate in the extracellular fluid. The kidneys also increase their formation and excretion of ammonia, which uses more hydrogen ions and results in hydrogen carbonate production. The serum bicarbonate concentration increases, correcting the carbonic acid:hydrogen carbonate ion ratio, and the pH moves towards normal. These renal compensatory responses require one or more days to be effective, provided that there is adequate blood circulation. The compensation is of greater value in acidosis associated with chronic respiratory diseases, such as emphysema and bronchiectasis.

METABOLIC ACIDOSIS

This occurs as a result of an excessive production or ingestion of acid or depletion of the hydrogen carbonate base. For example, a patient in a diabetic coma (hyperglycaemic) will metabolize fats to produce energy, producing ketones which are acid, and hence a metabolic acidosis may arise.

An adaptive response to the increased hydrogen ion concentration is to increase pulmonary ventilation. Respirations are increased in rate and volume to promote carbon dioxide elimination.

Table 7.15 outlines the causes of acidosis and common presenting conditions (signs and symptoms). A list of associated patient health problems is included.

ALKALOSIS

This is an acid–base imbalance in which there is an increase in the pH in excess of 7.45 due to a carbonic acid deficit or an excessive amount of bicarbonate. It may be classified as respiratory or metabolic.

RESPIRATORY ALKALOSIS

This disorder is due to an excessive loss of carbonic acid by hyperventilation. Carbon dioxide is being excreted by the lungs in excess of its production. The pH of the blood and the ratio of carbonic acid to bicarbonate are increased. If the condition is prolonged, large amounts of base are excreted by the kidneys, resulting in increased losses of sodium and potassium.

Table 7.15 The person with alteration in acid–base balance: Acidosis

Acid–base imbalance	Cause	Clinical characteristics	Associated health problems
Respiratory acidosis	Hypoventilation related to: • acute or chronic respiratory disease • circulatory failure • impaired alveolar perfusion • depression of respiratory centre • neuromuscular disturbances	• Serum pH < 7.36 • Serum $[H^+]$ > 45 nmol/l • Increased serum bicarbonate • Increased serum potassium • Increased $PaCO_2$ • Decreased PaO_2 • Hypoventilation • Increased urine acidity • Restlessness, weakness • Headache, confusion • Apprehension • Coma	• Breathing pattern ineffective • Alteration in tissue perfusion • Thought processes impaired • Knowledge deficit related to the disease process, treatment regimen, dietary plan, signs and symptoms of acid or base imbalance and actions to take if symptoms develop • Anxiety related to the illness
Metabolic acidosis	Increased acid production: • uncontrolled diabetes mellitus • starvation diet (fat catabolism) • alcoholism • lactic acidosis Increased acid ingestion: • excessive administration of ammonium chloride or acetylsalicylic acid Decreased urinary output of acid: • renal disease • dehydration, shock • hyperkalaemia Depletion of bicarbonate stores: • vomiting, diarrhoea • intestinal fistula • gastrointestinal suctioning • administration of carbonic anhydrase inhibitors (aceta-zolamide-Diamox)	• Serum pH < 7.35 • Serum $[H^+]$ > 45 nmol/l • Decreased serum bicarbonate • Increased anion gap (or normal) • Decreased $PaCO_2$ • Normal PaO_2 • Hyperventilation—increased rate and depth • Increased urine volume • Increased urine acidity • Nausea and vomiting • Headache, weakness • Drowsiness, confusion • Coma	• Breathing pattern ineffective • Alteration in tissue perfusion • Thought processes impaired • Alteration in pattern of urinary elimination • Knowledge deficit related to the disease process, treatment regimen, dietary plan, signs and symptoms of acid or base imbalance and actions to take if symptoms develop • Anxiety related to the illness

There is a corresponding decrease in the excretion of chloride and hydrogen ions.

METABOLIC ALKALOSIS

This decrease in hydrogen ion concentration and increase in pH may develop as the result of an abnormal loss of hydrochloric acid from the stomach in vomiting or gastric suctioning, excessive ingestion of alkaline substances (e.g. sodium bicarbonate) or a potassium deficit. The plasma concentration of bicarbonate is elevated with a corresponding increase in the pH and carbonic acid:bicarbonate ratio.

Respirations become slow and shallow in an effort to increase the carbonic acid content of the blood. If this is prolonged, it may produce an oxygen deficiency and the patient becomes cyanotic.

Kidney compensation is by conservation of hydrogen and chloride ions and by increased excretion of hydrogen carbonate. If the alkalosis is caused by vomiting, there is likely to be an associated dehydration which leads to decreased urinary output and reduced renal compensation.

ASSESSMENT OF THE PERSON WITH ACID–BASE IMBALANCE

Table 7.16 lists the most common causes of alkalosis. The development of an imbalance is influenced by the person's age, any pre-existing health problems, and the rate, severity and circumstances of the onset. The rate of onset is particularly important because of the rapidity of events which follow acute respiratory disturbances. When the onset is severe and sudden, the body's compensatory mechanisms may not be able to respond adequately. Renal responses require one or more days to effectively compensate for acute acid–base changes. When the disturbance is long-term in nature, such as

Table 7.16   Assessment of acid–base imbalance: Alkalosis

Acid–base imbalance	Cause	Clinical characteristics	Associated health problems
Respiratory alkalosis	Hyperventilation related to: • anxiety states • central nervous system disease which produces overstimulation of the respiratory centre • high fever • hypoxia • severe pain • high altitude • excessive mechanical ventilation	• Serum pH > 7.44 • Serum [H^+] < 35 nmol/l • Decreased serum bicarbonate • Decreased serum potassium • Decreased $PaCO_2$ • Cardiac arrhythmias • Hyperventilation: increased rate and depth • Decreased urine acidity • Tetany, cramps • Tingling in extremities • Convulsions • Dizziness, panic	• Breathing pattern ineffective • Alteration in tissue perfusion • Thought processes impaired • Knowledge deficit related to disease process, treatment regimen, dietary plan, signs and symptoms of acid or base imbalance and actions to take if symptoms develop • Anxiety related to illness
Metabolic alkalosis	Abnormal loss of acid: • vomiting or gastric suction • use of diuretics or mineralocorticoids Excessive ingestion of alkaline substances (i.e. sodium bicarbonate) is a contributing factor and not usually a primary cause	• Serum pH > 7.44 • Serum [H^+] < 35 nmol/l • Increased serum bicarbonate • Decreased serum potassium • Increased or normal $PaCO_2$ • Decreased PaO_2 • Cardiac arrhythmias • Hypoventilation: decreased rate and depth • Decreased urine acidity • Nausea, vomiting, diarrhoea • Tremors, twitching • Tetany, cramps • Tingling in extremities • Convulsions • Dizziness, apprehension, panic	• Breathing pattern ineffective • Alteration in tissue perfusion • Thought processes impaired • Alteration in bowel elimination: diarrhoea • Knowledge deficit related to disease process, treatment regimen, dietary plan, signs and symptoms of acid or base imbalance and actions to take if symptoms develop • Anxiety related to illness

occurs in individuals living in high altitudes or those with chronic obstructive lung disease or chronic renal disease, compensatory mechanisms play a major role in minimizing the effects. On the other hand, chronic disease states may result in decreased reserves and decreased ability to respond to further disturbances. The risk of functional and structural damage from acid–base imbalances is greatest in young children and the elderly.

Table 7.15 also outlines the clinical manifestations of a person with acid–base imbalance and the most common associated health problems.

NURSING INTERVENTION

Nursing actions for the person at risk of an acid–base imbalance focus on the prevention of deterioration, restoration of normal function and promotion of patient comfort.

PREVENTION OF ACID–BASE IMBALANCE AND MAINTENANCE OF OPTIMAL FUNCTION

The nurse has an important role in the identification of persons at risk for the development of an acid–base imbalance. This includes patients with acute health problems such as fluid and electrolyte imbalance, vomiting and diarrhoea, gastrointestinal drainage, renal dysfunction and metabolic disease such as diabetes mellitus. Patients with chronic health problems that may lead to acid–base imbalance require knowledge and skill to monitor their status, prevent the development of complications and maintain an optimal level of functioning. When narcotics are administered, the patient's respirations should be closely monitored and deep breathing and coughing should be performed at regular intervals to promote removal of respiratory secretions and adequate gas exchange.

Diuretic therapy increases the risk of acid–base disturbances because of fluid and electrolyte depletion. The specific action(s) and potential side-effects of the diuretic being administered should be familiar to nurses and the patient.

Knowledge deficit. The patient who has a chronic health problem in which an acid–base imbalance is a potential complication receives instruction so that early signs and symptoms of imbalance may be recognized and appropriate therapeutic measures initiated should the problem arise. Preventive measures should be stressed and the importance of following the prescribed treatment plan explained. For example, patients with chronic respiratory disease are taught deep-breathing and coughing techniques. Patients with diabetes and renal disease are taught to regulate their diets, administer drugs and modify living habits to prevent the development of acidosis. More specific information on prevention and maintenance measures for patients with specific health problems will be found in later chapters.

PROMOTION OF NORMAL OR COMPENSATED ACID–BASE BALANCE

Nursing interventions directed toward promoting the return of acid–base balance to normal or a compensated steady state include: (1) continuous assessment of changes in the patient's status; (2) communication of changes in the patient's condition to other members of the health team so that necessary adjustments or changes in the treatment can be made promptly; and (3) implementation of the nursing and medical plans of care.

Observations. Close observation of the patient with acidosis is important because the patient is critically ill; respiratory changes, either as a causative factor or as a compensatory response, may result in sudden changes in the individual's general condition.

The nurse should observe the vital signs, fluid balance, orientation and level of consciousness. Frequent collection of urine specimens may be required and may necessitate the use of a retention catheter. Blood specimens are taken at frequent intervals for serum hydrogen ion and electrolyte concentrations and pH estimations. Arterial blood gas determination will be done regularly and following any sudden changes in the patient's condition. The nurse should be alert for signs and symptoms of specific electrolyte deficits and excesses, especially potassium.

Early signs of disturbed neuromuscular functioning and tetany (e.g. muscle spasm and twitching) are noted and reported promptly. Trousseau's sign, which is characteristic of the onset of tetany, may be positive; it involves carpal spasm, which can be elicted by compression of the upper arm.

Fluids. If the patient is conscious, fluids should be encouraged. The fluids permitted vary with the cause of the acidosis or alkalosis. Parenteral fluids are usually administered to patients with acidosis or metabolic alkalosis. The solutions given and the rate of flow are based on the blood chemistry reports and kidney function. The patient with alkalosis may require potassium replacement either orally or intravenously if the serum potassium concentration is low. When potassium is added to an intravenous infusion, the rate of flow is very carefully regulated; it must be administered slowly and well diluted, with the dilution being specified by the doctor due to its potentially toxic effects on the heart. Close observation for signs of hyperkalaemia is neces-

sary; these include a slow weak pulse, restlessness and muscular weakness.

Oxygen/carbon dioxide administration. The rate, depth and characteristics of the patient's respirations should be observed closely. Oxygen may be administered to treat hypoxia, especially if the underlying cause is of respiratory origin. Oxygen must be administered with caution to patients with hypercapnia due to chronic airflow limitation as the oxygen promotes further retention of carbon dioxide and respiratory acidosis. A higher concentration of oxygen slows the respirations and less carbon dioxide is eliminated.

The patient with respiratory alkalosis related to hyperventilation is directed to rebreathe his own carbon dioxide by breathing into a paper bag.

PROMOTION OF COMFORT AND PREVENTION OF COMPLICATIONS

1. *Mouth care.* Frequent mouth care is especially important because of hyperpnoea, mouth breathing, vomiting and dehydration that frequently accompany acid–base imbalances.
2. *Safety.* Safety precautions are necessary if the patient manifests disorientation or confusion. If comatose, nursing measures applicable to an unconscious patient are required (see Chapter 2).

EMOTIONAL SUPPORT

The patient and family require support and reassurance that everything necessary is being done. They should be kept informed about the patient's progress and advised of treatment procedures. Time is taken to listen to their concerns and to answer their questions.

NURSING MEASURES FOR THE MAINTENANCE AND RESTORATION OF FLUID, ELECTROLYTE AND ACID–BASE BALANCE

The role of the nurse has four major components:

1. Identification of persons at risk for fluid and electrolyte abnormalities.
2. Implementation of nursing measures to prevent the development of a fluid, electrolyte or acid–base imbalance.
3. Provision of ongoing assessment to promote early identification of any imbalances.
4. Collaboration with other heath care professionals to provide interventions which restore the fluid, electrolyte or acid–base balance.

Identification of Persons at Risk

The onset of any illness or trauma can precipitate a fluid, electrolyte or acid–base imbalance. Factors which influence the development and the patient's ability to respond to imbalances include the rate, severity and circumstances of the onset, pre-existing conditions which may interfere with adaptive responses and the individual's age. When the onset is severe and sudden, the body's compensatory mechanisms may not be able to respond adequately. When the disturbance is long term in nature, compensatory mechanisms play a major role in minimizing the effects. On the other hand, chronic disease states may result in decreased reserves and decreased ability to respond to further disturbances. Illnesses such as diabetes mellitus and insipidus, kidney diseases, ulcerative colitis, congestive heart failure, cirrhosis and liver failure, respiratory diseases and hormonal imbalances can all lead to changes in the body's fluid and electrolyte balance. There are a number of special situations which also predispose a person to fluid or electrolyte abnormalities. These include extreme debilitation or illness, chronic malnutrition, coma, inability to swallow or lack of access to water, the use of diuretics or laxatives, surgical procedures, burns or massive injuries, copious suctioning or wound drainage, the use of concentrated tube feedings, and intubation and mechanical ventilation. Nurses must also be aware of the potential for fluid and electrolyte abnormalities in persons presenting with fever, vomiting or diarrhoea, haemorrhage or hyperventilation.

The effects of any trauma or illness are magnified in young children and the elderly. Infants and young children have a greater vulnerability to fluid imbalances as their fluid reserves are small, the younger the child the greater the risk. An infant requires a proportionately larger intake of fluid because: (1) insensible losses are greater as a result of the increased body surface to body mass proportion; (2) infants have an increased basal metabolic rate, and (3) the infant's immature kidneys require a larger proportion of water to excrete the metabolic wastes. An infant requires 70–100 ml/kg per 24 hours, whereas a healthy adult requires only 30–40 ml/kg per 24 hours. When stressed, the infant's immature renal tubules are unable to compensate for fluid or electrolyte disturbances as effectively as those of an adult.

The elderly are also at high risk for the development of fluid or electrolyte imbalances. There is a loss of functioning nephrons and renal mass with ageing. This, coupled with a decrease in renal blood flow, results in a reduced glomerular filtration rate and reduced creatinine clearance. The elderly demonstrate slower response to acute changes in fluid and electrolyte balance. The kidney is less responsive to antidiuretic hormone and aldosterone, contributing to an inability to conserve or excrete sodium and water appropriately. Fluid balance can be maintained if the elderly person can take in enough fluids to balance the output (at least 2000 ml per 24 hours). This is often not possible as the thirst mechanism is frequently blunted or absent in the elderly and many are physically unable to indicate their need for fluids. The physically disabled or institutionalized elderly may not have ready access to the fluids they require.

Prevention of Fluid, Electrolyte or Acid–Base Imbalance

When a patient has been identified as being at risk of a fluid, electrolyte or acid–base imbalance, the nurse should teach the patient, family, or other care-givers:

- The manifestations of the patient's underlying disease.
- The complications that can occur.
- The specific plan for management of the health problem.
- The actions and side-effects of all medications.
- The content and preparation of prescribed diets.
- The importance of maintaining an adequate fluid intake.
- The signs and symptoms of the specific imbalance(s) the patient is at risk of developing.
- Actions to take should symptoms develop.

For example, patients with diabetes or renal disease are taught to regulate their diets, administer medications and modify their life-style to prevent the development of fluid or electrolyte imbalances. More specific information on prevention and maintenance measures for patients with specific health problems will be found in later chapters.

Early Identification of Imbalance

The nurse can prevent a patient's condition from deteriorating through careful, ongoing observations and assessment. The most important nursing actions include the following:

- Intake and output
  —Careful measurement of all fluid intake.
  —Careful measurement of all fluid loss including urine, gastric losses, wound drainage, diaphoresis.
- Daily weight
  —Weigh the patient daily on the same scale, in the same clothing.
  —A gain of 1 kg indicates retention of 1 litre of fluid.
- Blood pressure
  —Blood pressure usually increases as extracellular fluid increases.
  —A fall in systolic blood pressure to less than 100 mmHg generally indicates volume depletion.
- Pulse rate
  —A full bounding pulse can be seen in fluid excess, a weak thready pulse in fluid depletion.
  —Electrolyte abnormalities may result in irregular pulse rates.
- Respiratory rate
  —Tachypnoea with or without dyspnoea may be present in fluid overload due to pulmonary oedema.
  —Rate, depth and regularity of breathing vary with acid–base imbalances.
- Temperature
  —Increased temperature indicates an increased metabolic rate and potential for increased fluid loss leading to dehydration.
- Neurological assessment
  —Assess level of consciousness.

—Assess muscle tone and strength, reflexes.

—May be altered with any electrolyte imbalance.

- Laboratory results

  —Review laboratory results, report abnormal results promptly.

Restoration of Fluid, Electrolyte and Acid–Base Balance

In general, nursing actions include the administration/ restriction of fluids as prescribed, monitoring and teaching of dietary prescriptions, and administration of medications. Specific interventions for each fluid, electrolyte or acid–base imbalance are detailed throughout this chapter.

Supportive nursing care. The patient with fluid, electrolyte or acid–base imbalance may experience a number of associated health problems (outlined in the text under the specific imbalance). Most nursing actions are

targeted towards the promotion of patient comfort and safety. Of importance are maintaining skin integrity through positioning, skin care and mouth care, promoting normal bowel and urinary elimination, maximizing patient activity tolerance, and providing psychological support. Nursing interventions specific to these problems are discussed in detail in Chapter 26 (skin), Chapter 16 (bowel elimination) and Chapter 20 (urinary elimination).

SUMMARY

In health, fluid, electrolyte and acid–base balance are maintained by the body's homeostatic mechanisms. When age or illness interfere with normal functioning, a fluid, electrolyte or acid–base imbalance can develop. The nurse is in a unique position to identify those persons at risk for the development of such an imbalance, and to institute nursing measures to prevent or promote resolution of the fluid, electrolyte or acid–base imbalance.

LEARNING ACTIVITIES

1. Fluid balance charts usually record a cup of tea or coffee as an arbitrary amount of fluid (typically 150, 180 or 200 ml). Measure the volume of fluid held by a standard ward cup. How much fluid might a patient leave behind after drinking a cup of tea or coffee? How many cups might not be touched or only a mouthful or two consumed, yet a full cup is recorded? What sort of difference might the above errors make to a person's actual daily intake compared to that recorded?
2. Role play with a colleague on how you would explain to a patient the link between being short of breath and having oedematous ankles. Teach your 'patient' how diuretics work and when they should be taken.
3. An 80 year old widower who lives alone is admitted to your ward in a confused, drowsy and dehydrated condition. What signs might lead you to suspect dehydration? Why do you think this patient may have become dehydrated? What advice would you give him prior to discharge to help prevent this occurring again.
4. Draw a chart to summarize the causes of respiratory/metabolic acidosis/alkalosis. The following format is suggested:

	Acidosis	Alkalosis
Respiratory		
Metabolic		

REFERENCES AND FURTHER READING

Carpenito LJ (1989) *Nursing Diagnosis: Application to Clinical Practice* 3rd edn. Philadelphia: Lippincott.

Francombe P (1988) Intravenous filters and phlebitis. *Nursing Times* **84(26):** 34–35.

Guyton AC (1986) *Textbook of Medical Physiology* 7th edn. Philadelphia: Saunders, Chapters 30, 32 and 33.

Hecker J (1988) Improved technique in i.v. therapy. *Nursing Times* **84(34):** 28–33.

Hinchcliffe S & Montague S (1988) *Physiology for Nursing Practice.* London: Baillière Tindall.

Kim MJ, McFarland GK & McFarlane A (1984) *Pocket Guide to Nursing Diagnosis.* St Louis: Mosby.

Leggett A (1990a) IV infusion pumps. *Nursing Standard* **4(28):** 24–26.

Leggett A (1990b) IV infusion pumps (contd). *Nursing Standard* **4(30):** 29–31.

Luken J & Middleton J (1990) IV infusion pumps. *Nursing Standard* **4(29):** 30–32.

Miller J (1989) Intravenous therapy in fluid and electrolyte imbalance. *Professional Nurse* **Feb.:** 237–241.

Pitt M (1989) Fluid intake and urinary tract infection. *Nursing Times* **85(1):** 36–38.

Walsh M and Ford P (1989) *Nursing Rituals, Research and Rational Action.* Oxford: Heinemann.

Temperature Regulation

OBJECTIVES

On completion of this chapter the reader will be able to:
- Describe the physiological mechanisms of thermoregulation
- Explain the impact of age-related changes on thermoregulation in the elderly
- Recognize causative and related factors and characteristics of the health problems of hyperthermia and hypothermia
- Describe the nursing assessment of persons with potential for and actual alteration in body temperature
- Describe nursing interventions to promote, maintain and re-establish thermoregulation
- Teach the individual and family to:
  - monitor body temperature
  - identify factors influencing thermal regulation
  - implement measures to promote, maintain and re-establish thermoregulation

BODY TEMPERATURE

Temperature reflects the heat content of the body, and provides information that contributes to the identification of relevant health problems and nursing intervention. Sudden alteration in body temperature may signal a change in the person's health status and indicate a need for immediate nursing and medical intervention. On the other hand, the temperature changes associated with hypothermia may be insidious in onset but with potentially fatal consequences if unrecognized and allowed to progess unchecked. Normally, the *internal* or *core body temperature* is maintained within narrow limits in persons of all ages. The temperature of the skin and subcutaneous tissues is referred to as the *surface temperature* and may vary with the temperature of the environment.

Body temperature results from the balance between the heat produced and acquired by the body and the amount lost. Normally, the body maintains a relatively constant core temperature within the range of 36–37°C, regardless of the environmental temperature. For this reason, man is classified as homothermic or warm-blooded as opposed to the poikilothermic or cold-blooded species whose body temperature fluctuates with variations in the environmental temperature.

Heat Production and Dissipation

Constancy of a temperature of 36–37°C, which favours normal cellular activity, is maintained by physiological processes that preserve a balance between heat production and heat dissipation. Increased production of heat (e.g. after exercise) is compensated by increasing heat loss (sweating), while a fall in body temperature leads to increased heat production and attempts to conserve heat.

Heat is generated in the body by chemical reactions within the cells. The more active the tissue, the greater is its production of heat; as a result, especially large amounts of heat are produced by the muscles and liver. A small amount may be acquired from external sources by radiation and conduction. Heat production is dependent upon cellular activity, and biochemical reactions (metabolism) increase as body temperature increases. A decrease in body temperature slows the rate of cellular activity, decreasing heat production. Body temperature may also be increased by the hormones thyroxine, adrenaline, noradrenaline and progesterone.

Normally, an excess of heat is produced within the body and must be eliminated to maintain a normal temperature. The excess is dissipated by the physical processes of radiation, conduction, and evaporation. Most of it is lost through the skin and the remainder is eliminated by the processes of respiration and excretion.

Radiation is the process by which radiant energy is transmitted from one object to another without direct contact. *Conduction* is the transfer of heat between two objects that are in contact; in practical terms this occurs most when skin is exposed to the air. *Conduction* depends upon a temperature gradient existing between the warmer and cooler objects and also the physical properties of the materials involved. If air in contact with skin is in motion, heat loss is more rapid, as the warmed air rapidly moves away from the body to be replaced by cooler air, maintaining a larger temperature gradient. The use of a fan cools the skin partly by this mechanism and also by increasing evaporation from the skin. In addition, sweat glands pour their secretion on to the skin surface; the heat of the blood in peripheral vessels is utilized in evaporating the secretion. Some vaporization takes place constantly, but the amount taking place on the skin varies. If there is a need to increase the heat loss, the sweat glands increase their secretion and peripheral vasodilatation occurs, resulting in increased vaporization. If there is a need to conserve body heat, less moisture is released on to the skin surface and vasoconstriction reduces circulation to the periphery.

Heat loss depends on a temperature gradient. If the environmental temperature is equal to or greater than that of the body, heat dissipation becomes completely dependent on the evaporation process.

Temperature Regulation

Temperature regulating mechanisms are essential to prevent the damaging effects on body tissues by extremes of heat and cold.

Regulation of body temperature is co-ordinated by the hypothalamic *thermostat*. Body temperature is maintained at a constant level, or set point, which varies only about 1°C throughout the day. Responses to changes in body temperature are evoked by sensory nerve impulses that originate in temperature receptors in the skin and by the direct effect of the blood temperature on the preoptic area of the hypothalamus, and possibly from other receptors in the body core.

Receptor cells that are sensitive to heat and cold are located in the skin. It is suggested that since there are far more cold receptors than heat receptors, peripheral detection of temperature mainly concerns detection of cold. When changes in the cutaneous temperature occur, the receptors give rise to nerve impulses that are delivered to the cerebral cortex and hypothalamus of the brain. Those that reach the cerebral cortex make the individual conscious of the temperature change. Be-

havioural responses to aid in correcting the change may then be produced. For example, if experiencing the sensation of cold, the individual may voluntarily increase muscle acivity to generate more heat, seek a warmer environment and add clothing to reduce the heat loss. In a hot environment, the behavioural responses might be to decrease activity in order to lower the heat production and to change to lighter clothing to permit more radiation.

In the anterior portion of the hypothalamus is a group of neurones that is referred to as the thermostatic or heat-regulating centre. This centre responds to cutaneous temperature impulses and to changes in the temperature of the blood. When the body temperature rises above normal, noradrenergic impulses responsible for peripheral vasoconstriction are reduced, resulting in passive dilatation of the cutaneous blood vessels; pseudomotor nerves stimulate the sweat glands. Heat loss is increased by evaporation of the additional sweat, as well as by radiation from the larger volume of blood brought to the surface. Heat production is decreased by the inhibition of shivering and decreased production of thyroxine, adrenaline and noradrenaline.

If the normal body temperature is threatened by a reduction in body heat, the centre initiates impulses which reduce heat loss and increase the production of heat. Superficial blood vessels constrict, secretion by the sweat glands is inhibited, shivering and non-shivering thermogenesis occur (Table 8.1).

Factors Related to Alteration in Body Temperature

The body temperature shows slight variations within the normal range from one individual to another and under certain circumstances. Variations within the normal may occur as a result of viological or circadian rhythms, age, physical activity, hormonal variations and environmental factors. Alteration in temperature results from extremes of these factors as well as from disease, compromised

Table 8.1 Summary of temperature regulation.

	Heat loss	Heat production
Response to cold	Heat loss is decreased by: Seeking a warmer environment Adding warmer clothing Changing posture to decrease effective surface area of body Vasoconstriction of cutaneous blood vessels	Heat production is increased by: Increased muscle activity (shivering and voluntary activity) Increased secretion of thyroxine, adrenaline, noradrenaline and progesterone
Response to heat	Heat loss is increased by: Wearing lighter clothing Seeking cooler environment Use of fans Vasodilatation of cutaneous blood vessels Increased sweating	Heat production is decreased by: Decreased physical activity Decreased muscle tone Decreased production of thyroxine, adrenaline, noradrenaline and progesterone

physical and mental status, and adverse socioeconomic factors.

To assess a person experiencing changes in body temperature and to plan relevant nursing care, the nurse requires an understanding of how physiological and environmental factors can alter body temperature.

Time of day

As with many biological activities, there is an evident diurnal pattern of change in body temperature or circadian rhythm. It decreases between 2 and 6 a.m. and slowly rises throughout the day, reaching a peak between 6 and 10 p.m. This rhythm is not directly related to activity, but its pattern may be altered in persons who are active during the night and sleep during the day.

Physical activity and exposure to heat produce a transient elevation in body temperature which is normally readily dissipated by the skin and lungs.

The fever associated with illness tends to follow the normal circadian rhythm; the fever is greatest in the evening and lower through the night unless the disorder involves the temperature-regulating centre and mechanism.

Age

Infants have a higher normal temperature. Their heat production is greater owing to the higher metabolic rate associated with their growth and activity. Also, the ability to regulate heat loss and production is not sufficiently developed in the early years to regulate temperature efficiently.

Older people have a somewhat lower normal temperature because of their slower metabolic rate and reduced muscular activity. The elderly are at greater risk of problems of thermoregulation. Changes in the vascular system, the loss of subcutaneous fat, the atrophy of sweat glands, and the lowered metabolic rate that occur with age, impede adjustment to changes in environmental temperature. The development of hypothermia is greater in the elderly as a result of diminished cutaneous sensitivity to temperature change and impaired ability to produce body heat. Social isolation, poverty and poor housing exacerbate these factors.

Exercise

Strenuous exercise may cause an elevation to 40°C core temperature, but it quickly returns to normal when the activity ceases. Women in labour frequently show an increase in temperature, attributed to their increased muscular activity.

Menstrual cycle

A variation in temperature is characteristic of certain phases of the menstrual cycle. There is an increase of 0.3–0.5°C when ovulation occurs, which is usually about the middle of the cycle. This is attributed to the increased activities of the endometrial cells, initiated by the secretion of progesterone. The slight increase is maintained until a day or two before the onset of menstruation, when it falls to the previous normal level.

Pregnancy

A slight increase in temperature occurs in the first 3–4 months of pregnancy and is followed by a gradual fall of 0.5–1°C. The lower temperature continues to full term and returns to the individual's normal level after parturition.

Environment

Extremes of heat and cold in the environment affect body temperature. The body acclimatizes to cold through adaptive changes, including increased thyroid activity and metabolism and reduction in visible shivering. Heat acclimatization is achieved through increased effectiveness of the sweat mechanism.

Disease, illness and trauma

Infection is the most common cause of elevated body temperature. Mental confusion, cardiovascular, neural, endocrine and respiratory disorders, dehydration and physical trauma all interfere with thermoregulation. Exposure to extremes of environmental temperature may exacerbate existing disease and further impair temperature control. Severe brain damage in head injury may also lead to a loss of thermoregulation and elevated temperatures over 40°C.

Drugs and alcohol

Antipyretic or aspirin-like drugs decrease elevated body temperature when it is caused by fever and thus related to alteration in the set point. Pyrogen produced as a result of an infection or inflammation stimulates the hypothalamus to release prostaglandins that increase the set point. Aspirin-like drugs act by blocking the production and release of prostaglandins and thus cause the set point to return to normal. Use of these drugs may mask symptoms of an underlying disorder and cause a delay in seeking treatment. Antipyretic drugs do not lower body temperature resulting from exposure to extreme heat or excessive physical activity.

Alcohol and anaesthetic, antipsychotic, antihypertensive, diuretic and anticholinergic agents may raise or lower body temperature. The central nervous system effects of many of these drugs make the person unaware of or unconcerned about the change in temperature. This is of particular concern with the elderly who often take one or more of these medications.

Hyperthermia

Hyperthermia is an elevation of body temperature above normal. It is a manifestation of tissue injury or a disorder that results in an increase in heat production in excess of the rate of dissipation, or in an impairment of the heat-dissipating or control mechanisms.

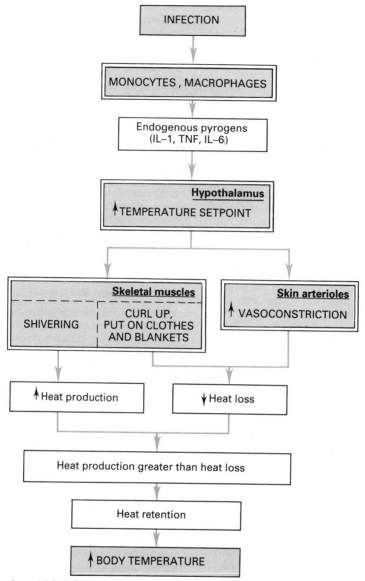

Figure 8.1 Pathway by which infection causes fever. IL-1, interleukin-1; TNF, tumour necrosis factor; IL-6, interleukin-6.

CAUSES OF HYPERTHERMIA

The imbalance in body heat content may be caused by malfunction of the temperature-regulating centre, the response of the centre to a pyrogen, exposure to a very high environmental temperature, or impaired dissipation.

Fever is a specific type of hyperthermia caused by a resetting of the thermostat in the hypothalamus. Disturbances in the regulation of the thermostat may be the result of the direct action of brain disease or increased intracranial pressure, or by the action of a substance that is released into the blood at the site of tissue injury or disintegration anywhere in the body. The substance, which may be referred to as a pyrogen, reacts first with leucocytes to form a second substance called endogenous pyrogen.

Stimulation of the hypothalamic heat centre by endogenous pyrogen is analogous to the setting of the thermostat of an automatic heating system to a higher level; heat is produced until the set level of temperature is achieved. The higher temperature is maintained as long as the pyrogen is present. As the concentration of the pyrogen is reduced, the level of the thermostat is lowered, and there is a corresponding decrease in the fever by activation of the heat-dissipating responses, peripheral vasodilatation and sweating (Figure 8.1).

In the case of hyperthermia due to exposure to a high temperature, the body cannot dissipate heat as fast as it is being received from the exterior.

Hyperthermia occurring because of inefficient heat-dissipating mechanisms is seen most often when severe dehydration develops. The secretion of sweat is reduced, resulting in a marked decrease in heat loss by evaporation.

CHARACTERISTICS OF HYPERTHERMIA

The onset of hyperthermia or fever may be sudden and rapid, or the rise in body heat may develop gradually without the individual being aware of it. The initial manifestations of fever vary with the degree of disturbance in the thermostatic centre. If the elevation is moderate and gradual, the patient may experience slight chilliness for a brief period, general malaise, headache and anorexia. With a sudden and greater degree of stimulation of the centre, the patient has a chill in which he or she shivers and feels very cold, even though the temperature may already be above normal. Adrenaline is released which accelerates metabolism, increasing heat production. In turn, the rise in temperature further accelerates the metabolic rate and heat production. The skin becomes pale and is cold to the touch because of peripheral vasoconstriction. The shivering is increased muscular activity for the purpose of producing heat; it may be severe enough to cause chattering of the teeth and shaking of the whole body. Small elevations of skin (goosepimples) appear and the small fine hairs become erect, owing to the contraction of small muscles attached to the hair follicles. The chill lasts until the temperature reaches the level set by the stimulated thermostatic centre in the hypothalamus. Then, as long as the pyrogen is effective, a balance between the heat production and dissipation maintains the temperature at approximately this higher level.

Frequently the onset of fever in infants and young children is accompanied by a convulsion which is due to the immaturity and instability of their nervous systems.

With subsidence of the chill, the patient's skin becomes hot and flushed, and he or she complains of feeling hot. Disorientation and delirium are not uncommon when the fever is high, especially in older persons.

The basal metabolic rate is increased in proportion to the elevation of temperature. With a fever of 40.5°C there is an increase in metabolic rate of approximately 50%. A negative nitrogen balance develops with the increased destruction of body protein in metabolism, and there is a loss of weight. Respiration and the heart rate are accelerated. There is a greater loss of fluid by evaporation from the hot skin and in the increased respiration.

If the temperature rises above approximately 40.5°C there is danger of cellular damage. The hypothalamus may lose its capacity for temperature regulation, resulting in a progressive increase in fever until death occurs. The limit to which the temperature may rise before causing death is about 43.4–44.4°C.

When the pyrogenic factor is suddenly removed, the mechanisms that contribute to heat loss are set in operation. There is marked peripheral vasodilatation and profuse sweating (diaphoresis); heat is lost rapidly by radiation and vaporization. This sudden lowering of the temperature is referred to as the *crisis of fever*. If the temperature returns to normal gradually over a period of several days, the process is known as *lysis*.

Hyperthermia inhibits the growth of some pyrogenic organisms and makes others less virulent. Antibody production is increased when body temperature is elevated. Hyperthermia also slows the growth of some tumours.

HEAT STROKE

A heat stroke occurs with relatively long exposure to extreme heat. At first the individual may experience headache, visual disturbances, nausea and vomiting. Weakness, flaccidity of the muscles, a rapid bounding pulse and rapid respirations are manifested. The individual becomes delirious, collapses and lapses into coma. The skin is hot and dry, and there is an absence of sweating due to dehydration and central nervous system damage. The temperature progressively rises to 40.6–43.3°C. Unless the condition is discovered in the early stages and the body is rapidly cooled, circulatory failure develops and the patient dies.

ASSESSMENT OF THE PATIENT WITH ALTERED BODY TEMPERATURE

This requires the nurse to apply knowledge of physiological, pathological, social and environmental factors. In other words there is more involved than monitoring body temperature; other vital signs may need recording, together with a background health history and relevant social factors, depending upon the patient's circumstances.

Taking a patient's temperature may seem a simple enough procedure but, as Walsh and Ford (1989) have shown, there are many examples of nurses performing this inaccurately. A clinical thermometer may take between 8 and 10 minutes to reach a stable recording in the sublingual pocket (below the tongue), however the increase in temperature shown between 4 and 10 minutes is too small to be clinically significant (i.e. whether a temperature of 38.4°C or 38.7°C is recorded will make no difference to treatment). It seems reasonable therefore to leave a thermometer in situ for 4 mintues before recording the temperature, less than that period of time and measurements significantly under the real temperature will result. Such errors are unacceptable.

The nurse should ensure the patient has not just had a hot or cold drink, nor is smoking or mouth breathing as these factors significantly alter oral temperature measurement. A delay of 10 to 15 minutes after drinking or smoking seems reasonable to allow oral temperature to return to normal.

Temperature may also be measured in the axilla or rectum. The axilla is recommended if the patient is mouth breathing or has recently had a fit but if the peripheral circulation is shut down (see p. 357) a meaningful recording will not be possible. Axillary measurement requires the thermometer to be left in for a longer period, up to 10 minutes, but even then temperatures are usually 0.5°C lower than oral recordings. The rectal route requires the use of a specially marked thermometer to avoid the risk of it later being used for oral measurement and usually gives a reading closest to core body temperature. The rectal route tends to be used with infants and also with patients suffering profound hypothermia. Continuous electronic temperature measurement is possible with the use of probes inserted into the rectum or oesophagus, although this usually only occurs in intensive therapy units.

It is important that temperatures be recorded consistently in the same site and for the same length of time so that any variations represent real changes in the patient's clinical condition and not spurious errors due to poor observation techniques. Thermometers must be cleaned after use as a preventative measure against cross-infection, although it should be noted that transmission of HIV by saliva alone has never been recorded and this is not felt to be a risk.

The patient with Hyperthermia

If the patient's temperature is above normal (pyrexial) this is most likely to be due to an infective process. The nurse should enquire about the patient's general health, checking for evidence of likely causes, such as a respiratory or urinary tract infection, and also looking at any obvious potential sites of infection, such as a wound, or, if the patient has a catheter, examining the urine for signs of infection. Respiratory and pulse rates should be recorded as these may be elevated. The patient's mental status should be checked to see if he or she is alert and oriented in time and space. Mental functioning may be impaired in severe infections or if the patient is hypoxic due to a chest infection. Fluid intake should be assessed as dehydration due to increased fluid loss may develop in patients who are pyrexial. It should be remembered that there are other possible causes for a pyrexia, e.g. brain damage associated with a head injury, heatstroke.

Once the nurse has identified hyperthermia as a problem, the logical goal is to return the patient's temperature to within normal limits. An initial time scale might be 24 hours, although this will vary with the condition of the individual patient.

NURSING INTERVENTION

Nursing interventions include increasing the rate of heat loss from the body, intervening where possible to deal with the cause of the pyrexia, and providing support for the other systems of the body that are affected (e.g. ensuring hydration). Psychological support is also required.

Increasing the rate of heat loss

Surface cooling is the method most readily employed. Exposing the patient with a minimum of clothing and bedding increases heat loss by radiation while allowing sweating to occur with minimum discomfort. A fan helps further cooling, while the process of tepid sponging also promotes heat loss as the body evaporates the residual water left on the skin.

Source of infection

Ensuring the patient receives the prescribed antibiotic regimen accurately is a key nursing intervention. Other interventions will depend upon the source of the infection, e.g. if it is a septic wound, a good aseptic technique and appropriate dressing agent (e.g. Iodosorb followed by Granuflex) are required to clean the wound out before wound healing can occur.

Antipyrexial drugs

Aspirin is commonly given to lower temperature. It works by reducing the sensitivity of the heat-regulating centre.

Psychological support

General feelings of malaise may lead to anxiety and unhappiness. It is important to find out how the patient feels and what is his or her view of the situation. The patient can readily see the response to treatment by looking at the 'obs chart' at the foot of the bed; if the temperature remains high, the patient may become very distressed and worried, feeling he or she will never get better. Time should be set aside to talk to the patient, allowing for the expression of anxieties and raising of questions, which should always be answered honestly. Excessive sweating may also be embarrassing to the patient and every effort should be made to ensure comfort, including frequent changes of linen and nightwear. Explanations concerning nursing care such as tepid sponging and increasing fluid intake (see below) should always be given to promote patient involvement in care.

Supporting systems

Substantially increased fluid loss requires a fluid balance chart to be maintained to ensure adequate fluid intake; a minimum of 3 l/day is suggested. The increase in metabolism associated with pyrexia places extra demands upon the patient's resources; food intake is therefore important and steps should be taken to ensure that the patient is receiving a good diet. An increase in calorie and protein intake is particularly important. Pain is commonly associated with sepsis and should be assessed and appropriate steps taken to ensure the patient is pain free (pp. 129–40). Mouth care is important as the patient may develop a dry mouth, which is prone to infection with candida (thrush).

EVALUATION OF CARE

Care should be evaluated by accurately recording temperature 4-hourly, monitoring the process of sepsis resolution where appropriate, and keeping an accurate fluid balance chart. Problems such as pain and anxiety should also be kept under frequent review. If the patient fails to respond to therapy, changes such as a different antibiotic regimen or more vigorous cooling methods may be needed.

The patient with Hypothermia

This is a condition in which, in response to exposure to

a cold environment, the patient's temperature falls below normal. This process may be exacerbated by a loss of thermoregulation, typically seen in neonates or the elderly (p. 119). Prolonged exposure to severe weather, particularly in mountainous areas with a high wind chill factor, or immersion in cold water can induce hypothermia in otherwise fit and healthy adults. Homeless people sleeping rough are also prone to hypothermia in winter conditions. One other risk group are patients undergoing lengthy surgical procedures, particularly the elderly. White et al (1987) showed that prolonged exposure in cool operating theatres led to hypothermia in eight out of a sample of 21 elderly patients undergoing surgery for hip fractures. Hypothermia may also be deliberately induced during cardiac surgery to reduce tissue oxygen demand while the patient is on bypass.

The familiar response of shivering is associated with the early stages of hypothermia but, as core temperature falls below 34°C, this mechanism ceases as progressive muscle weakness ensues. This, coupled with a steady deterioration in mental status, makes the person less able to care for himself or herself. Drowsiness lapses into coma at around 30–32°C and further falls in temperature make the person liable to serious cardiac arrhythmias. It seems that if a person's temperature drops significantly below 28°C, the condition becomes irreversible and death ensues as the body loses its ability to generate heat. Circulatory collapse and shock is associated with hypothermia, and at 18–22°C the heart stops beating completely.

Assessment of a patient with hypothermia requires a clear social history which may have to be obtained from others (ambulance crew, neighbours, relatives) to assess the social conditions in which the person is living and, if possible, how long the patient may have been hypothermic. In cases of hypothermia the patient's skin over the trunk area of the body is strikingly cold to the touch, even if clothed. A low-reading rectal thermometer should be used for measurement of core temperature. Collapse and shock may develop, hence the need for frequent vital signs monitoring, including blood pressure. The patient should have a 12-lead ECG and rhythm strip taken and continuous ECG monitoring may be requested by medical staff in view of the risk of cardiac arrhythmias, while an initial level of consciousness should be determined as a baseline against which to measure progress (p. 302).

It is important to stress that if a patient is found in a collapsed hypothermic state, an assessment of the whole patient is essential. The question to be asked is: Why did this person become hypothermic? Did the patient fall, leading to a head injury or fractured hip which rendered them immobile and unable to seek help, or has the person suffered an acute medical disaster such as a stroke or myocardial infarction? The assessment should look at the whole body, checking for signs of injury or assault, paying particular attention to pressure areas and obtaining a general impression of how well cared for the person is.

The immediate goal for such a patient is to return the body temperature back to normal without any cardiovascular or other complications. This requires a slow and gradual warming. A long-term goal is to prevent such an episode occurring again.

NURSING INTERVENTION

Rewarming

This should be carried out gradually because too rapid rewarming can result in circulatory collapse. A rate of 0.5°C per hour should be aimed for. The safest way of achieving this is by conserving the heat being generated by the body; this involves the initial use of a reflective aluminium foil 'space blanket' which reflects heat radiation back into the body and should therefore be close to the skin for optimum effect. A disproportionate amount of heat is lost through the scalp which should therefore also be covered. External sources of heat are to be avoided (e.g. hot water bottles) because of the danger of burns and also because the need is to raise core temperature, not superficial skin temperatures. Rapid peripheral warming may lead to vasodilatation and provoke circulatory collapse. Intravenous infusions prewarmed to body temperature may also be given.

Avoiding complications

Pressure area care is crucial during the rewarming phase if the patient is immobile. Continual ECG monitoring has already been mentioned and frequent observations of vital signs are needed in order that any other cardiovascular complications are detected as early as possible. Level of consciousness should be monitored to assess how alert and orientated the patient is; the safety of the patient should never be forgotten and a confused, disorientated elderly patient is clearly at risk. Oxygen therapy may be required and an accurate fluid balance chart should be maintained to ensure hydration.

Psychological support

The patient may have suffered a very frightening experience, lying on the floor, in pain, perhaps thinking of death, before being found. This distress should be recognized and if able, the patient encouraged to talk about how he or she feels. Psychological warmth is every bit as important as physical warmth in this situation. If the patient is confused, simple explanations and reorientation are needed until the patient becomes more lucid. If the core temperature is below 28°C, recovery is extremely unlikely and the patient will probably die without recovering consciousness. At all times nursing staff should be honest and considerate with the family, who should be informed of the prognosis, while maintaining the highest standards of care and support for the patient.

Future prevention

If recovery occurs it is important to discuss the patient's health and social problems in depth with family and patient. Teaching about hypothermia should take place, explaining what it is and how its onset is so insidious that the patient will probably not recognize it. The importance of wearing layers of clothing, keeping the head covered and trying to maintain at least one room in the house at a temperature of 21–23°C should be stressed. A good calorie intake and plenty of warm drinks will also help. The patient may, however, argue with reason that these sort of measures cannot be afforded. The electricity supply to the house may already have been cut off. The patient may not even have a home to go to. The weakness of concentrating on life-style modification in health education is clearly shown!

Social service staff may need to be involved in obtaining extra financial assistance for heating. It may be necessary to consult the general practitioner and community nursing services to ensure that the patient can manage at home, or if this is not thought advisable, to explore with the patient the possibilities of moving to more appropriate accommodation. The shortage of single person hostel accommodation makes the homeless patient particularly difficult to help, especially if there are significant mental health problems.

EVALUATION OF CARE

Frequent monitoring of core temperature is needed to check progress (at least hourly during rewarming). This may be done rectally, but research by Mravinac et al (1989) on postoperative patients who had hypothermia induced preoperatively indicated that the rectal temperature lagged behind continuously-monitored pulmonary artery temperatures during rewarming. This suggests that rectal readings might be a slight underes-timate of true core temperature during rewarming.

The nurse must realize that the patient with hypothermia is suffering a serious, life-threatening illness and that even small changes in their condition could herald a potentially fatal outcome. Very close observation of progress is therefore essential during the acute stages, hence the importance of monitoring vital signs, level of consciousness and fluid balance.

It is important to check how much the patient has learnt about steps to avoid hypothermia before discharge and to try and arrange a visit by a community nurse post discharge to evaluate the home situation.

SUMMARY

Pyrexia can occur in a wide range of patients in response to infection, less commonly after serious head injury or in extreme environmental conditions. Age-related changes and socioeconomic factors make the elderly most at risk of developing hypothermia, although people of all ages may develop this condition. The basic aim of nursing care is to restore body temperature to within normal limits by either increasing heat loss or conserving heat, as necessary. A wide range of supportive measures are also necessary to deal with the various effects of an abnormal temperature on the body.

LEARNING ACTIVITIES

1. Measure the temperature of a colleague by leaving a thermometer in situ (orally) for 30 seconds, shake the mercury back down and repeat, this time for 1 minute. Repeat this exercise, shaking the mercury down each time, lengthening the period by 30 seconds at a time until three consecutive observations are the same. How long does it take to achieve a steady reading? If your colleague had a temperature of 38.5°C, what effect do you think this would have on the time needed to record a steady temperature?

2. Record a colleague's temperature orally. Now give a hot drink and immediately after several mouthfuls have been taken record the temperature again; repeat with an ice cream. What are the different temperatures you recorded?

3. What practical advice could you give to (a) an elderly person; (b) a homeless person to avoid hypothermia in winter?

4. Find out what the policies are of your local gas and electricity companies towards arrears. Do they check the age and social circumstances of customers before cutting off the supply for non-payment?

REFERENCES AND FURTHER READING

Mravinac C, Draceys K & Clochesy J (1989) Urinary bladder and rectal temperature monitoring during clinical hypothermia. *Nursing Research* **38(2):** 73–76.

Walsh M & Ford P (1989) *Nursing Rituals, Research and Rational Action.* Oxford: Heinemann.

White E et al (1987) Body temperatures in elderly surgical patients. *Research in Nursing and Health* **10(5):** 317–321.

Pain: Prevention and Care

9

OBJECTIVES

On completion of this chapter the reader will be able to:
- Appreciate the significant role nurses play in the assessment and management of pain
- Understand the physiological mechanisms and psychological factors involved in an individual's perception of and response to pain
- Identify the necessary data for nursing assessment of pain
- Recognize the importance of patient cooperation in the formulation of a pain management plan
- Identify pharmacological and non-pharmacological nursing interventions for pain relief
- Identify the need for on-going evaluation of the effectiveness of pain management strategies

PAIN

Pain is a complex, distressing experience involving sensory, emotional and cognitive components. The quality and intensity of pain vary with the individual and are influenced by psychological and sociocultural factors. Pain plays an important protective role; one progressively learns from early childhood to avoid situations which cause pain. When sensation is lost in an area of the body, as it is in spinal cord injury, the lack of awareness of injury and the absence of normal protective responses may lead to extensive tissue damage.

Nurses encounter people experiencing pain in a variety of health care settings: the community, acute hospitals, hospices and long-term care facilities. Pain is one of the most compelling symptoms that prompt an individual to seek medical or nursing advice. Pain may indicate a disease process and thus provide information that aids in making a medical diagnosis. Pain may also be secondary to treatment, diagnostic procedures or a process such as childbirth. Working alongside other health professionals, nurses are in key roles to work with patients and their families to achieve good pain control.

Pain Mechanism

The structures essential for the pain sensation are receptors that are sensitive to pain stimuli, impulse pathways to and within the central nervous system (brain and spinal cord), and areas within the brain for perception, interpretation and the initiation of responses. The body also has an inbuilt natural analgesic system which is capable of modulating and controlling pain.

PAIN STIMULI

A wide variety of stimuli evoke pain; these stimuli may be classified as mechanical (e.g. pressure from a blow or distension), thermal (extremes of heat or cold) or chemical (e.g. chemicals released by injured cells or micro-organisms). Prostaglandins are chemical agents released by damaged tissues which act as powerful pain stimuli.

Many stimuli are non-specific but elicit pain through their intensity. For instance, light pressure produces an awareness of touch, but increasing the intensity of the pressure causes pain. Similarly, heat and cold must reach a certain intensity to stimulate pain receptors.

PAIN RECEPTORS

Stimuli that cause pain sensation are received by freely branching bare nerve endings which form a diffuse network in the tissue. The concentration of these receptors varies throughout the body; they are abundant in the skin and on joint surfaces, but there are relatively fewer in the deeper tissues and viscera.

Some pain receptors respond to specific stimuli; most are 'polymodal' as they respond to any stimulus threatening tissue integrity. Research into the activity of polymodal nociceptors (pain receptors) has identified substance P as a neurotransmitter for pain.

PAIN IMPULSE PATHWAYS

The sensory, or afferent, nerve fibres, whose bare terminal branches form the pain receptors, provide pathways to conduct the impulses into the spinal cord or brain stem. (Sensory, or *afferent*, nerve fibres carry impulses toward the central nervous system (brain and spinal cord). *Motor*, or *efferent*, nerve fibres transmit impulses away from the central nervous system to peripheral structures.) These sensory nerve fibres are of two types; some have a fatty insulating sheath (myelin) and are classified as A delta fibres; the others are non-myelinated and designated C fibres. The myelinated fibres transmit the impulses very rapidly. A sudden, pain-producing stimulus causes two pain sensations. The impulses transmitted by the myelinated fibres produce

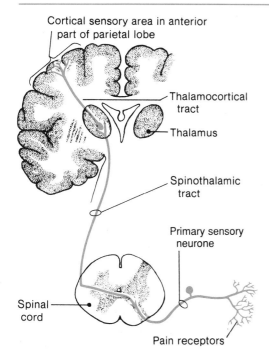

Cortical sensory area in anterior part of parietal lobe

Thalamocortical tract

Thalamus

Spinothalamic tract

Primary sensory neurone

Spinal cord

Pain receptors

Figure 9.1 Diagram illustrating a pathway of pain impulses.

the sharp, pricking, localized pain that is felt immediately when the injury occurs. The non-myelinated fibres conduct more slowly and are responsible for the more diffuse, throbbing, burning type of pain or ache that follows the immediate sharp pain associated with the initial injury.

Various theories have been presented to explain the physiology of pain, none of which has proved entirely satisfactory. The specificity theory and the gate control theory have been the more prominent theories.

The *specificity theory of pain* proposes that there are specific structures (afferent nerve fibres and central nervous system pathways and neurones) concerned with the pain sensation. Pain impulses are transmitted by specific sensory nerve fibres from the stimulus site and enter the spinal cord via the dorsal and ventral spinal roots to neurones within the posterior column or horn of grey matter. Some impulses may be passed directly to motor neurones to initiate impulses that are carried out of the cord along motor or efferent nerve fibres to skeletal muscles. These motor impulses produce a reflex response, such as withdrawal of the injured part from the object producing the pain stimulus (as seen in the withdrawal of the finger that receives a pin prick or touches a very hot object). The other pain impulses cross to the other side of the cord and ascend the anterolateral spinothalamic pathway to the brain (Figure 9.1).

Although current research indicates conduction of pain impulses is more complex than originally proposed, the recognition of the specific pain pathways inherent in the specificity theory provides the basis for surgery in intractable pain. The procedure interrupts the pain pathway and impulses do not reach conscious level.

The *gate control theory* advanced by Melzack and Wall (1965) proposes that pain impulses can be regulated, modified or blocked by certain cells within the central nervous system. It is thought that impulses can be prevented from reaching the transmission cells of the posterior column by the action of the substantia gelatinosa cells, which are said to 'close the gate'. Whether or not the gate is open to permit the conduction of impulses through the posterior horn cells and hence to higher levels is dependent upon the nature of the impulses delivered to the substantia gelatinosa, which is an area of special neurones located close to each posterior column of grey matter and extending the length of the spinal cord. It has been indicated that when cutaneous impulses aroused by such stimuli as vibration, scratching, cold and heat are transmitted by large fibres in the afferent nerve they can negate the input of the fibres of smaller diameter. That is, they close the gate. It remains open to impulses transmitted by small fibres if there is 'relatively little activity in the large fibres'. The activity of the gating mechanism may also be affected by emotion and impulses in descending tracts from areas of the brain (brain stem, thalamus and cerebral cortex). Thus, the gate control theory expanded the role of the spinal cord: it is not just a relay station, but a centre for filtering and integrating incoming sensory information.

The gate control theory establishes a basis for the following procedures in lessening pain and suffering: (1) use of sensory input such as distraction and guided imagery; (2) reducing fear and lowering the level of anxiety; (3) patient teaching about the cause and relief of pain; (4) local counterirritants, massage and heat applications; (5) electrical stimulation; and (6) acupuncture.

PAIN CONTROL MECHANISM

Current research supports the gate control theory and has provided new information on the mechanisms of pain modulation and control. In addition to the previously described gating mechanism, a natural pain control or analgesic system exists within the brain and spinal cord. Three components of this analgesic system have been identified: descending pathways, opioid receptors, and endogenous analgesics.

It is believed that activation of the pain receptors and ascending fibres by a harmful stimulus activates the pain control or analgesic system. This involves special receptors referred to as opiate receptors, which are found primarily in three central nervous system sites: midbrain periaqueductal grey matter, costroventral medulla and the dorsal horns of the spinal cord. Three classes of opioid receptor sites have been identified and these sites have practical application for the effective use of opioid analgesics such as morphine, for it is these receptors that opioid analgesics bind to chemically to produce their effect. Table 9.1 lists the three opioid receptor sites and their activities.

The brain produces endogenous analgesics in the form of enkephalins and endorphins which possess morphine-like action. The enkephalins, like the opiate receptors, are found mainly in the areas of the brain and spinal cord associated with pain control. Enkephalins are short-acting and probably act at the synaptic level. The endorphins, which are longer-acting (half-life 4 hours), have been isolated from the pituitary gland and the hypothalamus. The enkephalins and the endorphins are presumed to function as excitatory transmitter substances that activate portions of the brain's analgesic system. The concentrations of enkephalins and endorphins increase following electrical stimulation of the brain stem.

Knowledge of the opiate receptors, the endogenous analgesics and other neurotransmitters in the nervous system provides direction for more effective pharmacological control of pain and provides rationale for physiological and psychological techniques of pain management.

The pain sensation has two components: perception and responses.

Pain Perception and Pain Tolerance

Pain perception may be defined as the least experience of pain that a person can recognize. Simply, it is the point at which a given stimulus is felt as painful, and the amount of pain felt beyond that point. Qualifying the type of pain and relating it to various stimuli are learned experiences. The child gradually learns to associate the unpleasant feeling with objects and situations that cause pain.

From the previous descriptions of pain mechanisms, it is evident that pain perception is a complex process with a number of influences affecting impulse transmission and ultimately perception. Both physical and mental (thoughts and feelings) responses contribute to pain perception as well as pain tolerance.

Pain tolerance is the duration or intensity of pain that a person is willing to endure (McCaffery and Beebe, 1989). Pain tolerance varies between patients, and in an individual patient from one situation to another. Pain tolerance may decrease with prolonged exposure to

pain; pain tolerance may increase in response to an individual's concerns about analgesia. For example, a mother may tolerate pain during childbirth.

Pain Responses

Individuals vary not only in pain perception and pain tolerance, but in their response to pain. These responses or expressions of pain may be physical (skeletal muscle and autonomic nervous system), behavioural (changes in ambulation or sleep pattern), vocal (crying or calling out), as well as verbal descriptions of pain.

MUSCLE RESPONSES

Skeletal muscle reaction may be the immediate withdrawal reflex (cited previously), involuntary contraction, or increased tone in an attempt to splint or immobilize the affected part (e.g. rigidity of the abdomen). The individual may support or rub the part, change position frequently, clench fists, rock or pace back and forth or toss about. Voluntary muscle activity may also be involved in correcting the situation when the individual removes the offending object, treats the site or seeks assistance.

AUTONOMIC NERVOUS SYSTEM RESPONSES

The physiological responses seen most commonly in acute pain are mediated by sympathetic innervation and the secretion of adrenaline. Superficial vasoconstriction occurs; the blood supply to the skeletal muscles and brain is increased as a defence mechanism; the blood pressure, pulse and respirations increase; salivary secretion and gastrointestinal activity decrease; perspiration increases, and the pupils dilate. The individual manifests pallor, cold clammy skin and dry lips and mouth.

If the pain is deep, severe and prolonged, the above reactions may not develop and the patient may exhibit

Table 9.1 Summary of actions at opioid receptor sites.

Opioid receptor site	Activity	Drug Action	
		Agonist (on)	Antagonist (off)
Mu (μ)	Analgesia, respiratory depression, physical dependence, tolerance, constipation, euphoria	Pure: e.g. morphine, methadone, codeine, pethidine Partial: buprenorphine (Temgesic)	Pure: naloxone (Narcan) Partial: nalbuphine (Nubain), pentazocine (Fortral)
Kappa (κ)	Analgesia, sedation, no physical dependence, no respiratory depression	Buprenorphine (Temgesic), nalbuphine (Nubain), pentazocine (Fortral)	Pure: naloxone (Narcan)
Sigma (σ)	Vasomotor stimulation, psychomimetic effects (e.g. hallucinations, paranoia)	Pentazocine	Antagonists not very effective at this site.

Modified from McCaffery and Beebe (1989) with permission.

shock and extreme weakness; the blood pressure falls, the pulse weakens and nausea and vomiting may occur. In chronic pain, the body adapts and these physiological indicators of pain are often absent, thus limiting the value of physical measures in assessing chronic pain.

BEHAVIOURAL, VOCAL AND VERBAL RESPONSES

Even if the intensity and the nature of the pain stimulus could be determined as the same for several persons, the type and degree of response is likely to vary considerably because of individual differences in psychological makeup. The nature of a person's psychological reactions is determined, to a large extent, by past experiences and the degree of threat and frustration inherent in the pain. Some may cry or call out or use verbal expressions of suffering and fear and may further indicate their distress by restlessness and purposeless movements. Others may be very stoical, remain still and 'suffer in silence'.

Factors which may influence patients' responses include the following:

1. *Meaning of the pain.* The most important factor affecting an individual's reaction to pain is the meaning the individual ascribes to the experience. In a frequently cited study by Becher (1946), wounded soldiers' reduced analgesic needs were related to the meaning of their injury and subsequent removal from battle. The patient who fears he or she has cancer may manifest greater pain reaction until it is learnt that the biopsy report is negative.

2. *Emotional state.* Anxiety and depression can lower the pain threshold, increasing the patient's perception of the pain. Antidepressants can be used to help reduce the pain in a patient who is clinically depressed. Anxiety may be related to the illness or treatment, to the anticipation of pain to come, or to other problems not related to the illness, such as home or work concerns. Providing information about a patient's condition and treatment can help reduce anxiety; Hayward (1975) showed that requirements for postoperative analgesics can be reduced in patients who are given specific information about the nature of the pain they are likely to experience postoperatively.

3. *Distraction.* Reactions as well as perception are influenced by the amount of the patient's attention that is focused on the pain. If a situation commands considerable concentration on the part of the individual or creates pleasurable emotion, pain responses are minimized. The person actively engaged in competitive sport may not even be aware of the pain of an injury received. But if the patient focuses the whole attention on the discomfort, reactions are more pronounced.

4. *Sociocultural background.* An individual's responses are conditioned by social and cultural attitudes to pain. Some learn from those around them that pain is to be endured without obvious emotional reactions. If others have been accustomed to persons in pain exhibiting outward responses which are accepted and which receive attention, they consciously or unconsciously develop a similar pattern of response. Although cultural patterns may be identified, it is important to recognize individual differences and not stereotype.

5. *Previous pain experience.* Responses may be either increased or decreased by the memory of previous pain. Fear of a repetition of former severe suffering may produce marked outward reactions. With some, a greater tolerance and resignation may develop.

6. *Physical condition.* Psychological reactions are usually greater in weak and fatigued persons. For instance, the obstetric patient whose labour is prolonged may be quite calm and uncomplaining at first, but as she becomes tired and anxious that something is wrong, her pain becomes less tolerable.

7. *Intensity and duration of pain.* If the pain stimulus is very intense, the individual feels more threatened and may find it difficult to control emotional responses, even become quite disorganized. Similarly, pain of long duration is wearying and may initiate more overt reactions; on the other hand, the patient may become more resigned to the pain and take the attitude that it has to be lived with.

INTERDEPENDENCE OF PHYSIOLOGICAL AND PSYCHOLOGICAL RESPONSES TO PAIN

The emotional components of pain are interdependent with the physiological mechanisms of pain transmission and control. Both may aggravate the pain and increase the complexity and intensity of the responses. Anxiety can result from pain and in turn anxiety may intensify the pain and a vicious circle develops. Physical and social functioning may be altered by the pain experience, leading to feelings of helplessness, isolation, fear and anxiety. Unless the cycle is interrupted these factors, singly or collectively, will continue to increase pain perception and intensity.

Chronic pain leads to endorphin depletion, which results in a decrease in the pain perception threshold and the tolerance threshold. Persistent pain may also cause loss of sleep and appetite, leading to general fatigue and disability. Uncontrolled pain frequently leads to disruptions in the family, social life and work; physiological changes lead to inefficient function and increased psychological responses to pain.

Types of Pain

Some of the more common terms used to classify pain are as follows:

Acute pain is time-limited and generally has a defined cause and purpose. It may be mild, moderate or severe in nature and is usually sudden in onset.

Chronic pain is a complex physiological and psychological phenomenon that causes varying degrees of disability in a large portion of the population. It may begin as acute pain but it persists over an extended period of time, usually at least 6 months. The pain may be mild, moderate or severe and may be intermittent or continuous. Chronic pain is classified as malignant or non-malignant in origin. The cause may be unknown or if identified cannot be eliminated. The associated disruption in the individual's functions and life-style frequently leads to extreme fears, depression and debilitation.

Acute and chronic pain are quite different; acute pain may serve as a warning of disease or damage, chronic pain has no useful function. As mentioned earlier, responses to these two types of pain may be quite different. The principles of management for acute and chronic pain are different.

Superficial pain occurs when the receptors in surface tissues are stimulated. Conversely, *deep pain* arises from deeper tissues. Deep pain is divided anatomically into *splanchnic*, which refers to pain in the viscera, and deep *somatic* referring to pain in deep structures other than the viscera, such as muscles, tendons, joints and periosteum.

Localized pain arises directly from the site of the disturbance. *Referred pain* is that which is felt in a part of the body which is remote from the actual point of stimulation. The impulses usually arise in an organ, but the pain is projected to a surface area of the body. A classic example of referred pain is that associated with angina pectoris; the pain originates in the heart muscle as a result of ischaemia, but it may be experienced in the midsternal region, the base of the neck and down the left arm. Pain arising in the gallbladder or bile ducts may be referred to the epigastrium and the right scapular region. Referred pain may also be secondary to reflex muscular spasm. The muscle spasm originates as a reflex response to pain signals elsewhere in the body, as seen when lumbar muscles go into spasm as a result of severe ureteric pain.

It is suggested that the fibres carrying the pain impulses from the viscera and those from peripheral tissues converge upon the same neurone within the spinal cord. The impulses are then interpreted as coming from the superficial area because of previous pain experience.

Projected pain occurs when impulses are set up at some point along the pain pathway beyond the peripheral pain receptors. The pain is perceived as arising at the site of the pain receptors served by the pathway in which the pain originated. A person who has had an amputation may experience what is referred to as *phantom limb pain*. Stimuli arising from the stump may be localized on the basis of the previously established body image, and as a result the pain is projected to the portion of the limb that was removed.

Persistent, severe pain that cannot be effectively controlled by the usual medications is referred to as *intractable pain*.

Headache is a frequent discomfort experienced by many persons, and applies to the pain sensation that is perceived as being in the cranial vault (i.e. facial pain, toothache and earache are excluded). Headache is a common complaint in many illnesses in which the primary disturbance is quite remote from the head.

The pain receptors within the cranium occur in the walls of the arteries and in the meninges. The actual brain tissue is devoid of pain receptors. Headache may originate with tension or spasm of associated muscles at the back of the neck. Extracranial pain is usually well localized to the area where superficial pain receptors are being stimulated.

Psychogenic pain is that experienced when there is no detectable organic lesion or peripheral stimulation. It is thought that the pain is the conversion and physical expression of a distressing psychic disturbance or problem. It must be remembered that the discomfort is very real to the individual and that efforts must be made to provide relief. Psychogenic pain is thought to be very rare.

NURSING MANAGEMENT

The nurse plays an important role in the identification of pain and pain management. As Copp (1985) states:

'Pain is a bond between nurse and patient. Pain management is a pact between them. All too often, the physician does not hear the pleading as he exercises his option to leave the scene. The patient and nurse cannot leave as much as both of them might like to do so. How they work out pain management agreeable to both is the essence of nursing care.'

Although we tend to focus on the management of the pain itself, nursing has an important role in anticipating and preventing pain, and in supporting patients who have been through a physically painful experience. It is the work of Hayward (1975), referred to earlier in this chapter, that has helped to highlight the importance of providing patients with information about anticipated pain. Appropriate information effectively communicated can do much to help provide a sense of control and minimize anxiety.

Advances in knowledge of the physiological and psychological dimensions of pain provide a challenge for the nurse to critically examine nursing practices in pain assessment and management. McCaffery and Beebe (1989) identify several misconceptions that hamper assessment of the patient with pain. Awareness of these misconceptions and of the facts as presently understood provides guidelines which promote effective, comprehensive care of the patient with pain (Table 9.2). Despite an increased emphasis on pain management and the important contributions of nurses like McCaffery, nurses continue to have deficits in their knowledge and misconceptions about pain assessment and management.

Assessment

Assessment is essential for diagnosis and for planning of pain control measures. Pain is difficult to measure because it is a subjective phenomenon. Only the person experiencing the pain knows its nature, intensity, location and what it means to them. Thus nursing has generally adopted McCaffery's definition of pain as 'pain is whatever the experiencing person says it is, existing whenever the experiencing person says it does' (McCaffery and Beebe, 1989).

Table 9.2 Misconceptions about assessment of patients who indicate they have pain.

Misconception	Correction
1. The health team is the authority about the existence and nature of the patient's pain sensation	The person with pain is the only authority about the existence and nature of that pain, since the sensation of pain can be felt only by the person who has it
2. Our personal values and intuition about the trustworthiness of others is a valuable tool in identifying whether a person is lying about a pain	Personal values and intuition do not constitute a professional approach to the patient with pain. The patient's credibility is not on trial
3. Pain is largely an emotional or psychological problem, especially in the patient who is highly anxious or depressed	Having an emotional reaction to pain does not mean that pain is caused by an emotional problem. If anxiety or depression is alleviated, the intensity of pain will not necessarily be any less
4. Lying about the existence of pain, malingering, is common	Very few people who say they have pain are lying about it. Outright fabrication of pain is considered rare
5. The patient who obtains benefits or preferential treatment because of pain is receiving secondary gain and does not hurt as much as he or she says or may not hurt at all	The patient who uses pain to advantage is not the same as a malingerer and may still hurt as much as stated
6. All real pain has an identifiable physical cause	All pain is real, regardless of its cause. Almost all pain has both physical and mental components. Pure psychogenic pain is rare
7. Visible signs, either physiological or behavioural, accompany pain and can be used to verify its existence and severity	Even with severe pain, periods of physiological and behavioural adaptation occur, leading to periods of minimal or no signs of pain. Lack of pain expression does not necessarily mean lack of pain. How must the patient act for us to believe he or she has pain?
8. Comparable physical stimuli produce comparable pain in different people. The severity and duration of pain can be predicted accurately for everyone on the basis of the stimuli for pain	Comparable stimuli in different people do *not* produce the same intensities of pain. Comparable stimuli in different people will produce different intensities of pain that last different periods. There is no direct and invariant relationship between any stimulus and the perception of pain
9. People with pain should be taught to have a high tolerance for pain. The more prolonged the pain or the more experience a person has with pain, the better is the tolerance for pain	Pain tolerance is the individual's unique response, varying between patients and varying in the same patient from one situation to another. People with prolonged pain tend to have an increasingly low pain tolerance. Respect for the patient's pain tolerance is crucial for adequate pain control
10. When the patient reports pain relief following a placebo, this means that the patient is a malingerer or that the pain is psychogenic	There is not a shred of evidence anywhere in the literature to justify using a placebo to diagnose malingering or psychogenic pain

From: McCaffery and Beebe (1989) with permission.

The assessment process should provide the nurse with an understanding of the patient's pain, as well as establishing the nurse as a partner in the patient's search for pain relief. Patient teaching is an integral part of assessment, as information is provided in clarifying the nurse's questions or responding to the patient's concerns. As patient discomfort is a source of stress to the family, it is important to involve the family and other members of the patient's support network in the pain assessment. If the patient's ability to speak for himself or herself is limited, it is imperative to involve the family.

A number of pain assessment tools have been described in the literature (Bagley et al, 1982; Melzack, 1987; McCaffery and Beebe, 1989) and there is some evidence that consistent use of these tools does improve pain control (Raiman, 1986; Walker et al, 1987; McMillan et al, 1988); in her study looking at the management of chronic cancer pain, Walker found the use of a pain chart to be a valuable tool for pain assessment for both patients and nurses.

As pain assessment is an ongoing process, a pain chart needs to include both a section for initial assessment and a section for continuing assessment. Pain assessment forms part of the overall nursing assessment of a

TO USE THIS CHART ask the patient to mark all his or her pains on the body diagram below. Label each site of pain with a letter (i.e. A, B, C etc.)

Then at each observation time ask the patient to assess:
1. the pain in each separate site since the last observation. Use the scale above the body diagram, and enter the number or letter in the appropriate column.
2. the pain overall since the last observation. Use the same scale and enter in the column marked OVERALL.

Next record what has been done to relieve the pain:
3. note any analgesic given since the last observation — stating name, dose, route, and time given.
4. tick any other nursing care or action taken to ease pain.

Finally, note any comment on pain from patient or nurse (use the back of the chart as well, if necessary) and initial the record.

Excruciating	5
Very severe	4
Severe	3
Moderate	2
Just noticeable	1
No pain at all	0
Patient sleeping	S

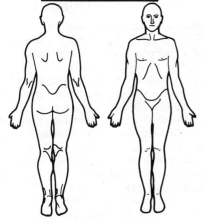

TIME	PAIN RATING		OVERALL	MEASURES TO RELIEVE PAIN	Specify where starred									
	BY SITES			ANALGESIC GIVEN (Name, dose, route, time)	Lifting	Turning	Massage	Distracting activities	Position change*	Additional aids*	Other*	COMMENTS FROM PATIENTS AND / OR STAFF	Initials
	A B C D E F G H												

Figure 9.2 The London Hospital Pain Chart. From the London Hospital.

patient, and the documents used to assess pain need to be integrated with other nursing assessment documents. It is important to avoid unnecessary, time-consuming duplication of material.

Pain assessment tools are biased towards verbal expression of pain. In situations where the patient cannot provide this information (e.g. unresponsive patients, infants, patients who do not speak the language, etc.), the nurse endeavours to gather the necessary information from discussion with the family and observations of the patient's physical condition and vocal and behavioural responses to pain, bearing in mind that chronic pain may alter these responses. It is also important for the nurse to appreciate that people in severe pain cannot respond to prolonged questioning about their pain and that a more detailed pain assessment can only be done when pain is relieved.

The information required for pain assessment include the following items.

Location
The location should be identified as specifically as possible. For example, abdominal pain may be localized to the lower or upper left or right quadrant, epigastrium or mid-abdomen. The site may be well defined or diffuse or the pain may radiate, involving a wide area. Encourage the person to identify the location of all the pains that are being experienced as people are often reluctant to disclose more than one or two 'pains'. Observing the pain locations on the patient's body will help localize the sites of pain as well as identify any physical changes at the site, such as swelling or discoloration.

Intensity
The intensity or severity of the pain experienced by the patient should be translated into words or numbers that can provide objective data for on-going assessment. Numerical scales such as 0–10 or 0–5 (Figure 9.2), with or without written descriptions, are often used. Also see Figure 10.6 in the next chapter. If patients have difficulty relating to these scales, descriptions of pain which are meaningful for the person can be developed and used consistently. For patients who speak a language

unfamiliar to the nursing staff, scales can be translated. The intensity of pain at present as well as the worst and the best level of pain in the past 24 hours, with accompanying circumstances, is required.

Quality

A description of the pain, using the patient's own words, is helpful in determining the origin of pain and possible pain relief measures. If the patient is unable to provide such descriptors, the descriptors used in the McGill Pain Questionnaire may be helpful (Melzack, 1987); for example, words such as throbbing, stabbing, cramping, hot-burning and aching.

Onset and duration

When the pain first began and how the pain has changed over time should be determined. If the pain varies over the course of a day, this variation and the circumstances surrounding the variation are described. The pattern of pain may be constant, intermittent, variable, etc.

Relief measures

The efficacy of measures used by the patient to relieve pain should be identified. This includes both those activities suggested by the medical and nursing staff, such as the use of analgesics, as well as measures employed by the patient himself, such as distraction, visualization, rubbing, etc. All drugs used by the patient for pain relief, including the exact amounts and the frequency, should be identified.

Exacerbating factors

Often patients may be comfortable at rest, but have difficulty moving due to pain. Activities which exacerbate the pain should be identified, as additional pain relief may be required at these times.

Associated symptoms

The impact of pain on the person's physical functioning should be explored. Associated symptoms can include nausea and vomiting, profuse perspiration, fainting, inability to perform usual functions, dulling of senses, apathy, clouding of consciousness, disorientation and inability to rest and sleep.

The meaning of pain

The nurse cannot assume that the patient who does not talk about pain is comfortable or that the patient who claims to be 'uncomfortable', 'feeling bad' or 'suffering' is referring to pain. It is important to have the patient clarify the meaning of the terms used.

A nursing history identifies social, cultural and religious beliefs that may influence responses to pain, past experiences with pain, how the pain has changed social and physical activities of daily living, and perceptions of how the pain may affect future plans. The medical diagnosis and its meaning to the patient should also be determined.

With chronic pain, patient's responses to pain will change depending on the stage of their disease and with the development of different patterns of coping. During the initial stages of a disease process patients may talk freely of their pain and discomfort, but with time and progression of the disease they may refrain from discussing it, either as a result of coping with their prognosis or in response to social pressure from others who stop listening to repeated descriptions.

Coping patterns

Information should be collected on how the patient is coping with the present pain and how the individual has coped with pain in the past. It is important for the nurse to know what measures have worked for this patient and if any measures have been taken that have not been effective in relieving pain.

Patient goals

Identification of the expectations and goals of the patient with regard to pain management and control is necessary before effective patient care can be planned. What information about the analgesic regimen does the patient require? Does the patient want to know about the pain associated with planned procedures? Is the patient motivated to acquire the knowledge, skills and changes in behaviour necessary to manage pain?

Planning

The information gathered in the nursing assessment is used to identify patient problems, for example: 'Alteration in comfort: pain'. Other problems may be identified related to either the pain itself or secondary to the management of the pain, such as constipation related to use of opioid analgesics. The problem statements, goals and interventions constitute the nursing care plan for the patient. Some hospitals are using standard care plans which can be individualized for each patient, but provide the nurse with a general framework for developing a care plan. Communication of the nursing care plan is important. The plan needs to be accessible, current, and individualized so it can be implemented by each nurse caring for the patient. Interventions performed by the patient should be included in the plan so that the nurse is aware and can support the patient. Including both non-pharmacological as well as pharmacological interventions is a challenge for nursing as we tend to rely heavily on pharmacological means of pain control (Anderson, 1982).

Although the nursing care plan emphasizes the nursing interventions, the plan should reflect the health care team's understanding of the cause of the patient's pain and the team's goal for pain control. As the patient is the most important member of this team, these goals need to be established with the patient. The interventions used and their expected outcomes will of course vary with the patient and the different types of pain. A patient embarking on a rehabilitation process after prolonged immobility with the expectation that total or partial function will be regained may tolerate more pain on movement than a patient with terminal malignant disease. The patient's definition of satisfactory pain control, including the desire to tolerate some pain in exchange for less analgesia, needs to be respected and supported by the use of alternative measures which the patient finds beneficial. Goals may need to be staged such that a patient in severe pain first achieves a pain-free night's sleep; secondly, is pain free at rest; and finally, is pain free upon movement.

GOALS

The Vancouver General Hospital has set patient outcomes for nursing interventions for pain control (Vancouver General Hospital, 1988):

1. The patient and family will demonstrate knowledge regarding the aetiology of the pain.
2. The patient will state that he or she is pain free or that the pain is tolerable.
3. Responses to pain decrease, as evidenced by:
   (a) Heart, respiratory rates and blood pressure within normal ranges for the patient.
   (b) Relaxation of skeletal muscles.
   (c) Absence of body postures associated with pain.
   (d) Absence of verbal responses such as crying, groaning or silence.
4. The patient and family will demonstrate knowledge of measures which minimize the development and perception of pain.
5. The patient and family will demonstrate knowledge of measures to manage the side-effects of interventions such as analgesia.

Although these outcomes will help the nurse in planning care for many patients, it must be remembered that for patients with chronic pain some of these outcomes will not be appropriate.

Nursing Intervention

Nursing interventions for the patient in pain can be broadly grouped into the following categories: (1) teaching activities to enhance the patient's understanding of the significance and meaning of the pain; (2) measures which alter either the sensory input or the patient's perception of pain; and (3) patient teaching to develop skills in self-management of pain.

All nursing interventions take place in the context of a nurse–patient relationship. Trust is an essential ingredient in this relationship. The patient must feel the nurse believes the descriptions of pain and is committed to helping. If necessary, the nurse should act as an advocate for the patient in relation to other members of the health team. The patient's family and significant others should be aware of the management plan and its expected outcomes. Their questions and concerns are also addressed; for example, encouraging social activities for distraction is not devaluing the pain, or explaining that long-term opiate use in malignant pain does not lead to drug addiction.

The patient in pain may feel isolated and cut off from the world around. The physical presence of the nurse can be reassuring. Sitting quietly with the patient can be helpful; if the nurse cannot be physically present for extended periods of time, family members or friends are encouraged to be with the patient. The nurse can also assure the patient of frequent return visits and encourage the use of the call-bell to summon help.

Listening to the patient allows the expression and sharing of fears and permits the patient to offer suggestions and participate in care planning and management. The effectiveness of listening and personal contact in decreasing pain perception depends on the quality of the nurse–patient relationship. Patients in acute pain may not have the energy to talk about it but may wish to do so once the pain has passed. Some patients, such as those with migraine headaches, may benefit most from quiet and isolation. The need for and the effectiveness of contact should be assessed on a continuous basis.

The confidence of the nurse in her ability to assist the patient is reflected in positive statements regarding the action and effectiveness of interventions such as medications. This positive attitude enhances cognitive control over pain perception, as demonstrated by the effectiveness of placebos in relieving pain in some situations. Nursing statements can influence a patient's subjective assessment of an experience.

KNOWLEDGE OF THE PURPOSE AND MEANING OF PAIN

The nurse should provide information about the patient's actual and anticipated pain and his physical condition and safety. Discussing this with the patient helps decrease anxiety, alleviate the actual pain, and alter its influence on future pain experiences. These factors promote the individual's well-being and security. Table 9.3 outlines objectives, rationale and possible content areas that the nurse should include in teaching patients about the significance and meaning of pain. Teaching strategies include identification of the meaning and significance of actual and anticipated events with the patient, exploration of the patient's feelings, and providing the patient with specific information. Assessment of the patient's level of anxiety and attention span enable the nurse to provide the needed information in simple, concise terms, the content being relevant to the patient at that time. As anxiety blocks learning, information provided in the teaching session may need to be repeated on several occasions.

INTERVENTIONS TO ALTER SENSORY INPUT AND REDUCE PAIN PERCEPTION

These interventions will be grouped and discussed using two broad categories: non-pharmacological and pharmacological interventions.

NON-PHARMACOLOGICAL INTERVENTIONS

The non-invasive non-pharmacological pain management techniques which may be offered by nurses are often used as adjuncts to the analgesic regimen, not alternatives.

Methods of anxiety reduction and altering perception of pain

Perception of pain and the anxiety associated with it are useful reactions to acute pain. They serve to protect the

Table 9.3 Patient teaching: the purpose and meaning of pain.

Objective	Rationale	Content
To promote patient safety and prevent further injury and pain	Pain has a protective purpose in signalling tissue damage. Prompt medical treatment may be life saving for the patient with an acute myocardial infarction. Preventative measures can avert further tissue damage for the patient with certain conditions	Factors precipitating the onset of pain The purpose and origin of the pain Specific techniques and measures to take to prevent pain, e.g. proper body mechanics Actions to take when pain occurs What to do if the pain becomes severe
To enable the patient to assume some control over the pain	Anticipation of the unknown leads to feelings of helplessness, isolation and fear Patient communciation and participation promotes understanding of the meaning of pain for the individual patient	What activities and situations are going to happen What the activities involve What will be expected of the patient What the patient can expect from the nurse and others What pain control measures are available to the patient The importance of communication of onset of pain and requesting intervention before the pain is intense Exploration of the patient's expectations, fears, anxieties and perceptions of anticipated events
To decrease anxiety	Prior knowledge of sensory experiences decreases fear and anxiety during the procedure Decreasing anxiety is thought to promote endorphin release, thus decreasing pain	Type and duration of sensations the patient may experience during procedures What will be expected of the patient What will be done to prevent and alleviate pain
To alter the impact of pain on future pain experience	Past experience with pain is known to influence individual responses to actual and anticipated pain	The cause and purpose of the pain The patient's actual reaction to the pain Measures which were effective and not effective in alleviating the pain Patient's feelings about the experience

patient from further injury, motivate the person to seek medical advice and help in diagnosing the cause of pain. Anxiety associated with chronic pain increases the pain responses, so the goal is to decrease the perception of the pain and the distress associated with it.

Measures taken to alter perception of pain and related anxiety are directed towards supporting the body's natural pain control mechanisms by stimulating endorphin release and modifying variables that influence the individual's tolerance to pain. In those situations where pain can be anticipated, nursing care is directed towards decreasing the anxiety associated with anticipation of pain. Prevention and control of pain are the goals when pain is present while alleviation of future pain is the aim afterwards.

Measures used to alter the perception of pain and reduce anxiety are relaxation, promoting sleep, distraction and imagery.

Relaxation
Pain perception may be modified by relaxation, which decreases secondary sources of pain such as muscle tension and fatigue. Relaxation techniques include: alternate tightening and relaxation of specific groups of muscles; breathing techniques; meditation; yoga; autogenic techniques; and biofeedback. (Biofeedback techniques provide the individual with sensory evidence, usually visual or auditory, of a body function.) Benson (1975) identified four elements essential to achieving relaxation, regardless of the technique used: a quiet environment, a mental device such as repeating a word, a passive attitude, a comfortable position. Muscular relaxation may also be promoted by massage, warm baths, ice packs, comfortable room temperature and quiet relaxing music for some persons. Knowledge of what has worked for the patient in the past helps the nurse and patient to select relaxation measures that are effective for that patient. Some hospitals and hospices have cassettes and videos on relaxation for patients to use.

Rest and sleep
Fatigue slows mental processes and decreases the energy available for coping strategies and repair

processes. Relaxation techniques and sedatives are helpful in promoting rest and sleep.

Care should be planned so that the patient is disturbed as little as possible. Consideration is given to the location of the patient in the ward, and noise in the environment is kept to a minimum; the more the patient is alerted, the more acutely he is aware of pain.

The bedtime routine to which the patient is accustomed should be followed as closely as possible to promote night sleep. Activities such as brushing the teeth, bedtime drinks, warm baths can be encouraged.

Distraction

Distraction helps focus attention away from the pain and, to some extent, any contact the nurse has with the patient which is not focused on the pain *per se*, for example, teaching relaxation, serves as distraction. It is very important for the nurse to demonstrate to the patient and family that the patient's ability for self-distraction does not indicate absence of pain. Distraction serves to increase pain tolerance; that is, it makes the pain more bearable. Naturally-occurring activities such as meals, radio, television and the arrival of visitors, etc. can be used as distraction. Humorous books and videos can be particularly useful as laughter may be helpful for pain control beyond just being a distraction. As well as activities, distraction can take the form of focusing on internal or external stimuli. If the pain is severe, the patient will need to exert considerable effort to achieve self-distraction; focusing on a familiar song or picture in the room can be done for a limited period of time, e.g. during venepunctures or childbirth. Using distraction during painful episodes can increase the patient's sense of control over the pain.

Imagery and visualization

Imagery is the process of using one's imagination to create mental images or internal representations through the senses of sight, sound, taste, smell and touch. Imagery can be used for distraction, relaxation, or to produce an image of pain relief. Imagery for pain relief can take many forms, including mentally replacing the sensation of warmth for burning or more elaborate visualizations such as the ball of healing energy (McCaffrey and Beebe, 1989). Consideration needs to be given to the appropriateness of imagery for the patient; for example, patients who are hallucinating should not use imagery.

Removal of the cause

Although most nursing interventions are directed at altering sensation or modifying perception of pain, the goals of medical intervention, when possible, are the diagnosis and treatment of the causes of pain (an alteration in body structure and function) and/or modifying the body responses producing pain. For example, angina due to coronary artery disease might be corrected by coronary bypass surgery and drugs to enhance coronary circulation. In those situations, where medical intervention can remove the cause of pain, this approach is the most effective means of altering sensory input. Physical removal of a splinter, bowel protocols to relieve discomfort due to constipation, or the removal of distending gas by means of a rectal tube may be the only measures necessary in some situations.

Positioning

A change of position may provide some relief for the patient by reducing the pressure and tension on the affected area. Venous and lymphatic drainage are promoted in order to decrease the accumulation of fluid in the tissue and thereby relieve pain. Adequate assistance and extreme gentleness are necessary when turning or moving the patient. The patient should be moved slowly, and support provided for the painful area. It is often helpful to ask the patient how the movement can be made least distressing for him. Good body alignment contributes to comfort by eliminating tension and hyperextension. A turning programme developed with the patient and posted at the bedside can ensure frequent turns take place. Support and elevation of a painful limb on a pillow or the use of support bandages or plaster casts will be helpful.

There are a number of specialized beds, such as Clinitron and alternating pressure mattresses, and wheelchair seats available which enhance comfort and reduce the risk to pressure areas. The input of health team members such as occupational therapists and physiotherapists is very helpful in determining proper positioning, transfer techniques and assistive devices.

Cutaneous stimulation

Cutaneous stimulation is defined as 'stimulating the skin for purposes of relieving the pain' (McCaffery and Beebe, 1989). Although the exact nature of the method by which cutaneous stimulation provides pain relief is not known, it is generally accepted that the gate control theory provides a rationale for its use. That is, stimulation activates large diameter fibres, thus inhibiting small diameter fibre transmission. These measures also increase the body's natural mechanisms for pain modulation and control. McCaffery and Beebe describe several methods of cutaneous stimulation including massage, application of heat and cold, menthol application and transcutaneous electrical nerve stimulation (TENS). In a few circumstances cutaneous stimulation may be medically contraindicated and advice should be sought from the patient's doctor before embarking upon a programme of pain relief which includes one of these techniques. Any of these techniques, however, can be carried out by the nurse and none are difficult to use. In selecting the most appropriate type of cutaneous stimulation, the nurse would consider the type and location of pain; feasibility in terms of time, cost, etc; and patient preferences. An open mind and a willingness to experiment on the part of the nurse and patient are important. Cutaneous stimulation can be applied by the patient and/or family as well as the nurse and thus can provide for increased patient control and family participation in care. Focusing on these techniques may also provide distraction and promote relaxation. Thus the therapeutic effects and advantages of cutaneous stimulation, as with other techniques, are multifaceted and evaluation of the techniques is thus difficult.

Massage

Rubbing a painful part occurs instinctively. The immediate response to striking an elbow is to hold it and rub the part. The nurse can effectively utilize this technique to help alleviate a patient's pain and teach the technique to the patient and family. Massage may involve a local partial area such as the elbow or cover areas of skin such as the back, feet and hands. Techniques include long, smooth, firm strokes or circular motions, or light, brisk movements. The hands should be warm and an oil used to facilitate movement. Massage is contraindicated for abdominal pain, over open skin lesions and when a thrombus is suspected such as in phlebitis or when there are extensive bony metastases.

Pressure

The application of pressure over the injury or at acupuncture points produces a numbing effect as well as decreasing the blood supply to the area. Pressure may be applied using the hand, firm objects or using the thumb and fingers to apply pressure and massage over acupuncture or trigger points. The services of a trained acupuncturist are now available in certain hospitals and hospices.

Thermal applications

The application of moist or dry heat or cold may produce relief of pain. The effects of heat are the relaxation of muscle tension or spasm and the increased rate of blood flow through the area. Precautions should be taken to prevent burning, since the patient in pain may be less sensitive to excessive heat.

Cold applications stimulate constriction of the local blood vessels and reduce the amount of blood in the area and the accumulation of tissue fluid (lymph). This diminishes the painful swelling and congestion in the affected area. Cold also reduces the sensitivity of the pain receptors. For these reasons, it is better to apply cold immediately after an injury. Both heat and cold are helpful for muscle spasms, and in some situations are used alternately.

Menthol application

Menthol acts as a counterirritant and therefore relieves pain by creating a cutaneous sensation of either warmth or coolness. Commercial preparations containing menthol can be purchased and are generally used for arthritis or muscular aches and pains.

Electrical stimulation

Electrical stimulation of peripheral nerves is used for the relief of musculoskeletal pain and a variety of chronic pain conditions. This is referred to as TENS (transcutaneous electrical nerve stimulation). Electrodes are applied to the surface of the skin or implanted in an area of contact with a major sensory pathway. An electric current is discharged into the electrode and produces stimulation of large afferent nerve fibres. Endorphin release is activated and small fibre transmission is blocked. Most TENS machines are designed to be operated by the patient, giving him control over his pain and its management. Symptom-control specialist nurses, physiotherapists and pain clinics can often provide specialist knowledge for nurses and patients on the use of TENS machines.

Electrical stimulation may be used for relief of chronic pain by implanting the electrode in the spine so that the impulses enter the posterior column directly. The operative procedure for implanting the electrode of the posterior column stimulator involves open surgery and a laminectomy.

PHARMACOLOGICAL METHODS OF PAIN CONTROL

The drugs used to relieve pain work by altering pain sensation, depressing pain perception or modifying the patient's response to pain. As the nurse has considerable control over and responsibility for the effective use of medicines to reduce pain, knowledge of the drugs used in pain control, their routes of administration and side-effects is needed. General principles for effective use of medications include: selecting drugs based on the cause and intensity of pain, use of a preventive approach, use of oral preparations whenever possible and titrating doses to achieve effective analgesia. The preventive approach is critical to effective pain control; if pain is constant, analgesia needs to be given routinely at intervals based on the drug's particular duration of action. 'PRN' prescriptions are not appropriate for continuous pain. If pain is episodic and a 'PRN' approach is appropriately being used, analgesia must be given as soon as pain begins rather than waiting until pain is severe.

Drugs used in pain control can be broadly categorized into analgesics and adjuvant therapy. Analgesics are drugs which directly induce a state of analgesia (being pain free), adjuvants have different actions in relieving pain. Analgesics can be divided into two broad groups, non-opiates and opiates. Non-opiate analgesics, for example paracetamol, tend to be milder pain killers, and opiates, for example morphine and papaveretum (Omnopon), are stronger pain killers. It is not possible in this chapter to discuss all of the very many analgesics available; pharmacy departments and the British National Formulary can be used to ensure that the nurse is adequately informed about the analgesics being administered. However, this chapter will look in more detail at some of the important groups of drugs used in pain control: opiate analgesics, adjuvant therapy and non-steroidal anti-inflammatory drugs (NSAIDs).

Non-steroidal anti-inflammatory drugs

The non-steroidal anti-inflammatory drugs are effective for mild–moderate pain and have three usual effects: analgesic, anti-inflammatory, and antipyretic. Although NSAIDs do not act in identical ways, they are generally

Table 9.4 Equal analgesia chart (equivalent dose compared to standard morphine 10 mg IM).

Drug/trade name	IM/sc dose (mg)	PO dose (mg)
Morphine sulphate	10	20–30
Hydromorphone —Dilaudid	2	4
Anileridine —Leritine	25	75
Oxycodone with ASA—Percodan with ACET—Percocet	—	10–15
Levorphanol tartrate —Levo-Dromoran	2	4
Codeine phosphate	120	200
Oxymorphone —Numorphan	1.5	—
Meperidine —Demerol	75	300
Methadone	10	20
Diamorphine —Heroin	5–8	10–15
*Nalbuphine —Nubain	10	—
*Pentazocine —Talwin	60	180

* Agonist/Antagonist

N.B. Equivalent Oral Morphine Doses
Dose of MS Contin q12h
= 3 × q4h dose of immediate-release morphine
= 4 × q3h dose of immediate-release morphine
= 6 × q2h dose of immediate-release morphine

considered to work at a peripheral level by inhibiting prostaglandin synthesis and thereby preventing sensitization of pain receptors to pain. NSAIDs are used as general analgesics as well as specifically for treatment of pain due to bony disease or damage, e.g. arthritis and bone metastases. There are a number of NSAIDs available such as aspirin, ibuprofen, naproxen (e.g. Naprosyn), ketoprofen and indomethacin (Indocid). The drug paracetamol has similar analgesic and antipyretic properties as NSAIDs, but does not have an anti-inflammatory effect. The general side-effects of NSAIDs include gastric irritation and ulceration, bleeding and renal insufficiency, thus limiting their use in some medical conditions. Medications to reduce gastric irritation such as antacids, cimetidine or ranitidine are often given concurrently with NSAIDs. The choice of a particular NSAID is usually based on the known side-effects and the desired route and frequency of ad-

ministration. Most NSAIDs are taken orally, in either short-acting or slow-release preparations, however, indomethacin and aspirin are available in suppository form. As NSAIDs have dosage ceilings, if the drug is ineffective at the optimal dosage this indicates a need to either change to another NSAID and/or combine the NSAID with a more potent analgesic.

Opiate analgesics

Opiate analgesics are used for the treatment of moderate to severe pain, and may be used in combination with a NSAID and/or a co-analgesic. Opiates work by binding to the opiate receptors in the central nervous system. As mentioned earlier, opiate analgesics vary in opiate receptor site binding (see Table 9.1) and thus vary in their action and side-effects. Titrating the dose of opiates is very important; there is no maximum dosage; the dose is limited by side-effects.

The opiate analgesics can be classified into three groups: the naturally-occurring opium derivatives (morphine, papaveretum and codeine), the semi-synthetic derivatives (oxycodone and diamorphine), and the entirely synthetic analgesics (pethidine and methadone). The most commonly used drugs for severe pain are morphine, diamorphine, pethidine and papaveretum and each of these potent analgesics will provide adequate analgesia if the appropriate dose is given at the proper interval. Opiate analgesics vary considerably in their potency and considerable care must be taken when converting a patient from one opiate to another or when changing the route of administration. Equianalgesia charts are available to help (Table 9.4). The choice of opiate analgesic is based on the type of pain (acute or chronic), ease of administration (both route and dosing interval), individual patient response to the drug, known side-effects and the length of anticipated use. Pethidine is not recommended for prolonged episodes of acute or chronic pain due to its short duration of action (2–3 hours), high incidence of side-effects due to the toxic metabolite norpethidine, and the need for high oral doses to achieve effective analgesia.

As individual titration for pain control is necessary, a wide range of dosage possibilities exists and ease of administration of the necessary dose is an important consideration. Morphine in particular is available in varying concentrations of short-acting tablets, sustained-release tablets, and liquid preparations which can be used for oral administration. Oxycodone and morphine suppositories are available. Diamorphine, morphine and papaveretum are all available for parenteral routes: subcutaneous injections or infusions via a syringe driver (which are preferable to intramuscular injections) and intravenous injections or continuous infusions via an intravenous infusion pump. Although oral administration is still the preferred route. The opiate analgesics may produce side-effects, the incidence and nature of which vary from one patient to another. Nausea, vomiting and constipation are common side-effects. The principle of laxative prescription should comprise a stool softener and a bowel stimulant to prevent constipation. Nausea and vomiting, if they occur, are most common during the first 2–3 days following the start of opiate therapy. Patients who experience nausea may require an antiemetic or a change to another opiate.

The more potent opiate analgesics can cause some depression of the respiratory centre. The rate and volume of respirations should be noted following the administration of these drugs, particularly in the cases of older patients, those known to have respiratory dysfunction and immediately postoperatively. However, patients on opiates develop tolerance to the respiratory depression and rarely develop problems. Naloxone can be used to reverse this side-effect, if necessary, although it should be noted that the patient's pain may return as naloxone blocks the pain receptor sites. Drowsiness may result from overdosage or may co-exist with pain; adequate analgesia without drowsiness is the optimal goal for pain management, although not always achievable.

The possibility of addiction (physical and emotional dependence on a drug) when a patient is receiving repeated doses of analgesics or sedatives is largely overestimated. Repeated doses of opiate analgesics, over 10 days, probably account for less than 1% of patients becoming addicted. Myths also abound with regard to prolonged use of opiate analgesics in patients with chronic pain. These patients are more likely to make repeated requests for analgesia if inadequate doses are given. Long-term use of analgesics may lead to a decreasing response to the prescribed dose (drug tolerance) as well as physical dependence; neither of these indicate addiction. Tolerance is managed by increasing dosage or switching to another analgesic, and physical dependence can be managed by slow withdrawal if pain should subside.

Adjuvant therapy

Adjuvant therapies used for pain relief may not have analgesic properties in their own right, but when used with conventional analgesics may significantly help in alleviating pain. Commonly used adjuvant therapies for pain relief include antidepressants, tranquillizers, anticonvulsants, muscle relaxants and steroids; it is only under a certain set of specific circumstances that the use of any one of these drugs is indicated.

Earlier in this chapter the fact that depression and anxiety can lower the patient's pain threshold, increasing the experience of pain, was discussed. Antidepressants such as imipramine (Tofranil) and anxiolytics such as diazepam (Valium) may be very effective in these circumstances. Similarly, lack of sleep can lower the pain threshold and a night sedative such as temazepan can be a useful adjuvant therapy in such cases.

When the cause of pain is known to be muscle spasm, a preparation that produces relaxation of the muscle tissue may be prescribed. For example, spasm of the smooth muscle tissue of the gastrointestinal tract, the urinary tract and biliary tract may be relieved by antispasmodic preparations, such as hyoscine butylbromide (Buscopan), atropine sulphate and propantheline bromide (Pro-Banthine). These drugs produce their effect by reducing the parasympathetic impulses to the visceral muscle.

Corticosteroids are used to relieve pain caused by raised intracranial pressure and nerve compression. Anticonvulsants, antihistamines and antibiotics may be used for pain relief for specific types of pain. Anaesthetic agents such as Difflam mouthwash provide relief for pain in the oral cavity. Entonox, a pain-relieving gas that acts rapidly (optimal effect within 2 minutes) is useful for brief, painful episodes.

'Co-analgesic' is an alternative term for drugs used as adjuvant therapy for pain relief.

Certain physical measures such as radiotherapy and nerve blocks can be used as adjuvants in pain control. Radiotherapy is very effective in helping relieve certain types of cancer pain, particularly pain caused by metastases in the bone.

MANAGEMENT OF ONE'S OWN EXPERIENCE OF PAIN

THE PATIENT WITH ACUTE PAIN

The patient with acute pain can influence the course of management and participate in the planning, implementation and evaluation of specific pain control measures. As has been established, knowledge of planned procedures and pain control measures, and the sensations anticipated during and after the procedures, not only decreases the patient's anxiety but also decreases the sense of helplessness and loss of control such situations present. Patients can influence management by communicating pain responses and informing carers of measures which have worked for them in the past and what has not been effective. Patients should be encouraged to participate in planning pain control measures and to evaluate the effect of these.

THE PATIENT WITH CHRONIC PAIN

Chronic pain frequently leads to major disruptions in all aspects of the individual's life. To effectively manage chronic pain, patients require knowledge of the pain, the pain management plan and coping skills.

Pain management, to be effective, must be multidimensional in approach. Pain clinics have been established to provide expertise in the management of chronic pain; for patients with chronic malignant pain, the resources of a support care/palliative care/hospice team may be extremely helpful. Working in the community, the Marie Curie and MacMillan nurses visit patients with advanced cancer at home to advise on pain relief and to offer support to the patient and family.

A teaching plan may be developed for the patient with chronic pain; selection of the content depends on the assessment of the patient, the patient's goals, and ability and willingness to participate. Examples of the content of the teaching plan and teaching–learning approaches follow.

Knowledge that the patient should receive

Pain

- Characteristics of the pain experience including the onset, duration, location, quality and intensity of the pain
- Factors that precipitate pain
- Patterns of pain

- Behavioural responses to pain
- Effects of the pain and pain responses on daily life and functioning
- The meaning of the pain, including recognition that the existence of chronic pain and impairment of bodily functions do not necessarily prevent the individual from living a meaningful and self-fulfilling life

Pain relief

- The technique and mode of action of various pain relief measures including medications, relaxation techniques, massage, biofeedback or electrical stimulation
- Alternative relief measures available
- The purpose of and expectations related to the psychological aspects of treatment
- The specific plan for pain relief developed for the patient
- Resources available to faciliate implementation of the plan
- Roles and responsibilities of health care professionals
- Expectations and responsibilities of the patient in implementing the plan

Rest and sleep

- The importance of receiving adequate rest and sleep
- Individualized plan to promote rest and establish or maintain a pattern for night sleep

Physical activity

- The benefits of increasing physical activity where possible
- Specific physical activities to be increased
- Physical activities to be decreased and avoided

Information may be provided to individuals or groups of patients. Group teaching is directed to patients with pain of similar aetiology and manifestations. Patients being taught in a group may share experiences and learn from others with similar problems. Individual sessions are also necessary for those participating in group classes to provide an opportunity to make the information applicable to the particular patient and situation, to discuss feelings, answer questions and set goals.

Skills

Many patients with chronic pain need to develop skill and dexterity in carrying out the planned pain relief techniques and to implement changes in their sleeping habits and physical activity. The physiotherapist and occupational therapist have major roles in rehabilitation, and it is the nurse's responsibility to involve these professionals at an early point in the physical rehabilitation programme.

The patient's day should be structured and focused on one step at a time. When one step has been successfully completed, the patient works towards achieving the next skill. Goals and expectations for each step are deter-mined by the patient, with mutual agreement of the health team. Active physical participation may not be possible or appropriate for some patients. Goals must be realistic and recognize the need to conserve the patient's energy and enhance his quality of life.

Feedback and reinforcement

Positive relationships between the patient and the nurse, the patient and other members of the health team, and within the health team promote an environment of trust and openness that is essential for the development and reinforcement of positive coping behaviours by the patient. The patient's rights to make decisions, whether one approves of the decisions or not, must be respected. The person who regains some control over his daily activities is usually more motivated to exert some control over his pain. Ongoing feedback and support are provided as the patient takes the initiative to learn new skills, increase activity and increase social interaction. The long-term treatment programme must include opportunities for the patient to practise at home and in the work environment, and the physiotherapist and occupational therapist will be involved in co-ordinating these major steps in the patient's rehabilitation programme.

Family members and relatives play an important role in reinforcing and encouraging behaviour conducive to improvement in daily functioning. They are given support and guidance as to how to best help the patient.

Evaluation

Evaluation of the effectiveness of nursing care provided to people in pain takes place on various levels:

- Firstly, the ongoing evaluation of care to the individual patient as an integral part of the nursing process. The nursing care plan is either continued or modified based on this evaluation.
- Secondly, evaluation of standards of care set as part of a unit or hospital's ongoing quality assurance programme. Hockley (1988) describes setting standards for pain control which include structure (characteristics of the organization, staffing patterns, etc.), process (the nursing actions, including teaching), and outcomes. Audits have been developed to review the adequacy of pain management.
- Thirdly, research concerning the effectiveness of interventions to improve pain management. Examples of areas of nursing research include pain assessment (Camp, 1987), effectiveness of nursing tools such as standard care plans (Donovan and Dillon, 1987) and patient education.

Ethical issues

Nurses can experience a number of ethical dilemmas in pain management. One of the most frequently cited is the concern that in order to provide adequate pain relief for terminally ill patients, nurses may be shortening the patients' lives. There is, however, no evidence to support this fear. The Hastings Centre has provided clear guidelines for nurses involved in providing palliation to terminally ill patients:

'Providing large quantities of narcotic analgesics does not constitute wrongful killing when the purpose is not to shorten the lives of these patients, but to alleviate their pain and suffering, and the alternatives have been carefully evaluated and this course found to serve the patient best ... There are no sound moral grounds for failing to provide adequate relief from pain to those who are dying and wish such relief.' (Hastings Centre Report, 1987)

SUMMARY

This chapter has emphasized the important role that nurses play in caring for the person in pain, identifying patients experiencing pain, facilitating communication with other members of the health care team, and encouraging patient participation in the decision making process. This chapter provided basic information on pain assessment and nursing interventions for pain management.

LEARNING ACTIVITIES

1. Review the pathways of pain transmission and their relevance to pharmacological and non-pharmacological approaches to pain management.
2. Consider your own biases about pain behaviour: how do you react when in pain and how do you expect others to act?
3. Complete a pain assessment on a patient experiencing pain, using either a standardized tool or developing your own tool.
4. Develop a nursing care plan for your patient experiencing pain including the patient's own techniques for managing pain.
5. Practise using a relaxation technique and then practise teaching the technique to a colleague.
6. Identify what patient education materials for pain management are available.

REFERENCES

Anderson J (1982) Nursing management of the cancer patient in pain: a review of the literature. *Cancer Nursing* **Feb.:** 33–41.

Bagley CS et al (1982) Pain management: a pilot project. *Cancer Nursing* **June:** 191–199.

Becher HK (1946) Pain in men wounded in battle. *Annals of Surgery* **123:** 96–105.

Benson T (1975) *The Relaxation Response.* New York: Avon.

Camp LD (1987) Comparison of medical, surgical and oncology patients' descriptions of pain and nurses' documentation of pain assessments. *Journal of Advanced Nursing* **12:** 593–598.

Copp LG (ed.) (1985) *Perspectives on Pain.* New York: Churchill Livingstone.

Donovan MI & Dillon P (1987) Incidence and characteristics of pain in a sample of hospitalized cancer patients. *Cancer Nursing* **10:** 85–92.

Guyton AC (1986) *Textbook of Medical Physiology.* 7th edn. Philadelphia: WB Saunders.

Hastings Centre Report (1987) *Guidelines on the Termination of Life-Sustaining Treatment and the Care of the Dying.* Hastings Centre.

Hayward J (1975) *Information: A Prescription Against Pain.* London.

Hockley J (1988) Setting standards for pain control. *Professional Nurse* **3:** 310–313.

McCaffery M & Beebe A (1989) *Pain: Clinical Manual for Nursing Practice.* Toronto: Mosby.

McMillan SC et al (1988) A validity and reliability study of two tools for assessing and managing cancer pain. *Oncology Nursing Forum* **15:** 735–741.

Melzack R (1987) The short-form McGill Pain Questionnaire. *Pain* **30:** 191–197.

Melzack R (1990) The tragedy of needless pain. *Scientific American* **262:** 27–33.

Melzack R & Wall P (1965) Pain mechanism: a new theory. *Science* **150:** 971–979.

Mohide EA et al (1988) Assessing the quality of cancer pain management. *Journal of Palliative Care* **4:** 9–15.

Raiman J (1986) Towards understanding pain, and planning for relief. *Nursing* **11:** 411–423.

Vancouver General Hospital (1988) Nursing protocol: Care and management of the patient with chronic cancer pain. Vancouver: Vancouver General Hospital.

Walker VA et al (1987) Pain assessment charts in the management of chronic cancer pain. *Palliative Medicine,* vol. 1. pp. 111–116.

Caring for the Patient with Cancer

10

OBJECTIVES

At the end of this chapter the reader should be able to:

- Identify the differences between benign and malignant neoplasms in terms of growth patterns, ability to recur and threat to the patient
- Describe the process and routes of metastasis
- Discuss the genetic, environmental, life-style and viral factors which are components of carcinogenesis
- Explain the role of nursing in primary and secondary cancer prevention; and the seven warning signs of cancer
- State the primary treatment modalities for cancer and their role in the treatment of cancer
- Discuss the common side-effects and toxicities of chemotherapy, radiotherapy, biological therapy and bone marrow transplantation
- State the nursing assessments and interventions for common side-effects and toxicities related to cancer therapies
- Differentiate between acute and chronic pain; list the components of a pain assessment
- Describe the principles of pharmacological and non-pharmacological management of pain
- Discuss the grief reaction and its implications for nurses
- Identify common psychosocial responses to cancer and the applicable nursing interventions
- Discuss the role of palliation in the care of the patient with advanced cancer; and supportive nursing behaviours
- Delineate the goals of rehabilitation in the care of cancer patients

---

Cancer is a disease but it is also a series of experiences that profoundly affect the daily living of both the person who has the cancer and those who share the experience. Nursing involvement in the care of the patient with cancer and the family encompasses patient education, assessment, monitoring, treatment and support, and requires knowledge of both the biomedical and psychosocial components of cancer care.

THE NATURE OF CANCER

An understanding of the biological principles involved in the development and spread of cancer and of their therapeutic implications is important for all professionals involved in the care of the patient with cancer and the family. A strong foundation in the principles of cancer biology facilitates understanding of cancer-related literature, interaction with other health care personnel, interpretation or reinforcement of explanations to patients, and effective decision making about nursing care.

Normally, the production of cells is a regulated process which allows for growth in early life and for the replacement of worn-out or damaged cells throughout life. The mechanisms for the initiation of

cell reproduction, and the control of that reproduction so that it does not exceed the needs of the organism, are not understood. Occasionally, the control of cell reproduction is lost in some cells in a particular area of the body and an excessive production occurs, forming an abnormal mass that is referred to as a neoplasm or new growth. The cells of the neoplasm serve no useful purpose and use nutrients and oxygen, causing deprivation in the host's normal tissues.

BENIGN NEOPLASMS

A benign neoplasm is considered much less of a threat to the host's life because it does not spread to other sites. It is usually possible to cure benign neoplastic disease by surgical removal of the mass.

Growth of a benign neoplasm is slow and tends to be expansive rather than invasive; the mass remains localized and is frequently encapsulated, and the cells may show little abnormality compared with those of the normal tissue from which they originated. When excised, it rarely recurs. Since a benign neoplasm is a space-occupying lesion, it may cause serious effects on neighbouring structures, depending on its size and location; in some instances it may obstruct blood vessels or a passageway or may cause pressure on vital tissues, leading to serious malfunction. Some benign lesions

Table 10.1 Differences between benign and malignant neoplasms.

	Benign	Malignant
Cells	Relatively normal and mature	Little resemblance to normal; poorly differentiated, atypical in size and shape, non-uniform, and immature
Growth	Slow and restricted. Non-invasive of surrounding tissue; expansive, pushing aside normal tissue	Usually rapid and unrestricted. Invasive of surrounding tissue
Spread	Remains localized. Usually encapsulated	Metastasizes via blood and lymph streams
Recurrence	Rarely recurs	Frequently recurs
Threat to host	Prognosis favourable. The effect depends on the size and location. May cause pressure on vital organs or obstruct a passageway, which is usually corrected by surgical excision of neoplasm	Threatens life by reason of its local destructive proliferation and formation of secondary neoplasms in other structures. Prognosis more favourable with early diagnosis and treatment, when cells show less departure from the normal and there is no metastasis

tend to become malignant if left untreated; examples are polyps in the intestine, papillomas of the bladder and larynx, and pigmented moles. Furthermore, some tissues may display cytological changes of malignancy but without any invasion of other structures, e.g. carcinoma-in-situ of the cervix.

MALIGNANT NEOPLASMS

A malignant neoplasm is a distinct threat to life by virtue of its ability to proliferate destructively into surrounding tissue and to other parts of the body. Some of the cells become detached from the primary mass and are carried via the blood or lymph to a distant area of the body where they set up colonies of the malignant cell (metastases). The neoplastic cells tend to grow and reproduce rapidly and change in structure and activity in varying degrees. Table 10.1 summarizes some of the differences between benign and malignant neoplasms.

In addition to being classified as malignant or benign, a neoplasm is also named according to the type of tissue involved.

CANCER

Cancer is a term commonly used to designate any disease that is a malignant neoplasm. Cancer is a group of diseases in which the mechanism within the cell and its microenvironment responsible for restraint of growth is defective, and therefore the cancer cell reproduces without regard for need (Marino, 1981a).

Malignant neoplasms have certain common characteristics, but there are also marked differences from one type to another because of the type of tissue involved, the location, and the degree to which the cells in the neoplasm depart from normal. They also differ as to signs and symptoms, effects on the host, rate of growth, metastasis, form of treatment used and their response to treatment.

Cancers are classified according to the type of tissue or cells from which they arise. The four main groups are those arising from the epithelium; connective tissue (including lymphoid and haemopoietic tissues); muscle; and nervous tissue. In addition, there are some neoplasms whose origin is uncertain, and anaplastic neoplasms whose cells bear no resemblance to any normal tissue.

Cancer begins as a localized disease, but when the cells commence invasion of surrounding tissues it may be referred to as invasive cancer. In the more advanced stages of the disease, cells become detached from the neoplasm and are carried by lymph or blood vessels to other parts of the body, where more cancer develops. Malignant cells may also spread by implantation or seeding within a body cavity. The serous fluid in the pleural or peritoneal cavities carries the tumour cells through the cavity. This process is described as metastasizing. Some tumours such as basal cell carcinomas and gliomas rarely metastasize, while others such as melanomas and lung carcinomas metastastize widely and are less invasive. The cells carried in the lymph may be trapped in lymph nodes near the original site, producing disease in the nodes and causing what is known as regional involvement. Eventually these areas of disease disseminate cancer cells to other parts.

Recent experimental studies have supported clinical observations that certain tumours consistently metastasize to particular organs. Although lung, liver, bone and brain are the most common sites of metastasis, many tumours have been observed to have unique patterns of metastasis that may include not only those common target organs but some more unusual sites as well.

The preferential distribution of metastasis is not random and is probably related to tumour cell characteristics that promote growth in some organs and not in others. Certain properties on the surfaces of tumour cells are probably responsible for the organ specificity of metastatic cells. In addition, it is thought that, although tumour cells may lodge in the capillary beds of multiple organs, certain microenvironmental characteristics determine whether tumour growth will be supported.

Specific and predictable patterns of lymphatic and/or haematogenous spread have been identified clinically for many tumours. For example testicular tumours generally favour the lymphatics as an initial route of spread. Once entry into the lymphatic channels has occurred, vascular spread follows, and the lungs are the most common distant target organ for this particular tumour.

Malignant neoplasms are graded according to the degree of differentiation of the tumour cells and the estimated rate of growth of the tumour. A numerical system of three or four grades is commonly used, with the higher numbers indicating a greater degree of undifferentiation and a more aggressive type of tumour. Staging refers to the clinical evaluation of the extent of the cancer. The staging system takes account of primary tumour size; local and regional lymph node involvement; and evidence and extent of metastatic deposits. Roman numerals I to IV are used to indicate the stage, with the highest numerals indicating most extensive disease.

CANCER AS A CHRONIC ILLNESS

Advances in the treatment of cancer, together with the general application of the concept of a health–illness continuum, has resulted in a changing perception of the illness cancer. No longer is cancer regarded as a universally fatal disease, but rather a group of chronic diseases with clinically distinct presentations and differing biological behaviour and clinical manifestations, for which effective treatment exists. These diseases are still very serious and life-threatening, but the hopelessness that prevailed in earlier periods is not as generally evident today.

HISTORY

Malignant diseases are older than man, and they are known to affect not only the animal kingdom but plant life as well. Evidence of cancer has been noted and recorded since as long ago as 2500 BC. The first reported 'chemically induced' tumours were scrotal cancers in chimney sweeps in England. Sir Percival Potts provided the classic description of these tumours in 1775. In 1827 Meckel traced the origin of buccal carcinoma to the oral epithelium. Johannes Müller established that there were cellular differences in tumours in 1838, and in 1839 Schwann established the cell theory of animal structure.

Although chemotherapy has been recognized since the early days of medicine, it was not until the late 1940s that investigations led to the development of chemotherapeutic agents that were effective in the treatment of primary and disseminated disease. Since then a programme of worldwide research has been established to accelerate progress in the treatment of cancer with chemotherapy and, of course, radiotherapy.

Modern techniques in anaesthesia, the development of broad-spectrum antibiotics, and perfected surgical techniques have all been instrumental in lowering mortality from cancer. Continued improvements in prosthetic devices have enabled patients who have undergone laryngectomy, mastectomy or colostomy to live more normal lives.

INCIDENCE AND TRENDS

Cancer diseases account for a large number of deaths each year. They are second only to heart disease as a killer in the United Kingdom, and it is estimated that one out of every four persons develops cancer. In 1985, 119 960 men and 133 150 women in the UK were newly registered as having cancer. Figure 10.1 shows the ten most common cancers for both men and women. During 1988, over 160 000 people died from cancer (Cancer Research Campaign, 1988). Figure 10.2 shows the ten most common causes of cancer deaths. Statistics indicate that cancer accounts for an increasing number of deaths. Factors which have probably contributed to the increase include: (1) a greater number of persons living to an older age, which increases cancer susceptibility; (2) the increased risk of developing certain cancers because of greater exposure to specific carcinogens (e.g. cigarette smoking); (3) new and improved diagnostic procedures; and (4) a decrease in deaths from diseases such as pneumonia, scarlet fever and other acute infections.

Statistics of the incidence of certain types of cancer may provide clues to predisposing factors and causes in relation to the environment, occupations, health habits and customs, and may also indicate the value of preventive and early detection programmes. For instance, in the United States, the decrease in uterine cancer may be correlated with the increasing practice of an annual Papanicolaou cervical smear (Pap test). The increase in cancer of the respiratory tract, particularly lung cancer, is attributed to increased cigarette smoking in both sexes.

The incidence of cancer varies with age. It occurs in infants and children as well as adults, but increases with advancing age. Leukaemia and neoplasms of the central nervous system account for many of the malignancies occurring in children up to 5 years of age. Between the ages of 5 and 15 years there is a lesser incidence, but from age 15 on there is a steady increase.

Although the overall incidence of cancer has increased, the survival rate of individuals diagnosed as having cancer has also increased over the past 20 years. This increase in survival of 5 years following diagnosis is attributed primarily to improved treatment and management of patients and to early diagnosis of the cancer. Figure 10.3 shows the relative survival for males and females diagnosed in 1981.

CARCINOGENESIS

Although a number of theories have been proposed, no single unifying hypothesis has been offered to explain carcinogenesis, and the exact cause of most human cancers remains unknown. Neoplastic transformation is thought to be a multistep process, and researchers have been successful in identifying risk factors and agents that may act as cofactors in this process.

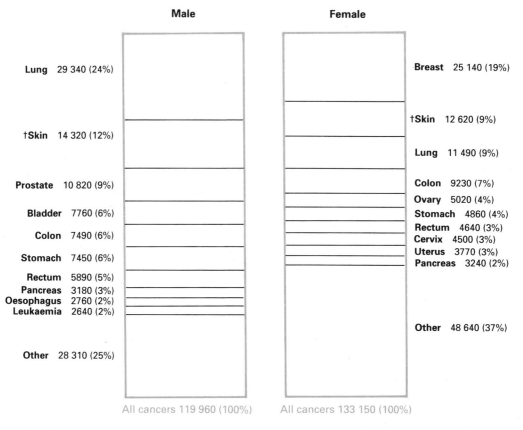

Figure 10.1 Ten most common cancers per new cases registered in the UK in 1985. From Cancer Statistics–Registrations, 1985, HMSO, 1990.

It has been generally accepted that neoplastic transformation results from some genetic alteration in the cell, which in turn deregulates the control of cell proliferation. The controversey has centred around the question of what stimuli induce the necessary transformation in the DNA of a cell. Genetic, environmental, life-style and viral factors have all been implicated as components of carcinogenesis.

Smith and Thier (1985) indicate that chromosomal disorders involving the absence, duplication or rearrangement of long segments of the genetic materials may influence the development of cancer. For example, the risk of leukaemia is 11 times greater in individuals with Down's syndrome (each cell contains an extra chromosome). The incidence of retinoblastoma is greater in children born without part of a chromosome. Single-gene disorders are known to predispose to neoplasia of the haematopoietic and lymphoreticular system. Risks among relatives of patients with certain cancers have been shown to be statistically higher than in comparable control families or in the general population. The influences of environmental factors have been difficult to separate from a possible genetic aetiological component but, in general, these familial patterns appear to reflect the genetically transmitted susceptibility to neoplasia. Research on oncogenes,

which have the potential to cause cancer when activated, will hopefully provide answers on the aetiology of cancer and lead to more effective preventive, diagnostic and treatment techniques.

An excessive concentration of certain hormones appears to influence the change of some normal cells to malignant ones. Such cancers are said to be hormone dependent and manifest changes in growth activity when the concentration of certain hormones is altered. For instance the ovarian oestrogenic hormones favour the growth of some breast cancers, while androgens (male hormones) tend to suppress their progress. Cancer has been produced experimentally in mice by the injection of oestrogen. Whether the hormone is the primary incitant in hormone-supported cancer in humans or whether it simply produces a tissue susceptibility to viral, chemical or physical carcinogens is not known.

In the last decade there has been renewed interest in cancer immunology. Considerable attention and support are being given to the concept that the abnormal cells contain substances that are foreign to the host's normal body cells and are therefore antigenic. These neoplastic antigens prompt an immune response in the host that controls the development, growth and spread of the disease. There is evidence that spontaneous regression and disappearance of the neoplasm have occurred when

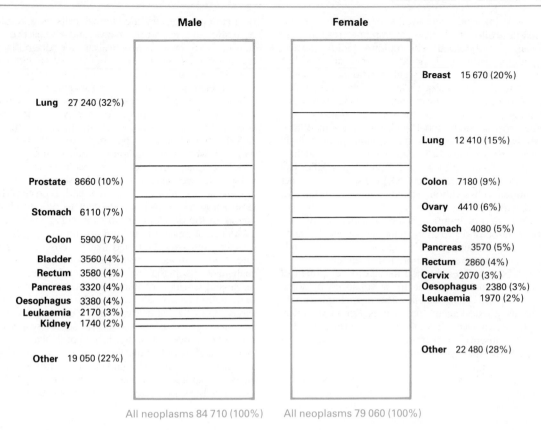

Figure 10.2 Ten most common causes of cancer deaths registered in the UK in 1989. From Cancer Research Campaign Annual Report 1990.

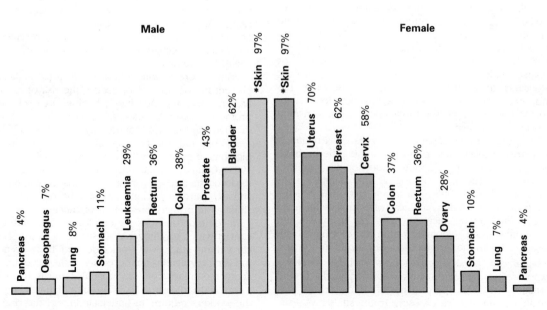

Figure 10.3 Five-year relative survival %—England and Wales 1981 (adjusted for non-cancer deaths). From Cancer Research Campaign, 1988.

the host's immune mechanisms have destroyed the neoplastic cells. If the host's immune response is deficient, the abnormal cells multiply rapidly, invade surrounding tissues and spread to distant areas. It has been observed that there is a higher incidence of cancer in persons with an inadequate immune response, which may be partly due to primary immunodeficiency disease, immunosuppressive drugs, radiation exposure or the ageing process (Smith and Thier, 1985; Sabiston, 1986).

Sabiston (1986) suggests that tumour immunity is mediated by a variety of immune mechanisms, including: humoral antibodies; T and B lymphocytes; killer (K) lymphoid cells; natural killer (NK) cells, which can act on tumour cells without specific immunization; and macrophages.

Investigation of immune factors in cancer continues, with the hope of determining why the patient's defence mechanisms fail and of providing information that aids in cancer prevention, detection and treatment.

It has been well established that the development of most cancer diseases is due to or enhanced by some factors in the environment. These include certain chemicals, physical agents and viruses. Certain chemical and physical agents and some viruses are recognized as having a causative or contributory role. A number of chemicals in the environment are being studied as possible carcinogens and a number have been determined to be offenders. The latter include asbestos, vinyl chlorides, aniline dyes and benzene. Many of these have been recognized through the high incidence of cancer associated with occupational exposure to the specific chemical. For example, persons working with an aniline dye, which may be absorbed through the skin and excreted in the urine, show a high incidence of urinary bladder cancer. A causative relationship has also been established between asbestos and lung cancer. Insecticides and herbicides are highly suspect, and animal growth-stimulating hormones and some food additives are being investigated as potential carcinogens. Cigarette smoking as a cause of cancer of the respiratory tract, and a contributor to cancer of the bladder, has also been well documented. Air pollutants and involuntary or passive smoking (second-hand smoke) are also suspect, especially in relation to lung cancer. Research has indicated that there is usually a relatively long latent period between exposure to chemical carcinogens and cancer development.

The study of nutritional carcinogenesis is a relatively new area of investigation, and researching the problem of diet as a factor in tumour induction is a difficult process. To date, epidemiological and animal studies have provided the bulk of available information. High levels of dietary fat, nitrosamines, coffee, and deficiencies of fibre and certain micronutrients (e.g. vitamins A and C, riboflavin and selenium) within the diet have been associated with the development of cancers in humans.

Significant physical carcinogens include excessive exposure to the sun's rays, radiation and chronic irritation. A large percentage of skin cancers are attributed to excessive exposure to the sun's rays. Fair-skinned individuals with less natural pigmentation of the skin, and those whose occupation keeps them outdoors (e.g. farmers), appear to be more susceptible to neoplastic changes in the dermal cells as a result of excessive sun exposure. X-rays and radioactive substances have proved beneficial in the diagnosis and treatment of some diseases but repeated and heavy radiation exposure may lead to malignant neoplasia. The adverse effects may not be seen for quite a long period following irradiation, since the effects can be cumulative. Repeated exposures to even very low doses may eventually be of pathological significance. This was unfortunately found to be the case with personnel working with X-ray equipment before the need for more adequate shielding was recognized; many developed leukaemia or cancer of the skin.

Chronic irritation of an area and repeated tissue destruction and repair are thought to be contributory factors in the development of cancer. For example, the incidence of cancer of the lip is greater in pipe smokers.

Scientists have established that various types of RNA and DNA tumour viruses produce some forms of malignant neoplasia in experimental animals. The successful isolation of human viruses in some patients with leukaemia strongly supports the aetiological role of viruses in malignant disease, but the exact viral action in producing cancer is not known. Viruses are suspected in the development of some forms of leukaemia, lymphomas and nasopharyngeal cancer, as well as Hodgkin's lymphoma. Viruses are known to cause warts and mucosal papillomas in man, and the human papilloma virus has been associated with cancer of the cervix.

PREVENTION AND EARLY DETECTION OF CANCER

Cancer nursing is directed towards the prevention and early detection of neoplasms as well as the care of the patient in treatment, recovery or advanced stage of cancer. At present, it is not possible to prevent all types of cancer but some cancers can be prevented by avoidance of recognized carcinogens and by altering health behaviours.

Primary prevention of cancer is activity taken to prevent the occurrence or reduce the risk of cancer in healthy persons. Activities in this area of health promotion include identifying risk factors for individuals and groups; counselling regarding risk factor reduction and cancer prevention activities; and implementing cancer prevention programmes (Park et al, 1985). Counselling individuals regarding the hazards of tobacco use, alcohol consumption, inadequate nutrition and exposure to sunlight are specific nursing responsibilities in primary prevention of cancer.

In some occupations the employees may have direct contact with a carcinogenic substance, such as asbestos, chromium, ether, vinyl chloride and benzyprene. In industry, regulations are necessary to protect employees and communities from carcinogenic hazards. In addition to protective measures for those in a high-risk situation, the workers require an understanding of the risks and the precautions that should be observed. They should be aware of early symptoms that must be reported promptly, and receive regular examinations. Some

Table 10.2   Early detection and screening activities.

Cancer	Detection and screening activity
Cervix/endometrium	Pap smear and pelvic examination
Breast	Mammography and breast examination
Colorectal	Digital rectal examination Stool occult blood test Proctosigmoidoscopy
Oropharyngeal	Self-examination of oral cavity Annual oral examination by dentist
Testicular	Testicular self-examination Testicular examination by physician
Skin	Self-examination for skin changes, especially moles
Prostate	Digital rectal examination

From Glasel (1985).

industries may produce and release hazardous substances that could affect many citizens in the community. Governments are becoming more aware of such hazards and are requiring protective measures. Individuals who develop cancers as a result of industrial exposure may be eligible to receive compensation via government compensation schemes.

All industries should be encouraged by their occupational health department to provide cancer education. An attempt should be made to identify high-risk individuals such as heavy smokers and those with a family history of the disease, and to establish measures for prevention and early detection.

In recent years, government bodies and cancer societies have instituted intensive campaigns to alert the public to high-risk factors and to behaviour changes which may modify their risk of developing cancer.

Secondary cancer prevention is focused on early diagnosis, of which early detection and screening are the major components. Screening and detection programmes are concentrated on some of the most common cancers, including cancers of the breast, cervix, colon/rectum, prostate, skin and oropharynx. Table 10.2 outlines the major methods that are available for the screening and detection of these cancers.

A person with an early sign of cancer may delay seeking health care because of fear. Most malignant neoplasms begin as a localized disease; if all the cancer cells are confined to their source of origins, most cancers may be successfully treated. Delay in detection and treatment diminishes the chance of cure and survival, since it permits the growing neoplasm to invade surrounding tissues, with cells becoming detached and carried to other body areas. Important early symptoms that are stressed in public education are: *unusual bleeding or discharge from any body orifice; a lump or thickening in the breast or elsewhere; a sore that does not heal; a persistent change in bowel or* *bladder habits; a persistent cough or hoarseness; indigestion or difficulty in swallowing; and an obvious change in a wart or mole.*

In order to assume the expected role in cancer prevention and early detection programmes, the nurse must keep informed about the trends in the incidence of cancer and advances being made. Members of the public should be aware of the environmental and lifestyle factors which predispose to cancer; know the seven early symptoms of cancer; identify community resources for information about cancer, cancer prevention and early detection; and utilize services for the detection of cancer appropriately.

Webb (1988) describes the value of reinforcing verbal information-giving and teaching by the use of written booklets.

DETECTION AND DIAGNOSIS OF CANCER

Most cancers remain undetected until the patient begins to experience signs and symptoms secondary to the cancer, such as weight loss, bleeding, an unexplained lump, a sore that does not heal, pain or fatigue. A wide variety of diagnostic procedures may be used in determining the presence, type and extent of a cancer.

IMAGING OF TUMOURS

The detection and staging of cancers through various imaging techniques has become progressively more refined and of greater diagnostic value with the introduction of new techniques. Common methods are listed below and described elsewhere in the text.

- Plain X-ray examinations
- Mammography
- Barium studies
- Computerized tomography (CT)
- Ultrasound examination
- Nuclear medicine imaging
- Magnetic resonance imaging (NMR)

BIOPSY AND HISTOLOGICAL EXAMINATIONS

A biopsy obtains tissue for histological examination and thereby allows a pathological diagnosis. The confirmation or exclusion of malignancy is the most common indication for biopsy; however inflammatory and infective tissue may also have characteristic microscopic appearances. When malignant tissue is found, the type of cancer and the degree of differentiation of the cells can be determined. Samples of tissue may be obtained by aspiration (a technique which involves removing a small plug of tissue using a needle and syringe) or by open excision of a section of tissue under local or general anaesthesia. For those lesions that are impalpable, biopsies are easily performed under CT or ultrasound guidance.

Histological examination of tumour tissue may be done periodically to determine the effectiveness of treatment or to monitor progression of the patient's disease.

Clonogenic assay involves the growth of human tumour cells on a special culture medium to predict specific chemotherapy for the individual patient. Culture and sensitivity assays of human tumour cell responsiveness to chemotherapeutic agents provides for more effective drug treatment of cancer.

Exfoliative cytological tests involve the microscopic examination of smears of secretion or fluid taken from a body cavity. Cells are continuously shed from the epithelial surface tissue of the body cavities; this process is referred to as exfoliation or desquamation. Neoplastic cells may be detected before there are any other recognizable signs or symptoms, resulting in early successful treatment. Specimens may be taken from the cervix, vagina, respiratory tract, mouth, oesophagus, stomach, urinary tract, prostate and the pleural and peritoneal cavities.

ENDOSCOPY

This is the introduction of a lighted tube (endoscope) into a body passage or organ for direct inspection of the area. At the same time a biopsy may be obtained. This method of examination may be used in the larynx, bronchi, oesophagus, stomach, colon, sigmoid, rectum and bladder.

LABORATORY STUDIES

Some haematological and serological tests are used to refine the diagnosis or to follow the progress of the malignancy. For example, the serum acid phosphatase level is used in investigation for carcinoma of the prostate; it is elevated when the disease is present. Blood and plasma cell evaluations are important in diagnosis and assessment of malignant disease of the bone marrow and reticuloendothelial system.

Tumour markers

Tumour markers are substances produced by tumours or by the host in response to the presence of tumour. Tumour markers are useful in staging disease, following response to treatment and in predicting recurrent disease. A broad range of tumour markers exist, including antigens, antibodies, genes, enzymes and hormones. Limitations in the clinical usefulness of most tumour markers are the lack of sensitivity and lack of proportionality, i.e. presentations of the marker are irregular or fail to reflect the true tumour burden (Lovejoy et al, 1987).

Some of the more useful markers used today are β human chorionic gonadotrophin (β-hCG), which is elevated in women with choriocarcinoma and men with testicular carcinoma. β-hCG is useful in following tumour size and in detecting recurrent disease. Cancer antigen 125 (CA 125) is present in women with ovarian cancer; it is proportional to tumour burden and is used to follow patients with disease and in detecting recurrence.

TREATMENT OF CANCER

Surgery

The role of surgery in the treatment of cancer includes tissue diagnosis through biopsy; staging of disease; treatment through excision, amputation or surgical diversion; palliation; and reconstruction. Surgery may be a primary curative treatment for some forms of cancer; it is increasingly used in combination with other treatment modalities to improve treatment results.

Establishing a tissue diagnosis through biopsy can be done by incisional biopsy, where a small portion of tissue is removed and examined. Excisional biopsies involve removing the whole tumour. An example of excisional biopsy is a breast biopsy done under local anaesthesia. Needle biopsies use a needle to aspirate fluid or tissue and are easily done under local anaesthesia.

Surgery can be utilized to determine the stage of disease where other diagnostic methods are not satisfactory. A diagnostic laparotomy is the most common example. Second-look procedures are follow-up procedures done after original surgery to establish the presence or absence of disease. With the advent of more sophisticated diagnostic testing and tumour markers this type of surgical intervention is being done less frequently.

Surgery can be a definitive treatment for some cancers. Skin cancers can be removed and cured by local excision. More radical block dissections involve removal of tumour, regional lymph nodes and any other involved contiguous structures. Examples are radical neck dissection, radical mastectomy and radical nephrectomy. Radical excisions may involve diversions of bladder or bowel and creation of stomas. Cancer in situ can be treated with cryosurgery, endoscopy or carbon dioxide laser.

Ablative surgery is done to remove hormonal influences on tumour growth through procedures such as oophrectomy, adrenalectomy and orchiectomy.

Palliative surgery is performed to improve the quality of life for the patient, rather than as a curative procedure. Examples of palliative surgery include neurosurgical management of pain (cordotomy, nerve blocks); bypass of an obstruction in the bowel; drainage of abscesses; and management of oncological emergencies such as haemorrhage and cord compression.

In recent years, major strides and improvements have been made in reconstructive surgery. Reconstruction utilizing skin, tissue and bone grafting is now often done simultaneously with the excisional procedure. These advances have dramatically improved the appearance and functioning of patients undergoing head and neck, orthopaedic and radical abdominal and pelvic surgeries. There are also improved options for breast reconstruction.

The nursing management of the patient receiving surgical treatment offers unique challenges. Patients in the diagnostic phase are frequently anxious and need opportunities to express their fears. They also require information regarding diagnostic procedures and the possible treatment options should a diagnosis of cancer be confirmed.

The person who is receiving definitive treatment may experience radical changes in functioning and/or appearance as a result of surgery and requires extensive support and teaching both preoperatively and postoperatively. Definitive treatment may occur close to the time of diagnosis, when patients are only just beginning to cope with the impact of diagnosis on physical and emotional health. Nursing care should include exploration of reactions and concerns; provision of information on disease and treatment; and teaching for self-care in relation to postoperative recovery and alterations in functioning.

Equally important is comprehensive discharge planning and referral to appropriate resources. Patients with urinary and bowel diversions require the resource of a care nurse either in hospital or community, and ongoing access to a supplier of ostomy equipment. The woman who has had a mastectomy will need referral for fitting of a breast prosthesis. Community support groups may assist in coping with cancer and life-style adaptation. Patients who have had an amputation may require referral to a rehabilitation service. With progressively shorter stays in hospital, nursing is playing an increasingly important role in planning and co-ordinating continuing care in the community.

Chemotherapy

Chemotherapy is the use of chemicals or drugs (cytotoxic agents) in the treatment of cancer. A relatively recent development in cancer care, this modality is becoming an increasingly more prominent cancer treatment.

HISTORY AND DEVELOPMENT

During World War II accidental exposure of soldiers to nitrogen mustard gas produced bone marrow hypoplasia and atrophy of the lymph glands. In the next few years nitrogen mustard was developed as a chemical and, when given to patients with lymphoma, resulted in short-term therapeutic responses. These results stimulated further development and testing of chemicals in the treatment of cancer. In the late 1940s nitrogen mustard and methotrexate were the first two drugs recognized as chemotherapeutic agents. Since then many thousands of chemicals have been tested for antitumour effects and currently there are a few dozen chemotherapy agents commonly used in the treatment of cancer.

ROLE OF CHEMOTHERAPY IN THE TREATMENT OF CANCER

Chemotherapy may offer a cure, provide long-term control, improved survival and palliation. It may be used as a primary form of treatment or in combination with surgery or radiation. As a systemic treatment, chemotherapy is often used for cancers that are disseminated in the body.

Chemotherapy is a primary and potentially curative mode of treatment for some forms of cancer, such as Hodgkin's lymphoma, testicular cancer, acute lymphocytic leukaemia in children, Ewing's sarcoma and choriocarcinoma.

Temporary remissions, long-term control and improved survival have resulted from the use of chemotherapy for patients with leukaemia, breast cancer, lung cancer, lymphoma, prostate cancer and multiple myeloma. Often chemotherapy may be used in combination with radiation and surgery. This is usually referred to as adjuvant chemotherapy.

Palliative chemotherapy may be used in a treatment of patients whose cancers cannot be controlled or cured but where benefit to the patient can be in the control of pain or other distressing symptoms. Attempts are made to temporarily shrink tumour masses which are causing obstruction or pressure on nerves or the lymphatic system.

MECHANISM OF ACTION

All cells have a life cycle of five phases, which is the process of cellular reproduction (Figure 10.4) G_0 is the resting phase when cells carry out normal cell functions for which they have been genetically programmed. In this phase the cells are not actively involved in reproduction. The next phase is G_1 when the cells begin to produce the many enzymes required for DNA synthesis. Cells then progress into the S (synthesis) phase, when DNA is duplicated in preparation for division of the mother cell. In G_2 there is production of proteins, RNA and the mitotic spindle. Finally in the M (mitosis) phase the mother cells divide as they pass through four brief phases: prophase, metaphase, anaphase and telophase. The amount of time required to complete the process of cellular reproduction varies greatly between different types of cells. The phase which accounts for most of the variation in time is the G_0 phase.

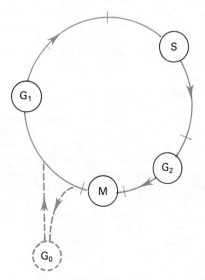

Figure 10.4 The cell cycle.

Cancer cells tend to divide and proliferate more quickly than normal cells because cancer cells lack the normal mechanisms for inhibition of cell division. Cytotoxic drugs act by interfering with the process of cellular growth and division, usually by interfering with DNA synthesis. Cancer cells which are in the process of reproduction are the cells most likely to be affected by chemotherapy. Unfortunately the growth and division of all cells in the body can be affected by chemotherapy. The effects are most obvious on the rapidly dividing cells such as those of the hair, mucous membranes and the haematopoietic system.

The action of chemotherapy is either cell cycle specific or cell cycle non-specific. Cell cycle specific agents sustain their major cytotoxic effect during a particular phase of the cell cycle, such as mitosis. Cell cycle non-specific agents act on resting and dividing cells, making the cells unable to divide or repair damage.

The method and time of action of individual agents has important implications for the combination of drugs used in chemotherapy treatment regimens.

CLASSIFICATION OF CHEMOTHERAPY AGENTS

Cytotoxic drugs may be classified as alkylating agents, antimetabolites, plant alkaloids, antibiotics, hormones, steroids, immune agents or miscellaneous. They may be used in combination or as single agents. Repeated administration of these drugs is often more effective in reducing the size of neoplasms than a single course of treatment.

The alkylating agents, also known as antimitotic drugs, act within the nucleus of the cell and alter the DNA molecules, resulting in inhibition of cell growth and reproduction. Their activity is not specific to any one stage of the cell cycle, although reproducing cells are more vulnerable.

The antimetabolites resemble substances that are essential to cellular activities, and which are therefore taken up by cells. These preparations are sufficiently different from normal metabolites to alter metabolism and inhibit growth and reproduction. They function at a specific phase of the life cycle of the cell.

The plant alkaloids currently in use are derived from periwinkle plants. They block cell reproduction during metaphase.

Certain antibiotics have been found to be of value in inibiting some types of neoplastic cells. They act by interfering with DNA and/or RNA synthesis of the cells.

The hormones used in the treatment of cancer alter the synthesis of RNA and protein in the tissues that contain steroid binding receptors. Adrenal cortico-steroids are commonly used because they suppress cell reproduction through inhibition of cellular protein synthesis.

New drugs are introduced frequently, and the search continues for a drug that will be selective and prove toxic to malignant cells without damaging normal tissues.

SIDE-EFFECTS AND TOXICITIES

Because chemotherapy has a systemic action and therefore affects the growth and division of cancer cells and normal cells, a wide variety of generalized side-effects and toxicities are experienced by patients receiving chemotherapy. The side-effects most commonly associated with chemotherapeutic agents include bone marrow depression leading to leucopenia, thrombocytopenia and anaemia; mucositis; nausea and vomiting; diarrhoea and constipation; hair loss; and fatigue. Since the side-effects vary with different drugs, it is essential that the nurse knows the chemotherapeutic agent given, the possible side-effects of that particular drug, their significance, how they are manifested and the appropriate nursing management. Table 10.3 outlines the side-effects and toxicities of the most commonly used chemotherapeutic agents.

Haematopoietic system

The cells of the haematopoietic system are among the most rapidly dividing cells of the body, and therefore the bone marrow is susceptible to the cytotoxic side-effects of chemotherapy. Evidence of bone marrow depression is observed by blood counts falling below the normal range, particularly the white blood cells and platelets. The usual pattern is a decreasing count of 1–2 weeks post chemotherapy. The lowest point the patient experiences in the white blood cell count is referred to as the nadir. The nadir may last several days, after which the bone marrow gradually recovers over a number of days from the effects of the chemotherapy. In most patients recovery is seen within 14 to 21 days after chemotherapy. The degree of bone marrow depression caused by chemotherapy varies greatly among the various agents. Patients may experience only a slight, transient decrease in their blood counts with one drug, while another may cause dramatic decreases and expose the patient to potential complications such as bleeding and infection.

Alopecia

Chemotherapy may cause alopecia (hair loss) as the epithelial cells of the hair follicle are damaged or destroyed. Patients may have thinning of the hair or complete hair loss depending on the agent used and the dose and frequency of chemotherapy administration (Welch and Lewis, 1980). Hair loss is more apparent on the scalp because of the large percentage of dividing epithelial cells, but patients may also lose eyebrows, eyelashes, pubic and axillary hair, as well as hair on the trunk and extremities. Alopecia is a temporary side-effect and regrowth usually begins within several weeks following the last chemotherapy treatment.

Nausea and vomiting

Two of the most common and distressing side-effects of chemotherapy are nausea and vomiting. Nausea and vomiting generally occur within 2–6 hours following administration. Duration of symptoms may last several days or, rarely, weeks (Lazlo, 1983).

Anticipatory nausea and vomiting (ANV) is a phenomenon that occurs prior to treatment with chemotherapy.

Table 10.3 Chemotherapy agents: side-effects and toxicities.

Columns grouped as **Side-effects** (Bone marrow depression, Nausea and vomiting, Mucositis, Diarrhoea, Alopecia) and **Toxicities** (Dermatological, Hepatic, Cardiac, Pulmonary, Renal, Haemorraghic cystitis, Neurotoxic, Ototoxic, Reproductive, Irritant, Vesicant).

Chemotherapy agent	Bone marrow depression	Nausea and vomiting	Mucositis	Diarrhoea	Alopecia	Dermatological	Hepatic	Cardiac	Pulmonary	Renal	Haemorraghic cystitis	Neurotoxic	Ototoxic	Reproductive	Irritant	Vesicant	Other
Alkylating agents																	
Cyclophosphamide	+++	++	+		++					+	+			+			• IADH
Busulphan	+++	++	+		+	+			+					+			• Addisonian-like syndrome
Melphalan	+++	++	+		++				+					+			
Chlorambucil	+++	++			+				+					+			
Cisplatin	+	+++			+					+		+	+++	+			• Anaphylaxis-like reactions
Dacarbazine	+++	+++	++	+	+	+								+	+		• Flu-like syndrome starting 7 days post-treatment
Mechlorethamine	+++	+++	+	++	++	+								+		+	• Tinnitus, thrombophlebitis
Thiotepa	++					+								+	+		
Ifosfamide	+++	+++			++					+	+	+		+			
Antimetabolites																	
Cystosine arabinoside	+++	++	++	+	++							+		+			
5-Fluorouracil	+++	++	+++	+++	++	+	+					+		+			• Conjunctivitis
6-Mercaptopurine	++	++	+	+	+	+	+							+			• Fever
Methotrexate	+++	++	+++	+++	+	+	+		+	+				+			• Photosensitivity
6-Thioguanine	+++		+	+++	+++	+	+	+						+		+	
Nitrosureas																	
BCNU	+++	+++	+		++	+			+	+				+			• Facial flushing
CCNU	+++	+++	++	+	+	+											
Streptozocin	++	+++	+	+	+	+				+						+	• Glucose intolerance
Antibiotics																	
Actinomycin D	+++	+++	+++	+++	+++	+										+·	
Bleomycin	+	+	++		++	+			+					+			• Fever, anaphylaxis
Daunorubicin	+++	++	++		+++			+									• Red urine
Doxorubicin	+++	++	+++	++	+++	+		+								+	• Red urine, flare reaction at site of injection
Epirubicin	+++	+	++	++	+++	+		+								+	• Red urine, flare reaction at site of injection
Mithramycin	+++	+++	++	++	+	+	+			+				+			
Mitomycin C	+++	++	+		++	+			++					+			
Plant alkaloids																	
Vinblastine	+++	+	+		++							+			+		
Vincristine	+	+	+		++							+			+		• IADH
Vindesine	+++	++	++		+++	+						+			+		• Fever, malaise
VP-16	+++	++	+	+	++							+				+	• Hypotension, allergic reactions
Miscellaneous																	
L-asparaginase		+	+		+		+					+		+			• Pancreatitis, anaphylaxis
Hydroxyurea	+++	++	+	+	++	+		+						+			
Procarbazine	+++	+++	++	+	+	+						+		+			
Mitoxantrone	+++	++	+	+	++	+	+							+			

+++, Major toxicity; dose limiting; ++, less frequent or less severe; +, rarely causes or mild.
IADH, increased secretion of antidiuretic hormone.

While the exact mechanisms involved with the development of ANV are not completely understood, it is widely accepted that other stimuli in the environment that are associated with the experience of chemotherapy can become paired with the occurrence of nausea and vomiting. These learned stimuli become signals that can elicit a learned or conditioned response of nausea and/ or vomiting. Examples of learned stimuli are the chemotherapy clinic, sights of needles, or characteristic odours. ANV usually begins to be experienced after a number of treatment sessions (4–5) and a regular pattern of response has been established (Nesse et al, 1980). Several treatment factors increase the chance of developing ANV, including receiving chemotherapeutic agents with a high emetic potential and inadequate use of antiemetics before and after chemotherapy.

Stomatitis

Stomatitis is a result of chemotherapeutic suppression of epithelial cell renewal in the oral cavity. Patients may develop inflammation, desquamation and ulceration. Early evidence of stomatitis is erythema, oedema, dryness and burning of the oral tissues. Progression to ulceration increases the pain experienced by the patient, and also increases the risk of fungal, viral and Gram-negative bacterial infections in the mouth.

Diarrhoea

Diarrhoea may occur as a result of chemotherapy because of impaired cell renewal of the epithelial lining of the intestinal tract. The villi and microvilli are denuded and there is increased mucous production, which stimulates rapid transit of intestinal contents. Nutrients, electrolytes and water are insufficiently absorbed. Antimetabolites cause diarrhoea which may be severe enough to interrupt therapy.

Sexual and reproductive changes

Chemotherapy can cause changes in fertility, sexual response and fetal development. The alkylating agents are the agents which most commonly cause infertility, as well as cytosine arabinoside, 5-fluorouracil, vinblastine, vincristine and procarbazine.

In men, chemotherapy causes depletion of the germinal epithelium which lines the seminiferous tubules. Oligospermia and azoospermia result in infertility. Certain chemotherapy regimens, such as MOPP (mustine, vincristine (Oncovin), procarbazine, prednisone), cause infertility in a greater proportion of patients than other regimens. Fertility may improve with time, depending on the dose and duration of chemotherapy. Treatment with oestrogens can cause a decrease in libido, and impotence.

Chemotherapy in women causes ovarian failure, hormonal alterations and destruction of ova and follicles (Feldman, 1989). Women may experience dryness of the vaginal mucosa due to decreased oestrogen levels, irregular menses or amenorrhea, and temporary or permanent sterility. Decreased sexual desire, decreased sense of sexual fulfilment and decreased level of sexual

excitement are also common responses.

Chemotherapy, particularly alkylating agents and antimetabolites, causes alterations in fetal development (Yasko, 1983). Chemotherapeutic agents can cross the placental barrier and cause cellular damage. During the first trimester, congenital abnormalities can result from chemotherapy exposure. Second or third trimester exposure may result in premature birth or low birth weight.

Neurotoxicity

Neurotoxicity results from only a few chemotherapy agents. The most common presentation is peripheral neuropathy: the patient experiences paraesthesias of the fingers and toes, weakness and loss of deep tendon reflexes. Autonomic neuropathy is evidenced as constipation and colicky abdominal pain. Generally neurotoxicity resolves over several weeks to months following cessation of treatment.

Nephrotoxicity

Nephrotoxity results from agents that cause damage to tissues in the kidneys, and can be permanent. Prevention of renal damage includes aggressive hydration, diuresis, alkanization of the urine and careful monitoring of renal function.

Pulmonary toxicity

Fibrotic changes in the lungs caused by chemotherapy are usually irreversible and progressive. Patients commonly experience dyspnoea, dry cough and tachypnoea. Severe pulmonary toxicity may be fatal.

Hepatic toxicity

Many chemotherapeutic agents are metabolized by the liver and some are hepatotoxic. Evidence of toxic effects on the liver ranges from temporary increases in liver enzymes to cirrhosis. Patients receiving agents which are hepatotoxic must have their liver function tests monitored on a regular basis.

Bladder toxicity

Bladder toxicity may result from treatment with cyclophosphamide, which causes haemorrhagic cystitis. Preventative management includes aggressive hydration and frequent urination.

Cardiotoxicity

Cardiotoxicity is a dose-limiting effect of two commonly used drugs: doxorubicin and daunorubicin. Effects on the heart range from mild electrocardiographic changes to severe congestive heart failure. Permanent damage to the heart muscle may occur, and be life threatening to the patient. As there is no treatment for cardiotoxicity, the total dose of either of these drugs is restricted to an amount that usually prevents permanent damage.

Ocular toxicity

Ocular side-effects of chemotherapy can include cataract formation, diplopia, blurred vision, increased lacrimation, conjunctivitis, photophobia and retinal haemorrhages. These side-effects are not common and in most cases dissipate with cessation of treatment.

Ototoxicity

Tinnitus and hearing loss are ototoxic effects of chemotherapy, particularly of cisplatin. Hearing loss may be permanent.

Secondary malignancies

A rare long-term effect of treatment of cancer is the development of a second primary malignancy. Although it is an infrequent occurrence, this phenomenon has been documented in patients treated with chemotherapy for Hodgkin's disease, multiple myeloma, ovarian and non-Hodgkin's lymphoma. The most common secondary malignancy is acute non-lymphocytic leukaemia (Fraser and Tucker, 1988). The chemotherapy agents that have been associated with secondary malignancies are the alkylating agents: cyclophosphamide, melphalan, nitrogen mustard and chlorambucil.

Combination treatment with chemotherapy and radiation may also influence this process. The evolution of secondary malignancies has led to the re-evaluation and design of new chemotherapy protocols which seek to maximize the antitumour effect, while minimizing the exposure of patients to drugs and treatments which may induce a second malignancy.

COMBINATION CHEMOTHERAPY

In the treatment of cancer with chemotherapy, two or more agents are generally used together in a combination. Clinical research trials have demonstrated that combinations of chemotherapy agents are more effective than using a single agent. The principles determining the selection of a combination of agents are: each agent is active against the disease when used alone; synergism is evident; the agents differ in mechanism of action; and differ in the site, severity and duration of side-effects. Multiagent chemotherapy protocols are given to patients on a predetermined sequence and schedule while maximizing tumour cell kill. A protocol such as CMF (cyclophosphamide, methotrexate, 5-fluorouracil) which is used in the treatment of breast cancer (Figure 10.5) may be repeated for several courses. Within a course, there is usually a scheduled non-treatment period which allows recovery from the side-effects of the chemotherapy.

Adjuvant chemotherapy is the administration of chemotherapy following primary treatment with surgery or radiotherapy. The aim of adjuvant chemotherapy in the treatment of possible micrometastases which are undetectable in order to prevent recurrence. Some cancers that potentially benefit from adjuvant chemotherapy are breast and testicular cancer.

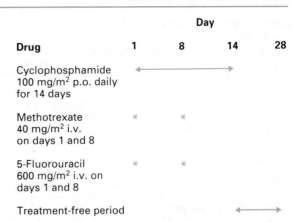

Figure 10.5 Chemotherapy protocol. CMF is a treatment protocol for breast cancer. The cycle frequency is 4 weeks. Within each cycle there is a 14-day treatment period and a 14-day treatment-free period.

Clinical research trials are utilized to determine the effectiveness and side-effects of new drugs and combinations of drugs. Experimenting with different schedules, dosages and combinations continues in order to improve treatment outcomes. All new chemotherapy agents undergo rigorous testing before general use of the agent is approved. Phases of testing include new agent screening for antitumour activity, evaluation of side-effects and toxicities, determination of optimal dosage and scheduling, evaluation of new therapy versus standard therapy, and evaluation of new agents in combination with other therapies.

ADMINISTRATION OF CHEMOTHERAPY

Dose determination

Determining the dose of the chemotherapy is done by multiplying the body surface area of the patient by the recommended dose of the chemotherapy agent per metre^2 of body surface area. Body surface area is calculated from the patient's weight and height using a graph called a nomogram. The calculated dose may then be adjusted by the physician if necessary. If adjustments are made, it is usually a decrease in the dose because of factors such as delayed bone marrow recovery or other severe side-effects.

Preparation, handling and disposal

Rigorous preparation, handling and disposal of chemotherapeutic agents is necessary because of the biohazardous nature of these chemicals. Drugs used in the treatment of cancer are very toxic. Specific instructions as to the preparation, handling and disposal of agents should be identified by the nursing and pharmacy departments and guidelines prepared by the health authority. Current safety guidelines for the preparation of chemotherapeutic agents recommend the use of a laminar airflow hood and protective clothing in order to prevent exposure to the agents of the person preparing the drugs. Personnel who are administering chemotherapy must also take precautions to prevent self-exposure or environmental contamination. It is recommended that, at a minimum, personnel administering chemotherapy wear surgical latex or polyvinyl chloride gloves. All materials used in the preparation and administration of chemotherapeutic agents must be disposed of as biohazardous waste.

Methods of administration

Chemotherapy agents may be administered by several routes: oral, topical, intravenous, intramuscular, subcutaneous, intra-arterial, intraventricular, intrathecal and intracavitary.

Intravenous administration of chemotherapeutic agents requires careful selection of the vein because of the need for repeated administration. Many chemotherapeutic agents are extremely irritating to tissue and may cause thrombosis of the vein. Some agents which are classified as vesicants may cause necrosis of tissue if infiltration occurs. Agents classified as irritants will cause irritation and pain in the vein if not diluted sufficiently before administration, and if infiltrated into the tissue will cause pain without necrosis. Table 10.3 indicates which agents are vesicants and irritants. The injection site should be observed closely and frequently for signs of redness or swelling and the patient questioned as to pain, tenderness or burning. Prompt identification and management of site infiltration is important to prevent excessive and unnecessary tissue damage. Treatment of extravasation includes the administration of specific antidotes for the drug, and the application of ice packs to the site to decrease the spread of the drug.

Intra-arterial administration of chemotherapy is used to deliver chemotherapy directly into an artery that supplies the malignant area. The drug circulates through the affected part in high concentration before it becomes diluted in the general circulation. An arterial catheter is introduced into the appropriate artery under fluoroscopy. For example, in liver cancer, the organ may be infused with the drug of choice via a small catheter introduced into the hepatic artery. Since it is intra-arterial, pressure is required to overcome the arterial blood pressure. Normally, a pump is used to deliver the drug at a prescribed rate. For patients receiving a series of intra-arterial treatments, an arterial port may be surgically implanted rather than introducing a temporary catheter for each treatment.

Intrathecal administration may be given when there are tumour cells in the central nervous system. Chemotherapy given by other routes is not usually able to cross the blood–brain barrier, and therefore tumour cells present in the central nervous system (CNS) are unaffected by the drugs. Presence of tumour cells in the CNS is documented by examination of spinal fluid. Intrathecal therapy may also be given prophylactically to leukaemia patients who are at high risk for development of CNS disease. This type of therapy may be given either by lumbar puncture or through a ventricular reservoir called an Ommaya reservoir, which is surgically implanted in the right frontal region of the skull.

Intracavitary administration of chemotherapeutic agents is usually done following aspiration of fluid from a body compartment such as the intrapleural space or the peritoneal cavity. Patients who develop malignant pleural effusions may have chemotherapy instilled in the pleural cavity through a thoracotomy tube. The resulting sclerotic changes in the lining of the pleural cavity may prevent the reaccumulation of fluid in the pleural space. Intraperitoneal chemotherapy allows direct contact of the drugs with tumour in the peritoneal cavity. Direct delivery of the chemotherapy to tumour cells maximizes the effect of the chemotherapy while minimizing the systemic side-effects of the drugs. Intraperitoneal chemotherapy is most commonly used in the treatment of ovarian cancer.

Alternative devices for administration of chemotherapy
For patients receiving long-term or repeated courses of chemotherapy a right atrial catheter may be inserted. Long-term right atrial catheters are inserted through the chest wall and into a large vein. A portion of the catheter remains outside the body and the exit site is covered with an occlusive dressing. The greater blood volume in the large vein and right atrium dilutes the medication, and thus decreases irritation to the vessel walls. The risk of extravasation into tissue is decreased and the peripheral veins are preserved. A right atrial catheter such as a Hickman catheter allows for greater patient mobility as it can be left in indefinitely and sealed with a cap between treatments. Venous access is assured for both chemotherapy, intravenous fluids and medications, as well as blood products. Patency of the line is maintained by flushing with a dilute solution of heparin on a daily basis when the catheter is capped off (see Chapter 13).

An alternative to central venous catheters is the more recent introduction of totally implanted central venous ports. These ports are implanted under the subcutaneous tissue and the catheter attached to the port is inserted into a central vein. Access to the port is established by inserting a needle through the skin down into the port. As with the external catheters, patency is maintained by flushing with heparin before the needle is removed from the port. Ports only require flushing once a month. Implanted ports are advantageous to patients as much less self-care is required. There is no need for a dressing and there is no interference in activities of daily living as a result of having a port. Most recently, an even smaller version of implanted ports is available for implantation in the small veins of the forearm.

Radiation Therapy

Radiation therapy is viewed by some health professionals and members of the public alike as mysterious, magical and frightening. Radiation is associated with burning, mutilation, sterility, pain, loss of social acceptance and death. Many people think that the person receiving external radiation is radioactive and therefore can cause harm to others if close contact is made. This of course is not true. Radiation is also generally thought of as being given only to those who are going to die of cancer, and may be perceived as signalling a poor prognosis. However, one-half of all cancer patients receive radiation therapy sometime in the course of their overall treatment. The nurse who is knowledgeable about this treatment modality can develop a comprehensive plan of care to support the patient and family during this important phase of treatment, and return patients to their optimal level of functioning.

HISTORY

Radiation therapy for cancer began shortly after the discovery of X-rays at the turn of the century. Unfortunately, in the early era of radiation therapy, it was a rather crude treatment. The measurement of tissue dose, time–dose fractionation, and the concepts of radioresistant and radiosensitive tissues were not known. The outcome was often fatal, at worst, with recurrence from under-radiation occurring at the other extreme. Other consequences of erroneous treatment did not appear for years as late effects of treatment. Thus, evaluation of this modality in the early stages of cancer was never really possible. Since that time, research has greatly expanded the knowledge and development of radiation as an effective treatment modality for cancer. Today, radiation therapy is precisely calculated to deliver the correct dose to the area treated, while sparing the surrounding normal tissues.

CURRENT USE OF RADIATION THERAPY IN THE MANAGEMENT OF CANCER

Radiation therapy is one of the three most commonly used cancer treatment modalities. It is used alone as the treatment of choice for certain early-stage malignant lesions, preoperatively and postoperatively to enhance local tumour control, concurrently with surgical intervention or chemotherapy, and for palliation of pain or pressure in advanced disease.

The aim of radiation therapy may be *curative*, as in skin cancer, carcinoma of the cervix, Hodgkin's disease or seminoma. For certain other lesions, cure or eradication is not possible, and *control* of the cancer for periods ranging from months to years may be the aim. Recurrent breast cancer, some soft tissue sarcomas, and lung cancer are examples of cancer controlled by radiation therapy in combination with surgery or chemotherapy. *Palliation* may be another goal of radiation therapy. Relief of pain, ulceration or bleeding, prevention of pathological fractures, and return of mobility can be achieved with radiation to metastatic lesions from a variety of tumours including breast, lung and prostate tumours. Palliative radiation therapy is also given for the relief of central nervous system symptoms caused by brain metastasis or spinal cord compression. Haemorrhage, ulceration and fungating lesions can be effectively reduced and in some cases eliminated by palliative radiation therapy. Palliative radiation therapy may also be used to prevent the emergence of potentially symptomatic lesions before they become a problem. Examples include the treatment of a mediastinal mass that threatens to produce superior vena cava obstruction, and treatment of a vertebral lesion when spinal cord compression is impending.

The type, duration and method of delivery of radiotherapy depends upon many factors and is tailored to individual requirements. Curative regimens may continue over many weeks and be very exhausting for the patient, whereas doses given for palliation may only need to be very low and are sometimes delivered in a single treatment.

The nursing care of cancer patients undergoing radiation therapy involves education about the purpose, method of administration, prevention of complications, and the management of unavoidable local or systemic toxicity. In order to meet the physical and psychosocial needs of the patient receiving radiation therapy, the nurse must have an understanding of the physical and biological principles of radiation therapy, usual treatment approaches, the onset and character of commonly encountered side-effects, and the measures that should be initiated to ameliorate toxicity.

PHYSICAL EFFECTS OF RADIATION

We often visualize radiation as a beam that travels directly from the treatment unit through the body to the tumour. Actually, the beam is not a single source of energy but a series of chain reactions. When the radiation beam strikes an atom, it frees electrons from that atom. This is ionization. The process of releasing those electrons requires energy; thus the radiation beam loses energy. The energy has been transferred to the newly released electrons. These freed electrons strike other nearby body atoms and cause further ionizations until their energy has been depleted. In this way, one single ionization disrupts many neighbouring atoms.

UNITS OF RADIATION MEASUREMENT

In the field of radiation physics, specific units are used to express certain concepts about radiation. The *unit of radiation dose* is called a gray (Gy). This term was officially adopted in 1985; replacing the term rad (an acronym for radiation absorbed dose): 1 Gy = 100 rad; 1 cGy = 1 rad.

BIOLOGICAL EFFECTS OF RADIATION

Tumour growth and tumour control or destruction take place at the cellular level. Radiation alters the cellular environment, producing chemical and physical changes incompatible with successful cell cycling processes. First, radiation damages the chemical bonds necessary for the reproduction of DNA within the cell (Moss et al, 1979; Berger, 1980). The changed atoms no longer fit into the DNA pattern resulting in cellular death at the time of mitosis (Berger, 1980). Radiation also causes fatal changes in cell membrane permeability and functional changes in enzymes and fatty acids (Berger, 1980). Radiation further contributes to cell damage by causing ionization in the water component of the cytoplasm. Since the cell is approximately 75% water, radiation forms ions from water molecules, producing $H_2O_2^-$, HO_2, OH^-, and H_2^-. These ions cause further chemical reactions within the cell. In some cases the exact amount of free ions produced depends on the amount of oxygen present. For this reason it is therapeutically desirable to increase the oxygenation of the cells to promote a response to irradiation of tumours (Lowry, 1974).

The effects of radiation on the chromosomes can be described in several different ways (Rubin, 1983). First, the chromosomes break into pieces, reunite haphazardly or incompletely, or remain apart; or second, they can be injured, resulting in the unequal divison of chromosomes at the time of mitosis. Cells in the resting phase of the cell cycle may appear uninjured but will later die when mitosis occurs. Mutation may also occur without visible chromosomal damage, resulting in irreparable changes appearing in later generations.

While cells in all phases of the cell cycle can be damaged by radiation, the lethal effect of radiation may not be apparent until after cell division occurs. In some instances, irradiated cells can successfully undergo five or six cell divisions before the lethal effects of the radiation kill the cells and their progeny. The effectiveness of radiation therapy depends on the proportion of cells actively dividing in the tumour mass, the histological characteristics of the cells, the oxygenation of the cells, and the dose and frequency of radiation.

Several critical conditions are involved in tumour shrinkage: (1) cell loss must exceed cell reproduction; (2) phagocytic processes must be intact to promote absorption of cellular debris; and (3) the dose fractionation of radiation must be sufficient to damage a large number of proliferating cells (Moss et al, 1979).

TUMOUR SENSITIVITY

Tumours can be defined as radiosensitive or radioresistant. Tumour cells and normal cells that are undergoing cell division are more sensitive to radiation. Such tissues include bone marrow and lymphoid tissue, testes, ovaries, and intestinal crypt cells. Moderately radiosensitive tissues are composed of cells that divide regularly, mature, and differentiate between mitotic cycles, namely, spermatagonia and spermatocytes. Showing a lesser degree of radiosensitivity are growing bone and connective tissue and vasculature cells with long individual life spans, such as those of the liver, thyroid and kidneys. The least radiosensitive tissues are composed of cells that cannot reproduce, such as those of the brain, spinal cord and muscles (Battles, 1981).

Virtually all cancer cells can be destroyed by radiation. The dose required to destroy some types of cancer cells is so high, however, that normal cells in the radiation fields are also irreversibly damaged. Such cancers are designated radioresistant.

As previously mentioned, the sensitivity of cells to the biological effects of radiation is highly dependent on the presence of oxygen, and thus vascularization of the tumour itself can influence tumour sensitivity to radiation. Generally the greater the vascularization and oxygenation of the tumour, the higher the degree of radiosensitivity. Hypoxic cells require a dose of radiation 2–3 times higher than that required to achieve the same therapeutic effect in well-oxygenated cells. This is

one reason the total dose of radiation therapy is delivered in fractions. As each fractionated dose of radiation causes tumour shrinkage, cells that were hypoxic are brought closer to the vascular supply. This increases the level of oxygenation and thus the effect of each successive radiation treatment. Fractionation of radiation over time is also designed to allow maximal repair of sublethal damage to normal cells. Therefore, the dosage of radiation administered to a patient is stated with reference to the daily fraction administered and the total time course (e.g. 4000 cGy at 200 cGy/day for 5 days/week over 4 weeks). Variations such as hyperfractionation (more than one treatment per day) are currently being tested in clinical trials.

RADIOSENSITIZERS AND RADIOPROTECTORS

Certain chemicals may have the capacity to sensitize hypoxic, and therefore radioresistant, tumour cells to the cytotoxic effects of radiation exposure (Noll, 1990). These substances are referred to as radiosensitizers. Such drugs mimic the sensitizing effects of oxygen. Attempts are also being made to develop chemicals that can provide protection of normal tissues from radiation-induced damage but afford no protection to malignant tissue (Noll, 1990). These are called radioprotective agents.

HYPERTHERMIA

The use of hyperthermia to achieve a synergistic effect with radiation therapy has been studied and applied in clinical situations with considerable enthusiasm. Although researchers are uncertain whether hyperthermia actually sensitizes tumour cells to radiation or whether the modalities simply combine to produce a greater effect than either has on its own, this treatment method is receiving increased attention (Guy and Chou, 1983; Bicher et al, 1986). Hyperthermia may act in several ways. First, heat is cytotoxic to cancer cells, particularly hypoxic cells. In addition, heat is also known to inhibit the repair of radiation damage, thus increasing the therapeutic ratio. Hyperthermia may be achieved through immersion of the local area in a heated bath, ultrasound, microwaves, and perfusion techniques. Side-effects of combined hyperthermia and radiation include local skin reaction, pain, fever and gastrointestinal effects (Wojtas, 1990).

A number of chemical and thermal modifiers of radiation are currently being studied in clinical trials. Development of such approaches could make many tumours now considered radioresistant amenable to control with radiation therapy (Guy and Chou, 1983; Bicher et al, 1986; Noll, 1990; Wojtas, 1990).

METHODS OF ADMINISTERING RADIATION THERAPY

Various methods are available for delivering the prescribed dose of radiation. A large radiation therapy centre will have available a selection suitable for the treatment of almost any malignancy in any part of the body. The methods are external radiation (radiation from a source at a distance from the body) or internal application (radiation from a source placed within the body or a body cavity). Radiation may also be administered via radioactive isotopes in a liquid form, e.g. iodine-131.

External radiation

This method requires the patient to lie immobile on a firm treatment table, alone, in a room behind a closed door, while a large machine emits radiation that penetrates the body over a period of seconds or minutes. Simulation is the pretreatment process of developing a treatment plan. The radiation oncologist and physicist use an array of sophisticated computers and diagnostic equipment to determine the exact dose of radiation to be delivered to the tumour volume as well as to the various adjacent anatomical areas. During simulation the patient is placed in the projected treatment position on a device called a simulator. A simulator is actually a type of diagnostic X-ray machine that can reproduce the geometrical arrangement of the treatment unit. Contrast media may be used during simulation in an attempt to visualize soft tissue structures and their exact locations.

As part of the pretreatment workup it may be decided that an immobilization device is necessary. Such devices are commonly fabricated from thermoplastic. Immobilization shells are used during treatment to prevent movement and provide a reproducible geometry from one treatment to the next. These devices are limited to use in external radiation therapy.

Treatment portals have traditionally been marked on the skin with indelible ink or black tattoo dots. Field markings may be placed on the plastic immobilization shell, thus avoiding conspicuous marks. It is important to irradiate the same tissue volume throughout the course, thus the rationale for the emphatic directions to patients not to wash away the markings. If, during the course of treatment, tumour shrinkage is evident, a technique of shrinking the portals is also employed.

The selection of the treatment units is determined by the location of the tumour. The *kilovoltage* units (e.g. Maxitron) were the first machines developed for therapeutic use. Treatment units in this category produce rays that deliver their maximum dose to the skin surface or 1–2 cm beneath it. Skin tolerance becomes the limiting factor in the amount of radiation that can be delivered to the malignant lesion. Consequently, these units are now used only for superficial skin lesions or tumours located very near the skin surface. *Megavoltage* units (e.g. cobalt, betatron, and linear accelerators) have a much wider range of energies, from 2 to 40 MeV and have distinct advantages over kilovoltage units, including deeper beam penetration, more homogeneous absorption of radiation, and greater skin sparing.

Intraoperative radiation therapy was developed in the United States during the late 1970s and was initially used for unresectable tumours. In recent years this approach has been used in combination with resection of primary tumours for locally advanced colorectal carcinoma, pancreatic, gastric and bladder cancers, and soft tissue sarcomas (Erickson et al, 1989).

After surgically exposing the target area, a single large fraction of radiation is delivered directly to the tumour site by a specially built cone attached to the therapy unit. The surgical procedure is then completed and a further postoperative course of conventional radiation therapy is given. Despite the technical difficulties in performing intraoperative radiation therapy, it appears to have potential for further development and application in cancer management (Erickson et al, 1989).

Internal radiation

The second technique, internal radiation, or brachytherapy, is the placement of radioactive material within or near a tumour so as to administer treatment to a local area. Internal radiation is frequently used in combination with external radiation, and also may be used preoperatively and postoperatively.

Radioactive isotopes such as caesium-131 and iridium-192 may be utilized in the form of wires, capsules, or needles and placed via an applicator directly into or adjacent to the tumour. Isotopes in this form are designated sealed sources, whereas the radioactive isotope iodine-131 in liquid form is administered systemically and is thus an unsealed source. The uptake of iodine-131 is highly selective to thyroid tissue and in cases of well-differentiated thyroid cancer both primary and secondary deposits may be effectively treated in this way. Tumours of the head and neck, particularly lesions of the tongue, may be irradiated via caesium needles and iridium-192 may be used in wire form to treat breast tumours and the surrounding breast tissues.

The placing of needles and wires needs to be exact to ensure an even dose of radiation to the tumour and requires good co-operation between the radiotherapy and surgical teams.

Internal radiation is most often employed in the treatment of gynaecological lesions. A variety of techniques and types of equipment have been designed to provide a desired dosage to the tissues around the radiation source. Many of these applicators are the afterloading type that can be positioned in the operating room and loaded with the radioactive source at a later time after the proper position has been checked by radiograph and the patient returned to the ward. The afterloading method is most desirable because it prevents unnecessary radiation exposure to personnel. The radioactive source is usually caesium-131 but in some centres radioactive cobalt is used at a fast dose rate.

EFFECTS OF RADIATION ON BODY TISSUES AND ORGAN SYSTEMS

Several specific components determine the effect of radiation on tissues: the *dose*, the *fractionation*, *time* and *volume*, and the *area* treated. Dose–time–volume interrelationships are as follows: (1) the greater the dose, the shorter the time of onset of any reaction; and (2) the larger the treatment area, the more potentially severe the reaction.

Except for those systemic effects that will be described, radiation side-effects are seen only in the tissues and organ systems that are within or immediately adjacent to the treatment field. Thus, an individual receiving treatment to the mediastinum will not develop radiation-induced diarrhoea, nor will an individual receiving treatment to an abdominal field lose scalp hair. Similarly, those individuals undergoing brachytherapy will develop reactions to treatment that vary with the site, dose, volume and energy of the source. It is important to remember that the side-effects from radiation will vary from individual to individual, and therefore an individualized plan for teaching and care must be planned for each patient.

Both the immediate or acute effects of treatment and the late effects must be considered in any discussion of the effect of radiation on tissues. In general, acute effects are seen within the first 6 months following treatment and are due to cell damage in which mitotic activity is altered in some way. If acute effects are not reversible, late or permanent tissue changes occur. These late effects can be attributed to the organism's attempt to heal or repair the damage caused by the radiation.

To assess pathophysiological changes, the nurse must think in terms of cross-sectional anatomy (external radiation enters the body at the portal, passes through all tissues and organs encompassed in the treatment volume, and exits on the opposite side of the body); review normal anatomical and physiological features of organs and tissues encompassed in the treatment volume; and review the known biological responses to radiation. These factors contribute to a strong knowledge base for assessing and managing the side-effects of radiation.

The skin

The outer layer of skin (epidermis) is composed of several layers of cells, with mature, non-dividing cells at the surface and immature, dividing cells at the base. Normal mature cells are constantly being shed from the skin surface and replaced by new cells from the basal layer. This continuous state of reproductive activity accounts for the high radiosensitivity of skin. Although the skin may be the primary site of radiation (as in skin cancer), it is also irradiated when any other site within the body is treated because radiation must pass through whatever tissues it encounters before reaching the target site.

Acute radiation reactions begin after a dose of 450–500 cGy. Erythema, which acts and feels like a sunburn, can occur within hours or up to one week after the first treatment, depending on the daily dose and the type of machine used. Depending on the equipment used, skin at the exit portal may also be affected. It usually reaches its peak of severity near the completion of treatment.

Radiation skin reactions are caused by the inflammatory response that results from the breakdown of basal cells in the epidermis. Erythema may be the only manifestation, or the skin reaction may progress to dry and then moist desquamation. A dry desquamation is characterized by drying and scaling of the skin, while wet desquamation is characterized by a weeping of the skin. This reaction is due to the upper layers of the skin

having been shed, leaving the derma exposed. Healing may be slow, but is usually complete and leaves minimal evidence of the acute damage except for the changes in pigmentation. Fibrosis and atrophy may occur after high doses, as may ulceration and necrosis, although such changes are uncommon with modern equipment and techniques.

It is important to note that skin in certain areas such as the groin, gluteal fold, axilla, and under the breasts, usually exhibits a greater and often earlier reaction to radiation due to the natural warmth, moistness and friction in these areas.

An inappropriate term for this type of reaction is a radiation 'burn' since this term implies accidental or unexpected damage, neither of which should take place in a controlled therapeutic setting.

Radiation affects all rapidly growing cells: the hair roots are no exception. Hair, after receiving threshold doses, becomes loose and may be pulled out painlessly or fall out spontaneously. Generally this occurs during treatment or shortly thereafter; regrowth generally occurs in 2–3 months. Hair loss may be permanent if high doses of radiation are given to the area. The loss of hair is traumatic to most people regardless of whether they are prepared for this change in body image. The needless fear of this loss is equally traumatic and if patients are receiving treatments to areas that do not include the scalp, they should be reassured that hair loss will not occur as a result of treatment.

Haematopoietic system

Bone marrow and lymphoid tissues are highly radiosensitive. The greatest effect is on the stem cells, while mature, non-dividing blood cells in the circulating blood stream are relatively insensitive to radiation. When large areas of bone marrow in the adult are irradiated, including the ilia, vertebrae, ribs, skull, long bones and sternum, the number of circulating mature red blood cells, white blood cells and platelets decreases because production is suppressed. This reaction is more severe if prior or concomitant chemotherapy has been given. It is sometimes necessary to interrupt treatment for a few days to allow the bone marrow to recover.

Gastrointestinal system

The gastrointestinal tract, from mouth to rectum, is lined with mucous membrane that contains layers of cells. A large proportion of these cells are undifferentiated and mitotic and are thus extremely sensitive to radiation.

Oral mucous membrane may develop mucositis, usually after 2–3 weeks of fractionated radiation therapy. The mucous membrane will initially have increased redness, which will progress to yellowish-white patches. These patches will eventually become a pseudomembrane covering large areas of the mucosa. Salivary function is altered, and the patient may experience soreness, pain on swallowing, hoarseness, dryness, or changes in the sense of taste. If the oesophagus, stomach or bowel are within the irradiated field, the patient may experience nausea, vomiting or diarrhoea. When the oesophagus is within the field, painful swallowing, dryness and spasms may occur. Abdominal irradiation is frequently associated with nausea, with greater exposures causing vomiting, abdominal cramping and diarrhoea. These can lead to electrolyte imbalances, dehydration and weight loss. If the anal sphincter is in the field of radiation and distressing symptom of tenesmus (painful ineffectual straining) also sometimes occurs.

Respiratory system

Acute radiation pneumonitis may be asymptomatic or cause a hacking cough or mild chest discomfort. With moderate levels of radiation acute changes such as shortness of breath may subside after 3 or 4 weeks. Large doses (75% of lung tissue exposed to 2000 cGy or more) will often cause permanent damage, with the degree of disability related to the amount and condition of remaining untreated lung tissue.

Reproductive system

The germinal cells of the testes are very sensitive to even small doses of radiation. Small doses will cause temporary halting of sperm production; 500–1000 cGy will probably cause permanent sterility. The secretion of testosterone is not affected, thus sexual characteristics are unchanged.

Radiation to the ovaries produces either temporary or permanent sterility, depending on the age of the person being treated and the dose of radiation. Permanent sterilization will occur at doses of 600–1200 cGy, and older women are sterilized at lower doses than younger women. In addition to sterility, hormonal changes (especially loss of oestrogen production) and early menopause may occur.

SYSTEMIC EFFECTS OF RADIATION THERAPY

Generalized symptoms which commonly appear during radiation treatment are fatigue, weakness, headache, nausea and anorexia. These symptoms are more frequently discussed in the nursing literature than the medical literature, and their aetiology is not well understood. One suggested cause of generalized symptoms is the rapid breakdown of cells destroyed by radiation. Cell breakdown would release toxic metabolites and endproducts that accumulate faster than they can be excreted (Haylock, 1979). Walter suggests that these chemicals may act as toxic foreign proteins, causing some degree of shock (Walter, 1977). Others suggest that these symptoms result from an increased metabolic rate, from the body's attempt to restore homeostasis, or from the emotional stresses of daily treatment for a life-threatening illness (Walter, 1977; Haylock, 1979; Welch, 1980; Yasko, 1982).

LATE EFFECTS

The late effects of radiation therapy can be attributed to the organism's attempt to heal or repair the damage caused by radiation. These complications may appear several months to a few years after the completion of treatment. Most late complications reflect diminished

Table 10.4 Late effects of radiation therapy.

Organ/system	Reaction
Skin	Fibrosis, atrophy, and tanning over irradiated areas; telangiectasia Acute recall reaction may occur after the administration of certain antineoplastic drugs such as dactinomycin
Gastrointestinal system	Oral fibrosis, decreased taste acuity or the loss of taste sensation, xerostomia, dental caries, chronic enteritis, intestinal fistulae formation
Lung	Radiation pneumonitis (acute/chronic)
Blood and bone marrow	Anaemia, leukaemia
Eyes	Cataracts
Thyroid	Hypothyroidism, thyroid cancer
Reproductive system	Temporary or permanent sterility. Premature menopause in women. Fertility may return to normal depending on the dose of irradiation administered to the gametes and age
Urinary system (bladder)	Reduced capacity, chronic bleeding
Central nervous system	Transient or widespread demyelination

vascular supply and increased fibrosis in heavily irradiated areas. Unlike acute reactions, these complications are often chronic, and nursing management is symptomatic and based on the degree of functional impairment. The late complications of radiation therapy are summarized in Table 10.4.

NURSING CARE OF THE PATIENT RECEIVING EXTERNAL RADIATION

The nurse caring for the patient receiving external radiation requires some understanding of how radiation is administered and its effects on body tissues. This knowledge is essential for providing comprehensive nursing care for each individual before, during and after radiation therapy.

It is important that the patient is given precise information about the purpose of treatment and its duration and method of delivery. It should be emphasised that all treatment is prescribed and planned on an individual basis. Often the patient has heard about other patients' experiences with radiation therapy and may be convinced that the same problems will develop. Of course, side-effects do occur but their severity depends on such factors as treatment site, treatment volume, fractionation, total dose, and so on, and especially on the individual being treated. Most individuals respond best to a reassuring pretreatment discussion in which side-effects specific to their treatment are discussed, stressing the symptomatic relief that is available. Knowing what to expect usually helps prevent the person from worrying that a treatment-related side-effect represents a worsening or reoccurrence of the disease. At this time, the nurse can also mention briefly the reactions that will not occur, since most people are reassured to know, for example, that they will not lose their hair or be nauseated, if this is the case.

Nurses also have a role in helping patients to prepare for the physical surroundings, and sensory experiences they may encounter at the radiation treatment centre. A brief description of the treatment unit, which may appear rather ominous, will help to reduce anxiety. The patient is advised that, although alone in the room, there will be constant observation by the radiographer, with whom he or she may communicate. The patient should also be informed that the treatment period will be brief, that there will be no pain or sensation felt as the rays penetrate, and that it is important to maintain the position in which placed by the radiographer. It should be made clear to all concerned that the patient will not be radioactive following the treatment. Time should be taken to talk with the patient and family, to answer questions and to provide support. The inclusion of the family will help them cope with their feelings and support the patient. Nurses working in oncology settings or regularly caring for individuals with cancer should make it a part of their own education to visit and familiarize themselves with radiotherapy departments.

SPECIFIC NURSING CARE MEASURES FOR PATIENTS RECEIVING EXTERNAL RADIATION THERAPY

During a course of radiation therapy, certain treatment-related side-effects can be expected to develop, most of which are site specific as well as dependent on volume, dose fractionation, total dose, and individual differences. Many symptoms do not develop until approximately 10–14 days after the start of treatment, and some do not subside until 2 or more weeks after treatments have ended. Patients should be assessed regularly by the nurse while on treatment. The skin of the area receiving radiation as well as the exit portal should be examined regularly, and the patient observed for fatigue, weakness and nutritional problems.

Nursing care measures and medical management described in the following sections reflect the general consensus from the literature (Battles, 1981; Yasko, 1982) and the authors' clinical experience. Alternatives exist for the management of these problems, and specific approaches may vary from institution to institution.

Skin reactions

Because moisture may enhance skin reactions, the person being treated should be advised to keep the skin in the treated areas as dry as possible. Bathing or showering is permissable, but long periods of soaking are inadvisable. Treated skin should be bathed gently with tepid water and gently patted (not rubbed) dry. Lines or markings placed on the skin at simulation should not be removed until the radiographer advises the patient to do so. It may therefore be necessary to take sponge baths rather than tub baths or a shower for some time to avoid washing off the markings.

General guidelines to follow for care of the skin within the treatment site include:

1. Keep the skin dry.
2. Avoid using soaps, powders, lotions, creams, alcohol and deodorants on skin over the treatment area. (As well as being an irritant, many such preparations contain metallic elements that may cause scattering of radiation beams.)
3. Wear loose-fitting, cotton clothing next to the treatment area.
4. Do not apply tape to the treatment site if dressings are applied.
5. Shave with an electric razor only. Do not use preshaves or aftershaves.
6. Protect the skin from exposure to direct sunlight, chlorinated pools and temperature extremes (avoid cold packs, hot-water bottles or heating pads).

Such precautions are necessary throughout the course of treatment and until any skin reaction has disappeared afterwards.

Specific measures that are useful in treating skin reactions include the use of a light dusting of cornflour for pruritus from erythema and dry desquamation. If moist desquamation and denuded areas appear, a thin layer of an appropriate topical agent, e.g. hydrocortisone cream may be applied, followed by a nonstick dressing to protect the clothing and the skin. The radiation oncologist or oncology clinical nurse specialist should always be consulted regarding general skin care measures or those appropriate to the individual experiencing a skin reaction. Out-patients should be given explicit directions for managing at home, and written directions are very helpful in addition to the verbal instructions.

It should also be remembered that individuals are often treated by parallel opposing portals and that only one of these portals may be marked to indicate the field. This means that in addition to the clearly marked portal on the person's abdomen or chest (for example), there may be a corresponding field on the posterior that needs the same careful attention.

Care of the hair and scalp while receiving radiation to the scalp includes very gentle brushing and combing and infrequent shampooing. Some radiation oncologists request that patients not shampoo at all, whereas others will suggest a once a week cleaning. Permanent waves or hair colouring are contraindicated because of the potential harm to the irradiated skin of the scalp. Individuals being treated in the neck and facial areas should also avoid any procedures on the hair that involve the use of harsh chemicals because such substances may run down on to treated skin. As with irradiated skin in general, the scalp should be treated with care and caution for several months to a year or more after all healing has taken place. The top of the head, forehead, ears and neck may exhibit sensitivity to the sun and should be protected from sunburn with a cap or wide-brimmed hat.

Bone marrow depression

When large volumes of active bone marrow are irradiated (especially the pelvis or spine in the adult), the effect on the marrow can be quite significant. Other areas of concern when large fields are treated include the sternum, ribs, long bones, skull. During simulation and treatment planning, provision is made for shielding as much of this active marrow as possible without compromising the treatment; thus the majority of people receiving therapy are able to tolerate a course of treatment without experiencing bone marrow depression. None the less, complete blood cell counts should be done at regular intervals on all individuals receiving radiation therapy. Particular attention should be paid to this when individuals are receiving concomitant chemotherapy or those who have had extensive chemotherapy before radiation. More detailed information about the nursing assessment and management of the patient with bone marrow depression is given on p. 170.

Mucositis, xerostomia

Mucositis is an alteration in the mucous membranes of the oral cavity which manifests as inflammation, desquamation and overt ulceration. The mucous membranes of the oral cavity sustain a great degree of trauma on a daily basis. The cells of these tissues must be highly proliferative to replace the cells which are continually damaged by thermal, mechanical, chemical and microbiological stressors. Radiation has the greatest effect on cells that have a rapid rate of cellular division. Because cells are damaged and cell replication is disrupted due to the effect of radiation, there is an inadequate supply of new cells to maintain the integrity of the oral mucosa, and signs and symptoms of mucositis appear. Factors such as poor nutritional status, poor oral hygiene, or any other factor that causes dryness and/or trauma of the mucous membranes, increase the severity and the duration of mucositis. Xerostomia (dry mouth) may result from radiation to the salivary glands or portions of them. Xerostomia results in difficulty talking, eating and swallowing, and can be quite distressing. Further information about the nursing assessment and management of the patient experiencing oral symptoms is given later on in this chapter.

Radiation caries

Although it is a potential late effect of irradiation to the mouth and oropharynx, radiation caries can be greatly reduced or avoided by proper care before, during and after a course of treatment. Absence of or a decrease in saliva and the altered pH produced by treatment promote decay. Before the start of therapy, a thorough dental examination and prophylaxis should be carried out. If extensive decay and general poor dentition exist,

full mouth extract is usually the treatment of choice. However, if teeth are in good repair, a vigorous preventative programme is begun to protect them from the late effects of radiation. This can include brushing the teeth with a soft-bristled brush several times daily, and a daily application of fluoride gel. Nursing support and encouragement are necessary in helping to ensure continuation of this preventive treatment when radiotherapy is completed.

Oesophagitis, dysphagia

When the oesophagus is located in the treatment field, inflammation and ulceration of the mucous membranes may occur. This condition produces difficulty in swallowing as well as a great deal of discomfort for the patient. Patients describe the discomfort of oesophagitis as a pain located in the substernal area that is severe and constant.

Nausea and vomiting

Of the potential side-effects from radiation therapy, nausea and vomiting are probably the most distressing to the person being treated. Although nausea and vomiting are not common, the fear that they will occur causes great stress in many individuals. As with other side-effects, treatment site and dose are the variables to be considered, along with pre-existing conditions related to chemotherapy and sites of disease. The patient's emotional state and apprehension about the disease and treatment are sometimes responsible for nausea when treatment is unlikely to be the cause. Generally the person receiving radiation therapy can be expected to experience some degree of nausea when treatment is directed to any of the following: abdomen, large pelvic fields, whole brain irradiation. However, the majority of patients experience little or no difficulty with this side-effect. When nausea does occur, it can usually be controlled by antiemetics administered on a regular schedule and by adjusting the eating pattern so that treatment is given when the stomach is relatively empty. Delaying intake of a full meal until 3–4 hours after treatment is also helpful because nausea, if it occurs, will usually appear from 1–3 hours after treatment.

Diarrhoea

Diarrhoea, like nausea and vomiting, is not an expected side-effect in most individuals receiving radiation therapy. However, it does occur if areas of the abdomen and pelvis are treated after about 200 cGy have been given. Some individuals experience only an increase in their usual number of bowel movements, whereas others develop loose, watery stools and intestinal cramping. For most individuals with radiation-induced diarrhoea, a low-residue diet (e.g. starchy foods, white bread, bananas or apples, avoiding caffeine, whole grains, high fibre, most fruits and juices, and fried, spicy or pickled meats) and perhaps a prescription of loperamide hydrochloride are usually sufficient.

Anorexia

Anorexia occurs frequently among individuals receiving radiation therapy, regardless of the treatment site. Like fatigue, anorexia is probably related to the presence in the person's system of the waste products of tissue destruction. Other possible causes for anorexia include anaemia, inactivity, medications, alterations in the person's ability to ingest and digest foods, and psychological factors. The cause often cannot be identified clearly, and therefore the symptom must be treated by utilizing all the techniques known to encourage adequate intake. A self-perpetuating cycle of anorexia, weight loss, weakness, inactivity and more anorexia can develop if the symptom is untreated. Fluid intake should be encouraged to promote elimination of the products of tissue breakdown.

Fatigue

Fatigue or malaise is common among most individuals during the course of radiation therapy and for varying periods after treatment is completed. More detailed information on the nursing assessment and management of fatigue in the individual with cancer is given on pp. 175–176.

Table 10.5 Preparative teaching for patients receiving internal radiation.

Preparation for internal radiation should include the following elements:

- General
  —Ensure that patient demonstrates knowledge and understanding prior to treatment
  —Explain why nurse can spend only limited time with patient
  —Use booklets, audiovisuals, demonstrations with instruments and models if appropriate
  —Reassure concerning fears of radiation
  —Stress importance of adhering to safety regulations and regulations governing visiting time and proximity to patient
  —Explain guidelines for visitors to patient and family
     Visitors should check at nursing station before entering the room
     No visitors under twelve years of age
     No pregnant visitors
     Visitors are restricted to a thirty minute period each day
     Visitors should sit at the end of the bed to decrease their exposure to the radiation
  —Provide explanation to patient regarding removal of the applicator:
     Explain to patient that there is little or no discomfort associated with removal
     Radioactive material is removed first and placed in a portable lead safe
     There may be a noticeable odour from the gynaecological packing when it is removed. Explain that this is always expected
     Inform patient that they will be helped with their first attempt to get out of bed as they may feel weak or dizzy
     if they have been lying flat for several days. Reassure them as their energy increases they will be able to get up as much as they wish
- Description of the procedure for inserting applicators and sources
- Possible change in appearance
- Anticipated pain or discomfort and measures available for relief
- Potential short-term and long-term side-effects and complications
  —Example: oedema, swelling, dysuria, sterility, formation of adhesions
- Restrictions on activity while the radioactive sources are in place
- Visiting restrictions
  —Help patient to prepare for the possible isolation and boredom that are sometimes the most difficult part of treatment with radioactive source by planning for suitable activities such as reading, listening to music, handwork, television, etc.
- Radiation precautions observed by hospital personnel
  —Reassure patient that personal care needs will be met but that the nurses' time at the bedside and in the room will be restricted because of the presence of the radioactive sources
  —Explain need for patient to perform as much self-care as possible

---

Tenesmus, cystitis, urethritis

Although infrequent, tenesmus, cystitis and urethritis do occur in some individuals receiving pelvic irradiation. Tenesmus of the anal or urinary sphincter produces a persistent sensation of the need to evacuate the bowel or bladder. Relief can sometimes be obtained from gastrointestinal and urinary antispasmodic and anticholinergic agents. The problem may persist, however, until after the course of treatment has ended. Cystitis and urethritis resulting from radiation to the bladder areas is distressing to the person being treated. A clean voided urine specimen for culture and sensitivity should be obtained and appropriate antibiotic therapy instituted if indicated. Usually, infection is not found and treatment consists of urinary antispasmodics for symptomatic relief. High fluid intake is encouraged.

NURSING CARE OF THE PATIENT RECEIVING INTERNAL RADIATION

Patients who are receiving internal radiation therapy need careful, detailed explanations of the treatment and subsequent care in order to participate responsibly in that care. They need to know what they will experience when the radiation source is applied or administered. The reasons nursing care is planned for minimal exposure time need to be explained. Any restrictions on physical activities need to be explained and planned for. Table 10.5 outlines the points to be considered in designing preparative teaching programmes for the patient who will receive internal radiation.

In addition to experiencing fears related to the radiation treatment itself, the patient receiving internal radiation therapy will have to cope with a brief period of social isolation. Although measures must be taken to minimize exposure of all hospital personnel to radiation, nursing care should be planned in such a way that communication is maintained and the patient feels supported. The nurse can accomplish this by frequent, brief stops at the doorway of the patient's room or by providing care at intervals throughout the day, rather than giving care all at one time and then staying away for the rest of the shift. Patients who have internal sources of radiation are usually very sensitive to the fact that they can cause harm to others. This causes an increase in anxiety, especially since they have no way of detecting that this harm is occurring. They are also anxious about the harm the radiation is doing to their own normal tissues. This anxiety can be decreased by explaining the controls designed to protect others. It is also important for patients to know that they are no longer radioactive when the source has been removed.

Family members also often have a difficult time during internal radiation because of the enforced separation. They frequently benefit from increased information and support. The radiation may be so fearful that some family members will avoid the patient completely. Explanations of safeguards and limiting time of contact can be helpful to these family members. If they are still reluctant to go near the patient, telephone communication can be encouraged.

Table 10.6 General nursing care measures for the patient receiving internal radiation.

- Pain
  —Assess for type of pain, intensity and location
  —Use special mattresses to promote comfort and minimize skin lesions
  —Administer analgesics as required and monitor effectiveness
  —Plan pain management strategies incorporating psychological, cultural and spiritual factors that may influence pain
  —Ensure that patients who have difficulty sleeping because of pain or position required by implants obtain sleep medications
  —Minimize dysphagia and mucositis through use of soft or liquid diet, pain medications or topical anaesthetic as ordered, and careful oral hygiene after removal of head and neck implant
  —Teach relaxation and imagery to cope with pain, discomfort and isolation
- Nausea and vomiting
  —Prevent nausea and vomiting wherever possible by use of antiemetics, administered regularly if required, and appropriate diet
  —If vomiting occurs, monitor head and neck patients for dislodgement of radiation sources or aspiration of vomitus; monitor patients with cervical or uterine implants for dislodgement

- Psychological issues
  —Provide support and comfort as much as possible within restrictions of radiation safety precautions
  —Avoid showing fear of radiation; avoid making patient feel 'untouchable'
  —Make time spent with patient quality time and focus complete attention on patient in this period
  —Encourage open communication and exploration of fears of altered body image, loss of sexual function, fear of death, etc, and provide specific sexual instructions (where appropriate)
  —Consider referral to clinical nurse specialist, social worker, psychologist or religious adviser, as indicated
- Dislodgement
  —Patients with gynaecological implants must remain in bed
  —Prevent bowel movements during implant (gynaecological only) by ensuring clean bowel prior to procedure and providing a low-residue diet and antidiarrhoeal agents. Ensure patient not constipated prior to return home (laxative may be needed)
  —Avoid vomiting, constipation or diarrhoea
  —If dislodgement occurs, notify radiation safety officer immediately; follow radiation safety procedures
- Long-term complications (fibrosis, stricture, adhesions, dyspareunia, etc)
  —Head and neck implant: provide saliva substitute and encourage consumption of fluids prior to eating. Gradually advance diet from liquid to soft to solid foods
  —Gynaecological implant: teach use of topical creams and lubricants to affected areas; teach use of vaginal dilators after implants. Inform patients about when to resume sexual intercourse and alternative sexual positions to decrease/eliminate painful intercourse

---

Table 10.6 outlines the general nursing measures for the care of patients receiving brachytherapy. Interventions specific to the care of patients receiving various types of internal radiation can be found in the suggested readings at the end of the chapter.

RADIATION SAFETY PRINCIPLES

Radiation safety is not a concern for nurses caring for patients who are receiving external beam therapy; radiation is not being released by their body after treatment. However, when caring for a patient with an internal radiation source the nurse must practise in a manner that will reduce his or her exposure to radiation. Hospitals that have an extensive programme of radiation therapy may have specially designed facilities for patients receiving brachytherapy. The point should also be made that the degree of safety precautions necessary during use of internal sources is dictated by the energy of the isotope. Therefore, it is important that the nurse check with the radiation safety officer to determine the specific radiation safety precautions required.

Personnel are provided with monitoring badges which measure the amount of radiation to which the worker is exposed. Some people unconsciously believe that these badges are a form of protection against radiation and they may be less cautious when wearing one. The badge provides no protection at all; it simply measures exposure. The dose received is calculated at regular intervals, with records kept of the cumulative dose. Accurate reading of the badge requires that the badge be kept on the nursing unit to which the nurse is assigned; it should not be loaned to another nurse, worn on the street or at home, and so on.

Three factors are important in taking adequate radiation precautions: *time*, *distance* and *shielding*.

The safety principle concerning *time* dictates that the nurse should spend a minimal amount of time with a patient who has a radioactive source in place. Necessary treatments and care should be well planned and expedited to minimize the time spent at the bedside, while still providing for the patient's needs.

In addition, the greater the *distance* from the source, the less radiation will be received. The intensity of radiation decreases as the square of the distance from the source of radiation. The further away the nurse is from the source, the smaller the dose of radiation he or she will be exposed to over a given time. For example, if the distance from the source is doubled, the radiation dose intensity will decrease to one-quarter of the dose intensity at the original point.

The principle of *shielding* is more readily employed by the nurse in the handling of displaced radioactive sources, excreta collection and disposal, and required disposition of linen, dressings and equipment contaminated with radioactive solutions. Because shielding from gamma radiation requires 6-mm thick lead or 10-cm thick concrete, it is usually impractical to expect that much physical care can be given from behind such a shield. The lead aprons used in diagnostic radiology are not of sufficient thickness to stop gamma rays and cannot protect the care-giver from exposure when caring for individuals with radium or caesium sources, for example. In the rooms of patients with encapsulated sources there should be a special container into which the sources can be placed if they become dislodged. If a source does dislodge, nurses must use 12-inch forceps and not the hands to place it in the container provided. Contaminated linen, equipment, dressings and excreta are usually a safety hazard only when metabolized radiation therapy is employed (e.g. ^{131}I). The decontamination of these items is necessary prior to disposal or reuse. Since the procedures to be followed vary with the isotope employed, the radiation safety officer should provide specific instructions as to storage and disposal.

Some other ways of reducing exposure include: preparing meal trays outside of the person's room instead of at the bedside; positioning the bedside table, call bell, and television controls within each reach of the patient to avoid return trips to the bedside; and using appropriate radiation precaution signs, wristbands and tags.

In concluding this discussion of radiation safety principles it should be noted that a pregnant nurse is never assigned to care for patients undergoing internal radiation therapy.

Bone Marrow Transplantation

Bone marrow transplantation (BMT) has evolved over the past 30 years from an experimental procedure to an established and effective treatment for selected patients. In the last decade, the number of recipients of marrow transplantation has increased and BMT is now being used as a treatment for an expanding list of malignant and non-malignant haematological diseases.

Conventional treatment of cancer consists of the use of surgery, chemotherapy and/or radiation therapy to eradicate all tumour cells. Doses of chemotherapy and/or radiation therapy are often limited because of toxicity to the patient's bone marrow. Many believe that if bone marrow toxicity could somehow be minimized, chemotherapy doses could be increased to levels that would cure the patient of the malignancy (Santos and Kaizer, 1982; Parkman, 1986). If the patient's own marrow or that of a compatible donor can be introduced into the body and successfully engrafted, then doses far higher than those conventionally used become possible (Thomas et al, 1975). This is the rationale for BMT.

DISEASES TREATED WITH BONE MARROW TRANSPLANTATION

BMT provides two potential therapeutic advantages over more standard therapy. It makes it possible to increase the intensity of cytoreductive therapy without regard to haematopoietic toxicity, and it is thought that post-transplant changes in immunological responses may provide an immunotherapeutic effective against residual tumour cells (Santos and Kaizer, 1982; Parkman, 1986). With this rationale in mind, BMT is currently the treatment of choice of some patients with acute and chronic leukaemia, hairy cell leukaemia, preleukaemic states, lymphoma, multiple myeloma see Chapter 13, neuroblastoma, and selected solid tumours. BMT is also used to treat non-malignant disorders of the bone marrow, such as acquired aplastic anaemia, Fanconi's anaemia, thalassaemia and sickle cell anaemia. In addition, immunodeficiency diseases such as severe combined immunodeficiency (SCID) and Wiskott–Aldrich syndrome are being treated with BMT (Thomas, 1985).

SOURCES OF DONOR BONE MARROW

There are three sources of donor bone marrow: autologous, syngeneic and allogeneic. The source of bone marrow is dependent on the disease being treated and the results of histocompatibility typing of potential donors (Santos, 1984; Freeman, 1988).

Autologous BMT uses the patient's own bone marrow that has been stored for use for haematopoietic reconstitution at a later date; thus donor and recipient are the same. Using the patient's own bone marrow is advantageous because there is no risk of incompatibility. However, relapse following autologous BMT is a frequent problem and may be from failure of the pretransplant therapy or from reinfusion of tumour cells at the time of transplant (Santos and Kaizer, 1982). Treating the autologous bone marrow with monoclonal antibodies or chemotherapy in an effort to rid the marrow of residual tumour cells before reinfusing it are currently being studied (Feldman, 1989). Autologous transplants are only performed for malignant diseases; the patients are usually in a state of remission when the marrow is collected (Gorin, 1986; Yeager et al, 1986).

Syngeneic BMT is the use of bone marrow from an identical twin; a perfect histocompatible match. Syngeneic BMT eliminates the problems of bone marrow rejection and graft-versus-host disease (GVHD). Mortality secondary to treatment complications is also reduced; however, death due to leukaemic relapse increases (Thomas et al, 1975; Santos and Kaizer, 1982). This is thought to be due to the absence of a graft-versus-leukaemia effect provided by mild GVHD (Kamani and August, 1984).

The most common source of bone marrow is *allogeneic*. The donor is most often a sibling, but occasionally an unrelated person. Unrelated but tissue-type identical allogeneic transplants have been made possible through the use of computer generated lists of volunteer blood donors who have been tissue typed in North America and Europe (Hansen et al, 1980; Cheson and Curt, 1986).

TISSUE TYPING

In marrow transplantation, as in any other organ transplant, histocompatibility testing must be carried out. Histocompatibility is determined by two tests: human leucocyte antigen (HLA) typing and the mixed lymphocyte culture or reaction (MLC or MLR).

HLA typing can only identify the antigens located on the A, B or C locus of chromosome 6. Compatibility at the HLA-D and HLA-DR loci is determined by the mixed lymphocyte culture (MLC). The MLC establishes compatibility by combining lymphocytes from the potential donor with those of the recipient in a culture medium for several days. If a disparity exists between the antigens, the potential donor's lymphocytes react against the recipient's foreign antigens. A *non-reactive* MLC signals compatibility (Dudjak, 1984).

Donors may have identical HLA typing and be MLC-non-reactive, yet have different ABO blood types. This ABO incompatibility does not preclude BMT. With the use of plasmapheresis and immunoadsorption techniques, the removal of A or B antibodies from recipients is possible.

OVERVIEW OF THE BONE MARROW TRANSPLANTATION PROCESS

Once a source of donor bone marrow has been identified the recipient is prepared for the transplant. Pretransplant preparation includes a comprehensive physical assessment, baseline studies and a family assessment to identify families that may need special support. Patients also have an indwelling central line inserted for long-term venous access. Venous access is crucial for the infusion of hyperalimentation, antibiotics and blood products, and for frequent blood sampling.

The high-dose chemotherapy and total body irradiation used in preparative regimens cause gonadal failure; consequently, sperm banking should be considered before admission to the hospital in patients with adequate sperm counts.

A protocol or treatment plan for pre-BMT immunosuppression must be chosen. Pretransplant immunosuppression serves three purposes: (1) it destroys the patient's own immune system and therefore decreases the risk of graft rejection; (2) it removes malignant cells; and (3) it prepares space in the bone marrow for engraftment of the new marrow (Kamani and August, 1984). The type of preparation chosen is influenced by the underlying disease. For non-malignant conditions the preparation is directed at immunosuppression, whereas in malignant disorders therapy must also eradicate the malignant cells (Thomas et al, 1975). Conditioning regimens typically last 4–8 days. Common protocols combine total body irradiation (TBI) in either single dose or multiple fractionated doses with very high doses of chemotherapy (Thomas et al, 1976; Hansen et al, 1980; Dudjak, 1984; Gringrich et al, 1985; Cheson and Curt, 1986).

Cyclophosphamide is a common alkylating agent used for intensive cell destruction. It is most effective on the rapidly dividing cells of the marrow. Other drugs that may be used include busulphan, thioguanine, cytarabine, etoposide and lomustine (Cheson and Curt, 1986). Total body irradiation adds to the immunosuppressive effect of the chemotherapy and is able to penetrate such chemotherapy-resistant sites as the central nervous system and the testicles (Gringrich et al, 1985). After this preparation the patient is ready to receive the donor marrow.

The major-side effects of the pretransplant conditioning regimens are nausea and vomiting, diarrhoea, stomatitis, skin reactions and alopecia (Hutchison and King, 1983). Low grade fever and parotid gland tenderness and swelling are often seen following TBI (Thomas et al, 1975).

Although risks to donors are minimal, donors are carefully evaluated for tolerance of general anaesthesia for marrow harvest. Marrow donors are usually admitted to the hospital shortly before the surgery and discharged 24–48 hours after surgery.

Bone marrow harvesting

The purpose of marrow harvesting is to collect enough stem cells (pluripotent cells) to fully reconstitute the haematopoietic system after infusion. The stem cell is able to reproduce itself as well as serve as precursor to the various blood components found in the marrow and peripheral blood. The majority of stem cells are found in the marrow but some can be found in the peripheral circulation.

Allogeneic BMT. The collection of bone marrow from the donor is done in the operating room, usually under general anaesthesia. Marrow is aspirated from the posterior and sometimes the anterior iliac crests. Approximately 150–200 aspirations are done although only 6–10 skin punctures are made because the aspiration needles are redirected to different sites under the skin. Approximately 400–800 ml of bone marrow, or a total of approximately 10–15 ml/kg of recipient body weight, is collected. However, the actual number of stem cells obtained is more important than the quantity of marrow collected; the number of nucleated marrow cells required for consistent haematopoietic reconstitution is 0.5×10^8 cells per kilogram. Most centres obtain three to four times this amount to ensure reconstitution in all patients. The bone marrow is filtered to remove bone chips and fat particles, mixed with heparinized saline to prevent clotting, and transferred to a blood transfusion bag for delivery to the recipient within 2–4 hours.

Autologous BMT.   Aspirations for autologous transplantation are obtained in a similar manner. The marrow may be incubated with chemotherapeutic drugs, immunotoxins, or monoclonal antibodies to purge tumour cells, cryopreserved for up to 3 years, or immediately infused after completion of the high-dose preparative regimen (Schryber et al, 1987).

Bone marrow infusion

The transplant itself, the actual infusion of bone marrow, is often an anticlimatic event. The marrow arrives in a large blood transfusion bag and is infused intravenously over 2–3 hours through one of the patient's indwelling central lines. Cryopreserved bone marrow for autologous transplantation is rapidly thawed at the bedside and infused immediately. Complications that have been seen with the infusion of marrow include volume overload and pulmonary abnormalities secondary to fat emboli. Symptoms similar to blood transfusion reaction, such as chills, urticaria and fever, are seen occasionally (Hutchison and King, 1983; Kamani and August, 1984).

Postinfusion/engraftment period

Following the ablative chemotherapy and/or radiation therapy, severe pancytopenia occurs. Once the marrow is infused the stem cells circulate through the patient's blood and repopulate the bone marrow. This constitutes bone marrow regeneration and is usually detectable within 2–4 weeks after transplantation. When bone marrow engraftment is complete, while blood cells, red blood cells and platelets are produced and are deposited into the peripheral bloodstream. Until this occurs, however, the patient has no marrow function, and production of white blood cells, platelets and red blood cells is halted.

Both allogeneic and autologous transplant necessitate a period of 4–6 weeks hospitalization in protective isolation. Complications which may arise from the immediate or delayed effects of the transplant include: infection; stomatitis; bleeding; graft-versus-host-disease (in allogeneic transplants); inadequate engraftment (in autologous transplants); relapse from disease; or hepatic, cardiac, renal, neurological and psychological complications. Physical and psychological convalescence requires at least 1 year and can be extremely stressful for both the patient and the family.

GVHD occurs when immunologically competent T lymphocytes are introduced into a host who is immunologically incompetent and therefore incapable of

rejecting this foreign invasion. The donor T lymphocytes elicit the response of GVHD in the host. Since the host is immunosuppressed the lymphocytes of the graft proliferate and mount an attack against various host cells. Thus, after BMT, when the donor's immunocompetent lymphocytes come in contact with an immunosuppressed recipient, they proceed to attack and kill selected host cells.

There are also psychosocial problems associated with BMT. Patients and families are often treated at centres far from home. The stresses of being treated for an otherwise fatal illness, long-term isolation and frequent, painful procedures often cause patients to become anxious, depressed or angry. Refusal to co-operate with staff as well as overdependence often occur.

Biological Response Modifier Therapy

In the past, the care of patients with cancer required an understanding of three treatment modalities: surgery, radiation therapy and chemotherapy. Over the past two decades medical technology has developed a group of agents whose primary site of action is the immune system. Collectively known as biologics or biological response modifiers (BRMs), these agents now comprise the fourth type of cancer therapy. Some predict that in the 1990s biologics will be used increasingly in the treatment of cancer.

As the need for health care professionals to know about biologics has grown, so has the expectation that they should be able to interpret the available information for the patient and family. A complete description of the functioning of the immune system and how it relates to biological response modifier therapy is beyond the scope of this chapter. (The reader is referred to several excellent sources for more information: Oldham and Smalley, 1983; Suppers and McClamrock, 1985; Abernathy, 1987; Irwin, 1987; Moldawer, 1988; Carter et al, 1989; Yasko and Dudjak, 1990). However, the following sections provide an overview of the therapeutic effects of biologics in the treatment of cancer and the organ/system toxicities and side-effects commonly encountered with this therapy. See also Chapter 6.

BIOLOGICAL RESPONSE MODIFIER THERAPY IN THE TREATMENT OF CANCER

Biological response modifiers, or biologics, are agents or approaches to cancer treatment that modify the individual's own biological response to the tumour (Oldham and Smalley, 1983). A BRM is defined as any soluble substance that is capable of modifying the immune system with either a stimulatory or a suppressive effect (Huffner et al, 1985). Depending on the BRM, one or more therapeutic effects may be noted:

1. Regulation and/or augmentation of the immune response.
2. Cytotoxic or cytostatic activity directed toward cancer cells.
3. Inhibition of metastasis, differentiation or maturation.

Table 10.7 Biological response modifier therapy: actions, potential indications and side-effects

	Postulated mechanism of action	Potential indications	Toxicities/side-effects
Colony stimulating factors (CSFs)	• GM-CSF: stimulates production of neutrophils, macrophages, eosinophils and, in the presence of erythropoietin, red blood cells • G-CSF: stimulates neutrophil production • M-CSF: stimulates macrophage production • EPO—erythropoietin: stimulates maturation of erythrocytes	• Not directly tumoricidal. Research indicates they may be useful for cancer treatment because they: 1. Decrease duration of neutropenia that often results from chemotherapy 2. Enable higher doses of chemotherapy to be given since CSFs can alter the dose-related toxicity of myelosuppression 3. Decrease bone marrow recovery time following bone marrow transplants or radiation therapy-related suppression of marrow In clinical studies, CSFs have shown activity in the treatment of leukaemias, including chronic lymphocytic leukaemia, hairy cell leukaemia, myelodysplastic syndrome, and neutropenia secondary to chemotherapy	• Flu-like syndrome: fever, chills, fatigue/weakness, myalgia/arthralgia, headache • Gastrointestinal: nausea, diarrhoea, vomiting, anorexia • Other: facial flushing
Tumour necrosis factor (TNF)	• In vitro: binds to receptors on tumour cells and is directly tumoricidal or tumoristatic • In vivo: precise mechanism of action is unclear. TNF may be directly cytotoxic or it may cause vascular endothelial damage in tumour capillaries resulting in haemorrhage and necrosis of tumour cells. TNF may also work through immune cell activation as it has been found to augment natural killer T-cell activity and to enhance B-cell proliferation	• Many clinical trials are underway to determine the efficacy of TNF. TNF may be helpful in treating metastatic adenocarcinomas including colorectal, hepatic, and bladder carcinomas	• Flu-like syndrome: fever, chills, fatigue/weakness, myalgia/arthralgia, back pain • Gastrointestinal: nausea, vomiting, diarrhoea, anorexia • Non-specific: severe pain at tumour site
Monoclonal antibodies (MoAbs)	• Application of MoAbs is based on the knowledge that all cells (including tumour cells) have antigens present on their surface that are specific to that cell type • MoAbs may be used alone or bound to radioisotopes, toxins, or chemotherapeutic drugs to stain, destroy or identify cells with specific antigens on their cell surface	• May be used in the treatment of cancer as well as for diagnostic purposes. In clinical trials MoAbs have shown activity in the treatment of leukaemia, lymphoma, metastatic breast and colorectal cancer, ovarian, renal, bladder and prostate cancer	• Flu-like syndrome: fever, chills, headache, fatigue, malaise, myalgias • Gastrointestinal: nausea, diarrhoea, vomiting • Skin: generalized erythema, urticaria, pruritus • Anaphylaxis (rare but severe and life threatening)
Interferons (IFNs)	• *Antiviral:* IFNs stimulate cells infected with viruses to produce proteins that interfere with viral replication • *Antiproliferative:* IFNs slow the reproduction of cells. Although	• Has shown some activity in the treatment of Hairy cell leukaemia, AIDS-related Kaposi's sarcoma, multiple myeloma, nodular cutaneous T-cell lymphoma and chronic granulocytic	• Flu-like syndrome: fever, chills, headache, fatigue, malaise, myalgias • Gastrointestinal: nausea, diarrhoea, vomiting, anorexia, taste alterations, xerostomia

Table 10.7 *Continued*

	Postulated mechanism of action	Potential indications	Toxicities/side-effects
	the mechanisms are not well understood, possible contributing factors include inhibition of DNA and protein synthesis of cancer cells and prolongation of the cell cycle • *Immunomodulatory:* depending on the type of IFN, different aspects of the immune system are stimulated or augmented. Examples include: T-cell activation, increased phagocytic and cytotoxic activity of macrophages and mature natural killer cells	leukaemia	• Neurological/psychological: mild confusion, somnolence, irritability, poor concentration • Haematological: neutropenia and thrombocytopenia
Interleukins (ILs)	• Interleukins are among the most important regulatory substances produced by lymphocytes and monocytes. Seven types of ILs have been isolated and identified; however, other than IL-1, IL-2 and IL-3, little is known about their biological effects. Presently only IL-2 and IL-3 are being studied actively in clinical trials • The ILs appear to act by causing proliferation and stimulation of T and B lymphocytes, assisting in the synthesis and secretion of lymphokines (e.g. interferon, CSFs) and/or enhancing natural kill T-cell activity	• Has shown some activity in the treatment of metastatic renal cell carcinoma, malignant melanoma, and non-Hodgkins lymphomas	• Administration of interleukin results in multisystem toxicities that may be life threatening. Toxicities are related to dose and schedule • Flu-like syndrome: fever, chills, headache, fatigue, malaise, myalgias • Gastrointestinal: nausea, diarrhoea, vomiting, anorexia, taste alterations, xerostomia • Skin: dryness, erythematous rash, pruritus, desquamation • Neurological/psychological: confusion, irritability, impaired memory, sleep disturbances, depression • Cardiovascular: capillary leak syndrome, peripheral oedema, ascites, arrhythmias, hypotension • Pulmonary: dyspnoea, pulmonary oedema, ascites, arrhythmias, hypotension • Renal: oliguria, anuria, azotaemia, elevation of serum creatinine and blood urea nitrogen levels

Due to advances in recombinant DNA technology, highly purified biologics are now produced in large quantities and are available for use in cancer therapy. This process involves isolating a portion of the DNA gene that codes for a specific BRM (e.g. the DNA responsible for the production of interferon) from the chromosome of a human cell and fusing it to the DNA of a bacterial cell. This is recombinant DNA. The hybrid DNA is then reinserted into a bacterium or a yeast cell that acts as a host cell. When the host cell divides and replicates, it copies itself and the recombinant DNA. The new gene directs the host cell to make a new protein product such as interferon. The rapid reproduction of the host cells allows mass production of the BRM protein. Biologics produced in this manner are designated as recombinant.

Biologics are unique in their ability to regulate or enhance the immune response. The cytotoxic or cytostatic effects of chemotherapeutic agents and radiation therapy are primarily a result of direct interaction with cancer cells. In contrast, biologics can activate the body's natural defences. Consequently, compared with more conventional forms of treatment, biologics have potentially greater antineoplastic activity and reduced toxicity. However, biologics are still under investigation and additional information is needed.

Table 10.7 summarizes the principal actions, potential indications and commonly reported toxicities and side-effects for several of the biologics. Because the majority of BRMs are still under investigation, this information continues to evolve. Also, because optimal dosages have not been determined, recommended dose ranges are not included.

The side-effects associated with biologics are variable in their onset and intensity. Side-effects and toxicities vary with the agent, the dosage schedule, the dose and the patient. It is important to note that not all BRMs, or even the same BRM at the same dose, produce the same side-effects. The side-effect most unique to the BRM therapy is a set of symptoms collectively known as flu-like syndrome. These symptoms include fever, chills and rigors, fatigue, anorexia, hypotension, myalgias, arthralgias and headache. Collectively, biologics have the potential to manifest toxicities in virtually every body system. Table 10.8 lists some suggested nursing measures for patients receiving biologics. Several excellent references describing the nursing assessment and management of symptoms experienced by patients receiving biological response modifier therapy are listed at the end of the chapter.

Unproven Therapies

Many unproven methods of cancer treatment are available to the person with cancer. Such methods range from true quackery to the still unproven. It is essential that nurses are aware of and knowledgeable about such methods as patients frequently have questions about unproven treatments or may be actually engaged in a treatment.

The common characteristics of unproven methods are that the treatment provider lacks formal training in cancer therapy or has meaningless credentials; detailed information about the treatment is not shared with the public or health care professionals; and frequently the promoter of an unproven method will attack the medical and scientific community (Miller and Howard-Ruben, 1983).

While a patient may or may not experience any harm from using an unproven method, they may be at risk from being given unrealistic hope, and being financially burdened by the costs associated with unproven methods.

The types of unproven methods include machines; drugs and chemicals, particularly herbs and vaccines; nutritional programmes; and psychological techniques. Some well-known treatments include laetrile, macrobiotic diets, the Simonton method and the Greek cure. However, in fairness it should be said that many conventional practitioners show a marked reluctance to acknowledge that anything other than orthodox medical treatments can be of benefit to individual patients.

It is also important to differentiate between alternative *medicine* and complementary therapies, e.g. relaxation, massage, aromatherapy, stress reduction techniques. The former may lead an individual to reject conventional therapy, with potentially adverse consequences, whereas the latter may serve as a source of comfort and support and enable a person to adapt more easily to the effects of disease and treatment.

It is understandable that a person faced with a

Table 10.8   Suggested nursing measures for patients receiving BRMs.

- Observe for presence and severity of symptoms
- Provide information and reassurance
  —Encourage and answer questions
  —Provide support and clarification of information to assist in decision-making process
  —Reinforce explanation of specific agent, including mode of action, method of administration, side-effects and self-care strategies
  —Provide written materials
  —Include family/significant other in teaching session
  —Help patient to anticipate and deal with flu-like symptoms
  —Educate patient and family to report subtle symptom changes
  —Participate with other team members in evaluating patient's understanding of and ability to participate in a clinical trial
- Minimize discomfort and maintain optimal mobility level and nutritional status
  —Administer narcotics, antihistamines, and prostaglandin inhibitors as ordered to manage flu-like symptoms
  —Teach patient coping skills such as relaxation, imagery
  —Teach patient measures to maintain level of mobility, pattern of daily activities, appropriate use of medications, application of heat
  —Provide warmth during chills
  —Allow for rest periods throughout the day
  —Assess nutritional status and evaluate dietary intake regularly
  —Provide specific suggestions for managing anorexia, nausea and vomiting, and taste changes

---

potentially life-threatening disease should seek out any avenues that appear to offer hope and survival. For many individuals, complementary therapies and alternative treatments give an opportunity to regain some choice and control over lives disrupted by disease.

Nurses have a responsibility to be knowledgeable about alternative and complementary therapies in order to discuss options and help patients to make informed decisions. By giving patients sufficient time to communicate fears and anxieties, nurses may play a key role in guiding the patient away from desperate measures and towards helpful coping strategies.

NURSING ASSESSMENT AND MANAGEMENT OF DISEASE AND TREATMENT RELATED PROBLEMS

The nursing care assessment and management of the most common disease and treatment related problems of cancer are discussed in this section.

BONE MARROW DEPRESSION

Leucopenia makes the patient very susceptible to infection. A marked decrease in white blood cells below

Table 10.9 Nursing care of the person with bone marrow depression.

Assessment	Patient problems/Goals	Intervention
A. Leucopenia and infection		
• Assess the patient for signs and symptoms of infection: —Fever >38°C, hypotension, chills —Monitor the respiratory and genitourinary systems, skin and mucous membranes, and sites of peripheral and central venous catheters for infection —Monitor white blood cell counts and the differential daily. A neutrophil count of less than 10^6/l substantially increases the risk of infection —Monitor for signs and symptoms of sepsis	• The major problem is the potential for infection and consequently the patient goal is that infection will not occur • The onset of infection will be identified as soon as defining signs and symptoms appear • Patient/significant other will identify appropriate member of the health team when symptoms occur • Patient/significant other know the signs and symptoms of infection and is able to monitor and report on them • Patient will be protected from nosocomial infection during the period of hospitalization	• Monitor temperature 4-hourly or more frequently • Minimize exposure to potential sources of infection —Persons with transmissible diseases —Stagnant water (flower vases, respiratory equipment, humidifiers) —Faeces of animals • Instruct the patient in maintaining good hygiene —Handwashing after toileting and before meals —Daily shower or bath • Maintain integrity of skin and mucous membranes —Prevent injury of rectal mucosa by avoiding enemas, suppositories and rectal thermometers —Promote oral hygiene and prevent injury to oral mucosa by avoiding heavy brushing —Use an electric razor —Avoid injections if at all possible • Avoid use of invasive equipment such as indwelling urinary catheters • Practice protective measures —Wash hands before and after caring for neutropenic patients —Keep equipment in contact with the patient clean —Institute protective isolation (single room, strict handwashing, exclude fresh fruits and vegetables from diet, no potted plants) when the neutrophil count is <1000/mm^3 • Administer antibiotics, antifungal and antiviral agents on time • Instruct the patient on signs and symptoms of infection, self-care measures, how to take an oral temperature, and to notify health care providers if infection is suspected
B. Thrombocytopenia and bleeding		
• Monitor the platelet count daily • Monitor for signs and symptoms of bleeding, especially petechiae; bleeding gums; bruising; epistaxis; blood in urine, stool emesis; heavy menstruation; intracranial bleeding; oozing from i.v. sites or other wounds	• The principal potential problem is that of bleeding and the patient goal is therefore that bleeding will not occur • Signs and symptoms of minor and serious bleeding will be detected and reported • Patient/significant other can list measures to prevent bleeding	• Avoid use of medications that alter platelet production and function, i.e. aspirin and aspirin-containing products, anticoagulants, non-steroidal anti-inflammatory agents • When the platelet count is <50 000/mm^3 institute measures to prevent trauma and possible bleeding: —Avoid activities that could cause physical injury —Use electric razors to shave —Avoid rectal manipulation including enemas, suppositories, rectal temperature —Blowing of the nose should be gentle to avoid epistaxis • Avoid injections. If necessary, use a small needle and apply pressure after the injection for 3–5 minutes or until bleeding stops.

Table 10.9 *Continued*

Assessment	Patient problems/Goals	Intervention
		Minimize venepunctures as much as possible
		• Administer platelet transfusions as prescribed

a normal range must be identified and nursing measures instituted to minimize the risk of infection. Patients with severe leucopenia are in a potentially life-threatening situation. The most common sites of infection are the blood, respiratory tract, alimentary tract, skin and the genitourinary tract. The use of invasive procedures, and breaks in the normal protective mechanism such as the skin and mucous membranes, may potentiate the risk of infection. An increase in temperature above 38°C is the most common sign of infection in a neutropenic patient. In most situations antimicrobial treatment is initiated immediately and continued until the patient has recovery of the bone marrow and is afebrile.

Anaemia may be manifested by weakness, tiredness, pallor and shortness of breath. Chemotherapy-induced anaemia is usually a gradual process and may not be evident for several weeks after initiating chemotherapy. If patients are symptomatic due to anaemia, transfusion of packed red cells will be given until marrow recovery.

Thrombocytopenia increases the risk of the patient bleeding because of the impairment of the blood clotting process. Signs of thrombocytopenia include ecchymoses, petechiae, blood in the urine or stool, vaginal bleeding or evidence of bleeding of other organs or systems. The sclera is a common site of haemorrhage. When the platelet count drops below 50×10^6 platelets/l spontaneous haemorrhage may occur, and this risk increases when the counts drop below 20×10^6 platelets/l. Platelet transfusions are given to support the patient until his or her own bone marrow starts to produce adequate platelets.

Nursing management of bone marrow depression includes prevention and management of infection and bleeding, patient education, close monitoring, and implementation of preventive nursing care measures. Table 10.9 describes the specific nursing care of patients with bone marrow depression.

GASTROINTESTINAL PROBLEMS

Nausea and vomiting

Nausea and vomiting are two of the most common and distressing sequelae of cancer and cancer therapy. Inadequate control of nausea and vomiting results in complications such as dehydration, anorexia, malnutrition and metabolic disturbances. The distress associated with nausea and vomiting may cause patients to be unable, unwilling or to refuse to continue treatment. In recent years there has been increased effort to develop pharmacological and non-pharmacological methods to prevent and to control nausea and vomiting.

The precise physiological mechanism of nausea and vomiting is not entirely clear. The act of vomiting is integrated and co-ordinated by the true vomiting centre (TVC). This centre is located bilaterally in the medulla. The TVC receives afferent impulses from the chemoreceptor trigger zone (CTZ) located in the medulla at the base of the fourth ventricle. Administration of certain drugs directly stimulates the CTZ which then activates the TVC. The CTZ also receives impulses from the labyrinth in the middle ear, which is the mechanism related to motion sickness. Distension and irritation of the stomach and duodenum will cause vagal visceral afferent stimulation of the TVC. Inflammation, irritation and obstruction of the gastrointestinal organs and other viscera also cause sympathetic visceral afferent stimulation of the TVC. The role of the higher brain stem and cerebral cortex in nausea and vomiting is the most complex and least understood. The higher brain centres are stimulated by all senses (particularly smell and taste), anxiety and pain. Noxious psychosensory stimulation such as disagreeable sights and odours can directly stimulate the TVC. It is thought that such mechanisms are responsible for anticipatory nausea and vomiting.

The symptoms of nausea and vomiting may result from a wide variety of physiological causes other than cancer chemotherapy. Causes include mechanical obstruction of the gastrointestinal tract (bowel, biliary); increased intracerebral pressure due to tumour; fluid and electrolyte imbalances (hypercalcaemia, hyponatraemia, hypokalaemia, volume depletion); radiation therapy (particularly to the abdomen, pelvis, back and brain) and pharmacological agents (antibiotics, narcotics).

Nursing care is directed at the prevention and aggressive management of nausea and vomiting, as well as management of nutrition, hydration and comfort while the patient experiences nausea or vomiting. See Table 10.10 for the specific nursing care measures for the patient with nausea and vomiting.

Mucositis

Impaired mucosa manifests as inflammation, desquamation and ulceration of the oral mucous membrane (stomatitis). Oesophagitis may also develop if the effects of treatment result in damaging or destroying epithelial cells in the oesophagus. Nursing care is directed at managing comfort, nutrition and hydration, preventing infection and promoting oral hygiene.

Careful assessment of the oral cavity is essential when mucositis is an expected side-effect of treatment. An oral assessment includes inspection of the lips, mucous membranes, gingiva and tongue for evidence of inflammation, desquamation, ulcers and infection, as well as moistness and evidence of debris. Note the amount and viscosity of the saliva, as it becomes thick, ropy and

Table 10.10 Nursing care of the person with nausea and vomiting.

Assessment	Patient problems/Goals	Intervention
• Assess factors which may be causing or contributing to nausea and vomiting • Assess the onset, duration, frequency and intensity of nausea and vomiting: —Amount and character of emesis —Impact of nausea and vomiting on nutrition and fluid and electrolyte balance • Assess previous response to emetic therapies • Monitor intake, output and fluid balance • Monitor effectiveness of antiemetic therapy	• The potential problem of nausea and vomiting leads to a patient goal stating that nausea and vomiting will not occur • Patient will be able to maintain adequate hydration and nutrition	• Administer antiemetic drug therapy at least 1 hour before emetic treatments and at regular intervals around the clock as long as the nausea persists in order to prevent or minimize nausea and vomiting. If the patient is unable to tolerate oral antiemetics, administer antiemetics by rectal suppository, intravenously or sublingually. Commonly-used antiemetics include phenothiazines, butyrophenones, steroids, metoclopramide, benzodiazepines and cannabinoids • Use combinations of antiemetics with different mechanisms of action when one agent is not effective • Maintain adequate hydration either orally or intravenously • Encourage a bland, cold diet or a clear liquid diet • Counsel the patient to avoid eating 1–2 hours before and after chemotherapy or other treatments which cause nausea and vomiting • Eliminate noxious sights, smells or other stimuli that may exacerbate nausea • Provide frequent oral hygiene using water or normal saline • Utilize techniques such as visual imagery, relaxation and hypnosis to prevent and control nausea and vomiting • Educate the patient and family regarding self-care measures to relieve nausea and vomiting

Table 10.11 Nursing care of the person with mucositis.

Assessment	Patient problems/Goals	Intervention
• Assess the lips and oral cavity daily using a light source: —Inspect for red inflamed areas, ulcerations, bleeding and oedema —Note degree of moistness of tissues; amount and viscosity of saliva —Note presence of pain, difficulty eating or swallowing, difficulty talking —Assess for evidence of infection (fungal, viral, bacterial), particularly in areas of ulceration, and on the tongue and palate	• When the problem of mucositis occurs the goal should be that the patient will have a normal oral mucosa and experience no discomfort • Patient will verbalize understanding of oral hygiene measures and perform them after meals and at bedtime	• Teach the patient an oral hygiene regimen or assist if the patient is dependent —Self-inspection of the mouth and oral cavity —Follow regimen a minimum of 4 times a day or every 4 hours while awake —Brush teeth with a soft toothbrush and floss once daily —If platelets <50 × 10^6/l, or gums are bleeding or painful, utilize a foam-tipped applicator or gauze to clean and discontinue flossing —Use a non-irritating toothpaste or baking soda to brush —Avoid commercial mouthwashes as they contain alcohol and are drying and irritating to oral mucosa. Do not use lemon and glycerin as this combination is drying and irritating —Use normal saline or diluted baking soda

Table 10.11 *Continued*

Assessment	Patient problems/Goals	Intervention
		(5 ml in 500 ml water) as a mouthwash; increase frequency of rinsing if oral tissues are dry or if saliva production is decreased
		—A solution of 1:4 hydrogen peroxide and normal saline or water may be used as a mouthwash to help clean debris from the mouth
		—Lubricate the lips using a water soluble lubricant or lanolin
		• Control pain:
		—Use a topical analgesic such as Xylocaine. Use as a mouthwash or apply to painful areas with a swab. Numbness lasts approximately 20 minutes which may aid the patient with eating and drinking. Ensure foods and drinks are not hot as sensation is impaired with topical analgesics
		—Utilize systemic analgesic therapy when the patient experiences continuous, severe pain. A continuous, intravenous infusion of morphine will ease pain until healing begins
		• Promote adequate hydration and nutrition. Counsel the patient to:
		—Alter diet to soft or liquid to reduce mechanical irritation
		—Avoid salty, spicy, acidic or hot foods as they are chemically irritating
		—Try high protein nutritonal supplements
		—Maintain hydration of 3000 ml per day. If the patient is unable to swallow, intravenous hydration may be necessary
		• Manage infection
		—Monitor temperature 4-hourly if the patient has ulcerations or signs of infection
		—Increase frequency of oral hygiene to at least every 4 hours
		—Administer topical and systemic antibiotics and antifungal agents as prescribed

viscid with severe mucositis, contributing to the dryness of the oral cavity and difficulty in eating. The patient's ability to eat, speak, swallow or wear dentures may be severely impaired. While the patient may experience mild burning at the onset of stomatitis, a severe case is extremely painful and may require systemic narcotic analgesic management, usually a continuous morphine infusion.

Infection is a potentially serious problem when mouth ulcerations exist. The *Candida albicans* fungus is frequently the cause of lesions and inflammation, or may be a secondary infection when the oral mucosa is damaged by chemotherapy or radiation. Candidiasis presents as white patches on the tongue and buccal mucosa. When the patches are scraped off, a reddened ulcerated surface is apparent. Herpes simplex infection on the lips develops into painful vesicles which rupture

and become encrusted. Gram-negative infections may occur in the mouth, as well as pseudomonas. The risk of systemic infection is of great concern. Ulcerated areas act as a port of entry for pathological organisms into the body which may cause sepsis. Therefore maintenance of good oral hygiene during periods of mucositis is essential in order to minimize the risk of infection. Refer to Table 10.11 for specific nursing measures in the care of the patient with mucositis.

Anorexia

Anorexia and weight loss are common problems with many cancer patients. Many factors may contribute to anorexia, including side-effects of therapy, nausea, taste changes, pain, fatigue and stomatitis. Clearly, inadequate intake results in nutritional deficiencies which impair

Table 10.12 Nursing care of the person with taste alterations.

Assessment	Patient problems/Goals	Intervention
• Assess for the presence, type, onset, degree and duration of taste alterations • Assess for contributing factors (poor oral hygiene, oral infection) • Assess for any change in nutritional status and, in particular, which foods cause dysgeusia	• The problem of taste alterations leads to the goal that the patient will report normal taste sensations or an absence of unpleasant tastes	• Eliminate foods which cause the patient unpleasant taste sensations. High-protein foods such as meat commonly cause dysgeusia. Use other sources of protein such as eggs, cheese, fish, nuts, legumes and milk products • Experiment with seasonings and flavourings to enhance taste. Experiment with foods that mask bitter or metallic tastes (mint, lemon) • Promote adequate oral hygiene; keep the oral mucosa moist

the body's ability to repair and heal, as well as affecting the patient's quality of life.

Taste alterations

Alterations in taste can occur as a result of cancer treatment. The types of taste alterations include dysgeusia, which is an unpleasant taste perception; ageusia, an absence of taste; and hypogeusia, a decrease in the acuity of taste sensation.

Surgical treatment for cancer in the oral cavity, particularly the tongue, salivary glands, nasal area and trachea, may cause hypogeusia and ageusia. Mucositis and infections in the oral cavity may also contribute to alterations in taste. Taste alterations caused by chemotherapy include metallic and bitter taste sensations, and an increased threshold for the sweet sensation (DeWys and Walters, 1975). The chemotherapy agents most commonly associated with taste alterations include cyclophosphamide, nitrogen mustard, 5- fluorouracil, vincristine, methotrexate and decarbazine. Taste alterations vary widely amongst patients in terms of severity and duration. Changes due to chemotherapy and radiation usually return to normal within weeks to months.

Nursing care is directed towards maintaining nutrition and hydration and assisting patients to adapt their diet during periods of taste alteration. Assessing the presence of taste changes and informing patients of this possibility are important nursing actions in order to assist with coping with taste alterations. Refer to Table 10.12 for the detailed nursing care of the patient with taste alterations.

Constipation

Constipation may be induced by a variety of causes, including nutritional deficits, particularly a lack of fibre; immobility, or by the administration of the chemotherapy agents, vincristine and vinblastine (Cimprich, 1985). The vinca alkaloids cause smooth muscle neurotoxicity, and consequences in the bowel range from mild constipation to paralytic ileus. Chemotherapy treatment is usually interrupted during periods of ileus. Opioid analgesics frequently cause constipation due to decreased peristalsis in the bowel. Patients should be

given stool softeners and bulk laxatives in order to prevent constipation; and increase their fluid and fibre intake as much as possible.

Diarrhoea

Diarrhoea may cause fluid and electrolyte imbalances and contribute to the weakness and fatigue that patients experience. Nutrition may be severely hampered. Diarrhoea is also irritating to the perianal skin surfaces and may cause skin breakdown. Nursing actions are focused on maintaining adequate hydration and nutrition, promoting comfort and hygiene, and returning bowel function to normal. Refer to Table 10.13 for the specific nursing care measures for the patient with diarrhoea.

ALOPECIA

Alopecia or hair loss is a side-effect of some chemotherapy agents and of radiation therapy to the head. While hair loss is temporary, the emotional impact on the patient is considerable because of the visibility of the change. The protective functions of hair are also lost: conservation of heat, protection from the sun, and the filtering out of airborne particles from the eyes and nose.

Efforts to prevent hair loss due to chemotherapy have focused on the use of scalp hypothermia and peripheral restriction. Utilizing a tourniquet or inflatable cuff around the scalp causes peripheral restriction; while application of a cooling cap causes hypothermia. Both of these methods restrict circulation and the ability of the drug to be taken up by hair follicles. The efficacy of such methods is difficult to evaluate and experience has shown that results are not very predictable and cannot be guaranteed (Tierney, 1987). Use of either method is not recommended in patients who have the potential for skin metastases, especially leukaemia and lymphoma.

Nurses play an important role in preparing patients for hair loss, to cope with partial or complete alopecia, and in educating the patient regarding changes in self-care during periods of alopecia. Refer to Table 10.14 for specific nursing care interventions for the patient with alopecia.

Table 10.13 Nursing care of the person with diarrhoea.

Assessment	Patient problems/Goals	Intervention
• Monitor the pattern of diarrhoea: onset, duration, frequency, amount and character • Note presence of blood, which may indicate ulceration in the intestinal tract • Monitor the degree of discomfort (gas, cramping) • Assess the perianal region for irritation and breakdown • Monitor fluid balance (intake and output) and adequacy of nutrition • If diarrhoea is severe, monitor electrolyte levels, particularly potassium	• The problem of diarrhoea leads to a goal that the patient will return to the normal bowel habit and show no signs of dehydration	• Alter diet to low residue or fluids. Eliminate foods which irritate or stimulate the bowel • Maintain oral intake of 3000 ml per day • Perform skin care to perianal skin regions after each episode of diarrhoea. Cleanse with water and mild soap or skin cleanser and/or have the patient use a sitz bath. Apply a barrier cream or other creams for perianal use. Avoid thick, sticky creams which are difficult to clean off the skin • Administer antidiarrhoeal agents as prescribed

Table 10.14 Nursing care of the person with alopecia.

Assessment	Patient problems/Goals	Intervention

• Assess the patient's understanding of the potential for hair loss and expected timeframe for regrowth
• While the patient has hair loss, inspect the scalp for dryness; and the eyes and nasal area for irritation
	• Patient/significant other will verbalize an understanding of hair loss and its temporary nature
	• Patient/significant other will verbalize feelings regarding hair loss and demonstrate continued interest in self-care/grooming
		• Inform the patient of the possibility of hair loss, including the expected onset, duration and severity
		• Instruct the patient in self-care measures:
		  —Regular cleansing of the scalp with a mild shampoo
		  —Restrict the use of harsh chemicals on the hair as well as extreme heat or brushing
		  —While in the sun use a sunscreen, hat or scarf
		• Discuss with the patient the possibilities for coping with hair loss: wigs, turbans, scarves and hats. A net or turban may be helpful during periods of heavy hair shedding. A photograph taken before hair loss may assist the patient in selecting a wig most suited to them
		• Alterations in application of make-up help to create eyebrows and improve appearance when eyebrows and eyelashes are lost
		• Provide the patient with opportunities to discuss feelings and reactions to hair loss

FATIGUE

Fatigue or lack of energy are symptoms that occur frequently and are ones that virtually every person with cancer experiences. Fatigue is well known to individuals with cancer and can precede or accompany the illness and can serve as a marker of disease progression and recurrence. A multitude of factors may contribute to fatigue, including surgery, chemotherapy (Cassileth et al, 1985), radiotherapy (Haylock and Hart, 1979; Cassileth et al, 1985; King et al, 1985; Kobashi-Schoot et al, 1985), disturbances in sleep and rest patterns (Knoff, 1986), inadequate nutrition, mood disturbances (McCorkle and Young, 1978; Knoff, 1986; Wickham et al, 1990), and symptom distress. While a relationship between anaemia and fatigue has been postulated, research has failed to show a consistent relationship (Maxwell, 1984).

Nursing care of the patient experiencing fatigue focuses on adaptation of lifestyle, maintaining optimum activity, promoting adequate nutrition and rest, and ameliorating factors which are contributing to fatigue. Refer to Table 10.15 for the detailed nursing care for fatigue.

SHORTNESS OF BREATH

Dyspnoea is an uncomfortable awareness of breathing, a sensation similar to pain. It serves as a stimulus for relieving respiratory insufficiency: clearing the airway, removing constrictive clothing, or breathing rapidly and deeply. As in managing chronic cancer pain, the

Table 10.15 Nursing care of the person with fatigue.

Assessment	Patient problems/Goals	Intervention
• Assess factors which may be contributing to fatigue: nutrition, sleep/rest patterns, treatment, symptom distress • Assess pattern of fatigue: onset, duration, severity, ameliorating and exacerbating factors and impact on life-style	• The problem of fatigue leads to the setting of a goal, in conjunction with the patient, that the patient will achieve adequate periods of rest	• Assist patient to pace activities according to energy level. Include periods of mild activity in daily routine. Obtain assistance for activities which are fatiguing, e.g. housework, child care • Promote adequate rest and sleep pattern • Control symptom distress, particularly pain, nausea and vomiting, fever, diarrhoea • Meditation, progressive muscle relaxation and guided imaging may promote relaxation and increase energy

symptom should be viewed first as a warning of disease, a signal to investigate and treat the underlying medical condition. Second, dyspnoea is a discomfort that can be relieved regardless of its pathophysiological basis.

Respiratory failure, particularly pneumonia, is a frequent cause of death among cancer patients, and dyspnoea may also occur with a variety of other terminal conditions (e.g. sepsis, cardiac failure, severe anaemia and hypovolaemic shock). The cause of this symptom is often multifactorial. Anxiety often accompanies dyspnoea; the patient may fear they will choke or will just stop breathing and die. The family may also fear that the patient will suffocate or suddenly stop breathing or that the breathlessness will become insufferable. Suggested nursing measures for the patient experiencing shortness of breath are listed in Table 10.16.

Table 10.16 Suggested nursing measures for the patient with shortness of breath.

• Reduce need for exertion
  —Plan activities in advance to minimize expenditure of effort. Include planned rest periods, particularly with more demanding activities. Schedule more demanding activities at hours of the day when breathing is the easiest. Set priorities (what is really important to the patient, including something really pleasant) and omit low priority activities
  —Give smaller, more frequent meals of soft, easy-to-chew foods
• Position patient for maximal respiratory excursion using pillows, i.e. sat upright
• Improve air circulation with fans, open windows
• Maintain adequate humidity to decrease dry airway and thick secretions
• Administer chest physiotherapy selectively
• Treat anxiety, give assurance
  —Sit with patient
  —Educate on significance of symptoms
• Administer low doses of narcotics, sedatives, bronchodilators, oxygen therapy, as ordered. Steroids or antimuscarinic agents (such as atropine) may be helpful in some situations

PAIN

Pain is the symptom most frequently associated with cancer and one of the most feared consequences of the disease and treatment. Studies suggest that moderate to severe pain is experienced by one third of cancer patients receiving active therapy, and by 60–80% of patients with advanced cancer (Bonica, 1980). These statistics support observations from clinical practice that the assessment and management of pain and other symptoms in cancer patients is one of the major activities of the oncology nurse. In order to assess and assist in planning a treatment regimen for cancer patients experiencing pain, nurses must have sound knowledge of the pathophysiology of cancer pain, pain assessment strategies and pain management principles. For further details see Chapter 9.

Definition and description

Even though a person may experience pain and knows how it feels to hurt, it is difficult for both the observer and the sufferer to define and describe pain adequately.

Pain is commonly divided into two subtypes: acute and chronic. Acute pain is characterized by a well-defined time of onset and is associated with subjective and objective signs indicating activation of the sympathetic nervous system (e.g. sweating, pale, tachycardiac, hypertensive, grimacing, crying and anxiety). Chronic pain, on the other hand is defined as the persistence of pain for longer than six months. In general, the onset of chronic pain is less well defined. In addition, patients with chronic pain no longer exhibit the signs and symptoms usually associated with pain. In fact the patient with chronic pain often shows very few signs of distress; often the suffering is hidden beneath a brave, stoic face. After long periods of unrelieved pain, the face no longer reveals anxiety, but exhaustion and depression. The lack of outwardly obvious signs and the depressed, sleepy face is often misinterpreted and the patient's complaints of severe pain discounted.

Cancer patients can experience either acute pain, chronic pain, or acute pain superimposed on chronic pain. The type of pain the patient is experiencing is determined by the stage of the disease, the type of treatment the patient is receiving, and any other predisposing medical or surgical conditions.

Nature of cancer pain

In order to focus attention on the complexity of pain as a somatic and psychological experience, Cicely Saunders coined the term 'total pain'. The suffering experienced by the patient with cancer pain is derived from a variety of sources. Anger, anxiety, depression, isolation, fearful memories, boredom and other psychosocial factors can in fact lower a patient's pain threshold. On the other hand, a positive outlook, a supportive family, empathy from nurses and doctor, forgiveness, diversion and sleep will all raise the pain threshold and decrease the pain experience.

Aetiology of cancer pain

As shown in Table 10.17, the pain of cancer can have multiple causes, including the cancer itself, the treatment, and concomitant non-malignant disease or factors unrelated to cancer or therapy.

Table 10.17 Pain syndromes in cancer patients.

Pain caused by cancer
Bone metastasis
Compression or infiltration of nervous structures
Compression or infiltration of veins, arteries, lymphatics
Rapid tumour growth causing stretching of pain-sensitive structures
Obstruction of a hollow viscus, such as bowel
Ulceration of pain-sensitive mucosal surfaces

Pain causes by anti-cancer therapy
Surgery
Chemotherapy
Radiation therapy

Coincidental pain
General debility
Joint stiffness
Pressure sores
Constipation

Assessment

The phase of assessment is possibly one of the most important steps in good pain management, and accurate assessment is based on trust. We must trust the patient's assessment of the pain and believe that pain is what the patient says it is, and not what we expect it to be or think it ought to be (McCaffery, 1979). The extent of disease shown on examination, X-ray or scan does not tell us the extent of pain. When we distrust the reliability of a patient's report of pain, the patient usually can sense our lack of belief and this can accentuate the patient's feelings of helplessness and hopelessness. This may lead to the patient stoically underreporting pain or anxiously overreporting the experience. Either reaction aggravates the spiral of mistrust, anxiety and pain.

At the initial pain interview and as part of an ongoing nursing assessment, the key elements of a pain history listed in Table 10.18 should be known.

Table 10.18 Components of the pain history.

- Site(s) and radiation
  Where is the pain? Does it spread anywhere?
- Timing
  How long have you had it? Does it come and go, or is it always there? How long does each spasm last?
- Quality
  Describe the pain in your own words (e.g. dull, sharp, aching, throbbing, burning)
- Severity
  How severe is the pain? (Consider using an instrument such as a 5 or 10 point rating scale to assist the patient in describing the intensity of pain and to track response to pain management strategies over time. See below)
- Aggravating factors
  What brings on the pain or makes it worse? (e.g. posture, movement, eating, time of day).
- Relieving factors
  What makes the pain better?
- Impact of pain on daily life
  On sleep: Does pain disturb your sleep: (N.B. Patients with pain may adapt to it so they sleep)
  On mood: Does the pain cause you to be depressed or discouraged?
  On activity: How has pain affected your activities: ambulation, self-care, job, social life, etc.?
- Knowledge and/or fears about use of analgesics to treat chronic pain
- Meaning of pain:
  What does patient think is causing the pain? What does patient think should be done about it?
- Previous therapies:
  Which drugs (or other therapies) have helped and which ones have failed to relieve the pain?
  Analgesic history should include:
  dose, frequency, regular or p.r.n., patient's view of drug efficacy, duration of use, side-effects, reason for discontinuation

Measurement. Although the experience of pain is not open to direct external measurement, several instruments have been developed to assist the patient in describing the intensity of pain. Measurement tools are advantageous because they facilitate:

- Clarity and consistency in interpretation and communication of the pain. (Verbal or written statements of a patient's exact numerical pain ratings are likely to be more consistently reported among health team members than a word description, e.g. 'a lot of pain'.)
- Quantification of the effectiveness of an intervention. (For example, if a patient's pain is the most severe at 9 and the least severe it gets is a 7 two hours after analgesia, it is quickly evident that more effective interventions are needed.)

Examples of some instruments are given in Figure 10.6. The type of scale used is less important than the consistency with which it is used, the patient's understanding of the scale and the clarity with which the scale assigns a score to the pain experience. For example, a

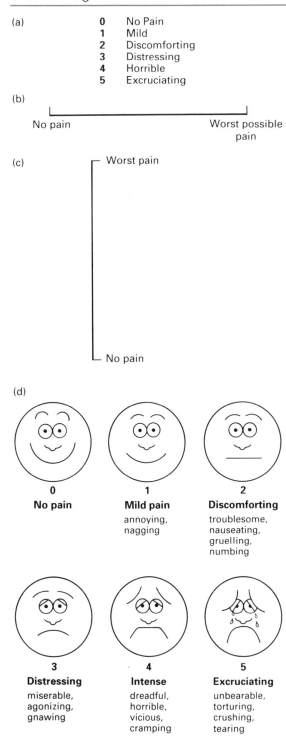

(a)

0	No Pain
1	Mild
2	Discomforting
3	Distressing
4	Horrible
5	Excruciating

(b)

No pain ———————————— Worst possible pain

(c)

— Worst pain

— No pain

(d)

0	**1**	**2**
No pain	**Mild pain**	**Discomforting**
	annoying, nagging	troublesome, nauseating, gruelling, numbing

3	**4**	**5**
Distressing	**Intense**	**Excruciating**
miserable, agonizing, gnawing	dreadful, horrible, vicious, cramping	unbearable, torturing, crushing, tearing

Figure 10.6 Pain scales. (a) McGill–Melzack Present Pain Intensity (PPI). (b) Linear Analogue Scale Assessment (LASA). (c) Vertical Visual Analogue Scale. (d) Wong–Baker Faces Rating Scale (Wong & Baker, 1988).

rating of 5 is meaningless unless it is following by a statement of the scale used, e.g. 5 on a scale of 0 to 10 (0 = no pain, 10 = worst pain) or 5 on a scale of 0 to 5 (0 = no pain, 5 = worst pain).

Some patients are unable to use a numerical scale to rate their pain; the numbers do not make sense to them or it is too hard for them to apply numbers to their experience. In this case, the following choice of descriptive words may be helpful for the patient to use:

No pain
A little pain
A lot of pain
Too much pain

These four phrases may then be converted to a 0 to 3 scale for documentation and communication among health team members; 0 = no pain, 1 = a little pain, 2 = a lot of pain, 3 = too much pain.

Some form of recording or tracking the characteristics of the patient's pain and the response to therapy is essential for adequate management of the problem (see Figure 9.7). Not keeping pain records when dealing with a patient in pain is like trying to treat hypertension without recording blood pressure.

The flow sheet allows ongoing evaluation of pain. The only safe and effective way to administer an analgesic is to monitor the patient's response to the medication and make changes based on these responses. The flow sheet is a tool that allows quick documentation of such responses along with easy retrieval of information for continuous evaluation. An example of a flow sheet that may be used by the patient or by the nurse is given in Figure 10.7.

Pharmacotherapeutics

Administration of systemic analgesics, psychotropic drugs and anti-inflammatory agents is probably the most practical and widely used method for relieving cancer pain (Bonica, 1980). Twycross has suggested a realistic clinical plan for 'graded pain relief': initially, a pain-free, sleepful night; next, comfort at rest in bed or a chair during the day; and finally, freedom from pain on movement (Twycross and Lack, 1984).

The choice of analgesic will partly depend on whether the cancer patient is suffering chronic or acute pain or a combination of both. Acute pain in a cancer patient (e.g. postoperative, recent fracture, painful diagnostic procedure) might call for an i.m. injection of a standard dose of a relatively short-acting narcotic. Further analgesia would be on a p.r.n. basis since pain intensity is likely to change rapidly.

Chronic cancer pain on the other hand demands a different approach. Analgesics should be given regularly (around the clock) with the dose and choice of medication matched to pain intensity. Pain severity is determined by listening to the patient's report of pain and observing the degree of relief obtained from previous drugs (Lipman, 1980).

As part of the Worldwide Cancer Pain Relief Program, the World Health Organization (WHO) has advocated a three step-analgesic ladder. This concept is illustrated in Figure 10.8.

NAME:

DATE/TIME	PAIN RATING ON A SCALE OF_____	RESPIRATORY RATE	ACCOMPANYING SYMPTOMS/ LEVEL OF CONSCIOUSNESS/ OTHER OBSERVATIONS	ANALGESIC

CODE KEY FOR ACCOMPANYING SYMPTOMS:

1. Nausea   3. Vomiting   5. Constipation   7. Drowsiness
2. Confusion   4. Hallucinations 6. Fatigue/weakness

Figure 10.7 Pain flow sheet.

Principles of therapy

1. *Use the oral route whenever possible.* The oral administration of narcotics gives more consistent and prolonged analgesia and avoids the toxicity that may occur with parenteral administration. The oral route eliminates parenteral injections, enables the patient to maintain control of the drugs and allows for mobility for home care and travel.

2. *'Round the clock' dosing.* Most narcotics have a duration of analgesic action of 4–6 hours; therefore control of chronic pain requires 4–6 doses spaced equally throughout the 24-hour period.

3. *Never p.r.n.* Continuous pain requires continuous analgesia. The aim of therapy is to prevent the resurgence of pain rather than to repeatedly treat

it. This anticipation breaks the vicious cycle of pain–despair–more pain which causes dose escalation. While p.r.n. orders may be needed for 'breakthrough' pain, the basis of control must be regular scheduling. Teach the patient and family members the rationale for using a preventive approach.

4. *Wake the patient.* A patient with chronic pain often sleeps despite severe pain. Sleep does not indicate pain control. On initiating therapy, the patient should be woken until pain has been consistently controlled for 2–3 days and the patient's confidence has been restored. Once pain is well controlled some centres give a larger dose at bedtime (e.g. one and a half times or twice the daytime dose), often allowing the

Step 3
FOR SEVERE PAIN

Use strong narcotics:
Morphine (drug of choice)

Plus or minus NSAIDs or other adjuvant drugs, as needed

Step 2
FOR MODERATE PAIN

Use weak narcotics:
Codeine (drug of choice)
Codeine and aspirin
Codeine and paracetamol

Plus or minus NSAIDs or other adjuvant drugs, as needed.

If pain persists or increases, go to Step 3.

Step 1
FOR MILD PAIN

Use non-narcotics:
Aspirin
Paracetamol
Non-steroidal anti-inflammatory drugs (NSAIDs) such as ibuprofen, indomethacin or naproxen

If pain persists or increases, go to Step 2.

Figure 10.8 Analgesic ladder.

patient to sleep throughout the night free of pain.

5. *Titrate dose individually.* There is no standard or set dose of narcotics in cancer pain. There is great variation between individuals in analgesic efficacy. The correct dose of a narcotic is that which gives pain relief for at least three or preferably four or more hours. As pain changes through various stages of disease and treatment, narcotic dosage must be adjusted to match pain intensity.

6. *Consult.* Consult with nursing and medical experts in pain management when usual interventions are unsatisfactory and before pain becomes intractable.

Co-analgesics. Several drugs, while not true analgesics in the pharmacological sense, act to relieve pain, either alone or in combination with analgesics. These co-analgesics may be used in the treatment of all types of cancer pain but are particularly important for those pains which are relatively unresponsive to morphine. Even when a narcotic is being used, the addition of a co-analgesic may often result in better pain control with fewer side-effects. Examples of co-analgesics include the steroids (e.g. prednisone, Decadron), major tranquilizers (e.g. haloperidol), tricyclic antidepressants (e.g. amitriptyline) and anticonvulsants (e.g. carbamazepine).

Non-pharmacological measures. Usually cancer pain requires systemic analgesic therapy. However in many

Table 10.19 Co-analgesics and non-pharmacological measures in cancer pain.

- For bone pain
    Full doses of NSAIDs (e.g. indomethacin, naproxen, aspirin), if tolerated
    Radiation therapy
- For nerve compression
    Corticosteroids
    Anaesthetic nerve blocks
    Transcutaneous electrical nerve stimulation (TENS)
- For nerve destruction
    Anticonvulsants
    Tricyclic antidepressants (e.g. amitryptyline)
    Corticosteroids
    Nerve blocks/epidural blocks
    TENS
- Other modalities
    Positioning
    Massage, warm or cold compresses
    Air fluidized therapy (e.g. Clinitron)
    Physiotherapy and occupational therapy; collars, corsets, splints, slings (for extra support), elastic stockings, compression cuffs, transfer aids, walking aids, hydrotherapy, etc.)
    Distraction, relaxation, imagery
    (Note: The response to these modalities may be limited when used alone, but they can be useful when most pain has been controlled by other means, as above)

situations non-drug measures may be extremely important adjuncts. Table 10.19 lists some of the co-analgesic and non-pharmacological measures that may be helpful in relieving cancer pain.

It is very important to periodically reassess the adequacy of pain control and to consider reasons for loss of previously adequate pain control. Cancer pain is seldom static: new pains develop and old pains re-emerge. Changes in the site or intensity of pain require thorough reassessment and possibly more than an increase in the dose of analgesic.

Control of narcotic side-effects
Constipation. If not carefully monitored and prevented, constipation may be just as difficult to control as the pain itself. The constipation associated with narcotics is caused because the morphine binds to receptors in the gastrointestinal tract, causing decreased peristalsis and diminished secretions. In cancer patients, decreased liquid intake, less exercise and low fibre diet all aggravate the problem. As in pain control, the aim of bowel care should be to prevent rather than treat the problem. Some suggestions for preventing and managing this problem are given in Table 10.20.

Nausea and vomiting. When strong narcotics are initiated, nausea and vomiting may occur. Narcotics may induce nausea and vomiting via several mechanisms, and the taste of the oral morphine solution, fear of being started on morphine, and other forms of anxiety may also contribute.

When a patient is first started on oral morphine an order for an antiemetic should be obtained in case nausea or vomiting develop. The risk of nausea and vomiting often decreases a week or two after morphine is started so that the antiemetic may be phased out in some patients.

Drowsiness/sedation. When morphine is initiated, transient sedation frequently occurs. This is partly a direct drug effect on the central nervous system, but the exhaustion and sleep deprivation of chronic pain is another major factor. When pain is finally relieved, the patient may sleep for long periods. Drowsiness usually clears 2–5 days after a steady dose is achieved.

Continuing drowsiness may indicate a need to decrease the narcotic dose and/or to add less sedating co-analgesics. Sedation may also be a sign of disease progression and not always a side effect of therapy.

Management of Oncological Emergencies

TUMOUR LYSIS SYNDROME

Patients with cancer of all types may present with emergency conditions releated to their disease or treatment. The appropriate management will depend upon the nature of the underlying disease, previous therapy and likely long-term prognosis. Tumour lysis syndrome can occur in the treatment of tumours which have a large number of tumour cells, such as acute

Table 10.20 Management of common side-effects associated with narcotic analgesics.

- Constipation
  - —Record bowel movements daily
  - —Rectal examination to rule out impaction (in presence of diarrhoea or faecal incontinence, this also rules out over-flow impaction)
  - —Start patients on a bowel regimen containing appropriate doses of bowel stimulants and faecal softeners. Avoid bulk laxatives
  - —Maintain adequate fluid intake; encourage prune juice if liked
  - —Provide increased fibre in patient's diet as tolerated
- Nausea and vomiting
  - —Pre-empt nausea. Use prochlorperazine 6.25–12.5 mg with every dose or every other dose of narcotic
  - —Nausea is worst when beginning narcotics and as the dose is increased. After a stable dose is reached, anti-emetic medication may be decreased
- Sedation
  - —Sometimes this is a difficult side-effect to avoid
  - —The patient/family should be taught that transient sedation frequently occurs when narcotics are commenced. This is partly a direct drug effect on the CNS, but the exhaustion and sleep deprivation of chronic pain may be another major factor. When pain is finally relieved the patient may sleep for long periods. Drowsiness usually clears 2–5 days after a steady dose is achieved
  - —Continuing drowsiness may indicate a need to decrease narcotic dose or change to less sedating co-analgesics (e.g. anti-inflammatory agent)

leukaemia or lymphoma, which are very sensitive to chemotherapy. As large numbers of malignant cells are killed by the chemotherapy, cell lysis releases large amounts of nucleic acids and intracellular ions into the bloodstream. This can cause hyperuricaemia (raised levels of uric acid in the blood) which, when excessive, leads to hyperuricaemic nephropathy and severely affects renal function. Other metabolic imbalances such as hyperkalaemia, hyperphosphataemia and hypocalcaemia may also occur as a result of massive cell lysis. Patients at risk for tumour lysis syndrome are those who are over the age of 65, who have pre-existing renal disease or are being treated with nephrotoxic drugs. Prophylactic treatment includes careful monitoring of renal function and biochemistry parameters in conjunction with increased fluid administration, diuresis, alkanization of the urine and administration of allopurinol.

HYPERSENSITIVITY REACTIONS

Hypersensitivity reactions can occur in response to some chemotherapeutic agents. The agents which most commonly produce hypersensitivity reactions are bleomycin and L-asparaginase. Patients with lymphoma who are receiving bleomycin have about a 6% incidence of hypersensitivity reactions which may be as severe as anaphylaxis. Non-lymphoma patients tend to have milder reactions. L-asparaginase produces mild reactions in about 25% of patients but about one-third of patients will have more severe reactions after they have had five doses or more. Intramuscular administration of L-asparaginase has been shown to decrease the incidence of hypersensitivity reactions. The administration of test doses for bleomycin and L-asparaginase to assess patient sensitivity is recommended.

HYPERCALCAEMIA

Hypercalcaemia is a potentially fatal metabolic condition that occurs in approxiamtely 8–20% of cancer patients (Dietz and Flaherty, 1990). Hypercalcaemia is caused by increased bone resorption which results from tumour invasion of bone; increased levels of parathyroid hormone (PTH); prostaglandin; or osteoclast activating factor. Patients at greatest risk are those with bone metastases (commonly from breast, prostate, lung and kidney tumour) which cause extensive bone destruction and release of calcium into the extracellular fluid.

The effects of hypercalcaemia in the body are seen in the gastrointestinal, neuromuscular, cardiac and renal systems. Gastrointestinal changes include anorexia, nausea, vomiting, constipation, abdominal pain and dehydration. Neuromuscular changes are confusion, lethargy, convulsion and hyporeflexia. The heart may be affected, leading to rhythm disturbances such as brady-cardia, and tachycardia. Polyuria, polydipsia and renal failure are signs of renal dysfunction. Diagnostic studies will show an elevated serum calcium level. A calcium level greater than 13 mg/dl requires emergency inter-vention, including aggressive hydration, in order to promote renal excretion of calcium, and diuretic therapy and intravenous mithramycin or calcitonin to inhibit bone resorption. Oral phosphate may be used to control chronic or mild hypercalcaemia.

Monitoring of early signs and symptoms of hypercal-caemia is an important nursing function in patients at risk for hypercalcaemia. Patients and families should be watching for these signs and symptoms as well. Patients should be encouraged to drink 3 litres per day to maintain hydration and promote excretion of calcium. In the acute phase, close monitoring of intake and output, weight, oedema, respiratory distress, serum calcium and electrolytes is essential.

SPINAL CORD COMPRESSION

Early detection and management of spinal cord com-pression is essential in order to preserve and maintain neurological functioning. Spinal cord compression is usually caused by metastatic tumours (95%) and by primary tumours of the spine (5%) (Bruckman and Bloomer, 1978). Metastatic spinal tumours of the breast, lung and prostate are the most common cancers causing cord compression. Signs and symptoms include central back pain close to the site of compression which is not relieved by lying down, motor weakness (weakness, foot drop, ataxia), sensory loss (parasthesias, numbness, tingling), and abnormal bladder and bowel sphincter control. The degree of sensory and motor loss is dependent on the level of the cord compression.

Treatment must be instituted rapidly in order to preserve as much neurological function as possible. Radiation therapy, surgical decompression or a com-bination of both may be recommended. Steroids are used immediately after diagnosis to decrease inflamma-tion, relieve pain and increase neurological function. Chemotherapy may be used for extremely chemosensi-tive tumours where a rapid effect may be seen.

Nursing care includes monitoring and evaluation of neurological status (sensory and motor function), vital signs and degree of pain. Assistance with self-care may be necessary if the patient is experiencing motor and sensory deficits. Assessment of skin integrity and instituting measures to prevent skin breakdown are essential with patients experiencing sensory and motor deficits. Maintenance of regular bowel habits may require starting a bowel maintenance regimen (laxa-tives, suppositories). Loss of voluntary micturition control may result in distension, retention, urinary overflow and urinary tract infections. Patients may require intermittent catheterization if unable to void. Checking of residual urine after voiding is necessary. Rehabilitation following the acute phase may be indi-cated if the patient suffers permanent deficits.

Other emergencies may occur related to the car-diovascular system, e.g. cardiac tamponade, pericarditis or superior vena cava obstruction. Erosion of major arteries may result in sudden catastrophic haemorrhage unless vascular surgery can be undertaken very swiftly.

A rare but life-threatening and distressing emergency is that of upper airways obstruction. Gradual onset may be followed by symptoms of acute breathlessness and stridor. A combination of radiotherapy and steroids is usually the most effective form of treatment, or possibly laser therapy to an obstructing lesion in the trachea.

In any such emergency the nurse needs to combine efficient clinical skills with understanding and empathy for the distress and anxiety of the patient and concerns of family and friends.

COMMON ISSUES IN COPING WITH CANCER

Coping with cancer is a complex, multidimensional and ongoing process for the person with cancer and their family. From discovery of disease, through complex treatment regimens, rehabilitation and dying, many challenges are faced by patients and their care-givers. An individual's perception of the threat posed by their disease is an important factor in determining their adjustment to disease. There is an increasing amount of evidence to suggest that a positive mental attitude may have a significant effect on disease outcome, particularly in patients with early non-metastatic cancers. The reader is referred to the work of Mooney and Greer (1989) for further discussion on this point.

GRIEF AND LOSS

Grieving by the patient with advanced cancer may be due to the loss of a body part or body function, loss of independence, loss of role in the family and/or society, and the threat to life.

The patient's and family's responses to loss and death may be categorized according to the stages of grieving. Knowledge of these various stages of behaviour help the nurse to understand the patient's responses. It should be remembered that all individuals do not necessarily progress through these phases progressively or within a given period of time. Individuals fluctuate in their reactions, varying in the time spent in any given phase. Labelling of behaviours does not help the patient, but it may be useful to guide the nurse to recognize what is happening to the patient. Hine states that perhaps the most useful expectation is that what ought to be happening with the patient and family is what is happening at any given moment (Hine, 1982).

The five stages of grieving described by Kubler-Ross (1973) are: denial, anger, bargaining, depression and acceptance. Behaviour characteristic of the various stages include: shock, disbelief, denial, crying, rage, frustration, anger, sorrow, detachment, acceptance, calmness and return to realistic functioning and reattachment.

Nursing interventions begin with awareness that the patient and family are grieving. The nature and cause of the grief are identified; it cannot be assumed that a patient with advanced cancer is grieving because of the possibility of death. The patient may have adapted to this possibility but grief may now be related to loss of independence or the effect illness and death will have on the family. The nurse may help the grieving patient by showing awareness of what he or she may be experiencing.

The nurse may help the patient to express feelings of grief, sorrow, anger or frustration by listening and providing opportunities for quiet discussion, and the use of touch. The patient and family may wish to share their grief together. Support by the nurse and other health professionals may make it easier for them to express their concerns and feelings of loss.

Grieving is a normal process that requires understanding and support but rarely direct intervention. Counselling and help from skilled, experienced workers may be necessary when grieving is delayed or one stage is prolonged or the patient is not able to resolve grief. Problems may also arise when the patient and family members are at different stages of the grieving process at a given time. They may require help to understand the responses and feelings of each other and why conflicting emotions are occurring.

NEED FOR INFORMATION AND KNOWLEDGE

Advances in cancer treatment are encouraging; patients are living longer and the occurrence and duration of remissions of the disease are increasing. The period of hospitalization for most oncology patients is relatively short in relation to the overall illness experience. Responsibility for day-to-day care of the cancer patient rests to a large extent with the individual and the family, who require knowledge, skills and resources to manage the patient's home care successfully. Understanding of the care plan and reasons for it also facilitates patient

and family participation in decision making regarding treatment and care and provides them with a sense of control and involvement in what is happening to them.

The nurse can further enhance the delivery of care by explaining patient care to the family and encouraging the family to participate in decision making. Home care courses are helpful in increasing families' skill and confidence in providing care in the home. Conferences with the patient and family provide the opportunity to advise them of changes and progress in the patient's condition and enables them to express their questions and concerns. Family members should receive information directly; information delivered second-hand may be incomplete or altered because of differences in perceptions and priorities.

A teaching plan for health management must take into account the patient's and family's perspectives. What are their major concerns about hospital and homecare management? What knowledge and skills do they possess? What resources exist within the family and neighbourhood? What health care and social services are available in the community? How does the patient learn best? What barriers exist to learning?

Teaching sessions should include supervised practice of care as well as information giving. The patient and family can carry out care procedures during the period of hospitalization or with guidance from a visiting nurse in the home. The development of a teaching plan to be achieved within a definite time ensures that necessary content and skills are taught and opportunity is provided for discussion practice and repetition. Explanations about basic care and treatment should be repeated each time care is delivered. Dodd and Mood demonstrated that information provided once about chemotherapy to adult oncology patients was not retained. Follow-up information visits by a nurse resulted in increased accuracy and retention of the information (Dodd and Mood, 1981).

Written information given to the patient and family enhances learning and facilitates recall. The use of videos, slides and pictures helps the patient and family to envisage a technique or problem being discussed. Group sessions are useful to provide basic information and to promote sharing and discussion of experiences. All patients and families require some individualized learning sessions for them to acquire knowledge and skills unique to their particular situation.

A referral may be made to the community nursing services. The community nurse should be informed of the patient's and family's progress in developing self-care skills and of specific needs for continuous help and guidance. Volunteers may be able to assist with transport, social visits and day to day activities. Visiting nurses can also arrange for the loan of equipment such as hospital beds and wheelchairs. In most areas, specialist nursing services and hospital or community-based symptom control teams are available to advise and support patients and the staff involved in home care.

SEXUAL AND REPRODUCTIVE CHANGES

Biopsychosocial alterations in sexuality of the person with cancer may be influenced by: altered body structure and function resulting from the disease process and/or therapy; change in self-concept, body image or sense of attractiveness; lack of knowledge; prolonged hospitalization; and lack of privacy.

Surgery may alter reproductive capabilities if there is removal of the uterus, ovaries or testes. Surgery involving the colon, rectum and genitourinary structures may cause physiological changes such as impotence, retrograde or lack of ejaculation, dyspareunia, sterility and decreased libido. Chemotherapy and radiotherapy can cause changes in function in relation to sexual response, fertility and fetal development.

Lamb and Woods (1981) point out that living with cancer may enhance some aspects of sexuality as well as impinge on others. Fatigue, pain, decreased physical mobility, sterility, impotence and alterations in body structures resulting from the cancer or therapy may be barriers to sexual expression. Confrontation with a potentially fatal disease encourages some couples to reassess their values and relationship. They may find that sexual expression enhances the feelings of being alive and human, and that it may serve to allay fears and provide comfort to each partner.

Open communication regarding sexuality is enhanced when trust and respect are part of the nurse–patient relationship. Discussions on sexuality should begin with the initial nursing assessment to establish its importance and convey a willingness to discuss the topic. Privacy should be provided for the patient and partner.

Discussions with the patient and partner should identify and correct any misinformation. Patients should be aware of the effects of cancer and treatment on fertility so that they can make informed choices about treatment and anticipate possible problems. Sperm banking can be offered to men whose treatment plan may result in sterility. Effective birth control should be used during treatment and for 2 years after treatment to avoid teratogenic effects of treatment.

Information on measures available to compensate for the changes resulting from the disease or treatment (e.g. use of a lubricating gel when vaginal secretions are decreased) should be made available to patients.

Alternative ways of expressing physical love may be discussed with the patient and partner. Limitations affecting sexual intercourse may be identified and other possible methods of sexual gratification suggested. Complex problems may be referred to an appropriate consultant, and counselling should be provided for the patient and partner.

ALTERED BODY IMAGE

Physical changes may result from the cancer itself, surgical removal of a body part, or the effects of chemotherapy or radiation treatment. The loss of a limb, a mastectomy, mandibular resection, loss of hair, changes in skin pigmentation, skin rashes and weight loss are examples of visible changes in the body with which many cancer patients are faced. Body image is an adaptive mechanism that maintains equilibrium among the physiological, psychological and sociocultural components of the body (Marino, 1981b).

Actual changes in body structure and function can be assessed but how the individual perceives these changes and how they influence his or her responses is subjective, individual and difficult to measure. The patient with a disturbance in body image may exhibit: decreased socialization; denial of the changes and avoidance of looking at the affected body part or of looking into a mirror; refusal to touch the affected part; avoidance of physical contact with close family members or friends; expression of fears of rejection; expression of feelings of hopelessness and helplessness; or preoccupation with the change.

Grieving for the lost part or previous physical appearance occurs before the patient can adjust to the changes, whether they are temporary, permanent, actual or perceived. During the grieving process, the nurse accepts the patient's responses and acknowledges that his or her feelings and responses are normal.

The cause of the physical changes and what may be expected should be explained and suggestions made as to ways of improving physical appearance. Patients are encouraged to use make-up and to wear a wig or clothing that will cover the defect or scars so long as this is acceptable to them.

Social contact is encouraged and the family is helped to understand and accept the patient's feelings and behaviour. The attitude of those giving care can do much to promote a feeling of self-worth and acceptance of the physical change on the part of the patient. The nurse who is comfortable handling and looking at the patient's colostomy or breast scar, yet aware of the patient's feelings, promotes confidence and encourages the patient gradually to look, touch and talk about the incision and participate in care and future planning.

NURSING ASSESSMENT AND MANAGEMENT OF SPECIFIC PSYCHOSOCIAL RESPONSES TO CANCER

The aim of this section is to provide guidelines for the assessment and management of some specific psychosocial responses to cancer. By increasing their own knowledge and understanding of the complexity of emotional responses, nurses may be able to assist the patient towards a greater understanding of his or her feelings and behaviour. Tables 10.21–10.24 give details of some nursing interventions which may be useful as the basis for formulating individualised patient care plans.

ANGER AND HOSTILITY

Anger is a common and appropriate response to the insults imposed by cancer and its treatment on bodily and personal integrity. Anger can have enormous adaptive value, allowing patients to mobilize inner resources of strength, determination and hope. Adaptive anger is generally not directed at anyone in particular. Dysfunctional anger, on the other hand, is more diffuse and intense, and may feel out of control to the patient.

Dysfunctional expressions of anger may include self-destructive behaviour, refusal of treatment, and displacement on to family members, health-care providers and others. Such exaggerated anger can isolate the patient from important sources of personal support. Rather than trying to soothe the patient's anger, the nurse should encourage the patient to talk about it, understand it and accept it. Defensive responses to anger directed at the medical establishment (e.g. 'There's no reason to be angry at me, I didn't cause your cancer') should be avoided. Pointing out the brighter side is also likely to be ineffective and alienating. Providing quality nursing care to an angry patient is not easy. Table 10.21 details the nursing intervention approaches for patients experiencing anger.

Table 10.21 Patient problem: anger.

Aetiology
Fear, guilt, anxiety, repressed resentment, grief, powerlessness, thwarted needs or goals, threat to need for security control or belonging, threatened self-concept

Nursing intervention
- Assist patient in identifying sources of anger. Give the patient a role in solving the problem that has provoked the anger. Encourage patient to verbalize frustrations and anger, and listen to these actively
- Structure a stable, predictable environment with predictable limits and consequences so that the patient can retain control over his or her own behaviour
- Involve the patient in treatment to decrease feelings of helplessness and dependency
- Do not shout or argue with the angry patient. Do not touch the patient or invade personal space, since these actions may be perceived as threatening and can escalate the anger

Nurses may become afraid and defensive and withdraw from the angry patient. This increases the patient's anger and a vicious circle begins. The patient manifesting anger is not likely to feel grateful or express gratitude for the care given.

The nurse must accept and tolerate the anger and work with the patient to clarify and validate its sources. Since anger is usually a defence against deeper feelings of hurt and fear, this area must be approached gently and compassionately. Explaining that the anger is a reasonable reaction to the patient's situation can also be helpful when the anger is expressed.

The patient needs to be encouraged to move beyond the anger to problem-solving strategies in order to cope with the situation that caused the feelings; however these actions will not magically eliminate the patient's feelings of anger. The patient will continue to need to express anger as it is experienced.

Some patients are so angry that trust is not possible. This usually occurs when the anger is not dealt with and a very unhealthy system of interaction develops. Some patients have had such negative experiences in other institutions or situations that trust develops very slowly, if at all. Great care must be taken not to abandon the

Table 10.22 Patient problem: anxiety and fear.

Definition
Anxiety is a sense of uneasiness, apprehension or tension which is caused by a threat to one's security
Fear is a feeling of dread related to an identifiable source which the person validates

Nursing intervention
- Assist patient in identifying threats, stresses, and fears that might be removed. It is often very useful to ask the patient what he or she thinks would help
- Let the patient know you are aware of this anxiety and that you take it seriously. Listen respectfully to what the patient has to say. Encourage the expression of thoughts and feelings about illness, dependency and other concerns, rather than inappropriately reassuring the patient. Often the intervention of exploration will result in the ability of the patient to focus on the threat or to appraise the stimuli in a different way, thus reducing anxiety
- Since perceptions are narrowed when anxiety is increased, realize that the patient may have difficulty making decisions, problem solving, attending or remembering
- Explain all treatments and procedures simply and concisely
- Maintain a calm manner, using short declarative sentences and utilizing a soft but firm voice
- Be available to the patient, checking in with him or her often if this seems to ease anxiety. Allow time for the development of rapport/trust
- For anxiety that is mild to moderate, teach the patient to use breathing and relaxation techniques

patient. Staff should attempt to provide as much continuity as possible in patient assignment; assigning the angry patient to a different nurse every day only serves to increase the patient's sense of abandonment. The patient should be allowed as much choice and control as possible rather than setting strict limits.

ANXIETY AND FEAR

Anxiety has been described, with depression, as the most common psychosocial reaction experienced by persons with cancer. Anxiety is an unpleasant feeling of dread, and may be caused by an unconscious conflict between an underlying drive and the reality of the environment; the anxious person is unaware of the specific cause of his or her feelings. Anxiety is a different emotion from fear. Fear is an unpleasant feeling caused by a threat in the environment that is specific and can be identified.

Patients with cancer are justifiably fearful and anxious about many things: pain, death, abandonment, dependency, recurrence. Some fears are based on inaccurate information and can be relieved by proving that information. Other fears, such as the anticipation of unrelieved pain, will require reassurance and a description of measures that will be taken to ensure the relief of pain. Some suggested nursing interventions for minimizing fear and anxieties are detailed in Table 10.22.

Death is a real possibility for many patients, and must be worked through philosophically. However, many patients are more afraid of the process than of death itself. Patients often benefit from reassurances that they will not be abandoned by staff.

DEPRESSION

Depression, sadness, despair and hopelessness in response to losses can be thought of as natural consequences of the actual or potential disruption of a close attachment or important goals. Since cancer represents the potential loss of not only life, but also body parts and functions, roles and relationships, depression has been identified as one of the most common responses to cancer.

The depressed patient often moves, thinks and speaks slowly, motivation and energy are often very low. Patients who are extremely depressed will have little desire or energy to express feelings or make decisions.

Other people tend to avoid the depressed person. The desire is often to try and 'cheer up' the depressed patient with happy, bubbly, enthusiastic talk. This does not work and may drive patients further within themselves. The nurse can verbally reflect the feelings that the patient's behaviour expresses. The appropriateness of the sadness needs to be recognized. Patients can be encouraged to talk about their thoughts and feelings. If the patient is very withdrawn, remaining silently with the patient for periods interspersed throughout the day can sometimes be helpful. Suggested nursing interventions for patients experiencing depression are given in Table 10.23.

Sometimes patients can feel very depressed and conceal the feeling behind a facade of 'normal' happy behaviour. This type of depression is a serious drain on the patient's available energy. Signs of this depression will be much more subtle but many of these patients will admit to feeling depressed if asked.

UNCERTAINTY AND LOSS OF CONTROL

The uncertainty and unpredictability of the course of terminal illness can create enormous stresses. Most people are accustomed to a certain amount of predictability in their daily lives and in the way their bodies function. Cancer creates havoc. How will treatment turn out? When will new symptoms develop? How and when will death come? Uncertainty places enormous constraints and demands on the patient.

The feeling that one's internal environment is out of control often generates a frightening sensation of helplessness and vulnerability. Deep shame may arise from concerns about loss of physiological control. Some patients fear that they will not be able to control their emotions under the stress of cancer.

Serious illness like cancer often serves to diminish, at least temporarily, a patient's sphere of control. In addition, the patient is often required to give up certain usual roles and responsibilities and to accept the care of others. For those patients whose self-esteem and personal worth derives from attending to others, the need to be taken care of may cause great conflict. In

Table 10.23 Patient problem: depression.

Definition
A universal mode of interaction manifested by sadness, poor self-concept, and inability to act for self

Nursing intervention
- Teach skills to help patient gain control over emotions and cope effectively with anger and loss
- Teach techniques that assist the patient to deal with stress more effectively: progressive relaxation, visual imagery
- Encourage physical exercise such as walking or other motor activities
- Encourage activities that increase self-esteem and promote a realistic and positive self-concept
- Avoid cheerfulness and reassurances that primarily reassure the nurse, not the patient. Superficial reassurances are countertherapeutic
- Teach problem solving skills by asking the patient to list alternative actions, consider the rationale of each action, and evaluate which action might be in the best interest of the patient
- Refer to appropriate mental health practitioners for evaluation and consideration for medication if symptoms deepen or fail to improve
- Provide accurate information about the plan of care
- Assisting the patient to focus on immediate goals of care often reduces the overwhelming feelings of helplessness. Focus on positive abilities of the patient, negotiate goals for increasing independence in self-care and decision making, contract short-term goals of care that the patient can achieve, and reinforce patient attempts and successes to meet established goals
- Reinforce small gains with praise, discussion, recognition

addition, work, finances and family issues may be negotiated without the patient's involvement. Nursing interventions to reduce the impact of uncertainty and powerlessness and to promote feelings of control in the situation are outlined in Table 10.24.

FAMILY ISSUES

The patient's family suffers as a result of temporary or permanent changes in the patient's capacity to fulfil family and career roles, the increased stress on family members, role transitions, and changes in responsibilities.

Northouse's review (1984) of the impact of cancer on the family provides a framework for understanding family responses and problems in coping with cancer.

In the initial phase the three major potential problems for family members are: feeling excluded from the receiving of care and participation in care; communicating with hospital staff and others; and managing emotional distress. Family members may feel despair, isolation, vulnerability and helplessness, uncertainty, confusion and shock (Giaquinta, 1977; Thomas, 1978). Feeling excluded from care may occur as professional care-givers focus on the care of the patient.

Table 10.24 Patient problem: powerlessness.

Definition
Perception of a person that his or her own behaviour cannot influence or determine the desired outcome and there is a lack of control over situations and events

Nursing intervention
- Gather data on needs and desire for control, areas in which control is particularly important, and any discomfort with giving over some measure of control for a period of time
- Based on patient concerns, discuss areas in which it is possible to negotiate for maintaining control, and the rationale for relinquishing control in other areas where health care providers or the system require control
- Allow the patient to make as many decisions as possible in planning and scheduling (e.g. when pain medication is needed, the number and timing of visitors, and environmental choices such as timing of personal care activities)
- Increase the patient's capability for self-care by providing appropriate patient/family education in regard to the course and management of the disease, the signs and symptoms that warrant seeking medical intervention, and the kinds of self-care strategies that the patient should perform. Prepare individual for any procedures, diagnostic tests, transfers, etc. Encourage the asking of questions
- Help the patient maintain dignity. Being sensitive to the patient's privacy needs, asking permission to move personal belongings, showing consideration for embarrassment in certain situations, and giving assistance only as needed, but not excessively, will help to convey respect for the patient as a person
- When the patient voices concerns of dependency, loss of control, etc., encourage the expression of these feelings rather than simply giving reassurance as this often feels like discounting the feelings. Avoid rescuing behaviours which reinforce sense of helplessness and powerlessness. Promote identification/reaffirmation of inner strengths
- Offer intervention approaches that may increase the sense of mastery (e.g. relaxation exercises, imagery, contracts, keeping journal, etc.)

Families may encounter difficulty obtaining information from professionals and are frequently in the position of having to initiate contact and requests for information. Communication within the family may be affected as it is common that family members are unsure how to discuss a diagnosis of cancer and their concerns. Emotional tension in the family may be exhibited by anxiety, agitation or guilt. A sense of helplessness and loss of control is common at this time.

During the adaptation phase the family deals with adjusting to changes in roles and life-styles, meeting the needs of well family members, and living with uncertainty. Changing role responsibilities in the family may cause the patient to feel dependent on others and to worry about being a burden, while other family members may have had little preparation to assume homemaking or extended parenting roles. Financial resources may be affected by the loss of ability to work. The needs of well family members may be neglected because of the focus on the ill member. Coping with uncertainty about the future is a challenge for all family members. Some families may have open communication about fears and uncertainties, while others may be closed in order to try and prevent worry.

During the terminal phase the family deals with communicating about death among family members; providing care and support to the dying person; and dealing with feelings of loss and separation. Very little discussion about death may occur among family members. Vachon et al (1977) suggest that non-discussion may be an effective coping mechanism for some people.

Caring for the dying family member may cause considerable strain on the family in terms of physical care and emotional support (Rose, 1976). Families have learning needs in terms of physical aspects of care, pain control and increased dependency. Feelings of grief and loss are paramount in this phase. Family members may feel helpless, abandoned and anxious.

Intervention strategies for families fall into three categories: assessing the needs of the family members; providing support to families; and providing families with information and assistance (Northouse, 1984). Many studies have identified family members' needs for help with the physical and emotional care of the ill member and an emphasis on the need for health care professions to provide excellent personalized care for the patient (Freihofer and Felton, 1976; Edstrom and Miller, 1981; Googe and Varricchio, 1981; Grobe et al, 1981; Welch, 1981; Lewandowski and Jones, 1981).

The family can be informed of available community resources for patient care and social services. Referral for counselling may be appropriate when the family is facing long-term disruption and when the ability of the family to cope is actually or potentially inadequate. Family members are encouraged to seek help from those they consider to be helpful and appropriate for them. Continuing help and support should be readily available from the nurse, doctor, social worker, pastoral counsellor, hospital chaplain, friends and relatives. Continuity in those giving care does much to facilitate communication and long-term planning.

It is important that family members spend time together as well as resuming socialization outside the home. In the hospital setting, measures are taken to provide privacy and opportunity for the family to be together as a unit.

CARE OF THE PATIENT WITH ADVANCED DISEASE

Hospice or palliative care of the patient with advanced cancer is directed towards the relief of symptoms and improving the quality of life, as opposed to quantity of life. Caring for the person who is terminally ill is to provide a holistic approach to care, focusing not only on the physical symptoms of disease but the psychosocial and spiritual needs of the patient as well, and extending this care to the family and significant others (Scanlon, 1989). Such care may be provided in an institution or in the home, the preferred locale being the choice and preference of the patient and family.

Problems which are common to patients with advanced disease are alterations in comfort and symptom distress. The increasing severity of pain may be perceived as signifying advance of the cancer. The pain contributes to the physiological and psychological factors that enhance its severity. Loss of sleep and rest due to pain increases the patient's fatigue. Anorexia, nausea and vomiting associated with the pain contribute to nutritional deficiencies and weight loss. Mobility is restricted by the pain, increasing the potential for skin breakdown, constipation, muscle weakness and chest complications. The patient may exhibit anxiety, irritability, anger and withdrawal. Adequate pain control requires the co-operative efforts of the patient and nursing and medical personnel. Assessment of the patient's pain and the effectiveness of interventions must be continuous.

Persons who are terminally ill respond and cope in a variety of ways. Patients are grieving for a range of actual and potential losses, while still trying to maintain hope. While the hope is not likely to be for a cure, hope remains to achieve short-term goals, to have a painless death, or to see the family again tomorrow. Frequent emotional responses are denial, anxiety, fear, depression, withdrawal, acceptance, resignation and anger.

Denial may assist the individual to protect himself or herself from the painful reality of dying and to preserve hope. There are certainly degrees of denial and, while it is a useful protective response, it may also interfere with problem solving and communication between patient and family or patient and care-givers. Fear is a response to perceived danger, while anxiety is a feeling of distress and discomfort. Sources of anxiety for the patient may be spiritual in nature, fear of death or fear of the dying process and what may lie ahead. The person may respond to a terminal illness by withdrawal and depression as he or she disengages from relationships and surroundings. Acceptance and resignation to disease may fluctuate over time. They are dynamic in nature and may be observed in concert with other responses. Sadness and a sense of aloneness may be apparent at this time. Anger may be felt in response to actual and expected losses, and the helplessness that patients sometimes experience.

The needs of families in the terminal phase of illness are well documented in the literature (Hull, 1989). Families consistently identify the need for information about their dying relative that is clear and honest (Googe and Varricchio, 1981). They particularly need to be informed when death is imminent, and to be called at home if changes occur. Families want to be assured of patient comfort (Freihofer and Felton, 1976). Families may wish to be physically close to the dying person and to spend as much time as possible with them (Wright and Dyck, 1984). Information is needed on how to provide physical care to the person at home (Grobe et al, 1981).

Nurses need to be realistic about how far they can actually help and support family care-givers in their grief and loss. Popularly-held beliefs that nurses can assist patients by encouraging the sharing and ventilation of feelings, encouraging crying and talking about negative feelings may not be perceived as supportive behaviours by those they are supposed to help (Freihofer and Felton, 1976). This is not to say that the opportunity to express such feelings may not be of great value to certain individuals at certain times, but respect for privacy is equally important. Open communication is the key to providing appropriate support and there is much evidence to suggest that many nurses have less than optimum skills in this area. Macleod, Clark and Sims review some of the relevant literature and suggest ways in which nurses can enhance their own skills and confidence. This may also help to reduce the undoubted stress that is experienced by nurses caring for dying patients, as relationships can become very intense.

Following the death of a person at home, the withdrawal of previously frequent community nursing services may be an additional loss for those that are left to sustain. Continued visits by the primary community nurse may be helpful in re-establishing daily life and expressing grief. Referral to specialist bereavement counselling services may be appropriate for some individuals to provide support and guidance during the period of mourning and reorganization.

SPIRITUAL ISSUES

Distress of the human spirit can be defined as a disruption in the life principle that pervades a person's entire being and that integrates and transcends one's biological and psychological nature (Kim et al, 1984). Spirituality involves the individual's attempt to find meaning and purpose in life and encompasses the concepts of faith, hope and love.

Factors related to the spiritual distress of the patient with cancer may include: challenged belief and value system; loss of sense of purpose; a feeling of remoteness from God; loss of faith; questioning of moral–ethical nature of therapy; a sense of guilt or shame; intense mental suffering; unresolved feelings about death; and anger toward God (Kim and Moritz, 1982).

Expression of distress of the human spirit is very individualized. Behaviour which may indicate spiritual distress includes: struggles with the meaning of life and death; seeking of spiritual assistance; expressions of anger and/or guilt; crying; withdrawal; sleep disturbances; questioning the meaning of suffering; fear of ability to endure suffering; views of illness as a punishment from God; questioning or refusing therapy; and seeking unorthodox therapy (Kim and Moritz, 1982).

Some patients may find the confrontation with their values and religious beliefs to be a rewarding and reassuring experience. The significance of spirituality and religious observances in the patient's life should be assessed.

The nurse may function as a listener and counsellor in encouraging the patient to express feelings of support or conflict related to spiritual needs. The practice of religious observances can be facilitated by providing privacy for prayers or personal discussions, encouraging attendance at a place of worship, and arranging for bedside religious observances. A religious advisor known and respected by the patient should be sought when possible. Pastoral counsellors or chaplains from within the hospital or from the community may also provide counselling.

REHABILITATION

The principal goal of cancer nursing is to assist the patient and family to adjust maximally to their circumstances. In other words, nursing intervention with the patient with cancer and the family seeks to promote adaptation and maximal rehabilitation. However, until recently, the term 'cancer rehabilitation' was seldom found in cancer nursing literature. Perhaps the view of cancer as a terminal disease has conflicted with the concept of rehabilitation. Often little thought is given to rehabilitation of the patient with cancer as compared with those with other conditions such as cardiac disease or stroke. Rehabilitation needs in the patient with cancer are frequently not identified, or the appropriate resources are not mobilized. This occurs despite the fact that the 5-year survival rate of cancer patients has improved to 50% of all those diagnosed with cancer, while 30% of coronary patients will not survive their convalescent periods and 50% of stroke patients will have died by the end of the first year after the stroke (Dudas and Carlson, 1988).

Rehabilitation is a process that maintains or restores a person to an optimal level of function and effectiveness within the limitations of their disease or disability in terms of their physical, mental, emotional, social and economic potential, and affords an opportunity to redefine what is a meaningful life (Dietz, 1981; Gruca, 1984; Gunn, 1984; Watson, 1986; Wells, 1990). In order to accomplish rehabilitation goals, preventive, restorative and palliative approaches may be used (Dietz, 1981).

The preventive aspects include such things as aggressive pulmonary hygiene to prevent pneumonia in a patient undergoing chemotherapy, or thorough, systematic oral care to decrease discomfort and the chance of infection with stomatitis. For a patient receiving radiation therapy, for example, preventive rehabilitation may also include teaching realistic expectations for daily energy expenditure so that unnecessary fatigue is avoided and so that the daily plan can meet the individual's priorities. For the family, support through the period of bereavement can assist family members in integrating the loss within the larger context and re-establishing meaning in their lives.

The restorative aspects of the rehabilitation process may include ambulation training and prosthesis fitting after an amputation of a leg because of an osteosarcoma, or bowel and bladder management after a cord compression from spinal metastases. Bowel and bladder management after a colostomy or urostomy would also be restorative care as the individual learns to manage a new way of meeting elimination needs. Counselling can assist with adjustment to the changes imposed by illness, and family adjustment, and can restore a sense of self-esteem, coherence and emotional balance.

The palliative aspects of the rehabilitation process are those measures used to provide comfort, symptom control, emotional support and family support during the terminal phase of the illness.

A variety of disease and cancer treatment-related problems amenable to rehabilitation approaches have been identified, including decreased mobility, problems with activities of daily living (including weakness), pain, nutritional problems, financial and vocational problems, appearance, lymphoedema, respiratory difficulties, swallowing disorders, communication, transportation, and difficulties in individual and family psychological adjustment (Lehman et al, 1978; Romasaas et al, 1983).

The rehabilitation team may include a doctor, rehabilitation nurse, physiotherapist, occupational therapist, speech therapist, orthotist, prosthetist, vocational counsellor, nutritionist, psychologist, social worker and religious adviser. Not every or even most patients will need all the resources available. However, it would seem that almost all cancer patients will need the services of at least one of the team members.

Nursing assessment and intervention relative to many of the rehabilitation needs of the patient with cancer have been addressed in other sections of this chapter. As increasing numbers of cancer patients survive, nurses can contribute to the quality and satisfaction of their patients' lives by developing a philosophy that incorporates rehabilitation principles as an integral part of their practice.

SURVIVORSHIP

Early detection and effective multimodal therapies have increased significantly the numbers of cancer survivors. Historically, cancer survivors have been defined as individuals 'cured' of their disease, with the 'cured' state commencing 5 years after diagnosis. The burgeoning population of survivors has given emphasis to the need to address quality of survival and the psychosocial consequences of cancer and its treatment. Long-term survivors may experience problems ranging from minor short-term difficulties to major psychosocial crises (Schmale et al, 1983; Cella and Tross, 1986; Fobair et al, 1986; Cella, 1987; Loescher et al, 1989).

Fear of recurrence is probably the most common concern for all cancer survivors. Fear of relapse may present in a variety of forms, ranging from general uneasiness about the aetiology of mild to moderate or intermittent symptoms, to pronounced anxiety that interferes with daily life. As time passes, anxiety concerning recurrence may decrease, however a heightened sense of vulnerability to illness is often a feature of the survivor's experience (Northouse, 1981; Maher, 1982; Schmale et al, 1983; Cella and Tross, 1986). Not knowing when and if cancer will reappear often negatively affects the survivor's sense of control over his or her life (Northouse, 1981; Welch-McCaffrey, 1985).

The need for close, ongoing evaluation following the

cessation of therapy mandates an ongoing relationship between the patient and the health care team. These relationships may engender both ambivalence and anxiety. As patients are nearing the end of treatment, they may feel elated over the prospect of discontinuing therapy, while at the same time feeling fearful of distancing themselves from the team who has helped them to get to this extended survival stage. Fear of detecting recurrence or other problems can lead to hypochrondriasis, avoidance of doctors and pronounced anxiety about attending follow-up examinations.

Attempts to minimize memories of the treatment experience and to return to usual life tasks may not be easy. The transition from a sick role to a healthy role may be challenged by physical symptoms, negative expectations from those within the patient's work and social circle, and social stigma (Maher, 1982). The survivor's family may also experience worry about the possibility of relapse and the difficulties of social reintegration and may respond with overprotectiveness and pervasive anxiety. On the other hand, family members may be hesitant to discuss mutual concerns about the recurrence of cancer since these concerns can trigger their own sense of insecurity about the future (Welch-McCaffrey, 1985).

Many survivors encounter ongoing socioeconomic impediments to full recovery, including difficulties regaining financial and work-related stability and maintaining insurance coverage (Stone, 1975).

Because of the prevailing perception that cancer results in a painful, lingering death, most patients' immediate reaction to the diagnosis is the expectation of a shortened life span. Once successful completion of therapy is achieved, hope for continued survival often supersedes thoughts of death. Many survivors experience a greater appreciation of life, value reprioritization and a greater sense of generalized well-being as a reaction to the possibility of dying younger than expected (Loescher et al, 1989).

The availability of wellness-orientated follow-up clinics, education, counselling, and supportive services, as well as advocacy, community action and policy development are crucial to the achievement of quality survival. Further research is required to identify needs, and develop and evaluate model programmes encompassing both professional and peer support.

SUMMARY

Cancer nursing is and will continue to be one of the most challenging fields in the entire health care system. This chapter has provided an overview of the many ways that nurses intervene with people experiencing a cancer diagnosis. Knowledge from the basic sciences such as anatomy, pathology, pathophysiology, epidemiology and psychology were used as part of the knowledge base needed to generate nursing diagnoses and describe the nursing assessment and management of cancer-associated problems in daily living. As the body of knowledge continues to expand, with new discoveries in cancer aetiology, prevention and treatment, nursing care will also change and expand. Nurses must keep abreast of the latest trends in the field of cancer care, medical intervention, surgical intervention, prevention, community awareness, psychosocial needs, supportive care, patient education and other methods of treatment.

Cancer remains a major health care problem and a very fearsome, isolating illness for the patient and family to confront individually. Medicine has shown the significant contributions that can be made in the diagnosis and treatment of the numerous forms of cancer. New approaches to early diagnosis of cancer, new techniques to treat cancer, new measures to ameliorate distressing manifestations of cancer and its treatment, and new approaches to improve the quality of life for cancer survivors will continue to emerge, and nurses will continue to be integral to these developments.

LEARNING ACTIVITIES

1. Determine the cancer prevention activities in your community and the availability of screening services.
2. Select a chemotherapy protocol and delineate the expected side-effects. Determine for each side-effect the appropriate elements of a nursing assessment and a nursing care plan.
3. Visit a hospice and observe the care of patients in this setting, particularly pain and symptom management.
4. Conduct a pain assessment with a patient experiencing pain due to cancer. How may this pain be relieved?
5. Identify the patient resources for education about cancer and its treatment available in your nursing setting and community.

REFERENCES

Abernathy E (1987) Biotherapy: an introductory overview. *Oncology Nursing Forum* **14(6):** 13–15.
Battles CSE (1981) Nursing management of the radiation therapy client. In Marino LB (ed.) *Cancer Nursing*, pp. 260–286. St Louis: Mosby.
Berger PS (1980) Principles of radiobiology. In Sokol G &

Maichel R (eds) *Radiation–Drug Interactions in the Treatment of Cancer*, pp. 21–39. New York: Wiley.

Bicher H, Wolfstein R, Lewsinsky B et al (1986) Microwave hyperthermia as an adjunct to radiation therapy: summary experience of 256 multifraction treatment cases. *International Journal of Radiation Oncology, Biology and Physics* **12**: 1667–1671.

Bonica J (1980) Cancer pain. In Bonica J (ed.). *Pain*, pp. 335–362. New York: Raven.

Bruckman JE & Bloomer WD (1978) Management of spinal cord compression. *Seminars in Oncology* **5**: 135–140.

Carter P, Engelking C, Rumsey E et al (1989) *Biological Response Modifier Guidelines: Recommendations for Nursing Education and Practice*. Pittsburgh: Oncology Nursing Society.

Cassileth BP, Lusk EJ & Bodenheimer BJ (1985) Chemotherapeutic toxicity—the relationship between patients pre-treatment expectation and post treatment results. *American Journal of Clinical Oncology* **8**: 419–425.

Cella D (1987) Cancer survival: psychosocial and public issues. *Cancer Investigation* **5**: 59–67.

Cella DF & Tross S (1986) Psychological adjustment to survival from Hodgkin's disease. *Journal of Consulting and Clinical Psychology* **54**: 616–622.

Cheson BD & Curt GA (1986) Bone marrow transplantation: current perspectives and future directions. *Journal of the National Cancer Institute* **76**: 1265–1267.

Cimprich B (1985) Symptom management: constipation. *Cancer Nursing* **8(1)**: supplement, 39–43.

DeWys WD & Walters K (1975) Abnormalities of taste sensation in cancer patients. *Cancer* **36**: 1888–1896.

Dietz J (1981) *Rehabilitation Oncology*. New York: Wiley.

Dietz KA & Flaherty AM (1990) Oncologic emergencies. In Groenwald SL et al (eds) *Cancer Nursing Principles and Practice* 2nd edition. Boston: Jones & Bartlett.

Dodd MJ & Mood DW (1981) Chemotherapy: helping patients to know the drugs they are receiving and their possible side effects. *Cancer Nursing* **4(4)**: 311–318.

Dudas S & Carlson C (1988). Cancer rehabilitation. *Oncology Nursing Forum* **15(2)**: 183–188.

Dudjak L (1984) HLA typing: implications for nurses. *Oncology Nursing Forum* **11**: 30–36.

Edstrom S & Miller MW (1981) Preparing the family to care for the cancer patient at home. A home care course. *Cancer Nursing* **4**: 49–52.

Erickson S, Ochran T & Edel E (1989) Intraoperative radiotherapy. *Dimensions in Oncology Nursing* **3(4)**: 5–8.

Feldman JE (1989) Ovarian failure and cancer treatment: incidence and interventions for the premenopausal women. *Oncology Nursing Forum* **16(5)**: 651–657.

Fobair P, Hoppe R, Bloom J et al (1986) Psychosocial problems among survivors of Hodgkin's disease. *Journal of Clinical Oncology* **4**: 805–814.

Fraser MC & Tucker MA (1988) Late effects of cancer therapy: chemotherapy related malignancies. *Oncology Nursing Forum* **15(1)**: 67–77.

Freeman S (1988) An overview of bone marrow transplantation. *Seminars in Oncology Nursing* **4(1)**: 3–8.

Freihofer P & Felton G (1976) Nursing behaviour in bereavement. *Nursing Research* **25**: 332–337.

Giaquinta B (1977) Helping families face the crisis of cancer. *American Journal of Nursing* **77**: 1585–1588.

Glasel M (1985) Cancer prevention: the role of the nurse in primary and secondary cancer prevention. *Cancer Nursing* **8(1)**: supplement, 5–12.

Googe MC & Varricchio C (1981) A pilot investigation of home health care needs of cancer patients and their families. *Oncology Nursing Forum* **8**: 24–28.

Gorin N (1986) Autologus bone marrow transplantation in acute leukaemia. *Journal of the National Cancer Institute* **76**: 1281–1287.

Gringrich RD, Howe CWS & Ginder GD (1985) Autologous marrow transplantation (AMT) without total body irradiation in refractory lymphoma. *Blood* **66(5)**: abstract 251A.

Grobe ME, Ilstrup DM & Ahmann DH (1981) Skills needed by family members to maintain the care of an advanced cancer patient. *Cancer Nursing* **4**: 371–375.

Gruca J (1984) Oncology rehabilitation. *Rehabilitation Nursing* **9(3)**: 27–30.

Gunn AE (1984) *Cancer Rehabilitation*. New York: Raven.

Guy A & Chou CK (1983) Physical aspects of localized heating by radiowaves and microwaves. In Storm F (ed.) *Hyperthermia in Cancer Therapy*, pp. 279–304. Boston: GK Hall.

Hansen JA, Clift RA & Thomas ED (1980) Transplantation of marrow from an unrelated donor to a patient with acute leukaemia. *New England Journal of Medicine* **303**: 565–567.

Haylock PJ & Hart LK (1979) Fatigue in patients receiving localized radiation. *Cancer Nursing* **2**: 461–467.

Hine VH (1982) Holistic dying: the role of the nurse clinician. *Topics in Clinical Nursing* **3**: 45–54.

Hull M (1989) Family needs and supportive nursing behaviours during terminal cancer: a review. *Oncology Nursing Forum* **16(6)**: 787–792.

Hutchison M & King A (1983) A nursing perspective on bone marrow transplantation. *Nursing Clinics of North America* **18(3)**: 511–522.

Irwin M (1987) Patients receiving biological response modifiers: overview of nursing care. *Oncology Nursing Forum* **14**: 32–37.

Kamani N & August C (1984) Bone marrow transplantation: problems and prospects. *Medical Clinics of North America* **68**: 657–674.

Kim MJ & Moritz DA (eds) (1982) *Classification of Nursing Diagnosis*. New York: McGraw Hill.

Kim MJ, McFfarland GK & McLaine AM (1984) *Pocket Guide to Nursing Diagnosis*. St Louis: Mosby.

King KG, Nail LM, Kreamer K, Strohl RA & Johnson J (1985) Patient descriptions of the experience of receiving radiation therapy. *Oncology Nursing Forum* **12(4)**: 55–61.

Knoff MT (1986) Physical and psychological distress associated with adjuvant chemotherapy in women with breast cancer. *Journal of Clinical Oncology* **4(5)**: 678–684.

Kobashi-Schoot JAM, Hanewald G, Van Dam F & Bruning PF (1985) Assessment of malaise in cancer patients treated with radiotherapy. *Cancer Nursing* **8(16)**: 306–313.

Kubler-Ross E (1973) *On Death and Dying*. New York: Macmillan.

Lamb MA & Woods NF (1981) Sexuality and the cancer patient. *Cancer Nursing* **4(2)**: 137–144.

Laszlo J (1983) *Antiemetics and Cancer Chemotherapy*. Baltimore: Williams & Wilkins.

Lehmann J, Delisa J, Warren G et al (1978) Cancer rehabilitation: assessment of need and developoment of a model of care. *Archives of Physical Medicine and Rehabilitation* **59(9)**: 410–419.

Lewandowski W & Jones SL (1988) The family with cancer

nursing interventions throughout the course of living with cancer. *Cancer Nursing* **11(6):** 313–321.

Lipman A (1980) Drug therapy in cancer pain. *Cancer Nursing* **3:** 39–48.

Loescher L, Welch-McCaffrey D, Leigh S et al (1989) Surviving adult cancers. Part 1: Physiologic effects. *Annals of Internal Medicine* **3:** 411–432. Part 2: Psychosocial sequelae. *Annals of Internal Medicine* **3:** 517–524.

Lovejoy NC, Thomas ML, Halliburton P & Mimnaugh L (1987) Tumour markers: relevance to clinical practice. *Oncology Nursing Forum* **14(5):** 75–82.

Lowry S (1974) *Fundamentals of Radiation Therapy and Cancer Chemotherapy.* London: English Universities Press.

McCaffery M (1979) *Nursing Management of the Patient with Pain.* Philadelphia: Lippincott.

McCorkle R & Young K (1978). Development of a symptom distress scale. *Cancer Nursing* **1:** 373–378.

Maher EL (1982) Anomic aspects of recovery from cancer. *Social Science and Medicine* **16:** 907–912.

Marino LB (1981a) The nature and scope of the cancer problem. In Marino LB (ed.) *Cancer Nursing.* St Louis: Mosby.

Marino LB (ed.) (1981b) *Cancer Nursing.* St Louis: Mosby.

Maxwell MB (1984) When the cancer patient becomes anemic. *Cancer Nursing* **7:** 321–326.

Miller NJ & Howard-Ruben J (1983) Unproven methods of cancer management. Part I: Background and historical perspectives. *Oncology Nursing Forum* **10(4):** 46–52.

Moldawer N (ed.) (1988) The biotherapy of cancer. *Oncology Nursing Forum Supplement* **15(6):** 1–40.

Moss WT, Brand WN & Battifora H (1979) *Radiation, Technique, Results.* St Louis: Mosby.

Mullan F (1984) Re-entry: the educational needs of the cancer survivor. *Health Education Quarterly* **10:** 88–94.

Nesse RM, Carli T, Curtis GC & Kleinman PD (1980) Pretreatment nausea in cancer chemotherapy: a conditioned response. *Psychosomatic Medicine* **42(1):** 33–36.

Noll L (1990) Chemical modifiers of radiation therapy. In Hassey K & Hilderley L (eds) *Nursing Perspectives in Radiation Oncology.* Albany, NY: Delmar Publishers.

Northouse L (1981) Mastectomy patients and the fear of cancer recurrence. *Cancer Nursing* **4:** 213–220.

Northouse L (1984) The impact of cancer on the family: an overview. *International Journal of Psychiatry in Medicine* **14(3):** 215–242.

Oldham R & Smalley R (1983) Immunotherapy: the old and the new. *Journal of Biological Response Modifiers* **2:** 1–37.

Park D et al. Principles and methods of cancer screening and early detection. C. Reed Ash (editor). Memorial Sloan Kettering Cancer Center, New york, 1982, in Glasel M (1985) Cancer Prevention: the role of the nurse in primary and secondary cancer prevention. *Cancer Nursing* **8(1):** supplement, 5–12.

Parkman R (1986) Current status of bone marrow transplantation in paediatric oncology. *Cancer* **56:** 569–572.

Romasaas EP, Juliani LM, Briggs AL et al (1983) A method for assessing the rehabilitation needs of oncology outpatients. *Oncology Nursing Forum* **10(3):** 17–21.

Rose MA (1976) Problems families face in home care. *American Journal of Nursing* **76:** 416–418.

Rubin P (1983) *Clinical Oncology for Medical Students and Physicians: A Multidisciplinary Approach* 6th edition. Rochester: American Cancer Society.

Sabiston DC (1986) *Davis–Christopher Textbook of Surgery* 13th edn, chap. 21. Philadelphia: WB Saunders.

Santos G (1984) Bone marrow transplantation in leukemia: current status, *Cancer* **54:** supplement, 2732–2740.

Santos G & Kaizer H (1982) Bone marrow transplantation in acute leukaemia. *Seminars in Haematology* **19:** 227–239.

Scanlon C (1989) Creating a vision of hope: the challenge of palliative care. *Oncology Nursing Forum* **16(4):** 491–496.

Schmale A, Morrow GR, Schmitt MH et al (1983) Well being of cancer survivors. *Psychosomatic Medicine* **45:** 163–169.

Schryber S, Lacasse C & Barton-Burke M (1987) Autologus bone marrow transplantation. *Oncology Nursing Forum* **14(4):** 74–80.

Smith LH & Thier SO (1985) *Pathophysiology: The Biological Principles of Disease* 2nd edition, pp. 271–286. Philadelphia: WB Saunders.

Stone R (1975) Employing the recovered cancer patient. *Cancer* **36:** 285–286.

Suppers VJ & McClamrock EA (1985) Biologicals in cancer treatment: future effects on nursing practice. *Oncology Nursing Forum* **12:** 27–32.

Thomas ED (1985) High-dose therapy and bone marrow transplantation. *Seminars in Oncology* **12:** supplement 6, 15–20.

Thomas ED, Storb R & Clift RA (1975) Bone marrow transplantation. *New England Journal of Medicine* **292:** 832–843, 895–902.

Thomas ED, Storb R & Buckner CD (1976) Total body irradiation in preparation for marrow engraftment. *Transplantation Proceedings* **8:** 591–593.

Thomas S (1978) Breast cancer: the psychosocial issues. *Cancer Nursing* **1:** 53–60.

Tierney AJ (1987) Preventing chemotherapy-induced alopecia—is scalp cooling worthwhile? *Journal of Advanced Nursing* **12:** 303–310.

Twycross R & Lack S (1984) *Therapeutics in Terminal Cancer.* London: Pitman.

Vachon ML, Freedman K, Formo A, Rogers J, Lyall W & Freemen S (1977) The final illness in cancer: the widow's perspective. *Canadian Medical Association Journal* **117:** 1151–1153.

Walter J (1977) *Cancer and Radiotherapy: A Short Guide for Nurses and Medical Students.* New York: Churchill Livingstone.

Watson PG (1986) Rehabilitation philosophy: a means of fostering a positive attitude toward cancer. *Journal of Enterostomal Therapy* **13(4):** 153–156.

Webb P (1988) Patient teaching. In Faulkner A (ed.) *Oncology.* London: Scutari.

Welch D (1980) Assessment of nausea and vomiting in cancer patients undergoing external beam radiotherapy. *Cancer Nursing* **3:** 365–371.

Welch D (1981) Planning nursing interventions for family members of adult cancer patients. *Cancer Nursing* **4(5):** 365–370.

Welch D & Lewis K (1980) Alopecia and chemotherapy. *American Journal of Nursing* **80:** 903–905.

Welch-McCaffrey D (1985) Cancer anxiety and quality of life. *Cancer Nursing* **8:** 151–158.

Wells R (1990) Rehabilitation: making the most of time. *Oncology Nursing Forum* **17(4):** 503–507.

Wickham R, Blesch KS, Paice J et al (1990) Fatigue and its correlates in breast and lung cancer patients. *Oncology Nursing Forum* **17(2):** supplement, 146.

Wojtas F (1990) Hyperthermia and radiation therapy. In Hassey K & Hilderley L (eds) *Nursing Perspectives in Radiation Oncology*. Albany, NY: Delmar.

Wright K & Dyck S (1984) Expressed concerns of adult cancer patients' family members. *Cancer Nursing* **7(5)**: 371–374.

Yasko J (1982) *Care of the Client Receiving External Radiation*. Reston, VA: Reston Publishing.

Yasko JM (1983) Sexual and reproductive dysfunction. In Yasko JM (ed.) *Guidelines for Cancer Care: Symptom Management*, pp. 269–287. Reston, VA: Reston Publishing.

Yasko J & Dudjak L (1990) *Biological Response Modifier Therapy: Symptom Management*. University of Pittsburgh: Cetus Corporation.

Yeager AM, Kaizer H, Santos G et al (1986) Autologous bone marrow transplantation in patients with acute non-lymphocytic leukemia, using ex vivo marrow treatment with 4-hydroperoxycyclophosphamide. *New England Journal of Medicine* **315**: 141–147.

FURTHER READING

PREVENTION AND DETECTION

Bragg DG (1989) State of the art assessment: diagnostic oncology imaging. *Cancer* **64**: 261–265.

GENERAL CANCER NURSING

Brown M, Kiss M, Outlaw E & Viamontes C (1986) *Standards of Oncology Nursing Practice*. New York: Wiley.

Donovan M & Girton S (1984) *Cancer Care Nursing*. Norwalk, CT: Appleton-Century-Crofts.

Faulkener A (ed.) (1990) *Oncology*. London: Scutari.

Groenwald SL, Frogge MH, Goodman M & Yarbro CH (eds) (1990) *Cancer Nursing Principles and Practice* 2nd edn. Boston: Jones & Bartlett.

Johnson BL & Gross J (eds) (1985) *Handbook of Oncology Nursing*. New York: Wiley.

McIntire S & Cioppa A (1984) *Cancer Nursing: A Developmental Approach*. New York: Wiley.

Tiffany R (ed.) (1989) *Oncology for Nurses and Health Care Professionals* 2nd edn. Volume 1. Pathology Diagnosis and Treatment; Volume 2. Care and Support; Volume 3. Cancer Nursing. London: Harper & Row.

Ziegfeld CR (ed.) (1987) *Core Curriculum for Cancer Nursing*. Philadelphia: WB Saunders.

CHEMOTHERAPY

Brager BL & Yasko J (1984) *Care of the Client Receiving Chemotherapy*. Reston, VA: Reston Publishing.

Schulmeister, L (1989) Developing guidelines for bleomycin test dosing. *Oncology Nursing Forum* **16(2)**: 205–207.

Holmes S (1990) *Cancer Chemotherapy*. The Lisa Sainsbury Foundation Series. London: Austen Cornish.

Valanis B & Shortridge ? (1987) Self protective practices of nursing: handling antineoplastic drugs. *Oncology Nursing Forum* **14(3)**: 23–27.

Weiss RB (1982) Hypersensitivity reactions to cancer chemotherapy. *Seminars in Oncology Nursing* **9(1)**: 5–13.

RADIATION

Bucholtz J (1987) Radiolabeled antibody therapy. *Seminars in Oncology Nursing* **3(1)**: 67–73.

Dudjak L (1987) Future directions of brachytherapy. *Seminars in Oncology Nursing* **3(1)**: 74–77.

Hassey K & Hilderley L (1990) *Nursing Perspectives in Radiation Oncology*. Albany, NY: Delmar.

McCarthy C (1987) The role of interstitial implantation in the treatment of primary breast cancer. *Seminars in Oncology Nursing* **3(1)**: 47–53.

Maddock P (1987) Brachytherapy sources and applicators. *Seminars in Oncology Nursing* **3(1)**: 15–22.

Shell J & Carter J (1987) The gynaecological implant patient. *Seminars in Oncology Nursing* **3(1)**: 54–66.

Smith D & Chamorro TP (1978) Nursing care of patients undergoing combination chemotherapy and radiation therapy. *Cancer Nursing* **1**: 129–134.

Strohl R (1987) Head and neck implants. *Seminars in Oncology Nursing* **3(1)**: 30–45.

Welch D (1979) Radiation-related nausea and vomiting: a review of the literature. *Oncology Nursing Forum* **6**: 8–11.

Welch D (1980) Assessment of nausea and vomiting in cancer patients receiving external back radiotherapy. *Cancer Nursing* **3**: 365–371.

Wood HA (1985) Radiation therapy implants. In Johnson B & Gross J (eds) *Handbook of Oncology Nursing*. New York: Wiley.

BONE MARROW TRANSPLANTATION

Champlin R & Gale R (1987) Bone marrow transplantation for acute leukemia: recent advances and comparison with alternative therapies. *Seminars in Hematology* **24(1)**: 55–67.

Cogliano-Shutta N, Broda E & Gress J (1985) Bone marrow transplantation: an overview and comparison of autologous, syngeneic, and allogeneic treatment modalities. *Nursing Clinics of North America* **20(1)**: 49–66.

BIOTHERAPY

Crum E (1989) Biological response modifier induced emergencies. *Seminars in Oncology* **16(6)**: 579–589.

Gallucci B (1987) The immune system and cancer. Oncology Nursing Forum **14(6)**: 3–12.

Glaspy J & Ambersley J (1990) The promise of colony-stimulating factors in clinical practice. *Oncology Nursing Forum* **17(1)**: 20–24.

Haeuber D (1989) Recent advances in the management of biotherapy-related side effects: flu-like syndrome. *Oncology Nursing Forum* **16**: 35–41.

Haeubner D & DiJulio J (1989) Hemopoietic colony stimulating factors: an overview. *Oncology Nursing Forum* **16(2)**: 247–254.

Hahn M & Jassak P (1988) Nursing management of patients receiving interferon. *Seminars in Oncology Nursing* **4**: 95–101.

Hood LE (1987) Interferon. *American Journal of Nursing* **87**: 459–465.

Huffner TL, Kanapa DJ & Stevenson HC (1985) *Basic Immunology for Professionals*. National Cancer Institute.

Jassak P (1987) Future trends in biotherapy. *Oncology Nursing Forum* **14(6)**: 38–40.

Jassak P & Sticklin L (1986) Interleukin-2: an overview.

Oncology Nursing Forum **13:** 17–22.

Lynch M (1988) The nurse's role in the biotherapy of cancer: clinical trials and informed consent. *Oncology Nursing Forum* **15:** 23–27.

Moldawer N & Figlin R (1988) Tumour necrosis factor: current clinical status and implications for nursing management. *Seminars in Oncology Nursing* **4:** 120–125.

Moldawer N & Murray J (1985) The clinical uses of monoclonal antibodies in cancer research. *Cancer Nursing* **8:** 207–213.

Padavic-Schaller K (1988) Nursing applications in a developing science. *Seminars in Oncology Nursing* **4:** 142–149.

Simpson D, Seipp C & Rosenber S (1988) The current status and future applications of interleukin-2 and adoptive immunotherapy in cancer treatment. *Seminars in Oncology Nursing* **4:** 132–141.

Strauman J (1988) The nurse's role in the biotherapy of cancer: Nursing research of side effects. *Oncology Nursing Forum* **15:** 35–39.

UNPROVEN METHODS

Brigden ML (1987) Unorthodox therapy and your cancer patient. *Postgraduate Medicine* **81(1):** 271–280.

Greek Cancer Cure (1990) *CA—A Cancer Journal for Clinicians* **40(6):** 368–371.

Hiratzka S (1985) Knowledge and attitudes of persons with cancer toward use of unproven treatment methods. *Oncology Nursing Forum* **12(1):** 36–41.

Holland JC (1982) Why patients seek unproven cancer remedies: a psychological perspective. *CA—A Cancer Journal for Clinicians* **32(1):** 10–14.

Howard-Ruben J & Miller NJ (1984) Unproven methods of cancer management. Part II: Current trends and implications for patient care. *Oncology Nursing Forum* **11(1):** 67–73.

Jarvis W (1986) Helping your patients deal with questionable cancer treatments. *CA—A Cancer Journal for Clinicians* **36(5):** 293–301.

Lerner IJ (1981) Laetrile: a lesson in cancer quackery. *CA—A Cancer Journal for Clinicians* **31(2):** 91–95.

Simonton OC, Mathews-Simonton S & Creighton IL (1978) *Getting Well Again.* London: Bantam Books.

SYMPTOM MANAGEMENT

Burish TG, Cavey MP, Redd WH & Krozely MG (1983) Behavioural relaxation techniques in reducing the distress of cancer chemotherapy patients. *Oncology Nursing Forum* **10(3):** 32–35.

Dodd M (1987) *Managing Side Effects of Chemotherapy and Radiation Therapy: A Guide for Nurses and Patients.* Norwalk, CT: Appleton & Lange.

Hunt JM, Anderson JE & Smith IE (1982) Scalp hypothermia to prevent adriamycin induced hair loss. *Cancer Nursing* **5(1):** 25–31.

Kennedy M, Packard R, Grant M, Padilla G, Presant C & Chillar R (1983) The effects of using Chemocap on occurrence of chemotherapy induced alopecia. *Oncology Nursing Forum* **10(1):** 19–24.

Royal Marsden Hospital Manual of Clinical Nursing Policies and Procedures (1988) 2nd edition. London: Harper & Row.

Strohl R (1984) Understanding taste changes. *Oncology Nursing Forum* **11(3):** 81–84.

Welch D & Lewis K (1980) Alopecia and chemotherapy. *American Journal of Nursing* 903–905.

Wickham R (1989) Managing chemotherapy related nausea and vomiting: the state of the art. *Oncology Nursing Forum* **16(4):** 563–574.

Yasko J (1983) *Guidelines for Cancer Care: Symptom Management.* Reston, VA: Reston Publishing.

Yasko JM (1985) Holistic management of nausea and vomiting caused by chemotherapy. *Topics in Clinical Nursing* **7(1):** 26–38.

PAIN

Bagley C, Falinski E, Garnizo N & Hooker L (1982) Pain management: a pilot project. *Cancer Nursing* **5:** 191–199.

Baker S (1988) Symptom management and quality of life. *Dimensions in Oncology Nursing* **2(4):** 20–22.

Cleeland C (1984) The impact of pain on the patient with cancer. *Cancer* **54(11):** 2635–2641.

Cleeland C (1987) Barriers to the management of cancer pain. *Oncology* **April**, special supplement.

Donovan M (1982) Cancer pain: You can help! *Nursing Clinics of North America* **17(4):** 713–728.

Jacox A (1977) *Pain: A Source Book for Nurses and Other Health Care Professionals.* Boston: Little Brown.

Levy M (1985) Pain management in advanced cancer. *Seminars in Oncology* **12(4):** 394–410.

McCaffery M & Beebe A (1989) *Pain: Clinical Manual for Nursing Practice.* St Louis: Mosby.

McGuire D & Yarbro C (1987) *Cancer Pain Management.* New York: Grune & Stratton.

Steitz A (1987) Analgesic utilization patterns in a hospice. *Oncology* **April**, special supplement.

Walsh T (1987) Control of pain and other symptoms in advanced cancer. *Oncology* **April**, special supplement.

Wong D & Baker C (1988) Pain in Children: Comparison of Assessment Scales, *Paediatric Nursing* **14(1):** 9–17.

COPING AND CHRONIC ILLNESS

Miller JF (1983) *Coping with Chronic Illness.* Philadelphia: FA Davis.

Mooney S & Greer S (1989) *Psychological Therapy for Patients for Cancer. A New Approach.* Oxford: Heinemann Medical.

Strauss AL, Corbin J, Fagerhaugh S et al (1984) *Chronic Illness and the Quality of Life* 2nd edn. St Louis: Mosby.

Thorne SE (1988) Helpful and unhelpful communications in cancer care: the patient perspective. *Oncology Nursing Forum* **15(2):** 167–172.

Weisman AD (1979) *Coping with Cancer.* New York: McGraw Hill.

FAMILY

Hinds C (1985) The needs of families who care for patients with cancer at home: are we meeting them? *Journal of Advanced Nursing* **10:** 575–581.

Hull MM (1989) Family needs and supportive nursing behaviours during terminal cancer: a review. *Oncology Nursing Forum* **16(6):** 787–792.

Leahey M & Wright LM (1985) Interviewing with families with chronic illness. *Family System Medicine* **3(1):** 60–69.

Stetz KM (1987) Caregiving demands during advanced cancer. *Cancer Nursing* **10(5):** 260–268.

Thorne S (1985) The family cancer experience. *Cancer Nursing*
  8(5): 285–291.

TERMINAL ILLNESS

Amenta MO & Bohnet NL (1986) *Nursing Care of the
  Terminally Ill.* Boston: Little Brown.
Saunders C & Baines M (1983) *Living with Dying.* Oxford:
  Oxford University Press.
Twycross RG & Lack SA (1984) *Therapeutics in Terminal Care.*
  London: Pitman.

Caring for the Patient Undergoing Surgery

11

OBJECTIVES

On completion of this chapter the reader should be able to:

- Describe the principal types of anaesthesia used.
- Identify common potential problems associated with anaesthesia and surgery.
- Discuss the preoperative nursing interventions and patient teaching required to ensure these complications do not occur.
- Discuss the psychological preparation of the patient for surgery.
- Identify the principal aspects of the nursing role during the perioperative phase.
- Discuss the nursing interventions required for a safe patient recovery in the immediate post operative phase.

Surgery may be described as the treatment of disease, injury or deformity by manual or instrumental procedure. This indicates the special feature that categorizes the patient as being surgical, but the care that contributes to the restoration and maintenance of optimum physiological status before and after the operation comprises a large portion of the total surgical treatment and is extremely important in determining the patient's progress and recovery.

Surgical operations may be classified as elective, essential or emergency. An *elective operation* is not necessary for the patient's survival but is expected to improve the patient's comfort and health. *Essential surgery* is considered necessary to remove or to prevent a threat to the patient's life. An *emergency operation* is one which must be done with a minimum of delay in the interest of the patient's survival.

Operative procedures vary greatly. They range from one that is quite simple and uncomplicated, taking only a brief period, to a prolonged, complex, major procedure that has severe traumatic effects. Many necessary considerations and nursing measures are common to the care of all surgical patients, regardless of their particular type of surgery. The basic components of the plan of care may require modification and/or additional specific details, according to the particular operation, the individual's psychological or physiological status and the type of anaesthetic used.

PREPARATION OF THE PATIENT FOR SURGERY

The preoperative period, which begins with the decision that surgery is to be performed, may extend over an hour to several days or weeks. Whenever the patient's condition permits, sufficient time is taken for assessment and treatment so that the patient goes to the operation in the best condition possible. Intelligent, conscientious preoperative nursing may contribute much to having the patient achieve an optimum condition that favours a satisfactory postoperative progress and minimizes the possibility of complications. When the surgery is elective or essential, there is usually a period of several days or weeks during which the patient is at home awaiting admission to the hospital. A district nurse may contribute to the patient's physical and psychological preparation during this time. Some of the patient's and family's questions may be answered, psychological support provided and advice given on such matters as nutrition and rest. Possible solutions to social and economic problems that are precipitated by the impending surgery may also be suggested by the district nurse.

Psychological Preparation

IDENTIFICATION OF PATIENT PROBLEMS

Potential problems common to the patient preoperatively include: (1) anxiety; and (2) lack of knowledge.

Preoperative *goals* are for the patient to be able to state that the level of anxiety has been reduced and to show a satisfactory level of knowledge about the operation and measures that will promote recovery. Nursing interventions are as follows.

1. To decrease anxiety by:
   (a) Identifying the patient's fears and concerns.
   (b) Assessing effectiveness of adaptive responses.
   (c) Supporting effective adaptive responses.
   (d) Answering questions and providing information.
2. Patient teaching. The nurse should:
   (a) Assess the patient's understanding of the operation and events that will occur pre- and postoperatively.

(b) Inform the patient about the surgical procedure and the pre- and postoperative procedures and activities.

(c) Teach the patient to perform deep-breathing, coughing and leg exercises, explaining the purpose of each.

(d) Provide information relating to the expectations of the patient and explain the nurse's pre- and postoperative role.

ANXIETY

Few patients face surgery without some degree of anxiety. The concerns and fear vary from one person to another: some may be anxious about the pain and discomfort, others fear possible disfigurement and incapacity, loss of control of self, or death. They may be worried because of absence from work, lack of support for dependants, lack of care for the family or disruption of plans. Many are disturbed because they simply don't know what to expect; the unknown tends to be more threatening than the known.

The patient's emotional state and physical condition should receive equal consideration. Psychological stress evokes physiological responses (release of adrenaline and noradrenaline) which may have an unfavourable effect, especially if prolonged. The emotionally disturbed patient may experience a greater problem with vomiting, urinary retention, pain and restlessness during the postoperative period.

Assessment

The patient's concerns, perception of the surgery and usual patterns of dealing with stress should be identified. Understanding the meaning of religion to the patient may help in the selection of appropriate support for the patient and family. We live in an increasingly multiracial society so language barriers merit consideration. Most hospitals have access to a list of available translators. It may not be necessary to involve a translator when a member of the patient's family would be more suitable, given the nature of some clinical questions and/or explanations. Through more prolonged and intimate contact, the nurse has the opportunity to assess the patient's perception of the situation and identify attitudes and concerns. Many fears may be unrealistic, based on misinformation and misconceptions about the surgery. Sexual barriers also bear recognition: it should be borne in mind, for example, that women from a strict Muslim background prefer, when possible, to be examined and treated by women.

The level of the patient's anxiety may be assessed by observation of behaviours such as hyperactivity, increased talking, repetition of questions, crying, physical withdrawal, decreased social interactions and insomnia. Objective signs of stress include increased heart and respiratory rates, elevated blood pressure, moist palms and restless movements.

Nursing intervention

The patient is encouraged to reveal fears and concerns, which the nurse should show are accepted, reasonable and to be expected. The problems are explored and, through expressing them and receiving some explanation or available assistance, some of the apprehension may be allayed. The fact that someone expects the patient to have some qualms and is sufficiently interested to listen is in itself a comfort. Some patients may be reluctant to express their fears because they think of them as a personal weakness, but they may be manifesting their insecurity in other ways, such as tenseness, restlessness or withdrawal. The nurse, recognizing the problem, may initiate a discussion by saying, 'I am sure you are concerned about your operation; there may be something I could clarify for you if you would like to talk about it'. There may be the occasional patient who displays a total lack of concern; this person may have considerable deep underlying concern which for some reason he is denying. Effective adaptive responses and available family and helpful community resources are discussed.

Unrealistic fears based on misinformation and misconceptions can be alleviated by providing factual information (Boore, 1978). The patient should be kept informed as to the purpose of the operation and what is involved in the investigative and preparatory procedures. What may be expected on the day of operation and in the postoperative period is discussed. Ignorance of what is going to happen usually causes more fear and mental suffering than being advised of the facts.

Any anticipated permanent change in body function or appearance is explored, and the patient is advised as to the available assistance and how life may be managed in future; emphasis is placed on the positive aspects. For example, a patient who is being prepared for a permanent colostomy may be encouraged to see and talk with a person who has had the same operation and is living a relatively normal, active life. Patients should be referred, where possible, to nurses who have specialized in these particular problems.

It is an established practice in some institutions for an operating theatre nurse who will be involved with the patient's surgery to visit the ward before the day of operation. This has distinct advantages for the patient. It tends to lessen 'the fear of the unknown'. The visit means that when the patient is received in the operating theatre, the nurses will not all be complete strangers. It also indicates an interest on the part of the staff, which is reassuring. The nurse reviews the patient's history, talks with the ward nurse and advises the patient of the purpose of this visit. The discussion includes such matters as transport to the operating theatre, the type of room the patient will be in, any pre-anaesthetic checks, why staff are gowned and masked, the anaesthetic and the postoperative return to the recovery room or the surgical ward. The patient is encouraged to ask questions. Even if theatre staff do not make such visits, ward staff should be exploring these areas with the patient. The visit to the ward and patient provides the theatre nurse with information about the patient that enables the theatre staff to be more fully prepared for this particular patient. For example, the patient may have a disability that necessitates preparation for placement in a different position to that normally used.

Consideration should be given to placement on the ward by selecting a bed that is quiet and nearer to those less likely to increase anxiety in the patient. Long periods in which the patient is entirely alone should be avoided; relatives are encouraged to visit and the nurse should 'drop in' at frequent intervals. Some form of interesting diversion may be provided. The patient may find a minister of religion a source of strength and courage. In some instances help beyond that which the nurse can provide is needed to reduce the patient's fear. It may be necessary to consult the surgeon, anaesthetist or social worker and have one of them talk further with the patient.

Visits with other patients and socializing in the dayroom are encouraged. Most patients tend to talk readily to each other about their problems and share their preoperative fears. The fact that many of the same concerns are experienced by others seems to put them in proper perspective and make them less ominous.

Family members are kept informed, and time is taken to talk with them, answer their questions, and advise them as to how they can offer support to the patient.

PATIENT TEACHING

Assessment

The identification of learning needs includes an assessment of the patient's understanding of the surgical procedure and perceptions of the pre- and postoperative experiences. The fact that surgery is scheduled motivates most patients to seek information, and their receptiveness to the information provided is increased. In emergency situations, life-threatening needs receive priority over detailed extensive explanations, but the patient always has the right to some information and to make *informed* decisions. A moderate degree of anxiety enhances learning, but when anxiety increases, the attention span and receptiveness decrease.

Nursing intervention

The surgeon will have discussed the operation with the patient and family: why it is necessary, what it involves and the expected results. Frequently the patient and the family are so emotionally overcome at the time that they do not grasp all that has been said. Later, they want clarification of what has been said, and they usually have a number of questions. The nurse determines what information was given to them by the doctor and, in simple, understandable terms, repeats necessary information and answers their questions.

Preoperative procedures and what will be expected of the patient are discussed. Expectations for the postoperative period are outlined. The patient is advised as to where he or she will be after the operation has taken place; that is, whether he or she will be taken to a recovery room or the intensive care unit or returned to the present location.

A description of the recovery room and what occurs there is given to the patient, and the family is told that they will be permitted to visit when the patient returns to the ward. When the patient is very young, a parent should be allowed to participate in the recovery phase by being there as the child recovers consciousness. The reasons for the *frequent assessment of vital signs*, alertness and responses should also be explained.

Deep breathing is demonstrated and taught; maximal inspirations, which are held for 3–5 seconds and practised several times an hour, increase arterial oxygen saturation and prevent postoperative pulmonary complications. The technique should be demonstrated and the patient given the opportunity to practise it prior to surgery. Use of a respirometer, to show the patient how much air is taken into and expelled from the lungs, provides incentive to practise the exercises and provides evidence of the effectiveness of the patient's efforts. The patient is taught to *cough* by supporting the area where the incision will be, taking a deep breath and expelling the air forcefully through the mouth. Coughing is encouraged postoperatively to facilitate the removal of bronchial secretions. Table 11.1 lists deep-breathing and coughing techniques. The patient is assured that necessary assistance and support will be provided. Emphasis should be placed on *non-smoking* during the preoperative and postoperative periods; any irritation of the respiratory tract predisposes to pulmonary complications.

Postoperative *lower limb exercises* to prevent circulatory stasis and thrombosis are described and demonstrated. The patient is advised that he or she will be expected to get out of bed, sit in a chair and walk around the room for brief periods in the early postoperative period; early ambulation promotes normal body functioning and reduces problems such as vomiting, wind pains and urine retention. If the use of drainage tubes (e.g. chest or gastric) or special equipment such as a suction machine is anticipated, preoperative preparation includes an explanation of the purpose and procedure and what will be expected of the patient.

Information is also given about any postoperative pain that may be expected, the cause of the pain and what will be done to control it. The patient is told how to participate in pain control by asking for medication before the pain becomes severe and by practising relaxation, leg exercises, ambulation and other techniques that may have worked previously in relieving pain. Relaxation techniques may be taught if the patient is very anxious, requests it or if severe, prolonged pain is anticipated. Anxiety exacerbates pain, and fear of the unknown leads to anxiety. It should be apparent therefore that giving information and explanations together with answering patient questions can make a major contribution to reducing postoperative pain and promoting recovery (Hayward, 1975).

Group instruction in deep breathing, coughing, leg exercises and pain management can be an effective method of teaching. Group instruction saves nursing time and provides opportunity for patients to practise techniques together and share anxieties and fears. Individual instruction is necessary to provide specific information related to the surgical experience of the individual and the family.

Table 11.1 Instructions given to patients about breathing and coughing exercises.

Sustained maximal inspiration	Coughing
From a sitting or standing position: 1. Take a deep breath through the mouth, pushing the diaphragm down and distending the abdomen as the chest expands 2. Hold breath for 3–5 seconds 3. Breathe out slowly 4. Repeat several times each hour	From a sitting position: 1. Support incision with hands or pillow 2. Take a deep breath through the mouth pushing the diaphragm down and distending the abdomen as the chest expands 3. Immediately force the air from the lungs out through the mouth 4. Expectorate secretions into a sputum pot 5. Repeat several times every 2–4 hours if secretions are present

Physical Preparation

PHYSICAL ASSESSMENT

Common concerns with all surgical patients are cardiac, pulmonary and renal function, blood volume and composition, nutritional status and fluid and electrolyte balance. Basic laboratory tests for all preoperative patients include urinalysis, haematocrit, urea and electrolytes, haemoglobin, white cell count, and bleeding or clotting time. An electrocardiogram is often done, and the chest is examined by auscultation and probably X-ray. Other laboratory tests, functional studies and X-rays may be done, as well as specific investigative procedures relevant to the patient's particular disorder and physiological status. These studies should be understood by the nurse so that the necessary explanation, support for the patient and the appropriate adaptations to the nursing care plan can be made.

The nurse is constantly alert for signs and symptoms that might indicate a condition or change in the patient which could interfere with progress and predispose to complications. Such factors as the following are promptly reported to the doctor: a raised temperature; a significant change in pulse, respirations or blood pressure; a rash; a cough; complaint of sore throat or nasal discharge that might point to a respiratory infection; bleeding gums, which may indicate a vitamin C deficiency; onset of menstruation; diarrhoea; nausea and vomiting; and a deficient food or fluid intake.

PATIENT HISTORY

The patient's history includes information that may be significant in responses to surgery and recovery.

Infants, young children and the elderly are less able to tolerate the stress of surgery. Obesity and nutritonal deficiencies interfere with wound healing and predispose to cardiovascular and pulmonary problems. Smoking irritates the respiratory tract and increases secretions, predisposing to respiratory complications; platelet function and blood coagulation are also altered. Existing cardiovascular, renal and liver disorders and diabetes increase the potential for the development of complications postoperatively.

A detailed drug history related to both prescription and non-prescription medications is obtained. Acetylsalicylic acid preparations prolong bleeding. The nurse should be aware of the potential effects of prior drug therapy so that potential risks may be identified and plans made for postoperative observations and interventions for the prevention and prompt identification of problems.

History of any allergic reactions is recorded and an allergy alert bracelet may be placed on the patient's wrist and the chart marked appropriately to alert the surgeon, anaesthetist and nursing personnel.

NUTRITION

The patient who is malnourished tolerates surgery less well. Protein deficiency delays healing and decreases the resistance to infection because of a slower response in antibody formation. Vitamin C also plays an important role in healing since it is necessary for the laying down of collagen fibres. It also contributes to capillary integrity. Optimum amounts of the vitamin B complex are necessary for normal glucose metabolism and for the maintenance of cellular enzymes. A deficient intake of carbohydrate depletes the liver glycogen, leaving the body without a reserve source of glucose during the period when food intake is decreased, which leads to catabolism of the body tissues.

If the patient is not obese and can tolerate it, he is given a high-calorie high-carbohydrate diet and vitamin supplements; this is individually assessed. The patient is more likely to cooperate if advised of the significant role nutrition plays in postoperative progress. Feeding or providing some assistance with feeding may be necessary if the patient is weak or uncomfortable. Frequent small meals may prove more successful than three large meals. When possible, the patient is consulted as to food preferences.

If the patient's condition is such that the ordinary solid food cannot be taken, fluids containing commercial protein concentrates and glucose may be tolerated. When oral intake is insufficient or not possible, intravenous solutions of glucose, protein preparations, plasma or whole blood may be administered.

There is considerable increase in the risk of surgery

on obese persons. They have a greater tendency to develop cardiovascular, pulmonary and wound complications. The excessive fat tissue frequently makes the operative procedures more difficult. The patient who is overweight is advised of the need to lose weight before operation and may be given a diet assessed on an individual basis.

FLUIDS AND ELECTROLYTES

A normal fluid balance is extremely important in the surgical patient: dehydration predisposes to shock, a retention of metabolic wastes and disturbances in electrolyte concentrations. The patient who has been ill for some time, particularly if the disorder is gastrointestinal, frequently has a fluid and electrolyte deficit. A record of the fluid intake and output is kept and the patient is observed for signs of dehydration (see Chapter 7). A minimum intake of 2500–3000 ml is encouraged unless contraindicated. Blood biochemistry studies are done to determine electrolyte concentrations, and any deficiencies are corrected by oral or parenteral preparations.

REST AND EXERCISE

The patient awaiting an operation may find it difficult to rest and sleep because of anxiety and decreased activity. The patient's accustomed presleeping habits are determined and measures which promote relaxation, such as massage, warm drinks, reading or soft music, are instituted. The doctor may be consulted regarding a prescription for a mild sedative to promote relaxation and the necessary rest.

When the patient is well enough, exercise should be encouraged. This prevents general weakness, contributes to normal fatigue and rest, and diminishes the probability of circulatory complications later.

SPECIFIC THERAPY

Certain treatments to correct secondary physiological disturbances or coexistent diseases may comprise a large part of the preoperative preparation. The patient who has developed anaemia because of a loss of blood or a nutritional deficiency may receive one or more blood transfusions. A course of an antimicrobial drug may be necessary to clear up some infection. A diabetic patient may require dietary and insulin therapy to bring the disease under control, lower the blood sugar, and have the urine free of sugar and ketones. The purpose of any such treatments and their significance to the surgery should be explained to the patient and family.

Informed Operative Consent

Informed consent implies that the patient has been given information by the doctor about the nature of the surgery to be done and that the patient understands that information. A *consent form* signed by the patient is also necessary for some major and invasive diagnostic procedures. It also implies that consent is given freely and that the patient has not been put under undue pressure (Mason and McCall-Smith, 1987).

In seeking consent the doctor is required to provide sufficient details and information about what is proposed to enable the patient (or parent or guardian in the case of a minor or a person suffering a disability such as mental handicap) to form a proper decision and so give an informed consent.

The extent of the explanation given, when seeking consent, will depend on factors such as the patient's age and maturity, physical and mental state and the reason for the operation, and will also be influenced by the questions asked by the patient. Some patients request far more information than others about side-effects, complications, etc.

There is no requirement in English law that every possible complication and side-effect should be explained to the patient. The purpose of informed consent is to protect the hospital, surgeon and anaesthetist against claims of unauthorized anaesthesia and surgery and claims related to possible adverse sequelae to the patient, and to protect the patient against unauthorized procedures (Palmer, 1985).

When asked to sign the consent form the patient must be rational, alert and not under the influence of any drugs or alcohol that might impair comprehension and judgement.

The signing of an operative consent form must be witnessed by a medical practitioner who attests to the fact that in his or her presence the statement has been read by the signatory, who stated that he or she understood and then signed the consent. If the patient is mentally competent, but unable to write, an 'X' indicating a consent is acceptable if witnessed by two signatories.

In the UK any person of sound mind who has attained the age of 16 years may give a legally valid consent to surgery. A minor's capacity to make his or her own decision depends upon the minor having sufficient understanding and intelligence to make the decision, and is not determined by any fixed age limit. Until the child achieves the capacity to consent, consent must be obtained from a parent or legal guardian.

In the case of a genuine emergency the doctor may safely proceed to do what is reasonably necessary without a formal consent, acting in good faith and in the immediate interests of the patient's health and safety. If the emergency arises in an unconscious patient the doctor should, if time permits, endeavour to obtain the consent of the next of kin.

When the patient is mentally ill or impaired (handicapped), a valid consent can only be given if the matter concerned is within his or her understanding. The relatives or responsible medical officers have no legal power to consent on the patient's behalf though their approval should be obtained.

Immediate Preoperative Preparation

The following preparatory measures receive consideration the day before and on the day of operation.

FOOD AND FLUIDS

The patient's stomach should be empty when going to the operating theatre to prevent the possibility of aspiration of vomit. All food and fluids are withheld for at least 4–6 hours before the scheduled time for surgery and an explanation is given to the patient (Hamilton-Smith, 1972). Essential oral medication (with a small amount of water) may be given during this time. If the patient's mouth becomes dry and uncomfortable, a mouthwash is given. When a patient inadvertently takes food or fluid, the anaesthetist should be promptly notified. It will probably necessitate a postponement of the operation or the passing of a gastric tube to evacuate the stomach contents.

When the patient is an infant or small child, the doctor may stress the giving of clear sweetened fluids for 24 hours up to 4–6 hours before operation. This is to promote an optimum glycogen reserve in the liver, since it is normally proportionately less than in the adult and will be depleted quickly.

If the patient is to receive a local anaesthetic, a light breakfast may be permitted by the doctor.

ELIMINATION

The doctor's orders may or may not include giving the patient an evacuation enema. If the patient has had a normal bowel movement the day before operation, it may not be considered necessary. Some surgeons prefer all patients having major surgery to have an evacuation enema the evening before surgery to prevent constipation following the operation, when diet and activity are restricted. If the surgery involves the bowel, a thorough preparation is essential in order to ensure the bowel is empty during surgery. This may involve a special diet (low residue) and bowel washouts, depending on the wishes of the surgeon.

The bladder should be empty when the patient goes to the operating theatre in order to prevent incontinence during the anaesthetic induction and operation. In the case of low abdominal or pelvic surgery, a full bladder may interfere with the surgical procedure by making the site less accessible, and it may also increase the risk of accidental injury to the bladder wall. The patient is asked to void just before the preoperative medication is administered. If the patient is unable to void, the staff in the operating theatre are informed and, if necessary, catheterization is performed in the operating room prior to the surgery. If an indwelling catheter is needed it is usually inserted in the operating room, unless otherwise ordered by the surgeon.

LOCAL SITE PREPARATION

Although the details of the preparation of the site of the operation vary according to the area and the surgeon's preference, the principles are the same. Preoperative skin care is to have the skin as free as possible of dirt particles, hair, desquamated cells, secretions and organisms. Prior to surgery the patient takes a warm bath or shower. Hair may be safely removed by depilatory cream but abrasions and lacerations in the skin caused by a razor serve as an entry for microorganisms. If hospital policy insists that hair is shaved from the skin, it is recommended that it be done with a wet shave 1–2 hours prior to surgery. When the skin is to be shaved the surgeon usually specifies the extent of the area to be shaved and the time it is to be done in relation to the surgery. Some research now indicates that not shaving or using a depilatory cream reduces the risk of postoperative wound infections. Walsh and Ford (1989) have discussed this research and the whole preparation for theatre, coming to the conclusion that much care is ritualistic, with little basis in sound research. Shaving skin preoperatively is one such ritual.

If a patient is discovered to have acne or infected lesions, the operation may be delayed until the condition is corrected. Daily antiseptic baths or the application of an antimicrobial preparation may be prescribed.

Special preparation extending over several days may be ordered by the surgeon for some operations such as skin grafts and orthopaedic procedures. Specific instructions for local preparation are received for any surgery on the head, face and eye.

For rectal and lower bowel surgery, the patient is usually given a bowel clearance preparation such as Picolax, followed by evacuation enemas or rectal washouts until the return fluid is clear. Rectal washouts are given high and slowly, and the patient is allowed to rest following each one. They should also be given early enough to make sure all fluid is expelled before the patient is taken to the operating theatre. The perineum and surrounding area are thoroughly cleansed with water and detergent following the final evacuation.

In the case of operations on the mouth or throat, unless specific preparatory instructions are given, the teeth are cleaned and the mouth rinsed well with an antiseptic mouthwash the night before and the morning of the day of operation.

PERSONAL CARE

The patient has a bath, shower or bed bath on the evening prior to surgery or the morning of surgery, using an antibacterial preparation. Prior to surgery the patient is given a clean hospital gown.

The teeth are cleansed and an antiseptic mouthwash may be used the night before and the morning of the day of operation to make sure all food particles are removed. Dentures are removed because they may become displaced and interfere with respiration. They should be placed in an appropriate container, labelled with the patient's name, and put in the patient's locker. Any prosthesis, such as an aritifical eye or limb, is removed and safely stored. If the patient uses a hearing aid, it is usually left in place until arrival in the anaesthetic room. It is then removed and safely stored.

The hair is combed, neatly arranged back from the face, left free of hairpins, and may be secured under a cap so that it does not become soiled or interfere with the administration of anaesthetic. Coloured nail polish and make-up are removed, since checking of the colour of the lips and nail beds for cyanosis is necessary. All jewellery is removed for safekeeping. The identification wristlet should be checked to make sure it is clearly legible, secure and the name is correct.

SPECIAL PROCEDURES

Some special procedures may be ordered before certain operations. A nasogastric or duodenal tube may have to be passed or an intravenous infusion started. The nurse sees that the necessary equipment is available and that the procedure is completed by the time the patient receives the preoperative medication.

MEDICATION

When the immediate preoperative orders are written, the nurse should ascertain whether there are any preceding orders for medications and, if so, ask the doctor whether these preparations are to be withheld or given. The patient may have been receiving a cardiac drug, insulin or other important drugs and the omission of such could have serious effects.

A sedative is usually given the night before operation to ensure a good night's sleep for the patient. A benzodiazepine such as temazepam or a chloral derivative such as dichloralphenazone (Welldorm) or triclofos sodium are commonly used. All patients receiving hypnotic preparations are instructed not to get up after taking the drug but to signal for the nurse if they want something or are unable to sleep. Frequently, simple nursing measures such as a back rub, change of position, turning the pillow or staying with the patient briefly may reduce tension and apprehension and promote sleep.

Approximately 45–90 minutes before operation, the patient usually receives a drug to produce relaxation and allay anxiety; this is known colloquially as the 'premed', i.e. premedication before the anaesthetic. The doctor's choice of drugs is based mainly on the patient's condition and age. Mild sedatives such as trimeprazine (Vallergan) or droperidol are used for children. At this stage a local anaesthetic paste may be placed on the dorsal aspect of a child's non-dominant hand so that by the time the patient arrives in the anaesthetic room the area is anaesthetized and the insertion of a venous cannula is a painless procedure.

If a general anaesthetic is to be given, the patient may also receive an anticholinergic preparation such as atropine or hyoscine hydrobromide (scopolamine) to reduce salivary and respiratory secretions and to block vagal impulses that cause the bradycardia and hypotension associated with some anaesthetic agents. Scopolamine tends to make the respiratory secretions less tenacious than atropine. It may be administered alone without a sedative to young children, since it depresses mental activity as well as secretions.

All preparatory procedures should be completed before the preoperative medication is given. The patient is then left undisturbed and quiet is maintained. A relative may remain in the room to provide comfort and security for the patient.

A final check and recording may be made of the pulse, respirations and blood pressure about 30 minutes after the preoperative drug has been given.

PATIENT'S CHART

Treatments and any pertinent reactions of the patient are recorded, and the complete chart including the nurses' notes, diagnostic reports, progress notes, patient's history, relevant X-rays and/or scans and the operation consent form are put together and taken to the operating theatre with the patient. A sheet on the front of the chart should list any factors that may be considered particularly important for the anaesthetist, surgeon and theatre staff to note. Examples are allergies, drug sensitivity, coexisting disease and limitation of joint movement in a limb. The latter may be significant in relation to positioning the patient on the operating room table. The patient's blood type is also noted.

Relatives are normally advised to go home whilst the patient is in theatre and to telephone the ward after the operation has taken place.

Emergency Preoperative Preparation

Preoperative preparation in emergency surgery is limited to basic essentials. When the patient is in shock or is bleeding, the haemoglobin is checked and the blood typed immediately. An intravenous infusion is started using normal saline or a plasma expander (e.g. Haemaccel) until compatible whole blood is available.

If the patient is to have an inhalation anaesthetic and is likely to have taken food and fluid within the last 6–8 hours, a gastric tube is passed to evacuate the stomach contents. In the case of intestinal obstruction, a nasogastric or duodenal tube is passed and intermittent suction started in order to keep the stomach and duodenum free of fluid and gas.

As soon as possible, the patient is asked to void to obtain a specimen for urinalysis and to have the bladder empty for surgery. If the patient is unable to void, the doctor may ask for the patient to be catheterized, as it is important to know before operation whether the urine contains sugar or abnormal constituents that might indicate diabetes mellitus or impaired renal function.

The consent form for operation is signed, and preoperative medication is given. Any dentures or prostheses and jewellery are removed, and the hair may be covered with a cap.

If the patient has just been admitted and is not accompanied by a relative, the nurse should be sure to obtain the name and telephone number of a family member and should notify the person as soon as possible.

Evaluation of Preparation for Surgery

1. The patient identifies concerns related to surgery.
2. The patient will acknowledge feeling less anxious and show a relaxed posture and ability to sleep the night before surgery.
3. Physical preparation of the patient is completed safely.

4. The patient expresses an understanding of the surgical procedure and the pre- and postoperative events.
5. The patient demonstrates the ability to perform deep-breathing, coughing and leg exercises and can state their significance.

INTRAOPERATIVE PHASE

Operating theatre procedures vary greatly from one hospital to another. The information that follows is generally applicable to most situations and may prove helpful to the nurse caring for the patient experiencing surgery. No attempt is made to present the detailed knowledge and techniques essential to nurses who are members of the operating theatre team. Anticipating surgery is a threatening and fearful experience for the patient. Some fear may be allayed if the nurse at the bedside can give the patient some information as to what will take place in the operating room. It is also important that the nurse caring for the patient in the postoperative period has some understanding of what the patient has experienced.

The operating theatre is located, constructed and equipped to promote safety and quiet, prevent infection and facilitate surgical procedures. It is located near the recovery room. The temperature of the room is readily controlled according to the patient's needs as well as those of the operating personnel. Windows may be absent in the operating room; air conditioning is provided by a special ventilation system which filters the air before it enters the room to remove dust and organisms and reduce the risk of infection. It also provides a higher atmospheric pressure within the operating theatre. The higher atmospheric pressure means that when doors into the theatre are opened, air flows out of the theatre rather than in, thereby reducing the risk of airborne infection. Equipment, for example lights and tables, is designed to withstand frequent disinfection and to facilitate aseptic technique and the surgery. Entry to the operating room is controlled to reduce potential transmission of organisms from the wards or outside the hospital.

All operating theatre personnel wear operating room gowns or suits which are laundered by the hospital. Street clothing or ward uniforms are not permitted in the operating theatre. Personnel wear caps to cover their hair, a mask that is impervious to moisture over their nose and mouth, and covers over their shoes or antistatic footwear. A staff member with an infection (respiratory infection, local skin infection) is excluded from the operating theatre.

The incision and exposure of underlying tissues and viscera place the patient at serious risk of infection, demanding the practice of strict surgical asepsis. Everything that comes in contact with the patient's operative site must be sterile. Table covers, drapes, instruments, sutures, ligaments and sponges are sterilized and are handled only by members of the surgical team who have scrubbed their hands and arms and are dressed in sterile gowns and gloves. Tables, lights and other equipment that do not come in contact with the wound are kept surgically clean by cleansing with a disinfectant between operations. Floors are similarly cared for.

Transfer to Operating Theatre

At the appropriate time, the patient is taken to the operating theatre, either in bed or on a trolley.

Before leaving the ward, the personnel responsible for transporting the patient to the operating theatre check the patient's identification bracelet with the ward staff and operating room list to be sure they have the right patient. The patient is lifted on to the stretcher and adequate covers provided to keep the patient warm. Woollen blankets are not allowed within the operating theatre; wool is a potential source of static electricity. This point is particularly important as many of the gases used in anaesthesia are highly inflammable and therefore the risk of any static sparks must be avoided. Cot sides are used on the trolley. The patient is disturbed as little as possible; preoperative medication has usually been given to reduce anxiety and induce drowsiness.

Reception of the Patient

The patient is taken to a waiting or holding room or area and introduced by name to the operating theatre personnel; it is important not to leave the patient unattended. An operating theatre nurse introduces him- or herself and proceeds to check the following data:

- The patient's response (drowsy, alert, anxious).
- Name and age. Identification is made both verbally if the patient is responsive and by the identification bracelet, and the name is also checked with the operating room list.
- The operation consent form. Is it correctly signed? The type of anticipated surgery is compared with the operating theatre list and any exceptions are indicated.
- If the surgery to be performed is to be on one of paired organs (e.g. kidneys, lung) or limbs (e.g. leg, arm) or a specific unilteral area (e.g. hernia), is the correct unilateral area clearly identified?
- Special problems (e.g. allergy, rash, joint problem and limited range of motion which may interfere with positioning).
- Laboratory reports; serum electrolytes Ca^{2+} (2.2–2.6 mmol/l or 4.5–5.5 mEq/l)
  K^+ (3.5–5.5 mmol/l or 3.5–5.5 mEq/l)
  Na^+ (135–145 mmol/l or 140–145 mEq/l)
  (Further information on the tests required can be found in Chapter 13.)
  Prothrombin time (PT) 11–15 seconds
  Blood type.
- Preoperative medication; what was given and the dose? Medication may be given to: allay anxiety, induce drowsiness, which lessens the amount of anaesthetic needed in the induction phase; reduce respiratory secretions; or to diminish undesirable

reflex responses during induction (nausea and vomiting).

- Vital signs; these are entered on the operation sheet as base-line data.

Any significant observations (e.g. anxiety state; abnormal finding that is recorded, such as allergy, increased prothrombin time; or abnormal vital sign, such as tachycardia) is brought to the anaesthetist's attention before any anaesthetic is administered. A final check is made to make sure the patient has no dentures. The hair is covered with a cap if this has not already been done.

If sufficiently alert, the patient is advised of the waiting period; the nurse remains close by and communicates by calmly speaking to the patient, or simply by touch if the patient is drowsy. The waiting area should be quiet; loud noises, talking and confusion arouse the patient and heighten anxiety. An overheard conversation may be misinterpreted because of drowsiness and preoperative medication.

Anaesthesia

The type of anaesthesia to be used for each patient is decided by the anaesthetist, in consultation with the patient and surgeon. The term anaesthesia implies loss of sensation; that produced may be classified as general or regional. *General anaesthetic* agents produce reversible depression of the cerebral neurones that are responsible for awareness and responses; there is loss of sensation, consciousness, reflex responses and skeletal muscle tone. The muscle relaxation facilitates the surgery. *Regional anaesthesia* temporarily blocks the sensory receptors in the surgical area or the nerve impulses in an area of the sensory impulse conduction pathway. The patient remains conscious but may be drowsy due to preoperative sedation.

METHODS OF ANAESTHETIC ADMINISTRATION

General anaesthesia may be produced by agents administered by inhalation or intravenous infusion. Most frequently, the current practice involves induction of anaesthesia by the intravenous injection of an anaesthetic agent such as thiopentone sodium (Intraval), followed by the inhalation administration of one or more anaesthetic agents. Endotracheal intubation is almost routinely done when an inhalation anaesthetic is to be given. Using a laryngoscope, a cuffed tube is introduced into the trachea by the anaesthetist, following the intravenous induction; the chest is observed for rise and fall and is auscultated for air entry to make sure the tube is in the respiratory tract and not the oesophagus. When the tube is in the desired position, the cuff is inflated with air to maintain an airtight seal. Overinflation is guarded against; excessive pressure may cause necrosis of the mucosa. The tube is attached to the anaesthetic machine. The inhalation method has the advantage of the control which the anaesthetist can maintain on the amount given. Its disadvantage may be irritation of the respiratory tract and increased secretions. Suction must be readily available. Following the

removal of the endotracheal tube, there may be hoarseness or loss of voice due to temporary impairment of the vocal cords, and laryngeal oedema or spasms may occur.

Regional anaesthesia is produced by the following methods.

1. *Local infiltration.* This involves the injection of an anaesthetic agent into the surgical site or into the area to be manipulated. The agent makes the local receptors unresponsive to stimuli. It is used principally for minor superficial surgical procedures.
2. *Peripheral nerve block.* This regional anaesthesia is produced by the injection of an anaesthetic agent into the area of a large nerve trunk or plexus, or into the tissues surrounding the operative site. The conduction of sensory nerve impulses is interrupted. This type of anaesthesia may be used, for example, for a tonsilectomy.
3. *Spinal anaesthesia.* This method entails the injection of the anaesthetic agent into the subarachnoid space in the lumbar region of the spine (usually between the second and fourth lumbar vertebrae). The agent blocks impulses at the origin of peripheral nerves. The area anaesthetized is determined by the level to which the drug rises in the spinal canal as well as by the amount of the drug used. This type of anaesthesia may be used in low abdominal and lower limb surgery. Chest and high abdominal surgery would require the agent to be carried to higher levels which would place the patient at risk of respiratory insufficiency as a result of blocking of impulses to the respiratory muscles.
4. *Epidural or caudal anaesthesia.* This regional anaesthesia is induced by the injection of an agent into the extradural space of the lower part of the vertebral canal (the sacrococcygeal region). The drug blocks impulses carried along the fibres of the cauda equina. Epidural anaesthesia may be used in rectal and perineal operative procedures and is commonly used in obstetrics during labour and delivery. Thoracic epidural anaesthesia can be appropriate for selected patients.
5. *Topical or surface anaesthesia.* This is produced by the application of the agent to the skin or mucous membrane. Absorption of the agent results in a blocking of the sensory receptors. It is used principally in nose and throat procedures.

ANAESTHETIC AGENTS

A variety of drugs are used as anaesthetic agents. Table 11.2 gives examples of anaesthetic agents used according to the method of administration. The choice depends upon the method of administration to be used, the surgery to be performed, the anticipated time for the procedure, and the physiological and psychological condition of the patient.

The inhalation agents commonly used may be in the form of a gas or a rapidly evaporating (volatile) solution. They are absorbed from the lungs and reach the brain quickly via the circulation. The liquid preparations are vaporized in the anaesthetic machine

Table 11.2 Examples of commonly used anaesthetic drugs.

Type of anaesthesia	Method of administration	Agent

General	Inhalation	Volatile liquids:
		  Halothane (Fluothane)
		  Enflurane (Ethrane)
		  Isoflurane (Forane)
		  Trichloroethylene (Trilene)
		Gas:
		  Nitrous oxide

	Intravenous	Solutions:
		  Thiopentone sodium (Intraval)
		  Methohexitone sodium (Brietal Sodium)
		  Ketamine (Ketalar)
		  Etomidate (Hyponomidate)

Regional	Local infiltration	Solutions:
		  Lignocaine (Xylocaine)
		  Prilocaine (Citanest)

	Spinal	Prilocaine (Citanest) Cinchocaine (Nupercaine) Bupivacaine (Marcain) Lignocaine (Xylocaine)
	Epidural	Lignocaine (Xylocaine) Bupivacaine (Marcain)
	Topical or surface	Cocaine Lignocaine (Xylocaine) Benzocaine Amethocaine (Anethaine)

and usually combined with oxygen for inhalation. For many years, ether and cyclopropane were popular inhalation agents but were extremely hazardous because of their inflammability and explosive potential. They have been almost entirely replaced with safer agents. Cyclopropane is still occasionally used on infants for speed of effect.

The intravenous anaesthetic agents take effect quickly and recovery is rapid. They are used for induction and for very brief surgical procedures (e.g. incision for drainage of an abscess). A disadvantage of the intravenous method is the greater difficulty in controlling the degree and depth of anaesthesia.

Spinal anaesthetic agents depress motor and autonomic innervation as well as sensory innervation. The patient's blood pressure must be monitored at frequent intervals. A spinal anaesthetic is contraindicated for the patient whose blood pressure is labile or unstable, is in shock or likely to develop it, or has a respiratory problem. Respirations are observed closely for early recognition of the innervation block going to a level that results in impaired function of respiratory muscles. Assisted respiration may be necessary. For administration of a spinal anaesthetic, the patient is placed in a lateral position and the spine arched to increase the interver-

tebral spaces. The patient is then turned on to his back and the head of the table lowered.

The agents used in local anaesthesia are frequently combined with adrenaline, which constricts the blood vessels in the area. This reduces the rate at which the anaesthetic agent is absorbed into the bloodstream and the amount of bleeding in the area. The slower absorption maintains anaesthesia in the area for a longer period and prevents undesirable side-effects from rapid absorption. Local and regional anaesthesia are not usually used when there is infection in the area; insertion of the needle tends to spread the infection and breaks down localization.

Epidural anaesthetics may be administered over several hours. A special blunt needle is used to guard against passing through the dura mater into the subarachnoid space.

MUSCLE RELAXANTS

Muscle relaxation is important in many surgical procedures. Deep anaesthesia, sufficient to produce complete muscle relaxation, may place the patient at risk of cardiac and respiratory failure. To facilitate surgery and lessen the amount of anaesthetic required, a muscle relaxant such as suxamethonium (Scoline), pancuronium (Pavulon) or tubocurarine may be given intravenously by the anaesthetist. If given, it is brought to the attention of the nurse in the recovery room; the patient is observed closely for respiratory depression as the muscle relaxant paralyses *all* muscles, including those required for breathing.

Surgical Team

The personnel required for an operation includes the anaesthetist, anaesthetic nurse or operating department assistant (ODA), surgical or 'scrub' nurse(s), circulating nurse, surgeon and surgeon's assistant. The number of personnel required depends upon the surgical procedure being carried out. For example, a radiologist or pathologist may be needed.

The *anaesthetist* assesses the patient's condition and must also check all anaesthetic equipment for efficient function of all components. Having done this, anaesthesia is induced and maintained and the patient's vital signs are monitored throughout the procedure. If special monitoring devices are to be used, the anaesthetist puts them in place before the sterile drapes are applied and prescribes necessary support during surgery, as indicated (e.g. drug to correct cardiac arrhythmia, intravenous solution).

The *scrub nurse* performs the sterile nursing activities. These include the following:

- The setting-up and organization of the necessary tables, drapes, instruments, needles, sutures, ligatures, and special equipment appropriate to the particular surgical procedure.
- Assisting with the application of sterile drapes over the patient.
- During the operation, anticipating the necessary supplies (e.g. sutures, instruments) and having them readily available for the surgeon.
- On completion of the main surgery and before wound closing, checking instruments and needles with the circulating nurse to make sure all are accounted for.
- When the wound is closed and area is cleansed of blood, applying the sterile dressing.
- Assisting with the transfer of the patient to the trolley.

The *circulating nurse* carries out non-sterile nursing activities which include:

- Assisting with the preparation and setting-up for the operation.
- Reception of the patient and the checking of the necessary data (see section on Reception of the Patient).
- Providing necessary emotional support for the patient.
- Assisting with the safe transfer of the patient to the operating room table, ensuring a minimum of exposure and securing a wide strap above the knees and placing the arm(s) in the appropriate restraining straps. One arm (the one on the same side as the anaesthetic machine) is usually placed on a padded

arm board and a blood pressure cuff applied so it is readily accessible to the anaesthetist.

- Being available to provide necessary equipment, drugs, etc. throughout the operation.
- Positioning of the patient for surgery and exposing the area to be prepared and draped.
- Observing for possible breaks in aseptic technique. This can occur without the personnel carrying out the sterile activities being aware of it.
- Checking needles and other instruments with the scrub nurse.
- Preparing the patient for transfer to the recovery room.
- Accompanying the patient to the recovery room.
- Giving a report of the surgery and patient's condition to the recovery room nurse who takes over the care of the patient.

The *anaesthetic nurse* is available to assist the anaesthetist as follows:

- Assisting the anaesthetist and anaesthesia induction (e.g. intravenous anaesthetic infusion) and the setting-up of monitoring devices to be used.
- Monitoring of the patient's condition throughout the surgery.
- Recording medications and intravenous solutions.

Positions Used in Surgery

The patient is positioned to:

1. Provide the necessary accessibility and exposure for the surgery.
2. Provide safety for the patient and prevent injury.
3. Promote normal respiration.
4. Facilitate anaesthesia and efficient monitoring.

The position required will depend on the surgery to be performed. The operating room table is designed so that sections of it may be elevated or lowered when necessary. The positions are shown in Figure 11.1 and include the following.

Supine position (Figure 11.1a). The patient lies flat on his back with a wide strap over the upper thighs. The arm on the side of the anaesthetic machine is extended on a padded arm board. A blood pressure cuff is applied and the arm secured. In positioning the arm on the board, hyperextension resulting in shoulder injury and discomfort must be avoided. The other arm is placed at the side of the patient, palm down and is secured.

Prone position (Figure 11.1b). Three or four persons are required to turn the patient on to the anterior body surface. The restraining strap is placed below the knees. The head is turned to one side. One arm is placed at the side, palm up and secured; the other arm is positioned on the arm board, palm up. The feet are elevated off the table by placing a pillow or roll under the ankles. A body roll may have to be placed under each side of the patient to raise the chest off the table and allow for free chest excursion in respiration.

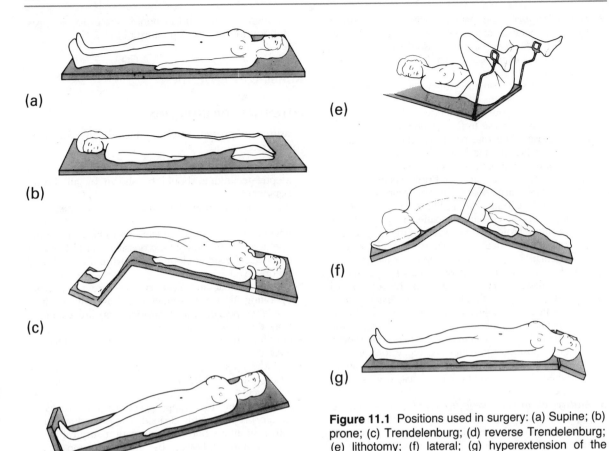

Figure 11.1 Positions used in surgery: (a) Supine; (b) prone; (c) Trendelenburg; (d) reverse Trendelenburg; (e) lithotomy; (f) lateral; (g) hyperextension of the head.

Trendelenburg position (Figure 11.1c). The patient is placed in the supine position with the knees at a break in the table. The table is adjusted so that the patient is on an incline of about 45°, the head being lower than the hips and knees. The end of the table is lowered so the legs are flexed at the knees. Shoulder supports are in place to hold the patient in the position. This position is used in low abdominal and pelvic surgery; the intestines move into the upper abdomen in the head-down position, providing accessibility and greater exposure of the operative organs.

Reverse Trendelenburg position (Figure 11.1d). In the supine position, the patient is placed on an incline with the feet lower than the shoulders and head. A support is in place at the foot of the table. This position may be used in gallbladder surgery.

Lithotomy position (Figure 11.1e). The patient is in the supine position with the buttocks at a break in the table. The thighs and legs are lifted and flexed and the feet placed in stirrups. The arms are supported on the chest or on arm rests. This position is used for perineal, vaginal and rectal surgery. On completion of the surgery, the legs are lowered slowly to prevent a rush of blood into them which could cause a sudden fall in blood pressure.

Lateral position (Figure 11.1f). The patient is turned on to the unaffected side; sand bags or bed rolls are used to support the patient and maintain the position. A wide strap is placed over the hip region. Precautions are used in positioning the arm and lower limb that are on the 'down' side to prevent hyperextension or prolonged pressure on them. The arms may be folded in front of the patient. This position may be used in chest or kidney surgery. In the latter, the patient is positioned so that the kidney elevator of the table lies between the lower ribs and the iliac crest. When the patient is secured in the lateral position the kidney elevator section of the table is raised.

Hyperextension of the head (Figure 11.1g). This is used for thyroid and neck surgery and may also be necessary for endoscopy (e.g. gastroscopy, bronchoscopy).

Potential Patient Problems

Table 11.3 lists the potential problems common to patients during surgery.

1. *Infection.* The patient is at risk of infection because of the surgical interruption of the integrity of the skin.

2. *Physical injury.* The patient's anxiety, drowsiness from preoperative medication and then the loss of sensation and consciousness due to anaesthesia produces risk of physical injury. The potential causes include:

(a) Lack of sides on the trolley, or of appropriate restraining straps.

(b) Leaving the patient unattended, which may result in a fall from the trolley or operating table.

(c) Malpositioning that produces nerve damage or the occlusion of a blood vessel by prolonged pressure on a part. For example, the ulnar nerve is at risk if the arm is firmly secured to an *unpadded* arm board; the sciatic nerve may be injured if both lower limbs are not flexed together when placing the patient in the lithotomy position. Prolonged pressure on the veins of the calf of the leg may interfere with venous circulation and cause thrombus formation.

(d) Hyperextension in positioning. For example, hyperextension of the arm on the arm board may injure the shoulder or hyperextension of the head may injure cervical nerves.

(e) Insufficent number of persons to transfer the patient from the trolley to the table or vice versa, or to position the patient correctly for surgery.

(f) Omission of a conduction pad under the patient when electrical equipment (e.g. cautery) is being used.

3. *Airway clearance ineffective and gas exchange impaired.* Endotracheal intubation and irritating inhalation anaesthetics place the patient at risk of respiratory dysfunction. The irritation may cause excessive secretions, laryngeal oedema or spasm or temporary impairment of the vocal cords with later hoarseness of loss of voice. Not all patients respond similarly to anaesthetic agents and some agents may depress respirations. If the patient has spinal anaesthesia, there is the risk of the solution going high enough in the subarachnoid space to suppress innervation of the respiratory muscles.

NURSING INTERVENTION

POTENTIAL FOR INFECTION

Measures to prevent infection include the following considerations.

- Knowledgeable and conscientious observance of aseptic technique should be shown by all theatre personnel.
- Entry of personnel into the operating theatre is restricted.
- Regulations regarding the clothing to be worn in the operating room to avoid the possible transmission of organisms by street clothes or ward uniforms should be observed.
- Periodic throat and nose cultures are taken from operating theatre personnel and those with positive results (especially for staphylococcus) are excluded from the operating theatre.
- Bedding from the ward is not brought into the theatre.
- Periodic spot-checking of sterile goods by a bacteriologist should be done to determine sterilization efficiency.
- A large skin area (appropriate to the particular surgery) is thoroughly cleaned. The procedure varies with institutions but cleansing with a surgical detergent solution followed by the application of an antiseptic may be the practice. In applying the antiseptic, the pooling of skin preparation solutions between two skin surfaces (e.g. the groin) is avoided because of the risk of irritation and skin damage.
- Any break in aseptic technique should be recognized and promptly corrected.

Table 11.3 Potential problems common to the patient during surgery.

Problem	Causative factors	Goals
Potential for infection	Surgical interruption of skin integrity	Infection will not occur
Potential for physical injury	Anxiety Altered level of consciousness Loss of sensation Preoperative sedation Anaesthesia Decreased mobility Altered positioning of a body part	The patient will maintain body functioning and prevent injury
Airway clearance ineffective	Endotracheal intubation Inhalation anaesthesia	The patient will maintain a clear airway and adequate respirations
Gas exchange impaired	Altered level of consciousness Increased respiratory secretion Laryngeal oedema or spasm	

- A sterile dressing is securely applied to the wound on completion of the surgery.
- In some institutions, a follow-up is made of surgical patients to determine if they remain free of infection. If infection develops, efforts are made to determine its origin. Potential sources include the operating theatre, instruments and materials used at operation, operating theatre staff and the patient's own skin flora.

POTENTIAL FOR PHYSICAL INJURY

Some degree of trauma is inevitable with a surgical procedure but nursing measures should aim to minimize that trauma and prevent unnecessary injuries.

- The patient should be lifted and positioned very gently, the limbs and head being adequately supported.
- The covering sheet is tucked in to support the arms and the cot sides are also in place on the trolley during transfer to and from the operating theatre.
- Similarly, when the patient is on the operating table, the appropriate restraints are necessary. A wide strap may be placed above the knees. A nurse remains with the patient during the induction and early stage of anaesthesia; extra restraint may be necessary because of restlessness. Less of this occurs with the rapid induction that is associated with the commonly-used intravenous anaesthetic administration.
- When positioning the patient, precautions are observed to avoid hyperextension or exposing vulnerable areas to excessive pressure and interference with blood flow. For example, having the arm board padded, correct positioning of the arm and lower limb that are on the side that the patient is on when in the lateral position, and having two persons available to lift and flex the lower limbs together when placing the patient in the lithotomy position are measures that prevent injuries and complications.
- In setting up before surgery, if the use of electric equipment such as the electrocautery is anticipated, placement of a conduction pad under the patient is necessary.

POTENTIAL FOR INEFFECTIVE AIRWAY CLEARANCE

The following nursing considerations contribute to the maintenance of respiratory function.

- The patient's record is checked for information that indicates the respiratory status (history, vital signs, blood gas analysis report). Auscultation of the chest is done before anaesthetic administration. Anything abnormal or questionable is brought to the anaesthetist's attention.
- Anaesthetic equipment is kept in good condition. The anaesthetic machine is tested at frequent intervals by the engineering department; tubes, valves, pressure regulators, flow meters, chemical (soda lime) to absorb carbon dioxide, filters and tubes are checked by engineers as well as by the anaesthetist in preparation for the operation.

- Airways, suction equipment, emergency drugs and an Ambu bag are readily available.
- The patient is received with a calm reassuring manner and the nurse introduces him- or herself. A quiet confident patient has a better reaction to anaesthetic than the anxious, fearful and restless patient.
- The patient's respirations are monitored throughout the administration of the anaesthesia and surgery. Equipment for taking a specimen for blood gas analysis may be required and should be at hand.

POSTOPERATIVE MANAGEMENT

All surgery has certain common effects that vary in extent and intensity with each particular individual and each specific operation. It produces tissue trauma, pain, psychological reactions and loss of blood. There is an increased possibility of invasion of body tissues by pathogenic organisms through a break in the continuity of the skin or by the introduction of foreign objects into the body. In addition, there are disturbances in body functions which are due directly to the surgical procedure or indirectly to the responses of the autonomic nervous system and the adrenal glands to the associated psychological and physical stresses.

The nurse who is caring for a patient following an operation must possess knowledge and understanding of the implications of the particular surgery for the patient, its possible effects on the patient's body functions and the care and support required to assist in the return to normal with a minimum of discomfort and pain. A constant watch of the patient's clinical progress is necessary. Adverse changes and their possible significance must be recognized promptly and the surgeon alerted. If possible, the nurse who is to care for the patient in the postoperative period will have had an opportunity to become acquainted with the patient and learn something of the condition before the operation. The patient may be more confident with a nurse who is not a complete stranger, and the nurse, knowing something of the patient, is better able to evaluate the patient's reactions and condition.

PREPARATION TO RECEIVE THE PATIENT

Most hospitals have a recovery room, either within the operating theatre department or adjacent to it, to which the patient is taken on completion of the surgery. In a few instances, the patient may be returned directly to the ward unit. The recovery room has several distinct advantages: constant surveillance is provided by a staff experienced in immediate postoperative care and whose attention is undivided; proximity to the operating theatre reduces the distance the patient is transported in this critical period; equipment necessary for emergencies is concentrated in the area and is in immediate readiness; and one nurse may care for two or three patients, a situation which would not be possible on the ward where each patient is in a different location. The patient remains in the recovery room until consciousness is fully regained and vital signs are stabilized.

Most hospitals have intensive care units apart from the recovery room in which critically ill patients and patients with a special problem, such as respiratory insufficiency, receive care. The patient who has had major surgery or who has developed serious complications may be transferred directly from the operating theatre to the intensive care unit, where the intensive type of care given in the recovery room may be extended for several days. The advantages of such a unit are similar to those of the recovery room, but the latter provides a briefer period of care. In a few situations, the two units may be combined, using the same staff and equipment.

In the surgical unit to which the postoperative patient is to go, certain basic preparations are made to receive the patient. The bed is made up and the top bedding folded to one side to facilitate the transfer of the patient; a draw sheet or transfer sheet may be placed on the bed to facilitate moving and turning of the patient. The bed has cot sides in place ready for use in the event that the patient becomes restless and confused during recovery from the anaesthesia.

Basic equipment to be assembled at the bedside includes a sphygmomanometer, stethoscope, thermometer, vomit bowl, tissues, face flannel, recording charts and drip stand. Suction apparatus, a portable emergency respirator (Ambu bag with oxygen), and an emergency tray with cardiac and respiratory drugs, sterile syringes and needles, tourniquet, alcohol swabs, oropharyngeal airway (e.g. a Guedal airway) and endotracheal tubes should be readily available.

Equipment most likely to be needed because of the nature of the surgery should also be assembled in readiness for prompt use. For instance, if the patient is having gastric surgery, equipment for gastric suction or aspiration will be necessary.

The bed area is tidied; unnecessary equipment and objects are removed, and daily cleaning is done in order to prevent disturbance of the patient later. The call button is tested to make sure it is in order should assistance be required.

TRANSFER OF THE PATIENT FROM THE OPERATING THEATRE

On completion of the operation, the patient is dried if the skin is moist with perspiration, and a clean gown and sheet are applied. The patient is then lifted, gently and without unnecessary exposure, by a sufficient number of persons to provide adequate support and prevent strain on any part, particularly the operation site. When the bed is used the patient is placed in the lateral or semiprone position, and the cot sides are raised. If the transfer is to a trolley, the dorsal recumbent position is more likely to be used and cot sides must be raised for safety. Sufficient covers are used to ensure warmth and protection from draughts. The head is extended and an oropharyngeal airway is probably in place to facilitate breathing. If the patient is on his back, the lower jaw must be held up and forward to prevent the tongue from obstructing breathing. The

anaesthetist and a nurse accompany the patient to the recovery room. Along with immediate treatment orders, the nurse taking over receives a report on what was done, the patient's condition and anything special for which to be alert.

Immediate Postoperative Care

The discussion presented here deals with general postoperative considerations applicable to most surgical patients. Modifications and additional care related to specific surgery are included in later sections.

The purpose of *nursing intervention* in the immediate postoperative period is to:

1. Assess cardiovascular and respiratory functions, level of consciousness, physical activity, emotional responses, level of pain, if any, and level of comfort.
2. Maintain adequate ventilation.
3. Maintain adequate circulation.
4. Identify and evaluate potential or actual complications and initiate emergency treatment promptly if indicated.
5. Protect the patient from injury.

ASSESSMENT

When the patient is received in the recovery room, an immediate check is made of the respirations, pulse, blood pressure, colour of the skin and mucous membranes, condition of the skin (warm or cold, dry or moist) and the level of consciousness. The wound area is examined for bleeding and drainage. If there is a catheter or other type of drainage tube, it is checked for patency. These initial observations and the patient's preoperative vital signs serve as a comparative baseline which assists the nurse later in recognizing favourable and unfavourable changes and in making decisions as to actions. Cardiac arrhythmia, weak pulse, a decrease or fluctuations in the systolic blood pressure, abnormal respiratory rate and volume, and bleeding in the wound area should be reported promptly to the doctor.

The vital signs are recorded every 15 minutes for a minimum of three recordings and observation is made of the patient's colour, skin condition and operative site for any untoward signs, and the patient's responses are noted at frequent intervals.

The fluid intake and output are accurately recorded until normal fluid and food intake and normal urinary elimination have been resumed.

MAINTENANCE OF ADEQUATE VENTILATION

Inadequate ventilation (hypoventilation) is a common problem in the immediate postoperative period for the patient who has had a general anaesthetic, and it may lead to serious respiratory complications. Hypoventilation implies that the volume of air being moved in and out of the alveoli (air sacs of the lungs) with each respiration is below normal. It leads to a decrease in the vital capacity and surfactant activity resulting in a decrease in blood oxygen concentration. Pulmonary secretions increase and if retained, may obstruct a bronchial tube, resulting in the collapse of a segment of the lung (atelectasis). Bronchitis or pneumonia may develop, since retained secretions provide an excellent medium for the growth of pathogenic organisms. Postoperative hypoventilation and airway obstruction may result from: (1) central nervous system depression by the anaesthetic agent(s); (2) the depression of respiratory muscle activity by a muscle relaxant; or (3) partial airway obstruction caused by the tongue or lower jaw blocking the pharyngeal area, excessive mucus secretion or laryngeal oedema. Laryngeal oedema may develop if endotracheal intubation was used by the anaesthetist.

Hypoventilation may be recognized by: (1) abnormally slow or shallow respirations; (2) audible moist, gurgling respirations, indicating excessive secretions; (3) wheezing, or 'crowing' respirations (stridor); (4) râles or non-entry of air into an area detected by auscultation; or (5) restlessness, cyanosis and rapid pulse rate that are characteristic of hypoxaemia.

Measures to promote adequate ventilation include the following:

1. During unconsciousness, unless contraindicated by the nature of the surgery, the patient is placed in a lateral or semiprone position without a pillow under the head. This position lessens the danger of aspiration of mucus and vomit, and of the relaxed tongue and lower jaw 'falling back' to block the pharynx. The head is hyperextended to facilitate free entry of air and expiration. A firm pillow may be placed at the patient's front and back, if necessary, to maintain the desired position. The knees are flexed to reduce strain, and the uppermost limb is flexed to a greater degree than the lower one. The arm that is uppermost is supported on a pillow so that chest expansion is not restricted. If the patient must be kept on the back, an oropharyngeal airway may be necessary during the unconscious period to prevent occlusion of the airway.

2. Excessive secretions may be removed by pharyngeal suction. The suction catheter is in place, the hole is occluded by the thumb and suction established. The catheter is rotated and withdrawn slowly. If the secretions are beyond pharyngeal suction, tracheal suction may have to be undertaken.

3. Oxygen may be administered as a supportive measure and to prevent hypoxaemia. It may be given by nasal cannulae, nasal catheter or mask (see p. 428). Oxygen therapy is usually continued until the patient is conscious and able to take deep breaths on command.

4. If hypoventilation persists, the concentration of blood gases is determined. Mechanical ventilatory assistance may be necessary (see pp. 429–30 for details).

Aspiration of vomit may occur in the unconscious patient. If vomiting occurs, the head should be kept low, turned to the side and the mouth and pharynx cleared of secretions by suctioning. If aspiration occurs, tracheal suctioning is done to remove the secretions.

MAINTENANCE OF ADEQUATE CIRCULATION

The patient's pulse, blood pressure, skin colour and activity are assessed every 5–15 minutes and the surgical area is checked for signs of bleeding. Hypotension, shock, cardiac arrhythmias and haemorrhage are complications that may occur in the immediate postoperative period and during the next few days.

Hypotension results from the anaesthetic agents, reactions to drugs, cardiac arrhythmias, inadequate ventilation and may also result from moving the patient. Following an operation it is common for the patient's blood pressure to be slightly lower than usual. Systolic pressures below 90 mmHg and pulse rates below 60 per minute or above 110 per minute require prompt intervention.

Shock is a circulatory failure that results in an inadequate perfusion of tissues and organs. This failure at the microcirculatory level reduces the delivery of oxygen and other essentials to a level below that required for normal cellular activities. It may develop during or immediately following the surgery, or it may develop more slowly and become evident several hours after operation (see Chapter 12).

Early manifestations of shock are a decrease in blood pressure, restlessness, inappropriate anxiety, ashen pallor, cold moist skin, rapid weak pulse and decreased pulse pressure. Shock is serious and immediately life threatening; prompt recognition and action are necessary to prevent the condition from becoming irreversible.

Haemorrhage may occur as a result of a slipped ligature, an increase in blood pressure opening up previously collapsed vessels, or the dislodgement of a clot that plugged a severed vessel.

The haemorrhage may become evident externally at the site of operation, or it may be concealed internally and only manifested and recognized by changes in the vital signs and the patient's general appearance and complaints of weakness. Loss of blood causes a fall in blood pressure, rapid thready pulse, deep rapid respiration (which is referred to as air hunger), pallor, apprehension, restlessness and changes of responses and level of consciousness.

The dressing should be checked frequently for signs of bleeding and the body area checked for swelling or distension. Blood from the incision may run down under the patient and not be apparent on the dressing; it is only discovered by sliding a hand under the patient in the area of the surgery. Any suspicion of haemorrhage must be immediately reported. The dressing should be reinforced and the patient returned to the operating theatre for ligation of the blood vessel(s).

A *cardiac arrhythmia* may develop and is usually caused by the anaesthetic agent or is secondary to cardiac surgery. If the arrhythmia was present preoperatively, usually no intervention is necessary. Ventricular arrhythmias may lead to cardiac arrest and require continuous monitoring and immediate intervention. Cardiac arrest, although rare, requires rapid, emergency treatment. A cardiac arrest trolley and emergency drugs are always kept available in the recovery room area. External cardiac massage and artificial respirations with an Ambu bag must be initiated immediately. The cardiac arrest is due to failure of the heart muscle to contract, or to ventricular fibrillation. In the latter, the normal synchronized contractions of the ventricular muscle fibres are replaced with rapid, weak, irregular, uncoordinated contractions that result in incomplete filling and emptying of the chambers and insufficient blood being pumped into the systemic circulation. A defibrillator, by which one or two electric shocks are delivered to the heart, may be used (see Chapter 14). For details of cardiopulmonary resuscitation see Chapter 14.

PROTECTION OF THE PATIENT FROM INJURY

While emerging from anaesthesia, the patient may be restless. Cot sides are used on the bed or trolley to protect the patient. The nurse remains until the patient is conscious and ensures that tubes and essential equipment are not dislodged. The patient is addressed by name and given a simple, direct explanation of where he or she is and what is happening in order to help orientation to the situation as well as reducing fear.

RETURN OF THE PATIENT TO THE SURGICAL UNIT

When the patient returns to the surgical unit, the nurse from the recovery room provides an assessment of the patient's condition and information about the surgical procedure and postanaesthetic events.

ASSESSMENT

The patient is immediately assessed for level of consciousness, pain and discomfort and status of vital signs. The dressing is checked for signs of bleeding, and drainage and tubes are observed for patency. Equipment is connected, the cot sides raised and the call button placed within reach of the patient. If the patient is alert and the vital signs are stable, an assessment is made half hourly and then extended to hourly intervals and then 2–4-hour intervals over the next 12–14 hours.

Fluid intake and output should be recorded until normal fluid and food intake and normal urinary elimination have been resumed.

The patient is positioned comfortably, maintaining normal body alignment. When a spinal anaesthetic has been given, the bed is kept flat and no pillow is used. This position should be maintained until sensation and motor ability have returned to the lower limbs and the systolic pressure is over 90 mmHg. The family may visit briefly if they wish.

TREATMENT

The surgeon's orders for specific treatment are noted immediately. For instance, oxygen, intravenous infusion, appropriate drainage system, special positioning and observations, and drug therapy may be ordered by the surgeon.

Any drainage tubes that are to be connected to appropriate bottle or a suction system must receive prompt attention as they are usually clamped during transit from the operating theatre. If drainage is not quickly established, the tube may become blocked, or sufficient pressure may be built up within the body cavity to cause serious effects. For example, if a gastrointestinal tube remains clamped following gastric or duodenal sugery, distension may cause a leakage of secretions into the peritoneal cavity and may result in peritonitis.

Evaluation

1. The patient is conscious, opens the eyes spontaneously and in response to speech, makes verbal responses which indicate orientation to time, place and person, and responds appropriately to commands.
2. Blood pressure, pulse and respirations are stable and within the normal range for the patient.
3. There are no complications, or if there were they have abated or are controlled.

Continuing Postoperative Care

Table 11.4 lists patient problems which might occur postoperatively.

Nursing interventions during the ensuing postoperative period may be summarized as follows:

1. Promote comfort and control pain.
2. Maintain fluid and electrolyte balance and adequate nutrition.
3. Promote a return to normal patterns of elimination.
4. Promote increasing levels of activity.
5. Promote wound healing.
6. Maintain ventilation.
7. Maintain circulation.
8. Decrease patient anxiety.
9. Prepare patient for discharge and self-management.

PROMOTION OF COMFORT AND CONTROL OF PAIN

Discomforts common to many postoperative patients include pain, nausea and vomiting, indigestion pains and apprehension.

Pain

Pain at the operation site is to be expected because of the unavoidable tissue trauma in surgery. Inadequate control of postoperative pain may cause restlessness and contribute to shock and injury to the operation site.

Assessment of postoperative pain includes data on the nature, duration and location of the pain and the patient's perception of the cause. Pain is not always incisional in origin; it may result from abdominal distension, a full bladder, decreased circulation due to immobility, pressure or muscle spasms. The most reliable guide to the severity of pain being experienced by the patient is what the patient says. The use of a simple scale from 0 to 5, where the patient rates the pain from 0, no pain, to 5, the most severe imaginable, is therefore recommended in assessing pain (see

Table 11.4   Potential problems common to the patient postoperatively.

Problem	Causative factors	Goals
Alteration in comfort: pain	Surgical intervention Nausea and vomiting Abdominal distension Anxiety	The patient will state he or she is free of pain
Alteration in fluid and electrolyte balance and nutrition	Decreased oral intake Fluid loss during surgery via drainage tubes Altered gastrointestinal activity	Fluid intake of 2.4 l/day minimum
Alteration in patterns of elimination	Decreased fluid volume Immobility Pain Surgical intervention Altered sensation	Patient will return to normal pattern of elimination once bowel function returns
Reduced mobility	Pain and discomfort Weakness Immobility	Short term. Patient will sit out of bed within 24 h; will not develop complications of immobility (DVT, pressure sores, chest infection); will walk to bathroom within 48 h (with assistance)
Potential for infection	Altered level of consciousness Ineffective airway clearance Decreased sensation Impaired skin integrity Decreased mobility	No infection will occur and wound will heal without complications
Airway clearance ineffective	Respiratory irritation from anaesthesia Pain and discomfort Decreased mobility	Respiratory rate 12–20 per minute; breathing to be of normal depth and pattern
Inadequate circulation	Effects of anaesthetic Surgical intervention Increased fluid loss Decreased mobility	BP systolic > 90; pulse regular, within range 60–90 bpm
Anxiety	Fear of unknown Lack of knowledge Pain and discomfort Diagnosis	The patient feels able to talk about concerns and fears
Insufficient knowledge about health care	Lack of knowledge and skill	The patient will verbalize an understanding of the factors involved in improving health after discharge

Chapter 9 and Figure 10.6). The surgeon usually orders an analgesic such as papaveretum (Omnopon), pethidine or buprenorphine (Temgesic) to be given every 4 hours if required (prn) for the first 24–48 hours or analgesics may be given by continuous infusion, using a pump which allows accurate control of the rate of infusion. The patient should be kept free of pain by the administration of analgesics before the pain becomes severe. The nurse needs to use judgement, however, in the administration of analgesics, since narcotics tend to depress respirations. When the pain is adequately controlled the patient tends to relax muscles and participate more effectively in deep-breathing and coughing exercises. The use of analgesics is more hazardous with older persons, patients with some respiratory insufficiency (e.g. patients with chronic bronchitis or emphysema) and with young children.

The patient's position is changed and deep breathing, coughing and necessary treatments are carried out following the drug administration so that the patient may derive maximum benefit. After the first day or two, the dose of the analgesic is usually reduced or a milder drug is substituted.

Prevention of strain on the operation site by good positioning and support with a pillow contributes to the prevention and relief of pain. For instance, a patient with a pendulous abdomen who has had abdominal surgery may suffer less discomfort if the strain on the wound is relieved.

Occasionally, a patient may complain of a backache or pain in a shoulder which may have been caused by prolonged immobilization during surgery. Gentle massage or local application of heat using a heat pad or pack may provide relaxation and relief. If the lower limbs are causing discomfort, the patient is encouraged to do a few simple movements such as flexing toes, feet and legs. Massage is never used, but a change of position and support under the full length of the limbs may be helpful. Massage of the lower limbs is discouraged because of the danger of dislodging a thrombus that may have formed as a result of venous stasis. Relaxation techniques, music, sensory stimulation by massage and guided imagery may also be used to lessen the discomfort.

The patient should be encouraged to practise techniques that were taught preoperatively and to inform the nurse about the type and severity of pain and the effectiveness of interventions. The patient who understands the course of the pain and participates in planning and carrying out pain control measures is usually less apprehensive and more tolerant of the discomfort.

Nausea and vomiting

Surgical patients may experience some nausea and vomiting immediately after the operation as a result of the toxic effects of the anaesthetic, pain, anxiety and the handling of viscera in abdominal surgery. Assistance is provided by having a kidney dish available, holding the patient's head, providing a mouthwash and wiping the patient's mouth. If the patient is still under the influence of the anaesthetic or drugs, precautions are taken to prevent aspiration by turning the patient's head to the side and if necessary using suction to make sure the vomit is removed from the mouth and pharynx. Oral fluids are usually withheld, and the patient is kept quiet and is disturbed as little as possible. An antiemetic drug such as metoclopramide (Maxolon) may be administered. Vomit bowls should be emptied promptly and soiled linen changed. Vomiting that persists beyond 24 hours after the operation should be reported as it may indicate a complication or intolerance to the analgesic being used. (For a fuller discussion of nausea and vomiting see Chapter 16).

Flatulence and abdominal distension

Patients who have had abdominal surgery may experience some pain and distension which are caused by an accumulation of gas in the gastrointestinal tract. Most of the gas is air that is swallowed during nausea or when the patient is tense and fearful. The depressing effects of anaesthetics and drugs, handling of the intestine during surgery and the lack of food intake in the tract may contribute to a reduction in peristalsis. Distension persists until bowel tone returns and peristalsis resumes. The discomfort may be relieved by the insertion of a rectal tube for a brief period or by an enema. When the distension is high, a nasogastric tube may be passed and suction decompression used (see Chapter 16). If the distension persists, it may indicate a serious complication such as paralytic ileus, bowel obstruction or peritonitis (see Chapter 16). Frequent turning, early ambulation and normal fluid and food intake are helpful in re-establishing normal peristalsis and preventing distension and gas pains. The patient is usually kept nil by mouth (NBM) until bowel sounds are audible on auscultation, indicating the return of peristalsis.

Mechanical intestinal obstruction, paralytic ileus and peritonitis are serious complications which may develop following abdominal surgery. Nursing care of patients with gastrointestinal complications is discussed in Chapter 16.

Apprehension

The postoperative patient may be apprehensive and concerned about his or her condition; this anxiety is likely to cause restlessness and aggravate discomfort and pain. An explanation of what has taken place and what may be expected may relieve some concern. The patient is also told that the nurse is close by and will be able to help. Having a family member visit or remain quietly by the bedside may be helpful. It may be necessary for the nurse to spend as much time as possible with the patient and to provide repeated explanations and reassurance until the patient regains sufficient confidence and control. If the patient is worried about the findings at operation, it may be helpful to have the surgeon advise as to the condition and the prognosis.

MAINTENANCE OF FLUID AND ELECTROLYTE BALANCE AND NUTRITION

A blood transfusion will probably be given during a major operation or immediately after to replace the blood loss or to combat shock if the blood pressure falls below 90 mmHg. Before the transfusion is started, the blood is checked by two persons to be certain that the label bears the patient's name, is the correct blood type and is within the expiry date. The blood bank labels the blood with the patient's name and identification number after making sure it is the right type and is compatible. The blood should be used within 30 minutes of being taken from the fridge and blood warming apparatus should therefore be used if the patient is to have a rapid transfusion of more than one unit of blood. The patient is observed for signs or symptoms of untoward reactions, such as a chill, fever, dyspnoea, pain in the lumbar region or chest, or a fall in blood pressure.

Symptoms of a reaction are usually manifested during the infusion of the first 50–100 ml of each unit of blood. The rate of flow will depend on the reduction in the patient's vascular volume, blood pressure and cardiac function. It is usually considerably slower in an elderly person.

If a reaction is manifested, the transfusion is stopped and the doctor is notified immediately. In some situations, the blood and equipment are then returned to the blood bank for examination to determine the cause of the reaction.

Oral fluid and food are restricted during the period of nausea and vomiting and following abdominal operations. Intravenous infusions of electrolyte and glucose and/or saline solutions are given to meet the patient's daily requirements and maintain normal fluid and electrolyte balance. Frequent rinsing of the mouth and cool, moist compresses laid over the lips will help with the patient's discomfort of thirst.

As soon as fluids are permitted, sips of water are given and gradually increased in amount. The intake is then progressively increased, as can be tolerated, through fluids and soft diet to general diet. The resumption of a normal diet as soon as possible promotes normal gastrointestinal functioning, and the patient is less likely to experience abdominal distension, gas pains and constipation. Normal nutrition also favours wound healing, maintenance of strength and a sense of well-being.

In the case of a patient who has had surgery on the alimentary tract (gastric or intestinal), all oral intake is withheld until peristaltic activity is established. Palpation and auscultation of the abdomen will reveal the return of peristaltic movement, as will passage of flatus and bowel sounds, usually about the second or third day following gastrointestinal surgery.

Electrolyte balance may be assessed by monitoring serum levels and determining the extent and type of fluid loss. Sodium and potassium depletion occurs with blood loss during surgery and through loss of gastrointestinal secretions in vomiting or nasogastric suctioning. Chloride is also depleted with a loss of gastric secretions. Potassium chloride is often added to intravenous solutions administered to the patient postoperatively.

The postoperative patient may be rather indifferent to food, but may be encouraged to take more by the offering of small amounts of those foods for which the patient has indicated a preference. Foods and fluids are often not taken simply because the patient is weak and finds the effort expended in reaching and feeding too exhausting. The necessary assistance should be provided until the patient regains sufficient strength. The amounts of food and fluid taken are recorded until a normal diet is resumed.

PROMOTION OF NORMAL ELIMINATION

The patient who is adequately hydrated will usually void within 6–8 hours of surgery. The total urinary output on the operative day will be less than the fluid intake because of fluid loss during surgery and vomiting and fluid retention; fluid retention is due to the increased secretion of antidiuretic hormone which occurs with major surgical trauma and stress. The fluid and electrolyte balance usually returns to normal by 48 hours postsurgery.

The postoperative patient may have a temporary inability to void because of a depression of the bladder sensitivity to distension; the impulses that produce the desire to void and the reflex emptying are not initiated. The inhibition may be due to the anaesthetic, drugs or trauma in the region of the bladder. The recumbent position, nervous tension and fear of pain may also contribute to urinary retention. The patient may have the desire to void but is unable to do so because of spasm of the external sphincter. When the bladder becomes distended, a small amount may be voided frequently, but the bladder is not emptied; this is referred to as retention with overflow. Restlessness, complaints of pain or of a feeling of pressure in the pelvic area, and a palpable fullness above the symphysis pubis are associated with retention.

Distension and stagnation of urine predispose to inflammation and infection of the bladder. If the patient has not voided for 12 hours, close monitoring is instituted and efforts are made to induce voiding. If possible, the patient is assisted out of bed to assume the normal, accustomed position. If the patient is not well enough to be out of bed, a bedpan or a commode by the edge of the bed may be used unless contraindicated. Opening taps to produce the sound of running water or pouring warm water over the vulva of the female patient may be helpful. The male patient may be permitted to stand at the side of the bed to use a urinal. The amount of fluid the patient has had since last voiding should be noted. Catheterization may be ordered if the patient's bladder is distended and retention is prolonged. Strict asepsis and gentleness are necessary in the passing of a catheter to avoid trauma of the mucous membrane and the introduction of infection.

In major abdominal and pelvic surgery, an indwelling catheter may be passed and left in place for 2 or 3 days to avoid pressure from a full bladder on the internal operation site. An indwelling catheter may also be used to determine hourly secretion of urine if the patient is in shock or has some renal insufficiency due to disease. There is concern if the output is less than 30 ml per hour.

Since the bowel is usually empty at the time of surgery and food intake is restricted for 2 or 3 days, bowel elimination is not an immediate postoperative concern. The patient, probably accustomed to a daily bowel movement, may be worried unless advised that the delay is to be expected and will not be harmful.

If a normal diet is quickly re-established, a laxative or enema may not be necessary. Some doctors order a mild laxative, glycerine suppository, or a small enema 2 days after operation. Early ambulation and being allowed to go to the toilet or use a commode help in re-establishing normal bowel elimination.

INCREASE LEVEL OF ACTIVITY

Bed rest and inactivity predispose to problems of flatulence and abdominal distension, retention of urine, loss of strength, joint stiffness, and respiratory and vascular complications. Gastrointestinal peristalsis is sluggish, venous stasis occurs, and respirations are shallow.

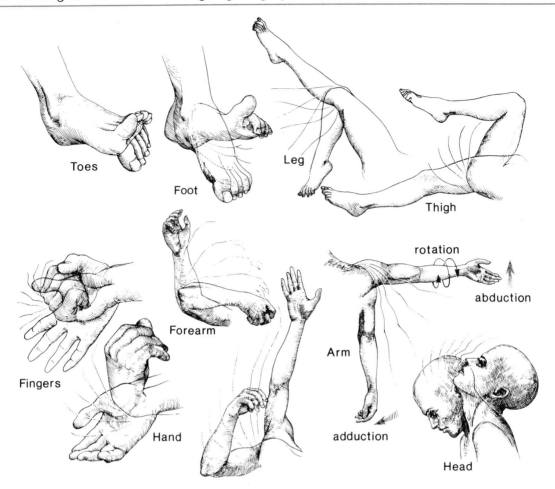

Figure 11.2 Bed exercises for postoperative patients.

To minimize these potential difficulties, some activity and frequent change of position are promoted. Venous stasis and the resultant danger of thrombus formation, particularly in the lower limbs, may be prevented by stimulating the circulation with foot and leg exercises. These are usually commenced 8–10 hours after the operation and done every 2–3 hours until the patient is up and walking. Alternating active flexion and extension of the toes, dorsal and plantar flexion of the feet, and flexion and extension of the legs and thighs are carried out under the direction of the nurse.

If early ambulation is not possible and the surgeon approves, self-care and the following exercises are included as soon as the patient's condition permits: (1) flexion and extension of the head; (2) flexion and extension of the fingers, hands, forearms and arms; (3) abduction, adduction and external rotation of the arms at the shoulders; and (4) contraction of the abdominal muscles. The purpose of self-care and the exercises are explained to the patient who may otherwise feel resentful and consider due care is not being offered. The proposed activities stimulate circulation and respirations and prevent contractures and loss of strength (Figure 11.2).

Early ambulation

Within 12–48 hours after surgery, if the vital signs are stable and the general condition satisfactory, the patient is assisted out of bed and encouraged to walk about. At first the patient may take only a few steps, but movement can be progressively increased as the patient feels stronger and more secure. This early ambulation promotes the return of normal physiological activities such as gastrointestinal peristalsis, reduces the incidence of respiratory and circulatory complications, prevents the loss of muscle tone, improves the patient's morale and shortens the period of hospitalization and convalescence.

The patient is likely to be cautious and weakened the first time out of bed and will need assistance and support. The height of the bed is lowered, and the patient is turned to a lateral position near the edge of the bed with the legs and thighs flexed. The patient is then slowly assisted to the sitting position and the legs are put over the side of the bed. A change in position from supine to sitting or standing may produce postural hypotension. The patient's pulse rate and rhythm and respirations are determined at this point and a check is made for pallor, feelings of dizziness or light-headedness. The patient remains in the sitting position until the pulse and respirations stabilize. The erect position may then be assumed, with the nurse available for support if needed.

Equipment such as an intravenous drip stand and suction machine should not interfere with ambulation. Intravenous bags can be placed on moveable stands and pushed by the nurse or patient. If the patient has a nasogastric tube on suction, the surgeon may indicate that it may be clamped for a brief period of ambulation. When equipment cannot be disconnected, the patient is assisted to walk within the confines of the bed area.

Sitting in a chair may be relaxing and more comfortable for the patient than lying in bed but does not replace ambulation and should not be prolonged. When sitting, patients are encouraged to elevate their legs to prevent venous stasis in the lower limbs and lower abdomen.

The patient is encouraged to use a commode or go to the toilet while up to promote normal bladder and bowel elimination. Precautions against overactivity are necessary when the patient is up more frequently for longer periods because the reparative processes are still going on within the body.

Early ambulation is contraindicated or delayed when there is shock, haemorrhage or cardiac insufficiency.

WOUND CARE

The objectives in wound care are for the wound to remain uninfected and heal firmly with a minimum of scar tissue. When the edges of a wound are in close apposition, healing usually takes place by primary intention. A mild inflammatory reaction with fluid and cellular exudate occurs during the first 24 hours. The patient's temperature is usually slightly elevated and the wound edges will be swollen, red and warm. The gap between the incised edges is bridged within 2 or 3 days as epithelial cells migrate across the wound and help to seal it. During the next 10 days, a collagen network forms and regeneration begins. The area will be highly vascular and red in appearance and the edges slightly elevated. The supportive network is usually adequate for the sutures to be removed in 5–10 days, unless absorbable sutures have been used for wound closure. The strength of the wound increases over the next few months and the tissue shrinks and becomes pale. With no complications, the scar will have the appearance of a thin, white line in about 6 months.

On completion of the surgery, the incision is covered with a sterile dressing, which is usually transparent, and the area is inspected frequently during the immediate postoperative period for signs of drainage or bleeding. If the dressing becomes moist with serous drainage, it is reinforced by the application of sterile pads without disturbing the initial dressing. Should bright blood be evident, the doctor is notified promptly. The sutures are removed in 5–10 days, depending on the type of suture, rate of healing, etc. If clips or staples have been used to close the wound, these may be removed slightly earlier.

A drain may have been inserted at the time of surgery to allow the escape of serum, or a body fluid such as bile. An accumulation of fluid within the tissues increases pain, delays healing and increases the risk of infection. The tube may pass through the incision or a separate small stab wound. Precautions are necessary when moving or bathing the patient in order to prevent dislodgement of the tube, particularly when it is attached to a drainage system. The drain is usually removed when the surgeon is satisfied that drainage has ceased; this is commonly about 24–48 hours postoperatively.

Infection

Infection is manifested by fever, increased pulse rate, general malaise and redness, swelling and tenderness of the wound area. Spontaneous purulent drainage occurs unless the infection is deep, in which case the surgeon may remove a suture and probe the area to facilitate drainage. A swab of the first discharge is taken for culture to determine the causative organism. An antimicrobial drug is administered. Even though the wound is infected, strict aseptic dressing technique is used to prevent the introduction of a secondary infection. When the soiled dressings are removed they are immediately placed in a bag for disposal, and precautions are taken to avoid contamination of the bedding and other objects in the environment so that the transmission of infection to others is prevented.

Haematoma

A small amount of bleeding around the wound site will be drained off if a wound drain has been left in situ. A collection of blood in the surgical wound may occur however and is usually due to impaired blood clotting. Patients receiving anticoagulant therapy or aspirin for a period of time preoperatively are more at risk of developing a haematoma. The wound edges are elevated and discoloured. If the haematoma is small and causing minimal discomfort, it may be left to be absorbed. If the swelling interferes with vital functions, causes discomfort and/or impairs healing, the surgeon evacuates the clot by needle aspiration or reopening the wound.

Dehiscence

Excessive strain on a wound, such as occurs in prolonged abdominal distension or severe coughing, wound infection, malnutrition, and general debilitation, may cause separation of the edges of the incision; this separation is called *dehiscence*. Resuturing or the application of adhesive strips (Steri-strips) may be used to pull the edges together.

Evisceration

If there is some separation of all the tissue layers (skin, fascia and peritoneum) in an abdominal wound, protrusion of a loop of intestine on to the surface of the abdomen may occur. This is referred to as *evisceration*. It is usually sudden, and the patient experiences 'something giving way' and a warm sensation on the skin surface due to the escape of peritoneal fluid and viscera. The surgeon should be notified and sterile dressings, moistened with sterile normal saline, are applied to the exposed intestine. If a large portion of the bowel is eviscerated, a sterile towel moistened with the saline will provide better protection. The patient is requested to lie very still and his head and shoulders and the lower limbs are slightly elevated to reduce the strain on the abdominal wall. Someone remains with the patient to provide reassurance. Since the patient will most likely be returned to the operating theatre, an anaesthetic and operation consent form is signed after the surgeon has explained what is necessary, and the family is notified. The anaesthetist or surgeon is advised as to when the patient last took food and fluid so that necessary precautions are taken to prevent aspiration. Lavage or induced vomiting are contraindicated since intra-abdominal pressure would be increased and more intestine eviscerated.

MAINTENANCE OF VENTILATION

As soon as consciousness is regained, the patient is encouraged to do the deep-breathing and coughing exercises which are taught preoperatively. Sustained, maximal inspirations are carried out several times each hour. The patient is positioned to allow for maximum chest expansion and is coached by the nurse to take a deep breath, hold it for 3–5 seconds and then breathe out slowly. Coughing exercises are carried out with the incision supported by the patient or nurse. A sitting position is best for both activities. The patient's level of pain is assessed prior to beginning coughing activities and medication is given to alleviate the pain if indicated. Pain, fear and lack of understanding of the importance of deep-breathing and coughing activities interfere with patient compliance. Alleviation of pain, provision of support and coaching of the patient in carrying out the exercises are necessary for effectiveness.

The patient is turned from side to side frequently to allow full expansion of both lungs and the drainage of secretions. Early ambulation is essential to promote respiratory functioning and prevent complications caused by hypoventilation and the retention of secretions.

Respiratory complications

The respiratory complications seen most often postoperatively are hypoventilation, atelectasis, pneumonia and pulmonary embolism. Whatever the disorder that develops, the common denominator is hypoxia and hypercapnia. An oxygen deficiency affects the entire body. Hypoxia may be manifested by headache, restlessness and irritability, and then apathy, dullness and clouded consciousness. The pulse rate increases and arrhythmias may develop. The respiratory rate increases as the carbon dioxide level rises.

As noted earlier in this chapter, *hypoventilation* occurs frequently in the immediate postoperative period as a result of respiratory centre depression by drugs or the anaesthetic agent. If the patient does not periodically hyperventilate, atelectasis may develop due to decreased vital capacity and surfactant activity. Suggestions for improving ventilation were presented in the earlier discussion.

Obstruction of a bronchial tube by aspirated material or a plug of mucus results in *atelectasis*, the collapse of the portion of the lung distal to the obstruction. If the collapsed area is large, the patient becomes dyspnoeic and cyanosed, the respirations are rapid and shallow, chest expansion is decreased on the affected side and intercostal retraction may be evident. The pulse rate and temperature are elevated. On examination there is percussion dullness and an absence of breath sounds in the area. Trapped secretions tend to harbour organisms, leading to infection (pneumonia) in the collapsed area.

A chest X-ray may be ordered to determine the extent of the area involved. Frequent deep breathing, coughing and turning are required. Percussion of the chest by a physiotherapist to dislodge the mucus is done several times daily. An increased fluid intake and humidification of the inspired air are used to promote liquefaction of the secretions so they can be raised more easily. Endotracheal (deep) suction may be used, depending upon the location of the collapsed area and the amount of secretions in the tracheobronchial tree. If the mucus plug cannot be dislodged, bronchoscopic aspiration may be necessary. An antimicrobial preparation is prescribed to combat infection.

Pneumonia may develop independently of atelectasis. Any secretions retained in the alveoli and bronchial tubes readily become infected. The patient usually develops a cough and may complain of chest pain. The temperature, pulse and respirations are elevated, and the sputum becomes purulent and streaked with blood. (See Chapter 15 for a detailed discussion of pneumonia.)

Prevention of postoperative respiratory complications begins with the preoperative preparation. Recognition of even a very mild respiratory infection is important and should be reported. Unless the surgery is an emergency, the operation is deferred until the infection is cleared up. A good nutritional status contributes to the patient's resistance to infection, and smoking should be discouraged. It is extremely important that the patient's stomach be empty when receiving an anaesthetic to decrease the danger of aspiration of vomit.

Postoperative nursing measures that contribute to the prevention of respiratory complications include the following:

- Lateral or semiprone positioning of the patient during recovery from general anaesthesia to prevent obstruction of the airway and promote drainage of secretions and vomit.
- Use of suction when necessary to remove secretions from the pharynx and mouth.
- Frequent deep breathing, coughing and change of position.
- Avoiding exposure to persons with a respiratory infection.
- Early ambulation.
- Prompt recognition and reporting of adverse signs and symptoms.

MAINTENANCE OF CIRCULATION

As soon as consciousness is regained and the vital signs are stable, the patient is encouraged to move about in bed, do limb exercises and begin ambulation. Hypotension may result from sudden changes in position during the immediate postoperative period; a change in position should be made slowly and the patient's responses monitored closely. Physical and emotional support are necessary. Leg and arm exercises and ambulation were discussed in an earlier section of this chapter. Circulatory complications including shock, haemorrhage, cardiac arrhythmias and hypotension were also discussed as they related to the postanaesthetic period.

Vascular complications that may develop during the postoperative phase include deep vein thrombosis, thrombophlebitis and embolism.

Deep vein thrombosis and thrombophlebitis

Deep vein thrombosis (DVT) is the formation of a clot in the veins due to a stasis of the blood. It develops most often in the lower limbs, hence the importance of early mobilization. Frequent foot and leg exercises play an important role in the prevention of DVT in the bed patient.

The thrombus formation is a 'silent' process; there may be some tenderness in the calf of the leg that is accidentally discovered on pressure, or a positive Homan's sign (pain on stretching of the calf muscle), but there are no evident signs or symptoms. If DVT is suspected or recognized, the patient is placed at rest with the foot of the bed elevated. An anticoagulant (e.g. heparin) is usually prescribed to prevent enlargement of the thrombus. The condition is very dangerous because the clot may be carried along in the bloodstream and eventually may block an artery in the lungs, causing what is called a pulmonary embolism, which may be fatal. As a precautionary measure the surgeon may order an elastic compression stocking (such as Thromboembolic deterrent stockings), which usually remain in place until just before the patient is discharged or resumes a normal amount of activity. The nurse removes and reapplies them twice daily to give the necessary skin care.

Thrombophlebitis is due to trauma, infection or chemical irritation of the wall of a vein, initiating a local inflammatory reaction and clot formation. In this instance the clot is fairly firmly attached to the wall of the vein. The condition is quickly recognized because the surrounding tissue becomes oedematous, reddened and painful, and there is an elevation of temperature and pulse.

The patient may be kept on bed rest with the affected limb elevated. External heat may help to relieve the pain caused by vasospasm, and an anticoagulant may be ordered to prevent enlargement of the thrombus. The affected limb is handled very gently and is never massaged, in order to avoid dislodging the clot and the possibility of an embolism.

Pulmonary embolism

This is a serious vascular postoperative complication that compromises the individual's gas exchange and the volume of blood returned to the left side of the heart. Embolism involves the transport by the bloodstream of a detached blood clot (thrombus) or mass of 'foreign' material (tissue, fat globules, air) to a site remote from its origin or point of entry into the vascular system. It is most often a thrombus which eventually lodges in a vessel, obstructing the flow of blood and causing an infarction in the area.

A frequent site of embolism is a pulmonary artery, and the size of the artery occluded determines what happens to the patient. If it is a large pulmonary artery, the patient may experience sudden severe chest pain and respiratory distress and collapse and die immediately. If a smaller pulmonary artery is blocked, the patient experiences chest pain, dyspnoea, coughing and elevation in temperature, pulse rate and respirations. Blood-streaked mucus may be expectorated. If it is a relatively large infarction, shock develops rapidly. In a few hours an area of dullness may be detected by percussion, and auscultation may reveal an area in which there are no breath sounds, as the alveoli in the infarct gradually collapse. A chest X-ray is done and the blood pH and gas (oxygen and carbon dioxide) concentrations are determined frequently.

Oxygen is administered and an analgesic such as morphine sulphate may be ordered to relieve the patient's pain and anxiety. An anticoagulant (heparin) is given by intravenous infusion.

Postoperative embolism occurs more often following pelvic surgery, prolonged bed rest, fractures and orthopaedic surgery. It develops more readily in elderly persons and in those with varicosities or a history of a recent leg injury. It is also suggested that women who have been using an oral contraceptive are predisposed to embolism.

Frequent foot and leg exercises and early mobilization are important measures in the prevention of embolism.

DECREASING PATIENT ANXIETY

Nursing measures to decrease the patient's anxiety should be specific to the individual patient. What does the surgery mean to the patient? How does the patient perceive the postoperative events and activities? What are the implications for the individual in terms of body image, future life-style changes and social and family functioning?

An opportunity should be provided to discuss the patient's concerns and perception of the surgical experience. Immediate and long-term problems are identified and assistance planned. An explanation of what to expect and what is happening at the present time and correction of misconceptions decrease the patient's anxiety and helps the development of realistic plans for the future.

When the patient is faced with new and unfamiliar activities, including getting out of bed for the first time or walking with complex equipment attached to the body, the nurse should stay with the patient and provide both physical and emotional support.

PREPARATION FOR DISCHARGE FROM HOSPITAL

Surgical patients remain in the hospital for a much shorter period now than they did a few years ago. Early ambulation, self-care and early resumption of a normal diet hasten recovery and help to maintain the patient's strength, making a shorter period of hospitalization possible.

Since the reparative processes continue, the patient and family receive instructions as to the amount of activity permitted and the necessary rest required. Instructions given will depend on the type of surgery but in general patients should be encouraged to take some exercise (e.g. walking) daily and will need more rest than usual. The nurse should give explicit advice to each patient, in terms the patient will understand, which should be specific for each patient's needs. 'Activity' and 'rest' mean different things to different people. If dressings or treatments are required, the patient and a family member are taught how these are carried out, or a referral may be made for a district nurse to visit. The doctor may give the patient some idea of when work may be resumed before discharge from hospital, or it may not be decided until the initial follow-up examination.

Evaluation of Postoperative Care

1. The patient is free from pain and discomfort, as shown by verbal expression and participation in physical activities and his ability to rest and sleep.
2. The fluid intake and electrolyte concentrations are normal for the patient.
3. The patient is taking a nutritionally balanced diet.
4. Urinary and bowel elimination are re-established and normal for the patient.
5. The patient is ambulatory, active and participating in care.
6. The incision is clean, dry and intact.
7. Vital signs are normal for the patient.
8. No manifestations of complications are present.
9. The patient and family demonstrate an understanding of the required care during convalescence and the resources available.

SUMMARY

Surgery and the effects of anaesthesia constitute major stressors to the person which affect not only physiological, but also psychological and social functioning. The nurse has a major role in preparing the patient for surgery and in ensuring the recovery from anaesthesia is safe and free from complications. Good preoperative care can greatly reduce potential postoperative problems while the role of the nurse in ensuring a pain free recovery is crucial.

LEARNING ACTIVITIES

1. Study a group of patients on your surgical ward, how long are they kept nil by mouth before the actual induction of anaesthesia and how does this compare with recommended times?
2. Carry out a postoperative analgesia audit on your ward. For each of the first 3 days post op, calculate the maximum amount of analgesia a patient may be given on a prn basis according to the drug chart and how much they actually were given. How big is the difference? Does this mean doctors overprescribe or nurses under administer pain relieving drugs?
3. Talk to some surgical patients when they are ready to go home, ask them what they were most anxious about when they were admitted and what surprised them most about their surgery. What implications do these answers have for nursing care?
4. Find a relative, friend or acquaintance who has had surgery. Ask them how long it was after discharge from hospital before they felt back to their normal selves and how well prepared they felt for coping after discharge.

REFERENCES AND FURTHER READING

Adams A (1990) *Theatre Nursing*. Oxford: Heinemann.
Boore J (1978) *Prescription for Recovery*. London: Royal College of Nursing.
Brigden R (1988) *Theatre Technique* 5th edn. Edinburgh: Churchill Livingstone.
Carrie LES & Simpson PJ (1988) *Understanding Anaesthesia*. London: Heinemann.
Carter DC (ed.) (1988) *Perioperative Care*. Edinburgh: Churchill Livingstone.
Farndale WAJ (1979) *Law on Hospital Consent Forms*. Beckenham: Ravenswood.

Gooch J (1984) *The Other Side of Surgery*. London: Macmillan.
Hamilton-Smith S (1972) *Nil by Mouth*. London: Royal College of Nursing.
Hayward J (1975) *Information: A Prescription Against Pain*. London: Royal College of Nursing.
Hosking J & Welchew E (1985) *Post Operative Pain*. London: Faber & Faber.
Keen G (1987) *Operative Surgery and Management*. Bristol: Wright.
Mason JK & McCall Smith R (1987) *Law and Medical Ethics*. London: Butterworth.

MDU, RCN & NATN (1988) *Theatre Safeguards* 2nd edn. London: Medical Defence Union, Royal College of Nursing and the National Association of Theatre Nurses.

Nightingale K (1987) *Learning to Care in Theatre*. London: Hodder & Stoughton.

Palmer RN (1985) *Consent, Confidentiality, Disclosure of Medical Records*. London: Medical Protection Society.

Tschudin V (1986) *Ethics in Nursing: the Caring Relationship*. London: Heinemann.

Walsh M & Ford P (1989) *Nursing Research, Rituals and Rational Action*. Oxford: Heinemann.

Westabys S (ed.) (1985) *Wound Care*. London: Heinemann.

Wilson M (1985) *Surgical Nursing*. London: Baillière Tindall.

OBJECTIVES

On completion of this chapter the reader will be able to:

- Describe the pathophysiological mechanisms of shock.
- Describe factors contributing to the development of shock.
- Describe the clinical characteristics of shock.
- Recognize the importance of identifying the early indications of shock.
- Assess the individual for risk factors, clinical characteristics of shock and related health problems.
- Plan, implement and evaluate nursing intervention for the person in shock.
- Recognize complications of shock.
- Describe measures to prevent the development of complications.
- Discuss the role of the nurse in relation to the early identification, control and management of the person in shock.

In order to sustain life, the body requires equilibrium or *homeostasis*. Virtually every organ system participates in maintaining homeostasis. Fundamental to the life of every cell are the homeostatic mechanisms that control the intake of atmospheric oxygen, the transport of this oxygen to all body cells and the utilization of oxygen in cellular metabolism. The lungs allow oxygen to enter the blood by the process of diffusion. The heart pumps the oxygenated blood out to the tissues. The blood acts as the vehicle to carry oxygen and the blood vessels provide the communicating pathways from the heart and lungs to the cellular sites. Oxygen, once delivered to the cells, diffuses across cellular membranes and participates in energy-generating metabolism. Waste products of metabolism diffuse back into the blood and are transported to excretion sites (e.g. carbon dioxide to the lungs). Dysfunction of the pump, the transporting vehicle, the communicating pathways, or the cellular membrane itself, characterizes the shock syndrome.

Definition. Shock is characterized by inadequate tissue perfusion leading to tissue hypoxia and altered cellular metabolism. Early recognition of the signs and symptoms of shock can prevent the deterioration that may result in serious complications or even death. As nurses provide continuous observation and assessment of patients' conditions long after other care-givers have left the bedside, it is imperative that they have the knowledge and skill necessary to recognize early indications of shock and to intervene appropriately.

PATHOPHYSIOLOGICAL MECHANISMS OF SHOCK

Although the visible features or presentation of shock will vary with the underlying cause of the syndrome,

certain properties characterize all types of shock. The problem, in all cases, is an insufficient supply of oxygen to meet the demands of the body. Shock will, therefore, always be manifested by evidence of cellular disturbances caused by a lack of oxygen. Any injury or stress that might cause shock will immediately provoke a response by the sympathetic nervous system. This system acts to compensate for early decreases in tissue perfusion.

One of the first actions of the sympathetic nervous system is to cause generalized *vasoconstriction*. The purpose of this response is to shunt blood to the heart and brain, which take priority over other less vital organs. Consequently, blood flow to the skin and to the gastrointestinal and renal systems is reduced. Through neural, hormonal and direct feedback mechanisms the heart rate and the strength of cardiac contractions increase. All of these mechanisms help to maintain a normal blood pressure and perfusion to the heart and brain. The remainder of the body, however, continues to experience reduced perfusion as a result of decreased oxygen availability causing increased tissue *hypoxia*. Hypoxia, in turn, will produce changes in the permeability of the cell membrane. Fluid, normally held within specific compartments, will shift out into the blood vessels in an effort to augment the circulating volume.

An increase in activity in the sympathetic nerve supply to the kidneys or a reduction in renal perfusion activates the renin–angiotensin system, which is one of the body's self-defence mechanisms. Renin is an enzyme released by the kidneys; it acts upon a plasma protein, angiotensinogen, to produce the substance known as angiotensin II. This increases peripheral resistance and hence systemic blood pressure, stimulates aldosterone release from the adrenal cortex and produces a sensation of thirst. Aldosterone, it will be recalled (pp. 89–90), leads to increased sodium reabsorption in the nephrons and hence water retention. In this way the body attempts to conserve fluid volume and maintain blood pressure.

Hypoxia disrupts the normal process of *aerobic* metabolism and switches cellular functioning to *anaerobic* metabolism. Anaerobic metabolism results in a decreased production of the energy source compound, *adenosine triphosphate (ATP)*. Reduced concentrations of this product cause immediate cellular swelling or *oedema*. Normally, sodium concentrations are maintained at relatively low levels within cells by means of an ATP-driven sodium pump. When ATP is depleted, the pump fails. Sodium enters the cell, drawing fluid with it by the process of *osmosis*. Swelling and fluid shifts damage the internal organelles of the cell, contributing to further deteriorations of cell function. Hypoxia also initiates the release of *vasoactive* substances such as *histamine*, *bradykinins* and *prostaglandins*. These substances further aggravate the problems of vasoconstriction and amplify the deleterious changes occurring within the microcirculation.

The above outline represents a general overview of the parallel pathophysiological reactions that signify shock. Figure 12.1 illustrates the cycle of events and compensatory mechanisms discussed. These reactions will be discussed in more detail in relation to the specific types of shock.

CLASSIFICATION OF SHOCK

A variety of classification schemes for shock can be found in the literature but all suggest a problem with the pump, the vessels (or pipes), or the volume. Shock is classified as: (1) hypovolaemic, (2) cardiogenic, (3) distributive.

Hypovolaemic Shock

Hypovolaemic shock occurs as a result of the loss of intravascular fluid volume. The pump and the vascular network may be intact, but due to internal or external losses the circulatory blood volume is inadequate. Hypovolaemic shock is present when 15–25% of the total blood volume is lost. If the normal adult blood volume is 5 litres, a loss of 1 litre would signify a loss of 20%, and, therefore, would constitute hypovolaemic shock. The degree of shock will depend on: (1) the volume lost, (2) the rate of loss, (3) compensatory mechanisms, and (4) the age and physical condition of the individual.

If fluid loss occurs internally, the cause and/or effects may not be immediately visible. In contrast, external losses are often more readily visible to the nurse. Table 12.1 outlines examples of internal and external fluid losses.

Whatever the mechanism, the loss of circulating volume leads to a reduction in venous return to the heart. Reduced venous return influences ventricular

Table 12.1   Factors causing hypovolemic shock.

Internal fluid loss	External fluid loss
Trauma, e.g. ruptured spleen	Gastrointestinal bleeding
	Burns
Long bone fractures	Diarrhoea
Lesions causing haemorrhage, e.g. perforated ulcer	Diuresis in hyperglycaemic diabetic coma

filling pressure and stroke volume, resulting in a decreased cardiac output.

Cardiogenic Shock

Cardiogenic shock occurs as a result of poor cardiac function. This can be referred to as pump failure. This type of shock is often associated with acute myocardial infarction, usually involving at least 40% of the left ventricle. The vascular system and circulating volume are intact, but the pump's action is inadequate to maintain tissue perfusion. Pump failure may result from factors other than muscle damage. When pump failure occurs as a result of pericardial tamponade, pulmonary embolism, or pulmonary hypertension, it can be referred to as *obstructive shock*. As with hypovolaemic shock, the end-result is decreased cardiac output, decreased blood pressure and a reduction in tissue perfusion.

Distributive Shock

Distributive shock can be defined as a relative hypovolaemia because of loss of vascular tone or integrity. The blood or fluid volume and the pump are intact, but the pipes are too large. As vessels dilate, the capacity of the venous system expands. A greater volume is required to fill this enlarged space. Distributive shock can be further classified into: (1) septic shock, (2) neurogenic shock, (3) anaphylactic shock.

SEPTIC SHOCK

Septic shock is a devastating syndrome with an average mortality rate of 50%. It is thought that the toxins produced by the pathogenic organism responsible affect the peripheral circulation in such a way that the capillaries become dilated and, due to damage affecting the capillary walls, permeable, so that plasma may leak out of the circulation. Patients in hospital may develop septic shock as a result of invasive diagnostic procedures, surgery, immunosuppressive therapy, and the presence of indwelling urinary and intravenous catheters. Nurses must maintain a high index of suspicion with regard to any patient in hospital who may be subject to such invasive interventions and treatments. The population most at risk are the very young and the elderly,

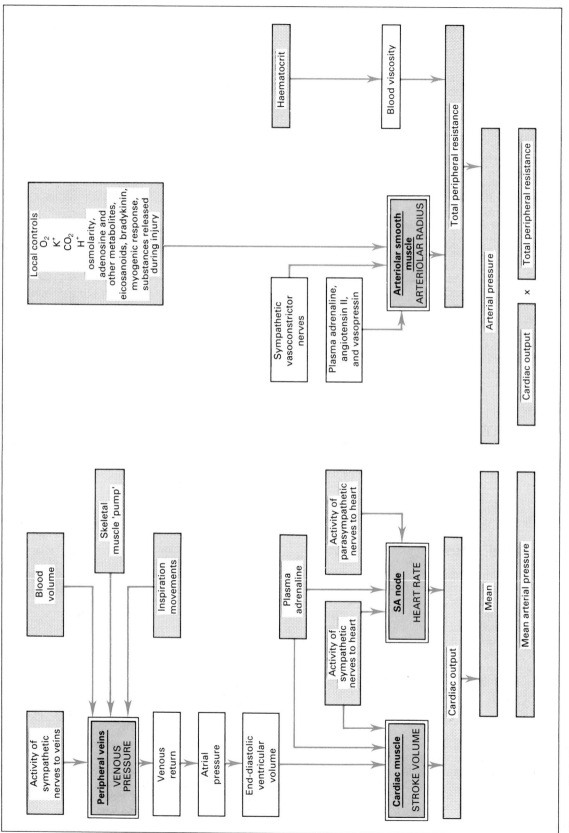

Figure 12.1 Summary of factors which determine systemic arterial pressure. Modified from Vander et al (1990) with permission.

the malnourished, and those suffering chronic health problems or complications of pregnancy.

Septic shock presents in a manner that is dissimilar to the presentation of other shock syndromes, and may, therefore, go unrecognized until a state of significant compromise has been reached. Instead of a cold, vasoconstricted appearance, the patient is more likely to demonstrate evidence of a hyperdynamic state, characterized by a warm, pink appearance. The most common organisms causing septic shock are Gram-negative bacteria, such as *Escherichia coli*, Klebsiella-Enterobacter-Serratia, and *Pseudomonas aeruginosa*. Gram-positive bacteria such as streptococci and staphylococci, viruses, fungi, and rickettsiae may also precipitate septic shock.

NEUROGENIC SHOCK

Continuous sympathetic nervous input normally maintains sufficient tone to arteriolar and venous systems to ensure perfusion. Increases or decreases in sympathetic stimulation are normal feedback mechanisms that respond to alteration in mean arterial pressure. By this means, blood pressure and perfusion to vital organs are manipulated to maintain homeostasis. If sympathetic stimulation is interrupted, vascular tone is lost. Diffuse vasodilatation results. This is the mechanism of neurogenic shock. Going back to the 'pipes and pumps' model used previously, neurogenic shock can be illustrated as a 'pipe' problem. The pump and the volume are normal. The volume of the pipes has increased to a capacity beyond that which the present volume of fluid can fill. Adding volume to the system can only improve the situation if it is of sufficient quantity to fill the space. The dilated vascular capacity is such that huge volumes might be required. Unless vascular tone is reestablished, it is doubtful that enough volume could be added to maintain mean arterial pressure within normal limits.

Neurogenic shock may be induced by spinal anaesthesia, spinal cord injury, or damage to the vasomotor centre in the medulla.

ANAPHYLACTIC SHOCK

Initial introduction of an antigen into the body results in the production of an antibody specific to that antigen. Subsequent presentations of that antigen may induce the physiological reactions that characterize anaphylaxis. Antibody response releases histamines, bradykinins, and other vasocative substances. In combination, these substances produce vasodilatation, increased capillary permeability and severe bronchoconstriction. As in neurogenic and septic shock, the vasodilatation creates an increased venous capacity. Decreases in venous return to the heart, ventricular filling pressure, stroke volume and cardiac output result. This syndrome is further complicated by bronchospasm that can interfere with gas exchange. If shock is a disruption in oxygen delivery and utilization, it is apparent that anaphylaxis presents a unique set of problems. Oxygen entry and transport are interrupted and must be reestablished in order to prevent cellular demise. Obviously, shock is a complicated syndrome and to delineate physiological mechanisms specific to each type would be beyond the scope of this text. It is recommended that the reader examine other resources, particularly for more information on septic shock.

COMPLICATIONS OF SHOCK

Alterations in tissue perfusion account for the overt complications of shock throughout the body. Damage to the larger organ systems as well as to the microcirculation may progress to the point where it is irreversible and death ensues. The complications associated with diminished perfusion, e.g. acute renal failure, will prolong hospital stay and may contribute to long-standing patient problems.

Disturbed cellular function results in a conversion to anaerobic metabolism. Energy supplies are diminished and all organ systems are affected according to the oxygen requirements of the composite organs.

Brain. The brain requires a constant supply of glucose and oxygen for normal function. Decreases in cerebral circulation leading to hypoxia and acidosis will be characterized by depressed cerebral function, beginning with restlessness and confusion and progressing to diminished consciousness and vasomotor centre dysfunction.

Myocardium. Perfusion of the coronary arteries is dependent on mean arterial pressure. The pressure required depends in turn upon many factors, including the patient's underlying cardiovascular status. The myocardium is extremely intolerant of any decrease in perfusion below that minimum required level. Poor perfusion manifests initially as angina. Changes on the electrocardiogram, indicating ischaemia and possible infarction, become progressively noticeable. Alterations in cellular electrolyte pumping mechanisms will contribute to poor contractility and the propagation of cardiac arrhythmias.

Gastrointestinal system. Decreased perfusion to the gastrointestinal system disrupts the integrity of intestinal mucosa, allowing the normal gastrointestinal bacteria to enter the circulation and cause sepsis. Necrosis of tissue leads to ulceration and intestinal bleeding.

Hepatic system. Metabolism of carbohydrates, fats, and proteins and detoxification of harmful materials, including those released by bacteria, will be significantly compromised in states of hypoperfusion of the hepatic system. Dysfunction of the reticuloendothelial system will diminish the patient's ability to resist further infection.

In addition to the systems mentioned above, the respiratory, haematopoietic, and renal systems are significantly affected by the hypoperfusion associated with shock. Three specific conditions that often result are:

1. Adult respiratory distress syndrome (ARDS): characterized by the presence of pulmonary oedema and hypoxia without underlying cardiac disease.
2. Disseminated intravascular coagulation (DIC): disruption of the normal coagulation process such that diffuse blood coagulation in capillaries results in a

widespread deficiency of clotting factors and, para-doxically, bleeding throughout the vascular system.

3. Acute renal failure (ARF: acute tubular or renocortical necrosis may occur secondary to hypoperfusion and will contribute to acid–base and fluid and electrolyte disturbances.

These syndromes contribute to the overall multisystem affects of shock.

ASSESSMENT

Patients experiencing the complications of shock will exhibit characteristics with which every nurse should be familiar. Nursing recognition of early signs and symptoms of impending shock can be pivotal in the prompt initiation of treatment and in averting serious complications. Assessment should begin with a review of the patient's health history, which may hold clues to the source of the problem. Table 12.2 outlines some conditions and associated factors that place patients at risk for development of shock.

Once the health history has been obtained and the risk factors have been identified, physical assessment should follow. Physical signs and symptoms of shock are those consistent with decreased organ perfusion.

TISSUE PERFUSION

Decreased tissue perfusion in the cardiovascular system is manifested by the following symptoms:

- Increased pulse rate, possibly irregular cardiac rhythm
- Decreased blood pressure (late)
- Cool, moist skin
- Mottled, pale or cyanotic colour.

The nurse at the bedside is most likely to recognize the rapid pulse and decreasing blood pressure as significant problems. As discussed earlier, however, the activation of sympathetic responses will result in maintenance of a normal blood pressure during the early phases of shock. When vasoconstrictive mechanisms are activated, cool, mottled or pale, moist skin is likely to be seen.

Remember that in septic shock, the picture may be one of a flushed, warm appearance. The presence of an elevated temperature should help to clarify this seeming ambiguity in findings. The routine recording of vital signs can show trends that should trigger the nurse's suspicion and encourage more frequent observation of the patient. For example, if on making rounds a patient is found to have a pulse rate of 95 per minute when 3 hours before the pulse was 70, it would be prudent to carry out a thorough assessment.

LEVEL OF CONSCIOUSNESS

Decreased perfusion of the nervous system is manifested as:

- Thirst
- Restlessness
- Anxiety
- Confusion
- Lethargy
- Unconsciousness.

Table 12.2 Patients at risk for development of shock.

Type of shock	Contributing factors
Hypovolaemic shock Haemorrhage	• Blood loss internally, e.g. gastrointestinal bleeding • Blood loss externally, e.g. post-partum bleeding
Dehydration	• May result from fluid and electrolyte or endocrine disturbances, e.g. vomiting, diarrhoea, diabetes mellitus
Third space loss	• Plasma lost as a result of injury to the cellular membranes, e.g. burns, oedema due to sepsis
Cardiogenic shock Pump failure	• Acute myocardial infarction, often associated with loss of ventricular wall function • Cardiac tamponade and mediastinal shift resulting in obstruction of pump function
Septic shock	Impaired immune status related to: • Age: under 1 year or over 65 years • Chemotherapy • Steroid therapy • Chronic health problems (diabetes, AIDS, liver disease, renal disease) • Bone marrow suppression Invasive procedures: • Parenteral therapy • Blood transfusion, total parenteral nutrition • Drug abuse • Abortion • Catheters: urinary, venous • Incision and drainage procedures • Delivery: risk for mother and infant

It should be noted that this list represents a continuum of symptoms. The patient may experience feelings of impending doom. It is at this point that the patient may require a creative and challenging approach to nursing management. The restlessness and agitation may make it difficult for the nurse to distinguish physiological signs that point to organic illness. In elderly patients particularly, confusion may be taken as 'normal' for that individual. In such circumstances, it is easy to overlook other signs that indicate that an acute problem exists.

Tachycardia may be attributed to restlessness rather than to a compensatory mechanism. It is always important to investigate the causes of restlessness or anxiety. If the change in the person's mental status is related to the development of shock, it will progress from a raised level of consciousness to one of diminishing response. This change represents an alteration in the amount of oxygen available to the brain. As mentioned earlier, compensatory mechanisms will maintain flow to the brain at the expense of other organs. Decreasing levels of consciousness represent a significant failure of compensation and must therefore be acted upon promptly.

GAS EXCHANGE

Respiratory signs and symptoms of shock include:

- Gasping respirations
- Increased rate and depth of respirations
- Cyanosis
- Depressed respirations (shallow, irregular)
- Changes in auscultatory findings (increased crackles and diminished breath sounds).

Efforts to obtain sufficient oxygen will cause the patient in shock to increase the rate and depth of respiration. Gasping can also signify 'air hunger'. Cyanosis is a late sign of inadequate tissue perfusion. If blood gases are drawn, one is most likely to see a low PO_2 with a correspondingly low oxygen saturation. An oxygen saturation of less than 90% indicates a very significant state of hypoxia. As shock progresses, changes in alveolar capillary membrane permeability may manifest as pulmonary oedema. In septic shock, pulmonary oedema may not be seen until 36–48 hours after the event that initiated the shock. In cardiogenic shock, pulmonary oedema may be an early sign of pump failure. Neurogenic shock can precipitate profuse, rapidly developing pulmonary oedema.

GASTROINTESTINAL FUNCTION

The most common symptoms of shock in the gastrointestinal system are reflections of decreased gastrointestinal motility due to the sympathetic response. They include:

- Nausea
- Vomiting
- Abdominal distention
- Decreased or absent bowel sounds.

Haematemesis and melaena will be associated with gastrointestinal haemorrhage, causing hypovolaemic shock. These symptoms may also appear in septic shock as a result of damage to mucous membranes caused by vasoconstriction and invading organisms.

PATTERNS OF ELIMINATION

As cardiac output falls renal perfusion and therefore glomerular filtration decreases, resulting in a urinary output of less than the normal 30 ml/h. Monitoring urinary output is most accurately done by using an indwelling urinary catheter. This enables the nurse to take hourly measurements. If the patient has no catheter and has not voided for several hours or voids dark concentrated urine, the nurse should assume that renal perfusion is inadequate if there is no evidence of urinary retention such as a palpable bladder.

The signs and symptoms of shock associated with dysfunction in each body system will vary as shock progresses from a potential to an actual and worsening problem. Table 12.3 summarizes patient parameters in early, mid, and late stages of shock.

Clinical Diagnostic Measurements

LABORATORY TESTS

Once the patient's clinical condition has been assessed, other, more technical, data should be obtained from the laboratory. Nurses should have a working knowledge of the common laboratory tests that can aid with the assessment of shock.

- Complete blood count: haemoglobin, haematocrit, white blood cell count, platelets
- Biochemistry: serum electrolytes, blood urea nitrogen, creatinine, lactate, glucose
- Blood cultures
- Electrocardiogram (ECG)
- Arterial blood gas measurements.

Table 12.4 indicates the changes in the biochemistry of the blood that might be expected in shock.

HAEMODYNAMIC MONITORING

Once an initial assessment has been made, other monitoring devices may be introduced to provide further information about the patient's status and progress. These include:

- Central venous pressure (CVP)
- Pulmonary artery pressure (PAP)
- Pulmonary artery wedge pressure (PAWP).

These three measurements will reflect the fluid volume status of the patient and help to determine whether the shock is of cardiac or non-cardiac origin. A low central venous, pulmonary artery, or wedge pressure is commonly found in hypovolaemic or septic shock. These pressures are likely to be elevated in cardiogenic shock. Measurement of pulmonary artery and wedge pressures requires the use of a pulmonary artery catheter and advanced haemodynamic monitoring equipment and is therefore confined to intensive care situations. Central venous pressure, however, can be monitored via a catheter inserted into a large central vein. Its use is, therefore, more common and practical on a general nursing unit. Normal CVP is 0–7 mmHg or 6–12 cmH$_2$O. CVP can supply the nurse with valuable information regarding volume status before the patient develops overt clinical signs.

Table 12.3 Assessment of the patient in shock.

	Non-progressive or compensated stage	Progessive stage	Irreversible or refractory stage
Subjective data	Restlessness, apprehension and anxiety Nausea Thirst	Listlessness or apathy Anorexia Confusion	Non-responsive
Objective data Skin and mucous membrane	Ashen, pale, cold, moist and clammy Mouth dry	Cyanotic, moist and clammy Mouth dry	Cyanotic, cold and clammy Jaundice, petechiae and bleeding from mucous membranes and lesions
Cardiovascular	Pulse rapid and thready ↑ Heart rate Blood pressure normal	Pulse weak, rapid and thready ↑ Heart rate Cardiac arrhythmias ↓ Blood pressure ↑ Pulse pressure	Pulse slow, irregular or imperceptible Cardiac arrhythmias ↓ Blood pressure: diastolic may be difficult to obtain
Respiratory	↑ Respiratory rate and depth	↑ Respiratory rate Shallow respirations	Respirations slow, shallow and irregular Crackles and wheezes heard
Temperature	↓ Body temperature or ↑ Body temperature (septic and toxic shock)	↓ Body temperature	↓ Body temperature
Urinary	↓ Urinary output	↓ Urinary output	↓ Urinary output or no urine output
Gastrointestinal	↓ Bowel sounds	↓ Bowel sounds or absent Haematemesis, melaena	Bowel sounds decreased or absent Abdominal distension Haematemesis, melaena
Level of consciousness	Confused as to time, place and person Judgement impaired	Confused or inappropriate verbal responses Flexion, extension, or no response to painful stimuli	Absence of verbal and motor responses to noxious stimuli

NURSING INTERVENTION FOR THE PERSON IN OR AT RISK OF DEVELOPING SHOCK

Once the clinical assessment has been made, the nurse must be prepared to intervene and prevent further deterioration. Primary responsibilities include patient assessment and monitoring the effects of interventions.

Patient Problems Associated with the Shock Syndrome

1. Altered tissue perfusion
2. Impaired oxygen and carbon dioxide exchange

3. Altered level of consciousness
4. Alteration in comfort
5. Impaired physical mobility
6. Altered nutritional needs
7. Alteration in patient and family relationships.

The basic goals are the maintenance and/or restoration of adequate tissue perfusion and homeostasis.

Goals

1. The circulating fluid volume will return to normal as indicated by the following:
   (a) Arterial blood pressure within 20 mmHg of preshock level.

Table 12.4   Summary of laboratory data in shock.

Laboratory test	Normal values	Changes in shock	Causative factors
Arterial blood gases			
pH	7.35–7.45	Elevated (compensatory) Decreased (progressive shock)	Respiratory alkalosis with hyperventilation Depressed respirations Metabolic acidosis
Pao_2	11–13 kPa (80–100 mmHg)	Elevated (compensatory) Decreased (progressive shock)	Hyperventilation Hypoventilation Ventilation–perfusion imbalance
$Paco_2$	4.8–6.0 kPa (35–40 mmHg)	Decreased (compensatory) Elevated (progressive shock)	Hyperventilation Hypoventilation
Biochemical levels			
Serum lactate	0.5–2.0 mmol/l	Elevated (progressive shock)	Tissue hypoxia, acidosis
Sodium	135–145 mmol/l	Elevated (compensatory) Elevated or decreased (progressive shock)	Decreased renal excretion Altered renal perfusion
Chloride	100–106 mmol/l	Decreased (compensatory) Elevated (progressive shock)	Alkalosis Acidosis
Potassium	3.5–5.5 mmol/l	Decreased (compensatory) Elevated (progressive shock)	Increased renal excretion Acidosis Decreased renal excretion
Calcium	2.2–2.6 mmol/l	Decreased (progressive shock)	Renal failure
Glucose	3.9–6.1 mmol/l	Elevated (compensatory) Decreased (progressive shock)	Sympathetic activity Depletion of glycogen stores Impaired liver function
Total serum protein albumin	60–80 g/l 40–50 gl	Decreased (progressive shock)	Leakage through capillaries
Blood urea	2.9–8.9 mmol/l	Elevated (progressive shock)	Decreased renal excretion
Creatinine	60–120 µmol/l	Elevated (progressive shock)	Decreased renal excretion
Haematology			
Haemoglobin	Males: 13–18 g/dl Females: 12–15 g/dl	Decreased	Blood loss
Haematocrit	Males: 40–50% Females: 37–47%	Increased	Fluid volume (loss) Plasma loss (burns)
White blood cell count	$4.0–11.0 \times 10^9$ per litre	Increased	Infection
Platelet count	$150–400 \times 10^9$ per litre	Decreased (progressive and irreversible shock)	Clotting disturbances
Prothrombin time (PT)	11–15 s	Prolonged (progressive and irreversible shock)	Clotting disturbances
Partial thromboplastin	60–70 s	Prolonged (progressive and irreversible shock)	Clotting disturbances

(b) Central venous pressure of 10–12 cmH$_2$O (0–4 mmHg).
(c) Pulmonary artery pressure of 10–20 mmHg.
(d) Pulmonary artery wedge pressure of 10–12 mmHg.
2. Urinary output will be greater than 30 ml/h.
3. Serum electrolytes will be within the normal range:

Sodium	135–145 mmol/l
Chloride	100–106 mmol/l
Potassium	3.5–5.5 mmol/l
Calcium	2.2–2.6 mmol/l
Phosphate	0.8–1.5 mmol/l
Magnesium	0.8–1.3 mmol/l
Glucose	3.9–6.1 mmol/l (fasting: 2.5–5.6 mmol/l).

4. Cardiac output will return to preshock level:
(a) Heart rate is ± 10 of the preshock rate.
(b) Heart rhythm is regular.
5. Blood gases will be within the normal range: Pao_2, 11–13 kPa; $Paco_2$, 4.8–6.0 kPa (35–40 mmHg).
6. Respiratory function will return to normal:
(a) Respiratory rate will be 16–22 per minute and regular.
(b) Lungs will be free of crackles or wheezes on auscultation.
7. Metabolic needs will be decreased as evidenced by:
(a) The patient will be able to rest and sleep.
(b) The body temperature will be normal (37°C).
(c) The patient will be comfortable and free of pain.
(d) The patient will be less anxious.
8. Acid–base balance will be restored:
pH 7.35–7.45
[H$^+$] 35–45 nmol/l
HCO$_3^-$ 24–28 mmol/l
Serum lactate 0.5–2.0 mmol/l.
9. Blood urea and creatinine levels will be normal: Blood urea, 2.9–8.9 mmol/l; creatinine, 100–120 mmol/l.
10. The patient will be alert and conscious:
(a) Eyes open spontaneously
(b) Verbal responses show orientation to time, place and person.
(c) Motor responses are coordinated and appropriate to command.
11. The skin will be warm, dry and normal in colour.
12. Complications from immobility will be absent:
(a) The skin is dry and intact.
(b) The limbs are free of contractures.
13. The patient and family will understand the reason for constant monitoring and therapeutic interventions.

ALTERED TISSUE PERFUSION

Alteration in tissue perfusion constitutes the major difficulty in shock. Tissue perfusion is compromised as a result of changes in the amount of blood flow reaching the periphery and because of changes occurring within the vascular structures that limit flow. Nursing intervention must therefore be aimed at the causes of poor perfusion. If the cardiac pump is the source of the failure, interventions will be aimed at improving pump

Table 12.5 Immediate nursing interventions for the person with diminished tissue perfusion (shock).

1. Stay with patient.
2. Assess level of consciousness.
3. Ensure adequate airway.
4. Apply pressure to bleeding sites.
5. Place patient with legs elevated above level of heart.
6. Assess vital signs: pulse, respirations, blood pressure.
7. Inform physician of unusual findings.
8. Prepare for fluid resuscitation.
9. Administer oxygen.

activity. If the volume of blood is inadequate, then replacement will be the priority. Similarly, if a vascular mechanism is the cause of limited flow, then interventions should be aimed at either dilating or constricting vessels to maximize perfusion.

Table 12.5 lists the immediate actions that a nurse should take when diminished perfusion manifests. These actions will promote perfusion of vital organs to protect the patient while other interventions are planned and instituted.

NURSING INTERVENTIONS IN THE EVENT OF SHOCK (DECREASED TISSUE PERFUSION)

1. Monitor circulatory status:
(a) Assess pulse rate and blood pressure every 15 minutes if necessary. Check for regularity of pulse.
(b) Report blood pressure <100 mmHg systolic. Consider elevating lower limbs to increase venous return.
(c) Check skin for cold, clammy feeling.
(d) Administer i.v. fluids as prescribed and maintain fluid balance chart.
(e) Take steps to control external haemorrhage by direct pressure over wound.
(f) Report urine output <30 ml/hour. In the event of cardiogenic shock the following extra interventions would also be necessary.
2. Administer and monitor effects of vasoactive medications/cardiac glycosides:
(a) Familiarize self with actions, side-effects of medications such as digitalis, β-blockers, calcium channel blockers, inotropes, vasodilators, diuretics.
(b) Note effectiveness of drug action.
(c) Assess for potential venous access problems, e.g. infiltration.
3. Minimize work load of the heart:
(a) Plan for sufficient rest periods for the patient.
(b) Group nursing tasks to accomplish care without tiring the patient.
(c) Provide explanations to patient and family to minimize anxiety.

ALTERATION IN OXYGEN AND CARBON DIOXIDE EXCHANGE RELATED TO VENTILATION IMPAIRMENT

1. Take measures to prevent impairment of gas exchange in all patients (see Chapter 15):
   (a) Turn and reposition at least every 2 hours.
   (b) Encourage deep breathing and coughing every 1–2 hours in any patient who is immobile, postoperative or at risk of developing atelectasis or pneumonia.
2. Monitor for signs of impaired gas exchange:
   (a) Note use of accessory muscles, tachypnoea (respiratory rate > 30), shallow respirations.
   (b) Assess level of consciousness hourly. Be aware that anxiety, confusion and restlessness may indicate poor gas exchange.
3. Ensure patent airway:
   (a) Suction if patient is unable to clear secretions.
   (b) If patient is unconscious, use head tilt, chin-lift manoeuvre or jaw thrust. Consider insertion of oral or nasopharyngeal airway. Nurse on the side.
4. Administer oxygen:
   (a) Provide oxygen at ordered level.
   (b) Continue to monitor assessment parameters, paying particular attention to levels of oxygenation.

ALTERED LEVEL OF CONSCIOUSNESS RELATED TO DIMINISHED PERFUSION OF THE CENTRAL NERVOUS SYSTEM

1. Assess for signs of altered level of consciousness (see Chapter 21):
   (a) Assess responsiveness and compare with normal level for that patient.
   (b) Question patient regarding orientation to person, place and time.
   (c) Note increasing restlessness, agitation, anxiety, confusion.
2. Protect patient with altered level of consciousness from injury:
   (a) Provide reassurance through speech, touch, reorientation.
   (b) Use padding to protect patient from injury from bed rails.
   (c) Stay with the patient.
   (d) Use sedation and analgesia to control agitation and pain. Note effects of medication on level of consciousness and vital signs.
3. Ensure patency of airway.

ALTERATION IN COMFORT RELATED TO PAIN, IMMOBILITY, ANXIETY

1. Administer analgesics and sedatives:
   (a) Assess levels of pain on scale of 1–5.
   (b) Note effectiveness of medication in diminishing pain or anxiety.
2. Provide physical comfort measures (see Chapter 9):
   (a) Turn and position patient every 2 hours if tolerated.
   (b) Provide hygiene measures.

ALTERATION IN MOBILITY RELATED TO DIMINISHED CARDIAC OUTPUT AND POTENTIALLY LIFE-THREATENING CONDITION

1. Provide skin care measures:
   (a) Turn and position at least every 2 hours, if tolerated.
   (b) Check for reddened areas over pressure points and attempt to reposition patient so that pressure is redistributed away from those areas.
   (c) Consider use of pressure relieving devices, e.g. ripple mattress.
2. Maintain joint and muscle mobility:
   (a) In consultation with physiotherapist, participate in range of motion exercises.
   (b) Encourage patient to assist in whatever activities can be tolerated.
   (c) Plan for increasing levels of activity as patient condition improves.

ALTERED NUTRITIONAL STATUS RELATED TO DECREASED PERFUSION OF GASTROINTESTINAL SYSTEM

1. Promote early reestablishment of nutritional intake by consulting with dietary/nutritional services to maximize intake of nutrients while maintaining fluid balance.
2. Consider placement of nasogastric tube to decrease abdominal distinction/discomfort/vomiting.

ALTERATION IN PATIENT AND FAMILY RELATIONSHIPS

1. Explain interventions to patient and family prior to implementing.
2. Communicate with patient verbally and through touch.
3. Provide reassurance and support to patient and family.
4. Ensure consistent communication between health care professionals and patient and family.
5. Allow family participation in patient care as much as possible.

EVALUATION

The efficacy of immediate nursing intervention should be evaluated by changes in the patient's condition occurring within a short time following the intervention. Immediate actions are taken to restore as great a level of perfusion as possible to prevent irreversible complications and to provide adequate cerebral perfusion. These early measures can be life saving. Achievement of the goals would be assessed by comparing the patient response to the outcome criteria. After the initial goals have been achieved, further measures are instituted to alleviate the underlying cause of shock and to reestablish perfusion to the less vital organs.

SUMMARY

Shock is a devastating cycle of compensation/decompensation that may progress to an irreversible state wherein death may occur in an otherwise healthy individual. It is the responsibility of every nurse to be aware of the factors that may precipitate shock, to anticipate the development of shock and to take measures to prevent and treat this syndrome in its early phases. The nurse as the first responder can provide support to the vital functions and provide a basis from which more advanced measures can be taken. Although complex biochemical and haemodynamic monitoring is often only available after transfer to the intensive care unit, much of the initial resuscitation must occur on the primary nursing unit. Rapid assessment and the ability to put problems in order of priority, communicate findings and institute emergency interventions remain the key components of an appropriate response to shock.

This chapter does not explore the impact of an episode of shock on the patient and family. The reader is referred to Chapter 5 for a discussion of the responses of the individual and family to illness. The clinical situations given below are presented to illustrate the application of the assessment and therapeutic measures described in this chapter and to provide some insight into the possible impact of the situation on the person and family.

LEARNING ACTIVITIES

Using the information in this chapter and in the following clinical situations, formulate a nursing plan of action. For each situation, consider the following:

1. What data indicates that the patient may be at risk of developing shock?
2. What are the potential and actual patient problems in order of priority?
3. What nursing interventions would you initiate first?
4. What type of shock is the most likely cause of the patient's symptoms?
5. What secondary nursing measures might be implemented. What medical measures might be anticipated?
6. How would you evaluate the outcome of your nursing interventions?
7. What nursing strategies would you consider implementing to identify and to alleviate the patient's and family's anxieties?

CLINICAL SITUATION—1

Mrs D. Rideout is a 52-year old woman admitted to hospital for removal of a large intestinal mass. Her previous medical history is unremarkable. A bowel resection is required to remove the large tumour. On arrival in the recovery room, the patient is lethargic but rousable. Her skin is pale and cool to touch. The abdominal dressing is dry. When awake, Mrs Rideout complains of abdominal pain and extreme thirst. A urinary catheter inserted preoperatively reveals an hourly urinary output of 20 ml/hour for the past 2 hours. Mrs Rideout's vital signs are:

- Temperature: 35.8°C (rectally)
- Pulse: 118 beats per minute
- Respirations: 22 per minute
- BP: 96/60 (preoperatively: 136/90).

The anaesthetic record does not indicate blood loss. Intraoperative fluid replacement is recorded as 2 litres of Ringer's lactate.

Mrs Rideout's husband and son are in the waiting room anxious for information about her and the outcome of the surgery.

CLINICAL SITUATION—2

Mr Omer Heart was admitted 3 days ago to a general medical unit for investigations related to his diabetes. One evening, he awakes and complains of severe chest pain. He is pale, diaphoretic, anxious and dyspnoeic. He has a previous history of myocardial infarction and hypertension. On assessment, his vital signs are:

- Temperature: 36°C
- Pulse: 120 beats per minute
- BP: 100/70.

Twenty minutes later, his level of consciousness deteriorates. His blood pressure drops to 80/50 and pulse rate increases to 150/minute.

CLINICAL SITUATION—3

Neil Young is an 18-year-old motor cyclist brought to the Accident and Emergency Department after colliding with a tree at 7.45 am. He is alert and orientated, though very distressed. His left thigh is tense and swollen and there is bruising over the left side of his abdomen, which is very tender. His leg is causing him severe pain, which was particularly marked when he was transferred from ambulance to trolley. Clinically he probably has a fractured left shaft of femur (see p. 877). Initial vital signs are:

- Pulse: 100 beats per minute
- Respirations: 22 per minute
- BP: 125/80.

REFERENCES AND FURTHER READING

Billings DM (ed.) Shock update. *Critical Care Nurse Quarterly* **11(1)**: 1–85.

Hinchcliffe S & Montague S (1988) *Physiology for Nursing Practice*. London: Baillière Tindall.

Holloway NM (1988) *Nursing the Critically Ill Adult* 3rd edn. Menlo Park PA: Addison-Wesley.

Holloway NM (1989) *Critical Care Plans*. Springhouse PA: Springhouse.

Rice V (1984) Clinical continuum of septic shock. *Critical Care Nurse* **4(5)**: 86–109.

Rice V (1984) Shock management: I. Fluid volume replacement. *Critical Care Nurse* **4(6)**: 69–82.

Rice V (1985) Shock management: II Pharmacologic intervention. *Critical Care Nurse* **5(1)**: 42–57.

Thelan LA, Davie JK & Urden LD (1990) *Textbook of Critical Care Nursing: Diagnosis and Management*. St Louis: Mosby.

Vander AJ, Sherman JH & Luciano DS (1990) *Human Physiology: The Mechanisms of Body Function* 5th edn, pp. 404–405. New York: McGraw-Hill.

Caring for the Patient with a Haematological Disorder

OBJECTIVES

On completion of this chapter, the reader will be able to:

- Describe the composition and functions of the blood
- Assess individuals for manifestations of erythrocyte disorders
- Plan, implement and evaluate nursing intervention for the person with erythrocyte disorders
- Assess individuals for manifestions of leucocyte disorders
- Appreciate the impact of malignant blood disorders on the individual and family
- Plan, implement and evaluate nursing intervention for the person with leucocyte disorders
- Assess individuals for manifestations of platelet disorders
- Describe first aid measures to control bleeding
- Plan, implement and evaluate nursing intervention for the individual with platelet disorders
- Recognize the patient and family as active participants in the control and management of the patient's blood disorder
- Safely administer blood and blood products to clients

COMPOSITION AND PHYSIOLOGY OF BLOOD

Blood is a red fluid tissue that is pumped through the vascular system by the heart. It transports cellular requirements and products from one part of the body to another. There is a continuous exchange between the fluid surrounding the cells (interstitial fluid) and the blood; this exchange serves to maintain a suitable cellular environment that varies only within narrow limits and is vital to the maintenance of homeostasis.

Blood is opaque; whole blood has a viscosity 3.5–5.4 times that of water, while plasma has a viscosity of 1.4–1.8 times that of water. Its colour is dependent on the pigment in the haemoglobin of the red blood cells and varies with the amount of oxygen combined with the haemoglobin. A higher concentration of oxygen produces a brighter red. Blood has a slightly alkaline reaction, with a pH of 7.35–7.45. The average volume in the adult is 5–6 litres, or approximately 70–75 ml/kg of body weight. The volume remains remarkably constant.

Functions of the Blood

The blood performs several important functions:

1. Transportation of oxygen from the lungs to the cells and carbon dixoide from the tissues to the lungs for excretion.
2. Transportation of absorbed nutrients from the alimentary tract to the cells.
3. Conveyance of metabolic wastes from the cells to the organs of excretion (kidneys, lungs, liver and skin).
4. Distribution of hormones, enzymes and other endogenous chemicals that regulate many body activities.
5. Exchange of heat between body tissues and the surface of the body.
6. Protection of the individual against excessive loss of blood by coagulation and against injurious agents, such as bacteria, viruses and toxins, by its leucocytes and antibodies.
7. Maintenance of fluid, electrolyte and acid–base balance (see Chapter 7).

Blood Components

Fifty-five to sixty per cent of the blood is a straw-coloured fluid called plasma, in which the formed elements of the blood (blood cells and platelets) are suspended (Figure 13.1).

PLASMA

COMPOSITION

The constituents of plasma are water (90–91%) and a wide variety of solutes. The latter include all the substances which cells take in and use, as well as many substances produced by the cells. Examples are the organic solutes which include the plasma proteins, the most abundant solutes (albumin, globulins and fibrinogen); the nutrients (amino acids, glucose and lipids); metabolic end-products; and the inorganic solutes of mineral electrolytes and salts. In addition, there are anticoagulants, clotting factors and antibodies.

The concentration of the solutes remains relatively

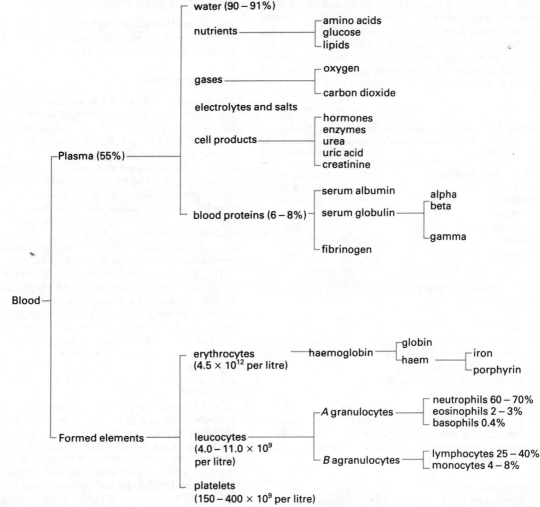

Figure 13.1 Composition of blood.

constant even though water and solutes are continually being added and removed. There are temporary variations but, under normal conditions, complex interactions and mechanisms function quickly to restore the plasma to normal. A good example of a quick readjustment that is made to preserve homeostasis is the maintenance of the plasma concentration of glucose between 3.9 and 6.1 mmol/l. Following a meal, the blood sugar becomes elevated but within 1–2 hours the level returns to normal. Liver cells remove excess glucose, converting it to glycogen and storing it, while insulin stimulates facilitated diffusion of glucose into all the body cells, except the brain, where it is oxidized to produce energy. Conversely if blood glucose levels are falling, glycogen is converted to glucose in the storage depots and released into the blood to maintain a normal plasma concentration.

BLOOD PROTEINS

Three types of proteins comprise the greater part of the solutes of the plasma. These are referred to as the plasma or blood proteins and are *serum albumin*, *serum globulin* and *fibrinogen*. The normal concentration of the plasma proteins is about 60–80 g/l. They are large in molecular structure and do not readily diffuse through the capillary walls. The resulting concentration of these non-diffusible substances within the capillaries is responsible for what is referred to as the colloid osmotic pressure or oncotic pressure of the plasma. A pressure gradient results between the tissue fluid and the blood that promotes the movement of the fluid from the interstitial spaces back into the capillaries (see Chapter 14). An abnormal decrease in the plasma proteins, especially albumin, due to excessive loss or diminished production, reduces the oncotic pressure, resulting in an accumulation of fluid in the tissues known as oedema. The proteins contribute to the viscosity of the blood, which influences circulation.

The plasma proteins are formed from the amino acids of ingested foods but in protein starvation they may be synthesized from tissue protein. Serum albumin and fibrinogen are formed by the liver.

α-Globulins and β-globulins are made by hepatic

cells, while the γ-globulins are produced by B lymphocytes and plasma cells in lymphatic tissues (spleen, lymph nodes, liver and bone marrow). The γ-globulin fraction contains antibodies. For this reason it may be administered to provide a temporary immunity against measles or other infections. (See Table 13.1 for normal blood protein values.)

Table 13.1 Normal values of the plasma proteins.

Plasma protein	Concentration (g/l)
Total plasma proteins	60–80
Albumin	40–50
Globulins	20–30
α globulin	4.6
β globulin	8.6
γ globulin	7.5
Fibrinogen	3.0

In summary, the functions of the plasma proteins are as follows:

Albumin
- Albumin exerts an intravascular oncotic pressure that influences fluid exchange between the interstitial and intravascular compartments.
- Albumin increases blood viscosity.

γ-Globulin
- γ-Globulin contributes to the immune response. It is the antibody fraction of the blood which binds to antigenic material, and inactivates microbial agents and toxins.

Fibrinogen
- Fibrinogen plays a role in blood coagulation which protects the individual from an excessive loss of blood.
- At the site of inflammation or injury, fibrinogen forms an insoluble mesh in which the various tissues can grow and repair themselves.

General
- Plasma proteins will combine with both alkalis and acids and can act as buffers to maintain a normal pH of body fluids. They may accept hydrogen ions from acids or, when necessary, donate hydrogen ions to reduce excessive alkalinity.
- The proteins bind some substances such as hormones, enzymes, lipids, fat-soluble vitamins and essential ions during their transport in the blood. This prevents too rapid escape of these substances by filtration in the renal glomeruli.
- Many exogenous substances are also bound to plasma proteins. Drugs bound in this way (e.g. warfarin) may be biologically inactive until the protein reservoir is saturated or until they are displaced by a more strongly bound substance.
- Amongst the plasma proteins are a group known collectively as the complement system. These enhance the inflammatory and immune responses.

FORMED ELEMENTS OF THE BLOOD

The formed elements include the *red blood cells* (erythrocytes), the *white blood cells* (leucocytes) and the *blood platelets* (thrombocytes).

ERYTHROCYTES

The normal red blood cell is an elastic biconcave disc. The approximate number of erythrocytes contained in the blood is $4.5–6.3 \times 10^{12}$ per litre in the adult male and $4.2–5.5 \times 10^{12}$ per litre in the adult female. The volume percentage of erythrocytes in whole blood is 45–50, and is expressed as the packed cell volume (PCV) or haematocrit. (The packed cell volume percentage of erythrocytes is determined by centrifuging a blood sample, which separates the cells from the plasma. Erythrocytes normally occupy 45–50% and the plasma 55–60% of the volume of the blood.) Each cell has a nucleus when first formed, but the normal mature circulating erythrocyte is devoid of a nucleus.

The *function* of red blood cells, by virtue of their composition, is the transportation of oxygen and carbon dioxide between the tissue cells and the lungs. The major constituent of the cell is *haemoglobin*, which is made up of the protein globin and an iron-containing pigment called haem. Haem is formed by the union of iron and the pigment porphyrin; each haem group combines with a polypeptide chain, the globin portion, and four of these units bind loosely together to make up the complex haemoglobin molecule. Oxygen has an affinity for this compound; four molecules of oxygen combine with one molecule of haemoglobin to form *oxyhaemoglobin*. Approximately 1 g of haemoglobin combines with 1.34–1.36 ml of oxygen. There is a loose combination, so when there is little or no free oxygen in the red cells' environment (plasma), oxygen is freed from the red blood cell and diffuses out of the cell into the plasma, leaving what is known as *deoxyhaemoglobin*.

Some of the carbon dioxide in the blood (approximately 27%) is carried by the red blood cells in the form of the compound carbaminohaemoglobin. When the haemoglobin takes on oxygen in the lungs, the carbon dioxide is released into the plasma and then diffuses into the alveoli.

Haemoglobin is produced by the red blood cells themselves before they are released into the circulation from their site of production, the red bone marrow. Because of its pigment content, haemoglobin gives the red colour to the blood. The *normal concentration of haemoglobin* is 14.0–18.0 g/dl in men and 12.0–16.0 g/dl in women.

Production of erythrocytes (erythropoiesis)
After birth, erythrocytes are produced exclusively by the red bone marrow. In the developing fetus they are produced by the yolk sac until the 11th week and then by the liver, and to a lesser extent the spleen, kidney, lymph nodes and thymus. The liver is the major site from the 9th to the 24th weeks. During the remaining months the red bone marrow develops and gradually takes over the role. During infancy and childhood most of the bones contain red bone marrow that participates in erythropoiesis. (*Poiesis* is the Greek word meaning

Table 13.2 Production of erythrocytes.

Stages of development	Description
Proerythroblast/pronormoblast ↓	A nucleated cell with no haemoglobin that divides into two smaller nucleated cells
Basophilic normoblast (early) ↓	A large nucleated cell with no haemoglobin that divides into two cells. The nucleus is smaller than it was in the previous stages and the cytoplasm is more abundant
Polychromatophilic normoblast (intermediate) ↓	A nucleated cell that divides. The nucleus becomes smaller and more dense and a small amount of haemoglobin appears
Orthochromatic normoblast (late) ↓	A cell in which the nucleus becomes compressed and eventually is ejected from the cell; the haemoglobin content of the cytoplasm increases. No cell division
Reticulocyte ↓	A non-nucleated cell with an increasing amount of haemoglobin. The cytoplasm has a reticular network. Reticulocytes mature to red blood cells over 2–4 days. Some maturation takes place in the bone marrow, some after release during sequestration in the spleen
Erythrocyte	The mature red blood cell from which the nuclear remnants have disappeared. It is almost completely filled with haemoglobin

From Hoffbrand and Pettit (1984).

formation or production.) When the growth process is completed, the red blood cells are produced by the red bone marrow of the cancellous (spongy) tissue of the skull bones, vertebrae, ribs, sternum, pelvis and proximal ends of the femora and humeri.

The red blood cells, the white blood cells produced by the marrow, and the platelets (thrombocytes) develop from common primitive stem cells which differentiate to become either red or white blood cells, or platelets. In erythropoiesis, the proerythroblast goes through a series of nuclear and cytoplasmic changes, becoming progressively smaller. These changes are outlined in Table 13.2 and compose what is referred to as the maturation process of red blood cells.

Regulation of erythropoiesis

Under normal conditions the rate of production and maturation of red blood cells approximates the rate of removal of the old cells from the circulation and their destruction. The red blood cell count and the amount of haemoglobin remain relatively constant, sufficient to meet the tissues' oxygen needs but, at the same time, controlled in order to prevent a concentration of cells that would impede the blood flow.

The oxygen concentration of the blood is the essential factor in the regulation of the production of erythrocytes. If the rate of cell destruction is increased or if there is a loss of red blood cells, as in haemorrhage, the concomitant decrease in the oxygen level brings about a prompt increase in erythropoiesis if the bone marrow is normal and the essential substances are available. At high altitudes where the oxygen concentration of the air is low, the body compensates by producing more red blood cells.

The red bone marrow does not respond directly to the hypoxaemia (lowered concentration of oxygen in the blood). The stimulation is brought about by a hormone called *erythropoietin*, or *haemopoietin*, which is produced in response to the hypoxaemia. Most of the erythropoietin is produced by the kidneys and to a lesser extent the liver. It is secreted in response to a decrease in tissue oxygen.

Erythropoietin stimulates primitive stem cells to differentiate along erythroid lines.

Protein, iron, vitamin B_{12} (cyanocobalamin), folic acid (pteroylglutamic acid, a member of the vitamin B complex), vitamin C (which is necessary for the maintenance of folic acid reductase, an enzyme necessary to keep folic acid in its active form) must be available to the bone marrow to ensure an adequate production of normal erythrocytes. *Protein* is a necessary element in the structure of the cell and its haemoglobin. *Iron* is essential for the formation of haemoglobin. Only a limited amount of iron is absorbed from the small intestine; it is then loosely combined with transferrin to be transported in the blood plasma. Excess iron is deposited in the liver and other cells where it combines with a protein (apoferritin) to form ferritin, which is referred to as storage iron. Ferritin occurs in the spleen, bone marrow, kidney, heart, pancreas, intestine and placenta. It is released as iron is needed by the bone marrow. Much of the iron used in the formation of haemoglobin is derived from the breakdown of worn-out erythrocytes. Only a small amount of dietary iron is necessary to maintain that required under normal circumstances. When transferrin and apoferritin are saturated, absorption of iron by the small intestine is inhibited. If erythropoiesis is increased, as it is in haemorrhage, pregnancy or other conditions causing hypoxaemia, more iron is absorbed. In persons who have a normal haemoglobin concentration and a normal amount of iron in storage, extra dietary iron and medicinal iron preparations do not increase the absorption; the excess iron is simply eliminated in the faeces. With increased demands on the bone marrow, the iron stored in the intestinal mucosa and liver is reduced and absorption by the intestine is increased accordingly.

Vitamin B_{12}, which is referred to as the *extrinsic factor* or *antianaemic factor*, is essential to normal erythropoiesis. It acts as a catalyst, promoting the synthesis of nucleic acids to form normal red blood cells. The extrinsic factor is especially abundant in liver

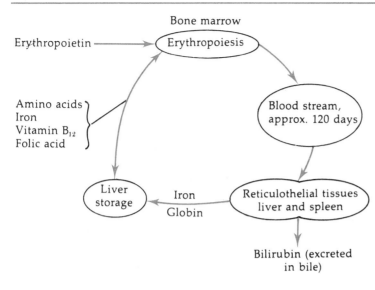

Figure 13.2 Life cycle of erythrocytes.

and red meats and is only absorbed in the presence of a factor or enzyme that is secreted by the gastric mucosa. This substance, essential for the absorption of vitamin B_{12}, is known as the intrinsic factor. The vitamin is then stored in the liver and released as it is needed. In the absence of either the extrinsic factor or the intrinsic factor, the number of erythrocytes is reduced, and many that are in circulation are abnormal.

Folic acid (pteroylglutamic acid), acting as a catalyst, also influences the production and maturation of erythroblasts and is sometimes used in the treatment of a deficiency of red blood cells (Bouchier et al, 1984). The richest dietary sources of this vitamin are liver, kidney and fresh green vegetables. Vitamin C is also needed to maintain the active form of folic acid.

Life span and normal destruction of erythrocytes

The average length of life of the red blood cells is 120 days (Guyton, 1991). The ageing process of the cells is not fully understood but enzyme systems degrade and cannot be replaced and the erythrocyte becomes fragile and less flexible. As they squeeze through the small capillaries the cells rupture. Haemoglobin is engulfed by macrophages, and the globin and iron fractions are reclaimed for use. The porphyrin molecules are converted to bilirubin and excreted in bile (Figure 13.2).

LEUCOCYTES

The white blood cells are less numerous and larger than the erythrocytes, and have nuclei. There are several types, which differ in structure, origin, function and staining reaction. Normally, the blood contains $4.0–11.0 \times 10^9$ per litre (4000–11 000 per µl). The count tends to be lower after a period of rest and increases following a meal or activity. There is a rapid increase to above normal in most infections in defence of the body.

Types of leucocyte

The leucocytes are divided into three types: granulocytes, lymphocytes and monocytes (Table 13.3).

Table 13.3 Types and normal values of leucocytes.*

Type	Percentage of total	Number ($\times 10^9$/l)
Granulocytes		
neutrophils	40–75	2.5–7.5
eosinophils	1–6	0.04–0.44
basophils	< 1	0.015–0.1
Lymphocytes	20–50	1.5–3.5
Monocytes	2–10	0.2–0.8

* The total leucocyte count is normally $4.0–11.0 \times 10^9$ per litre.

Granulocytes (polymorphonuclear leucocytes)
The granulocytes are formed in the red bone marrow and have lobulated nuclei. Three types are recognized by the staining quality of their cytoplasm: neutrophils, eosinophils and basophils.

1. *Neutrophils* stain with a neutral dye, and their nuclei may have several lobes. The latter characteristic results in the neutrophils also being called *polymorphonuclear* neutrophils. They may comprise 60–70% of the total white blood cells.
2. *Eosinophils* stain with eosin, a red acid dye, and normally constitute about 2–3% of the white blood cells.
3. *Basophils* stain with basic dyes and comprise about 0.4% of the total leucocytes.

Lymphocytes
The lymphocytes are smaller than the granulocytes and have a larger spherical nucleus that fills most of the cell. Lymphocytes are formed in the bone marrow. Some immature lymphocytes migrate to the thymus gland where they become immunocompetent and develop into T lymphocytes. Subsets of T cells exist, including helper, suppressor, cytotoxic and natural killer cells (see Chapter 6). B lymphocytes acquire immunocompetence

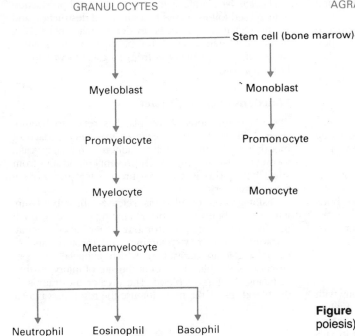

GRANULOCYTES   AGRANULOCYTES

Figure 13.3 Formation of white blood cells (leucopoiesis).

in the bone marrow. Mature lymphocytes circulate in the blood and become entrapped in lymphoid tissues. Of the total white blood cells, 25–40% are lymphocytes.

Monocytes
The monocytes are larger than the lymphocytes and have a kidney-shaped nucleus. They are produced in the red bone marrow. Ganong (1989) indicates that they circulate in the blood for 10–20 hours, and then enter the tissues and become macrophages. (*Macrophages* are large phagocytic cells that engulf and destroy microorganisms and foreign substances.) Monocytes make up about 4–8% of the total number of leucocytes.

Leucocyte count
When a white blood cell count is requested, an estimation is made of the total number of cells per litre. Frequently, a differential white cell count is done, since it is known that certain types of cells are increased in certain disease conditions. For example: in acute infections the neutrophils increase rapidly; in chronic infections, the lymphocytes are increased; the number of monocytes are increased in protozoal infections such as malaria; and the eosinophil count is known to rise in allergic reactions and with parasitic invasion of the body. In a differential count the percentage of the various types of leucocytes is determined.

The various types of white blood cells are produced by the stem cells in the blood cell-forming organs in three primitive forms: the myeloblasts, monoblasts and lymphoblasts (Figure 13.3). The *myeloblast*, which is produced by stem cells in the red bone marrow, is agranular and the nucleus is not divided into lobules. Successive changes occur and are characterized by the appearance of granules in the cytoplasm; the myeloblasts become promyelocytes, which change to myelo-

cytes. The latter differentiate to form neutrophils, eosinophils and basophils. Following this, nuclear changes develop, resulting in lobulation and the release of the cell into the blood.

The *monoblast* undergoes mitotic division to form the promonocyte. The cell remains large and agranular, but the nucleus changes, becoming oval and then kidney-shaped.

The *lymphoblast* goes through developmental phases comparable to the other leucocytes. The lymphoblast divides by mitosis and the cells progressively become condensed to form mature, small lymphocytes.

Factors in leucopoiesis

Little is known about the physiological stimulus responsible for the production and maturation of leucocytes. It has been observed that the breakdown of white blood cells is followed by the appearance of numerous young white blood cells in the blood. This suggests that a chemical which stimulates leucopoiesis may be released from the disintegrated cells.

Increased leucopoiesis occurs in infection, haemorrhage and tissue destruction. The nutrients, protein and vitamins which are essential to all cells of the body are necessary for the production of leucocytes. Some drugs may depress the production of leucocytes; for example, sulphonamides, gold and many cytotoxic drugs may result in a low white blood cell count.

Characteristics and functions of leucocytes

The leucocytes serve as an important body defence. They destroy many injurious substances such as microorganisms and the products of degenerating tissues. This is made possible by certain special properties the cells possess: diapedesis, mobility, chemotaxis and phagocytosis.

Diapedesis is the ability of the leucocytes to squeeze through the capillary walls and escape into the tissues. They are capable of amoeboid movement which takes them through the tissues to the source of irritation. (Amoeboid movement is achieved by the cell protruding a protoplasmic extension into which the remaining cell substance streams.) The neutrophils are especially mobile; they are attracted by a chemical substance which is liberated by bacteria or by the irritated tissue cells. This process of chemical attraction is known as chemotaxis.

Phagocytosis is the engulfing and digesting of particles and is the most important function of the neutrophils and monocytes in protecting the body against microorganisms.

The lymphocytes play an important role in immunity, discussed in Chapter 6.

Life span and destruction of leucocytes

The life span of the white blood cells varies greatly with the body's protective needs and with the types of white cells, ranging from a few hours to as long as several hundred days. Guyton (1991) suggests that granulocytes may circulate in the blood for 4–8 hours and survive in the tissues for 4–5 days. In the presence of an infection this life span may be reduced to a few hours. Monocytes spend 10–20 hours in the blood before migrating into the tissues, where they can exist for months as tissue macrophages. Lymphocytes circulate between the blood, the tissues and lymph and may survive for months or even years.

It is thought that the white blood cells that are destroyed or die are disposed of by phagocytosis by the macrophages of the reticuloendothelial tissues.

BLOOD PLATELETS (THROMBOCYTES)

The third and smallest of the formed elements of the blood are the platelets. They are oval, non-nucleated granular structures, numbering $150–400 \times 10^9$ per litre of blood (150 000–400 000 per µl). They are produced in the red bone marrow. The stem cells develop into giant cells called megakaryocytes which may extend parts of their membrane and cytoplasm; these separate from the parent cells to form the platelets. The cell contains important substances, including calcium, potassium, several clotting factors, serotonin, adrenaline, adenosine diphosphate (ADP) and enzymes. When an injury occurs to the wall of a blood vessel, platelets adhere to the injured area, especially where collagen is exposed. As they adhere, the platelets start swelling and their fragile membranes readily permit the escape of platelet content. It is suggested that chemicals released are responsible for the vasoconstriction that occurs at the site of injury. The substances released also cause nearby platelets to become sticky, resulting in more of them adhering to the original clump and contributing to the formation of a 'haemostatic plug'. The clotting factors released from the thrombocytes promote coagulation (Ganong, 1989).

Platelets have a life span of 8–12 days and production is increased following tissue trauma and destruction and in hypoxaemia. There is evidence that there is a humoral substance called thrombopoietin which affects the production of platelets from megakaryocytes in the bone marrow.

Functions of blood platelets

The major functions of the platelets relate to haemostasis. With any slight damage to the inner surface of blood vessels the platelets adhere and aggregate, forming a platelet plug which prevents blood loss from small holes. This is a normal process that occurs very frequently every day.

Disintegration of platelets releases thromboplastin, which contributes to the blood clotting process through the activation of prothrombin. They also liberate serotonin (5-hydroxytryptamine) and thromboxane A_2 (a prostaglandin derivative), which enhance vasoconstriction of the blood vessel at the site of injury, further reducing the loss of blood. The greater the trauma to the blood vessel, the more intense the resulting vascular spasm.

Blood Groups

Blood may differ from one individual to another according to the presence or absence of specific antigens (agglutinogens) on the surface of the red blood cells and the presence or absence of specific antibodies (agglutinins) in the plasma. For this reason, the blood of a person taken at random cannot be used in transfusion since the bloods might be of different types and could cause a serious reaction. The blood groups of greatest clinical significance are the ABO and Rh (Rhesus) types.

ABO BLOOD GROUPS

In the ABO system (Table 13.4) an individual's blood is typed as A, B, AB, or O, depending on the presence or absence of agglutinogens, termed A and B, on the erythrocytes. If a person has A or B or both A and B naturally occurring agglutinogens, the plasma will not contain antibodies that will agglutinate the individual's own erythrocytes. Type O is the most common blood type, occurring in 46% of the general population. Type A occurs in 42% of Caucasians. While the incidence of blood group antigens varies from race to race, types B and AB are found less frequently than types O and A.

In blood that is *typed as A*, the erythrocytes contain *agglutinogens A*. The plasma has anti-B agglutinins which only cause clumping of erythrocytes that have agglutinogens B. Blood that is *typed as B* has erythrocytes containing *agglutinogens B* and, in the plasma, *anti-A agglutinins*, which only cause clumping of red blood cells with agglutinogen A. In blood that is *typed as AB*, the erythrocytes bear both *agglutinogens A and AB*. The plasma is free of anti-A and anti-B agglutinins; otherwise, the individual's own red cells would be attacked. In blood that is typed as O, both agglutinogens are absent, but the plasma contains both anti-A and anti-

Table 13.4 ABO system.

Blood type	Agglutinogen in erythrocytes	Agglutinins in plasma	Plasma agglutinates erythrocytes of blood type:
A_1	A_1	Anti-B	B, A_1B and A_2B
A_2	A_2	Anti-B	B, A_1B and A_2B
B	B	Anti-A	A_1, A_2, A_1B and A_2B
A_1B	A_1B	None	None
A_2B	A_2B	None	None
O	None	Anti-A_1, anti-A_2 and anti-B	A_1, A_1B, A_2, A_2B and B

B agglutinins. Antigen A is subdivided into A_1 and A_2. It is suggested that A_2 cells have fewer antigen sites than A_1 cells (Smith and Thier, 1985).

The type of blood is determined by adding specially prepared serum, containing either anti-A or anti-B antibodies. The procedure is as follows:

Anti-A serum is added to a sample of the blood to be typed; if clumping of the red blood cells occurs, the blood is type A.

Anti-B serum is added to a sample of the blood to be typed; if clumping occurs, the blood is type B.

If clumping of the red cells occurs with the addition of anti-A and anti-B sera, the presence of both A and B agglutinogens is indicated, and the blood is type AB.

When there is no agglutination with the addition of either anti-A or anti-B serum, it indicates the absence of both A and B agglutinogens in the erythrocytes. The blood type is O.

The blood type of a person is determined genetically: a gene received from each parent influences the type of blood of the offspring. There are three possible alleles that determine the ABO blood types. The genes for A and B agglutinogens are co-dominant. The genotype of an individual who is blood group A may be AA, where the gene for the agglutinogen is inherited from both parents, or AO if they have inherited the gene for the A agglutinogen from one parent and no agglutinogen from the other. Similarly, a person who is blood group B may have the genotype BB or BO. In the case of a person whose blood group is AB their genotype will also be AB, and if blood group O their genotype will be OO.

RHESUS (Rh) BLOOD GROUPS

This system involves several antigens (agglutinogens) having varying degrees of antigenicity. The D factor is the strongest antigen and is of greatest clinical significance. Approximately 85% of Caucasians possess the D factor and are classified as Rh positive. The remaining 15% are said to be Rh negative.

Plasma antibodies (agglutinins) against the D factor do not occur naturally. They only develop in the plasma of Rh(D) negative blood when the D factor is introduced. The anti-D agglutinins will clump erythrocytes containing the D factor. The formation of anti-D antibodies may be evoked within an Rh negative person receiving a transfusion of Rh(D) positive blood, or by the development of an Rh(D) positive fetus within an Rh(D) negative mother. In the case of the blood transfusion, usually no clumping of the Rh positive donor's cells in the Rh negative recipient's blood occurs with the first transfusion because the anti-D antibodies are developed slowly and may not reach sufficient concentration before the foreign positive cells are terminated. But, if a second transfusion of Rh(D) positive blood is given, a reaction occurs, causing agglutination of the donor's cells.

When an Rh positive fetus develops within an Rh negative mother, some of the fetal red blood cells, or D factors released by worn-out erythrocytes, pass through the placenta into the maternal circulation. The mother then forms anti-D agglutinins which diffuse into the fetal circulation and cause agglutination of the fetal erythrocytes. The clumped cells are ultimately disintegrated, and the haemoglobin is broken down and converted to bilirubin, causing jaundice (yellowness of the skin and conjunctivae). This condition is known as erythroblastosis fetalis and intrauterine management can prevent the complications of Rh-incompatibility in the infant. Maternal sensitization can be prevented by giving an Rh negative woman anti-Rh antibodies in the form of immunoglobulin following a spontaneous or induced abortion, amniocentesis, at about 28 weeks gestation and following the first delivery, and in subsequent pregnancies (Llewellyn-Jones, 1986).

The Rh blood group factors are inherited, and the gene for the D agglutinogen is always dominant (Figure 13.4). Someone who is Rh positive may be homozygous (DD) having inherited a gene for the D factor from each parent, or may be heterozygous (Dd), having inherited a gene for D from one parent only. If the developing fetus is Rh negative, there is no problem, even if the mother is Rh positive, because there is no corresponding d agglutinogen.

Haemostasis and Blood Coagulation

Any rupture or severance of a blood vessel is normally followed by certain responses in an effort to reduce the loss of blood. These responses are local vasoconstriction, the formation of a temporary plug, coagulation of the blood and the formation of scar tissue to close the opening in the vessel. These defence responses occur frequently in the body without the individual being aware of them. During normal day-to-day activities and in minor injuries, minute blood vessels are ruptured

		Rh-negative mother	
		d	d
Rh-positive	D	Dd	Dd
father	D	Dd	Dd

(homozygous)

Offspring: all heterozygous Rh positive

		Rh-negative mother	
		d	d
Rh-positive	D	Dd	Dd
father	d	dd	dd

(heterozygous)

Offspring: 50% chance of being Rh positive; 50% chance of being Rh negative

		Rh-negative mother	
		d	d
Rh-negative	d	dd	dd
father	d	dd	dd

(homozygous)

Offspring: all Rh negative

Figure 13.4 Rh factor: genetic possibilities for agglutinogen D. The Rh factor (agglutinogen D) is dominant. If the mother is Rh negative and the offspring is Rh positive, the mother will form anti-Rh antibodies.

and the loss of blood is controlled by these mechanisms. If a large vessel, especially an artery, is interrupted, coagulation and vasoconstriction may not be adequate in checking the bleeding. Ligation, pressure or cautery may have to be used.

VASOCONSTRICTION IN HAEMOSTASIS

Local vasoconstriction reduces the blood flow to the injured site and is brought about by direct vascular muscular tissue reaction to the injury and by reflex nerve impulses that occur as a result of the trauma to the vessel. In the latter, sensory impulses arising in the injured vascular wall are transmitted into the central nervous system, causing impulses to be sent to the musculature of the vessels, and stimulating contraction. This vascular spasm is augmented by the release of serotonin (5-hydroxytryptamine), adenosine diphosphate, and the powerful vasoconstrictor thromboxane A_2 by the platelets at the site of injury.

HAEMOSTATIC PLUG

Injury and interruption of a vascular wall results in a clumping of platelets at the site. The aggregation serves as a loose temporary plug in the opening and is the forerunner of blood coagulation and the formation of a clot.

BLOOD COAGULATION

Coagulation of the blood is the formation of a jelly-like mass in the blood by the conversion of the soluble plasma protein fibrinogen to an insoluble mass of thin threads called fibrin. Blood cells are enmeshed in the fibrin to form the mass known as a clot. The conversion of fibrinogen to fibrin is dependent upon a chain of reactions between a series of clotting factors (procoagulants) that are designated by numbers. A list of these, their synonyms and their role in the blood clotting process are found in Table 13.5 and Figure 13.5. Thromboplastin and calcium are indicated by name rather than numerals. Clot formation may be initiated by an extrinsic or intrinsic mechanism. The extrinsic mechanism is initiated by tissue injury and release of tissue thromboplastin. The intrinsic pathway is more complex and may be initiated by factor XII, the direct action of platelets or by platelet aggregation on blood vessel walls.

The major steps in coagulation are:

1. Conversion of prothrombin to thrombin, which occurs in the presence of calcium ions, either as a result of the extrinsic coagulation pathway in the presence of thromboplastin (Figure 13.5) or activation of the intrinsic pathway in the absence of thromboplastin.
2. Conversion of fibrinogen to fibrin by thrombin.
3. Stabilization of the fibrin clot by factor XIII.

Prothrombin is normally present in the blood and is the inactive form of thrombin. Vitamin K is essential for its production by the liver.

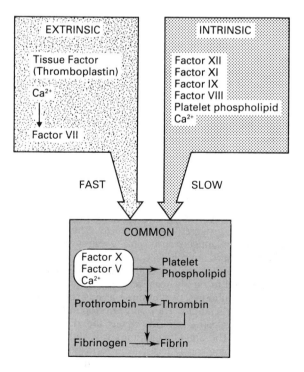

Figure 13.5 The process of blood coagulation. Modified from Hirsh and Brain (1983).

NORMAL ANTICOAGULANTS

A remarkable property of blood is its ability to remain fluid in the blood vessels; this is necessary for its circulation. Under normal circumstances, small amounts of thromboplastin are released by the disintegration of some platelets and tissue cells and could initiate coagulation. In order to counteract this, two important physiological systems exist. One involves the presence of naturally occurring anticoagulants. The other involves a system whereby fibrin is broken down, the *fribrinolytic system*.

Naturally-occurring anticoagulants include antithrombin III, heparin cofactor II, α-macroglobulin, Protein C, Protein S, C1-inhibitor and α₁-antitrypsin.

The fibrinolytic system involves plasminogen activators, synthesized by and released from endothelial cells, which convert the plasma protein plasminogen to plasmin. Plasmin has the capacity to hydrolyse fibrin and some other pro-coagulant proteins. The fibrinolytic system also has naturally occurring inhibitors, including antiplasmin and plasminogen activator inhibitor.

CLOT RETRACTION AND ORGANIZATION

Clot formation is normally completed within 3–6 minutes of damage. Clot retraction occurs as a result of contraction of contractile proteins found in the platelets. These exert a pull on the fibrin strands and the plasma that was trapped along with the blood cells is extruded. This fluid is referred to as *serum* and differs from normal plasma because it lacks fibrinogen, clotting factors II, V and VIII and has a high serotonin content. The fibrin strands of the clot are attached to the edges of the injured area of the blood vessel; as they shrink they pull the edges of the opening closer together, helping to check the loss of blood.

The opening in the vessel is repaired by a process called *clot organization*. Fibroblasts proliferate in the clot and, as they mature, the area is filled in by fibrous tissue. Macrophages (large reticuloendothelial phago-cytes which develop from monocytes) clear away the trapped blood cells. Endothelial cells of the intima proliferate to replace the vessel lining in the area.

MANAGEMENT OF THE PERSON WITH A BLOOD DISORDER

To summarize, physiological functions of the blood and its components include: internal respiration, cellular nutrition and excretion and defence of the body against infectious organisms or foreign antigens.

Blood disorders (dyscrasias) may affect the *erythrocytes*, *leucocytes*, *platelets* or the *coagulation process*. The problem may be due to a defect originating in the blood-forming organs, the deficiency of an essential element, or the abnormal destruction of cells. The disorders may be primary or secondary to another disease.

Diseases of the blood-forming organs may involve the red bone marrow or reticuloendothelial tissue.

The clinical manifestations of blood dyscrasias are varied and frequently are non-specific. The patient's health history, physical examination, results of diagnostic procedures and knowledge of the haematopoietic system form the database on which the nurse and doctor formulate their assessment of the patient's problems and develop specific plans for medical and nursing intervention.

DATA COLLECTION

History

The patient's history includes information about *family history* of any haematological disorders, a drug history and a history of exposure to *toxic substances*. Drugs of specific importance are the cytotoxic drugs used in the treatment of some cancers, immunosuppressive drugs

Table 13.5 Blood clotting factors and their roles in blood coagulation.

Factor number	Synonym	Role in blood coagulation
I	Fibrinogen	Forms fibrin
II	Prothrombin	Forms thrombin which converts fibrinogen to fibrin
V	Labile factor (accelerator globulin AcG, proaccelerin)	Necessary in the formation of active thromboplastin
VII	Proconvertin (stable factor, serum prothrombin conversion accelerator, SPCA)	Accelerates the action of tissue thromboplastin
VIII	Antihaemophilic factor, AHF (anihaemophilic globulin, AHG), antihaemophilia A factor	Promotes the breakdown of thrombocytes and the formation of active platelet thromboplastin
IX	Christmas factor, antihaemophilia B factor	Similar to factor VIII
X	Stuart–Prower factor	Promotes the action of thromboplastin
XI	Plasma thromboplastin antecedent (PTA)	Promotes clumping and breakdown of thrombocytes and the release of thromboplastin
XII	Hageman factor	Similar to factor XI
XIII	Fibrin-stabilizing factor (FSF), Laki-Lorand factor (LLF)	Converts the loose fibrin mesh to a dense tight mass
Pre K	Prekallikrein, Fletcher factor	Component of the intrinsic pathway
HMW-K	High molecular weight Kininogen, Fitzgerald factor	Non-enzymatic cofactor in intrinsic pathway

including antibiotics, and drugs affecting blood coagulation. An occupational history may provide clues to possible exposure to toxic chemicals.

The most common presenting symptoms are fatigue, lethargy, weakness and weight loss. The history should include details of any fever, night sweats, repeated infections or any indications of unusual bleeding that the patient may have experienced.

Physical assessment

The patient's *general appearance* should be noted for weight loss, pallor and lethargy; the latter two signs in particular indicate a decrease in red blood cells and oxygen carrying capacity (anaemia). The patient's *skin* and *mucous membranes* should be inspected for pallor, petechiae, bruises, dryness and texture, as blood disorders may manifest themselves by an increased tendency for the patient to bleed.

Blood pressure and pulse rate and rhythm are recorded and compared with normal values for the particular patient. The respiratory rate and rhythm are also assessed; chest expansion and the characteristics of respirations are noted as part the of patient's general health assessment. The patient's mental status should also be assessed for evidence of hypoxia, such as confusion.

Investigative procedures used in blood disorders

Tests used to assess erythrocytes, leucocytes and haemorrhagic disorders are discussed in Table 13.6.

Table 13.6　Laboratory tests for assessing blood disorders.

Test	Normal values	Description
Assessment of erythrocytes		
Red blood cell count	Males:　4.5–6.3 × 10^{12} per litre Females: 4.2–5.5 × 10^{12} per litre	The normal red blood cell count varies with sex, age, altitude and exercise. It will increase with hypovolaemia and decrease with hypervolaemia
Haemoglobin content of erythrocytes	Males:　14–18 g/dl (8.1–11.2 mmol/l) Females: 12–16 g/dl (7.4–9.9 mmol/l) Children (3 months to puberty): 10–14 g/dl	The normal values for haemoglobin vary with age, sex, altitude and exercise. Elevated levels occur with hypovolaemia and decreases are found with excess blood volume
Packed cell volume (haematocrit)	Males:　40–50% Females: 37–47%	The volume of red blood cells in one decilitre of blood (volume percentage of erythrocytes)
Erythrocyte indices	MCV 76–96 fl (femtolitres) MCH 27–32 pg (picograms) MCHC 30–35 g/dl	Mean corpuscular volume (MCV) is the average size of individual red cells Mean corpuscular haemoglobin (MCH) is the average amount of haemoglobin per red cell Mean corpuscular haemoglobin concentration (MCHC) is the average weight in grams of haemoglobin in one decilitre of red blood cells
Reticulocyte count	0.5–1.5%	The percentage of circulating non-mature, non-nucleated red blood cells. Results are indicative of bone marrow activity
Haemoglobin electrophoresis Haemoglobins A$_1$, A$_2$, F, C and S	Adult: HbA$_1$ 95–98% total Hgb 　　　HbA$_2$ 1.5–3.5% 　　　HbF$_1$ <2% 　　　HbC 0% 　　　HbS 0% Newborn: Hb F 40–70% of total Hb Infant: Hb F 2–10% total Hb Child (over 6 months): Hb F 1–2% total Hb	The diagnosis of haemolytic anaemias that are resistant to usual therapy requires the separation and identification of the different types of haemoglobin present in the red blood cells. Normal adult haemoglobin and fetal haemoglobin may be identified as well as abnormal haemoglobin. Haemoglobin S is the most common of the abnormal haemoglobins. It is found in sickle cell anaemia, in combination with other variations of haemoglobin or in a symptomatic sickle cell trait
Sickle cell test	Adult: 0 Child: 0	This test demonstrates the presence of haemoglobin S. A reducing agent is used to deoxygenate the erythrocytes and the cells are observed under a microscope for evidence of sickling. Red blood cells containing haemoglobin S become distorted and crescent or sickle-shaped when deprived of oxygen

Table 13.6 *continued*

Test	Normal values	Description
Vitamin B$_{12}$	118–959 pmol/l	B$_{12}$ is necessary for red blood cell production. It requires intrinsic factor for its absorption from the gastrointestinal tract. It is tested to diagnose macrocytic anaemia
Folic acid (folate)	3.0–2.5 nmol/l	Folic acid is required for the normal production of red and white blood cells and DNA. Its absorption is dependent on a normally functioning intestinal mucosa. It is tested to diagnose macrocytic anaemia
Red-cell mass	Males: 20–33 ml/kg Females: 20–27 ml/kg	Performed by labelling the red cells with chromium-51 (^{51}Cr). This is used in the diagnosis of polycythemia
Plasma volume	Males: 31–55 ml/kg Females: 36–50 ml/kg	Measured with iodine-125 (^{125}I) labelled human albumin
Bone marrow examination by aspiration or biopsy	Normal values differ with the source used, age of patient and test method. Differential counts are done on each type of cell	Specimens of red bone marrow are obtained by aspiration or percutaneous needle biopsy, usually from the sternum or iliac crest. Smears are made of the marrow specimen and the cells are examined. The number of cells in the various developmental and maturational phases, and the size, shape and characteristics of cell content are noted. The skin is cleansed and a local anaesthetic introduced prior to the test. Discomfort occurs from the pressure needed to pass the needle through the cortex of the bone into the marrow and with aspiration of the marrow fluid

Assessment of leucoytes

Test	Normal values	Description
White blood cell (leucocyte) count	4.0–11.0 $\times$ 10^9 per litre	The number of white blood cells in a microlitre of blood
Differential count	Neutrophils (polymorphonuclear leucocytes) 40–75% (2.5–7.5 $\times$ 10^9 per litre) Eosinophils 1–6% (0.04–0.44 $\times$ 10^9 per litre) Basophils <1% (0.015–0.1 $\times$ 10^9 per litre) Monocytes 2–10% (0.2–0.8 $\times$ 10^9 per litre) Lymphocytes 20–50% (1.5–3.5 $\times$ 10^9 per litre)	
Bone marrow aspirate and biopsy		See above
Leuocyte alkaline phosphatase (LAP) stain	Quantitative method 15–100 units	Alkaline phosphatase is an enzyme active in neutrophils. The test demonstrates the rate of intracellular metabolism within neutrophils and is useful in diagnosing chronic granulocytic leukaemia

Assessment of haemorrhagic disorders

Test	Normal values	Description
Blood platelet (thrombocyte) count	150–400 $\times$ 10^9 per litre	The number of platelets in a microlitre of blood
Bleeding time	2–5 minutes (varies with method used)	This is the time it takes bleeding to stop naturally—that is, the period of time blood continues to escape from an 'open' area
Prothrombin time (PT) or International Normalized Ratio (INR)	11–15 seconds 2–4	This is the time it takes for coagulation following the addition of thromboplastin and calcium to the specimen. The INR is designed to produce consistent results in all laboratories regardless of reagents used

Table 13.6 *continued*

Test	Normal values	Description
Partial thromboplastin time (PTT) to activated partial thromboplastin time (APTT)	PTT 40–100 seconds APTT 30–45 seconds	The partial thromboplastin time is a general test of coagulation used for screening and to monitor anti-coagulant therapy. Clotting deficiencies other than factor VII, XIII and platelets can be detected. The activated partial thromboplastin time (APTT) involves the addition of activators to the regular test reagent to shorten the clotting time
Plasma fibrinogen	2–4 g/l	This indicates the fibrinogen concentration
Other tests Coombs' test	Direct—negative (no agglutination) Indirect—negative	The erythrocytes are examined for the presence of immune bodies (agglutinins) that adhere to the red blood cells and lead to clumping and haemolysis. In vivo sensitization is measured by the direct Coombs' test. An indirect method which assesses in vitro sensitization, is done on serum to test for the presence of the antibodies to the erythrocyte antigens The Coombs' test may be used in identifying haemolytic anaemia or erythroblastosis fetalis
Lymph node biopsy	Negative	A tissue specimen of a lymph node that has undergone some change is obtained. The change may be associated with an alteration in the patient's leucocytes, especially the lymphocytes

The Person with Erythrocyte Disorders

A deficiency or an excess may occur in the number of circulating red blood cells, or the cell composition may be abnormal. Variations in the size, shape and haemoglobin content may be present. Certain descriptive terms are used to denote some of these characteristics.

Erythrocytes that are larger than the normal are referred to as *macrocytes*; if they are smaller than the normal, they are *microcytes*. Cells that possess a normal amount of haemoglobin are said to be *normochromic*, but if it is deficient, they are described as *hypochromic*. Those with a volume of haemoglobin greater than the normal are *hyperchromic*. If the cells present have abnormal shapes, they are described as *poikilocytic*.

ERYTHROCYTE AND HAEMOGLOBIN DEFICIENCY (ANAEMIA)

The term anaemia implies a reduction in the oxygen-carrying capacity of the blood as a result of fewer circulating erythrocytes than is normal or a decrease in the concentration of haemoglobin. It may sometimes be classified according to the characteristics of the erythrocytes. For example, in anaemia which is due to an iron deficiency, the cells are hypochromic and microcytic; the disease may be referred to as hypochromic-microcytic anaemia.

CAUSES

The abnormal reduction in the number of erythrocytes may be due to decreased production (erythropoiesis) or excessive red blood cell destruction. Anaemia may be primary, but frequently is secondary to some other disorder, and because of this the patient may undergo extensive investigation to determine the cause. Anaemia due to decreased erythropoiesis may be caused by a deficiency of factors essential for normal production, e.g. deficiency of erythropoietin, as in chronic renal failure, or by depressed bone marrow activity. Excessive destruction of the red blood cells may be associated with intracorpuscular defects or extracorpuscular factors such as blood loss.

GENERAL EFFECTS AND CHARACTERISTICS

Although there are various causes and types of anaemia, they present a common problem, that of a decrease in the capacity of the blood to transport oxygen. The patient, regardless of the cause or type of anaemia, manifests signs and symptoms attributable to tissue and organ hypoxia and the ensuing reduced metabolism. The occurrence and severity of these manifestations depend on the degree of anaemia present and its rapidity of onset. A gradually developing anaemia can be tolerated without significant incapacity, whereas a relatively small but rapid loss of blood may produce marked symptoms. Table 13.7 lists the clinical characteristics of anaemia.

Table 13.7 Signs and symptoms manifested by a patient with anaemia.

Body structure	Objective and subjective data
Skin	Pallor Brittle nails and dry hair
Mucous membranes	Pale (e.g. conjunctivae)
Respiratory	Shortness of breath on exertion Increased respiratory rate Fluid in base of lungs (with severe anaemia)
Cardiac	Increased pulse rate Cardiac palpitation Cardiac enlargement Angina pectoris (with severe anaemia) Increased stroke volume
Neuromuscular	Headache, dizziness General fatigue Tingling or 'pins and needles' in extremities (vitamin B_{12} deficiency) Fainting Decreased attention span
Gastrointestinal	Anorexia
Metabolism	Increased sensitivity to cold

A. ANAEMIAS SECONDARY TO DECREASED ERYTHROPOIESIS

1. Nutritional deficiency anaemias

An essential nutrient for erythrocyte production, such as iron, vitamin B_{12}, folic acid, ascorbic acid or protein, may be lacking in the diet, or there may be defective absorption of an essential factor. In some instances, there may be an increased demand within the person which the normal supply cannot meet. The deficiency anaemias seen most often are those resulting from iron, vitamin B_{12} or folic acid deficiency.

When considering the following types of anaemia it will become apparent to the nurse that a healthy diet is the key to preventing such problems occurring. Health education in the community should therefore focus on the importance of avoiding conditions such as anaemia, as well as the more obvious targets of a healthy eating campaign such as the obese. The nurse should be sensitive to individual dietary preferences, some of which may be culturally determined, but also be aware of the trap of stereotyping i.e. assuming that because a person belongs to a particular group they will automatically eat a certain diet or be likely to have a specific health problem.

The issue of diet and health promotion raises the specific question of whether the person can actually afford a healthy diet. It is one thing for the nurse to educate a person in what constitutes a healthy diet, but if that person cannot afford certain foods, the nurse is left in a difficult ethical dilemma. The issue moves to a different level, that of society as a whole and its responsibility for ensuring that all members of our society can afford a healthy diet that will prevent any individual from developing diseases such as the deficiency anaemias. This is a professional responsibility that the nurse cannot avoid.

(a) Iron deficiency anaemia

Anaemia due to a deficiency of iron is characterized by small red blood cells with less than the normal content of haemoglobin (microcytic-hypochromic). There is usually some slight reduction in the total number of red blood cells. The deficiency of iron may be due to: (1) chronic blood loss, (2) an insufficient dietary intake, (3) impaired intestinal absorption, or (4) an increased requirement. The most common cause in adults is chronic blood loss. It is not uncommon in women during their reproductive years because of menstrual blood loss and because of the increased demands during pregnancy and lactation. Anaemia due to an iron deficiency is uncommon in adult males unless there has been a loss of blood or the development of hypochlorhydria secondary to gastric disease or atrophy of the gastric mucosa.

In addition to the general symptoms of anaemia (Table 13.7), the patient with iron deficiency anaemia may experience soreness and inflammation of the mouth and tongue. The tongue may be very red and may have a smooth, glazed appearance due to atrophy of the papillae. Rarely, the patient with a severe anaemia complains of dysphagia (difficulty in swallowing). The combination of dysphagia, stomatitis (inflammation of the mouth) and atrophic glossitis (inflammation of the tongue with atrophy of papillae) in anaemia may be referred to as the Plummer–Vinson syndrome. Changes in the fingernails are common in prolonged iron deficiency. They become brittle and concave or spoon-shaped.

Treatment. Treatment of iron deficiency anaemia depends on the cause. If a source of blood loss is identified, then steps should be taken to correct or remove the lesion (i.e. peptic ulcer disease, colonic carcinoma). When iron supplementation is required, medicinal iron is usually given orally in the form of a ferrous salt. Examples of preparations commonly used are ferrous sulphate and ferrous gluconate.

(b) Vitamin B_{12} deficiency anaemia (pernicious anaemia)

Vitamin B_{12} (cyanocobalamin) is essential for the production of normal red blood cells and may be referred to as the extrinsic antianaemic factor. When it is not available to the red bone marrow, excessively large cells called megaloblasts are formed. The number of red blood cells produced is less than normal, and they show marked variation in size and shape. The megaloblasts contain a greater than normal amount of haemoglobin, but the deficiency in the total number of erythrocytes results in an inadequate oxygen-carrying capacity of the blood. The condition may be referred to as *megaloblastic anaemia*.

The cause of vitamin B_{12} deficiency anaemia is usually

non-absorption of the vitamin. Rarely, vitamin B_{12} deficiency occurs because of an inadequate dietary intake (Table 13.8).

Table 13.8   Possible causes of vitamin B_{12} deficiency anaemia.

A. Non-absorption of vitamin B_{12}
   1. Deficiency of intrinsic factor
      (a) Gastric secretory defect
      (b) Gastrectomy (partial or total)
      (c) Autoimmune mechanism
   2. Intestinal resection
   3. Intestinal disease (e.g. regional ileitis, steatorrhoea, intestinal parasites)

B. Malnutrition
   1. Inadequate dietary intake of foods containing vitamin B_{12}
   2. Totally deficient food intake

As cited earlier in this chapter, an intrinsic factor secreted by the gastric mucosa is essential for the absorption of vitamin B_{12}. Non-absorption of the vitamin results from a deficiency of the intrinsic factor, which may be due to a gastric secretory defect, gastrectomy or an autoimmune mechanism. Failure of absorption of the vitamin may also occur as a result of extensive resection of the small intestine or intestinal disease such as ileitis, steatorrhoea and parasitic infestation. Blind or stagnant loops in the small intestine may develop following intestinal surgery or with multiple diverticula (sacs or outpouchings in the walls) and may cause a proliferation of bacteria that use up the available vitamin B_{12} before it can be absorbed.

The most common cause of vitamin B_{12} deficiency is associated with pernicious anaemia and a decreased production of intrinsic factor. It is a hereditary autoimmune disorder that was historically associated with individuals of Scandinavian or northern European ancestry and is now seen in various other ethnic groups. It is more common in females, has an insidious onset and usually develops between 35 and 65 years of age.

Clinical characteristics. In addition to the general symptoms of anaemia cited previously, the patient may experience gastrointestinal and nervous system changes. The tongue is sore and smooth. There is loss of appetite and some intolerance for food, but the person does not always show a corresponding loss of weight. The lack of vitamin B_{12} may cause myelin and nerve fibre degeneration in the spinal cord and peripheral nerves. As a result of this degeneration, the patient may develop symmetrical tingling or 'pins and needles' or coldness and numbness in the extremities. Unless the deficiency is corrected, serious motor disturbances may develop in the form of muscular weakness, ataxia (loss of coordination and staggering) and paralysis. In prolonged, severe deficiencies, degeneration of the optic nerves may occur, resulting in serious impairment of vision. When degenerative changes occur in the spinal cord,

the condition is referred to as *subacute combined degeneration of the cord.*

In severe pernicious anaemia, the skin may show some jaundice, a result of increased haemolysis or erythrocyte breakdown. Laboratory examination of the blood reveals a deficiency of erythrocytes. The cells are unusually large with more than the normal amount of haemoglobin (macrocytic-hyperchromic). Gastric analysis demonstrates hypochlorhydria even after stimulation with histamine. Bone marrow aspirated by sternal puncture shows hyperplasia of the bone marrow and failure in normal erythropoiesis. Vitamin B_{12} assay shows a deficiency.

Treatment. Pernicious anaemia is treated by intramuscular injections of vitamin B_{12}. Since the deficit of vitamin B_{12} is primarily due to malabsorption, intramuscular administration is the method used to achieve adequate blood levels of the vitamin. Oral preparations of vitamin B_{12} and intrinsic factor should not be used because of the propensity to develop antibodies to these formulations. A daily dose may be prescribed for a period of time; then, the interval between injections is gradually increased and the dosage is reduced to a maintenance level according to the patient's response. The patient will require regular maintenance doses of vitamin B_{12} for the rest of his or her life. The majority of those with pernicious anaemia require 1 mg of hydroxocobalamin monthly to maintain normal haemoglobin and erythrocyte levels. Regular red cell counts and haemoglobin estimations are necessary. Initially, the rapid regeneration of erythrocytes in response to treatment may deplete the iron stores, resulting in insufficient haemoglobin production. Ferrous sulphate may be prescribed for a period of time in addition to the vitamin B_{12}. Hypokalaemia may also develop during the initial phase of therapy; the potassium level should therefore be monitored. The haematological response to treatment is usually rapid. Neurological symptoms, if present, take much longer to improve and may never completely disappear.

Regular medical examinations are necessary so that early and insidious regressive changes may be recognized before serious degenerative changes develop.

In contrast to pernicious anaemia, the anaemia associated with a dietary deficiency of vitamin B_{12} or intestinal disease does not manifest hypochlorhydria or degenerative changes of the nervous system. The dietary deficiency of vitamin B_{12} (extrinsic factor) is rare and usually occurs when the diet lacks animal protein and consists mainly of carbohydrates and vegetables. When the anaemia is secondary to intestinal disease, care of the patient includes treatment of the initial cause as well as parenteral administration of vitamin B_{12}. Oral or parenteral preparations of folic acid may also be prescribed.

(c) Anaemia due to deficiency of folic acid and vitamin C
A lack of folic acid or ascorbic acid may interfere with the production of normal erythrocytes. Either deficiency may result from inadequate intake or a malabsorptive problem. It is also more likely to develop during

pregnancy because of the increased demand. Laboratory tests reveal the same haematological changes as appear with vitamin B_{12} deficiency, but the patient does not manifest nervous system involvement, achlorhydria or a decreased vitamin B_{12} absorption.

Folic acid may be given orally or intramuscularly to correct the deficiency. A person with megaloblastic anaemia, before it is determined whether it is due to B_{12} or folate deficiency, should receive both B_{12} and folate. If someone with B_{12} deficiency receives folate alone, there may be an initial haematological response to the administration but the neurological sequelae of B_{12} deficiency may be precipitated. Food sources include dark green leafy vegetables, asparagus, liver and kidney.

Vitamin C enhances the catalytic action of folic acid in erythropoiesis. If the folic acid dietary intake is satisfactory, the administration of vitamin C in anaemia will assist in increasing red cell production.

2. Aplastic anaemia

This type of anaemia is the result of depressed bone marrow activity. There may be an actual reduction in the amount of blood-forming marrow, or the marrow may have a functional defect. Aplastic anaemia usually results in a deficiency of leucocytes and thrombocytes as well as insufficient red blood cells. Rarely the disorder may involve only failure of the bone marrow to produce erythrocytes, causing anaemia alone, without leucopenia or thrombocytopenia. When all three formed elements of the blood are reduced, the condition is referred to as *pancytopenia*.

Causes

Depression of bone marrow activity may be the result of the toxic action of certain drugs or industrial chemicals, excessive exposure to radiation, chronic infection or invasion by malignant cells. Drugs capable of suppressing bone marrow function include sulphonamides, antineoplastic agents (e.g. nitrogen mustard, busulphan, cyclophosphamide, methotrexate, mercaptopurine), gold salts (sodium aurothiomalate, Myocrisin), chloramphenicol (Chloromycetin) and phenylbutazone (Butazolidin). Examples of industrial chemicals that may depress erythropoiesis include benzene, aniline dyes, lead, mercury and arsenic. Some insecticides and plant sprays may also be offenders in bone marrow failure. In relation to radiation, drugs and chemicals, there appears to be no direct correlation between the dosage and the development of the anaemia. Sensitivity of the individual seems to be a contributing factor. With some patients their aplastic anaemia may be idiopathic; the cause remains obscure.

Clinical characteristics

The person with aplastic anaemia is critically ill and, as well as suffering severe hypoxia, is usually susceptible to infection because of the deficiency of leucocytes (leucopenia). Spontaneous bleeding is also a problem when the platelet count falls to 20×10^9 per litre or less. With a platelet count of 10×10^9 per litre the tendency to bleed is very high (Napier, 1987). The onset of the anaemia may be sudden and prostrating, or it may be insidious and gradual. The patient manifests the general symptoms of anaemia (see Table 13.7), oral and throat lesions, fever, infection and haemorrhagic areas.

Treatment

Exposure to any toxic agent is discontinued and supportive therapy is given in the form of frequent transfusions of packed red cells and platelets, antibiotic administration to control infection and occasionally a corticoid preparation such as prednisone. The latter is thought to have a stimulating effect on the bone marrow. Packed cells are transfused in preference to whole blood to prevent fluid overload. Platelet transfusions are given at the same time or immediately following red cell transfusions to prevent haemorrhage. Platelet counts may be low prior to transfusions and fall during transfusions of red cells either due to a dilutional effect or to immune complex formation (Napier, 1987).

Bone marrow transplantation is the treatment of choice for patients under 50 years of age with severe aplastic anaemia when a suitable donor is available. Immunosuppressive treatment with antilymphocyte globulin (ALG) has been shown to be of benefit to some patients. Treatment with bone marrow transplantation and immunosuppressive therapy provide some hope of a cure or a remission for selected patients. Supportive nursing care is very important.

B. ANAEMIAS SECONDARY TO INCREASED DESTRUCTION OF ERYTHROCYTES (HAEMOLYTIC ANAEMIAS)

Excessive haemolysis (disintegration of red blood cells) causes anaemia if the rate of destruction exceeds the erythropoietic ability of the red bone marrow. Premature haemolysis may result from (1) *intracorpuscular (intrinsic) defects* that reduce the ability of the cells to survive the normal life span in circulation, or it may be due to (2) an *extracorpuscular (extrinsic to the erythrocytes) factor or mechanism.*

The patient's symptoms depend on the rate, severity and duration of the cell destruction. As well as the symptoms produced by the reduced oxygen-carrying capacity of the blood, there is an increased concentration of unconjugated bilirubin in the blood; this may cause jaundice, which is evident first in the sclerae. An increased amount of urobilinogen appears in the urine and faeces and, rarely, free haemoglobin is detected in the plasma and urine. Laboratory examination of the blood reveals an increased number of reticulocytes in circulation (reticulocytosis) because of the constant demand for new cells, as well as a deficiency in the total number of red cells. Examination of a bone marrow specimen demonstrates hyperplasia and hyperactivity of the marrow. Acute haemolytic anaemia may cause a chill followed by a high temperature, prostration, headache and pain in the back and legs.

The haemolytic anaemias caused by a congenital corpuscular defect include hereditary spherocytosis, sickle cell anaemia and thalassaemia. Haemolysis due to extracorpuscular factors may be caused by some infective agents, an autoimmune reaction or certain drugs.

1. Haemolytic anaemias due to intracorpuscular defect

(a) Hereditary spherocytosis

This type of haemolytic anaemia is also known as congenital haemolytic jaundice, familial haemolytic anaemia and acholuric jaundice. The erythrocyte defect is an abnormal cell membrane that is excessively permeable to sodium. The influx of sodium increases the demand on the 'sodium pump', adding to the total metabolic work of the cell. The high sodium content of the cells also leads to the entrance of more than the normal amount 'of water through osmosis, which accounts for the characteristic spherical shape of the cell rather than the normal biconcave disc. This spherical shape predisposes the cells to entrapment in the spleen and their marked fragility results in ready destruction.

The disorder is inherited from an affected parent. The gene with the abnormal trait is dominant; that is, to have the disorder expressed, one need only receive a gene for the trait from one parent. The age at which the disease is recognized varies, depending on its severity. The patient may have little difficulty and go undiagnosed until adulthood. The enlarged spleen may be discovered during a routine examination. It is usually the jaundice or the symptoms of anaemia that prompt the patient to seek medical assistance. Occasionally, the increased bilirubin leads to the development of gallstones.

Treatment is removal of the spleen, which reduces the excessive destruction of the abnormal red blood cells and relieves the anaemia. The abnormal erythrocytes persist, but the majority survive a normal life span in the absence of the spleen.

(b) Haemoglobinopathy

The complex haemoglobin (Hb) molecule is a combination of globins (protein) and the red pigment haem (porphyrin and ferrous iron). Three forms of haemoglobin occur normally; the type is determined by slight variations in the globin portions of the four subunits. The haemoglobin in the erythrocytes of the fetus is type F (Hb-F) and consists of two α- and two γ-globin chains. During the first few months of life this is replaced. About 97% of the haemoglobin that develops after birth is known as type A (Hb-A), and the remainder as type A_2 (Hb-A_2). Hb-A consists of two α- and two β-globin chains, and Hb-A_2 has two α- and two δ-chains.

The term haemoglobinopathy indicates the presence of red blood cells containing an inherited abnormality of haemoglobin, the result of a genetic mutation which causes a disorder in haemoglobin synthesis. This results in structural variations in one or more of the globin chains, which may cause premature haemolysis of the erythrocyte or a decreased production of haemoglobin. The most common haemoglobinopathies are sickle cell disease and thalassaemia. The haemoglobin in the former disease is designated as Hb-S; in the latter there is a decreased production of structurally-normal haemoglobin.

Sickle cell disease. This recessive, hereditary blood disorder is characterized by erythrocytes that contain Hb-S. It occurs in two forms, sickle cell trait and sickle

		Mother	(sickle cell trait)
		O	S
Father	O	OO	OS
(sickle cell trait)	S	OS	SS

Offspring: 25% chance of being normal; 25% of having sickle cell anaemia; 50% chance of having sickle cell trait

		Mother	(normal)
		O	O
Father	O	OO	OO
(sickle cell trait)	S	OS	OS

Offspring: 50% chance of being normal or having sickle cell trait

		Mother	(sickle cell trait)
		O	S
Father	S	OS	SS
(sickle cell anaemia)	S	OS	SS

Offspring: 50% chance of having sickle cell anaemia or sickle cell trait

Figure 13.6 Examples of inheritance of sickle cell disease. S, gene for Hb-S; O, gene for normal haemoglobin.

cell anaemia. *Sickle cell trait* is a heterozygous state; the individual has inherited the Hb-S gene from only one parent. Only a small amount of the individual's haemoglobin is type Hb-S. The person with sickle cell trait usually does not manifest symptoms of sickling except in some very stressful situations, especially those that cause hypoxia (e.g. high altitude, unpressurized flights, or poor general anaesthesia). He or she is a carrier, and there is a 50% chance that offspring will inherit the sickle cell gene (Figure 13.6).

Sickle cell anaemia occurs because the individual is homozygous for Hb-S; that is, a gene for the abnormal haemoglobin has been inherited from each parent (Figure 13.6). A large amount of haemoglobin S is present.

The disease affects both males and females and occurs mainly in Afro-Caribbean people, the incidence being 1:400–1:500, although those of Mediterranean, Middle-Eastern or Asian Indian ancestry may also be affected.

Haemoglobin S is less soluble than normal haemoglobin, especially when it gives up its oxygen to become deoxyhaemoglobin, and when the pH is below normal firm crystals form within the cells which are distorted and become crescent-shaped (like a sickle). Sickle cells increase the viscosity of the blood which then will not flow as readily through the capillaries. Circulatory stagnation and thrombosis may result, leading to a greater reduction of the oxyghaemoglobin and ensuing local metabolic acidosis (reduced pH). Sickle cells are more fragile and haemolyse readily. Their life span is about 26–35 days as compared with the 120-day life span of normal erythrocytes. Sickling and vascular occlusion resulting in an infarcted area may occur in any tissue or organ; the severity and site are not predictable. Frequent sites are the lower limbs, joints, kidneys, mesentery, lungs and brain.

The individual usually has symptom-free periods alternated with exacerbations. There is a continuous premature destruction of red blood cells, resulting in a haemoglobin level of approximately 7–10 g/dl, increased bilirubin in the blood, reticulocytosis, enlargement of the spleen and liver and hyperplasia of the red bone marrow. At intervals, an exacerbation or acute episode, referred to as a sickle cell crisis, occurs. It is frequently precipitated by an infection, stress, dehydration, exposure to cold, acidosis, or any situation in which the individual experiences hypoxia. The acute episode is characterized by sickling, circulatory stagnation and thrombosis. Pain, swelling and impaired function develop in whatever area suffers the interrupted blood supply. The individual is irritable and weak and develops a fever. Jaundice is evident with the increased haemolysis. The symptoms may be quite similar to those of many diseases; for example, if the vascular occlusion occurs in the mesentery, the condition may be mistaken for appendicitis because of the acute abdominal pain and tenderness unless the individual is known to have sickle cell disease. Occlusion of kidney vessels may destroy some nephrons, resulting in renal insufficiency. Obstruction of a cerebral artery may cause some paralysis or reduced mental ability. Growth is retarded and the individual tends to develop a thin short trunk, long extremities, narrow shoulders and hips and increased anteroposterior diameter of the chest. Symptoms do not usually appear within the first 6 months of life because the individual is protected from sickling during this period by the haemoglobin F that is still present in the erythrocytes.

Thalassaemia. Synonyms that may be used for this type of anaemia are Mediterranean anaemia, homozygous anaemia and heriditary leptocytosis.

This disease occurs in several forms and is seen most frequently in persons of the Mediterranean countries and Southeast Asia. The common feature is of a genetically determined defect in the cellular synthesis of the globin fraction of the haemoglobin which affects either the α- or β-chains. The red blood cells are smaller than normal, fragile, irregular in shape and deficient in haemoglobin. A percentage of the haemoglobin may be of the fetal type (Hb-F).

Thalassaemia major, also referred to as Cooley's anaemia, is a homozygous state; a gene for thalassaemia having been received from each parent. The disorder is manifested in infancy or early childhood. Fortunately, this form of the disease is of lesser incidence than thalassaemia minor. It produces very severe anaemia and marked hyperplasia of the red bone marrow and may cause pain in the bones. Reticulocytosis occurs and immature nucleated red blood cells may appear in the circulation. The spleen and liver are enlarged as a result

of the rapid haemolysis of the abnormal red blood cells, and jaundice may be apparent. The serum bilirubin level is elevated. Growth and development are retarded and the child does not usually survive beyond early childhood. Treatment consists mainly of blood transfusions and splenectomy if the spleen is enlarged.

Thalassaemia minor is a heterozygous state and is less severe. The red blood cells are smaller than normal but are less deficient in haemoglobin than those of the major type and there is less premature haemolysis. The degree of anaemia varies greatly in affected persons; some may be asymptomatic and live a normal life, with their disease only being detected by a blood cell examination. Others may be handicapped to some degree by anaemia.

The heterozygous state can be detected for both sickle cell disease and thalassaemia and genetic counselling can be offered. Antenatal diagnosis to detect an affected fetus is available and may be offered when both parents are carriers.

The worldwide distribution of these two haemoglobinopathies has been found to closely resemble that of the malaria parasite. It has been suggested that the heterozygous form of both conditions conveys some resistance to the erythrocytes which renders them less susceptible to the malaria parasite.

2. Haemolytic anaemia due to extracorpuscular factors

Extrinsic mechanisms that may cause haemolysis include (a) some infections, (b) immune bodies, and (c) certain drugs and chemicals.

(a) An increased rate of erythrocyte destruction may be associated with severe infections caused by the haemolytic streptococci, *Staphylococcus aureus*, pneumococcus, *Clostridium perfringens (Bacillus welchii)* and some viruses. Excessive haemolysis may also acompany malaria. The red blood cells may be damaged by the pathogenic organisms or their toxins.

(b) Haemolytic anaemia may be caused by antibodies which may be acquired or may be developed in response to an endogenous or exogenous antigen. Erythroblastosis fetalis (haemolytic disease of the newborn) is an example of haemolytic anaemia occurring as a result of acquired antibodies.

When a person develops antibodies that result in the destruction of his or her own erythrocytes, the condition is referred to as autoimmune haemolytic anaemia. Frequently, the cause of this condition is not known. In many instances, it is secondary to a collagen disease (e.g. lupus erythematosus) or to a disease involving lymphoid tissue (e.g. Hodgkin's disease). The agglutinins adhere to the red blood cells, predisposing them to entrapment and destruction, especially in the spleen and liver.

Treatment of autoimmune haemolytic anaemia includes blood transfusions, splenectomy to reduce the trapping and destruction of the red blood cells, and the administration of a corticoid preparation such as prednisone to decrease sensitivity and antibody formation.

(c) Haemolytic jaundice may develop in some persons receiving preparations of quinine, or sulphonamide. Its incidence has also been reported in persons exposed to insecticides, arsenic and coal tar products such as aniline dyes and toluene. The mechanism by which certain drugs and chemicals produce haemolysis in some persons is not known.

C. ANAEMIA SECONDARY TO BLOOD LOSS

The loss of blood removes erythrocytes from the circulation, reducing the oxygen-carrying capacity of the blood. A blood count taken immediately after a haemorrhage does not reflect the degree of anaemia since the total intravascular volume is reduced. Over a period of 24–48 hours, the intravascular volume is restored by the entrance of extracellular fluid into the vascular compartment and probably by intravenous infusion. The red blood cells at this time are those that remained after the blood loss and are now dispersed in a greater volume of plasma. The count (per litre) now gives a more accurate indication of the severity of the anaemia.

Normally, the bone marrow responds quickly to the tissue hypoxia, and the erythrocyte count returns to normal over a period of 4–5 weeks. At first, more than the normal number of reticulocytes are in circulation and some immature nucleated normoblasts may also be released. Since a considerable amount of iron is lost from the body in haemorrhage, haemoglobin production may lag behind red blood cell production. The administration of an iron preparation may be necessary to bring the haemoglobin concentration back to normal.

If the blood loss is 20% or more of the total blood volume, rapid replacement by means of a blood transfusion is necessary to prevent renal failure and endocrine and sympathetic nervous system responses which can lead to cardiac, renal, respiratory and gastrointestinal problems (see Chapter 12). This quickly increases the total circulating volume as well as the number of erythrocytes available to carry oxygen.

In cases of chronic blood loss in which there is a continuous loss of a relatively small amount over a long period, the bone marrow may keep the erythrocyte count close to normal. The continuous loss of iron, however, creates a deficiency of that essential element, and the erythrocytes in circulation are small and lack a full complement of haemoglobin. The anaemia may be described as microcytic-hypochromic. Treatment includes correction of the cause of the bleeding and the administration of an iron preparation such as ferrous sulphate.

NURSING MANAGEMENT OF THE PERSON WITH ANAEMIA

The care required by the anaemic patient varies with the severity and cause of the disease. Anaemia is a symptom of an underlying disorder. Most persons with anaemia are treated as out-patients. The anaemia may be chronic, as in pernicious and sickle cell anaemia, resulting in the patient's need for continuous treatment and supervision and modification in his or her way of life. With some,

the anaemia may be entirely cured by correction of the cause. Depending on the causative factor, there may be symptoms and problems in addition to those attributable to anaemia. For example, in haemolytic anaemia there may be the problem of jaundice; in the sickle cell type there is the serious problem of vascular obstruction. Regardless of the type of anaemia, the patients have one common difficulty: namely, a decreased capacity of their blood to transport oxygen.

ASSESSMENT

Health history

Information collected begins with the patient's perceptions of the symptoms of anaemia experienced, which will vary from very mild to extensive disruption of daily activities. The clinical characteristics that the person may demonstrate are listed in Table 13.7 and the nurse should be aware of any of these signs appearing in the patient's history. The patient is asked about gradual or sudden changes in daily activities, changes experienced with exertion and increased need for rest and sleep.

The history includes information about any family history of anaemia, exposure to chemical agents, including the nature of the work environment, a complete drug history, any history of bleeding disorders, renal disease, liver or gastrointestinal disorders.

A nutritional history may be obtained and the diet assessed for essential nutrients, especially an adequate intake of iron and vitamin B_{12}.

The history also includes an assessment of the patient's knowledge of the anaemia and prescribed therapeutic measures.

Physical examination

This begins with observation of the patient's posture, drooping of the shoulders, slow movements or other signs of fatigue. The *skin* and *mucous membranes* are inspected for pallor and in the case of haemolytic anaemia for initial or increasing jaundice. The nails are inspected for brittleness and the hair for thinning and dryness. The *respiratory* and *heart* rates are recorded and any changes on exertion noted.

The patient with pernicious anaemia is observed for signs of degenerative changes in the nervous system. Any complaint of tingling, numbness and sensations of 'pins and needles' in distal portions of the extremities, loss of finer movements, difficulty in holding small objects, weakness of limbs, ataxia and impaired vision are recorded.

If the patient has sickle cell anaemia, frequent close observation is made for swollen, tender and painful areas, and changes in body functions or the patient's mental and physical abilities that may indicate areas of thrombotic disease.

Reports of laboratory studies are followed and nursing measures adapted to indicated changes. For example, a decrease in the haemoglobin, packed cell volume or erythrocyte count may be such that the patient's activity should be reduced.

PATIENT HEALTH PROBLEMS RELATED TO ANAEMIA

The reduced capacity of the blood to carry oxygen may give rise to some or all of the following:

1. Inability to sustain the usual level of activity
2. Potential risk of tissue damage and injury
3. Pain due to tissue ischaemia or hyperplasia of the bone marrow
4. Impaired thought processes

The person may also experience problems such as:

5. Inability to maintain an adequate dietary intake of nutrients essential for red blood cell production
6. Lack of knowledge concerning the disease process, treatment and measures to promote health

NURSING INTERVENTION

1. Goal: the person will achieve an acceptable level of activity while maintaining vital signs within the normal range

Energy expenditure should be reduced in order to decrease the demand for oxygen; nursing care is planned to achieve this. An explanation of the basis of the fatigue and weakness experienced and emphasis on the importance of balancing rest and activity may help the person to understand what is happening and to accept limitations on activity. Activity is encouraged but the importance of resting before becoming fatigued and breathless is explained. Assisitance may be required to enable the person to perform essential activities, such as maintaining personal hygiene and dressing, with the minimum of effort.

Severe anaemia may cause shortness of breath or dyspnoea, even at rest, and the person may be less distressed with the head of the bed raised or in a sitting position, and with good ventilation. Oxygen administration may be necessary during the acute period. Prolonged use is inadvisable as increasing the concentration of oxygen in the blood suppresses erythropoiesis. A blood transfusion of packed cells may be administered. Individuals may have questions about the safety of blood transfusions and wish to explore problems associated with this treatment, especially if they are required regularly on a long-term basis.

In the long term, if the person is active and employed it may be necessary to encourage adjustments to the normal life-style. The nurse should help the individual and family to evaluate the usual daily routines and identify activities that are priorities so that a plan may be developed which aims at avoiding sudden strenuous activity and scheduling rest periods. The person's activity tolerance is reviewed regularly and, taking the clinical condition into account, activity is increased or decreased accordingly.

2. Goal: the person's skin and mucosal tissues will remain intact and no accidental injury will be experienced

The reduced oxygen supply to the tissues renders the skin more susceptible to pressure and increases the risk of pressure sore development, especially if activity is limited. The person with anaemia should be carefully assessed, using a risk assessment scale such as Norton or Waterlow, and the appropriate precautionary measures instituted. This may range from 2-hourly changes of position to the use of special beds such as the Mediscus or Clinitron systems.

People with haemolytic anaemia who are jaundiced often experience pruritus (itching). Warm or tepid water is used for bathing and use of soap is avoided. Calamine lotion may be applied to relieve itching; the fingernails should be kept short and clean to prevent excoriation and infection should the patient scratch the irritated areas. Skin creams and emollients are useful in keeping skin supple and preventing dry, cracked skin.

In pernicious and iron deficiency anaemias ulcerative lesions of the oral mucosa and a sore, raw tongue may occur. Regular cool, mild mouthwashes may be soothing. A soft toothbrush is advised for cleaning the teeth. Hot spicy foods are best avoided and the mouth should be cleaned after taking nourishment.

The person who is very weak and dizzy as a result of their anaemia may be at risk from falls. It is important to assess this risk and remove from the patient's immediate environment any object that might cause injury. The person who has sensory loss as a result of anaemia may demonstrate poor co-ordination and be at risk of injury from dropping objects.

If the person with anaemia is also susceptible to infection, additional safety precautions may be required. These are discussed later in the chapter.

3. Goal: the person states he or she is pain free

The person with anaemia may experience angina-like pain, headache, pain due to marrow hyperplasia or pain due to vascular occlusion and ischaemia as a result of a sickle cell crisis. Whatever the cause the pain should be fully assessed, using a pain chart if appropriate, and analgesia administered as required to achieve pain relief. The person in a sickle cell crisis may require 4-hourly narcotic analgesia, but non-invasive measures such as rest of the affected part, local heat application, use of a bed cradle and relaxation techniques may also be valuable.

4. Goal: the person and family report improvement in thought processes

The person with anaemia should be observed for signs of confusion and slow intellectual responses. The person and family should be reassured that mental disturbance and a reduced concentration span are associated with the condition and should improve, as treatment, generally aimed at increasing the oxygen-carrying capacity of the blood, will also improve cerebral oxygenation.

5. Goal: the person is able to select appropriate foodstuffs and maintain an adequate dietary intake, as indicated by improvement in laboratory blood results

When nutrition has been identified as a problem the

nurse and dietician should discuss with the person and family the importance of diet. Food preferences are identified and help given to plan menus that will provide the necessary nutrients in an acceptable form. Foods should be light, easily digested and provide protein, iron, vitamins B_{12} and C and folic acid. Dietary sources of iron include red meats, liver, eggs, fish, green leafy vegetables, enriched whole grain cereals and bread and dried fruits. Meat is an excellent source of protein. Sources of B_{12} include red meats, liver, eggs and dairy produce. Folic acid is present in meat (especially liver), whole grain cereals, leafy vegetables, beans, brewer's yeast and dairy products. Citrus fruits and other fruits and vegetables are good sources of vitamin C.

Anorexia may be an accompanying problem and may be exacerbated if the person has a sore mouth. Small frequent meals and avoidance of certain foods may help. Mouth care is important and food should be presented attractively. Help with feeding and social contact at mealtimes should be provided as necessary. Elderly people at home may require a home help or meals-on-wheels, arranged with the assistance of the social worker. Social contacts can be provided through local authority luncheon clubs.

Extra fluids are important for the person with a haemolytic anaemia, especially sickle cell anaemia. The person who is hospitalized during a sickle cell crisis should have fluid intake recorded and may require intravenous hydration if unable to maintain a good oral intake (2–3 litres per 24 hours for an adult).

Dietary intake may be supplemented by prescription of oral iron preparations, folic acid or vitamin C. Vitamin B_{12} injections are administered intramuscularly for deficiency of intrinsic factor.

6. Goal: the person is able to describe the cause and characteristics of the anaemia and the treatment plan and discuss plans to modify lifestyle and minimize risk of complications

A full explanation of the nature of the disorder and reasons for symptoms experienced should be made to the individual and the family/members. The person is advised of changes that might indicate a recurrence of the disorder and a need to seek medical help.

Information should be provided about the prescribed treatment and plan of care and the person's understanding evaluated by having him or her carry out procedures such as medication administration and the planning and preparation of diet. Explanations should be provided about any prescribed drugs and possible adverse effects. For example, the person prescribed iron should be warned to expect dark stools and possible gastrointestinal irritation. Long-term iron therapy has a tendency to cause constipation and thus the importance of a high-fibre diet should be stressed. The necessity of getting regular maintenance doses of vitamin B_{12} should be stressed to the person with pernicious anaemia and a district nurse referral made to facilitate this if attendance at the clinic for the injections is not possible.

In the case of sickle cell anaemia, parents should receive an explanation of the disease and factors that predispose to crises. Children and parents can be advised of the importance of prophylactic care during remission. This involves living as normally as possible but avoiding chilling, contact with people with infections, high altitudes, overfatigue and stressful situations. A well-balanced diet, plenty of fluids and adequate rest are important. Proper dental care and immunization against infectious diseases are stressed, as well as attendance at clinics for regular physical and haematological assessment.

In the case of the schoolchild, parents are encouraged to inform the teacher and school nurse of the child's problem. Identification indicating that the person has sickle cell disease (e.g. a Medic Alert bracelet or pendant) should be carried at all times, as symptoms of a crisis may mimic other conditions. Referral to a support group or association (e.g. Sickle Cell Society) may provide additional help and support.

Individuals with a hereditary form of anaemia should be advised of genetic counselling opportunities for themselves and for their families.

Persons with haemolytic spherocytosis who have had a splenectomy, and persons with sickle cell anaemia or thalassaemia who have impairment of splenic function require teaching regarding the potential for post-splenectomy sepsis. Pneumococcal vaccine may be administered as a preventive measure.

EVALUATION

Objective measurement of the effectiveness of nursing intervention for the person with anaemia is provided by ongoing laboratory results which show that the haemoglobin, red blood cell counts, haematocrit, B_{12} and folate levels are within the normal range for the individual. The person will report a decrease or absence of the clinical symptoms previously identified.

Evaluation of patient and family teaching is based on assessment of their knowledge of dietary and treatment measures and their verbalization of strategies to control symptoms and resume usual daily activities. Questions regarding the therapeutic plan should be answered and the person should be aware of community resources for ongoing health care.

POLYCYTHAEMIA (ERYTHROCYTE EXCESS)

An excessive number of erythrocytes and a corresponding increase in the concentration of haemoglobin is referred to as polycythaemia. The red blood cell count may be $7–10 \times 10^{12}$ per litre (7–10 million per µl) with a haemoglobin concentration of 18–25 g/dl. The condition may be primary or secondary.

Secondary polycythaemia may be a physiological compensatory increase in the number of erythrocytes by the red bone marrow in response to a low concentration of oxygen in the blood and an increase in erythropoietin. It occurs normally at high altitudes where the atmospheric oxygen tension is low, and in pathological conditions in which there is tissue hypoxia. Examples of the latter are congenital malformations of the heart which lead to blood bypassing the pulmonary circulatory system, pulmonary conditions that interfere with normal gas exchange (e.g. emphysema, chronic bronchitis) and cardiac failure.

Primary polycythaemia is known as *polycythaemia vera*; it is a rare malignant disorder of the red bone marrow in which there is an uncontrolled production of an excessive number of red blood cells and haemoglobin. It may be accompanied by some overproduction of myeloctyes (leucocytes produced by the marrow) and platelets. The cause is unknown. The onset is usually in middle-aged persons, with a higher incidence in males and Jewish persons.

CLINICAL CHARACTERISTICS

Polycythaemia vera increases the total volume and viscosity of the blood. The blood pressure is elevated and the work-load of the heart is increased. The rate of flow through the vessels is reduced and, with the increased number of erythrocytes and blood viscosity, predisposes to the development of thrombi. Occlusion of a vessel may occur, causing a cerebral vascular accident, coronary thrombosis, pulmonary infarction or gangrene of a limb. Heart failure may develop insidiously as a result of the increased cardiac demands. The spleen enlarges because of the increased number of red blood cells to be destroyed.

Symptoms vary greatly; the individual may not experience any discomfort and be totally unaware of any problem until the excessive number of erythrocytes are discovered during the course of a regular physical examination. Symptoms may include headache, dizziness, a full feeling in the head, weakness and ready fatigue. The patient may complain of pruritus, especially after a hot bath, and pain in the bones as a result of hyperplasia of the red bone marrow. A high colour (deep dusky red) is manifested in the lips, nose, cheeks, ears and neck. The distal parts of the limbs (especially lower) may be cyanotic at times, owing to the sluggish circulation incurred by the increased viscosity of the blood. These patient's also have a tendency to develop a peptic ulcer which is attributed to an associated increase in gastric secretions. The person with secondary polycythaemia is usually cyanosed because of underlying cardiac or respiratory disease.

TREATMENT AND CARE

Treatment and care of patients with polycythaemia vera depends upon the age of the individual. A phlebotomy (venesection) is done at regular intervals to provide a temporary reduction in the blood volume. Five hundred to 1000 ml may be withdrawn each time. The normal blood donor equipment for the collection of blood is used. Additional therapy includes the use of myelosuppressant drugs or radioactive phosphorus (^{32}P) in the elderly. These agents are usually not used in younger persons because of the concern about their leukaemogenic potential. Red and glandular meats and iron-containing foods may be restricted in the patient's diet. Allopurinol is administered daily to lower the excessive serum uric acid level and relieve the inflammation and pain in the joints of the extremities.

These people are not usually treated as in-patients until a complication such as thrombosis, peptic ulcer or cardiac insufficiency develops. A reasonable amount of activity is encouraged to prevent circulatory stasis. They are advised of the need for regular, frequent visits to their general practitioner or the haematology clinic for close supervision. The family and patient are alerted to early indications of impending complications and advised of the importance of promptly contacting their general practitioner.

The Person with Leucocyte Disorders

Alterations in the number of leucotyes may involve an increased or decreased production of the cells.

LEUCOCYTOSIS

The number of leucocytes in circulation increases to a level in excess of the normal $4.0–11.0 \times 10^9/l$ in defence of the body in most infections and in response to necrotic tissue. This increase is referred to as leucocytosis and is usually predominant in one type of white cell. Information as to which type of leucocytes are in excess of the normal provides significant information for the doctor, since some leucocytoses are known to be associated with certain pathological conditions. For instance: neutrophil leucocytosis normally develops quickly in response to most infections (e.g. appendicitis, pneumonia) and tissue destruction (e.g. myocardial infarction); lymphocytosis is characteristic of certain infections such as measles, mumps, pertussis and infectious hepatitis; and an increase in eosinophils (eosinophilia) accompanies many allergic conditions. The white blood cell count returns to normal when the infection is controlled, the necrotic tissue is disposed of, or the initiating factor, such as an allergen, is removed.

LEUKAEMIA

Normal leucocytes progress from differentiated, proliferating blast cells (myeloblasts, lymphoblasts, monoblasts) to mature, non-proliferating, functioning white blood cells. Leukaemia is a disease in which there is an excessive uncontrolled production of leucocytes in blast form. They continue to proliferate and remain immature, and consequently are unable to perform their normal functions. The cell production is comparable to the uncontrolled production of cells in malignant neoplastic disease. For this reason leukaemia is sometimes referred to as cancer of the blood.

There is usually a marked increase in the number of leuocytes in circulation, and many of these are immature and abnormal. Their inability to perform their normal role in body defence makes the individual very susceptible to infection. Hyperplasia of the haemopoietic tissue, the accumulation of leucoblasts within it and disturbance of the normal regulatory mechanisms hamper the formation and maturation of erythrocytes and thrombocytes, leading to anaemia and thrombocytopenia. The circulating leukaemic cells infiltrate organs and tissues and cause dysfunction in these areas. The liver, spleen and lymph nodes are often enlarged.

The enlargement of viscera causes discomfort, pain and interference with neighbouring structures, and hyperplasia of the bone marrow causes tenderness and pain, especially in the long bones.

The marked overproduction of leucocytes and the rapid rate of other destruction result in an increase in the body's metabolic rate. The use of certain substances in the proliferation of these cells deprives other cells of essential metabolic elements (amino acids, vitamins, etc.) and results in wasting and weight loss as the disease progresses.

TYPES OF LEUKAEMIA

The leukaemias are divided into two basic types, each of which may be acute or chronic, depending on the rapidity of onset. Lymphoblastic leukaemia (LL) begins in the lymphocytic precursors of the lymph nodes or other lymphogenous tissue. Non-lymphoblastic leukaemia (NLL) or myelogenous leukaemia (ML) begins in the myelogenous cells of the bone marrow and then spreads to other areas of the body.

Acute lymphoblastic leukaemias (ALL)

These can be classified morphologically, or by using immunological markers, into three types: common ALL, which accounts for about 70% of cases of ALL, T-cell and B-cell ALL (Soutami and Tobias, 1986). Special techniques for testing markers which provide further subsets of ALL cells are now being used. Identification of cell characteristics are useful in diagnosis, treatment and predicting outcomes.

Acute myeloid leukaemia (AML) or acute non-lymphoblastic leukaemia (ANLL) is subdivided as follows (Eastham, 1984)

1. Classification M_1 to M_3 designates myeloblastic leukaemia which differs in the extent of maturation of the white blood cells. Type M_1 cells are immature while M_2 cells are predominantly myeloblasts and promyeloblasts. Type M_3 cells are mostly abnormal promyeloblasts with extensive granulation
2. M_4—myelomonocytic leukaemia
3. M_5—monocytic leukaemia with monoblasts predominating
4. M_6—erythroleukaemia
5. M_7—megakaryoblastic leukaemia

INCIDENCE

Leukaemia occurs in all age groups. Below 15 years of age ALL accounts for 80% of all cases and AML for most of the rest. Over 15 years of age 85% of cases are AML, and its incidence increases with age, especially over 50 years of age (Soutami and Tobias, 1986).

While extensive research for the cause of leukaemia and for a means of preventing and curing the disorder continues, chemotherapeutic agents used in recent years have produced remissions and prolonged the life of those with acute leukaemia. The therapeutic regimen is directed toward reducing the production of leukaemic cells and preventing associated complications, such as infection, anaemia and haemorrhage. The chronic forms of the disease progress slowly, are less malignant and manifest more normal mature leucocytes in the blood.

AETIOLOGY

Leukaemia, although highly treatable, is considered to be a fatal disease of unknown aetiology in most instances. Factors within the patient that predispose to leukaemia include: chromosomal abnormality (e.g. Down's syndrome), chronic marrow dysfunction (e.g. aplastic anaemia), immunodeficiency and inherited genetic disorders, e.g. Fanconi's anaemia and Bloom syndrome. Environmental factors contributing to the development of leukaemia include: radiation, chemicals and viruses (Gillis, 1988). There is significant evidence that overexposure to ionizing radiation is the causative factor in some cases. This is substantiated by the high incidence of leukaemia found in the survivors of the Hiroshima and Nagasaki atomic bombing, radiologists, and patients with ankylosing spondylitis (arthritis of the spine) who were treated by X-ray radiation. Absorption of the chemicals benzol, pyridine and aniline dyes have been strongly suspected of being leukaemogenic. Previous treatment with cytotoxic drugs, especially alkylating agents, predispose to the development of acute leukaemias. A human T-cell leukaemia virus, called HTLV-1, has been isolated. This causes a specific type of leukaemia that is distinct from other T-cell cancers. It is rare in North American and European populations but is found in the Caribbean, Japan, Africa and South America. Regardless of the initial cause, the uncontrolled production of leucocytes is the result of a cancerous mutation of a myelogenous or a lymphogenous cell (Guyton, 1991). Studies have shown that chromosomal abnormalities are frequently present in the leucocytes involved.

CLINICAL CHARACTERISTICS

Acute leukaemia usually has an abrupt onset that is frequently accompanied by weakness, general malaise and non-specific complaints. Fever, excessive perspiration, lowered heat tolerance, tachycardia and weight loss develop because of the increased metabolic rate. Bone marrow dysfunction and the resulting anaemia are manifested by pallor, shortness of breath, extreme fatigue, weakness and palpitation. External and internal bleeding may occur due to the reduced production of thrombocytes. Bleeding of the gums, nose and gastrointestinal tract is common. Petechiae or ecchymoses may appear as further evidence of the reduced ability of the blood to coagulate. The patient with myelogenous leukaemia will most likely complain of tenderness and pain in the long bones and sternum from the hyperplasia and crowding in the bone marrow.

Although there is an excessive number of leucocytes, they are immature and do not provide the normal defence against infection. The patient may complain of a sore mouth and throat which exhibit infected necrotic ulcers. An acute infection such as pneumonia, septicaemia or perirectal abscess may develop. The spleen and liver enlarge and, in the later stages, infiltration of the leukaemic cells into the kidneys may cause renal insufficiency. Renal dysfunction also occurs as a result of the excessive blood concentration of uric acid produced by the rapid destruction of the leucocytes. Urate crystals may form and obstruct renal tubules. Sensory and motor disturbances, severe headache, convulsions or disorientation may occur, indicating central nervous system involvement. Lymph nodes enlarge and are tender, owing to infiltration by the leukaemic cells. This may be readily detected in the axillary, cervical and inguinal lymph nodes.

The leucocyte count varies greatly but is usually above normal and may exceed 100×10^9 per litre. In some instances, the count is within normal levels or may even be below normal. This is attributed to the bone marrow retaining the leucocytes because of their immature state; normally, they are not released until mature. The erythrocyte and thrombocyte counts are abnormally low. A specimen of aspirated bone marrow demonstrates the proliferation of leukaemic cells.

The *chronic forms of leukaemia* have an insidious onset, but are slowly progressive. They may go unrecognized for a lengthy period. The disovery is often made when the individual undergoes a regular physical checkup or is being investigated for some unrelated condition.

Chronic myelocytic (granulocytic) leukaemia (CML) is manifested by a progressive development of weakness, loss of weight, anaemia and thrombocytopenia. The granulocytes are in excess and upon examination reveal a deficiency of alkaline phosphatase and glycogen and an increased histamine content. A chromosomal abnormality (the Philadelphia chromosome) is detectable in the cultured marrow cells of up to 90% of people with CML. In the advanced stage of the disorder, the enlarged spleen may cause considerable discomfort; an infarction within it may precipitate acute, severe pain in the upper left abdomen. Large ecchymoses and other signs of bleeding appear. The person with CML becomes progressively weaker because of the increased anaemia. In this later stage the number of immature granulocytes (myeloblasts) in circulation shows a marked increase and may result in leucostasis, a medical emergency causing visual defects, priapism, confusion and coma. Pain is experienced in the sternum and long bones owing to marrow hyperplasia. Within 3–6 years following diagnosis the disease may evolve into acute leukaemia (acute blastic crisis) which resembles AML (Soutami and Tobias, 1986).

CML can occur at any age but is more common in middle and old age.

Chronic lymphocytic leukaemia (CLL) is a disease of the elderly and the rate at which it progressively develops varies with patients. Some remain free of symptoms and in relatively good health with only mild anaemia and a moderate increase in lymphocytes for several years. In others the leukaemic process slowly but steadily increases in severity. The blood picture is one of an increased leucocyte count, with small atypical B-lymphocytes predominating. There is a variable degree of anaemia and thrombocytopenia. The person experiences recurring infections because the immune

and defence mechanisms are impaired; antibodies are not formed in antigenic response to organisms. The spleen, liver and lymph nodes enlarge; pressure on neighbouring structures may cause impaired function, discomfort and pain. In the advanced stage many more immature lymphocytes (lymphoblasts) appear in the circulation and the anaemia and deficiency of thrombocytes become severe.

TREATMENT OF THE PATIENT WITH LEUKAEMIA

The treatment and care of the patient with leukaemia are directed toward suppressing the abnormal cell production, the prevention of complications (infection and haemorrhage), and supporting the patient physiologically and psychologically. A person who has normal blood counts and normal bone marrow with no signs and symptoms following treatment is said to be in *remission*.

Chemotherapy is the main treatment modality used for acute leukaemias. The first phase of treatment aims to induce remission within a few weeks. This may be consolidated with further courses of treatment and additional drugs to prevent early relapse. In ALL, intrathecal chemotherapy and whole brain irradiation are used to prevent recurrence in the central nervous system. Maintenance therapy is continued on an outpatient basis for up to 2 years to eliminate any residual disease.

Drug therapy

The chemotherapeutic programme for the patient with acute leukaemia involves a variety of drugs which are given in combinations or singly. Selection of the drugs depends on accurate identification of the type of leukaemia. The chronic leukaemias are treated much less aggressively. Symptomatic control may be achieved using single-agent therapy. Antileukaemic agents act by interfering with cell mitosis and the synthesis of the leucocyte cellular substance, and by depressing the red bone marrow. Unfortunately they affect normal cells, especially those which reproduce rapidly (e.g. mucous membrane, erythrocytes), in addition to leukaemic cells, and produce serious side-effects with which the nurse must be familiar as they necessitate physiological and psychological supportive measures. Table 13.9 lists common antileukaemic agents. The most common side-effects associated with these chemotherapeutic agents are nausea, vomiting, stomatitis and ulceration, alopecia (loss of hair), change in bowel habit (diarrhoea or constipation) and bone marrow suppression that predisposes the individual to infection and haemorrhage.

Nursing responsibilities associated with drug therapy include the following. It is important that the nurse be familiar with the expected action, route of administration used and the potential side-effects of the antileukaemic agents. The patient is advised of the possible effects, that support will be provided and that those drugs now available do bring about a remission and permit the individual to leave the hospital and resume many former activities. Opportunities should be provided for the patient and family to ask questions and

Table 13.9   Antileukaemic agents.

Agent	Classification	Administration	Potential side-effects
Vincristine (Oncovin)	Plant alkaloid Inhibits mitosis of leukaemic cells	Intravenous	Mild alopecia Abdominal cramps Constipation Nervous system disturbances: hyporeflexia, abnormal gait, loss of coordination, stumbling, paresthesia, peripheral neuritis, paralytic ileus Tissue necrosis with extravasation
Prednisone	Hormone—an adrenocorticosteroid Retards leukaemic cell reproduction	Oral Intravenous	Gastric distress and ulceration Decreased immune responses and increased susceptibility to infection Retention of fluid Diabetes mellitus Hypertension
L-Asparaginase	Enzyme Deprives leukaemic cells of amino acid, L-asparagine	Intramuscular Intravenous	Anaphylactic shock Allergic reactions Impaired liver and pancreatic functions (hyperglycaemia) Depression (psychological)
Methotrexate	Folic acid analogue Deprives leukaemic cells of folic acid	Oral Intravenous Intrathecal	Bone marrow depression Oral and gastrointestinal ulceration and bleeding Nausea, vomiting, diarrhoea Dermatitis Impaired liver function and failure CNS effects: dizziness, blurred vision
6-Mercaptopurine	Purine analogue Deprives leukaemic cells of essential purine	Oral	Bone marrow depression Nausea and diarrhoea (with large doses) Stomatitis (with large doses)
Cyclophosphamide (Endoxana)	Alkylating agent Suppresses leukaemic cell reproduction	Oral Intravenous	Nausea and vomiting Bone marrow depression Haemorrhagic cystitis Alopecia Amenorrhoea/reduced spermatogenesis
Daunorubicin (daunomycin, rubidomycin)	Antibiotic Inhibits synthesis of normal cellular substance (DNA)	Intravenous	Nausea and vomiting Stomatitis Fever Alopecia Bone marrow depression Cardiac toxicity Tissue necrosis with extravasation
Doxorubicin (Adriamycin)	Antibiotic Inhibits DNA synthesis and DNA-dependent RNA synthesis	Intravenous	Nausea, vomiting Bone marrow depression Stomatitis Alopecia Liver and cardiac toxicity Tissue necrosis with extravasation

Table 13.9 *continued*

Agent	Classification	Administration	Potential side-effects
Cytarabine (cystosine arabinoside ara-C, Cytosar)	Pyrimidine analogue	Intravenous Intrathecal Subcutaneous	Nausea and vomiting Bone marrow depression Stomatitis Neurotoxicity with intrathecal use Cerebellar toxicity with high dose Transient influenza-like syndrome
Thioguanine (6TG)	Purine analogue	Oral	Bone marrow depression Diarrhoea Hepatitis
Etoposide (VP-16)	Prevents mitosis Interferes with DNA synthesis	Oral Intravenous	Bone marrow depression (leucopenia, thrombocytopenia) Nausea and vomiting Alopecia Immunosuppression Severe hypotension if infused too rapidly
Busulphan (Myleran)	Aklylating agent Interferes with mitosis	Oral	Bone marrow depression Alopecia Nausea, vomiting, diarrhoea Pulmonary fibrosis Hyperpigmenation of the skin Amenorrhoea/reduced spermato-genesis
Chlorambucil (Leukeran)	Alkylating agent Antimetabolic action	Oral	Nausea and vomiting Bone marrow depression Amenorrhoea/reduced spermato-genesis
Hydroxyurea	Antimetabolic	Oral	Nausea and vomiting Bone marrow depression Skin reactions Diarrhoea
Amsacrine (Amsidine)	Inhibits DNA synthesis	Intravenous	Bone marrow depression Mucositis Nausea and vomiting Headache, dizziness Alopecia, skin rash Liver and cardiac toxicity
Vinblastine (Velbe)	Plant alkaloid Inhibits mitosis of leukaemic cell	Intravenous	Bone marrow depression Mild alopecia Neurotoxicity: mild paraesthesia, constipation, jaw pain Tissue necrosis with extravasation

discuss feelings about therapy and reactions to it. If the individual's need for information and assurance are not met, he or she cannot participate fully in decisions regarding care.

A frequent assessment is made of the patient for changes and manifestations of reactions to the drug(s). Nursing measures should be instituted promptly to provide necessary support and relief. For example, nausea may be prevented by administering an antiemetic before the antileukaemic drug is given and throughout the course of the infusion; relaxation techniques, reducing external stimuli by dimming the light and disturbing the patient as little as possible are helpful.

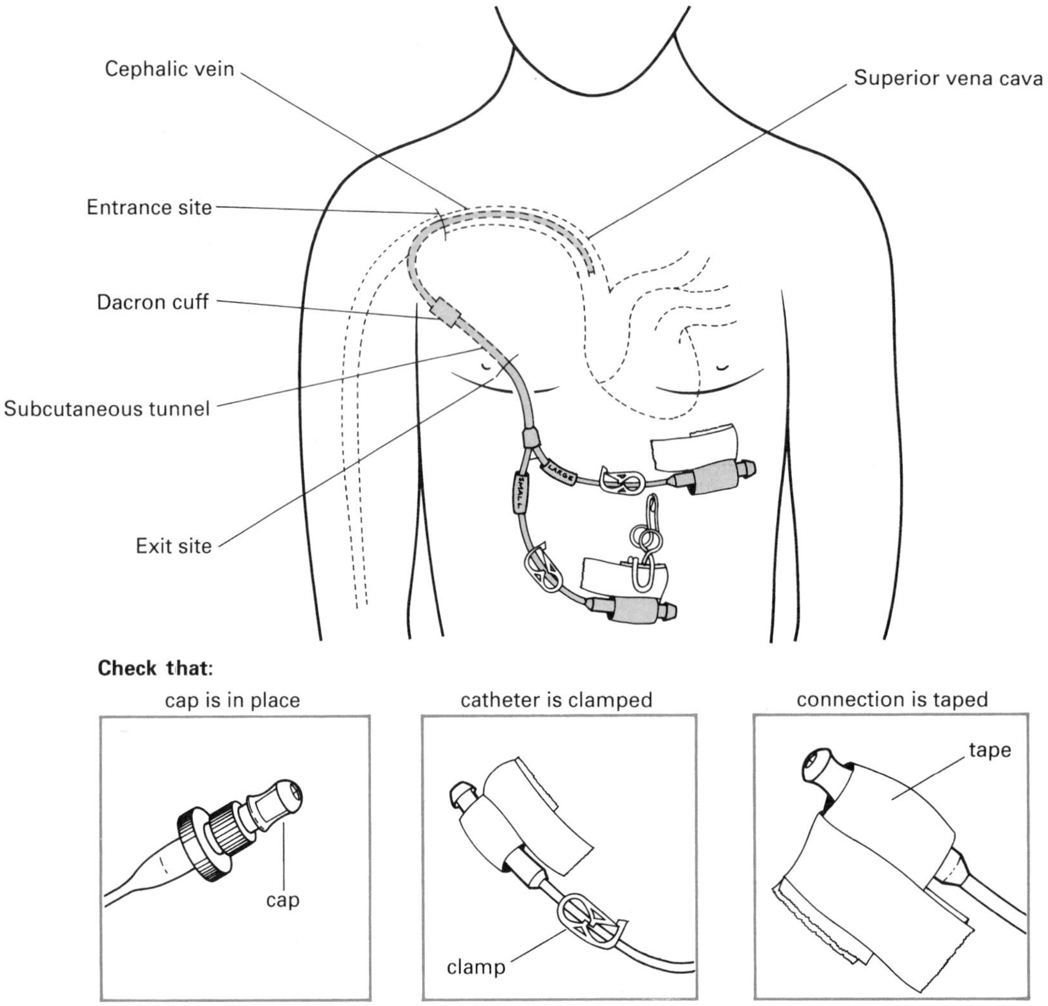

Check that:

Figure 13.7 Central venous catheter: placement and safety precautions to be observed.

Since most patients receive repeated courses of intravenous chemotherapy and also require many laboratory tests necessitating withdrawal of blood samples, care must be taken to preserve the integrity of the patient's veins. The need for tests should be reviewed and if necessary withdrawal of blood specimens should be done when the intravenous line is being started to decrease the number of venepunctures. A central venous catheter (Figure 13.7) may be inserted and can be used for drug administration, blood product support and nutritional supplementation. Multiple lumens in the central venous catheter facilitate the administration of several infusions at one time. Patients may be receiving total parenteral nutrition, antibiotics, antiemetics, packed red blood cells, platelets and chemotherapeutic agents intravenously. The larger lumen of the catheter is reserved for the withdrawal of blood and the administration of blood and blood products. Precautions include the use of Luer–Lok connections on all intravenous tubing, the taping of all connections and

use of clamps when changing equipment. Each line of the catheter has a coloured marker to facilitate identification. Care must be taken not to confuse the lines of the catheter and intravenous solution and the tubing connected to each line. The catheter is capped when not in use allowing the patient to participate in most daily activities. Each lumen of the catheter is flushed regularly with normal saline or a solution of heparin to keep it patent when it is not being used. Clinical studies, although of varying degrees of rigour, show saline flushes at either 8-hour or 24-hour intervals to be equally as effective as heparin flushes in maintaining patency of closed central venous lines (Dunn and Lenihan, 1987). A second study reported twice as many restarts and a higher incidence of phlebitis at the catheter insertion site when saline flushes were used instead of the usual heparin flushes (Cyganski et al, 1987). There is a need for further trials to evaluate clinical practices which have developed quickly in response to new technology. Evidence related to the effectiveness of dressing procedures is also lacking, although there is strong support for the continued use of povidone–iodine solutions and ointments to decrease the incidence of infection at the catheter insertion sites. The patient or a family member is taught to irrigate the catheter lines regularly with a

solution of heparin or a referral is made to the district nurse. Table 13.10 lists the content for a programme to teach patients and families to care for the central venous catheter, to prevent complications and what to do if problems occur. Table 13.10 also lists patient goals for the patient teaching programme.

Table 13.10 Patient goals for self-care and management of long-term central venous catheters.

- *Patient Information.* The patient and/or family members will be able to:
  - (a) State the purpose and use of central venous catheters
  - (b) State three essential safety points that should be checked several times daily
  - (c) State the purpose of flushing the catheter
  - (d) State the frequency of performing the heparin or saline flush procedure
- *Practice.* The patient and/or family members will be able to:
  - (a) Demonstrate ability to fill a syringe with solution safely
  - (b) Demonstrate ability to flush the central venous catheter safely

- *Safety precautions.* The patient and/or family members will be able to:
  - (a) State actions to take if the catheter cap comes off
  - (b) State action to take to prevent puncture of the catheter
  - (c) State actions to take if the catheter is punctured
  - (d) State actions to take if the catheter becomes blocked
  - (e) Describe signs which may indicate infection at the catheter site
  - (f) State actions to take if signs of infection are present
  - (g) State plans to obtain a Medic Alert identification
- *Use of community resources.* The patient and/or family members will be able to describe plans for community nursing services

PATIENT INFORMATION

What is a long-term central venous catheter?
The central venous catheter is a narrow, silicone rubber tube which is inserted through the skin and into a vein on your upper chest or shoulder. The tip of the catheter is situated in a large vein near the heart. The outer end is tunnelled a few inches along the chest wall just under the skin and then comes out to the surface. This is the section you can see.

The catheter has one or more *lumens* or lines. Each line has a cap and a clamp at the end of it. The cap is taped in place and the clamp is kept closed when the line is not in use.

The purpose of the catheter
The long term central venous catheter provides a ready access to the circulation. It can be used to give medications, blood products or nutritional therapy. It can also be used to withdraw blood samples.

Routine care of the catheter
When the catheter is not being used, there are three important points you should check to ensure that the catheter is completely closed off.

Check to see that:
1. Each cap is in place
2. The clamp is closed on each line
3. Each connection is taped at the cap

Observations should be done:
1. When you get up in the morning
2. Before and after bathing (showering)
3. When dressing
4. Before going to bed

Routine maintenance of the catheter
Flushing of the catheter (lines):
When the catheter is not in use, each line must be flushed with heparin or saline regularly to prevent clotting in the

lines. You will be told how often to flush your catheter and how much solution to use in each catheter line.

How to flush each line
1. Gather the equipment. You will need:
   - Syringe and needle for each line
   - Alcohol wipes
   - Heparin or saline solution (*heparin should be stored in refrigerator*). Check the label on the heparin bottle.
2. Wash your hands. *Hands should be thoroughly washed using soap and running water and scrubbing for 3 minutes.*
3. Connect the needle to the syringe, without touching the connecting ends with your fingers.

PRACTICE

To fill syringe with heparin (saline)
1. Vigorously clean the top of the heparin (saline) bottle with an alcohol wipe for about 30 seconds.
2. With the cap on the needle, pull back on the syringe to the designated ml mark.
3. Remove the cap from the needle. Be sure you *do not touch* the needle.
4. Holding the bottle on a firm surface, insert the needle into the rubber cap of the bottle.
5. Push the plunger down to inject the air into the bottle.
6. Invert the bottle and syringe. Be sure the tip of the needle is in the solution.
7. Pull back on the plunger and fill the syringe to the __ ml mark with the heparin (saline) solution.
8. Check that there are no air bubbles in the syringe. If there are, tap the syringe to force the bubbles to rise to the needle. Push plunger to rid syringe of air bubbles. Re-fill syringe to __ ml mark with solution.
9. Withdraw needle from bottle.
10. Replace cap on needle and return solution to refrigerator

Table 13.10 *continued*

How to inject heparin (saline) into the line
1. Vigorously clean the end of the cap with alcohol for about 30 seconds.
2. Insert the needle of the syringe into the cap.
3. Release the clamp.
4. Inject the heparin (saline) slowly up to the last ½ ml.
5. Replace the clamp.
6. Gently press on the plunger of the syringe to check that no more solution goes in.
7. Remove the needle from the cap.
8. Check that the cap is secure and taped and that the clamp is closed.
Repeat the flushing procedure for each catheter line.

SAFETY PRECAUTIONS

What problems can occur?
If you follow the instructions to check your catheter several times a day and to flush each line, you should not encounter any problems. Problems that might happen are:
- The cap could loosen.
- The tubing could be punctured.
- The tubing could become blocked.
- Infection could develop at the exit site.

These problems are quite simple to handle. But it is important that you take immediate action should any of these situations occur.

What to do if the cap comes off
1. Check that the clamp is closed. If it is open, close it immediately.
2. Vigorously clean the end of the catheter with an alcohol swab.
3. Put a new sterile cap on the catheter. You will be given an extra cap that you should keep with you at home.
4. Retape the cap in place.
5. Recheck to be sure the clamp is closed.

Puncture of the catheter
The catheter is made of silicone rubber and can be easily punctured by a needle, pin or other sharp objects.

To prevent puncture of the catheter:
1. Take care when flushing the line. Hold the catheter straight and insert the needle into the centre of the cap and line. If the catheter is bent or at an angle, the needle

could possibly puncture the side of the catheter.
2. Avoid wearing jewellery, pins or other sharp objects on your clothing over the area of the catheter.

If the catheter should be punctured, close the clamp immediatley. If the damage is between the clamp and your chest, clamp the catheter with your metal bulldog clamp. Place the clamp between your chest and the damaged area. Go to the Emergency or Outpatient Department of the hospital where the catheter was inserted, or call your visiting nurse.

What to do if the catheter is blocked
If your catheter should become blocked and you are not able to inject the heparin (or saline) first check that the catheter is not kinked, then check that the clamp is released when you are injecting the solution.
Next change your position; take a deep breath and lift both your arms.
If you are still not able to inject the solution, clamp the catheter and call the visiting nurse or go to the Outpatient or Emergency Department of the hospital where the catheter was inserted.

How to watch for signs of infection
The exit site to the catheter should be checked daily through the transparent dressing for any signs of infection.
Changes that might indicate an infection at the exit site are: Redness, tenderness, swelling and drainage.
If an infection is present at the exit site or anywhere else in your body, you may also have an increase in your temperature.
Report these changes immediately to your doctor, visiting nurse or clinic.

Medic Alert identification
The presence of a central venous catheter is not apparent under your clothing. In case of an emergency it is advisable to wear a Medic Alert identification bracelet or necklace and carry a card describing the catheter.

USE OF COMMUNITY RESOURCES

When you are at home your general practitioner and district nurse will be able to help you obtain further equipment (syringes, solutions, etc.). Should you have any concerns, questions or problems, discuss them with the community team. Show them this booklet so they will know what you have been taught.

Modified from *Self Care Management of Long Term Central Venous Catheters*, St Joseph's Hospital, Hamilton, Ontario (revised March 1989).

Supportive therapy during periods of bone marrow depression may consist of the administration of red blood cells to combat the associated anaemia and platelets to control bleeding. Packed red blood cells are administered if the patient's haemoglobin is less than 10 g/dl. Platelets may be administered to prevent bleeding as well as to treat active bleeding. During periods of severe bone marrow depression from the induction chemotherapy, platelet transfusions may be required daily to maintain a platelet count greater than 20×10^9 per litre. During and immediately following any administration of blood products, the patient is

observed closely for adverse reactions; examples of these are outlined later in the chapter. The patient may receive corticosteroids, paracetamol (Panadol) or antihistamines prior to the transfusion of platelets or packed red blood cells to reduce the possibility of reaction.
A combination of antibiotics, including an aminoglycoside (gentamycin) and a semisynthetic penicillin, are administered promptly if signs of infection appear. The neutropenic patient with an altered immune system is very susceptible to infection, which can be life threatening. Antibiotic therapy is continued until the

patient's white blood cell count rises following chemotherapy. Granulocyte transfusions may also be prescribed.

Total parenteral nutrition may be administered if the patient has severe stomatitis and is unable to swallow or retain nutrients. Care of the patient receiving total parenteral nutrition is discussed in Chapter 16.

BONE MARROW TRANSPLANTATION

A bone marrow transplant consists of the intravenous administration of marrow cells. It is used in the treatment of persons with acute lymphoblastic leukaemia, acute and chronic myelogenous leukaemias, aplastic anaemia, and severe combined immune deficiency syndrome. While still experimental, success rates are continuously increasing. Bone marrow transplantation offers a potential cure for many persons and should be discussed as a treatment option. There are two types: *allogenic* transplants, which use bone marrow from a compatible and healthy donor, usually a family member, and *autologous* transplants, which use the person's own marrow, obtained during a period of remission in the disease process and cryopreserved and stored for transplantation. The patient receives high-dose chemotherapy, with or without total body irradiation, prior to the bone marrow transplant. This not only destroys leukaemic cells but also suppresses the immune system; the patient must therefore be cared for in a pathogen-reduced environment. Long-term survival of patients receiving bone marrow transplants is greatest in patients who achieve a complete remission of the disease following induction therapy. When making a decision related to bone marrow transplantation, the patient and family should be aware of alternative treatment, and consideration should be given to the patient's age and personal wishes (Milliken et al, 1988).

Nursing care of the patient receiving a bone marrow transplant focuses on the prevention of infection, maintaining nutritional status, prevention and control of bleeding (see p. 169) (Edwards, 1989).

Graft-versus-host disease, in which the donor T lymphocytes immunologically attack host tissue, is a major complication in allogenic transplants. All blood products administered to the patient, with the exception of the donor marrow, are irradiated prior to use. Treatment of the syndrome includes the administration of corticosteroids, cyclosporine or methotrexate. Relapse is a major problem encountered with autologous transplants.

NURSING IMPLICATIONS

Leukaemia is a life-threatening disease. Like other people with cancer, people with leukaemia require frequent and often prolonged episodes of hospitalization, causing stress to the individual and family. Nurses have a vital part to play in enabling the person with leukaemia to come to terms with diagnosis and treatment and its sequelae. Nursing measures for the person with cancer are discussed in Chapter 10. Nurses are in close and prolonged contact with the patient and are pivotal members of the multidisciplinary care team. They may be concerned as much with the person's psychosocial problems as with the physical problems.

When the person with leukaemia is a child, creation of a trusting partnership between the child, parents and siblings and the nursing staff is essential. Given good psychosocial support, parents may be encouraged to be the primary care-givers, if they so desire.

CLINICAL SITUATIONS

The following clinical situations illustrate differences in symptoms, disease progression, treatment protocols and individual responses to therapy for two people with different types of leukaemia. The situations have been adapted from actual clinical situations (with the permission of Denise Bryant, Clinical Nurse Specialist).

1. Ms Susan Rees, A young woman with acute lymphoblastic leukaemia

Susan Rees, a 17-year-old female student experienced left flank pain for 1 month prior to admission. One week prior to admission she developed headaches, weakness and lethargy. On admission to hospital she was febrile.

Clinical and diagnostic findings
- Temperature of 39.4°C (infected finger likely cause of fever)
- Tachycardia with a heart rate of 100/minute
- Blood pressure: 100/70 lying, 90/60 standing
- Normal neurological examination
- Palpable liver and spleen (splenomegaly was the likely cause of left flank pain)
- Full blood count: haemoglobin 6.6 mmol/l; white blood cell count 1.0×10^9/l with 38% abnormal blast cells
- Platelets 90 000.

Immediate care for Susan included hydration and the administration of broad-spectrum antibiotics.

Further investigations included:

- Bone marrow biopsy and aspirate
- Computerized tomographic (CT) brain scan to rule out central nervous system (CNS) disease
- Abdominal ultrasound examination
- Chest X-rays (posteroanterior and lateral views)
- Lumbar puncture to rule out CNS disease.

Results
- Bone marrow studies showed acute lymphoblastic leukaemia
- CT scan: brain normal
- Abdominal ultrasound: negative for enlarged liver and spleen as well as negative for abdominal and pelvic lymphadenopathy
- Chest X-rays negative for mediastinal adenopathy
- Lumbar puncture: pressure normal, cerebrospinal fluid clear, no abnormal cells.

Treatment
Susan was started on the current UK all treatment protocol which uses multiple combinations of intravenous, oral and intrathecal (into spinal fluid) chemotherapy in several phases, including induction, consolidation and maintenance treatment over a period of 2 years.

Evaluation

After 1 month of treatment she was in remission. Susan completed 2 years of treatment successfully; however, 6 months after her treatments, she relapsed, showing reinvolvement of the central nervous system and bone marrow. She has now gone into a second remission as a result of further treatment with second-line chemotherapy. Plans are in progress for an unrelated donor bone marrow transplant or an autologous transplant, with purging of Susan's own marrow with monoclonal antibodies. However, her prognosis is guarded for the long term.

2. Mr Brian Peters, a man with acute myeloid leukaemia

Mr Brian Peters is a 36-year-old man who is married and has three children. He was employed as a labourer in a wiring factory where he had been exposed to several chemicals.

Brian presented at the haematology clinic with a 3-month history of fatigue and headaches. Full blood count (FBC) done at the onset of his illness was normal, with the exception of a mildly decreased platelet count.

Clinical and diagnostic findings

Brian had experienced fevers, rigors (acute episodes of shivering), and night sweats over the previous 2 weeks. He had a 5-kg weight loss. He also complained of shortness of breath and a pressure sensation in his chest. His FBC on admission to hospital showed:

- Haemoglobin 8.7 mmol/l
- White blood cell count $2.96 \times 10^9/l$
- Platelet count of 51 000
- Erythrocyte sedimentation rate (ESR) elevated to 107 mm/hour
- Bone marrow tests showed acute myeloid leukaemia.

Treatment

Brian received standard induction chemotherapy and his disease went into remission. He had two subsequent courses of consolidation chemotherapy. All courses of chemotherapy were complicated by sepsis. Post chemotherapy, Brian developed herpes zoster.

Evaluation

Approximately 11 months after diagnosis, Brian had a recurrence of his acute leukaemia. He chose to receive chemotherapy to attempt a second remission but suffered multiple problems, with sepsis and bleeding, and died before completing the course of chemotherapy.

LEUCOPENIA

Leucopenia may be defined as a reduction in the number of leucocytes below the normal lower limit of 5.0×10^9 per litre. It may be due to a decreased production or excessive destruction of leucocytes. The deficiency occurs most often in the granulocytes, especially in neutrophils. Lymphopenia, a deficiency of lymphocytes, occurs rarely but is seen occasionally in patients receiving an adrenocorticoid preparation or adrenocorticotropic hormone (ACTH) and in those with uraemia.

AGRANULOCYTOSIS (NEUTROPENIA)

Agranulocytosis is characterized by a marked reduction in neutrophils.

CAUSES

In most instances, this blood disorder is the result of the toxic effects of certain drugs in persons with a sensitivity or idiosyncrasy. The drugs found most frequently to be offenders include gold salts, sulphonamides, amidopyrine, phenylbutazone (Butazolidin) and chlorpromazine (Largactil). The condition may also be associated with typhoid fever, malaria, miliary (widespread throughout the body) tuberculosis or any severe, overwhelming infection (e.g. septicaemia).

Neutropenia may be an integral part of the aplastic anaemia that may develop with radiation and anticancer drug therapy, or it may be due to an excessive destruction of the neutrophils by the spleen (hypersplenism). The disease has a higher incidence in females than in males.

CLINICAL CHARACTERISTICS

Neutrophils play an important role in defending the body against infection because of their ability to ingest and destroy organisms. Neutropenia lowers the normal resistance to infection, resulting in prompt invasion of the mucous membranes and skin by pathogenic organisms. The source of the infecting organisms may be the individual's own body flora.

The disease usually has a sudden onset and is manifested by chills, fever and hypotension. A pyrexia and rigors often develop without any obvious infective focus. The mouth, throat, skin and perineum are all potential sources of infected lesions. Urinary tract and respiratory infections may also develop, so a chest X-ray and midstream specimen of urine are usually obtained. Some patients complain of severe joint pain (arthralgia). The neutrophil count may be less than 1.5×10^9 per litre of blood.

TREATMENT AND NURSING CARE

Goals for the patient with neutropenia are to: (1) avoid infections occurring and, should an infection develop, (2) be able to recognize the signs immediately and seek medical help.

Treatment of neutropenia includes prompt elimination of any suspected cause. Intravenous antibiotic therapy in large doses is commenced promptly to prevent infection and blood cultures are taken to identify the infective organism. If the infection can be prevented or controlled and supportive care provided, a gradual increase in the number of neutrophils and improvement in the patient's condition may be expected in 1–2 weeks.

Nursing intervention for the patient with neutropenia is directed toward controlling the patient's environment in order to decrease contact with infectious agents and prompt identification and treatment of infections. The assessment, goals, identification of problems, nursing intervention and expected outcomes for the patient with an increased potential for infection are presented in Chapter 6.

PREVENTION OF NEUTROPENIA

All drugs that might have contributed to an affected person's neutropenia should be discontinued. It is important to inform people that drugs should only be taken under medical supervision and according to specific directions. It is not uncommon to learn of someone who has been taking a potentially dangerous drug unsupervised over an abnormally long period of time. Equally dangerous is the situation in which a family member, neighbour or friend share a drug. They do not appreciate that a drug may affect one person quite differently from another and that it is prescribed by the doctor on an individual basis following a careful study of the patient's condition. Reactions and side-effects to drugs are unpredictable, but if the drug prescribed is likely to cause neutropenia, careful supervision is necessary and the person should be taught to recognize early toxic manifestations.

The Person with Disorders of the Plasma Cells

MULTIPLE MYELOMA (MYELOMATOSIS)

Multiple myeloma is a malignant disease characterized by a proliferation of abnormal plasma cells in the bone marrow. Plasma cells are involved in the synthesis of the immunoglobulins that function as antibodies. In multiple myeloma the malignant plasma cells proliferate in the bone marrow, producing abnormal immunoglobulins known as paraproteins and forming diffuse, multiple solid tumours. It occurs in middle to late age and affects both sexes.

CLINICAL CHARACTERISTICS

Diffuse areas of bone destruction develop; these areas may coalesce and leave large 'punched out lesions'. The breakdown in bone structure frequently results in pathological fractures, especially in weight-bearing bones such as the vertebrae. The patient experiences pain in the areas of the bone lesions, which worsens with movement, jarring and pressure. The vertebrae are a common site of involvement, and pressure on nerve roots by the tumours and/or collapsing vertebrae causes severe back and/or lower limb pain; interruption of nerve impulses may give rise to paraplegia. Changes in posture and stature become evident. The ribs and skull bones are frequently affected. As tumours and areas of bone destruction develop in the skull, soft subcutaneous masses may be palpated. As the disease progresses, the patient has more and more pain and becomes increasingly incapacitated and deformed. Skeletal X-rays show areas of bone destruction.

The excessive production of abnormal plasma cells results in a decrease in the synthesis of normal immunoglobulins. This decrease in normal antibodies predisposes the patient to infections which are usually respiratory, but bladder infection and skin lesions are not uncommon.

The production of leucocytes, erythrocytes and thrombocytes diminishes as the bone marrow is crowded and replaced by the myeloma. The reduction in white blood cells further predisposes the individual to infection. Symptoms of anaemia (shortness of breath on exertion, pallor, chilliness, weakness) and a bleeding tendency (bleeding gums, petechiae, ecchymoses, melaena) may be manifested.

The breakdown of bone tissue give rise to the release of calcium and hypercalcaemia develops (normal calcium: 2.2–2.6 mmol/l). The excretion of the serum calcium by the kidneys entails an increased loss of water. If the fluid intake is not correspondingly increased, the patient manifests dehydration, the serum calcium is retained and the urinary output falls. Nausea, loss of appetite, impaired cardiac function, constipation and disorientation may occur with hypercalcaemia.

Urinalysis may record proteinuria, and electrophoresis of urine may demonstrate the presence of an abnormal protein, referred to as Bence Jones protein which is excreted by the kidneys. In high concentration this protein may be precipitated in the renal tubules, forming casts and damaging the tubules and possibly resulting in renal insufficiency. The high serum urate (normal: 250 μmol/l or 3–7 mg/dl) incurred by the rapid destruction of cells further contributes to impaired renal function; precipitation of the uric acid in renal tubules can obstruct and destroy them. Another factor that contributes to impaired renal function is the hypercalcaemia cited above.

Laboratory blood tests reveal an elevation in erythrocyte sedimentation rate, erythrocyte, leucocyte and platelet counts below normal, and elevated serum calcium and uric acid levels. Examination of a bone marrow specimen shows the presence of abnormal plasma cells. Serum electrophoresis demonstrates the presence of abnormal globulin.

TREATMENT

Care of the patient with multiple myeloma involves the administration of chemotherapeutic agents, radiation therapy and supportive care to relieve symptoms.

Drug therapy

The chemotherapeutic agents used in the treatment of multiple myeloma are melphalan (Alkeran), cyclophosphamide (Endoxana), prednisone and vincristine (Oncovin). Melphalan is given orally; it causes nausea and bone marrow depression. Cyclophosphamide may be substituted for patients who do not respond to melphalan, but it is more toxic. Combination chemotherapy and high-dose chemotherapy are sometimes used for patients who relapse; interferon has also been used. The bone marrow depression caused by the chemotherapy contributes to the anaemia, haemorrhagic tendency and leucopenia that are also caused by bone marrow crowding and replacement by the abnormal plasma cells. The blood cell counts are followed closely; the dosage or protocol for the drug administration may have to be readjusted.

Allopurinol may be prescribed to decrease uric acid production and prevent impaired renal function. Steroids and calcitonin are often prescribed to reduce serum calcium levels in patients with hypercalaemia.

Radiation therapy

Radiotherapy to local areas of involvement may be used to reduce the tumour mass. It is of great value to people with painful bone deposits, especially if there is a likelihood of pathological fractures or spinal cord compression.

Supportive care

The patient's anaemia and thrombocytopenia may necessitate blood and platelet transfusions. If the fluid balance is negative, whole blood is used. If the oral intake has been adequate, packed red blood cells and platelets are transfused to prevent overtaxing the heart by overload. The patient is observed closely for reactions during and following the transfusion.

NURSING CARE

The person with multiple myeloma needs to be assessed frequently as significant changes may occur in a very short period of time. Laboratory data are noted so that the nurse may make the necessary modifications in the care plan according to the findings. For example, it is important to know if the patient's anaemia is worsening or improving, to be aware of the leucocyte count in order to judge susceptibility to infection, and to ascertain whether the platelet count is such that there is a predisposition to haemorrhage. The specific gravity of the urine is noted; if it is high, it may indicate an increase in serum calcium and/or urate and the need to increase the fluid intake. The fluid intake and output are recorded and the balance noted.

The patient should be observed frequently for signs of infection; the temperature is taken, respirations noted and the skin and mouth checked for lesions.

Posture, the degree of freedom or difficulty with which the patient moves and the amount of incapacity and pain are evaluated constantly. Any numbness or loss of movement is promptly reported to the doctor. Observations are also made for the possible toxic effects of the chemotherapeutic agent(s) that the patient is receiving.

The Person with Disorders of the Lymphatic System

INFECTIOUS MONONUCLEOSIS

This is a benign infectious disease involving the lymphatic system and is seen most commonly in adolescents and young adults. The causative organism is the Epstein–Barr virus (EBV). The disease is not highly infectious, but may be transmitted by close personal contact.

CLINICAL CHARACTERISTICS

The symptoms vary from one patient to another. Common complaints are sore throat, gingivitis, headache, tiredness, anorexia and general malaise. The patient has a fever which may be intermittent, and there is enlargement and tenderness of the superficial lymph nodes (cervical, axillary and inguinal). The spleen is usually enlarged and tender, and palpation may also reveal abdominal tenderness due to involvement of the mesenteric lymph nodes. Some patients develop an erythematous or maculopapular rash. Some patients are jaundiced as a result of the development of hepatitis.

The total leucocyte count is elevated and may range from $10.0–20.0 \times 10^9$ per litre. A differential count reveals an increase in lymphocytes and monocytes, and many of the lymphocytes are atypical. The percentage of granulocytes may be below normal. The patient may experience anaemia due to increased haemolysis. Diagnosis may be confirmed by a positive Paul–Bunnell test. Heterophile antibodies appear in the serum of patients with infectious mononucleosis; these antibodies cause the agglutination of sheep blood cells, which is the basis of the Paul–Bunnell test. The Paul–Bunnell reaction does not usually become positive until after the first week of infection. A mononucleosis spot test (Monospot test) is easier to carry out and is considered to be more specific.

TREATMENT AND NURSING CARE

Goals for the patient with infectious mononucleosis are to:

1. Obtain adequate rest until the temperature returns to normal
2. State satisfaction with the degree of comfort
3. Avoid the spread of the infection to others
4. Avoid secondary infections

The disease usually runs a self-limited course of 2–4 weeks and is managed at home. The treatment is symptomatic and supportive. The patient is in bed or rests until the temperature is normal. Aspirin or aspirin compound (e.g. aspirin, caffeine and codeine) or co-proxamol is usually prescribed to relieve the headache, general body discomfort and sore throat. Warm saline throat irrigations may also help to relieve the sore throat. A high-calorie, high-protein diet is recommended to support the patient's resistance. The patient may become discouraged and depressed as the illness continues for weeks, and may become fearful of the outcome. The nurse should convey understanding to the patient, accept these reactions and provide reassurance that although improvement appears slow, normal function will return. Convalescence is usually prolonged. Contact sports are avoided because of the enlarged spleen and danger of injury.

The patient may develop a secondary throat infection; frequently it is due to β-haemolytic streptococci and is treated with an antibiotic.

MALIGNANT LYMPHOMAS

This is a term that may be applied to a group of neoplastic diseases that primarily affect lymphoid tissue (nodes and spleen). They are characterized by painless, progressive enlargement of lymph nodes and spleen. In some the proliferating cells invade extralymphatic tissues and organs. These diseases are usually described as Hodgkin's disease, which is the most common lymphoma, and non-Hodgkin's lymphomas.

NON-HODGKIN'S LYMPHOMAS

Non-Hodgkin's lymphomas are proliferative disorders primarily of B and T lymphocytes. They usually originate in the peripheral lymphoid tissues and are often widespread at diagnosis. They are less predictable in terms of pattern of spread than Hodgkin's disease.

Causes

Although the cause is unknown, non-Hodgkin's lymphomas are considered to result from a combination of factors, including damage to the immune system by radiation, immunosuppressive drugs and environmental chemical hazards. Viral infections are also believed to contribute to the complex aetiological process and non-Hodgkin's lymphomas sometimes occur in individuals with AIDS.

Clinical characteristics

The symptoms vary from person to person. Enlarged, often painless, lymph nodes may be the first indications of a problem although generalized disease is not uncommon. This results in a wide variety of problems, including respiratory difficulty, superior vena cava obstruction, abdominal swelling and ascites, lower limb oedema and intestinal obstruction.

Recurrent fever, night sweats, weight loss and fatigue are other general symptoms that may occur. Diagnosis must be confirmed by biopsy.

HODGKIN'S DISEASE (LYMPHADENOMA)

Hodgkin's disease is a disease of unknown aetiology that involves lymphoid tissue of the immune system. It may develop at any age but usually occurs in adolescents and young adults. There is a higher incidence of the disorder in males. Until recently Hodgkin's disease was considered a fatal condition. It is now considered to be potentially curable. Impressive advances have been made in assessing the extent of the lymph node involvement and treating the affected areas with radiation and chemotherapeutic agents.

Classification

Hodgkin's disease can be divided histologically into four subtypes. This is known as the Rye classification:

- Lymphocytic predominant
- Nodular sclerosing
- Mixed cellularity
- Lymphocyte depleted.

Large atypical cells known as Reed–Steinberg cells are characteristic of Hodgkin's disease and are seen in different numbers in the various subtypes.

Clinical characteristics

The disease has an insidious onset and is manifested by painless enlargement of one group of lymph nodes (usually cervical at the beginning). The disease spreads progressively to other lymphoid tissues throughout the body and a variety of symptoms develop, depending upon the lymphoid tissue involved. The enlarging lymph nodes may cause pressure on nerves, resulting in pain, or may impose on neighbouring organs, causing dysfunction. Axillary and inguinal nodes frequently interfere with venous and lymph drainage, leading to oedema in the arms and legs. Enlarged mediastinal nodes may produce a distressing cough, dyspnoea or difficulty in swallowing (dysphagia). The spleen becomes enlarged, causing abdominal discomfort.

Constitutional symptoms are not prominent until the later stages. The patient gradually develops fatigue, weakness, fever, anorexia, loss of weight and pruritus.

The leucocyte count varies with the patient; it may be increased or it may be normal or below normal. Diagnosis is established by biopsy of an affected lymph node.

INVESTIGATION AND STAGING OF MALIGNANT LYMPHOMAS

When a diagnosis of Hodgkin's disease or non-Hodgkin's lymphoma has been confirmed, a series of investigations is organized to determine the extent of the disease. These include: full blood count, bone marrow aspiration and biopsy, blood urea, electrolyte, liver function and immunoglobulin estimations and chest X-ray, together with CT scans, lymphangiography, gastrointestinal radiography, isotope scans, ultrasound and lumbar puncture, as indicated. Some individuals with Hodgkin's disease may undergo a staging laparotomy, liver biopsy and splenectomy or a laparoscopy.

Lymphangiography is an invasive procedure and requires explanation. Lymphatic vessels on the dorsum of each foot are identified by the subcutaneous injection of a small quantity of blue dye. Under a local anaesthetic, suitable lymphatic vessels are cannulated and a contrast medium is injected over a period of several hours. X-rays are then taken to visualize the lymphatic pathways and nodes. Sutures are inserted in the feet. Follow-up X-rays are taken over a period of time and since the contrast medium remains in the nodes for several months, the effects of treatment can be assessed without repeating the procedure.

Malignant lymphomas are staged according to the spread of the disease using the Ann Arbor classification (Table 13.11). People with non-Hodgkin's lymphomas rarely have localized disease at presentation; the treatment and prognosis of people with Hodgkin's disease is, however, critically dependent on accurate staging.

TREATMENT AND NURSING CARE

Treatment may consist of radiation therapy, chemotherapy or a combination of both. The patient requires psychological and physiological supportive care.

Table 13.11 Ann Arbor staging criteria.

Stage	Extent of disease
I	Involvement of a single lymph node region
IE	Involvement of a single extralymphatic region
II	Involvement of two or more lymph node regions on the same side of the diaphragm
IIE	Localized involvement of an extralymphatic site and of one or more lymph node regions on the same side of the diaphragm
III	Involvement of lymph node regions on both sides of the diaphragm
IIIE	As stage III but with localized extralymphatic involvement
IIIS	As stage III but with splenic involvement
IIISE	As stage III but with both extralymphatic and splenic involvement
IV	Disseminated involvement of one or more extra-lymphatic organs with or without lymph node involvement

Each stage will also be subdivided according to absence (A) or presence (B) of any or all of the following symptoms: weight loss of more than 10% of body weight in 6 months; unexplained fever above 38°C; night sweats.

Treatment of non-Hodgkin's lymphoma

The choice of treatment depends on the person's medical history and the classification and characteristics of the disease. Radiation therapy and chemotherapy are used singly or in combination. For low-grade tumours, single-agent treatment may be adequate. For persons with intermediate-grade disease, combinations of chemotherapeutic agents, with or without local radiation, are used. Prognosis is favourable, with a 30–60% cure rate and 80% chance of significant prolongation of survival. For persons with high-grade tumours, cures are seen in approximately 30%. Treatment involves intensive combination chemotherapy, and possibly radiotherapy. Chemotherapeutic agents may include cyclophosphamide, vincristine, prednisone, doxorubicin, bleomycin, etoposide, procarbazine, methotrexate and 6-mercaptopurine.

Clinical situation: Mrs June Bell a woman with peripheral T-cell lymphoma (adapted with permission of Denise Bryant, Clinical Nurse Specialist)
June Bell is a 27-year-old woman, married with a 7-year-old daughter. She works part-time as a cashier in a fast-food restaurant.

She was admitted to hospital with a 3-month history of a small bowel obstruction, including chronic abdominal pain with eating, nausea, vomiting and weight loss. She had been able to tolerate only fluids for the previous 2 months. June had been investigated prior to admission for what was thought to be a hiatus hernia, and then possibly Crohn's disease.

Clinical and diagnostic findings:
- Weight loss of 17 kg
- No palpable adenopathy and no hepatosplenomegaly
- Chest X-ray showed a large mediastinal mass
- FBC showed a mild microcytic anaemia
- Barium swallow showed a small-bowel obstruction
- Bone marrow biopsy and aspirate was normal
- Lumbar puncture results were negative for lymphoma
- June underwent a small bowel resection and biopsy of the small bowel which showed infiltration of the bowel with peripheral T-cell lymphoma.
  Treatment. June was started on an intense protocol using multiple oral, intravenous and intrathecal drugs over 15 months.
  Evaluation. June's disease is currently in remission 2 years after completion of all therapy. Her prognosis is excellent.

Treatment of Hodgkin's lymphoma

Radiation therapy
A person with stage I or II disease is usually treated with a course of radiotherapy. The area treated includes contiguous nodal areas. Side-effects of treatment will vary according to the field of treatment and all patients will need information and opportunities to discuss treatment, potential side-effects and how these may be minimized.

A person having irradiation above the diaphragm may experience a dry mouth, altered taste, dysphagia, vocal changes, and hair loss in the treatment area. These affects are temporary and usually completely reversible. A person having irradiation below the diaphragm is likely to experience gastrointestinal disturbances, colic, flatulence and diarrhoea and will require dietary advice. Women who wish to remain fertile should be offered oophoropexy (repositioning of the ovaries) to allow the ovaries to be shielded during treatment. Men normally have their testes shielded to protect testicular function.

With both radiation fields, haemoglobin concentration and blood cell counts are determined frequently, since bone marrow depression may occur. Nausea and persisting fatigue are the most common problems. The patient is advised to plan for rest periods during the day and to retire early. Antiemetics and small, frequent, selective meals may be necessary to relieve the nausea. The patient is reassured that these problems will be temporary.

Chemotherapy
Chemotherapy with or without radiotherapy is used to treat stage III or IV disease. The drugs used include mustine hydrochloride (nitrogen mustard), vincristine (Oncovin), prednisone, procarbazine (Natulan), vinblastine, cyclophosphamide (Cytoxan), doxorubicin and bleomycin. A combination of three or four drugs is usually given. Some drug combinations are less likely than others to cause infertility, which is a consideration for most persons when selecting a treatment plan. Potential side-effects of these drugs are given in Table 13.12.

Nursing intervention

The potential patient problems, goals and nursing interventions for the patient with a malignant lymphoma are similar to those for the patient with leukaemia. Following the investigational procedures and initial therapy, the patient (especially one with stage I, II or III disease) returns home and is encouraged to resume, as much as possible, a normal lifestyle. The patient and family should be fully involved in discussing care, factors such as prevention of infection, the importance of regular visits to the doctor or clinic for reassessment; the need for extra rest, medications and coping with therapy reactions are emphasized. Literature for patients can be obtained from the Hodgkin's Disease Association, BACUP and the Royal Marsden Hospital, London.

Nursing Management of the Person with Disorders of White Blood Cells

White blood cells or leucocytes are composed of granulocytes (neutrophils, eosinophils and basophils), lymphocytes and monocytes. The major function of the leucocytic system is protection of the body against foreign invasion. When the leucocyte count is decreased or the cells are abnormal, the neutrophils are decreased in number and the lymphocytes and monocytes are also affected. The body's defences against infection are impaired.

RESPONSES OF INDIVIDUALS TO MALIGNANT DISORDERS OF WHITE BLOOD CELLS

The diagnosis of a malignant disorder of white blood cells, such as leukaemia or lymphoma, has a dramatic impact on the person and the family. The emotional and psychological impact of the diagnosis is only the beginning of a long and very challenging road to acceptance and adjustment. Their lives are forever altered.

The following dialogue is condensed from an actual nurse–patient interaction (the names have been altered). James Adams is a 22-year-old man who was in his second year of college when he was diagnosed as having leukaemia. During the interview he recalled many of his experiences from the time of his diagnosis to this 2-year interview. He shared his perceptions of the impact his diagnosis had on himself, his parents and his younger brother and how his family and health professionals helped him to cope.

Clinical situation: James Adams, a young man with leukaemia (Broadfield, 1988)

James: 'When I was first diagnosed I felt that I was the only one who had this disease. I thought once you had it, it was the end. Slowly I began to realize there was a chance that this thing could be beaten through chemotherapy.

I went through the stages of anger, denial, and acceptance. I let the stages take their course, but it was very hard to accept and took a long time. I remember people coming up to me and saying "you have cancer", and I would say, "No, I don't, I have leukaemia. There is a difference". That was just another way of denying it even though cancer and leukaemia are the same thing. I could not believe it was happening to me. I was the healthiest person in the world.'

Cheryl (nurse): 'You have told me about the support and encouragement you have received during this time.

How have your family, friends and the health care workers helped you in coping and adapting to your diagnosis of leukaemia?'

James: 'My family and friends were always very supportive. There were times when I was very irritable and told them that I did not want anything to do with them. They always managed to give me a "sort of shake" and put things back into perspective. When I was at my lowest point, they would drag me out of the house, even though I did not want to go, and take me for a drive. They made me look at things in a different perspective—to open my eyes—and say "What am I doing sitting here feeling sorry for myself".

The nurses taught me how to deal with all the different things I was exposed to like needles, hospitals, and dealing with things mentally and emotionally. The nurses could provide more support if they had more time for each patient—the time they have sometimes is not quite enough.

The chaplain made me look at things in a different light. The doctor, of course, helps with the treatments and all the side effects. I think it takes a very caring and special individual to work on a haematology ward because you develop close relationships with the patients. I have known some of the nurses for two years. The nurses are aware of everything the patients are going through and know what each patient likes and dislikes.

When you spend as much time in hospital as I do, you like to have a sense of independence. That is something the nurses on haematology allow me to have. It does a lot for me psychologically.'

Cheryl: 'How has your leukaemia altered your life?'

James: 'There are many restrictions. At certain times I cannot drink alcohol. I have to be in hospital a lot. I am in for one week each month and if there are complications, I am in longer. Following treatments you do not feel well and therefore are not up to doing what you would like to do. I have a Hickman (central venous) Catheter and therefore cannot be as athletic as I would like to be. I cannot play contact sports. If I was injured it would cause a lot of problems for me. But, the goal is to get through therapy and hopefully get back to a normal lifestyle.'

Cheryl: 'Do you have any comments you would like to make to a newly diagnosed leukaemic patient?'

James: '1) Try to lead as normal a life as possible.
2) Your attitude is important. If you let it beat

you mentally, then you have not got a hope.

3) It is good to talk to people—that has been my experience. I speak to the nurses, the chaplain, the doctors—as many people as possible. They help you put things in perspective when you are really upset and you cannot look at things logically.

4) Speak to someone who has gone through a similar experience. When I spoke with a volunteer from the Cancer Society, I thought "How come you are okay?" People with this disease do not have a chance? Seeing this young man and realizing that he had gone through some hard times and was okay now. I thought "well if he can do it, I can do it too".

As a result of my experience, I appreciate little things more and take advantage of every minute. The time I spend with family, friends and nurses I appreciate a lot more. I take things one day at a time.'

ASSESSMENT

Assessment of the person with disorders of white blood cells, is continuous during the acute phases of illness and treatment and during periods of remission. The patient and family are taught the importance of early identification of infections and to assess changes in the person's health status that may indicate infection.

HEALTH HISTORY

The person is questioned regarding the presence of risk factors for disorders of white blood cells: exposure to chemicals and/or radiation; medications that may suppress white cell formation and the dose and length of time the medication has been taken. Immunosuppressive drugs such as corticosteroids and anti-inflammatory agents may also mask signs of infection.

The health history includes information about past and present illnesses that may indicate a white blood cell disorder.

Emphasis is placed on past and present infections: a history of repeated infections and factors that may contribute to the development of infections. The person is asked specific questions about any signs of infection: (1) redness, swelling, warmth, drainage; (2) fever, chills, shivering; (3) general malaise, or weakness; (4) white patches in the mouth, skin rashes; (5) pain and discomfort in the abdomen, joints, rectal and perineal areas, throat, eyes or ears; (6) changes in the character or colour of stools, diarrhoea; (7) nausea or vomiting.

A major component of the health history is identification of the responses of the patient and family to the illness, diagnosis and treatment. Anxiety and fear are common responses, as are denial and anger. Most persons are aware of the life-threatening nature of the disorders and their treatment. The treatment regimens as well as the disease processes place the person at risk for infections when their body defences are impaired. Emotional responses of the patient and the family will change as the person's clinical situation and health status alter.

PHYSICAL EXAMINATION

1. The person's blood pressure, pulse, respirations and body temperature are assessed for baseline data.
2. The person's skin and all body sites with high potential for infection are inspected for baseline data. The nurse inspects skin-fold areas (buttocks, axillae, perineum, breasts) and sites of intravenous infusions, central venous catheters, bone marrow aspirations, parenteral injections, lumbar punctures or other invasive procedure for signs of redness, warmth, swelling or drainage. The mouth is inspected for white patches or redness, (signs of *Candida albicans* infection).
3. The person's respiratory status is assessed. The presence and nature of any cough and sputum is noted as well as any dyspnoea or alteration in breathing pattern.
4. The frequency and nature of urinary elimination are observed. The urine is observed for cloudiness and blood.
5. Patterns of bowel elimination and the colour and consistency of stools are noted.
6. The person's hydrational status is assessed by determining skin turgor and measuring the fluid intake and output.

LABORATORY TESTS

The person's white blood cell and differential white blood cell counts are monitored regularly. Neutropenia is present if the neutrophil count is less than 2×10^6 per cubic litre. The person is at high risk for infection if the count is below 1×10^6/l.

PATIENT PROBLEMS

The primary health problem is:

- Potential risk of local or systemic infection due to white blood cell deficiency or dysfunction, altered immune response or bone marrow depression

Other problems may include some or all of the following:

- Anxiety related to diagnosis of a malignant disorder, fear of the unknown, loss of control of life events and uncertainty of the future
- Lack of knowledge of the disease process and treatment
- Pain due to the disease process (marrow infiltration, bone destruction, etc.) and to treatment (e.g. stomatitis)
- Inadequate fluid and food intake due to the disease process and treatment
- Ineffective individual and family coping strategies related to altered roles and relationships, prolonged treatment and hospitalization

In addition there may be very specific problems caused by treatment-related toxicity and concurrent anaemia and thrombocytopenia.

GOALS

1. The person will demonstrate an absence of infection as indicated by:
   - Body temperature within normal range
   - Absence of pain, tenderness, redness, swelling, warmth and drainage
   - Intact skin and oral mucosa.
2. Changes in the above will be promptly identified and reported by the patient
3. The person will describe self-care measures to prevent infection and actions to be taken if signs of infection occur.

INTERVENTION

PREVENTION OF INFECTION

Environment
In hospital the person should be nursed in a single room or protective isolation, if available, so that a pathogen-reduced environment can be maintained. Staff and visitors entering the person's room should be kept to a minimum. Equipment and supplies should be kept for the sole use of the patient to reduce the risk of cross-infection.

Patient and family teaching
The patient and family are kept informed of the patient's laboratory test results and taught the normal ranges for white blood cell and neutrophil counts and the significance of variations from normal. The nurse also explains the functions of white blood cells and the causes of the patient's decreased white blood cell counts.

The person and family are advised to caution anyone with a current or recent infection to refrain from visiting the patient in hospital or at home.

Meticulous hand washing is essential to decrease the potential for transmission of infection to patients. The patient, family and visitors are taught good hand washing technique and the importance of washing hands before any direct contact between the patient and others.

The patient and family are taught to assess and identify signs of infection and to inform the nurse or contact the doctor if the oral temperature is over 38°C.

The patient's usual activities and interests while at home are reviewed and the patient is instructed to avoid situations where exposure to infections may occur. Extra caution is advised when the neutrophil counts are below $1 \times 10^6/l$. Exposure to people with respiratory infections, herpes infections, varicella, herpes zoster or infectious mononucleosis is to be avoided. Situations requiring mingling or contact with large groups or crowds should also be avoided whenever possible.

Personal hygiene
Meticulous personal hygiene is promoted. The person is urged to shower daily, establish an oral hygiene routine, and practice good perineal care.

Particular attention is given to the perineum, groin, axillae and skin folds when showering or bathing. The patient is taught to note any redness, tenderness, swelling, lumps or unusual skin lesions and to report these to the nurse and/or doctor.

Deodorants containing antiperspirants are avoided as they can lead to blockage of the sweat glands and subsequent infection.

Men should be advised to use electric razors to decrease the potential for causing breaks in the skin while shaving.

Oral hygiene
The prevention of trauma to the oral mucosa is necessary in the prevention of infection. Oral hygiene should be practised after each meal using a soft toothbrush or foam sticks and a mouthwash composed of a mild solution of saline or sodium bicarbonate if there is thick mucus or food debris. Mouthwashes containing alcohol, which may be drying and irritating to the gums and oral mucosa, are avoided. Dental floss should not be used while white cell and platelet counts are low. The person is taught the importance of regular dental checks at least every 6 months. The dentist and doctor should discuss the person's needs before the dental examination. Appropriate antibiotics may be prescribed if invasive procedures are necessary. Dentures should be checked to ensure that they fit properly. Ill-fitting dentures should not be worn.

Bowel care
The patient is taught the importance of avoiding constipation and rectal straining that may damage the rectal mucosa and provide entry for organisms found in the gastrointestinal tract. A bowel routine using stool-softeners and mineral oils or other mild, non-irritating laxatives should be established with each patient as needed and implemented on a regular basis. Maintenance of regular bowel habits is promoted. Enemas and rectal tubes should not be used.

If constipation or diarrhoea are problems, the person's diet and fluid intake are reviewed. The diet should be high in fibre and a fluid intake of 3000 ml per day is recommended unless contraindicated.

The person is advised to wipe from front to back when performing perineal cleansing after each bowel motion and to observe for rectal itching, pain and tenderness or abnormal discharge during and after bowel movements. Changes should be reported immediately to the health care team.

Food and fluids
The patient is encouraged to maintain a nutritionally balanced diet containing adequate calories for increased metabolic needs, adequate protein and vitamins. Daily calorie counts may be carried out periodically to evaluate caloric intake. Topical analgesics may be prescribed and used prior to eating if the person is experiencing pain and tenderness as a result of the oral lesions found with leukaemia or the stomatitis from the chemotherapy. Increased fluid intake of 3000 ml per day is recommended unless contraindicated by pre-existing cardiovascular or other health problems. The patient and family are instructed that the patient should not share eating utensils, drinking cups or glasses.

Approximately half the infections in persons with neutropenia are caused by hospital-acquired organisms that have colonized the gastrointestinal tract. (The administration of prophylactic non-absorbable oral antibiotics to sterilize gastrointestinal bacteria and antifungal agents to prevent proliferation of yeasts is controversial.) The role of food and water as a major source of these organisms is not well appreciated. The protective mechanisms of the gastrointestinal tract are impaired in persons who are neutropenic, either by the underlying disease mechanisms which affect all immune responses or by chemotherapeutic agents or antibiotic therapy. Fresh fruits and vegetables are a source of Gram-negative bacteria and dairy products and water are sources of Gram-negative rods. Ice machines are further sources of contamination. Low-bacteria diets are often prescribed when the patient is in hospital. They are easily followed by patients in the community. The diets eliminate foods of high bacterial count: all dairy products, including ice creams, puddings made with milk, or cakes with cream fillings; raw fruits and vegetables and reconstituted juices; raw meats and fish; cultured cheeses, blue cheese, Roquefort and Camembert; egg whites and foods with raw egg whites; and any foods made with tap water such as jelly. Ice is not used in beverages. Drinks may be cooled by placing the container in ice rather than placing the ice in the liquid. Beverages made with boiled water, cooked meats, vegetables, fruits, nuts and sweets are all allowed. Water and other beverages should be changed regularly and not left to stagnate.

A recent literature search did not produce any prospective controlled studies on the effectiveness of low-bacteria diets in preventing infections in persons with low white blood cell counts or neutropenia. Arguments for use of low-bacteria diets include recognition that food is a major source of pathogenic organisms, that the diets do no harm to the patient and appear to provide some benefits, and that the diets are easy to implement and follow and do not interfere with the person obtaining a nutritionally balanced diet.

Avoidance of invasive procedures
Invasive procedures are avoided or their need reviewed before being instituted. Rectal thermometers are avoided. Suppositories should not be used. Women are instructed not to use vaginal tampons or douches. The use of indwelling urinary catheters should be avoided. Intermittent catheterization is preferable to the use of indwelling catheters if catheterization is deemed essential. Strict aseptic technique is maintained and the smallest lumen catheter that will be effective is used. The closed drainage system should be disrupted as little as possible.

Subcutaneous, intramuscular, venous and arterial punctures are avoided if possible. Long-term central venous catheters are preferable to avoid the need for reinsertion of peripheral intravenous lines and provide a ready access for drugs, fluids, blood products and nutritional support. The risk of infection is minimized by appropriate skin care. The skin is cleansed prior to each puncture with an alcohol preparation followed by povidone-iodine solution. Insertion sites are inspected

at least every shift and cleansed with the same antiseptic agents prior to removal of the lines. The exit site of long-term central venous catheters is cleansed with alcohol and then povidone-iodine and povidone-iodine ointment is applied prior to an occlusive dressing. The transparent dressing permits inspection of the site for signs of inflammation. Swabs are taken for culture if inflammatory changes are present. Strict asepsis is required.

Intravenous tubing and all solutions should be changed every 24 hours.

Bone marrow and lumbar puncture sites are covered with sterile dressings for 24 hours. The sites are inspected for signs of infection.

Delivery of nursing care
The nurse and other care-givers should take precautionary measures to prevent transfer of infection from themselves to the patient. Meticulous hand washing is important prior to any contact with the patient. If the care-giver has an indication of a potential or actual infection, a change in patient allocation should be requested. The least number of care-givers should be used to provide care and the nurse should always review allocated patients and ensure that persons at risk for infection are cared for first. Patients with known infections should be cared for separately by another nurse whenever possible.

EARLY IDENTIFICATION OF INFECTION

The individual is assessed for risk of infection. If the patient is neutropenic, assessment takes place at least every 4 hours and whenever changes occur. The doctor is notified immediately (by the nurse if the person is in hospital or by the patient if in the community) if: the oral temperature rises above 38.0°C; the person experiences chills, rigor, tachycardia, cyanosis, cold clammy extremities, or unexplained abdominal or rectal pain or tenderness; or the person becomes irritable, restless or shows an alteration in the level of consciousness.

Blood will usually be drawn for aerobic and anaerobic cultures, and urine specimens, sputum, wound and throat swabs or swabs from any obvious skin lesion will be sent to the laboratory for culture as indicated. Intravenous antibiotic therapy is then initiated as soon as possible if any of the above signs of infection are present. It is continued, as prescribed, on a 24-hour basis in order to maintain therapeutic levels of the drug in the blood.

EVALUATION

Review of care should demonstrate that assessment for signs of infection has been continuous and that the patient and family have been taught and understand measures to decrease the potential for infection, identify signs of infection and know what to do if infection develops. Persons with disorders of white blood cells should be able to alter their life-styles to decrease the risks for infection and still participate in social activities.

The Person with Haemorrhagic Disorders

An abnormal tendency to bleed may be due to a disorder of the clotting mechanism, an excess of anticoagulant, a low platelet count or dysfunctional platelets, or a vascular defect. A haemorrhagic disorder is characterized by: prolonged bleeding following tissue damage; spontaneous bleeding into mucous membrane, skin and organs; and bleeding in more than one area of the body.

Failure of the clotting mechanism may result from a deficiency of any of the essential factors in the coagulation process. These disorders include haemophilia, hypoprothrombinaemia and thrombocytopenia.

When a haemorrhagic disorder is suspected it is important to note the form in which the bleeding presents: purpural areas, haematoma, ecchymoses, oozing or free flow from wound, and whether from single or multiple sites.

DISORDERS OF PLATELETS

Platelet function may be impaired because of a decrease in the number of platelets (thrombocytopenia) or the presence of dysfunctional platelets (thrombopathia). A platelet disorder without associated disease is referred to as a primary disorder and may be inherited or acquired. Secondary platelet disorders result from a related clinical disease. The major characteristics of platelet disorders are (1) abnormal bleeding, and (2) a prolonged bleeding time in a person with a normal platelet count.

THROMBOCYTOPENIA (THROMBOCYTOPENIC PURPURA)

Failure of the coagulation process may be due to a deficiency of circulating thrombocytes (blood platelets), known as thrombocytopenia. Thrombocyte deficiency may be due to failure in the production of thrombocytes, pooling of platelets in splenomegaly, dilutional loss resulting from excessive blood transfusions within a short period or increased destruction of thrombocytes.

Insufficient thrombocyte production may be associated with leukaemia or lupus erythematosus or may be caused by bone marrow suppression resulting from drugs or radiation. Destruction of thrombocytes may result from excessive intravascular coagulation, damage to thrombocytes from abnormal blood vessel walls or from an antigen–antibody reaction in which the person develops antibodies (agglutinins) which destroy the thrombocytes. The latter is referred to as immune thrombocytopenia which may be idiopathic (cause unknown) or caused by drugs, transfusions of platelets carrying PLA–1 antigen, or transfer of maternal antibodies across the placenta to the neonate. The normal life span for platelets is approximately 8–10 days; in idiopathic thrombocytopenia their survival time is only 1–3 days. The cause of the antibody production is not known, but in most cases of idiopathic thrombocytopenia antibodies can be detected.

Clinical characteristics

The disorder manifests by bleeding in any site. Petechiae and purpuric areas may appear in the skin or mucous membranes and bleeding from the nose or from the gastrointestinal or urinary tract may occur.

Treatment

Treatment is directed toward removing the cause of the thrombocytopenia (e.g. withdrawal of drugs that suppress the bone marrow) and protecting the patient from trauma and ensuing bleeding with transfusions of fresh blood and platelets.

The patient with idiopathic thrombocytopenia is treated with immunosuppressive drug therapy to reduce the number of circulating antibodies. If the patient does not respond favourably to these measures, splenectomy may be performed. Although the spleen does not become enlarged, it appears to be active in thrombocytopenia. It separates out and harbours the platelets and is suspected of producing some antibody.

PLATELET FUNCTION DISORDERS

Defects of platelet function may be hereditary or acquired. If the bleeding time is prolonged and the platelet count is normal, the impairment may result from:

- Failure of the platelets to adhere to the subendothelium of the blood vessel walls, as seen in von Willebrand's disease, Bernard–Soulier syndrome and hypergammaglobulinaemia.
- Failure of platelets to release adenosine diphosphate.
- Failure of the platelets to synthesize thromboxane A_2.
- Failure of the platelets to aggregate with adenosine diphosphate.
- Defective platelet coagulation activity.
- Mixed defects seen in persons with renal failure, hypergammaglobulinaemia and myeloproliferative disorders.

BLOOD CLOTTING FACTOR DEFICIENCY

Deficiencies of blood clotting factors may be inherited/congenital or acquired. Failure of the coagulation process may result from a decrease in the quantity or abnormal function of any one of the factors which promote the blood clotting process. A deficiency of some factors occurs rarely and symptoms of factor deficiencies vary from mild to severe. The disorders include haemophilia (A and B) caused by factor VIII and factor IX deficiencies.

HAEMOPHILIA

Haemophilia is a coagulation disorder that occurs in males as a result of a deficiency of factor VIII (the antihaemophilic factor) or factor IX (the Christmas factor). If the bleeding tendency is the result of a deficiency of factor VIII, the disease is referred to as *haemophilia A*; if it is the result of a deficiency of factor IX, it is known as *haemophilia B* or *Christmas disease*. It

Normal male

		X	Y
	X	XX	XY
Female carrier	X^h	X^{h}X	X^{h}Y

XX   Normal female
XY   Normal male
X^{h}X   Female carrier
X^{h}Y   Male with haemophilia

Male with haemophilia

		X^h	Y
	X	XX^h	XY
Normal female	X	XX^h	XY

XX^h Female carrier
XY   Normal male

Figure 13.8 Genetic possibilities in haemophilia.

is inherited as a sex-linked recessive trait. The defective gene is carried on an X chromosome and is transmitted from mother to son.

The female has two X sex chromosomes, and the male has one X and one Y. If a female inherits an X chromosome bearing the haemophilic gene, she becomes a carrier. The disorder is not manifested in her because the X chromosome with the abnormal gene is dominated by the normal X chromosome. If the carrier marries a non-haemophiliac, there is a 50% chance her daughters will be carriers. Her male progeny have a 50% chance of being haemophilic (Figure 13.8). The sons of a haemophilic father receive only a Y chromosome from him, so the disorder is not passed on to them or their descendants. All daughters of a haemophilic male carry the trait since the father's genetic contribution to each is an X chromosome, which in his case bears the defective gene (Figure 13.8).

Clinical characteristics

Haemophilia is usually recognized within the first year or two of life. Excessive bleeding from the umbilical cord does not occur because of the transplacental transfer of the mother's clotting factors to the fetus. Occasionally, persistent bleeding when the infant is circumcised leads to early diagnosis of the disorder.

The severity varies in individuals; some bleed excessively with very slight trauma and others bleed only with a more severe injury or during incidents such as tooth extraction or surgery. The important characteristic feature of the bleeding is its persistence rather than the amount. Most children experience some bleeding into joints, especially the knees, ankles and elbows. With some, this may be so severe that, as well as causing pain, it produces crippling deformities. As the blood clot organizes, fibrous adhesions may cause ankylosis. Haematomas and haematuria may be manifested. Early death may occur as a result of the pressure of a haematoma (collection of blood within tissue) on a vital structure, or from the loss of blood. The latter is rarely fatal since blood and plasma have become so readily available.

Laboratory blood studies indicate a prolonged whole blood clotting time (normal: 5–11 minutes when glass tubes are used); the bleeding time (normal: 2–9 minutes), blood platelet count (normal: 150–400 × 10^9 per litre) and prothrombin time (normal 11–15 seconds) are normal. The activated partial thromboplastin time is prolonged (normal: 30–45 seconds). Quantitative assays of factors VIII and IX are performed.

Treatment and care

The patient (if old enough) and the family are alerted to the need for continuous ongoing care.

Treatment of episodes of bleeding
Control of bleeding will depend on the level of the clotting factors in the blood. If factor VIII is low, it can be replaced by factor VIII concentrate or cryoprecipitate (fibrinogen and factor VIII). If the patient is factor IX deficient it can be replaced, although it is only available as a commercial product. Mild forms of haemophilia A may be treated with synthetic vasopressin (DDAVP), which raises circulatory factor VIII by releasing it from storage sites.

The advantage of the commercial concentrates and cryoprecipitate is that either can be infused in a small volume; this prevents overloading of the individual's cardiovascular system. A hazard of factor replacement therapy is the increased risk of hepatitis and HIV infections because the concentrates are prepared from the plasma of many pooled donations. During the early 1980s many haemophiliacs were exposed to infected concentrates and have themselves been infected with HIV virus. Some have developed AIDS and have died. Since 1985, clotting factor concentrates have been heat treated. This, together with serological testing of donations and exclusion of high-risk donors and their sexual partners, should prevent further infection in this group (Napier, 1987).

During an episode of bleeding the patient is confined to bed. If there is bleeding into a joint, the joint is immobilized and attention is given to positioning with good alignment to reduce possible deformity. The patient may be fearful of using the joint after the bleeding has been arrested in case of further haemorrhage; he must be encouraged to resume activity as soon as possible to prevent ankylosis. Full range-of-motion exercises are started 48 hours after the bleeding has been controlled.

Prophylactic and supportive measures
Nursing responsibilities including planning and implementing instruction for the patient and family about the nature of the disorder, safe activities, necessary precautions, recognition of the need for factor replacement, and appropriate action when bleeding occurs. In some instances one or two members of the family may be taught the administration of the prescribed concentrate so that treatment can be given at home, avoiding hospital delays.

Patients are urged to seek prompt treatment following trauma and on the earliest symptoms of bleeding; for example, replacement of the deficient factor is recommended as soon as the patient experiences slight tightness or pressure in a joint, especially if he knows it has received a bump.

It should be emphasized that the person with haemophilia should always carry some form of identification indicating the disorder and blood type.

The patient and family are advised to carry on as normal a life as possible. The severity of the disease determines the restrictions placed on the individual's activities; they must be consistent with safety but there are non-traumatic sports, occupations and forms of recreation in which he may and should be encouraged to participate. Parents and siblings are warned against overprotection and promoting dependency. If of school age, the child is usually able to attend a normal school. The teachers should be informed of the condition, the necessary restrictions and precautions and what to do if he receives an injury or bleeding commences. For the child whose disease is severe, arrangements may be made for him to pursue his education at home or to attend special classes. The problem must be kept in mind when selecting toys and sport equipment.

During the teaching sessions the patient and family are informed that individuals with haemophilia must not be given aspirin because of its tendency to promote bleeding. Parenteral administrations must also be kept to a minimum; usually the introduction of a needle is restricted to the administration of the antihaemophilic factor.

Good dental hygiene is stressed so that extractions may be avoided. A very soft brush to clean the teeth is recommended to prevent trauma and bleeding of the gums. The patient's dentist is advised of the disorder on the initial visit so that the necessary precautions can be taken. Antifibrinolytic agents (aminocaproic or tranexamic acid) are usually administered if dental procedures are required.

A referral should be made to the district nurse and health visitor so that home visits may be made to provide necessary assistance and supervision. The patient and family are acquainted with the resources of a local haemophilia society.

The genetic possibilities in offspring are reviewed with parents and young adults in the family. A referral may be made to the appropriate clinic for genetic counselling. Opportunities are available for prenatal testing and antenatal diagnosis of affected fetuses.

Complications
Some patients, after receiving several doses of a factor concentrate, develop antibodies to the factor. Precautions and activity restrictions have to be reassessed and are usually made more rigid. If a bleeding episode occurs, a much larger dose of the antihaemophilic preparation may be prescribed in an effort to counteract the antibody activity.

Repeated haemarthroses (bleeding into joints) may lead to serious restriction of movement and deformity in the affected joints.

VON WILLEBRAND'S DISEASE

This disorder resembles haemophilia but occurs in both sexes. It is characterized by prolonged bleeding, bruising and nosebleeds.

This is an autosomally transmitted disorder caused by a deficiency of a protein, the von Willebrand factor. This factor is necessary for normal platelet function and interacts with another protein involved in factor VIII production. The patient therefore has a deficiency of factor VIII and defective platelet adhesion, resulting in a prolonged bleeding time. The platelet count is normal. Bleeding is controlled by the administration of cryoprecipitate or DDAVP (desmopressin).

PROTHROMBIN, FACTOR VII, FACTOR IX AND FACTOR X DEFICIENCIES (VITAMIN K DEFICIENCY)

Vitamin K is essential in the production of prothrombin and factors VII, IX and X by the liver. A deficiency may result from a deficient supply, impaired absorption or defective utilization of vitamin K. If the diet does not supply an adequate amount, it is synthesized by the bacteria which normally inhabit the intestinal tract. The bleeding tendency in the newborn is attributed to the lack of bacterial synthesis of vitamin K during the first 2–3 days of life when the tract is free of organisms. Sterilization of the bowel by the oral administration of antibiotics may produce a vitamin K deficiency.

Bile salts are essential in the intestine for the absorption of vitamin K. A frequent cause of a deficiency of prothrombin and factors VII, IX and X is obstruction to the flow of bile into the small intestine. An insufficient production of prothrombin may also occur in liver disease, such as chronic cirrhosis.

Vitamin K deficiency due to impaired synthesis or absorption is treated with a synthetic preparation of vitamin K [phytomenadione, (Konakion)] which may be administered parenterally or orally. When the deficiency is due to liver disease, the patient may receive blood transfusions to supply prothrombin and the deficient factors.

EXCESS OF ANTICOAGULANT (HEPARIN/ WARFARIN TOXICITY)

Haemorrhage may be a complication of excessive anticoagulant drug therapy. The products most commonly used are heparin and warfarin. Heparin interferes with clotting factor activations in both the intrinsic and extrinsic pathways of thromboplastin generation; it also has a strong affinity for antithrombin III, increasing its inhibitory action on thrombin and other activated coagulation factors (II, IX, X, XI and XII). Warfarin interferes with the ability of vitamin K to activate clotting factor precursors, causing a decrease in factors II, VII, IX and X.

If bleeding occurs, anticoagulant therapy is stopped and, if necessary, fresh frozen plasma or whole blood is administered. For heparin overdoses, protamine sulphate, a specific antidote for heparin, may be required. For bleeding associated with warfarin, administration of vitamin K will antagonize the anticoagulant effect.

Prolonged administration of acetylsalicylic acid (aspirin) may also affect coagulation. Acetylsalicylic acid decreases plasma prothrombin levels, inhibits platelet aggregation and prolongs the bleeding time.

VASCULAR PURPURA

In some instances, bleeding into tissues and organs occurs because of damage to or a defect in the small blood vessels. The result may be increased permeability or inadequate vasoconstriction, predisposing to blood loss. This type of disorder may be associated with an allergic reaction, septicaemia or a vitamin C deficiency (scurvy) and vasculitis.

A rare herediary bleeding disorder known as hereditary haemorrhagic telangiectasia is characterized by dilated, thin-walled vessels (especially veins) that lack the normal amount of muscular tissue. Angiomas (tumours composed of blood vessels) appear on the skin and mucous membrane surfaces, and normal vasoconstriction does not take place in the affected vessels.

DISSEMINATED INTRAVASCULAR COAGULATION (DIC)

Disseminated intravascular coagulation (DIC) is a potentially fatal condition that is a secondary development in a serious primary illness. It is characterized by two phases. In the first phase multiple diffuse microthrombi develop within the vascular system. This widespread coagulation depletes the blood of thrombocytes and several clotting factors to the extent that haemorrhage occurs. This is the second phase of the disorder. Contributing to the haemorrhagic phase is the fibrinolysis that occurs.

DIC may be seen as a complication in many disorders, which include any condition associated with extensive tissue damage, shock, severe infections (especially those associated with Gram-negative organisms), severe trauma, burns, extensive metastatic disease, surgery involving extracorporeal shunts, obstetric complications (toxaemia and abruptio placentae) and amniotic embolism.

Factors involved with the onset of DIC include hypotension, usually associated with shock acidaemia, and stasis of capillary blood (Gobel, 1990). The process involves diffuse traumatization of tissue cells and/or blood platelets by the primary disorder; thromboplastin is released which triggers the clotting process. The blood clots may seriously interfere with the blood supply to some tissues and organs, resulting in impaired function. Respiratory insufficiency and renal failure are common ensuing problems.

Plasminogen is activated during the pathological clotting and forms the enzyme plasmin, which breaks down the fibrin of clots and fibrinogen. The degradation products of this dissolution process inhibit the thrombin–fibrinogen reaction which yields fibrin. They cause a prolonged thrombin time and retard the production of thromboplastin. Obviously, these reactions inhibit coagulation and cause haemorrhage.

Disseminated intravascular coagulation differs from normal clotting in that: (1) it is diffuse rather than localized; (2) it damages, rather than fulfils the normal protective role; and (3) it consumes prothrombin, fibrinogen, platelets, factor V and factor VIII faster than they can be produced and so bleeding occurs (Eastham, 1984).

CLINICAL CHARACTERISTICS

Diffuse bleeding occurs in various areas and may be evident by petechiae, ecchymoses, haematuria, gastrointestinal bleeding, vaginal bleeding, epistaxis, or persistent oozing from a surgical wound or needle puncture. The patient may complain of pain as a result of bleeding into tissues. Oliguria and respiratory distress may develop.

Laboratory blood studies indicate a marked decrease in the number of blood platelets, decreased levels of fibrinogen and factors V and VIII, and prolonged prothrombin, thrombin and partial thromboplastin times.

TREATMENT AND NURSING CARE

Treatment is directed toward reversing the primary disorder and arresting the diffuse coagulation process. It is based on the replacement of consumed clotting factors with fresh frozen plasma and cryoprecipitate plus platelet transfusions. Intravenous heparin may be administered in very selected situations.

The patient is usually critically ill and the nurse is concerned with the primary condition as well as the blood disorder. Care includes: (1) maintaining blood pressure and volume, (2) preventing trauma that could initiate further bleeding, and (3) preventing stasis and correcting hypoxaemia and acidosis (Gobel, 1990). Close observation is made for bleeding, and frequent assessment of the patient's vital signs and general condition is necessary. The hourly urinary output is noted to monitor fluid balance and detect early signs of renal failure. Continuous cardiac monitoring may be set up and, if respiratory insufficiency occurs, the patient may be put on a mechanical ventilator (see p. 429).

Nursing Management of the Person with Haemorrhagic Disorders

ASSESSMENT

HEALTH HISTORY

The nurse should enquire what initiated the bleed and get the patient to describe any rashes, bruising, swelling tenderness or areas of discoloration in the skin or mucous membranes. It is important to determine:

- If the individual has a history of bleeding; that is, has this type of response been occurring since early childhood, or is this the initial incidence?
- How long the bleeding has been taking place.
- If there is anyone in the family with a history of a similar problem.
- What precipitated this bleeding (e.g. trauma, visit to the dentist).

It is also important to ascertain the circumstances and degree of any trauma and past responses to physical trauma or injury. Answers to these questions help to identify if the disorder is hereditary or acquired or if it is a result of physical injury and not a defect in haemostasis.

PHYSICAL EXAMINATION

The individual is examined for signs of bleeding. Clinical characteristics of bleeding that may be identified by inspection and palpation of the skin, mucous membranes and joints include:

- *Haemorrhage.* This is the loss of blood from a ruptured blood vessel. The bleeding may be external or internal. The amount of blood lost will depend on the size of the blood vessel(s), whether an artery or vein has been ruptured, and the effectiveness of the body's clotting mechanisms. External bleeding can be assessed by direct observation and estimation of the amount of blood which has soaked into a person's clothing or pooled on or under the affected part.
- *Petechiae.* These are small red spots about the size of the head of a pin and may be seen in crops over various parts of the body. They are a result of an increased permeability of blood vessels which enables blood to extravasate into the surrounding tissue.
- *Purpura.* Purpuric spots are caused by the same mechanism but are larger than petechiae.
- *Ecchymosis or bruise.* This is a large area of extravasated blood which usually occurs as a result of trauma or platelet disorders.
- *Haematoma.* This is a large bruise caused by infiltration of blood into the subcutaneous or muscle tissues as a result of a coagulation defect or an overdose of an anticoagulant. It is characterized by discoloration of the skin and swelling and deformity of the tissue.
- *Telangiectasis, angioma.* These are red spots or patches resulting from blood in abnormally dilated blood vessels. The lesions do not blanch on pressure.
- *Haemarthrosis.* This is a haemorrhage into a joint, usually caused by a severe coagulation disorder such as haemophilia. It is characterized by pain, tenderness and swelling of the affected joint.

Additional observations are made for signs of:

- *Haematuria,* or blood in the urine, which usually occurs with kidney lesions or a severe coagulation disorder such as haemophilia or an overdose of anticoagulants.
- *Epistaxis,* or nosebleed, which may be caused by mild trauma to dilated blood vessels in the anterior nares, or a platelet defect.

It is important to note the sites and extent of bleeding. If the person has a haemostatic defect, the bleeding will probably occur at multiple sites. Bleeding at individual sites usually results from local factors, including trauma.

The person's blood pressure, pulse and respiratory rates should be recorded every few minutes during episodes of acute bleeding. (See Chapter 12 for an account of shock.)

NURSING INTERVENTION

FIRST AID

Frank bleeding is controlled by the application of direct pressure and elevation of the affected part. There is no indication for the use of tourniquets or pressure points, which can cause tissue ischaemia; direct pressure will control bleeding. A realistic assessment of blood loss is useful information for accident and emergency staff receiving the patient later. It must be remembered that, however dramatic blood loss may appear, airway and breathing remain the priorities in a first-aid situation.

Specific nursing needs of patients with haemorrhagic disorders vary with each individual and with the cause, associated symptoms, and severity of the disease, but there are some common problems and general considerations applicable to all. These are presented in the patient care plan in Table 13.12.

TRANSFUSION OF BLOOD AND BLOOD PRODUCTS

An infusion of blood or blood components may be given to: (1) replace blood lost during surgery or in haemorrhage; (2) replace a deficiency of specific blood components, such as erythrocytes, platelets and clotting factors; (3) increase the oxygen-carrying capacity of the blood, as in anaemia; and (4) to increase the intravascular volume in shock.

When blood is taken from the donor, it is received in a special sterile container that contains anticoagulant. The anticoagulant most frequently used is a mixture of sodium citrate, citric acid and dextrose (acid citrate dextrose). The sodium citrate prevents clotting, the citric acid serves as a preservative and the dextrose prolongs the life of the erythrocytes. Heparin is used as an anticoagulant in blood that is to be transfused within 24 hours of procurement. Heparinized blood is necessary for extracorporeal shunts (as in open heart surgery). The heparin is less damaging to platelets and to the enzyme 2,3-disphosphoglycerate (DPG), which promotes the release of oxygen from oxyhaemoglobin.

The blood is labelled clearly to indicate donor number, blood type, whether Rh negative or positive, anticoagulant used, and expiry date. The blood may be given as whole blood or some of the components may be separated out for administration. Blood is stored at a temperature of 2–4°C and may be used within 21 days of having been obtained, except that which is heparinized.

Table 13.12   Patient care plan: the person with a haemorrhagic disorder.

Problem: Potential risk of bleeding due to a platelet disorder, deficiency of clotting factors, excess anticoagulant or a vascular defect

Goal	Nursing intervention
1. Bleeding will be limited due to prompt identification	• Inspect the skin for appearance of petechiae and purpura • Record any change in size or new areas of petechiae and purpura • Observe open lesions, incisions, and intravenous and intramuscular injection sites for oozing or haematomas • Test urine, stools and vomit for blood • Examine joints for oedema, tenderness and limited movement • Assess symptoms of internal bleeding by recording changes in vital signs 4-hourly or as condition indicates • Observe for signs of cerebral dysfunction, confusion, disorientation or restlessness
2. Bleeding will stop with minimal blood loss and vital signs will be within normal range	• Control overt bleeding with pressure and elevation of affected part if possible • Estimate and record blood loss in vomit, nasogastric drainage, stools and on dressings and sanitary pads • Keep the person at rest in bed • Administer blood products and medications as prescribed, observing for potential reactions • Monitor and record vital signs regularly as indicated by person's condition • Maintain an accurate fluid balance record • Immobilize limbs or joints if bleeding is present in these areas
3. Patient will experience no further bleeding or long-term complications	• Move the person gently to avoid causing tissue trauma • Ensure cot sides are padded • Remove sharp objects from the patient's immediate environment • If there is bleeding into joints immobilize in the optimum alignment • Provide a bed cradle to keep the weight of bedding off the affected part • Begin range of motion exercises 48 hours after bleeding stops • Use pressure relieving aids on beds and chairs • Avoid invasive procedures, injections, etc. and minimize number of venepunctures • Apply direct pressure to venepuncture sites for 10 minutes • Take blood pressure only when essential and rotate sites
4. Patient will express decreased fear and anxiety and actively participate in the treatment plan	• Assess person for behaviour indicative of anxiety and fear (restlessness, hyperactivity, withdrawal, crying, expression of anger) • Acknowledge acceptance of person's fear • Explain all procedures and reinforce information given • Encourage questions and expression of anxieties • Encourage participation in decisions concerning treatment and care
5. Patient will describe signs of bleeding, preventive measures and action to take if bleeding occurs	• Inform the patient about causes, signs and symptoms of bleeding disorders (epistaxis, bleeding gums, petechiae, bruising, haematuria) • Instruct patient and family to seek medical advice immediately if these occur • Discuss measures aimed at preventing tissue trauma, e.g. use of soft toothbrush, avoidance of constrictive clothing, use of electric razors for shaving, need to keep nails short and clean, need to prevent constipation and injury to rectal mucosa, need to avoid self-medication with any aspirin-containing drug • Advise on safety of occupation and recreational interests and identify activities that are safe to continue and those to be avoided, e.g. contact sports • Provide information on community support available, self-help and support groups, etc. • Inform patient of genetic counselling opportunities if appropriate • Suggest need to wear a Medic Alert identification in case of emergencies if condition is prolonged

Donor blood is tested for:

- ABO and Rh typing of the red blood cells;
- Antibody screening for antibodies capable of reacting with the clinically important antigens that may be present in the recipient's red blood cells;
- Transmittable infections: AIDS, hepatitis, syphilis and possibly cytomegalovirus.

The recipient's blood is tested for:

- ABO and Rh typing of the red blood cells;
- A 'major side' crossmatch to detect antibodies that could react with the donor red blood cells;
- Antibody screening for selected antibodies.

A compatibility chart is shown in Figure 13.9.

Preparations used in transfusions (Table 13.13)

1. Whole blood. Whole blood is administered to replace blood loss or to increase the intravascular volume in shock.

2. Packed red cells. A large portion of the plasma is removed from whole blood by centrifuging. The remaining cells are given to increase the oxygen-carrying capacity of the recipient's blood. The advantage of packed cells is that a lesser volume is added to the patient's intravascular volume, thus preventing the risk of overload. The cells may be administered in a small volume of normal saline or plasma.

3. Plasma. Plasma may be used fresh, fresh frozen or dried. It contains all the labile clotting factors and is used to control bleeding when specific concentrates are unavailable or the precise deficiency is unknown.

4. Thrombocytes. Platelets may be concentrated and given in a small volume to avoid the administration of a large volume of fluid. This avoids the risk of overtaxing the recipient's heart and overloading the circulatory system. Transfusion of platelets is used to control bleeding in patients with thrombocytopenia. ABO compatibility is not essential but the development of alloimmunization is a complication of platelet transfusions. The rate of platelet destruction is increased in the sensitized individual. Rh immunoglobulin is administered to Rh-negative persons who receive platelets from an Rh-positive donor to prevent Rh sensitization.

5. Granulocytes. White blood cells from an ABO compatible donor are prepared by leucophoresis. They are administered to neutropenic patients with an infection that has not responded to antibiotic therapy.

6. Albumin is prepared from plasma and is available in 5% and 25% solutions. It is used to rapidly expand plasma volume in severe hypovolaemia.

7. Clotting factors. Concentrates of certain clotting factors (e.g. VIII, IX) are prepared from fresh frozen plasma to control bleeding in haemophilia A and B or in fibrinogen deficiency. Preparations include cryoprecipitates and specific factor preparations.

Donor blood group	Recipient blood group			
	A	B	O	AB
A	✓	✗	✗	✓
B	✗	✓	✗	✓
O	✓	✓	✓	✓
AB	✗	✗	✗	✓

Figure 13.9 ABO blood group compatibility. ✓, compatible; ✗, non-compatible.

Nursing responsibilities

1. The patient should be fully informed about the procedure and any questions should be answered.
2. The patient's mobility may be restricted during transfusion, patient comfort should therefore be ensured.
3. The patient's blood type has been determined and the blood crossmatched with donor blood for compatibility. Before the matched blood is given, a check is made by two persons to ensure that the blood that has been received is for this particular patient, and is of the correct type. The expiration date on the blood label should also be checked and contents examined for abnormal cloudiness and particles.
4. The rate of administration depends upon the patient's condition; if the blood volume has been markedly depleted by haemorrhage or if the patient is in severe shock, it may be delivered at a faster rate than is used if the intravascular volume is normal. A rate commonly used is the delivery of a unit (500 ml) over 4 hours. If the blood volume has not been depleted or if there is a risk of overtaxing the patient's heart, the rate should be reduced and a diuretic is often administered. Blood should be administered within a 4-hour period because of the potential for bacterial contamination. If the transfusion has not been completed within 4 hours it is discontinued and a new unit set up. The patient should be observed closely throughout the administration for signs of circulatory overload (dyspnoea, coughing, pink frothy sputum, weak pulse).
5. Precautionary measures are used. The blood is infused through a filter and is *gently* mixed at intervals to keep cells suspended throughout the plasma. A normal saline infusion is started so that the tube can be flushed before and after the blood is administered.

No medication should be given into the blood that is being administered; if a drug must be given, the blood is temporarily stopped and the normal saline infusion restarted.

The nurse remains with the patient for a period of 15–20 minutes following the beginning of the blood transfusion, or until at least 100 ml has been delivered; the patient may be very apprehensive at first and most reactions usually develop within that period. The patient is assessed frequently for possible reactions and the rate

Table 13.13   The administration of blood and blood products.

Blood/blood product and composition	Administration	Common complications
Whole blood Red blood cells, leucocytes, plasma, platelets, clotting factors, (500 ml/unit)	1. Warm blood 20–30 minutes at room temperature before administering 2. Check labels carefully according to hospital policy 3. Use a parenteral administration set with a blood filter inside the drip chamber 4. Use only normal saline (0.9% NaCl) solution for intravenous infusion 5. Fill the drip chamber to cover the filter with the blood 6. Agitate the blood bag gently before and during administration 7. Begin the tranfusion at a slow flow rate of approximately 1 ml/kg/per hour and observe patient constantly for the first 15 minutes Adjust rate if there are no adverse reactions 8. Record vital signs before each unit, every 10 mins for 30 mins then every hour until complete 9. Complete transfusion in 2–4 hours 10. Discard any blood not transfused within 4 hours	Transfusion reactions include: fever chills headache restlessness back pain dyspnoea tachycardia palpitation hypotension cold clammy skin thready pulse altered level of consciousness risk of circulatory overload haemoglobinurea
Packed red cells Fresh—red blood cells, 20% plasma, some leucocytes and platelets (300 ml per unit) Frozen—red blood cells, no plasma and few leucocytes or platelets (200–300 ml/unit)	1. Use a Y-connector set with normal saline solution to improve infusion rate 2. Use blood administration set with blood filter 3. Fill drip chamber to cover filter 4. Agitate bag before and every 20–30 minutes during administration 5. Administer over 4 hours	Transfusion reactions are the same as with blood but are less frequent
Plasma Fresh, frozen or dried—all plasma proteins and clotting factors (no RBC, WBC or platelets) (200 ml/ unit)	1. Use a standard intravenous administration set 2. Administer as rapidly as necessary and tolerated for volume replacement 3. Administer fresh, frozen plasma promptly after thawing to prevent deterioration of clotting factors 4. Requires ABO compatibility	Greater risk of allergic reactions and viral hepatitis than with whole blood because of multiple donors Risk of fluid overload with rapid infusions
Platelets Platelets, lymphocytes and some plasma (40–50 ml/unit)	1. Use a platelet transfusion set 2. Administer as rapidly as tolerated (½–1 hour) 3. Use Y-set with normal saline	Chills, fever Alloimmunization producing rapid destruction of transfused platelets
Granulocytes White blood cells and plasma with some red blood cells, platelets and other white blood cells (200–300 ml per suspension)	1. Use a standard blood filter infusion set 2. Use a Y-connector set with normal saline solution only 3. Administer first 50–75 ml slowly and observe for transfusion reaction 4. Administer over 2–4 hours 5. Use within 24 hours of collection	Chills, fever Allergic reactions (urticaria, wheezing) Hypotension, shock Respiratory distress
Albumin Albumin with plasma and normal saline (5% in 250–300 ml units, 25% in 25–50 ml units)	1. The rate of administration depends on the reason for administration. It is administered rapidly for volume expansion but is usually given slowly 2. Use administration set with filtered air inlet	Fluid volume overload
Clotting factors Cryoprecipitated antihaemolytic factor	1. Administer by standard intravenous drip set 2. Administer promptly on thawing 3. Multiple units are usually administered	Chills and fever Risk of hepatitis Bleeding if infusions are not

Table 13.13 *continued*

Blood/blood product and composition	Administration	Common complications
Factor VIII concentrate		repeated because of short half-life of product
Factor IX concentrate	1. Administer by syringe as intravenous bolus 2. Use within 30 mins of preparation	Chills and fever Allergic reactions Risk of hepatitis

of flow is checked. Observations should continue for at least 1 hour after stopping the infusion.

Ethical issues: patient refusal of transfusion

Although blood transfusion is a commonly-used therapeutic procedure, it is necessary to bear in mind that a transfusion may be refused because of religious beliefs or other considerations. Refusal of blood and blood products on religious grounds is usually associated with Jehovah's Witnesses. Most courts have recognized the right of adult Jehovah's Witnesses to refuse blood and blood products for themselves. However, it has usually been judged that parents and guardians do not have the right to refuse life-saving therapy (including blood transfusions) for their minor children and a court order may be applied to protect a child. Whenever it becomes apparent that a patient is a Jehovah's Witness, the use of blood and blood products should be discussed with the patient, with a clear explanation of the consequences of refusing transfusion treatment. It is advisable to obtain a signed and witnessed statement if treatment is refused (Napier, 1987).

Reactions

The transfer of blood or any component of it carries a risk of a reaction. The blood or its components may act as a foreign protein or antigen that prompts an immune response or tissue reaction.

Unfavourable responses to transfusions include the following:

1. Acute haemolytic reaction

This is agglutination of the donor's red blood cells followed by their haemolysis, which occurs as a result of incompatibility. Antibodies within the recipient's blood attack the donor's erythrocytes. Haemoglobin and other products of the haemolysis are circulated throughout the body.

Early manifestations of incompatibility include local pain at the infusion site, chills, headache or full feeling in the head, anxiety, restlessness, pain in the kidney area (backache), and/or chest, dyspnoea, tachycardia and palpitation. Anaphylactic shock may develop; the patient's blood pressure falls, the skin becomes cold and clammy, respiratory distress is increasingly more severe, the pulse weakens and consciousness is clouded. In anaesthetized patients a haemolytic reaction can be difficult to detect.

After several hours, even though the patient's general condition has improved markedly, haemoglobinuria and/or oliguria may appear. The haemoglobin released by the haemolysed cells is excreted in the urine, colouring it red. The haemoglobin may be precipitated in the renal tubules by the acidity of the urine. The tubules become blocked and are damaged, reducing the urinary output. Acute renal failure and anuria may develop if the haemolysis is extensive as a result of the patient receiving approximately 100 ml or more of the incompatible blood.

Complications associated with a haemolytic reaction are hyperkalaemia and hypocalcaemia. The haemolysis of the donor's red blood cells releases potassium. The impaired renal function results in retention of the potassium, and its serum concentration exceeds the normal level. Hyperkalaemia may develop when the whole blood that is being given has been stored for 5 days or more. Some red cells are broken down and the serum potassium concentration of the donor blood is increased.

Treatment. The administration of the blood or blood component is stopped promptly with the initial manifestation(s) of reaction. The normal saline is started again slowly to maintain an open intravenous line in case medications may have to be administered intravenously.

If the patient complains of shortness of breath and 'tightness' in the chest, adrenaline 1:1000 (0.5–1 ml) subcutaneously or intramuscularly may be prescribed. A marked fall in blood pressure (hypotension) may be treated by increasing the intravascular volume with a plasma substitute such as Haemaccel.

Treatment is instituted to promote urinary output and reduce impairment of renal function by the haemoglobin released through haemolysis. The fluid intake and output must be accurately measured and recorded. An indwelling catheter may be passed so the urinary output may be measured hourly. Fluids containing potassium must be avoided. Intravenous solutions are administered and may include mannitol (25 g), an osmotic diuretic. If the urinary output progressively decreases, the fluid intake is limited to insensible fluid loss and losses by other channels (vomiting, bowel elimination). Anuria and renal failure may develop, necessitating haemodialysis.

2. Febrile reaction

A fairly common reaction to a transfusion is fever preceded by a rigor. It is attributed to the recipient's sensitivity to the donor's leucocytes, thrombocytes or plasma proteins. It may also develop as a result of a pyrogenic material in the equipment or solution used. The transfusion is slowed to relieve the discomfort of the febrile reaction and chills. If the person has had multiple transfusions or experienced this type of reaction before, hydrocortisone and chlorpheniramine (Piriton), an antihistamine, may also be prescribed.

A febrile reaction may be the first sign of an acute haemolytic reaction or it may indicate that the blood or blood product was infected with live bacteria or bacterial toxins.

3. Allergic reaction

A component of the donor's blood may act as an antigen and initiate an allergic response. It is also suggested that the cause of an allergic reaction may be the response of antibodies in the donor's blood to an antigen within the recipient. The most common manifestations are urticaria and asthma. Severe bronchospasm and anaphylaxis occur less frequently. Anaphylaxis occurs in persons who are IgA deficient. When such persons are sensitized, either by a previous pregnancy or transfusion, an anaphylactic reaction may occur with a transfusion of plasma containing blood products. An antihistamine preparation, such as diphenhydramine hydrochloride (Benadryl), may provide relief. If the bronchospasm is severe or anaphylaxis develops, adrenaline 1:1000 may be administered parenterally as well as a corticosteroid preparation.

4. Circulatory overload

The giving of a transfusion too rapidly, or the administration of whole blood or plasma to someone with a normal intravascular volume or who has or is predisposed to cardiac or renal insufficiency, is dangerous. The resulting increased intravascular volume places too great a demand on the heart. Heart failure and pulmonary oedema ensue. The patient develops severe dyspnoea, coughing, anxiety, weak pulse and cyanosis. A pink frothy sputum is expectorated.

Circulatory overload may be prevented by the slow administration of packed red cells while the central venous pressure is monitored carefully. (See p. 306 for central venous pressure monitoring).

Non-cardiogenic pulmonary oedema or adult respiratory distress syndrome (ARDS) may also occur. This is likely to be due to a reaction to the HLA antibodies in the donor plasma.

5. Infection

Infected blood often causes chest and abdominal pain, and hypotension may occur (septicaemic shock). If this is suspected, antibiotic therapy is prescribed.

Hepatitis is the most common infectious problem associated with transfusions. Donors' blood is tested in blood banks for the hepatitis B antigen, but the transmission of hepatitis is still a possibility. The onset of manifestations of the infection may occur many weeks after the transfusion.

Syphilis, malaria, AIDS and hepatitis B, non-A and non-B may be transmitted by transfusion, but the possibility is minimal because of the screening of donors and the tests that are performed on all donor blood.

If a transfusion reaction occurs

1. The transfusion should be stopped promptly; slow infusion of normal saline is resumed to maintain an open line, and the doctor is notified.
2. The remaining blood or blood component is returned in the container with the tubing to the blood bank for analysis and determination of the cause of the reaction.
3. The blood bank is notified of the nature of the reaction.
4. Blood specimens are taken from a vein other than the one that was used to administer the blood. They are sent to the laboratory for retyping, culture and estimation of free plasma haemoglobin.
5. A nurse remains with the patient; vital signs are monitored frequently and continuous assessment of the patient's condition is necessary. The patient is likely to be very apprehensive and fearful and will require some information about what is happening and reassurance that everything possible is being done.
6. A urine specimen is collected from the patient as soon as possible and sent to the laboratory for haemoglobin determination.

Autologous blood transfusion (ABT) involves collecting and infusing the patient's own blood. It may be an acceptable alternative for Jehovah's Witnesses and has the specific advantage of involving no risk of transmission of viral infections such as HIV and hepatitis. There is no risk of a haemolytic reaction and ABT is useful for elective surgery if there is a shortage of donated blood. ABT involves collection of blood prior to surgery, or intraoperative salvage involving special recovery systems. These techniques are relatively uncommon and unlikely rapidly to replace the existing system of blood donation (Zugic, 1990). Human recombinant erythropoietin is currently being evaluated as a means of reducing the need for blood transfusion in some anaemic patients and for increasing the amount of autologous blood that can be collected prior to elective surgery.

SUMMARY

Persons with disorders of the blood experience various acute and chronic symptoms and disruptions in the quality of their daily lives as a result of changes in one or more of the components of the haematological system. This chapter focuses on the person with common disorders of the red blood cells, white blood cells and platelets. Nursing management of the person with disorders of the haematological system is described in detail in relation to the major health problems experienced by patients. Potential associated health problems are identified but discussed in less depth. Several clinical situations are presented to illustrate the impact of the disorders on the person and family and to emphasize some of the options available to them and the decisions they are faced with regarding therapy and the quality of their lives.

Nursing measures related to the safe administration of blood and blood products are discussed and ethical issues relevant to transfusions of blood and blood products are presented.

LEARNING ACTIVITIES

1. Mrs Jones is a 76-year-old woman who lives alone in a small flat. During your visit as a district nurse, she tells you that she has been feeling very tired lately. On further exploration you discover that she has been falling asleep during her favourite afternoon soap opera on television. She is receiving adequate sleep at night and reports that she eats very well and does her own cooking. When pushed for details she says she has tea and toast with jam each morning and tea and biscuits in the afternoon and evening. Further questioning reveals that she has decreased her social activities significantly.
   Describe the goals, outcome criteria and plan of care you would develop with Mrs Jones.
2. Explore the availability of and services provided by self-help groups in your community for patients with bleeding disorders and their families.
3. Ask your tutor to arrange a visit to your Regional Blood Transfusion Service headquarters.
4. Is it right that patient's blood should be tested, without their knowledge, for HIV, and, if positive, that this information is withheld from the patient? Discuss the issues around these two questions.

REFERENCES AND FURTHER READING

Barnard DL, McVerry BA & Norfolk DR (1989) *Clinical Haematology*. Oxford: Heinemann.

Borley D (ed.) (1989) *Oncology for Nurses and Health Care Professionals. Vol. 3 Cancer Nursing* 2nd edn. Beaconsfield: Harper & Row.

Bouchier IAD, Allan RN, Hodgson HJF & Keighley MRB (1984) *Textbook of Gastroenterology*. Eastbourne: Baillière Tindall.

Chanarin I, Brozovic M, Tidmarsh E & Waters DAW (1985) *Blood and Its Diseases* 3rd edn. Edinburgh: Churchill Livingstone.

Cyganski JM, Donahue JM & Heaton JS (1987) The case for the heparin flush. *American Journal of Nursing* **87(6):** 796–797.

Dunn DL & Lenihan SF (1987) The case for the saline flush. *American Journal of Nursing* **87(6):** 798–799.

Eastham R (1984) *Clinical Haematology* 6th edn. Bristol: Wright.

Edwards J (1989) Nursing patients with acute and chronic leukaemias. In Borley D (ed.) *Oncology for Nurses and Health Care Professionals. Vol. 3 Cancer Nursing* 2nd edn. Beaconsfield: Harper and Row.

Ford R & Eisenberg S (1990) Bone marrow transplant: recent advances and nursing implications. *Nursing Clinics of North America* **25(2):** 405–422.

France-Dawson M (1986) Sickle cell disease: implications for nursing care. *Journal of Advanced Nursing* **11(6):** 729–737.

Ganong WF (1989) *Review of Medical Physiology* 14th edn. Norwalk CT: Appleton & Lange.

Gillis C (1988) The epidemiology of human cancer. In Pritchard P (ed.) *Oncology for Nurses and Health Care Professionals. Vol. 1 Pathology, Diagnosis and Treatment* 2nd edn. Beaconsfield: Harper & Row.

Gobel BH (1990) Plasma and plasma derivative therapy for coagulation disorders. *Seminars in Oncology Nursing* **6(2):** 129–135.

Gurevich I & Tafuro P (1986) The compromised host: deficit-specific infection and spectrum of prevention. *Cancer Nursing* **9(5):** 263–275.

Guyton AC (1991) *Textbook of Medical Physiology* 8th edn. Philadelphia: Saunders.

Hinchliff S & Montague S (1988) *Physiology for Nursing Practice*. London: Baillière Tindall.

Hirsh J & Brain EA (1983) *Haemostasis and Thrombosis: A Conceptual Approach* 2nd edn. New York: Churchill Livingstone.

Hoffbrand AV & Pettit JE (1984) *Essential Haematology*. Oxford: Blackwell.

Llewellyn-Jones D (1986) *Fundamentals of Obstetrics and Gynaecology. Vol. 1 Obstetrics*. London: Faber & Faber.

McElwain TJ & Selby P (eds) (1987) *Hodgkin's Disease*. Oxford: Blackwell.

Marieb EN (1989) *Human Anatomy and Physiology*. Redwood City CA: Benjamin/Cummings.

Milliken S, Lakhani & Powles R (1988) Bone marrow transplantation. In Pritchard P (ed.) *Oncology for Nurses and Health Care Professionals. Vol. 1 Pathology, Diagnosis and Treatment* 2nd edn. Beaconsfield: Harper & Row.

Napier JAF (1987) *Blood Transfusion Therapy: A Problem Orientated Approach*. Chichester: Wiley.

Pritchard P (ed.) (1988) *Oncology for Nurses and Health Care Professionals. Vol. 1 Pathology, Diagnosis and Treatment* 2nd edn. Beaconsfield: Harper & Row.

Pritchard AP & David JA (eds) (1988) *The Royal Marsden Hospital Manual of Clinical Nursing Procedures* 2nd edn. London: Harper & Row.

Redheffer G (1989) Treating wounds at the scene. Part 1. *Nursing 89* **19(7):** 51–57.

Richardson A (1987) A process standard for oral care. *Nursing Times* **82(20):** 1086–1088.

Royal Marsden Hospital (1985) *Care of a Skin-Tunnelled Catheter*. Patient Information Series No. 3. London: Royal Marsden Hospital.

Royle J & Green E (1985) Right atrial catheters: a patient and family education program. *Cancer Nursing* **81(3):** 51–54.

Smith LH & Thier SO (1985) *Pathophysiology* 2nd edn. Philadelphia: Saunders.

Soutami R & Tobias J (1986) *Cancer and Its Management*. Oxford: Blackwell.

Trentor RP & Creasun N (1986) Nurse administered oral hygiene: is there a scientific basis? *Journal of Advanced Nursing* **11:** 323–331.

Tschuden V (ed.) (1988) *Nursing the Patient with Cancer*. London: Prentice-Hall.

Zugic VE (1990) Autologous blood transfusion (ABT). A study of clinical applications and a literature review. *Intensive Care Nursing.* **6:** 30–37.

Caring for the Patient with a Disorder of the Cardiovascular System

OBJECTIVES

On completion of this chapter, the reader will be able to:
- Describe the anatomy and physiology of the cardiovascular system
- Describe a complete assessment of a person's cardiovascular system
- Identify risk factors for cardiovascular disease and recommendations for life-style modifications which prevent or relieve these risk factors
- Discuss the various pathophysiological processes which a person can develop or sustain in relation to the cardiovascular system
- Discuss the nursing management of people who have cardiovascular diseases, and their families

CIRCULATION

Normal cellular activity is dependent upon a constant supply of oxygen, nutrients, and certain chemicals, as well as the removal of metabolic waste products. The unicellular organism is in direct contact with the outside environmental source of its essentials, but in complex multicellular organisms cell needs are not as simply met. Specialized organs are necessary for the processes of oxygenation, nutrition and excretion, as well as a transportation system between these organs and the cells throughout the body. This transportation of materials to and from tissue cells by the propulsion of blood through a closed system of tubes is the process referred to as circulation.

Circulatory Structures

The circulatory system consists of the heart and the vascular system.

HEART

The heart is a hollow, cone-shaped, muscular organ lying obliquely in the thoracic cavity. Approximately two-thirds of it is situated to the left of the midline. The upper border (or base) lies just below the second rib. The lower border (or apex) is directed downward, forward and to the left and lies on the diaphragm at the level of the fifth intercostal space in the left midclavicular line.

Pericardium
The pericardium is a strong, non-distensible sac which loosely encloses the heart and attaches to the large blood vessels at the base of the heart and to the diaphragm at the apex. It consists of two layers. The outer one forms the fibrous pericardium, and the inner one, the serous pericardium. The latter is also divided into two layers: one layer lines the sac, and the other is

reflected over the surface of the heart as the epicardium, or visceral pericardium. The space formed between the sac and the heart is normally only a potential space. The surfaces are in close contact, and thin, clear pericardial fluid is secreted to keep them moist and to prevent friction between the heart and the sac. The fibrous pericardium, because of its inextensible nature, prevents overdistension of the heart. It also supports the heart, preventing alteration of its position during postural changes. Although the pericardial sac is firm and considered non-extensible, it does extend in response to the gradual, sustained stretching imposed by enlargement of the heart (hypertrophy).

Heart walls
The walls of the heart are composed of three layers of tissue. The epicardium forms the outer layer of the heart and is the visceral layer of the pericardium. The myocardium is the middle layer of tissue. This is composed of involuntary striated muscle fibres which interlace, branch and anastomose. This arrangement produces a very firm, closely related mass of tissues through which an excitatory impulse for contraction spreads very quickly. This layer of muscle is responsible for the heart's contractile force. The endocardium is a thin layer of endothelial cells lining the interior surface of the heart's chambers and covers the heart's valves. This layer creates a smooth surface, reducing friction between moving blood and the walls of the heart.

Heart chambers
From shortly after birth, the human heart is divided longitudinally by a partition into two halves between which there is no direct communication. The cavity of each side is divided horizontally by an incomplete partition which results in two upper chambers, called the right and left atria, and two lower ones, which are the right and left ventricles (Figure 14.1). The atria serve primarily as receiving chambers for blood, while the ventricles act as pumping chambers.

The atrial myocardium is much thinner than that of the ventricles and the left ventricular wall is thicker than

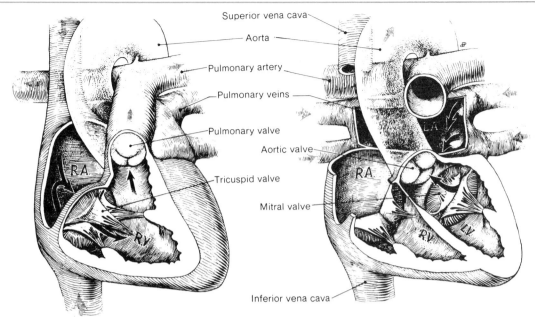

Fig. 14.1 The heart.

Figure 14.1 The heart.

that of the right. These differences can be correlated with the force that must be given to the contained blood. The atria are receiving chambers and are only required to deliver the blood to the ventricles, which discharge blood from the heart. The right ventricle pumps blood through the lungs to the left atrium, forming the circuit referred to as the pulmonary circulatory system. The left ventricle must provide sufficient pressure to carry blood through all parts of the body and return it to the right atrium. This latter circuit is referred to as the systemic circulatory system.

Cardiac valves
Normal circulation requires the flow of the blood in one direction only. This is maintained in the heart by a set of four valves: two atrioventricular and two semilunar.

The atrioventricular (AV) valves are formed of fibrous cusps, or leaflets, which derive from the fibrous ring that encircles each atrioventricular opening. They are covered with endothelial tissue which is continuous with the endocardium. The right AV valve is located between the right atrium and ventricle. It has three cusps and is called the tricuspid valve. The left AV valve, situated between the left atrium and ventricle, has two cusps and is called the mitral valve. These valves open into the ventricles but are prevented from opening into the atria by fine tendinous cords (chordae tendineae) which insert on the free border of the leaflets and originate in small pillars of muscle projecting from the ventricular walls (papillary muscles). When the ventricles fill, the valve cusps are forced up in the direction of the atrioventricular opening. They meet, closing off the opening and, with the contraction of the papillary muscles, sufficient tension is exerted by the chordae tendineae to prevent the valves from opening into the atria (Figure 14.1).

The semilunar valves guard the openings from the ventricles into the pulmonary artery and aorta and are called the pulmonary and aortic valves, respectively. Each consists of three pocket-like pouches arranged around the origin of the artery, with the free borders being distal to the ventricle (Figure 14.1). During the contraction of the ventricles and ejection of blood into the aorta and pulmonary artery, the valve cusps offer no resistance to the flow of the blood. When the ventricles relax and there is a reversal in the direction of pressure, blood fills the semilunar pouches, bringing their surfaces together. This closes off the opening into each ventricle, preventing backflow of blood.

ELECTRICAL CONDUCTION SYSTEM

The heart is a unique organ because it has an electrical conduction system to maintain its rate and rhythm of activity.

The sinoatrial (SA) node is a small mass of specialized tissue located in the upper portion of the right atrium near the superior vena cava inlet. It is responsible for initiating impulses for a rhythmic heartbeat.

The atrioventricular (AV) node lies in the lower part of the right atrium in the interatrial septum. It conducts electrical impulses from the atria to the ventricles. A bundle of fibres called the bundle of His proceeds from junctional tissue at the AV node into the ventricular septum, where it divides into two, forming the left and right bundle branches. The left bundle branch further divides into the anterior (superior) and posterior (inferior) divisions (Figure 14.2). As it descends, each bundle branch gives rise to a network of fine fibres which are known as the Purkinje fibres. They are distributed to the ventricular myocardial cells.

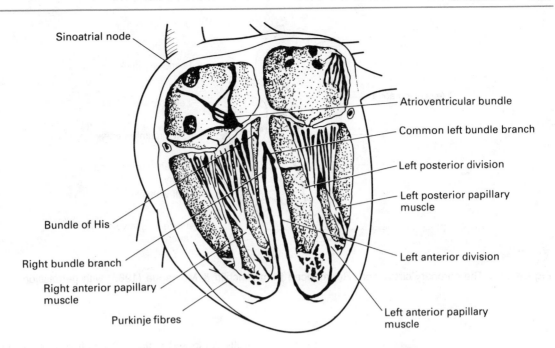

Sinoatrial node

Atrioventricular bundle

Common left bundle branch

Left posterior division

Left posterior papillary muscle

Bundle of His

Left anterior division

Right bundle branch

Right anterior papillary muscle

Purkinje fibres

Left anterior papillary muscle

Figure 14.2 The impulse conduction system. Modified from Wyper and Walsh (1989) with permission.

CORONARY ARTERY SYSTEM (FIGURE 14.3)

The coronary artery system provides the myocardium with its blood supply. The coronary arteries arise from the sinus of Valsalva in the root of the aorta and sit on the epicardial layer of the heart, radiating inward through the myocardium to the endocardium. There are two main coronary arteries, the left and right. The left main coronary artery divides into the anterior descending artery (LAD) and the circumflex artery. The LAD is distributed to the anterior part of the left ventricle and portions of the right ventricle. In addition to the anterior wall of the left ventricle, the LAD supplies the anterior papillary muscle of the left ventricle, the anterior two-thirds of the interventricular septum, and distal parts of the conduction system. The circumflex artery carries blood to the lateral and lower posterior, left ventricular walls and to the left atrium. Branches of the right coronary artery supply the remaining portions of the myocardium. The right coronary artery nourishes the SA node in approximately 55% of people and the AV node in 90% of people. At other times, the blood supply to these structures is provided by the left circumflex artery. The large arteries divide and subdivide to form a network of smaller arteries and capillaries throughout the heart muscle. The blood is returned to the right atrium through a system of progressively enlarging veins which terminate in the coronary sinus.

The myocardium requires a large blood supply since it must work continuously and adapt its activity to the varying needs of tissues throughout the body. The coronary vessels dilate to increase the supply when demands are increased. For example, during vigorous activity, coronary artery blood flow can increase to help ensure adequate oxygen supply to the myocardium.

They also dilate when there is an increase in the carbon dioxide concentration of the blood and a decrease in the pH.

The flow of blood through the coronary system is dependent upon the pressure of the blood in the aorta; a reduction in blood pressure will result in a smaller volume entering the coronary arteries. The coronary volume is greater during myocardial relaxation. In systole, with the myocardium contracted, the vessels are compressed and their volume is reduced. When a person is at rest, the blood entering the coronary system is approximately 4% of the total cardiac output. The coronary blood supply can be increased, but to a lesser degree than the cardiac output. That is, the work of the myocardium can be increased to a greater extent than its blood supply.

VASCULAR SYSTEM

The blood travels from the heart through arteries, arterioles, capillaries and veins back to the heart (Figure 14.4). The structure of each type of vessel is modified according to its function and location. One common structural characteristic of all the vessels is the smooth endothelial lining, known as the intima. The arteries and arterioles form a high-pressure distributing system; the capillaries are structured and organized for exchanging substances between the blood and interstitial fluid; the venules and veins serve as a low-pressure collecting system which returns the blood to the heart.

ARTERIES AND ARTERIOLES

The large arteries carry blood away from the heart and

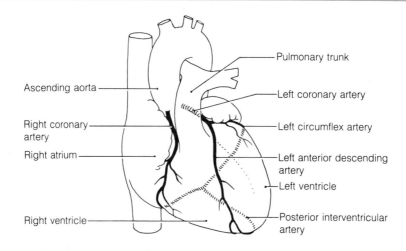

Figure 14.3 The coronary circulation. Reproduced from Hinchliff & Montague (1988) with permission.

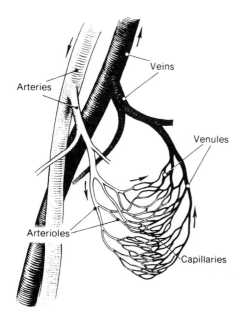

Figure 14.4 Artery-arteriole-capillary-vein sequence in the circulation.

branch and subdivide many times. Their structure varies with their size, the larger ones being more elastic and less muscular. Elasticity is an important property of these vessels; with the ejection of blood from the heart, the vessel distends and on recoil exerts a slight pressure on the contained fluid, helping to force it forward. If resistance is offered to the flow of the blood, normally the arteries can stretch to accommodate the increased volume of blood, and the pressure of the blood remains within the normal range.

The smallest arteries emerge as arterioles, which have walls composed mainly of a well-developed muscular coat over the endothelium. The muscle tissue may contract or relax to decrease or increase the amount of blood through the arterioles (vasoconstriction or vaso-dilatation). This feature of the arterioles gives them an important role in determining arterial blood pressure and in controlling the blood flow into the capillaries.

CAPILLARIES

Each arteriole channels its content into microscopic endothelial tubes, the capillaries, which anastomose with each other to form a capillary bed. These vessels are the principal functional unit of the cardiovascular system. The exchange of fluids, gases and nutrients to maintain and regulate cell activity takes place as the blood passes through the thin capillary walls, usually by diffusion.

Not all the capillaries are open at all times. There are wide variations in the amount of activity in some tissues such as skeletal muscle, while in others such as brain tissue a more constant blood supply is necessary. Similarly, when an area is irritated, more blood is brought to that part in its defence (e.g. inflammation). The number of capillaries through which blood is passing at any given time is adjusted locally to meet the needs of the tissues in the area. A small proportion of the blood is located in the capillaries in resting states; the volume increases as tissue activity increases. This adjustment is possible because some capillaries have at their origin a ring of plain muscular tissue which forms a precapillary sphincter allowing for closure of its capillaries when they are not needed.

VENULES AND VEINS

The collecting part of the vascular system originates in venules which drain the capillaries and progressively unite and enlarge to form veins. They differ from arteries in several ways: (1) they carry blood toward the heart; (2) their walls are much thinner and less elastic with the result that they collapse when empty; (3) the contained blood is under a much lower pressure; and (4) many of the veins have valves.

The structure of veins changes as they increase in size; more muscle and fibrous tissue appear in the walls but, in comparison with arteries, the muscle fibres are sparse. Most of the pressure of the blood created by the heart is dissipated in the arterioles and capillaries and, in order to maintain the flow in one direction, valves similar in structure to the semilunar valves of the heart occur at intervals in many of the veins. They are particularly numerous in the lower extremities where the blood is flowing against gravity. The thinner walls of the veins are readily compressed by skeletal muscle contraction; this assists the blood along its course toward the heart, since backflow toward the capillaries is prevented by one-way valves.

Physiology of Circulation

Normal circulation through the cardiovascular system is dependent upon an appropriate pressure gradient throughout the system, an adequate volume of blood, a closed system of unobstructed tubes and a set of valves to ensure flow in one direction only.

PRINCIPLES APPLICABLE TO THE FLOW OF FLUIDS THROUGH TUBES

Since circulation is the continuous flow of blood in a pressure system composed of a pump and a series of tubes filled with the blood, it might be as well at this point to consider some physical factors which govern the flow of any liquid through tubes. The rate at which a fluid moves through a tube depends upon the pressure gradient and the resistance to flow.

PRESSURE GRADIENT

Fluids flow from an area of high pressure to one of lower pressure. The pressure of fluid at any given point in the system must be greater than that in the succeeding area into which it is to flow. This difference is referred to as the pressure gradient, or driving force. If the pressure should become the same throughout the system, no movement of fluid takes place.

The pressure gradient which maintains the normal flow of blood through the vessels is the difference between the pressure of the blood in the arterial system and that of the venous system. The main source of the driving force is the pumping action of the heart which produces a relatively high pressure in the arteries.

RESISTANCE TO FLOW

The amount of resistance offered to the flow of fluid is determined by the dimensions of the tube and the viscosity of the fluid.

The pressure of a fluid progressively decreases as it flows through a tube because of the friction between the fluid and the walls of the tube. This friction, which is referred to as peripheral resistance, causes a loss of energy. Fluid flows more slowly through a tube of smaller diameter since more friction is created between the walls and the fluid, resulting in an increase in resistance. As the blood flows through blood vessels having a lesser radius (arterioles and capillaries) resistance is increased, causing a decrease in the rate of flow and blood pressure.

Similarly, resistance is increased as the length of the tube increases, since the greater amount of surface provides more friction.

If the volume of fluid remains the same in a system of tubes, the rate of flow decreases as the tubular space (capacity) increases. This factor contributes to the marked decrease in the velocity of the blood in the capillaries. Although the radius of the capillaries is extremely small, the total cross-sectional area of the vast number of these minute tubes exceeds the total area of all the other vessels combined.

The viscosity of a fluid is the internal resistance to flow created by the friction between the molecules of fluid and their tendency to adhere. Obviously, a greater concentration of particles in a fluid produces an increased internal resistance. For example, an excessive number of blood cells, particularly erythrocytes, increases the viscosity of the blood and retards its rate of flow.

In summary, resistance to flow is inversely proportional to the diameter of the tube, directly proportional to the length of the tube, and directly proportional to the viscosity of the fluid. If the volume of fluid remains the same, the rate of flow decreases as the diameter of the tube increases.

The preceding principles are based on the flow of fluids through rigid tubes. Some modification is necessary in applying them to circulation. The blood vessels are not rigid tubes and their diameters are variable. Branches, division and curves occur at frequent intervals in the blood vessels. Blood is viscous and its flow is pulsatile, rather than steady, in a large part of the circulatory system.

The Role of the Heart in Circulation

The pressure that keeps the blood in continuous movement through the circulatory system originates in the heart and is augmented slightly by the elastic recoil of the large arteries. A continuous succession of alternate myocardial contractions and relaxations, occurring rhythmically on an average of 60–70 times per minute, pumps the blood through the body.

IMPULSE ORIGIN AND CONDUCTION IN HEART CONTRACTION

The cells of the myocardium are of two types, those which contract when stimulated and those which originate and conduct impulses. The ability to originate and conduct impulses is referred to as the electrical activity of the heart. The heart has three electrical properties: (1) automaticity, or the ability to initiate an electrical impulse; (2) excitability, or the ability to respond to an electrical impulse; and (3) conductivity, or the ability to transmit an impulse from one cell to another. The muscle fibres have an absolute and a relative refractory period. The fibres are unresponsive to any stimulus during the absolute refractory period, which immediately follows a contraction. The relative refractory period is the interval in which the muscle fibres gradually recover their excitability but will respond to a stimulus if it is stronger than the usual. The refractory period in cardiac muscle is longer than in other muscle tissue. Excitability is more slowly regained, giving the heart chambers time to fill effectively.

Contraction of the myocardium is dependent upon impulses which arise within the myocardium itself. The structures capable of generating and conducting impulses within the myocardium form the conduction system. They are the SA node, tracts of conducting fibres originating with the SA node, the AV node, the bundle of His, bundle branches and the Purkinje fibres. Several areas of the conduction system are capable of the spontaneous generation of impulses, namely the SA node, the junctional tissue where the conducting fibres join the AV node, the bundle of His and the Purkinje fibres. The rate at which impulses are normally fired varies in the different areas: the SA node originates approximately 60–80 impulses per minute; the junctional tissue, 50–60 impulses per minute; the bundle of His, 40–50 impulses per minute; and the Purkinje fibres, 30–40 per minute. Since the region which is producing the highest rate of impulses sets the heart rate (number of contractions per minute), the SA node is referred to as the dominant pacemaker.

Impulses arising in the SA node are quickly conducted through the atria, initiating their contraction. At the same time, impulses are transmitted to the AV node where they are delayed; this delay allows for completion of atrial emptying and ventricular filling. From the AV node and junctional tissue they travel through the bundle of His and along the right and left bundle branches and the widely distributed Purkinje fibres to the ventricular contractile fibres, initiating their contraction.

ELECTROPHYSIOLOGY

Electrical currents in cardiac cells are produced by ion movement across the cell membrane. There is a marked difference in the intracellular and extracellular concentrations of ions, the most important of which are sodium and potassium. In the resting state the potassium concentration is approximately 30 times greater inside the cell than outside, and the sodium concentration is approximately 30 times less within the cell than outside. During the resting state the inside of the cardiac cell is negatively charged while the outside is positively charged, and the membrane is referred to as polarized. By inserting microelectrodes inside the cardiac cell, researchers have been able to measure the potential difference in voltage across the membrane. In the resting state, the potential is −90 millivolts, as shown in

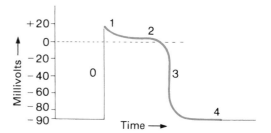

Figure 14.5 The electrophysiology of the cell.

Figure 14.5 and is called the resting membrane potential.

During depolarization, the cell membrane becomes permeable to sodium, which rapidly shifts inside the cell. This sudden influx of sodium reverses the transmembrane potential and potassium moves out of the cell.

In Figure 14.5 the resting or polarized phase is shown as the straight line at −90 millivolts. The change in transmembrane potential is represented by the upstroke, phase 0. After excitation the action potential rapidly declines and then levels off for a short period, as represented by phases 1 and 2. This time is referred to as the absolute refractory period and further stimulation produces no response.

Repolarization, or return to the normal resting potential, occurs during phase 3, the relative refractory period. The inside of the cell gradually resumes its negative electrical charge. During this time a stimulus of greater than normal intensity could reactivate the cell. Phase 4 shows a period of stable resting potential which remains until the next wave of excitation.

During depolarization ions move into and out of the cell because of differences in concentration gradients on either side of the cell membrane. During repolarization, however, an active transport system is required to pump out the sodium which has entered the cell and to pump in an equivalent amount of potassium. This mechanism is known as the 'sodium pump' and requires energy.

THE CARDIAC CYCLE

The succession of events which occurs with each heart beat is called the cardiac cycle. It consists of the relaxation and contraction of the atria and ventricles and the opening and closing of the cardiac valves in a sequence that permits the filling and emptying of the heart chambers. Contraction of the atria or ventricles is called systole; their relaxation is known as diastole. In referring to contraction or relaxation of the atria or ventricles, the terms used are atrial or ventricular systole or atrial or ventricular diastole, respectively. If systole or diastole is used alone, it refers to ventricular performance only.

The sequence of events of the cardiac cycle is as follows (Figure 14.6). The atria in diastole fill with blood received from their inlet vessels. In the early part of the relaxation period, the AV valves are closed but, as pressure builds up in the atria, it becomes greater than that in the ventricles, forcing the AV valves open, and the blood starts to flow through into the ventricles. Atrial

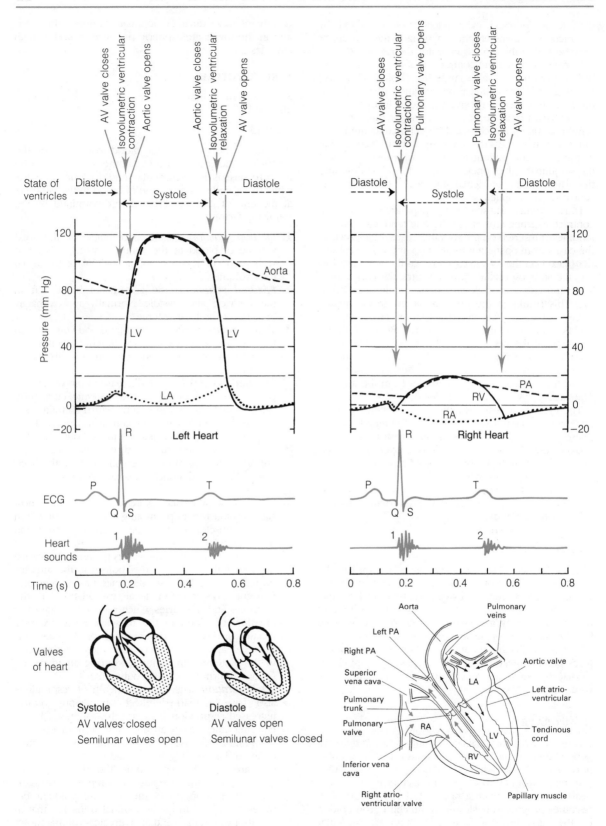

Figure 14.6 Diagrammatic illustration of the cardiac cycle. Key: RA, right atrium; LA, left atrium; RV, right ventricle; LV, left ventricle; PA, pulmonary artery.

diastole is followed in a fraction of a second by contraction, to complete the emptying of the two upper chambers, and the atria again enter their diastole.

During the filling and contraction of the ventricles the blood floats the AV valve cusps up, closing off the AV openings and preventing a regurgitation of blood into the atria. In order to receive the blood from the atria, the ventricles must be in diastole and, at this time, the semilunar valves are closed. With ventricular filling the intraventricular pressure builds up until it exceeds that in the aorta and pulmonary artery, with the result that the semilunar valves open, allowing blood to flow into the arteries. The ventricular muscle contracts, and the ventricles are emptied.

During ventricular systole, the papillary muscles also contract, exerting tension on the fine tendons (chordae tendineae) inserted on the AV valve cusps. This prevents the cusps from opening into the atria. If this control was not placed on the AV valves, there would be a backflow into the atria, especially with the ventricular contraction. The ventricles relax following their systole and empty-ing. This results in the pressure being greater in the arteries than in the ventricles, thus favouring the backflow of blood into the ventricles. But flow in the direction of the heart brings about the closure of the semilunar valves by the filling of the semilunar pouches; their free borders are brought together, preventing the blood from re-entering the ventricles from the arteries. The cardiac cycle is now completed.

The cycle in a heart beating approximately 70 times per minute is completed in 0.7–0.8 s. The length of each phase of the cycle varies; atrial diastole lasts ap-proximately 0.7 s, while its systole is approximately 0.1 s. Ventricular diastole is about 0.4–0.5 s, and its systole takes about 0.3 s. Following the ventricular contraction there is a brief period, approximately 0.4 s, in which the entire myocardium is relaxed. The ventricular diastole overlaps the atrial diastole.

CARDIAC OUTPUT

The performance of the heart as a pump can be described in terms of cardiac output (CO). This is the volume of blood pumped by each ventricle in 1 minute. It is equal to the stroke volume (SV) or the volume of blood pumped by a ventricle in one beat, multiplied by the number of heart beats in a minute (HR) (CO = SV × HR). In an adult, the CO varies from 3 to 6 litres per minute, and the SV averages 60–80 ml. Thus, cardiac output is dependent on heart rate and stroke volume.

HEART RATE

The number of heart beats per minute varies in different people and under different conditions. The average normal rate for an adult is 70 beats per minute, but it may range from 60 to 90. Several factors influence the heart rate. In the infant a rate of 110–130 is normal. It becomes progressively slower as the child grows older; by the early teens it is usually about 80. Muscular exertion will produce a marked increase, especially in an individual unaccustomed to physical exercise. The rate usually increases during emotional reactions, with fever, and in the lower atmospheric pressures found at high altitudes.

STROKE VOLUME

Stroke volume is influenced by preload, contractility and afterload.

Preload

Preload is the pressure of blood contained in the ventricle at the end of diastole. Another term to describe this pressure is left ventricular end-diastolic pressure, which is related to the volume of blood in the ventricle at the end of diastole. Preload is determined by the following factors:

1. *Ejection fraction* is the percentage of the total volume of blood in the ventricle which is ejected with each contraction (about 56–72% of the usual total volume).
2. *Residual volume* is the amount of blood left in the ventricle after systole. Normally approximately 28–44% of the total volume.
3. *Venous return* is affected by total blood volume, and by exercise and respirations which influence the distribution of that volume within the circulatory system.
   (a) *Total blood volume.* A decrease in the volume or pressure of the blood in the systemic circulation causes a decrease in the venous return. Certain areas of the body normally contain a relatively large volume of blood which may be moved out when the normal circulating volume is threatened. These areas are referred to as blood reservoirs and are the liver, spleen, large abdominal veins and venous plexuses of the skin.
   (b) *Exercise.* Muscular exercise is one of the most significant factors in promoting venous return. When skeletal muscles contract, veins are compressed, and more blood is forced out of them. It must move toward the heart since the valves prevent a backward flow. Also, the increased metabolism in the muscles during exercise increases their need for oxygen and nutrients, resulting in local vasodilation of the arterioles and capillaries which reduces resistance to the flow of blood in the muscles. Since exercise usually involves a large number of muscles, this causes an appreciable decrease in the total resistance in the systemic circulation, favouring an increased venous return and cardiac output.
   (c) *Respiration.* The rate and depth of respirations also have a marked effect on venous return; increased respirations increase the volume of blood entering the right atrium. On inspiration, the diaphragm descends, compressing the abdominal cavity and increasing the pressure on the veins in that area. At the same time the thoracic cavity enlarges and the pressure on regional veins is reduced. This increases the pressure gradient be-tween the blood in the abdominal veins and that in the thoracic veins so that a greater volume flows from the abdominal veins into the thoracic vena cava and on into the heart.

Contractility

The contractile or inotropic state of the myocardium is the ability of the heart to contract. Normal heart structures, absence of disease and an adequate supply of nutrients and oxygen are important factors in the heart's ability to produce the necessary force to eject the contained blood.

If the heart is undamaged and is in a condition to respond, the strength of the heart beat is determined mainly by the length of the muscle fibres when contraction begins. Stretching of muscle fibres, within limits, increases the strength of their contraction. The length or stretching of the myocardial fibres is dependent upon the volume of blood entering the heart. This principle is known as Starling's law of the heart and may be expressed thus: 'the energy of contraction is proportional to the initial length of the cardiac muscle fibres.'

The inotropic state of the heart is also affected by local and circulating catecholamines, the rate and rhythm of ventricular contractions, physiological depressants such as acidosis or myocardial hypoxia, the amount of ventricular substance and certain drugs such as digoxin and/or caffeine.

Afterload

Afterload describes the force against which the ventricle is working, or the resistance to the ejection of blood. This resistance is also called impedance and is reflected in the tension which ventricular muscle develops during systole. Left ventricular afterload is affected by the following factors:

1. *Functional state of the aortic valve.* If the aortic valve functions competently, it poses little resistance to the emptying of the left ventricle. However, if the aortic valve has extensive stenosis, this will increase afterload.
2. *Systemic vascular resistance (SVR).* This is the resistance imposed by the peripheral vasculature on the blood leaving the ventricle. Conditions such as arterial vasodilatation caused by septic shock can profoundly reduce systemic vascular resistance. Atherosclerosis can increase the resistance imposed on the left ventricle.
3. *Characteristics of the blood.* The viscosity of blood will influence the afterload required to move it through the circulatory system.

CARDIAC RESERVE

The ability of the heart to increase its output commensurate with increased tissue activity and needs is called cardiac reserve. The normal heart is capable of forwarding the volume of blood delivered to it and of responding to an increased demand without difficulty. It does this without causing prolonged breathlessness, tachycardia or palpitations.

For example, in strenuous exertion, the cardiac output may increase to a volume 13 times greater than the output during rest. This is achieved by an increase in the heart rate and the stroke volume. An increase in the

cardiac output also occurs in high environmental temperature, emotional responses such as fear, anger or other excitement, after a heavy meal and in the later months of pregnancy.

REGULATION OF CARDIAC ACTIVITY

Certain nervous, chemical and mechanical factors play an important role in the action of the heart.

NERVOUS INFLUENCE

The heart muscle is capable of generating its own impulses for contraction, but nerve impulses from the parasympathetic and sympathetic divisions of the autonomic nervous system may modify the rate and strength of the contractions. Nervous regulation is mediated by impulses which arise in the medulla oblongata in a group of neurones known as the cardiac centre. Parasympathetic impulses reach the heart by way of branches of the vagus nerve (Xth cranial nerve) and are delivered to the SA and AV nodes and to the atrial muscle. Vagal or parasympathetic innervation has an inhibitory effect on cardiac activity; it slows the heart rate and decreases the force of the atrial contraction by reducing the excitability of the pacemaker (SA node) and the conductivity of the AV node and conducting system.

Sympathetic impulses enter the heart by the cardiac accelerator nerves, originating in a cervical ganglion. These impulses are transmitted to the SA node, the conducting system, and the atrial and ventricular muscle. Sympathetic stimulation increases the heart rate and the strength of the heart contractions.

Parasympathetic innervation predominates in heart action. Normally, it exerts a fairly constant check on the heart rate, thus conserving the heart's strength.

The cardiac centre may be stimulated by impulses originating in higher levels of the brain or in some part of the body which is outside the central nervous system (brain and spinal cord). One need only recall the change experienced in one's own heart action during fear, anger or other excitement. The response of increased or decreased heart activity is due to impulses being discharged by the cerebral cortical level to the cardiac centre.

Sensory impulses from outside the central nervous system enter the cord or brain and may be relayed to the cardiac centre, resulting in changes in cardiac activity. The response of the heart to peripheral sensory impulses may be referred to as a cardiac reflex. The most significant of these are the vasosensory impulses originating in the baroreceptors and chemoreceptors. A group of sensory nerve endings in the aortic arch and in the carotid arteries at their bifurcation are sensitive to changes in the blood pressure and are called baroreceptors. In the same areas are nerve endings that are sensitive to changes in the carbon dioxide and oxygen concentration and the pH (hydrogen ion concentration) of the blood. These are known as the chemoreceptors. Impulses initiated in these receptors enter the brain or cord and are relayed to the cardiac centre.

An increase in blood pressure produces a response in

the cardioinhibitory centre. Vagal stimulation of the heart is increased and the heart rate decreases. (Marey's Law: the pulse rate is inversely related to the arterial blood pressure.) A decrease in the oxygen concentration, an increase in carbon dioxide concentration and a decrease in the pH of the blood result in stimulation of the cardioacceleratory centre and in elevation of the heart rate.

CHEMICAL INFLUENCE

Normal, rhythmic heart contractions are greatly dependent upon an optimal concentration of potassium, sodium and calcium in the extracellular fluid. (Optimal serum concentrations: K^+, 3.5–5.5 mmol/l; Na^+, 135–145 mmol/l; and Ca^{2+}, 2.2–2.6 mmol/l.) These minerals play an important role in the excitability of the cardiac muscle cells and their contraction.

If the potassium level is greater than its normal concentration in the extracellular fluid, an impairment in conduction and contraction occurs. It causes a prolonged relaxation of the heart with abnormal dilatation of the chambers. The heart rate slows. A decrease below the normal concentration of sodium results in weaker contractions. The pulse is rapid and weak, and there is a fall in blood pressure. An excess sodium concentration does not directly affect cardiac action. An excess of calcium produces a stronger and prolonged systole. Conversely, a lack of calcium prolongs the diastole.

Other chemicals of significance in heart action are oxygen and carbon dioxide. Any deficiency of oxygen is quickly reflected in a deterioration of heart action. The myocardium is much more sensitive to oxygen lack than skeletal muscle. The pulse becomes rapid, weak and irregular. With an excess of carbon dioxide in the blood, as may occur in respiratory insufficiency, heart action is impaired. Conduction is slowed, the relaxation period is prolonged and the contraction is briefer than normal.

MECHANICAL INFLUENCE

The principal mechanical influence on cardiac activity is the stretching of the myocardial fibres by the volume of blood entering the chambers. As previously stated, stretching of muscle fibres increases the strength of their contraction. An increase in arterial blood pressure also demands a greater force of contraction; the heart muscle must release a greater amount of energy to perform its function because of meeting greater resistance.

Blood Pressure and Pulse

BLOOD PRESSURE

Blood pressure may be defined as the pressure exerted laterally on the walls of the blood vessels. It varies in different parts of the circulatory system, being greatest in the large arteries, with a progressive decrease as the blood continues on through the smaller arteries, arterioles, capillaries and veins. The pressure is highest in the aorta and lowest in the large caval veins which enter the heart. Blood pressure at any point in the vascular system is dependent upon the force with which the heart pumps the blood out of the ventricles, the volume of blood in the system, the elasticity of the arteries and the amount of resistance to the flow of the blood from one portion of the circulatory system to the next.

ARTERIAL BLOOD PRESSURE

The blood pressure of greatest clinical interest is that in the arteries. The pulsatile nature of heart activity causes fluctuations in the pressure. With each contraction of the left ventricle a volume of blood is pumped into the aorta, which is already filled with blood. This causes an appreciable increase in the pressure of the blood and stretches the aortic walls. If the aorta were not elastic, the rise in pressure would be much higher and sharper. During the ventricular diastole, the elastic walls of the aorta recoil, exerting a pressure on the contained blood. If the aorta were a rigid tube which did not recoil, the pressure of the blood would fall more rapidly and to a much lower level than it does normally. The higher pressure produced by the ventricular systole is referred to as the *systolic blood pressure*. The lower pressure that occurs during the ventricular diastole is dependent upon the recoil of the large arteries and is known as the *diastolic blood pressure*. The difference between these two pressures is called the *pulse pressure*. Pulse pressure varies inversely with the elasticity of the arteries. Rigid vessels with a loss of ability to distend and recoil produce a higher systolic pressure and a lower diastolic pressure, resulting in an increased pulse pressure.

Factors which determine arterial blood pressure

Arterial blood pressure is influenced by the strength of the heart beat, volume of blood, elasticity of the vessels and the resistance offered to the flow of blood.

Strength of the heart beat
If the myocardial strength is weakened by disease, lack of essential materials or a deficiency in stimulation, it follows that the pressure under which the blood is ejected into the arteries and the volume of blood emitted would be reduced. The arterial pressure is directly proportional to the cardiac output.

Blood volume
Any reduction in the intravascular volume will reduce the head of pressure and the stretch and recoil of the arteries, resulting in an appreciable decrease in the pressure of the blood. Small decreases in the volume are compensated for by the contraction of vessels but, in some conditions (e.g. haemorrhage, severe dehydration, burns), the loss may be beyond compensation. In some instances, vasodilatation may occur (e.g. anaphylaxis), increasing the capacity of the system beyond that of the

contained volume, and the blood pressure falls. A disproportion between the volume of blood and the capacity of the vascular system due to widespread vasodilatation or a diminished blood volume, as in haemorrhage, reduces the venous return to the heart. This is an important factor in determining the cardiac output, the strength of the heart beat and the blood pressure.

Aldosterone, a hormone secreted by the adrenal cortex, produces an increase in the intravascular volume and a corresponding increase in blood pressure by its effect on kidney activity. It promotes absorption of sodium by the kidney tubules. The increased sodium concentration of the blood in turn causes more water to be absorbed by the renal tubules, increasing the total vascular volume and, as a result, the blood pressure. Conversely, a reduction in aldosterone secretion will reduce the intravascular volume, and the blood pressure falls. The mechanism that regulates the amount of aldosterone secreted by the adrenal cortices is not yet established.

Elasticity of the vessels

The elastic quality of the large arteries has an important role in determining blood pressure. It allows for an increase in the capacity of the arteries when the blood is ejected by each heart beat. The stretch factor reduces the resistance offered to the flow of blood from the heart, thus reducing somewhat the demand on that organ. With ventricular diastole and the run-off of blood into succeeding vessels, the elastic arterial wall recoils. This provides some pressure on the contained blood to augment its forward movement, and helps to maintain a continuous flow of blood between ventricular contractions. The pressure of the blood at this time (i.e. during arterial recoil and between ventricular contractions) represents the diastolic blood pressure. If the elasticity of the arteries is reduced, as in arteriosclerosis, the blood is pumped into rigid, non-distensible tubes; the systolic pressure is increased because of the lack of vascular stretching and the diastolic pressure is reduced because of the reduced force of recoil.

Resistance to blood flow

The amount of resistance with which the blood is met as it flows through the vascular system depends mainly on the calibre of the arterioles and the viscosity of the blood.

Calibre of the arterioles. The relatively large lumen of the arteries offers little peripheral resistance to the flow of blood, but their subsequent branching into numerous arterioles introduces more surface contact for the blood, which increases friction and resistance to the flow. This resistance determines the rate at which blood can flow from the arteries into the arterioles, which in turn influences the volume of blood confined in the arteries and, hence, the arterial blood pressure.

Normally the arterioles are in a constant state of partial contraction, referred to as the basic level of tone, but the calibre of the vessels may be modified by contraction or relaxation of the well-developed, circular, smooth muscle in the walls in response to various factors. Obviously, with relaxation, the increased diameter of the arterioles will offer less resistance, more blood will pass from the arteries through the arterioles to the capillaries and the arterial blood pressure will tend to be normal or below normal. Conversely, with contraction of the arterioles, the decreased diameter increases the resistance to the blood flow, less blood escapes from the arteries and arterial blood pressure is maintained at a normal or above normal level. The calibre of the arterioles is controlled by nerve impulses delivered to the musculature of the arterioles and by certain chemical changes in the extracellular fluids. The latter may exercise their influence directly on the vessels or indirectly through the autonomic nervous system.

Neural control of vascular tone is exerted by the autonomic nervous system. The vessels are supplied by two types of nerve fibres: those whose impulses cause contraction of the muscle tissue of the vessel are the excitatory or vasoconstrictor nerves, and those which cause relaxation are the inhibitory or vasodilator nerves. All vasoconstrictor nerves derive from the sympathetic division of the autonomic nervous system and are thought to act on the alpha (α) receptor sites of smooth muscle. Sympathetic vasoconstrictors are located in the kidneys, skin, gut and spleen. Vasodilatation may be initiated by a decrease in sympathetic innervation which allows a relaxation of the smooth muscle of the vessel or, in some instances, dilatation results from impulses delivered by nerves to the vessel walls. The vasodilator, or inhibitory, nerves in some areas of the body belong to the parasympathetic division; in others the vasodilator as well as the vasoconstrictor nerves originate in the sympathetic nervous system. Sympathetic vasodilators are distributed to the vessels of skeletal muscles, the intestines, the coronary system and some areas of the skin. Parasympathetic vasodilators supply the vessels in the tongue, sweat and salivary glands, external genitalia and possibly the bladder and rectum.

The principal source of the impulses that regulate the calibre of the blood vessels is the vasomotor centre in the medulla. Some impulses may arise from spinal cord neurones in the thoracolumbar areas. These areas may be influenced by impulses received from the blood vessels themselves, the baroreceptors and chemoreceptors of the carotid sinus and aortic arch, the cerebral cortex, the hypothalamus and various other regions of the body, such as the skin, muscles and viscera.

Chemical influence on the smooth muscle in the vessels may be direct or may be indirect through the nervous system. Certain chemical changes in the composition of the extracellular fluid may result in the initiation of nerve impulses which influence the blood vessels. Increased carbon dioxide or decreased oxygen tension results in vasoconstriction and a corresponding increase in resistance. Similarly, an increase in the hydrogen ion concentration (decreased pH) causes vasoconstriction.

A direct effect on the arterioles may be produced by metabolites and hormones. Metabolites produce the opposite effect locally to that caused indirectly through the nervous system. An increase in the concentration of hydrogen ions and carbon dioxide and a diminished oxygen tension in an area cause dilatation of the arterioles in that area. The indirect action of the nervous system produces a more general vasoconstriction and a rise in blood pressure, increasing the rate of flow through the locally dilated arterioles, when there is an increased need for more oxygen and nutrients, and for the removal of more metabolites.

When tissue cells are irritated or injured, chemical substances are released which produce relaxation in the local arterioles and capillaries, resulting in more blood in the area. One of these substances is identified as histamine, a strong vasodilator.

Still another chemical substance, renin, stimulates vasoconstriction and increases arterial blood pressure. It is produced by kidney tissue in response to a diminished blood supply (renal ischaemia). Renin is a proteolytic enzyme which, when released into the bloodstream, acts upon a globulin fraction, producing the vasoconstrictor angiotensin (hypertensin) that acts directly on the arterioles. It would appear that angiotensin has no significant role in the maintenance of normal blood pressure, since it is quickly destroyed in the healthy person. It remains active for a longer period in persons with a blood pressure higher than normal and is receiving some attention in relation to the disease of hypertension.

The hormones associated with vasomotor activity are adrenaline and antidiuretic hormone (ADH). Adrenaline, secreted by the adrenal medulla or administered parenterally, has a direct vasoconstricting effect on the arterioles in the skin, mucous membranes and the splanchnic area. At the same time, it inhibits the tone in the arterioles of the skeletal muscles and the coronary system. The effect of adrenaline on the coronary system may be indirect, since the hormone stimulates metabolism which causes the local metabolic regulatory system to increase blood flow.

The secretion of the neurohypophysis, or posterior lobe of the pituitary gland, contains ADH. It excites the smooth muscle of most blood vessels, but its effect is slower than that of adrenaline.

It may be seen from the foregoing discussion of vasomotor regulation that peripheral resistance is a complex affair. Resistance is directly proportional to the length of vessels and inversely proportional to the diameter, and many factors may influence the diameter. A moderate degree of vasoconstriction is essential; most of the arterioles must be in a partial state of constriction at all times. If too many vessels relax at one time, blood pressure falls to dangerously low levels and circulation becomes seriously impaired.

Frequent and quick readjustments in the calibre of the arterioles are necessary to maintain a relatively constant level of blood pressure and to meet the changing needs of tissue cells. Increased activity of structures or areas demands more blood in those parts and vasodilatation occurs. To compensate for the increased volume in one area, vasoconstriction must occur in other parts of the body to maintain a forward movement of the blood and a normal cardiac output and blood pressure. For example, when a person moves from the recumbent to the upright position, the blood tends to collect in the lower part of the body because of gravity. This causes a decrease in the blood pressure in

the aorta and carotid arteries, and the baroreceptors then initiate the reflex response of vasoconstriction in the arterioles. This response maintains an adequate circulation throughout the upper parts of the body.

Blood viscosity. The second factor on which the resistance to the flow of blood depends is the viscosity of the blood. It is a much less significant factor than the calibre of the arterioles. Viscosity is the resistance to flow created within the fluid itself by the friction and cohesiveness between its molecules. Resistance of a fluid is directly proportional to its viscosity.

Blood viscosity is mainly dependent on the concentration of the red blood cells and blood proteins. It is approximately 2.5–5 times the viscosity of water. An increase above the normal number of red blood cells (polycythaemia) impedes the flow of blood and may cause an appreciable increase above normal in the arterial blood pressure. The calibre of the arterioles is subject to frequent fluctuations, but usually viscosity only changes when blood is diluted or when there is an increase or decrease in the number of red blood cells.

Normal variations in arterial blood pressure

Age, exercise, emotions and weight influence blood pressure.

Blood pressure changes with age. During infancy and childhood, blood pressure is lower than later in life. In the newborn infant systolic pressure is approximately 55–90 mmHg; the diastolic is approximately 40–55 mmHg. This gradually increases throughout childhood, reaching adult level about puberty. Usually in the fifties, the systolic pressure begins to show a slight increase which progresses with age, corresponding to the loss of elasticity and to the thickening of the walls of the arteries characteristic of the ageing process.

Physical exertion is accompanied by a rise in the arterial blood pressure due to the increased venous return and the increased production of metabolites such as carbon dioxide and lactic acid. The systolic pressure may increase by as much as 60–70 mmHg in strenuous exercise.

Emotions may also cause an elevation in blood pressure; the more excited, anxious, angry or fearful a person becomes, the higher the blood pressure goes. Vasoconstriction is increased due to sympathetic innervation and the release of adrenaline into the bloodstream.

Blood pressure increases with increased body weight, especially after middle age. This is of significance in our present-day society in which overweight and hypertension have a high incidence.

VENOUS BLOOD PRESSURE

The pressure of the blood is reduced slowly but progressively from the time it leaves the capillaries until it reaches the right atrium.

Venous blood pressure is influenced by cardiac strength, blood volume, respirations and posture. Venous pressure is actually the force that remains of that created by the left ventricular contraction. The blood enters the venous system under a pressure of approximately 10 mmHg. The walls of the veins continue to offer some resistance and the blood, particularly in the lower parts of the body, must travel a considerable distance before reaching the heart. (Pressure is inversely proportional to frictional resistance and the length of the tube.) As a result, the pressure is dissipated progressively, and by the time it reaches the right atrium is very low, 0–10 cmH$_2$O (0–1 mmHg). Obviously, if the left ventricular systole is weak and the blood starts out at a lower than normal arterial pressure, it will tend to move more slowly in the veins towards the heart.

Cardiac strength

Maintenance of normal pressure and flow of the venous blood are influenced by the ability of the right heart chambers to empty sufficiently to receive the volume of blood being forwarded by the large veins. If the heart cannot pass on the blood it receives, the normal volume cannot enter and there is a damming back in the veins. The resulting increased volume causes an increase in the blood pressure. Normal emptying of the right atrium actually promotes venous flow; in diastole, the empty right atrium tends to produce an aspirating effect on the large veins.

Blood volume

The greater the volume of blood flowing into the veins from the arterioles and capillaries, the greater will be the venous pressure. If the arterioles are constricted, the pressure in the veins will be lower. If the arterioles are dilated, as in muscular exercise, the greater volume escaping into the veins will increase the venous pressure. Normally, marked changes do not occur since the veins have the ability to adjust by either vasoconstriction or dilatation to the volume of blood being received. This is accomplished mainly in the smaller veins.

Respiration

On inspiration there is a decrease in intrathoracic pressure and an increase in intra-abdominal pressure. Abdominal venous pressure increases while that in the thoracic veins is lowered, causing a larger volume of blood to move into the thoracic veins. On expiration, intrathoracic pressure increases, compressing the veins and raising the pressure within them, thus helping to move the blood into the atria.

Posture

Due to gravity, the upright position favours an increase in venous pressure in the lower parts of the body, but continuous venous return is preserved by compensatory mechanisms. The baroreceptors initiate reflex vascular constriction, which usually preserves an adequate blood pressure. In spite of the compensatory vasoconstriction, a greater volume of blood is likely to accumulate in the lower veins during long periods of standing. This may be seen in persons who faint when required to stand for a relatively long period.

PULSE

Each ventricular contraction ejects a volume of blood into the aorta, producing an increase in the blood pressure which causes an expansion of the artery. During ventricular diastole, the elastic recoil of the aorta moves the blood into the next portion of the artery, which stretches and then recoils. This alternating expansion and recoil spreads along the whole arterial system, producing a pulse wave. Each pulsation corresponds to a heart beat and is the result of the impact of the ejected volume of blood on the arterial wall. The pulsations occur in the arteries of the pulmonary circulatory system as well as in the systemic circulation.

For assessment of arterial pulse see p. 301.

PREVENTION OF CARDIOVASCULAR DISORDERS

Heart disease is a national health problem of considerable proportions. It is a leading cause of death in the UK. Many nursing hours in hospitals, homes and clinics are devoted to patients with heart disease.

The Nurse's Role in Prevention of Heart Disease

The nurse has many opportunities to contribute to the prevention of cardiac insufficiency. Whether the work is in the hospital, clinic, home, industry or school, the role may be participation in health screening, education or provision of care. In order to recognize and fulfil the responsibilities in the preventive programme, the nurse must be informed and must make a personal effort to keep abreast of new knowledge. In addition to an understanding of the role of the heart in supplying all the cells throughout the body with materials essential to their survival and activities, a knowledge of how this function may be impaired by various pathological processes is necessary. This information serves as the basis for the recognition of excessive demands on the heart, significant signs and symptoms and the need for medical attention. It also provides the basis for explanations and appropriate health education as well as for the planning and giving of safe and effective care.

Risk factors have been identified in large scale epidemiological studies as clinical variables which are statistically associated with the manifestation of heart disease, particularly ischaemic heart disease (IHD). These factors are presumably involved in the pathogenesis of atherosclerosis of the coronary arteries. The presence of multiple risk factors increases exponentially the likelihood of developing IHD, although individuals may live for many years with multiple risk factors and no manifestations of heart disease.

The nurse can play a very important role in facilitating health promotion, assessing potentially detrimental health patterns and identifying and undertaking strategies to prevent or correct these behaviours.

Risk factors can be classified as non-modifiable and modifiable. Non-modifiable risk factors are age, sex and family history. Modifiable risk factors are hypertension, hyperlipidaemia, cigarette smoking, diabetes mellitus, obesity and personality characteristics.

NON-MODIFIABLE RISK FACTORS

1. *Age*. Ischaemic heart disease is more prevalent in older people. Thus, the older the individual, the greater the likelihood of developing cardiovascular disease.

2. *Gender*. Men have a higher incidence of IHD than women, although this difference diminishes as age increases. Women have a dramatically increased incidence of IHD after the menopause.

3. *Family history*. A history of IHD among blood relatives is associated with an increased risk of cardiovascular disease and a poorer prognosis when it develops.

MODIFIABLE RISK FACTORS

1. *Hypertension*. Elevated systolic and diastolic blood pressure is a significant risk factor for cardiovascular disease including IHD, stroke and heart failure. In British men there is a twofold risk of heart attack in the top 40% of the distribution of systolic blood pressure and a threefold risk in the top 20% of diastolic blood pressure (Shaper, 1987). Discussion of the nurse's role in management of hypertension can be found later in this chapter.

2. *Hyperlipidaemia*. Blood lipids include cholesterol, triglycerides, phospholipids and free fatty acids. Cholesterol and triglycerides are of clinical significance and are transported in plasma as lipoproteins. There are four major classes of lipoproteins, which are chylomicrons and pre-β-, β-, and α-lipoproteins; each contains varying proportions of protein and the three blood lipids. The lipoproteins may be separated by the process of electrophoresis.

Chylomicrons are mainly of dietary origin. Pre-β-lipoproteins contain a large amount of triglycerides, primarily of hepatic origin, synthesized from fatty acids and carbohydrate. β-Lipoproteins carry one-half to two-thirds of the total plasma cholesterol. α-Lipoproteins carry little triglycerides but larger amounts of protein and an appreciable amount of cholesterol. Certain studies have suggested that high levels of high density lipoproteins (HDL) may protect against the development of coronary atherosclerosis, although it is uncertain how this occurs.

Hyperlipoproteinaemia may be classified as type I, II, III, IV or V. Types I and V hyperlipidaemia are rare. Types II, III and IV are associated with an increased incidence of ischaemic heart disease. Hyperlipoproteinaemia may be secondary to another disease such as obstructive liver disease, due to an excessive intake of saturated fats and cholesterol in the diet, or may result from a primary or familial disorder. Determination of serum cholesterol and triglyceride levels will detect hyperlipoproteinaemia in most cases and is less costly than other laboratory procedures. However, in some instances, further studies may be warranted. Control of hypercholes-

teraemia is directed toward lowering the serum cholesterol levels by diet and in some instances by medications.

Studies suggest that by modifying the dietary intake of fats, carbohydrate and calories, the blood lipid levels of most patients with primary hyperlipidaemia can be lowered (Lipid Research Clinics Coronary Primary Prevention Trial, 1984). The contribution of diet to the prevention of coronary atherosclerosis is not clear but evidence suggests that this approach might be worthwhile.

The purpose of the diet is to reduce body weight when required and to lower the intake of total fat, saturated fatty acids and cholesterol, while increasing the intake of unsaturated fatty acids (see Table 14.1). Saturated fat and cholesterol are found in high-fat meats and dairy products and in some commercially baked goods. Polyunsaturated fats are contained in vegetables and fish oils.

The modified diet emphasizes substitution of lean meat, poultry and fish for fattier meats (pork, visible meat fat). It also includes non-fat products such as corn oil, margarine, skimmed milk and low fat cheese, whole grain or enriched flour products, fruits, vegetables and polyunsaturated vegetable oils.

The degree of dietary restriction depends upon the type of hyperlipidaemia and the age and condition of the patient. Dietary teaching is a combined function of the doctor, nurse and dietitian. The dietitian is the primary person involved if the diet is complex, but the nurse also needs to be informed so that teaching can be reinforced. Some patients may require much support and understanding to continue on their diets, especially if drastic changes in eating habits are needed. Compliance will probably be greater if the diet is adjusted as much as possible to individual tastes.

Lipid-lowering drugs may be ordered for selected patients who do not respond to diet therapy alone. These include clofibrate, nicotinic acid and cholestyramine. The King's Fund Forum Consensus Statement (1989) recommends cholesterol testing for offspring of any person who develops symptomatic heart disease and who has a high blood cholesterol.

Table 14.1 Recommendations for dietary modification.

---

1. Total fat should not exceed 35% of energy intake.
2. Saturated fatty acids should not exceed 11% of energy intake. Reducing the intake of foods containing saturated fatty acids will usually reduce cholesterol intake as well, but in addition patients should restrict their intake of foods high in cholesterol.
3. Fibre intake should be an average of 18 grams per day.
4. Refined sugar should not exceed 11% of food energy – no more than 60 grams per day.

From Department of Health (1991).

3. *Cigarette smoking.* For both men and women, cigarette smoking is one of the major risk factors for cardiovascular disease. The risk of morbidity and mortality is dramatically greater for smokers than for non-smokers, particularly in people under the age of 50 and those who have other risk factors.

Research has indicated that there are a number of compounds in cigarette smoke which are harmful. Nicotine stimulates catecholamine secretion which, in turn, promotes platelet aggregation, increased heart rate, blood pressure and oxygen consumption. Carbon monoxide also appears to increase platelet adhesiveness and reduce oxygen supply, which in the presence of coronary lesions, may increase the incidence of angina pectoris.

Various studies have shown that nurses' knowledge about the effects of smoking is limited (Haverty et al, 1987) and they need to increase their confidence and skills in order to practise as educators in relation to smoking.

There are a number of strategies to facilitate smoking cessation:

(a) Providing information which is tailored to the individual's needs (Table 14.2). A patient who has already experienced a recent cardiac condition may be more receptive to messages on the impact of smoking on the heart and health.

(b) Eliciting social support can be beneficial. Family members and friends can discuss their roles in helping the person stop smoking.

Table 14.2 Advice for smokers.

1. Tell patients that they are making a major decision: i.e. a 65-year-old who smokes two packets of cigarettes a day may forfeit six years of life but can regain four of those years by stopping smoking.
2. If a patient resumes smoking, provide reassurance that stopping smoking is like any other new skill: several tries may be necessary.
3. If the patient has one cigarette, inform the patient that it does not mean immediate dependence; however, emphasize that it should not become habitual.
4. Inform patients that withdrawal symptoms are generally most severe 2–4 days after stopping and symptoms slowly subside during the following week, but reach a second peak about 10 days after stopping, before slowly tapering off permanently. Emphasize that symptoms will be short-lived and can often be countered by planning for them.
5. Advise patients that any weight gain almost never exceeds 2.5–3 kg (5–10 lb.) and that very few ex-smokers maintain the added weight for more than one year. Suggest an exercise programme.

(c) Self-help efforts can be beneficial. Discussing with the individual behaviours which are associated with the activity and how to avoid these situations, at least initially when attempting to stop, can be helpful. Social and psychological reinforcers contributing to smoking behaviours can be very powerful in preventing successful cessation.

(d) Gradual reduction of number of cigarettes smoked can be a successful strategy. Not all smokers can stop the habit suddenly on a particular day. Reducing the number of cigarettes smoked on a daily basis, with an established target day, can be successful for some people. This gradually reduces the dependence on the substance.

(e) Pharmacological strategies, including the use of nicotine chewing gum, can be useful when a strong addiction is present. When chewed, this gum replaces the nicotine provided by cigarettes to a certain extent.

(f) Cessation programmes are often available in the individual's community. The nurse should be aware of these programmes and facilitate the patient's referral as appropriate.

4. *Diabetes mellitus.* Cardiac disease is prevalent in individuals with glucose intolerance, particularly women. In post-mortem studies, people with adult-onset diabetes have been found to have more extensive coronary artery lesions, which are more diffuse and involve a greater number of vessels than those found in gender-matched controls. Previously-undetected diabetes is found in about 5% of coronary patients admitted to hospital (Oswald et al, 1984). The management of diabetes mellitus is discussed in detail on pp. 598–603.

5. *Obesity.* Being overweight is a weak independent risk factor for IHD. However, obesity is a major indicator for increased risk of cardiovascular disease as it is associated with many other risk factors. The presence of overweight or obesity in British men also denotes an increased likelihood of hypertension, hyperlipidaemia and diabetes mellitus (Shaper, 1987). These risks can be improved by weight loss, indicating the important role weight control has in improving one's risk profile.

6. *Personality characteristics.* The risk of IHD is thought by some researchers to be increased in association with a person displaying characteristics of the type A behavioural pattern, including aggressiveness, competitive drive and a chronic sense of time urgency. However, a number of methodological difficulties in measuring these psychological characteristics have led to the results being viewed with caution. An extensive study in the UK failed to show any relationship between type A behaviour and the incidence and prevalence of ischaemic heart disease (Johnston et al, 1987). Research studies to determine if reduction in type A behaviour reduces mortality

and morbidity from IHD are being conducted. Interventions directed at group counselling have indicated that this may be an effective strategy in modifying type A behaviour.

THE PERSON WITH ALTERED CARDIOVASCULAR FUNCTION

Assessment

Assessment of the individual's cardiovascular function provides data needed to identify actual and potential health problems, guide nursing intervention and evaluate care. A cardiovascular assessment includes:

- Health history
- Physical examination
- Diagnostic procedures
- Knowledge of manifestations of cardiovascular disorders.

The nurse collects and analyses the assessment data, formulates patient-centred problems and develops a goal-orientated plan of care with the patient and family, which is then implemented and evaluated.

HEALTH HISTORY

The health history will assist the nurse in defining the patient's health problems. The depth and manner in which this information is collected will depend on the patient's clinical status and availability of family or significant others.

If the patient is acutely ill, then brief, direct questions should be used to identify essential information during admission procedures. If the patient's status is stable, the nurse may sit at the bedside and conduct a formal interview using more open-ended questions.

The health history includes data concerning the patient's primary health problems, history of present illness, past health history, family history, and social and personal history.

1. *Primary health problem.* The patient identifies the chief concern or reason for contact with the health care system. Common cardiovascular health problems include chest discomfort, dyspnoea, syncope, palpitations and intermittent claudication.
2. *History of present illness.* This is a detailed investigation of the patient's primary health problem and previously prescribed treatment plan. It is important to use a systematic approach when gathering this data to ensure it is comprehensive. One method of organizing this data collection is using the PQRST mnemonic (Table 14.3).
3. *Past health history.* Assessment includes the patient's general state of health, major health problems and treatment plans, hospital admissions, surgical procedures and injuries. The patient's response to these events provides data concerning coping strategies

Table 14.3 PQRST mnemonic for symptom assessment.

Letter	Aspect	Sample questions
P	Precipitators	What were you doing when the _____ started? Have you ever had this before?
Q	Quality Quantity	What does it feel like? On a scale of 1 to 10, where would you rate this?
R	Region Radiation	Point to where it hurts. Does it move anywhere?
S	Signs and Symptoms	Have you had any other symptoms?
T	Time	When did it start? Is it constant or does it come and go? Did it come on suddenly or gradually?
	Treatment	What have you done to make it go away? Did it help?

From Holloway (1988). Reproduced with permission from Addison-Wesley.

utilized. Allergies to food, medication and environmental agents are identified and allergic reactions described.

4. *Family history.* Information concerning the patient's blood relatives may suggest a specific cardiac problem. The patient may be questioned if any one in his family has ever had hypertension, diabetes mellitus, ischaemic heart disease, vascular disease or hyperlipidaemia.
5. *Social and personal history.* This data facilitates an understanding of the person's uniqueness as an individual and suggests needs for health teaching and discharge planning. Data is gathered in the following areas:
   (a) *Personal characteristics.* Include patient's age, marital status, education, occupational experiences, socioeconomic status and religious beliefs.
   (b) *Life-style.* Information concerning the individual's daily activities is collected, including dietary, bowel and sleep habits and usual activities, and data concerning use of tobacco, alcohol, caffeine and social drugs. Identification of these factors can help facilitate planning in the areas of health promotion and prevention of progression of disease.
   (c) *Patient's perception of the illness and ability to cope.* What does this illness mean to the patient? This provides information as to the patient's level of understanding about the condition and the impact on his or her life. How the patient has coped with other problems may identify coping strategies which the nurse can facilitate when planning care with the individual.

(d) *Relationships with others.* The patient is questioned about the network of family and friends to assess social support systems available. The family and significant others' perceptions of the patient's condition and coping will provide information as to their levels of understanding and their abilities to handle the situation.

(e) *Home environment.* Who is living with the patient? Describing the physical characteristics of the home including stairs, location of bathroom (toilet facilities), etc. will help start discharge planning. This is particularly important for the individual with reduced activity resulting from cardiac dysfunction as daily routines will need to be modified to accommodate changes in function.

(f) *Knowledge of cardiovascular function.* The patient's understanding of the condition and the treatment plan is important for planning health education. Does the patient know the current medical diagnosis and what this means in terms of treatment and life-style? For example, does the patient who had a myocardial infarction understand activity limitations and medication schedules?

BASIC PHYSICAL EXAMINATION OF THE CARDIOVASCULAR SYSTEM

In this section, basic physical examination techniques for assessing the person's cardiovascular system will be described. The more specialized techniques are beyond the scope of this text and the nurse is referred to specialized cardiovascular sources. Certain of the techniques described are normally carried out by the doctor. However, it is necessary for nurses to understand the principles of these techniques in order to gain a wider appreciation of the patient's experience and to be equipped to explain the nature of the techniques to patients.

Basic physical examination is a cornerstone of the nurse's methods of data collection. Performing a physical examination facilitates gathering the objective data on the person's cardiovascular system which is necessary to establish a baseline of the person's condition and to assess ongoing changes in health status.

GENERAL APPEARANCE

1. *Facial expressions.* Does the patient appear alert, anxious, distressed, exhausted? Grimacing, biting of lips are noted as they may be signs of pain.
2. *Posture.* Does the patient appear comfortable, restless, agitated? Is he sitting, lying supine?
3. *Skin and mucous membranes*
   (a) Colour: Examine skin in symmetrical areas, noting any increase or loss of pigmentation, redness, pallor, cyanosis and jaundice. Ask the patient if there have been any recent changes in the colour of the skin. Observe for signs of bleeding such as petechiae, bruising or haematomas.
   (b) Moisture: inspect skin for dryness, oiliness or

sweating (diaphoresis).
   (c) Hair pattern: note hair distribution on limbs, glossy shiny appearance of skin surface.

PALPATION

This method of examination is used to assess skin and peripheral pulses.

Skin

1. *Capillary refill.* This is noted by applying pressure to the nail-bed and releasing quickly. A normal response is for the nail-bed to blanch on pressure and to quickly reperfuse and become pink when pressure is released. An abnormal response is a delay of more than 3 seconds in the return to pink.
2. *Temperature.* The skin is palpated symmetrically to establish the temperature of the skin using the back of the hand and noting generalized warmth or coolness of any localized areas.
3. *Turgor.* A fold of skin is lifted and the speed with which it returns into place is noted.
4. *Oedema.* Assessment is made for oedema in symmetrical locations, including feet, ankles, lower arms and the sacrum. Three fingers are pressed firmly over symmetrical bony surfaces for 5 seconds and released. Pitting oedema, which is continued depression of the skin and underlying tissue after pressure is released, is noted.

Peripheral arterial pulses

Arterial pulses are assessed for pressure rate, rhythm and amplitude (volume) at symmetrical locations on the body. The carotid, brachial, radial, femoral, popliteal, dorsalis pedis and posterior tibial pulses can be included.

The heart rate can be assessed by counting the pulse rate. The radial or carotid pulse rate can be palpated and counted for 60 seconds to establish heart rate.

The heart rhythm can be initially assessed using the pulse. The radial or carotid pulse is palpated to identify if the rhythm of pulses is regular. If it is irregular, any pattern present is noted.

The pulse amplitude may be graded and recorded as follows:

    0 — not palpable
   +1 — barely palpable, weak, thready
   +2 — decreased, moderate impairment
   +3 — full
   +4 — bounding

AUSCULTATION

Arterial blood pressure

Arterial blood pressure is an important predictor of morbidity and mortality and is therefore one of the most important clinical observations, yet there is considerable confusion concerning its measurement (Thompson, 1981).

Arterial blood pressure is most frequently measured in millimeters of mercury (mmHg) by means of a sphygmomanometer and a stethoscope, using the brachial artery. The rubber cuff of the blood pressure apparatus is applied to the upper arm just above the elbow and is inflated with air, which compresses the brachial artery. The pressure in the cuff is transmitted to the column of mercury of the manometer. The stethoscope is applied over the brachial artery just below the cuff.

When the cuff pressure becomes greater than the blood pressure, no pulse is heard. The air in the cuff is slowly released and the height of the mercury on the manometer is noted when the pulse is first heard. This corresponds to the systolic blood pressure.

With further slow deflation of the cuff, the pulse gradually becomes softer. The level of the mercury is again noted just before the pulse becomes inaudible or when there is a pronounced change in the sound heard, known as muffling. This represents the diastolic blood pressure. If the blood pressure is recorded as 100 mmHg, it simply means that the pressure of the blood on the walls of the vessel is sufficient to raise a column of mercury to a height of 100 mm. The normal systolic pressure in a healthy young adult in a sitting position is 100–135 mmHg; the normal diastolic pressure is 60–80 mmHg.

When the person has a history of fainting or dizziness when changing position or of hypertension or may be dehydrated, the blood pressure should be taken in three positions if possible: supine, sitting and standing. Under normal conditions, the systolic pressure will either drop slightly or stay the same when the person rises, while the diastolic pressure rises slightly.

Blood pressure may also be determined by a more direct method, the arterial line. A needle or a cannula is placed in an artery and connected to a transducer for electronic recording on a continuous basis.

Heart sounds

Auscultation of the heart involves listening to the heart with a good stethoscope using a systematic approach. Heart sounds are assessed considering the following characteristics: frequency, intensity, duration and location.

Two sounds are produced in quick succession in each cardiac cycle. These are followed by a brief pause before being repeated in the next cycle. Through a stethoscope the heart sounds will be heard as a lubb-dubb and are produced by closure of the heart valves.

The first heart sound, S_1, is a prolonged low-pitched sound (lubb). It is produced by the closing of both atrioventricular valves, the mitral and the tricuspid, just before ventricular systole. Although closure of the two valves occurs almost simultaneously, the mitral valve closes slightly before the tricuspid valve. Therefore, the mitral component is heard slightly before the tricuspid and is the main component of the first heart sound. S_1 is heard best in the tricuspid and mitral areas using the diaphragm of the stethoscope.

The second sound, S_2, is briefer and higher pitched (dubb). It is produced by the closing of both semilunar valves, the aortic and the pulmonary, just before diastole. Since the aortic valve closes slightly before the pulmonary valve, the aortic component of S_2 will be heard slightly before the pulmonary. The components of the second sound are normally affected by respiration. During inspiration, closure of the pulmonary valve is delayed because of the increased venous return to the right heart. The difference in the two components of S_2 is therefore more apparent. This is referred to as physiological splitting and disappears during expiration. S_2 is best heard in the aortic and pulmonic areas using the diaphragm of the stethoscope.

CLINICAL DIAGNOSTIC STUDIES

The cardiac patient may require a number of diagnostic studies to evaluate disease processes and treatments. The nurse requires an understanding of these procedures and their implications to manage patient care effectively and to teach patients who wish to be more knowledgeable about their own care. Blood tests, non-invasive and invasive diagnostic procedures will be discussed.

BLOOD TESTS

A number of blood tests are conducted when investigating heart disease; these are discussed elsewhere in this book.

NON-INVASIVE DIAGNOSTIC PROCEDURES

Non-invasive diagnostic procedures include electro-cardiography, echocardiography, nuclear magnetic resonance imaging and chest radiography.

Electrocardiography

Electrocardiography is the study of the electrical activity associated with heart contractions. The electrocardiogram (ECG), which produces a graphic recording of heart activity, provides one of the most dependable aids in assessing heart function and in diagnosing heart disease.

Each heart contraction results from electrical currents which spread from the heart and can be monitored from the surface of the body. These currents, which reflect the electrical activity of the heart, are detected when electrodes are placed on the external surface of the body. An application of contact jelly is made to the skin beneath the electrodes in order to facilitate conduction. The ebb and flow of the electrical forces result in a specific pattern, called a complex or cardiac cycle. Each part of the complex represents the electrical pathway of a specific part of the heart and normally occurs over a specific period of time.

The electrical complexes are recorded on special graph paper (see Figure 14.7). The horizontal axis of the graph paper represents time. Each small horizontal square indicates 0.04 s. Each large square is composed of five small squares and is therefore equal to 0.20 s.

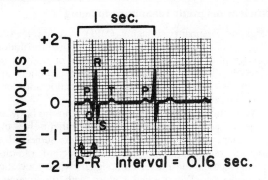

Figure 14.7 A normal electrocardiogram.

The vertical axis of the graph indicates voltage. Each small vertical square represents 0.1 millivolt, while a large square composed of five small squares equals 0.5 millivolt.

The deflections for each cycle are identified as P, Q, R, S and T, as shown in Figure 14.7.

The baseline of the graph paper represents zero electrical potential. Deflections above the baseline are considered positive, and deflections below the baseline are considered negative. When a wave form has both a positive and negative component, it is considered biphasic.

The P wave, or first rounded contour, represents atrial depolarization. It begins when the electrical impulse leaves the SA node and initiates atrial depolarization. The P wave can be positive, negative or biphasic, depending on the monitoring lead, and should be no more than 2 or 3 mm high.

The P–R interval is the time interval from the beginning of the P wave to the beginning of the QRS complex. The normal P–R interval is 0.12–0.20 s. The P–R interval represents the time for an impulse to travel from the SA node to the ventricular Purkinje fibres.

The QRS complex represents ventricular depolarization. The Q wave is the initial downward (negative) deflection following the P wave, the R wave is the initial upward (positive) deflection following the Q wave, and the S wave is the downward deflection following the R wave. The QRS complex should not exceed 0.10 s in duration and the normal amplitude varies significantly depending on the monitoring lead.

The ST segment is an interval of zero potential, the period between completion of depolarization and the beginning of repolarization (recovery) of the ventricles. Usually it is isoelectric, but it may normally deviate 2.0 mm above or below the baseline.

The T wave represents the recovery phase after contraction or return of the ventricular muscular fibres to their resting state. Normally, the T wave is slightly rounded, asymmetrical and not more than 5–10 mm in height, depending on the lead.

A *standard 12-lead ECG* records electrical conduction events from 12 different angles or leads, six recordings from the limb leads and six recordings from the chest leads. The ECG tracing is studied for deviations by comparing it with a tracing made by a normal heart; the direction, contour and timing of the waves and segments are noted. Information is obtained that is related to impulse formation and conduction and to the condition and response of the myocardium.

The patient should be given a brief explanation of the procedure and told that it takes approximately 5 minutes and that it is important to lie still during the procedure to produce good tracing. The patient should be aware that the electrical recording will not cause any discomfort and there is no danger of electrocution.

In some coronary care units the nurse is responsible for obtaining the ECG. Nurses working in these specialty areas interpret ECG patterns and changes in the ECG tracings of patients connected to cardiac monitors. Nurses may not be responsible for the interpretation of recordings, but are expected to be aware of the results and their significance for the individual patient.

Bedside monitoring. While on a specialized cardiac unit, the patient's cardiac functioning may be monitored by bedside equipment. This equipment allows continued surveillance of the patient's ECG tracing, with rapid identification of abnormal or changing rhythms and prompt treatment. Thompson et al (1986) found that the vast majority of the 100 patients they studied did not seem to mind being attached to a cardiac monitor, and seemed to find the presence of the monitor reassuring.

A *telemetry monitoring system* can be used in hospital to monitor an ambulant patient's cardiac activity. This method incorporates a transmitter (a small battery powered unit), which can fit into a pocket, and a receiver and monitor, which are commonly housed in the coronary care unit. The patient, attached to the transmitter by means of chest electrodes, can be in a ward in another part of the hospital as long as he or she is within the working radius of the transmitter and receiver. The cardiac rhythm can thus be monitored in the coronary care unit by nurses who are able to recognize cardiac arrhythmias.

Ambulatory electrocardiography
The Holter technique of electrocardiography is a means of studying, over a prolonged period of time, the electrical activity of the heart during a person's normal daily activities. The ECG is continuously recorded on a magnetic tape while the patient performs normal activity, usually for 24 hours. The patient keeps a diary of activities and symptoms over the recorded period. The tape is then analysed by computer for arrhythmias which can be correlated with activities and symptoms.

This technique can be used to detect and document suspected or known cardiac rhythm disturbances and to assess cardiac function during symptoms such as syncope, palpitations or chest pain.

The nurse should determine that the patient understands electrodes will be applied to the chest and that a light-weight tape recorder will be carried while the test is being conducted. As the machinery cannot be immersed in water, the patient will not be able to have a bath or shower during the test. It is very important that the patient maintains a normal level of activity during the test and records all symptoms and activities in the diary.

Exercise electrocardiography

An exercise ECG, also known as a stress test or graded exercise test, is used to detect and evaluate ischaemic heart disease while the individual exercises. Exercising increases myocardial oxygen demand and this test assesses the ability of the coronary arteries successfully to meet the increased demand. Thus it is useful in the evaluation of chest pain and the assessment of cardiac reserve or presence of IHD following myocardial infarction or cardiac surgery. Electrodes are attached to the patient, who is monitored continuously during the procedure. Periodically, recordings are printed.

The patient exercises on a treadmill or rides a bicycle at gradually increasing speeds against a regulated amount of resistance, according to an established protocol. The exercise continues until the patient reaches a predetermined maximal heart rate according to age and sex. The test is discontinued earlier if the patient develops chest pain, hypotension, severe ventricular arrhythmias, marked ST depression, undue dyspnoea or fatigue. The exercise ECG is considered positive if the ECG shows an ST segment displacement of 1 mm or more.

The nurse should be aware that the patient may have nitrates, calcium channel blockers and β-blockers withheld 48 hours prior to the test.

The day of the test, the patient should have a light meal and should not smoke for 2 hours prior to the procedure. The patient should come to the test prepared to exercise, wearing loose-fitting trousers or shorts and lace-up walking shoes, with socks to prevent blisters. It is important that the patient knows that he or she can stop the test at anytime and that any symptoms, including chest discomfort, light headedness, leg cramping and weakness, must be reported to the staff. After the test, the patient should be encouraged to rest and not to take a hot shower within 2 hours of completing the test.

Echocardiography

This is a non-invasive test used to detect ventricular dysfunction, valvular abnormalities, pericardial effusions, intracardiac masses and congenital defects.

High frequency sound waves are aimed at the heart. Some sound waves reflect or 'echo' off thoracic structures, are picked up by a transducer, visualized on a screen and recorded on videotape or on a strip chart recorder for analysis.

Doppler echocardiography is a valuable adjunct to the conventional echo examination. This technique, using ultrasound waves, provides information concerning blood flow patterns by assessing blood velocity at multiple locations of the heart or great vessels. Doppler colour flow mapping provides information concerning direction of blood flow. Doppler imaging is especially useful in evaluating valvular heart disease and the presence of septal defects.

Patients should be aware that they will need to lie quietly in a dimly-lit room for 20–30 minutes while the technician performs the echocardiogram. They will also be asked to change position several times during the procedure.

Nuclear magnetic resonance imaging

Magnetic Resonance Imaging (MRI) is a non-invasive diagnostic technique used to obtain high-resolution, tomographic, three-dimensional images of body structures. It allows visualization of cardiac chambers and blood vessels to determine structure, function and tissue characteristics.

When the nuclei of certain atoms within the body are subjected to a magnetic field, they align themselves in a particular pattern, which changes when subjected to another radiofrequency. When the second radiofrequency ceases, the nuclei emit signals while they align themselves to the original pattern with the magnetic field. The MRI scanner records these signals and translates them into detailed pictures of body tissues without lung or bone interference. These images are produced without the use of radiation and are therefore considered safe for pregnant women and children. Contraindications for MRI include the presence of internal surgical clips, pacemakers or other fixed metallic objects in the body, claustrophobia or acutely-ill, unstable patients.

Patients should be aware that they will be enclosed in the MRI scanner for about 30 minutes. No discomfort is felt during the procedure.

Chest radiography

An X-ray of the chest provides valuable information about the heart and lungs. Heart size may be assessed relatively accurately; the normal heart should be less than 50% of the width of thoracic cavity and not exceed 16 cm. Cardiac enlargement is an early sign of cardiac failure but an enlarged cardiac shadow may be seen in other conditions, such as valvular disease, cardiomyopathy, cardiac aneurysm and pericardial effusion. The location of invasive catheters, such as pacemaker or pulmonary artery catheters, can also be identified.

A brief explanation by the nurse will allay any apprehension on the part of the patient, particularly if he or she is unfamiliar with the X-ray procedure.

INVASIVE DIAGNOSTIC PROCEDURES

Radionuclide imaging techniques

Nuclear cardiology includes a group of diagnostic tests in which tracer substances called radionuclides are injected into the bloodstream and their distribution in cardiac chambers is measured using a computer and a gamma camera. Tracer substances are composed of two components: the radionuclide and the substance to be tagged. The measurement to be made determines the choice of nuclide and substance to be tagged.

Tracers are characterized by their chemical behaviour, their physiological and biological half-life and by the type, number and energy of radiation emitted. For example, tracers that emit gamma radiations are used to make most of the measurements in nuclear cardiology. Gamma rays can usually be detected externally and have the greatest chance of penetrating tissues.

Gamma rays emitted from the patient are detected by a gamma camera and an image of the distribution of radioactive isotope in the area of interest is obtained. This information on isotope distribution and the relative amounts of isotope present can be obtained in fractions of a second and stored in a computer for subsequent analysis.

Nuclear cardiology techniques are non-invasive except for a peripheral intravenous injection and are considered safer and are more easily repeated than invasive techniques. Some measures are carried out while the patient is at rest and others during exercise.

Information provided varies with the test performed. Some tests estimate myocardial blood flow: others, cardiac haemodynamics such as cardiac output, stroke volume or ventricular performance. Radionuclide techniques may be divided into two general types: (1) first-pass techniques, in which only the first transit of a radionuclide bolus through the circulation is analysed, and (2) equilibrium studies in which serial studies can be obtained over time.

Two nuclear myocardial imaging techniques will be described: the thallium and technetium scans.

Thallium myocardial imaging
Thallium-201 is an element with properties similar to potassium and is the radiopharmaceutical of choice for myocardial perfusion scintography. Clearance from the blood is rapid and extraction by the myocardium is high.

Thallium-201 scanning provides an assessment of myocardial tissue perfusion. Normally, coronary blood perfusion is equal throughout the myocardium, and thallium-201 would be distributed evenly in the tissue. In areas of myocardial ischaemia or necrosis, little or no thallium would be picked up. These areas of no perfusion would be seen as dark or 'cold' spots on the composite computerized image. In some patients, myocardial perfusion may be normal at rest, even with severe coronary disease. With exercise, however, the blood supply will differ in the area supplied by the diseased vessels to that supplied by normal vessels. Thus thallium imaging can be paired with exercise stress-testing to evaluate myocardial perfusion at rest and when stressed.

After the heart is stressed, exercise-induced ischaemia or previous myocardial infarction with a non-viable scar will produce a perfusion defect or cold spot. A second myocardial scan (or reperfusion image) is usually done 3 hours later. During the rest period, the exercise-induced ischaemic tissue will be reperfused and will no longer show as cold spots. This is called the redistribution pattern.

Patient preparation for this procedure is the same as for an exercise ECG (see p. 304).

Technetium myocardial imaging
The radioactive substance in this procedure is [^{99m}Tc] pyrophosophate. This test detects the size, location and approximate age of myocardial damage within 7–10 days of damage. The technetium-99m is absorbed by injured myocardial cells and images obtained of the heart will show these areas as 'hot' spots or bright areas. The scanning to obtain images takes approximately 30 minutes to perform.

Cardiopulmonary angiography

There are various techniques whereby the pulmonary and cardiac circulation can be assessed. The most widely used method involves the selective placement of a suitable catheter in the vessel or cardiac chamber proximal to the region being investigated. Injected radiopaque contract medium flows away from the catheter tip and its path may be recorded either with cine, video or rapid sequential radiographs.

Cardiopulmonary angiography may be used to investigate and diagnose a number of abnormalities, including valvular lesions, such as stenosis or regurgitation, pulmonary emboli, cardiac tumours, myocardial dysfunction, coronary artery stenosis or occlusion.

Cardiac and pulmonary angiography is invasive and not without complications; as with all investigations, the potential benefit from making a correct diagnosis must exceed the risk from the diagnostic procedure. The indications for the test must be clear and the patient fully informed of what to expect. It is the doctor's duty to discuss the procedure with the patient and to gain consent, but the nurse must have sufficient understanding to respond to additional questions and be reassuring, thereby reducing anxiety. Teaching the patient relaxation techniques prior to the procedure reduces stress (Rice et al, 1986). Patients are likely to be less anxious if they are told what sensations to expect, although some respond better if they are not told in so much detail what the procedure is like (Watkins et al, 1986).

It is the policy of most hospitals that informed, written consent be obtained prior to angiography. Food and fluids are withheld for the preceding eight hours and opiate premedication is advisable. There are few contraindications to the administration of radiopaque contrast media. Although most patients experience a sensation of warmth with the injection, major side-effects, which include respiratory distress, hypotension, urticaria, nausea and vomiting, are fortunately rare. Treatment will depend on the severity of the reaction, but intravenous fluids, antihistamines, steroids, adrenaline and oxygen should be available.

Right heart and pulmonary catheterization
This investigation provides information about the right side of the heart and the pulmonary circulation. Under local anaesthetic and sterile technique, the common femoral vein (usually the right) is punctured using a stiletted needle. The stilette is withdrawn and, once venous backflow occurs, a guide wire is threaded through the needle into the vein as far as the inferior vena cava. The needle is removed and an appropriate catheter is passed over the wire until it is in a satisfactory position, as judged by fluoroscopy. A small injection of contrast medium will confirm the position of the catheter tip.

The indication for the examination will determine where the doctor places the catheter; if a pulmonary

Table 14.4 Range of normal resting haemodynamic values.

	Mean	Systolic	End Diastolic
Pressures (mmHg)			
Right atrium	0–8		
Right ventricle	9–16	15–30	0–8
Pulmonary artery		15–30	3–12
Pulmonary artery wedge and left atrium	1–10		
Left ventricle		100–140	3–12
Systemic arteries	70–105	100–140	60–90

Grossman, W. & Barry, W. (1988), p. 250.

angiogram is required, for example for suspected pulmonary emboli, the catheter is guided through the tricuspid and pulmonary valves. In the assessment of right ventricular function, valvular disease or congenital defects, the catheter will be placed in the appropriate cardiac chamber.

Left heart and coronary artery catheterization
The femoral or brachial artery is used for evaluation of the left heart and coronary arteries. The technique of catheter introduction is similar for arterial studies, but more care is required because the pressures are higher. The catheter is passed retrogradely up the aorta. Crossing the aortic valve usually causes very little disturbance to cardiac or valve function; however, arrhythmias may be induced, so continuous cardiac monitoring is mandatory. Preshaped catheters facilitate the cannulation of the coronary ostia.

Cardiac catheterization also allows haemodynamic measurements and other parameters, such as the degree of oxygenation of blood within the various chambers, to be recorded (Table 14.4). This may be valuable in the investigation of congenital heart disease. For example, with an arterial septal defect, an increased oxygen tension may be found in the right side of the heart.

The nurse has a major role in preparing the patient for cardiopulmonary angiography. As indicated above, informed written consent is required. The patient is informed of the equipment that may be seen during the procedure, the sterile precautions that will be taken, and some of the physical sensations that will be experienced, such as a feeling of pressure when the catheter is introduced and the warm flush which immediately follows the injection of the contrast medium. Although each step is usually explained during the procedure, the patient's anxiety is often decreased when given this information beforehand. Some institutions may provide leaflets describing the experience.

The patient's reaction must be observed closely during the procedure. The ECG tracing is constantly monitored. Irritation of the myocardium by the catheter may rarely precipitate ventricular fibrillation, so a defibrillator is close at hand. The patient experiences little discomfort but may complain of a fluttering or irritation in the chest, especially during movement of the catheter. He is advised that this is a temporary sensation.

Following the catheterization, which may have taken 2 or 3 hours, the patient is given fluids and nourishment and is allowed to rest. The pulse below the catheter insertion site is checked at frequent intervals: every 15 minutes for the first hour and then at gradually increased intervals if it remains normal. An irregular, rapid or weak pulse is promptly reported to the doctor. If the catheter was passed through a femoral artery the patient remains in bed for 22–24 hours, and the site where the catheter was inserted is examined frequently for possible bleeding. A pressure dressing is applied in some institutions. The wound is observed for redness and tenderness which may indicate irritation or phlebitis.

Patients frequently wish to discuss their feelings following the procedure. Although one probable reaction is relief that the procedure is completed, anxiety about the findings and their implications is often evident.

Electrophysiology studies

An electrophysiology study (EPS) is an invasive procedure used to assess and facilitate management of recurrent symptomatic arrhythmias. The heart is deliberately provoked in an attempt to identify the existence, type and severity of the rhythm disturbance. The heart is stimulated using pacing catheters. The pacing catheters may be introduced by the oesophageal route by getting the patient to swallow them. The catheters are positioned behind the left atrium, which will receive the stimuli. The pacing catheters may also be introduced into the heart by the percutaneous route. This procedure is very similar to that described for a cardiopulmonary angiogram (see above). Once the pacing catheter(s) are in place (Figure 14.8), programmed stimulation is used to induce the rhythm disturbance.

If the arrhythmia is induced, medications and various manoeuvres may be attempted to prevent or treat it. A long-term treatment regimen can thus be established.

Preparation and postprocedure management of the patient undergoing EPS by the percutaneous route are similar to those described for a cardiopulmonary angiogram. However, postprocedure, the patient will require telemetry heart monitoring. The patient with significant arrhythmia disturbances may require ongoing evaluation using EPS.

Measurement of venous blood pressure

Venous blood pressure is an important parameter in the care of seriously ill patients. It reflects the intravascular volume and the ability of the heart to forward the blood it receives. Measurement of the venous pressure may be made in a peripheral vein, such as the medial basilic, or in a large central vein, such as the superior vena cava.

Central venous pressure
Central venous pressure (CVP) is more reliable than the peripheral, and is being used clinically more often in assessing the patient's condition. It may be used as a

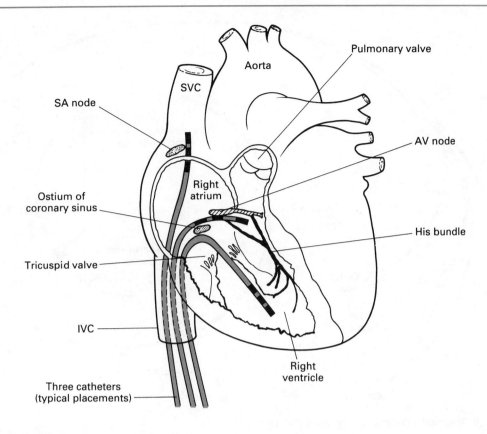

Figure 14.8 Placement of catheters in electrophysiology studies. SVC, superior vena cava; IVC, inferior vena cava. Modified from Vacek et al (1984) with permission.

guide for fluid replacement for the dehydrated or postoperative patient, or for a critically ill patient.

An intravenous catheter is passed into the superior vena cava via the subclavian or internal jugular veins, or occasionally into the inferior vena cava via a femoral vein. The catheter is attached to a three-way stopcock which is also connected to a water manometer and intravenous infusion. An alternative and more frequently used method employs a pressure transducer in the CVP cannula and electronic monitoring of the CVP reading. In setting up the CVP line the zero level of the manometer is positioned at the level of the right atrium, which is approximately in line with the midaxillary and suprasternal notch. The most important factor is that the equipment is at the same level for each recording, so the initial level is usually marked on the patient's skin. In most instances the changes in the venous pressure are more significant than the actual level. The patient must be in the same position for each reading. The pressure is generally recorded hourly. When the catheter is introduced, the stopcock is adjusted to allow fluid to flow to the patient. Then, to determine the venous pressure, the stopcock is turned to direct the fluid up into the manometer to a level of 30–35 cm. The valve is then adjusted to close off the flow from the

intravenous bag and to establish a flow line between the manometer and the catheter. When the fluid reaches the level of the venous pressure it remains at a relatively stationary level, rhythmically rising and falling 1–2 cm with respirations. Following the recording the stopcock is readjusted to allow the intravenous solution to flow to the patient.

The normal central venous pressure is approximately 5–10 cmH$_2$O. This varies with the patient's size, position and state of hydration. The significance of the pressure is determined in conjunction with the arterial blood pressure, the hourly output of urine, pulse rate and volume, and ECG. The nurse needs to know the levels at which the doctor is to be informed, and the type, volume and rate of flow of the infusion must be prescribed.

Other nursing responsibilities include observation for complications such as inflammation at the insertion site. This may be prevented by the use of aseptic technique during catheter insertion and during the application of dressings. Interference with flow may be minimized by periodic flushing with a solution of heparinized saline to prevent clotting and loosely coiling the tubing to prevent it from kinking.

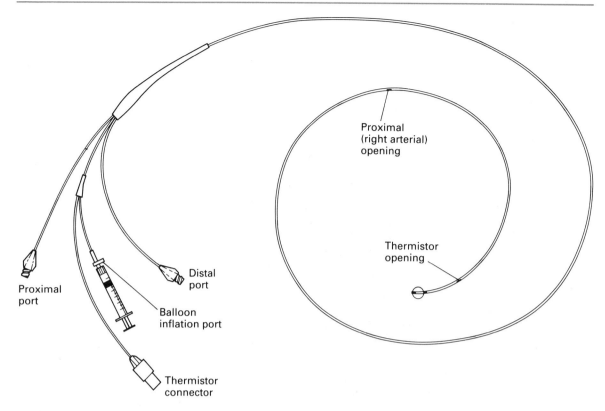

Figure 14.9 Thermodilution pulmonary artery catheter.

Measurement of pulmonary artery pressure (wedge pressure)

To obtain more specific information about the functioning of the left side of the heart, pulmonary artery and pulmonary capillary pressures are measured. This procedure is used for critically ill patients in whom early detection of left ventricular dysfunction is important.

A flow-directed (Swan–Ganz) catheter is inserted into a peripheral vein (Figure 14.9). A balloon at the tip of the catheter is partially inflated and the catheter floats into the right atrium, right ventricle and pulmonary artery at which time the pulmonary artery pressure may be measured. The catheter is then advanced into a branch of the pulmonary artery until it becomes wedged in a pulmonary capillary. Pressure measurements are obtained which reflect pressures in the left atrium. The balloon is then deflated until the next pressure reading.

The nurse is responsible for monitoring pressures, reporting abnormalities and preventing complications. The normal pulmonary artery pressure is 25/10 mmHg, and the normal pulmonary capillary wedge pressure is 4–12 mmHg.

CLINICAL CHARACTERISTICS OF IMPAIRED CARDIAC FUNCTION

Any impairment in circulation due to an abnormal heart condition is reflected in signs and symptoms which are produced by various factors: (1) a reduced blood supply to the heart and tissues throughout the body, causing a reduced nutrient and oxygen supply and an accumulation of metabolic wastes; (2) malfunctioning of the conduction system; and (3) the inability of the heart to eject the blood it receives. The last factor results in an excessive volume in the venous system, creating congestion and increased pressure that interfere with the function of tissues and organs.

The signs and symptoms of cardiac conditions vary with the degree to which circulation is impaired and with the form and location of the heart condition. Those which are discussed here do not necessarily all occur in every patient, nor are they all inclusive but are the more common problems presented by cardiac patients.

Abnormal pulse
The pulse rate may be abnormally fast or slow and the intervals between the heart beat may be unequal. The volume may vary. Some specific abnormalities of the arterial pulse are as follows:

Pulsus alternans. With pulsus alternans, the heart beats are regular but vary in amplitude. This condition is produced by changes in the left ventricular contractile force and is often precipitated by a premature ventricular beat. It is frequently associated with left ventricular failure resulting from hypertension, cardiomyopathy or aortic valve disease.

Pulsus bigeminus. Premature contractions alternating with normal heart beats result in variation in the strength of the heart beats. This alteration in pulse volume from beat to beat is called bigeminal pulse. It differs from pulsus alternans in that the weaker beat occurs regularly after a stronger, normally conducted beat.

Pulsus paradoxus. Normally, the strength of the arterial pulse falls during inspiration because of pooling of blood in the pulmonary vascular system. This occurs because of the more negative intrathoracic pressure and expansion of the lungs causing a reduced left ventricular stroke volume. If the blood pressure falls more than 10 mmHg (the normal fall during inspiration), the pulse is called pulsus paradoxus. Causes include cardiac tamponade, chronic constrictive pericarditis, emphysema and bronchial asthma.

Blood pressure

Arterial blood pressure is an important indicator of the patient's circulatory status. The systolic pressure depends on the cardiac output and, obviously, will fall with a reduced output by the left side of the heart. Venous pressure is frequently used to assess the ability of the heart to accept the inflow into the right side of the heart. A venous pressure in excess of the normal may indicate cardiac insufficiency or failure or an excessive intravascular volume, i.e. there is more blood returning to the right side of the heart than it can cope with.

Dyspnoea

The patient may experience shortness of breath or laboured breathing only on exertion, or it may be present even at rest. This is due to pulmonary congestion. The left side of the heart may not be forwarding all the blood it receives, and the blood is dammed back in the pulmonary veins. The pulmonary congestion and hypertension resist alveolar expansion, increasing the work of breathing and decreasing the vital capacity. If the congestion is long standing, alveolar tissue changes occur; the elastic tissue is replaced with fibrous tissue, and normal gas exchange is disturbed.

Dyspnoea that occurs when the patient is recumbent is referred to as orthopnoea. It may be relieved when the patient sits upright.

Cough

Fluid escapes into the alveoli from the capillaries in the congested pulmonary system and acts as a cough stimulus. This collection of transudate in the alveoli may be referred to as pulmonary oedema. The fluid may be expectorated as a frothy sputum and in severe heart failure may contain blood.

Hypoxia

Any impairment in circulation will create an oxygen deficiency in tissues. The cardiac output may be reduced, or a disturbance in pulmonary circulation may reduce the exchange of gases in the lung. Symptoms of an oxygen deficiency are many and varied, since the function of all structures is affected. The brain quickly reflects oxygen deprivation and reduced mental ef-ficiency, restlessness, apathy and disorientation are manifested. If the deficiency is severe, consciousness is lost and, unless the supply to the brain is promptly re-established, there is likely to be permanent tissue damage.

Severe pain occurs when muscle tissue, such as the myocardium, is deprived of adequate oxygen. Hypoxia may also cause cyanosis, a bluish colour, which is usually seen first in the lips and nail beds.

Oedema

Excess fluid accumulates in the interstitial spaces of the tissues in cardiac disease when the heart cannot forward the blood it receives. The blood backs up in the veins and venules, raising the venous blood pressure. Normally, at the venous end of the capillaries, the colloidal osmotic pressure exceeds the hydrostatic pressure of the blood, and interstitial fluid moves into the capillary. However, if the hydrostatic pressure of the blood in the distal portion of the capillaries exceeds the blood protein osmotic pressure, interstitial fluid will not be moved into the capillaries.

The retention of sodium ions also contributes to the formation of oedema in the cardiac patient. The decreased sodium excretion is promoted by the reduced blood flow through the kidneys which results from the impaired circulation. It is also suggested that some mechanism may exist which causes an increased secretion of aldosterone by the adrenal cortices. This hormone promotes reabsorption of sodium in the kidney tubules.

Oedema is a very characteristic sign of some weakening in heart function. Considerable fluid accumulates before the oedema becomes apparent; a person may retain 4.5–7.0 kg (10–15 lb) of excess fluid before the oedema becomes evident. It appears first in the dependent parts of the body where the venous and capillary blood pressures always tend to be greater. If the patient is ambulant, it becomes evident first in the ankles and feet but, if in bed, it appears initially in the sacral region.

Pain

Chest pain may result from a variety of conditions. Non-cardiac causes include: musculoskeletal disorders such as cervical arthritis; gastrointestinal disorders such as reflux oesophagitis and gallbladder disease, pulmonary conditions such as pulmonary embolus, and psycho-logical states such as severe anxiety.

The discomfort may mimic in both severity and description that of cardiac origin. For example, the pain of oesophageal spasm is usually burning in nature, located substernally and may be relieved by glyceryl trinitrate (GTN). Non-cardiac disease is ruled out by a careful history, physical examination and specific diag-nostic tests such as gastric or gallbladder investigations. The chest pain which cardiac patients experience is usually due to the deficiency of oxygen in the myocardium. It is important to determine the location, nature and precipitating or contributing factors of chest pain in order to distinguish the specific cause. The pain may be described as sharp, aching, squeezing, a feeling of heaviness or weight on the chest or a sensation of

Table 14.5 Chest pain profiles.

P Precipitating factors	Q Quality Quantity	R Region and radiation	S Associated symptoms and signs	T Time and response to treatment
A. Cardiac				
Angina				
Physical exertion Emotional stress Environmental factors Eating	Pressure Tightness Squeezing Burning Mild to moderate pain	Substernal Unable to pin- point Radiates to arms, throat, jaw, back, upper abdomen	Sweating Nausea, vomiting Dyspnoea Syncope Uneasiness	Gradual onset Duration < 30 minutes Relief with rest or GTN
Acute myocardial infarction				
Same; more likely to occur with no precipitators	Same descriptions Severe pain Worsened by fear and movement	Same region and radiation	Same, plus: Apprehension more severe Extra heart sounds Pulmonary congestion	Sudden onset Duration > 30 minutes No relief with rest or nitroglycerin Relief with narcotics
Dissecting aortic aneurysm				
Hypertension	Tearing sensation Excruciating pain worse at onset	Substernal Radiation to back and abdomen 'Travelling' sensation	Dyspnoea Apprehension Sweating BP differences between arms Absence of pulse unilaterally Hemiplegia or paraplegia Murmur of aortic regurgitation	Sudden onset No relief with rest or GTN Relief with narcotics
Pericarditis				
Myocardial infarction Uraemia Trauma Infections	Sharp Stabbing Knife-like Mild to severe Deep or superficial Worsened by inspira- tion, coughing, muscle movement, lying on left side	Precordial (left of chest midline) Retrosternal Radiation to neck, arm, or back	Dyspnoea Friction rub	Sudden onset Continuous No relief with rest or GTN Relief with sitting forward or aspirin
B. Pulmonary				
Pulmonary embolism				
Prolonged sitting or lying down Phlebitis Long-bone fracture	Crushing Deep ache Shooting Increased by deep inspiration or coughing	Lateral chest (over lung fields) Radiation shoulder, neck	Dyspnoea Pallor or cyanosis Syncope Cough with haemoptysis Apprehension Sinus tachycardia Pleural rub Fever	Sudden onset No relief with rest or GTN Relief with narcotics

Table 14.5 *Continued*

P Precipitating factors	Q Quality Quantity	R Region and radiation	S Associated symptoms and signs	T Time and response to treatment
Spontaneous pneumothorax				
Chronic obstructive pulmonary disease None	Tearing Increased by breathing	Lateral chest	Dyspnoea Decreased breath sounds Tachycardia Agitation	Sudden onset
Pneumonia				
Respiratory infection	Moderate ache Increased by coughing, inspiration, movement	Over lung fields Radiation shoulder, neck	Dyspnoea Tachycardia Pleural rub Fever Productive cough	Gradual onset Continuous duration Relief with sitting up

From Holloway (1988). Reproduced with permission from Addison-Wesley.

pressure within the chest. It may be mild or excruciating. It may be localized to one area or may radiate across the chest, and into the back, neck, jaw, shoulders and/or arms. It may be precipitated or aggravated by activity, breathing cold air, or certain bodily positions, and may be relieved by resting or a change of position. Table 14.5 describes some cardiac problems and the pain often associated with them.

Palpitation
Change in heart function may cause the person to be conscious of heart beats. Palpitation may be due to the apex of the enlarged heart striking the chest wall with each contraction, or it may occur with an increased stroke volume in extrasystole, or ectopic beats (see Arrhythmias, p. 334).

General debilitation, loss of strength and decreased mental and physical efficiency
Weakness, loss of appetite and weight, general apathy and reduced efficiency occur as the result of the reduced nutrient and oxygen supply, venous congestion and the accumulation of metabolic wastes.

Abnormal heart sounds
Cardiac murmurs are abnormal sounds caused by small jets of blood which create eddies in the bloodstream. Movements of these currents produce audible vibrations which are referred to as murmurs. The most frequent causes of heart murmurs are stenosed and incompetent valves and openings between the right and left sides of the heart. Murmurs may also occur in an aneurysm, a localized saccular dilatation of an artery.

The doctor, in determining the significance of a murmur, considers when it occurs in the cardiac cycle, its intensity, quality of sound, duration, factors which alter the sound (such as respiration and change of position) and the patient's history. Murmurs in some persons may have no great significance.

Occasionally a third heart sound becomes audible, producing a quick sequence of three sounds during each cardiac cycle. This phenomenon is referred to as gallop rhythm and is an unfavourable sign since it indicates a weakening and dilatation of the heart and often indicates heart failure.

Classification of Patients with a Cardiac Condition

The required care is not the same for all patients with a cardiac condition, since there are varying degrees of heart impairment and reduced efficiency, in addition to different pathological conditions.

There are those individuals who have a slight abnormality or who have had a condition which has been cured. The heart may carry some structural change or scar, but the cardiac efficiency and reserve are such that no restrictions on activities are necessary. Some of these people have unwarranted fears and restrict their activities unnecessarily, even though they have been advised by their doctors to live a normal, active life. The role of the nurse with these patients is to try to dispel their unsound fears and encourage them to be active. In some instances, overprotection by the family may be a problem.

A second group of people whom the nurse may help are those who are not ill but who have a reduced cardiac reserve. The heart condition has resulted in adaptive changes (dilatation, hypertrophy and/or acceleration) to compensate for the defect in order to maintain circulation. Energy expenditure must be restricted to correspond to the functional capacity of the heart in order to avoid failure. Obviously, the limitations vary with the extent of pathology and physiological changes in the heart and its resulting capacity. For some it may mean only giving up strenuous competitive sports; for others, greater restrictions are necessary. The aim of the care of these people is to have each one live within his compensatory limits and, at the same time, live as useful and satisfying a life as possible. Continuous treatment may be necessary for some to remain asymptomatic. The doctor assesses each patient's capacity, and the nurse helps the patient and family accept and adjust to the necessary restrictions. Positive emphasis is placed upon certain activities; suggestions are made as to what the patient can do, remembering that appropriate amounts of work, recreation and rest are more satisfying and beneficial.

The functional capacity of some cardiac patients may be so limited that they cannot participate in any physical activity without experiencing symptoms of cardiac insufficiency. They may be restricted to self-care activities or may be confined to a chair or bed, completely dependent upon others. The nurse's role with these patients is to provide the prescribed treatment and necessary care.

The doctor may use the functional and therapeutic classifications developed by the New York Heart Association and published by the American Heart Association or other methods of assessing cardiovascular disability. These serve as general guides to the type of care required and may influence the choice of suitable employment for the patient.

Common Health Problems Related to Cardiovascular Function

Analysis of data gathered during assessment may identify a number of health problems related to the individual's cardiovascular status, emotional response to disease and alterations in life-style. The most common problems are:

- Decreased cardiac output
- Activity intolerance
- Chest discomfort
- Altered family process
- Anxiety
- Alterations in life-style and self-care.

See Table 14.6.

DECREASED CARDIAC OUTPUT

Patient goals

1. The patient will experience no rhythm disturbances.
2. The patient will have improved contractility of the heart.
3. The patient will reduce workload on the heart.

Intervention

1. *Provide rhythm monitoring and treatment*

- *Cardiac rhythm monitoring.* Provide continuous ECG monitoring (see p. 303). Identify and document changes in cardiac rate and rhythm which cause alteration in cardiac output in collaboration with the doctor. Notify the doctor of rhythm disturbances, as appropriate.
- *Administer antiarrhythmic medications* as per protocol to treat rhythm disturbances, as appropriate.
- *Administer medications* that improve myocardial contractility, and monitor impact on cardiac output. These may include positive inotropes such as digoxin, dopamine and dobutamine.

2. *Reduce workload of the heart*

- *Rest.* Rest is important in the treatment of the patient with decreased cardiac output since it reduces the demand on the heart by reducing body requirements for oxygen. For the patient with an acute decrease in cardiac output, bed rest may be required to reduce workload on the heart. The patient could be advised to be on 'complete bed rest' or simply 'bed rest'. These usually mean something different, and the nurse must determine exactly what is meant by each in the particular situation. Generally, 'complete bed rest' is interpreted as absolute minimal activity on the patient's part, with the nurse doing everything possible for him. The patient is fed, bathed, turned, and assisted on and off the commode or bedpan; the teeth are cleaned and the hair combed. 'Bed rest' usually means that the patient may participate to some degree in personal care, and the nurse observes the effects of such activities on the patient. If they produce shortness of breath, an increase in pulse rate and excessive fatigue, activities are reduced.

  Once the acute episode has passed, the patient is allowed out of bed for gradually increasing intervals. Intermittent rest periods during the day and following activities are arranged, and the patient rests before and after meals and between procedures.

- *Positioning.* The position the patient with decreased cardiac output finds most comfortable in bed may be determined by his or her breathing. If the patient is experiencing a profound decrease in cardiac output and little dyspnoea, the supine position is preferable. This position facilitates venous return to the heart and reduces the heart's workload. The patient who is experiencing dyspnoea will be more comfortable with the head of the bed elevated, but the height of elevation should only be that at which the dyspnoea is minimal.

  Patients may manifest orthopnoea, that is, less difficulty in breathing with the trunk in the upright position. This position increases the vital capacity and tends to reduce the volume of blood returned to the heart and to the pulmonary system. Pressure of abdominal viscera on the diaphragm is reduced. Some patients may be still more comfortable in a

Table 14.6 Common problems related to cardiovascular dysfunction.

Problem	Related factors	Defining characteristics
Decreased cardiac output	• Cardiac arrhythmias • Impaired contractility of myocardium • Changes in preload • Altered afterload • Coronary vasospasm • Changes in myocardial automaticity	• Altered level of consciousness • Changes in blood pressure • Changes in cardiac output, pulmonary capillary wedge pressure • Arrhythmias • Jugular venous distension • Decreased or absent peripheral pulses • Increased body weight • Altered rate and depth of respirations • Crackles in lungs • Changes in skin colour • Decreased or absent urine output • Fatigue
Activity intolerance	• Immobility • Imbalance between oxygen supply and demand • Generalized weakness • Sedentary life-style • Impaired myocardial contractility • Impaired nutritional status • Limited cardiac reserve • Arrhythmias • Lack of knowledge about energy conservation	• Statement of fatigue, weakness • Inactivity • Dyspnoea on exertion • Chest pain on exertion • Expression of decreased energy • Significant changes in heart rate, blood pressure on exertion
Chest discomfort	• Decreased myocardial perfusion • Increased myocardial oxygen requirements	• Statement of chest pain • Facial grimacing • Clenched fist on chest • Changes in rate and depth of respirations • Altered blood pressure • Changes in heart rate, rhythm • Diaphoresis (sweating)
Altered family process	• Disruption of family functioning due to patient's illness, hospitalization, treatment • Lack of knowledge of cardiovascular disease process, management plan • Altered sexual functioning	• Decreased family involvement in social and community affairs • Failure to participate in usual family activities • Lack of family participation in patient's care
Anxiety	• Prognosis • Diagnosis • Treatment plan	• Complaints of anxiety • Sleeplessness • Restlessness • Abnormal rate/rhythm of pulse • Abnormal rate of respirations • Elevated blood pressure

true sitting position, that is, with the lower limbs down. A special cardiac bed on which the foot of the bed can be lowered to provide a chair-like support is available. Alternatively the patient may find comfort from sitting in a chair. The sitting position promotes the formation of peripheral oedema in the dependent parts but relieves the pulmonary congestion to some extent; peripheral oedema is much less serious than pulmonary oedema.

In the sitting position a pillow placed longitudinally at the patient's back may help provide some comfort. Pillows should be used at the sides to support the arms and relieve the fatiguing pull on the shoulders. A change may be effected by arranging a table and pillow over the bed, upon which the patient may rest the head and arms. Cot-sides may be kept up on the bed to safeguard the patient when in the upright position, since he or she may become drowsy and fall to the side, or may experience cerebral hypoxia which causes disorientation. The sides are also useful when a change of position is made since they may be grasped by the patient and used for added support. Patients in the upright position are encouraged to assume the recumbent position for periods to help reduce circulatory stasis and oedema in the lower parts of the body. However, patients should not be forced to do this if they are suffering from severe dyspnoea.

In patients with heart conditions, as with all patients, the general principles of positioning apply. Good body alignment is respected to prevent contractures, hyperextension and circulatory stasis. *Even a slight change in position* every 1–2 hours is helpful. A footboard is used to prevent foot drop.

- *Prevention of constipation.* Constipation should be prevented and the patient cautioned against straining at stool because of the stress it places on the heart. A mild laxative or stool softener may be given as necessary.

3. *Provide haemodynamic monitoring*

- *Monitor haemodynamic status.* Monitor the patient's cardiac output by physical examination and by utilization of specialized techniques such as pulmonary artery catheterization (see p. 308) when available. Document findings and notify the doctor of changes requiring medical treatment.
- *Administer treatments* which return to normal patient's preload and/or afterload and monitor the effectiveness of these treatments: (a) treatments which increase preload include administration of fluid, such as saline, blood and blood products, and medications such as vasoconstrictors; (b) interventions which decrease preload include medications such as diuretics, vasodilators, venodilators, restrictions of fluids and sodium, and, rarely, phlebotomy; (c) interventions which increase afterload including administration of fluids such as blood, blood products and saline; and (d) treatments which decrease afterload include administering medications such as vasodilators and venodilators.

Evaluation

Evaluate the effectiveness of nursing care by assessing if the patient:

1. Experiences no rhythm disturbances
2. Has improved contractility of the heart muscle
3. Reduces workload on the heart.

ACTIVITY INTOLERANCE

Patient goals

1. The patient will be able to perform planned activities without increased dyspnoea and fatigue.
2. The patient will understand and participate in planned activity programme.

Intervention

Activity progression

An acute episode of cardiovascular dysfunction will often confine the patient to bed until symptoms abate.

This means the patient is dependent on the nurse to facilitate care. It is important to discuss this necessary dependence with the patient so that its purpose, importance and temporary nature are understood.

The patient is allowed mild activities such as cleaning teeth, washing face and hands and feeding, as long as reaching is avoided. Exercising of the lower limbs to prevent venous stasis is commenced. Most patients are permitted to use a bedside commode, since this demands less energy than using a bedpan. Undisturbed rest periods are provided following short periods of activity, for instance after eating and after bathing.

As the patient's condition improves, activities and ambulation are gradually increased. An important principle in gradual ambulation is pacing activities. Rest periods are alternated with activities, and certain activities may be avoided for a period of time. These may include pushing, pulling, lifting or straining.

When a patient learns that he or she has a heart condition or recovers from an acute cardiac illness, he or she is advised as to whether former activities may be resumed or if it will be necessary to curtail some activities. The amount of activity and necessary restrictions are defined by the doctor on the basis of the functional capacity of the heart. Many of these people consider themselves doomed to complete invalidism and an early death. They may have an unjustified fear of another attack or of participating in any activity and may become helpless and dependent, creating unnecessary problems and hardships for themselves and their families.

Heart disease does not differ from many other diseases in that the patient may recover and resume a normal life. Some may find that a few simple adjustments in their pattern of living are necessary, while others are more restricted.

The doctor has several ways of assessing the patient's capacity for activity and any limitations. The doctor may observe the patient's responses to a gradual increase in energy expenditure. This will probably begin with self-care activities which are progressively extended to include more strenuous efforts. The assessment programme may go on over several weeks or months, and the patient may require considerable encouragement to persevere.

The nurse may assist in the assessment of the patient by observing and recording responses to various activities. Any complaint of shortness of breath, palpitation, fatigue or an undue increase in the pulse rate are reported, and the effort is discontinued until the patient is checked by the doctor.

It is sometimes helpful to have the patient list the accustomed pattern of activities. The doctor may then indicate what changes, if any, are necessary. This is useful in getting the patient to think and talk about how much he or she will be able to do. It encourages the patient to plan independently and to reach a compromise between activity and restrictions.

Once the patient is free of pain and other early symptoms and feels quite well, activities must still be restricted. Time may drag, so some effort is made to provide suitable diversions in which the patient is interested. Reading and radio and television programmes may occupy the patient. Some hobby may be pursued without overtaxing the heart. Visitors are restricted at first, but later they help relieve the patient's boredom. Visitor selection should be made by the family to avoid those who might excite or distress the patient. Visitors should be made aware of time limitations as it may be difficult for the patient to ask them to leave if he or she becomes tired.

Evaluation

Evaluate the effectiveness of nursing care by assessing if the patient:

1. Is able to perform planned activities without increased dyspnoea or undue fatigue.
2. Understands and participates in planned activity programmes.

CHEST DISCOMFORT

Patient goals

1. The patient will acknowledge and report chest discomfort as appropriate.
2. Appropriate interventions will be undertaken by the patient to reduce and eliminate chest discomfort.
3. The patient will engage in activities to prevent chest discomfort.

Intervention

1. *Early detection of chest discomfort*
The patient needs to be taught to acknowledge when signs and symptoms of chest discomfort are experienced and communicate this to others. If the patient is in hospital, chest discomfort should be reported immediately to the nurse so that it can be assessed and appropriate treatment begun. Studies have shown that nurses' assessments of patients' pain are not always reliable (Bondestam et al, 1987). When the patient is at home, chest discomfort should be acknowledged to others present so they can facilitate additional treatment if necessary.

2. *Elimination of chest discomfort*
- *Administration of nitrates.* Nitrates act by relaxing vascular smooth muscle. This results in decreased peripheral vascular resistance and venous return, with a subsequent decrease in heart size, stroke volume and cardiac output. The net effect is a decrease in the oxygen consumption of the heart.

    Glyceryl trinitrate (GTN) is a short-acting vasodilator administered in tablet or spray form. The tablet is placed under the tongue where it is absorbed very quickly. The patient may experience a tingling feeling on the tongue at first and should obtain relief in 1–2 minutes. Patients should not take multiple doses to get quick relief of pain. If relief is not apparent after 3 tablets taken at 5-minute intervals and the patient is outside the hospital, he or she should come to the hospital as soon as possible. If the patient is in hospital, the nurse will initiate therapy as ordered by the doctor. Initial dosage of GTN should be 0.3 mg. This reduces the likelihood of severe headaches, which often occur in the initial stage of treatment. People who suffer attacks of angina are advised to carry the drug at all times. It should be replaced periodically so that a fresh supply is available when required. Tablets should be kept in a dark glass container and those not being carried should be stored in a cool, dark place, since GTN is affected by both light and heat. The patient is advised that there may be a mild fullness, warmth or throbbing in the head, but fortunately with continued use these side-effects usually diminish.

    In emergency situations GTN may be administered intravenously.
- *Administration of analgesics.* An analgesic such as diamorphine is usually given to relieve severe pain not relieved by nitrates. The drug is administered intravenously in small doses in the accident and emergency department and in the coronary care unit. Intramuscular injections elevate creatine phosphokinase readings, as this enzyme is also present in skeletal muscle and diagnosis of a myocardial infarction may be obscured. The effect of the drug on the respirations should be noted, since depression of the respiratory centre may occur.

    This drug will reduce preload, afterload, sympathetic tone and the patient's anxiety.
- *Administration of oxygen.* Oxygen is usually administered in order to increase arterial oxygen tension, which may help to relieve the myocardial pain caused by hypoxia and prevent extension of the infarction. Observations are made of the patient's response to the oxygen. Its effectiveness will be indicated by reduced pulse rate, less dyspnoea, improvement in colour and less restlessness. (For details of administration of oxygen, see p. 428.)
- *Activity reduction.* Reduction of physical activity to bed rest will decrease the demand for oxygen on the myocardium. Elevate the patient's head 30° to promote physical comfort. Decrease environmental stimulus such as lights and noise to promote rest.

3. *Prevention of chest discomfort*
- *Administration of nitrates.* GTN ointment is used prophylactically to prevent attacks of angina but is not used for treating them.

    The ointment is measured out in 1–5-cm lengths and spread over the application paper, providing an application area of approximately 5–8 cm^2. The paper is then applied to the patient's skin and may be covered with any commercial plastic covering to facilitate maximum absorption. GTN ointment may be applied to skin on the arms, legs, chest or abdomen. Sites should be rotated. It is best to keep the size of the application site constant, to prevent the side-effects which may occur when it is enlarged. Side-effects are the same as those of GTN tablets.

    Transdermal GTN patches have now been developed which deliver glyceryl trinitrate into the bloodstream at a constant rate for 24 hours. They are less messy and difficult to use than ointment and may enhance patient compliance.

Isosorbide dinitrate is a slower- and longer-acting nitrate given sublingually in small doses or orally in larger doses. It is ordered for patients experiencing regular attacks of angina. Since it reduces vascular tone, some patients may experience hypotension on standing, especially when taking larger doses. The patient is usually started on small doses, which are gradually increased as the drug becomes tolerated.

- *Reduction of workload on the heart.* The reduction of workload on the heart is important so that there is sufficient oxygen available to the myocardium to meet the demands placed upon it. Pacing of activities to ensure adequate periods of rest between periods of activity can facilitate balanced supply and demand on the heart.
- *Modification of risk factors.* To prevent further progression of underlying ischaemic heart disease, the patient and family need to be instructed as to how to modify their life-style. This is discussed extensively on pp. 298–300.

Evaluation

Evaluate the effectiveness of nursing care by assessing if the patient:

1. Acknowledges and reports chest discomfort as appropriate.
2. Undertakes appropriate interventions to reduce and eliminate chest discomfort.
3. Engages in activities to prevent chest discomfort.

ANXIETY

Patient goals

1. Patient will be able to verbalize feelings of anxiety.
2. Manifestations of anxiety are reduced or absent.

Intervention

Patients with heart disease are frequently anxious. Serial measurements of the anxiety levels of coronary patients have shown that anxiety is highest on admission to the coronary care unit and immediately after transfer to the ward, falling rapidly over the following week and rising just before discharge (Thompson et al, 1987).

The common knowledge that the heart is a most vital organ and that heart disease is a frequent cause of death produces a great emotional reaction in the person advised of a diagnosis of a heart disorder. The patient becomes fearful and apprehensive; life, job, family security and the whole future are threatened. Rarely does any other condition, even though it may be an equally severe threat, engender as much fear and concern.

The nurse who understands the patient's condition, knows what to look for and what to do, usually displays calm and composure which contribute to the patient's confidence and security. Brief and precise explanations

of all equipment, routines, tests and procedures prove very helpful. A quiet, controlled atmosphere may do more toward allaying fear than verbal reassurance.

Patients may pose direct questions about their condition, such as 'Is it serious?' or 'Will I recover?' Answers should be honest and supportive. Each patient must be helped to find a coping strategy appropriate to his or her personal situation and own strengths and weaknesses. This is done through effective communication with the patient. Effective communication includes listening to the patient and responding to any cues, introducing statements to which the patient might respond and allowing the patient to discuss feelings. Considerable help and peace of mind may be derived from a vicar, priest or other religious leader.

If the patient is very upset the nurse remains until the patient is less apprehensive, and confirms that someone is close by and will be in and out frequently. The presence of a close member of the family who will not disturb the patient may provide additional comfort. Occasionally, diazepam or another anti-anxiety drug may be prescribed.

There may be a problem at home that contributes to the patient's unrest which should be discussed if appropriate or arrangements made for assistance from the social services or primary health care team.

Evaluation

Evaluate the effectiveness of nursing care by assessing if the patient:

1. Detects early signs and symptoms of anxiety.
2. Participates in activities to reduce or eliminate anxiety.
3. Actively engages in activities to prevent anxiety.

ALTERED FAMILY PROCESS

Patient's family goals

1. The family will express feelings of support and awareness of available resources.
2. The family will be able to participate in the patient's treatment as appropriate.

Intervention

Members of the patient's family experience shock and anxiety in response to the patient's diagnosis. Seeing someone close to us in pain and seriously ill is a very frightening experience. Relatives of patients have described their initial reaction as 'feeling numbed and dazed'. As reality sets in, anxiety about the patient's survival and future increases.

The doctor and nurse speak to a member of the family shortly after the patient's admission to the hospital, explaining the suspected diagnosis and the treatment to be given during the next few hours. The nurse then attempts to speak to close family members whenever they visit to answer any questions and to show understanding of the anxiety they are experiencing. Relatives as well as patients are reassured by simple explanations of equipment, procedures and routines. In talking to the family, the nurse may elicit information about the patient's habits, likes and dislikes and emotional reactions, which are helpful in planning care.

Alleviating the anxieties of relatives and/or close family friends allows them to be more supportive of the patient. As with the patient, concern may prevent the members of the family from absorbing all that they are told. Explanations and instructions may have to be repeated. The family should be included in teaching programmes provided for the patient or in programmes specifically designed for them to ensure they understand the patient's condition.

The nurse also assists the family to assess their need for community resources to facilitate coping with their altered situation. Support groups for families coping with cardiovascular disease may be available. The community nurse may be required.

There is evidence that professional support, particularly of the spouse, may be inappropriate or inadequate (Thompson and Cordle, 1988). The main need is to feel that there is hope (Norris and Grove, 1986). A simple programme of in-hospital counselling for coronary patients and spouses has a number of benefits, including a reduction of anxiety and depression (Thompson, 1990b).

Evaluation

Evaluate the effectiveness of nursing actions by assessing if the patient's family:

1. Expresses feelings of support and awareness of available resources.
2. Participates in the patient's treatment as appropriate.

ALTERATIONS IN LIFE-STYLE AND SELF-CARE

Patient goals

1. *The patient will show knowledge of the disease process*
In order to make the best possible adjustment to illness and recovery, the patient must have some understanding of the illness and how he or she can assist in recovery. Providing this information helps give the patient some control over the situation. Teaching programmes are adjusted to specific patient needs and capabilities, since learning capacity varies among individuals. Patients experiencing cardiovascular conditions often have many misconceptions of their condition and how it will affect their future. It is useful for the nurse to find out what the patient already knows and to obtain information about life-style. The nurse has many opportunities to reinforce and elaborate on explanations given by the doctor and to respond to further questions.

During the acute stage, the patient is often too anxious to absorb much information. *Simple* explanations of equipment being used and procedures common to coronary care units are usually adequate. Following

transfer to the general ward, the patient is usually better able to participate in a planned programme. Written as well as verbal instruction can be provided. Visual aids such as heart models or diagrams help to enhance learning.

Short teaching sessions are necessary, as many patients with cardiovascular conditions tire easily. It is helpful if one of the family can be present in the teaching session. Acknowledgement is made of the feelings that the patient has in response to the illness. The patient may wish to express verbally the feelings being experienced, such as discouragement, fear, anger and/or depression; the nurse should provide opportunities for free expression and should be a willing listener.

The nurse should have a copy of the many useful pamphlets and booklets available from the British Heart Foundation. Many of these deal with rehabilitation, and appropriate copies may be given to the patient to read.

2. *The patient will engage in life-style modification to reduce risk*
Several areas where modification may be necessary are discussed. These are further elaborated on p. 298.

Since smoking, particularly cigarettes, is found to be vasoconstricting, the patient is advised to discontinue smoking.

Clarification of the prescribed diet is made. Many patients are advised to continue with a low sodium intake and a limited number of calories. Foods allowed, those restricted and meal planning are discussed. The importance of keeping the weight normal and avoiding large meals is explained. Preferably, the discussion of the diet should be with the family as well as the patient. Directions and suggestions are given to the patient in writing, and an appropriate diet booklet can be obtained from the British Heart Foundation or the Health Education Authority.

The medications that are to be continued are discussed, and written instructions are provided. Early signs of untoward reactions are cited, and included with these are directions about what to do if they develop. For example, if an anticoagulant such as warfarin is to be continued, the patient and a family member are advised of the action of the drug and the necessary observations to recognize bleeding. They are told that bleeding from body orifices, discoloured areas of the skin (bruises and petechiae), bleeding gums, and persistent bleeding from minor cuts or injuries are to be reported immediately to the doctor or clinic. If there is dental work to be done, the patient should advise the dentist that he or she is receiving warfarin. The patient is given an identification card to carry which states that he or she is receiving warfarin. A weekly visit to clinic for prothrombin time evaluation is usually requested by the doctor.

Many patients with heart conditions are required to take digoxin continuously and should understand that loss of appetite, nausea or diarrhoea may indicate the need for some adjustment in the dosage of the drug. If the patient is an elderly person who lives alone, it is advisable for a calendar to be kept available with the days that a medication is to be taken clearly marked. It is stressed that the patient should adopt the habit of marking off the medication as soon as it is taken.

Progressively increased activity is encouraged and directed by the nurse to condition the patient to the level of activity that corresponds to the heart's ability.

Changes may be necessary at home if the patient is not allowed to use stairs. It may be helpful to have a member of the primary health-care team or an occupational therapist or social worker assess the home situation before the patient returns to it. Suggestions may be made in the interests of the patient and care-givers. For example, a bedroom and bathroom may have to be provided on the ground floor. Distance from public transport and work may be factors that require consideration for some patients.

It should be pointed out to the patient and family that moderation in everything is a good rule for persons who have had a heart illness. Some work, exercise, rest and recreation are important for everyone. Situations that are likely to add undue strain should be anticipated and avoided. Enough time should be allowed to prevent rushing. For example, rather than run the risk of running for a bus, the patient should plan to leave earlier. Climbing, walking against a strong wind, lifting, pushing and fatigue are to be avoided. Constipation, infections and emotional upsets also tend to increase the demands on the heart. The patient should strive for equanimity and develop the philosophy that what cannot be changed must be accepted. Suitable recrea-tional activities, which meet both interests and cardiac functional capacity, may be suggested. Some exercise is beneficial and appropriate forms are discussed. Walking is considered a good exercise. Regular hours of rest at night and, if necessary, a rest period during the day are recommended.

The doctor, a social worker or the nurse may discuss necessary adjustments in the person's work situation with the employer or the occupational health nurse. Assistance might be given to find suitable employment or to obtain retraining if a change in occupation is indicated.

Some follow-up service is important. The patient and family are advised of the resources outside the hospital, and a referral may be made to the hospital cardiac rehabilitation programme, general practitioner and district nurse. Home visits by a nurse can be very helpful; they provide an opportunity for the patient and family to ask questions and receive counselling on the various aspects of care. At the same time the patient's condition and progress are noted.

Evaluation

Evaluate the effectiveness of nursing care by assessing if the patient:

1. Discusses accurately the disease process and management.
2. Engages in life-style modifications which may reduce risk of further cardiovascular health problems.

CAUSES AND TYPES OF HEART DISORDERS

Heart disorders may be classified as congenital or acquired. Various subclassifications may be used in acquired heart disease. Some authors concentrate on structure, such as pericardium, myocardium and en-docardium. Others highlight the causes of heart disease, such as trauma, infections, degenerative processes, and hyper- and hypometabolic processes. This text classifies heart disorders as:

1. Congenital cardiovascular defects
2. Disorders of cardiac muscle
3. Disorders of myocardial blood supply
4. Disorders of electroconduction
5. Disorders of myocardial pumping capacity
6. Disorders of the vascular system.

Discussion of the person with each of these disorders will follow.

CONGENITAL CARDIOVASCULAR DEFECTS

Congenital cardiovascular defect implies a structural abnormality that was present at birth in the heart or the large proximal blood vessels. It has only been within the last two to three decades that many of the congenital cardiovascular defects have been identified and success-fully treated by surgery. Many are recognized shortly after birth if the infant survives. Others may go undiscovered for months or years because the heart maintains an adequate circulation by compensation. As in so many congenital deformities, the cause remains obscure. In some instances it is thought that a viral infection, such as German measles, occurring in the mother in the first trimester of pregnancy, may cause the defect. Frequently, cardiovascular malformations accom-pany other congenital defects such as cataract, mental handicap and deaf–mutism.

Many types of heart malformations occur. They may be classified into three main groups: (1) those which produce a left-to-right shunt of blood; (2) those which offer resistance to the blood flow; and (3) those which cause a right-to-left shunt (Figure 14.10).

Anomalies which Cause a Left-to-Right Shunt

Several malformations occur which produce an abnor-mal pathway that permits a direct flow of blood from the left side of the heart or aorta to the right heart or pulmonary artery, creating a bypass of the systemic circulation and an overloading of the pulmonary circulation. These anomalies include patent ductus arteriosus and septal defects.

ATRIAL SEPTAL DEFECT

An opening between the two atria may be due to failure of the foramen ovale to close after birth or to a gap in the septum, either above or below the foramen ovale. Blood in the left atrium will flow through the opening into the right atrium, increasing the volume of blood in the pulmonary system. The right atrium, right ventricle and pulmonary artery enlarge. Pulmonary hypertension develops and causes dyspnoea, particularly on exertion. The reduced systemic circulatory volume retards physical and mental development and efficiency. The size of the opening may be so small that it goes undiscovered, and the patient may not experience any respiratory or circulatory difficulty.

Surgical repair of an atrial septal defect is usually accomplished by open heart surgery. Some defects may be closed simply by suturing while others may require a patch of Teflon, an inert material to which tissues do not react.

VENTRICULAR SEPTAL DEFECT

An opening in the ventricular septum results in a left-to-right shunt and produces problems similar to those cited in atrial septal defect: pulmonary hypertension, enlargement of the right ventricle and pulmonary arteries, and a deficient systemic circulation. If the defect is small and the patient is asymptomatic, surgery is not indicated. Moderate to severe defects may be closed by patching with either pericardial tissue or Teflon. Occasionally the defect closes spontaneously in the young child.

PATENT DUCTUS ARTERIOSUS

Normally, after birth, a gradual spontaneous constriction and atrophy of the ductus takes place. If it remains open the blood in the aorta, under a pressure approximately 5–6 times that in the pulmonary artery, is shunted into the pulmonary artery. This increases the volume of blood entering the lungs, resulting in a high pulmonary blood pressure and dilatation of the pulmonary vessels. The patient experiences dyspnoea, particularly on exertion. There is a corresponding increase in the venous flow into the left atrium and left ventricle, causing dilatation and hypertrophy of the left side of the heart. The volume of blood in the systemic circulatory system is less than normal, and the resulting oxygen and nutritional deficiencies retard normal mental and physical development.

The patent ductus arteriosus is corrected by surgical division and suturing of the two ends of the vessel.

Anomalies which Cause Resistance to Blood Flow within the Circulation

The seriousness of the resistance is determined by the degree of constriction or stenosis which may be found in the pulmonary artery or the aorta.

PULMONARY STENOSIS

A stenosis of the pulmonary valve or artery offers resistance to the outflow of blood from the right side of the heart. The right ventricle enlarges and the pressure in both the right ventricle and atrium is above normal. Blood may be backed up in the venous system, while the blood volume entering the pulmonary system is below normal. The latter creates an oxygen deficiency throughout the body which is manifested by fatigue, shortness of breath and, less frequently, cyanosis. Symptoms may not be present for several years.

This malformation may be treated surgically by incision of the constricted ring.

AORTIC STENOSIS

A defect comparable to pulmonary stenosis may occur in the aorta and offer resistance to left ventricular outflow. The left side of the heart enlarges and the pressure in both left chambers is above normal: this may be reflected in an increased pulmonary pressure if the restriction is severe. The cardiac output is lower and reduces arterial blood pressure and the systemic circulation as well as the blood supply into the coronary arteries. The defect may be treated by surgery, using an extracorporeal pump-oxygenator (cardio-pulmonary bypass) during the procedure.

COARCTATION OF THE AORTA

Coarctation is a stricture in a segment of the aorta. Postductal coarctation occurs just beyond the obliterated ductus arteriosus and distal to the origin of the left subclavian artery. The second type, preductal coarctation, develops in the segment of aorta before the entrance of the ductus arteriosus. With this latter type the ductus usually remains patent.

Blood volume and pressure are increased behind the stricture, and the work of the left side of the heart is increased greatly. The blood volume and pressure are high in the upper extremities and head, but are abnormally low in the body parts which derive their blood supply from below the stricture. A difference in growth and development may be seen between the areas supplied from behind the stricture and those supplied from the aortic flow distal to the stricture. The patient may experience headaches, epistaxis, dyspnoea on exertion, leg cramps and fatigue.

Surgical treatment of the condition involves resection of the constricted area and an end-to-end anastomosis or, in some instances, the area is excised and a graft of inert material introduced.

Anomalies which Cause a Right-to-Left Shunt

A shunting of blood from the right side of the heart to the left involves a combination of two or more anomalies. Normally, the pressure is much higher in the left side of the heart than in the right side. A stenosis which offers resistance to flow from the right ventricle

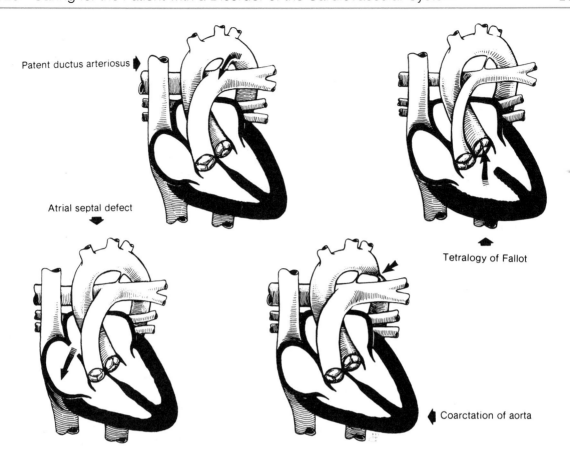

Patent ductus arteriosus

Atrial septal defect

Tetralogy of Fallot

Coarctation of aorta

Figure 14.10 Congenital cardiac defects.

may increase the pressure in the right side to a level exceeding that in the left side. If a septal defect coexists with this increased pressure, blood is shunted from the right to the left side of the heart.

One of the most frequently seen combinations of anomalies which produces a right-to-left shunt is the tetralogy of Fallot. Tetralogy denotes a set of four conditions: pulmonary stenosis, ventricular septal defect, dextraposition of the aorta which causes it to override the septal defect, and right ventricular hypertrophy. The pulmonary stenosis produces an increased pressure in the right ventricle, causing a right-to-left shunt. The volume of blood flowing through the pulmonary system for oxygenation is reduced. Unoxygenated blood escapes into the aorta and a general systemic hypoxia occurs, manifested by cyanosis and dyspnoea, especially on physical exertion, and by clubbing of the fingers. Compensatory responses to the oxygen deficiency develop in the form of polycythaemia, high haemoglobin level and increased pulse and respiratory rates.

Correction of these defects is possible by means of open heart surgery and the use of the pump-oxygenator. The septal opening is patched, and the pulmonary stenosis is relieved. Occasionally the surgeon may decide not to perform corrective surgery but will proceed with a palliative surgical procedure, referred to as a 'shunt'. This consists of an anastomosis between the

subclavian and pulmonary arteries (Blalock's operation) or between the aorta and pulmonary artery (Potts' operation). The purpose of the anastomosis is to divert a larger volume of blood through the lungs for oxygenation.

Miscellaneous Congenital Cardiac Anomalies

Only the more common anomalies that are recognized and treated have been presented here. A wide variety of anomalies can occur, many are not yet amenable to treatment, and others may be so severe that the infant cannot survive. Transposition of the great vessels is relatively common and may be treated surgically. In this anomaly, the pulmonary artery originates from the left side of the heart and conducts the oxygenated blood back to the lungs, and the aorta rises from the right ventricle, carrying unoxygenated blood into the systemic circulation.

Rarely, transposition of the pulmonary veins to the right of the heart is seen, and transplantation of the veins to the left atrium may be attempted.

Valvular atresia (absence of an opening) is another form of anomaly which occurs most frequently with the tricuspid valve but may also develop with the aortic valve. Tricuspid atresia raises the pressure within the right atrium to a level exceeding that in the left atrium, and blood flows through the foramen ovale. This anomaly is frequently accompanied by a ventricular septal defect which permits some blood to enter the right ventricle and pass into the pulmonary artery. Either the Blalock or Potts operation (see above) or an anastomosis between the superior vena cava and the pulmonary artery may be done to increase the volume of blood through the lungs.

THE PERSON WITH DISORDERS OF CARDIAC MUSCLE

In this section, discussion will focus on cardiomyopathies and inflammatory disorders of the heart, including rheumatic fever, infective endocarditis and pericarditis, as well as the nurse's role in caring for people with these disorders.

Cardiomyopathy

Cardiomyopathy is a term used to describe diseases which affect the myocardial layer of the heart and have no obvious cause.

Three types of cardiomyopathies have been identified, based on their pathophysiological abnormalities: (1) dilated or congestive, (2) hypertrophic, and (3) restrictive or obliterative.

DILATED CARDIOMYOPATHY

This is the most common of the three types. It is characterized by dilated, usually thin-walled ventricles which produce poor systolic function and low cardiac output. A variety of conditions have been associated with this disorder, including viral infections (polio virus, coxsackie B virus), immunological disorders, systemic hypertension and exposure to toxic agents (particularly alcohol).

Symptoms of this disorder include congestive heart failure, particularly left-sided failure, fatigue, activity intolerance, chest pain and tachyarrhythmias. As a result of relative status of blood in the ventricles, patients may experience systemic or pulmonary emboli.

The medical treatment of dilated cardiomyopathy is palliative in nature. The goal of treatment is to improve cardiac output by increasing contractility and reducing workload.

Positive inotropes such as digitalis and amrinone may be used to strengthen the myocardial contractility. Diuretics may be used to decrease circulating blood volume and decrease preload. Vasodilator therapy such as captopril may be used to improve cardiac output and improve activity tolerance. Antiarrhythmics may be used to prevent arrhythmias. Anticoagulants may be used to prevent systemic and pulmonary emboli. Supportive measures including restricted activity, low sodium diets

and abstinence from alcohol may also be advocated.

End-state dilated cardiomyopathy may be treated surgically with cardiac transplantation.

HYPERTROPHIC CARDIOMYOPATHY

This has been identified by a variety of names including idiopathic hypertrophic subaortic stenosis and muscular aortic stenosis. It is characterized by a hypertrophied left ventricle, particularly the septum, with no dilatation of the chamber. Thus the left ventricle has thickened walls but there is no enlargement of the chamber size. This results in supernormal systolic function and impaired diastolic filling of the ventricle.

Symptoms of hypertrophic cardiomyopathy include dyspnoea, palpitations, syncope, angina pectoris and activity intolerance. The first sign of this disorder may be sudden death.

Medical management of hypertrophic cardiomyopathy focuses on improving cardiac output by enhancing diastolic function, reducing contractility and preventing ventricular arrhythmias. β-Adrenergic blocking agents, most commonly propranolol, are used to decrease the rate and force of ventricular contraction and improve diastolic filling time. Calcium channel blockers such as verapamil may be used instead of β-adrenergic blockade for long-term management.

Ventricular arrhythmias may be controlled by antiarrhythmics such as amiodarone. Surgical management may be indicated, with a septal myotomy-myorectomy being performed. This procedure involves removal of a portion of the hypertrophied septum, thus widening the outflow track from the left ventricle to the aorta.

Several medications are generally contraindicated in the treatment of hypertrophic cardiomyopathy, although they may be used with careful supervision. Digitalis is contraindicated because it increases contractility and increases outflow obstruction. Nitrates and diuretic therapy are avoided because they cause decreased venous return to the heart, increased contractility and increased outflow obstruction.

RESTRICTIVE/OBLITERATIVE CARDIOMYOPATHY

This is the least common of the three types of cardiomyopathies. It is characterized by rigid, hypertrophied ventricular walls and impaired diastolic filling, leading to decreased cardiac output. This loss of compliance may be a result of myocardial infiltration and/or fibrosis.

This disorder may manifest as pulmonary congestion, activity intolerance and chest pain. Atrial arrhythmias, particularly atrial fibrillation, are common.

Medical management of this disorder is also palliative in nature and involves managing the symptoms of heart failure by diuretic therapy, and fluid and sodium restriction. Antiarrhythmics may be necessary to control atrial arrhythmias. Surgical resection of thickened endocardial tissue has been performed.

Nursing management of patients with cardiomyopathy

of any sort may focus on the following problems:

- Activity intolerance related to fatigue, limited cardiac reserve
- Decreased cardiac output related to poor cardiac function
- Ineffective coping related to fear of chronic disease and death. (See Chapter 5 for a discussion of these problems.)

Further discussion of these nursing problems can be found on p. 312.

The Person with Inflammatory Disorders of the Heart

In any tissue, the inflammatory process may result in destruction of normal functional tissue followed by its replacement with scar tissue, which is fibrous in nature and less specialized.

Diseases which produce inflammatory heart lesions and impaired function include rheumatic fever, infective endocarditis and pericarditis.

RHEUMATIC FEVER

This is the most common cause of inflammation in the heart structures. Although any or all parts may be affected by rheumatic fever, the valves and the myocardium are the most frequent sites and tend to sustain greater permanent damage. The disease is a complication of a group A streptococcal infection which is usually respiratory. A period of 1–5 weeks may lapse between the infection and the onset of the rheumatic fever, during which time the patient may have recovered completely from the infection.

The inflammatory response, which may occur in the joints as well as in the heart, is thought to be due to a sensitivity of the affected individuals to the antibodies that were formed in response to the invading bacteria. The antistreptococcal lysin titre is found to be high in these people at the onset of rheumatic fever. This sensitivity is only present in certain individuals, since not all those with streptococcal infection develop rheumatic fever. The symptoms of the acute stage vary in intensity and may be so mild that they go unrecognized. In some, joint involvement and fever may be predominant with no evident symptoms referable to the heart, and it is not until much later that it becomes known that cardiac tissue was involved and received permanent damage.

Rheumatic fever may cause acute myocarditis with subsequent scarred areas that reduce myocardial efficiency and impair the conduction system.

The valves are the most common area of the heart to be affected, and the mitral and aortic valves are the most susceptible. They frequently become scarred, distorted and functionally impaired. Both the valve ring at the opening and the valve cusps may be affected. Following the acute inflammation scarring occurs, the orifice is diminished and the edges of the cusps may fuse. These changes result in resistance to the forward movement of

the blood, thus increasing the work of the heart chamber behind the obstruction. Damage of this type is referred to as a stenosis. Normally, the mitral opening in an adult is large enough to admit three fingers; in severe stenosis it can become so restricted that only one finger may be introduced.

In some instances, the scarring of the valvular cusps produces a thickening and loss of tissue that prevents them from coming together to close off the opening completely. This incomplete closure allows a regurgitation or backflow of blood through the valve, and is called valvular incompetence or regurgitation. An added strain is placed on the heart chamber behind the incompetent valve. Many patients with rheumatic heart disease have a combined stenosis and incompetence in the affected valve. If the mitral valve is involved, the left atrium develops dilatation and hypertrophy to compensate for the resistance of stenosis and the backflow of valvular incompetence (i.e. the leaking of the blood back through the valve). In the case of aortic valvular damage, the left ventricle dilates and hypertrophies. Prolonged strain created by a damaged valve, increased demands on the already weakened heart, or further progress of the initial rheumatic disease process may result in decompensation or heart failure.

Treatment of rheumatic fever includes drug therapy (antimicrobial preparations, salicylates, corticosteroids), rest and possible surgery.

In the acute stage of rheumatic heart disease the patient may receive large doses of penicillin to destroy any haemolytic streptococci which may still be active in the body. Reactivation of the disease occurs very readily with any subsequent streptococcal infection. Patients with rheumatic fever, particularly children, continue on prophylactic doses of oral penicillin or on a monthly intramuscular injection of a large dose which is slowly absorbed. Anti-inflammatory drugs may be used to decrease inflammation.

Nursing management of patients with rheumatic fever may focus on:

- Knowledge deficit related to prophylactic antibiotic use
- Activity intolerance related to fatigue
- Ineffective coping related to managing of disease process.

INFECTIVE ENDOCARDITIS

Infective endocarditis is inflammation of the endocardium, primarily the heart valves. Factors predisposing to infective endocarditis include parenteral drug use, valvular abnormalities either congenital or acquired in origin, rheumatic fever, minor infections, dental procedures and cardiac surgery. Infective endocarditis may be classified into acute or subacute forms, based on the causative organism and the rapidity of disease onset. Acute infective endocarditis is caused by organisms of higher virulence including *Staphylococcus aureus*, *Streptococcus pneumoniae* and *Neisseria meningitidis*. This form of the disease has a rapid onset and progression, usually affecting normal heart valves. The subacute form is most commonly caused by *Streptococ-*

cus viridans and *Staphylococcus epidermidis*. The onset of symptoms may be insidious and more commonly affects previously damaged heart valves.

In infective endocarditis, the organisms, transient in the blood, implant on areas of the endocardium, and clusters of vegetative structures form consisting of inflammatory exudate, fibrin, platelets and bacteria. As the infection subsides, the affected areas become scarred; if a valve was involved, incompetence is likely to develop, and the patient then has the same problems as mentioned in relation to the patient with rheumatic fever.

Symptoms may include signs of infection such as fever, malaise, chills, joint tenderness and petechiae. Valvular destruction usually produces a cardiac murmur, heard on auscultation, and signs of embolism, caused when fragments of vegetative lesions break away and lodge downstream in an artery. Diagnosis is confirmed by blood cultures which identify the causitive organism. Echocardiography may be useful in visualizing vegetations on heart valves.

Treatment of infective endocarditis includes eradicating the infecting organism by long-term antimicrobial therapy. Surgical repair of damaged valves may be required.

Nursing management of the patient with infective endocarditis may focus on the following problems:

- Knowledge deficit related to the disease process, need for antibiotic prophylaxis and treatment
- Activity intolerance related to fatigue
- Anxiety related to the disease process and length of the recovery period.

PERICARDITIS

Pericarditis is an inflammation of the pericardium and is most commonly caused by bacterial and viral infections, cardiac injury or an autoimmune reaction. Fluid accumulates in the pericardium as part of the inflammatory response, causing a pericardial effusion. The pressure exerted on the heart by this fluid may prevent its normal filling, creating a condition referred to as cardiac tamponade. In some instances, extensive scarring of the visceral pericardium may prevent normal stretching and filling of the heart chambers.

Symptoms of pericarditis may include chest pain, which is exacerbated by movement and dyspnoea. A pericardial friction rub may be heard on auscultation. A paradoxical pulse may be present if cardiac tamponade has occurred. Electrocardiographic changes characteristic of pericarditis include elevation of ST segments, followed several days later by T wave inversions. Chest X-rays and echocardiography may be used to identify a pericardial effusion.

Treatment goals for the patient with pericarditis include relieving pain, controlling the underlying cause and preventing complications.

Medical treatment includes non-steroidal anti-inflammatory agents, such as salicylates and indomethacin, and occasionally corticosteroids to combat inflammation.

Antibiotics will be prescribed for bacterial pericarditis. The patient must be observed carefully for complications such as cardiac tamponade.

Nursing management of the patient with pericarditis may focus on the following problems:

- Chest pain related to pericardial inflammation
- Anxiety related to illness
- Knowledge deficit related to the disease process and management.

THE PERSON WITH DISORDERS OF MYOCARDIAL BLOOD SUPPLY

Coronary Atherosclerosis

A narrowing or obstruction in the coronary arteries reduces the blood supply to the myocardium, and causes what is called ischaemic heart disease. It results in a deficiency of oxygen and nutrients to the muscle. The reduced oxygen supply is most significant and is quickly reflected in reduced myocardial efficiency. The heart muscle can withstand only a very small oxygen debt, as it is much more susceptible to a reduced oxygen supply than skeletal muscle. In most instances the decreased blood supply to the myocardium is due to degenerative changes in the arteries that produce a narrowing of the lumen of the vessels. Fatty substances, which include cholesterol, are deposited within the intima of the arteries to cause *atherosclerosis*. These fatty plaques interfere with the nutrition of the cells in the intima, leading to necrosis, scarring and calcification, which leave the surface rough and the lumen reduced. These roughened constricted areas allow less blood through and predispose to thrombus formation and occlusion of the vessel.

Atherosclerosis usually develops gradually. While the blood supply through the artery is being reduced, a collateral circulation develops in an effort to increase the supply to the myocardium, but this supplementary circulation is rarely sufficient to provide enough oxygen to the heart muscle during strenuous physical exertion.

Angina Pectoris

The term angina pectoris describes a clinical syndrome characterized by chest pain. 'Pectoris' indicates the general location (chest) and 'angina' refers to the choking, suffocating nature of the pain. This condition arises because of a discrepancy between the oxygen being supplied to the myocardium and the energy being expended. The pain, arising from heart muscle fibres which are deficient in oxygen, is usually precipitated by physical exertion or emotional stress which increases the work-load of the heart. There is a need for a greater

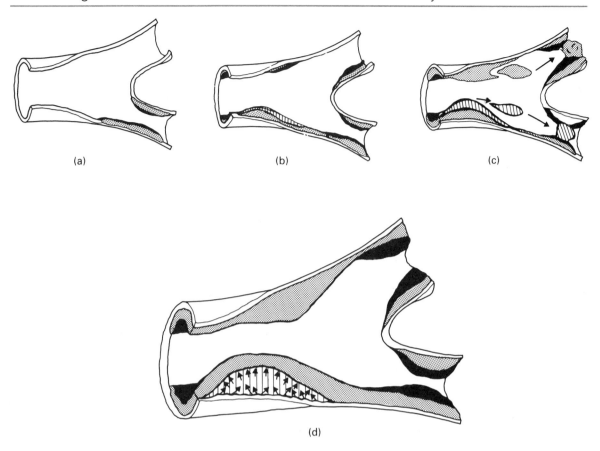

Figure 14.11 Coronary artery obstruction by (a) plaque formation, (b) clot formation around plaque, (c) thrombi on top of fixed plaque formation, and (d) vessel haemorrhage.

blood supply than is being delivered by the coronary circulation.

The patient suddenly develops chest discomfort retrosternally, which may radiate to the left or both shoulders and arms and occasionally up the neck to the jaws. The pain may, however, be atypical and arise only in the arms, jaw or neck and not in the chest. It is usually relieved within a few minutes by resting and/or by glyceryl trinitrate (GTN) but may last as long as 30 minutes. The patient may become short of breath.

Angina may remain a stable condition brought about by predictable precipitating factors with no change in the severity or frequency of the attacks. Stable angina is usually associated with fixed obstructive coronary artery disease (Figure 14.11a). It is then controlled by limiting those activities or situations known to cause pain, and by medication. However, the pain may progress in frequency and intensity if the atherosclerosis process in the coronary arteries proceeds more rapidly than the development of collateral circulation. This condition is known as unstable angina pectoris. Activities may then need to be curtailed greatly and the patient may even experience pain at rest.

Unstable angina is distinguished from stable angina by four characteristics:

1. The syndrome has developed within the previous month.
2. A pattern of stable exertion-related angina pain becomes less predictable, more prolonged, frequent or severe.
3. The syndrome occurs at rest.
4. The pain is not relieved as promptly with glyceryl trinitrate as it is with stable angina.

Unstable angina frequently precedes myocardial infarction and may be referred to as preinfarction syndrome or crescendo angina. The pathology of unstable angina involves varying amounts of fixed obstructive coronary disease and dynamic obstruction caused by platelet activation and thrombosis (Figure 14.11c).

Prinzmetal angina refers to a type of unstable angina in which the pain occurs at rest and at the same time each day. It is not precipitated by exertion. The underlying cause is spasm of the coronary arteries and obstructive coronary artery disease may or may not be present.

Diagnosis of angina pectoris is made using a thorough history, resting electrocardiogram, exercise stress test and/or radionuclide imaging. The most reliable diagnostic procedure to evaluate angina pectoris is cardiac angiography.

MEDICAL MANAGEMENT

Management of angina pectoris is focused on balancing myocardial oxygen supply and demand to ensure the supply is greater than or equal to the demand. Interventions focus on immediate care, reducing or eliminating risk factors, activity management, medications, percutaneous transluminal coronary angioplasty (PTCA) and intra-aortic balloon pump.

Immediate care
At the onset of an anginal episode, the patient stops whatever activity he or she may be engaged in and the prescribed medication is administered [e.g. glyceryl trinitrate (GTN)]. If the person is in hospital, the pulse, respirations and blood pressure are checked during the episode. The doctor may want a 12-lead ECG taken while the patient is experiencing pain.

Risk-factor modification
Altering life-style to reduce the progression of coronary artery disease is discussed in detail on p. 298.

Activity management
The patient is advised that strenuous physical activity and emotional outbursts should be avoided. Moderate exercise below the point of producing pain is encouraged. Walking is excellent exercise and should be done on a regular basis. The individual should begin with short walks on level ground, gradually increasing the distance over a period of weeks. Regular, medically supervised exercise programmes are recommended for some patients. Regular exercise improves muscle tone and general well-being and stimulates the development of collateral circulation in the myocardium. Normal weight is more easily maintained. The psychological benefit of exercise to the patient cannot be overestimated.

Medications
One of the cornerstones of management of angina is pharmacological therapy. The medications commonly used are presented in Table 14.7.

Percutaneous transluminal coronary angioplasty (PTCA)
PTCA provides an alternative for some patients who might otherwise require coronary artery bypass surgery. PTCA is a non-surgical method of dilating stenotic or occlusive lesions in the coronary arterial system. Thomas (1991) recommends that patients should be prepared as for cardiac catheterization. However, as 1% of patients may require subsequent surgery due to complications such as tamponade, PTCA is only carried out on sites with a cardiothoracic surgical capability.

Criteria for selection of patients include: (1) recent onset of angina pectoris; (2) angina refractory to medical treatment; (3) angina symptoms of sufficient severity to compromise the quality of life of the patient; (4) single vessel disease with the lesion situated high in the vessel so that it is easily accessible to the catheter; and (5) the patient is an acceptable candidate for bypass surgery.

Table 14.7 Drugs used in the management of angina.

Medication	General action with angina
Nitrates	
Short acting e.g. Glyceryl trinitrate	• Vasodilate vascular smooth muscle • Decrease preload, decrease afterload • Vasodilate coronary arteries
Long-acting e.g. Isosorbide dinitrate GTN ointment	• As above
β-Blockers	
e.g. Propranolol Atenolol	• Decrease heart rate, automaticity • Decrease force of contraction • Decrease myocardial oxygen consumption
Calcium channel blockers	
e.g. Nifedipine Diltiazem	• Dilate coronary and peripheral vessels
Antiplatelet agents	
e.g. Aspirin	• Decrease platelet aggregation • Decrease thrombosis formation

Diagnostic testing prior to this procedure is similar to that for coronary bypass surgery and includes coronary angiography. Nursing care includes giving both physical and emotional support to the patient, as the procedure is often frightening. Educational responsibilities include an explanation of ischaemic heart disease, if this has not been given, and of all the tests carried out prior to the procedure. The doctor will explain the procedure, the risks involved, the possible need for bypass surgery and the expected results of this treatment. The nurse reinforces and gives further information as required.

PTCA is performed using local anaesthesia in the cardiac catheterization laboratory. A guide catheter is introduced into the right or left femoral or brachial artery. This catheter is advanced under fluoroscopy to the affected coronary artery. Once through the stenotic narrowing in the coronary artery, a dilating catheter is slipped through the guide catheter. When positioned within the atherosclerotic lesion, the dilating balloon is inflated. The resultant stretching of the coronary arterial muscle wall widens the lumen of the artery, allowing blood to flow more freely. In addition, research is being conducted into the application of laser energy in this treatment of atheromatous disease.

Possible complications include bleeding or thrombosis of the affected artery due to injury of the vascular endothelium, coronary artery spasm and rupture of the artery, causing cardiac tamponade. These complications may result in acute myocardial infarction.

Medications such as nifedipine and β-blockers may be given either prior to or during the procedure to prevent coronary artery spasm. Intravenous glyceryl trinitrate may be administered to promote vasodilatation. Generally patients receive an anticoagulant such as heparin, which may be followed by treatment with warfarin or antiplatelet drugs.

Following the procedure, ECG monitoring is maintained continuously and the patient is observed closely for signs or symptoms indicating bleeding, myocardial ischaemia, impaired left ventricular function or electrolyte imbalance.

Bed rest is maintained for 24 hours and the patient is gradually mobilized and usually discharged within 2–4 days. Prior to discharge, instruction is given on risk factor modification, medication and activity regimens, and medical follow-up.

Intra-aortic balloon pump

Occasionally counterpulsation with the intra-aortic balloon pump is utilized for the patient with unstable angina prior to coronary artery surgery. The intra-aortic balloon is inserted into the aorta from one of the femoral arteries; it is inflated during diastole and is deflated as the heart ejects its contents during systole. In this way it reduces afterload and myocardial oxygen demand, decreases myocardial ischaemia and relieves angina. The intra-aortic balloon pump is an invasive method of treatment; consequently, the patient and his family require a great deal of support from nursing and medical staff. Further discussion of this intervention is beyond the scope of this text.

NURSING MANAGEMENT

The nursing management of a patient with angina focuses on the following health problems.

- Knowledge deficit
- Activity intolerance
- Potential for chest discomfort
- Anxiety.

These problems are discussed in detail on p. 312. A clinical scenario will be used to illustrate care of a person with angina.

Clinical situation: Mrs Carter, a woman with angina

Mrs Carter was a 70-year-old woman diagnosed with stable angina 6 months ago. She had been referred to the community nurse to be monitored for her ability to manage her angina. Mrs Carter lived with her daughter and son-in-law in a bungalow. When visited in her home, Mrs Carter expressed anxiety related to her inability to cope with chest pain when it occurred. She was concerned that she would not do the 'right things'.

Mrs Carter's primary health problem was identified as *knowledge deficit* related to her disease process and management. The *goals* of care for Mrs Carter were that she could:

- Recognize symptoms of myocardial ischaemia.
- Undertake appropriate interventions to reduce and

eliminate myocardial ischaemia if it occurred.
- Engage in activities to prevent myocardial ischaemia.

Intervention

- Mrs Carter was asked to describe the signs and symptoms of myocardial ischaemia which she had experienced. Descriptors which described myocardial ischaemia were reinforced and other possible symptoms were discussed.
- The patient was questioned as to her understanding of the cause of her angina. The concept of myocardial ischaemia was clarified. The heart's need for enough oxygen to meet its demands was emphasized and the impact of ischaemic heart disease was discussed. This was done using straightforward language, reinforced with diagrams.
- Mrs Carter was prompted to discuss what she did when she experienced chest pain. The use of rest and correct administration of glyceryl trinitrate were reinforced. She was encouraged to tell whomever she was with that she was experiencing chest discomfort so they could assist her as needed. If the chest pain was not relieved by rest and glyceryl trinitrate in the prescribed time, Mrs Carter was advised to ask to be taken to the nearest hospital where she could be assessed by health care professionals.
- Preventive strategies to avoid angina were also discussed. Mrs Carter indicated that she did not get overtired. The need to alternate activity and rest were reinforced. Use of glyceryl trinitrate prophylactically when Mrs Carter engaged in activities which caused angina was encouraged.
- An educational booklet which described the contents discussed was given to Mrs Carter to read at leisure. This provided her with a reference so she could review any concerns.

Evaluation

At the end of the visit, Mrs Carter could describe signs and symptoms of myocardial ischaemia, actions she would take if she developed chest pain and how she planned to pace herself. On a follow-up visit, 2 weeks later, Mrs Carter described how she had managed an episode of chest discomfort, which was appropriate. She also had paced her activities, incorporating more quiet periods into her life. Mrs Carter expressed feelings of increased confidence in her ability to manage further episodes.

Acute Myocardial Infarction

Acute myocardial infarction (MI) (also known as coronary occlusion or thrombosis) is the most serious and acute form of ischaemic heart disease. A coronary artery becomes blocked and the myocardial area which it supplies suffers oxygen deficiency and cell necrosis. This occurs suddenly, and compensation through collateral channels is inadequate to maintain the myocardial cells. The resulting area of necrotic tissue is referred to as an infarction.

The extent of the infarction varies from patches of 1 or 2 cm in diameter to widespread areas of necrosis. One or more layers of the heart may be involved. The area of infarction becomes soft and then eventually fills in with firm, fibrous scar tissue. Survival and the extent of subsequent restrictions depend upon the amount of myocardial damage and the area of the heart affected. Death may occur immediately or within a few hours. Obviously, the remaining viable heart tissue must compensate for the loss of functional tissue.

Occlusion may be preceded by some manifestations of coronary insufficiency such as angina, or it may occur suddenly without any previous warning.

TYPES OF MYOCARDIAL INFARCTION

It is difficult to delineate the precise area of the myocardium which is affected, but general areas can be identified from the 12-lead ECG. This is important to know because damage to each area can produce different complications. Although other areas of the heart may be involved, most infarctions occur in the left ventricle.

Anterior wall infarction. The anterior wall of the left ventricle is infarcted due to an occlusion of the left anterior descending artery. The papillary muscles of the left ventricle and the intraventricular septum may also be involved. In the latter instances, the infarction would be referred to as anteroseptal.

Lateral wall infarction. An infarction in the lateral wall of the left ventricle is associated with an occlusion of the lateral branch of the left circumflex artery. Occasionally both the anterior descending and the left circumflex branches are obstructed, and the infarction is designated anterolateral.

Inferior wall infarction. This term implies an infarction of the part of the left ventricle which rests on the diaphragm. It is usually due to occlusion of the right coronary artery.

Posterior wall infarction. This type is usually due to occlusion of the posterior branch of either the right coronary or left circumflex artery. It is sometimes called a true posterior infarction to distinguish it from an inferior infarction.

Right ventricular infarction. The right ventricle may infarct in conjunction with an inferior or posterior left ventricular infarction. It is usually caused by occlusion of the artery that perfuses the posterior ventricular wall, either the right coronary artery or less commonly, the left circumflex artery.

SYMPTOMS

- *Pain.* The most common presenting complaint of patients with myocardial infarction is severe chest pain. The pain may last for several hours or until relieved by analgesics. It should not persist for days; prolonged pain may be an indication of pericarditis or an extending infarction.
- *Dyspnoea.* Dyspnoea may be due to pulmonary congestion or pain. It may also occur as activity is increased. Relief of pain and congestion may relieve the dyspnoea. It is important to note whether shortness of breath is present at all times or, if intermittent, how it is precipitated and what measures relieve it.
- *Skin.* The skin may be cool, moist and a greyish colour in response to the decreased cardiac output.
- *Nausea and vomiting.* Nausea and vomiting may be experienced at the time of the attack, lasting from several hours to 2 or 3 days. Occasionally, nausea and vomiting occur in response to the opiates being administered.
- *Weakness and tiredness.* Extreme weakness may be experienced and may persist for many days. Many patients complain of tiredness for weeks after their infarction. The exact cause of this is not clearly defined. Some suggest it results from decreased oxygen perfusion of the tissues due to a lowered cardiac output. It has also been attributed to weakened skeletal muscles as a result of even a brief period of immobilization. The patient may have been in a state of physical exhaustion prior to the attack or may be emotionally exhausted from the experience.
- *Heart rate.* The pulse becomes rapid and weak and may be imperceptible at the time of the attack. Initially, a few patients may exhibit bradycardia, followed by tachycardia.
- *Blood pressure.* Due to the decreased pumping efficiency of the heart, the blood pressure falls but may be elevated in the first few hours following an attack due to an augmented sympathetic response.
- *Temperature.* Myocardial necrosis causes an elevation of body temperature ranging from 37.7 to 39 °C. The temperature usually rises within 24–48 hours and returns to normal by the sixth or seventh day. If the increased temperature persists for longer, it may be due to complications.
- *Psychological reactions.* A heart attack carries the threat of death or invalidism for the patient. The sudden change in well-being leaves feelings of vulnerability and helplessness. The patient is required to make very rapid adjustments to both the illness and change in environment.

Anxiety is the most common psychological response. It is manifested by various overt and covert behaviours, such as tenseness, restlessness, short attention span, inability to concentrate, crying, constant talking and expression of feelings of anxiety. The patient may appear generally relaxed but may exhibit more subtle manifestations of anxiety such as darting eye movements. Patients may also show denial, refusing to acknowledge the seriousness or even the presence of symptoms and may be angry and/or depressed. These emotional responses may appear in varying degrees and at any time during hospitalization or may not become evident until after discharge from the hospital. The individual's interpretation of the experience and personal coping pattern influence responses. Continuing restlessness and apprehension are noted and reported.

DIAGNOSIS

Medical diagnosis of an acute myocardial infarction is made using the clinical history, changes in the 12-lead ECG and serum enzymes.

Changes in the electrocardiogram

Theoretically, three types of changes are present in the myocardium when an infarction develops. These define three areas, referred to clinically as the area of infarction, the area of injury and the zone of ischaemia, resulting in a distinctive electrocardiographic pattern. In the infarcted area, irreversible structural changes occur with resulting necrosis of the tissue. Since electrical impulses cannot be conducted through this tissue, electrical energy is lost, causing a relative gain of electrical activity directed away from the necrotic area. These developments produce a negative deflection (Q wave) in electrodes facing the infarcted area, indicating that electrical activity is not being directed toward it but away from it. An increased positive deflection (R wave) will be seen in leads facing the opposite surface of the heart, indicating electrical activity moving toward the leads and away from the infarcted area.

Surrounding the zone of infarction is an area of injury which suffers a decreased blood supply, but the damage is not permanent. Although specific abnormal electrocardiographic changes are produced, these may revert to normal if the blood supply is restored. Electrodes placed over the injured area will record an ST segment elevation.

The zone of ischaemia surrounds the area of injury and may also return to normal once the blood supply is restored. Inverted T waves indicate ischaemia.

ST elevations appear within several hours following an infarction and disappear in a few days. In the early stages T waves become taller and appear as an extension of the elevated ST segment. They later become inverted. Q waves appear within 1–2 days and persist (Figure 14.12). The area of infarction will be reflected in leads which view that portion of the heart. Thus, inferior infarctions can be identified in leads II, III and AVF, anterior infarctions can be identified in the anterior leads V_1 to V_4 and lateral wall infarction in leads I, AVL, V_5 and V_6. Since under normal conditions no leads face the posterior wall of the heart, diagnosis is based upon reciprocal changes in leads facing the opposite wall; that is, increased R waves in leads V_1 and V_2.

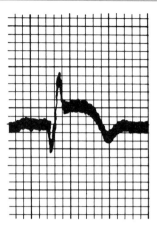

Figure 14.12 Electrocardiographic changes indicating acute myocardial infarction: Q wave, ST elevation, and T wave inversion.

Changes in serum enzyme levels

Certain intracellular enzymes known to be persistent in myocardial cells are released into the blood when the cells are damaged or destroyed. Serial determinations of the serum concentrations of these enzymes can provide information concerning the presence and degree of cardiac damage. The normal values of serum enzymes vary depending on laboratory techniques and sampling methods.

In the coronary care unit, the most commonly ordered enzyme level estimations are creatine phosphokinase (CPK), aspartate aminotransferase (AST) and lactic dehydrogenase (LDH) (see Table 14.8). Diagnosis of a myocardial infarction can be confirmed by elevations of these enzyme levels.

Creatine phosphokinase (CPK). CPK is present in cardiac and skeletal muscle and brain tissue. CPK levels begin to rise in the serum 4–8 hours post myocardial infarction, peak in 12–24 hours and return to normal in 3–4 days.

A rise in CPK levels can also be caused by pericarditis, severe congestive heart failure, electrical cardioversion and intramuscular injections. Thus, in order to determine the source of elevated CPK, electrophoresis or radioimmunoassay can be used to separate CPK into three fractions or isoenzymes. The MB isoenzyme has been found predominantly in the myocardium. Studies have shown that CK-MB (or MBCPK) is very sensitive and specific for the diagnosis of acute myocardial infarction, provided that it is determined between 6 and 36 hours after the suspected myocardial infarction.

Thus, in assessing the presence of an acute myocardial infarction with CPK levels, it is important to ensure that blood samples are drawn on admission and every 8 hours for the 24 hours after the onset of chest pain.

Aspartate aminotransferase (AST). The concentration of AST rises within 8–12 hours after a myocardial infarction, reaching a peak in 18–36 hours and usually returning to normal within 3–4 days. Elevated AST levels are also seen in patients with hepatic and skeletal

Table 14.8 The elevation of serum enzyme levels in one patient following a myocardial infarction (units/litre).

Enzyme	Day of admission	Day 2	Day 3	Day 7
CPK	6	162	5	5
AST	14	177	201	23
LDH	151	513	789	419

muscle disease, pulmonary embolism and pericarditis. This is a problem for diagnosis of a myocardial infarction because there are no cardiac specific isoenzymes of AST. Thus, the routine use of AST in diagnosis of acute myocardial infarction is debatable.

Lactic dehydrogenase (LDH). LDH is present in most body organs including the heart, kidneys, lungs, liver and skeletal muscle. After an acute myocardial infarction, the LDH level becomes elevated in 8–24 hours, peaks in 3–6 days and returns to normal in 8–14 days.

A rise in total LDH may also be present in patients with pulmonary embolism, neoplastic disorders, hepatic disease and shock. Thus, it is important to assess LDH isoenzyme levels to assess if cardiac damage is causing enzyme elevation. LDH has five isoenzymes and cardiac muscle contains primarily LDH_1. A rise in the percentage of LDH_1 exceeding 40% of the total LDH value and an increase in the ratio of LDH_1 to LDH_2 is considered a sensitive indicator of myocardial infarction. Thus, when a patient has a suspected myocardial infarction that occurred more than 2 days previously, LDH isoenzyme analysis can be more revealing than CPK analysis.

Other diagnostic procedures which may be used to assess the extent of myocardial infarction include echocardiography, radionuclide imaging and thallium stress electrocardiography.

MEDICAL MANAGEMENT

Management of an acute myocardial infarction focuses on the areas of control of symptoms, acute myocardial reperfusion and recognition and management of complications.

Control of symptoms

- *Relief of chest discomfort.* Management of chest discomfort is discussed on p. 315. See Table 14.7 for medications used to control and/or prevent angina.
- *Prevention of arrhythmias.* Prophylactic treatment of ventricular arrhythmias in the acute phase of myocardial infarction is used in some institutions. Lignocaine administered as a continuous intravenous infusion is the drug of choice. This may be used after thrombolytic therapy to prevent reperfusion ventricular arrhythmias.

Acute myocardial reperfusion

- *Thrombolytic therapy.* Evidence that coronary thrombosis is a very early event in acute myocardial infarction, recognition of the prognostic importance of infarction size, and evidence that infarction size might be reduced by early intervention have resulted in thrombolytic therapy becoming the most significant recent development in the management of the patient with acute myocardial infarction. Several agents which lyse clots are currently being used in patients who have sustained an acute MI; these agents include streptokinase and tissue plasminogen ac-

tivator (tPA). Research to evaluate the impact of these agents on morbidity and mortality, as well as to establish the most effective management protocols, is ongoing.

Therapy needs to be initiated as soon as possible after the onset of myocardial infarction to give maximum benefit. Thus, enabling patients experiencing chest pain to attend units which can promptly administer these agents has become increasingly important.

Nurses need to be aware of the possible complications of bleeding, arrhythmias, allergic reaction, drop in blood pressure, as well as anxiety and lack of knowledge, that might accompany the administration of thrombolytics.

- *Anticoagulants.* Heparin therapy is routinely used by some cardiologists when there is evidence on echocardiograms of left ventricular thrombus, active deep vein thrombosis or anterior wall myocardial infarction. It may also be used prophylactically for a patient with an inferior wall MI experiencing atrial arrhythmias, and also those having congestive heart failure and left ventricular wall motion abnormalities. Heparin may also be administered after thrombolytic therapy. Low dose heparin may be used for patients with high risk of venous thromboembolism.
- *Antiplatelet drugs.* Multiple clinical trials are being undertaken to evaluate the role of aspirin in the management of acute myocardial infarction. Daily dosing with aspirin significantly reduces the risk of reinfarction and death.
- *Percutaneous transluminal coronary angioplasty (PTCA)* and *coronary artery bypass surgery (CABG).* These procedures may be indicated for the acutely unstable individual who requires aggressive therapy to prevent mortality after coronary angiography is conducted. Discussion of PTCA can be found on p. 325.

Recognition of complications

Doctors and nurses share the responsibility of assessing and recognizing complications of an acute myocardial infarction. It is important for the nurse to have a sound understanding of the possible complications so that rapid identification and initiation of treatment, as required, is conducted. Complications following myocardial infarction include arrhythmias, congestive heart failure, pericarditis, mitral regurgitation, myocardial rupture, aneurysm and systemic or pulmonary emboli.

- *Arrhythmias.* Arrhythmias usually occur early following a myocardial infarction (see p. 332 for a discussion of arrhythmias). The most serious arrhythmia that may be seen is ventricular fibrillation: this is treated by cardiac defibrillation. Bradyarrhythmias, such as sinus bradycardia, first-degree atrioventricular block and Wenckebach heart block are most often associated with inferior wall infarctions. Since the SA node and the AV junctional tissue are most often supplied by the right coronary artery, occlusion of this vessel will lead to their decreased functioning. Anterior myocardial infarctions are more prone to heart failure and arrhythmias that accompany it, such as sinus tachycardia and rapid atrial arrhythmias, and to intraventricular conduction disturbances, such as Mobitz type II block. Complete AV block (third-degree or complete heart block) can follow either inferior or anterior wall infarction.

- *Heart failure.* Mild congestive heart failure occurs in many patients due to the decreased efficiency with which the heart contracts. Gross left ventricular failure is more common following an anterior infarction. Heart failure is diagnosed by the presence of crackles on chest auscultation, complaints of shortness of breath and a chest X-ray.

- *Pericarditis.* Pericarditis following a myocardial infarction is thought to be due to an autoimmune reaction in which antigens originate from the injured myocardial tissue, initiating inflammation of the pericardium. It may occur as early as 24 hours after the infarction. The pain which accompanies pericarditis is similar to that of a myocardial infarction but is sometimes more excruciating. It is alarming to the patient, who may think that he or she is having another heart attack. A distinction may be made if the pain is increased by deep breathing or twisting the trunk, or if it is relieved by leaning forward, lying on the right side or sitting in an upright position with the trunk straight. A friction rub may be heard on auscultation but is not always present in the early stages. The patient's temperature may remain elevated for more than 1 week. Treatment is usually with non-steroidal anti-inflammatory drugs such as indomethacin or soluble aspirin. A cortico-steroid preparation may be used.

- *Mitral regurgitation.* This complication may occur when a papillary muscle dysfunctions or ruptures, causing the valve to become incompetent. This is a grave complication which may be corrected by surgery. Less severe mitral insufficiency may be due to infarction of the papillary muscle.

- *Myocardial rupture.* Myocardial rupture, when present, usually occurs within 7 days. It is more often seen in patients with transmural infarctions. Rupture of the interventricular septum usually occurs within the first 2 weeks and is a very grave prognostic sign. Instead of flowing normally from the left ventricle into the aorta, blood is re-routed to the right ventricle, increasing the demands on it and flooding the lungs.

- *Aneurysm.* An aneurysm is a ballooning out of the infarcted myocardial tissue, causing the heart to contract in a disruptive fashion. If large, it seriously impedes the maintenance of normal cardiac output. The extent of the aneurysm may be determined by a myocardial scan and in some instances may be corrected by surgery.

- *Emboli.* Emboli occur because clots formed in the healing area of the myocardium break loose and escape into the circulation. Pulmonary emboli may arise in the leg veins due to circulatory stasis, and may be prevented by exercising the limbs. The treatment for emboli includes anticoagulant drugs.

NURSING MANAGEMENT

The nursing management of a patient who has sustained a myocardial infarction in the acute phase will be illustrated using a clinical example.

Clinical situation: Mr MacGregor with myocardial infarction

Mr MacGregor was a 57-year-old man, married with two grown-up children. He was admitted to hospital via ambulance with the diagnosis of acute anterior wall myocardial infarction. On the day of admission, he was shovelling snow when he developed 'crushing' chest discomfort which radiated down his left arm. He felt nauseated and sweaty and was short of breath. He sat down on the steps and called his wife. She telephoned the ambulance service and Mr MacGregor arrived at the hospital approximately 1 hour after his chest pain started.

Mr MacGregor's past medical history included no cardiovascular disorders or bleeding problems. He had sustained several injuries to his left knee which had required surgical correction. Mr MacGregor had several risk factors for ischaemic heart disease, including his age, sex and habit of smoking a pack of cigarettes a day for 40 years. He did not know his cholesterol levels and did not have hypertension. Mr MacGregor considered his position as an executive to be stressful. His father had died of a heart attack in his seventies.

Care in the coronary care unit
Mr MacGregor's initial assessment indicated that he was medically stable. His vital signs were stable and he was in normal sinus rhythm. Interventions included:

- Oxygen via nasal cannulae at 4 litres per minute was commenced.
- Intravenous line was set up.
- 12-lead electrocardiogram showing changes consistent with an anterior wall myocardial infarction was recorded.
- Cardiac enzymes were obtained.
- Glyceryl trinitrate was given sublingually three times without relief of chest discomfort. Diamorphine hydrochloride 2.5 mg i.v. was given with good relief of chest pain.
- Thrombolytic therapy was commenced to reduce the size of the myocardial infarction as there were no contraindications. Streptokinase was administered via intravenous infusion.
- The doctor and nurse met with Mrs MacGregor to discuss her husband's condition and to provide reassurance.

Mr MacGregor was somewhat restless and fully conscious. He indicated that he had no discomfort in his chest and that he was worried about his wife. Mr MacGregor knew that he had had a heart attack. His respiratory rate was 14 breaths per minute and he remained on 4 litres per minute oxygen via nasal cannulae. His blood pressure was equal in both arms and was 120/60 mmHg. The cardiac monitor showed Mr MacGregor remained in normal sinus rhythm, 72 beats per minute with ventricular ectopic beats (VEB) approximately 5–10 per minute.

The doctor was notified that Mr MacGregor was having the VEBs and lignocaine was commenced via intravenous line. The streptokinase infusion was complete and a heparin infusion was started.

Three priority health problems were identified in the provision of nursing care for Mr MacGregor:

1. Potential decrease in cardiac output
2. Anxiety
3. Potential for haemorrhage.

Potential decrease in cardiac output

This was related to damaged myocardium, as evidenced by 12-lead electrocardiogram changes, presence of ventricular arrhythmias, clinical history and cardiac enzymes.

The *goals* in caring for Mr MacGregor were that:

1. The patient would reduce workload on his heart.
2. No further ventricular arrhythmias causing haemodynamic instability would be experienced.
3. Mr MacGregor would report any episodes of myocardial ischaemia.

Intervention

- Mr MacGregor's vital signs were monitored every 4 hours for any changes in blood pressure. His heart rate and rhythm were monitored continuously for any changes. Close attention was paid to ventricular arrhythmias as the patient had had VEBs. Initial damaged ventricular muscle predisposed him to lethal ventricular arrhythmias. Lignocaine was administered to treat his VEBs.
- Mr MacGregor was encouraged to report any episodes of chest discomfort to ensure rapid treatment. Glyceryl trinitrate was placed at his bedside to facilitate rapid treatment, if needed.
- The patient was placed on bed rest to limit cardiac workload. His activity level was gradually increased over several days to allow the heart time to recover and to facilitate assessment of his activity tolerance.
- The importance of avoiding straining and of performing isometric exercises was stressed. A laxative was given, as necessary, to avoid constipation.
- A quiet environment was provided to facilitate rest. Mr MacGregor was encouraged to rest for an hour after each meal to reduce myocardial workload.
- Supplemental oxygen via nasal cannulae was administered continuously for the first 24 hours and if the patient had chest pain. This ensured additional oxygen was available to improve myocardial oxygen supply if required.

Evaluation. Mr MacGregor experienced no further arrhythmias and the lignocaine was tapered off 24 hours later. He reduced his cardiac workload by resting quietly in bed and performing gentle exercises. The patient reported that he experienced no episodes of chest discomfort.

Anxiety

Anxiety was related to diagnosis and admission to hospital, as evidenced by inability to concentrate, apprehension and difficulty in sleeping.

The *goals* in treating this problem were that:

1. Early signs of anxiety would be detected.
2. Mr MacGregor would participate in activities which would reduce or eliminate his anxiety.

Intervention

- Reassurance and comfort were provided for Mr MacGregor. The nurse stayed with him frequently, speaking calmly and providing competent, efficient care.
- A quiet environment was provided and sensory stimulation was reduced. The door was partly closed and the lights were dimmed during rest periods to facilitate sleep.
- Mr MacGregor was informed of the procedures and treatments he could expect. He was kept up-to-date, with the use of language he could understand. The patient was encouraged to ask questions about his environment and condition. Honest, concise information was provided to clarify his understanding of heart disease. As Mr MacGregor liked to read, he was given a pamphlet to reinforce information provided. He was informed that many patients find it difficult to concentrate while in hospital, so he should not be alarmed by his poor concentration span.
- Visitors were limited to immediate family. Mrs MacGregor was encouraged to visit her husband and was kept informed of his condition. She was encouraged to attend the cardiac family support group to meet other spouses and receive support from them.
- Mr MacGregor took a mild sedative in the evening to encourage sleep.

Evaluation. Mr MacGregor indicated that he felt less anxious and more in control of his environment when he was well informed. He eagerly asked questions about his condition and prognosis. The booklet was helpful as he recorded questions he wanted to ask the doctor in it so he would not forget them. Mrs MacGregor enjoyed the family support group and found it helpful.

Potential for haemorrhage

There was a potential for haemorrhage related to thrombolytic agent and concurrent administration of anticoagulant.

The *goals* were that there would be an:

1. Absence of all subjective and objective signs of gastrointestinal, vascular and soft tissue haemorrhage.
2. Early detection of bleeding, within 15 minutes of commencement.

Intervention

- Vascular punctures were kept to a minimum.
- All intravenous and puncture sites were observed frequently for bleeding. Any bruising was outlined

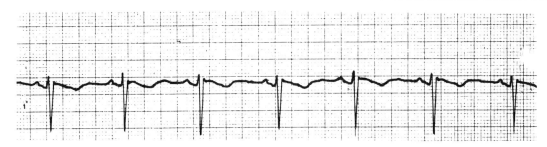

Figure 14.13(a) Sinus rhythm.

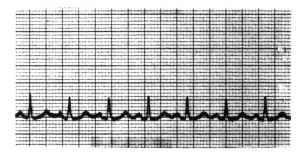

Figure 14.13(b) Sinus tachycardia: rate over 100 per minute; P wave and QRS are normal in 1:1 relationship.

and assessed more frequently for increasing size.
- All bodily excretions were visibly inspected for signs of blood.
- Mr MacGregor was informed of the risk of bleeding and was encouraged to report immediately any signs of bleeding to the nurse.
- Mr MacGregor used his own electric razor and soft toothbrush.

Evaluation. Mr MacGregor showed no signs of haemorrhage during his stay in the coronary care unit.

When Mr MacGregor improved and was transferred from the coronary care unit to the general medical ward, several other health problems became more important. These included activity intolerance, potential for chest discomfort and alteration in life-style and self-care. These health problems are discussed in detail on pp. 312–317.

THE PERSON WITH DISORDERS OF ELECTROCONDUCTION

Normally, the rate and rhythm of the heart contractions are established by impulses generated in the SA node at a rate between 60 and 100 beats per minute (Figure 14.13a). A disorder of rate or rhythm is referred to as a cardiac arrhythmia, and is due to some disturbance in the formation or conduction of impulses. The arrhythmia may be of short duration or persistent, and may be

functional in origin, result from organic heart disease or be associated with an electrolyte imbalance, such as hypokalaemia.

An arrhythmia may have significant haemodynamic consequences. For example, an excessively slow or fast heart rate may decrease the cardiac output and blood pressure, thus compromising the perfusion of vital organs such as the brain, kidneys, liver and heart itself. Arrhythmias may also predispose the patient to thrombus formation. It is important for nurses to have a sound knowledge of arrhythmias and their management in order to plan and provide care for patients with these health problems.

Common irregularities include tachycardia, bradycardia, ectopic beats (extrasystoles), flutter, fibrillation and heart block. The arrhythmia is further defined by the site of its origin; sinus arrhythmia originates in the SA node, atrial originates in an atrium, junctional originates in the AV junctional area, and ventricular originates in a ventricle.

Tachycardias

SINUS TACHYCARDIA

In this rhythm the heart rate is greater than 100 beats per minute, and the impulse originates in the SA node. It is not always an abnormal rhythm, since it occurs during and after exercise and in response to emotional stress. It may be due to an abnormal state, such as fever, anaemia, infection, hyperthyroidism, myocardial infarction and heart failure. It also may result from medications: for example, atropine, adrenaline, isoprenaline hydrochloride and thyroid extract, or other drugs such as alcohol and nicotine (Figure 14.13b).

Tachycardia is significant for two reasons: coronary blood flow occurs predominantly during diastole. With tachycardia, the diastolic time is shortened, reducing the time for perfusion of the myocardium. Also, an increased heart rate increases the need of the myocardium for oxygen. In someone with narrowed coronary arteries, tachycardia may precipitate myocardial ischaemia.

Treatment may be directed at correcting the underlying cause or it may be necessary to reduce the rate by giving a drug such as a digitalis preparation or propranolol.

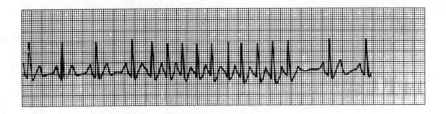

Figure 14.13(c) Paroxysmal atrial tachycardia.

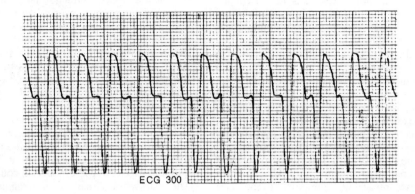

Figure 14.13(d) Ventricular tachycardia.

PAROXYSMAL ATRIAL TACHYCARDIA (PAT)

This is an abrupt onset of a very rapid heart rate, usually 150–250 beats per minute, initiated in the atria. It may last a few seconds or longer. Such attacks cannot be explained in some persons; in others they may be related to organic heart disease (Figure 14.13c).

A rapid heart rate of this type is serious if imposed on a diseased heart. When this arrhythmia occurs, the patient is advised to rest and the doctor is notified. If the patient is subject to recurring attacks, he or she is encouraged to recognize and avoid possible precipitating factors such as fatigue, emotional stress, reaching, or excessive smoking or coffee drinking. In some instances an attack may be relieved by measures that increase parasympathetic (vagal) innervation to the heart. Among those suggested is pressure on the carotid sinus. *Caution must be used in relation to the manoeuvre.* Carotid sinus massage applied injudiciously may result in asystole. This is performed by the doctor. The Valsalva manoeuvre, which involves an inspiration followed by voluntary closure of the glottis and an effort to exhale, may prove helpful. This reduces the venous return from the extremities and head, thus reducing the volume of blood entering the heart, which in turn decreases the cardiac output and the arterial blood pressure. An antiarrhythmic agent such as verapamil, a β-blocker or digoxin may be used. Disopyramide or amiodarone may be useful. Long-acting quinidine preparations are sometimes prescribed.

VENTRICULAR TACHYCARDIA

The term ventricular tachycardia usually refers to a run of rapidly repeated ventricular beats, essentially regular in rhythm, at a rate of 100–210 per minute. Any rate above 60 per minute which is initiated in the ventricles might be considered tachycardia because the ventricles normally do not initiate impulses at more than 25–40 beats per minute. However, rates between 60 and 100 per minute are usually distinguished from the faster rates. They are usually referred to as 'accelerated idioventricular rhythms' but are also called 'slow ventricular tachycardia' (see Figure 14.13d).

Ventricular tachycardia is a serious arrhythmia as there is always the danger it will lead to ventricular fibrillation. It is usually due to ischaemia heart disease and is frequently present following a myocardial infarction (see p. 329).

Treatment includes electrical defibrillation and/or antiarrhythmic drugs such as intravenous lignocaine. Other drugs that may be used include intravenous procainamide or bretylium tosylate.

Bradycardias

SINUS BRADYCARDIA

Sinus bradycardia is discharge of the SA node at a rate less than 60 beats per minute (Figure 14.13e).

Circulation may be adequately maintained by an increased stroke volume in a person with sinus bradycardia. With fewer contractions more blood collects in the heart chambers to produce greater stretching of the myocardial fibres, resulting in a stronger contraction and increased output. Obviously this can only occur if the myocardium is in good condition. If the heart rate is less than 30–40 per minute circulatory insufficiency is likely to occur, especially with physical activity.

The most common causes of sinus bradycardia are a decreased blood supply to the SA node, increased vagal tone, head injury, amyloidosis and obstructive jaundice. Circulatory reflexes may initiate a compensatory increase in the heart rate but, if the cause persists and becomes progressively severe, the heart muscle will gradually become weaker and less responsive, producing fewer contractions. Any disturbance which initiates an increase in vagal nerve impulses to the heart will produce a decrease in the heart rate. An example of this would be bradycardia produced by carotid sinus massage or, in some people, by vomiting. Other examples of conditions in which slowing of the heart rate may be secondary are increased intracranial pressure and myxoedema (a deficiency of thyroid secretion).

The pulse rate may normally be slower in those with well-developed cardiac reserve, such as well-trained athletes. In such people, the venous return is of greater strength, producing an increased stroke volume with each contraction.

Sinus bradycardia does not require treatment unless the individual is symptomatic. Atropine sulphate may be administered to decrease vagal tone. If the arrhythmia is due to medication administration, this should be withheld and re-evaluated.

Ectopic beats

When impulses which influence the heart rate and rhythm are generated elsewhere than in the SA node, the contractions are called *ectopic* or *premature beats* or *extrasystoles*. The ectopic or premature beat occurs when the myocardial fibres are in the relative refractory period following a normal contraction. The impulse from the SA node for the succeeding normal contraction is ineffective, since it arrives when the muscle fibres are in the absolute refractory period following the premature beat, and no contraction takes place. This causes a longer than normal pause before the next normal contraction and the heart 'misses' a beat. The next normal contraction may be stronger because of the prolonged filling period. The time between the normal heart contraction which precedes the extrasystole and the one that follows is equal to two normal cardiac cycles. The subject usually describes the experience as his heart 'missing a beat'.

Extrasystoles, or premature beats, may be due to ischaemic areas or to inflammation in the heart muscle. The fibres may also become irritated and hypersensitive as a result of certain toxic conditions, such as may occur with the excessive use of tobacco, coffee, tea or alcohol. The extrasystoles may occur irregularly, with varying lengths of time between them. The incidence may be so rare as to have no clinical significance but they should be investigated if persistent, even though they occur irregularly and at relatively long intervals. Premature beats may arise regularly and at a rate in excess of that of the normal SA pacemaker, resulting in tachycardia.

ATRIAL ECTOPIC BEATS

The ectopic focus is in the atria and the complex occurs earlier than expected. Atrial ectopic beats are significant because, if they occur during the vulnerable period of the atria, they may precipitate more serious atrial arrhythmias, such as atrial flutter or atrial fibrillation. They may or may not be conducted to the ventricles, depending upon the state of conduction through the AV node and the refractory period at which they occur.

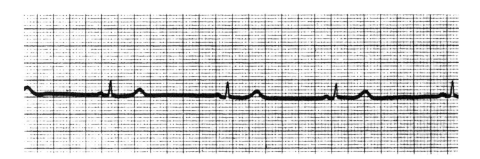

Figure 14.13(e) Sinus bradycardia.

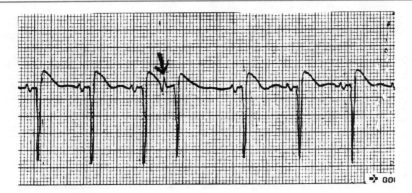

Figure 14.13(f) Atrial ectopic beat.

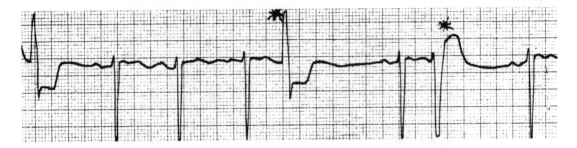

Figure 14.13(g) Ventricular ectopic beat.

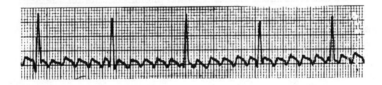

Figure 14.13(h) Atrial flutter.

Treatment is not usually required unless they occur with great frequency or unless progression to more serious arrhythmias is feared, as may occur following a myocardial infarction. If a precipitating cause is recognized, it should be eliminated (Figure 14.13f).

VENTRICULAR ECTOPIC BEATS (VEBs)

The ectopic focus is in the ventricle, and therefore there will be no related P wave on the electrocardiogram. Occasional ventricular ectopic beats may be innocuous but they may also precipitate ventricular tachycardia and/or fibrillation. If they occur in a diseased heart, in groups of three or more, more frequently than five per minute, arise from more than one focus (multifocal) or are on the T wave of the preceding complex, they are considered serious and require treatment. The usual immediate treatment is lignocaine given by bolus intravenous injection followed by a continuous intravenous drip. An oral drug such as disopyramide might be given when the lignocaine infusion is gradually tapered off; however, many patients do not require this (see Figure 14.13g).

Flutter

ATRIAL FLUTTER

As with atrial tachycardia, atrial flutter is due to a rapidly firing ectopic focus in the atria. The atrial rate usually falls between 250 and 350 beats per minute and a characteristic sawtooth pattern is seen on the ECG. AV block is usually present, so that the ventricular response may vary from 150 to 175 beats per minute (Figure 14.13h). Atrial flutter may occur with mitral stenosis, ischaemic heart disease and chronic obstructive airways disease. The usual treatment is cardioversion when the patient is haemodynamically unstable. Digoxin is the drug of choice to slow the ventricular rate by blocking impulses at the AV node. It may convert the flutter to atrial fibrillation which is easier to manage. Quinidine may be used after digoxin to convert the rhythm to normal sinus rhythm. Verapamil may be used to slow the ventricular rate.

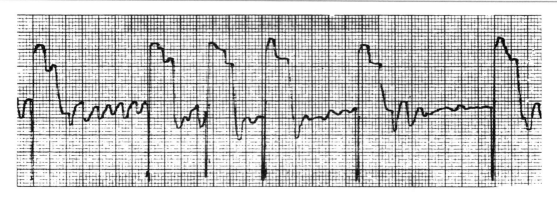

Figure 14.13(i) Atrial fibrillation with varying ventricular responses.

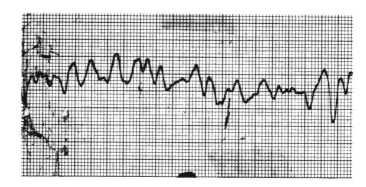

Figure 14.13(j) Ventricular fibrillation: chaotic ventricular activity.

Fibrillation

This is an arrhythmia in which the normal rhythmic contractions of the myocardium of either the atria or ventricles are replaced by extremely rapid (250–500 per minute), ineffective contractions, irregular in force and rhythm. Some area of the heart gives rise to very rapid and irregular impulses, and the myocardial contractile fibres do not achieve the contraction and relaxation that permit normal emptying and filling of the chambers.

ATRIAL FIBRILLATION

Atrial fibrillation is a fairly common arrhythmia in which electrical activity in the atria is totally disorganized. It is due to myocardial disease which may be the result of coronary insufficiency, valvular heart disease, congestive heart failure or acute infection. The atria are never completely empty, and normal filling cannot occur. Since little pressure is created by the atrial contractions, the flow of blood into the ventricles is due mainly to the pressure created by the volume of blood. Circulation may become seriously impaired. Only a proportion of the impulses arising in the atria are conducted through the AV node to the ventricles, but those that do pass through may far exceed the normal in frequency, and are irregular (Figure 14.13i). Normal filling and emptying of the ventricles do not take place, cardiac output is reduced, arterial blood pressure falls and the blood is backed up in the large veins. If the ventricular response is rapid, cardiac output may fall further as a result of decreased ventricular diastolic filling time. The pulse may be weak and irregular.

To control the ventricular response, digoxin, verapamil and β-blockers such as propranolol may be used. To decrease atrial tissue irritability, quinidine is most commonly used. Procainamide and amiodarone may be used in more resistant cases. Cardioversion may be used with the patient who is haemodynamically unstable (see p. 344).

A complication that may follow atrial fibrillation is embolism. The blood that was not forwarded into the ventricles during fibrillation may have formed a thrombus in an atrial chamber and then, when normal heart action is re-established, the thrombus may be moved out into the circulation.

VENTRICULAR FIBRILLATION

In ventricular fibrillation very rapid, asynchronous quivering arises in the ventricular myocardium because

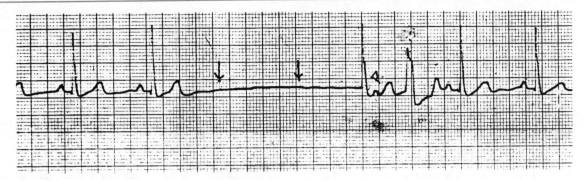

Figure 14.13(k) Sinoatrial block.

the electrical activity occurs in a totally disorganized sequence (Figure 14.13j). The contractions are so ineffective in pumping that the condition very quickly proves fatal. The pulse and blood pressure become unobtainable in a few seconds, the patient quickly loses consciousness, pupils dilate, reflexes are lost and cyanosis is likely to develop. Prompt emergency treatment may re-establish circulation. If the patient is being monitored in a coronary care unit, the arrhythmia may be identified immediately at onset and treatment would consist of immediate defibrillation (see p. 344 for a discussion of this procedure). In many coronary care units nurses who are taught this procedure implement it. *Hospital policy will dictate who may defibrillate a patient, as it constitutes part of the nurse's extended role.* An important guideline is that it must be initiated very quickly. The role of the nurse in a cardiac arrest is discussed on p. 339.

Ventricular fibrillation may occur with irritation of the heart during heart catheterization, because of coronary occlusion by the catheter or when conditions such as myocardial infarction, hypothermia, hypoxia, hypokalaemia and electrical shock exist. Very frequently ventricular fibrillation is preceded by ventricular premature beats. Prompt administration of an antiarrhythmic drug such as lignocaine may prevent serious ventricular tachycardia and fibrillation.

Heart Block

This is a condition in which impulse formation is depressed or impulse conduction is blocked. Although conduction may be interrupted between the SA node and the atria, the term 'heart block' usually refers to a disorder of conduction at the junctional tissues, which are the atrioventricular node and the common bundle (bundle of His). The SA node or the conduction pathway may be damaged by inflammatory disease such as rheumatic fever, coronary insufficiency, pressure from scarred or calcified tissue, or surgical trauma.

SINOATRIAL BLOCK

In sinoatrial block, impulses either are not formed in the SA node, fail to be conducted from it or emerge very

slowly. If sinoatrial impulses are not received by the atria, occasional beats may be dropped, cardiac standstill may occur, or the ventricles may respond to impulses arising from a lower pacemaker, such as the junctional tissue. In the latter instance a junctional rhythm will result (Figure 14.13k).

The seriousness of an SA block depends on the extent to which the heart rate is slowed and cardiac output is decreased. A slow rate may precipitate other arrhythmias. Specific precipitating causes include drugs such as digoxin and some antiarrhythmic drugs, salicylates, ischaemic heart disease, myocardial infarction and increased vagal tone.

Treatment is directed at removing the cause, when possible, and improving conduction between the SA node and the atria by drugs such as atropine and isoprenaline. If drug therapy is not effective, artificial pacing may be required.

Heart block at junctional tissues occurs in varying degrees of severity and may be categorized as first degree, second degree (type I and type II) and third degree, or complete atrioventricular block. Conduction may be impaired in the bundle branches, referred to as right or left bundle branch block.

FIRST DEGREE ATRIOVENTRICULAR BLOCK

First degree heart block is usually due to delayed conduction through the AV node, and the interval between atrial and ventricular contractions is lengthened. This is exhibited on the ECG by a prolonged P–R interval (greater than 0.20 s) (Figure 14.13l). It may be caused by increased vagal tone, digoxin toxicity, inflammatory heart disease or coronary artery disease. First degree atrioventricular block may progress to second and third degree block but in the absence of evidence of disease requires no treatment. Digoxin may be discontinued or the dosage reduced.

SECOND DEGREE ATRIOVENTRICULAR BLOCK

Second degree or partial block refers to a more advanced disturbance in which some of the sinus impulses fail to get through and activate the ventricles. It may be divided into Mobitz type I or Wenckebach and Mobitz type II.

In Wenckebach block the period of time between atrial and ventricular conduction becomes progressively longer, until finally an atrial impulse is completely blocked. The ECG shows progressively longer P–R intervals, until finally a P wave is not followed by a QRS complex. The P–R interval following this dropped ventricular beat is close to the normal range, but with each successive beat it lengthens and the cycle repeats itself. The patient may be conscious of a decreased ventricular rate if the change occurs suddenly but may exhibit no physical symptoms (Figure 14.13m).

Type II, second degree block, is more serious than type I. At specific intervals impulses are blocked at the AV node and an atrial beat fails to be followed by a ventricular beat. The ratio of atrial to ventricular beats may vary, for example 2:1, 3:1, 4:3, 3:2. The P–R interval is constant. The patient may experience syncopal (fainting) attacks (Figure 14.13n).

Both second degree blocks may be due to inflammatory or fibrotic processes, ischaemic heart disease,

infarction, or drugs such as digoxin, β-blockers or verapamil. Atropine sulphate may be required to increase the heart rate and temporary cardiac pacing may be needed if the ventricular rate is slow (see p. 341).

COMPLETE ATRIOVENTRICULAR BLOCK

In this arrhythmia conduction is so disturbed that no impulses reach the ventricles and the atria and ventricles beat independently at their own inherent rhythms. The block may occur at the AV node, or the bundle of His. It is a more advanced block and may be caused by any of the disorders responsible for type II partial blocks. Since atrial impulses are unable to penetrate the AV node, a lower pacemaker takes over and controls the ventricles. If this 'rescuing' pacemaker is initiated in the junctional tissue, the ECG will show a QRS complex which is normal in appearance and not wide unless there is an associated bundle branch block. If the pacemaker is in the ventricles, the QRS complexes will be wide and abnormal in shape (Figure 14.13o).

This condition may be managed with an infusion of isoprenaline if the patient shows signs of decreased cardiac output. A temporary cardiac pacemaker may be required and evaluation of the need for permanent cardiac pacing conducted to manage this arrhythmia.

Cardiac Arrest

Cardiac standstill or arrest means the sudden cessation of effective ventricular contraction. It includes ventricular tachycardia when there is no pulse, ventricular fibrillation and asystole. Possible causes are myocardial ischaemia, respiratory insufficiency, heart block, electric

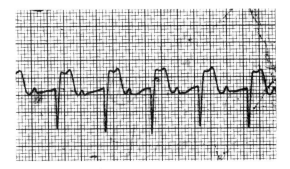

Figure 14.13(l) First degree heart block.

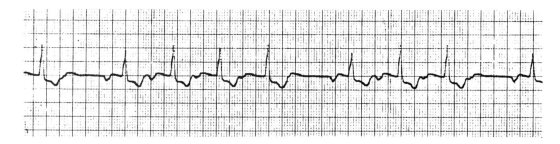

Figure 14.13(m) Wenckebach block.

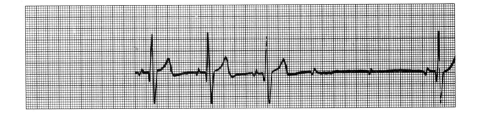

Figure 14.13(n) Type II second degree block.

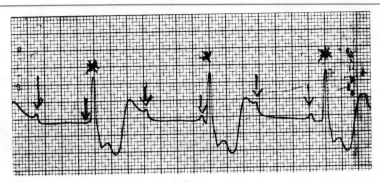

Figure 14.13(o) Complete heart block.

shock, metabolic acidosis and adverse reactions to medications.

Cardiac arrest must be recognized as a critical emergency. This condition is diagnosed when the individual is assessed as unconscious, not breathing and having no carotid pulse. It is imperative that oxygen supply be re-established to the brain within 4 minutes of cardiac arrest to prevent irreversible anoxic brain damage.

Basic cardiopulmonary resuscitation (CPR) must be commenced as soon as cardiac arrest is diagnosed. The ABC steps of CPR are Airway, Breathing and Circulation (Figure 14.14). It is every nurse's responsibility to be prepared and well versed in conducting basic CPR.

A. Airway
After unresponsiveness has been determined, the airway is opened using the head-tilt/chin-lift manoeuvre.

B. Breathing
After the airway is opened, assessment for respiration is conducted. Once absence of breathing is determined, artificial respiration using the mouth-to-mouth method is started. The rescuer gives two initial breaths, ensuring the patient's nose is pinched closed. In a hospital or clinic, resuscitation should be performed using a self-inflating (Ambu) bag attached to an oxygen source rather than mouth-to-mouth as a greater volume of oxygen is delivered under more controlled conditions.

C. Circulation
Circulation is checked by palpating the carotid pulse. If no pulse is found, external chest compression is started immediately. This consists of the regular application of vertical pressure at a point one-third up the sternum from its tip (xiphoid process). Both hands should be used, with the fingers interlocked, applying pressure with the heels of the hands and maintaining the elbows locked in an extended position so that the arms are straight. The increase in intrathoracic pressure produces a limited circulation of blood which, to be effective, must force enough blood into the arteries to produce pulsation in the carotid and femoral arteries. The pressure should depress the sternum 2–4 cm. The thoracic cage is quite flexible in an unconscious person and the possibility of injury to the ribs is therefore reduced. This technique of resuscitation is simple,

requires no special equipment and may be done anywhere.

If one rescuer is present, compressions are interrupted every 15 compressions for the lungs to be ventilated twice. If two rescuers are present, one ventilation is delivered every five compressions. The aim should be to deliver at least 12 respirations per minute, whichever ratio is used.

Basic CPR is enhanced by the provision of advanced cardiac life support by trained personnel who are prepared to diagnose and provide definitive therapy. One member of the team attaches electrodes to the patient and continuous cardiac monitoring is begun to determine the underlying cardiac rhythm. Another member of the team inserts an intravenous line for the infusion of medications. If ventricular fibrillation has caused the arrest, an electric defibrillator is used to deliver an electric current through electrodes into the chest wall. Emergency drugs are given as required.

Every institution has written policies governing the responsibilities of medical and nursing personnel and members of the cardiac arrest team. The nurse should review and be aware of which responsibilities and procedures she is expected to assume.

CARE FOLLOWING RESUSCITATION

The patient who has been resuscitated requires constant observation of the vital signs. If possible, the patient is transferred to an intensive care unit and continuous monitoring of heart action is established. A pacemaker may be applied to deliver a stimulus to the heart in the event of recurring asystole. Peripheral pulses are checked for volume, rhythm and rate.

Respirations and blood pressure are noted and recorded at frequent intervals (every 15 minutes); the temperature is checked hourly. The defibrillator and mechanical ventilator are kept nearby and ready for immediate use.

The patient will be very apprehensive and must be advised of improvement in condition and of the importance of rest and minimal emotional stress, and is assured that someone will either be present or close by so that treatment may be quickly instituted should it be needed.

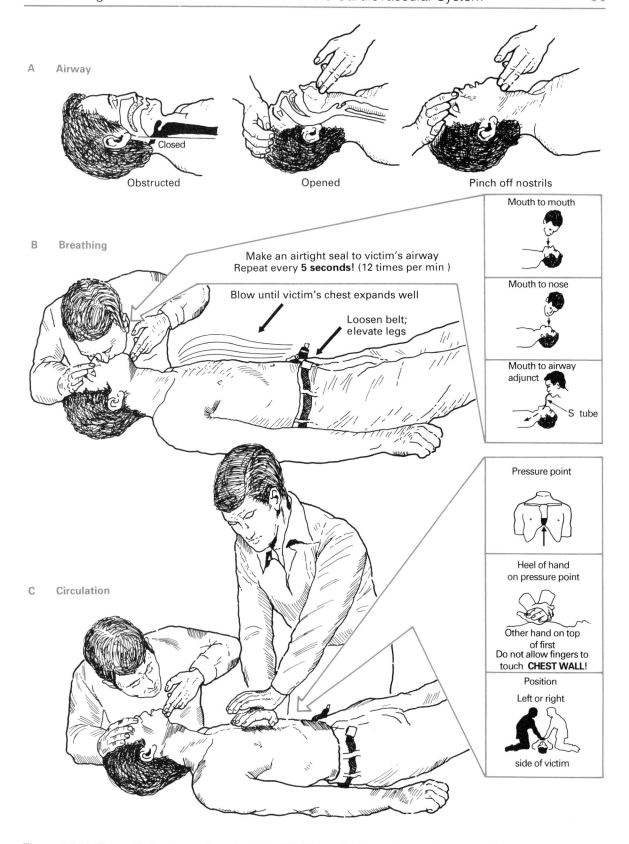

A   Airway

Closed

Obstructed

Opened

Pinch off nostrils

Mouth to mouth

B   Breathing

Make an airtight seal to victim's airway
Repeat every **5 seconds**! (12 times per min)

Blow until victim's chest expands well

Loosen belt;
elevate legs

Mouth to nose

Mouth to airway
adjunct

S tube

Pressure point

C   Circulation

Heel of hand
on pressure point

Other hand on top
of first
Do not allow fingers to
touch **CHEST WALL!**

Position
Left or right

side of victim

Figure 14.14 Resuscitation in cardiac arrest. Modified from the Resuscitation Council of Guidelines.

ETHICAL ISSUES: DECISIONS TO WITHHOLD CARDIOPULMONARY RESUSCITATION

Although decisions to withhold CPR have been debated extensively during the past two decades, such decisions remain a common and difficult ethical problem for most health care providers. The usual presumption in any instance of cardiac arrest is that CPR will be attempted. However, there are situations in which CPR does not appear to be appropriate. The main difficulties in trying to determine whether or not CPR is appropriate can be reduced to three: determining in *which* situations CPR should be withheld, determining *who* should make that kind of decision, and determining *how* the decision should be made and implemented. A typical situation might be described as follows:

Mrs Jones is an 86-year-old woman who has been admitted to hospital with increasing shortness of breath. Tests show that she has lung cancer which has metastasized throughout her chest. she has been an active woman until recently and agrees to a trial of radiotherapy to control the malignancy to a certain extent. After a week she starts to deteriorate.

If Mrs Jones has a cardiac arrest, should she be resuscitated? How should such a decision be made?

Background

Deciding not to resuscitate is of course a controversial issue (Gillon, 1989). Like many technological advances, CPR raises ethical issues that previous generations of health care providers did not have to face. The imperative to extend a life-sustaining technology to an ever wider range of patients brings eventually with it the need to set limits to the use of the technology. When CPR was introduced in 1960 its goal was to prevent sudden and unexpected death from cardiac arrest. Before long it was applied to almost anyone who suffered cardiac arrest (i.e. anyone who died). Now, in most hospital practice, and in most hospital policies, it is presumed that in the event of cardiac arrest CPR will be performed unless a specific decision not to resuscitate is made. In the 1960s, any decisions not to resuscitate were made by doctors verbally at the time of making rounds.

As practitioners were confronted with increasing and sometimes inappropriate use of CPR, and as nurses became more uncomfortable at being left with only verbal orders, attempts were made to establish guidelines for making decisions about CPR. The nurse has an obligation to determine if there are advance directives.

Although limitation of treatment decisions are usually couched in terms of the principle of autonomy, or 'patient wishes', other principles are involved in actually coming to the decision. A decision to forgo CPR is usually guided by balancing the benefits and the burdens of the treatment for a patient. When the burdens of a treatment such as CPR appear to be disproportionate to the benefits that may be obtained, it is important for the care-givers to initiate a discussion of the appropriateness of CPR for the individual. In evaluating a decision, the benefits and the burdens are both considered from the point of view of the patient. At present, most policies require that decision making on this issue include the patient or relatives, and that decisions be made only after discussion with the patient or relative.

A further issue which might be considered is balancing the benefit to the patient with the burdens that the treatment will place on family members or society in general.

Certain types of underlying disease and other characteristics of the patient are associated with reduced survival, and for some associated complications, e.g. pneumonia, the chances are practically zero. It may be possible, with further study, to define circumstances in which CPR would be definitely futile, and would therefore not even have to be offered. Until then, the patient or patient's family should be involved in the decision making.

Communication

While there has been increased awareness of the ethical aspects of decisions regarding CPR, actual practice does not seem to have kept pace with our understanding. Thus, although it is common for institutions to have policies on the subject, the level of communication on this subject between patient and doctor is still disappointing.

Although it is still considered the role of the doctor to carry out the discussions and make the decisions regarding CPR with patients and families, it is often the nurse who makes the initial assessment that the appropriateness of CPR should be questioned and who assumes the role of facilitator of the decision-making process. It is important, therefore, that the nurse has a clear understanding of the principles on which decisions regarding the withholding of CPR should be made.

Treatment of Cardiac Arrhythmias

Treatment of heart arrhythmias includes the use of a pacemaker, medications and/or defibrillation.

ARTIFICIAL CARDIAC PACEMAKERS

In serious conduction defects, and sometimes in the treatment of tachyarrhythmias, electrical stimulation may be provided by an electronic battery-operated pacemaker to stimulate or control cardiac contractions.

An artificial pacemaker generates an electric stimulus used to send a specific electrical current to the myocardium to control or maintain a minimum heart rate. Every pacemaker consists of a pulse generator, which emits and senses electrical impulses, and a wire catheter with one or more electrodes which conduct the impulses to the heart. This electrode or lead system may transmit impulses by contact with the endocardium established through the venous route into the right atrium and/or ventricle; or by contact with the epicardium established by thoracotomy. Contact may also be made by the transthoracic approach when the pacing stimulus is delivered through electrodes applied on the external anterior and posterior chest wall in an emergency.

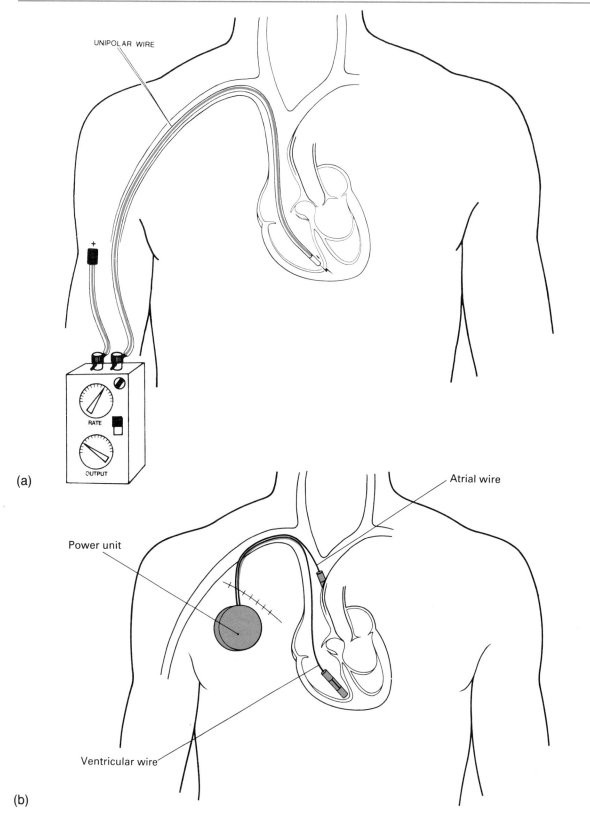

Figure 14.15 Pacemakers: (a) temporary invasive;
(b) permanent dual chamber.

Table 14.9 Positions describing pacemaker functioning.

Position	I	II	III
Category	Chamber(s) paced	Chamber(s) sensed	Mode of response
Letters used	V—ventricle A—atrium D—dual (atrium and ventricle)	V—ventricle A—atrium D—dual (atrium and ventricle) O—none	T—triggered I—inhibited D—dual O—none

If the conduction defect is transient, a temporary pacemaker is used. A pacing electrode is introduced through the external jugular, subclavian, antecubital or femoral vein and advanced into the right ventricle under fluoroscopy. The electrode wire is connected to an external battery-operated pacemaker. The site of insertion of the electrode is secured with a sterile dressing (Figure 14.15a).

When the conduction defect is irreversible, a permanent pacemaker is implanted within the body. The electrode is introduced transvenously, usually through the right cephalic or the right external jugular vein, and the battery unit is implanted subcutaneously in a supermammary pouch on the chest wall. Alternatively, it is implanted beneath the muscle of the upper abdominal wall. This requires a small incision (Figure 14.15b). In order to standardize description of pacemaker functioning, the Intersociety Commission of Heart Disease (ICHD) established a five-position code. Using this code, pacemaker functioning can be easily described based on: (1) the heart chamber paced, (2) the chamber in which the heart's intrinsic electrical impulse is sensed, (3) the mode of pacemaker response, (4) its programmable characteristics, and (5) the antitachyarrhythmic features. Often, only the first three positions are used to describe a particular pacemaker's functioning (Table 14.9).

There are several modes of pacemaker, categorized according to their pattern of activity. The pacemaker may be preset to discharge at a fixed rate, by demand or at a rate that corresponds to cardiac activity. Fixed rate pacing is asynchronous, meaning that it does not sense the heart's own impulses. The pacemaker therefore delivers a predetermined rate of impulses, even if the heart is generating its own spontaneous rhythm. A second mode of pacing is the demand mode. In this mode, the pacemaker is programmed to sense the heart's intrinsic electrical activity and fire only when the intrinsic rhythm falls below a preset rate.

Several common pacing modalities include the following:

VVI: Ventricular Synchronous Demand Pacing. The ventricle is paced, the ventricle is sensed and the pacemaker is operated by being inhibited by the heart's intrinsic QRS impulse. The pacemaker will fire when the patient's own ventricular rate falls below a preset level.

DVI: Atrioventricular Sequential Pacing. Both the atria and ventricles are paced, the ventricle is sensed. The pacemaker operates by being inhibited when the heart's intrinsic ventricular depolarization is sensed. The pacemaker monitors the ventricle for intrinsic activity. If ventricular activity is sensed within a prescribed time, the pacemaker is inhibited and does not fire. If no ventricular activity is sensed during that time, the pacemaker fires in the atria. It then waits for the passing of the impulse through the atrioventricular node. If no spontaneous ventricular activity occurs, the pacemaker fires in the ventricle.

DDD: Fully Automatic or Universal Stimulation. Both the atria and ventricles are paced, both are sensed and the pacemaker is operated both by being inhibited and triggered.

NURSING CARE OF THE PATIENT WITH A PACEMAKER

Nursing care involves assisting in the preparation of the patient for implantation. The patient may be apprehensive because of the symptoms being experienced, such as dizziness and fainting, and may also be fearful of the procedure and being dependent upon a mechanical device. When explaining the need for a pacemaker the doctor reviews the procedure with the patient. The nurse reinforces this explanation and answers any further questions before the patient signs the consent form. Explanations are also given to the family.

The patient receives a sedative before the implantation. Temporary pacemakers are usually implanted under local anaesthetic in the angiography department, in the radiology department or occasionally, in an emergency, at the bedside. Permanent pacemakers are inserted in the operating theatre or the angiography department.

Following the implantation of a permanent pacemaker, the patient is monitored continuously until it has been established that the pacemaker is functioning properly. Bed rest is indicated for the remainder of the day. If a temporary pacemaker has been inserted, mobility is restricted, depending upon the site of insertion as well as the patient's general condition. Cardiac monitoring may be continued as long as the temporary pacemaker is being used.

The nurse is responsible for monitoring and reporting the patient's rhythm, for checking the operation site and cleansing the wound as necessary, for assessing and reporting any complications and for supporting the patient and providing any information needed.

Complications which could occur include mechanical malfunction of the pacemaker, perforation of the myocardial wall by an electrode, breakage or dislodgement of the electrodes, thrombus formation, and infection, such as phlebitis, endocarditis or septicaemia. Mechanical malfunctions may occur because the pacemaker fails to fire, fires too rapidly or fires erratically. Malfunctioning may be detected by cardiac monitoring or by an ECG, as well as by the presence of certain physical signs and symptoms, such as decreased pulse rate, dizziness and/or fainting.

Following perforation of the myocardium blood seeps into the pericardium, causing cardiac tamponade. The resulting compression of the heart causes low blood pressure, tachycardia, increased central venous pressure and distended neck veins. The electrode may also stimulate innervation to the upper abdominal or lower chest muscles, resulting in spasm. Breakage or dislodgement of the electrode will result in a change in the shape of the QRS complex and in the heart rate.

The nurse is also alert to electrical hazards in the environment. Electrical equipment in the patient's environment must be properly earthed and the external pulse generator of temporary pacemakers must be kept dry.

Caution regarding electrical hazards includes avoiding close contact with large electrical motors; for example, in a machine shop the patient may develop arrhythmias as a result of the electrical interference (Sager, 1987). Microwave ovens may cause similar interference with some pacemakers if the oven is faulty with an inadequate door seal. Small home appliances, if properly grounded, produce no untoward effects. Contact sports might be allowed on the doctor's advice. The patient's dentist should be advised that the patient is wearing a pacemaker before any electrical equipment is used.

The amount of information given to the patient depends upon the interest shown and the capacity for learning. Certain points are reviewed with the patient and a member of his family. Basic information is given on the functioning of the heart, the way in which the pacemaker works, activities allowed, battery changes, and precautions regarding electrical hazards. A follow-up appointment is made for the patient to visit the pacemaker clinic or the outpatient department and it is stressed to the patient that regular checks are necessary.

The patient should carry an identification card indicating the type of pacemaker being worn and the doctor to be notified in case of difficulty. Before travelling, the patient should obtain the name of a local doctor or hospital in case of an emergency.

DRUGS USED TO MANAGE ARRHYTHMIAS

Drugs commonly used to manage cardiac arrhythmias are described in Table 14.10.

DEFIBRILLATION AND CARDIOVERSION

Although an electrical shock may cause fibrillation, it may also be used to stop it. In defibrillation two electrodes ('paddles') are placed on the chest wall, one on each side of the heart or one on the ventral wall with a second on the dorsal wall. A strong electrical discharge (approximately 200–400 J) is passed through the electrodes for a brief period. All the muscle fibres of the myocardium are thrown into contraction together and then enter a refractory period simultaneously. This quiescent period may give the normal pacemaker, the SA node, an opportunity to take over. It is important to make sure that no one is touching the bed or the patient

Table 14.10 Drugs commonly used to manage cardiac arrhythmias.

Drug	General actions	Clinical uses
Cardiac glycosides e.g. Digoxin	• Increase force of contraction without significantly increasing oxygen utilization • Decrease conduction through AV node	• Atrial arrhythmias
Sodium channel suppressors e.g. A. Quinidine sulphate Procainamide	• Depress automaticity • Slow conduction • Decrease myocardial contractility	• Atrial arrhythmias • Ventricular arrhythmias
B. Lignocaine	• Depress ventricular ectopic foci	• Ventricular arrhythmias, ventricular ectopic beats
β-Adrenergic blockers e.g. Propranolol	• Decrease ventricular ectopy • Decrease heart rate • Increase PR interval • Decrease myocardial contractility • Decrease myocardial oxygen demand	• Ventricular arrhythmias
Prolong repolarization e.g. Bretylium Amiodarone	• Decrease ventricular conduction • Increase duration of the action potential	• Atrial arrhythmias • Recurrent ventricular fibrillation
Calcium channel blockers e.g. Verapamil	• Prolong refractory period of AV node	• Atrial arrhythmias

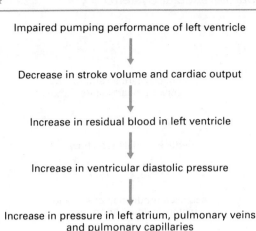

Impaired pumping performance of left ventricle

↓

Decrease in stroke volume and cardiac output

↓

Increase in residual blood in left ventricle

↓

Increase in ventricular diastolic pressure

↓

Increase in pressure in left atrium, pulmonary veins
and pulmonary capillaries

↓

Clinical manifestations of overt left ventricular failure

Figure 14.16 Events leading to left ventricular failure.

during the electrical discharge to prevent their receiving a severe shock.

Cardioversion differs from defibrillation in only one important aspect. It is a synchronized procedure designed to deliver smaller amounts of electrical energy to the heart at a set time in the cardiac cycle. The same equipment is used to perform cardioversion as defibrillation but a synchronization circuit is activated to allow for timing of the cardiac cycle. After the machine is discharged, the shock is held until the next QRS complex is tracked and then it is discharged. This prevents the shock from being delivered during ventricular depolarization and causing ventricular fibrillation. Cardioversion is used to treat ventricular tachycardia and rapid atrial arrhythmias, such as atrial fibrillation and flutter, when the patient is haemodynamically unstable.

THE PERSON WITH HEART FAILURE

Heart failure can be defined as insufficient cardiac output to meet the metabolic demands or needs of the body. This syndrome can be caused by any condition which impairs cardiac function, including ischaemic heart disease, myocardial infarction, hypertension, valvular heart disease, cardiomyopathy and arrhythmias.

Heart failure may involve either side of the heart. However, since both sides of the heart work in series, one side does not usually fail for long before the other is affected.

In left-sided heart failure, the left side of the heart cannot forward all of the blood it receives to the systemic circulation. As a result, blood backs up in the pulmonary circulation (Figure 14.16). The pulmonary vessels become congested and the alveoli gradually fill with serous fluid.

A serious consequence of left-sided heart failure may be acute pulmonary oedema. This condition occurs when the alveoli fill up with serous fluid and the exchange of respiratory gases is impaired. A patient in acute pulmonary oedema will manifest symptoms of acute respiratory distress including dyspnoea and cough. Rapid treatment is necessary to prevent further deterioration of respiratory function. Management may include reduction of preload, afterload and augmentation of contractility to improve cardiac output.

Right-sided heart failure may be secondary to that of failure of the left side, or it may occur independently. When the right side of the heart fails, it cannot effectively forward blood to the pulmonary arteries and lungs. As a result, increased pressure is placed on the venous system. This leads to venous congestion and oedema developing in tissues and organs (Figure 14.17).

SYMPTOMS OF HEART FAILURE

- *Respirations*. Dyspnoea is the most common symptom of heart failure. Pulmonary oedema impairs gas exchange and may induce hypoxia. In mild or early failure, dyspnoea may only be experienced with exertion. With severe heart failure, it is present at rest. With acute pulmonary oedema, it is severe. The respirations are checked every ½–1 hour in acute failure and every 4 hours in moderate or mild failure. With breathlessness related to activity, the degree of exertion is noted.
- *Cough*. Due to congestion and fluid in the alveoli and bronchial tubes, cough may be present. The frequency, characteristics and amount of sputum are noted. Frothy, colourless sputum occurs in pulmonary oedema, and blood may appear from the rupture of capillaries and arterioles in severe congestion.
- *Pulse*. The pulse may be rapid, weak and irregular, as tachycardia frequently accompanies severe heart failure. The strength, rate and rhythm of the pulse are noted frequently and in relation to activities.
- *Blood pressure*. The blood pressure is checked frequently since it reflects the cardiac output.
- *Body temperature*. Many patients with cardiac insufficiency register a subnormal temperature since their heat production is reduced because of inadequate circulation, deficiency in oxygen and resulting decrease in metabolism.
- *Colour*. The colour of the lips, nail beds and skin is observed, and any changes noted. There may be cyanosis of lips and nail beds. The skin may show pallor due to generalized vasoconstriction.
- *Generalized oedema*. Failure of the right side of the heart causes fluid to accumulate in the systemic venous circulation. The reduced venous return to the heart leads to a reduction in left ventricular output and compensatory mechanisms occur in an attempt to maintain adequate perfusion of vital organs. This causes further retention of fluid. Systemic venous and capillary pressures are raised due to the inability of the heart to receive the blood. Fluid escapes from the vascular system into the interstitial tissues, resulting in oedema.

One looks for oedema in the dependent areas of the body. If the person is mobile, swelling first

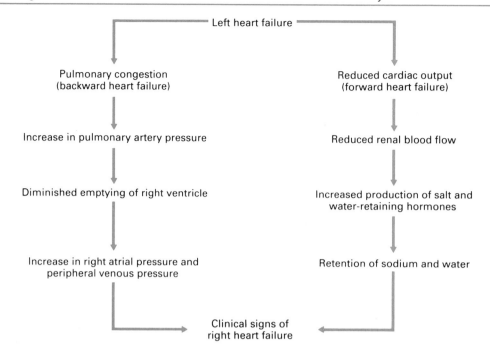

Figure 14.17 Sequence of events leading to right heart failure.

appears in the feet and ankles, but, if confined to bed, oedema may first become apparent in the back and sacral region. As it becomes more severe all body tissues become affected, and even ascites may develop.

The most accurate method of observing the patient for oedema is by weighing daily if the patient's condition makes this possible. Weighing should be at the same time each day with the same weight of clothes. Before oedema becomes apparent, 4.5–7.0 kg (10–15 lb) of water may be retained.

- *Fluid balance*. An accurate record is kept of the patient's fluid intake and output. A positive balance is brought to the attention of the doctor, particularly if the urinary output is decreased to 20–25 ml per hour. The amount of sweating is noted as a large amount of fluid may be lost in this manner.
- *Chest or abdominal pain*. Chest pain and any apparent precipitating causes are observed and reported immediately. Abdominal pain may be due to the congestion and poor perfusion of internal organs. Abdominal distension may be associated with reduced peristalsis as a result of congestion and reduced blood supply.
- *Anorexia*. The patient may not eat because of lack of strength or because of dietary restrictions which make meals unpalatable. Congestion of internal organs due to oedema may contribute to loss of appetite. Anorexia may also result from drug toxicity (e.g. digoxin). The amount and type of food the patient eats should be observed at every meal.
- *Fatigue*. The degree of fatigue is noted at rest as well as in relationship to specific activities.

- *Orientation and level of consciousness*. When circulation and/or the oxygen content of the blood perfusing the brain is inadequate, the patient's cerebral functioning may decrease. Observations are made as to the patient's level of consciousness, orientation to person, time and surroundings, and response to stimuli such as questioning.
- *Anxiety*. It is very important to observe the patient for fear and apprehension. Anxiety may initiate the release of adrenaline, which increases the demands on the heart. The patient's apprehension may indicate a need for information, explanations or sedation.

DIAGNOSIS

Diagnosis of heart failure can be made using the history, physical examination, chest X-ray, arterial blood gas levels and result of two-dimensional echocardiogram. Haemodynamic monitoring may be initiated to assess the patient's preload, contractility and afterload.

MEDICAL MANAGEMENT

Management of a patient with heart failure focuses on two areas. The cause of heart failure must be determined and corrected if possible. Often the underlying cause is lack of adequate functioning myocardium related to myocardial infarction which cannot be cured without a heart transplant. The second focus of treatment is improving the functional ability of the heart. This is accomplished through the following interventions.

- Decrease myocardial workload. This focuses on facilitating the patient's physical and mental rest. This will decrease the resting heart rate, reduce myocardial oxygen consumption and improve myocardial oxygen supply.
- Afterload and preload reduction. Reduction of afterload can improve stroke volume, reduce myocardial workload and decrease oxygen consumption. The use of vasodilator medications can be very effective in managing heart failure. Arterial and venous dilators such as sodium nitroprusside and the converting enzyme inhibitors (e.g. captropril) may be used. Direct arteriolar dilators with no venous effects such as hydralazine can be beneficial. Nitrates which are good venous dilators and poor arteriolar dilators may be useful in reducing preload.
- Improve cardiac contractility. Medications utilized to enhance myocardial contractility are positive inotropes. These include digoxin, which is the traditional medication for heart failure. Digoxin improves myocardial efficiency by improving contractility with only a moderate increase in oxygen consumption. Phosphodiesterase inhibitors such as amrinone, a relatively new agent, can be used to treat patients critically ill with heart failure.
- Reduce fluid accumulation. A diet restricted in sodium may be useful in decreasing fluid retention. Diuretics, including the thiazide and loop groups, are cornerstones in the treatment of heart failure.

NURSING MANAGEMENT

Nursing management of the person with congestive heart failure focuses on several specific health problems. These include:

1. Decreased cardiac output
2. Fluid volume excess
3. Anxiety
4. Alteration in life-style and self-care.

Decreased cardiac output

Goals

1. The patient will demonstrate signs of improved cardiac contractility.
2. The patient will show signs of improved oxygenation.
3. The workload of the heart will be reduced.

Intervention

1. *Improving cardiac contractility.* Heart contractility is improved by pharmacological agents ordered by the doctor. The nurse is responsible for administering them and observing their effects and possible side-effects. Drugs commonly used to improve cardiac contractility are inotropic agents such as cardiac glycosides, sympathomimetic agents and phosphodiesterase inhibitors.

2. *Oxygenation of the tissues.* Oxygen may be administered by mask or nasal cannulae to increase arterial oxygen concentration. It will only be effective if delivery to the tissues is improved.

The nurse should explain the procedure to the patient briefly and remain until the patient is accustomed to the mask or nasal cannulae. Observations are made of the patient's response to the oxygen. Its effectiveness will be indicated by reduced pulse rate, less dyspnoea, improvement in colour and less restlessness.

In severe pulmonary oedema, the doctor may administer oxygen under positive pressure to counteract the movement of fluid from the capillaries into the alveoli.

3. Reducing work-load of the heart

- *Administration of medication* which reduces cardiac work-load (including vasodilators) is undertaken when ordered by the doctor (see Table 14.11). The nurse will monitor the effectiveness of these medications.
- *Promotion of rest.* Rest is important in the treatment of the patient with heart failure since it reduces the demand on the heart by reducing body requirements for oxygen. For the patient in failure, rest in bed is necessary until the oedema is decreased.

  Once the acute episode has passed, the patient is allowed out of bed for gradually increasing intervals. Intermittent rest periods during the day and following activities are arranged, and the patient rests before and after meals and between procedures.

  Physical comfort will contribute to the patient's rest and may be promoted by change of position, bathing, warmth, etc. Anticipation of need and the planning and provision of undisturbed rest periods are important. Co-operation is sought from the laboratory, dietary and house-keeping staffs to control the interruptions.
- *Activity.* Rest has been emphasized as an important phase of the treatment of cardiac patients, but it is well known that there are certain disadvantages inherent in bed rest. The limbs should be put through passive movements to promote venous drainage and prevent phlebothrombosis. Gentle massage will also be helpful. If the patient's condition permits, it may be suggested that he or she gradually commences foot, leg and arm exercises. The patient is also encouraged to take five to ten deep breaths every 1–2 hours. As soon as possible the patient is allowed to get out of bed to use a commode, since the use of a bedpan for defecation places considerable strain on the patient.

  Observations are made of reactions to any activity so that undue stress on the heart may be avoided. These will also assist the doctor in defining the patient's future activities and the amount of rest and restriction that will be necessary.
- *Positioning.* The position that the patient with heart failure finds most comfortable in bed is determined by the breathing. The patient who is experiencing dyspnoea will be more comfortable with the head of the bed elevated, but the height of elevation should only be that at which the dyspnoea is minimal.

  Patients with congestive failure manifest orthopnoea, that is, less difficulty in breathing with the trunk in the upright position. Semi- or upright position increases the vital capacity and tends to reduce the volume of blood returned to the heart and to the pulmonary system. Pressure of abdominal viscera on the diaphragm is reduced. Some patients may be still more comfortable in a true sitting position (i.e. with the lower limbs down). A special cardiac bed on which the foot of the bed can be lowered to provide a chair-like support is available. Alternatively the patient may find comfort from sitting in a chair. The sitting position promotes the formation of peripheral oedema in the dependent parts but relieves the pulmonary congestion to some extent; peripheral oedema is much less serious than pulmonary oedema.

In the sitting position a pillow placed longitudinally at the patient's back may help provide some comfort. Pillows should be used at the sides to support the arms and relieve the fatiguing pull on the shoulders. A change may be effected by arranging a table and pillow over the bed, upon which the head and arms may rest. Cot-sides may be kept up on the bed to safeguard the patient when in the upright position, since the patient may become drowsy and fall to the side, or may experience cerebral hypoxia which causes disorientation. The sides are also useful when a change of position is made since they may be grasped by the patient and used for added support. Patients in the upright position are encouraged to assume the recumbent position for brief periods to help reduce circulatory stasis and oedema in the lower parts of the body. However, patients should not be forced to do this if they are suffering from severe dyspnoea.

In patients with heart conditions, as with all patients, the general principles of positioning apply. Good body alignment is respected to prevent contractures, hyperextension and circulatory stasis. *Even a slight change in position* every 1–2 hours is helpful. A footboard is used to prevent foot drop.

- *Elimination.* Constipation and straining at defecation are to be avoided because of the undue strain placed on the heart. A mild laxative may have to be given to keep the stool soft. Abdominal distension is also to be avoided, since it raises the diaphragm and further inhibits the patient's breathing. The use of the bedpan requires more energy than getting out of bed and using a commode. Therefore it is preferable for the patient to use a bedside commode for defecation.

When a patient receives a diuretic it will mean frequent use of the urinal, bedpan or commode, which can be very exhausting. The nurse provides the necessary assistance, and the patient is allowed to rest undisturbed between voidings.

Evaluation
The effectiveness of interventions will be evaluated by assessing if the patient:

1. Demonstrates signs of improved cardiac contractility.
2. Shows signs of improved oxygenation.
3. Decreases work-load of the heart.

Fluid volume excess

Goals

1. The patient will demonstrate a decrease in weight.
2. The patient will reduce dietary sodium and fluid as appropriate.

Intervention

1. *Administer medications* to produce diuresis as ordered by the doctor (Table 14.11) and monitor the effectiveness of these.
2. *Nutrition and fluids.* Modifications in the diet for patients with heart failure are based first on their retention of an excess of sodium which causes the formation of oedema, and secondly on the knowledge that overeating and overweight increase the work load of the heart.

Low-sodium diets may be prescribed to reduce oedema and to prevent further accumulation of fluid in the tissues. The sodium restriction varies with patients, depending upon their heart efficiency and amount of oedema. Normally the average daily salt intake is 10–12 g. If no salt is added to food either at the table or in cooking and no salted foods are used, the intake may be reduced to approximately 3 g. With the advent of the newer and more potent diuretic drugs, severe dietary sodium restriction is not as mandatory as it was previously for the average patient with heart failure.

The normal daily salt intake may be reduced by half by eliminating salt-rich foods and salt added at the table. This reduction would be required for the patient with mild or moderate heart failure. Omitting all salt from cooking reduces salt intake to one quarter of the normal. Even further reductions to between 500 and 1000 mg may be obtained for the patient in severe heart failure by eliminating milk, cheese, bread, cereals, canned vegetables and soups, some salted cuts of meat and fresh vegetables such as spinach, celery and beets that have a high sodium content.

Low-sodium diets are unpalatable, and the patient finds it difficult to adhere to the prescribed restriction. Frequently the result is that the patient does not take sufficient food to meet nutritional needs. The nurse should explain the purpose of the diet and relate it to symptoms the patient is experiencing. There are many spices and foods allowable that help to make a low-sodium diet more palatable.

If the patient with heart failure is overweight, the caloric intake is reduced in an effort to reduce the weight to normal. A maintenance diet is then prescribed. The lower-calorie diet should contain less fat but enough of the other foods to meet nutritional requirements.

In addition, curtailing the fluid intake to about 1500 ml daily can be advantageous. It is unusual, however, to find that a more rigorous restriction is warranted.

Table 14.11 Medications used in the treatment of heart failure.

Medication	General action related to heart failure

Reduce myocardial workload
 Vasodilators
  e.g. Nitrates
   Angiotension inhibitors
	• Reduce preload and/or afterload
	• Reduce systemic vascular resistance
	• Improve cardiac output

Improve cardiac contractility Cardiac glycosides e.g. Digoxin	• Increase force of contraction • Increase cardiac output
Sympathomimetic agents e.g. Dobutamine	• Increase force of contraction • Systemic vasodilatation • Reduce ventricular filling pressures
Phosphodiesterase inhibitors e.g. Amrinone Milrinone	• Increase force of contraction • Systemic vasodilatation • Improve cardiac output

Reduce fluid accumulation
 Diuretics
  e.g. Loop
   Thiazide
	• Reduce venous return to heart
	• Vasodilatation

3. *Daily weight.* Instruct the patient to weigh at the same time each day, record the result on a calendar and notify the doctor if more than 1.5 kg in 2 or 3 days or more than 2.5 kg in a week is gained.

Evaluation
Evaluate the effectiveness of nursing care by assessing if the patient:

1. Demonstrates a reduction in weight.
2. Reduces dietary sodium and fluids as appropriate.

Anxiety and altered life-style

The nursing care of the patient with anxiety, alterations in life-style and self-care are discussed in detail on pp. 316 and 317.

NURSING THE PERSON HAVING CARDIAC SURGERY

Significant advances have been made in the field of cardiac surgery in correcting acquired heart defects. Correction of acquired heart disease includes surgery for coronary artery disease and for stenosed or incompetent cardiac valves. The fact that the heart must function immediately after the surgery presents a problem different from that in many areas of the body. It must heal while continuing to maintain adequate circulation. This creates the need for greater support and for minimizing physiological demands.

Progress in this area of surgery was delayed until the introduction of the pump-oxygenator. This machine permits extracorporeal oxygenation of the blood and maintenance of circulation while the heart is arrested and opened to provide a direct approach to defects within the heart. Circulation bypasses the heart and lungs. The venae cavae are cannulated, and the blood passes from them into tubes leading to the mechanical oxygenator, which takes the place of the lungs. It is then pumped through a heat exchanger and filtered back into the arterial system, generally via the aorta. Sufficient blood enters the coronary system to sustain the myocardial cells. The blood is heparinized in order to prevent coagulation and thrombus formation. On completion of the cardiopulmonary bypass, the heparin is neutralized by the administration of protamine sulphate.

Hypothermia is used to reduce the metabolic activity of the heart so the cells can survive interruption of the coronary circulation. Reducing the body temperature to within a range of 20–30 °C (hypothermia) is used in heart surgery as an adjunct to the extracorporeal circulation. It reduces the metabolic activity of cells throughout the body and therefore their oxygen and nutritional needs. Hypothermia prevents damage to the brain and other vital organs when an interruption of circulation or a reduction in oxygenated blood to a dangerously low level is anticipated.

SURGERY FOR ISCHAEMIC HEART DISEASE

Both direct and indirect methods are used to revascularize the myocardium. The indirect method involves implanting the internal mammary artery into the myocardium and is rarely used. Collateral circulation develops over a period of months; revascularization is not immediate. Consequently, infarction and mortality rates are higher during this period than with direct revascularization procedures.

The most popular procedure is the aortocoronary bypass surgery, in which one end of a resected saphenous vein is anastomosed to the aorta and the other to the coronary artery beyond the point of obstruction. The left internal mammary artery may also be used as a grafting vessel. The blood supply to the myocardium is immediately improved.

Angioplasty may also be used in coronary artery disease (see p. 325).

SURGERY FOR DISEASED VALVES

The surgeon can significantly enlarge the size of the orifice of stenosed valves in some individuals by dilating the valve. Others, however, may require valve replacement.

Certain patients with regurgitation of the aortic, mitral and/or tricuspid valves, who no longer respond to medical treatment, require total replacement. This is accomplished with an artificial valve prosthesis or the use of tissue homografts.

Preoperative Nursing Care

The preoperative preparation for cardiac surgery may extend through days to weeks, while the patient is thoroughly investigated and physical and mental conditions are improved.

Assessment

During the preoperative period, vital signs, fluid intake and output, daily weight and reactions to any exertion are noted. The patient is also observed closely for indications of any condition, such as a cold or skin infection, which could cause serious postoperative complications. A detailed knowledge of the patient and the patient's vital signs serves as a basis for comparison postoperatively.

Cardiac and respiratory functional tests as well as complete blood studies, are done to further assess the patient's condition. The blood work will include typing and crossmatching so that compatible blood will be available at the time of operation. Serum electrolytes, cardiac enzymes, serum creatinine and blood urea determinations are also performed, and blood clotting tests such as prothrombin time and partial thromboplastin time are done. A preoperative urinalysis is carried out.

The nurse explains the tests to the patient and provides the required preparation and aftercare applicable to each one. For several hours following the more complex cardiac tests, such as heart catheterization, close observation is necessary for manifestations of reactions or complications. Bleeding or irritation at the site of entrance into the blood vessel, reaction to the radiopaque substance, ventricular fibrillation and cardiac arrest occur rarely.

For most patients, tests such as cardiac catheterization are done several weeks preoperatively, and the patient may re-enter the hospital 1–3 days prior to surgery.

PSYCHOLOGICAL PREPARATION

In most instances, heart surgery carries more than the ordinary risk. The incision may be midsternal, which avoids entrance into the left pleural cavity and collapse of the left lung, or it may be through the left chest and may result in collapse of the left lung. Because of the tremendous emphasis placed on the heart by most people, it is understandable that the patient and family will be very apprehensive. The surgeon describes the patient's condition to the patient and family, and the likely prognosis if he or she continues untreated. An explanation is then made of what can be done surgically and the inherent risk.

It takes courage to face heart surgery; patients may find it difficult to arrive at a decision. They require a great deal of emotional support. The nurse assesses the patient's anxiety and fears, and efforts are directed towards minimizing them, since they will affect the patient's reaction to surgery and postoperative progress. The patient is encouraged to talk about concerns and to ask questions. Worries may become less significant through talking about them and being able to share them. Socioeconomic problems may come to light which should be referred to the social worker. The patient may fear death and may wish to talk about this. A visit from the patient's minister of religion may provide considerable support.

Acquainting the patient with what to expect when going to the operating theatre and after the surgery will reduce some of the fear of the future (McCauley, 1988). As the patient talks more and more about the whole major event, he or she will begin to accept it with less stress. Nursing research has demonstrated that when appropriate information is given to patients preoperatively, postoperative pain and stress are reduced (Boore, 1978). In all discussions with the patient and family, what is said should be informative, in understandable terms, and judiciously selected to prevent inducing unnecessary anxiety. Sincere interest and understanding of the problems are frequently better expressed by feeling tones than by words.

To prevent unnecessary concern, the patient is advised of the multiple and complex equipment that will be seen after the operation. It may be helpful with some patients to actually let them see some of the equipment in this preoperative period. The patient is told that there will be a tube in the throat (endotracheal) for oxygen ventilation, which will reduce the work of breathing; that the blood pressure, heart rate and rhythm will be continuously monitored for information; and that there will be a tube in the chest as well as an intravenous tube and an indwelling catheter. The nurses will be making frequent checks of these tubes and the drainage. The patient is told that there will probably be discomfort from the chest incision and is reassured that the staff will do everything possible to provide relief. In many hospitals, the patient is visited the day before surgery by the nurse who will be providing care in the intensive care unit. This pre-operative visit establishes a contact for the patient as well as helping the nurse to know him or her better.

PHYSICAL PREPARATION

Optimum nutritional status is important; attention is directed to having the patient take adequate meals. Protein and vitamin C are particularly important, for they contribute to tissue repair. If the patient has been having a low-sodium diet previously, this will be continued. Optimum hydration is desirable; a daily intake of 2000–2500 ml is encouraged as long as the output is adequate and the patient is not in cardiac failure.

The patient is advised that it will be necessary to cough, take five to ten deep respirations, change position and do some simple leg and foot exercises frequently, for several days after the operation. Arm and shoulder exercises will also be necessary later. The purposes of these activities should be explained. Instructions are given on how to cough and do the exercises, and the patient is encouraged to practise. To cough, the patient is instructed to take a deep breath, contract the abdominal muscles and then cough with the mouth and throat open. Postoperative coughing and deep breathing promote expansion of the lungs, the removal of secretions from the respiratory tract and the removal of air and fluid from the thoracic cavity. The foot and leg exercises are to prevent phlebothrombosis. The arm exercises promote a return to the full range of motion of the arms, since the patient will tend to be reluctant to move them following the operation.

FAMILY

Consideration is given to the relatives during this stressful situation. A spouse, parent or someone close whom the patient wishes to have may be allowed to visit before the preoperative medication is administered. The family may wish to remain at the hospital during the operation, or may decide to return home to await word by telephone. If they remain, they are shown to a sitting room and are given emotional support during the long wait (Cozac, 1988). The nurse should take a few moments at intervals to go and speak with them and to see that they have refreshments. Recognition on the part of the nurse or others that this is a difficult time will help. Many surgeons, knowing the family's stress, may forward a message from time to time to reassure them.

Postoperative Nursing Care

The patient who has had cardiac surgery is cared for in an intensive care unit where the necessary special equipment is assembled for 1–3 days postoperatively. Continuous observation and constant, expert nursing care are required. The patient becomes very anxious and fearful if left alone for even a very brief period the first day or two.

The care must be adapted to the patient's particular needs and the surgeon's directives. The following points

of care may not be applicable nor complete in all situations, but may serve as a guide to the nurse who is planning and providing care for the surgical cardiac patient.

RECEPTION OF THE PATIENT

The closed chest drainage, urinary drainage, intravenous infusion, arterial line, and central venous and pulmonary arterial pressure lines are checked for function. The endotracheal tube is attached to the mechanical ventilator and respiratory support and the administration of oxygen are continued as ordered. Limbs with infusions are secured and continuous cardiac monitoring is started.

Assessment

A constant monitoring of the heart action is used so that cardiac arrhythmias and change of rate may be quickly detected. Blood pressure, radial pulse and apex beat, respirations and colour are checked and recorded every 15 minutes at first and every hour once the vital signs become stabilized.

CVP readings are taken as an indication of intravascular volume and right heart function. Pulmonary artery and pulmonary capillary wedge pressures, when ordered, are measured as an indication of left heart functioning. These measurements may be continued for at least 24 hours following surgery.

Initially the patient is supported by mechanical ventilation. The adequacy of this ventilation is assessed by measurement of arterial blood gases as well as by observation of the patient's responses, which include colour, blood pressure, mental status and pulse rate. Arterial blood specimens are collected from the interarterial line when the patient is first admitted to the intensive care unit and periodically thereafter. Observations related to the ventilator are discussed in Chapter 15. The arterial line is flushed with normal saline hourly.

Movement of both sides of the chest is noted; unequal expansion of the two sides, audible moist sounds and dyspnoea should be reported.

Continuous recording of the temperature by an electric thermometer may be used for the first day or two. The wounds are observed at frequent intervals for possible bleeding.

Level of consciousness including orientation, restlessness and anxiety are significant and should be noted. Stasis of circulation during surgery may have resulted in the formation of a thrombus which later may move out as an embolus. Also, a small amount of air left in the heart on closing may cause an air embolism. For these reasons the patient's ability to move the limbs and the speech are tested every 1–2 hours. Any weakness or loss of function is promptly reported. Peripheral pulses in the limbs, as well as the radial pulse, are checked (dorsalis pedis, femoral and posterior tibial). The absence of one of these may point to a thrombosis or embolism.

Fluid intake and output are recorded. When the condition permits, the patient is weighed daily to detect possible retention of fluid.

Respiratory tests may be required at frequent intervals; the expiratory volume per minute may be estimated by the use of a spirometer. Blood specimens are collected for determination of blood gases, electrolyte concentrations, haemoglobin, and haematocrit.

NURSING INTERVENTION

Assisting respiratory function

As mentioned, the patient's endotracheal tube is attached to a mechanical ventilator. While the endotracheal tube is in place the patient is given suction every hour, or more often if necessary. The secretions are assessed for amount, colour and consistency. Suction can be a very frightening experience for the patient, so the procedure is explained before it is carried out. Careful aseptic technique is observed and each suction should not exceed 10 seconds.

After approximately 12–24 hours the patient is assessed to see if he or she can breathe spontaneously and adequately. As soon as lung expansion is adequate and arterial blood gases are within acceptable limits, the endotracheal tube is removed. The patient then receives warm, humidified oxygen.

Coughing every 1–2 hours is started as soon as the blood pressure is stabilized. The nurse assists the patient by elevating him to a sitting position and supporting the chest, back and front. If the coughing is not productive, and it is evident that secretions are present, suction is used.

Intermittent positive pressure ventilation may be used prior to chest physiotherapy to help loosen and moisten secretions and to help in lung expansion. When the patient is not being ventilated, he is encouraged to take five to ten deep breaths every 1–2 hours.

Deep breathing, coughing, turning and skin care are done at one time in order to provide a longer, undisturbed period for the patient.

Management of fluid loss

Drainage tubes are inserted into the thoracic cavity at the end of surgery to promote the drainage of blood and secretions. These tubes are connected to a tube which extends into the fluid in a drainage bottle. Keeping the end of the tube submerged in the water allows fluid and air to escape from the chest cavity but prevents air from entering the chest. (For details of closed, water-sealed drainage in chest surgery, see Chapter 15.) The system is observed at frequent intervals for functioning; the level of the fluid should fluctuate in the tube in the bottle, with respirations and with coughing. To prevent blockage by a clot the tubes are 'milked' at least hourly for the first 24 hours. If the tubes are not draining it is reported promptly, since an accumulation of fluid in the thoracic cavity could cause serious cardiac embarrassment. The drainage is examined for possible bleeding, and the volume is measured. The tube must be clamped with two clamps close to the chest wall in the event of any disruption of the system.

The urine drainage is checked hourly for the first 24–36 hours, particularly if the blood pressure is low. An hourly output of 30 ml or less is brought to the doctor's attention since it may indicate the onset of a renal shutdown.

The total 12–hour or 24–hour output is recorded and the fluid balance determined.

Nutrition and fluids

For the first 24–48 hours the patient is maintained with intravenous fluids. The maximum amount to be given in an hour is specified and the rate of flow carefully controlled to prevent overloading the circulatory system and increasing the demand on the heart.

Sips of water may be permitted to relieve the thirst sensation once the endotracheal tube is removed and the patient is able to swallow. Frequent mouth care also helps and is necessary to prevent infection. All fluid intake is measured and recorded. A positive balance may necessitate restricting the fluid intake to a prescribed volume.

The diet progresses from fluids to soft foods and then to light solid foods as tolerated. Frequent small amounts are more acceptable than larger amounts less often. Gas-forming foods are to be avoided, and sodium restriction may be indicated.

Rest

Uninterrupted periods of rest are important to reduce the demands on the heart. The various observations that must be made and the treatments, tests and doctors' visits sometimes make it difficult for the patient to get sufficient rest. The nurse should be alert to the problem and plan care to facilitate rest periods.

Psychological care

The patient who has had considerable preparation for what will follow the operation tends to accept the postoperative situation with less anxiety than patients who have not had a similar preparation. It is important that questions are answered and that information is freely given about progress. Brief explanations of what is going to be done are appreciated by the patient and a visit from a family member is also reassuring.

It is not uncommon for the patient's spirits to fluctuate; there may be brief periods of depression and the patient may become very irritable. It is important that the patient feels able to talk about fears and anxieties, something that men in particular, may be reluctant to do, which means the nurse must convey the message of being able and willing to listen.

Medications

Analgesics and sedatives are used with care after the patient has been extubated and is self-ventilating, since they tend to depress respirations and the cough reflex.

A small dose of papaveretum may be prescribed for the relief of pain. Close observation of the patient's response to the drug is necessary; respirations are checked before the administration and during the period following. Very judicious use of these drugs is necessary; to withhold the drug unnecessarily may be harmful, since pain and the patient's response to it may increase the demands on the respiratory system and the heart. The narcotic ordered by the doctor should be used only for pain, not for restlessness. The latter condition indicates the need for increased observation to determine its cause; it may be due to hypoxia or haemorrhage and should be reported.

A prophylactic antibiotic may be administered for a period of 5–10 days. The number of days will depend on the patient's history; if there is a history of rheumatic fever and rheumatic heart disease the antibiotic will probably be given for a longer period to prevent reactivation of the rheumatic disease.

Digoxin may be prescribed to strengthen the heart. If the patient experiences cardiac arrhythmias cautious use of antiarrhythmic drugs may be advised.

Exercises and mobility

The patient is kept flat until the blood pressure is stable, then raised gradually and the responses noted. Unless otherwise directed, the position is changed every 2 hours from back to left side to back and to right side, etc. Precautions are necessary to avoid dislodging any tubes when turning the patient.

To prevent circulatory stasis and thrombus formation some activity is desirable. Passive movements of the limbs are initiated first and are followed by active foot and leg exercises when indicated by the doctor. Later, active exercises are extended to include the arms and shoulders. A pull cord by which the patient may pull up may be attached to the foot of the bed. The next move will be to the side of the bed, then to a chair, and finally to self-care activities and walking.

The patient tends to immobilize the shoulders and arms and may develop 'frozen shoulders'. Gentle passive movement is all that may be tolerated at first, but as soon as possible he is encouraged to use arms and put them through a full range of motion as instructed preoperatively.

The starting of exercises and the rate of progression and degree of mobility will be decided for each patient. For example, the patient who has had surgical correction of a coarctation of the aorta must remain inactive for a much longer period than many other patients. The patient's responses will also be a factor in determining the amount of activity and when it should be started.

The family

When the operation has been performed, the family will be seen. They will be informed about what was done and advised about the patient's condition. It is then helpful if they may see the patient without disturbing him or her. Before taking them to the patient's room, a brief description of some of the equipment in use may reduce their concern when they enter the room. A close family member may wish to remain in the hospital for most of the day and may be allowed to look in on the patient briefly at intervals. The nurse who stops to speak briefly with the family and inform them of the patient's condition conveys to them an understanding of their anxiety.

Transfer from the intensive care unit

When patients are moved to various wards as their condition changes, the problem arises in the patient's adjustment to different environments and variations in the nursing care provided. Patients experience discomfort and anxiety upon leaving the intensive care unit where they receive more frequent observation and attention. The adjustment required may seem abrupt to the patient. Although requiring less monitoring and technical support, patients still need measures for relief of pain and fatigue, assistance with personal hygiene, teaching and guidance regarding activity, medications and diet, and opportunities to express emotional reactions to the experience of heart surgery. To make the transition as smooth as possible, communication is required between the staff of the units involved as to the patient's progress, individual reactions and needs.

Convalescence and rehabilitation

While the patient's physical activity is increased, tolerance is noted. Any shortness of breath, cardiac pain, significant increase in heart rate or oedema is promptly reported and activity is stopped until the doctor has seen the patient.

Prescribed exercises are continued throughout convalescence and rehabilitation. A member of the family and the patient are given instructions about care after discharge. How long the patient must curtail activities and to what extent will depend on the condition before and after the operation and on responses to activity.

Planning for the return home and rehabilitation should include consideration of the factors discussed on p. 312, recognizing of course that every programme must be determined on an individual basis.

THE PERSON WITH DISORDERS OF THE VASCULAR SYSTEM

Disturbance of circulation within the vascular system may originate in the arterial system (arteries and arterioles) or in the veins. In the case of the former, a partial or complete occlusion reduces the volume of blood into the part which the vessel supplies, and the tissues suffer oxygen and nutritional deficiency. Hypertension is an arterial vascular condition with a sustained elevation in blood pressure. If the site of the vascular problem is the veins, there is interference with the normal outflow of venous blood, causing congestion and oedema within the tissues. Vascular conditions may be chronic, developing slowly over a considerable period of time, or they may be sudden and acute.

Diastolic Blood Pressure (mm Hg)	Systolic Blood Pressure (mm Hg)		
	Less than 140	140 to 159	160 or greater
Less than 85	Normal Blood Pressure	Borderline Isolated Systolic Hypertension	Isolated Systolic Hypertension
85 to 89	High Normal Blood Pressure		
90 to 104	.... MILD HYPERTENSION		
105 to 114	.... MODERATE HYPERTENSION		
115 or greater	.... SEVERE HYPERTENSION		

* The average of two or more measurements on two or more occasions.

Figure 14.18 Recommended scheme for arterial blood pressure categorizing in individuals aged 18 years and over. (Report of Joint National Committee, 1984.)

The Person with Hypertension

Hypertension is a condition in which there is a sustained elevation of the arterial blood pressure. The level at which the normal blood pressure becomes abnormally high is not firmly established. Borderline hypertension is a term used for those readings consistently between 140/90 and 160/95 mmHg. Readings above 160/95 mmHg are termed definite hypertension. These readings may be further classified as mild, moderate and severe: the diastolic pressures being 95–104 mmHg, 105–114 mmHg and 115 mmHg or greater (Figure 14.18). The diastolic pressure is the more significant since it reflects the degree of peripheral resistance.

Sustained hypertension is a serious condition. Sustained elevation in blood pressure results in vascular disease. The changes in the arterial walls involve thickening and sclerosis which alter the blood supply to tissues and ultimately may reduce their functional ability. The arteries may develop necrotic areas that weaken and tend to rupture under the high pressure of the blood, or they may thicken and narrow the lumen, predisposing to thrombosis.

Four organs which are the most frequent targets for damage are the heart, kidneys, brain and eyes. The sustained elevation in the arterial blood pressure seriously increases the work-load of the heart. The myocardium hypertrophies in response to the increased demands but there is not an adequate increase in the coronary blood supply and eventually some pump failure develops. Hypertension is a major risk factor for developing coronary disease. Thickening and sclerosis of the coronary arteries may cause ischaemic heart disease, the patient may experience angina pectoris or suffer a myocardial infarction. Kidney function becomes impaired as the result of sclerosing haemorrhage or thrombosis of the renal arteries which destroys functional tissue. Retinal haemorrhages and oedema of the optic disc occur frequently, resulting in degenerative changes in the eyes.

TYPES OF HYPERTENSION

Hypertension may be classified by aetiology as primary (essential) or secondary. Approximately 90% of people with hypertensive disease are said to have essential hypertension; the remaining 10% have secondary hypertension.

Primary or essential hypertension

Primary hypertension is most frequently referred to as essential or idiopathic hypertension. The cause of this type of hypertensive disease is not known; no initial disturbance in the areas commonly associated with secondary hypertension has been established. It may cause cardiac or kidney disease but is not preceded by either. Heredity is thought to be a factor, since most persons with the condition have a history of a parent or grandparent having had it.

Essential hypertension may be classified according to the degree of severity of the disease. The numerical grading is based on changes in the ocular fundi, the response to treatment, the amount of cardiac hypertrophy and the effect on kidney function. Grades 3 and 4 are considered serious, and the patient with a Grade 4 hypertension as well as papilloedema may be said to have a malignant hypertension.

Secondary hypertension

Secondary hypertension is distinguished from essential hypertension by having an identifiable cause. Common causes include renal diseases, endocrine disorders and medications.

Renal disease

Any condition which reduces the blood flow through the kidneys or destroys renal functional tissue causes hypertension. Examples of such conditions are sclerotic changes or stenosis of a renal artery, nephritis and polycystic disease. The ischaemic kidney reacts by secreting a proteolytic enzyme called renin. In the bloodstream, renin acts upon a plasma protein to produce angiotensin I which is then converted to angiotensin II by another enzyme. This angiotensin II causes widespread vasoconstriction of the arterioles and increased peripheral resistance, leading to an elevation of arterial blood pressure. Angiotensin II is also alleged to increase the secretion of aldosterone by the adrenal glands, which, as previously cited, increases the blood pressure through its influence on sodium and water retention.

Endocrine disorders

A phaeochromocytoma is a tumour of the adrenal medulla. Tumours may be single or multiple. The tumour cells secrete adrenaline, in the same way as normal medullary cells, which produces vasoconstriction and an increased cardiac output with a corresponding elevation in arterial blood pressure. Removal of the tumour restores a normal blood pressure.

An increased output of aldosterone by the cortex of the adrenal glands may also be responsible for hypertension. The increased secretion may be idiopathic or may be due to a tumour. Aldosterone increases the reabsorption of sodium by the kidney, leading to water retention and an expansion of the intravascular volume, increasing the arterial blood pressure. It is suggested that aldosterone may also have a direct vasoconstricting effect. A general increase in the secretion of all of the adrenocorticoids causes Cushing's disease, which is also accompanied by hypertension.

Medications

Some women taking oral contraceptives may develop hypertension. It is thought that the oestrogen component of the pills may be responsible by stimulating hepatic synthesis of angiotensinogen which leads to increased amounts of angiotensin. The contraceptive agents are discontinued for 6 months and the blood pressure usually returns to normal.

SYMPTOMS

A person may have an abnormally high arterial blood pressure for a long period without symptoms. The condition is often discovered on a routine physical examination of blood pressure. Those who do experience symptoms may complain of a throbbing occipital headache or migraine. The headache may be accompanied by weakness, dizziness, visual disturbances, epistaxis, palpitations, angina pectoris and dyspnoea. Symptoms of emotional instability, memory lapses and personality changes may indicate cerebral vascular damage. Later, other manifestations appear as the heart, kidneys, brain or eyes become damaged by the persisting hypertension. The person who manifests even a slight elevation above the normal in both systolic and diastolic blood pressures should undergo careful investigation to determine a possible primary cause.

DIAGNOSIS

Hypertension should not be considered on the basis of a single blood pressure measurement. Initial elevated readings should be confirmed on at least two subsequent occasions, with average levels of diastolic pressure of ≥ 90 mmHg or systolic pressure of ≥ 140 mmHg for diagnosis. Repeated blood pressure measurements will determine whether initial elevations persist and require prompt attention or if they have returned to normal and need only periodic remeasurement.

Several systems may be investigated in an attempt to identify the cause of hypertension. The renal and endocrine systems are the more important of these.

MEDICAL TREATMENT

If the hypertension is secondary, treatment is directed toward correcting the primary condition. In essential hypertension, treatment is directed at: (1) lowering the blood pressure in an effort to prevent serious complications; and (2) having the patient adjust life to reduce the demands on the cardiovascular system and kidneys. The treatment depends on the height and constancy of the blood pressure and the signs and symptoms of impaired function in vulnerable organs. The patient with mild hypertension may simply be advised to reduce weight to normal, avoid overwork and overexcitement, and decrease salt intake to a prescribed level in order to prevent the development of hypertension.

People with more severe hypertension may receive a drug to lower blood pressure (Table 14.12) and are likely to be more restricted in activities and diet.

NURSING CARE

The most common health problem encountered by people with hypertension is managing the disease process. Thus, it is important for nursing care to focus on this concern.

Goals

1. The patient's blood pressure is within normal limits.
2. The patient can describe the disease process and the factors contributing to disease management.
3. The patient can describe the health behaviours needed to manage the hypertension.
4. The patient actively participates in a disease management programme.

Nursing intervention

Diet

- Discuss with patient and family the need to achieve and maintain a normal body weight as this may facilitate lowering of blood pressure.
- Reduction of sodium intake may be required as excess sodium expands intravascular volume and aggravates hypertension. The degree of restriction depends on the severity of disease. A 'no-added salt' diet may be recommended.
- Reduction of alcohol intake is recommended because alcohol increases the risk of obesity and may cause a rise in blood pressure. The recommended intake is less than 60 ml spirits, 240 ml wine or 720 ml beer per day.

Table 14.12 Oral medications used in management of hypertension.

Group	Example	General action
Diuretics		
• Thiazides	Hydrochlorothiazide	• Reduce interstitial fluid volume causing decreased vascular wall stiffness
• Loop	Frusemide	
• Potassium sparing	Spironolactone	
Converting enzyme inhibitors	Captropril	• Reduce peripheral arterial resistance
Vasodilators		
• Predominantly arteriolar	Hydralazine	• Relaxes arteriolar vascular smooth muscle
Drugs acting on central nervous system		
• Centrally acting	Methyldopa	• Displace noradrenaline from receptor sites, decreasing sympathetic nervous system activity
• Post-ganglionic blockers	Guanethidine	• Block release of noradrenaline from adrenergic nerve endings
• α-Cell blockers	Prazosin	• Peripheral arteriolar vasodilator
• β-Cell blockers	Propranolol	• Blocks β-adrenergic receptors of sympathetic nervous system
Calcium channel blockers	Nifedipine	• Potent arteriolar dilator

Exercise

• Discuss with the patient a plan of regular exercise which should be undertaken once hypertension is under control. Regular physical activity is a beneficial strategy to achieve and maintain a satisfactory weight.
• Exercise such as weight lifting is contraindicated for people with hypertension because of the tremendous rise in blood pressure during the activity.

Stress management

The relationship between stress and hypertension has not been clearly defined. However, stress reduction is advocated as a health promotion activity.

• Encourage the person to express feelings of stress and to identify stressors in the environment which are both avoidable and unavoidable. Facilitate the patient's planning of strategies that can be used to reduce or eliminate the available stressors in a defined time.
• Teach the patient relaxation techniques which can be used to reduce stress in a variety of settings. There are a number of resources available in the community to teach relaxation techniques, as well as books and cassette tapes which can be purchased. Encourage the patient to utilize these resources as required.

Medications

• Medications required to control hypertension need to be taken regularly for long periods of time. Ensure that the patient and family have accurate perceptions of the use and need for these drugs.
• Assist the patient to develop a simple, convenient schedule to take medications which is tailored to fit personal schedule and habits. Ensure that the patient has a record of the medication plan.
• General knowledge of side-effects can prepare the patient to deal with these, if and when they occur. Discuss the most common side-effects of the patient's medications and encourage the patient to seek advice from the doctor if they occur.

Evaluation

Evaluate the effectiveness of care by assessing if the patient:

1. has blood pressure within normal limits identified for him or her.
2. can describe hypertension and the factors contributing to disease management.
3. can discuss the health behaviours being engaged in to manage the hypertension.

The Person with Arterial Disorders

AORTIC ANEURYSM

An aneurysm is a saccular dilatation of the wall of an artery and develops as a result of weakness in the wall of the vessel in that area. The weakness in the majority of cases is due to atherosclerosis but may also be caused by an infectious disease (e.g. syphilis), congenital defect or trauma. The aorta and cerebral arteries are the most common sites of aneurysms.

The aneurysm that does not extend completely around the artery is referred to as a *saccular aneurysm*.

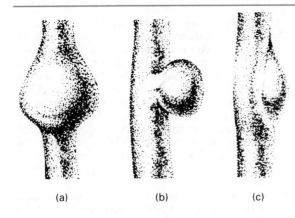

|(a)|(b)|(c)|

Figure 14.19 Types of aneurysm: (a) fusiform, (b) saccular, and (c) dissecting.

If it involves the complete circumferences, it is classified as a *fusiform aneurysm* (Figure 14.19).

Separation of the layers of the aorta is referred to as a *dissecting aortic aneurysm*, even though no dilatation may be present. The tear is often in the intima and may be due to bleeding in the medial layer from the vasa vasorum. The dissection may extend lengthwise for a considerable distance and may involve branches of the aorta. The aortic aneurysm may also be classified according to the section of the artery in which the defect is located; for example, it may be designated as a thoracic or abdominal aortic aneurysm. The former may be further categorized as an ascending thoracic aortic aneurysm, a transverse thoracic aneurysm or a descending thoracic aortic aneurysm.

A serious threat to any patient with an aneurysm is rupture of the weakened vascular area; the rapid loss of blood almost always proves fatal.

MANIFESTATIONS

Signs and symptoms may be absent until the aneurysm is large enough to compress adjacent structures. The patient with a thoracic aneurysm may experience chest pain, dyspnoea, hoarseness due to vocal cord paralysis and/or congestion of the veins in the neck because of pressure on the superior vena cava. With an abdominal aneurysm, the patient may complain of midabdominal, lumbar or pelvic pain, often severe. Physical examination may reveal an expansile, abdominal mass. Femoral pulses may be reduced. Careful physical examination, X-rays, echocardiograms and/or aortography are means of confirming the diagnosis.

Symptoms of a dissecting aortic aneurysm include pain, often described as ripping or tearing in nature, and may involve the chest, back and/or abdomen. Blood pressure drops and there may be a discrepancy in pulses in various locations in the body.

TREATMENT

In recent years, encouraging advances have been made in the surgical treatment of aneurysms. If a small blood vessel is affected, it may be tied off and the flow of blood is diverted to another artery. In treating an aortic aneurysm, the area is resected and replaced with a graft of inert synthetic material such as Teflon or Dacron which does not cause tissue reaction.

Nursing management of the patient is similar to that for the patient having heart surgery (see p. 349).

ACUTE ARTERIAL OCCLUSION

Acute occlusion occurs suddenly as a result of external compression, thrombosis or embolism. It is serious because there is a lack of collateral circulation to the tissues supplied by this artery.

Arterial thrombosis occurs with the formation of an abnormal blood clot (thrombus) within an artery, usually as the result of narrowing of the lumen of the artery by atherosclerotic changes. The stasis in the blood flow predisposes to the formation of the clot, partially or completely blocking the vessel. If the vessel is not completely blocked, treatment is directed towards preventing the clot from enlarging to occlude the vessel and toward keeping it at the site of formation to prevent an embolism.

Arterial embolism is the blocking of an artery by a foreign mass that has been carried by the bloodstream until it reaches an artery too small for it to pass through. The foreign mass is referred to as an embolus.

Most frequently it is a thrombus that breaks loose from its site of origin, but it may consist of air, fragments of vegetations from diseased cardiac valves, fat, atherosclerotic plaques or small masses of tissue or cancerous cells. The effects of an embolism are determined by the localization of the embolus. The vessel which the embolus obstructs depends upon the size of the embolus, its origin, and whether the artery blocked is an end-artery or one that anastomoses above the block with smaller vessels in the part supplied. Obviously, if it is an end-artery, the tissue entirely dependent upon it becomes necrotic. An embolus originating in a vein or the right side of the heart is likely to cause a pulmonary embolism (see Chapter 15). One arising from the left side of the heart or a large systemic artery may produce a cerebral embolism or may plug a smaller artery. The site of arterial occlusion by an embolus may also be a lower extremity.

CHRONIC ARTERIAL OCCLUSION

This most frequently develops as a result of gradual changes in the walls of the vessels, causing narrowing of the lumen. It may also be of functional origin due to a hyperactivity of the sympathetic nervous system, causing an excessive vasoconstriction. Gradual occlusion of the vessels allows for collateral circulation to be established, lessening the problem of deprivation in the tissues distal to the occlusion.

The most common causes of chronic occlusion are atherosclerosis and arteriosclerosis. The arteries in any area of the body may be affected, but the coronary, cerebral and renal arteries are frequent sites. The problems caused by their insufficiency are discussed under disorders of the relative structures. When the abdominal aorta and/or medium- and large-sized arteries are involved, the condition may be referred to as *arteriosclerosis obliterans*. The arteries of the extremities are also a relatively frequent site of chronic occlusion that may be referred to as *peripheral vascular disease*.

In this condition there is progressive loss of the blood supply to the legs, leading to intermittent claudication and the appearance of necrotic tissue, usually on the toes and feet. Patients are typically of late middle age to elderly, have a history of smoking, and are often diabetic. Amputation may be necessary and this is discussed in detail in Chapter 24.

Two other forms of peripheral vascular disease are Raynaud's disease and thromboangiitis obliterans.

Raynaud's disease is a condition in which episodes of excessive vasoconstriction occur in the digits of the hands and/or feet. The cause is obscure, but the episodes are most frequently precipitated by cold or emotional stress. The disease is more common in females, usually develops before the age of 40–45 years and is bilateral.

Thromboangiitis obliterans (Buerger's disease) is a chronic occlusive disease in which there is an inflammation and thickening of the walls of limb arteries, predisposing to thrombosis. It has a higher incidence in young males and in Jewish people. The parts are very tender and painful, and necrotic areas develop in the distal portions of the digits. The condition is seriously aggravated if the person smokes. The cause of this disease is unknown.

MANIFESTATIONS OF ARTERIAL INSUFFICIENCY IN THE EXTREMITIES

These manifestations are due to the deficiencies in oxygen and nutrients to the tissues resulting from the decreased blood supply through the limb. If there is complete tissue deprivation, the cells die, and necrosis occurs in the form of ulceration or gangrene.

- *Intermittent claudication*. This is leg pain that occurs with exercise and is relieved by rest. The blood supply is sufficient to meet the tissue needs when the part is at rest. However, with exercise, oxygen demands cannot be met and metabolic wastes are not readily removed from the muscle tissue. The result is ischaemic muscle pain. Rest allows increased supply of oxygen to tissues and removal of metabolic waste, thus relieving the discomfort.
- *Rest pain*. Muscle leg pain at rest indicates advanced peripheral vascular disease. This pain may be described as burning or numbing and may become more prominent at night.
- *Peripheral pulses*. Absent or unequal peripheral pulses may be present indicating peripheral vascular disease. An oscillometer or Doppler flowmeter may be used to palpate the pulsation of arteries in an area where the vessels are deeper and cannot be palpated by the fingers. A comparison is made of the pulse in the different arteries and would reveal a partial block if one were present. Complete occlusion would be indicated by an absence of the pulse.
- *Colour*. A difference in the colour of the two

extremities or an abnormal change in both extremities, if both are involved, will most likely be present. The skin may become white and blanched, or it may become a dusky red or mottled, depending on the amount of blood in the capillaries and the amount of reduced haemoglobin in the blood. On being raised, the limb becomes even paler as the venous drainage increases but, on being lowered, it fails to increase its colour quickly as the normal limb would do with the rush of arterial blood into it. The superficial veins are slow in filling when the limb is lowered; normally, they fill in approximately 5 seconds.

- *Skin changes*. The skin temperature and moisture may be different in the two limbs. The affected one exhibits a coldness to the touch and may be unusually moist. Limb tissues may atrophy, causing the affected limb to become smaller than the other. The skin becomes dry and shiny and loses its hair. Nails thicken and become brittle and ridged.
- *Necrosis*. Ulcerated or gangrenous areas may develop, denoting areas of tissue completely deprived of blood supply. Ulceration is a superficial area of devitalized tissue; gangrene is a more massive area of dead tissue.

DIAGNOSIS

In most instances, a thorough history and an adequate vascular physical examination result in an accurate diagnosis of occlusive arterial disease. Various tests may be used to diagnose and assess vascular disease.

- *Exercise tolerance*. The patient is required to walk or perform some form of exercise until intermittent claudication occurs. The length of time from the start of activity until the occurrence of pain is noted.
- *Duplex ultrasound*. The combination of real-time ultrasound and Doppler studies are being used increasingly in the evaluation of patients with arterial disease. The great advantage is that it is non-invasive and in some parts of the body, e.g. carotid vessels, its accuracy in assessing the degree of stenosis is comparable to arteriography. Furthermore, the Doppler aspect of the study yields valuable information about the haemodynamic significance of any stenosis identified.
- *Angiography*. The method frequently used to locate the site of occlusion precisely is angiography, either aortography or selective arteriography. A radiopaque contrast medium is introduced into the arteries, and X-rays are made of the vessels. The site of narrowing or obstruction may be located in this way, and some information as to the amount of collateral circulation present may also be obtained.
- *Reactive hyperaemia*. In this test, the flow of blood into the limb is reduced by the application of a tourniquet or blood pressure cuff for 2–3 minutes. On release, vasodilatation normally follows, and blood flows in very quickly to produce warmth and flushing of the skin. In arterial insufficiency the flow of blood into the part is delayed.

MEDICAL MANAGEMENT

Vasodilating and anticoagulant drugs have been used to treat patients with arterial occlusive disease.

Although many drugs are promoted as agents capable of increasing peripheral blood flow, many are universally ineffective. Any α-adrenergic blocking drug will increase the flow through the skin but no drug can increase flow to muscles when the underlying disease is atherosclerosis of a major artery.

Anticoagulant drugs may be prescribed to prevent and treat thrombosis. The most widely used anticoagulants are heparin and warfarin. Aspirin or sulphinpyrazone may be used. Heparin is given parenterally since it has no effect orally. It is thought to block the effect of thrombin on fibrinogen, thereby preventing clot formation. Heparin begins to be effective within minutes after administration and is prolonged for 3–4 hours. It may be given in a continuous intravenous infusion or at regularly spaced intervals. Heparin therapy is usually extended over several days and then gradually replaced by a warfarin preparation given orally. Warfarin takes effect in approximately 48 hours, so it is started before the heparin is withdrawn.

The dosage and frequency of warfarin administration is dependent upon the prothrombin time. The dosage of heparin is decided by the partial thromboplastin time (PTT). A therapeutic level is generally considered to be one and one-half times to twice the normal values for the PTT. A clotting time is done when PTT cannot be measured.

These drugs produce the risk of bleeding but their therapeutic value may be considered to outweigh this risk.

The nurse's responsibilities include close observation for signs of haemorrhage. Profuse bleeding from minor cuts, bleeding gums, haematuria, haematemesis, blood in the stool, petechiae and abnormal vaginal bleeding are reported promptly. In the event of bleeding the drug is discontinued, and vitamin K and a blood transfusion may be given to counteract the reduced coagulation. Protamine sulphate, a heparin antagonist, is given if severe bleeding occurs as a result of heparin administration.

The prothrombin or partial thromboplastin time is determined by the doctor before the anticoagulant drug is administered. Patients outside the hospital taking anticoagulants are usually required to report to the clinic weekly for a prothrombin time check. More recently, drugs which prevent platelet aggregation, such as aspirin and sulphinpyrazone are being used to prevent arterial thrombosis.

SURGICAL MANAGEMENT

A direct surgical approach may be employed in which the surgeon chooses to do an endarterectomy, a bypass or a graft. An endarterectomy is the removal of the thickened intima and atheromatous plaques from the artery and is used when the disease is localized to a relatively small area. The establishment of a bypass channel in order to reduce the arterial insufficiency may be achieved by transplanting one end of another artery into the occluded artery below the site of obstruction or by an autogenous venous graft. The latter consists of the removal of a section of vein (usually the saphenous), reversing it (because of the valves) to ensure flow in the right direction and attaching it to the affected artery above and below the occlusion. The surgeon often elects to resect the affected segment of the artery and replace it with an inert synthetic (Teflon or Dacron) graft. This type of graft is relatively porous and is eventually incorporated into host tissues. An intima develops within it fairly quickly as cells proliferate through the interstices and from the host intima of the artery at each end of the graft. A layer of fibrous tissue also develops on the exterior surface, reinforcing the tube.

The most frequent site of major vascular surgery for occlusive disease is the aorta and the iliac and femoral arteries. Failure of surgical intervention may lead to amputation of the affected limb as ischaemic pain becomes continuous and gangrene may develop.

NURSING CARE

Arterial occlusive disease (peripheral vascular disease) is a chronic condition, and the patient will most likely have to continue with the prescribed care and precautions indefinitely. It may create considerable hardship for the patient and family, depending on the severity of the disease and the limitations it imposes. Adjustments may have to be made in occupational and social life; the patient may become partially or completely dependent financially and for personal care and will certainly find it difficult to accept the situation. The nurse must be alert to the possible implications for the patient and family and should provide the necessary assistance and guidance.

The patient and a member of the family are instructed in the necessary care. They should understand that commitment to the plan of care is all important in preventing serious complications. Common health problems and nursing care will be discussed below.

IMPAIRED SKIN INTEGRITY RELATED TO ISCHAEMIA

Goals

1. The patient will have intact skin.
2. The patient will inspect the skin daily.

Nursing intervention

1. The patient is taught to inspect the skin daily for signs of irritation or injury. The presence of neuropathy may reduce the person's awareness or perception of pain, thus daily inspection may be the only reliable indicator of skin integrity.

   Daily bathing in comfortably warm (not hot) water using a mild soap is recommended. Gentle and thorough drying is important, and special attention is given to the areas between the digits. If the skin is dry, the limbs may be gently massaged with lanolin or some light emollient. Nails are cut straight across but not right down to the soft tissue. A pumice stone may be used on calluses, but corns should be removed by a chiropodist; the patient should not undertake to 'pare' them with sharp instruments.

2. *Clothing*. The patient is advised of the importance of well-fitting shoes and socks or stockings. Socks should be loose and are changed daily. The patient is instructed to avoid walking about in bare feet; a cut, abrasion, sliver or infection could be quite serious, since the tissue resistance is lowered and healing is poor due to the impaired blood supply. If injury does occur, even of a minor nature, it should receive prompt medical attention. Anything tight or restricting must not be worn.

3. Good general nutrition is essential to promote tissue healing and prevent tissue breakdown.

Evaluation

Evaluate the effectiveness of nursing care by assessing if the patient:

1. Inspects skin daily for signs of irritation or injury.
2. Has a daily skin routine.
3. Wears appropriate clothing.
4. Reports eating according to general nutritional guidelines.

DECREASED TISSUE PERFUSION RELATED TO REDUCED BLOOD FLOW TO AREA

Goals

The patient will have:

1. Extremities warmer to touch.
2. Improved colour of skin.
3. Reduced oedema of extremities.

Nursing intervention

1. *Positioning*. The horizontal position is used when the patient rests. Occasionally, raising the head of the bed may be used to encourage the flow of blood into the lower limbs by gravity. Position should be changed at frequent intervals throughout the day, and long periods of standing must be avoided. The patient is advised not to cross the legs and, when sitting, pressure on the popliteal region is avoided. If ambulatory, the patient sits or lies down every 2–3 hours and elevates the feet for 10–15 minutes.

2. *Exercise*. Many authorities indicate the most effective treatment for intermittent claudication is physical exercise, especially walking. It is suggested that the patient should walk 20–30 minutes daily at a slow to moderate pace on a level surface. The patient may do this by walking to the point of intermittent claudication, stopping until the discomfort disappears, and then continuing to walk until the distress develops again. The patient repeats this process for the prescribed period. The underlying theory is that exercise increases collateral circulation.

Passive and active exercises may also be prescribed; flexion and extension of the legs, feet and toes may be used for lower limbs, and similar exercises may be employed for the arms and fingers if these are the sites of the arterial insufficiency. Exercises promote emptying and filling of the vessels and stimulate the development of collateral circulation.

3. *Protection from cold*. Exposure to cold with lowering of normal body temperature produces undesirable responses: peripheral vasoconstriction and increased metabolism. Special precautions are necessary in cold weather. Extra, warm clothing should be worn. If exposure to cold precipitates an episode, the patient is advised to take a warm drink and seek a warm environment. Local heat applications to the affected parts are discouraged because the tissue resistance is lowered and, frequently, there is a reduced nerve sensitivity leading to the risk of localized tissue damage. The patient is advised to wear warm socks or to wrap the feet in a warm blanket rather than applying a hot-water bottle.

4. *Smoking*. The use of tobacco is discontinued, since it promotes vasoconstriction and aggravates the disease.

Evaluation

Evaluate the effectiveness of nursing care by assessing if the patient:

1. uses appropriate positioning.
2. engages in a daily exercise programme.
3. protects himself from cold.
4. does not smoke.

The Person with Venous Disorders

As stated earlier, interference with the flow of blood through the veins reduces venous return from the part, including congestion and oedema which interfere with normal cell function and eventually prevent a normal arterial volume from reaching the tissue cells. Common venous conditions are varicose veins, thrombophlebitis and phlebothrombosis.

VARICOSE VEINS

When venous blood meets with increased resistance to its forward flow, the walls of the veins become dilated and tortuous, the valves become damaged and incompetent and the blood tends to pool and stagnate. The condition may be referred to as varicosities, or as varicose veins. The superficial veins of the lower extremities are most susceptible. Because of our upright position, the venous pressure in the lower limbs is increased by gravity. Other common sites of varicosities are the veins of the anal canal (haemorrhoids), spermatic veins (varicocele), oesophageal veins (oesophageal varices), and the vulvar veins in pregnant women due to pressure from the enlarging uterus.

Although resistance to the flow of blood is the main cause of varicosities, an inherited weakness of the valves of the veins is said to be a factor. Long periods of standing also predispose to the development of varicose veins in the lower extremities.

MANIFESTATIONS

Varicose veins cause local oedema of the tissues, crampy pains or aching, and a full, heavy feeling in the affected area. The congestion and oedema in the tissues interfere with the normal supply of oxygen and nutrients reaching the cells, leading to fibrosing of subcutaneous tissues and, in some instances, necrosis of superficial tissue, producing what is referred to as a varicose ulcer. The affected area appears swollen and discoloured, and the veins are seen as tortuous, bulbous protrusions. These veins readily develop phlebitis, and occasionally the vessel wall ruptures, causing haemorrhage.

The test most frequently done for varicosities in the lower limbs is the Trendelenburg test. While the patient is in the horizontal position, the leg is elevated above the level of the pelvis until the superficial veins appear to be empty. The patient then stands, and the veins are observed as they fill. Normally they fill relatively slowly from below; in varicosities, the incompetent valves allow them to fill from above as well.

CONSERVATIVE MANAGEMENT

The patient is instructed to avoid situations and factors that tend to increase the resistance to venous flow, to provide support to the veins and tissues by bandages or elastic compression stockings, and to assist drainage by elevation of the limb at intervals.

If the varicosity is not extensive, the doctor may inject a sclerosing agent (e.g. sodium tetradecyl sulphate or ethanolamine oleate) into the veins. The varicosed segment becomes inflamed, scarred and thrombosed by the sclerosing agent. Antihistamines and the emergency drug tray are kept readily available in the event of a reaction.

SURGICAL TREATMENT

With more severe varicosities in the lower limbs, surgical treatment in the form of ligation and stripping of the veins may be employed, usually under general anaesthesia. The affected vein is ligated above the varicosity, its connecting branches are severed and tied, and the vein removed. The venous blood then returns via the deep veins. The great saphenous vein is the one most frequently ligated and removed from the groin to the ankle. This necessitates several small horizontal incisions along the course of the vein. Elastic bandages are applied from the foot to the groin after the operation, and the foot of the bed is elevated.

THROMBOPHLEBITIS AND PHLEBOTHROMBOSIS

Phlebitis is an inflammation of the walls of a vein and may be caused by injury, prolonged pressure or infection. The endothelial lining is damaged and a thrombus develops·at the site of inflammation, producing a secondary condition known as thrombophlebitis.

Phlebothrombosis is the formation of a blood clot within a vein with no associated inflammation and for this reason may be referred to as a bland or silent thrombosis. It is nearly always due to slowness or stasis of the circulation, such as occurs with prolonged bed rest, inactivity or pressure causing resistance to the venous blood flow. The serious factor in both phlebothrombosis and thrombophlebitis is the blood clot, which becomes a potential embolus. The silent thrombus or that associated with inflammation may be carried along in the bloodstream and may eventually lodge in an artery to cause an embolism. Phlebitis and venous thrombosis may occur in any vein, but the most frequent site is the saphenous veins of the legs.

MANIFESTATIONS

Thrombophlebitis in superficial veins produces local pain, tenderness and swelling. The pain may vary from moderate discomfort on touching the limb to severe cramping. If the leg is involved, there may be calf pain during dorsiflexion of the foot (Homans' sign). Systemic symptoms such as fever, headache, and general malaise develop. If the vein is superficial, the overlying skin becomes red and hot. It may be taut and shiny.

With deep vein thrombosis, the process may be silent. No symptoms may be present until the thrombus is swept along and causes an embolism. In either phlebothrombosis or thrombophlebitis, the thrombus may become large enough to block the vein, causing severe congestion, oedema and pain.

SUMMARY

Cardiovascular disease is one the most important single causes of death in the UK. Although it is of multifactorial origin so there is no one single preventative measure that would reduce its incidence dramatically, several key components in its causation have been identified. The role of the nurse as a health educator is of prime importance in reducing the current mortality rate. However so too is the role of government in health promotion and recently, considerable interest has been shown by the government in targetting heart disease. This may go some way to addressing the issue of why Britain's mortality statistics from cardiovascular disease are amongst the worst in Europe.

LEARNING ACTIVITIES

1. A large scale reduction in cigarette smoking in the UK would mean major redundancies in the industry, however a successful marketing drive in Eastern Europe and the Third World would allow the tobacco companies to sustain productivity, growth, profits and jobs. Consider the moral issues in this statement, debate them with your colleagues.
2. Prepare a discharge leaflet for patients who have suffered myocardial infarction which advises them about sexual activity.
3. Role play with a colleague talking to a middle aged man about the benefits of increasing physical exercise and changes in diet.

REFERENCES AND FURTHER READING

Bondestam E, Havgren K, Gaston Johansson F et al (1987) Pain assessment by patients and nurses in the early phase of acute myocardial infarction. *Journal of Advanced Nursing* **12**: 677–682.

Boore JRP (1978) *Prescription for recovery*. London: RCN.

Cozac J (1988) The spouse's response to coronary artery bypass graft surgery. *Critical Care Nurse* **8(1)**: 165–174.

Darovic G (1987) *Hemodynamic Monitoring: Invasive and Noninvasive Clinical Application*. Philadelphia: Saunders.

Department of Health (1991) *Report on Health and Social Subjects 41*. Dietary reference values for food energy and nutrients for the United Kingdom. Report of the Panel or Dietary Reference Values of the Committee on Medical Aspects of Food Policy.

Gillon R (1989) Deciding not to resuscitate. *Journal of Medical Ethics* **15**: 171–172.

Grossman W & Barry W (1988) Cardiac catheterization. In E Braunwald (ed.) *Heart Disease* 3rd edn. Toronto: Saunders, pp. 243–267.

Haverty S, Clark JM & Elliot K (1987) Helping people to stop smoking. *Nursing Times* **83(28)**: 45–49.

Hinchliff S & Montague S (1988) *Physiology for Nursing Practice*. London: Baillière Tindall.

Holloway N (1988) *Nursing the Critically Ill Adult* 3rd edn. California: Addison-Wesley.

Johnston DW, Cook DG & Shaper AG (1987) Type A behaviour and ischaemic heart disease in middle aged British men. *British Medical Journal* **295**: 86–89.

Jowett NI & Thompson DR (1988a) Basic life support: the forgotten skills. *Intensive Care Nursing* **4**: 9–17.

Jowett NI & Thompson DR (1988b) Advanced cardiac life support: current perspectives. *Intensive Care Nursing* **4**: 71–81.

Jowett NI & Thompson DR (1990) *Comprehensive Coronary Care*. London: Scutari.

King's Fund Forum Consensus Statement (1989) *Blood Cholesterol Measurement in the Prevention of Coronary Heart Disease*. London: King's Fund.

Kinney MR, Packa DR, Andreoli KR et al (1991) *Comprehensive Cardiac Care* 7th edn. St Louis: Mosby.

Marrie T (1987) Infective endocarditis: a serious and changing disease. *Critical Care Nurse* **7(2)**: 31–46.

McCauley K (1988) Preoperative instruction: nursing assessment and teaching guide. In K McCauley, A Brest & D McGoon McGoon's Cardiac Surgery: An Interprofessional Approach to Patient Care. Philadelphia: FA Davis, pp. 237–249.

Norris LO & Grove SK (1986) Investigation of selected psychosocial needs of family members of critically ill adult patients. *Heart and Lung* **15**: 194–199.

Ockene JK, Sachs D & Solberg L (1988) Sure-fire smoking cessation. *Patient Care* **22(20)**: 83–116.

Oswald GA, Corcoran S & Yudkin JS (1984) Prevalence and risks of hyperglycaemia and undiagnosed diabetes in patients with acute myocardial infarction. *Lancet* **i**: 1265–1267.

Report on the Joint National Committee on Detection, Evaluation and Treatment of High Blood Pressure (1984) NIH Publication no 84–1088. National Institute of Health.

Rice VH, Caldwell M, Butler S et al (1986) Relaxation training and response to cardiac catheterization: a pilot study. *Nursing Research* **35**: 39–43.

Sager D (1987) Current facts on pacemaker electromagnetic interference and their application to clinical care. *Heart and Lung* **16**: 211–221.

Shaper AG (1987) Risk factors for ischaemic heart disease. *Health Trends* **19**: 3–8.

Stanton B, Savageau JA & Aucoin R (1984) Perceived adequacy of patient education and fears and adjustments after cardiac surgery. *Heart and Lung* **13**: 525–531.

Stokes P & Jowett NI (1985) Haemodynamic monitoring with the Swan–Ganz catheter. *Intensive Care Nursing* **1**: 3–12.

Thomas S (1991) Coronary angioplasty. *Nursing Standard* **5(42)**: 47–48.

Thompson DR (1981) Recording patients blood pressure: a review. *Journal of Advanced Nursing* **6**: 283–290.

Thompson DR (1990a) Intercourse after myocardial infarction. *Nursing Standard* **4(43)**: 32–33.

Thompson DR (1990b) *Counselling the Coronary Patient and Partner*. London: Scutari.

Thompson DR & Cordle CJ (1988) Support of wives of myocardial infarction patients. *Journal of Advanced Nursing* **13**: 223–228.

Thompson DR & Meddis (1990a) A prospective evaluation of in-hospital counselling for first time myocardial infarction men. *Journal of Psychosomatic Research* **34**: 237–248.

Thompson DR & Meddis (1990b) Wives' responses to counselling early after myocardial infarction. *Journal of Psychosomatic Research* **34**: 249–258.

Thompson DR, Bailey SW & Webster RA (1986) Patients' views of cardiac monitoring. *Nursing Times* **82(9)**: 54–55.

Thompson DR, Webster RA, Cordle CJ et al (1987) Specific

sources and patterns of anxiety in male patients with first myocardial infarction. *British Journal of Medical Psychology* **60**: 343–348.

Toth J (1984) The person with coronary artery disease and risk factors. In C Gazzelta & B Dossey (eds) *Cardiovascular Nursing: Body Mind Tapestry*. St Louis: CV Mosby

Underhill S, Woods S, Sivarajan Froelicher E et al (1989) *Cardiac Nursing* 2nd edn. Philadelphia: Lippincott.

Vacek J, Smith W & Philips J (1984) Cardiac electrophysiology. An overview. *Practical Cardiology* **10(4)**: 83–97.

Watkins LO, Weaver L & Odegaard V (1986) Preparation for cardiac catheterization: tailoring the content of instruction to coping style. *Heart and Lung* **15**: 387–389.

Wyper S & Walsh E (1989) The patient with cardiovascular problems. In B Lang & W Phillips *Medical Surgical Nursing*. 2nd edn. St Louis: CV Mosby.

Caring for the Patient with a Disorder of the Respiratory System

15

OBJECTIVES

On completion of this chapter the reader should be able to:
- Describe the structure and functioning of the respiratory system
- Describe the main causes of respiratory health problems
- Assess the person with a disorder of the respiratory system
- Plan, implement and evaluate care for a person with respiratory health problems
- Discuss the role of the nurse in patient teaching with regard to the above
- Be aware of the psychosocial effects of respiratory disorder
- Discuss strategies for helping the patient and family cope with the above

RESPIRATION

A constant exchange of oxygen and carbon dioxide between the living organism and its environment is essential for survival. Respiration is the process which performs this function. The exchange takes place between the total organism and the external environment and between the tissue cells and the blood. The former involves pulmonary ventilation and diffusion of the gases through the alveolar membrane of the lungs. The exchange between the cells and the blood (sometimes called internal or tissue respiration) requires transportation of the gases by the blood and an exchange of oxygen and carbon dioxide between the capillaries and tissue cells.

Pulmonary ventilation or breathing consists of the movement of air into and out of the lungs (inspiration and expiration). Diffusion involves the movement of gases between the air in the pulmonary air sacs (alveoli) and the blood in the pulmonary capillaries in the direction of the lower pressure or concentration.

Respiratory Structures

The structures concerned with ventilation are the upper and lower respiratory tracts, respiratory muscles, thorax and portions of the nervous system. (Figure 15.1).

UPPER RESPIRATORY TRACT

The upper airway is formed by the nose, mouth, pharynx and larynx. It serves as a passageway for air being inspired and expired, filters, warms and moistens the inhaled air, and provides the protective reflexes of sneezing and the closing off of the larynx to prevent aspiration of fluid and solids. Irritation of the pharynx and larynx may also initiate the cough reflex.

NOSE

The nose has a highly vascularized and ciliated mucous membrane lining which serves to moisten, warm and filter inhaled air. The nasal cavities and their connecting sinuses act as resonating chambers in sound production. The posterior portion of the cavities contains olfactory receptors concerned with the sense of smell (olfactory sense). The external orifices are called the nostrils, or anterior nares.

PHARYNX

The pharynx, a muscular tube lined with mucous membrane, provides a common passageway for air entering the larynx and food entering the oesophagus. Air reaching the pharynx passes readily into the larynx, but the presence of food or fluid stimulates a reflex contraction of the pharyngeal tube. The posterior nares (openings into the nasal cavities) are then blocked off and the larynx is closed off by a lowering of the leaf-shaped structure, the *epiglottis*. These closures prevent the entrance of food or fluid into the nose and lower respiratory tract. As a result of the contraction, the pharyngeal content is directed into the oesophagus.

LARYNX

The larynx is composed of muscle tissue and cartilage and is lined with mucous membrane. It functions as an air passage and contains the *vocal cords*, which are responsible for sound production. The laryngeal passageway is narrowed in one area by membranous folds reflected over the vocal cords. The slit-like space between these two folds is referred to as the *glottis* and is varied in size to produce the different levels of pitch in voice production. In normal quiet inspiration and expiration the vocal cords are relaxed and the glottis is open.

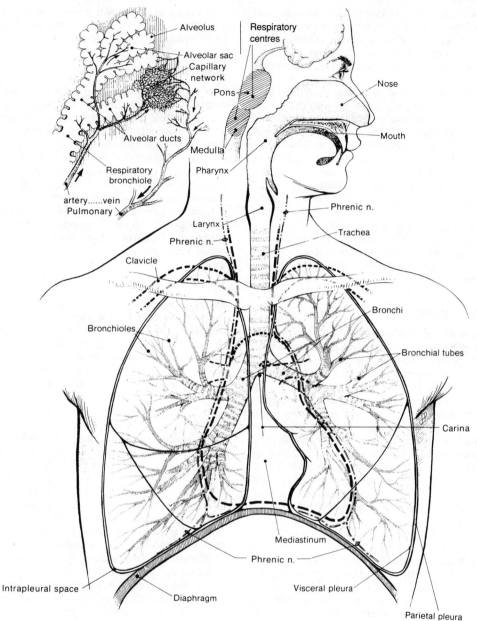

Figure 15.1 The respiratory system.

LOWER RESPIRATORY TRACT

The lower tract consists of the trachea, bronchi and two lungs.

TRACHEA

The trachea is a continuation of the inferior end of the larynx and divides into two tubes: the right and left bronchi. The right bronchus is shorter and more vertical than the left; this accounts for aspirated foreign particles entering the right bronchus more often than the left.

The tracheal walls are composed of fibroelastic tissue in which incomplete cartilaginous rings are imbedded to prevent collapse of the tube. The trachea simply serves as an air passageway.

BRONCHI, BRONCHIAL TUBES AND BRONCHIOLES

Each bronchus enters a lung where it branches like a tree to form the bronchial tubes and, eventually, the very small tubes, the bronchioles. As the branches become more distal, the lumen of the tubes narrows and the walls change structure. The bronchi and bronchial tubes are similar in structure to the trachea except for the addition of plain muscle tissue in their walls. In the bronchioles, the cartilaginous tissue disappears and the smooth muscle tissue becomes more abundant.

The trachea and bronchial air passages are lined by a ciliated mucous membrane continuous with that of the upper air passages. The cilia are hair-like projections of protoplasm which alternately bend in one direction and straighten, providing a sweeping motion to remove the mucus secreted and any foreign particles that may have been inhaled. Excessive secretions may initiate the cough reflex, which is a defence mechanism to rid the tract of such substances (see p. 373). The bronchi conduct air between the external environment and terminal structures where gas exchange takes place. These conducting airways constitute the anatomical dead space because they take no part in gas exchange. The bronchioles divide and subdivide, becoming progressively smaller.

RESPIRATORY ZONE

Each bronchiole eventually gives rise to a spray of microscopic tubes known as *alveolar ducts*. Microscopic sacs called *alveoli* (singular: alveolus) increase in number along the terminal bronchioles and completely line the alveolar ducts and terminate in alveolar sacs containing alveolar projections. Collectively, these structures are referred to as the *terminal respiratory units*. The walls of the alveoli consist of thin epithelial cells, elastic connective tissue and a network of capillaries. The air in each alveolus is separated from the blood in the capillaries by a very thin semipermeable tissue which permits diffusion of the oxygen and carbon dioxide through it. The respiratory zone makes up most of the lung. It has a volume of about 3000 ml.

LUNGS

Each lung is made up of conducting airways comprising: the bronchial tubes, with their successive branches; the respiratory zone, composed of respiratory bronchioles, alveolar ducts and alveoli; and the many blood vessels of the pulmonary circulatory system. The right lung is divided into three lobes, and the left is divided into two lobes. Each lung is enclosed in an adherent serous membrane called the *visceral pleura*, which is continuous from the hilum of the lung with a similar layer that lines the thoracic wall—the *parietal pleura*.

Blood supply to the lungs

Blood from two sources enters the lungs. The bronchial arteries convey blood from the aorta to nourish the conducting airways (from the main bronchi to the terminal bronchioles). The pulmonary artery delivers the blood from the right side of the heart to the walls of the alveoli to be oxygenated. Blood from both sources is then collected from the capillaries around the alveoli and other structures into veins and is returned to the left side of the heart by the four pulmonary veins. Some blood from the bronchial arteries, around the area of the hilum, enters bronchial veins, which empty into larger veins, to be transported to the right atrium.

Lymphatic drainage

Two pulmonary lymphatic systems exist: the superficial network located within the connective layer of the visceral pleura, and the deep or parenchymal system which surrounds the airways, arteries, veins and terminal respiratory units. Lymphocytes and plasma cells are found throughout the tracheobronchial structures. Small lymph nodes are also found in the lungs. The lymphatic system of the lungs plays a vital role in defence against infection; lymphoid tissue in the mucous membrane of the tracheobronchial tree provides antibody- and cell-mediated immune responses. Pulmonary lymphatic dysfunction causes pulmonary oedema and infection.

Thorax

The lungs are well protected by the bony thoracic cage which is formed by the sternum, ribs and thoracic vertebrae. The apices of the lungs extend about 2.5 cm above the clavicles. The thorax acts as an airtight box in which the lungs are suspended and in which pressure can be varied by contraction of respiratory muscles, altering the thoracic cavity dimensions.

SECRETIONS

The respiratory tract produces two secretions: *mucus* and *surfactant*. The inner surfaces of the alveoli and alveolar ducts are covered with a film of surfactant (or surface active substance), a phospholipid compound synthesized by special epithelial cells in the walls of the alveoli. The composition of this solution is such that it reduces the surface tension, facilitating inflation and preventing collapse of the alveoli on expiration. Surfactant also prevents the movement of fluid from the capillaries into the alveoli (pulmonary oedema) by reducing the surface tension.

The *mucus* which is secreted by the mucus glands and goblet cells of the mucous membrane lining of the respiratory tract serves to protect the organism in several ways. It provides a protective barrier against inhaled irritants and traps foreign particles, facilitating their removal by the cilia. It also waterproofs the surface, thus diminishing the loss of body water, as well as setting up a barrier to inhaled organisms. Insufficient secretion of mucus or the production of a thick tenacious mucus prevents the action of the cilia, predisposing to infection and partial or complete obstruction of bronchial tubes and bronchioles.

CHEST CAVITIES AND THEIR PRESSURES

The spaces between the visceral and parietal pleurae form the intrapleural or *pleural cavities*. (Each lung has its own closed pleural cavity.) Each pleural cavity is only a potential space, since the visceral and parietal pleurae are normally separated by just a thin film of fluid that moistens the surfaces. The surfaces of the lungs are in close apposition with the chest walls. The pressure within the pleural cavities is approximately 5 mmHg less than atmospheric pressure, which is 760 mmHg at sea level. It may also be expressed as a negative pressure equal to that exerted by a column of water 10 cm in depth.

The *intrapulmonary cavity* is the space within the lungs. If the pressure within this cavity is lower than atmospheric, air will be sucked into the lungs (inhalation); if it is greater, air will be exhaled. The mechanics are discussed below.

The space in between the two lungs and their pleurae is known as the *mediastinum*. It contains the large blood vessels, heart, oesophagus, trachea, bronchi, and lymphatic ducts and nodes.

RESPIRATORY MUSCLES

The muscles used in normal breathing are principally the diaphragm and the intercostal muscles. The *diaphragm* is a dome-shaped muscular partition between the thoracic and abdominal cavities and is the most important respiratory muscle. When the diaphragm is relaxed, its thoracic surface is convex. On contraction, the convexity is reduced and the thoracic cavity is lengthened. The diaphragm also functions in coughing and sneezing and, in conjunction with the abdominal muscles, is used in defecation, vomiting and parturition.

The *external intercostal muscles* increase the lateral and anteroposterior diameters of the thoracic cavity by elevating the sternum and moving the ribs into a more horizontal position.

Accessory muscles may be used to facilitate breathing. In laboured and forced inspiration, the sternocleidomastoid muscles elevate the sternum, and the scalene and pectoralis muscles contract to raise the upper ribs. At the same time the nostrils dilate and the glottis widens. Forced or difficult expiration involves the abdominal and internal intercostal muscles. The abdominal muscles contract to raise the relaxed diaphragm higher in order to compress the lungs and facilitate expiration.

Respiratory Functions

MECHANICS OF PULMONARY VENTILATION

Figure 15.2 illustrates the steps of respiration. On inspiration, air enters the lungs; gas exchange occurs between the alveoli and the blood and between the blood and the tissues; expiration returns the used air to the atmosphere.

Each respiration involves inspiration and expiration. Inspiration is an active phase during which air moves into the lungs. Expiration, in normal breathing, is a passive phase during which air moves out of the lungs. Pulmonary ventilation is made possible by rhythmic variations in the dimensions of the thoracic and intrapulmonary spaces brought about by the alternating contraction and relaxation of the respiratory muscles.

Gases possess certain physical properties which explain the movement and exchange of respiratory

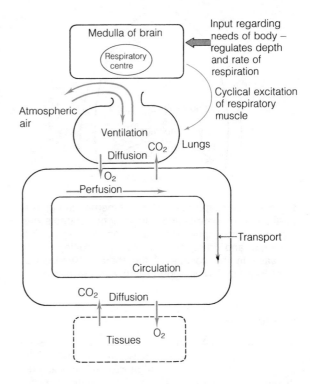

Figure 15.2 Schematic representation of the processes involved in respiration. Reproduced from Hinchliff & Montague (1988) with permission.

gases. They differ from fluids in that their molecules spread out to fill the space available to them. The molecules of a gas are in ceaseless movement and strike the walls of the container, creating a pressure. Within a given space, the greater the number of molecules of gas, the higher is the pressure produced. *The pressure of a gas varies inversely with the space in which it is contained if the temperature remains constant* (Boyle's law). If the space in which the volume of gas is confined is reduced, more gas molecules strike a smaller area of the container, increasing the pressure. Conversely, if the space is increased, the pressure of the gas is decreased. *Gas molecules move from an area of higher pressure to one of lower pressure.*

According to Dalton's law of partial pressure, *each gas in a mixture of gases exerts the same pressure that it would exert if it were not in a mixture, and that pressure is proportional to its concentration.* The pressure of the mixture is the sum of the pressures of the constituent gases. The pressure of each gas in the mixture is termed the partial pressure of that gas, and is indicated by a 'P' preceding the gas symbol. For example the pressure of oxygen in a mixture of gases is recorded as Po_2.

The amount of a gas absorbed by a fluid (i.e. its solubility) is directly proportional to the partial pressure of the gas. The fluid will absorb the gas until the pressure of the gas is the same as that at the surface. This is referred to as Henry's law of the solution of gases.

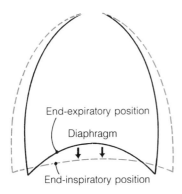

Figure 15.3 Diaphragmatic movements during respiration. The dome-shaped diaphragm contracts during inspiration, pressing down on the abdominal contents and lifting the rib cage, resulting in an increase in the volume of the thorax. Reproduced from Hinchliff & Montague (1988) with permission.

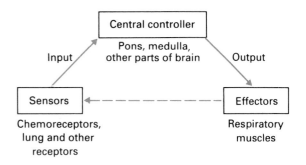

Figure 15.4 Basic elements of the respiratory control system. Information from various sensors is fed to the central controller, the output of which goes to the respiratory muscles. By changing ventilation, the respiratory muscles reduce perturbations of the sensors (negative feedback).

INSPIRATION

When the diaphragm and external intercostal muscles contract, the effect is to increase the volume of the thoracic cavity as the chest wall moves outwards and the diaphragm downwards. The parietal pleura expands with the chest wall and, as the visceral pleura adheres to the parietal pleura by surface tension, this also expands. Contraction of the diaphragm reduces its convex curvature towards the thoracic cavity. It is a combination of these two effects that produces the volume increase and a consequent pressure decrease of 4–5 mmHg within the thoracic cavity, which sets up a pressure gradient between atmospheric and intrapulmonary air. The result is that air is sucked into the lungs, where pressure is now below atmospheric, and inspiration takes place (Figure 15.3).

EXPIRATION

Relaxation of the respiratory muscles reverses the inspiratory process. As the intrathoracic space decreases with the muscular relaxation, the pressure within the cavity increases. The elastic alveoli, which were stretched, now also recoil, diminishing the intrapulmonary space. The pressure of the air within the lungs is increased to a level above that of the atmospheric air. This causes air to move out until the intrapulmonary pressure is equal to that of the atmosphere, thus producing an expiration. Normally, this cycle of inspiration and expiration is completed 14–18 times per minute in the adult.

THE WORK OF BREATHING

The inspiratory phase of breathing requires energy to overcome the elastic forces in the lungs (compliance work), the flow-resistant forces within the air passages (airway resistance work) and the viscosity of the lungs and thoracic cage (tissue resistance work). Owing to their elastic property, the lungs and chest wall constantly tend to maintain the position they occupy at the end of a normal expiration. When the respiratory muscles contract to expand the intrathoracic and intrapulmonary spaces to provide inhalation, they must overcome this elastic resistance. *Compliance* is the term used to indicate the distensibility of the lungs and the thorax, or the ease with which they are stretched.

Some energy is also necessary to overcome the frictional and viscous resistance offered by the surface tissues in the air passages.

CONTROL OF VENTILATION

Figure 15.4 illustrates the three basic elements of respiratory regulation: *Sensors* gather information and feed it to the *central controller*, the respiratory centres in the brain. The information is processed and impulses are sent to the *effectors* or respiratory muscles which cause ventilation. Respirations are regulated by both nervous and chemical mechanisms.

Neural regulation

Inspiration and expiration are dependent upon alternate contraction and relaxation of muscles which are subordinate to impulses initiated by groups of neurones in the medulla and pons of the brain stem. These groups of neurones make up the *respiratory centres* (see Figure 15.1).

The *medullary centre* is considered responsible for spontaneous, rhythmic respiration. Some neurones in this centre discharge impulses that result in contraction of the respiratory muscles and inspiration; others discharge impulses that cause relaxation of the muscles and expiration. The rhythmic discharge of the neurones in the medulla may be modified by impulses generated by groups of neurones (centres) in the pons (*pontine centre*) and by impulses transmitted to the medullary centres by afferent (sensory) nerve fibres of the vagus nerves. These nerve fibres transmit impulses from receptors in the lungs that are sensitive to stretching (pulmonary stretch receptors), irritation (irritant receptors), possibly capillary distension and increased interstitial fluid volume (juxtacapillary receptors). Stretching of the lungs by inflation produces impulses that have an inhibitory effect on the neurones that generate inspiratory impulses (the *Hering–Breuer reflex*). Stimulation of the irritant receptors causes bronchoconstriction and hyperpnoea, while the juxtacapillary receptors are believed to play a role in the sensation of dyspnoea and in producing rapid, shallow breathing.

Impulses from the respiratory centre descend into the spinal cord. Those carried to the diaphragm are transmitted by the phrenic nerves, which originate with the third, fourth and fifth cervical spinal nerves. The impulses to the intercostal muscles are delivered by the intercostal nerves that arise from the spinal cord with the third, fourth, fifth and sixth thoracic spinal nerves. Mental alertness and wakefulness normally have a stimulating effect on breathing, but sleep, sedatives and anaesthesia tend to reduce the rate and volume of ventilation.

Respiratory muscle activities may be modified by impulses originating in the cerebral cortex that are delivered to the respiratory centres. For example, breathing may be controlled voluntarily for a limited period, as in breath-holding or the taking of large deep breaths. Voluntary control and a high level of central nervous system coordination and integration are needed in speaking and singing. Changes in the rhythm, rate and depth of respirations are frequently associated with emotional states (e.g. excitement, laughing, crying, depression, fear).

Certain sensory impulses may influence respirations. Severe pain produces faster and deeper respirations. Muscle activity increases respirations; this is attributed both to an increase in carbon dioxide production and to impulses originating in the stretch and pressure receptors of muscles, tendons and joints.

Chemical regulation

The major chemical factors that control respiration are the partial pressures of carbon dioxide and oxygen in blood ($P\mathrm{co}_2$ and $P\mathrm{o}_2$) and the hydrogen ion concentration in the bloodstream (pH). The hydrogen ion concentration is a way of measuring how acid or alkaline a liquid is, a value of 7 is neutral (e.g. pure water), while as the value drops below 7 it becomes more acid and conversely values above 7 are more alkaline. For example, urine typically has a pH of 5 to 6 (acid), while the norm for arterial blood is 7.4 (slightly alkaline). Life is only possible with a range of blood values between 7.0 and 7.8 (Hinchcliffe and Montague, 1988).

An increase in $P\mathrm{co}_2$ above normal makes the blood more acid (pH falls). The high carbon dioxide level stimulates the respiratory centres, producing an increase in both rate and depth of respiration in an attempt to remove excess carbon dioxide from the body. Any other mechanism which makes the blood more acid (e.g. the production of ketone bodies in a diabetic coma) will stimulate extra respiratory effort as the body tries to restore pH to normal values by removing carbon dioxide from the blood. Variations in $P\mathrm{o}_2$ appear to

have less effect on respiration, except in those individuals who have suffered chronic lung disease and whose respiratory centres seem to have become used to permanently high carbon dioxide levels. In this situation, a falling $P\mathrm{o}_2$ level may act as a respiratory stimulant.

Changes in the pH (or hydrogen ion concentration) and tensions of carbon dioxide and oxygen in the blood bring about respiratory changes through *respiratory chemoreceptors*. These are groups of cells that are sensitive to certain changes in the chemistry of the blood. According to their location in relation to the nervous system the chemoreceptors are of two types, peripheral and central.

Central chemoreceptors are located in the medulla and respond to changes in the hydrogen ion concentration in the extracellular fluid surrounding the receptors. An increase in the $P\mathrm{co}_2$ in the blood results in carbon dioxide diffusing into the cerebrospinal fluid from the cerebral blood vessels. Hydrogen ions are then liberated and stimulate the chemoreceptors; the resulting increase in the rate and volume of respirations reduces the $P\mathrm{co}_2$ in the blood and in the cerebral spinal fluid. A decrease in the hydrogen ion concentration in the surrounding extracellular fluid inhibits the central receptors.

The peripheral chemoreceptors are located in the carotid bodies (lying in the bifurcations of the carotid arteries) and the aortic bodies (on the wall of the aortic arch) and are sensitive to decreases in the arterial $P\mathrm{o}_2$ and to a lesser extent to increases in $P\mathrm{co}_2$. The carotid bodies also respond to decreases in the pH or increases in the hydrogen ion concentration. Impulses are initiated in these receptors and are then transmitted to the respiratory neurons via the glossopharyngeal and vagus nerves, resulting in changes in the rate and volume of respirations.

When body metabolism increases, more oxygen is used by the tissues and more carbon dioxide and acid metabolites are produced. Normally, this decreases the $P\mathrm{o}_2$ and increases the $P\mathrm{co}_2$ and hydrogen ion concentration in the blood, and a corresponding increase in the rate and volume of respirations occurs.

RATE OF RESPIRATION

Respiratory rate varies with age; it is more rapid in the young, decreasing with age. The rate at birth may be 40–70 respirations per minute, at 5 years of age it is approximately 25–30 per minute, at 10 years it is 20–22 per minute, and at 15 years of age and older it is 16–20 per minute.

COMPOSITION OF INSPIRED, EXPIRED AND ALVEOLAR AIR

INSPIRED AIR

Dry, inspired or atmospheric air at sea level is composed of nitrogen, oxygen and carbon dioxide in the following proportions:

oxygen	21%
carbon dioxide	0.04%
nitrogen	79%

Various quantities of water vapour, dust particles, and insignificant amounts of rare gases, such as argon, neon and ozone, may be present. Oxygen and carbon dioxide are the respiratory gases; nitrogen is not of concern since it is inert in the body.

EXPIRED AIR

This shows a reduction in oxygen and an increase in the carbon dioxide as compared with atmospheric air. It is a mixture of alveolar and atmospheric air from the passages above the alveoli. No exchange of gases is made in the air passages above the terminal respiratory units. This non-respiratory area is called the *anatomical dead space*. If any alveoli are not perfused by capillary blood flow, those alveolar spaces combined with the anatomical dead space compose the *physiological dead space*. If a person breathes through a tube, the dead space is increased; less of the inspired air reaches the alveoli.

ALVEOLAR AIR

Air that moves into the alveoli with each inspiration is a mixture of newly inspired air and air that moved into the dead space from the air sacs on previous expirations. In other words, as inspiration begins, alveolar air which had moved into the dead space on expiration is drawn back into the alveoli mixed with a portion of newly inspired air. Thus air entering the alveoli does not have exactly the same composition as inspired atmosphere air.

Alveolar ventilation may be increased by increasing the inspiratory volume and the frequency of respirations per minute. The latter will only be effective if the inspiratory volume is increased at the same time. Rapid shallow respirations simply ventilate the dead space and expend considerable muscular energy to no avail.

DIFFUSION AND TRANSPORT OF RESPIRATORY GASES

DIFFUSION

The diffusion component of pulmonary respiration is the interchange of oxygen and carbon dioxide across the alveolar and capillary membranes. Gases move rapidly from areas of higher to lower pressure. The rate of transfer of gases across the alveolar membrane is 'proportional to the tissue area and the difference in gas partial pressure between the two sides and inversely proportional to the tissue thickness' (Fick's law). The alveolar area is very large and thin and the tissue characteristics are ideal for promoting the transfer of gas. Gas characteristics relevant to diffusion include solubility and molecular weight; carbon dioxide diffuses more rapidly than oxygen because it is more soluble, even though the molecular weights of the two gases are similar. A pressure differential occurs between the oxygen in the alveolar air and that in the blood in the

Table 15.1 Partial pressures of respiratory gases.

	P_{O_2} (kPa)	P_{CO_2} (kPa)
Alveolar air	13.0 (100)	5.3 (40)
Venous blood	5.3 (40)	6.0 (46)
Arterial blood	12.6 (95)	5.3 (40)

Figures given in brackets are values for mmHg.

pulmonary capillaries and, as a result, oxygen moves from the alveoli into the blood. Carbon dioxide moves in the opposite direction for the same reason.

Blood enters the vast number of pulmonary capillaries with the P_{O_2} at about 5.3 kPa (40 mmHg) and the P_{CO_2} at approximately 6.0 kPa (46 mmHg). Alveolar air has a P_{O_2} of approximately 13.0 kPa (100 mmHg) and a P_{CO_2} of about 5.3 kPa (40 mmHg). As a result of the diffusion exchange that quickly takes place as the blood flows through the pulmonary capillaries, blood enters the pulmonary veins with a P_{O_2} of 12.6–13.0 kPa (95–100 mmHg) and a P_{CO_2} of approximately 5.3 kPa (40 mmHg) (Table 15.1 and Figure 15.5).

TRANSPORT OF RESPIRATORY GASES BY THE BLOOD

Oxygen. Very little oxygen is carried by the blood in solution, most of it enters red blood cells where it combines loosely with the haemoglobin to form the compound oxyhaemoglobin. If the haemoglobin has its normal complement of iron, each gram can carry 1.34 ml of oxygen and is about 97% saturated. The chemical process that produces oxyhaemoglobin is reversible so that as oxygen is used up by the tissues, more is made available by the dissociation of the unstable oxyhaemoglobin ($Hb + O_2 \leftrightarrows HbO_2$).

The rate at which haemoglobin combines with oxygen and the rate of dissociation of oxyhaemoglobin are influenced by the P_{O_2} and P_{CO_2} of the plasma (Figure 15.6). An increase in the P_{O_2} and a decrease in the P_{CO_2} hasten the formation of oxyhaemoglobin. Conversely, a decrease in the P_{O_2}, and an increase in the P_{CO_2}, as occurs in the systemic capillaries, promote the release of oxygen from haemoglobin; the saturation of haemoglobin declines. The pH of the blood has a significant effect on the dissociation of oxygen and haemoglobin. A decrease in the alkalinity below the normal (i.e. a decrease in the pH) promotes release of oxygen from the haemoglobin molecule. Body temperature also influences oxygen–haemoglobin dissociation; an elevated temperature also promotes the release of oxygen from oxyhaemoglobin.

Carbon dioxide. This is produced within the body by cellular metabolism and diffuses out of the cells through the tissue fluid into the blood, where it is carried in several forms. Only a very limited amount remains in solution in plasma; the larger proportion is carried in the form of hydrogen carbonate (HCO_3^-) and in

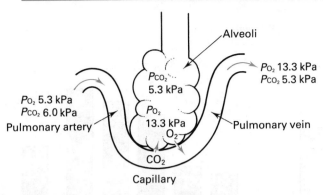

Figure 15.5 Oxygen and carbon dioxide exchange through alveolar–capillary membranes.

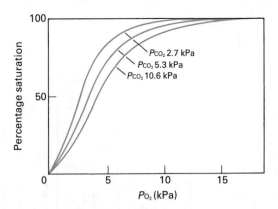

Figure 15.6 Oxyhaemoglobin dissociation curve.

combination with haemoglobin and plasma proteins (carbamino compounds). About two-thirds (70%) of the total blood carbon dioxide is carried as sodium bicarbonate ($NaHCO_3$) in the plasma and serves to maintain the normal blood alkalinity (pH 7.4). Carbon dioxide diffuses from the tissues into the plasma and on into the red blood cells where the enzyme carbonic anhydrase rapidly promotes a reaction with water to form carbonic acid.

$$CO_2 + H_2O \xrightarrow{\text{carbonic anhydrase}} H_2CO_3 \quad (1)$$

This is a very unstable acid and readily ionizes to hydrogen and hydrogen carbonate ions.

$$H_2CO_3 \rightarrow H^+ + HCO_3^- \quad (2)$$

If the hydrogen ion concentration were to increase unchecked within the red blood cell, this would disrupt its function; however, haemoglobin reacts with the H_2CO_3 to form potassium hydrogen carbonate and a reduced form of haemoglobin which is a much weaker acid than H_2CO_3. This reduced haemoglobin tightly binds its hydrogen ions; consequently, the hydrogen ion concentration remains stable.

$$
\begin{array}{ccccc}
H_2CO_3 & + & KHb & \rightleftharpoons & HHb & + & KHCO_3 \quad (3) \\
\text{Carbonic} & & \text{Potassium} & & \text{Reduced} & & \text{Potassium} \\
\text{acid} & & \text{haemoglobin} & & \text{haemoglobin} & & \text{hydrogen} \\
& & & & & & \text{carbonate}
\end{array}
$$

Any system such as this which acts to limit changes in hydrogen ion concentration (pH) is known as a *buffer*.

TISSUE RESPIRATION

The exchange of carbon dioxide and oxygen which takes place between the cells and the blood in the systemic capillaries throughout the body comprises tissue or internal respiration. The basis of the gaseous exchange is the pressure gradient of each of the respiratory gases. The PO_2 of the arterial blood when it enters the systemic capillaries is approximately 12.6 kPa (95 mmHg) and is much higher than that of the interstitial fluid, so oxygen diffuses from the plasma into the tissue fluid. The higher PO_2 of the tissue fluid results in a movement of oxygen into the cells. As the oxygen

tension is reduced in the plasma, the loosely combined oxyhaemoglobin dissociates to free oxygen. By the time the blood again reaches the pulmonary capillaries the oxyhaemoglobin has given up considerable oxygen.

The chemical activities of the cells (metabolism) produce carbon dioxide. Its concentration in the cell produces a pressure gradient that results in its movement into the tissue fluid. From here, because of the pressure difference, it moves into the capillary blood and gradually accumulates a higher concentration in the venous blood than that of alveolar air. This promotes the diffusion of carbon dioxide from the pulmonary capillary blood into alveolar air.

The respiratory system allows the pH of blood, or acid–base balance, to be regulated within the narrow limits necessary for normal metabolism. Consideration of equations (1) and (2) together leads to the following equation:

$$CO_2 + H_2O \rightleftharpoons H_2CO_3 \rightleftharpoons H^+ + HCO_3^- \quad (4)$$

In practice, sodium and potassium are closely involved with these reactions. Reduction of carbon dioxide levels is possible by increased ventilatory effort; this would have the effect of reducing H_2CO_3 levels, which in turn would reduce H^+ concentrations and hence make the blood less acid. This equation can proceed the other way so that metabolic changes which made the blood more acid (metabolic acidosis) can be corrected by increased respiratory effort removing carbon dioxide from the body.

If through disease the patient experienced respiratory difficulty which increased carbon dioxide levels, this would increase the acidity of the blood (respiratory acidosis). Conversely, changes which led to the person reducing carbon dioxide levels below normal, such as overbreathing or hyperventilation, would lead to the blood becoming too alkaline (respiratory alkalosis).

Respiratory Health Problems

Health problems affecting breathing and the respiratory system strike at the very root of human well-being and, as the student will quickly learn, are all too common in

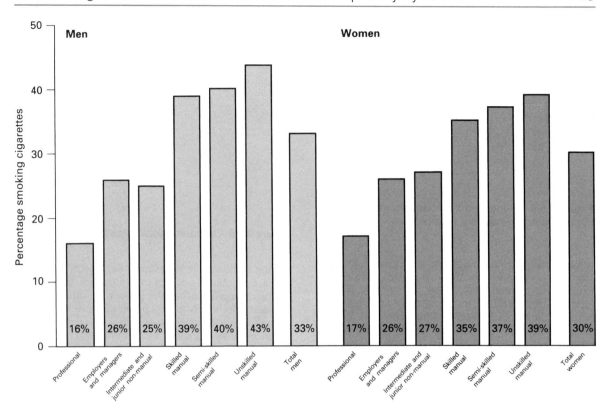

Figure 15.7 Cigarette smoking prevalence by sex and socioeconomic group: 1988. (Source: OPCS 1990.)

a wide range of patients. Illness affecting the respiratory system can range from acute, life-threatening episodes (e.g. an acute asthmatic attack) to long-term debilitating conditions such as chronic obstructive airways disease. Other systems of the body, particularly the cardiovascular system, are often involved. The consequences of such health problems are not only physical: severe psychological distress can also occur and be accompanied by major social disruption.

The prevalence of respiratory illness may be gauged from the fact that the Hospital In-Patient Enquiry (OPCS, 1985) reported that of a 1 in 10 sample of all hospital patients in 1985 in England and Wales, 46 023 were suffering from respiratory illness and a further 5499 were suffering from cancer of the bronchus or lung. This suggests that about half a million admissions per year involve disorders affecting the respiratory system if these figures are extrapolated to the whole hospital population.

Mortality statistics show that in 1986 there were 32 999 male and 30 053 female deaths in England and Wales from respiratory illness, while cancer of the bronchus and lung accounted for a further 25 235 male and 10 022 female deaths (OPCS, 1986). Cancer of the lung is the second most common neoplasm to cause death in women, after cancer of the breast (13 641 deaths in 1986). Current trends illustrate it is set to overtake cancer of the breast in the near future as the

gap between them has been steadily narrowing over the last 15 years. Within the non-malignant respiratory mortality figures there is a marked contrast between genders. Chronic obstructive airways disease (COAD) accounted for 20 148 male but only 9755 female deaths; however pneumonia and influenza show the reverse pattern: 10 320 male and 17 891 female deaths.

Table 15.2 Regional variation in mortality for respiratory illness.

Area	Sex	Cancer of lung and bronchus	Other respiratory illness
Wales	M	97	106
	F	89	102
Yorks	M	104	115
	F	109	108
North	M	129	112
	F	141	111
East Midlands	M	94	100
	F	89	91
East Anglia	M	86	83
	F	79	81
All South East	M	96	94
	F	101	98

Table 15.2 *Continued.*

Area	Sex	Cancer of lung and bronchus	Other respiratory illness
Greater London	M	107	107
	F	111	106
South West	M	80	74
	F	80	77
West Midlands	M	103	102
	F	83	101
North West	M	117	124
	F	117	122

Standardized ratio = 100 for England and Wales.
M, male; F, female.
Source: OPCS (1987).

Table 15.2 shows there are marked variations in respiratory illness in England and Wales, with the poorer industrial areas having a higher than expected death rate compared with the more prosperous areas, which are below the national norm; this clearly shows the effects of social factors on illness. The work of Black et al (1982), referred to earlier in this book, showed very strong links between social class and mortality rates for respiratory illness: the poorer a person, the more likely he or she was to die from a respiratory disease. It should also be remembered that lung disease may be associated with work in rural settings as well as urban environments, e.g. 'farmer's lung' (Kane, 1989).

Smoking is a well-known major cause of respiratory disease. Figure 15.7 illustrates the relationship between smoking and socioeconomic group; and while the overall proportion of smokers has reduced from 46% of the population aged 16 and over in 1972 to 32% in 1988 (OPCS, 1990), it is interesting to note that many more men than women have given up smoking. The figures reveal a fall from 52 to 33% for men during that period, but a more modest decline from 41 to 30% for women. The policy that the tobacco companies have pursued of targeting women with their advertising is paying off, with the result that we may soon have more women than men smoking, a major concern for health in general and women's health in particular.

While there is no dispute that stopping smoking will improve a person's respiratory function and general health, it must be realized that there are many subtle and interrelated social factors, other than a simple lifestyle change, that need to be tackled if the nurse is to promote good health in this field. Smoking and health is also discussed in Chapter 14.

Whatever the process of the respiratory disease it is possible to discern three principal ways in which the patient may be affected. These may be summarized as:

- Obstruction of varying degrees to the airway, which leads to ineffective airway clearance.
- Alterations in the normal breathing pattern.
- Disturbance of the normal gas exchange process.

INEFFECTIVE AIRWAY CLEARANCE

The patient faces the actual or potential problem of being unable to clear the airway in order that normal ventilation of the lungs may occur. The airway may be obstructed by either an inhaled foreign body, part of the patient's own anatomy (e.g. the tongue, if the patient is unconscious), constriction of part of the respiratory tree, or by body fluids such as blood, vomitus or secretions resulting from various pathological or non-pathological processes affecting the respiratory system.

Increased secretions are also found in response to most of the mechanisms listed above and, together with a cough, constitute the most common sign of ineffective airway clearance. Abnormal breath sounds are present and the person's respiratory rate, rhythm and depth change. Localized pain and discomfort may be present and the person experiences fatigue and lack of energy. The work of breathing increases and dyspnoea may be present (see Table 15.4).

COUGH

A cough is a sudden, expulsive expiration for the purpose of removing an irritant from the air passages. It is a protective reflex that indicates the presence of some irritation in the tract.

Mechanism

The cough mechanism involves stimulation of receptors in the mucous membrane of the bronchial tubes, trachea, larynx or pharynx or stimulation at a point along the vagus nerve. The impulses travel via afferent fibres of the vagus nerve or the glossopharyngeal nerve to the cough centre, formed by a group of neurones in the medulla of the brain. Responsive impulses are initiated in the centre and travel to the respiratory muscles and the larynx, producing, in succession, a quick inhalation, closure of the glottis, relaxation of the diaphragm and contraction of the abdominal and internal intercostal muscles to increase the intrathoracic and intrapulmonary pressures. The latter is exerted against the closed glottis which opens suddenly, releasing a forceful gust-like expiration. A review of the sequence of activities shows three phases: inspiratory, compressive and expulsive. During the compressive phase, pressure is placed on the alveoli and their secretions are moved into the small bronchial tubes. The increased velocity of the airflow in the expiratory phase results in secretions being expelled from the air passages.

The cough is generally an involuntary response, although some voluntary control may be exerted to inhibit it or produce it. If a cough is unproductive, it may be helpful to instruct the patient to make an effort to inhibit the cough in order to conserve his energy and prevent exhaustion. In other instances, the patient may be required to initiate a series of coughs at regular intervals to prevent the accumulation of secretions in the air passages. The strength or vigor of a cough is determined by the volume of the precough inspiration, the strength of the compression and the rate of expulsion of air.

Causes

The origin of the cough stimulus may be within the respiratory tract or may be extrinsic to it. *Intrinsic stimuli* include inflammation, secretions, fluid, scar tissue which causes traction on the nerve endings, bronchial hyperreactivity, new growths, inhaled or aspirated particles of dust, irritating gases and foreign bodies and very cold or very hot air. *Extrinsic stimuli* are abnormal conditions in neighbouring structures which exert pressure on some area of the tracheo-bronchial tree. Pleurisy and cancer of the oesophagus are examples of extrinsic causes.

Implications for nursing

A persistent cough should always be considered as an indication of something abnormal that requires investigation.

SECRETIONS

Normally, the adult produces about 100 ml of mucus daily. This is increased when there is some irritation in the air passages and may change in colour and consistency. The expectoration of blood occurs in many respiratory disorders and in varying degrees of severity. There may be only a slight streaking of the mucus with blood or there may be expectoration of frank blood. The latter is referred to as *haemoptysis*. Blood in the sputum is commonly associated with inflammatory conditions and lesions which cause erosion and necrosis of the tissues and blood vessels, such as bronchitis, pneumonia, tuberculosis, carcinoma and pulmonary infarction.

BREATH SOUNDS

Normal respirations present characteristic sounds as air enters and leaves the lower respiratory tract. Absence of such sounds or the accompaniment of other sounds may indicate excessive secretions in an area or constriction or blockage of a section of the system.

Vesicular breath sounds are heard in normal respirations. They are a soft, low pitched sound and are heard over all the lung areas except over the apex of the right lung. This is because of the proximity of the large bronchial tubes to the chest wall. The inspiratory phase of a vesicular sound is longer and louder than the expiratory phase. The differences may be attributed to the movement of inspiratory air into progressively smaller air passages (and vice versa in the case of the air being exhaled).

Bronchial breath sounds are associated with a short inspiratory phase and a longer expiratory phase. The sounds are higher pitched and equally loud in both phases. They are abnormal, and indicate some disease process such as pneumonia in the lung.

Adventitious sounds are abnormal sounds superimposed on breath sounds as a result of a disease process within the tracheobronchial tree and/or lungs. These include crackles, wheezes and pleural friction rub.

Crackles may also be called *rales* or *crepitations* and are described as fizzing or popping sounds created by the equalization of airway pressures during the explosive reopening of previously closed terminal respiratory units.

Wheezes (rhonchi) are whistling, musical sounds associated with spasm of the bronchial walls and tend to occur on expiration.

Stridor is a distinctive sound heard on inspiration when there is partial airway obstruction; a totally obstructed airway is usually silent as there is no air movement to produce any sound.

Pleural friction rub is a characteristic rough, grating sound produced when inflamed roughened pleurae rub against each other on inspiration. It becomes audible during the latter part of the inspiratory phase.

CHEST PAIN

Pain associated with respiratory disorders originates mainly in the upper air passages or in the pleurae. Inflammation of the trachea or bronchial tubes causes a burning 'raw' type of pain which is not affected by respirations but becomes worse on coughing. Pleural pain tends to be localized to one side of the chest and is due to the stretching of the affected pleura. It is sharp and stabbing on inspiration, causing the patient to take shallow breaths.

Pain originating in the chest wall itself is usually a result of trauma, e.g. a fractured rib.

RELATED FACTORS

Maintenance of a patent airway is dependent upon the normal defence mechanisms of the upper and lower airways, including the warming, humidification and filtering of inspired air. Effective clearance of the lower airways requires a functioning mucociliary system, alveolar macrophage activity and an effective cough.

Factors which make it more difficult to maintain a clear airway include increased production of respiratory secretions due to infection; thickening of secretions with dehydration; ineffective cough mechanisms; fatigue and decreased energy; confusion and disorientation; and trauma or impairment to the airway structures as seen in persons with artificial airways (see Table 15.5). Thompson (1990) points out that many of these factors are associated with immobility, emphasizing the need for regular changes of position and breathing exercises to prevent the serious respiratory complications that may occur if a patient is immobile.

Assessment of the Person with Ineffective Airway Clearance

Assessment of normal and altered respiratory status begins with an overview of the individual's general appearance followed by a specific health history and examination of respiratory function.

GENERAL APPEARANCE

On first meeting the patient the nurse should take an overview of his or her general appearance in order to gain a feeling for the overall health status of the patient. The facial expression might give clues as to mood; colouring should be noted to check for signs of a flushed, red appearance that might indicate pyrexia. Cyanosis (a bluish discoloration around the lips that is a late sign of severe respiratory failure) may be noted. The patient's posture should be observed to note if it indicates a sense of ease and relaxation or anxiety and tenseness, associated perhaps with difficulty in breathing.

HEALTH HISTORY

The nurse conducts the health history to obtain information about the person's respiratory function, past history related to respiratory disorders and treatment programme, in order to identify factors which contribute to the promotion as well as any impairment of airway clearance. The information the nurse obtains from the patient and/or family members includes:

- The symptoms which prompted the patient to seek health care.
- A description of the precipitating events.
- Duration of the symptoms.
- The person's perception of the causes and implications of the symptoms.

The symptoms manifested by the patient may include:

- *Cough.* The presence, frequency and depth of the cough are noted as well as the nature and sound of the cough. It may be hard and racking, croupy, hacking, shallow, deep and rattling or may have a whooping sound. The cough may be worse at certain times of the day and the patient should be asked if pain accompanies the cough. It is noted if the cough is productive of sputum. Finally, it is important to assess the effect of the cough on the patient; does the exertion exhaust the patient, create anxiety or disrupt sleep or daily activities?
- *Sputum.* It is necessary to determine the consistency (mucous, watery, purulent, tenacious, frothy, caseous or blood-streaked), colour, amount and if the amount has increased recently.
- *Breathlessness.* The patient may complain of breathlessness and the history should reveal if it occurs with usual activity, increased effort or when at rest, and whether it interferes with daily activities and sleep pattern. It should be noted if the patient's speech is audible, clear and effortless, or if the responses are weak, short and jerky phrases with apparent effort. The patient is questioned as to what was done to prevent or modify the breathlessness and if the suggested actions were effective in preventing or alleviating the breathlessness.
- *Fever.* The patient may have a fever and give a history of having night sweats.
- *Pain and discomfort* may be associated with the chest, breathing activities or coughing; the nature, severity, duration and precipitating factors are noted.

The patient's understanding of the respiratory problems should be carefully explored. If the patient is severely distressed, questions should be kept to a minimum and if possible asked in such a way that they may be answered by a nod or shake of the head. More detailed discussions may be more appropriate later when the patient's breathing is easier.

Observation of whether the airway is patent, followed by assessment of respiratory rate, depth and rhythm, may identify serious problems immediately, and in all patients provides a vital basic record which can be used as a baseline to monitor subsequent progress. The tongue of an unconscious patient may, for example, block the airway. If the brain is deprived of oxygen, serious damage occurs within 3 minutes. Any obstruction to the upper airway is potentially fatal within minutes, hence the importance of always beginning an assessment by checking that the upper airway is clear. Only then may breathing be assessed. To avoid the patient being conscious of having the breathing monitored, which may affect the rate, it is suggested that the respiratory rate is taken immediately after the pulse, while still holding the patient's wrist.

ASSESSMENT OF RESPIRATION

The healthy adult breathes 12 to 18 times per minute at rest, although this rate is much quicker in infants, 40 breaths per minute being typical of a new born baby. A rapid respiratory rate (tachypnoea) in an adult may indicate anxiety, pain, pyrexia, metabolic disorders (e.g. acidosis) or may be the result of the body attempting to compensate for inadequate oxygenation due to a wide range of cardiovascular and respiratory disorders (e.g. heart failure or shock). Slower breathing rates are associated with sleep or with disorders and drugs that depress the respiratory centre, e.g. narcotics.

Observation of the thorax should also be carried out to note its shape, size and symmetry, in addition to forming an impression about the amount of effort involved in breathing. Long-standing respiratory disease leads to a characteristic 'pigeon chest' shape. Unequal chest movements (i.e. one part of the chest wall appears to move in the opposite direction from the rest of the chest wall) indicate ribs fractured in two places, known as a flail segment. This is potentially fatal as the ensuing lung collapse that occurs may make it impossible for the patient to achieve sufficient ventilation to be compatible with life (p. 409).

Although respiratory rhythm is normally regular, whatever the rate, a striking exception is provided by Cheyne–Stokes breathing: typically, a brain-damaged, unconscious patient appears to stop breathing for periods of up to 20 seconds (apnoea) before taking very deep breaths and hyperventilating. This continues in a cyclical pattern and is thought to occur in patients whose breathing has become controlled by Po_2 rather than Pco_2. The respiratory centre appears to be less sensitive to changes in Po_2 than it is to changes in Pco_2; consequently, after hyperventilation which raises Po_2, a lengthy period of apnoea ensues while Po_2 drops low enough to stimulate breathing again.

One final method of assessment which the nurse may

use is to measure peak flow rates for the patient. This is a test of the maximum rate of exhalation a patient can achieve (in litres per minute) by the patient blowing as hard as possible into a simple instrument. It assesses the degree of impairment in respiratory function due to airway narrowing in diseases such as asthma.

MEDICAL DIAGNOSTIC PROCEDURES

The nurse may be required to assist with the examination of the patient's chest. Medical staff will also wish to carry out a series of tests and investigations to help them arrive at their medical diagnosis. If they are to be able to assist and support the patient through these procedures, nursing staff need to understand what is happening to the patient and why. Luke (1989) has provided a useful summary of respiratory investigations.

RADIOLOGICAL EXAMINATION

X-ray of the chest. Radiological studies of the chest may reveal a lesion in the respiratory tract or thoracic cavity, its location, the size of the area involved and something of the nature of the lesion. They also provide information about the mediastinum, the structure of the thorax, the size of the heart and aorta and the level of the diaphragm.

The procedure is explained to the patient and clothing is removed to the waist to prevent the possibility of objects such as buttons obscuring the X-ray films. If the patient is wearing an identification tag or a necklace, it is also removed; a gown is provided. The patient is advised to take a deep breath and hold it while the X-ray is being taken in order to ensure the lungs are fully expanded and that there is no movement to blur the image formed on the film. The patient is then told to breathe normally.

BACTERIOLOGICAL AND CYTOLOGICAL STUDIES

Specimens of sputum, throat secretions, pleural fluid or tissue may be examined for pathogenic organisms and malignant cells.

Sputum is examined microscopically in a smear or by culture for disease organisms, bronchial casts, eosinophils and cancer cells. Tests are also done to identify the antimicrobial drug(s) (usually antibiotics) to which the infecting organisms present in the sputum are sensitive. This denotes the drugs that will be effective for the patient.

The sputum specimen should be collected first thing in the morning, since the secretions that accumulate during the night may have a higher concentration of organisms. The mouth should be clean and free of residual food particles. The patient is given a small sputum container and is instructed to cough deeply to raise the sputum from the lungs. When the specimen is obtained, the container is labelled and delivered to the laboratory. Sputum specimens may be collected during or following postural drainage. They may also be obtained by tracheal aspiration if the patient is uncon-

scious or too weak to cough. The sputum specimen container is attached to the suction catheter, which allows the sputum to flow directly into the container.

Bacteriological studies may also be made of secretions from the *throat* and *pleura*.

Skin tests for tuberculosis. A tuberculin skin test is used in the diagnosis of tuberculosis and to identify those who have been exposed. The test involves an intradermal injection of tuberculin bacillus extract using a syringe and needle (Mantoux test) or a multiple puncture apparatus (Heaf, Tine or Mono-Vac). Tuberculin extract preparations include purified protein derivative (PPD) and old tuberculin (OT) which are available in several strengths. The forearm is the usual site of innoculation. Results are interpreted in 48–72 hours. A positive reaction is characterized by an area of induration of 10 mm or greater.

BLOOD STUDIES: LEUCOCYTE COUNT

A total and differential count of the white blood cells may be ordered since this information may be useful in confirming infection and distinguishing between an acute disease, such as pneumonia, and a chronic one, such as tuberculosis. A leucocytosis, with the increase being mainly in the polymorphonuclear granulocytes is generally associated with an acute infection. In chronic infection there is usually only a slight increase above the normal in the total number of leucocytes, and it is usually the lymphocytes that account for any increase. The eosinophils are increased in allergic asthma. The normal leucocyte count value is $4.0–11.0 \times 10^9$ per litre.

Nursing Intervention for the Person with Ineffective Airway Clearance

The *goal* is to maintain a patent airway. This may be measured by the following criteria:

- The person's respiratory rate, depth and rhythm will be within normal range.
- Abnormal breath sounds will be absent.
- The person will demonstrate effective deep breathing and coughing.

The maintenance of a patent airway so that air can reach the lungs requires passages free of foreign objects and secretions. The removal of a foreign object from the upper respiratory tract is discussed on p. 408. When mechanical obstruction occurs, an artificial airway must be established (see p. 384).

REMOVAL OF SECRETIONS

The methods used to promote the removal of secretions include (1) coughing, (2) suction, (3) chest physiotherapy, (4) postural drainage, (5) hydration, and (6) humidification.

Coughing

Coughing is a primary defence mechanism of the lung for the removal of secretions from the trachea and bronchial tree. The retention of pulmonary secretions predisposes to infection, atelectasis and reduced alveolar ventilation and gas exchange. Therapeutic coughing has been shown to increase mucocilliary clearance, increase the volume of sputum expectorated and improve airway function (Kirilloff, 1985). It has been emphasized that coughing is an expiratory manoeuvre that produces alveolar deflation, a reduction in lung volume and increased pleural pressure which reduces venous return to the heart. The purpose of the cough manoeuvre should be explained to the patient and instruction is given as to how to cough effectively. The patient assumes the sitting position, if possible, and a deep breath is taken through the mouth. The patient is instructed to hold his breath to the count of three, contract his abdominal muscles and forcibly exhale. Effectiveness of the cough depends on the volume of air and the force of the expiration. Repetition of the cough procedure helps the patient to expel the secretions that were mobilized by the initial cough.

Staged coughing is taught to patients with cardiovascular disorders who cannot tolerate the increases in vascular pressure from forceful coughs, and to patients with severe airflow limitation who cannot generate a full, effective cough. It involves a slow deep inspiration and then the patient is asked to cough in three short 'bursts'. Short coughs use less energy and are less likely to cause wheezing or airway collapse. Coughing is performed clinically only when the presence of audible crackles and gurgling sounds are demonstrated so the patient is not fatigued unnecessarily.

If the patient has difficulty in producing a cough, stimulation of the pharynx with the tip of a suction catheter may precipitate the desired response. Coughing by the surgical patient may be facilitated by the application of firm support over the incision to lessen the pain. 'Huff' coughing is another technique that is believed to facilitate mobilization of secretions while stabilizing the airways and preventing airway collapse. The patient is instructed to breathe in as much air as possible and to exhale sharply and rapidly while whispering the word 'huff' two to three times. The glottis remains open during this manoeuvre and explosive forces are avoided. This procedure is contraindicated during acute asthmatic attacks.

During coughing the patient is observed for signs of fatigue and allowed to rest when indicated.

Suction

This is a very important procedure used to remove secretions from the oropharynx, trachea and bronchi (Allen, 1988). A sterile disposable catheter, connected to a wall source of negative pressure, or to a suction machine, may be gently passed directly into the oropharynx or trachea or through an endotracheal or tracheostomy tube into the trachea or proximal portion of either bronchus. The dominant hand of the nurse is gloved prior to picking up the catheter.

Suction of the oropharynx. This involves the use of a catheter with an open-tip or a whistle tip which is connected to a tube leading to the source of negative pressure. A suction catheter has a 'built in' vent (thumb valve) that is normally open until a finger or thumb is placed over the opening. The patient is informed of what is to be done and its purpose. The catheter may be passed through the mouth or a nostril to the pharyngeal region. When the tip of the catheter is in position, a finger or thumb is placed over the vent to establish suction. The catheter is gently rotated and withdrawn.

The introduction of the catheter frequently initiates the cough reflex, resulting in the removal of deeper secretions in addition to those in the pharynx.

Intratracheal suction. Deeper suction is used to remove pulmonary secretions or aspirated material (food or vomitus). The procedure requires considerable skill and is usually performed by critical care nurses via a tracheostomy or endotracheal tube.

Chest physiotherapy

This is used to loosen secretions so that they can be coughed up. Percussion or clapping and vibration of the chest are the manual procedures used. There is currently no data to indicate the effectiveness of chest percussion and vibration (Kirilloff, 1985). These techniques are used along with therapeutic coughing and postural drainage. The affected lung areas requiring chest physiotherapy are identified by auscultation or chest X-ray. Chest percussion may be used routinely over the lung bases or the complete chest during the postoperative period, or if the patient is immobilized over a long period, especially when there is a history of obstructive pulmonary disease or repeated chest infections.

Chest percussion is applied by clapping the chest with cupped hands over the area to be drained. The chest wall is struck rhythmically using both hands rapidly and alternately with uniform force for 1 or 2 minutes. The therapist's shoulders are relaxed, the wrists are flexed and extended in rhythmical movements producing a hollow sound. Obviously, surgical or injured areas are avoided, as are bony prominences, kidney areas and female breasts.

Chest vibration may be used after 30–40 seconds of percussion or as an alternative in patient's pulmonary physiotherapy. The procedure is performed by placing one hand flat over the other on the chest area to be vibrated and, while exerting moderate pressure, uniform vibratory movements are made to dislodge and mobilize secretions. The vibration is done to coincide with an exhalation, and pressure is relieved during inhalation. It is repeated three or four times.

Chest physiotherapy is usually used in conjunction with deep breathing and coughing. Postural drainage may also be used as an adjunct.

Postural drainage

This requires the patient to be placed in certain positions to promote the elimination of pulmonary secretions. The position assumed initiates gravitational movement of fluid and mucus to a level of the tracheobronchial tree that favours its removal by coughing or suctioning. As cited above, postural drainage may be accompanied by percussion and/or vibration to dislodge the secretions in the lung segment requiring drainage.

The position assumed depends upon the lung segment or particular area to be drained. To promote the movement of secretions out of *upper lobes*, the patient is placed in a sitting position and alternately leans forward and to each side to drain different segments. For drainage of the *middle lobe, lower lobes* and *lingula* (the small projection from the lower portion of the upper lobe of the left lung), various side-lying, prone and supine positions are used. The patient may be horizontal or, to remove accumulations in lower segments, may be tilted so that the head and chest are lower (Table 15.3).

An explanation is made before commencing chest physiotherapy and/or postural drainage so that the patient will know what to expect and that he or she will be required to cough. The patient's condition and the treatments being used (e.g. intravenous infusion) may necessitate modification of some positions, but the nurse should be familiar with the one appropriate to the drainage of various lung segments. The patient is made as comfortable as possible in whatever position is used; for example, in the lateral positions at a 45° angle a pillow is placed in front of the patient to provide support.

The treatment usually lasts for 20–30 minutes, if possible. The patient is then encouraged to cough, and suction may also be necessary to assist in elimination of the dislodged secretions.

Hydration therapy

Liquefaction and raising of respiratory secretions are facilitated by a generous fluid intake as well as by humidification of the air. The nurse assesses the patient's hydrational status, fluid intake and output, and the existence of cardiovascular, renal or other disorders that might contribute to fluid overload. The elderly are usually unable to tolerate large increases in fluid intake. The nurse helps the patient to adjust the fluid intake to an optimum level. Oral intake of fluids is preferable but critically ill patients in hospital may receive intravenous fluid therapy.

Humidification

Normally the inspired air is adequately moistened within the respiratory tract by moisture evaporated from the mucosal surface and the cilia. If the mucosa is irritated and depleted of water, the mucus becomes viscous and crusted, and ciliary activity is depressed. The ensuing retention of the tenacious secretions increases airway resistance and promotes infection.

Various methods are used to humidify the air or gas to be inspired. The method used depends mainly upon: (1) whether or not the upper airway is bypassed: (2) the degree of dehydration of the mucosa and secretions: (3) the equipment available, and (4) the flow rate of oxygen administration. Humidification is not required when oxygen is administered at low flow rates (e.g. 3 or 4 l/min) or by Venturi mask.

EVALUATION

Effective airway clearance is demonstrated by a patent airway. The individual's respirations are regular, rhythmic, and of normal rate and depth. Normal breath sounds are heard on auscultation, and breathing is quiet and effortless. The patient is able to demonstrate the techniques of deep breathing and coughing. Sputum is absent or scant, and thin and colourless in nature.

Table 15.3 Postural drainage positions.

Areas to be drained	Posture
Apical lobes	
Apical segment	Sitting position; patient alternately leans forward and to each side
Anterior segment	Supine position
Posterior segment	Right/left lateral, about 45° angle
Lingula	
Superior and inferior segments	Foot of bed elevated 35–40 cm; turned slightly to right
Middle lobe	
Medial and lateral segments	Foot of bed elevated 35–40 cm; turned slightly to left
Lower lobes	
Superior segment	Prone position with hips elevated on a pillow
Medial basal segment	Right lateral with hips elevated or foot of bed elevated 40 cm
Anterior basal segment	Supine position with hips elevated or foot of bed elevated 40 cm
Lateral basal segment	Lateral right/left with hips elevated or foot of bed elevated 40 cm
Posterior basal segment	Prone position with hips elevated or foot of bed elevated 40 cm

Ineffective Airway Clearance Related to Infection of the Respiratory Tract

Most adults experience several episodes of respiratory tract infection annually. Clearance of secretions is the most common health problem seen in patients with respiratory infections. The severity of the problem ranges from an annoying, watery nasal discharge experienced with rhinitis to a productive cough, the accumulation of secretions in the lower airways and impairment of gas exchange in patients with pneumonia.

RESPIRATORY INFECTIONS

RHINITIS

Rhinitis is an acute or chronic inflammation of the nasal mucous membrane caused by infection or an allergic reaction. It may also result from nasal polyps or a deviated nasal septum. Symptoms are those of the common cold. The nasal mucosa is red and oedematous and there is a clear nasal discharge which becomes purulent with some infections. The individual breathes through the mouth (see below for treatment).

SINUSITIS

Sinusitis is an acute or chronic inflammation of the sinus cavities resulting from infection or allergies. It is accompanied by rhinitis because the mucous membranes of the sinuses are continuous with those of the nose. As secretions accumulate in the sinuses feelings of heaviness, discomfort and headache develop. General malaise and fever accompany the local symptoms when infection is present.

Treatment of rhinitis and sinusitis is usually symptomatic. Anti-inflammatory drugs such as aspirin or a decongestant may be taken by adults to decrease inflammation and secretions and promote comfort. Fluid intake is increased, a balanced diet eaten and adequate rest obtained. If the problem persists or becomes severe, a general practitioner's advice should be sought.

PHARYNGITIS (SORE THROAT)

Pharyngitis is a common respiratory inflammatory disorder caused by allergies, viral or bacterial infections. Symptoms include dryness, soreness of the throat, difficulty swallowing, fever and general malaise. Sore throats of bacterial origin are treated with antibiotic therapy. Other measures include rest, increased fluid intake, warm saline gargles and mild analgesics.

TONSILLITIS

Tonsillitis is usually of bacterial origin and is most common in children and adolescents. Swabs are taken of the throat to identify the causative agent and antibiotic therapy is prescribed for acute tonsillitis.

Symptoms include a sore throat, difficulty swallowing, chills, fever and malaise. The white blood cell count will be elevated. Complications include acute otitis media, acute rhinitis and sinusitis and peritonsillar abscess. Tonsillitis usually resolves spontaneously in 5–7 days. Acute peritonsillar abscess (quinsy) requires treatment with antibiotics, and incision and drainage of the abscess may be necessary. Adequate analgesia (e.g. pethidine or papaveretum for adults) should be administered. Airway obstruction can be life threatening if treatment is not instituted promptly.

Surgical removal of tonsils and adenoids is usually indicated only when the individual experiences recurrent, incapacitating infections.

PNEUMONIA

Pneumonia is the term generally used to indicate infection and inflammation of lung tissue. Pneumonitis is a synonymous term but is used less frequently than pneumonia. Guyton (1986) defines pneumonia as 'any inflammatory condition of the lung in which the alveoli are usually filled with fluid and blood cells'.

Pneumonia caused by pneumococci is a common type of pneumonia, but other bacteria or viruses may be the cause. Non-bacterial and non-viral causes include: aspiration of gastric secretions, food, fluids or lipoids (aspiration pneumonia), and retention of secretions, which occurs frequently in the immobilized elderly or debilitated individual (hypostatic pneumonia).

It should be remembered that the most common respiratory complication faced by individuals with HIV infection is *Pneumocystis carinii* pneumonia (PCP). The individual with PCP may be critically ill and is likely to present with a dry, non-productive cough, shortness or breath, high fever, and night sweats. PCP may be difficult to diagnose as the individual may have a normal chest X-ray and breath sounds. Bilateral infiltrates are likely to be present in an abnormal chest X-ray. Diagnosis is usually made by cultures obtained by bronchoscopy. PCP is readily treated with antibiotic regimens. Combinations of drugs such as trimethoprim sulphamethoxazole (TMP/SMX) and dapsone or pentamidine may be used to treat the infection. These drugs must be used with caution because of their side-effects. For example TMP/SMX may cause severe rash. Pentamidine given intravenously can cause nausea, orthostatic hypotension and hypoglycaemia. Prophylactic regimens are also effective in preventing PCP. Prophylaxsis is available to patients using a decreased amount of the above medications. Pentamidine when used for prophylaxis is given in aerosol form, generally with a hand-held nebulizer. Prophylactic regimens are usually initiated when the patient's T_4 count drops below 200 000 cells/l. The patient is taught to assess for signs of infection and learns to monitor respiratory rate and function. Nursing care is similar as for other patients experiencing respiratory impairment.

Manifestations

The onset, symptoms and course of disease vary with

different types of pneumonia. Infection of the alveoli results in their filling with inflammatory exudate (plasma, blood cells, pathological organisms and cellular debris) that readily overflows into other alveoli, extending the infection. A whole lobe of lung tissue may become consolidated or the consolidation may be patchy; pulmonary ventilation and diffusion are impaired, and the oxygen tension of the blood is reduced to below normal. The Pco_2 level generally remains normal or may be decreased. The increased respiratory rate caused by the initial increase in the Pco_2 results in increased amounts of carbon dioxide being excreted by the normal areas of the lung. In a few days the exudate becomes more liquid and may be gradually eliminated from the alveoli by expectoration and absorption. This process is referred to as *resolution*. The disease may clear up with dramatic rapidity when specific antibacterial drugs are administered. It may run a course of 5–10 days; untreated, it may rapidly prove terminal.

The onset of some infective pneumonias may be very sudden; they frequently begin with a chill, followed by fever (e.g. pneumococcal and Friedlaender's). Hypostatic, staphylococcal and atypical (viral) pneumonias have a gradual onset (less abrupt than the pneumococcal type). The last two may be associated at the onset with upper respiratory infection.

The pulse rate and respirations increase. The latter may be shallow and accompanied by an audible grunt characteristic of pleuritic pain. The nostrils flare on inspiration and the face may be flushed. Cyanosis of the lips, tongue and nail beds may develop. The patient's cough may be hacking, painful and unproductive at first; later, it becomes less painful and is productive. In bronchopneumonia the sputum is tenacious, blood-streaked and mucopurulent. In pneumococcal pneumonia, the sputum is usually rust-coloured and becomes purulent as resolution takes place. In Friedlaender's pneumonia the pulmonary secretions are dark, reddish-brown and very tenacious.

The patient experiences general malaise, weakness, headache and aching pains. The leucocyte count is elevated in some types (e.g. pneumococcal, staphylococcal) and normal or below normal in others (e.g. atypical). Sputum examination and culture and blood culture are used to identify the causative organism. Specific antimicrobial therapy is determined by culture and sensitivity tests.

PULMONARY TUBERCULOSIS

Tuberculosis is an infectious disease that is caused by the tubercle bacillus. The organism may attack other tissues in the body, but in Europe and North America the lungs are most frequently the primary site of invasion.

Infection is usually by inhalation of droplets bearing tubercle bacilli. The droplets have been expelled into the air by the sneezing or coughing of a person with active disease.

Tuberculosis is a disease of poverty, readily taking advantage of those with weakened resistance due to poor nutrition and general health. Social conditions therefore play a large part in determining a person's susceptibility to the disease. Homeless persons and the elderly, together with members of ethnic communities originating from the Indian subcontinent, are perhaps most at risk in the UK. Redfearn (1989) illustrates this latter point with statistics from the Blackburn area of Lancashire which witnessed substantial immigration in the 1960s. In 1960 45 new cases of tuberculosis were notified amongst Caucasians, but there was only one non-Caucasian case. In 1980 the figures were 22 and 103 new cases respectively. It is estimated that some 6500 new cases of tuberculosis occur each year in England and Wales (Redfearn, 1989), while mortality statistics for 1986 indicate that 471 people (mainly elderly) died of tuberculosis in England and Wales.

Disease process

Small, rounded nodules, with a tendency toward central necrosis, develop at the site of tissue invasion by the bacilli. These are referred to as *tubercles* and are composed of lung tissue cells, leucocytes, other phagocytic cells, fibroblasts and tubercle bacilli. If the body defences are strong enough to destroy the organisms the lesion heals and may calcify.

In some instances, the reproduction of the tubercle bacilli may be minimal; a few continue to survive within the tubercle but remain confined and dormant. This person, having been infected and still harbouring live bacilli, will show a positive tuberculin test in approximately 2–10 weeks after the initial infection; defensive cells have become sensitized and tend to inhibit or slow up the growth of tubercle bacilli. At a later date, if resistance is lowered, the reproduction of the tubercle bacilli may be accelerated and active disease develops. When the bacilli continue to multiply, the tubercle necroses centrally, producing soft, caseous material that may eventually be discharged from the tubercle, leaving a cavity. This caseous discharge is highly infective.

The initial infection does not affect pulmonary function. The later stages of tuberculosis, which are becoming again more common in Britain and Europe, produce systemic and local symptoms. The constitutional symptoms are vague and non-specific; they include lassitude, fatigue, malaise, loss of appetite and weight, fever (usually low grade) in the latter part of the day, tachycardia and night sweats. Symptoms produced by the local disease process at the site of the lesion in the lungs are cough, sputum, haemoptysis, dyspnoea and chest pain if the pleura is involved.

Diagnostic investigation

The investigation of a patient for pulmonary tuberculosis involves tuberculin testing, chest X-ray and bacteriological examination of sputum (see p. 376).

Treatment

Patients remain at home and continue to work and live normal and useful lives during the course of their treatment. The principal factors in the plan of patient care are prolonged chemotherapy, rest, and patient and family education.

The administration of specific antimicrobial drugs over a long period of time has proved very successful in the prevention and treatment of tuberculosis. Preventive therapy for susceptible individuals usually involves the administration of isoniazid for a period of 6 months to 2 years. Treatment regimens for individuals with tuberculosis initially include two, three or four antitubercular drugs. After several months of treatment this may be decreased to two or three drugs. It is important that the individual adhere to the drug programme for the prescribed duration of up to 2 years. The nurse should be familiar with the treatment plan and with the actions and possible side-effects of the drugs so that adverse reactions can be recognized early and the patient can be taught what to look for and what to do if side-effects occur.

- *Isoniazid.* This is taken orally. This drug is usually well tolerated. Patients are instructed to report any signs of hepatitis, such as fatigue, weakness, malaise, nausea, vomiting or anorexia, to the nurse and doctor. Malnourished persons are at risk of developing neuritis.
- *Ethambutol.* This is given orally. It inhibits the synthesis of RNA and cellular phosphate, and so destroys and arrests the reproduction of the tubercle bacilli. Patients receiving ethambutol should be assessed for visual acuity prior to treatment and monitored for changes.
- *Rifampicin.* This is taken orally 1 hour before or 2 hours after the ingestion of food to promote maximum absorption. However, the adverse gastrointestinal effects of heartburn, epigastric distress, nausea and diarrhoea may be minimized by administering the drug with food. Patients should be helped to establish a routine that best suits their responses. Patients should be aware that rifampicin may impart a red-orange colour to the urine, faeces, sputum, sweat and tears. Soft contact lenses may become permanently discoloured. The patient's liver function is monitored regularly.
- *Streptomycin.* This antibiotic may be administered intramuscularly for a shorter period than the other antitubercular preparations—usually not longer than 4 or 6 months. Serious side-effects of this drug are damage of the auditory nerves and consequent loss of hearing.
- *Para-aminosalicylic acid* (PAS). This drug was one of the earliest antitubercular preparations used but is poorly tolerated for prolonged administration. Side-effects include anorexia, nausea, vomiting, diarrhoea, chills and fever and skin rash.
- *Pyrazinamide.* This drug is often added during the first 2 months of therapy. It occasionally causes hepatitis, hyperuricaemia, gastrointestinal disturbances or arthralgia.

Resistant strains of the tubercle bacillus can develop in time; however, recent reports from the USA indicate that HIV patients may be more likely to develop a drug-resistant tuberculosis (Nursing Standard, 1990). In this report the frequencies of resistance to isoniazid were found to be 7.0%, to rifampicin 4.1%, and to a combination of both drugs 5.7%. It was found that almost all the rifampicin-resistant patients were HIV positive and all but one were reported by the same medical centre. Drug-resistant tuberculosis within an already immunosuppressed group of people is a cause for major concern and shows the importance of all staff pursuing vigorous infection control methods to prevent further spread of the disease.

In view of the lengthy courses of chemotherapy required to treat tuberculosis, there is a significant risk of patients failing to take their medication correctly or simply stopping altogether. Close supervision and reinforcement of teaching about the importance of completing the full course are therefore required in the community care setting.

CLINICAL SITUATION: MR FLEMING, AN ELDERLY MAN WITH PNEUMONIA

Mr Fleming was an emergency admission to the medical unit with a diagnosis of right lower lobe pneumonia. Upon admission, a thorough nursing history and assessment were completed. Further data was obtained from his daughter and from the results of diagnostic tests and additional assessments as they became available on his health record. Relevant findings included:

- *General appearance.* A well-nourished man in his mid-seventies, with obvious respiratory distress and diaphoresis.
- *Vital signs.* Respirations were rapid at 32 per minutes; apical pulse was increased to 110 per mintue; and oral temperature was elevated to 38.2°C.
- *Respirations* were laboured with moderate retraction of the intercostal spaces. Crackles and wheezes were heard over the right middle and lower chest on auscultation. No abnormal breath sounds were heard over the left lung.
- *Cough* was dry and hacking, producing a small amount of blood-streaked sputum.
- *Pain/discomfort.* The patient experienced occasional episodes of 'stabbing' chest pain that increased with respirations and travelled to his right shoulder.
- *Cognitive/perceptual status.* The patient was orientated to person but was confused as to time and place.
- *Chest X-ray* results demonstrated consolidation in the right lower lobe.
- *Sputum analysis* showed a positive Gram stain for bacterial pneumococci.
- *White blood cell count* was increased to $17\,000/\mu l$.
- *Arterial blood gas* analysis showed an elevated $Paco_2$ of 52 mmHg, a decreased Pao_2 of 70 mmHg, and a decreased oxygen saturation level of 86%.
- *Psychosocial history:* Mr Fleming is retired. He lives alone in the home he and his wife occupied until her death 3 years ago. His only daughter lives nearby.

The patient's daughter stated that her father was normally bright, alert and orientated. He was an active participant in planning and organizing events for the local senior citizens' group. He had complained of a cold and 'flu-like' symptoms a few weeks ago, but seemed to be improving. His present illness came on suddenly.

Patient problems

Based upon an analysis of available data the following major patient problems were identified:

1. The patient is unable to achieve normal lung ventilation due to the retention of respiratory secretions secondary to infection, i.e. ineffective airway clearance.
2. The patient is confused and disorientated in time and space probably due to cerebral hypoxia as a result of problem 1.
3. The patient has severely limited activity due to shortness of breath.

4. The patient is lacking in knowledge about how to improve his airway clearance.

Patient care plan

Table 15.4 illustrates the plan of care devised to deal with each of these problems. More than one goal may be devised and a time should be stated by when the goal is to be achieved. In this plan, where there are two goals for each problem the interventions apply to both.

Table 15.4 Patient care plan: Mr Fleming, an elderly man with pneumonia.

Patient problem	Goals	Nursing intervention	Rationale
1. Ineffective airway clearance related to retention of respiratory secretions secondary to inflammation of respiratory passages as a result of infection	• Respiratory rate will be 20–24 per minute within 3 days (date . . .)	• Assess respiratory rate and depth, breathing pattern and breath sounds 2-hourly	• Ongoing objective data provides a basis for planning further nursing interventions and identification of signs of respiratory failure
	• Breathing pattern will be regular, requiring minimal effort, and breath sounds normal within 3 days (date . . .)	• Monitor body temperature 4-hourly	• Provides objective data on disease progress and response to therapy
		• Obtain a sputum specimen for culture and sensitivity as ordered	• Antibiotic therapy alters sensitivity of organisms
		• Administer i.v. antibiotics 6-hourly as prescribed	• Treatment of infection
		• Administer oxygen at 24% by mask as prescribed	• To promote gas exchange and decrease respiratory effort
		• Ensure patient is sitting upright	• To facilitate lung expansion
		• Demonstrate and supervise deep breathing and coughing techniques 2-hourly during day and when awake at night	• To improve breathing pattern; promote removal of secretions
		• Provide anti-inflammatory analgesic preparation 4-hourly as prescribed until temperature within normal range	• To reduce body temperature and promote comfort to facilitate lung expansion
		• Offer apple juice, warm tea or water 2-hourly or more often. Leave fluids within reach. Monitor fluid intake and maintain at 2 litres daily or greater	• Adequate hydration facilitates movement of secretions
		• Cleanse mouth with diluted mouthwash after coughing (2–4-hourly)	• With increased expectoration of secretions, more frequent mouth care is required

Table 15.4   Patient care plan: Mr Fleming, an elderly man with pneumonia.

Patient problem	Goals	Nursing intervention	Rationale
2. Confusion and disorientation in time and space due to cerebral hypoxia	• Mr Fleming will be orientated to time and place as well as person within 4 days (date . . .) • Mr Fleming will participate in interactions with nurses, family and other visitors	• Assess cognitive status 4-hourly • Call Mr Fleming by name and introduce yourself on each encounter • Provide repeated explanations of all care activities prior to and during the procedures • Engage Mr Fleming in conversations during all activities • Encourage daughter to talk to him during visits • Ask daughter to leave family photographs at bedside	• To evaluate changes in hypoxic state • To promote orientation and decrease confusion and anxiety
3. Severely limited activity due to dyspnoea	• Mr Fleming will gradually resume self-care and other activities of daily living, becoming independent in 7 days (date . . .)	• Plan care activities to allow for uninterrupted rest periods. Adjust assessment and care to be completed when he is awake • Assist Mr Fleming with all aspects of self-care initially. Increase his participation gradually as tolerated • Assess daily for bowel function. Obtain order for stool softener if straining occurs • Sit Mr Fleming upright	• To promote maximum rest • To prevent exhaustion • Constipation is a side-effect of analgesic medications and dehydration. Straining at stool increases energy expenditure • To depress diaphragm and decrease effort of breathing
4. Knowledge deficit related to home care	• Mr Fleming and his daughter will state a plan for home care and maintenance of respiratory function	• To teach Mr Fleming and his daughter to observe for signs and symptoms of respiratory distress • Assist them to develop a plan for Mr Fleming to obtain regular and adequate nutrition and fluids and adequate rest when he returns home • Make a referral to the community nurse for follow-up care	• Mr Fleming and his daughter will recognize complications quickly and seek help • Mr Fleming and his daughter will be informed about his needs • Resources will be available within the community to ensure continuity of care

Evaluation

After 7 days the patient was able to feed, wash and dress himself, walk to the bathroom independently and describe plans for his discharge. He was alert and orientated. Due to pressure on beds he was discharged a day earlier than planned; this caused considerable inconvenience for his daughter who had to take him home at very short notice. A community nurse visit was arranged as part of the follow-up but this was later than planned due to the premature discharge. Local social services promised that a home help would be able to visit once a week, but due to staff shortages nobody came in the first week after discharge. Despite these problems the patient recovered fully.

CARE OF THE PATIENT WITH AN ARTIFICIAL AIRWAY

When there is an actual or potential obstruction of the upper airway, intervention is needed to secure efficient and reliable ventilation of the lungs.

ENDOTRACHEAL INTUBATION

An oropharyngeal airway is useful in emergency and post anaesthesia to safeguard the airway against blockage by the tongue, should the patient be unconscious and have therefore lost the gag reflex and the ability to cough. The airway should be introduced inverted and then rotated into the correct position over the back of the tongue. Once in situ, it should be left until the patient recovers consciousness sufficiently for the gag reflex to return; at this stage the patient will cough the airway out spontaneously.

The site of the obstruction may be lower than the oropharynx, there may be severe facial trauma threatening the airway, or the patient may require artificial ventilation. In cases such as these a different solution is required and the patient will either have an endotracheal tube introduced as a temporary measure, or a tracheostomy may be performed, which could be temporary or permanent.

Common clinical situations in which an endotracheal tube is passed include emergency airway management (e.g. trauma, cardiac arrest), preoperatively to facilitate artificial ventilation and anaesthesia, and to allow efficient airway management for artificially ventilated patients in intensive care units.

The tube is usually passed (this is called intubation) through the mouth into the trachea, although the nasal route may also be used. If the patient is conscious, a quick-acting anaesthetic drug and a muscle relaxant (e.g. suxamethonium) are usually administered intravenously to permit intubation. The patient's airway is totally dependent upon the endotracheal tube thereafter; if muscle relaxant drugs have been used the patient will be unable to breathe spontaneously as all muscles in the body will be paralysed. Maintaining ventilation, and hence the life of the patient, is therefore totally in the hands of the medical and nursing staff.

The endotracheal tube bypasses the upper airway where warming, humidification and filtration occurs; it also bypasses the vocal chords so that the patient cannot speak. If the tube is to be in situ for any length of time it is important that the artificial ventilation system in use permits air to be warmed and humidified. The patient cannot drink, which means regular oral toilet is needed, otherwise the patient's mouth will become dry and candida infection is possible.

If the patient is conscious, communication will be a major problem and aids such as a pencil and paper are vital. Ashworth (1980), in a classic piece of nursing research, showed how nurses failed to communicate with patients who could not talk back; every effort therefore should be made to communicate with such patients. If at all possible the patient should have been informed beforehand that he or she would not be able to speak after intubation, and the temporary nature of this should have been explained.

For intubation, any dentures should be removed and the patient should be positioned on the back, with the head extended and slightly supported to ensure correct alignment of the mouth, pharynx and larnyx. Using the laryngoscope, the doctor introduces the endotracheal tube, and the proximal portion of the tube is secured to the patient's face. The tube, made of soft plastic, is more pliable and less traumatizing to tissue than a rubber tube (Figure 15.8). The tube is equipped with an inflatable cuff a short distance above the distal end. The cuff, which when inflated, remains soft, and reduces the pressure on the tissue and the possibility of ischaemia and trauma. When inflated it prevents the aspiration of vomitus and oral secretions. It also permits more effective ventilation by preventing the escape of gases being delivered under pressure.

When the tube is in position the cuff is inflated with air if the patient is to receive mechanical ventilatory assistance. Near the proximal end of the fine tube leading to the cuff, and through which the air is introduced, there is a small balloon-like dilatation which remains inflated when the tube is clamped. It is observed frequently and as long as it remains inflated the cuff is also inflated.

Immediately following insertion of the tube, and then at regular intervals, the chest is auscultated to determine if air is entering both lungs. If the tube is too low, the inflated cuff could completely block off a bronchus and cause atelectasis of the respective lung. An X-ray may be made to check the position of the tube.

The endotracheal tube is distressing and a source of discomfort to the conscious patient. Prolonged use may cause damage to the vocal cords and ulceration in the trachea. If an artifical airway is necessary for a prolonged period, a tracheostomy is done and the endotracheal tube removed.

Periodic deflation of the cuff should not be necessary if a large-volume low-pressure cuff is used. The inspired gas is humidified before entering the endotracheal tube to liquefy secretions and prevent encrusting within the tract and tube. Frequent deep suction through the endotracheal tube is necessary. The procedure involves hyperoxygenation, oropharyngeal suction, tracheal suction, and hyperoxygenation.

Suctioning may deplete the amount of oxygen reaching the alveoli. The patient may be given oxygen prior to suction, and again following suction. The patient's pulse is monitored for possible cardiac

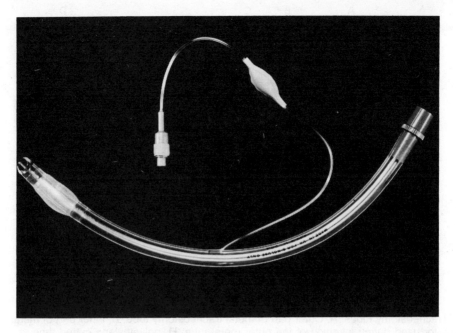

Figure 15.8 An endotracheal tube with inflatable cuff which provides a seal between the trachea and tube. After the tube is inserted, the cuff is inflated by the introduction of a specified volume of air through the fine, attached tube, which is then clamped.

dysfunction and arrhythmias (due to hypoxia) during and after the suctioning. If any irregularity occurs, suctioning is immediately discontinued and oxygen is administered with the self-inflating bag and mask.

Using sterile gloves, the nurse passes a sterile catheter, through the tube into the trachea. Suction is not applied while the catheter is being introduced. When in position, suction is applied intermittently and the catheter is rotated and withdrawn. If the airway is not clear of secretions, the catheter is not allowed to become contaminated and may be reintroduced into the trachea. It will likely be necessary to ventilate the patient with the self-inflating bag before passing the catheter again. If the secretions are tenacious, 5–10 ml of a sterile saline solution may be introduced into the tube, followed by immediate suction. Following suction the patient is hyperoxygenated.

Frequent mouth care is necessary, and suctioning of the oropharyngeal area at frequent intervals is done to remove the secretions that may form in response to the presence of the tube.

When the patient is to be *extubated*, the emergency (resuscitation) trolley should be accessible so the patient can be quickly reintubated if necessary.

Before the cuff is deflated and the doctor removes the tube, secretions are suctioned from the oropharynx to prevent aspiration. Following the removal of the tube, the patient is observed for respiratory distress and insufficiency. A nurse remains in attendance, constantly monitoring the patient's respirations, pulse and colour. The patient is usually apprehensive and needs the nurse's presence and reassurance.

TRACHEOSTOMY

Tracheostomy tubes are similar to endotracheal tubes but are inserted through an incision in the neck, directly into the trachea. The artificial airway bypasses the larynx and air passages above.

Indications for a tracheostomy include:

1. An upper airway obstruction (e.g. laryngeal tumour).
2. Prolonged, mechanically assisted ventilation where a seal is necessary to prevent loss of ventilatory gas that is under pressure.
3. The need for more efficient access to retained pulmonary secretions which, unless removed, may cause serious respiratory problems such as atelectasis and pneumonia.
4. The prevention of recurrent aspiration of oral secretions and vomitus.

Since endotracheal intubation has been more commonly used and can be performed very quickly, tracheostomy is rarely used in an emergency situation. The current procedure is generally elective, and is performed with an endotracheal tube in position and under aseptic conditions in an operating room. It may be necessary as an emergency measure if the patient cannot be intubated because of facial injuries or burns, laryngeal oedema or severe upper airway infection. If the tracheostomy is associated with laryngectomy, it becomes permanent.

The *operative procedure* is undertaken with the patient in the dorsal position, head and neck hyperextended. A pillow or folded sheet is placed under the

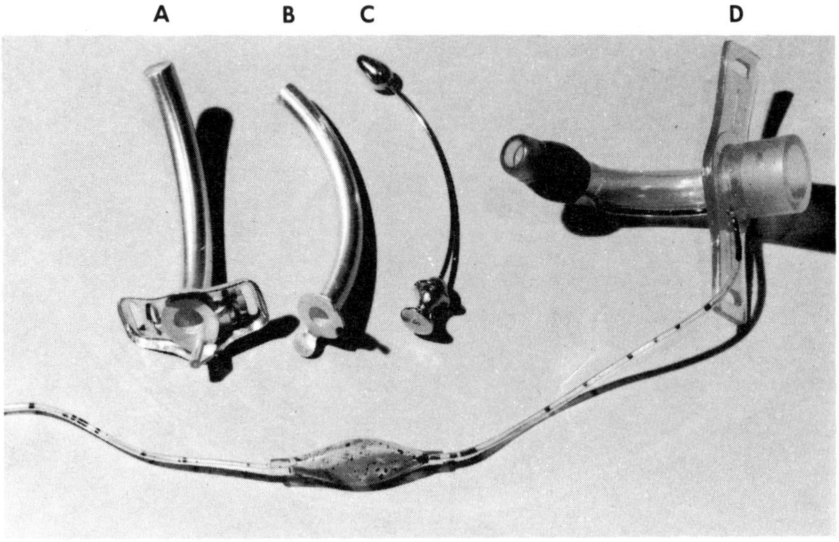

Figure 15.9 Tracheostomy tubes. A, Outer part of metal tracheostomy tube; B, inner part of metal tracheostomy tube; C, obturator used during insertion of the outer metal tube; D, polyethylene cuffed tube.

shoulders. A vertical or horizontal incision is made about 2 cm above the suprasternal notch to expose the upper part of the trachea. This is then opened, usually at the level of the second and third cartilaginous rings, and a tracheostomy tube is introduced. The tube is held in position by laterally attached tapes which are tied securely around the patient's neck.

Tracheostomy tubes are available in various sizes. The diameter and length of the tube selected depends upon the size of the trachea, and is slightly smaller in diameter than the trachea. They may be made of plastic, silver or nylon and may be single or consist of two parts, an inner and outer cannula (Figure 15.9). When a double-lumen tube is used, the outer cannula is fitted with an obturator that extends beyond the distal end of the tube. Its end is blunt and smooth which facilitates the introduction of the tube. As soon as the tube is in position, the obturator is removed and the inner tube is inserted and secured.

The tube with an inner cannula provides a more efficient means of clearing the airway of secretions, since the inner tube can be removed and readily cleansed without the risk of compromising the patient's airway. The single tube (without an inner cannula) must be changed about every 3 days or more often if secretions accumulate within the tube. The tube with an inner cannula may be left for a longer period.

Most synthetic tubes now in use have a high-volume, low-pressure cuff which encircles the lower part of the outer tube. After the tube is in position, the cuff is inflated by introducing a small amount of air via a fine tube that leads into it. The cuff creates a seal between the trachea and the tube and prevents air from entering or escaping around the tube, in addition to preventing the aspiration of secretions or fluid into the tract below.

This type of tube is used most frequently in patients who require mechanical assistance in breathing. A disadvantage of the cuff is possible ulceration of the tracheal mucosa due to pressure at the site. The cuff therefore may be deflated at frequent, regular intervals.

The amount of air required to produce a seal without unnecessary pressure on tracheal tissue varies from 2–10 ml. While introducing the air, the nurse listens and tests for the escape of air from around the tube. The tracheostomy tube may be blocked off momentarily while testing for leakage around the tube. When the inflation is completed, the end of the fine tube is clamped. The amount of air used in inflating the cuff is recorded each time; any significant change observed from one time to another is reported. A decreased amount of air used may indicate swelling and oedema in the 'air passage' tissues.

Near the proximal end of the fine inflating tube is a small balloon-like dilatation. This is inflated and, since it is visible, may be checked frequently to determine if the tube and the cuff below remain inflated. Obviously, if the small pilot balloon becomes deflated, a leak in the system is indicated and the cuff will be deflated, thus losing the intratracheal seal.

A variety of tubes are available which facilitate upper respiratory breathing or speaking and are used when weaning patients from mechanical ventilation.

Tracheostomy care

This is very important. The nurse should appreciate that the patient is dependent upon the patency of the tracheostomy tube for getting air in and out. Constant attention and meticulous care are necessary to prevent serious complications and to reduce the patient's fear of 'choking'. Sensitivity to the patient's fears and needs is important, since he or she cannot communicate verbally.

Preparation for the tracheostomy
The doctor explains the procedure to the patient and family and an informed consent is obtained. The nurse assesses the patient's understanding of the procedure. The patient is assured that someone will be in constant, close attendance and that provision will be made for communication by writing. A similar explanation is given to the family. Opportunities are provided for the patient and family members to ask questions and to receive further clarification.

Preparation to receive the patient
This includes assembling sterile suction equipment, ventilator if indicated, adapter to fit tracheostomy tube, oxygen, sterile tracheostomy tray with various sizes of tracheostomy tubes in case the one inserted becomes dislodged, sterile tape for securing the tube in place, gauze squares, tracheal dilator and artery forceps, sterile syringe to inflate the cuff, humidifier (the type will depend upon whether or not the patient is to receive mechanical ventilatory assistance; if not, a nebulizer may be available which fits over the opening of the tube), equipment for frequent mouth cleansing, and a pencil and slate or pad.

Position
The head of the bed is usually elevated to approximately a 45° angle if the patient is conscious and the blood pressure and pulse are stable.

Assessment
Frequent monitoring of the patient's blood pressure, respiratory rate and sounds, pulse and colour is necessary. An increase in the respiratory rate, crackles and wheezes and an increased pulse rate may indicate the need for suction. The patient may still experience respiratory insufficiency due to obstruction in the tract below the tracheostomy. This could be evidenced by marked respiratory effort, unequal movement of the sides of the chest and retraction of the soft tissues in the intercostal and supraclavicular spaces. Cyanosis and distress not relieved by suctioning are reported promptly. Increasing restlessness, especially if accompanied by a rapid pulse rate, may indicate hypoxia or bleeding.

The neck and area around the incision are inspected for possible interstitial emphysema due to air leaking into the subcutaneous tissue. The wound is observed for bleeding in the immediate postoperative period and then checked daily for signs of infection and sloughing.

The tube is checked frequently for patency and the characteristics (consistency, colour, amount) of the tracheobronchial secretions are noted. Increased secretion occurs in response to the tracheal trauma and is usally coloured by blood at first, but the blood content should gradually diminish and disappear.

Suction
The patient's cough is less effective in clearing the airway, so suction is necessary. Frequency of suction is determined by assessment of the patient's breathing and auscultation of the chest for wheezes and crackles. The frequency is decreased as the secretions become less. One has to be sure they are less and not thick and tenacious and retained because of lack of fluids and humidification. Sterile saline may be instilled into the tube and followed immediately by suction.

If the patient is receiving mechanical ventilatory assistance or oxygen, he or she is hyperoxygenated before suction (O_2, 100% for 3–5 minutes). Suction removes air and oxygen from the respiratory tract, as well as removing secretions, and may cause hypoxaemia and ensuing cardiac arrhythmia. It has been demonstrated that the development of hypoxaemia is related to the duration of suctioning and the frequency of passing the suction catheter (Shekelton and Nield, 1987).

The trachea is suctioned using a sterile glove and a sterile suction catheter moistened in sterile water or normal saline. The negative pressure is not applied during the insertion of the catheter but is applied when it is in position and intermittently during withdrawal. Suction must be brief, not longer than 10–15 seconds. If it must be repeated, the patient is allowed several breaths or is given oxygen again.

Secretions and suction may initiate coughing. Secretions escaping from the tracheostomy tube are gently wiped away with sterile unfrayed gauze (free of lint and absorbent). The mucus and exudate must be cleaned away quickly before being drawn back into the tube with a breath.

Tube and wound care
The wound and surrounding skin are kept as dry and free of secretions as possible; moisture predisposes to infection and maceration of the tissues. The wound and area under the tube are protected with sterile dry gauze to fit around the tube. The gauze should be unfrayed and free of lint and absorbent to prevent possible aspiration of a loose thread or particle. If the tapes securing the tube become soiled they are replaced with fresh sterile tapes.

The inner cannula of the tracheostomy tube is carefully removed and cleansed every 3–6 hours, or as often as necessary (perhaps even hourly). Hydrogen peroxide or sodium bicarbonate solution may be used to soak the tube to loosen crusts of mucus, and the cannula is then cleansed using a small tube brush or applicator. It is then rinsed in water and sterilized. The outer cannula is suctioned if necessary before the inner cannula is reinserted. Precautions must be taken not to displace the outer tube; the tapes which secure it are checked frequently.

Single tubes are usually changed by the surgeon or an experienced, trained nurse, as often as necessary to ensure patency. The tube with an inner cannula may be changed weekly. A tray with sterile replacement tubes and the necessary equipment is kept at the beside.

Should the tube come out of the trachea because of vigorous coughing or carelessly tied tapes, the tracheal opening closes and the patient is threatened with asphyxia. Prompt action is necessary. The tracheal wound is quickly reopened with the sterile tracheal dilator or artery forceps which are always kept at the bedside in the event of such an emergency. The opening is held open until the doctor (or specialist nurse) arrives and inserts the sterile tracheostomy tube.

Humidification

Adequate humidification of the inspired gas is very important to prevent encrustations forming within the trachea and the tube, which increase airway resistance. As cited above, the method used will depend upon whether or not mechanical ventilation is necessary. Equipment which provides a nebulized solution is more efficient.

Fluids and nutrition

A minimum fluid intake of 3000 ml is recommended to help liquefy pulmonary secretions, unless contraindicated by cardiac insufficiency and oedema. An accurate record is kept of the intake and output. The patient is not usually permitted any fluids or food by mouth; they are administered intravenously. Some patients receive feedings via a nasogastric tube (see Chapter 16).

If the tracheostomy is going to be permanent, or if the patient is not on a ventilator, oral fluids are introduced gradually; if tolerated, a soft diet is given and increased gradually to a regular diet. The nurse remains with the patient until sufficient confidence is gained.

Mouth care

Oral hygiene is important for the patient's comfort and to reduce the possibility of infection. The mouth is cleansed and rinsed every 2 hours until the patient is taking normal meals, at which time regular cleansing of the teeth and rinsing of the mouth after each meal and at bedtime suffice.

Communication

The patient is likely to be fearful of choking and concerned about his inability to cough up the secretions and to communicate. When the nurse leaves the bedside the patient is advised of the errand and how long it will take. A call-bell is given to the patient, who will be more secure knowing that someone can be called if necessary.

The nurse talks to the patient, informs him or her of progress and what is going to be done, and endeavours to anticipate information the patient might want to have but cannot ask for verbally, especially information about how long the inability to breathe and communicate normally is likely to last. A pad and pencil are kept readily within reach, and the patient is encouraged to communicate feelings and needs. Hand signals are developed to enable the patient to communicate 'yes' or 'no' or make routine requests by raising one or more fingers. Family members are encouraged to talk to him.

Extubation

If the patient has been receiving mechanical ventilatory assistance, removal of the tracheostomy tube is not considered until he or she is successfully weaned from the ventilator. When the tracheostomy is a temporary measure, the patient is gradually returned to breathing through the upper tract. In order to lessen tracheal injury and scarring the tube is removed as soon as possible, but without compromising adequate ventilation. The protective reflexes should be responsive; the epiglottis and glottis should be closed to prevent aspiration, the gag reflex should be present and the patient should be able to swallow fluids and food without risk of aspiration.

If a cuffed tube has been used, the cuff is deflated for 24–48 hours before the tube is removed and the patient's ability to keep upper tract secretions out of the lower tract is observed.

A sterile tracheostomy tray with tubes of several sizes is kept at the bedside in case a tube may have to be reinserted after extubation. Sterile suction equipment should also be available.

When the tracheostomy tube is removed, the wound is cleansed, the wound edges are approximated and taped and a firm dressing is applied. Healing occurs spontaneously; sutures are not considered necessary. The patient is advised to place a hand over the area and exert some pressure when coughing. He or she may be fearful of not being able to breathe when the tube is removed, so is assured beforehand that breathing is adequate via the normal route. A nurse remains following removal to be certain that no difficulty is experienced. Following discharge, the doctor or clinic keeps track of the patient who has had a tracheostomy for at least a year and the patient is checked for possible scarring and tracheal stricture resulting from irritation and trauma.

Home tracheostomy care

If the tracheostomy is permanent, the patient is instructed about the care of the tube and the stoma (the artificial opening to the surface). This is done as soon as the patient is well enough to undertake the care in the hospital so confidence will be developed. A member of the family also receives instructions about the necessary care and precautions.

The patient and family are referred to the district nurse who is able to obtain the necessary suction equipment and dressing supplies, and also give instruction in the use and care of the equipment.

The patient and family are advised how to conceal the site of the tracheostomy. The shirt will cover the stoma in a man; a woman may wear a scarf or high-necked blouse or dress. Small 'bibs' can be made or may be available from the district nurse.

An explanation is made of the danger of aspirating water through the tracheostomy tube; this precludes swimming or immersion in water to a high level. Precautions must also be used when taken a shower.

The patient is advised to return to the outpatient department or to the general practitioner at regular intervals, as directed, for changing the tube and examination of the stoma. Eventually, when the stoma is firmly healed and the tracheal opening remains patent, the patient or a member of the family may be taught to change the outer cannula, or the tube may be removed permanently. Precautions should be used to avoid close contact with those in the environment with respiratory infection.

Ineffective Airway Clearance Related to Laryngectomy/Cancer of the Larynx*

Cancer of the larynx is primarily a disease of males aged between 50 and 65 years of age. The ratio of male to female patients is about 7:1. In recent years there has been an increased incidence in this type of cancer.

CONTRIBUTING FACTORS

Cancer of the larynx is associated with life-style habits of cigarette smoking and alcohol consumption. Factors increasing the risk for this disease are heavy use of tobacco and alcohol and frequent exposure to pollutants and environmental irritants. To date there is no evidence that alcohol alone is carcinogenic but it has been suggested that alcohol may aid in the absorption of tobacco carcinogens, irritate tissues or facilitate the conversion of normal squamous cells to malignant cells. Heavy alcohol intake contributes to poor nutrition and dietary deficiencies. Other substances including inhaled asbestos fibres, irritate the larynx and may lead to histological changes.

CLINICAL CHARACTERISTICS

The most frequent and important characteristic of laryngeal cancer is progressive hoarseness. Hoarseness is a result of direct tumour pressure on the vocal cords. Earache is common due to 'referred pain' from the tumour. Referred pain occurs because the nerves in the larynx connect with nerves in the ear region and the brain therefore interprets the pain stimuli as coming from the ear. Other symptoms include localized throat pain, vague neck pain, lump in the neck, blood-tinged sputum, dysphagia and difficulty in breathing.

DIAGNOSTIC INVESTIGATIONS

The person with suspected cancer of the larynx will undergo a complete medical history and physical examination, indirect laryngoscopy, direct laryngoscopy, biopsy, X-ray and fluoroscopic examination, and computerized tomography (see pages 400–401).

LARYNGOSCOPY

Direct examination of the larynx is done with a flexible fibreoptic bronchoscope.

Preparation of a patient for a laryngoscopy includes an explanation of the procedure and the signing of a consent form. The patient is advised of the purpose of the procedure, that he or she will be on their back with the head hyperextended and will remain conscious throughout, since only topical anaesthesia is used to introduce the instrument. The patient should know that the room will be darkened and the eyes covered.

Food and fluids are withheld for the 6–8 hours prior to the scheduled examination time to avoid

* With permission Marietta Pupo, Clinical Nurse Specialist.

vomiting and aspiration. Dentures are removed and atropine may be prescribed to reduce secretions. Some sedation may also be ordered to promote relaxation and reduce the patient's anxiety.

Following the examination the head of the bed is elevated, and the patient is encouraged to breathe deeply. The swallowing and gag reflexes are usually absent for a few hours because of the local anaesthesia used; fluids and food are withheld until these reflexes return. The patient is usually able to take a soft diet in 8 hours and a regular diet by the end of 24 hours. The patient is encouraged to rest quietly and not attempt to talk, cough or clear the throat.

Trauma of the larynx may produce hoarseness or loss of the voice; the patient needs reassurance that either is only temporary, and a pencil and paper for communication is provided.

The sputum may be streaked with blood if a biopsy was done but should clear in 24–48 hours. Any excessive amount of blood is reported promptly as it may manifest haemorrhage from the biopsy site.

A tracheostomy tray is kept close at hand following a laryngoscopy because, occasionally, laryngeal spasm or oedema and difficulty in breathing develop. The patient is kept under close observation for several hours. Any indication of respiratory distress is brought to the doctor's attention immediately.

MEDICAL MANAGEMENT

The two main types of treatment are radiation and/or surgery. The medical management of the person with cancer of the larynx is specific to the characteristics of each patient: the exact site, size and type of tumour and the patient's general health.

TOTAL LARYNGECTOMY

This includes the complete removal of the larynx alone or with two or more of the tracheal rings and the epiglottis. With the larynx removed there is no longer a connection between the trachea below and the pharynx above. The trachea is sewn to the skin of the neck to form a permanent tracheostomy. A radical neck dissection is usually performed at this time.

After a total laryngectomy, normal speech is no longer possible. The patient breaths through a permanent tracheostomy. Aspiration does not usually present a problem because there is no connection between the upper and lower respiratory tracts (Figure 15.10).

RADICAL NECK DISSECTION

A radical neck dissection involves removal of the regional lymph nodes, the deep cervical lymph nodes, their lymphatic channels, and the muscles and the vessels that contain tumour cells.

CLINICAL SITUATION: MR SHASTRI HINDOCHA, A MAN WITH CANCER OF THE LARYNX

Mr Hindocha is a 59-year-old man admitted to hospital with a diagnosis of cancer of the larynx for a total

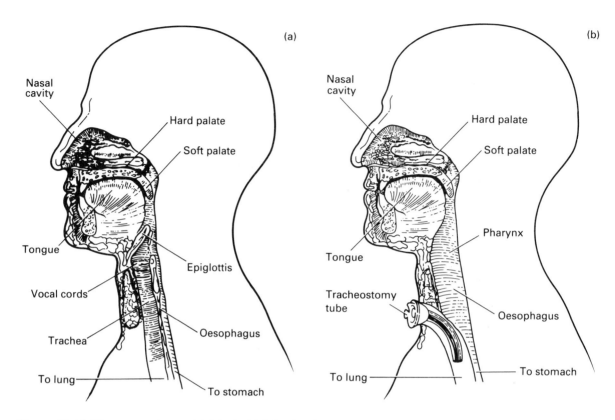

Figure 15.10 The upper airway. (a) Intact; (b) following laryngectomy.

laryngectomy and right neck dissection.

Mr Hindocha, a very independent man, is aware of his general health status and the implication of the planned surgery. He states that he has been happily married for 35 years and that his wife and married daughter are very supportive. He works as a Customs official but is presently on sick leave and hopes to return to work as soon as possible, Mr Hindocha has been physically active. He enjoys life, his family and friends and plans to take an early retirement.

Over the last 4 months he has experienced laryngitis, persistent hoarseness and difficulty swallowing. In the last 2 weeks he had occasional breathing difficulties, a burning, painful sensation on swallowing and has coughed up some blood-tinged sputum. He had severe pain in his right ear and general discomfort in his throat. Mr Hindocha has smoked 1–1½ packets of cigarettes per day for over 35 years. Alcohol intake includes 2–3 drinks per day and wine with supper.

Mr Hindocha is devastated by his diagnosis and the realization he will never speak normally again. He indicated to the nurse that he usually deals with stress by maintaining a positive attitude, by obtaining as much information as possible and discussing his options with his wife and daughter, and makes decisions based on facts.

Table 15.5 describes the plan of care devised to deal with Mr Hindocha's problems.

Table 15.5 Patient care plan: Mr S. Hindocha, a person with a laryngectomy.

Patient problem	Goals	Nursing intervention	Rationale
1. Knowledge deficit related to: (a) Surgical procedure (b) Altered breathing pattern post-operatively and altered ability to	• Mr Hindocha and his family will be knowledgeable about the outcomes of surgery: —altered form of breathing	• Explain the difference between the normal method of breathing and altered method of neck breathing postoperatively using anatomical	• Providing knowledge and an illustration of the expected postoperative anatomical changes, including the laryngectomy stoma and methods of breathing,

Table 15.5 *Continued*

Patient problem	Goals	Nursing intervention	Rationale
communicate effectively secondary to laryngectomy	—changes in body image	diagrams or models	assists Mr Hindocha to maintain some control during the preoperative period
	• Mr Hindocha and his family will be aware of the alternative methods of communication	• Reassure Mr Hindocha and his family that removal of the larynx eliminates only one anatomical structure of speech production	
		• Arrange for Mr Hindocha and his daughter to meet the speech therapist pre-operatively	• Information related to altered methods of communication demonstrates to Mr Hindocha that he will communicate independently postoperatively
		• Refer to loss of speech as temporary. Negotiate a plan for communication in the immediate postoperative period (i.e. pen and paper, magic slate, communication booklet with diagrams)	
		• Assess Mr Hindocha's literary level	
		• Assess Mr Hindocha's ability to see and hear	• Assessment data related to literacy level and functional status of seeing and hearing is needed to plan for the most effective communication method
		• Consider a visit from a person with an existing laryngectomy	• To provide a 'real' illustration of the changes the surgery will produce
2. Anxiety related to fear of the surgery	• Mr Hindocha will verbalize a decrease in anxiety prior to surgery	• Explain preoperative care to Mr Hindocha: —skin preparation —nothing by mouth for 12 hours	• Discussion of the care and demonstration of the postoperative tubes alleviates Mr Hindocha's fears of the unknown
	• Mr Hindocha will verbalize his fears and concerns related to surgery and hospitalization	• Explain postoperative nursing care routines: —suctioning —humidification via tracheostomy collar —laryngectomy stoma care —mouth care —drainage tubes —ambulation —breathing exercises —nasogastric tube	

Table 15.5   *Continued*

Patient problem	Goals	Nursing intervention	Rationale
		• Explain the involvement of other members of health care team: —speech therapist —physiotherapist —nutritionist —social worker —home care co-ordinator —pastoral care worker	• Individual members of the health care team make specific contributions to the rehabilitation of the laryngectomy patient and family
		• Encourage Mr Hindocha and his family to verbalize their fears and concerns	• Helps to decrease anxiety which subsequently assists in postoperative adaptation
3. Ineffective airway clearance related to laryngectomy	• Mr Hindocha's airway will be patent	• Suction laryngectomy stoma frequently immediately postoperatively then when mucus present	• Facilitates removal of secretions
	• He will demonstrate no signs of cyanosis	• Elevate the head of the bed 30° or more at all times	• Prevents an obstructed airway and allows Mr Hindocha to cough up secretions
	• His respiratory rate will be regular	• Encourage Mr Hindocha to deep breath and cough frequently	
		• Use humifidied air with a tracheal collar and/or a 'Roger's spray' (pump action aerosol spray, similar to an old-fashioned perfume spray, which can be filled with any liquid, usually normal saline or sodium bicarbonate solution)	• Normal humidification through nose is now non-existent
		• Clean laryngectomy tube every 4 hours and p.r.n. (If no laryngectomy tube is present ensure that the laryngectomy stoma is free from mucous crusts using a flashlight and bayonet forceps)	• Prevents build up of secretions and crusts which can narrow or obstruct the airway
		• Instill 3–5 ml of sterile normal saline into the tube to dislodge mucous plugs and then apply suction	• Saline liquifies secretions and allows for removal of deep crusts and mucus that can cause an airway obstruction
		• Mr Hindocha should have the call bell in reach to alert the nurses of breathing problems	• Mr Hindocha is unable to call for help. Call bell decreases his anxiety
		• Monitor respiratory rate, rhythm and volume and listen to breath sounds	• Consistent observation and assessment prevents complications —narrow or obstructed airway —pneumonia

Table 15.5 *Continued*

Patient problem	Goals	Nursing intervention	Rationale
4. Alteration in comfort: pain related to laryngectomy incision and surgical swelling	• Mr Hindocha will verbalize minimal or no pain	• Administer analgesia on a regular schedule during the first 24–72 hours post-operatively and then as requested by Mr Hindocha	• Provides comfort to Mr Hindocha and allows for early ambulation and ease in deep breathing and coughing
		• Assess the pain in head and neck area, throat and upper chest	• Information related to location, duration and intensity provides data from Mr Hindocha's perspective
		• Assess the effectiveness of the analgesia	• Goal is pain relief thereby allowing Mr Hindocha to become involved in his own care and facilitate independence
		• Encourage Mr Hindocha and his family to communicate feelings and concerns about pain and pain management	• A collaborative plan improves chances for pain control and decreases his fears about pain
		• Elevate the head of the bed 30° or more at all times	• Postoperative swelling in the head and neck area is minimized when the bed is elevated and as a result pain is decreased
		• Teach Mr Hindocha to support head and neck when going from a lying to a sitting position	• Neck weakness and loss of muscle control can be expected postoperatively. Prevent tension and strain on incision lines
5. Altered nutrition: less than body requirements related to surgical intervention and surgical swelling	• Mr Hindocha will maintain or improve his pre-operative nutritional status, including his normal weight	• Start tube feedings as ordered	• Swallowing normally in immediate postoperative period causes muscle activity that may strain the suture line
		• Explain the importance of maintaining adequate nutrition to Mr Hindocha	• Helps Mr Hindocha understand the need for proper nutrition to promote wound healing
		• Have nutritionist assess and counsel Mr Hindocha and his family	• Nutrition assessment provides data base related to caloric needs
		• Document calorie counts as required	
		• Ensure that Mr Hindocha has 2.5 l/day fluid intake; this may include alcohol if wanted	• Additional liquids via tube increases Mr Hindocha's morale and improves hydration. Many of these patients are used to a high alcohol intake which need not be discontinued at this time
		• Encourage Mr Hindocha and his family to express feelings and concerns about nutritional intake	• Facilitates Mr Hindocha's and his family's understanding of the role of diet in recovery

Table 15.5 *Continued*

Patient problem	Goals	Nursing intervention	Rationale
		• Reassure Mr Hindocha that eventually he will be able to eat again	• Feeding via tube is essential postoperatively for the incisions to heal and to prevent complications of fistula formation
		• When ordered, start Mr Hindocha with water to swallow first then gradually increase to soft diet	• Fluids are easier to swallow. Assess for signs and symptoms of aspiration. Soft diet is essential until pharyngeal muscle activity is at its optimal
		• Allow Mr Hindocha to have some control over his nutritional intake i.e. —allow him to choose when he wants his feeds —teach him self-administration of his tube feedings —allow him a choice of additional liquids	• Increases Mr Hindocha's sense of autonomy and independence
6. Altered communication pattern related to laryngectomy	• Mr Hindocha will be able to communicate effectively using alternative methods	• Immediately postoperatively supply Mr Hindocha with prenegotiated method of communication, i.e. pen and paper, magic slate and/or pictorial booklet	• Decreases anxiety and allows for self-control in expressing his needs. Protect Mr Hindocha's privacy and destroy notes as required
		• Be patient when Mr Hindocha is responding and utilize good communication skills	• An unrushed manner and the provision of adequate time allows Mr Hindocha to express himself. Do not attempt to finish his sentences. A caring attitude and acknowledgement of non-verbal communication enhance his self-worth and dignity
		• Encourage Mr Hindocha to express his feelings and concerns about communicating	
		• Arrange for speech therapist to work with Mr Hindocha	• Allows Mr Hindocha to select the most appropriate method of communication: external larynx/ oesophageal speech/ neoglottic reconstruction if available and appropriate
		• Involve family and other support systems in speech therapy	• Learning a new method of communication may be a frustrating experience for Mr Hindocha
		• Reassure Mr Hindocha that the loss of speech is temporary and convey an attitude of support and acceptance	
		• Encourage Mr Hindocha to wear a Medic Alert bracelet	• Provides vital information in an emergency situation

Table 15.5 *Continued*

Patient problem	Goals	Nursing intervention	Rationale
7. Disturbance in body image related to laryngectomy stoma and impaired communication	• Mr Hindocha will acknowledge his feelings about the changes in his body image • Mr Hindocha will socialize with his family and others	• Utilize good communication techniques and establish a trusting relationship • Encourage Mr Hindocha and his family to communicate feelings and concerns about alterations in body image • Monitor Mr Hindocha for signs of depression: —loss of appetite, —flat affect, —isolation, —and/or sleeplessness Acknowledge/confirm these signs with Mr Hindocha • Arrange for Mr Hindocha to meet another laryngectomy patient who has accepted his or her altered body image • Provide Mr Hindocha with the contact address of his local laryngectomy association (see Useful Addresses) • Establish a plan with Mr Hindocha for re-establishing social contacts following discharge • Provide Mr Hindocha with laryngectomy bibs prior to discharge • Encourage Mr Hindocha to learn self-care	• Allows Mr Hindocha to express his feelings of loss and/or grief which ultimately hastens adaptation • Mr Hindocha was fearful of unacceptability related to his appearance • Dealing with the permanent loss of his normal voice caused intense feelings of grief • Former patients who have adapted will provide encouragement for Mr Hindocha • Support groups provide opportunities to share fears and hopes • Mr Hindocha will not view himself as an invalid or as dependent or rejected by others • Covering the laryngectomy stoma is aesthetically and physically beneficial • Promotes autonomy and independence. Mr Hindocha will not consider himself an invalid
8. Potential for complications: (a) Infection (b) Inadequate wound healing related to surgical intervention	• Mr Hindocha's surgical wounds heal without infection and/or other complications	• Monitor incisions for signs and symptoms of infection and if infection is suspected swab incision for culture and sensitivity • Cleanse incisions with sterile normal saline or other appropriate solution, using aseptic technique • Maintain the patency of drains and observe drainage	• Prevent and/or promptly detect infections from any site • Asepsis promotes wound healing • Drainage tubes must be patent or collection of fluids will build up with possible wound dehiscence

Table 15.5 *Continued*

Patient problem	Goals	Nursing intervention	Rationale
		• Report any purulent and/or serous drainage	• Purulent drainage indicates infection. Serous drainage indicates a potential wound dehiscence
		• Administer antibiotics as ordered	• Antibiotics are the first choice of treatment for infection
		• Observe for oedema • Elevate head of bed 30° or more	• Following radical neck dissection oedema is usually present due to blockage in the lymphatic system. Elevated bed promotes lymphatic drainage
		• Encourage Mr Hindocha to do mouth washes or mouth irrigations routinely with laryngectomy care. As soon as possible re-establish brushing of teeth and re-stimulation of gums	• Frequent mouth care is necessary to maintain integrity of oral mucosa
		• Observe mucous membranes for signs and symptoms of infection, and/or discomfort	• Prevent and/or detect infection by reporting observations
		• Ensure that Mr Hindocha has adequate nutritional intake of at least 2500 ml of fluid daily	• Proper nutrition promotes wound healing and adequate fluid intake promotes liquidification of respiratory secretions preventing complications
9. Knowledge deficit related to postoperative care	• Mr Hindocha and his family will verbalize steps and rationale of laryngectomy care • Mr Hindocha and his family will demonstrate the correct care prior to discharge	• Provide an environment which is conducive to learning and respect Mr Hindocha's privacy	• Teaching–learning principles must be applied. Ventilation of Mr Hindocha's feelings is essential if learning is to occur
		• Assess Mr Hindocha's ability to learn	• Data base as to how Mr Hindocha learns best is beneficial for planning effective teaching strategies
		• Instruct Mr Hindocha and his family in self-care measures and reinforce each time care is given • Allow time for Mr Hindocha and his family to ask questions and to verbalize concerns and fears about self-care	• Knowledge and skill may need to be explained, demonstrated and re-enforced many times prior to discharge. Fluctuation in Mr Hindocha's mood may affect his readiness to learn. Family members can provide assistance and re-enforcement related to self-care activities

Table 15.5 *Continued*

Patient problem	Goals	Nursing intervention	Rationale
		• Give written information and self-care pamphlets to Mr Hindocha and his family	• Reinforces information related to laryngectomy care. Proper care decreases incidence of complications. Self-care promotes independence and facilitates overall adaptation

INEFFECTIVE BREATHING PATTERN

The North American Nursing Diagnosis Association (1989) states that: 'Ineffective breathing pattern exists when an individual's inhalation and/or exhalation pattern does not enable adequate pulmonary inflation or emptying'.

Characteristics of Ineffective Breathing Pattern

Changes in the respiratory rate or pattern are the major symptoms experienced by persons with impaired respiratory function related to an ineffective breathing pattern. Dyspnoea and use of the accessory muscles of respiration are usually present. The person assumes the sitting posture and leans forward, often breathing through pursed lips. Expirations are prolonged and difficult. Activity intolerance develops as the work of breathing increases and oxygenation of the blood is impaired while carbon dioxide levels increase (Table 15.6).

Table 15.6 Patient health problem: ineffective breathing pattern.

Defining characteristics	Related factors
• Altered rate and depth of respirations	• Neuromuscular impairment
• Dyspnoea	• Musculoskeletal impairment
• Use of accessory muscles	• Pain
• Pursed-lip breathing; increased duration of expiration	• Perceptual/cognitive impairment
• Altered arterial gases, pH and electrolytes	• Anxiety
• Increased anteroposterior chest diameter	• Decreased energy/fatigue
• Cyanosis	• Decreased lung expansion
• Cough	• Tracheal or bronchial obstruction
• Nasal flaring	
• Altered chest excursion	

ABNORMAL BREATHING PATTERN

Normal involuntary respirations are regular, effortless and quiet. Irregularities in breathing may relate to rate, volume, rhythm or the ease with which the person breathes. The following terms are used to indicate characteristic breathing patterns.

Eupnoea is quiet normal breathing at the rate of about 12–18 times per minute in the adult. Respirations are more rapid and shallow in the infant and preschool child; they vary from 30–50 per minute in infancy, gradually decreasing to adult levels by the age of 10–12 years.

Tachypnoea is rapid breathing with the volume of the respirations usually below normal.

Bradypnoea is an abnormally slow rate of respirations.

Hyperpnoea is an increase in the volume of air breathed per minute due to either an increase in the rate or depth of respirations or to both.

Dyspnoea refers to a subjective awareness of a disturbance in breathing. The patient experiences discomfort and/or the need for increased effort or work in ventilation. The individual's perception of difficult breathing or shortness of breath may be due to physiological or psychological stress. The experience is anxiety provoking, since the person knows that breathing is essential to life; the emotional reaction tends to aggravate and perpetuate the problem further. The individual may describe it as 'tightness in the chest', 'shortness of breath', 'unable to get enough air', or 'suffocating'. The dyspnoeic patient frequently has a distressed appearance, is restless and may be perspiring. The difficulty may only be present on exertion and may be episodic. The frequency of the episodes and whether their occurrence is related to a particular time of day, activity or certain situations or factors are noted.

Orthopnoea is dyspnoea which is present in the recumbent position but is relieved to some extent by elevation of the trunk.

Cheyne-Stokes respirations are characterized by a few seconds of apnoea followed by respirations that gradually increase in frequency and volume to a peak intensity and then gradually subside to a period of apnoea. This pattern is cyclic.

Biot's pattern of breathing is characterized by a few

respirations varying in volume, followed by a prolonged period of apnoea.

Kussmaul's respirations are rapid and very deep.

ABNORMAL CHEST MOVEMENTS

Unequal participation of the two sides of the chest in respiratory movements may be evident, or unusual retraction or ballooning of the intercostal spaces may occur. For example, in atelectasis or pneumothorax, in which a part or all of the lung is not being inflated, there is diminished movement of the chest wall on the affected side. Similarly, this may occur if a large section of alveoli is consolidated with fluid or secretions. Excessive retraction or ballooning is associated with extreme difficulty in getting air in or out of the air passages.

RELATED FACTORS

Ineffective breathing patterns usually develop in response to a combination of associated factors (Table 15.6). Factors which alter the structures of respiration, especially the chest wall and the strength and movement of the respiratory muscles, interfere with lung expansion and with the flow of air into and out of the alveoli. Intrapulmonary factors include narrowing and obstruction of the airways and the accumulation of air and fluid in the pleural space and thorax.

Assessment of the Person with Ineffective Breathing Pattern

Nursing assessment of the individual experiencing breathing impairment includes identification of the characteristics of the breathing pattern and of the factors contributing to the problem.

HEALTH HISTORY

Past history of respiratory disorders and treatment programme. The person is asked if there has been any recent trauma or surgery to the chest or respiratory passages, or any respiratory infections. The existence of any associated health problems is also determined. Information is obtained about all prescription and non-prescription drugs the person has been taking regularly or intermittently. The name, dosage, frequency, purpose and perceived effectiveness of each drug is noted (if the patient is able to supply this information).

Health promoting behaviours and risk factors.
Assessment includes data about factors in the person's life-style and health habits that promote respiratory efficiency or increase the person's risk for problems. What is the person's usual daily routine and exercise pattern? What is the quality of diet? Is the individual

overweight? Are appropriate health care services utilized? Information is also obtained about possible exposure to infectious agents; smoking habits including what is smoked, how often and for how long; the existence of any known allergies, the name of the agent and the nature of the reaction when exposed to it; and any risk factors or irritants to which the person is exposed at work, home or in the community.

The person's perceptions of and responses to altered respiratory status. How does the person perceive his/her present health status? Is he/she aware of the significance of related risk factors? What has been done to eliminate risk factors such as smoking, inactivity and other lifestyle factors that are amenable to change? It is important to also recognize which factors are beyond the control of the patient, such as working conditions, air pollution or poverty, and consider ways in which their effects may be reduced. Giving up work or moving away from a city may not be feasible or acceptable to the patient. The nurse also assesses the individual's and family's understanding of previously prescribed treatment and their perceptions of their ability to follow the plan. It is important to determine why the person sought health care and what his or her goals are for care. What does the individual state as the priority for care? Many respiratory problems are chronic in nature and it is therefore important that the person recognizes the long-term nature of the illness and the implications of this. Family support should be discussed to discover something of the social setting the patient has come from and will return to, as that setting may have significant influence over his or her health.

PHYSICAL EXAMINATION OF THE CHEST AND BREATHING PATTERN

Inspection

Thorax. Normally, the thorax is symmetrical. It is important to note any difference on either side and any apparent abnormality in the shape or bony framework of the thorax. Scoliosis or kyphosis may interfere with normal breathing. If the chest is barrel-shaped (slight kyphosis with the ribs in a horizontal position, the sternal angle prominent and the anterior posterior diameter enlarged) it may indicate chronic airflow limitation. A funnel-shaped chest is characterized by depression of the sternum while a 'pigeon' chest involves an outward location of the sternum and inward depression of the first few ribs with minimal impairment of breathing.

Chest movements associated with respirations. The frequency, rhythm and depth of respirations are noted by observing the chest. The thorax is normally symmetrical. On inspiration, as the diaphragm descends the lower rib cage moves slightly outward and upward. The upper rib cage simultaneously expands slightly. Expiration is passive and of slightly longer duration than inspiration. A short pause occurs prior to the next inspiration. If the individual's breathing is laboured, the intercostal spaces are observed for any 'ballooning out' during exhalation or retraction during inspiration.

Accessory muscles. Rhythmic movement of the diaphragm is observed with normal respiration. Use of the accessory muscles indicates some degree of respiratory distress and is characterized by retraction of the supraclavicular and suprasternal areas and elevation of the shoulders during inspiration. Enlargement of the accessory muscles, particularly the sternocleidomastoid muscles, occurs with chronic airflow limitation.

Palpation

This method of examination is used to assess chest excursion, symmetry, structural abnormalities and tenderness.

Chest excursion and symmetry. The chest excursion on inspiration reflects the extent of expansion and depth of respiration. It may be assessed by placing the hands on the chest with the fingers slightly outspread and the thumbs just meeting at the midline (Figure 15.11). As the patient breathes in, the hands are normally separated by the chest expansion. Whether the range of the chest excursion is the same on both sides is also noted; if it is equal, the thumbs will be moved an equal distance from the midline on each side. Normally the movements of the two sides are symmetrical.

Functional assessment

Functional assessment and investigations of the patient's effort tolerance are carried out to determine how energy expenditure in performing various activities can be reduced and how the environment can be modified to facilitate functioning:

1. What is the patient's usual level of daily activity?
   (a) Is he or she eating?
   (b) Can he or she dress, shave or shower without assistance?

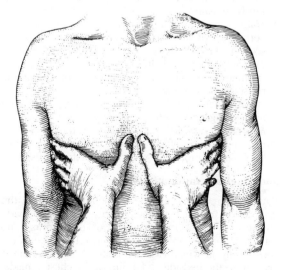

Figure 15.11 Assessing the chest excursion on inspiration.

(c) Can he or she climb stairs?
(d) What household activities can be performed, for example, vacuuming, making beds, preparing food?
(e) What occupational activities is the patient capable of performing (e.g. sedentary or physical)?

2. When does breathlessness occur? Is it:
   (a) With simple daily tasks such as shaving, dressing, tying shoe-laces?
   (b) With extra effort such as climbing stairs?
   (c) During the night?
   (d) On getting up in the morning?

3. Can the breathlessness be prevented by modifying the breathing pattern or by taking a bronchodilator before the activity?

4. *Effort tolerance* may be assessed by the use of a 'treadmill'. A chair should be available if the patient should have to stop and rest. The resting heart rate is recorded as well as the pulse rate on completion of the test. An ear oximeter is used to determine the changes in the arterial oxygen saturation associated with the exercise. The test estimates the patient's horizontal walking capacity.

   This information about the patient's energy assists in planning an acceptable daily routine and an exercise programme to increase the effort tolerance.

5. Further data are obtained to identify how the patient perceives the respiratory dysfunction.
   (a) What does it mean to the patient?
   (b) What losses in functioning are most relevant to the patient?
   (c) What losses is he or she able to accept?
   (d) How does he or she feel about it?
   (e) Is the attitude one of hopeless resignation or unrealistic denial?
   (f) Is the patient motivated to pursue a self-care programme?

DIAGNOSTIC MEASUREMENTS OF BREATHING PATTERN EFFECTIVENESS

The nurse functions in collaboration with the physician to identify the need for specific diagnostic tests, to co-ordinate patient activities related to the tests, and to prepare the patient for the tests. Knowledge of the findings from diagnostic procedures is used by the nurse to plan nursing care, set priorities for care and to assist the patient and family to develop a realistic health care regimen.

Pulmonary function tests

Measurements of lung volumes (Table 15.7). Lung volumes may be determined by spirometry at the bedside, in the clinic, doctor's surgery or patient's home. (Spirometry is the measurement of air taken into and expelled from the lungs.) Changes in lung volumes provide the best objective measurement of airflow limitation. Lung volume determinations are used to identify potential risks of respiratory complications in preoperative patients and to monitor changes in the postoperative period. Vital capacity and timed forced

Table 15.7 Summary of pulmonary function measurement.

Test	Symbol	Description	Comments
Vital capacity	VC	The maximal volume of air exhaled following a maximal inspiration (normal: 3500–5000 ml)	Reduced in restrictive airway disease because of limited lung expansion. In obstructive airway disease, the total lung capacity is increased but vital capacity may be reduced due to air trapping with increased residual volume
Tidal volume	V_T	The volume of air exhaled following a normal breath (normal: 450–500 ml)	
Forced vital capacity	FVC	The maximal volume of air that can be forcibly and rapidly exhaled following a maximal inspiration	Reduced in obstructive airway disease due to air trapping
Timed vital capacity	FEV_T	The percentage of vital capacity that can be expelled in 1 second (FEV_1), 2 seconds (FEV_2) and 3 seconds (FEV_3) (normal ranges: FEV_1, 80%; FEV_2, 90%; FEV_3, 95%)	Reduced in obstructive airway disease because of increased airway resistance; usually normal in restrictive airway disease
Maximal voluntary ventilation	MVV	The maximal volume of air that can be breathed in a given time interval (normal: about 40–70 breaths per minute breathing half of the vital capacity with each breath)	The least accurate of timed breathing tests. Useful indication of exercise tolerance
Residual volume	RV	The volume of gas remaining in the lungs at the end of a maximal expiration (normal: 25–40% of total lung capacity, e.g. 1500 ml)	Increased in obstructive airway disease
Functional residual capacity	FRC	The volume of air remaining in the lung after a passive exhalation in normal breathing (normal: about 3000 ml)	Increased in obstructive airway disease

expiratory volume are used most frequently at the bedside.

The normal values for the different lung volumes have been established from studies made on normal subjects. They vary with height, age and sex; tables of normal values are available.

- *Vital capacity* (VC) is represented by the maximal volume of air exhaled following a maximal inspiration. To determine the VC, the individual breathes through a mouthpiece which is connected to a tube leading to a spirometer. The normal VC ranges from 3500–5000 ml.

  The VC provides information about the compliance, since the person made an effort to expand his lungs fully when taking the maximal inspiration.
- *Tidal volume* (V_T) is the volume of air exhaled following a normal breath. The normal is usually stated as being 450–500 ml with the individual at rest, but varies with individuals and their activities. *Minute ventilation* (or minute respiratory volume) is determined by multiplying the tidal volume by the number of respirations per minute.
- *Forced vital capacity* (FVC) is the maximal volume of air that can be forcibly and rapidly exhaled following

a maximal inspiration.
- *Peak flow* measures the maximum rate at which air can be exhaled.
- *Timed forced expiratory volume* (FEV_T) records the percentage of vital capacity that can be expelled in 1 second (FEV_1). Normally about 80% of the vital capacity is expired in 1 second. Timed forced expiratory volumes provide information about the resistance to expiratory airflow.
- *Residual volume* (RV) is the volume of gas remaining in the lungs at the end of a maximal expiration.
- *Functional residual capacity* (FRC) is the air remaining in the lung after passive exhalation in normal breathing; no forceful or increased effort is used.

Radiological examinations

X-rays of the chest are done to identify lesions in the respiratory tract or thoracic cavity and to provide information about the structure of the thorax. The patient may be too ill to be moved to the X-ray department, in which case a portable X-ray machine is brought to the bedside and a film of the chest is made. Staff members leave the room while the X-ray is taken to avoid unnecessary exposure to radiation.

Radiological investigation may include making a series of films of the lungs at different planes. This type of radiology is referred to as *plain film tomography*. In these films the lung tissue is visualized at different depths. They provide details that are not revealed in ordinary X-rays because of overlying structures. Tomographs are helpful in recognizing solid or calcified lesions and cavitations.

Computerized tomography is a cross-sectional imaging modality which provides unique information about the lung fields and mediastinum. It is particularly useful in identifying small pulmonary nodules (e.g. early metastases), calcified foci and the degree of invasion of a malignant lesion (e.g. mediastinal involvement from a primary bronchial carcinoma). Such information may not be detected by other techniques.

Fluoroscopic examination (direct viewing by X-ray) of the chest may be done to view lung expansion and the respiratory excursion of the diaphragm.

Pulmonary and bronchial angiography. A pulmonary arteriogram may be performed via a catheter suitably placed in a large systemic vein (superior or inferior vena cava), the right side of the heart or the pulmonary artery (see Chapter 14). An injected radiopaque contrast medium will depict the pulmonary circulation and confirm or exclude the presence of pulmonary emboli. The nature and extent of arteriovenous malformations can also be delineated.

The bronchial arteries arise from the thoracic aorta; they may be selectively catheterized and their circulation studied. The usual indication is to establish the site of bleeding from a chronic cavity. Once found, the radiologist has the facility to embolize the main feeding artery, occluding the vessel and thereby controlling the haemorrhage.

Histological examinations

Bronchial biopsy. Bronchial tissue can be visually examined through a bronchoscope and samples of tissue and cells obtained by brushing or aspirating secretions from the involved areas.

Lung biopsy. A lung biopsy may be necessary to confirm a diagnosis when radiological studies reveal pulmonary infiltration or lesions. Lung tissue can be obtained for examination by open thoracotomy, bronchoscopy or percutaneous needle biopsy. Transbronchial biopsy involves the introduction of a bronchoscope, using fluoroscopy, and the insertion of long flexible forceps into the involved area. Small samples of tissue may be obtained in this manner. Percutaneous needle biopsy involves the insertion of a needle into the diseased area to obtain a small sample of tissue. The procedure is useful when the lesion is localized but other diseased areas may be missed.

Lymph node biopsy. The scalene lymph nodes, which are situated in a pad of fat anterior to the scalenus anterior muscle in the neck, drain the lungs and mediastinum. The nodes are examined histologically to help determine the spread of a bronchogenic carcinoma and the indications for surgical resection or the prognosis in diseases such as sarcoidosis, tuberculosis or lymphomas such as Hodgkin's disease.

Pleural biopsy. Pleural fluid and tissue may be obtained during open thoracotomy but is usually obtained by thoracentesis. A specially designed needle is inserted into the pleura and samples are taken. Tissue from several sites may be required to confirm a diagnosis of tuberculosis or a malignancy.

Nursing Intervention

The *goal* is that the patient will increase the effectiveness of breathing by maximizing ventilation and increasing airflow. This may be shown by the patient demonstrating:

- A decreased rate and increased depth of respiration.
- Awareness of factors contributing to impaired breathing pattern.
- Increased lung volume measurements.
- The ability to perform planned breathing techniques.
- Increased activity tolerance.

Nursing measures for the individual with an ineffective breathing pattern include: (1) positioning the person to increase lung inflation and emptying and to decrease respiratory effort; (2) teaching the individual the techniques of diaphragmatic breathing and pursed-lip breathing; (3) the use of relaxation techniques; (4) nutritional assessment and management; and (5) teaching the person effectively to utilize prescribed medications to manage their breathing impairment. These interventions are relevant regardless of the cause of the altered breathing pattern. Other measures specific to the aetiological factors are discussed with each problem.

POSITIONING

Individuals experiencing dyspnoea will usually assume a position that best facilitates lung expansion and minimizes the work of breathing, even though this posture may appear uncomfortable to the observer. Sitting, leaning forward from the waist facilitates movement of the diaphragm and is usually the position of choice. Resting the arms and shoulders on a fairly high table or other solid object provides support and decreases effort.

DIAPHRAGMATIC BREATHING

Increasing diaphragmatic excursions and reducing the use of accessory muscles achieves the following objectives: ventilation of the lung bases is improved by improving breathing efficiency and reducing upper alveolar overinflation; the work of breathing is reduced; uncoordinated breathing patterns are eliminated; activity tolerance improves; and the patient learns to control breathing when dyspnoeic, reducing the anxious feelings and panic.

Diaphragmatic breathing involves:

1. Placing the patient's or instructor's hands on the patient's abdomen below the ribs
2. Relaxation of the shoulders

3. Taking a deep breath through the nose while pushing the abdomen outward against the hands
4. Holding the breath for 1 or 2 seconds to keep the alveoli open
5. And breathing out slowly through the mouth while applying gentle pressure to the abdomen with the hands.

The exercise is repeated several times and the patient is encouraged to concentrate on the abdominal movement.

PURSED-LIP BREATHING

Pursed-lip breathing involves taking a deep breath and exhaling slowly and fully through pursed lips. The aim of this technique is to minimize airway collapse on exhalation, especially in emphysema.

RELAXATION

The use of progressive relaxation techniques and biofeedback help to reduce the respiratory rate, increase tidal volumes and decrease carbon dioxide production in patients with chronic airflow limitation. Patients are taught to use relaxation techniques during periods of high anxiety or 'panic attacks' and to plan periods of relaxation into their daily routine.

DRUGS TO PROMOTE VENTILATION AND IMPROVE AIRFLOW

1. *Bronchodilators* are administered to prevent or treat bronchoconstriction (Smith, 1985; Lindell and Mazzocco, 1990). Examples of these are:
  (a) *β₂-Adrenergic agonists.* These include salbutamol (Ventolin), terbutaline (Bricanyl), fenoterol (Berotec) and adrenaline. The metered-dose inhaler is the most commonly used form of these drugs. A specific amount of the drug is delivered each time the inhaler is activated (see Figure 15.12). The dose usually prescribed is two puffs 3–4 times a day. Salbutamol and terbutaline are also available for oral administration and salbutamol may also be given parenterally but these routes of administration are associated with increased adverse effects such as tremor and palpitations. In most patients, parenteral administration is no more effective and may be less well tolerated than inhalation of the drug.
    Adrenaline is a quick and powerful bronchodilator but its adverse cardiac effects limit its use. It is usually given subcutaneously. Following administration, the patient is observed closely for a rapid, irregular, weak pulse, tremors, anxiety and restlessness.
  (b) *Anticholinergic agents.* Ipratropium (Atrovent) is the most commonly used agent in this category of bronchodilators. It is usually given by inhalation using a metered-dose inhaler or in nebulized solution as additive therapy to salbutamol. It may cause dryness of the mouth.

  (c) *Theophylline.* This drug may be administered as theophylline or as aminophylline or oxytriphylline. It is effective given orally or intravenously. Side-effects include headache, cardiac arrhythmias, palpitations and hypotension.
2. *Corticosteroids* may be given in conjunction with a bronchodilator to reduce bronchial reactivity. Steroids are most commonly given by metered-dose inhaler. Examples of corticosteroid preparations are beclomethasone dipropionate (Beclovent, Becloforte, Beconase), budesonide (Pulmicort), flunisolide and triamcinolone. Administration by inhalation minimizes the side-effects characteristic of long-term systemic administration of corticosteroids. For acute respiratory manifestations, corticosteroids may be given orally or intravenously. The dose must then be tapered gradually and the patient placed on inhaled steroid therapy.
3. *Antibiotics.* A broad-spectrum antibiotic (e.g. co-trimoxazole, amoxycillin (Amoxil)) is given when the earliest signs of infection appear. These may be purulent sputum, general malaise, fever, decreased activity tolerance and shortness of breath. A sputum specimen may first be collected so that the organism may be identified and sensitivity tests made in order for a specific antimicrobial drug to be prescribed and administered.

Patient teaching related to drug therapy

Since there are no cures for the many chronic respiratory disorders, treatment programmes and drug therapy are planned for each individual according to personal goals, life-style situation, respiratory status and response to drugs and other therapeutic measures. The patient usually assumes responsibility for self-management of the therapeutic regimen and therefore requires the knowledge and skill necessary not only to administer the drugs but also to make decisions regarding the plan. The individual learns to monitor responses to medications, determine when adjustments are desirable and when to seek further professional assistance.

The teaching plan should include:

● Information about the action, duration of effect, method of administration and side-effects of prescribed medications.
● Instruction and practice in the proper use of metered-dose inhalers for optimal delivery of the medication into the bronchial tree. For individuals who have difficulty manipulating the metered-dose inhaler, an aerosol holding chamber (Aerochamber) may be used.
● Participation in the development of the medication schedule to meet the individual's needs. The duration of action of bronchodilators is approximately 4 hours; therefore, these drugs are usually administered four to six times per day. Administration may be planned to coincide with the beginning of specific activities to promote optimal functioning. The dose of corticosteroid preparations is adjusted so that the smallest dose necessary to maintain improvement in airflow is administered. Inhalation preparations are

used to minimize systemic effects; also, a smaller dose is required.

The effectiveness of nurses teaching patients with chronic respiratory disease is demonstrated by two studies in particular. Howard (1987) showed that a structured teaching programme had the effect of reducing hospital admissions, and the lengths of such admissions when necessary, in a sample of 115 patients (predominantly white males). The effect was a reduction of between 15 and 25% in the number of days this group would have been expected to spend in hospital. Nursing time spent on such activities is cost effective when consideration is given to the substantial savings that could be made by hospitals, and clearly the improvement in health that occurred is very beneficial to the patients.

A community based approach to patient teaching and support was used successfully by Heslop and Bagnall (1988) who studied the benefits patients might derive from monthly home visits by nurses. The major problems that were identified were patients' lack of knowledge and the great deal of fear and anxiety that was generated by breathless attacks which severely restricted the patient's activity. Patients were encouraged to set their own goals and met with a great deal of success in achieving them. However, psychosocial problems proved very resistant to change and caused major difficulties for many of the patients in this study.

Ineffective Breathing Pattern Related to Chronic Airflow Limitation

CHRONIC OBSTRUCTIVE AIRWAYS DISEASE (COAD)

This refers to a persistent limitation to airflow in the bronchial tree which, even after treatment, is greater than expected for the person's age, height and sex. As the limitation in airflow increases, breathing patterns change and become less efficient and eventually are unable to meet the ventilatory needs of the body. The accompanying dyspnoea and activity intolerance result from as well as contribute to the deterioration in breathing pattern. COAD occurs in a variety of conditions (chronic bronchitis, emphysema, bronchiectasis and asthma) but, more commonly, in association with a combination of these conditions. Roberts (1988) estimates about one million people in the UK are affected, 40 000 so seriously that they require help with daily living due to the limitations imposed on them by COAD. It is most common in the elderly and amongst the poorer sections of society.

Chronic bronchitis

This disease is characterized by hyperactivity of the mucus-secreting glands of the bronchial mucosa in response to prolonged or frequently recurring irritation (Duffy, 1985). The common irritants are tobacco smoke, infection and atmospheric pollutants such as dust, industrial fumes and smoke. The most frequent offender is tobacco smoke. The person experiences frequent, productive coughing. A higher incidence is seen in older persons and in persons of poor socio-economic circumstances. Dampness, wind and winter cold are considered to be aggravating factors.

The bronchial mucosa undergoes a chronic inflammatory process, together with hypertrophy and an increase in the number of mucus-secreting glands. Airway obstruction results from the narrowing of the bronchial lumen due to the hyperplasia of the mucus-secreting glands and the increased production of sputum. Clinical symptoms are characterized by an increase in sputum and coughing.

Pulmonary emphysema

Emphysema is the Greek word meaning inflation. In medicine, it implies a swelling or distension due to an accumulation of air. It may occur in any tissue. Pulmonary emphysema is a chronic disorder characterized by overdistension of the terminal respiratory units or pulmonary lobules by entrapped air. The connective tissue of the lung is damaged, resulting in enlargement of the alveolar spaces and loss of gas exchange surface. Destruction of the pulmonary lung units occurs with ageing in all lungs but is accelerated in some, leading to clinical emphysema. The damage is not uniform. It may affect only the central portion of the pulmonary lobules (centralobular emphysema) or it may result in destruction of most of the structures within a terminal unit, including the alveolar ducts and alveoli (panlobular emphysema). In some individuals, the incidence of panlobular emphysema is related to a hereditary deficiency of a protease inhibitor which normally protects the respiratory tissue from proteolytic enzymes. The disease process is accelerated by smoking.

The onset is insidious but, once initiated, is progressive and non-reversible. The lung damage cannot be repaired but the patient can be helped to breathe more effectively and live with less disability.

Bronchiectasis

This disorder is a chronic dilatation of bronchial tubes resulting from destruction of elastic and muscular tissue of the walls. It may involve any part of the lung, but the lower dependent segments are the areas affected most often.

The cause of bronchiectasis is repeated or prolonged pulmonary infection, bronchial obstruction by extrinsic pressure, a mucus plug or an aspirated foreign body. The dilatation occurs above the obstruction.

Dilatation of the tubes results in the retention and pooling of secretions which readily become infected. The infection is perpetuated and extends, causing further tissue damage. The degree of impairment of pulmonary ventilation and oxygen uptake depends upon the amount of chronic infection and lung damage. Retention of secretions causes bronchial obstruction and inadequate aeration of the bronchioles and alveoli distal to the bronchiectatic area, altering pulmonary ventilation and perfusion. In severe cases surgical removal of part of the lung may be needed (lobectomy). Glen (1986) has given a good account of the care such a patient may need.

The incidence of bronchiectasis has decreased with the prevention and antibiotic treatment of broncho-pneumonia. The decrease in childhood communicable diseases which predispose to respiratory infections has been an important contributory factor to the lesser incidence.

Asthma

Scadding (1977) defines asthma, in terms of patho-physiology, as a disease characterized by wide variations over short periods of time in resistance to flow in intrapulmonary airways. The use of the term 'asthma' without further specification should imply no more than clinically important variability in airflow resistance.

The reaction of the overresponsive airway to stimuli is oedema and thickening of the mucosa, hypersecretion by the mucous glands and contraction of bronchial and bronchiolar muscle tissue. This causes diffuse narrowing of the tracheobronchial tree and obstruction to airflow. The bronchoconstriction is attributed to: (1) the action of chemical mediators such as histamine, and other slow-reacting substances of anaphylaxis, and prostaglandins released in response to an antigen; they act on receptor sites on the membrane of smooth muscle cells, producing contraction of the smooth muscle; or (2) an abnormality in the neural regulation of the smooth muscle tissue of the airway. It is considered possible that both mechanisms may play a role in causing bronchoconstriction. Narrowing of the airway in asthma also results from the changes that take place in the mucosa of the airways.

Stimuli which may precipitate the asthmatic response include allergens, infection, irritating inhalants (chemicals, air pollutants), cold air, acetylsalicylic acid (aspirin), emotional stress, physical exercise and laughing. Frequently, there is a personal and/or family history of one or more allergies. Asthma often begins in childhood but may develop at any age. Warning signs of increasing bronchial reactivity include frequent awakening at night, decreased physical effort tolerance, shortness of breath on getting up in the morning and cough.

During an acute asthmatic attack the patient experiences tightness in the chest, wheezing and dyspnoea. The accessory muscles of respiration are used and expiration is prolonged. The patient appears distraught and assumes an upright sitting position. The sputum is scant and thick and the pulse is rapid.

Patients suffering severe asthmatic attacks may require intubation and artificial ventilation for a period if they do not respond to aerosol and intravenously administered bronchodilator therapy. Repeated peak flow measurements and arterial blood gas values are good guides to progress, together with vital sign monitoring. The importance of psychological support during acute episodes of respiratory distress cannot be overemphasized.

Asthma accounts for some 2000 deaths per year in England and Wales and will affect 1 in 5 children and 1 in 15 adults (Nocon and Booth, 1990) at some time in their lives. The number of general practitioner consultations for asthma has increased from 380 000 in 1955 to 875 000 in 1981–1982, while the cost of treating asthma in 1987 is estimated at £100m (Office of Health Economics, 1990). The increased incidence may partly reflect an increased awareness of, rather than a real increase in, the disease (Nursing Standard, 1990).

The effects upon families or patients with asthma can be devastating, as Nocon and Booth (1990) have shown, with the disease causing major practical and emotional problems for everyone, not just the unfortunate sufferer. These workers have found a great lack of knowledge amongst the patients they have seen, and comment upon how ideally placed nurses are to help. A lack of response to a bronchodilator is a vital warning sign of an impending serious attack, a sign that is often missed. Many authors (Walsh, 1989a) have advocated the use of routine peak flow monitoring at home, in the same way that diabetic patients monitor blood sugar. Deterioration in peak flow is another warning sign which, if acted upon, could avert a major medical emergency. There is a great deal of scope for patient teaching about practical physical aspects of the illness, as well as the need to recognize the psychological stresses that asthma places upon both the victim and the rest of the family.

The practice of labelling children 'asthmatic' at school, and hence making them 'special cases' when it comes to activities such as games, can clearly hinder their normal development. Research by Mead (1990) has shown that a deliberate policy of education and encouraging exercise amongst a group of 10–13-year-old asthmatic children was very beneficial, making the children feel much more positively about themselves, without any harmful physical effects. Mead strongly believes that this is the way forward if the myth of childhood asthma as a debilitating illness is to be overcome, but points out the shortcomings of teaching staff to understand the illness. There is a major role for school nurses to play in promoting health and improving knowledge about asthma.

PATIENT PROBLEMS COMMON TO THOSE WITH COAD

Ineffective breathing pattern

The most frequent symptom of COAD is a prolonged expiratory phase, as demonstrated by an increase in the forced expiratory time. Other characteristics of the breathing pattern of a person with COAD are rapid, shallow respirations and use of the intercostal and accessory muscles. Shortness of breath is experienced by many, but not all patients, despite severe airflow limitation. Dyspnoea varies daily with changes in activity, increased effort and during sleep. Characteristics of the breathing pattern and changes in objective clinical measurements in individuals with COAD are listed in Table 15.8.

Activity intolerance

Respiratory muscle fatigue develops in persons with COAD in response to the increased airway resistance, which in turn increases the work of breathing. The inspiratory muscles have to generate greater pressures to ventilate the lungs. Muscle fatigue occurs when the

Table 15.8 Characteristics of the breathing pattern of persons with COAD.

Physical characteristics
Clavicles are prominent (sculpturing)
Hypertrophy of accessory muscles of respiration
Tracheal shortening
Tracheal descent on inspiration
Costal margins of the rib cage move inward on respiration
Diminished breath sounds
Sputum production increased in many but not all patients

Symptoms
Breathlessness
Weakness

Measurements
1. Lung volumes:
   Forced expiratory time (FET)—increased (greater than 4 seconds)
   Forced expiratory volume (FEV)—decreased
   Vital capacity—normal or slightly reduced
   Ratio of FEV/VC—decreased
   Peak flow reduced
2. Blood gases:
   Pao_2—less than 8.0 kPa (60 mmHg)
   $Paco_2$—greater than 6.0 kPa (45 mmHg)

From Robinson & Pugsley (1981).

inspiratory muscles are no longer able to maintain the force required for ventilation.

Activity intolerance increases with exercise and stress and impairs the individual's ability to perform usual activities. Eventually, the effort of breathing consumes all of the individual's energy.

Altered nutrition: less than body requirements
Weight loss and muscle wasting are recognized problems in persons with chronic lung disease. An increased caloric intake is needed because of the increased energy expended with breathing. Associated problems include a loss of appetite and decreased senses of taste and smell. Dyspnoea increases with eating because of the competition between eating and breathing.

Knowledge deficit related to promotion and maintenance of respiratory function
Long-term management of COAD requires the patient to be an active participant in the care process. The individual requires knowledge of the disorder, an understanding of the use, actions, administration and side-effects of the medications, the ability to perform breathing retraining techniques, information on factors influencing respiratory function, and information about community resources.

NURSING INTERVENTION

Although COAD is irreversible, patient care has improved sufficiently over the past few decades to enable patients to live useful and satisfying lives. The patient's *goal* is to achieve an effective breathing pattern so that greater levels of activity can be tolerated. This can be shown by the patient being able to:

● Demonstrate a decreased respiratory rate and increased depth of respirations.
● Demonstrate increased lung volumes.
● Report decreased episodes and severity of dyspnoea.
● Tolerate increased levels of activity.

Breathing pattern
Assessment of the individual's respiratory status is ongoing and focuses on the relationship of the deterioration in ventilation to the person's ability to function in daily living activities. Interventions to improve dyspnoea are limited. The person's home and work environments are assessed for possible respiratory irritants and the individual is directed to appropriate resources for help in altering the environment where this is possible.

The nurse can assist the individual to gain control over the respiratory pattern. During an acute episode, the nurse can provide emotional support and at the same time teach the person to relax and control breathing. The nurse stays with the person, placing the hands on the patient's shoulder and abdomen and quietly repeating instructions and encouragement to breathe slowly and deeply, gradually altering the breathing pattern and decreasing fear and panic. Patients are taught the techniques of breathing retraining and relaxation discussed on p. 402. Bronchodilators and corticosteroids are the medications most often prescribed for persons with COAD. The nurse works in collaboration with the patient, general practitioner, physiotherapist and occupational therapists and pharmacists to teach the patient and family to monitor and manage the respiratory care programme.

Activity
Once respiratory muscles become fatigued, they must be rested. Interventions are directed toward decreasing the work of breathing and increasing the individual's tolerance. Inhaled medications are administered to dilate the bronchial airways and to decrease inflammation, thus decreasing the effort of breathing. Postural changes such as sitting in the forward leaning position may also facilitate breathing. The use of general body exercises and respiratory muscle training shows promise in improving respiratory muscle strength and developing a more effective breathing pattern but evidence is not yet adequate to recommend routine application of these interventions.

Patients are helped to plan their daily activities to include periods of rest before and following activity and to learn more effective ways of performing daily living activities.

Nutrition
Although no randomized controlled longitudinal studies have been carried out to date to show that nutritional support alters the outcome for persons with chronic

respiratory disease, malnutrition is a recognized patient health problem.

A nutritional assessment should be carried out on all patients with COAD. Appropriate nutritional counselling should be provided as indicated and measures instituted to alter the cause of the malnutrition. Patients need to be knowledgeable about the effects of malnutrition on their breathing pattern and be assisted to develop a plan to improve their nutrition intake.

Teaching

Self-monitoring and self-care are essential components of the management programme. The patient must learn to cope with the limitations imposed by the disease, prevent complications and comply with the treatment plan if a satisfactory life-style is to be achieved. As with any chronic disorder, the individual must learn to live with the disease process and to manage his daily routine accordingly. A learning plan specific to an individual patient with COAD is presented with the following clinical situation.

CLINICAL SITUATION: MR JACKSON WHO HAS COAD*

Mr Jackson is a 68-year-old man who lives with his wife in their own home in a small city. They have been married for 40 years and have three adult children and eight grandchildren who all live within a 50-mile radius.

For about 10 years Mr Jackson has been aware that he becomes short of breath before others, and has gradually limited his activities to the extent that, when he was admitted to hospital 6 months ago, he had stopped dressing every day and spent a great deal of time indoors. Often, when their children invited him and his wife to their homes, he would refuse, saying it was 'too much' for him. This disappointed Mrs Jackson who really enjoyed her family and loved to spend time with them, but she would not leave her husband at home alone.

While Mr Jackson was in hospital, he and his wife were taught things that were really surprising to them, and Mr Jackson found he could do many things he had previously thought impossible.

Often it is at a crisis period, such as Mr Jackson's hospital admission, that the health care team first meets a person who has been suffering unnecessarily for months or even years. The teaching that was begun at this time, and continued once Mr Jackson was discharged, made a significant difference to the life he was able to lead. The areas that were emphasized during this teaching/learning process included: use of medications, what to watch for, helpful breathing techniques, life-style considerations.

Learning objectives

Mr and Mrs Jackson will be able to:

- Describe the effects of his medications on his respiratory function.
- Demonstrate the proper use of his inhaler.

* With permission of Lee Robinson, Clinical Nurse Specialist.

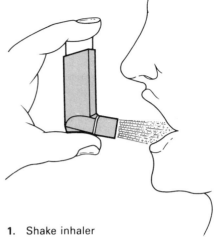

1. Shake inhaler
2. Exhale fully
3. Spray once into wide open mouth as you inhale fully
4. Hold breath for 5 seconds before exhaling
5. Repeat for each puff ordered

Figure 15.12 Using a metered dose inhaler.

- Implement his medication regimen with indirect supervision.
- Describe signs and symptoms of respiratory failure.
- State actions to take to prevent the recurrence of respiratory complications.
- Demonstrate effective use of breathing techniques.
- Develop plans to increase activity tolerance and participation in activities of daily living.

Use of medications

Mr Jackson has COAD. This has developed gradually in conjunction with his years of heavy smoking (he stopped smoking 3 years ago). For this reason, Mr Jackson takes an inhaled bronchodilator, salbutamol (Ventolin), on a regular basis throughout the day.

On his admission to the ward, the nurse noted his FEV/IVC before his four puffs of salbutamol was 0.8/2.0, but this rose to 1/2.6 after using the inhaler. This improvement was explained to him and the graphic recordings from the spirometer were shown to him and his wife so that they could appreciate the definite improvement achieved with his medication. The nurse also explained to them that the effects of this medication reduce after 3 hours and are almost gone by 4 hours, so it is important for Mr Jackson to use the inhaler every 4 hours while he is awake. He was also encouraged to use it during the night if he awakened. He was reassured there were no serious side-effects from salbutamol and he would not build up a tolerance by using it regularly.

In addition, the nurse explained correct inhaler use and watched as Mr Jackson took his inhaler to make sure he was using the correct technique (Figure 15.12).

Since an untreated respiratory infection precipitated Mr Jackson's need to be admitted to the hospital, he was taught to watch for changes in his cough, sputum colour or volume, as well as for systemic symptoms such as a sore throat, increased temperature or general malaise so that he might seek immediate medical treatment.

What to watch for (prevention of complications)

On admission, Mr Jackson was in respiratory failure, with an elevated arterial carbon dioxide level of 9.3 kPa (normal < 5 kPa) and a lowered oxygen of 5.4 kPa (acceptable if > 8 kPa). By the time he was discharged, his arterial blood gases did not indicate respiratory failure ($Paco_2$ 5.8 kPa, Pao_2 8 kPa), but he was in a high-risk category for developing it because of his severe airflow limitation and borderline arterial blood gases. For this reason, he was taught to recognize signs of respiratory failure.

The nurse reviewed with the Jacksons the signs and symptoms Mr Jackson had noticed before he came to hospital. Mrs Jackson pointed out that her husband was very restless and unable to sleep at night and that just the opposite occurred during the day, when he would be drowsy and uninterested in his surroundings and was always falling asleep. The nurse explained that this 'reversed sleep pattern' is common when respiratory failure develops and the carbon dioxide level in the blood rises. Mr Jackson remembered his legs were swollen and it had been difficult to move around because of that. The nurse explained this oedema was also the result of the build up of carbon dioxide. Mrs Jackson asked if the whole process of his 'decline' might have been prevented if he had been using his salbutamol more regularly and had seen his general practitioner for treatment as soon as he noticed his increased cough and yellow sputum. The nurse reassured her that she was right and Mr Jackson should be able to prevent the need for hospital stays in the future.

Other changes Mr Jackson had noticed were throbbing headaches, particularly on awakening, and a bluish appearance of his fingernails. The nurse emphasized that all of these observations were warning signs for him and that he would now know he needs to take action when his body tells him his respiratory problem is getting worse.

Techniques to improve breathing

Mr Jackson brings up a small amount of white sputum every morning. In addition to observing the colour and amount of this sputum, he was taught the importance of clearing the airways of sputum by deliberate coughing. A good time to cough is 30 minutes after his inhaled salbutamol, and particular efforts were encouraged in the mornings to clear any sputum that had not been coughed up during the night.

Mr Jackson was also taught to control his breathing pattern, particularly when anxious or exerting himself. The nurse explained that because there is obstruction to airflow, air cannot move quickly in and out of his lungs. This abnormality is most pronounced on expiration because the air tubes become smaller as the lungs shrink down. The tendency is for air to become trapped in the lungs, making them bigger and less efficient. This trapping can be reduced if he prolongs his expiration phase, making it twice as long as inspiration. Mr Jackson

was taught to slow his breathing pattern, to make his breath out twice as long as his breath in, and to breathe out through pursed lips, which will help to control the flow of expired air and to reduce the tendency for airways to collapse.

Since there is a natural tendency to hold the breath during activities which require extra effort or concentration, such as shaving, stair climbing and lifting objects, the nurse warned Mr Jackson to be conscious of his breathing pattern during these activities. One technique suggested was to do the heavier part of an activity during the breathe out.

Life-style considerations

Since Mr Jackson had reduced many of his activities, it was important to discuss his daily life and help him to plan to be more active. While on the ward he was given a programme of walking and stair climbing to help prepare him for more activity at home. In addition, he was taught how to anticipate shortness of breath and to offset severe symptoms by using his inhaler prior to activities which were likely to cause breathlessness. Most importantly, he was encouraged to be as active as possible and not be restricted in doing most things, as long as he modified his approach with consideration for his breathing.

Evaluation

Mr Jackson has been out of hospital for 5 months now. During that time, he has come into the out-patient clinic every 4–6 weeks to have his breathing and gas exchange evaluated with spirometry, rebreathing carbon dioxide and oximetry. He has seen his physician and the clinic nurse on these visits. The nurse has reinforced the teaching begun in hospital and has helped Mr Jackson to adapt the teaching to his daily life. He has successfully completed one course of antibiotic therapy and re-covered quite smoothly from this chest infection without needing admission to hospital. He has maintained a daily walking programme and has been able to go to his childrens' homes for visits. Both Mr and Mrs Jackson seem satisfied with their life and proud of their progress.

Ineffective Breathing Pattern Related to Localized Airway Obstruction

Localized obstruction of airflow is less common than chronic airflow limitation and causes less residual impairment.

OBSTRUCTION OF THE NASAL PASSAGES

The narrow nasal passages are particularly susceptible to obstruction. Obstruction may be the result of: trauma causing deviation of the septum and nasal fractures; foreign bodies in the nose, which are common in childhood; growths and polyps; and inflammation of the nasal mucosa as a result of irritation from pollution, allergies, smoking or infection. Signs and symptoms include assymetry of the nose from trauma, bleeding, and thin to thick, purulent drainage. The person breathes through one nostril or the mouth when obstruction is present.

OBSTRUCTION OF THE PHARYNX

Inflammation and enlargement of the adenoids in the nasopharynx and the tonsils in the oropharynx interfere with breathing and swallowing. Foreign bodies that are of sufficient size to lodge in the oropharynx are usually relatively easy to remove. Smaller objects that pass on to the larynx and bronchi pose a greater hazard.

OBSTRUCTION OF THE LARYNX

Oedema, laryngeal spasm, or aspiration of a foreign body may cause obstruction in the larynx. Any constriction or obstruction in the larynx is manifested quickly by hoarseness, dyspnoea, stridor (high-pitched crowing breath sound), cyanosis and increased but ineffective inspiratory effort, evidenced by the retraction of the intercostal spaces. Prompt emergency measures are necessary or death may ensue as a result of asphyxia.

OBSTRUCTION OF THE TRACHEA

Aspiration of a foreign body, scarring following trauma or surgery, or pressure from an aortic aneurysm or neoplasm of a neighbouring structure may narrow the trachea and offer resistance to the flow of air. Inspiratory and expiratory stridor result and hypoventilation leads to hypercapnoea and hypoxaemia.

Obstruction of the airway by an aspirated foreign body presents an acute emergency. The patient should be slapped vigorously between the scapulae. Alternatively, someone standing behind the individual places the arms around the victim's trunk just below the diaphragm, clasping the hands in front. Pressure is applied with the arms and hands (Figure 15.13). The compression (Heimlich hug or manoeuvre) forces air under pressure through the airway and may dislodge the aspirated mass. If this procedure does not dislodge the object, a laryngoscope may be quickly introduced by the doctor through which the offending object may be

retrieved. If the patient's breathing is completely obstructed, an emergency tracheostomy may have to be performed to establish an airway before the foreign body can be removed (see p. 385).

For *oedema* or *spasm*, intubation may be performed in which a tube is passed beyond the obstruction into the trachea to establish an airway, or the doctor may do a tracheostomy. If oedema of the larynx is due to an allergic response, the patient is given adrenaline 1:1000 subcutaneously. An adrenal corticosteroid preparation such as prednisone may be prescribed for a brief period to reduce tissue sensitivity. Local applications of ice to the neck may also be suggested.

When laryngeal muscle spasm is the cause of the obstruction, intravenous calcium chloride or calcium gluconate may be prescribed.

OBSTRUCTION OF A BRONCHUS

If a foreign body is inhaled, it may pass into either bronchus but most often it is the right one that is blocked. Localized obstruction may also be caused by enlarged lymph nodes surrounding the bronchus. Complete obstruction leads to atelectasis (collapse of the lung) beyond the obstruction.

Ineffective Breathing Pattern Related to Decreased Lung Expansion

Ineffective breathing pattern related to decreased lung expansion is a condition in which inflation of the lung is restricted, resulting in a reduction in lung volumes, particularly vital capacity (VC) and total lung capacity (TLC). Characteristics include (1) reduced lung volumes, (2) decreased maximal expiratory flow, (3) increased work of breathing and (4) maldistribution of ventilation.

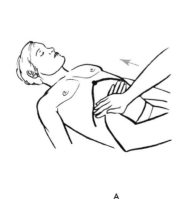

A

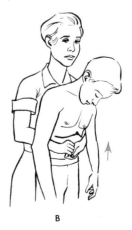

B

Figure 15.13 The Heimlich method of dislodging a foreign body from larynx or trachea.

CAUSES

CHANGES IN THE CHEST WALL

Ventilation may be restricted if the bony structure is abnormal or if there is rigidity of the wall. *Scoliosis* (a deformity in which the spine is S-shaped with one shoulder higher than the other) causes stiffness of the chest wall, as well as limiting the size. Surgical removal of ribs (*thoracoplasty*) results primarily in a reduction in the size of the thoracic cavity. Restriction to thoracic expansion may also occur following chest surgery when the patient tends to immobilize the chest and take shallow respirations to minimize the pain.

Blunt trauma to the chest wall may produce fractures of one or more ribs. The pain caused by such an injury may be severe and, as a result, the patient is reluctant to breathe deeply. If ribs are fractured in two places (a flail segment), that section of the chest wall becomes unstable and when negative pressure is created within the thoracic cavity for inhalation to occur, collapse of the chest wall inwards occurs (Fig. 15.14). This is known as paradoxical respiration. The result is that the lung is not adequately ventilated and life-threatening respiratory failure may ensue, particularly if the injury is associated with a haemopneumothorax. Wallis and Wells (1988), in an excellent review of chest injuries, point out that early death after chest trauma is usually due to hypoxia or hypovolaemia. Such injuries often require urgent positive pressure artificial ventilation, for which the patient needs intubation.

RESPIRATORY MUSCLE DYSFUNCTION

Restricted lung expansion may be the result of impaired innervation to the respiratory muscles, as occurs in the Guillain-Barré syndrome, poliomyelitis and amyotrophic lateral sclerosis, or it may be due to muscular weakness incurred by a chemical deficit at the myoneural junction (myasthenia gravis). The impaired muscle contraction causes dyspnoea and, if severe enough, respiratory failure. Involvement of the diaphragm increases symptoms and assisted ventilation is usually necessary. Severe obesity alters the mechanics of breathing by decreasing lung inflation, chest wall compliance and lung volumes.

DISORDERS OF THE PLEURAE

These include effusion and pneumothorax (collapse of the lung). Pleural effusion is an accumulation of an abnormal quantity of fluid in the interpleural space and is a symptom associated with a variety of conditions. The fluid may be a transudate or an exudate. A *transudate* may collect in the pleural space as a result of increased venous pressure incurred by congestive heart failure or an intrathoracic tumour which interferes with venous drainage in the area. Cirrhosis of the liver may cause a pleural effusion, as well as ascites. An accumulation of exudate in the pleural space indicates irritation and inflammation of the pleura associated with infection.

The patient with an effusion may experience some pleuritic pain, which is stabbing and is worse on inspiration before the excess fluid collects. The condition may develop insidiously and may go unrecognized until the increasing volume of fluid commences to compress the lung, causing dyspnoea and impaired pulmonary ventilation.

A chest aspiration (thoracentesis) is done to relieve the pressure on the lung and to obtain a specimen of fluid for examination (Mumford (1986). Treatment is directed toward the disease causing the effusion. A culture is made of the aspirated fluid for identification of the causative organisms and their antibiotic sensitivity. The patient receives antibiotics parenterally or orally, and the drug may also be injected into the thoracic cavity following aspiration. Surgical drainage may be necessary, especially if the pus is thick. Early breathing exercises to promote re-expansion of the lung are important, since the visceral pleura tends to become thick, fibrous and resistant to stretching, reducing lung compliance and the vital capacity.

Pneumothorax is a term used to describe a situation where a rupture in the visceral pleura allows air to accumulate in the pleural space, leading to collapse of part of the lung. This may occur after trauma or spontaneously. In *tension* pneumothorax the rupture acts as a one way valve so that air enters the pleural space on each respiration but cannot escape. This leads to a progressive build-up of air in the pleural space, collapse of the whole lung and displacement of the trachea away from the affected side. Major blood vessels become kinked and blood flow to the brain may be seriously impaired. Unlike a *simple* pneumothorax, which often resolves itself with the air in the pleural space being gradually reabsorbed, a tension pneumothorax is a life-threatening emergency. An accumulation of blood acts in the same way to compress the lung and is known as a *haemothorax*.

In order to expand the collapsed lung it is necessary to remove any blood or air from the pleura. This is done by introducing a drainage tube which is sutured in place and secured via an underwater seal drain to prevent air re-entering the pleural space (see p. 412). If the patient has a pneumothorax the chest drain is inserted high in the lateral chest wall, while to drain fluid and blood a site low down the lateral chest wall is selected. Drains may be inserted in both sites if blood and air need to be drained from the pleura (haemopneumothorax).

DISORDERS OF THE LUNG PARENCHYMA

Restriction of ventilation may be caused by a decrease in the lung tissue as seen with the surgical removal of a lung (pneumectomy) or by increased stiffness of lung tissue due to fibrosis.

Diffuse interstitial pulmonary fibrosis is frequently seen and is characterized by scattered areas of thickening of the interstitium of the alveolar walls. The respiratory bronchioles dilate and the alveoli coalesce forming larger air sacs. The cause is unknown in some patients. It may be associated with collagen–vascular diseases, prolonged occupational exposure to irritants or lung injuries. It has a higher incidence in older adults and results in dyspnoea and rapid shallow breathing on exertion. The larger airways, chest cage and respiratory

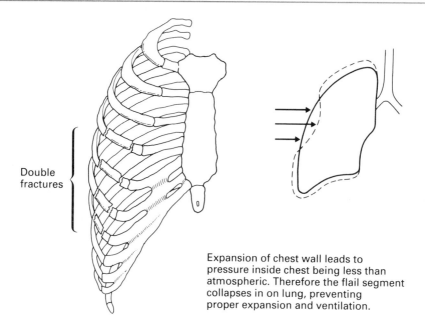

Double
fractures

Expansion of chest wall leads to
pressure inside chest being less than
atmospheric. Therefore the flail segment
collapses in on lung, preventing
proper expansion and ventilation.

Figure 15.14 A flail segment.

muscles remain normal. Distensibility of the lung is reduced, causing increased effort on inspiration and decreased lung volumes. Gas exchange is impaired and both the arterial Po_2 and Pco_2 are reduced.

Treatment usually includes corticosteroid therapy and breathing exercises to improve the patient's pattern of breathing and to establish more effective respirations.

ASSESSMENT

Nursing assessment focuses on the person's respiratory status and breathing pattern. The breathing pattern of an individual with decreased lung expansion resulting from impairment of one or more of the pulmonary components (chest wall, respiratory muscles, pleura and lung parenchyma) is characterized by decreased lung volumes, dyspnoea, use of the accessory muscles of respiration and rapid, shallow breathing. In non-emergency situations the nurse should ascertain the effect of the respiratory impairment on the patient's lifestyle and ability to carry out usual daily activities. Physiological measurements of pulmonary function are obtained, when possible, and the results used to validate the analysis of the health history and physical examination completed by the nurse. Additional data is collected from the patient, family and the health record to identify the factors contributing to the restrictive lung disorder.

The patient *goal* is to achieve a functionally effective breathing pattern with adequate gas exchange. The patient should demonstrate:

- Slower and deeper respirations
- Increased lung volumes
- Blood gases within normal range
- Modification of contributing factors, e.g. loss of weight, pain control.

NURSING INTERVENTION

Interventions are directed toward altering the factors contributing to the decreased lung expansion.

Extrapulmonary causes affecting the chest wall and respiratory muscles can be modified through use of breathing exercises and postural changes to decrease the work of breathing and strengthen the respiratory muscles. General body exercise and respiratory muscle training help to increase the individual's activity tolerance. A specific exercise programme may be planned by physiotherapists. The nurse assists the person to implement and evaluate the prescribed plan.

For the obese person, a long-term weight reduction programme should be established in collaboration with the patient. Nursing intervention for the obese person is discussed in Chapter 18.

Pain resulting from injury to the chest wall and pleura is controlled by the administration of analgesics. Narcotics depress respirations and the cough reflex, therefore close monitoring of the person's respiratory status is essential when they are administered. Entonox gas (50% oxygen, 50% nitrous oxide) is very useful in emergency situations. Intercostal nerve blocks may be carried out to provide pain relief and decrease the need for narcotics. Patients with rib fractures are usually more comfortable sitting upright. Analgesia is administered on a defined schedule of every 3–4 hours to maintain a relatively constant level of pain control. Deep breathing and coughing are encouraged during the period when the analgesic is most effective.

When the cause of the altered breathing pattern is *intrapulmonary*, involving the pleura and/or lung parenchyma, nursing interventions are generally planned in collaboration with the medical plan of care. Nursing and medical therapy focus on alleviating the symptoms of dyspnoea, hypoxaemia and hypercapnia.

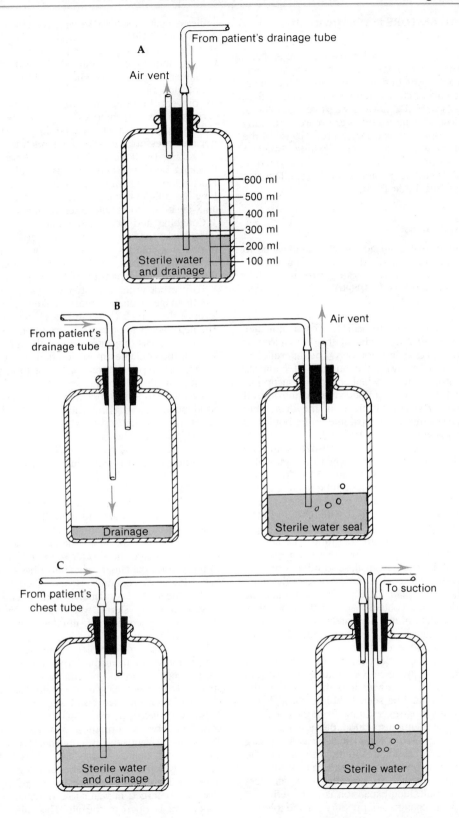

Figure 15.15 A, Water-seal chest drainage system using one bottle. B, Water-seal chest drainage system using two bottles. C, Water-seal chest drainage system using two bottles and suction.

MEASURES TO RESTORE INTRATHORACIC PRESSURE

The intrathoracic space is that between the visceral and parietal pleurae; the membranes are normally only separated by a thin film of fluid. Disruption of the pleura by disease, trauma or chest surgery results in air or fluid entering this space; the normal negative intrapleural pressure is lost. The increased pressure restricts lung expansion on inspiration and may cause collapse of the lung. Closed chest drainage is usually established. A thoracentesis (pleural aspiration) may be performed to remove fluid from the pleural cavity as well as for diagnostic test (see Table 15.10).

Closed chest drainage

A closed or water-seal drainage system is established to allow the escape of air and fluid from the pleural cavity and re-establish the normal negative pressure, while preventing any reflux (Walsh, 1989b).

Methods
Various methods are used to achieve closed drainage, but the principle is the same with all, that is, to allow air and fluid to pass in one direction only. The difference in the methods is generally in the number of compartments or containers used, whether or not suction is applied and whether or not a flutter valve is introduced into the system. The compartments of the disposable chest drainage systems are comparable to the bottles or containers described in Figure 15.15.

Water-seal drainage may be established with one container fitted with a two-holed stopper through which two glass or plastic tubes pass (Figure 15.15). The chest tubes are connected to a fairly long tube leading to the drainage container, where it is connected to a tube which has its distal end submerged at all times in sterile water or sterile normal saline to a designated depth (usually 3–5 cm). The depth of tube submersion determines the pressure exerted by the water; hence the term 'water-seal drainage'. A small, short tube, serving as an air vent, passes through the second hole of the tight-fitting, two-holed stopper. The water level must be marked clearly on the container so that the amount of drainage can be determined accurately.

With each expiration, the respiratory muscles relax, the intrapleural space is diminished and the pressure within the space is increased; this pressure exceeds that exerted by the water at the end of the tube, so fluid and air are forced from the cavity into the water in the container. The air may be seen bubbling through the water, from which it passes, escaping from the container through the vent. With inspiration the pleural space enlarges and the pressure within it decreases, causing water to rise several centimetres in the distal end of the tube. The evacuation of fluid and air from the intrapleural space results in greater space and less pressure. As a result, lung expansion is increased.

The alternating changes in pressure in the pleural cavity result in repeated fluctuations in the water level in the distal end of the drainage tube; these fluctuations correspond to the patient's breathing in and out and

indicate a patent system, serving as a guide to the nurse. If the water level does not oscillate, it may be suspected that the tube is blocked by a blood clot or fibrin. If this occurs, the tube is 'milked' toward the drainage container in an effort to relieve the blockage and, if this is not successful, the doctor is notified at once. In order to prevent blocking, the tube may be 'milked' or 'stripped' at stated intervals. This practice is controversial as stripping a chest tube may create excessive negative pressures. It is recommended that stripping of the tubing be done only when necessary to prevent blocking by clots when there is intrapleural bleeding. Fluctuation of the fluid level in the tube ceases when the lung has fully re-expanded. The doctor confirms this by an X-ray of the chest before removing the drainage tube.

Coughing and deep abdominal breathing alter the intrapleural space and pressure to a greater degree than normal respirations and, as a result, are important in promoting drainage of the cavity, removal of air and fluid and the re-expansion of remaining lung tissue.

To prevent water from being sucked into the chest, the drainage container must be kept well below the level of the patient (0.5–1 m below the patient's chest). The negative chest pressure is equivalent to 10–20 cm of water and sucks the water up into the tube only to that level. If the container must be lifted or moved, caution is observed to prevent traction on the tube, which might result in its dislodgement.

A safer method for preventing the possibility of water accidentally entering the chest cavity, and which also keeps the drainage separated from the water, is to use *two* containers. The second one contains the water, leaving the drainage container dry (Figure 15.15). When only one container is used, fluid drainage from the chest raises the level of the fluid, increasing the pressure at the distal end of the tube. More pressure is then required to force the fluid down on expiration and allow the escape of air and fluid. Blood and serum are more likely to collect and clot in the tube. In the two-container system, the first container is sealed and does not contain water; the shorter of the tubes is connected to the second container, which also has two tubes. The first (drainage) container is connected to the longer tube in the second container. The distal end of this tube is submerged in sterile water to a designated depth (3–5 cm). The second tube in container 2 is short and acts as an air vent.

If there is a considerable amount of air leaking into the pleural cavity from the intrapulmonary space, or if the patient's cough and respirations are not sufficiently strong to facilitate the clearance of fluid and air from the chest cavity, *continuous gentle suction* may be applied. This necessitates a two-container system; the first container serves as a drainage container and *water-seal*. The short air-vent tube in container 1 is connected to the second container which has a three-holed stopper through which two short tubes and one longer tube pass (see Figure 15.15C). The lower end of the longer tube is submerged in water to a designated depth. The upper end is open to the air. This tube controls the degree of suction applied to the pleural cavity. One short tube is connected to container 1; the second short tube is connected to a suction apparatus. The usual suction machine creates too strong a negative pressure to be applied directly to the pleural cavity. This may be reduced by a valve and meter (such as is used in 'wall suction') inserted between the suction and the water-seal container. If the portable suction machine is used, the negative pressure is controlled by the depth of submersion of the lower end of the open glass tube in container 2. A continuous bubbling in the control container (container 2) indicates that the suction is being maintained.

Disposable closed drainage receptacles with two compartments comparable to the two-container system are available. The receptacle is attached to suction and is suspended from the side of the bed, eliminating the danger of containers being knocked over and broken.

The water-seal system is cumbersome and also restricts patients' mobility. The nurse and patient are continuously apprehensive of such things as tubes becoming disconnected and containers being broken. As a safety measure and to permit greater freedom in turning and earlier ambulation, some surgeons prefer to introduce a plastic flutter valve into the system. It is placed between the chest drainage tube and the drainage container. Suction may still be applied. The system may be placed on a small cart or pole with wheels to allow the patient to move around the unit.

Responsibilities and precautions (Table 15.9)
When any method of water-seal drainage is used, nursing responsibilities include the following considerations.

Table 15.9 Nursing intervention in the management of the patient with water-seal chest drainage.

Patient problem: ineffective breathing due to air/fluid in the pleural space

Goals	Nursing intervention	Rationale
• The patient's respiratory rate, depth and pattern will be within normal limits • Deep breathing and coughing will be performed at regular intervals • Chest X-ray will demonstrate expansion of the lung prior to removal of the chest tube	*Connection of the closed drainage system* • Wash hands thoroughly and use sterile technique when opening the disposable or container drainage unit • Place the containers, a stand and disposable unit on a designated rack away from where it can be knocked over and below the level of the patient • Add sterile normal saline to the container or disposable system and adjust the tube in the container to designated depth (3–5 cm) of submersion • Check that the air vent tube or opening is open • Mark the fluid level on a strip of adhesive tape placed lengthwise on the container or indicate the calibration level on the disposable system • Connect extension tube to suction if ordered • Connect drainage tubing to the submerged tube in the container and attach the tube and connector to the chest tube • Tape all connections • Arrange tubing, coiling it loosely to prevent kinks and fasten it to the bedside • Place two clamps at the patient's bedside where they are readily visible and attainable	• To prevent contamination of the unit and spread of micro-organisms to the pleural space • To decrease the potential for accidental breakage or disconnection of the system, and to prevent fluid from being sucked into the pleural cavity • The depth of the tube determines the pressure exerted • To permit escape of air from the system • To provide a double check that the water level is adequate, and to enable measurement of the amount of drainage in single-container system • To promote drainage with low level suction • To connect the system • To make certain the system is airtight and to prevent accidental disconnection • To prevent kinks and obstruction of tubing and to prevent tubing from interfering with patient movement • To clamp the system in case of accidental disconnection and thus prevent air entry into the pleural cavity

Table 15.9 Nursing intervention in the management of the patient with water-seal chest drainage.

Goals	Patient problem: ineffective breathing due to air/fluid in the pleural space	
	Nursing intervention	Rationale
	Assessment	
	• Patency of the system as evidenced by fluctuations in the water level in the drainage container; air bubbling through the water	• To determine patency of the closed drainage system. Fluctuation in the water level will not occur when continuous suction is used
	• Safety: all connections are intact and taped; the containers/disposable system are below the level of the patient; the tubing is not kinked	• To ensure that all safety precautions are observed
	• The drainage is observed for volume, colour and consistency, especially during the first 24–48 hours	• To determine the effectiveness of the drainage system and to promptly identify complications such as bleeding
	• The patient is assessed for: rate, depth, pattern and frequency of respirations; signs of dyspnoea and cyanosis; and chest pain and rapid pulse. Lungs are auscultated for air entry and the presence of wheezes and rales	• Accumulation of air in the pleural cavity can cause collapse of the lung on the affected side
	Maintenance of the closed drainage system	
	• If blockage of the tubing is suspected, check for kinking and inspect tubing for clots. 'Milk' or strip the tubing in the direction of the drainage container	• 'Milking' of the tubing clears the tubing of clots. Since it creates excessive negative pressures it should be done only when necessary
	• Encourage the patient to deep breathe and cough at frequent, regular intervals	• Coughing and deep abdominal breathing increase the intrapulmonary and intrapleural pressures promoting drainage and preventing tension pneumothorax
	• Changing of the drainage container is done by an experienced person. Clamp each drainage tube close to the chest with two clamps and quickly disconnect the drainage container and connect the new sterile, calibrated container	• To prevent air being sucked into the pleural cavity and to prevent contamination with micro-organisms
	Accidental interruption of the drainage system	
	• Immediately clamp the tubing close to the chest wall with two clamps. A new sterile drainage system and tubing are connected	• To prevent air from entering the pleural cavity and collapse of the lung
	Discontinuation of the closed drainage system	
	• The patient is instructed to take a large breath and hold it as the doctor clamps the tube and removes it. A sterile occlusive dressing is simultaneously applied to the exit site and sealed with tape or a transparent adhesive dressing	• To prevent air from entering the pleural cavity
		• To protect the wound from micro-organisms

It is important that the nurse understands the purpose and operating principles of the system, as well as the precautions to be observed to prevent air and fluid from entering the chest cavity, which could cause a collapse of the lung and life-threatening respiratory insufficiency.

If the container system is used, the container should be calibrated so that the volume of water used is known and the drainage may be measured.

The system must be checked at frequent intervals for patency. This is determined by noting the oscillating water level in the submerged tube; this rises with inspiration and falls with expiration. When suction is employed, fluctuations of the water level do not occur because the continuous suction holds the water level in the tube at a fixed level. The suction may be interrupted briefly and the column of water observed for fluctuations. If the water level does not fluctuate in a closed system, the tube should be examined for possible kinks or compression caused by the patient lying on it. A clot may be obstructing the tube and may be dislodged by 'milking' or 'stripping' the tube toward the drainage container. If the system remains non-functional, the doctor is informed at once.

As a precaution, all connections are taped with adhesive to prevent their separation and to keep air from entering the system. The containers may be placed in a rack to prevent accidental moving or knocking over. Visitors and ward personnel are warned not to disturb them, and a warning sign placed by the containers is helpful.

The drainage tube is supported and lies free in a fold in the sheet, to which it is secured by a clip or tape. It should not be looped but should be long enough to avoid marked restriction of the patient's moving and turning.

The characteristics and volume of the drainage are noted and recorded frequently, especially during the first 24–48 hours. The drainage may be coloured by blood at first, but gradually clears and decreases in amount.

Changing the drainage container is done by someone who fully understands closed drainage. Each drainage tube is clamped close to the chest wall with two chest drain clamps, and the container is quickly replaced by a clean, calibrated sterile container.

If an interruption or break in the closed system should occur as a result of the disconnection of a tube or a broken container, the drainage tube(s) should be clamped off close to the chest wall immediately to prevent air from entering the chest cavity. An accumulation of air in the pleural cavity could cause a collapse of the lung on the affected side and produce compression of the unaffected lung, heart and large blood vessels. Associated symptoms are a complaint by the patient of tightness or pressure in the chest, dyspnoea, cyanosis and a rapid pulse. The doctor is notified promptly and the clamps remain in place until the integrity of the system is re-established. As a precaution, an extra set of sterile containers and connections should always be available.

Regular frequent staged coughing and deep breathing are important since they increase the intrapulmonary and intrapleural pressures, forcing air and fluid out of the cavity and promoting lung expansion. The patient should be ambulatory as soon as possible.

When turning the patient, or when giving any care, precautions are taken not to dislodge or disconnect the drainage tubes. A final check is made to make sure the patient is not lying on a portion of the tube and that there are no loops or kinks present to interfere with drainage.

Even if the system appears to be functioning satisfactorily, any patient complaint of pressure or pain in the chest, dyspnoea, cyanosis or a rapid, weak pulse is reported promptly.

When the lung is fully expanded and no fluid remains in the pleural cavity, the tubes are removed. The water in the closed drainage container will have stopped fluctuating, and the lung expansion is confirmed by the doctor by percussion, auscultation and a chest X-ray.

When the tube is withdrawn from the chest cavity, the wound is covered with a dry, secure dressing. In some cases a purse-string suture has been inserted around the tube and this is tightened off when the tube is removed and covered with a dry, secure dressing. The patient is observed closely for the next 24 hours for possible leakage of air into the chest and ensuing pneumothorax.

Evaluation

The person's breathing pattern will be more effective and dyspnoea, hypoxaemia and hypercapnia will be absent or sufficiently modified to permit optimal daily functioning. The individual's respirations will be regular, symmetrical and of usual rate and depth for the individual. There should be evidence that the causative and contributing factors are modified: if pain was present, the person will state absence of pain; injuries to the chest will demonstrate healing and repair and expansion of any impaired lung tissue will be shown by X-ray.

Thoracentesis (pleural aspiration) (Table 15.10)

A thoracentesis is the withdrawal of fluid or air from the pleural cavity. Normally pleural fluid serves to lubricate the pleura. Excessive fluid and air interfere with lung expansion. Chest expansion will be asymmetrical with distension and decreased movement present on the affected side. A thoracentesis is performed to remove excessive pleural fluid to facilitate lung expansion, for diagnostic purposes or to instil medication into the pleural cavity. Following preparation of the skin and injection of a local anaesthetic, the doctor inserts a needle through an intercostal space into the pleural cavity. A three-way adaptor (stop-cock) is attached to the needle to enable withdrawal of fluid through attached tubing or a syringe and closing of the system when fluid is not being aspirated. Care must be taken to maintain a closed system and to prevent air from entering the pleural space.

Table 15.10 Nursing intervention in the management of the patient having a thoracentesis.

Patient problem: ineffective breathing due to excess fluid in the pleural space		
Goals	Nursing intervention	Rationale
• The patient will verbalize understanding of the procedure and what to expect during the procedure • The patient's breathing will be regular, rhythmical and not laboured • Chest expansion will be symmetrical, with a usual degree of excursion	• The patient is informed of the procedure, and what to expect during the procedure • The nurse checks that the consent form has been signed following the doctor's explanation to the patient of the purpose of the test and expected and other possible outcomes, and that chest X-rays have been carried out • The prescribed sedation is administered prior to the start of the procedure • The patient is placed in a sitting position, leaning forward, with head and arms resting on a table or several pillows • During the procedure the nurse provides physical support for the patient and instructs him or her to remain still while the needle is being inserted and while it is in place • During the procedure the nurse provides ongoing explanations as to what is occurring. As the antiseptic solution is applied, the patient is told to expect a feeling of cold; injection of the local anaesthetic will be felt and a pressure will be experienced as the thoracentesis needle is inserted • A sterile transparent dressing or a gauze dressing sealed with tape is applied as the doctor withdraws the thoracentesis needle • The patient is assisted to a comfortable position in bed and assessed at least every 15 minutes for the first 2 hours. Observations include respiratory rate, depth and rhythm, pulse rate, presence of blood, frothy sputum, uncontrolled cough, dyspnoea, cyanosis, chest pain or tightness and feelings of dizziness or faintness. The site is inspected and the surrounding tissue palpated for puffiness or crackling • The volume, colour and consistency of the pleural fluid is determined and recorded. The specimen containers are labelled and sent promptly to the laboratory	• Knowledge of what to expect can reduce anxiety and opportunity is provided to answer the patient's concerns • X-rays provide information as to the exact anatomical location of the fluid and air in the pleural cavity • Sedation may be required to promote relaxation and decrease discomfort and anticipatory pain • Fluid is dependent and therefore accumulates in the lower portions of the pleural cavity when the patient is upright, making it easier to remove • To prevent spontaneous movement by the patient which may result in trauma to the pleura and lung • Patient co-operation increases and anxiety is decreased when he or she is aware of what is happening • To prevent air from entering the pleural cavity • To protect the site from micro-organisms • If a large amount of fluid is removed, lung expansion occurs suddenly and pulmonary and cardiac distress may occur. Spontaneous pneumothorax and subcutaneous emphysema may occur following thoracentesis. A portable chest X-ray is usually ordered to verify that a pneumothorax is not present • Accurate, prompt documentation is a legal requirement. Prompt labelling and discharge of specimens ensures identification of the specimen and that contamination of the specimen does not occur

Ineffective Breathing Pattern Related to Cancer of the Lung and Chest Surgery

LUNG CANCER

Lung cancer is the most common cancer in men and the primary cause of cancer deaths in both men and women (see p. 372). The incidence of lung cancer has been rising over the last 50 years but it is largely preventable. It is most common between the ages of 50 and 70 years.

RISK FACTORS

There is strong evidence that cigarette smoking is the major cause of lung cancer. About 80–90% of lung cancers occur in persons who smoke tobacco cigarettes. A clear dose–response correlation has been identified. The risk of developing lung cancer increases with the number of cigarettes smoked and the number of years the person has smoked. The risk declines consistently over time after stopping smoking. Non-smokers are placed at risk from exposure to mainstream smoke from burning cigarettes.

Carcinogenic agents found in atmospheric pollution, and exposure to asbestos, arsenic, nickel, radiation, chromates, mustard gas and coke-oven emissions in the work place, also contribute to the development of lung cancer.

Prolonged irritation of the respiratory mucosa, regardless of the irritant, results in a breakdown of the lung's defences. Cigarette smoke and polluted environments contain a large number of irritants. Although much is known about the actions of certain chemicals, there is still much to learn about their collective actions when mixed in cigarette smoke, or the work, home or community environments.

Knowledge of the effects of irritants on the respiratory mucosa is necessary for children and adolescents to develop healthy life-styles and to motivate adults to eliminate health hazards and establish positive health practices. However, when large, multinational corporations spend vast sums of money promoting, advertising and marketing their harmful products, the effects of such health education on individuals is bound to be limited. Bysshe (1989), in exploring the strong links between environmental factors and respiratory disease, comments upon the effects of smoking by pointing out that, of every 1000 young UK smokers, one will be murdered, six will die as a result of a road traffic accident and 250 will be killed by tobacco. The cost to the country of tobacco-induced disease was estimated by Bysshe at £370m. However, as the Government takes £1000m in taxes from tobacco, this leaves it with a profit of £630m. Financially, therefore, it makes sense for the Government to keep tax levels where they are and allow a large proportion of the population to smoke themselves to death(!).

The nurse should question the ethics and morality of this situation. It might be argued that freedom of choice is essential in our society, and smoking is an individual life-style choice. If tobacco was not addictive, this might have some value as an argument. However, given the addictive properties of the drug and the multimillion pound advertising campaigns that seek to persuade young people to take up the habit, the freedom of choice argument is significantly weakened. Social action is required to ban cigarette advertising altogether and to campaign for a substantial increase in the level of taxation on tobacco. In real terms, after allowing for inflation, cigarettes have become progressively cheaper over the last 20 years. Governments have failed to increase taxation, at least in line with inflation, to try and limit the increase in the retail price index, a short-term political goal that is damaging to the nation's health. As a final consideration, the nurse who smokes should think about his or her suitability as a role model for healthy behaviour.

Effects of smoking on respiratory function

Smoking affects respiratory function in the following ways:

1. It produces an allergic response. Tobacco glycoprotein is a specific antigen that produces an antigen–antibody reaction similar to asthma.
2. Movement of particles and mucus from the airways is impaired as a result of inhibition of the cilia. Mucus and particles from deeper portions of the lungs accumulate and are retained, providing a medium for infective organisms.
3. The production of mucus is increased in response to the irritation.
4. The airways narrow. Mucus-secreting glands increase in number and/or size, increasing the space they occupy in the airway. The walls of the smaller airways thicken and the muscle tissue in the walls contracts, adding to the constriction of the airways.
5. Destruction of the structures of the terminal respiratory units develops due to the release of enzymes from the macrophages when they are destroyed by the constituents in the smoke. Destruction of the macrophages also eliminates their protective action in engulfing and destroying particles in the alveoli.

CHARACTERISTICS OF CANCER OF THE LUNG

Early symptoms are usually absent or vague. The person may have a persistent, non-productive cough. Later, the sputum may be blood-streaked. Dyspnoea, localized chest pain and wheezing may develop. General symptoms include fever, chills, sweating (especially night sweats), anorexia, weakness, fatigue and weight loss. Symptoms are often insidious. Confirmation of the presence of lung cancer requires further diagnostic investigations.

PREVENTION OF CANCER OF THE LUNG

Stopping smoking

The World Health Organization and the National Cancer Societies emphasize that primary prevention is the key to reducing the incidence of and mortality from lung cancer. Smoking cessation is the major factor in prevention. The creation of a tobacco-free society by the year 2000 is the primary goal of the American National Cancer Advisory Board. To this end, they have recommended that tobacco be reclassified as a drug; that smoking be banned on airlines and on all forms of public transportation; that public buildings, the workplace and all schools be smoke-free; that the media should not glamorize smoking; that health professionals should actively recommend the non-use of tobacco to their patients and assist them to stop; and that smokeless tobacco products be subject to the same restrictions as tobacco.

Promotion of non-smoking should be directed to younger individuals before they begin to smoke. Programmes for this group are infrequent, yet there is some evidence that they can be successful. Social pressures not to smoke seem to be having some influence as fewer people are starting to smoke. The rights of non-smokers are being respected as smokers are being forced out of the work environment, restaurants and public buildings. Smoking outside (the new milieu for continuing smokers) loses its attraction on cold and rainy days. Individuals who have never smoked are less likely to put up with the difficulties encountered in finding a place to smoke than are the already addicted.

Smokers are faced with many difficulties when they attempt to stop. Tobacco is addictive; advertising campaigns try to glamorize it; and many smokers stop several times before completely succeeding. Numerous smoking cessation programmes are available to assist individuals who wish to stop. These programmes use a combination of tested and novel techniques including rapid smoking, gradual withdrawal, or 'cold turkey'; positive reinforcement; 'buddy' systems and/or group support; hypnosis; guided imagery; lectures and discussions. Nicotine gum may be prescribed to help motivated nicotine-dependent smokers give up. Although nicotine gum has some demonstrated benefits as a stop-smoking aid, use of the gum alone is not recommended.

The effectiveness of any single or combination of techniques is difficult to assess. Although most programmes claim success, evaluation methods vary and most studies are descriptive in nature. After reviewing the literature, Kramer (1982) concluded that no matter what treatment methods were used, only about 20% of the participants in smoking cessation programmes were still not smoking after one year. See p. 299 for further discussion on this topic.

The role of the nurse and other health professionals in antismoking activities has been the subject of several investigations. Saunders and colleagues (1986) found that although nurses reported that they had an important role in helping smokers to give up, only a few of the 369 questioned referred smokers to other agencies for help, recommended aids to stop smoking or used antismoking literature.

In summary, the individual who is likely to succeed in stopping smoking is one who is motivated, gives up 'cold turkey', has family, friend and social support and has made several previous attempts at stopping.

Nutrition

There is some evidence that vitamin A reduces the risk of lung cancer and can produce a decrease in laryngeal and oral cancers in smokers. β-carotene is also believed to be a significant antioxidant in reducing the risk of lung cancer. β-Carotene is found in yellow fruits such as peaches, cantaloupe and apricots and in green leafy vegetables. Liver, eggs, whole milk and butter are good sources of vitamin A, which is a fat-soluble vitamin. The vitamin A content of fruits and vegetables is linked to the β-carotene content. Present knowledge does not justify the use of high doses of vitamin A as a preventive measure. Smokers and others at risk for lung cancer should eat a balanced diet with adequate dietary intake of vitamin A and β-carotene.

Environmental and industrial pollution control measures

Control of atmospheric pollution requires the collective efforts of governments, industries, communities and individuals. Consumers should exert pressure for improved emission controls on all motor vehicles. Employers and employees should be requested to meet high standards of pollutant control.

The development of industrial health programmes which include frequent routine medical and radiological examinations and employee education should be encouraged, and every effort made to prevent inhalation of hazardous dust. Protection is achieved by damping systems, improved exhaust and ventilation systems and the use of masks and respirators by employees.

TREATMENT OF CANCER OF THE LUNG

Treatment of lung cancer usually involves a combination of chemotherapy, radiation and surgical resection. Small cell lung cancers, which are characterized by rapid cell growth and metastases, are usually sensitive to chemotherapy and radiation. The non-small cell variety are usually removed surgically. Most patients show some response to treatment but the 5-year survival rate remains poor.

Chemotherapy

Combinations of various chemotherapeutic agents may be prescribed for the 40% of patients who have metastatic disease on diagnosis and for those with recurrent disease. No effective drug regimen for cancer of the lung has been proven; the use of chemotherapy is therefore limited primarily to individuals with small cell lung tumours. Cyclophosphamide is usually used in combination with two other agents. The nursing care of persons receiving chemotherapy is discussed in Chapter 10.

Radiotherapy

Radiation is used as a primary treatment, in combination with surgery or for palliation. The total dose of and the schedule for radiation depends on the treatment goal.

Nursing care of the person receiving radiotherapy is discussed in Chapter 10.

Surgical treatment

Surgical resection is the treatment of choice for persons with non-small cell lung cancer with no evidence of extrathoracic metastases. Surgical treatment consists of a thoracotomy and resection of the involved lung tissue and regional lymph nodes.

Pneumonectomy, in which an entire lung is removed, involves the ligation of a large pulmonary artery, two large pulmonary veins and a bronchus. The phrenic nerve on the operative side is crushed or severed to permit the diaphragm to rise to reduce the size of the cavity that remains. Pneumonectomy is used when extensive tissue must be excised.

A *lobectomy* is the removal of a lobe of a lung and is used when the disease is confined to that particular lobe.

Segmental resection is used when the person's disease is localized to a segment of a lung, making it possible to conserve functional tissue and lessen the degree of overdistension in the other lung by removing only the affected segment.

Wedge resection is used when the disease is localized and small or when conservative treatment is indicated because of a poor prognosis.

NURSING CARE OF THE PERSON HAVING CHEST SURGERY

PREOPERATIVE NURSING CARE

Preoperatively the patient and family may be anxious and frightened. They may be denying the diagnosis of lung cancer and the severity of the prognosis, while at the same time be struggling to make decisions regarding treatment.

The patient is usually fatigued and restless and may appear thin and emaciated from recent weight loss and poor appetite. Chest pain and discomfort may not develop in the early stages. Respiratory function is usually impaired as a result of a history of heavy smoking and resulting chronic airflow disease as well as the lung cancer. The patient may experience a persistent non-productive cough and shortness of breath.

The patient's day is occupied with numerous diagnostic studies, including chest X-rays, cytological studies of sputum, bronchoscopy and pulmonary function studies.

The goals for nursing intervention during the preoperative period are to: (1) improve respiratory function prior to surgery; (2) to alleviate the anxiety of the patient and family by providing support during the decision-making process and in coping with the diagnosis and prognosis; and (3) to provide information about the operative procedure and expectations for the patient and family during the pre- and postoperative periods.

POSTOPERATIVE NURSING CARE (TABLE 15.11)

The arterial blood pressure, pulse and respirations are noted every 15 minutes for the first 2–3 hours and then the interval is increased to ½–1 hour for the succeeding 8–10 hours if the vital signs are stabilized.

The rise and fall of both sides of the chest in respiration should be noted. Dyspnoea, decreased movement of one side of the chest on inspiration (except in pneumonectomy), cyanosis or chest pain may manifest a pneumothorax and should be reported promptly to the doctor. This may develop as a result of

---

Table 15.11   Postoperative care plan for the patient with lung cancer.

Patient problem	Goals	Nursing intervention	Rationale
1. Alteration in comfort: pain related to thoracic incision and chest tubes.	• The patient will verbalize absence of pain • The patient will perform deep breathing and turning activities with minimal discomfort	• Narcotic analgesis given as prescribed with additional doses given for breakthrough pain as prescribed and as needed during the first 48–72 hours • Assess the patient's level of pain verbally on a five-point scale and administer medications as needed prior to deep breathing, coughing and turning activities • Assess the patient's breathing regularly, at least 2-hourly • See problem 5	• To maintain a constant level of pain control and to prevent episodes of severe pain • Shallow breathing may indicate increased pain. Slow respirations may result from the respiratory depressing effect of narcotic drugs

Table 15.11   *Continued.*

Patient problem	Goals	Nursing intervention	Rationale
2. Airway clearance ineffective related to anaesthesia, surgical procedure and incisional pain	• Patient will achieve adequate lung ventilation as shown by absence of signs of chest infection and normal blood gases	• As soon as the blood pressure is stabilized, the patient is asked to cough 1–2 hourly, or more often if there is evidence of retained secretions. It is important that the patient is wakened to cough at regular intervals throughout the night. Even with preoperative instruction and practice, the patient is usually fearful and may find the procedure difficult	• To promote airway clearance
		• Suction the mouth and pharyngeal area as indicated	• Suctioning loosens secretions in the lower tracheobronchial passages and raises them to the upper tract from which the patient may cough them up, or they may be reached by suction
		• The nurse assists the patient to a sitting position for coughing and, standing at the side of the bed which is opposite to the patient's incision, supports the operative side of the chest, back and front, with the hands. The patient is asked to take several deep breaths and to cough with expiration. If the cough and suctioning are not productive, listen to the chest for evidence of crackles and wheezes	
		• Physical therapy (vibration and percussion) may be used. A humidifier may be placed in the room	• To dislodge secretions from peripheral bronchial tubes and bronchioles. Humidity helps to liquify secretions
3. Breathing pattern ineffective related to anaesthesia, surgical procedure, pain and presence of fluid and/or air in the intrapleural space	• The person's respirations will be regular and symmetrical • Lung volumes will increase progressively • Chest tubes will be patent	• See problem 2 • *Deep breathing.* The patient is encouraged to take 5–10 deep breaths hourly and is given an explanation of the need to promote full expansion of the remaining lung tissue and the drainage of air and fluid from the thoracic cavity. Incentive spirometry may be used to encourage maximum inspirations	• To promote chest expansion. As the lung expands to occupy more space, the pressure increases within the pleural cavity, forcing air and fluid through the drainage tube

Table 15.11 *Continued.*

Patient problem	Goals	Nursing intervention	Rationale
		• *Positioning.* With the return of consciousness and stabilization of the blood pressure and pulse, the head of the bed is raised gradually to a 30–45° angle. The patient is turned 1–2 hourly and the doctor usually specifies whether he or she may be turned on either side or to one side only. In the case of a pneumonectomy, turning is from the back to the affected side only. With partial resection, the patient usually may be turned from back to left side, to back to right side, and so on. If a sternum-splitting incision is used, the patient is generally most comfortable on the back, but is encouraged to assume a lateral position for at least brief periods. During any moving or turning of the patient, precautions are necessary to prevent dislodging the chest drainage tubes	• This facilitates the patient's breathing by lowering the diaphragm • To avoid restriction on the remaining lung which is carrying the full respiratory load • To promote lung expansion and comfort
		• *Chest tubes and drainage.* All connections should be checked to make sure they are taped and airtight. Drainage receptacles are placed below the level of the patient. The system is checked regularly for functioning. The colour, volume and consistency of drainage is observed and recorded hourly initially and then every 2–4 hourly	• To prevent entry of air into the closed drainage system and possible collapse of the lung
4. Impaired gas exchange, related to anaesthesia, surgery, removal of lung tissue and pain	• Pulse and respiratory rates will be normal for the patient • The patient's colour will be good • Arterial blood gases will be within the normal range • The patient will be rational, orientated and will not complain of a headache	• *Oxygen administration.* The patient usually receives oxygen by mask, or nasal cannulae for at least the first 24–36 h. The administration is not prolonged unless the patient is experiencing some respiratory insufficiency	• To maximize available oxygen for gas exchange

Table 15.11   *Continued.*

Patient problem	Goals	Nursing intervention	Rationale
5. Fear and anxiety related to surgery and prognosis	• Patient will discuss fears and anxieties • Patient will talk realistically of the future	• Encourage patient to talk, give time to listen, be honest. Involve family in discussions where appropriate but allow patient privacy when needed • Give detailed explanations of all procedures • See problem 9	• Family and patient need to verbalize and recognize their fears • Prevents misunderstanding
6. Fluid volume deficit related to loss during surgery and decreased fluid intake	• Fluid balance will be achieved with a minimum daily intake of 3 l/day • B.P. systolic > 100	• The blood loss at operation is replaced by a blood transfusion, and fluids are usually given intravenously for the first 24–48 h. The rate at which the fluid is given must be closely monitored. The physician indicates the rate at which the intravenous fluid is to be administered • Clear fluids may be given orally as soon as there is no nausea and vomiting, and gradually are increased in volume as tolerated. The patient may have a soft diet the first postoperative day, as tolerated, and a regular diet the following day. Extra fluids are provided, unless contraindicated by increased venous pressure	• The rate of fluid administration is controlled to prevent too rapid filling of the reduced vascular compartment and subsequent pulmonary oedema, which is manifested by dyspnoea, bubbling sounds and frothy sputum • Adequate fluid intake is necessary to reduce the tenaciousness of the respiratory secretions
7. Impaired physical mobility related to chest/ sternal incision, pain, fatigue and decreased activity tolerance	• The patient will use affected arm to perform self-care activities • The patient will be up on the first postoperative day • The distance and duration of walking activity will increase each day	• Beginning the evening of surgery, assist the patient to a sitting position over the side of the bed and then into a chair. Monitor respiratory responses, pulse and blood pressure. Observe patient for signs of dizziness • When the patient's condition is stable, assist in walking around the room. Increase walking distance daily from the second postoperative day to include the ward corridor • Carry out passive range-of-motion exercises on affected arm and shoulder four times a day beginning the evening of surgery. Begin physiotherapy and active arm and shoulder	• Early ambulation promotes respiratory and circulatory function and helps prevent complications. Ambulation should not interfere with the functioning of chest drainage • To maintain range of motion of the arm on the affected side and to prevent contractures and restriction of function

Table 15.11   *Continued.*

Patient problem	Goals	Nursing intervention	Rationale
		exercises by the third day. Encourage the patient to use affected arm in self-care activities	
8. Wound healing incomplete, related to surgery and chest tube sites	• The incision and chest tube sites will be clean, dry and intact	• Observe dressing for signs of drainage or bleeding when the patient returns to the unit and 4-hourly during the first day	• Early identification of incis- ional bleeding enables prompt action by the surgeon as indicated and may prevent complica-tions
		• Observe incision and chest tube sites for signs of redness, tenderness, drainage and oedema during each dressing change and 8-hourly after the removal of the dressing. The dressing is usually removed within 48 hours	
		• Take a swab for culture and sensitivity if signs of infection are present	
		• When chest tubes are removed, cover the areas with occlusive dressings and seal tightly for about 48 hours	• To prevent entry of air into the thoracic cavity
9. Knowledge deficit related to postsurgical follow-up and planned treatment regimen	• Patient and family will demonstrate understand-ing of post-discharge care related to deep breathing and coughing, mobility exercises, rest, self-care activities, diet and fluids • Patient and family will verbalize plans for contin-ued physiotherapy and any additional radio-therapy or chemotherapy	• The rehabilitation must be adapted to each indi-vidual patient. Generally, the patient requires a fairly long period of convalescence during which he is encouraged to continue exercises and deep breathing. The patient is instructed to gradually increase daily activity. Referrals are initiated for social and occupational counselling as indicated	• Each patient's situation and response are unique. The body has to adjust to a reduced respiratory capacity, and the patient who has had a pneumonectomy will require a greater period of adjustment. The patient may not be able to resume the former occu-pation and may need help to find lighter work within the respiratory capacity
		• In preparation for going home, the patient receives instructions about the exercises, deep breathing and coughing which are to be continued. Plans are made for follow-up physiotherapy as an out-patient or at home	• Arm and breathing exercises are continued to maintain range of motion and to promote respiratory function
		• The patient is assisted in planning daily activities to allow for periods of rest and to rest when short-ness of breath develops	• General weakness and activity intolerance are expected initially. Over exertion aggravates res-piratory impairment

Table 15.11   *Continued.*

Patient problem	Goals	Nursing intervention	Rationale
		• The nurse explains that the patient may experience numbness, pain or heaviness in the operative area and reassures the patient that it is generally temporary	• Due to surgical interruption of the intercostal nerves
		• Plans for ongoing radiotherapy or chemotherapy are discussed with the patient. Treatment schedules and instructions are given to the patient in writing	• Understanding of the treatment regimen and awareness of schedules and plans facilitates compliance

Note: This care plan relates only to care specific to the surgery undergone; general care concerning pressure areas, hygiene, etc. is also required.

air or fluid collecting in the pleural cavity and compressing the lung. It must be treated quickly by chest aspiration (thoracentesis), or the patient may die of respiratory insufficiency. Respirations are also observed for audible moist sounds. A portable chest X-ray may be done daily for 2–3 days to determine lung expansion and detect the presence of fluid and air in the pleural cavity.

The wound area and chest drainage are examined frequently for any indications of bleeding. The sealed drainage system is checked frequently for functioning, and the tubing connections are examined for security. The volume of drainage is measured at regular 8-hour intervals. The intake and output are recorded, and the fluid balance is estimated.

The nurse measures the patient's tidal and minute volumes. Arterial blood specimens may be necessary for blood gas determinations which indicate possible respiratory insufficiency and the need for mechanical assistance and/or increased oxygen inhalation.

IMPAIRED GAS EXCHANGE

The North American Nursing Diagnosis Association (1989) states that: 'Impaired gas exchange is a state in which the individual experiences a decreased passage of oxygen and/or carbon dioxide between the alveoli of the lungs and the vascular system.'

Characteristics and Related Factors

The defining characteristics of impaired gas exchange develop as a result of inadequte oxygen supply and/or increased carbon dioxide in the blood. Confusion,

Table 15.12   Patient health problem: impaired gas exchange.

Defining characteristics	Related factors
• Confusion and irritability	• Ventilation–perfusion imbalance
• Lethargy and fatigue	• Shunting of blood
• Increased respiratory secretions	• Impaired transportation of gases
• Hypoxia	• Increased oxygen requirements
• Hypercapnia	• Inability of cells to utilize oxygen or exchange gases
• Cyanosis	

irritability and restlessness are the primary symptoms experienced by the person with impaired gas exchange. Table 15.12 lists the characteristics of and factors contributing to the health problem.

HYPOXIA

This means that the supply of oxygen available to the tissues is insufficient to meet cellular needs for normal metabolism.

Causes of hypoxia

The causes of hypoxia may be inadequate oxygenation of the blood, impaired delivery of oxygen to the tissues, increased oxygen demand by the body cells or inability of the cells to use the oxygen.

Inadequate oxygenation of the blood
This may be the result of:

- *Inadequate ventilation.* If less than the normal volume of air enters the alveoli, then obviously the exchange of gases is decreased. If the body's oxygen consumption is not correspondingly reduced, hypoxia results. This usually occurs as a result of a disorder of the central nervous system. Alveolar hypoventilation produces an elevation in P_{CO_2}, which responds to an increase in inspired P_{O_2} with the administration of oxygen.
- *Low atmospheric tension.* A decline in the oxygen tension in the atmosphere, as at high altitudes, is a cause of inadequate oxygenation of the blood.
- *Ventilation–perfusion mismatching.* Some alveolar capillaries may not be perfused; the alveoli are ventilated but inadequate blood perfusion results in a reduction in the oxygenation of the blood. This condition may be referred to as mismatching or inequality of perfusion and ventilation.
- *Diffusion defect.* Fibrosing changes or oedema of the alveolar walls produces a decrease in the amount of oxygen that diffuses from the alveolar air into the blood. Oxygen is less soluble than carbon dioxide, and is 20 times slower in its transfer to the blood than is carbon dioxide in its diffusion from the blood into the alveoli.
- *Venoarterial shunts.* A shunt within the circulatory system that causes a mixing of arterial (oxygenated) and venous (reduced oxygen) bloods lowers the oxygen tension of the blood delivered to the tissues. The blood that is shunted bypasses the lungs or ventilated areas of the lungs and therefore is not oxygenated. The P_{O_2} decreases but the P_{CO_2} is usually normal. Administration of oxygen does not raise the P_{O_2} level because the shunted blood which bypasses ventilated alveoli is not exposed to the increased alveolar oxygen concentration. The cause is usually a congenital cardiac condition which causes blood to move directly from the right to left side, or the blockage of a large pulmonary vessel by a pulmonary embolus.

Impaired transport of oxygen to the tissues
This may be due to:

- *Anaemia.* Fewer than the normal number of erythrocytes or less than a normal complement of haemoglobin reduces the amount of oxygen uptake by the blood.
- *Abnormal haemoglobin.* Hypoxia may be caused by a chemical alteration of the haemoglobin to a form that reduces its oxygen-carrying capacity (e.g. as seen in carbon monoxide poisoning). Certain drugs may also alter haemoglobin and prevent its combination with oxygen. Examples of these drugs are sulphathiazole and phenacetin.
- *Cardiac failure.* Failure of the heart to pump blood throughout body tissues results in stagnation. The oxygen becomes depleted and is not being replaced.
- Inadequate transportation of oxygenated blood may be limited to a certain area of the body (ischaemia)

as a result of thrombosis or embolism, and the tissues in that area experience hypoxia.

Increased oxygen requirement
This may develop in:

- *Severe hyperthyroidism.* The utilization of oxygen is increased in severe hyperthyroidism by the rapid rate of metabolism. Similarly, hypoxia may also develop in the person with a high fever; an excessive amount of oxygen is used by the cells in accelerated metabolism and the production of increased body heat.

Tissue cell impairment
This may result in the cells being unable to use the oxygen that is in the blood. The cellular defect is usually in the enzyme system, and is such that the normal oxidative processes are inhibited. This may occur in narcotic or cyanide poisoning.

Tissue oedema contributes to hypoxia by increasing the distances that gases must diffuse to reach the cells.

Classification of hypoxia

Hypoxia may be classifed according to the above causes as:

Arterial hypoxia, which indicates inadequate oxygenation of the blood.

Anaemic hypoxia, which is an oxygen deficiency in the blood due to a reduction in its oxygen-carrying power.

Circulatory hypoxia, which is characterized by a decline in the delivery of an adequate volume of oxygenated blood to the tissues.

Metabolic hypoxia, which is an imbalance between the oxygen demands of the tissue cells and the quantity of oxygen available.

Histotoxic hypoxia, which occurs when the cells become defective due to a toxic substance and, as a result, are unable to utilize oxygen.

Effects and symptoms of hypoxia

The effects and symptoms of hypoxia depend upon the severity of the hypoxia and the causative condition, and whether the oxygen deficiency is acute or chronic. If it is chronic, physiological adaptation by increasing the number of red blood cells (polycythaemia) may occur, such as when a person resides at a high altitude or has chronic airflow limitation.

General hypoxia produces some impairment of cellular activities throughout the body. The brain, heart, kidneys and liver are the most sensitive structures, and may suffer permanent damage due to the restricted oxygen supply. Metabolic processes are incomplete; the anaerobic situation results in an accumulation of lactic acid, producing tissue acidosis.

Initially, an acute deficiency of oxygen in the blood (hypoxaemia) induces an increased cardiac output and dilates the peripheral vessels. The pulse rate and blood pressure increase; then the pulse weakens as the myocardium suffers hypoxia. The patient may experience nausea and vomiting and complain of precordial pain.

The cerebral hypoxia and a consequent general reduction in metabolism produce a wide range of symptoms. Early manifestations may be headache, restlessness, weakness, muscle incoordination, and loss of visual acuity. If the oxygen deficit continues, reduced cerebral efficiency may progress through confusion and stupor to coma. Respirations may be increased, especially if there is a concomitant increase in the carbon dioxide content of the blood. They may be interspersed with sighing and yawning, and the patient may complain of dyspnoea. If the hypoxia persists, respirations gradually fail as the respiratory centres become depressed.

Cyanosis (bluish colour of mucous membranes and skin) is seen due to an excessive reduction of oxyhaemoglobin.

HYPERCAPNIA

Hypercapnia or hypercarbia is the retention of carbon dioxide in excess of the normal range (normal Pa_{CO_2}, 4.8–6.0 kPa (35–45 mmHg).

Causes of hypercapnia

Normally, the individual eliminates excess carbon dioxide by increasing the volume and rate of respirations. The respiratory centres and chemoreceptors are sensitive to the blood tension of carbon dioxide, which provides what may be referred to as the 'respiratory drive'.

The causes of retention of carbon dioxide are hypoventilation and mismatching of alveolar ventilation and perfusion.

Effects and manifestations of hypercapnia

The retention of an excess of carbon dioxide increases the respiratory drive and the respiratory rate and volume show a notable increase. If prolonged, the associated effort and energy expenditure may cause the patient to accept a higher level of P_{CO_2} and breathing becomes more dependent upon the hypoxic drive. If the hypercapnia is severe, the person becomes lethargic and the level of consciousness decreases. The retained carbon dioxide is hydrated to form carbonic acid $(H_2O + CO_2 \rightarrow H_2CO_3)$, the pH is decreased and the patient develops respiratory acidosis.

Circulatory changes include dilatation of peripheral and cerebral vessels. The skin is warm and flushed; the patient complains of headache and manifests apathy, reduced mental ability which may progress to confusion, and loss of muscle coordination. The cerebral vascular dilatation causes increased intracranial pressure, cerebral oedema and papilloedema.

The acidaemia associated with hypercapnia causes constriction of the pulmonary blood vessels, leading to aggravation of any pulmonary hypertension and existing heart complications.

CYANOSIS

A dusky bluish colour of the mucous membranes (central cyanosis) or of the skin and nail beds (peripheral cyanosis) may be associated with respiratory disease due to excessive deoxygenation of the haemoglobin.

The absence of cyanosis is not always a reassuring sign unless the haemoglobin level is known. In a person with 50% or less of the normal complement, the reduced haemoglobin may not be sufficiently concentrated to be reflected through superficial tissues.

CLUBBING OF THE FINGERS AND TOES

This unusual sign develops in some patients with primary pulmonary malignancies and occasionally in chronic respiratory disease and, although its cause is not known, it is thought to be due to increased vascularity in response to hypoxia.

PERCEPTUAL/COGNITIVE IMPAIRMENT

Confusion, somnolence, restlessness, irritability, visual disturbances, decreased co-ordination and impaired judgment are symptoms associated with the effects of hypoxia on the central nervous system. When hypoxaemia occurs, cerebral vascular resistance is reduced and cerebral blood flow increases. Despite these protective mechanisms, perceptual and cognitive changes are common manifestations of impaired respiratory function.

FATIGUE/DECREASED ENERGY

Increased airway resistance, decreased pulmonary compliance and the use of accessory muscles increase the work of breathing and energy expenditure. Increased energy demands result in accelerated metabolic activity and an increased demand for oxygen. The patient with chronic respiratory impairment experiences constant fatigue as the increased demand for oxygen further adds to the work of breathing. Activity tolerance is decreased and the person experiences increasing difficulty in meeting the demands of daily living activities.

Assessment of the Person with Impaired Gas Exchange

Nursing assessment of the person with impaired gas exchange includes identification of the effects of the hypoxia and hypercapnia on the individual. While taking the health history, the nurse identifies the severity and duration of the symptoms and their effect on the person's activity tolerance and daily living. Objective data are obtained from observations of the rate, rhythm and depth of the person's respirations, signs of cyanosis and pallor of the skin and mucous membranes and the results of clinical measurements of oxygen and carbon dioxide exchange.

DIAGNOSTIC MEASUREMENTS

Blood gas analysis

Impairment of respiratory ventilation and gas exchange are reflected in changes in the levels of blood gases. Normal values are:

PaO_2	11–13.3 kPa (80–100 mmHg)
$PaCO_2$	4.8–6.0 kPa (35–45 mmHg)
pH	7.35–7.45
$[H^+]$	35–45 nmol/l
Plasma CO_2	(20–32 mmol/l) (20–32 mEq/l)
Arterial oxyhaemoglobin saturation	95–97%

A blood specimen for gas analysis is withdrawn, usually from the femoral artery. The tube or syringe is placed on ice in a special, labelled container and sent promptly to the laboratory. Firm pressure is applied to the arterial puncture site for at least 7 minutes; it is then protected with a sterile covering.

Electrolyte concentrations

Determination of electrolyte values, particularly hydrogen carbonate ions (24–28 mmol/l) is necessary to interpret changes in acid–base balance.

Erythrocyte count and haemoglobin and haematocrit determination

It is important to know if the erythrocyte count is normal since erythrocytes contain the haemoglobin which carries the oxygen (normal: men, $4.5–6.5 \times 10^{12}$ per litre; women, $3.8–5.8 \times 10^{12}$ per litre). Similarly, an assessment of the patient includes a determination of the haemoglobin concentration (normal: men, 13–18 g/dl; women, 12–15 g/dl). Obviously, a deficiency of red blood cells or haemoglobin may produce an oxygen deficiency. The haematocrit represents the volume percentage of erythrocytes (normal: men, 40–50%; women, 37–47%).

Perfusion lung scan

This provides images in multiple views of the distribution of blood flow to the lung. Small aggregates of albumin 15–40 μm in size are labelled with technetium-99m and injected into a vein. These flow to and then stick in the first capillary bed they meet, which is the pulmonary capillary bed. Images of their distribution are made with a gamma camera. This is the most sensitive non-invasive test of decreased blood flow to small regions of the lung.

Ventilation scan

This provides images of the distribution of ventilation to the lungs. The patient inhales a radioactive gas such as xenon-133 or krypton-81m and an image is obtained with a gamma camera. More recently, inhaled submicronic aerosols of ^{99m}Tc-labelled agents are being used in place of radiogases. These are more readily available and are easier to use than radiogas. The ventilation scan helps to determine whether a defect seen on the perfusion lung scan is caused by pulmonary embolism or airway disease.

Nursing Intervention for the Person with Impaired Gas Exchange

The *goals* are that the patient will:

- Demonstrate arterial blood gas levels within his or her normal range.
- Be alert and orientated.
- Demonstrate ability to use home oxygen equipment safely, if relevant.

Nursing intervention (discussed previously) to promote airway clearance and an effective breathing pattern also improves gas exchange.

CHANGES OF BODY POSITION

Changes in body position affect ventilation and perfusion in healthy individuals and in persons with lung diseases. In the upright position the base of the lung is better ventilated and perfusion is greater than in the apex, producing regional differences in gas exchange. In the supine, prone and lateral positions, ventilation and perfusion are more uniform. Changes in body position significantly affect the rate of ventilation, the amount of lung capacity and the amount of physiological dead space.

Knowledge of the effects of position changes on pulmonary ventilation and perfusion in healthy subjects illustrates the need for nurses to assess the effects of various positions on patients with altered lung ventilation and perfusion. Studies have shown that in patients with chronic airflow limitation, differences in ventilation–perfusion ratios and gas exchange do not occur in the sitting position. Turning the patient with acute respiratory failure from the supine to prone position enhances gas exchange. Patients with disease predominantly affecting one lung showed improvement when turned from the supine position to a lateral position with the diseased lung uppermost. Measurements of lung volumes, blood gases and oxygen saturation by ear oximeter provide objective measures of ventilation and perfusion when evaluating a patient's response to changes in position. Pulse oximetry can be used in a wide range of clinical settings, for example in the intensive care or recovery units or in a rehabilitation ward (Schroeder, 1988). The nurse can also use the following parameters: observation of respiratory rate and depth; breath sounds; use of accessory muscles; pulse rate; skin colour; and the patient's general state of relaxation or tension.

Position changes for a patient with respiratory impairment are individualized and based on the assessment of the patient's responses to various positions. Awareness that position changes do affect oxygenation can assist the nurse in clinical decision-making related to position change in persons with respiratory impairment.

ADMINISTRATION OF OXYGEN

Oxygen is not usually prescribed for patients unless their PaO_2 is reduced to 8 kPa or the oxygen saturation is less than 85%. As with any medication, it should not be used indiscriminately. For instance, the administration of oxygen, except in a very low concentration, could be fatal to patients with hypoxia associated with chronic pulmonary disease. Normally, increased carbon dioxide tension stimulates the respiratory centres and elicits a ventilatory response that increases carbon dioxide elimination. The sensitivity of the chemoreceptors to hypercarbia is diminished in chronic hypercapnia and the patient becomes dependent upon hypoxia as a respiratory stimulus. If oxygen is given to correct the hypoxaemia, the patient's 'respiratory drive' is removed, hypoventilation develops and carbon dioxide retention is increased.

The concentration of oxygen administered to raise the oxygen level depends upon the patient's PaO_2, the effectiveness of the transportation of blood gases to the tissues, and on the tissue needs for oxygen and ability to utilize oxygen. Commonly, the flow rate per minute is set to deliver an oxygen concentration of about 30–40%. The doctor prescribes the concentration of oxygen to be administered. In an emergency situation, a nurse may initiate oxygen therapy after assessing signs of hypoxaemia, including rapid pulse, rapid shallow respirations, dyspnoea, use of accessory muscles of respiration, restlessness, confusion and cyanosis.

When using oxygen, it should be remembered that it is colourless, odourless, tasteless and heavier than air, and that it is hazardous because it supports combustion.

Methods of administering oxygen

The oxygen therapy device that is selected should be capable of delivering a consistent concentration of oxygen and be comfortable for the patient.

Oxygen delivery systems may be classified as *low flow* or *high flow*. Low-flow systems let the patient inhale room air which mixes freely with the oxygen. As the patient's ventilatory pattern changes so does the concentration of oxygen received. Low-flow systems are economical and comfortable but they do not provide a fixed concentration of oxygen. High-flow systems deliver a precise concentration of oxygen regardless of the patient's ventilatory pattern. Most of these systems use a Venturi mask which controls the amount of room air entering the system. The orifice size regulates the ratio of room air to oxygen, controls the velocity and directly affects the oxygen concentration being administered. Changes in the patient's respiration do not affect the inspired oxygen concentration as long as the correct litre flow is used and the mask fits snugly.

Low-flow oxygen therapy devices

Low-flow devices include the nasal cannulae (Figure 15.16), nasal catheter (rare), and the simple face mask.

Masks interfere with patient activities, especially talking and eating. They are less comfortable than the nasal cannulae but can deliver higher concentrations of oxygen.

Oxygen supplied from wall or tank systems lacks humidity and may cause drying of the mucosa. At low flow rates (e.g. 3–4 l/min) humidification of the oxygen is not needed and if supplied may cause 'feelings of suffocation'.

High-flow oxygen therapy devices/controlled oxygen therapy

These devices include Venturi masks and non-rebreathing masks.

Venturi mask (entrainment mask). This mask can deliver 24–40% oxygen which is fairly precisely controlled. When oxygen enters the mask, it passes through a narrow jet opening which increases the velocity of the flow. Room air is drawn through the entrainment ports into the stream of oxygen. Oxygen concentration is varied by changing the size of the jet or the size of the entrainment ports (Figure 15.17). The jets are calibrated which allows control of the ratio of oxygen to air. The larger the jet, the more room air inhaled. These masks are recommended for use by patients with chronic airflow limitation because oxygen concentrations can be controlled. However, like other masks, it interferes with patient activities. Humidifiers are not recommended with Venturi masks as the humidity may clog the jet openings and cause changes in the concentration of the oxygen delivered. Usually, enough room air is entrained to maintain sufficient humidity of the inspired gas.

Non-rebreathing mask. A bag is attached to the base of this mask to serve as a large reservoir for the oxygen. On inspiration, a one-way flap valve between the bag and the mask opens so that oxygen can be inhaled and one-way flap valves over the exhalation ports close to prevent entrainment of room air. If the mask fits

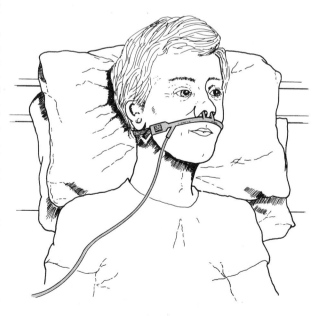

Figure 15.16 Plastic cannulae or prongs inserted into the nostrils to deliver oxygen.

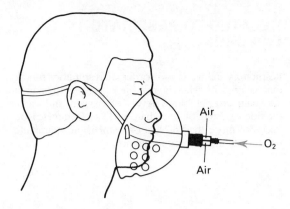

Figure 15.17 Venturi mask (entrainment mask).

securely, the patient breathes only the oxygen from the bag, permitting delivery of 90–100% oxygen concentrations. Exhaled air is directed through the exhalation ports and cannot enter the bag as the flap valve between the bag and the mask closes.

Humidifiers are not recommended for use with non-rebreathing masks as the water vapour condenses in the reservoir bag and interferes with the opening and closing of the flap valves. Generally these masks are used for only short periods of time.

Partial rebreathing mask. This mask also contains a reservoir bag but has no valve, therefore the patient's expired gas flows back into the bag.

The inspired oxygen concentration is slightly lower than that delivered by a non-rebreathing mask ranging from 60–90%.

Manual resuscitation bag (Ambu bag). This is part of the standard equipment on any ward emergency or resuscitation trolley. It is a portable ventilator that is operated manually (Figure 15.18). It consists of a self-inflating bag which connects with a source of 100% oxygen and has a short tube to which a mask is attached. A connecting adapter replaces the mask when the bag is used for a patient with an endotracheal or tracheostomy tube.

After applying the mask so that there is as tight a seal as possible, or after connecting the tube to the patient's artificial airway, the bag is squeezed with both hands. Collapse of the bag delivers an adequate tidal volume of oxygen into the patient's airway.

The self-inflating hand ventilator is useful for resuscitation in an emergency. It is kept at the bedside of a patient who is receiving mechanical ventilator assistance so it is readily available to ventilate the patient in case of malfunction of the respirator.

Oxygen toxicity

The nurse must be aware of additional precautions when administering oxygen. High concentrations of oxygen over prolonged periods can cause oxygen toxicity. Concentrations greater than 60% oxygen over

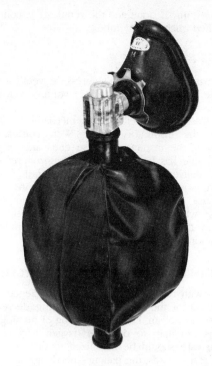

Figure 15.18 An Ambu resuscitator: a self-inflating hand-compressible breathing bag and mask.

24 hours can cause pathological changes in the lungs and central nervous system. The alveolar–capillary membrane is damaged, resulting in increased permeability and ensuing oedema of the interstitial tissues and alveoli. Oxygen and carbon dioxide diffusion is impaired. Some alveoli collapse. The PaO_2 falls and causes what is referred to as 'refractory hypoxaemia'. Retention of carbon dioxide and acidosis develop.

Neurological manifestations include muscular irritability that may progress to convulsions and impaired vision. Premature infants exposed to a high oxygen concentration develop vascular changes in their eyes that lead to blindness.

MECHANICAL VENTILATORS

When a patient is unable to ventilate the lungs effectively and maintain adequate alveolar–blood gas exchange, a mechanical ventilator (respirator) may be used to inflate the lungs and assist the individual's inspiratory effort. The ventilator introduces air or a mixture of air and oxygen intermittently into the patient's airway by producing a positive pressure (a gas pressure greater than that of the atmosphere). Expiration is passive when the inflow-regulating valve closes. The indications for ventilator use are ventilatory insufficiency, hypovolaemia and hypercapnia.

An artificial airway is necessary when a respirator is being used so that a seal is produced by a cuffed tube to prevent escape of the inspiratory gas. Initially, an endotracheal tube is generally used, but if mechanical respiratory support is necessary for a prolonged period, a tracheostomy is done and the ventilator is connected to a cuffed tracheostomy tube.

Types of ventilators

Three basic types of positive-pressure ventilators are available: (1) pressure-cycled; (2) volume-cycled; and (3) time-cycled.

The classification reflects the mechanism that terminates the inspiratory phase. With *volume-cycled ventilators*, the inspiratory phase ends after a preset tidal volume has been delivered. *Pressure-cycled ventilators* deliver the inspiratory gas until a preset pressure is reached which then terminates inspiration.

The use of ventilators is limited to intensive care settings, where nurses and doctors are skilled in adjusting the ventilator and where constant patient observation is assured.

DECREASED TISSUE DEMANDS FOR OXYGEN

Persons with respiratory limitations experience fatigue as a result of the hypoxia and ensuing decrease in cellular metabolism. Efficient planning of nursing interventions can help to decrease oxygen requirements. Nursing care should be organized to permit uninterrupted rest periods; the patient's needs are anticipated and objects that may be required are left within easy reach. Assistance is provided in turning and moving to minimize the patient's energy expenditure. Exercises can be performed passively by the nurse. Pain and discomfort are controlled before they become severe. Anxiety and apprehension are decreased by providing explanations of what is happening, communicating expectations for patient participation and reassuring the patient of his progress. Environmental stimuli, including noise and lighting are controlled.

If the patient is in an intensive care unit, where possible the usual day–night cycle is maintained. Lights are dimmed and noise and disruptions are kept to a minimum at night to promote sleep. The patient's usual pre-sleep habits are incorporated into his care if possible to reinforce familiar routines which promote relaxation and sleep.

Patients with chronic respiratory impairment are taught to organize their daily activities to allow for periods of rest and to carry out activities in ways that expend the least amount of energy.

If the patient experiences increased breathlessness following meals, he or she may find it easier to have smaller and more frequent meals, with rest periods before and after. Gas-forming foods should be avoided.

EVALUATION

The achievement and maintenance of adequate gas exchange is evaluated by the absence of signs of hypoxia and the alertness and orientation of the individual. The person's blood gas levels are within the usual range for the individual; the blood pH is within normal range; cyanosis is absent; the person is orientated and relates appropriately to the environment and is able to perform usual daily living activities.

IMPAIRED GAS EXCHANGE RELATED TO RESPIRATORY FAILURE

Respiratory failure is a disorder of respiratory function that is present when a person is unable to maintain adequate arterial blood levels of oxygen and carbon dioxide. A PaO_2 of less than 8.0 kPa (60 mmHg) or a $PaCO_2$ of more than 6.2 kPa (45 mmHg) are parameters used to define respiratory failure.

CAUSE

Respiratory failure may be encountered in any clinical area and may be associated with a variety of disorders, including: (1) trauma and surgery that incur shock; (2) intrapulmonary disorders, such as acute and chronic airway obstruction, resistive disorders and pulmonary vascular disorders; (3) central nervous system disorders, such as drug overdose, brain tumour, cerebral injury or haemorrhage; (4) neuromuscular disease that involves respiratory muscle innervation (e.g. myasthenia gravis and Guillain-Barré syndrome); (5) sepsis, especially if the organisms are Gram-negative; and (6) obstructive and central sleep apnoea.

Patients with a history of chronic obstructive pulmonary disease (asthma, chronic bronchitis) and cardiac or kidney disease, and those who are obese or debilitated are predisposed to develop respiratory failure.

Respiratory failure may be the result of alveolar hypoventilation, inadequate oxygenation of the blood (as occurs in ventilation–perfusion imbalance) or right-to-left shunt. In some instances more than one problem is present. Ventilation–perfusion inequality is the most frequent cause and is largely responsible for the low PO_2 in respiratory failure resulting as a complication of obstructive and restrictive diseases and adult respiratory distress syndrome. Alveolar hypoventilation is characterized by the retention of an excessive volume of carbon dioxide (hypercarbia), accompanied by hypoxaemia. The patient develops respiratory acidosis because of the elevated $PaCO_2$. It is frequently associated with general hypoventilation due to neuromuscular disturbances and chest wall injury. When diffusion is impaired the carbon dioxide retention is initially slight and hypoxia is usually minimal.

Failure to oxygenate the blood adequately may be due to abnormal distribution of the inspired gas, ventilation–perfusion inequality or shunting of the blood through unventilated areas of the lung. The alveoli may be filled with fluid, or the alveoli are not ventilated because of an airway obstruction or atelectasis. As a result, the blood may flow through the capillaries around the alveoli without gas exchange taking place. When blood enters the arterial system without going through ventilated areas of the lung, it is referred to as a shunt, such as occurs with a heart defect when the blood moves directly from the right side of the heart to the left. In other instances the alveoli may be ventilated but the respective capillaries do not receive an adequate blood supply or are occluded (ventilation–perfusion mismatching).

When respiratory failure is severe pulmonary capillary epithelium is damaged, which leads to haemorrhage and interstitial oedema. The oedema decreases diffusion because fluid lies between the alveoli and capillaries. Fluid infiltrates the alveoli; surfactant is destroyed by proteins which leak through the permeable capillaries, and functional terminal respiratory units collapse. The capillaries dilate, the alveolar walls hypertrophy and the lungs become fibrotic. Defective gas diffusion becomes extensive and very serious. This severe form of acute respiratory failure may be referred to as *adult respiratory distress syndrome* (ARDS) or *shock lung*. There is increased resistance to air entry in the airways and alveoli.

CHARACTERISTICS

The person may manifest the effects of hypoxaemia or hypercarbia, or both. Dyspnoea or tachypnoea may be present, or in ventilatory failure respirations may be depressed and are slow, irregular and shallow. The pulse rate increases and arrhythmias may develop. The patient may be restless and complain of headache or dizziness. Disorientation, apathy and slow responses develop as a result of the cerebral hypoxia, and may progress to unconsciousness. Periodic sustained contraction of a group of skeletal muscles (asterixis), slurred speech and mood fluctuations may occur if there is marked retention of carbon dioxide. The tidal and minute volumes are usually reduced.

Respiratory failure may develop quickly in a few hours after the initial insult, or the onset may be insidious over a few days or weeks. Serial monitoring of the patient's blood gases and tidal volume, and close observation of the characteristics of the respirations in circumstances where respiratory insufficiency may occur are important in early recognition of the problem.

TREATMENT

The underlying disorder which initiated the respiratory failure is treated and therapy is immediately directed toward improving ventilation and oxygenation of the blood. Airway obstruction is alleviated by removing retained secretions, through coughing, postural drainage and suctioning. A bronchodilator (e.g. salbutamol) is administered and respiratory stimulants may be given. Respiratory depressants are avoided. Corticosteroids are useful for some patients to improve their airflow.

Infections are treated promptly as they may produce respiratory failure in patients with chronic airflow limitation.

The aspiration of acid from the stomach into the lungs (acid reflux), occurs in many people with chronic respiratory failure, particularly when they are lying down. Measures to correct or modify the problem are developed in collaboration with the patient. Dietary measures include the avoidance of caffeine and eliminating evening snacks. The head of the bed is elevated on blocks. Antacid medications and H2 an-

tagonists may be used to minimize the effects of the stomach acid.

Diuretics are prescribed to decrease fluid overload in persons with cardiac complications. Changes in body weight are monitored and the person's ankles are observed for swelling.

Oxygen may be administered by Venturi mask to control the concentration delivered to the patient. The administration of uncontrolled oxygen via nasal prongs or a simple mask can depress respirations and increase the respiratory failure in individuals whose main respiratory stimulus is hypoxaemia. The number of hours of oxygen therapy per day is individually prescribed and will vary at different times for the same patient as the requirements fluctuate. A person who requires home oxygen for 14 hours a day when he is well, may require continuous oxygen therapy during a respiratory infection which has increased his/her respiratory failure.

Additional nursing measures include exercise programmes to strengthen respiratory muscles and the use of breathing techniques. Patients with chronic respiratory failure, are encouraged to remain active, eat a well-balanced diet, maintain their desired body weights and get adequate rest and sleep. Individuals and their families are taught to monitor their respiratory status and to adjust their therapeutic regimen to prevent complications and to treat them early when they do occur. Patient and family participation in preventing the development of respiratory failure was demonstrated in the clinical situation discussed on page 407. Tracheal intubation may be necessary (see p. 384).

When respiratory failure is acute and severe, intensive nursing care and constant monitoring are required.

SUMMARY

The constant exchange of oxygen and carbon dioxide between an individual and the environment is essential to life. Impairment of respiratory function threatens the individual's survival and either temporarily or permanently disrupts health and the quality of life. Respiratory disorders are common and familiar occurrences. Each of us has experienced the difficulties with airway clearance which result from acute respiratory infections. We can relate to the fear and apprehension demonstrated by persons with acute respiratory distress. It is much more difficult to appreciate fully the enormous personal impact chronic respiratory disorders have on the patient and family, their daily functioning and life-styles. Medical advances have been made in the management of acute and chronic respiratory disorders but medical cures do not exist for most respiratory diseases. Patients and their families must learn to live with the resulting health problems.

This chapter has been organized around the three interrelated health problems common to persons with altered respirations: *ineffective airway clearance; ineffective breathing pattern* and *impaired gas exchange*. The nursing care of persons with altered respiration includes the negotiation of long-term patient goals and outcomes as well as goals and outcomes for the current clinical situation. Nurses are assuming an increased role in helping patients with respiratory conditions and their families to acquire self-management skills and to achieve productive lives. Advances in nursing research related to respiratory function are providing scientific rationales for the selection of specific nursing strategies and helping nurses to evaluate the effectiveness of therapeutic measures. Nurses are becoming better prepared and able to assume greater responsibility for providing nursing solutions to patients' respiratory health problems. They play a key role in the promotion, maintenance and restoration of respiratory function. Nurses should be working collaboratively with other health professionals and the public to support health-seeking behaviours, the creation of a tobacco-free society and major reductions in atmospheric pollution.

LEARNING ACTIVITIES

1. Investigate a stop-smoking programme(s) in your community or health care agency. What techniques are used to help smokers give up? What are the immediate and 1 year post-programme success rates? How many of the participants are referred by a nurse?
2. Recall the circumstances of your last episode of acute respiratory infection.
   (a) How did this respiratory infection affect your usual activities?
   (b) What planned or spontaneous measures did you take to achieve a clear airway?
   (c) What actions hindered the maintenance of a patent airway?
3. Using the techniques described in this chapter, teach a colleague to cough effectively. Discuss the criteria you used to evaluate the outcomes of the learning that took place and the effectiveness of the person's coughing.
4. Attempt to explain the regional variations in death rates from cancer of the bronchus and respiratory conditions discussed on pp. 372–373.
5. Identify the major sources of atmospheric pollution within a 10 km radius of your workplace. What can be done to reduce the pollution they produce. What do you think is the relative importance of these sources in causing respiratory disease compared with smoking?

REFERENCES AND FURTHER READING

Allen D (1988) Making sense of suctioning. *Nursing Times* **84(9):** 46–47.

Ashworth P (1980) *Care to Communicate.* London: Royal College of Nursing.

Bysshe J (1989) Politics in the air. *Nursing* **3(38):** 15–18.

Duffy B (1985) Chronic breathing difficulties. *Nursing Mirror* **161 (Sept.25):** 40–42.

Guyton AC (1986) *Textbook of Medical Physiology* 7th edn, Philadelphia: Saunders.

Heslop AP & Bagnall P (1988) A study to evaluate the intervention of a nurse visiting patients with disabling chest diseases in the community. *Journal of Advanced Nursing* **13(1):** 71–77.

Hinchcliffe S & Montague S (1988) *Physiology for Nursing Practice.* London: Baillière Tindall.

Howard JE (1987) Respiratory teaching of patients, how effective is it? *Journal of Advanced Nursing* 12(2): 207–214.

Kane K (1989) The killing fields: farmer's lung disease. *Nursing Times* **85(8):** 40–44.

Kirilloff LH, Owens GR, Rogers RM & Mazzocco MC (1985) Does chest physical therapy work? *Chest* **88(3):** 436–443.

Kramer JF (1982) A one year follow up of participants in a smoke stoppers programme. *Patient Counselling and Health Education* **4(2):** 89–93.

Lindell KO & Mazzocco M (1990) Breaking bronchospasm's grip with MDIs. *American Journal of Nursing* **90(3):** 35–41.

Luke C (1989) Respiratory investigations. *Nursing* **3(38):** 5–8.

Mead D (1990) Asthma, children and physical exercise. *Nursing Standard* **4(36):** 28–31.

Mumford S (1986) Draining the pleural cavity. *Professional Nurse* **1(9):** 240–242.

Nocon A & Booth T (1990) Asthma: a hidden disease of our times. *Nursing Standard* **4(45):** 28–30.

North American Nursing Diagnosis Association (1989) *Taxonomy 1,* revised 1989. St Louis: NANDA.

Nursing Standard (1990) Clinical news. *Nursing Standard* **4(28):** 14.

Office of Health Economics (1990) *Asthma.* London: OHE.

OPCS (1985) Hospital In-Patient Enquiry. London: HMSO.

OPCS (1986) Mortality Statistics England and Wales: Cause. London: HMSO.

OPCS (1987) Mortality Statistics England and Wales: Area. London: HMSO.

OPCS (1990) Monitor: Cigarette Smoking 1972 to 1988. London: HMSO.

Piff C (1985) *Let's Face It.* London: Gollancz.

Pretty J & Whelan J (1989) Nursing patients with head and neck cancers. In Tiffany R (ed.) *Oncology for Nurses and Health Care Professions,* vol. 3, 2nd edn. London: Harper·& Row.

Pritchard AP & David JA (1988) *The Royal Marsden Hospital Manual of Clinical Nursing Procedures.* London: Harper & Row.

Redfearn S (1989) Pulmonary tuberculosis. *Nursing* **3(38):** 9–11.

Robinson LA & Pugsley SO (1981) Dealing with chronic airflow obstruction. In Anderson SVD & Bauwens EE (eds) *Chronic Health Problems*. St Louis: Mosby.

Roberts A (1988) Ageing lungs and airways. *Nursing Times* **84(37):** 49–52.

Saunders DJ, Stone V, Fowler G & Marzillier J (1986) Practice nurses and anti-smoking education. *British Medical Journal* **292:** 381–383.

Scadding JG (1977) *Definition and Clinical Categories in Asthma*. London: Chapman & Hall.

Schroeder CH (1988) Pulse oximetry: a nursing care plan. *Critical Care Nurse* **8(8):** 50–66.

Smith S (1985) How drugs act: drugs and the bronchi. *Nursing Times* 1985, 13 Feb: 50–51.

Thompson LF (1990) The hazards of immobility. *American Journal of Nursing* **90(3):** 47–48.

Towsend P (1988) *Inequalities in Health*. London: Penguin.

Wallis J & Wells F (1988) Chest injuries: diagnosis and management. *Care of the Critically Ill* **3(6):** 187–192.

Walsh M (1989a) Asthma: the Orem self-care nursing approach. *Nursing* **3(38):** 19–21.

Walsh M (1989b) Making sense of chest drains. *Nursing Times* **85(24):** 40–41.

Caring for the Patient with a Disorder of the Gastrointestinal System

16

OBJECTIVES

On completion of this chapter the reader will be able to:
- Describe the structures of the gastrointestinal tract
- Describe the processes of motility, secretion, digestion and absorption in the gastrointestinal tract
- Describe the protective and immunological functions of the gastrointestinal tract
- Appreciate the relationship between stress and gastrointestinal motility and secretion
- Describe the clinical characteristics of disorders of the gastrointestinal system
- Discuss the nursing assessment of the person with disorders of gastrointestinal function
- Plan, implement and evaluate nursing care for individuals with disorders of gastrointestinal movement, secretion, digestion and absorption.

THE ALIMENTARY CANAL

The alimentary canal, frequently referred to as the gastrointestinal tract, consists of a long hollow tube extending from the lips to the anus. It provides a non-sterile pathway for nutrients in the body and it is divided into the mouth, pharynx, oesophagus, stomach (Greek, *gaster*) and intestines (Greek, *enteron*). Modifications in structure occur in different parts of the tract, and are correlated with the particular functions featured in the respective area and the likely condition of the content when it reaches that part. The primary function of the gastrointestinal tract is to provide the body cells with a continual supply of nutrients, electrolytes and water in a form that is acceptable to the system. To do so it performs the functions of ingestion, digestion and absorption of food and fluid into the blood and elimination of residue and waste products. These functions are controlled by complex levels of integration. At the cellular level, each cell type has its own inherent properties, e.g. contractility, secretion or absorption. Within the gut wall itself, there is an intrinsic (enteric) nervous system with both sensory and motor nerves, as well as local endocrine circuits and mast and other cell types which respond to local intraluminal and intramural stimuli to influence the local secretomotor functions. Superimposed on this are the extrinsic neural and endocrine control systems. These extrinsic systems respond both to signals from the gastrointestinal tract and from higher centres. Thus a gastrointestinal response is one of the most common outcomes of a stressful situation, e.g. onlookers may vomit at the scene of an accident.

Food sustains life and determines an individual's nutritional status, which in turn plays a large part in determining overall health status, levels of achievement and resistance to and ability to cope with disease. It supplies the body with the energy required for all its activities (e.g. respiration, circulation of the blood, muscular activity and work). Food provides the materials for tissue growth and repair and those essential for the production of substances by the body cells (e.g. hormones and enzymes). Essential regulatory substances such as vitamins are also obtained from foods. Most foods are complex compounds: chemical and mechanical processes occur in the gastrointestinal tract to break them down into absorbable forms.

If food is withheld or a disorder within the tract interrupts the essential processing of the nutrients, the individual's survival is threatened.

STRUCTURAL DIVISIONS OF THE GASTROINTESTINAL TRACT

MOUTH

The mouth or oral cavity, the first part of the tract, is lined by a mucous membrane which secretes mucus to mix with the food, facilitating its movement through the pharynx and oesophagus. Although the mouth is primarily concerned with the ingestion of food, it also plays an important role in speech.

The tongue, teeth and salivary glands are contained within the mouth. The *tongue* is comprised of muscular tissue enclosed in mucous membrane. The upper surface is studded with numerous papillae and contains taste buds. The tongue functions in swallowing and speech as well as in taste.

Early in life, the human organism develops 20 primary deciduous *teeth*: 10 upper and 10 lower.

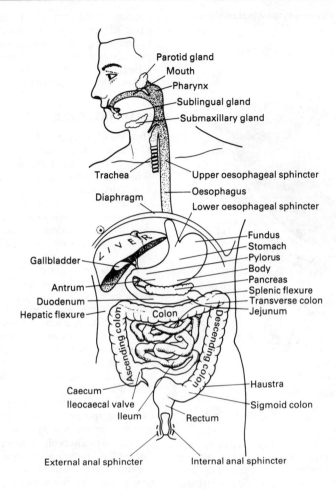

Figure 16.1 Structural divisions of the alimentary canal.

Beginning in the fifth or sixth year and continuing over a period of several years, the deciduous teeth are replaced by a permanent set of 16 in the upper jaw and 16 in the lower jaw. The front teeth are shaped for biting and tearing, and the remainder for grinding and masticating food. Hence, loss of teeth, or defects in them, can lead to malnutrition.

Each tooth consists of a crown and root (see Figure 16.4). The crown is the exposed portion which has a hard external covering of enamel and an internal substance called dentine. The root is the part buried in the jaw bone and has a covering of cementum, a substance softer and less smooth than the enamel. A central cavity running the length of the tooth contains nerves and blood vessels.

There are three pairs of *salivary glands* whose ducts open on to the surface of the mouth. The parotid glands lie in front of and just below the ear and produce a thin, watery secretion that includes an important digestive enzyme, ptyalin. The submaxillary and sublingual glands

are located in the floor of the mouth. The sublingual glands secrete only mucus; the submaxillary glands produce both a watery and mucous secretion. The secretions of the salivary glands and the oral mucosa collectively form the saliva. For the composition and functions of saliva see pp. 349–440).

PHARYNX

The second segment of the tract is the pharynx, which is a funnel-shaped muscular tube lined with mucous membrane that is continuous with that of the mouth, respiratory tract and oesophagus. It serves as a common pathway for food and air. When its muscular tissue contracts, the band of striated muscle known as the cricopharyngeal or upper oesophageal sphincter relaxes; food and fluid are directed into the oesophagus and the entrances to the larynx and the oral and nasal cavities are closed simultaneously.

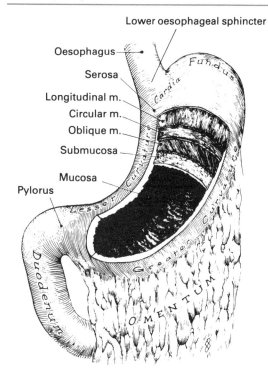

Lower oesophageal sphincter
Oesophagus
Serosa
Longitudinal m.
Circular m.
Oblique m.
Submucosa
Mucosa
Pylorus
Fundus
Cardia
Duodenum
OMENTUM

Figure 16.2 The stomach.

OESOPHAGUS

The oesophagus is a narrow muscular tube, approximately 10 inches long, that passes down behind the trachea and heart, through the mediastinum and diaphragm to the stomach. The upper third is striated muscle, the middle third is mixed striated and smooth muscle and the lower third smooth muscle. A thickened band of smooth muscle forms the lower oesophageal or gastrointestinal sphincter which opens when food is swallowed. It is lined with mucous membrane and has an outer protective coat of fibrous tissue.

STOMACH

The stomach and the intestines, the remaining portions of the digestive tract, lie within the abdominal cavity. The stomach is located just below the diaphragm and is the widest part of the alimentary canal which makes possible its retention of a considerable amount of food while it undergoes certain changes. The stomach is divided into three segments: the fundus, body and pylorus (Figure 16.1).

The gastric walls have three layers of muscle tissue; one in which the fibres run longitudinally, a second one in which they are circular, and a third in which they run obliquely to the others (Figure 16.2). The circular muscle layer is thickened at the opening of the oesophagus into the stomach to form the *cardiac* or *lower oesophageal sphincter*. Similarly, the opening into the small intestine is guarded by the *pyloric sphincter*.

The mucous membrane lining is thick and lies in folds to allow for distensibility as the stomach fills. It contains numerous minute glands made up of three types of secreting cells: the chief, or zymogen cells secrete the gastric enzymes, the parietal or oxyntic cells produce hydrochloric acid, and mucous glands provide mucus. The glandular secretions are poured out into the stomach to form collectively the gastric juice.

SMALL INTESTINE

The small intestine is the longest portion of the alimentary canal, being approximately 3.0–3.5 metres long, and is divided into the *duodenum, jejunum* and *ileum*. The duodenum is the short, proximal portion which originates with the gastric pylorus. It receives the bile and the pancreatic enzymes through a sphincter (sphincter of Oddi) at the junction of the common bile duct and the duodenum. The long jejunum and ileum lie in loops and fill the greater part of the abdominal cavity.

The mucosal surface of the small intestine is covered with many finger-like processes called villi, (Figure 16.3), each of which contains a central lymph channel, called a lacteal, and a network of capillaries. Each villus is covered with a single layer of specialized epithelial cells, the luminal surface of which is covered with small projections called microvilli (brush border). Digestion takes place in the lumen of the small intestine at the enterocyte brush border and within the absorptive cell itself, and in some cases is an integral part of absorption. The villi with their microvilli serve to greatly increase the absorptive area. This increased surface area ensures exposure of the luminal contents to the final digestive surface (the glycocalyx) before absorption across the microvillus membrane occurs. The small intestine contains many glands which secrete digestive enzymes (see p. 438) and hormones on to the glycocalyx, which covers the microvilli. The molecules of digested food are picked up by the blood in the capillaries and the lymph in the lacteals.

Lymph nodes appear in clusters throughout the small intestine and are referred to as Peyer's patches. Other lymphoid cells located in the intestinal mucosa and between the epithelial cells lining the villi, play an important role in the immunological defence of the body.

LARGE INTESTINE

The large intestine has a greater diameter than that of the small intestine and is divided into the *caecum, colon, rectum* and *anal canal*. The ileum opens into a pouch-like structure, the caecum, in the right lower abdominal quadrant. The *appendix*, a slender blind tube, is attached to the caecum and is a frequent site of inflammation and infection (appendicitis). At the junction of the ileum and caecum, an *ileocaecal valve* functions to allow contents to pass in one direction only: from the ileum to the caecum.

The large intestine ascends the right side of the abdominal cavity from the caecum as the ascending colon and flexes at the undersurface of the liver to form the transverse colon. The descending colon passes down the left side of the abdomen and, since it takes an

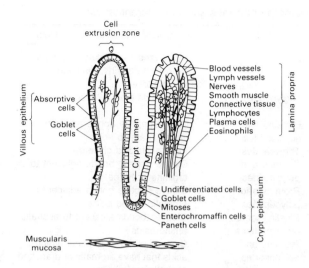

Figure 16.3 labels:
Cell extrusion zone

Absorptive cells

Goblet cells

Villous epithelium

Crypt lumen

Blood vessels
Lymph vessels
Nerves
Smooth muscle
Connective tissue
Lymphocytes
Plasma cells
Eosinophils

Lamina propria

Undifferentiated cells
Goblet cells
Mitoses
Enterochromaffin cells
Paneth cells

Crypt epithelium

Muscularis mucosa

Figure 16.3 Schematic diagram of two sectioned villi and a crypt to illustrate the histological organization of the small intestinal mucosa.

S-shaped course through the pelvis, becomes known as the sigmoid colon.

The mucosa of the large intestine has no villi but has many goblet cells which secrete mucus. The longitudinal muscle tissue is arranged in three strips that are shorter than the other tissues. This muscular arrangement, together with the contraction of segments of circular muscle, especially the transverse colon, forms small sacs along the tube which are referred to as *haustra* (see Figure 16.1).

The rectum is a continuation of the sigmoid along the anterior surface of the sacrum and coccyx. It is about 15–17 cm long and contains vertical folds referred to as rectal columns. Each column contains an artery and vein. The veins frequently become varicosed, forming haemorrhoids.

The short terminal portion of the alimentary tube, the anal canal, opens onto the body surface at the anus. The opening between the rectum and the anal canal is controlled by the *internal anal sphincter*, which is not under the control of the will. The anus is controlled by the *external anal sphincter* which, after infancy, is under voluntary control.

PERITONEUM

The outer protective coat of the stomach and intestines is serous membrane and is known as the *visceral peritoneum*. The abdominal cavity is lined with serous membrane called the *parietal peritoneum*. A fan-like expanse is reflected off the posterior abdominal wall and extends to the intestine where it becomes continuous with the visceral peritoneum. This portion of serous membrane is known as the *mesentery*; it

supports the intestine and transmits blood vessels, lymphatics and nerves. A sheet of peritoneum, the *great omentum*, is reflected off the stomach to lie like an apron in front of the intestines. The great omentum protects the intestines and, when infection or inflammation of the peritoneum (peritonitis) occurs, it makes an effort to wall off the affected area by surrounding it to prevent a spread of the infection; it can be used surgically to repair open wounds. The *lesser omentum* is a fold of peritoneum extending from the liver to the stomach.

BLOOD SUPPLY TO THE ALIMENTARY CANAL

The mouth, tongue and pharynx derive their blood supply from the external carotid arteries via the lingual and external maxillary arteries. The oesophageal artery arises from the thoracic aorta. Three main arteries supply the stomach, the left, right and short gastric arteries. The left gastric is a branch of the coeliac which is a large, shorter artery arising from the abdominal aorta. The other two gastric arteries originate from the other main branches of the coeliac, the hepatic and splenic arteries.

The remainder of the tract is nourished by the superior and inferior mesenteric arteries, direct branches of the abdominal aorta.

The blood into which the digested food products are absorbed is carried by the superior and inferior mesenteric veins into the portal vein, which transmits it to the liver. This makes the food products immediately available to the liver for its functions.

ACCESSORY STRUCTURES OF DIGESTION

THE BILE SYSTEM AND PANCREAS

The biliary system and exocrine pancreas are important contributory structures in digestion and absorption (see Chapter 17).

Digestion

Digestion consists of mechanical and chemical processes. The mechanical processes involve the neuromuscular tissues of the alimentary tract and have as their purposes the movement of food through the tract, the mixing of it with digestive secretions, and the repeated breaking up of the food mass to bring more of it in contact with the absorptive surface. These processes include mastication, deglutition (swallowing), movements of the stomach and intestines, and defecation. The chemical processes are chemical reactions catalysed by enzymes to reduce the food to simpler compounds.

The digestive enzymes are substances secreted by mucosal cells of the alimentary tract and by the associated digestive organs (pancreas and liver) (Table 16.1). Like all enzymes in the body they act as catalysts (i.e. they promote and speed up chemical reactions without becoming a part of them). All enzymes are specific and, in the case of the digestive enzymes, each is

Table 16.1 Principal digestive enzymes (with corresponding proenzymes shown in parentheses).

Source	Enzyme	Activator	Substrate	Catalytic function or products
Salivary glands	Salivary α-amylase	Cl⁻	Starch	Hydrolyzes 1,4α linkages, producing α-limit dextrins, maltotriose, and maltose
Lingual glands	Lingual lipase		Triglycerides	Fatty acids plus 1,2-diacylglycerols
Stomach	Pepsins (pepsinogens)	HCl	Proteins and polypeptides	Cleave peptide bonds adjacent to aromatic amino acids
	Gastric lipase		Triglycerides	Fatty acids and glycerols
	Trypsin (trypsinogen)	Enteropeptidase	Proteins and polypeptides	Cleave peptide bonds adjacent to arginine or lysine
	Chymotrypsins (chymotrypsinogens)	Trypsin	Proteins and polypeptides	Cleave peptide bonds adjacent to aromatic amino acids
	Elastase (proelastase)	Trypsin	Elastin, some other proteins	Cleaves bonds adjacent to aliphatic amino acids
	Carboxypeptidase A (procarboxypeptidase A)	Trypsin	Proteins and polypeptides	Cleaves carboxyl terminal amino acids that have aromatic or branched aliphatic side-chains
Exocrine pancreas	Carboxypeptidase B (procarboxypeptidase B)	Trypsin	Proteins and polypeptides	Cleaves carboxy terminal amino acids that have basic side-chains
	Colipase (procolipase)	Trypsin	Fat droplets	Binds to bile salt-triglyceride-water interface, making anchor for lipase
	Pancreatic lipase	—	Triglycerides	Monoglycerides and fatty acids
	Cholesteryl ester hydrolase	—	Cholesteryl esters	Cholesterol
	Pancreatic α-amylase	Cl⁻	Starch	Same as salivary α-amylase
	Ribonuclease	—	RNA	Nucleotides
	Deoxyribonuclease	—	DNA	Nucleotides
	Phospholipase A_2	Trypsin	Phospholipids	Fatty acids, lysophospholipids
	Enteropeptidase	—	Trypsinogen	Trypsin
	Aminopeptidases	—	Polypeptides	Cleave N-terminal amino acid from peptide
Intestinal mucosa	Dipeptidases	—	Dipeptides	Two amino acids
	Glucoamylase	—	Maltose, maltotriose	Glucose
	Lactase	—	Lactose	Galactose and glucose
	Sucrase*	—	Sucrose	Fructose and glucose
	α-Limit dextrinase*	—	α-Limit dextrins	Glucose
	Nuclease and related enzymes	—	Nucleic acids	Pentoses and purine and pyrimidine bases
Cytoplasm of mucosal cells	Various peptidases	—	Di, tri-, and tetrapeptides	Amino acids

* Sucrase and α-limit dextrinase are separate polypeptide chains that are subunits of a single protein.
From Ganong (1989) with permission.

secreted only by cells in a certain area of the digestive system. They are classified according to the food they act upon. An enzyme which promotes the breakdown of protein is called a *proteolytic enzyme* or *peptidase*; one that acts upon starches is an *amylase*; and a fat-splitting enzyme is known as a *lipase*.

Digestion takes place within the lumen of the alimentary canal or the cells lining the tract. The principal reaction in chemical digestion is hydrolysis, which is the breaking up of a large molecule of a substance into smaller molecules by combining it with water. For example, in the digestion of cane sugar, one molecule of sugar and one molecule of water yields two molecules of glucose that can be absorbed by facilitated or carrier-mediated transport.

$$C_{12}H_{22}O_{11} + H_2O \xrightarrow{\text{Enzyme}} 2(C_6H_{12}O_6)$$

Most food undergoes several chemical reactions before it is reduced to a form that can be absorbed. The steps in the digestive breakdown of protein, carbohydrate and fat follow.

Protein → proteoses → peptones → polypeptides → amino acids

Seventy to 80% of protein digestion is intracellular

therefore, only about 10–12% is broken down into amino acids within the intestinal lumen.

Carbohydrate

Starch (polysaccharide) → maltose → glucose
Disaccharides
    maltose → glucose
    sucrose → glucose and fructose
    lactose → glucose and galactose

Fat → glycerol and fatty acids

The motility and secretions vary from one area of the digestive tract to another. Digestion as it occurs in each of the different parts of the alimentary tract will now be discussed.

MOTILITY, SECRETION AND DIGESTION IN THE MOUTH, PHARYNX AND OESOPHAGUS

MOTILITY IN THE MOUTH, PHARYNX AND OESOPHAGUS

The mouth performs mastication and the initial part of swallowing. The pharynx and oesophagus are concerned only with swallowing.

Mastication

Most of the food entering the mouth undergoes biting and grinding by the teeth to reduce its size for swallowing and mixing with the saliva to produce a moist pulpy mass, called a bolus. Mastication is achieved by the contractions of the muscles of the lower jaw, lips, cheeks and tongue. Movement of the lower jaw is responsible for the biting and grinding done by the teeth.

Deglutition

Deglutition is the term applied to the transmission of food and fluid from the mouth to the stomach and is commonly referred to as swallowing. When mastication is completed, the food is moved to the posterior oral cavity by the tongue and cheeks and is then forced into the pharynx. Certain reflexes then occur in rapid succession. Muscles in the walls of the pharynx contract, drawing the soft palate up and back and closing off the entrance to the nasal cavities. The larynx is raised, bringing its opening against the epiglottis and the base of the tongue, thus preventing the food from entering the respiratory tract. The upper oesophageal sphincter relaxes and food cannot re-enter the mouth, for the back of the tongue is raised to block the opening. The pressure exerted on the bolus by the tongue and pharyngeal constriction forces the food into the only open route, the oesophagus.

The reflex responses of the pharynx to the entrance of food or fluid may be depressed by local anaesthetic. To prevent aspiration following anaesthetization of the pharynx, food and fluid are withheld until the swallowing reflexes have returned. This also applies following laryngoscopy, bronchoscopy, oesophagoscopy, gastrocopy and surgery on the mouth or throat. Depression of the swallowing centre in the medulla occurs with general anaesthesia, alcohol and drug intoxication, and following some cerebrovascular accidents, and can lead to aspiration of food and fluid.

When the bolus enters the oesophagus it is propelled forward under involuntary control by a complex series of reflexes controlled in the medulla. Contraction of the muscle section immediately behind the bolus, and relaxation (or inhibition) of the section preceding it, forces the food forward. This movement, called peristalsis, occurs progressively in a co-ordinated fashion. The lower 4 cm of the oesophagus, referred to as the cardiac (or gastro-oesophageal) sphincter, is normally contracted but relaxes when swallowing occurs, allowing the bolus to be propelled into the stomach.

The more liquid the bolus, the more rapidly it travels through the oesophagus. The passage of food through the oesophagus may be aided by gravity unless the person is in a horizontal position.

SECRETION AND DIGESTION IN THE MOUTH, PHARYNX AND OESOPHAGUS

Saliva is secreted by the salivary glands; added to it is a small amount of mucus produced by the mucous membrane of the oral cavity. The amount of saliva secreted varies from approximately 1–1.5 litres per day, depending on the quantity and quality of food taken. A greater volume of food requires an increased output of saliva, and appetizing foods also stimulate the output. The saliva is swallowed and much of the fluid is reclaimed by absorption. Any interference with swallowing or any condition that provokes loss of saliva from the mouth results in a considerable loss of body fluid, contributing to dehydration.

Saliva at rest has a pH of 6; with stimulation this increases to 7.8. The alkalinity helps to retain the calcium in the teeth. It consists of:

- Water (97–99%)
- Mucin
- Sodium, potassium, bicarbonate, calcium and chloride.
  (The bicarbonate salts of saliva are responsible for the formation of most of the tartar on the teeth. The salts, when exposed to air, release carbon dioxide and the bicarbonate is transformed to an insoluble carbonate.)
- Enzyme: salivary or alpha (α) amylase (formerly ptyalin)
- Organisms
- Epithelial cells from the mucosa
- Antibacterial agents: lysozyme, which has an antiseptic action, and immunogloblin (IgA), which has a defensive action. These agents prevent dental caries and halitosis.

Saliva contains *epidermal growth factor* which may facilitate the rapid turnover of epithelial cells.

Functions of saliva

One of the functions of saliva is to moisten the food and

lubricate the oral cavity in order to facilitate swallowing. Dry food is put into solution by saliva, making possible the taste sensation of sweet, sour, salt or bitter, since only food in solution reaches the taste buds which are recessed in small pits in the tongue. Speech is made more articulate when the oral structures are moist.

The enzyme salivary amylase acts on starches, reducing them to maltose. This is the only chemical digestive function performed by the saliva. The action of salivary amylase may be continued for some time in the stomach, as the saliva is swallowed with the food. Salivary amylase is only effective in an alkaline or very mild acid medium; in the stomach it is inactivated by the presence of the hydrochloric acid. The mucous covering of the bolus prevents acid from entering it and the action of salivary amylase continues until the whole bolus is acidified.

Saliva has a cleansing effect; it washes away food particles and other debris. If these are allowed to accumulate, they could act as a culture medium for organisms. Patients who are not secreting the normal amount of saliva require frequent cleansing mouth care. Disorders and a lack of the natural bacterial agents may lead to ulcers and tooth decay.

The salivary glands excrete certain substances from the blood into the saliva. Lead, sulphur and potassium iodide may be transferred to the saliva. Similarly, urea may be noticeable in the saliva of persons whose kidneys fail to excrete the normal amount of urea.

Finally, saliva has a role in relation to the water balance. The moisture of the mouth largely determines the sense of thirst. A reduction in salivary output occurs with dehydration and a sense of thirst accompanies the dry mouth. When the fluids are replenished, the mouth again becomes moistened by saliva and the sense of thirst is alleviated.

Regulation of salivary secretion

Control of the salivary glands is by the autonomic nervous system; each gland has both a parasympathetic and sympathetic nerve supply which deliver impulses from a salivary centre in the medulla of the brain stem. Sensory nerves conduct impulses from the mouth to the salivary centre to influence its action. The sensory impulses arise from taste and from pressure created by the presence of food or some instrument in the mouth.

Until recently, an increased output of saliva may have been considered a conditioned response to the sight, smell or thought of food. Current studies do not always support this notion (Davenport, 1982).

Parasympathetic innervation results in an increased volume of a watery secretion containing the enzyme salivary amylase; sympathetic innervation causes a scanty flow of a thick, viscous saliva. The generalized sympathetic innervation associated with fright or nervousness and stress frequently produces a dry, 'sticky' mouth. Release of vasoactive intestinal polypetide seems to complement the action of parasympathetic nerve stimulation in increasing salivation. Acetylcholine (ACh) is the parasympathetic neurotransmitter which brings about salivary secretion.

No enzymes are secreted by the pharynx and oesophagus; therefore, no chemical digestion is attributed to these areas. The mucous membrane produces mucus that facilitates the movement of food in swallowing. The mucus also protects the mucosa from any abrasive effect the food might have upon it and from tissue digestion by gastric juice that might escape into the oesophagus.

There is an oesophagosalivary reflex that increases salivation. A mass of bolus pressing on the walls of the oesophagus for any length of time gives rise to sensory impulses, resulting in stimulation of the salivary glands. The increased volume of saliva which is swallowed is an effort to 'wash down' the mass. Intense salivation is also associated with nausea and vomiting and may act to lubricate the vomitus and facilitate the emesis.

MOTILITY, SECRETION AND DIGESTION IN THE STOMACH

GASTRIC MOTILITY

The stomach retains the food and churns it about for a period of time until it undergoes certain chemical and physical changes. Each section of the stomach performs its own function. The fundus acts as a storage vessel by receptively relaxing with the entry of the food into the stomach. The body or corpus of the stomach contracts rhythmically about three times per minute to mix the food with enzymes, producing a mixture referred to as chyme. The gastric contraction is continuous from the antrum to the pylorus and through to the duodenum. The contraction pushes the liquid ahead of it and when it reaches the pylorus it closes it, preventing further emptying and regurgitation of the duodenal contents. The chyme is then forced back up into the relaxing corpus and antrum and the cycle is repeated.

Approximately 3–5 hours after the last meal, strong contractions which originate in the lower oesophagus and stomach, sweep the entire length of the small intestine at about 90 minute intervals. These waves of contractions are known as the interdigestive myoelectric complex. They expel undigested residue and seem to sweep debris along through the small intestines to the colon.

Gastric motility and emptying are regulated by gastric and duodenal factors and hormonal and nervous controls. The presence of food in the stomach stimulates volume-sensitive nerve receptors as well as chemical receptors. Increasing volume stretches the stomach wall which increases contractility force and secretion. The presence of proteins stimulates the release of gastrin and other polypetide hormones which increase motility and enhance antral contractions, forcing more chyme through the pylorus. At the same time, acid and enzyme secretion is stimulated. As the gastric content is liquefied, more chyme is forced into the duodenum.

The duodenum acts to slow down gastric motility and secretion, preventing overloading. Distension of the duodenum and the presence of increased acid and protein digestates or high fat content induces neural inhibition of gastric emptying and stimulates the release of duodenal hormones and secretions. These include cholecystokinin, vasoactive intestinal polypeptide and gastric inhibitory polypeptide, which act in various ways to inhibit both gastric motility and secretion.

To summarize, gastric emptying is controlled by the volume and consistency of the stomach content, the effects of gastrin in stimulating motor and secretory functions, and by neural and hormonal feedback from the duodenum.

GASTRIC SECRETION AND DIGESTION

The gastric glands secrete a clear, colourless, slimy fluid of high acidity (pH 0.9–1.5) that contributes to chemical digestion and changes the food to a more fluid consistency.

The constituents of gastric juice are:

* Water (97–99%)
* Hydrochloric acid (0.2–0.5%)
* Enzymes;
  pepsinogen (inactive pepsin)
  renin
  gastric lipase
* Inorganic salts of sodium, potassium and magnesium
* Haematopoietic or intrinsic factor (promotes absorption of Vitamin B_{12}
* Mucus

The hydrochloric acid and enzymes are the substances concerned with chemical digestion. Pepsinogen is activated to pepsin by the hydrochloric acid and the initial breakdown of proteins occurs. Pepsin reduces proteins to proteoses and peptones. Renin is a specific proteolytic enzyme that converts the soluble caseinogen of milk to insoluble paracasein. The paracasein, with the calcium of the milk, produces a curd, a more solid form that results in its retention in the stomach while it is digested by pepsin. Gastric lipase is produced in small amounts. Emulsified fats may undergo some reduction but fat digestion in the stomach is relatively insignificant.

The hydrochloric acid secreted by the parietal cells destroys many bacteria which are ingested with food. The acidity of chyme, due to the hydrochloric acid secretion, stimulates the secretion of the hormone secretin (prosecretin) by the duodenal mucosa. Secretin influences the pancreatic cells to release a fluid high in sodium bicarbonate.

Regulation of gastric secretion

The amount of gastric juice produced varies somewhat with the types of food taken, but with average meals, it is about 2 litres per day. With fasting, and during the night, the volume is reduced.

Secretion is influenced by mechanical, nervous and hormonal factors, and it is customary to describe gastric secretion as occurring in three phases: the cephalic, gastric and intestinal phases. The *cephalic (psychic) phase* of gastric secretion occurs before the food reaches the stomach. When food is anticipated, tasted and chewed, sensory impulses from the mouth enter the central nervous system and result in parasympathetic innervation via vagus nerve fibres, stimulating the gastric glands to pour out their secretions. The more appetizing the food is, the greater will be the vagal innervation and the response of the gastric glands. Psychic stimulation by the thought, smell or sight of appetizing food may produce the same effect. Conversely, excessive sympathetic innervation depresses the gastric glands and secretion is reduced. Emotional disturbances such as worry, fear and grief result in a decrease in gastric secretion.

Food reaching the stomach further stimulates its secretion, producing what is known as the *gastric phase*. The food causes a direct mechanical stimulation of the gastric glands and initiates sensory nerve impulses that are delivered via vagus nerve fibres to the medulla, resulting in return impulses, via vagal motor fibres that increase the activity of the gastric glands. Chemical stimulation is by a hormone, gastrin, that is released by the gastric mucosa into the blood. Distension of the stomach stimulates the long sensory pathways and the short enteric pathways to evoke the release of gastrin.

The question has always arisen as to why the pepsinogen activated by the hydrochloric acid (pepsin) does not digest the gastric tissue. A natural mucosal resistance includes the local release of prostaglandins, vasodilatation of the mucosal capillaries, the rapid extrusion and replacement of damaged cells and the secretion of alkaline mucous. Local sensory nerves are important for the maintenance of an intact mucosa. This mucosal barrier may be broken down by some substances, such as ethyl alcohol, acetylsalicylic acid and bile acids. The rapid repair mechanisms of the mucosa come into play when the agent breaking the barrier is removed.

Histamine which is produced, stored and released by enterochromaffin cells in the gastric mucosa, has been found to stimulate the parietal cells of the gastric glands, resulting in an increased output of hydrochloric acid. The gastric mucosal cells have a high histamine content. It is suggested that two types of histamine receptors, H_1 and H_2 are present, and the H_2 receptors initiate the release of histamine which stimulates the secretion of hydrochloric acid. The recent preparation of H_2 antagonists (e.g. cimetidine, ranitidine) aids in the treatment of ulcerative gastric disease by inhibiting histamine-stimulated acid secretion. Gastric acid secretion may be investigated by aspirating stomach contents after the patient has been given an injection of a histamine-like substance. There is a close interaction between the actions of histamine, gastrin and acetylcholine which act at the muscarinic receptors to regulate gastric acid secretion.

The *intestinal phase* of gastric secretion involves an increase in the concentration of various hormones which have a number of effects: they stimulate the parietal cells to produce gastric acid; they have a minor role in stimulating pepsinogen production; they induce enhanced contraction of the gastrointestinal sphincter, preventing reflux; they stimulate gastric and intestinal mucosal growth and the secretion of insulin and glucogon by the pancreas via the systemic circulation.

MOTILITY, SECRETION AND DIGESTION IN THE SMALL INTESTINE

MOTILITY OF THE SMALL INTESTINE

Food moves slowly through the small intestine so that digestion may be completed and the simpler molecules absorbed. The motor activities serve three functions: food is mixed with bile and with pancreatic and intestinal secretions, the mass is broken up to bring it into contact with the absorptive surfaces, and the unabsorbed content is moved into the large intestine.

Rhythmicity and automaticity are two notable features of the muscle tissue of this division of the alimentary canal; waves of contractions move down the tract at an orderly rate, appropriate to the stage of digestion and absorption. Approximately 16 rhythmic contractions per minute occur in the duodenum and about 11 per minute in the ileum. Contractions of the longitudinal and circular layers of muscle tissue produce two major types of movement, namely, *segmentation* and *mixing*. Segmentation occurs with areas of the circular muscle contracting and dividing the intestine into a series of alternating constricted and relaxed areas, giving the tube the appearance of a string of sausages. The mass of food stimulates the circular muscle of the section it is in, while those areas behind and ahead remain relaxed. The content in the contracted area is divided into two segments; one is squeezed into the relaxed portion of the intestine ahead and the other is forced back into the relaxed area behind the constriction. The area of contracted circular muscle relaxes and contraction occurs in the previously relaxed areas. Segmentation serves to break up the mass of content so it is mixed with the digestive juice and so more of it is brought into contact with the absorptive surfaces.

Mixing of the chyme and intestinal juice and absorption are facilitated by oscillations of the villi of the mucosa. The slow mixing and segmentation movements push the food along the tract. Any residue of a meal is cleared by the first wave of the interdigestive myoelectric complex as it moves along the tract.

Peristalsis is a wave-like muscular activity consisting of a wave of inhibition followed by a wave of contraction. The advancing portion of the wave involves relaxation of an area of the circular muscle and contraction of the longitudinal muscle, producing a sac-like dilatation. The posterior part of the wave consists of contraction of the circular muscle, producing a constricted area in the tube. The peristaltic waves vary in intensity and in the distance they travel. Some go only a short distance while others pass over a long section, pushing the content much further along the tract. Those that traverse a considerable length of the tract may be referred to as peristaltic rushes.

The small intestine terminates with the ileocaecal valve, which guards the opening into the caecum. The pressure in the small intestine forces open the valve and the fluid passes through into the large bowel.

Muscular and villous activity of the small intestine is regulated by both an intrinsic and extrinsic mechanism. The intrinsic control is by two neural plexuses (networks). One, the myenteric or Auerbach's plexus, is located between the longitudinal and circular layers of muscle tissue. The second intrinsic plexus lies between the circular muscular tissue and the submucosa. The receptors associated with the plexuses are sensitive to stretch or irritation of the mucosa. The reflex response is contraction of the muscle tissues which initiates segmentation, peristalsis and movements of the villi.

The extrinsic mechanism concerned with the motility of the small intestine is parasympathetic innervation via vagal nerve fibres and sympathetic innervation through splanchnic nerves. Parasympathetic impulses stimulate the muscle tissue and conversely sympathetic innervation tends to slow motility. Autonomic nerve impulses are not essential to intestinal motility but do influence it. The recent finding of multiple types of peptidergic nerves in both the myenteric and submucosal plexus has led to intense study of their involvement in the control of motility, blood flow and secretion in health and disease.

SECRETION IN THE SMALL INTESTINE

The digestive juice in the small intestine includes external pancreatic secretions and bile as well as the secretions of the intestinal mucosal glands.

Pancreatic juice and bile

Approximately 700–1200 ml of pancreatic secretions enter the duodenum daily and consist of:

- Water (97–98%)
- Enzymes:
  amylase (amylolytic)
  amylopsin
  proteinases (proteolytic)
    trypsinogen (inactive trypsin)
    chymotrypsinogen (inactive chymotrypsin)
    procarboxypeptidase (inactive carboxypeptidase)
  lipase (lipolytic)
    steapsin
- Salts: principal ones are sodium and potassium bicarbonate and sodium alkaline phosphate.

Because of the salts, the pancreatic secretion is alkaline, with a pH of 7.5–8.4, and neutralizes the acid chyme.

For the secretion and composition of bile, see Chapter 17. Bile does not contain a digestive enzyme, but the bile salts do facilitate the digestion of fat by the pancreatic lipase.

Regulation of pancreatic enzyme and bile secretion. Pancreatic secretion into the intestine is regulated mainly by hormones secreted by the intestinal mucosa. The entrance of the acid solution chyme into the duodenum causes the release of secretin (prosecretin) into the blood. When secretin reaches the pancreas, it activates the cells to secrete a fluid high in sodium bicarbonate. Failure to produce this alkaline solution may result in damage to the duodenum by the chyme, which is strongly acid and contains pepsin. The duodenal mucosa is not as well protected by mucus as the gastric mucosa.

A second hormone, cholecystokinin-pancreozymin (CCK), is also produced by the duodenal mucosa when food enters from the stomach. It is carried to the pancreas where it causes the cells to produce a thicker solution rich in enzymes. CCK also produces contractions of the gallbladder and enhances the action of secretin stimulating the alkaline pancreatic fluid. Secretion of CCK by the duodenal mucosa is stimulated by the presence of fatty acids and amino acids in the chyme.

Some control of pancreatic secretion is also exerted via the vagus nerve and local peptidergic nerves. It is suggested that this is part of the gastric reflex. Sensory impulses are initiated by food in the stomach and result in vagal stimulation of the pancreatic cells to produce enzymes.

The liver cells secrete bile continuously, but the amount is increased when food is taken, especially fat and protein. It is thought that the hormone secretin, which excites the pancreas, may also cause an increased output of bile. Probably the most effective mechanism is stimulation of the liver cells by bile salts. The bile salts are absorbed from the intestine and activate the liver cells to form bile. As noted above, CCK causes the gallbladder to contract and bile flows into the common bile duct. It also causes relaxation of the sphincter of Oddi, and bile that has been stored in the gallbladder enters the intestine. Bile salts are then available to be absorbed in the ileum and recirculated to stimulate the liver cells. In a fasting state, bile does not enter the duodenum and the secretion of bile is decreased.

Intestinal juice (succus entericus)

The mucosa of the small intestine produces 2–3 litres of fluid per day. The solution, called succus entericus, is rich in bicarbonate, and the pH varies from 7.0–9.0, depending on the region of the intestine. The composition of succus entericus is:

* Water
* Salts
* Mucin
* Epithelial cells
* Enzymes:
    entrokinase, which activates the trypsinogen and probably procarboxypeptidase

Sucrase, maltase and lactase act mainly on the glycocalyx (the sticky covering of the microvilli) and are shed into the intestinal lumen due to sloughing of the cells of the villi tips.

Regulation of secretion in the small intestine. The volume of fluid in the lumen of the small intestine is the net result of the movement of fluid between the mucosa and the serosa to maintain an isotonic state. Water moves passively with the active movement of material in either direction. The chyme entering the intestine from the stomach is hypertonic. Water diffuses from the serosa to the mucosa and into the hypertonic solution in the lumen. The presence of non-absorbable material in the lumen also moves water by osmosis. For example, mannitol, a non-absorbable sugar produces diarrhoea by holding water in the lumen of the intestine. Active absorption of nutrients and salts increases the net mucosal flow to the serosa, decreasing the fluid volume in the lumen.

Toxins such as those produced by a salmonella infection or cholera greatly increase water movement from the intestinal wall into the lumen as well as the active secretion of ions, producing diarrhoea, dehydration and metabolic acidosis.

Most of the polypeptide hormones located in the mucosa or enteric nerves of the small intestine influence either secretion or absorption. Of note is the secretory action of a vasoactive intestinal polypeptide which is produced in excessive amounts by certain tumours and results in diarrhoea. The opioid peptide enkephalin has an absorptive action which is a powerful antidiarrhoeal mechanism. This is probably the mechanism by which opiate drugs act to control diarrhoea.

DIGESTION IN THE SMALL INTESTINE

Most chemical digestion takes place in the small intestine.

Any polysaccharides which have not been reduced by salivary amylase to maltose are acted upon by the pancreatic enzyme amylase (amylopsin). Disaccharidases (enzymes) reduce disaccharides to monosaccharides by hydrolysis, producing the simple absorbable sugars, glucose, galactose and fructose. The intestinal enzyme maltase hydrolyzes maltose, lactase splits lactose, and sucrase breaks down sucrose. These enzymes are secreted by the absorptive cells and are an integral part of the sticky layer, the glycocalyx. The final splitting of the disaccharides takes place at the microvillous level.

Protein digestion initiated in the stomach by pepsin is completed by several pancreatic and intestinal enzymes. Trypsinogen is activated in the intestine by enterokinase and is then known as trypsin. Chymotrypsinogen is converted to the active form chymotrypsin by trypsin, and procarboxypeptidase becomes active carboxypeptidase. The proteolytic enzymes trypsin, chymotrypsin, carboxypeptidase and intestinal erepsin reduce proteins (polypeptides) to simpler forms of peptides. A considerable amount of ingested protein may be absorbed in the form of di- and tripeptides rather than amino acids. The latter are more slowly absorbed than the peptides.

The breakdown of fats into glycerol and fatty acids is done mainly by the pancreatic lipase, steapsin. The intestinal lipase is less effective. Fat digestion is greatly facilitated by bile, which emulsifies the fat.

Fats are absorbed in a multistep process; the fat globules are emulsified by bile which allows the triglycerides to be reduced to monoglycerides and fatty acids. These soluble products form micelles, or small polymolecular colloidal particles, which move toward the microvilli where the fats diffuse through the membrane and then are transferred to the systemic circulation via the lacteals of the lymphatic system. Within the absorptive cell the monoglycerides and fatty acids are reassembled into triglycerides and are covered with phospholipid and become chylomicrons.

MOTILITY, SECRETION AND DIGESTION IN THE LARGE INTESTINE

MOTILITY OF THE LARGE INTESTINE

Contractions of the muscular tissue in the large intestine mix and knead the content as well as move it through the large intestine toward the terminal portion. The mixing and kneading movements are performed in the ascending and transverse colons and facilitate the absorption of water.

Propulsion in the colon occurs as a mass movement three or four times a day, moving the content toward the rectum. When the content reaches the distal portion of the colon, it is then moved into the rectum. As the food proceeds through the mouth, stomach and small intestine, a large amount of water is added to it. Much of this water is reclaimed by absorption in the colon which changes the consistency of the remaining content. The latter becomes a soft, solid mass referred to as faeces.

Peristaltic movements in the large intestine are reflexly stimulated by the entrance of food into the stomach. This gastrocolic reflex, as it is termed, is usually most evident after breakfast when the stomach has been empty for a longer period of time. It results in the faeces being moved into the rectum, giving rise to the desire to defecate. Reflex stimulation originating with emotion, and distension or irritation of the colon, will also initiate movement.

Defecation is the term applied to the expulsion of faeces from the rectum and has both an involuntary and voluntary phase. Normally, the rectum remains empty until just before defecation. When faeces enter the rectum, the local distension and pressure give rise to sensory impulses that initiate reflex impulses to the internal anal sphincter and to the muscle tissue of the sigmoid colon and the rectum. The internal smooth muscle sphincter relaxes and the muscle tissue contracts, moving the faeces into the anal canal. The external anal sphincter is under voluntary control and must relax for evacuation of the rectum. Defecation may be assisted voluntarily by contracting the abdominal muscles and by forceful expiration with the glottis closed to increase the intra-abdominal pressure.

If the defecation reflex is ignored and the external sphincter is kept closed, the defecation desire soon wanes. Eventually, with repeated ignoring of the defecation reflex, local stimulation by distension and pressure is lost. Faeces accumulate in the rectum and lower colon, causing constipation.

Normally 8–10 hours are required for the chyme to pass through the small intestine and to reach the distal portion of the colon, where it accumulates until defecation. The content of the alimentary canal that is not absorbed may take 24 hours or longer to pass through the entire canal. Excessive mixing and local contractile motility of the colon lead to greater exposure of the material to the absorptive surface. This leads to dehydration of the contents and constipation. Material such as fibre holds water in the faeces and facilitates the mass movements. Lack of mixing contractions and diminished absorption combined with strong frequent propulsive contractile activity result in diarrhoea.

Faecal matter consists of unabsorbed food residue, mucus, digestive secretions (gastric, intestinal, pancreatic and liver), water and micro-organisms. The water content is progressively reduced by absorption as the faeces move through the large intestine so that, normally, on elimination the stool is a formed mass. If the faeces are moved rapidly through the large intestine, less water is absorbed and the stool is unformed and liquid. If movement of the faeces and elimination are delayed, an excessive amount of water is absorbed and the stool becomes hard and dry.

SECRETION AND DIGESTION IN THE LARGE INTESTINE

The large intestine is a major site of electrolyte and water absorption. It secretes a large amount of viscous alkaline mucus that lubricates the faeces, facilitating their movement through the large bowel. The mucus also protects the mucosa from mechanical and chemical injury, and its alkalinity neutralizes acids formed by bacterial action, which is considerable in the colon.

Irritation of an area of the large intestine results in an increased output of mucus as well as an outpouring by the mucosa of large amounts of water and electrolytes in an effort to dilute and wash away the irritant. This causes the condition known as diarrhoea (frequent liquid stools). The loss of fluid and electrolytes may cause dehydration and an electrolyte imbalance.

Intestinal micro-organisms

Many micro-organisms inhabit the intestine, and colon bacilli are present in large numbers. The tract is sterile at birth, but in a short time organisms which have been ingested with food are present in the intestine. These organisms are useful in that they synthesize vitamin K, which is essential to the production of prothrombin. A deficiency of vitamin K can result in uncontrollable haemorrhage. Intestinal bacteria also synthesize thiamine, riboflavin, and folic acid. The organisms normally found in the intestine are non-pathogenic to the tract but may cause disease if they are carried into other tissues.

Bacteria cause some fermentation and putrefaction of the intestinal content. The fermentation process breaks the content down into still simpler components and at the same time produces gas. The organisms may cause a breakdown of unabsorbed amino acids which may release poisonous substances such as histamine, indole, choline, ammonia, skatole and hydrogen sulphide. However, since this usually takes place in the large bowel, little of these toxic products are absorbed. If they are absorbed, the normal liver detoxifies them.

Absorption

Absorption is the movement of food, water, or drugs from the alimentary canal into the blood to make them available to the cells throughout the body. It is performed passively by the physicochemical processes of diffusion, osmosis and by active transport by the cells.

There are two channels by which food may be absorbed: the capillaries of the mucosa and the lacteals. That absorbed into the capillaries is carried via the portal vein to the liver. That absorbed into the lacteals is transported by the lymph to the thoracic lymphatic duct which empties into the junction of the subclavian and internal jugular veins. Water, salts, glucose, amino acids and some fatty acids and glycerol are absorbed into the capillaries. The larger proportion of the products of fat digestion is absorbed into the lacteals.

Like digestion, most absorption takes place in the small intestine. Its surface is especially adapted by the many circular folds in the mucous membrane to increase the surface area. The whole surface is also studded with millions of villi which contain epithelial mucosal cells that are specially adapted for both absorption and secretion. The network of capillaries and the central lymph channel of each villus take up much of the digested food.

ABSORPTION IN THE MOUTH

No food is absorbed from the mouth, but a few drugs may be taken into the blood through the buccal mucosa. Examples of these are glyceryl trinitrate and adrenaline.

ABSORPTION IN THE STOMACH

Absorption in the stomach is relatively negligible. The gastric mucosa does not actively transport food molecules across it but, if the concentration is high in the stomach (creating a considerable gradient between the blood and the stomach), glucose, water and electrolytes may be absorbed. Alcohol and some drugs are also absorbed from the stomach.

ABSORPTION IN THE SMALL INTESTINE

Minerals, vitamins, water, drugs, amino acids, simple sugars, fatty acids and glycerol are freely absorbed from the small intestine. Most absorption takes place in the upper part of the small intestine.

ABSORPTION IN THE COLON

Large amounts of water are absorbed in the colon. Approximately 500 ml of fluid pass from the small intestine into the colon daily. About 400 ml of water are absorbed from this, leaving 100 ml to be excreted in the faeces. Small amounts of glucose and salts are also absorbed by the large intestine, and a number of drugs may be administered by this channel. The absorptive capacity of the colon is seldom reached but water toxicity can be induced by excessive fluid introduced into the colon, especially in infants.

ABSORPTION OF VITAMINS

The water-soluble vitamins B complex and C are generally readily absorbed from the small intestine. The exception is vitamin B_{12}. For absorption of B_{12}, a substance called the intrinsic factor is necessary and is secreted by the mucosa of the stomach. A deficiency of the intrinsic factor or of vitamin B_{12} causes a deficiency in the production of mature red blood cells.

The fat-soluble vitamins A, D, E and K are absorbed from the small intestine if bile salts and pancreatic lipase are present.

Protective and Immunological Functions of the Gastrointestinal Tract

The gastrointestinal tract is a continuity of the skin and is formed by special endothelial cells. The material it receives does not have to be sterile. Bacteria are found in most foods ingested, yet rarely do these bacteria invade the system. This is in part due to the pH in the stomach and to enzymatic degradation of the bacteria themselves.

It has been shown that the gastrointestinal tract has its own immune system and the immunoglobulins produced in these areas differ from those produced elsewhere. These lymphoid cells are formed from precursor cells located in the Peyer's patches in the small intestine, and produce an immunity against antigens which enter the gatrointestinal tract. Oral poliomyelitis vaccine uses the immunological system of the gastrointestinal tract to produce local and systemic immunity to the poliomyelitis virus.

It is likely that the IgA antibodies found in breast milk are present through movement of the immunologically competent plasma cells of the intestine to the mammary glands. These antibodies protect the infant who is unable to produce antibodies immediately after birth. As with the systemic immune system, allergic reactions can occur in the gastrointestinal tract of sensitized individuals. For example, certain seafoods may be the offender. Recent evidence suggests that an immune or allergic response to an antigen may be classically conditioned to an accompanying stimulus and presentation of that stimulus at a later date will evoke an immune or allergic response.

THE PERSON WITH DISORDERS OF THE GASTROINTESTINAL SYSTEM

Disorders of the digestive system are many and varied; they may interfere with the ingestion, digestion, absorption of food and fluids, elimination of residue and/or with the immunological defence mechanism of the body. Any dysfunction threatens the well-being, functional capacity, and perhaps the survival of the person. The clinical characteristics depend largely on the location of the disorder in the system as well as the nature of the aetiological factor. Different diseases may cause similar disorders of function; that is, several manifestations that develop are non-specific.

Modern health education places much emphasis on nutrition, and any interference with the ability to take and retain food creates anxiety in the individual. The common knowledge of the high incidence of malignant disease in the gastrointestinal tract may cause considerable concern in anyone with any digestive upset. Fortunately, the digestive system has considerable reserve; parts of it may be removed and the patient, with some necessary adjustments in diet and living habits, may continue to live a useful life.

Frequently a disturbance of function in the alimentary tract is secondary to disease in another part of the body. For example, some disorders of the brain may be manifested first by vomiting or difficulty in swallowing. It may be a complaint of indigestion that brings the person with primary anaemia to the doctor. Fatigue or emotional stress may be the basis of malfunctioning of the gastrointestinal tract and most of us at some time have experienced functional disturbance in the stomach or bowel during a period of anxiety or grief. The person whose medical investigation rules out organic and structural disease still requires the nurse's understanding sympathy; efforts are made to identify problems that are causing emotional stress which may be the basis of the illness.

CLINICAL CHARACTERISTICS

In reading the following section which discusses some of the principal physical effects that gastrointestinal disorder has on the person, the nurse should consider how patient assessment may be influenced and guided by these pathological effects. Not only is it important to discover if any of these signs or symptoms are present, but it is also important to consider how they may affect the person's life and what fears and anxieties may be generated by these physical signs of disorder.

It is easy for the nurse to know that blood stained stools are often associated with disorder of the rectum and anus, often without any malignant disease being involved, however the patient may interpret this as a sign of cancer and understandably be very anxious and concerned. In addition there are powerful taboos and beliefs associated with the act of defecation which inhibit discussion of what is a very personal and embarassing bodily function for many people. The nurse must therefore display great tact and sensitivity in assessing the patient for evidence of any of the clinical manifestations discussed below and remember that how the patient feels about any sign is just as important as the sign or symptom itself. Such feelings and beliefs are crucial areas for nursing intervention ranging from helping the person to verbalize their fears and anxieties through to a whole range of patient teaching and health education activities.

PAIN

Pain caused by a digestive disorder may be due to strong contractions of muscle tissue, stretching of a viscus, chemical or mechanical irritation of the mucosa, inflammation of the peritoneum, or direct irritation or pressure on associated nerves. It may occur in any part of the abdomen or in some instances is referred to a site remote from its origin. For example, pain arising from a peptic ulcer or from the biliary tract may be referred to an upper area of the back.

Heartburn is a form of pain that is described as a burning sensation felt behind the sternum. It is usually attributed to irritation of the oesophageal mucosa by reflux of gastric acid fluid into the oesophagus and may be accompanied by regurgitation of some stomach content into the mouth. It may contribute to altered gastrointestinal function.

A person may complain of a sense of fullness, especially after eating. Normally the stomach relaxes and distends to accommodate food without increasing the intragastric pressure. This accommodation may not occur if there is a disease, such as carcinoma, or if the patient is in an anxious state.

Significant characteristics of the pain must be noted and recorded. Meaningful clues include the duration, location and the nature and onset of the pain as described by the patient. Aggravating factors such as activity, the taking of food or medicine, or some specific experience or emotional stress may exist. Nausea, vomiting, flatulence and defecation associated with the pain are pertinent observations. The effect of pain on each individual varies and also varies with the cause and nature of the pain. For example, the patient experiencing gallstone or kidney stone colic writhes in agony while the patient with peritonitis or paralytic ileus tends to remain immobile. The patient is observed for such changes as restlessness, pallor, perspiration, weakness and changes in the vital signs.

For a general and more detailed discussion of pain, the reader is referred to Chapter 9.

ANOREXIA

Anorexia is a loss of appetite for food and is a common complaint of patients with a digestive disorder but is also associated with disorders in practically all parts of the body. Anorexia is common in febrile conditions and with chemotherapy. It contributes to the general debilitation of patients. The individual may even express a revulsion to the odours of food. It may be functional in origin, resulting from an emotional upset. Persistent refusal of food due to psychological disturbance is referred to as *anorexia nervosa*. It may lead to emaciation and death (see Chapter 18).

NAUSEA AND VOMITING

Nausea is an unpleasant sensation in which one has a feeling of discomfort in the region of the stomach and the inclination to vomit.

Vomiting is the ejection of the gastric contents through the mouth and is usually preceded by nausea and hypersalivation. There may be nausea without vomiting, and vomiting may occasionally occur without being preceded by nausea. The involuntary muscular activity that precedes or accompanies vomiting is referred to as *retching*.

Nausea and vomiting are very common symptoms and are seen in a great variety of conditions. They can be manifestations of a digestive dysfunction, may represent hormonal changes such as occur in early pregnancy, or they may accompany practically any acute illness or stressful situation.

The vomiting process is initiated by a vomiting or emetic centre in the medulla oblongata. This centre may be excited by sensory impulses originating in the stomach or intestines, by impulses of psychic origin when fright, unpleasant sights, odours or severe pain are experienced, or by impulses from a group of neurons referred to as the chemoreceptor trigger zone in the floor of the fourth ventricle. The cells in the trigger zone are sensitive to certain chemicals in the blood and to impulses from the portion of the internal ear concerned with equilibrium. Vomiting in motion sickness, radiation therapy, toxaemia and as a side-effect of taking certain drugs such as digoxin results from impulses that arise from the chemoreceptor trigger zone. The sensitivity of the vomiting centre varies in different individuals; some vomit very readily and with little effort while others are not affected even though the stimulus may be similar and of equal intensity.

The impulses discharged by the vomiting centre result in excessive salivation, a quick, deep inspiration followed by closure of the glottis and epiglottis, closure of the nasopharynx by elevation of the soft palate, and relaxation of the oesophagus, cardiac sphincter and stomach. Vigorous contraction of the diaphragm and abdominal muscles increases intragastric pressure and simultaneously, strong reverse peristalsis begins in the stomach. The gastric contents are forced up through the relaxed oesophagus into the mouth. The retching or heaving that is experienced before and after vomiting results from the back-and-forth movement of the stomach contents between the negative pressure in the thorax and the positive pressure in the abdomen. The vomiting is accompanied by pallor, cold, clammy skin, increased heart rate and increased salivation and swallowing.

The nurse should be alert to the possible effects of vomiting, regardless of its cause. Considerable muscular energy can be expended in frequent vomiting and may result in exhaustion.

Obviously, nausea and vomiting interfere with normal nutrition and, if prolonged, malnutrition and loss of weight and strength occur. The reduced intake and loss of fluid may rapidly lead to dehydration. Loss of gastric secretion may deplete the body electrolytes and cause acid–base imbalance. Acidosis may develop as the patient becomes dependent on body fat as a source of energy. The patient may complain of abdominal soreness from the retching and muscular effort and may become increasingly anxious as a result of vomiting.

REGURGITATION

Ejection of small amounts of chyme or gastric secretion through the oesophagus into the mouth without the vomiting mechanism being employed is referred to as regurgitation. It may occur owing to some incompetency of the oesophageal–gastric (cardiac) sphincter, as seen in infants or those with hiatus hernia, or it may be a symptom of organic disease.

DYSPHAGIA

Dysphagia is defined as difficulty in swallowing. The patient may be able to swallow soft foods and liquids but may be unable to take firmer, more solid foods. Others may be able to swallow but complain of pain on doing so.

Dysphagia may be due to mechanical obstruction, dysfunction in the neuromucscular structures involved in swallowing or to diseases of the mouth, pharynx or larynx. Pain associated with swallowing frequently indicates an organic lesion such as an ulcer due to acid reflux from the stomach.

LOSS OF WEIGHT AND STRENGTH

If food cannot be taken, digested or absorbed, body tissue cells are deprived of their requirements for normal functioning. Body stores and actual tissues are mobilized to meet the needs, but eventually these may be depleted. The person manifests loss of weight, strength and efficiency.

If the problem is related to a specific food, symptoms characteristic of a lack of that particular food will appear. For example, effects of a protein deficiency include muscle wasting, weakness, hypoalbuminaemia, oedema, anaemia and, in the child, retarded growth and development. If there is a disturbance in the absorption of vitamin K due to a lack of bile salts in the intestine, the deficiency may be manifested by bleeding, since prothrombin, necessary for blood coagulation, will not be produced by the liver.

CHANGES IN THE MOUTH

Changes in the mouth may be of local origin or may be associated with digestive or general disorders. Disturbances may take the form of a coated or furry tongue, dryness, soreness, small ulcers (aphthous ulcers) and halitosis. Changes due to local conditions may be caused by inflammation, infection, neoplastic disease or injury of the tongue, buccal mucosa or lips. Any sore that does not heal in 2 weeks should be investigated.

HICCUP (HICCOUGH, SINGULTUS)

Persisting hiccups or frequent attacks of hiccups may be associated with organic disease of the digestive system. They are caused by intermittent spasms of the diaphragm due to digestive distension, irritation of the phrenic nerve or a metabolic disorder such as uraemia or toxaemia which affects the central nervous system. The frequency of the attacks and the effect of the hiccups on the patient should be noted. Dehydration, acid–base imbalance and malnutrition may develop, since hiccups may interfere with the taking of fluids and food. Disturbed rest and the expenditure of muscular energy may cause exhaustion. In many instances, the person becomes fearful because of the persistence of the condition.

A simple nursing measure is to have the person breathe into a paper bag held closely over the mouth and nose. Rebreathing the air in the bag gradually increases the carbon dioxide content of the air in the lungs and eventually the blood. The respiratory centres stimulate the diaphragm to contract normally in an effort to eliminate the carbon dioxide. The inhalation of a prescribed mixture of oxygen and carbon dioxide may be ordered. A sedative or tranquillizer may also be prescribed if the hiccups persist. Rarely, if they persist and are having serious effects on the person (exhaustion, dehydration, etc.) a phrenic nerve block or crush is done.

FLATULENCE

Flatulence is an excessive amount of gas in the gastrointestinal tract. The person may complain of a 'full, bloated feeling', pressure or actual pain. The abdomen may be distended and the person may eructate gas from the stomach through the mouth or may expel gas (flatus) from the bowel. Excessive gas in the stomach or bowel is frequently due to swallowed air. Aerophagia, or the unconscious swallowing of air, may be seen in nervous persons and in patients who are nauseated or experiencing some digestive stress. It is sometimes helpful to advise patients to make a conscious effort to avoid the swallowing.

Excessive gas in the intestine may result from the ingestion of excessive amounts of gas-forming foods (cabbage, turnips, onions, etc.) or from abnormal fermentation of the food due to bacterial action. Flatulence and distension occur with any obstruction in the tract and with paralysis of peristalsis. Another frequent cause is ingestion of milk in individuals who as adults do not possess the enzyme lactose. This can also occur in individuals who increase milk intake when they have been accustomed to very little.

Borborygmi (singular, borborygmus) is a term applied to the sounds made by the movement of a gas and fluid mixture in the intestines that are loud enough to be heard by the patient and others close by. The sound can be a significant observation, especially when there is some quesion of obstruction. The sounds do occur in the normal alimentary tract on occasion.

ABDOMINAL RIGIDITY

Rigidity of any area of the abdominal wall due to excessively tense muscle tone may be evident in patients with disease of the gastrointestinal tract. The muscle contraction is usually a response to irritation of an underlying structure. This symptom is usually noted by palpation of the abdomen when examining the patient.

CHANGE IN THE NORMAL PATTERN OF BOWEL ELIMINATION

A disorder of the intestine may cause a retarded or an accelerated movement of contents through the intestine. Delayed movement may cause *constipation* characterized by infrequent, hard, dry stools or may result in a complete failure of the passage of faeces. Acceleration of the content causes *diarrhoea*, which is frequent liquid or unformed stools. The person who experiences any persistent change in the normal pattern of bowel elimination should consult a doctor.

For a discussion on constipation and diarrhoea (see pp. 477–485).

FAECAL INCONTINENCE

Involuntary defecation is referred to as faecal incontinence. This form of incontinence is often preventable. Involuntary defecation may also be caused by underlying bowel disease or neurogenic impairment.

BLEEDING FROM THE GASTROINTESTINAL TRACT

Bleeding in the alimentary canal may be manifested by the vomiting of blood (haematemesis), by melaena (the passage of a black, tarry stool containing blood pigments), or by the passage of frank blood from the bowel. Haematemesis and melaena occur as a result of bleeding in the upper digestive tract. It should be remembered that blood is a gastric irritant, and swallowed blood (e.g. in a nosebleed) will lead to vomiting. The characteristic black tarry appearance of the stool is due to the effect of the digestive enzymes on the blood. Frank blood in the stool usually originates with bleeding in the colon, rectum or anal canal.

It may be necessary in some instances to examine the blood that has been ejected through the mouth to determine whether it has been coughed up (haemoptysis) or vomited. Blood from the respiratory tract is a brighter red and frothy because of the contained air; that from the stomach is usually darker and may contain small clots and food particles. Melaena may be so slight that it goes unrecognized unless a stool specimen is submitted for laboratory examination for *occult blood*.

The most frequent cause of haematemesis and malaena is peptic ulcer, but oesophageal varices, carcinoma, injuries or a blood dyscrasia may account for the bleeding. Any evidence of bleeding should be promptly reported to the doctor. The patient who has haematemesis or tarry stool is put on bed rest; blood pressure, pulse, respirations, colour and general state (e.g. strength and consciousness) are checked frequently to detect signs of shock.

Frank bleeding from the lower part of the tract may be due to erosion of the mucosa, a congenital malformation of arterioles, a neoplasm, ulcerative colitis, haemorrhoids or an anorectal fissure. The patient is advised to see a doctor immediately for early diagnosis and treatment.

THE PERSON WITH DISORDERS OF MOTILITY, SECRETION AND DIGESTION IN MOUTH, PHARYNX AND OESOPHAGUS

Disorders of the mouth and contained structures are numerous and may be of local origin or may be secondary to disease elsewhere in the digestive system or in some other system. Primary lesions may be due to bacterial, viral or fungal infection, chemical irritation, congenital malformation, injury or neoplastic disease. General diseases frequently accompanied by a mouth disorder include vitamin B complex or vitamin C deficiency, blood dyscrasias, metallic medication intoxication, infectious disease and any condition that

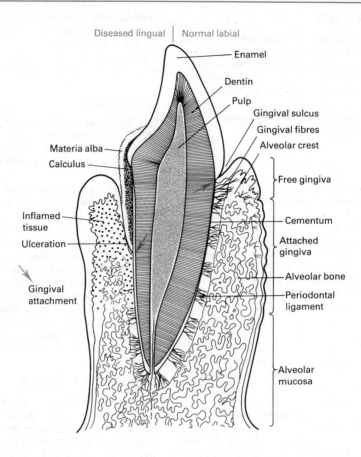

Diseased lingual | Normal labial

Enamel

Dentin

Pulp

Gingival sulcus

Gingival fibres

Alveolar crest

Free gingiva

Materia alba

Calculus

Inflamed tissue

Ulceration

Gingival attachment

Cementum

Attached gingiva

Alveolar bone

Periodontal ligament

Alveolar mucosa

Figure 16.4 Periodontal disease: diagrammatic representation of a tooth.

interferes with the normal fluid and food intake or salivary secretion.

Predisposing factors in mouth lesions are debilitation, poor dietary habits, poor oral and dental hygiene, dehydration, emotional stress and mouth breathing, and as a side-effect of chemotherapy.

Disorders of the Mouth

Manifestations of mouth disorders include discomfort or toothache, especially when taking food, and as a result the patient rejects adequate nutrition. There may be a palpable mass or a swollen area evident within the oral cavity or on the external surface. Bleeding of the gums or from a lesion may be present. An offensive breath may indicate sores or infection. Excessive salivation or dryness and/or disagreeable taste may be present. The individual may experience difficulty with clear speech or with swallowing.

DENTAL CARIES

Tooth decay is a major health problem caused by the action of organisms on ingested refined carbohydrates; acids are produced which eventually destroy the enamel surface of the teeth. Tooth decay, cavity formation, inflammation and eventual loss of teeth result if measures are not instituted to prevent progression of the process. Figure 16.4 illustrates the normal structure of a tooth and adjoining gum and the effects of build-up of debris on the tooth and gums.

PERIODONTAL DISEASE

This disorder affects the tissues that support the teeth. Development of periodontal disease is influenced by the build-up of plaque on the teeth, poor nutrition, poor oral hygiene, malocclusion of the teeth and by some metabolic disorders. Symptoms include inflammation, bleeding and tenderness of the gums and loosening of the teeth. Formation of plaque is prevented by regular brushing and use of dental floss and regular examination and care by a dentist.

ACUTE TOOTH INFECTION

Infection of the dental pulp or development of an abscess at the 'root' of a tooth is very painful and may cause an elevated temperature and general malaise. The person is advised to seek prompt treatment by a dentist. An opening or canal is made to provide drainage and an antibiotic preparation may be prescribed. In some instances, the tooth may be extracted. Frequent mouth-washes are recommended.

STOMATITIS

This is a term applied to inflammation of the oral mucosa. In some instances, it may involve the gums and the lips.

The *causes* are numerous, and include excessive smoking, dental sepsis, dehydration, vitamin deficiency, blood dyscrasia such as primary anaemia and leukaemia, local or systemic infection and a sensitivity to certain foods or drugs. A frequent cause is chemotherapy (see chapter 10). The mucosa is very red and tender and ulcerative areas may develop.

THRUSH (MONILIASIS)

Thrush is caused by the fungus *Candida albicans* and may also be referred to as *candidiasis*. It may develop in the vagina as well as in the mouth. It occurs most frequently in infants and children and in the very old, but may also appear in debilitated persons. Occasionally, it follows prolonged use of certain antibacterial drugs such as tetracycline (Achromycin) and chloramphenical (Chloromycetin). Areas of superficial ulceration occur in the oral mucosa or gums, and the membrane over the lesion becomes white and is easily detached. The lesions respond to the local application of 1% gentian violet or to an antifungal antibiotic solution such as nystatin. Attention is also directed to the person's diet in an effort to improve resistance and general condition.

GINGIVITIS (VINCENT'S ANGINA, TRENCH MOUTH)

This is an inflammation of the gums (gingivae) followed by ulceration and necrosis. It is thought to be caused by proliferation of specific fusiform bacilli and spirochetes which are present in only small numbers in normal mouths.

The gums are swollen and painful and bleed readily. Excessive salivary secretion and an offensive breath are usually present. There is a loss of marginal gum tissue and of the interdental papillae by the ulceration and necrosis. Lesions may develop on the buccal and pharyngeal mucosa. A smear may be made from the affected area to confirm the diagnosis. Predisposing factors are poor oral and dental hygiene, malnutrition and debilitation. It may be associated with dietary deficiencies, infections, mononucleosis, alcoholism or a blood dyscrasia.

Mouthwashes are given frequently. The person is advised not to smoke, and a soft, nutritious diet of non-irritating foods is recommended. The patient will require instrumentative treatment by a dentist as soon as the acute stage is over.

The condition is infectious and can be transmitted to other persons unless precautions are taken.

LEUCOPLAKIA

This condition is characterized by patchy, yellowish-white, firm, thickened areas of the oral mucous membrane or of the tongue. The lesion results from hyperplasia of surface epithelial tissue and keratinization.

The lesions are painless and are considered serious since they may be precancerous. They occur most frequently in men after the fourth decade of life. The lesions usually develop in response to chronic irritation that may be mechanical, chemical, thermal or infective in origin. The lesions may disappear with elimination of the irritation. In many instances, the cause is unknown.

Teeth are checked and defects corrected that may be causing irritation. Smoking should be discontinued and a high-vitamin diet is prescribed. If the area is fissured or ulcerated, a biopsy is done to determine if cancer has developed. If malignant changes have taken place, surgical excision and radiation therapy are used.

CANCER OF THE MOUTH

Carcinoma may develop on the tongue, floor of the mouth, oropharynx or buccal mucosa, but the most frequent site is the lower lip. It has a much higher incidence in males between the ages of 50 and 60 years, and is associated with heavy smoking and alcohol consumption.

The most common malignant lesion occurring in the mouth is squamous cell carcinoma. Smoking (especially pipe smoking in the case of lip cancer), excessive exposure to the sun, prolonged irritation by a jagged tooth or poorly fitting denture and chronic infection are considered to be predisposing factors. It usually appears first on the lip or mucosa as leucoplakia, as a roughened area or as a persisting ulcer.

The lesion in cancer of the tongue or buccal mucosa usually appears as a small firm lump. Later the area breaks down, leaving a painful ulcer. If the condition goes untreated, swallowing and speech become difficult, hypersalivation develops, the mucosa becomes infected and the malignant growth metastasizes to the jaw and to the lymph nodes in the neck.

As with all malignant disease, early recognition and treatment are extremely important; *any sore that resists treatment and persists for 3 weeks should receive prompt medical treatment.*

Treatment involves surgical excision of the cancerous tissue and radiation therapy. Irradiation may be by interstitial implantation of needles, seeds or moulds containing radium. When metastasis to lymph nodes is suspected, more radical surgery may be performed to include dissection of the cervical lymphatics and chemotherapy may be employed (see Chapter 10). Extension of the malignant disease into the jaw may necessitate extirpation of the jaw.

Table 16.2 Oral surgical procedures.

- *Lip resection* is the excision of a portion of a lip. It is usually done to remove a benign or malignant tumour.
- *Glossectomy* is the removal of the tongue for the treatment of carcinoma.
- *Hemiglossectomy* is the excision of a part of the tongue.
- *Mandibulectomy* is the removal of the lower jaw bone; it may be partial or complete.
- *Buccal resection* is the excision of a section of cheek (bucca).
- *Radical neck dissection* (en bloc dissection) involves the extensive excision of cervical lymph nodes and non-vital tissues on the side of a primary malignant neoplasm of the salivary gland, tongue or mouth.

INFLAMMATION OF THE PAROTID GLAND

Inflammation of a parotid gland is the most common disturbance of the salivary glands and may be due to infection by the specific virus that causes mumps, or it may develop as a result of any non-specific bacterial invasion of the gland. Non-specific parotitis may occur as a complication in febrile diseases or when dehydration is present and there is a lack of attention to oral hygiene. It tends to develop more readily in older and debilitated persons. The onset is sudden, the gland becomes swollen and painful and the patient develops a fever.

Preventive measures include frequent mouth care and keeping the mouth moist by ample fluid intake, sucking sour sweets (lemon) and chewing gum. The disorder is treated by the parenteral administration of antibiotics. If suppuration develops, surgical drainage is necessary. The fluid intake is increased and frequent mouth care is necessary. The local application of an ice bag to the area may be prescribed if pus has not formed.

OBSTRUCTION TO THE FLOW OF SALIVA

Obstruction of any one of the salivary glands may be due to *intrinsic* or *extrinsic* causes. Disease *within* the gland or duct may be infection, neoplasm or a calculus. In conditions that cause inflammation, the duct may be occluded by swelling and oedema or later by the resulting scar tissue. *Extrinsic* causes such as a tumour or infection in neighbouring structures may compress the duct, or scar tissue resulting from stomatitis may close off the duct orifice.

The obstruction is manifested by swelling of the affected gland. The swelling is most pronounced during meals because of the salivary stimulation and may subside between meals. Pain and tenderness may be due to the pressure or to the condition causing the obstruction. Fever and general malaise may accompany infection.

Constriction of the duct is treated by probing and dilatation. A calculus may be removed via the duct or, if this approach should fail, surgical removal may have to be undertaken.

A *tumour in a salivary gland* causes a more gradual swelling unrelated to salivary stimulation. It is treated by prompt surgical excision of the gland. The parotid gland is the most frequent site of salivary tumours; the submaxillary gland is next in order of incidence. If the doctor suspects the tumour is malignant because of its firmness, fixation and involvement of the facial nerve, a biopsy may be done to confirm the diagnosis. Surgery is the therapy of choice since malignant neoplasms of the salivary glands are radiation resistant. Carcinoma involves radical surgery. In the case of cancer of a parotid gland, removal of the mandible and dissection of the cervical lymphatics may be necessary. Surgical excision of the submaxillary gland for malignancy includes dissection of the cervical lymphatics and possible resection of the mandible. Following such disfiguring surgery as the extirpation of the lower jaw, a prosthesis may be constructed of a synthetic material which is physically and chemically inert and is implanted in the area to restore a normal appearance.

Following any surgery on the parotid gland, the patient is observed for signs of facial paralysis because of the close proximity of the facial nerve to the operative site. In some instances the facial nerve may be involved by a malignant tumour and is removed with the gland, leaving the patient with some permanent facial paralysis.

FRACTURE OF THE JAW

Fracture of the jaw is a relatively common injury in motor accidents, some sports and violent disagreements. Diagnosis may be made on crepitus, apparent deformity, and abnormal, painful movement of the mandible, and is confirmed by X-ray.

Treatment and nursing intervention for fracture of the jaw. If the fragments are displaced, they are approximated and the lower jaw is immobilized. The latter may be achieved by wiring the lower jaw to the upper jaw or by attaching soft metal bars to the upper and lower teeth. These bars have hooks from which rubber bands extend between the upper and lower jaws, applying traction and fixation.

Following immobilization of the lower jaw, the patient is placed in a semiprone or lateral position to promote oral drainage and prevent aspiration of secretions during recovery from anaesthesia. A wire cutter is kept at the bedside; if the patient vomits, the wire or bands that immobilize the lower jaw must be released immediately so the mouth can be opened to prevent aspiration. A nasogastric tube may be passed and attached to low suction to remove gastric contents and reduce the risk of aspiration. Pharyngeal and oral suctioning with a small catheter may be necessary to remove secretions; trauma and resulting oedema of pharyngeal tissues may interfere with swallowing.

The patient receives a high-calorie fluid diet. It may be given for a brief period via the nasogastric tube but as soon as possible it is taken orally through a straw.

The mouth is thoroughly cleansed every 2 hours after each feeding. Normal saline or a mild antiseptic mouthwash may be used. The buccal mucosa and exposed area of the gums are examined twice daily for lesions and sordes (deposits collected on teeth and lips consisting of food, micro-organisms and epithelial elements).

Early ambulation is encouraged and the patient may be discharged from the hospital as soon as he can care for himself. The nurse will be responsible for teaching the patient and/or a family member the importance of good oral hygiene and how to carry out the necessary cleansing and inspection. The diet, with suggestions for variation, and its preparation and digestion are discussed in detail. When the wires are removed the patient is urged to see a dentist.

HEALTH PROMOTION RELATING TO THE MOUTH

A person's sense of well-being, comfort, ability to maintain good nutrition, and personal attractiveness are all enhanced by effective mouth care. The nurse can play an effective role in educating individuals and groups of all ages to develop health habits which encourage good oral hygiene and ensure the early indentification and correction of problems. The aim is to promote healthy teeth, gums and oral mucosa.

ASSESSMENT

Health History

Information relating to current oral health practices:
- Frequency, method and tools employed.
- Does the individual smoke?
- Does the individual chew substances i.e. tobacco, etc?
- Does the individual regularly attend a dentist?

History of dental and oral disorders
Information relating to dental and oral problems:

- Has the individual experienced gum disease, oral infections, trauma, injury or surgery?
- Does the person wear dentures, bridge work or other dental appliances, and do they fit correctly?
- Has the individual experienced pain, tenderness, bleeding, swelling, lesions, sores, in the mouth, face or jaw.
- Does the individual have difficulty swallowing?
- Does the individual have restricted movement of the jaw, neck, tongue, etc.
- Does the person grind their teeth, or regularly bite their cheek or lip?

Nutritional status
Information relating to eating and drinking habits:

- Does the person take a balanced diet containing adequate food groups and vitamins and minerals?
- Is the individual able to maintain an adequate fluid intake?
- Does the person drink large amounts of alcohol?
- Does the individual consume large quantities of sugary foodstuffs or drinks?

General health status
Information relating to other health problems:

- Does the person have any chronic, or debilitating health condition?

- Does the individual suffer with allergic or sinus conditions?
- Does the person mouth breathe?
- What medications are taken, regularly or intermittently?
- Is the individual receiving any treatment which could effect oral health i.e. chemotherapy, antibiotic therapy, etc.?

Physical examination

A tongue depressor and light are needed to inspect the oral cavity and tongue. In a normal, healthy mouth:

- The lips are moist and intact.
- Breath is free from odour.
- Teeth are white, intact, firm and free from caries, jaggedness and plaque.
- The gums are moist, pink, intact and adhere to the teeth.
- The mucosa is moist, pink, soft and intact.
- The tongue is pink and moist with minute papillae on the superior surface.

Changes that occur with ageing include: (1) a decrease in saliva, leaving the mucosa dry; (2) the teeth becoming worn and chewing less effective; and (3) healing is slowed, therefore lesions may be more common.

The mouth and tongue are inspected for lesions, sordes, dehydration, bleeding and discoloured areas (e.g. leucoplakia). Whether or not the tongue is coated or is abnormally smooth is noted. The condition of the teeth and gums (gingivae) are also checked. The former are inspected for jaggedness and caries, and the gums for excessive redness, soft puffiness, recession and bleeding. The odour of the breath is noted to determine if it is offensive or is characteristic of that associated with a specific condition. For example, the odour of acetone may be associated with acidosis or starvation, that of urea with renal insufficiency and that of alcohol with alcoholism. Observation of the mouth may elicit significant information as to the person's state of hydration and nutrition as well as manifestations of systemic disease and local disorders. The tongue and mouth are the first sites to reflect dehydration; the mouth and tongue become dry and the latter may be furred. Dryness in some instances may be a side-effect of a drug that is being administered. Bleeding of the gums may indicate a deficiency of vitamin C or an infection. Excessive salivation (sialorrhoea) may be associated with a vitamin B deficiency or certain medications or a neoplasm in the mouth or neighbouring structure.

The lips are scrutinized for lesions (e.g. lumps, cracks, blisters, ulcers), dryness and abnormal colour and palpated if necessary to determine the presence and extent of a mass.

GOALS

The individual will demonstrate:

- Teeth that are white, intact and firm.
- Pink, moist, intact gums and oral mucosa.

- A pink, moist tongue with minute papillae on the surface.
- Understanding of the need for:
  —daily oral hygiene
  —dental check-ups every 6 months
  —maintaining nutritional and fluid needs.
- A plan to inspect mouth regularly for signs of irritation, inflammation and infection.
- Properly fitting dentures and/or repair/reconstruction of teeth.

NURSING INTERVENTION

- Use of a toothbrush is the method of choice.
- Foam sticks can be used by individuals who are unable to tolerate toothbrushing. These will not remove debris from the surface or between the teeth but will cleanse the oral mucosa. The stick, after immersion in appropriate mouthwash solution, should be rotated gently over the mucosa, teeth, gums and tongue, ensuring the whole surface is used.
- The choice of appropriate agent should be determined by assessing the person's needs and after assessment of the oral cavity. Toothpaste is satisfactory in many cases. Petroleum jelly can be used sparingly on the lips to create an oil film, preventing moisture loss.
- Provide artificial saliva and instruct the individual with a dry mouth or reduced saliva to use it to best effect.
- Frequency of mouthcare will be dependent on the needs of the individual and factors which increase mouth dryness, debris accumulation, and plaque formation, i.e. continuous oxygen therapy, intermittent suction, no oral intake, following anaesthesia, etc.

Evaluation

Evaluation of measures to promote oral hygiene and prevent the development of disorders of the teeth, gums and oral mucosa is based on achievement of the goals. Inspection of the person's mouth should show evidence of regular oral hygiene, dental care and self-assessment of the mouth, gums and teeth. The individual should be able to describe measures taken on a regular basis to promote oral hygiene.

ORAL SURGERY

The major surgical procedures are most frequently done for carcinoma. They include resection of the buccal mucosa, glossectomy, hemiglossectomy, mandibulectomy and radical neck dissection (Table 16.2). For *nursing management* of the patient requiring intra-oral or radical neck dissection, see Table 16.3. The reader is also referred to Chapter 11 for consideration of the care of the patient prior to surgery, and during the intraoperative and postoperative periods.

Rehabilitation exercises are used after a radical neck dissection. These exercises are started when the wounds are firmly healed. The type of exercises prescribed varies for each individual. The frequency of exercise is limited to start with and gradually increased as the patient's tolerance improves. They are commenced slowly and gently; quick, jerky movements are avoided.

Head exercises. The patient (1) turns the head to each side, (2) alternately flexes it laterally and forward, and (3) then extends it.

Shoulder exercises. The patient assumes the sitting position with arms and hands placed in front of the trunk. The arms and shoulders are drawn back, elevated and then rotated.

Further shoulder exercises are prescribed for the individual patient according to the extent of the surgery and the degree of wound healing that has occurred.

Disorders of the Oesophagus

Manifestations of oesophageal disorders include dysphagia (difficulty in swallowing), regurgitation, pyrosis (heartburn), substernal pain and bleeding.

CAUSES

Interference with the transmission of food and fluid from the mouth to the stomach may be due to an abnormal condition within the oesophagus or to an extrinsic disorder. Swallowing may be impaired by a disturbance in innervation to the oesophageal muscle tissue, a decrease in or an obstruction of the lumen or the tube or by mucosal irritation and inflammation.

Disease of neighbouring structures

Since the mouth, tongue and pharynx are involved in directing food and fluid into the oesophagus, it is obvious that disease in any one of these structures may interfere with the initial phase of swallowing. This may be seen in severe stomatitis, pharyngitis, tonsillitis, cleft palate and neoplastic disease of the mouth or tongue. The condition may actually interfere with the swallowing process or cause so much pain that the patient avoids swallowing.

Compression of the oesophagus by enlargement or neoplasms of neighbouring structures occurs rarely. Examples are goitre (enlargement of the thyroid), aortic aneurysm and enlargement of the mediastinal lymph glands.

Neurological disorder

Dysphagia may result from a nervous system disorder that affects innervation to the central striated muscle tissue of the oesophagus. Damage to the swallowing centre in the medulla or to nerve fibres of the tenth cranial (vagus) nerve concerned with the swallowing mechanism may cause a partial or complete paralysis. Paralysis may occur in the pharyngeal area owing to interference with normal innervation via the ninth (glossopharyngeal) cranial nerve. Failure of the normal pharyngeal phase of swallowing may result in food

Table 16.3 Plan of care for the patient undergoing oral surgery.

Patient problem	Goals	Nursing intervention
Preoperative preparation 1. Anxiety due to lack of knowledge of the disease process, impending surgical intervention, concern for potential deformity and disfigurement and loss of the ability to ingest food and communicate	• The patient will indicate understanding of the reasons for the surgery, the surgical procedures and what may be expected in the postoperative period regarding fluid and nutritional needs, pain management, communication, mouth and wound care and visits from the family	• Provide opportunity and privacy for the patient to express fears and concerns • Evaluate the patient's and family's understanding of the disease process, hospitalization, surgery and expectations for the postoperative period • Provide information about the disorder, surgery, hospital routines, pre- and postoperative care to be provided and expected patient participation • Correct any misconceptions the patient and family may have about the disorder and treatment • Excisions of the lip and tongue may interfere with speech and communication. Discuss communication measures that may be used such as writing with pad and pencil, hand signals or communication boards • If a hemiglossectomy is to be performed discuss alternative feeding methods that will be used, such as nasogastric tube feedings or total parenteral nutrition
2. Food intake less than body requirements, due to the discomfort incurred by oral lesions	The patient will demonstrate: • Maintenance of body weight • Fluid intake of 2.5 l/day	• Assess the patient's hydration and nutritional status • Provide oral fluids and nutrients as tolerated • Provide supplementary fluids and nutrients as prescribed by intravenous route, nasogastric feedings or parenteral nutrition through a central venous catheter • Record fluid intake and output
3. Alteration in oral mucous membrane related to interruption of normal defences of the mouth from the disease and impending surgery	• The patient will demonstrate lips, oral mucosa and tongue clean, moist and free of debris and crust	• Provide oral hygiene every 4 hours and following food and fluid intake
Postoperative care 1. Ineffective airway clearance, related to: oedema of the mouth, tongue and throat; impaired swallowing; and accumulation of secretions in the mouth and throat	• The patient will demonstrate respiratory rate and rhythm within the normal range, with no evidence of airway obstruction	• Extensive resection of the tongue and larynx may necessitate a tracheostomy (see care of patient with a tracheostomy Chapter 15) • Assess the respiratory status of the patient (constantly at first). Note: the respiratory rate, rhythm and pattern; pulse rate and volume; accumulation of oral secretions; and difficulty in swallowing. The face and neck are observed for swelling

Patient problem	Goals	Nursing intervention
		• Place the patient in a semi-prone or lateral position to facilitate drainage of secretions and prevent aspiration. As soon as the vital signs are stable, elevate the head of the bed
		• If secretions are excessive, place a gauze wick in the corner of the mouth to facilitate drainage. Suctioning should be performed gently to avoid trauma to suture line and sensitive tissues. Avoid suctioning if a hemiglossectomy was performed, as the tongue is very vascular and haemorrhage may occur
2. Potential postsurgical haemorrhage	The patient will demonstrate: • Absence of bleeding or oozing • Pulse and blood pressure within normal range • Absence of excessive swallowing and/or vomiting	• Observe tissues, dressings or drains for evidence of bleeding or oozing • Monitor pulse for increase in rate, reduction in volume and note any decrease in blood pressure • Observe for increased swallowing or blood stained vomitus • Inspect back of neck for accumulation of blood
3. Food and fluid intake less than body requirements, due to altered ability to ingest food and fluids	The patient will demonstrate: • Weight loss less than 2 kg • Fluid intake of 2.5 l/day	The method of supplying fluids and nutrition will depend on the nature and extent of the surgery: • Supply intravenously for the first few days • Nasogastric tube feedings are usually administered to allow healing of the mouth • If the patient has prolonged difficulty with swallowing or if reconstructive plastic surgery is undertaken, total parenteral nutrition is instituted • When oral fluids and foods are permitted, begin with a small amount of clear fluid to evaluate the patient's ability to swallow and to minimize the possibility of aspiration and regurgitation. Fluids are gradually increased as tolerated, and soft, puréed foods are introduced. Fluids and food should be at room temperature. There should be gradual progression to a soft then regular diet as tolerated. Consult dietician to ensure intake is nutritionally adequate and special requirements can be prepared
4. Impaired verbal communication, due to the surgical procedure, oedema and pain	The patient will demonstrate: • Ability to communicate by writing, hand signals or touch • Swallow and speak with minimal discomfort	• A pencil and paper, and/or a communication board are kept within the patient's reach while speech is impaired • Teach the patient hand signals so that he or she can convey needs and respond to questions

Patient problem	Goals	Nursing intervention
		• Administer analgesics regularly to control pain
		• The mouth is irrigated with sterile normal saline and artificial saliva is provided if indicated to lubricate the mouth to facilitate speaking and swallowing. Precautions are observed to prevent aspiration.
		• Place the patient's call-button within reach
		• Encourage family members to sit with the patient and encourage use of touch and other forms of communication in order to decrease the effort required by the patient in speaking.
		• Use statements requiring 'yes', 'no' or short answers when conversing with the patient
		• Arrange for speech retraining if extensive resection of the tongue has been performed
5. Alteration in oral mucous membrane, due to surgical intervention and interruption of normal defences of the mouth and oral mucosa	The patient will demonstrate: • A clean and moist mouth • An intact surgical incision	• Perform oral hygiene every 2–4 hours initially and following food intake when the patient begins oral feeding. Debris may be removed from uninvolved areas of the mouth with moistened foam sticks or cotton swabs. Teeth can be brushed with a small soft toothbrush unless contraindicated. The mouth may be irrigated using a small catheter, 'waterpix' or Higginson's syringe. Analgesic spray or gel may be used prior to performing mouth care to reduce discomfort • Inspect the mouth for healing of the surgical area and signs of redness, oedema, crusting and fluid accumulation
6. Disturbance in body image due to physical changes resulting from the surgical excision and reconstruction of tissues, and difficulty in speaking and swallowing	The patient will demonstrate: • The expression of concerns and feelings about appearance • Increasing social contact with family, friends and other patients	• Encourage the patient to express feelings and concerns • Provide information about the healing process and help the patient to set realistic expectations about how he or she will look when healing has taken place and the swelling has gone • Difficulty with swallowing and speaking may be temporary but if permanent changes are anticipated the individual should be informed of the nature of the disability and referred to the speech therapist for assessment, and retraining. Encouragement and reinforcement of the speech therapy programme will be important

Patient problem	Goals	Nursing intervention
		• Encourage social interaction by encouraging visits from significant others. Suggesting activities which involve interaction with fellow patients • Provide information regarding self-help groups and assist (if desired) in arranging a visit from a person with similar experiences • Encourage resumption of normal dress, make-up, hygiene, and personal appearance habits as soon as able. Provide information and advice regarding prosthetics • Provide information regarding altered sexual functioning, such as kissing and intercourse, to both the patient and partner. Encourage expression of concerns regarding sexuality and altered body image
7. Knowledge deficit related to health care needs, skills in performing care, and awareness of available resources	• The patient and family will describe a plan to meet nutritional needs and perform oral hygienic measures following discharge	• As soon as the patient is able, encourage participation in all aspects of care, i.e. oral hygiene, feeding, hygiene needs • Provide oral and written education regarding feeding and oral hygiene needs prior to discharge and ensure the individual understands the information • If supplementary feeding (enteral or parenteral) is required, teach the person and, if appropriate, significant other, the skills to self-administer and encourage practice under supervision. Provide appropriate supplies of equipment on discharge and information on how to replenish stocks • If necessary, refer person early to community nursing team to ensure continuity of care; provide contact telephone numbers and addresses • Provide information concerning further treatment programme, such as radiotherapy, speech therapy, physiotherapy, dental treatment, prosthetics. Discuss transport arrangements to attend therapy

passing into the trachea and the nasal cavities. The sphincter at the oesophageal opening may remain relaxed, allowing air to be drawn into the oesophagus during inspiration.

Conditions in which paralysis of swallowing is commonly seen include myasthenia gravis (failure of nerve impulse transmission at the neuromuscular junction), poliomyelitis that involves the motor neurones in the swallowing centre, and cerebrovascular accident (stroke).

Congenital abnormalities

A congenital abnormality may occasionally be the cause of impaired swallowing in the newborn infant. The most common malformations of the oesophagus include atresia, stenosis and tracheo-oesophageal fistula.

Reflux oesophagitis

The most common cause of oesophageal mucosal irritation is regurgitation of gastric content. Bacterial, viral or fungal infection may be imposed on the inflammation. Diagnosis is usually made on the basis of the patient's complaint of dysphagia, intolerance to hot, spicy foods and substernal pain and heartburn. X-ray, barium studies, and endoscopy may be performed to confirm the diagnosis. Biopsy and cytological examination of tissue of affected areas may be performed to exclude carcinoma.

In the case of chronic regurgitation of acid gastric content into the oesophagus, function studies are made. If the lower oesophageal sphincter is incompetent, gastric contents are allowed passage into the oesophagus, which leads to a burning sensation. The lower oesophageal sphincter is positioned within the abdomen (just below the diaphragm). When it is displaced into the thorax, as in a hiatus hernia, the lower oesophageal sphincter pressure is less than the intra-abdominal pressure, and reflux occurs. Sphincter incompetency also occurs in degenerative disorders of smooth muscle.

Treatment of chronic oesophagitis may include: elevation of the head of the bed to reduce the reflux of acid gastric content during sleep; administration of an antacid orally and inhibition of gastric secretion by a histamine H_2 receptor antagonist such as ranitidine (Zantac) or cimetidine (Tagamet). Regular meals of equal quantity and low fat are recommended as well as the avoidance of coffee, alcohol, spicy foods and smoking. The person is advised to remain upright for at least 2 hours following a meal and should avoid medication which could exacerbate the problem, such as salicylates, phenylbutazone and anticholinergics. Drinking milk is contraindicated as the high calcium content stimulates gastric acid secretion. A weight reduction programme in the obese may help in reducing symptoms. If the cause of persistent oesophagitis is an incompetent lower oesophageal sphincter, surgical repair to prevent reflux may be necessary. The operative procedure frequently used is a fundoplication, in which the fundus of the stomach is wrapped around the lower end of the oesophagus and sultured to it, or a modified form of this may be performed.

Chronic oesophagitis may incur progressive formation of scar tissue leading to stricture. This may be treated by intraluminal dilatation by the insertion of bougies at intervals over a period of time, or may necessitate surgical correction.

Oesophageal achalasia

This is the term used to describe the inability of the lower oesophageal sphincter to open in response to swallowing, accompanied by a lack of tone in the musculature above the sphincter and loss of peristalsis in that area. In the northern hemisphere the cause of achalasia is unknown. In South America it can be due to Chagas disease, caused by the parasite *Trypanosoma cruzi* which causes denervation of the gastrointestinal tract, probably by an autoimmune mechanism. The oesophagus gradually dilates above the denervated sphincter. The result is an accumulation and stagnation of food and fluids in the dilated segment.

The symptoms of the disorder are: a full, uncomfortable feeling in the substernal region, pyrosis (heartburn), inability to belch, dysphagia, regurgitation and eventually weight loss. The person may also experience coughing and dyspnoea due to pressure on the trachea by the distended oesophagus; a disturbance in normal cardiac functioning or pulmonary complications (aspiration pneumonia), due to inhalation of oesophageal contents, may be manifested.

Achalasia may be treated by the surgical procedure oesophagomyotomy which involves the division of the muscle fibres at the lower end of the oesophagus. The patient then tends to develop reflux oesophagitis. In some instances, the sphincter and lower end of the oesophagus may be dilated by the introduction of an inflatable bag under X-ray control.

If dysphagia is accompanied by severe chest pain, the patient may experience many cardiovascular examinations. A diagnosis of an oesophageal origin of the pain may reduce the anxiety and the dysphagia since emotional stress and anxiety tend to aggravate the disorder. When the innervation of the oesophagus is intact and the dysphagia is muscular in origin, multiple swallows in rapid succession may relieve the muscular hypercontractility of the sphincter and thus the pain.

Trauma of the oesophagus

Dysphagia or aphagia may occur as a result of the ingestion of a caustic substance, foreign objects or too large a mass of food.

When a *caustic substance* such as a strong acid (e.g. sulphuric or nitric acid) or base (e.g. household bleach) is swallowed, serious corrosive burning occurs in the oesophagus. The larynx may also be affected as well as the lips, mouth and pharynx. The mucosa manifests acute inflammation, blisters, oedema and possible ulceration. If the chemical is not removed or neutralized promptly, burning and corrosion of deeper layers of tissue occurs. Later with healing, scar tissue forms and the lumen of the oesophagus is constricted. Dysphagia progressively becomes more serious over several weeks as scar tissue is laid down.

There will be evident corrosive burns on the lips and in the mouth; the voice may be hoarse and the patient experiences dysphagia and probably dyspnoea and difficulty with speech due to laryngeal irritation and oedema. Shock may develop quickly.

Management of the person who has swallowed a caustic substance includes the following:

1. The chemical swallowed is immediately identified: the lips, mouth and clothing are examined if necessary for evidence. If a container of the chemical that was taken is available, the label is checked for suggestions as to an effective antidote. Milk may serve as a neutralizing agent.
2. Vital signs are assessed and treatment for respiratory insufficiency and shock promptly commenced.
3. An oesophagoscopy is done as soon as possible (within 12–24 hours) to determine the extent and depth of the burns.
4. An analgesic is prescribed for relief of pain.

5. Oropharyngeal suctioning may be necessary to prevent aspiration of secretions.
6. Sips of water may be permitted. Gastric lavage and induced vomiting are containdicated to prevent further damage to the oesophageal wall. An intravenous infusion is given to provide fluid and electrolytes.
7. A tracheostomy may be necessary if laryngeal oedema is indicated by respiratory distress and stridor. Blood gases are monitored.
8. A corticosteroid preparation is prescribed to reduce the inflammatory response and to lessen scar tissue formation and ensuing stricture. An antibiotic preparation is usually given to prevent serious infection.
9. A gastrostomy may be necessary in severe constriction in order to provide adequate food and fluids or the administration of parenteral feeding.
10. Stricture of the oesophagus is treated by bougienage; as soon as sufficient healing has taken place, bougies are placed into the oesophagus every day or two to dilate the lumen. The interval between treatment is gradually lengthened, but the bougienage may extend for over a period of a year or more. If a gastrostomy is necessary, it may serve for retrograde bougienage as well as for feedings. A very fine bougie is passed into the oesophagus and remains in place between treatments, one end protruding from the nose, the other from the gastrostomy opening. The two ends are then tied together. During dilatations, the larger bougie is attached to the lower end of the finer bougie and is then pulled up through the oesophagus.
11. If bougie therapy is not successful, surgical resection of the constricted area with end-to-end anastomosis may be performed. When the area is extensive, surgical reconstruction of the oesophagus may be undertaken. A plastic tube or a section of intestine may be implanted to provide a patent passageway.

Nursing intervention for the patient requiring surgery on the oesophagus is described in the plan of nursing care in Table 16.4.

The oesophagus may be injured by a rough or sharp foreign body (e.g. pen, nail, meat or fish bone, small toy). The object may cause dysphagia or aphagia. The person experiences choking and becomes frightened and agitated. An oesophagoscopy is done and the foreign body located and removed. The person may complain of soreness and dysphagia for a few days.

Occasionally a large mass of food may lodge in the oesophagus (meat is the most common offender) causing obstruction of the lumen and respiratory distress by pressure on the trachea. Oesophagoscopy may be done as a matter of urgency to locate and remove the mass and assess the injury to the oesophagus.

Neoplasms of the oesophagus

Benign neoplasms.
These occur rarely in the oesophagus. The most common of these are leiomyomas which are tumours of non-striated muscle tissue. Those encountered less frequently are polyps, cysts, fibromas, adenomas and fibrolipomas. As the tumour imposes itself on the lumen of the oesophagus or interferes with normal muscle activity, dysphagia occurs. Usually the patient first experiences difficulty in swallowing the more solid foods, such as meat and bread.

Carcinoma

Causes. Cancer of the oesophagus tends to develop more often in the older age group. Its incidence is mainly in males between 50 and 70 years of age, and the lower third of the oesophagus is the most common site. Although no definite cause has been determined, contributing factors include the ingestion of alcohol, tobacco and spicy foods and other carcinogens, injury to the oesophagus from corrosive agents, and possibly nutritional deficiencies of vitamins A and C and trace minerals such as zinc. A number of benign conditions have been associated with oesophageal cancer, including achalasia, Plummer–Vinson syndrome and reflux oesophagitis. The majority of malignant tumours of the oesophagus are squamous cell cancer (epidermoid cancer). Adenocarcinoma may occur but is most frequently secondary to gastric carcinoma.

Clinical Characteristics. The patient complains first of dysphagia with solid foods which gradually progresses to difficulty with liquids. Substernal discomfort and pain, regurgitation and loss of weight and strength are experienced with steadily increasing severity. In advanced states, bleeding may occur. Structures adjacent to the primary lesion may become involved: the disease may spread to the trachea, bronchi, stomach, diaphragm or associated lymph nodes, depending upon its location in the oesophagus.

Diagnosis is made by X-ray examination and an oesophagoscopy. A biopsy is obtained and a smear from the lesion is probably taken for cytological study during the endoscopic examination. Other investigations may be carried out, e.g. computerized axial tomography scans to determine the extent of the tumour and any infiltration into adjacent organs.

Treatment may be by surgical resection, chemotherapy, irradiation or a combination of these methods. Various surgical procedures are employed. The affected part of the oesophagus is resected with a wide margin of normal tissue as well as the regional lymph nodes. If the lesion is in the lower part, the upper portion of the stomach is also removed (oesophagogastrectomy). The remaining proximal portion of the oesophagus is anastomosed to the stomach which is drawn up into the thoracic cavity (oesophagogastrostomy). A nasogastric tube is passed and remains until the anastomosis is fairly well healed and peristalsis is established.

If the cancer is located in the middle or upper portions of the oesophagus, or if a large area is involved, it is more difficult to treat the patient surgically. A segment of the patient's intestine (jejunum or colon) may be implanted to replace the resected oesophagus.

Table 16.4 Postoperative plan of care for the person requiring surgery of the oesophagus.

Patient problem	Goals	Nursing intervention
1. Ineffective breathing pattern, related to the chest incision and the presence of chest drainage tubes	The patient will demonstrate: • Regular, rhythmic and deep respirations • Symmetrical chest expansion • Absence of wheezes and crackles • Arterial blood gas concentrations within normal range	• Care of the patient following general anaesthetic is discussed in Chapter 11 • Maximum inspirations are performed several times each hour. The nurse assists the patient to a sitting position and supports the incision • Staged coughing is performed to mobilize secretions; forced coughing is avoided because the increased pressure created presents a hazard to the oesophageal sutures
2. Potential for injury, related to surgical intervention and incomplete healing process	The patient will demonstrate: • The ability to swallow clear fluids without regurgitation when the nasogastric tube is removed in 4–7 days • Body temperature within the normal range	• If a nasogastric tube has been introduced in the operating room, it is usually attached to a collecting bag to drain gastric secretions by gravitation. Aspiration of the tube, using a syringe, may be performed 2–4 hourly to assess location of tube, its patency and to remove secretions which have not drained by gravity. The drainage may be coloured with blood for the first few hours but should gradually assume the characteristics of normal secretions. When normal gut functioning returns the nasogastric tube may be used for enteral feeding. • Alternatively, a temporary gastrostomy may be used for drainage and feedings; a nasogastric tube may simply be kept in position to maintain a patent oesophagus. (See care of the patient requiring gastric surgery) • A frequent check is made of the patient's temperature and pulse for any indication of infection. If either is increased to levels above the normal, parenteral administration of an antibiotic is ordered. In some instances prophylactic antibiotic therapy is given as a measure against infection. • Perform oral hygiene 2–4 hourly to promote comfort and prevent possible infection of the oral mucosa which could spread to the oesophagus.
3. Nutrition: less than body requirements due to inability to swallow, surgical intervention and nasogastric intubation	The patient will demonstrate: • Weight loss less than 2 kg over the postoperative period • Fluid intake of 2.5 l/day and urinary output within normal range • Oral fluids and soft foods taken and tolerated within 5 days	• The nasogastric tube may be removed in 4–7 days, and small amounts of water may then be given when peristalsis returns. Any difficulty in swallowing or regurgitation is promptly reported. The patient will find swallowing easier if sitting up. Fluids may be

Table 16.4 *Continued.*

Patient problem	Goals	Nursing intervention
		gradually varied and increased in volume. The diet gradually progresses through semiliquids, blended or soft foods and a normal diet. Parenteral fluids and gastrostomy feedings are continued until the patient is able to swallow adequate amounts of fluids and food. If the surgical procedure entailed an oesophagogastric anastomosis with the stomach being drawn up into the thoracic cavity, the patient may not be able to take the ordinary amount of food or fluid at one time without experiencing pressure in the chest and some dyspnoea. In this event, the patient is fed smaller amounts at more frequent intervals and should remain upright in the sitting position for 1–2 hours after eating. • A record is kept of the patient's fluid intake and output and the balance is noted until a normal intake by mouth is well established.
4. Alteration in comfort: pain, related to surgical intervention	The patient will demonstrate: • Absence of pain • Ability to relax and sleep	• Administration of analgesics; the person should be carefully monitored for respiratory depression • Simple nursing measures such as change of position, careful positioning of pillows, gentle back massage, diversion, and remaining with the person may help
5. Mobility is impaired as a result of surgery, decreased energy and the presence of tubes and suction equipment	The patient will demonstrate: • Intact skin with no areas of redness or oedema • Ability to move about freely. Ambulation progressively increases over the first few days postoperatively • Absence of complications of immobility, i.e. chest infection, pressure sores or deep vein thrombosis	• Assist patient to perform deep breathing 2–4-hourly and encourage compliance with programme initiated by the physiotherapist • Change the patient's position every 2–4 hours. Appropriate pressure area aids, i.e. Spenco mattress, alternating pressure (ripple) mattress, may be used. Assess condition of skin regularly to prevent breakdown • Encourage early mobilization. Gently increase activities from sitting on the side of the bed, to walking and sitting in a chair • If pressure gradient stockings (TED) are applied, ensure they fit correctly and are removed once daily to assess condition of skin. Encourage movement of limbs regularly when confined to bed
6. Knowledge deficit related to dietary modifications and post-hospital health management	The patient and family will: • Indicate a satisfactory plan to meet nutritional and other health needs at home • Exhibit an awareness of community resources for nursing care and social services	• Inform the patient of the expected length of the convalescent period and reasonable expectations of activities • Educate patient concerning dietary modifications and meal patterns. Involve significant others. Information

Table 16.4 *Continued*

Patient problem	Goals	Nursing intervention
		should include: eating small, well-chewed quantities and small, frequent meals, followed by rest periods; taking fluid after meals • Mobilize community services to ensure continuity of care and support on discharge. Provide contact telephone numbers and addresses • Ensure person understands any planned further treatment and establish transport arrangements (and organize if appropriate)

Relief from dysphagia, in those individuals with extensive disease, may be achieved by the palliative surgical approach of inserting a Mousseau–Barbin or Celestin tube through the constricted area.

Following diagnosis and investigation of the extent and spread of the tumour, it will be determined if the goal of therapy is curative or palliative. The tumour is considered curable if it has not extended into the wall of the oesophagus or metastisized to the regional lymph nodes. Radiation therapy may be used with some benefit. A nasogastric tube may be inserted through the constricted area and left in place so the patient can be given fluids and nourishment. Complications of ulceration and bleeding may develop with this latter palliative procedure. More often, a gastrostomy is employed by which nutrition is maintained for the remainder of the patient's life (see p. 476).

Oesophageal varices

This serious condition is associated with cirrhosis of the liver and is discussed in Chapter 17.

ASSESSMENT OF THE PATIENT WITH OESOPHAGEAL DISORDER

The patient admitted to hospital will probably have had a period of increasing difficulty in swallowing leading to undernourishment. It is important to discover how long the patient has been experiencing difficulties and what foodstuffs can still be swallowed in order that the patient be given an appropriate diet. Height and weight should be assessed and the patient asked whether they have lost weight recently. Serious undernourishment may be present which can significantly reduce the patient's prospects of recovery, consequently dietary supplements may be necessary.

The person's mood and feelings about their illness should be explored. The inability to eat and subsequent loss of weight may lead to great anxiety and fear. The person may suspect cancer but not have been told the diagnosis, clearly it is important to discover how the person feels about their illness and what questions are in their mind. The patient may also see a significant change in their body which constitutes a serious

challenge to their self concept. The nurse needs to know how successfully they are coping with this challenge and what methods are being used to adapt, e.g. making jokes about weight loss or withdrawal and denial in order to approach the patient sensitively and give support.

The nurse should obtain information related to the presence of any of the factors which may contribute to oesophageal disorders. The use of alcohol and tobacco is determined and the diet is assessed for adequacy of fresh fruits and vegetables and overuse of foods preserved with nitrates.

The nature of any symptoms related to swallowing, hoarseness, dryness or discomfort are identified.

Physical Examination

• *Swallowing.* Assessment of the individual's ability to swallow is achieved by asking them to sip from a glass of water with the head slightly tipped back. The nurse watches for any difficulties and for the larynx, trachea and thyroid to rise as the person swallows. The person is questioned regarding any discomfort experienced. If difficulties are observed, further assessment might include the use of soft, dry and formed foods to determine the degree and type of difficulties experienced.

Oesophagoscopy
The oesophagus may be examined and a biopsy specimen obtained by *oesophagoscopy* if the patient has complained of dysphagia, gastric reflux or regurgitation, or haematemesis. Oesophagoscopy is useful in localizing bleeding and is also used to remove a foreign body or a bolus that has lodged in the oesophagus (see Gastroscopy, p. 467).

NURSING CARE OF THE PERSON WITH SURGERY OF THE OESOPHAGUS

PREOPERATIVE CARE

Prior to surgery it is usually determined if the treatment goals are curative or palliative. The 5-year survival rate for persons with oesophageal cancer is only 5%.

Early involvement of other members of the health care team, such as dieticians, medical social workers, occupational therapists and physiotherapists, are of the utmost importance. The nurse may have an important role in co-ordinating the multidisciplinary team, ensuring continuity and encouraging the individual to participate in therapy.

Anticipatory grief and *anxiety* are real problems for both the person facing the surgery and significant others. The nurse must spend time assessing their understanding of the surgery and prognosis, provide information as indicated, identify their needs for emotional support, promote the development of coping strategies and help with the grieving process.

Preoperative preparation also includes emphasis on the promotion of *respiratory function* and teaching deep breathing and coughing techniques. Stopping smoking is essential for all patients who smoke.

The establishment of good *oral hygiene* and the alleviation of infections and potential causes of oral infections are important aspects of care. The person is referred for necessary dental repairs prior to surgery.

Optimal *fluid and nutritional status* is an important goal, involving the administration of oral, nasogastric and/or parenteral nutrition as indicated. Fluid intake should be adequate and deficits corrected.

POSTOPERATIVE CARE

Table 16.4 describes a postoperative plan for nursing care of the person following oesophageal surgery for cancer.

Principal patient *goals* in the postoperative period are that respiratory complications will be avoided, the wound will heal without complications, and the patient will be free of pain, having a fluid intake of 2.5 l/day, avoid weight loss and be able to discuss plans for discharge and self-care in a positive way. More general postoperative goals also apply (see Chapter 11).

HIATUS HERNIA

The openings of the diaphragm which accommodate the oesophagus and aorta are potential sites for the herniation of abdominal viscera into the thoracic cavity. The hiatus through which the oesophagus passes is the most vulnerable area; normally, when oesophageal content passes into the stomach it does not return to the oesophagus. If it does, it is referred to as reflux (a return flow).

CAUSES

The chief causes of the defect in the diaphragm are considered to be a congenital weakness and the ageing process. The former probably results from a defect in the fusion of tissues around the opening. The incidence of hiatal hernia is much greater in middle-aged and elderly persons, and is probably due to weakening of the diaphragmatic muscle. The weakness or gap that occurs results in imperfect closure of the hiatus around the oesophagus. Rarely, the hernia may be caused by trauma such as a fractured rib or perforating foreign object (e.g. bullet) or prolonged, extreme intra-abdominal pressure as occurs in ascites or pregnancy.

CLASSIFICATION

The hernia may be classified as sliding (oesophagogastric) or rolling (paraoesophageal) (Figure 16.5). A *sliding hiatal hernia* is one in which the oesophagogastric junction and a portion of the fundus of the stomach ride up into the thoracic cavity. In a sliding hernia, the lower oesophageal sphincter at the oesophagogastric opening (cardia) loses competency, resulting in reflux of the gastric contents into the oesohagus. In a *rolling* or *paraoesophageal hernia*, a sac-like portion of the peritoneum and stomach herniates through into the thorax alongside the oesophagus. A section of omentum may also be extruded. The cardiac sphincter usually remains competent but the displaced portion of the stomach occupies space within the mediastinum and may cause respiratory distress or impaired cardiac function by direct pressure on the heart. Distension of the herniated segment or strangulation may develop, which demands emergency surgery.

CLINICAL CHARACTERISTICS

The symptoms depend upon the size of the hernia and the amount of displaced viscus. Intermittent mild digestive disturbances only may be experienced. The patient may complain of substernal burning pain or discomfort (heartburn), regurgitation of acid fluid, belching, a feeling of fullness and shortness of breath. The symptoms are frequently precipitated by stooping over, straining associated with increased intra-abdominal pressure or a large meal. It may also be brought on when the patient is recumbent and may be relieved by sitting up.

Frequent reflux may cause oesophagitis, ulceration and bleeding. Scarring may develop that causes some constriction and probably dysphagia. Rarely, the herniated portion is so large that it becomes incarcerated and even strangulated. Respirations and cardiac function are likely to be compromised.

DIAGNOSIS

This is made by the person's history and by a barium meal or barium swallow. The pain of reflux oesophagitis associated with hiatal hernia is frequently similar to that associated with angina pectoris and myocardial infarction.

THERAPEUTIC MANAGEMENT

A slight hernia may be controlled and the patient kept relatively asymptomatic by loss of weight if obese, the avoidance of heavy lifting, and frequent, small, bland meals. Gas-forming foods, coffee and alcohol are avoided. An antacid such as aluminium hydroxide preparation is usually prescribed to be taken after meals and at bedtime. The person is advised to remain in an upright position for at least 2 hours after a meal. The head of the bed is elevated.

If a loop of the intestine or a portion of the stomach becomes confined in the thoracic cavity, surgical treatment is essential to return the viscus to the

A B

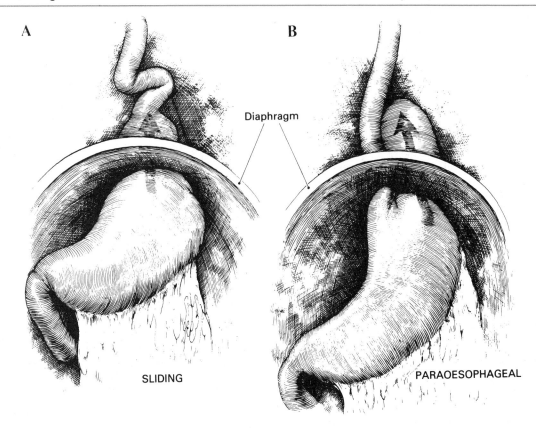

Diaphragm

SLIDING PARAOESOPHAGEAL

Figure 16.5 A, Sliding hiatus hernia. B, Paraoesophageal hernia.

abdominal cavity. The surgical approach is usually made through the chest but occasionally may be made via the abdominal cavity. Following replacement of the viscus, the hiatus hernia is repaired. A nasogastric tube is likely to be introduced, and mild suction is applied to prevent vomiting and intestinal distension. Fluids are administered by intravenous infusion for the first day or two, and then gradually introduced by mouth when the gastric suction is discontinued.

NURSING INTERVENTION

Dysphagia

Nursing measures to alleviate dysphagia include maintaining an adequate fluid intake to facilitate movement of food through the oesophagus and elevating the head of the bed at night to reduce gastric reflux during sleep. At home, the person can place a wedge under the upper portion of the mattress, place the head of the bed on blocks or use several pillows for sleeping.

Antacid medications such as magnesium trisilicate mixture may be administered orally at regular intervals during the day. Cimetidine (Tagamet) or ranitidine (Zantac) may be prescribed to inhibit the secretion of gastric acid if the cause of the dysphagia is acid reflux.

The patient with dysphagia of oesophageal origin is taught to swallow twice in rapid succession when symptoms occur. Fox has demonstrated that this simple manoeuvre of the double swallow may convert the painful oesophageal contractions into contractions of normal amplitude and duration and thus relieve the symptoms (Fox and Monna, 1980).

Identification of the foodstuffs which exacerbate the problem may be aided by encouraging the individual to maintain a diary of intake over a period of time. Since the pain of dysphagia is not constant, long pain-free periods are common. It is important to work with the patient to identify foods and stresses which exacerbate the symptoms and to help adjust eating habits and daily routines to avoid these factors. Citrus fruits, tomatoes and alcoholic beverages are likely to cause pain and discomfort in patients during swallowing. Education concerning positioning during eating, and standing following meals, may aid gravitational ingestion.

Stress has also been identified as a precipitating factor. Learning relaxation techniques such as deep breathing and visual imagery may be a useful strategy to enable the individual to cope with stressful periods. Gentle back massage during periods of discomfort may reduce pain. These techniques can be carried out before and after eating to promote muscular and emotional relaxation.

Care of the patient requiring surgery

Surgical intervention in oesophageal disorders involves entering the thoracic cavity in most instances. In planning care, the factors cited in the section on care in chest surgery are considered. Since surgery on the lower oesophageal sphincter also involves gastric surgery and the lower end of the oesophagus, the principles which apply to nursing in gastric surgery also apply.

A pre- and postoperative care plan for the patient requiring surgery of the oesophagus is outlined in Table 16.4. In clinical practice, the plan is adjusted to meet the needs of the individual patient.

THE PERSON WITH DISORDERS OF SECRETION, DIGESTION AND MOTILITY IN THE STOMACH AND DUODENUM

The gastric and duodenal disorders most frequently seen include gastritis, peptic ulcer and carcinoma.

GASTRITIS

The term gastritis implies inflammation of the stomach. The condition may be acute or chronic and the pathological process is usually limited to the mucosa.

CAUSES

The causes of *acute inflammation* may be the ingestion of large quantities of alcohol, contaminated foods, or foods to which the person is sensitive or allergic, such as seafood, mushrooms or salicylates (e.g. aspirin). Infective gastritis is most frequently due to the ingestion of foods bearing staphylococci or salmonella organisms.

CLINICAL CHARACTERISTICS

The patient with acute gastritis becomes ill suddenly and suffers severe epigastric pain, nausea, vomiting and fever.

The treatment includes keeping the patient nil by mouth, bed rest and parenteral fluids. Clear fluids are given when the symptoms subside and, if tolerated, a bland diet of soft foods is introduced and progressively increased until a normal diet is resumed.

Chronic gastritis occurs with prolonged and repeated irritation of the mucosa and results in atrophic changes in the mucosa and glands. The cause may be evasive, since the condition may be associated with other diseases such as pernicious anaemaia, and with the degenerative changes of ageing. It may result from constant subjection of the stomach to an ingested irritant, such as alcohol, and frequently accompanies a gastric ulcer or gastric carcinoma.

The symptoms of chronic gastritis are usually ill-defined but may include anorexia, discomfort and a full feeling after meals, flatulence, heartburn, nausea and occasionally haematemesis. The patient may lose con-

siderable weight as he or she tends to restrict food intake to avoid the distress it may precipitate. Attention is directed toward improving the general nutritional status by encouraging a well-balanced diet of non-irritating foods.

PEPTIC ULCER

A peptic ulcer is the erosion of a circumscribed area of tissue in the wall of the gastrointestinal tract that is accessible to gastric secretions. The actual erosion is caused by the digestive action of hydrochloric acid and pepsin. The most frequent sites of an ulcer are the stomach (*gastric ulcer*) and the proximal portion of the duodenum (*duodenal ulcer*) but the oesophagus or jejunum or any other part of the gastrointestinal mucosa may be susceptible if the surface comes in contact with gastric secretions.

The ulcer penetrates the mucosa and may invade the underlying submucosal and muscular tissues. Ulcers tend to recur; some heal promptly while others become chronic.

CAUSES

There is no consensus as to the initiating cause of peptic ulcer. Normally, hydrochloric acid and pepsin are secreted but ulceration does not occur. This is attributed to the following defensive factors. The mucosa secretes sufficient mucus to dilute the secretions and provides a protective coating that prevents mucosal digestion by the acid–pepsin action. The duodenum has the additional protection of the strong alkalinity of the bile and pancreatic and intestinal secretions which neutralize the acidic chyme. Still another defence is a healthy resistant mucosa which has a good blood supply and is capable of continuous rapid generation of the mucosal epithelial cells.

A peptic ulcer may develop when the secretory output of hydrochloric acid and pepsin is in excess of the normal or when the protective mechanisms are inadequate in relation to the amount of acid and pepsin produced. An ulcer is therefore caused by an imbalance between pepsin secretion and the body's natural defences. Stress is also involved as it causes capillary shutdown, decreasing the blood flow to the area, and a decrease in bicarbonate production, which results in an acid-base imbalance.

An increased acid level is not usually present in gastric ulcer, while duodenal ulcer is associated with a high acid level. The problem is: what causes a hypersecretion of acid and pepsin or lowers mucosal resistance? Factors that are suspect include individual physiological differences such as greater parietal cell mass, greater sensitivity of the cells to the stimulating hormone gastrin, excessive production of gastrin and more rapid passage of gastric contents into the duodenum, resulting in more free acid and pepsin being delivered to the duodenum. A disturbance in the autonomic nervous control of gastric secretion that results in increased vagal (parasympathetic) innervation causes prolonged secretion of hydrochloric acid and pepsin.

The following are considered to be potential contributing factors in the development of an imbalance between the secretion of hydrochloric acid and pepsin and the defensive mechanisms of the mucosa.

- *Emotional factors.* Emotional tension, anxiety, frustration and stress may cause an imbalance in the autonomic nervous system, resulting in increased vagal stimulation of gastric secretion.
- *Inflammation.* Gastritis and trauma of the mucosa reduces the resistance of the membrane to digestion. Cell destruction is accelerated and cell reproduction, which normally renews the superficial layers quickly, may be retarded.
- *Heredity.* Genetic factors appear to have a role, since studies on incidence show there is a tendency for peptic disease to occur in families and in persons of certain blood types. There is correlation between duodenal ulcer and the blood type O while gastric ulcer patients are more often of the blood group A.
- *Trauma and serious illness.* The patient with severe tissue injury such as that produced by extensive burns may develop severe peptic ulceration. It has been recognized as a complication frequently associated with any serious illness, especially if it is characterized by hypotension or respiratory insufficiency. These ulcers may be referred to as *stress ulcers.*
- *Certain drugs.* Some drugs, e.g. acetylsalicylic acid (aspirin), corticosteroids (cortisone), indomethacin (Indocid) and phenylbutazone (Butazolidin), are ulcerogenic in some persons.
- *Bile reflux.* The reflux of bile and pancreatic enzymes into the stomach due to an incompetent pyloric sphincter may lead to a gastric ulcer. The bile salts damage the gastric mucosa, predisposing it to ulceration.
- *Endocrine secretions.* Rarely, severe peptic ulceration is caused by marked gastric hypersecretion that occurs in response to an excessive gastrin concentration in the blood. The gastrin is produced by a tumour of the islets of the pancreas or the submucosa of the duodenum and stomach or regional lymph nodes (Zollinger–Ellison syndrome).
  Peptic ulceration also develops in hyperparathyroidism. The disturbance is attributed to the altered serum calcium level.
- *Histamine.* Histamine promotes stimulation of acid secretion; H_2-receptor antagonists which inhibit histamine action have been found in gastric parietal cells.
- *Sex.* Peptic ulcer has a much higher incidence in men than in women. It has been suggested that oestrogenic hormones in the female may account for this.
- *Other factors.* Poor dietary habits, particularly irregular meals, are thought to be an aggravating factor. Abnormally long periods between meals in persons with a prolonged hypersecretion of acid and pepsin leave the mucosa vulnerable. The protective mechanisms cannot withstand the acid–pepsin action without the diluting and neutralizing assistance of food. Smoking and excessive amounts of alcohol or coffee increase gastric secretion.

INCIDENCE

Peptic ulcer is a common disease and has a higher incidence in males between the ages of 40 and 55 years. Duodenal ulcer is much more common than gastric ulcer, and the incidence of gastric ulcer (not associated with cancer) is higher in females than in males. The patients frequently experience seasonal exacerbations in the spring and autumn.

CLINICAL CHARACTERISTICS

The prominent symptom of peptic ulcer is epigastric *pain* with definite characteristics. It may radiate to the back. The pain is usually described by the patient as gnawing or burning and of being rhythmic in its development and relief in relation to the ingestion of food. The onset of pain may be immediately or up to 4 hours after a meal, depending upon the location of the ulcer, and is relieved by taking food or an antacid. In the case of an *oesophageal ulcer*, the pain develops within a few minutes after the meal. It may be intermittent and the patient usually complains of heartburn and regurgitation. Pain associated with a *gastric ulcer* usually occurs ½–1 hour after the ingestion of food; that of a *duodenal ulcer* is delayed for approximately 2–4 hours. The patient's rest is frequently disturbed by nocturnal pain, especially with a duodenal ulcer. Although the ingestion of food generally provides relief, in a few instances it may be the initiating factor of the ulcer pain, particularly if the food is coarse or highly seasoned. The association of eating with relief of pain ensures that the patient is not usually undernourished.

Vomiting is not a common incident in peptic ulcer but may occur if the ulcer pain is very severe or if the ulcer is in the pyloric region. In the case of the latter, inflammation and oedema of the surrounding tissues, pyloric spasm or contracted scar tissue resulting from ulceration may narrow the lumen of the pylorus. This may delay the emptying of the stomach and may cause vomiting.

CLINICAL DIAGNOSTIC MEASUREMENTS

Investigation of the patient for peptic ulcer may include endoscopy, X-rays with a barium meal (see p. 493), gastric analysis to determine the hydrochloric acid secretion, gastroscopy, serum gastrin assays, exfoliative cytology and stool examination for occult blood.

Gastric secretory tests

Common gastric function tests used in the investigation of patients with symptoms of gastrointestinal disease include the measurement of the volume of secretions over a stated period and the determination of HCl secretion under basal conditions and then in response to a gastric stimulant. Gastric analysis in which a quantitative estimation is required involves the use of a nasogastric tube to aspirate the gastric contents. If the test is done only to determine whether HCl is being secreted or not, aspiration of the gastric contents is unnecessary. Radioisotope labelling techniques may also be used to measure the rate at which food leaves the stomach. The normal gastric emptying half-time is 45–90 minutes for solid food and 15–20 minutes for liquids.

Analysis of gastric contents

A fasting period of 8–10 hours precedes the test and the patient is instructed not to smoke, as smoking stimulates gastric secretion. Anticholinergic drugs (e.g. propantheline bromide) are also withheld for 24 hours prior to the test as they inhibit the histamine stimulation of gastric acid secretion. A tube is passed into the stomach and the gastric content is aspirated by a syringe. The volume of this aspirate is noted, recorded and labelled for determination of the acid concentration.

Following this initial specimen, the directions may be to aspirate the gastric secretion at intervals of 15 minutes for 1 hour. Each specimen is placed in a separate tube and numbered according to the order in which it is collected. These specimens provide information about the *basal secretory activity* of the stomach.

Occasionally, this fractional analysis procedure to evaluate secretory function includes the parenteral administration of a secretory stimulant such as pentagastrin, given intramuscularly, or (less frequently) insulin, given subcutaneously. The drug is administered after the initial aspiration. Aspiration specimens are then collected at intervals of 15 minutes for one hour.

If insulin is used as a secretory stimulant, the patient is observed closely for signs of hypoglycaemia. The doctor may start an intravenous infusion of normal saline before the insulin is given so that 50% glucose may be given without delay if hypoglycaemia develops.

The normal basal gastric secretion is 30–70 ml/h and the HCl production (basal acid output, BAO) is 2–5 mmol/h during the resting state. The normal maximum acid output (MAO) in response to a secretory stimulant is 10–20 mmol/h.

Achlorhydria indicates a deficiency in the gastric secretion of HCl. The term is applied when the pH of the gastric content is more than 6 following the administration of a secretory stimulant. Achlorhydria may be associated with cancer of the stomach, chronic gastritis, gastric ulcer or pernicious anaemia.

Hyperchlorhydria is a term used to describe an excessive secretion of HCl. An increase in acid secretion is seen in duodenal ulcer and the Zollinger–Ellison syndrome.

Serum gastrin level

Gastrin is a polypeptide hormone secreted by cells in the pylorus which stimulates the secretion of gastric acid and pepsin. An excessive release of gastrin may be associated with tumours of non-β-cell/islets in the pancreas. Normal serum gastrin levels are 40–150 ng/l.

Gastroscopy

This is usually used to obtain more detailed information about a lesion (e.g. ulcer) that has been identified as being present by previous barium X-ray. A biopsy is performed and pictures may be taken of the lesion. It may also be used to assess the healing of an ulcer.

The improvement in endoscopic instruments has made it possible in some instances to arrest haemorrhage by the direct application of electrocautery or a haemostatic preparation to the bleeding site.

The gastroscope may be passed through the pylorus to examine the duodenum. The ampulla of Vater may be cannulated and viewed, and a radiopaque dye injected to demonstrate the pancreatic and common bile ducts (cholangiopancreatography). Endoscopic examination may also be extended into the jejunum.

Nursing care in gastroscopy

Preparation for this diagnostic procedure should begin with an explanation to the patient of what to expect. The doctor may have described the examination and its values, but the patient will most likely still have questions. The nurse should have sufficient understanding of the procedure to be able to answer the patient's questions.

A written consent for the procedure is required. The oesophagus and the stomach must be completely empty. No food or fluid is given for 4–6 hours before the procedure. In gastroscopy, the doctor may request a gastric lavage to be done several hours before the examination in patients in whom some pyloric obstruction is suspected. The teeth are cleaned and a mouthwash provided before the procedure; dentures and jewellery are removed and kept safe.

An analgesic such as pethidine may be administered 30–60 minutes before the scheduled time as well as a sedative, or an analgesic may be administered intravenously during the procedure.

The pharyngeal area is sprayed with a local anaesthetic before the gastroscope is introduced. The patient is unable to speak when the endoscope is in position.

Following the examination, the patient is allowed to rest. All food and fluids are withheld until the effect of the local anaesthetic has worn off and the gag reflex returns (usually 4–6 hours). Before giving any fluid, the reflex may be tested by gently touching the back of the throat with an applicator or spoon. The patient may complain of a sore throat or soreness in midchest. Warm fluids may be soothing and may provide some relief. Any expectoration or vomiting of blood or severe pain should be reported promptly to the doctor.

ASSESSMENT OF THE PATIENT WITH PEPTIC ULCER

The nurse will generally encounter patients admitted with peptic ulcer in one of three situations; the person has been admitted for investigation and diagnosis, is having an acute exacerbation with possible severe bleeding, or has been admitted for planned surgery as the ulcer is failing to respond to medical treatment. Assessment will therefore tend to focus on different aspects of the patient in each of these situations.

The patient being admitted for investigations may be very anxious and have fears of cancer being diagnosed. It is essential therefore that in addition to the obvious physical parameters that are assessed, to consider how anxious the person is and what areas the person may wish further information. As health education about factors that predispose to ulceration will be a key part of the care plan, it is important to assess relevant areas of the person's lifestyle such as smoking and drinking habits, regularity and types of meals, stress levels, all of which are amenable to health education. It is also important to discover the person's level of understanding and attitudes towards health education as this will have a major influence upon the approach used.

In an acute emergency situation, physical parameters such as blood pressure and pulse are a high priority due to the risks of hypovolaemic shock and a major bleed that may be fatal. Close assessment of stools for melaena and vomit for the presence of fresh or altered blood are required. Pain must be carefully assessed so that appropriate relief can be given as required. The nurse should not lose sight of the patient's psychological condition however and carefully assess levels of both fear and understanding in what can be a very frightening situation.

The patient being admitted for surgery should be assessed along the lines discussed in the first scenario above. He or she may be optimistic as surgery is seen as a cure for a long term and distressing complaint. However lingering fears of cancer may be just below the surface along with all the fears that can be conjured up by the prospect of any surgery. Such topics need careful exploration during assessment as it is also important to discover whether the patient has a realistic view of the benefits surgery may bring and is aware of the various measures that will be needed to cope with the side effects of surgery in the long term. Successful health education prior to discharge will depend upon discovering such information.

MANAGEMENT

Treatment of the peptic ulcer patient is directed toward the relief of symptoms, healing of the ulcer and the prevention of complications and recurrence. A regimen of rest, non-irritating diet and various medications is designed to reduce gastric secretory and motor activity, dilute the gastric juice and neutralize much of the hydrochloric acid that is secreted in order to promote healing.

Hospitalization is not usually necessary.

Diet

Strict dietary control is not considered necessary. A regular well-balanced diet, free of foods which are upsetting to the individual, is recommended. Foods that patients usually find difficult to tolerate include coffee, tea, alcohol, highly seasoned foods and gas-forming foods. In the acute phase, small frequent meals will be more tolerable to the patient. These are gradually modified to the more customary three larger meals per day. In some instances five or six smaller meals may have to be continued.

Medications

The drugs used in the treatment of patients with gastric or duodenal ulcers include antacids, H2-receptor antagonists, prostaglandins and anticholinergic agents.

Antacids are used to neutralize the acid in the stomach. To be effective, antacids must be taken frequently throughout the day. Examples include aluminium hydroxide, magnesium hydroxide, calcium carbonate and sodium bicarbonate. Sodium bicarbonate increases the serum sodium level and should not be used. Magnesium and aluminium salts are absorbed minimally and should not cause any disturbances in electrolyte levels. Hypermagnesaemia and hyperaluminaemia, however, can occur in patients with renal failure. Magnesium hydroxide can cause diarrhoea and aluminium hydroxide tends to cause constipation. For this reason they are usually administered together as a combination product. Antacids may interfere with the absorption of certain drugs (e.g. ferrous sulphate, tetracycline, phenytoin) and it is usually recommended that the administration of antacids and other drugs be separated by at least 2 hours. Because of the availability of other drugs and the inconvenience of taking antacids so frequently, these drugs are usually used on a p.r.n. basis.

Sucralfate is a *sulphated polysaccharide* which acts directly at the ulcer site. Sucralfate binds with the gastric mucosa and forms a barrier which inhibits the diffusion of hydrogen ion and the local action of pepsin. It is poorly absorbed and hence has few side-effects. Occasionally constipation may occur. It should be administered 30 minutes prior to meals and at bedtime. If prescribed with antacids, administration should be separated by at least one hour.

Cimetidine and ranitidine are examples of *H2-receptor antagonists*. They block the H2 receptors in the parietal cells, inhibiting the secretion of acid, and have been proven to be effective in healing gastric and duodenal ulcers. When initially approved, cimetidine was recommended to be administered four times a day, ranitidine twice daily. Recent studies have shown that cimetidine and ranitidine may be given in a higher dose at less frequent intervals. When administered once daily, the medication should be given at bedtime to maximize the effect during nocturnal hours when acid secretion is the greatest.

Anticholinergic agents have many side-effects and hence have limited usefulness. They delay gastric emptying, which causes gastric distention and acid retention in the stomach, and should never be used for gastric ulcers. They may be useful for duodenal ulcers unresponsive to conventional therapy. However, the selective anticholinergic drug pirenzepine, which acts specifically by inhibiting gastric acid and pepsin secretion, may have a role in conjunction with H_2 antagonists in resistant cases.

Medications which are considered *ulcerogenic* may predispose the patient to gastrointestinal bleeding and should be avoided. Examples include acetylsalicylic acid, other non-steroidal anti-inflammatory agents, corticosteroids and potassium chloride.

Surgical treatment

If the symptoms persist and the ulcer becomes intractable, or if there has been bleeding or the ulcer has resulted in some obstruction in the gastric outlet, surgical treatment may be considered necessary. Various operative procedures are used in the surgical treatment of an uncomplicated ulcer in order to reduce the potential gastric acid secretion. Current operative approaches include the following procedures.

Gastric resection (subtotal gastrectomy) is the removal of a portion of the stomach, including the ulcer-bearing area and part of the parietal cell mass. An anastomosis is then made between the gastric stump and the duodenum (*gastroduodenostomy; Billroth I*) or jejunum (*gastrojejunostomy; Billroth II*) to restore gastrointestinal continuity.

Gastric resection plus vagotomy may be done. Vagotomy is a resection of the vagus nerve to reduce the stimulation of gastric secretion. It also reduces the motility of the stomach and may interfere with gastric emptying. For this reason it is rarely performed alone but is combined with a gastric resection or with a gastroenterostomy to provide effective gastric emptying.

A combined vagotomy and resection of the antrum of the stomach (antrectomy) may be performed. The vagotomy reduces the innervation that increases the gastric secretion; removal of the antrum removes the source of the chemical stimulus, gastrin.

Vagotomy with pyloroplasty involves a longitudinal incision made in the pylorus, which is then surgically closed transversely. This produces an enlarged outlet which compensates for the impaired gastric emptying resulting from vagotomy. In some instances a *gastroenterostomy* may be done instead of the pyloroplasty.

For nursing management of the patient who requires gastric surgery, see p. 476.

COMPLICATIONS OF PEPTIC ULCERATION

The complications that commonly occur with peptic ulcer are serious and usually account for the deaths attributed to peptic ulcer. They are haemorrhage, perforation, and pyloric obstruction.

Haemorrhage

Peptic ulceration is the most common cause of haematemesis and melaena. The loss of blood is due to erosion of a blood vessel at the ulcer site. Most of the patients who have a haemorrhage are known to have or to have had an ulcer but in a few it may be the first symptom that prompts them to seek treatment.

Vomiting of blood and the passing of black tarry stools are the prominent indications of serious ulcer bleeding together with the development of hypovolaemic shock. The patient experiences weakness, apprehension, dizziness and faintness, together with the classical signs of shock (p. 227). If a large vessel is eroded, the signs and symptoms appear rapidly and collapse occurs quickly.

Management of the patient with haemorrhage may be conservative or require surgery. The complication of haemorrhage is serious and demands prompt resuscitation and treatment of the site of bleeding.

Nursing Assessment. In assessing the patient with a haemorrhage, the blood pressure, pulse and respirations are monitored frequently and the level of consciousness, colour and body temperature are noted.

Blood typing and cross matching are done immediately. The haematocrit and haemoglobin levels are determined, initially to determine the extent of the

blood loss then later, at intervals, to assess the patient's response to treatment.

Accurate recording of the volume and characteristics of the emesis and drainage via the nasogastric tube is important. (Is the blood bright? Does the emesis contain clots?) An indwelling catheter may be passed so that urinary output per hour can be monitored.

It is important to assess the person's reaction to the situation, since fear and anxiety aggravate the condition. The principal problem facing the patient is shock and the main goals are that the patient's blood pressure and other vital signs will return to normal, indicating successful resuscitation and the cessation of bleeding.

Nursing intervention for a patient with haemorrhage includes the following:

- A plasma expander such as Haemaccel is given intravenously until compatible whole blood is available. The rate of flow is usually slowed as the patient's blood pressure increases; too rapid an increase in the blood pressure has the risk of increasing the bleeding. The blood pressure may need to be measured every 15–30 minutes.
- Rest should be promoted by reducing disturbances, keeping nursing interventions to a safe minimum. A sedative may be prescribed to promote relaxation.
- The patient and significant others should be kept informed to allay anxiety. Information should be presented in short segments, without excessive use of medical terms, delivered in a calm manner, and regularly reinforced.
- A nasogastric tube may be passed to remove blood and gastric secretions. Gentle aspiration of stomach contents will remove acid and pepsin which could further irritate tissues. Aspiration of blood may prevent vomiting (haematemesis), allow estimation of loss, and reduce trauma and discomfort.
- Gastroscopy is usually performed to locate the bleeding site; electrocautery, photocautery, or topical administration of a haemostatic preparation (pitressin) may be used to control bleeding. If this is unsuccessful emergency surgery may be necessary. If bleeding has ceased, close observation and maintained fasting is usually continued until the person's overall condition is stable.
- If treated conservatively, and when bleeding ceases and the cardiovascular state is normalised, oral intake is permitted. Once small volumes of water are tolerated by the person, intake is gradually increased to include clear fluids, liquid diet, soft food, and eventually an ordinary diet. Being able to take food and fluid again improves the patient's morale and lessens anxiety. A preparation of iron may be ordered to promote development of haemoglobin.
- Frequent mouth care is necessary because of the haematemesis, dehydration and the discomfort of extreme thirst. Analgesia may be necessary to relieve the pain caused by the ulcer.

Perforation

A peptic ulcer may progressively erode the submucosal, muscular and serous layers of the gastrointestinal wall. When the serous membranous layer is penetrated, some of the stomach or duodenal content escapes into the peritoneal cavity and causes a generalized peritonitis by chemical irritation and infection.

When perforation takes place, the patient immediately experiences sudden, incapacitating abdominal pain that begins in the epigastric region but spreads through the abdomen as more of the peritoneum becomes irritated by the intragastrointestinal content. Pallor, a cold clammy skin, rapid pulse, shallow grunting respirations and probably nausea and vomiting may be evident. The abdomen becomes rigid and board-like.

Perforation demands immediate treatment; emergency surgery may be performed to close the perforation or resect the affected area, or the patient's condition and history may be such that the perforation is treated by non-surgical conservative methods. The surgical procedure may consist of gastric resection or simple closure of the perforation by suturing the serous layer and reinforcing the area with a patch of omentum. The peritoneal cavity is cleared of the intragastrointestinal fluid that seeped through the perforation. In addition to the usual preoperative procedures for emergency surgery, preparation will include the insertion of a nasogastric tube and an intravenous infusion of electrolytes and fluids. An explanation of the need for surgery and what it entails will be made by the surgeon and reinforced by the nurse.

Non-operative treatment usually includes parenteral administration of an analgesic such as morphine, aspiration of the stomach content using a large tube, followed by the insertion of a nasogastric tube and continuous gastric suctioning, intravenous electrolytes and fluids (fluids may include whole blood) and antibiotic therapy. If the patient's condition is satisfactory, continuous gastric suctioning is replaced by intermittent aspiration after 30–48 hours.

Pyloric obstruction
This may be caused by inflammation, oedema and spasm when the ulcer is in the acute stage or by scar tissue which is formed as the ulcer heals. The ulcer may be gastric in the region of the pylorus, or it may be in the duodenum. The constriction causes gastric retention and dilatation.

The *symptoms* which the the patient complains of include a 'full feeling' which causes greater discomfort toward the end of the day. Pain may be experienced following eating as gastric contractions increase in intensity in an effort to overcome the obstruction. The contractions gradually decline and the stomach becomes atonic and dilates. Severe anorexia develops and the patient vomits large amounts irregularly. The loss of nutrients, water and electrolytes leads to loss of weight, weakness, dehydration and acid–base imbalance (alkalosis).

If the obstruction is due to the active ulceration process, it is treated medically by gastric aspiration and intravenous fluids.

Obstruction due to contraction of fibrous scar tissue is treated by surgery. A gastric resection with a gastroenterostomy or pyloroplasty may be performed. For a nursing care plan see pp. 475–477.

CANCER OF THE STOMACH

Although cancer of the stomach still accounts for a large number of deaths each year, there has been a significant decline over the last three decades. Incidence is slightly higher in males, rapidly rises from the age of 40, with the highest number of deaths occuring in the 55–60 age group.

CONTRIBUTING FACTORS

The cause of this cancer is unknown but certain conditions are considered predisposing. These include: pernicious anaemia, achlorhydria, atrophic gastritis, gastric polyps, and a possible relationship between benign gastric disease treated surgically (Eliis et al, 1979; Lawrence, 1986). There is also a higher incidence in individuals with the blood group A.

A link between dietary factors and gastric cancer has not been fully established. However, high intake of salt, alcohol and nitrate-preserved foods and low intake of fruits, vegetables and animal protein may predispose individuals to development of cancer at this site.

Any region of the stomach may be involved, but the most frequent sites are the pylorus and antrum.

CLINICAL CHARACTERISTICS

The manifestations are vague and insidious. At first, the person may complain of some mild discomfort after eating but, as the disease advances, belching, regurgitation, nausea and vomiting may be experienced, and there is a progressive loss of appetite, weight and strength. Blood may appear in the vomitus and stool when there is ulceration at the cancer site. Pain is usually a late symptom. Unfortunately, because the early symptoms are mild and vague, the person tends to delay seeing a doctor, and the disease becomes well advanced before there is medical intervention. Nurses should be aware of this problem and, on learning that a person is experiencing even mild 'digestive' disturbances, should stress the importance of seeking medical advice.

DIAGNOSIS

Investigation of the patient includes X-ray examinations, analysis of gastric content for acidity, cytological studies of gastric fluid, gastroscopy and biopsy, examination of the stool for blood, haemoglobin estimation and blood cell counts. Computerized axial tomography scan of chest and abdomen and liver ultrasound may be performed to establish the extent of the tumour and infiltration or development of metastases in other organs.

The gastric analysis is done to determine if there is a decrease in the secretion of hydrochloric acid as the majority of patients with cancer of the stomach demonstrate a hypochlorhydria or an achlorhydria. The blood examinations will probably show some deficiency of haemoglobin and red blood cells, as anaemia is a characteristic of gastric cancer due to the chronic bleeding, reduced production of the intrinsic factor by the gastric mucosa, reduced absorption of iron because of the hypochlorhydria and nutritional deficits.

METASTASES

Gastric carcinoma develops and metastasizes rapidly; all too often there has been a spread to some other structure(s) by the time of diagnosis. There may be direct extension to neighbouring organs (e.g. oesophagus, duodenum) or an indirect spread via the lymph and venous blood. The spleen, abdominal lymph nodes, peritoneum, liver, pancreas and lungs are frequent sites of metastases from gastric carcinoma. The left supraclavicular and axillary nodes may also be affected.

TREATMENT

Surgery, radiation therapy and chemotherapy, alone or in combination, are used to treat cancer of the stomach. Surgery is the treatment of choice but cure is possible only when the cancer is diagnosed in the early stages. The surgical procedure used will depend on the site of the cancer and its extension or possible course of extension. A subtotal gastrectomy or, rarely, a total gastrectomy is performed and may include resection of the duodenum, excision of the areas of lymphatic spread (omentum, spleen), resection of the pancreas or resection of the lower oesophagus. In subtotal gastrectomy, the stomach is anastomosed to the duodenum (gastroduodenostomy) or jejunum (gastrojejunostomy) if it has been the lower part of the stomach that has been removed. In the case of removal of the proximal portion of the stomach the operation is completed by anastomosis of the oesophagus to the remaining stomach (oesophagoantrostomy). Total gastrectomy and a resection of the oesophagus necessitate entrance into the thoracic cavity. Continuity of the alimentary tract is restored by an oesophagojejunostomy.

The preoperative and postoperative nursing care of the gastric surgical patient is presented on pp. 475–477. Care of the patient following a complete gastrectomy will include the care necessary for any patient who has had chest surgery (Chapter 15). The patient who has had a partial gastrectomy will require small frequent meals of easily digested foods due to the development of dumping syndrome (see below) and vitamin B_{12} injections.

Chemotherapy is usually employed in the management of gastric cancer for palliation. The agent 5-fluorouracil (5-FU), alone or in combination with adriamycin and mitomycin C (FAM), can produce a response, although this is often transient and far from curative. Radiotherapy is sometimes used to control severe obstruction, thereby improving quality of life (see chapter 10 for care of individuals receiving chemotherapy and radiotherapy).

DUMPING SYNDROME

Normally, the gastric content is delivered in small amounts into the intestine by the pylorus. Following a gastric resection, vagotomy or gastroentrostomy, the normal pyloric control of the volume moving from the stomach into the small intestine is absent. The dumping syndrome is caused by the precipitous passage into the small intestine of a relatively large amount of gastric content that has not undergone the usual dilution by gastric secretions and digestive changes. The exact mechanism by which the characteristic responses are initiated is not entirely clear; it is suggested that the following factors are implicated.

First, the sudden distension of the proximal portion of the small intestine initiates sympathetic reflexes. Second, the fluid that moved quickly out of the stomach is hypertonic, having a high concentration of sugar and/or electrolytes. The resulting hyperosmolarity on the intestine results in the movement of fluid from the intravascular spaces into the jejunum. Only a small percentage of patients develop the problem.

Nursing Care of the Person with Disorders of Secretion, Digestion and Motility in the Stomach and Duodenum

ASSESSMENT

Health History

The information obtained from the assessment will be enhanced and be more valuable for individualized care if it is focused on specific areas. The nurse may find it useful when recording information about pain to use a pain chart, recording site and location of pain and factors which increase and reduce the experience. The person may wish to participate by maintaining this themselves. The following areas should be explored:

Gastrointestinal functioning and factors which influence it
- What is the usual diet of the individual?
- How has the diet changed in relation to symptoms?
- What strategies have been adopted to relieve symptoms?
- Does the person smoke, take alcohol, or drugs such as aspirin or steroids?
- Has the individual experienced any particular stressful life events recently?
- Does the life-style vary, affecting diet, eating habits, etc?
- Do any activities increase symptoms?

Clinical symptoms
- Does the individual experience nausea, vomiting, epigastric fullness, discomfort or pain?
- Where is the pain located? Does it move to the back or shoulders?
- What factors appear to increase discomfort?
- What strategies has the individual adopted to relieve it?
- Is the pain or discomfort increased at night, when the stomach is empty or during any specific activities?
- Does the individual take antacids to relieve discomfort? Are they effective? How often are they taken, and are they taken?

- How long have the symptoms been experienced? Have they changed?

General health status
- Has the person lost weight recently and how much?
- Have there been any other health problems such as breathlessness, reduced mobility, poor healing, etc?

PATIENT PROBLEMS COMMON TO THOSE WITH DISORDERS OF THE STOMACH AND DUODENUM

- *Dehydration* due to nausea and vomiting.
- *Malnutrition* due to increased gastric secretions, gastrointestinal discomfort, nausea, vomiting, and possibly surgical intervention.
- *Ineffective individual coping* related to the role of stress on the gastrointestinal system.

GOALS

The person will demonstrate:
- Awareness of the factors contributing to the disorder of the stomach and duodenum.
- Absence or control of nausea and vomiting.
- Awareness of dietary measures to decrease gastric secretion.
- Ability to perform prescribed enteral feeding techniques.
- An adequate nutritional intake, as shown by progressive increase in body weight towards normal.
- Awareness of measures to decrease the effects of life stresses on the stomach and duodenum.

NURSING INTERVENTION

1. Alleviation of nausea and vomiting

Assessment
Assessment of the patient who is nauseated and is vomiting involves noting the following factors:
- Was the vomiting preceded by nausea?
- Was there retching or was the vomitus regurgitated without effort?
- Was pain associated with the vomiting?
- Was there any association with the ingestion of food or drugs?
- Do the nausea and vomiting occur at any time or are they more severe at a particular time of day?
- How frequent is the emesis?
- What is the quantity, consistency, colour and content of the vomitus?
- What are the effects (physical and emotional) on the patient?

The care must be individualized; what may prove helpful with one person may not be tolerated by another. The cause of the vomiting will also influence care planning.

Supportive measures
Sympathetic attention and understanding can mean a great deal to the patient. Since stress and fear can perpetuate nausea and vomiting, the patient is encouraged to express any concerns. The plan of care and any diagnostic and therapeutic measures should be explained to the patient; knowing that something is being done or going to be done provides reassurance.

Support is also provided by remaining with the patient, supporting the head or painful site (e.g. incision) holding the basin, cleansing the mouth and lips and making sincere efforts to relieve the discomfort.

Fluid and food
Oral intake is usually withheld for a period of time and is resumed gradually in small amounts. If vomiting is prolonged, an intravenous infusion of fluids may be necessary to prevent or correct dehydration and replace electrolytes. An accurate record is made of the fluid intake and output. The skin and oral mucous membrane are observed for dryness and skin turgor is assessed to identify dehydration. Laboratory reports of the concentration of plasma electrolytes (sodium, potassium, chloride) are followed closely so that imbalances may be corrected by appropriate intravenous fluids. The patient's weight is recorded daily.

Hygienic and comfort measures
The mouth is rinsed after each emesis and the basin emptied and disposed of promptly. Soiled bedding and clothing are changed and the room ventilated. The odour or sight of vomitus may contribute to the patient's discomfort and may cause repetitive vomiting. The patient may be reassured by having tissues and a clean basin always within reach, but it is less suggestive if covered with a clean towel.

Rest, quiet and a minimum of disturbance may reduce the incidence of vomiting. Encouraging the patient to take several deep breaths may help to lessen nausea and offset vomiting. Nausea tends to increase with motion; any change of position should be made slowly. Positioning should facilitate drainage of the vomitus from the mouth to prevent possible aspiration. Subdued lighting may reduce external stimuli and be conducive to rest.

Relaxation techniques including muscular relaxation, meditation, guided imagery and deep breathing exercises may help to decrease stress and relieve the nausea and vomiting.

Some individuals find food actually relieves nausea and prevents vomiting. Dry crackers, sips of soda water, and in some instances flat cola, can be helpful.

Medication
An antiemetic or a sedative may be prescribed. Diazepam (Valium) may be administered orally or parenterally for sedation. Prochlorperazine or metaclopramide are examples of antiemetics which may be given, usually via the intramuscular route.

The use of antiemetics or other drugs is restricted if there is any question of pregnancy to prevent any effects on fetal development. Anticipatory nausea and vomiting are also controlled by preventative and regular doses of

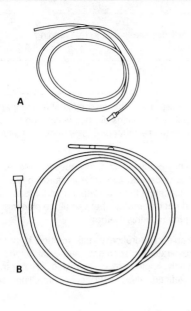

Figure 16.6 (A), Fine-bore tube. (B), Ryles tube.

antiemetics. Nausea and vomiting due to chemotherapy is prevented or controlled by the administration of antiemetics ½–1 hour prior to the chemotherapeutic drugs and throughout the infusion.

If the vomiting continues, gastric drainage by means of a nasogastric tube may be established.

2. Maintenance of adequate nutritional intake

When secretion, digestion and motility of the stomach and duodenum are altered, the nutritional intake is maintained by decreasing stimulation of certain secretions, adapting the person's diet to relieve the problem or by using alternative routes to administer nutrients.

Dietary measures
Measures to decrease stimulation of gastric secretions include withholding food for 24–48 hours to allow the stomach to rest. Fluids are given intravenously as even water taken by mouth will stimulate gastric acid secretion. Gastric intubation with aspiration may be used to remove gastric secretions to promote healing.

Recommended dietary modifications include the following principles:
- A nutritionally adequate diet.
- Substances which stimulate gastric secretion (e.g. coffee, strong tea, highly seasoned foods, especially those with pepper, citrus fruit and alcohol) are avoided.
- Meals are taken regularly at frequent intervals of about 3 hours to maintain the buffering action of food in the stomach.
- Meals should be small to avoid gastric distension which stimulates gastric acid secretion.

- Foods which the person recognizes as actually precipitating symptoms are avoided.
- The person should not smoke.
- Drugs such as acetylsalicylic acid (aspirin) which are known to damage the gatsrointestinal mucosa are avoided.

Alternative routes for the administration of nutrients
Oral intake of food is preferred, but when this is not possible nutrients can be administered intravenously or by nasogastric or gastric routes.

Nasogastric tube feeding. When a patient is unable to take fluid and foods by mouth, a nasogastric tube (Figure 16.6) may be passed, through which a specially prepared solution of essential nutrients is introduced directly into the stomach. This method of feeding a patient is known as enteral feeding.

Ethical issues related to the use of tube feedings are discussed in Chapter 18. The risk for aspiration should be assessed prior to instituting enteral feeds, especially with the elderly. There is no evidence that the use of small-lumen feeding tubes decreases the risk of reflux or aspiration.

Policies vary as to who is responsible for the insertion of nasogastric tubes. Often, small-bore, weighted tubes are inserted by a doctor. Careful preparation of the patient prior to insertion will help in reducing discomfort and facilitate ease of insertion. The individual should have the procedure explained in full, including the sensations they will experience and how they can assist by swallowing when they feel the tube touching the back of the throat. Measures which can reduce the unpleasant sensations include: application of sterile, water-soluble, lubricating jelly to the tube, deep breathing, relaxation techniques, and swallowing. A chest X-ray is usually taken following insertion of a fine-bore tube to ascertain its position before commencement of feeding.

Nasogastric tubes can be secured by applying hypoallergenic tape to the individual's nostril or by an adhesive patch to the cheek. Occasionally tubes are secured by a suture.

Enteral feeding involves close co-operation between medical, dietetic and nursing staff. The nurse has an important role in supervising the diet and teaching and supervising the individual (or carer) to achieve self-care.

Commercially prepared feeds are commonly used as they have a known nutrient content, flow easily through the nasogastric tube, and are easy to prepare. They come sterilized and can be administered from a sterile reservoir through an administration tube attached to the nasogastric tube, reducing the potential for the introduction of contaminants.

The regimen is determined according to the individual's nutritional and fluid requirements, based upon their age, sex, body weight, medical condition and biochemical measurements. Continuous delivery of enteral feeding is the ideal as it minimizes side-effects, such as distension and nausea, and maximizes absorption. Intermittent feeding may be more convenient for some individuals, especially when at home.

When evaluating a formula, consideration is given to its osmolality, caloric value and protein, carbohydrate,

Table 16.5 Summary of conclusions about the efficacy of commonly recommended measures to test feeding tube placement

Placement-testing Measures	Conclusions
Aspiration of visually recognizable gastrointestinal secretions	No published research data are available. However, this method is of questionable value as the visual characteristics of gatrointestinal secretions are not well defined. Cases have been reported in which fluid aspirated from the respiratory tract was mistaken for gastric fluid
Auscultation of air insufflated through tube	Efficacy of this method, at least as currently practised, is highly questionable, especially for small-bore tubes. Numerous instances of pseudo-confirmatory gurgling have been reported when tubes were inadvertently placed in the respiratory tract. Also, a descriptive clinical study indicated that nurses could not differentiate between tube placement in the oesophagus, stomach, duodenum or jejunum by this method
pH testing of aspirates	No published research data are available. Theoretically, this method is promising for differentiating between gastric and respiratory placement, and gastric and intestinal placement. Before it can be successfully implemented, expected pH parameters for various secretions need to be clinically defined. Also, methods for controlling confounding variables need to be described
Observing for coughing and choking	No research data are available. It is generally assumed that firm large-bore nasogastric tubes will induce coughing and choking in alert patients with normal tracheal irritability. However, if tracheal response is altered, these symptoms may be absent, even when large-bore tubes are used. Efficacy of this method is highly questionable for small-bore feeding tubes because there are numerous case reports of their inadvertent placement in the respiratory tract without observable symptoms
Testing ability to speak	No research data are available. It is generally assumed that large-bore tubes inadvertently placed in the trachea will interfere with phonation. However, even with large-bore tubes, this method is of no value if the patient is unable to speak for other reasons (such as unconsciousness or intubation). Efficacy of this method is highly questionable for soft small-bore tubes as there are case reports of patients able to speak during inadvertent respiratory placement
Observing for bubbling when tip of tube held under water	No research data are available. However, this method is thought to be unreliable as bubbles may emanate from the stomach as well as from the lung

From Metheny (1988).

fat, vitamin and mineral composition. Nutrients are present in simple forms, are easily digested and absorbed and leave minimal residue in the bowel. Patients with some malabsorption disorders may not tolerate some of the prepared formulae. Functioning of the patient's digestive tract and hydrational status are assessed before the preparation is selected.

Feeds can be administered cold or warm. In view of the fact that pathogens multiply in warm conditions and cold feeds have not been shown to have any major effect on gastric emptying and motility, it could be suggested that feeds should be administered as cool as can be tolerated (Pritchard and David, 1988). If this is the initial feeding, an explanation of the procedure is given to the patient. The head of the bed is elevated to 35–40°.

Testing feeding tube placement is a responsibility of the nurse prior to the administration of any feed. The usual methods of testing for placement do not work well with the newer small-bore nasogastric tubes. These tubes are more likely to become dislocated and it is more difficult to identify displacement of the tip into the respiratory tract. Table 16.5 summarizes conclusions

made following a review of the literature on the effectiveness of six commonly used clinical measures of tube placement. Metheny (1988) recommends waiting for radiological confirmation of initial placement prior to initiating feeds, and repeating X-rays after any event such as violent coughing or vomiting that might dislocate the tube. The most promising clinical tool to assess placement of nasogastric tubes seems to be pH determination of fluid aspirated from the tube. Standards need to be set for the interpretation of results, and interfering variables such as the administration of antacids must be identified.

A continuous infusion of the feed is given via a giving set attached to the nasogastric tube. The container with the liquid feed is hung on an intravenous stand. The fluid feed is given slowly, for example 500 ml over 6 hours, and the speed is regulated by a pressure regulator on the tubing.

The feed is administered slowly and allowed to flow into the stomach by gravity. To avoid air entering the stomach, a collapsible plastic feeding container is used. When the feed is completed, the tube is flushed with

30–40 ml of water and clamped. If regurgitation or vomiting occurs, it may be that the prescribed volume is too great. A smaller amount given more frequently may be tolerated.

Frequent mouth care is necessary and the nostril through which the tube passes requires attention.

The patient is encouraged to remain in a sitting position for at least one hour after each feed to decrease regurgitation and aspiration and to promote stomach emptying.

Gastrostomy. This is the establishment of an opening into the stomach through the abdominal wall and the insertion of a tube through which fluids and liquefied food may be introduced directly into the stomach. A general anaesthetic is not usually required as the tube is inserted by percutaneous endoscopy through the oesophagus, into the stomach and out through the abdominal wall through a small stab wound.

A gastrostomy may be a temporary procedure during a period of corrective surgery or it may be permanent when an oesophageal obstruction is considered inoperable or there has been an oesophagectomy.

The patient generally finds it difficult to accept a gastrostomy because the natural process of eating and its associated pleasures such as taste and sociability have been removed. Personnel caring for the patient, the family and friends should acknowledge to the patient that they understand any negative feelings this leads to.

Regular feeds are given according to the patient's needs. The food preparations used in gastrostomy are similar to those cited above for gastric tube feedings or are the person's normal diet liquidized. The required amount of feeds is given through an administration bag attached to the gastric tube. The patient's head and shoulders are elevated and he or she remains in this position for ½ hour after the feeding to prevent regurgitation into the oesophagus and leakage around the tube. The tube is cleansed following the feeding by flushing it with 30–40 ml of water and it is then clamped.

A gauze or transparent (Opsite) dressing is applied to the wound following inspection of the skin for excoriation. The escape of even a small amount of gastric juice from around the tube may irritate the skin because of its acid pepsin content. The gauze dressing is changed whenever there is drainage, and the skin is cleansed thoroughly with water and dried. A protective coating of petroleum jelly or a prescribed ointment or powder may then be applied. Should excoriation occur, application of a hydrocolloid dressing or wafer following cleansing of the skin may both promote healing and protect the skin from further damage.

The feeds may have to be adjusted from time to time. Too much fat or carbohydrate may cause diarrhoea. Complaints of a full feeling or abdominal discomfort may necessitate a decrease in the amount of feeds given. A record of the patient's weight is made which also serves as a guide in adjusting the caloric value of the feed's formula. This should be recorded twice weekly, and for greater accuracy the person should wear the same type of clothing whenever the weight is measured.

The patient's mouth will require special attention. Frequent cleansing and rinsing are essential.

If the patient is to be fed by gastrostomy over a long period while various stages of treatment are carried out or if the gastrostomy is permanent, teaching in the correct techniques is essential for both patient and family. Information should be provided regarding supplies of prescribed commercial feeding preparations and equipment. The nurse may direct the family to the appropriate community resources for the necessary assistance or make the contact for them.

Jejunostomy. A jejunostomy tube may be inserted and used for feedings when it is necessary to bypass the stomach as a result of surgery or reflux.

3. Promotion of coping and control of stress

Emotional and physical stress affect gastric function, and ill health of any type presents an additional stress to the individual. Whether stress is a contributing factor or a result of gatsrointestinal disorder, the nurse can play a role in identifying both the causes of the stress and the person's responses to it, and help that individual to explore, test and evaluate various coping strategies. Research on nursing measures to alter the stress–gastrointestinal relationship has not advanced sufficiently to provide direction for nursing practice. Nurses can facilitate the expression and exploration of feelings, provide information and teach patients self-management skills to alleviate the stresses imposed by the illness. The exploration of coping strategies that work for the individual and the development of relaxation and other stress management programmes with the patient and family fall within the role of the nurse. Nurses can teach muscle relaxation techniques and the use of guided imagery. They can inform the individual and significant others about resources available to them in their community and work setting. They can also help patients to identify stressors in their daily lives, to develop strategies to alter their life-styles to avoid these precipitating factors or to implement coping strategies when these situations occur.

Evaluation

The evaluation of the efficacy of nursing care for the person with disorders of secretion, digestion and motility of the stomach and duodenum should reflect achievement of the outcome criteria established for the individual and their unique situation. When evaluating the care delivered it is important to remember that it is not just the individual's response to management of illness which is important but also the life situation and personal expectations.

Nursing Care for the Person Requiring Gastric Surgery

Care of the patient requiring surgery is discussed in Chapter 11. The same general principles apply for the patient undergoing gastric surgery. Special considerations applicable to the patient experiencing gastric surgery are outlined below. The amount of gastric drainage obtained postoperatively and the extent of the nutritional deficit resulting from the surgical intervention vary according to the type and extent of gastric tissue excised during the surgical procedure. In clinical practice, the care plan is modified to meet the specific needs of the individual.

PREOPERATIVE CARE

The *goals* for the patient during the preoperative period are to:

- Improve fluid and nutritional status.
- Learn and practice deep breathing and coughing techniques.
- Reduce anxiety experienced by the individual and significant others.

If the patient's nutritional and fluid status are poor, enteral or total parenteral nutrition may be instituted. Intravenous solutions may be administered to increase the person's fluid volume and to correct electrolyte imbalances.

The incision will be in the upper abdomen below the chest; it is important therefore that the patient be competent at performing deep breathing and coughing techniques and understand the importance of performing these postoperatively.

Explanations about the surgery and hospital routines usually help to decrease anxiety in both the patient and family. The nurse should also take time to assess their learning needs and to determine their perceptions and expectations for the surgery and postsurgical outcomes.

POSTOPERATIVE CARE

Health problems common to persons undergoing gastric surgery include:

- *Altered fluid and electrolyte balance* related to gastric intubation and suction.
- *Malnutrition* due to preoperative nutritional deficits and decreased food intake postoperatively.
- *Pain* due to the surgical intervention.
- *Altered breathing pattern* due to incisional pain and the location of the incision.
- *Deficit of knowledge* related to postoperative care and skills required to achieve self-care.

GOALS

The patient will demonstrate:

- A patent gastric drainage system.
- Fluid volume intake of at least 2.5 l/day and output in balance.
- Absence of pain.
- A clean, dry, intact incision.
- Respirations, pulse and blood pressure within usual range.
- Maintenance of nutritional status as shown by a weight loss of less than 2 kg.
- Understanding of prescribed dietary regimen.
- Understanding of plans for follow-up care.

NURSING INTERVENTION

Gastric drainage

The patient will return from the operating room with a nasogastric, nasointestinal or gastrostomy tube in place.

The characteristics of the drainage fluid are noted and the total volume is recorded at regular intervals. Intermittent aspiration or free drainage will be ordered depending on the surgeon's preference. It is important that the patency of the tube be maintained to avoid a build up of secretions in the stomach. The drainage will probably be coloured by blood at first but usually clears in a few hours. The doctor is notified if large amounts of blood appear or if the drainage continues to be blood-coloured. The volume is an important factor in determining the fluid and electrolyte replacement needed. Loss of gastric secretions incurs a loss of hydrogen ions (H^+) and chloride ions (Cl^-) that may result in alkalosis. Loss of intestinal fluid may result in a severe loss of hydrogen carbonate (HCO_3^-) and potassium and cause acidosis. The number of days for which the nasogastric tube is left in and oral fluids are withheld varies with each surgeon and will also depend on the patient's progress. The nasogastric tube is usually removed when normal bowel sounds return.

Removal of the tube
Before removal, the tube may be clamped and left in place while oral fluid is introduced. If the fluid is tolerated, an order may then be given to remove the tube. The gastric tube is withdrawn gently and quickly. The patient is instructed to hold the breath to avoid possible apsiration of fluid or mucus that may escape from the tube into the oropharynx during removal.

The intestinal tube is removed slowly, a few inches at a time. The lumen into the air-inflated balloon is opened, and the air is allowed to escape. When slight resistance is encountered owing to the intestinal peristalsis, the tube is left for a few minutes and then withdrawal is resumed. The doctor should be notified if resistance to removal persists; force should not be used. If the tube has a mercury-filled bag at its distal end, the latter is brought out through the mouth and the bag removed. The remainder of the tube may then be pulled through the nostril. As with the removal of the gastric tube, the patient is asked to hold the breath as the terminal portion of the tube is drawn from the oesophagus.

The mouth should be cleansed and rinsed immediately following the removal of the tube. The patient may complain of soreness in the throat and nose which usually subsides in a day or two.

Pain management

Considerable pain is experienced by the patient who has had gastric surgery. Analgesics such as pethidine are usually prescribed to relieve discomfort. Analgesia should be given regularly for the first few days and administered prior to activities which could increase discomfort, such as physiotherapy, turning and mobilization. Analgesics are usually administered intramuscularly but continuous intravenous or sublingual routes are increasingly being used. Systems which allow self-administration of postoperative analgesia are used in some centres; these enhance patient control and increase participation in pain management. Continual assessment of pain levels is necessary in the postoperative period if the goal of a pain-free patient is to be achieved. Frequent regular change of position helps to relieve pain and discomfort.

Frequent cleansing and moistening of the mouth are necessary to lessen the patient's discomfort while the nasogastric tube is in place and oral fluids are restricted. The tube may cause irritation that results in mucus secretion which, if allowed to collect, might be aspirated. The nostril through which the tube is passed is cleansed and moistened and receives a very light application of mineral oil or water-soluble lubricant to prevent the accumulation and crusting of secretions.

Promotion of respiratory function

If a total gastrectomy was performed the incision may involve the thorax, and chest drainage tubes will have been established. Remind the patient hourly to take five to ten deep breaths and to cough several times using the staged coughing technique to prevent undue tension on the suture line. Provide necessary encouragement and support by holding a small pillow lightly over the operative site and placing a hand on the patient's back during the coughing. Acknowledge the patient's distress but at the same time emphasize the importance of deep breathing and coughing in the prevention of other problems.

When vital signs are stable, the head of the bed may be gradually elevated to promote deeper breathing and gastric drainage. Change the patient's position at regular frequent intervals: side-to-side to back-to-side. Ambulation usually starts on the first postoperative day.

Fluid and nutritional intake

Parenteral fluids are used to sustain the patient over the first few days. Different procedures are used to introduce the first fluids into the gastrointestinal tract; the surgeon may have the nasogastric tube removed and small stated amounts of water given every half hour or every hour. The amount is gradually increased if tolerated. The directive may be to introduce a specific amount of water at intervals through the nasogastric tube, which is then clamped.

If the patient tolerates the increased amounts of water without experiencing vomiting, pain or distension, liquids such as tea, fruit squash, soup and milk may be progressively introduced over 2–3 days but only when normal bowel sounds are heard on auscultation.

With normal progress, the patient is usually receiving a soft diet by the fifth to seventh day. The volume given at any one time remains small because of the reduced capacity of the stomach. Foods high in calories are selected and served frequently. The patient's weight is recorded regularly, and the doctor is advised if there is a loss or a failure to gain. Inability of the patient to take the prescribed diet, any regurgitation, vomiting, abdominal distension or complaint of pain is reported.

By the time the patient is ready to leave the hospital, a light diet of high-caloric foods divided into six meals is usually tolerated. Fluids may be omitted from the meals and taken in between so their volume will not prevent the patient from taking sufficient solid food. The patient is advised to gradually increase the amount taken at regular meals and, if no discomfort is experienced, eventually resume three or four meals with milk and other fluids taken between them.

Vitamins B complex and vitamin C and iron may be ordered, since the natural food sources of these will be restricted in the diet for a period of time.

Dumping syndrome

The patient is observed for signs of the 'dumping syndrome', which is precipitated by eating. These include: nausea, crampy abdominal pains, distension, diarrhoea, muscular weakness, dizziness, fainting, palpitation, sweating, rapid pulse and paleness. Explain to the patient and family that these symptoms occur when gastric surgery results in disruption or bypass of the pyloric sphincter.

Assess the patient for emotional factors which may contribute to the development of the dumping syndrome.

Measures to relieve the dumping syndrome include the avoidance of large meals and a reduced intake of salty and sweet foods; no fluids are given with meals. Six small, dry meals consisting mainly of proteins and fats are planned to meet the patient's caloric requirement. Liquids are taken between meals to maintain normal hydration but should be limited during the half hour preceding and following a meal. The patient is advised to eat slowly and to lie down for a half hour following each meal. The symptoms cause considerable emotional reaction in the patient. Encouragement to persevere with the suggested dietary regimen and reassurance that the condition will gradually subside as the gastrointestinal tract adapts to the structural changes is required. Anticholinergic drugs may be prescribed to decrease gastrointestinal motility.

Nutrional deficiency

Assess the patient for signs and symptoms of nutritional deficiencies, which include: the inability to maintain normal weight; insufficient food intake; feelings of satiety and overfullness following a small amount of food.

Assist the patient in developing a dietary plan that includes frequent high-caloric intakes (small amounts at first and gradually increased as tolerated).

Assess the patient's perception and responses to the necessary continuing dietary modifications following surgery. The need for a period of time for the digestive system to adjust to the changes is discussed.

Anaemia

Monitoring of the patient's red blood cell count and

haemoglobin is done regularly following gastric resection and information is elicited as to energy, fatigue and food elements in the diet. The patient may develop an iron deficiency as a result of decreased iron absorption. Normal absorption is facilitated by gastric acidity which is reduced if a gastrectomy is done. The bypassing of the duodenum by a gastrojejunostomy may also reduce the amount of iron absorption. The deficiency may in some instances be due to a poor dietary intake of foods that provide iron (red meat, liver, leafy vegetables, whole milk, eggs and certain cereals). A supplemental preparation of iron is prescribed and the diet corrected to contain the necessary sources.

Anaemia frequently develops as a result of a deficiency in the secretion of the intrinsic factor (due to the loss of gastric mucosa by the gastric resection) which promotes the absorption of vitamin B_{12}. It may develop within a few months or not until 2–3 years after the gastrectomy. The patient may be given weekly vitamin B_{12} by subcutaneous or intramuscular injections until a normal erythrocyte count is established. A maintenance dose is then given monthly throughout the remainder of the patient's life.

Postprandial hypoglycaemia

The patient who has extensive gastric surgery may develop hypoglycaemia 2–3 hours after taking a meal. Symptoms include: weakness, tremor, faintness, sweating and palpitation. The blood sugar level may fall to 2.7–3.3 mmol/l.

The hypoglycaemia is attributed to an abnormally rapid absorption of glucose from the intestine, causing a sudden hyperglycaemia. This stimulates a release of excessive insulin which rapidly lowers the blood sugar concentration to an abnormally low level. A high protein, low carbohydrate diet is recommended to eliminate the problem. Frequent small meals are helpful. Some forms of sugar (honey, lump sugar or orange juice) should be quickly available and taken when the early symptoms of hypoglycaemia are experienced.

Osteomalacia

This is characterized by decalcification of the bones and weakening of their structure, and is a rare complication following gastrectomy. This is attributed to decreased absorption of vitamin D and calcium. Associated symptoms include diarrhoea and steatorrhoea. Treatment involves administration of vitamin D and calcium supplements.

Patient and family teaching

The patient and family are helped to develop a plan to modify the diet and activity to accommodate temporary and long-term limitations imposed by the surgery. The importance of frequent small meals of non-irritating foods high in calories is explained. The size of the meals may be gradually increased when comfortably tolerated, as the remaining portion of the stomach progressively adapts to larger quantities. After several months, the person may find three regular meals can again be managed. Suggestions are made as to food selection and preparation. Written dietary instructions and outlines should be provided to reinforce verbal information. Involvement of the dietitian early in the patient's care will help in the dietary education process.

The patient is advised to weigh regularly and to report to the clinic or doctor on scheduled dates. If pain, vomiting, progressive loss of weight or other distressing symptoms occur the doctor is contacted promptly. Normal activities are resumed as tolerated and should not interfere with regularity of meals.

If a total gastrectomy has been done or a large section of the stomach removed, the patient will require regular parenteral administration of a maintenance dose of cyanocobalamin (vitamin B_{12}). The importance of receiving this is stressed and arrangments are made for the vitamin B_{12} administration at the scheduled times; it may be given by the individual's general practitioner or community nurse. Alternatively, a significant other may wish to be taught to administer the drug.

Information should be given to the patient and significant others concerning support available in the community. Early referral to the community nursing service will ensure continuity of care. Contact telephone numbers and addresses should be given to the patient.

EVALUATION

Evaluation is based on the goals determined for each patient. On discharge from the surgical unit, the patient and significant others should be familiar with the immediate dietary needs and what to expect as he or she adapts to the changes and gradually tolerates increases in the amounts and types of foods and liquids. The patient and significant others should be familiar with measures to take to alleviate the symptoms of dumping syndrome. They should be aware of community resources for dietary assistance and any required wound care. Follow-up medical supervision is planned, scheduled appointments are given to the patient and transport arrangements discussed.

THE PERSON WITH DISORDERS OF MOTILITY, SECRETION AND ABSORPTION IN THE INTESTINES

Disorders of the *small intestine* may cause disturbances in: the movement of the content along the alimentary canal; secretion, which may incur a problem in digestion or absorption; or absorption alone. A prolonged or serious dysfunction threatens the patient's nutritional status.

A disturbance in the function of the *large intestine* interferes with the excretion of bowel waste and, if the right half of the colon is involved, the normal absorption of water and salts may be reduced and cause dehydration.

A disorder in motility, secretion or absorption rarely occurs independently; a disturbance in one is usually accompanied by dysfunction in one or both of the other intestinal functions. For example, increased secretion may accelerate motility, decreased absorption causes dysfunction in motility and elimination, and inflammation usually causes a disturbance in all three functions.

Alteration in Bowel Elimination

Causative factors and defining characteristics for the assessment of problems *relevant to elimination* are listed in Table 16.6.

1. DIARRHOEA

The term diarrhoea implies an accelerated movement of content through the intestine with a decrease in mixing and absorptive processes resulting in frequent liquid or unformed stools. The faeces pass through the colon before the normal amount of water is absorbed.

Diarrhoea is a symptom of many different disorders which may be within the bowel or may be extrinsic to the intestine. Changes characteristic of organic disease may occur in the intestine and result in diarrhoea, or the bowel may be structurally normal with the hypermotility being functional. The most common causes of diarrhoea are presented here as intrinsic or extrinsic, although there are many different aetiological classifications in medical literature.

INTRINSIC CAUSES

Normally the stimulus for peristalsis arises within the intestine. It may cause direct stimulation of the muscle tissue, or it may initiate sensory nerve impulses that are transmitted into the central nervous system, resulting in parasympathetic nerve impulses being carried out to the intestine that then stimulate its motility. Disease or irritation within the bowel which may increase either direct stimulation or reflex hypermotility include the following:

Malabsorption. Impaired absorption of foods may be due to incomplete digestion or to a defect in the absorptive process of the small intestine. Obviously with reduced digestion and absorption, an increase in the bulk of the colon content results and is a stimulus to intestinal motility. The stools are bulky, have an offensive odour and usually contain large amounts of fats which are irritating to the bowel mucosa and initiate reflex peristalsis. The presence of unabsorbed osmotically active substances such as glucose or a disaccharide that cannot be split, causes osmotic diarrhoea. The increased intralumenal osmotic pressure causes water to move into the intestine, producing diarrhoea. General malnutrition is also evident.

Table 16.6 Potential problems of patients with altered bowel elimination.

Patient problem	Causes	Clinical characteristics
1. Diarrhoea	• Bacterial organisms and enterotoxins • Intestinal neoplasms • Diet high in roughage or spicy foods • Allergy to ingested foods • Malabsorption syndrome • Diverticulitis • Laxatives • Antibiotics • Inflammatory disorders of the intestinal tract • Emotional stress • Systemic diseases causing toxaemia (e.g. hyperthryroidism, uraemia, endocrine tumours) • Radiotherapy to the abdomen and pelvis • Chemotherapy (5-fluorouracil, cisplatin)	• Loose, watery stools • Several bowel movements per day • Dehydration: loss of skin turgor, weight loss, dry mouth • Abdominal cramping and pain • Weakness • Increased bowel sounds
2. Constipation	• Disease of the bowel • Decreased intestinal motility • Altered innervation to bowel and anal sphincter • Megacolon • Inadequate fluid intake • Lack of fibre or cellulose in diet • Physical inactivity • Medication (e.g. opiates) • Weakness of abdominal muscles and diaphragm	• Abdominal pain • Abdominal distension • Sensation of fullness and pressure in rectum • Loss of appetite • Headache • Dry, hard, formed stools • Infrequent bowel movements (less than three times per week) • Straining on defecation

Table 16.6 *Continued*

Patient problem	Causes	Clinical characteristics
	• Irregular habits of defacation • Loss of bowel tone from excessive use of laxatives • Haemorrhoids • Hypercalcaemia • Tumour mass in abdomen or pelvis • Alteration in mental state	
3. Impaction	• Altered tone, motility and sensation in bowel as a result of ageing process • Immobility • Central nervous system disorders	• Cramping pain • Oozing liquid stools • Headache • Loss of appetite • Abdominal distension • Dry, hard formed stools • Palpable hard rectal mass • Straining at defecation • No bowel movement for over three days
4. Incontinence	• Constipation • Faecal impaction • Excessive use of laxatives and enemas • Drugs (e.g. iron, methyldopa) • Diabetes • Diverticulitis • Proctitis • Carcinoma • Rectal prolapse • Regional enteritis (Crohn's disease) • Malabsorption syndrome • Ischaemic colitis • Neurogenic disorders	• Involuntary defecation • Constant soiling of clothing • Faeces soft and semiformed or loose • Absence of sensation or urge to defecate • Diminished propulsive contractions on rectogram

Inflammation. Chronic inflammatory bowel diseases (Crohn's disease, ulcerative colitis and diverticulitis) all cause inflammatory processes in different parts of the gastrointestinal tract. Crohn's disease and ulcerative colitis, while progressive in nature, are characterized by periods of remission and exacerbation. The problems resulting from diverticulitis are constant.

Diverticulitis. A pouch or sac may occur in the wall of the intestine and is known as a diverticulum (Figure 16.7). It may be congenital or may develop as a result of a weakening of an area of the muscle tissue in the wall. There may be several diverticula, or the defect may occur singly.

Diverticula of the large intestine are more likely to give rise to trouble, as the more solid faecal content tends to collect and be retained in the sac, setting up an inflammation that causes increased reflex peristalsis and diarrhoea.

Laxatives. Many laxatives act by direct irritation of the intestinal mucosa, resulting in the content being hurried through the colon before the normal amount of water is absorbed.

Infection. Food or fluid contaminated by salmonella, shigella or staphylococcal organisms is the most

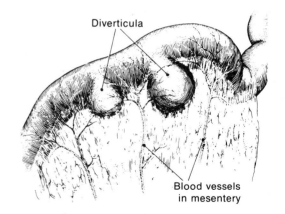

Figure 16.7 Intestinal diverticulum.

common cause of intestinal infection and may be referred to as bacterial food poisoning.

The shigella bacillia cause bacillary dysentery, and the primary source is usually the excreta of an infected person. This disease is rare, except under crowded and poor sanitary conditions.

The salmonella bacilli may inhabit the intestine of man, fowl and animals and may be the source of infection to others. It may be transmitted by the meat of infected animals and by food or water contaminated by the excreta of infected humans or animals. Sporadic outbreaks occur and may be due to a human carrier employed in the handling of food. Ingested salmonella or shigella organisms multiply, causing irritation and inflammation of the intestine, resulting in diarrhoea accompanied by crampy abdominal pain, fever, nausea and vomiting.

Hypersecretory bacterial diarrhoea may be caused by toxin-producing organisms such as staphylococci, salmonella, shigella and Vibrio cholera. The enterotoxins stimulate the release of excessive amounts of fluid and electrolytes by the small intestine.

Neoplasms. Diarrhoea may be a symptom of a malignant neoplasm of the colon and may be alternated with periods of constipation.

Dietary Factors. An excessive amount of coarse foods or highly seasoned irritating food may produce hypermotility of the bowel. Occasionally, allergy to a certain food may account for diarrhoea; if the intestinal mucosa is sensitive to the food, it becomes hyperaemic and oedematous and causes increased reflex hypermotility.

Antibiotics. Diarrhoea sometimes accompanies the oral administration of antibiotics. They may irritate the mucosa or alter the normal bacterial flora of the intestinal tract. The most frequent offenders are the tetracycline preparations.

Idiopathic inflammation. Patients with ulcerative colitis or regional enteritis experience severe diarrhoea. No specific cause has been recognized for either condition.

Extrinsic causes. Diarrhoea accompanies a variety of disorders in which the stimulus that results in increased parasympathetic innervation to the bowel originates outside the intestine.

Emotional stress. Anxiety or underlying tension may be associated with diarrhoea, producing a condition which is referred to as the irritable bowel or colon syndrome. On investigation, disturbances may be revealed that are secondary to the diarrhoea, but there is no organic disease in the intestine or elsewhere. Intestinal hypermobility and hypersecretion occur with both physical and mental stress. A study of the patient's total life situation may reveal a specific emotional conflict or ineffective coping that may account for the problem.

General or systemic disorders. Frequently, diarrhoea is associated with general diseases, particularly if they cause toxaemia. Examples of such conditions are acute infectious disease, hyperthryoidism and uraemia.

ASSESSMENT

It is important to obtain the following information:
- The patient's previous bowel habits.
- The number of bowel movements each day.
- The volume and consistency of the stools.

- Whether the stools contain abnormal components, such as blood and excessive mucus.
- Whether the patient experiences abdominal pain.
- Whether there is exacerbation with certain foods or activities.
- Whether the diarrhoea is worse during the day or the night. Functional diarrhoea tends to occur during the day, while that associated with organic disease is generally as disturbing at night as during the day.
- The systemic effects on the person:
  (a) What is the hydrational status?
  (b) Is the temperature elevated?
  (c) Is the person exhausted because of loss of sleep?
  (d) Is the person losing weight?
- Whether or not there are increased bowel sounds.
- The individual's perception of and reaction to the diarrhoea.
- The condition of the skin around the anus and over pressure areas.
- Fluid and electrolyte balances.

GOALS

The person will demonstrate:

- Formed stools
- A return to the usual frequency of bowel elimination
- Fluid balance and absence of signs of dehydration
- Integrity of skin.

NURSING INTERVENTION

Measures to decrease peristalsis

Peristalsis of the small and large intestines may be slowed by the following measures:
1. Removal of the cause of the diarrhoea. This may involve the administration of prescribed antibiotics for intestinal infection, avoidance of specific foods for the patient with a malabsorption disorder or an intestinal allergy, and avoidance of laxatives and treatment for systemic diseases such as hyperthroidism or uraemia.
2. Changing the diet to eliminate spicy foods, fruit juices, raw fruits and vegetables and gas-forming foods.
3. Use of drugs. Various medications may be used in the treatment of diarrhoea:
   (a) Drugs to reduce intestinal spasm and motility may be ordered. Examples are diphenoxylate hydrochloride (Lomotil) and loperamide hydrochloride (Imodium).
   (b) Opiates such as codeine phosphate are believed to increase absorption by acting on the opiate receptors, e.g. kaolin and morphine mixture.
   (c) Drugs to provide a protective coating on the intestinal mucosa or to provide an adsorbent, which condenses and holds irritating substances, are used. Examples are kaolin, aluminium hydroxide gel and bismuth subcarbonate.
   (d) An anti-infective drug may be ordered if the diarrhoea is of microbial origin. Sulphonamide preparations that are poorly absorbed, have a

local effect but are less frequently used orally; examples are calcium sulphaloxate, phthalylsulphathiazole and sulphaguanidine. Sulphasalazine (Salazoryrin) is indicated for the maintenance of remission in ulcerative colitis and Crohn's disease.

Rest

The patient with diarrhoea feels weak and fatigued. Rest periods are provided and the person is encouraged to relax and pursue sedentary activities such as reading or watching television. If necessary, the patient is assisted to the bathroom or a commode chair may be used at the bedside. The call-button should be answered promptly to avoid unnecessary effort or anxiety for the patient in attempting to reach the bathroom in time. Some people are unable to relax and rest because of a constant fear of not getting to the bathroom in time; in such instances it may be helpful to make an exception and leave a covered commode at the bedside within the patient's reach.

Fluids and nutrition

Fluids and electrolytes are replaced by intravenous infusions. If oral fluids are tolerated, water or clear soup may be given but carbonated drinks, whole milk, fruit juice and iced fluids are best avoided.

The diet is expanded as soon as possible to reduce the possibility of nutritional deficiencies. A high-calorie, high-vitamin and high-protein diet is gradually introduced, and the patient is observed as to the intestinal response. Roughage and gas-producing foods are restricted at first; whole grain bread and cereals, raw fruits and vegetables and highly seasoned and fried foods are not used. Concentrated sweets and fats are likely to be poorly tolerated. Fibre-containing foods and roughage are gradually introduced as tolerated. If the diarrhoea is due to malabsorption, a gluten-free diet may be ordered in which foods are avoided that contain any wheat, rye, and barley grains or flour.

The first few mouthfuls of a meal may initiate a mass peristaltic wave, and the meal is interrupted by defecation. The patient may require some persuasion to continue the meal due to fear of provoking another attack of diarrhoea.

Hygienic factors

The patient who is mobile should be located as near to the toilet as possible on the ward and, if confined to bed, privacy should be provided so the patient is less embarrassed by frequent use of the commode.

The anal region should be left clean after each defecation and, if the skin around the anus is irritated, it is washed and a protective cream applied. Soiled bedding or clothing is changed promptly. Provision is made for thorough washing of the patient's hands after each defecation while the nurse should also remember the importance of thorough handwashing. The patient may very well be embarrassed by the recurring episodes of diarrhoea. The nurse therefore should be sensitive

and supportive, being aware of the demoralizing effects this problem may have on the patient. It may help to provide distractions for the patient, particularly if confined to a side ward as a precaution against the spread of infection.

Control of infection

Cases of acute diarrhoea are considered potentially infectious until otherwise indicated. Precautions are used to prevent the possible spread of infection to others. The hands are scrubbed with soap and running water after each contact. Contaminated waste such as soiled dressings or swabs are put into bags which are sealed and labelled with a biohazard warning.

When performing any nursing care procedures requiring contact with the patient's faeces, disposable gloves are worn (see Chapter 6).

Acute infectious diarrhoea may readily spread throughout a family, school, hall of residence or neighbourhood because of a common source of infected food or water by the spread from an infected person. The nurse may play an important role in the prevention of diarrhoea by alerting people to the hazards of exposed and unrefrigerated foods, particularly meat and those with cream filling or topping. Opportunities may arise to emphasize the hygienic handling of food and the importance of thorough hand washing after going to the toilet and the handling of soiled clothing.

Carers should be informed of precautions they should take to prevent spread to others. Should other individuals who live with that person develop acute diarrhoea the likely source of the problem will need to be investigated.

If a large number of cases are found in a school or community, the local health authorities should be notified so that a systematic investigation as to the possible source may be instituted. Occasionally, acute diarrhoea may spread through the patients on one ward of a hospital. The primary source of such an outbreak should be sought. Ward personnel are urged to practice strict precautions, for infection may be carried from one patient to another or from a ward worker to patients through failure to thoroughly wash the hands between patients, after handling bedpans or linen, or after going to the toilet.

Evaluation

Evaluation of the goals and outcome criteria is based on examination of the person's stools, documented evidence of a decrease in the frequency of defecation and absence of fluid and electrolyte imbalances, as well as on the patient's reported perceptions that the diarrhoea is decreased or absent. For individuals with chronic bowel disease that causes diarrhoea, success of the interventions may be determined when they resume active participation in social and recreational activities.

Evaluation of the spread of infection may be determined on a particular nursing unit or by an infection control committee. All incidence of infection are reported and recorded. Quality assurance programmes provide objective data on which to measure success in preventing the spread of infection to other patients and to health care providers.

2. CONSTIPATION

The majority of persons normally defecate once every 24 hours but there is considerable variance in the frequency among healthy persons. Some persons have more than one bowel movement daily, while others may have an evacuation of a normal moist stool once every 2 or 3 days. Such variances in frequency of bowel elimination are compatible with health. An individual is considered to be constipated if bowel elimination is inexplicably delayed for several days or if the stool is so hard and dry that it is difficult to expel.

Constipation may be a delay in the passage of faeces through the colon, referred to as colonic constipation, or it may be a prolonged retention of the faeces in the rectum, designated as *rectal constipation* or *dyschezia*,

CAUSES

The causes of constipation are many and varied. It may be associated with organic disease, or it may be a functional disturbance.

Disease within the colon or rectum may narrow the lumen of the bowel and offer resistance to the forward movement of content. Common examples are: neoplasms of the intestine; inflammation, which causes spasm, scarring and adhesions; and partial volvulus (twisting of the bowel). Severe ascites (accumulation of fluid in the peritoneal cavity) or a tumour, such as an ovarian cyst or uterine fibroid, may compress the colon and delay the movement of intestinal content.

Failure of the normal propulsive movement may occur due to some disturbance or imbalance in the innervation of the intestine. The derangement may result in excessive tone and spasm in a segment of the bowel that retards the movement of the content. The spasm may be induced by a hypersensitivity of the colon or by anxiety. Constipation may be associated with injury or degeneration of the spinal cord or cauda equina, which affects the nerve supply to the colon and rectum.

Megacolon (Hirschsprung's disease) may account for constipation in infants. It is a congenital anomaly in which there is an absence of certain nerve structures (parasympathetic ganglia) in a segment of the colon, resulting in failure of peristalsis in the affected portion of the bowel. Surgical correction may be necessary.

Constipation may be associated with any illness in which there is diminished intake of food and fluid or in cases in which the diet is modified and lacks fibre, resulting in less residue. The lesser amount of food does not provide sufficient bulk to stimulate peristalsis. Dehydration causes a small, dry, hard stool that may irritate the colon, causing spasm, or may fail to stimulate normal colon motility.

Constipation is frequently secondary to physical inactivity or prolonged bed rest. It is a common complaint among persons with sedentary occupations who probably ride to and from work and do not

participate in any type of physical exercise.

Occasionally, drugs used in treatment may decrease intestinal motility and delay excretion. This increases mixing of the faeces and exposure to the absorptive surface, which dries out the faeces and produces constipation. Common examples of such drugs are opiates (e.g. codeine) and anticholinergic drugs (e.g. propantheline bromide (Pro-banthine)).

Expulsion of the faeces is aided by increasing the intra-abdominal pressure to compress the colon and rectum. This involves contraction of the muscles of the abdominal wall and of the diaphragm. Weakness of these muscles due to disease, ageing, malnutrition or inactivity may contribute to constipation. Similarly, lack of tone in the intestinal musculature or weakness of the levator ani muscles may impair peristalsis and expulsive power.

Frequent causes of constipation in persons who are not ill are faulty defecation habits, faulty diet and the habitual use of laxatives. If the urge to defecate is ignored and evacuation delayed, the reflex becomes weak as the rectal mucosa adapts to the pressure of the content. Repeated failure to respond to defecation reflex may eventually result in the rectum becoming insensitive to the presence of a faecal mass and the reflex is not initiated. The person may delay response to the defecation urge because it is inconvenient or because toilet facilities may not be available.

A deficiency of foods with cellulose and fibrous content in the diet may be the cause of constipation. Refined foods and those that leave little residue after absorption fail to produce sufficient bulk to stimulate colonic motility.

Many persons have an inordinate concern about bowel elimination and think they must have a daily bowel movement or a frequent purge and resort to unnecessary, repeated use of a laxative. Loss of intestinal tone and reduced peristaltic response to normal food residue follow the use of a laxative, and then too often the laxative is repeated. The colon is not allowed to regain its natural rhythmic response to the normal faecal mass.

Constipation may cause considerable discomfort; the person may experience abdominal pain, a full feeling and abdominal distension. There is a loss of appetite accompanied by headache and eventually nausea and vomiting. The hard dry masses of faecal matter may damage the intestinal mucosa and lead to a fissure. Haemorrhoids are frequently the result of chronic constipation.

The objectives are that the person will:
1. Relieve the constipation (short term).
2. Develop regular bowel elimination (long term).

ASSESSMENT

The nursing history includes information about:
- The person's usual bowel elimination habits.
- Any unusual effort or stimulation used to promote defecation including the use of laxatives or enemas.
- The person's perceptions of what is normal bowel elimination.
- The person's eating habits: types of foods taken and

the volume of fluid taken daily.
- The person's level of awareness of surroundings and bodily functions.
- The person's problem of constipation and potentially related factors:
  (a) The duration and severity of the problem.
  (b) Recent changes in usual eating habits, fluid intake and physical activity.
  (c) The person's perceptions of the problem.
  (d) Pain, abdominal cramps, passing of gas associated with constipation.
  (e) History of disorders or medication therapy that may have altered food intake, digestion or absorption of foods or bowel motility or sensation.
- The person's living arrangements and the availability of toilet facilities.
- The family's knowledge of: foods that contain fibre and the function of fibre in promoting bowel function; the need to maintain an adequate fluid intake; the benefits of exercise and activity; and the action and untoward effects of various types of laxatives.

The person may be asked to keep a record over 2–4 days to determine the frequency and time of bowel elimination, the volume and characteristics of the faeces. Any warning signs of constipation experienced by the patient, such as abdominal cramps or flatulence should be noted, along with the patient's own feelings about the problem.

GOALS

The person will demonstrate:

- Understanding of the role of dietary fibre and fluid intake in stool formation and defecation.
- Awareness of the role of regular physical activity in the promotion of bowel elimination.
- A plan to increase dietary fibre and fluid intake and to obtain regular physical activity.
- A planned schedule for defecation.
- Understanding and use of techniques to promote bowel elimination.
- Absence of use of laxatives.
- Regular bowel elimination.

NURSING INTERVENTION

Table 16.7 lists the steps to be implemented in formulating a plan to develop regular bowel elimination habits for a patient.

Establishing a regular schedule

It is helpful to explain to the person in simple terms the physiological mechanism of defecation so the significance of responding to the initial urge for defecation may be understood. The importance of establishing a regular time for bowel elimination is stressed, for most individuals about half an hour after breakfast is the usual time for defecation; the ingestion of food stimulates the necessary wave of intestinal peristalsis. The frequency of

Table 16.7   Steps to establish regular bowel elimination habits.

1. Identify factors contributing to constipation
2. Discontinue the use of laxatives and enemas
3. Develop a diet plan to increase fibre and fluid intake
4. Develop a plan to increase daily physical activity
5. Establish a schedule for daily bowel elimination
6. Implement diet, exercise plans and elimination schedule daily
7. Evaluate effectiveness of plan each day
8. Modify plan as necessary

bowel elimination varies with the individuals. It should be stressed to the patient that daily bowel elimination is not essential to health; defecation every 2–3 days may be normal for some persons.

Dietary modifications

The nurse and/or dietitian works with the patient and family to evaluate current dietary habits and then helps them to plan a diet that provides a liberal amount of fibre-containing foods, taking into consideration the person's food preferences, financial resources and daily routine. Emphasis is placed on whole grain cereals and bread, fresh fruits and vegetables and fruit juices. A daily fluid intake of 2000–2500 ml is recommended unless contraindicated by a cardiovascular or renal condition.

Peristalsis may be promoted by the drinking of a cup of hot water on rising in the morning (approximately one half hour before breakfast).

It has been demonstrated that regular bowel elimination can be achieved in the institutionalized elderly by adjusting the diets and adding a daily fibre supplement. Brown and Everett gave a daily 30 ml (2.2 g) serving of a fibre supplement made from bran cereal, apple sauce and prune juice to patients on a long-term geriatric unit. They found that the use of this recipe with an established bowel programme worked as well as laxatives, saved nursing time and was less expensive (Brown and Everett, 1990). Subsequent chart audits showed that patients who used the supplement continued to use fewer laxatives while maintaining their usual number of bowel movements.

Techniques to promote defecation

Table 16.8 lists various measures the person may use to promote regular bowel elimination: a scheduled time for defecation is stressed as is the importance of prompt response to the urge to defecate. Ensuring comfort and privacy during the defecation attempt, contracting abdominal muscles, leaning forward and bearing down to increase abdominal pressure and application of manual pressure to the abdomen may be helpful.

The person is instructed to implement these techniques daily until defecation occurs. If no bowel movement occurs in 2–3 days glycerine suppositories may be used. If this is still not effective, a stool softener or a bulk laxative may be administered. Once the person establishes a regular schedule, other laxatives or enemas should not be necessary.

Physical exercise. Some physical exercise is essential; walking is especially good. Good tone in the abdominal muscles is important; exercises to increase the strength of the abdominal muscles may be suggested. Examples of prescribed exercises are as follows: the person lies on the back on the floor or bed with the arms folded across the chest and rises to the sitting position, keeping heels on the floor. From the supine position, the person raises the lower limbs without bending the knees. These exercises are done two or three times daily, and the individual is also encouraged to contract abdominal muscles several times at frequent intervals through the day.

Laxatives and enemas. Laxatives, enemas and suppositories that the patient may be accustomed to using are discontinued. If increased dietary fibre, fluids and exercise are not sufficient at the beginning to establish normal bowel elimination, mild laxatives may be employed until the defecation reflex is restored and bowel irritability and spasm are reduced. Glycerine suppositories placed high against the wall of the anus may be used one half hour before the usual time of defecation to stimulate peristalsis. The suppository may be repeated daily for several days. If this is not effective a stool softener may be ordered to prevent severe straining at stool and injury to the rectal and anal tissues. The stool softeners in use are mineral oil and preparations of dioctyl sodium sulphosuccinate (Dioctyl). These latter preparations act as wetting agents, allowing water to penetrate and mix with the faecal mass. Mineral oil should not be used for prolonged periods because it may prevent normal intestinal absorption, especially of fat-soluble vitamins.

Bulk-forming laxatives may also be recommended. These preparations swell when combined with fluid in the gastrointestinal tract and have a stimulating effect. Examples of bulk-forming laxatives are bran and Fybogel. Use of these laxatives should be assessed carefully in the elderly if dehydration is present. Osmotic laxatives such as lactulose syrup are disaccharides that are not absorbed in the small intestine. They are broken down by bacteria in the colon and acidify the colonic contents, which then stimulates peristalsis and serves as an effective laxative for the elderly. Magnesium hydroxide (Milk of Magnesia) is a cathartic which is not completely absorbed in the small intestine and causes retention of water in the intestinal lumen, stimulating peristalsis. It is contraindicated for those with any renal insufficiency.

Evaluation

A programme of increased dietary fibre, increased fluid intake, regular physical activity and a schedule for defecation can promote effective regular bowel elimination for most adults as well as for the frail elderly. The use of laxatives is usually not necessary if a comprehensive bowel elimination programme is followed. Evaluation of the effectiveness of nursing intervention to promote bowel elimination is based on the assessment of the individual's bowel habits over time. In hospital and long-term care settings, the documentation of bowel patterns and laxative use on the same assessment tool facilitates regular review of the effectiveness of nursing intervention. Information from chart audits on a nursing unit as well as data provided by a quality assurance programme help nurses to analyse their clinical practice and to identify strengths and areas for change in relation to common health problems such as constipation.

3. FAECAL IMPACTION

Occasionally, faeces accumulate in the rectum, producing a hard dry mass that forms a partial or complete obstruction. It occurs most often in older persons and in those with central nervous system disorders. These patients frequently suffer a loss of intestinal musculature motility and sensation. It may be associated with dehydration, lack of dietary fibre and volume, immobilization or narcotics. Manifestations include crampy pain, the passage of liquid stools without expulsion of the hard palpable faecal mass. The patient may complain of headache, fatigue, loss of appetite and pressure and discomfort in the rectal and anal regions. Faecal impaction is identified by the presence of a palpable hard mass in the rectum, the oozing of liquid stools without passing the faecal mass and the absence of a bowel movement for over 3 days.

The objectives are that the patient will:
1. Relieve the impaction (short term).
2. Develop regular bowel elimination (long term).

GOALS

The patient will demonstrate:

- Regular bowel movements.
- Understanding of the role of dietary fibre and fluid intake in stool formation and defecation.
- Awareness of the role of physical activity in promoting bowel elimination.
- Application of a programme to promote regular bowel elimination.

NURSING INTERVENTION

Relief of impaction

The faecal impaction is treated by the administration of an oil-retention enema to soften the impacted stool and by oral administration of an emollient laxative such as dioctyl sodium sulphosuccinate which also softens the stools. The enema is followed in a few hours by digital breaking up and removal of the faecal mass. The nurse lubricates a gloved finger and gently inserts it into the patient's rectum to loosen the impacted faeces. A cleansing enema of saline or tap water is then given. This process is usually both embarrassing and exhausting; following the enema the patient is made comfortable and allowed to rest. Psychological support is very important.

Promotion of regular bowel elimination habits.

The patient experiencing faecal impaction should be assisted to develop a regular bowel elimination programme which includes dietary management, increased activity, a regular schedule, and the use of techniques to stimulate peristalsis. Glycerine suppositories, stool softeners or bulk laxatives may be required initially. Impaction occurs most often in the elderly who do not eat adequate fibre and who have problems with mobility and experience difficulties in getting to the bathroom. The patient's living environment is assessed and the accessbility of the toilet is taken into consideration. Assistance may be required from the district nurse, neighbours and friends to ensure the aged or incapacitated individual receives an adequate diet and necessary physical assistance. If the patient is in a hospital or a nursing home, a plan for bowel elimination is an integral part of the patient care plan. Excessive bed rest is avoided and physical activity encouraged.

Evaluation

Regular, spontaneous bowel movements will resume and further episodes of impaction will not occur. The patient will develop and implement a programme to promote regular bowel elimination.

4. FAECAL INCONTINENCE

ASSESSMENT

The nursing history is reviewed to determine the patient's usual bowel elimination habits. The problem of incontinence is assessed by observing and recording the frequency of defecation, the consistency of the stools, and warning signs experienced or expressed by the patient related to defecation. It is important to note if the patient experiences an urge to defecate, manifests abdominal discomfort, massages the abdomen, or provides verbal clues that defecation is occurring. The abdominal muscles are observed for tone, strength and voluntary control and the anus is digitally palpated to determine muscle control and sensation. Mental alertness is evaluated to determine the patient's ability to respond to the urge to defecate and to follow a bowel elimination schedule.

GOALS

The person will demonstrate:

- Controlled and regular bowel evacuation.
- Absence or decrease in episodes of faecal incontinence.

NURSING INTERVENTION

Establishment of a regular bowel routine

Faecal continence can be established by developing regular bowel elimination habits, as discussed for the patient experiencing constipation or by establishing a programme for regular bowel evacuation.

Programme to stimulate peristalsis

When the cause of the incontinence is constipation or faecal impaction, as commonly occurs in the elderly, a programme to adjust the diet and activity, maintain regularity and stimulate peristaltic activity is usually effective.

Prevention of reflex bowel emptying

When neuromuscular control is impaired, management of incontinence is directed to preventing reflex emptying of the bowel in response to rectal distension by faeces. If the patient has a predictable pattern of defecation such as after breakfast each morning, a schedule can be developed to ensure that the patient is assisted to the bathroom or to a commode each morning following breakfast. If the patient's pattern of defecation is irregular, attempts are made to establish a regular time for bowel evacuation. A daily routine is established similar to that described for the patient who is constipated. The techniques described in Table 16.8 to stimulate peristalsis are employed. If no bowel movement occurs, the routine is repeated the next day. A glycerine suppository may be used on the second or third day to further stimulate defecation. If the patient usually defecates every two days, this measure would be introduced on the second day prior to the expected involuntary defecation. A stool softener may also be used. Patients with spinal cord injury or neurological disease are usually able to establish a regular defecation

Table 16.9 Assessment of the patient with systemic manifestations of malabsorption

Patient problem	Causes	Clinical characteristics
1. Altered nutrition: less than body requirements	• Malabsorption of fat, carbohydrate or protein; calorie loss; and protein loss (albumin)	• Muscle wasting, weight loss and oedema
2. Altered bowel elimination	• Impaired absorption or increased secretion of water and electrolytes • Increased secretion of water and electrolytes with unabsorbed bile and fatty acids • Fluid and electrolyte load in excess of absorptive capacity of colon • Impaired carbohydrate absorption • Impaired fat absorption and increased loss of fat	• Diarrhoea, abdominal distension and flatulence • Pale, bulky, odorous stools
3. Altered urinary elimination	• Delayed absorption of water; hypokalaemia	• Nocturia and dehydration
4. Weakness and fatigue	• Impaired absorption of iron, vitamin B_{12}, folate; loss of electrolytes (potassium)	• Anaemia and weakness
5. Increased potential for bleeding	• Impaired vitamin K absorption; increased prothrombin time	• Ecchymoses and haematuria
6. Altered muscle tone and sensation	• Impaired calcium and magnesium absorption • Impaired potassium absorption	• Muscle cramps, tetany and prickling and burning sensations • Muscle flaccidity, weakness, decreased tendon reflexes and cardiac arrhythmia
7. Increased potential for injury	• Impaired absorption of calcium and protein; demineralization of bone	• Skeletal deformities and bone fractures
8. Altered sexuality patterns	• Impaired protein absorption; loss of calories	• Amenorrhoea • Decreased libido
9. Altered integrity of skin and oral mucosa	• Impaired absorption of iron, vitamin B_{12} and other vitamins	• Dermatitis, glossitis and dry fissures of the lips
10. Altered visual acuity	• Impaired absorption of vitamin A	• Night blindness

pattern and avoid episodes of incontinence. Routine enemas and laxatives are avoided. Patient participation in developing and implementing a bowel retraining programme is important if long-term results are to be achieved.

Personal hygiene

Until regular bowel evacuation is established, the incontinent patient is kept clean and dry, and skin irritation is avoided. Following faecal incontinence the skin is washed with soap, rinsed well and patted dry. Protective ointment may be applied to provide a coating over the skin. The clothing and bedding are changed as often as necessary to keep the patient clean. The nurse may reduce the patient's embarrassment and concern with reassurance that it is understood the patient cannot control the bowel movements but that this can be achieved with a bowel-retraining programme. Episodes of incontinence may still occur if the patient develops diarrhoea or if his routine is changed, but most patients

can achieve acceptable control if the programme is followed.

Evaluation

The patient will not experience incontinence, or episodes will occur infrequently. The person will state that he or she has acceptable bowel control and will resume social activities.

Disorders of Digestion and Absorption of the Small Intestine

MALABSORPTION SYNDROME

Malabsorption involves failure to transport nutrients from the intestinal lumen to the body fluids and loss of nutrients in the stool. It results from impairment of either the digestive or the absorptive process. Digestion involves the breakdown or hydrolysis of nutrients to smaller molecules which can be transported across the intestinal cells; it depends on the secretion of gastric acid and pepsin and on the actions of pancreatic enzymes and bile in the small intestine. Transportation mechanisms include facilitated active transport, which involves a carrier mechanism and energy to move substances across the cell membrane, and diffusion.

Nutrients are absorbed: (1) into the capillaries and from there are carried through the portal vein into the liver and then into the systemic circulation; or (2) through the lacteals into the thoracic lymphatic system and on into the systemic circulation. The absorptive cells of the intestinal villi are especially adapted for both absorption and secretion.

The causes of malabsorption may be: (1) a lack of normal intralumenal digestion, (2) dysfunction of the absorptive cells of the intestinal mucosa, or (3) impairment of the intestinal circulation or lymphatic system.

CLINICAL CHARACTERISTICS

The signs and symptoms of the malabsorption syndrome vary from severe to very mild; with the latter the disorder may go undetected for years. The major manifestations are: weight loss; abnormal stools which are bulky, soft, light yellow to grey in colour and have a rancid odour; abdominal distension; anorexia; muscle wasting; peripheral oedema; weakness and skeletal disorders. Table 16.9 lists the signs and symptoms of malabsorption with their aeteiological factors.

Digestive disturbances

Malabsorption due to *digestive disturbances* occurs with liver and biliary tract disease, following a gastrectomy and with bacterial overgrowth in the small bowel. With liver and biliary tract disease the primary symptom of inadequate digestion and absorption is the presence of steatorrhoea or undigested fat in the stool. Decreased synthesis or excretion of bile salts results in impaired digestion of fat and interferes with the absorption of vitamin D and calcium. Following a gastric resection, emptying of the stomach occurs more rapidly; the duodenum may be bypassed, decreasing the stimulation of pancreatic enzymes; mixing of bile salts may be inadequate; stasis of intestinal contents may occur and protein intake may be decreased.

Management includes the administration of pancreatic enzymes. Bacterial growth in the small bowel is controlled by normal peristalsis. When intestinal motility is impaired, bacterial proliferation occurs, resulting in changes in the action of the bile salts. Fat absorption is impaired and steatorrhoea is present. Vitamin B_{12} absorption is also decreased due to its utilization by the microorganisms. Treatment involves antibiotic therapy.

Dysfunction of absorbing cells

Malabsorption due to *dysfunction or destruction of the absorbing cells* may be due to an inadequate absorptive surface resulting from extensive resection of the small

bowel, intestinal bypass or extensive inflammatory disease. The extent and site of the area involved determines which nutrients are most affected. Iron, calcium, water-soluble vitamins and fats (monoglycerides and fatty acids) are absorbed in the proximal intestine. Sugars are absorbed in the proximal and mid-intestine. Amino acids are mostly absorbed in the mid-intestine and jejunum while bile salts and vitamin B_{12} are mostly absorbed in the distal portion of the small intestine. Water and electrolyte absorption occurs in the colon. Patient management includes a high caloric diet: high in carbohydrates and protein and low in fat. Vitamin and mineral supplements are administered. Drugs such as belladonna alkaloids and codeine may be given to decrease intestinal motility. Cimetidine or ranitidine may be given to decrease gastric acid secretion. Long-term parenteral nutrition may be required in very extensive resection or total removal of the intestine.

Enzyme deficiencies

The malabsorption syndrome may be due to *enzyme deficiences* in the intestinal mucosal cells. Adult lactase deficiency is a common disorder which causes an intolerance to lactose, the sugar found in milk. Hydrolysis of disaccharides takes place on the glycocalyx of the microvilli of the intestinal cells. When lactase is deficient, lactose is not hydrolysed to galactose, and glucose and is not absorbed; it remains in the intestinal lumen and draws water by osmosis into the lumen. Symptoms include abdominal cramps, distension, flatulence and diarrhoea following ingestion of milk. The diagnosis is made by taking a history and by a lactose tolerance test. The disorder is more common in Afro-Caribbean and Asian people than in Caucasians. Treatment consists of a milk-free diet; cheese contains a minimal amount of lactose and is tolerated by most patients.

Gluten-sensitive enteropathy

Gluten-sensitive enteropathy (coeliac disease) is an immunological disorder characterized by a reaction of the intestinal mucosa, particularly in the jejunum to gliadin, (a component of the gluten of wheat). The mucosa is damaged, the villi atrophy and absorptive cells are infiltrated by lymphocytes and plasma cells. Other enzyme alterations may occur. Mucosal damage results in decreased stimulation of pancreatic hormones, impaired absorption of water and electrolytes and the excretion of unabsorbed fats. Symptoms include weight loss, distension, diarrhoea and steatorrhoea.

A gluten-free diet is recommended; wheat, rye, barley and oats are avoided. Rice, corn, soy bean and potato flours are used as substitutes in the diet.

Lymphatic obstruction

Lymphatic obstruction as a cause of malabsorption occurs rarely and is associated with Whipple's disease (intestinal lipodystrophy). It is due to the invasion of the intestinal mucosa by an unidentified organism and impaired cell-mediated immunity. Characteristics of the disease include arthralgia, skin pigmentation, abdominal pain, diarrhoea, weight loss and impaired absorption. The patient receives antibiotic therapy.

Drugs

Certain drugs may also interfere with intestinal absorption. Examples of drugs which affect the absorption in the intestine include: antacids; anticonvulsants; biguanides and folic acid.

NURSING CARE OF THE PERSON WITH MALASBSORPTION SYNDROME

Assessment

Health history
Data collected from the patient during the health history focuses on the diet, bowel habits and the symptoms they are experiencing.

Problems commonly encountered by patients are listed in Table 16.9; these should be borne in mind during the assessment and form the basis for a patient interview. The patient's perspective is very important in considering these problems and the effects they may have on everyday life.

Physical examination
The nurse inspects the patient's skin for dryness, turgor and oedema. The gums are inspected for evidence of bleeding. The specific characteristics of the patient's stools are observed and documented. The person's height and weight are recorded and their desirable body weight is determined. The perianal area should be examined for soreness, excoriation, fissures and fistulae. Any episodes of faecal incontinence should be established, and how these were managed by the individual.

Goals

The person with malabsorption disorders, will demonstrate:

- Achievement and maintenance of a desirable body weight.
- A decrease in diarrhoea.
- Understanding of recommended dietary measures.
- Integrity of skin and oral mucosa.

Nursing intervention

Health problems common to persons with malabsorption syndrome are listed in Table 16.9.

Since malabsorption syndromes are usually not curable, care for the patient is directed towards control of nutritional deficiencies and alleviation of symptoms.

Diet
Dietary measures include elimination of the specific inabsorbable nutrient from the diet and administration of the unabsorbed nutrients by other routes if necessary.

The person with gluten-sensitive enteropathy should eliminate wheat, rye, barley and oats from the diet and substitute cornmeal and potato, rice and soya bean flour. The dietician may provide recipes which substitute these products for the traditional wheat, rye and oat flours used in breads, pastries, cakes and pastas. The patient is also advised about health food stores and other outlets which carry gluten-free products.

The person with lactose intolerance should avoid dairy products, prepared foods and baked goods containing milk, butter and cheeses, instant coffee and chocolate. Some individuals with lactose intolerance are able to tolerate fermented dairy products such as yoghurt and cheese. Commercial products that are low in lactose or lactose free, are available as substitutes for milk products in the diet or use as supplements.

Vitamins B_{12} and K are administered parenterally when deficiencies exist and persons with lactose intolerance may require calcium substitutes if dietary calcium is deficient.

Teaching
The nurse plays a major role in patient and family teaching about the malabsorption disorder and dietary measures to manage the syndrome and associated symptoms. The person is taught to identify foods and food products that contain the substances that cannot be tolerated and to avoid these in the diet. Skill and experience in reading product labels is emphasized. The individual is also taught ways to alter the diet to incorporate substitute foods for the ones that are not tolerated. The person also learns to identify their own symptoms and to evaluate their diet to identify contributing factors and then to readjust their diet accordingly.

Evaluation
Symptoms associated with the malabsorption disorder should decrease as the person responds to the dietary changes which eliminate the responsible elements. The person's understanding of the dietary changes and ability to implement them can be measured by the changes in the stools and a decrease in diarrhoea, as well as by the establishment and maintenance of a desirable body weight. The person's skin and gums will return to normal, menstruation will be more regular and the person will feel well.

Inflammatory Disorders of the Intestines

Inflammation may develop in any area of the small and large intestines and alter motility, secretion and/or absorption. The most prevalent inflammatory intestinal diseases include the acute condition of appendicitis and gastroenteritis, and the chronic disorders of Crohn's disease and ulcerative colitis.

APPENDICITIS

The appendix, a narrow blind tube extending from the inferior part of the caecum, is a common site of inflammation which may necessitate its surgical removal. The appendix has no essential function in the human and there is no change in body function when it has been removed.

CAUSES

The most common cause of appendicitis is obstruction of the lumen by a faecalith (a small, hard mass of accumulated faeces) or a solid foreign body, or by disease or scar tissue in the walls of the appendix. Secretion collects in the tube, causing distension that results in pressure on the intramural blood vessels. The mucosa becomes inflamed, ulcerates and readily becomes infected; the walls may become gangrenous because of the interference with the blood supply, and perforation is likely to occur. A ruptured appendix is serious; it allows the escape of organisms into the peritoneal cavity and may cause an abscess in the appendiceal region or a generalized peritonitis.

The disease may occur at any age but is more common in children over 4 years of age, adolescents and young adults. Early diagnosis and treatment of appendicitis is important to prevent serious complications.

CLINICAL CHARACTERISTICS

Manifestations of appendicitis are abdominal pain, nausea and vomiting, a moderate elevation in temperature and a leucocytosis with the increase being in the polymorphonuclear cells. At the onset, the pain may be diffuse or referred to the central portion of the abdomen or the lower epigastric region, and is described as crampy. As the inflammation involves the walls of the appendix, the pain becomes localized to the lower right quadrant or McBurney's point (the area about 5 cm from the anterior superior iliac spine on a line with the umbilicus which corresponds with the normal position of the appendix). The area is tender on palpation, and rigidity gradually develops in the muscles (muscle guarding). Rebound tenderness may be present which is determined by palpation of the left lower quadrant. With the sudden release of the pressure, the patient experiences pain or discomfort in the appendix region. The patient moves slowly and carefully to avoid jolting and movements that increase the pain, and tends to keep the right thigh flexed.

The omentum and adjacent bowel may become adherent to the inflamed appendix, walling off the area. If the appendix ruptures, an abscess will most likely form in the walled-off cavity. If perforation occurs before the area is walled off, a generalized peritonitis develops; the patient complains of pain and tenderness over the whole abdomen which becomes rigid (board-like) and distended. The distension is due to inhibited bowel motility, which may be referred to as paralytic ileus.

Examination of the patient includes palpation of the abdomen and a differential leucocyte determination. The doctor may also do a rectal examination, and a vaginal pelvic examination may be done on the female.

The *treatment* of appendicitis is surgical excision of the appendix.

NURSING INTERVENTION

The person with abdominal pain should be urged to seek medical advice and self-treatment is discouraged, particularly the taking of a laxative or an enema which could be serious, since either could cause perforation of the appendix through stimulation of peristalsis. The patient is also advised not to take food or fluid until seen by the doctor. This is in case immediate surgery is necessary. In most instances, surgery is performed as soon as the diagnosis is established unless perforation is suspected. If the appendix was intact at the time of removal, the patient usually makes a rapid, uneventful recovery with a short period of hospitalization.

If an abscess is present, a drain is placed in the abscess cavity at the time of operation. The collecting bag attached to the drain allows observation of the discharge and accurate measurement of the volume of fluid draining. Antibiotics are prescribed and the patient should receive a minimum of 2.5 l/day of fluids. An accurate record of the intake should be kept and, if the patient cannot take sufficient quantities by mouth, the administration of intravenous fluids may be necessary. Close observations are made for possible extension of the infection and generalized peritonitis, such as abdominal distension, nausea and vomiting, lack of bowel sounds, an elevated temperature and rapid pulse; these are brought promptly to the surgeon's attention.

PERITONITIS

Peritonitis is a localized or generalized inflammation of the peritoneum and is most often a secondary condition. It is usually acute but may be chronic.

CAUSES

The inflammatory response may be due to bacterial invasion or chemical irritation caused by bile, pancreatic, gastric or intestinal secretions, urine or blood escaping into the peritoneal cavity. A common infectious agent is *Escherichia coli* which has escaped from the intestinal lumen.

Intestinal motility is depressed and the intestine becomes distended with gas and fluid. The peritoneal serous membrane becomes hyperaemic and oedematous and there is an outpouring of fluid into the cavity that incurs serious fluid, electrolyte and protein imbalances.

CLINICAL CHARACTERISTICS

The patient experiences abdominal pain, nausea, vomiting and distension. The abdomen becomes rigid (muscle guarding) and progressively more distended. A leucocytosis and pyrexia may develop. The pulse becomes rapid and there is a decrease in blood volume due to loss of intravascular volume. The respirations may be shallow and rapid as a result of ventilatory interference by extreme abdominal distension. Unless quickly reversed, the patient shows signs of shock. Bowel sounds are absent as peristalsis ceases.

Treatment is directed toward the primary condition (e.g. surgery to close a perforated ulcer), relieving the distension and re-establishing peristalsis, combating infection and shock, and replacing fluids and electrolytes.

Gastric and intestinal intubation with continuous drainage are established. Nothing is given orally. An intravenous infusion is administered and the solutions used may be based upon laboratory determinations of serum electrolyte levels. A blood transfusion may be given to counteract shock and replace protein lost in the inflammatory exudate. An antibiotic is administered if organisms are the causative factor of the peritonitis. The patient is very ill and requires constant supportive nursing care.

GASTROENTERITIS

This is an acute inflammation of the stomach and intestines.

CAUSES

These include micro-organisms (e.g. salmonella bacillus, staphylococcus), parasites (e.g. roundworm) and chemical irritants (e.g. excessive alcohol). Rarely, the condition may be attributed to an allergic reaction to a certain food or drug.

CLINICAL CHARACTERISTICS

The patient experiences vomiting, diarrhoea, diffuse abdominal tenderness and pain, fever and leucocytosis.

CHRONIC INFLAMMATORY BOWEL DISEASE

Inflammatory bowel disease (IBD) is the term used to designate the two inflammatory gastrointestinal conditions of Crohn's disease and ulcerative colitis.

Crohn's disease is a chronic inflammatory disease which may affect any part of the gastrointestinal tract but has a predilection for the terminal portion of the ileum. Patches of granulomatous inflammation and ulceration develop in segments of the intestine and involve all layers of the wall. The bowel may perforate and form an internal or external fistula (an abnormal passage) into another loop of intestine or onto the skin. As the inflammation subsides, there is scarring and some stenosis which may lead to a partial obstruction.

Ulcerative colitis is characterized by severe inflammation and ulceration of the mucosa of the rectum and of a part or all of the colon. The process usually begins in the rectosigmoid area and spreads up the descending colon. There is marked inflammation and oedema in the affected area, followed by ulceration. The denuded areas result in infection, abscesses and a loss of fluid, electrolytes and blood.

INCIDENCE

Inflammatory bowel disease has a world-wide distribution, affects both sexes and all age groups. The incidence peaks between 15 and 30 years of age with a second peak occurring between 55 and 65. It is more common in Western countries than in Asia, Africa or South America. It affects Caucasians more frequently than Afro-Caribbeans. The incidence has been increasing but is now believed to have plateaued.

CONTRIBUTING FACTORS

The cause of inflammatory bowel disease is unknown. It is believed that Crohn's disease and ulcerative colitis are two distinct entities and not a progression of bowel disease, and that more than one mechanism contributes to the development of the disorders. There are many misconceptions about possible causes of inflammatory bowel disease such as dietary and personality factors. For example, personality characteristics attributed to patients with inflammatory bowel disease probably result from the disease and its pattern of exacerbations and remissions rather than contributing to its cause.

- *Immunological mechanisms* play a protective role in the gastrointestinal tract, which has its own immune system. To date, no immunological disorders have been identified as causes of either Crohn's disease or ulcerative colitis. However, raised levels of IgG and T lymphocytes in the active phase of inflammatory bowel disease do not revert to normal during remission, suggestive of the activation of an immulogical process.
- *Genetic factors* are thought to be involved because of the familial incidence of the disease. There does appear to be a relationship in some families between ankylosing spondylitis, the HLA phenotype B27, and inflammatory bowel disease.
- Infectious agents have long been considered to cause Crohn's disease. Investigators are currently studying the possible roles of anaerobic bacteria and of viruses. No organisms have been found to cause inflammatory bowel disease and there is no evidence of transmission from one person to another.
- *Environmental agents* have not been shown to cause inflammatory bowel disease, despite numerous investigations and evidence of its worldwide distribution.
- *Emotional factors and stress* have not been shown to cause inflammatory bowel disease, despite the demonstrated relationship between stress and bowel disorders. Emotional factors do contribute to the evolution and recurrence of ulcerative colitis and Crohn's disease (Myer, 1984). Further investigation is needed in this area.

CLINICAL CHARACTERISTICS

Ulcerative colitis

The major symptom of ulcerative colitis is diarrhoea, the severity and frequency of which depend on the extent of colon involvement. Stools are usually liquid, occur with tenesmus (painful, ineffective straining), and may contain blood, mucus and pus. The number of stools per day may vary from as few as four to as many as 24. Accompanying the diarrhoea is a sense of urgency and cramping abdominal pain. The pain is usually located in the lower left quadrant and is colicky in nature. After defecation, pain may subside.

Ulcerative colitis varies in intensity and severity of presentation, ranging from mild to severe. About 60% of patients have mild disease, 25% have moderate disease and 15% have severe disease. As the disease becomes more severe, malaise and fatigue occur. Anorexia is not common, but individuals may limit food intake in order to decrease bowel movements. In the more severe cases, tenderness in the left lower quadrant, guarding and abdominal distention may occur, as well as anaemia, leucocytosis, tachycardia, fever and dehydration.

Crohn's Disease

The patient with Crohn's Disease may have occasional acute episodes of illness but more often has mild and intermittent symptoms. Acute inflammatory symptoms include pain in the lower right quadrant, cramping, tenderness, spasm, flatulence, nausea, fever and diarrhoea. Unlike ulcerative colitis, there is often no visible blood in the stools. Borborygmus and increased peristalsis may also be present. The most severe pain may mimic acute appendicitis or bowel perforation. The more typical picture is the chronic type, which has more persistent but less severe symptoms. When the terminal ileum is involved, the pain is in the periumbilical region. Jejunal pain is in the upper and left abdomen. Initially the ileal pain is intermittent; later it becomes more constant and may be noticed in the lower right quadrant.

Pain or discomfort accompanied by diarrhoea are the most common symptoms. The pain is usually peristaltic and intermittent. Cramps of regional enteritis are not closely associated with defecation, and unlike cramps with colonic disease, relief does not occur after passing stool or flatus. A constant aching, soreness or tenderness usually indicates advanced disease.

Diarrhoea is usually less severe than that associated with ulcerative colitis. The usual consistency of the stool is soft or semi-liquid. If steatorrhoea is also present, the stools will be quite foul smelling and fatty. A large amount of flatus is also likely to be a problem.

Abscess formation is common and may be characterized by a spiking fever and leucocytosis. Perianal disease, including fistulas and fissures, can occur. Since Crohn's disease most often affects a portion of the small intestine, which then loses its ability to absorb nutritional matter, it can result in weight loss, malnutrition, cachexia, amenorrhoea in women and growth retardation in children.

Comparison of the two disorders shows differences as well as similarities. Crohn's disease may affect any part of the gastrointestinal tract. The lesions are patchy in distribution and transmural in nature, resulting in thickening of the wall, fistula formation and perforation of the bowel. Ulcerative colitis affects the large intestine, the lesions are continuous and as they progress the bowel thickens, narrows and shortens. There is an increased incidence of gastrointestinal cancer with both disorders. Both diseases may cause extracolonic manifestations, such as joint problems due to acute migratory polyarthritis, stiffness and pain in the back due to ankylosing spondylitis, jaundice and itching due to a chronic active hepatitis, and eye irritation due to episcleritis or uveitis.

Patients may suffer from weight loss, anaemia, debility, fatigue, nausea, vomiting, and fluid, electrolyte and metabolic disturbances. Ulcerative colitis and Crohn's disease are both characterized by remissions and exacerbations. Both are very disruptive to the lives of the patients and their families. They affect the person's ability to eat, participate in social and work activities, and personality.

DIAGNOSTIC INVESTIGATIONS

The diagnostic process can be prolonged and cause considerable discomfort and inconvenience to the patient. The preparation for and the procedures themselves further aggravate the already troublesome bowel problems.

Blood studies

Leucocyte count
An increase in the number of white blood cells (leucocytosis), particularly neutrophils, may indicate infection and an acute inflammatory process. Normal: leucocyte count $4–11 \times 10^9$ per litre.

Erythrocyte count, haemoglobin concentration and haematocrit
A deficiency in the number of red blood cells and in the amount of haemoglobin may indicate the loss of blood or nutritional deficiency and provide information as to the patient's condition.

Stool cultures

Stool cultures may be carried out to identify the presence of several micro-organisms that can mimic inflammatory bowel disease.

Sigmoidoscopy

A direct examination of the anal canal, the rectum and the sigmoid colon may be made by means of a sigmoidoscope. A tissue specimen (biopsy) may also be obtained at the same time.

An explanation of the procedure is given to the patient, including advice about the position that will be required. The knee–chest and the left lateral are the positions commonly used. The lower bowel should be empty; cleansing enemas are usually given 2–3 hours before the scheduled time. A low-residue diet may be prescribed for the preceding day.

Unnecessary exposure should be avoided by adequate

drapes. In the knee–chest position the patient lies face down and draws both knees up so that the body weight is borne by the chest and knees. The feet are extended over the end of the table, arms at the sides or at sides of the head, and the head is turned to one side. In the left lateral position the lower limbs are flexed, with the right one being drawn up further than the left. Suction is made available to remove any secretion or fluid faeces that interfere with visualization of the bowel mucosa.

After the examination, the perianal region is cleaned and the patient is encouraged to rest. The individual may experience discomfort during the examination as air is pumped into the bowel to distend the lumen.

Colonoscopy

The flexible fibreoptic colonoscope has made possible the visualization of the complete colon, the taking of a biopsy and pictures of a lesion and the removal of polyps. Insufflation of air is used during the procedure to distend the bowel, permitting better visualization.

The patient should be advised of the purpose of the examination and what to expect and is asked to sign a statement giving consent. The bowel must be absolutely clean. A low residue or clear-fluids only diet is usually given. On the day of the examination only a cup of black tea is allowed. Laxatives are given for 2 days prior to the colonoscopy to ensure that the bowel is empty. The regimen is modified if the patient is suffering from acute colitis or rectal bleeding.

The patient is told that it will be helpful during the examination to take deep breaths with the mouth slightly open and to relax the abdominal muscles. Sedation (pethidine or diazepam) may be given 30 minutes to 1 hour before the scheduled colonoscopy, or an intravenous infusion may be started and diazepam or pethidine administered intravenously during the procedure. The patient is requested to indicate pain during the examination. The patient is usually placed in the recumbent position on the left side and the nurse remains at the patient's head, providing necessary support.

Following the colonoscopy, the patient is allowed to rest and receives food and fluids. The patient is observed for signs of bleeding, pain and abdominal tenderness and rigidity. The intake may be restricted to fluids for a period of time, and then a low-residue diet is gradually introduced.

Radiological techniques and fluoroscopy

Introducing contrast medium into the lumen of the gastrointestinal tract allows it to be examined radiologically. Contrast medium may consist of a barium compound, an iodine solution, air or a combination of these. Barium sulphate is the most widely used and is very safe; however its use is contraindicated when perforation is suspected. In such cases a water-soluble solution of iodine should be used. The aim of the examination is to outline the lumen with barium, utilizing its coating properties so that any mucosal destruction, distortion or deviation from the normal contour can be assessed. Lesions extending into the lumen are shown as filling defects or as an abnormal extension to the line of the mucosa. Failure of the barium to progress with dilatation suggests obstruction.

The passage of barium may be followed in 'real time' by X-ray fluoroscopy. This yields useful information about function, e.g. the swallowing mechanism, and also facilitates the optimal position of the patient for a 'spot' radiography. The fluoroscopic image can be recorded on video for later analysis.

Barium may be used to examine the oesophagus (barium swallow), stomach and duodenum (barium meal), small bowel (small bowel meal or enema), colon (barium enema).

Patient preparation for the barium study will vary, depending on the part of the gastrointestinal tract being examined. Instructions are issued by the Radiology Department directly to patients in the case of out-patient investigations; to the ward in the case of in-patients. For barium swallows and meals the patient has nothing by mouth from the evening before, as residual food or fluid interferes with the technical quality of the examination and hinders interpretation. Mild to moderate laxatives are given prior to small bowel studies, to clear small bowel contents and help empty stool from the caecum, which facilitates the visualization of the ileocaecal region. More aggressive measures are needed for colonic cleansing prior to a barium enema, since even small amounts of faecal material can mimic polypoid lesions. These measures will vary from place to place, but they usually include food restriction for 24–48 hours prior to the examination and a purgative. Some centres also use colonic lavage. Frail, elderly patients may tolerate the bowel preparation poorly, e.g. they may become dehydrated and/or hypotensive. In these cases careful nursing supervision is required.

The majority of barium meals and barium enemas today are performed using double contrast; that is, using a combination of barium and gas. This achieves distension and a thin mucosal coating of barium, facilitating the identification of small mucosal lesions. Gas is given in the form of effervescent granules for barium meals; for barium enemas gas is delivered directly through the rectal tube. It has recently been shown that carbon dioxide is more rapidly absorbed and causes less discomfort to the patient than air.

After any barium study the patient should be warned that the stools will be clay-coloured until barium has been eliminated. Fluids are encouraged as barium may become dry and thick, causing constipation. Should the patient suffer constipation or impaction of faeces following barium studies, an evacuation enema may be prescribed to relieve discomfort.

COMPUTERIZED TOMOGRAPHY (CT)

This non-invasive examination of the abdomen is useful to locate neoplasms, abscesses and cysts by providing more specific information about changes in tissue density than is available with the standard X-ray procedures. In general, however, CT is not the first investigation for gastrointestinal tract lesions, except in those cases where a significant extralumenal or metastatic component is suspected.

Preparation of the patient for the scan includes an

explanation of what will take place. The person will be required to lie still during the scan. The investigation is not painful and normal activities may be resumed immediately after the test. It may be done on an out-patient basis. An abdominal CT scan requires that the gastrointestinal tract be opacified with dilute contrast (barium or iodine), since an unopacified loop of bowel can mimic a nodal or mesenteric mass. When scans are made through the pelvis, similar contrast in the rectum may help the interpretation of the images.

TREATMENT

The *goals* are that the patient with inflammatory bowel disease will achieve an optimum nutritional state, physical and emotional rest, and a return to an active and desirable life-style.

Drug therapy

Anti-inflammatory agents, immunosuppressants and antibiotics are used alone or in combination to treat inflammatory bowel disease. Other drugs may be prescribed for symptomatic treatment. These include anti-diarrhoeal agents, including narcotic preparations, such as codeine, which have a constipating effect.

1. *Corticosteroid preparations*. These (e.g. prednisone, prednisolone) are prescribed for their anti-inflammatory and immunosuppressant actions. Corticosteroids are often taken in both the oral form and applied per rectum in retention enema. Observations are necessary for side-effects such as retention of sodium and water, hypokalaemia and hypertension.
2. *Azathioprine (Imuran)*. This is anti-inflammatory and immunosuppressive. Although the prescribed dosage in regional enteritis is small, the patient's resistance to infection is lowered. The nurse and patient should observe the necessary measures to prevent infection.
3. *Sulphasalazine*. This is an anti-infective and anti-inflammatory drug. When prescribed, it is important that the patient takes a minimum of 2500 ml of fluid daily, as with any sulphonamide preparation. This is to prevent possible crystallization of the sulphonamide in the renal tubules.
4. *Antibiotics*. A fistula complicated by infection or a stagnant area or loop of intestine in which there is an overgrowth of bacteria may be treated with an antimicrobial agent (e.g. metronidazole).

Surgical intervention

Surgical intervention for persons with Crohn's disease is reserved for the patient with complications, as there is a high incidence of recurrence and operative mortality is about 3% (Myer, 1984). Complications include the partial or complete obstruction of the intestine by the scar tissue, the formation of abscesses, perforation of the bowel and the formation of fistulas.

About one-third of persons with ulcerative colitis require surgical intervention. The diseased colon and rectum are removed and the ileum is brought through the abdominal wall to form an ileostomy. A portion of the ileum may be used to form an internal continent pouch (see p. 502). Surgery is usually effective but prognosis depends on the rate of development, severity and extent of the disease process.

ASSESSMENT OF PATIENT FUNCTIONING

There are a number of instruments available to measure disease activity in Crohn's disease (Harvey and Bradshaw, 1980) and in ulcerative colitis. A major limitation of these indices is that they do not provide a detailed picture of the patient's subjective function, including the emotional and social problems associated with IBD. Assessment of a patient's quality of life provides insight into the problems that are most important for patients, allowing health workers better to deal with these problems. Obtaining such information, while important to understanding the patient's adjustment to IBD, may be difficult because of the embarrassment about discussing such topics as bowel movements and incontinence and because of fear of the disease. The process of raising difficult and embarrassing issues can be facilitated through the use of specially designed questionnaires such as the Inflammatory Bowel Disease Questionnaire (IBDQ) to evaluate quality of life in IBD patients (Guyatt et al, 1989).

Quality of life

Inflammatory bowel disease can have a major adverse impact on patients' lives. Numerous descriptions of the problems affecting IBD patients have documented limitations in work and social activities, home and married life, and emotional function (Mallett et al, 1978). In one study of 43 patients with ulcerative colitis and 54 patients with Crohn's disease, it was found that patients reported symptoms which fell into five major categories: bowel symptoms, systemic symptoms, emotional function, social impairment and functional impairment (Mitchell et al, 1988). Of the five categories, bowel symptoms, systemic symptoms and problems related to emotional function had the most profound impact on the lives of IBD patients.

Bowel Symptoms
Problems most frequently cited by IBD patients as having a significant impact on their lives include: frequent bowel movements, loose bowel movements, abdominal cramps, pain in the abdomen, abdominal bloating, passing large amounts of gas and rectal bleeding with bowel movements.

Systemic Symptoms
Systemic symptoms reported most often included fatigue, feeling unwell overall, tiring very easily, waking up during the night and feeling weak.

Emotional Function
Patients with IBD have sustained numerous losses, including loss of normal bowel habits, foods from the diet, body image, weight, relationships, work, valued leisure activities, familiar surroundings through hospitalization, income and self-esteem (Joachim, 1989). They report feeling frustrated, depressed, discouraged,

irritable, angry, anxious and impatient. They worry about not finding a toilet in time, about having to have surgery and about the next flare-up of symptoms.

Social Impairment
Loss of normal bowel habits resulting in bowel frequency, incontinence and embarrassment about sudden calls to the toilet can lead to a change in activities. IBD patients tend to avoid social events where toilets are not close to hand; social engagements may be cancelled if a flare-up occurs, and sporting activity may be severely curtailed.

Functional Impairment
Although some patients report an inability to attend work/school regularly, having to stop work/school and difficulty doing housework, most studies have found that the majority of people with IBD lose little or no time from work over the long term (Hendriksen and Binder, 1980; Joachim and Milne, 1985). When symptoms are flaring; many patients have to get up earlier than usual in the morning because bowel actions delay departure for work.

Further analyses indicate that Crohn's disease patients experience more systemic symptoms (most notably fatigue) than do patients with ulcerative colitis. Problems in one area are likely to cause problems in another area. Overall, systemic symptoms are a major determinant of functional impairment, social dysfunction and emotional problems, while bowel symptoms predict emotional problems.

Serious disruption of personal relationships is a problem for only a few IBD patients. Significant marital problems resulting from IBD have been found in less than 25% of IBD patients (Hendriksen and Binder, 1980). Mitchell et al found that less than one-quarter of the respondents complained of decreased interest in sex, or decreased ability to engage in sexual activities (Mitchell et al, 1988). Problems relating to the ability to communicate with the partner, or the partner's emotional support, were identified by less than a quarter of the patients.

The family may view the individual with IBD as a burden rather than as a capable, independent and functioning individual who needs understanding and support during flare-ups. However, it is not uncommon for family members to be so attentive and wrapped-up in the problems and needs of the individual with IBD that they tend to overlook their own personal needs. Such behaviour may result in increased family tension, fatigue, guilt feelings, resentment and a decreased ability to cope and offer support and reassurance over a long period of time.

In summary, symptoms of bowel disturbance such as frequent, loose bowel movements and abdominal cramps, as well as fatigue and malaise, have the most profound impact on the lives of IBD patients. Disturbances of emotional function, including frustration and irritability, depression and discouragement, are common in IBD patients. Impairment of social function is less frequent, with the majority of patients finding ways

to cope with their jobs, their social activities and their family relationships.

One articulate 45-year-old male with ulcerative colitis describes the impact of IBD on his life in the following way:
'During an attack (flare-up), it makes it almost impossible to carry on a normal social life. The major problem is you can't plan more than an hour or two in front of yourself. As a consequence, the way you and your family live through this period is radically altered from the norm.

You have to live through the problem for the weeks or months you have it and look forward to the time when the problem is in recession. It's not as simple as saying there is a toilet nearby and therefore we can go. You feel uncomfortable. There may not be a toilet there and if there is, it may be occupied, and I'm talking about minutes or less to get to the toilet. There's nothing worse than being somewhere and having the fear that you are not going to be able to get to a toilet.

Having IBD makes you irritable, probably because you're feeling so miserable and down and can't lead a normal life. Your mind is concentrating on *your* problem, *your* pain and *your* next visit to the toilet. It casts somewhat of a dampening effect on your personality. You tend to draw into yourself more … its the reluctance to get involved in a conversation and then have to dash off to find a toilet.

During an attack, there is an effect on work. First, I spend the first two hours after waking constantly in the bathroom passing stool, gas or pus. Then the problem of the journey to work … the 20-minute journey can be a nightmare. Once at work, I may visit the toilet 5–6 times before lunch … sometimes having to dash out of a meeting or away from a visitor. In the afternoon, I feel weak and find it hard to put an effort into what I should be doing.

Change can take place from day to day or within the same day. After a morning of constant visits to the bathroom, you can reach a point where the pain is gone away for 4–5 hours. At that stage, you can almost become a chameleon and change your personality. There is quite a distinction between the period of pain and those times of recession. If you don't get that period of pain relief, there is a constant draining of energy day after day.

IBD can have an effect on your holidays. Normally where one books a holiday 4–5 months in advance, you become reluctant to do that because you don't know if you will have an attack during that period. It affects your holiday and everyone you are with. In my case, we had planned a 2-week car trip during which I had an attack. The mornings became totally disrupted. I felt like I knew every toilet along the way.'

Kelly (1986) describes the subjective experience of living with ulcerative colitis and, using autobiographical data, explains the personal strategies for coping with the disease. In his account he describes adjusting to ill health using the processes of denial, normalization and accommodation, and proposes that these strategies can be both 'healthy' and problematic. He argues that some well-meaning counselling approaches which break down an individual's denial of their illness could promote adoption of the invalid or sick role, and cautions accordingly. His account also illustrates the miscommunication which can occur when the information given threatens the individual's personal construct of ill health and the disease. This paper provides the health care professional, caring for the person with inflammatory bowel disease, with insight into the experience of living with the condition and proposes approaches that can be adopted to encourage normal social development.

NURSING CARE OF THE PERSON WITH INFLAMMATORY BOWEL DISEASE

Patient problems

- *Malnutrition* due to the bowel inflammation, decreased absorption, diarrhoea, abdominal pain and lack of enjoyment of food.
- *Dehydration* due to diarrhoea and inadequate fluid intake.
- *Diarrhoea* due to the inflammatory process and disease complications.
- *Ineffective individual and family coping* related to the disease process, and the impact on quality of life and resulting personality changes.
- *Altered sexuality patterns* related to changes in body image, personality and sexual desires.
- *Deficit of knowledge* related to the disease process, disease management and coping strategies, and perceived misconceptions.

Goals

The person will demonstrate:

- Understanding of total parenteral nutrition.
- Gradual, consistent increase in body weight.
- Understanding of measures to promote adequate nutritional and fluid intake.
- Acceptible management of diarrhoea.
- Awareness of emotional responses.
- Recognition of positive coping strategies.
- Communication and sharing of significant others' concerns, and changes in sexuality patterns.
- Understanding of the disease process and its recurrent nature.
- Understanding of the treatment regimen and disease management.

Nursing intervention

Nutrition

Nutritional deficits and weight loss are common to persons with inflammatory bowel disease. When these are severe all oral intake is withheld to decrease the mechanical, physical and chemical activities of the gastrointestinal tract.

Total parenteral nutrition (TPN). Parenteral nutrition is the infusion, into a large central vein, of solutions of protein, glucose, electrolytes, trace amounts of essential minerals, vitamins, and lipids (fat emulsions) in sufficient concentrations to meet individual requirements for normal metabolism, tissue maintenance, repair and energy demands. It may also be used to supplement nutrition received orally.

Parenteral nutrition is used with patients who have Crohn's disease or a bowel fistula that requires that the intestinal tract be given a rest.

The successful management of total parenteral nutrition involves co-ordination of the efforts of all members of the multidisciplinary team. In some hospitals a special team, usually a specialist nurse, physician, dietitian and pharmacist, co-ordinate activities. Their responsibilities may include teaching and preparing the patient to manage the feeding regimen at home.

Strict surgical asepsis is mandatory throughout the insertion of the catheter, when handling the solutions and tubes, and when caring for the site of insertion. Infection causes a serious problem; the parenteral line serves as an excellent culture medium and, since it leads directly into the blood, bacterial invasion will cause septicaemia.

It is important to *prepare the patient*, especially if total parenteral nutrition is to be prolonged or permanent, with a detailed explanation of the procedure, its purpose and subsequent care. The patient and family are encouraged to ask questions and time is taken to answer them. They may require assurance that the patient will be able to eat normally after a period of being fed this way.

A large vein is used for administration of the highly concentrated (hyperosmolar) solutions, as they are irritating to the veins and can cause phlebitis in smaller peripheral veins. The rapid flow of blood in the large vessels dilutes the TPN solutions and lessens the risk of phlebitis.

The type of catheter inserted will vary from hospital to hospital and the patient's needs. When the TPN is to be used over an extended period of time, and particularly when the patient is to go home with the catheter in place, a long-term central venous catheter (e.g. Hickman or Cooke), is inserted and tunnelled under the skin on the chest wall to decrease the incidence of infection. Usually a multilumen catheter is inserted to provide flexibility of use.

The frequency with which the intravenous tubing and/or filter(s) are changed is indicated by hospital policy. If contamination occurs or is even suspected, a doctor is notified and the following investigations are performed:

- Blood cultures from the catheter and a peripheral vein
- Full blood count
- Midstream specimen of urine for microscopy, culture, and sensitivity
- Chest X-ray
- Other tests to eliminate potential sources of infection, e.g. wound swabs, throat swabs, etc.

All tubing changes are made quickly while the catheter is clamped to prevent air entry and the risk of embolism. If the catheter cannot be clamped, the patient is instructed to bear down and hold the breath before tubing is disconnected and to breathe again once the connection is made (Valsalva manoeuvre). The infusion line may contain one or two micropore filters. Tubing connections are always reinforced with adhesive to ensure maintenance of an intact line. Total parenteral nutrition solutions consist of an amino acid/dextrose solution and a fat emulsion solution which are infused at the same time.

The rate of flow of the solution prescribed by the doctor should be constantly supervised and no attempt should be made to 'catch up' if the fluid is running slowly. If the infusion is too rapid, glucose is not metabolized rapidly enough to maintain a normal blood sugar level. The latter is likely to exceed the glucose renal threshold and glucose is excreted in the urine, taking with it essential water and electrolytes. Ideally a volume control regulator (infusion pump) should be used to maintain a constant rate of flow. This is especially important if a 3-litre reservoir is used and avoids the problem of alteration in flow rate when patients change position.

On *dressing* the site strict aseptic technique is observed. Caution is necessary to avoid dislodging the catheter. The catheter site is inspected for redness, swelling or drainage; a swab is taken for culture if any irritation is observed. The skin is cleansed and re-dressed according to hospital procedure. A common regimen is: entry site cleaned with 0.5% chlorhexidine in 70% spirit; sprayed with povidone-iodine spray (waiting 2–3 minutes for it to dry); then application of a sterile semi-occlusive dressing (e.g. Opsite). The dressing of choice should be water- and bacteria-proof but permeable to air and water vapour. A transparent dressing permits frequent visualization of the area without disturbing the dressing, which can be left in place for as long as a week.

Frequent *mouth care* is essential. Regular, frequent cleaning of the teeth followed by a mouthwash is very important. The lack of oral food and fluid intake causes discomfort and favours the growth of organisms present in the mouth, producing inflammation and tooth cavities. If the parenteral nutrition is prolonged or permanent, the patient may be permitted boiled sweets to suck, or a small amount of food which may be chewed and then expectorated. Some patients may be able to take small amounts of clear fluids or specified nutrients if their gastrointestinal tract is intact.

When *assessing* the patient the following observations are very important.

The patient's blood pressure, pulse, respirations and colour are recorded frequently following the insertion of the catheter. Any complaint of pain or tightness in the chest or change in level of consciousness is reported promptly. Any such change may indicate air embolism or a pneumothorax or haemothorax.

The temperature, pulse and respirations are recorded one to four times daily. An elevation of temperature and increased pulse rate may indicate infection.

A urine specimen is usually examined daily for sugar and acetone. Blood specimens are usually taken daily for estimation of urea, electrolytes and glucose, and a full blood count, albumen, protein, magnesium, phosphate estimation and liver function tests may be performed twice weekly. Hyperglycaemia may develop,

necessitating the administration of regular insulin.

Blood cultures are done and checked for fungi as well as bacteria.

The patient's weight is recorded daily. The intake and output are recorded and the fluid balance noted.

The site of insertion is examined carefully each time the dressing is changed and is inspected daily through the transparent dressing for inflammation, oedema, sloughing or purulent discharge.

Psychological support is necessary as the patient receiving total parenteral nutrition for a prolonged period may report feeling 'very different'. Repeated explanations of the purpose and value of the feedings are necessary. As the procedure becomes more familiar and better understood, it becomes more acceptable to the patient. Activity is encouraged as exercise promotes protein synthesis as well as improving the patient's psychological well-being. Any weight gain should be reported to the patient as this may help morale; however, a failure to gain weight may have the opposite effect.

Bowel *elimination* decreases and the patient should be advised that as nothing enters the tract this is not surprising.

When TPN is *discontinued* the solutions are reduced gradually over 48 hours to prevent a sudden fall in blood glucose. Oral intake is gradually increased. The catheter tip is sent to the laboratory for culture.

Teaching must be given to the patient who requires long-term parenteral nutrition. Appetite decreases during parenteral feedings. This is attributed to the caloric intake, decreased gastric motility and underlying disease. Appetite remains suppressed when parenteral feedings are discontinued.

If this method of receiving nutrition is to be permanent or prolonged, carers and patient are pre-pared for discharge from the hospital. They are taught how to put up the solutions, the maintenance of asepsis, indications of problems (e.g. symptoms of infection), care of the site of catheter insertion, how often the tube is changed and by whom, and that the solution should not be frozen. They are advised of the necessary supplies and how they are obtained. They should also have contact telephone numbers and addresses in case of emergency. The patient is also taught to test urine for glucose and acetone and to make a daily record of weight.

Referral to the community nursing services is impor-tant on discharge. This will ensure early identification of difficulties or problems, monitoring progress, provision of support, and assistance if necessary with aspects of care.

Most patients not only feel attached to the intravenous poles they have been pushing around for a period of time, whether as an in-patient, out-patient or on home care; they also feel protective of and dependent on their TPN feedings. They may require help in dealing with their ambivalent feelings of wanting to discontinue the feedings and anxieties over the loss. The patient needs positive reassurance to deal with the change in health status and what it will mean.

Oral Intake. When oral intake is resumed, the patient may be given nutritionally balanced elemental feedings.

These preparations are bulk and residue free and low in fat making them easier to digest in the upper gastrointestinal tract. Palatability is enhanced by providing the feed chilled and in different flavours.

When food is permitted, a high-calorie, high-protein, non-irritating low-residue diet is given. Milk is usually poorly tolerated. Iced fluids, carbonated drinks, raw fruits and vegetables and all foods suspected of stimulating bowel activity are avoided. Recently, a more liberal diet with elimination of only those foods that the patient recognizes as increasing the diarrhoea has been recommended.

Nutrition of the patient requires a great deal of attention. The patient may develop serious nutrional deficiencies. Anorexia presents a problem, and there are serious losses of essential nutrients, fluid and electrolytes in the frequent stools. In many instances, the nurse must work at getting the patient to take sufficient nourishment; it may be necessary to provide frequent small meals. An effort is made to serve foods the patient likes, to provide variety, and to have the tray attractively arranged. A discouraging factor commonly encountered is that, as soon as the patient starts to eat, peristalsis is stimulated and he or she must get to the toilet.

Fluid and electrolyte replacement

An excessive loss of fluid in diarrhoea and a probable reduced intake by the patient because of abdominal pain and 'feeling sick' may lead to dehydration. The daily intake and output are recorded and the fluid balance is noted. The patient is encouraged and, if necessary, given assistance to take adequate amounts of fluid. Intravenous infusion may be necessary to correct dehydration and maintain sufficient intake. If the patient has TPN in progress, additional intravenous fluids and blood products should be given by a separate peripheral line to avoid contamination.

Serum electrolyte levels, especially potassium and sodium, are determined, as an abnormal amount may be lost in the stools or through fistula drainage. Replacement is made by intravenous fluids. A transfusion of packed red cells may be necessary to correct anaemia that has resulted from nutritional deficiencies. These develop due to insufficient food intake and/or impaired intestinal absorption.

Maintenance of skin integrity is an important role of the nurse when the patient is experiencing dehydration.

Bowel elimination: diarrhoea

The frequency, consistency, volume and colour of the patient's stools is recorded and the nurse and patient collaborate to identify foods, activities and emotional responses that increase or decrease the frequency and consistency of bowel movements.

Antidiarrhoeal medications may be given after each loose bowel movement. The rectal and perineal area are inspected for irritation and rĕdness. Should moist excoriation develop the area should be kept dry. Use of a hairdryer expelling cool air may help achieve this. Soreness may be relieved by the application of a local anaesthetic gel. A barrier cream can be used to protect the skin.

Individual coping

The nurse must appreciate that dependence and insecurity may be encountered in persons with IBD and a great deal of tact and sensitivity is required in giving care.

Family coping

Family members, like professional care givers, need help to understand the reasons for the person's changed behaviours and to appreciate the difficulties experienced in adjusting to a chronic illness that is probably progressive and definitely interferes with one's life. Awareness of the reasons for the behaviours and of the patient's needs provides a basis for understanding and the development of constructive coping strategies. The family may need assistance to identify and deal with their own needs as well as those of the patient.

Sexuality patterns

Issues arise related to sexuality, family planning, fertility and pregnancy. Questions still exist about a genetic contribution to the development of Crohn's disease. Family members need to be aware of these facts when planning a family. There is no evidence that inflammatory bowel disease affects fertility, and pregnancy is possible. Sexual desire is usually decreased by the disease and the unpredictable bowel habits, odours, fatigue and a possible ileostomy or colostomy raise additional barriers to healthy sex. The patient and partner may need support to discuss their concerns and to develop solutions to their particular situation. The disease process and outcomes affect feelings of sexuality and sexual function, necessitating effort and open communication between partners if they are to achieve a satisfactory relationship.

Patient and family teaching

Assessment of patient and family learning needs is ongoing as needs change throughout the disease process.

The possibility of a recurrence is reduced if the patient understands the illness and follows the advice discussed in this section. The patient is encouraged to return to work and to live as normal and useful a life as possible. A balance between rest, work and recreation is advisable. Assistance is given the patient in solving home or socioeconomic problems, since a relapse can frequently be associated with a psychosocial disturbance.

Referral to the medical social work department may be useful in resolving domestic or socioeconomic problems. Some hospitals have a clinical psychologist or counsellor whose role is to assist the person with inflammatory bowel disease and the family and significant others to explore the ramifications and meaning of the disease and develop positive coping strategies. Self-help groups can also be a useful resource to assist in adaptation, and have the added benefit of having members with similar experiences.

Emphasis is placed on the importance of a nourishing diet with the elimination of certain foods that are found to be irritating to the bowel.

Table 16.10 Causes of intestinal obstruction.

Mechanical	Non-mechanical
• Inflammation and oedema of the intestinal wall	• Neurogenic disturbances: Paralytic or adynamic ileus
• Scarring of the intestinal wall	Dynamic ileus
• Adhesions	• Interrupted blood supply: Mesenteric thrombosis
• Neoplasms (intramural and extramural)	Strangulation of blood vessels secondary to:
• Foreign body	Incarcerated hernia
• Incarcerated hernia	Volvulus
• Volvulus	Intussusception
• Intussusception	
• Congenital stenosis and atresia	

Evaluation

Inflammatory bowel disease is characterized by remissions and exacerbation which, together with prolonged treatment, interfere with the person's life and impact on the family and care-givers. Disease management and coping strategies vary according to the status of the disease and the person's responses and ability to cope with the chronic progressive illness. Evaluation is ultimately based on the patient's perceptions, how well they are feeling and how they perceive they are coping with the latest treatment, symptom, complication, remission or behavioral characteristics.

INTESTINAL OBSTRUCTION

Obstruction to the passage of intestinal content may occur in the small or large bowel and is a serious, life-threatening condition that demands prompt attention.

CAUSES

The cause of the obstruction may be within the wall or lumen of the intestine itself, or it may be extrinsic. It may be classified as mechanical, neurogenic or vascular and may be acquired or congenital (see Table 16.10).

Mechanical causes include inflammation, oedema and scarring of the intestinal wall; neoplasm of the bowel or of a neighbouring structure; adhesions, which are bands of fibrous scar tissue formed by the peritoneal tissue following inflammation and which may cause kinking and constriction of the intestine; occlusion by a mass, such as a hard, dry faecal accumulation, a large bolus of unchewed and undigested food, a gallstone or a foreign body; and intra-abdominal abscess.

Strangulated hernia, in which a loop of the intestine escapes from the peritoneal cavity through a defect in the abdominal wall, results in constriction of the lumen of the bowel and a blockage as well as compression of the blood vessels. The constriction may lead to

gangrene of the protruding segment of the intestine.

Obstruction may result from *intussusception*, a condition in which a segment of the intestine is invaginated into the segment immediately below. This telescoping results in compression of the attached mesentery between the layers of intestine in the intussusception and interference with the blood supply to the bowel. Intussusception occurs mainly in infants and young children.

Volvulus, which is a twisting of a loop of bowel on itself, interrupts the passage of intestinal contents and the blood supply to the involved segment. Older persons are more often affected, and the twisted section of bowel is usually the sigmoid colon.

Congenital malformations may be responsible for intestinal obstruction in the newborn. The anomaly may be a stenosis or atresia in an area of the small or large intestine, or it may be an imperforate anus. The infant fails to pass meconium.

In *neurogenic obstruction*, peristalsis is inhibited by a disturbance in the normal nerve supply to the intestine. Often this is an imbalance in the autonomic innervation which results in a cessation of peristalsis. It may develop with peritonitis, pancreatitis, severe toxaemia as in pneumonia and uraemia, shock, or spinal cord lesions, or occasionally after extensive abdominal surgery. An electrolyte imbalance in which the blood potassium is below normal also predisposes to intestinal immobility. The inhibition of peristalsis due to impaired innervation causes the condition known as *paralytic* or *adynamic ileus*. Dynamic or spastic ileus occurs rarely in some toxic conditions and is associated with intestinal hyperactivity. The spasm of a segment is severe enough to obliterate the lumen.

Obstruction of vascular origin is due to interference with the blood supply to a segment of the intestine and may be secondary to mechanical obstruction, or it may be primary and itself cause failure of bowel activity. Thrombosis and occlusion of a mesenteric artery may occur, blocking the blood supply to a large portion of the bowel and arresting peristalsis. The interruption in the blood supply may be secondary to an initial mechanical cause, as occurs in strangulated hernia, volvulus and intussusception.

CLINICAL CHARACTERISTICS

The symptoms and effects of obstruction depend on whether it is in the small or large bowel and whether or not the blood supply to the intestine is maintained.

The first symptom of mechanical obstruction is colicky abdominal *pain* due to the bowel spasms. The crampy pains are accompanied by high-pitched bowel sounds. In paralytic ileus, the pain is steady and is due mainly to the distension. There is an absence of bowel sounds in this type of obstruction. No faecal matter or gas is passed after that which was below the obstruction is evacuated.

In small bowel obstruction, *vomiting* begins earlier and is frequent; the vomitus at first consists of stomach content and then of fluid containing bile. Eventually it becomes dark brown and faecal in character as the intestine becomes distended with excessive fluids and gas which overflow into the stomach.

The *abdomen becomes distended* because of the accumulation of gas and fluids in the bowel. Intestinal secretions are increased and the loss of fluid and electrolytes in vomiting leads to *severe dehydration* and *electrolyte imbalance*. Extravasation of plasma from the capillaries adds to the accumulation of fluid in the intestine as the veins are compressed by distension. This depletes the circulating blood volume and causes *shock*.

The patient's general condition may deteriorate rapidly. Unless the bowel is decompressed and fluid and electrolytes are replaced, a serious state of *shock* develops, manifested by restlessness, anxiety, a rapid weak pulse, low blood pressure, subnormal temperature, greyish pallor and cold clammy skin.

If decompression of the intestine is not established, the pressure created within the intestinal lumen may increase until it exceeds venous and capillary pressure. This causes congestion, oedema and necrosis of the mural tissue and may lead to perforation of the intestine.

The colicky pain becomes continuous as peristalsis diminishes, and the intestine loses its tone because of the marked distension and strangulation. Bowel sounds diminish and the vomiting changes character; it is no longer preceded by nausea and retching; the vomitus comes up without effort (regurgitated).

Peritonitis may develop as the weakened intestinal wall becomes permeable to organisms. *Generalized abdominal tenderness* and rigidity become evident.

Obstruction of the large intestine is less acute, and the symptoms develop over a longer period of time. Complete constipation (obstipation) and crampy abdominal pain are the patient's first complaints. Distension of the large bowel develops more slowly since fluid is absorbed, but eventually the distension may be very marked as the segment of the bowel is closed off by the obstruction at one end and the ileocaecal valve at the other. The ileocaecal valve will permit the entrance of content from the ileum but not until the later stage does the content of the colon and caecum back up into the ileum. Vomiting and the attendant dehydration and electrolyte imbalance occur in this later stage.

MEDICAL DIAGNOSIS

Diagnostic investigation in intestinal obstruction may include an X-ray examination of the abdomen in which the presence and levels of gas and fluid may be apparent without a contrast medium.

TREATMENT

Intestinal obstruction other than that due to paralytic ileus is treated surgically. In simple mechanical obstruction without strangulation, the operation may be delayed for a brief period in which medical treatment is used to improve the patient's general condition. This treatment includes nasogastric and intestinal intubation and suctioning to remove the accumulation of gas and fluid and to relieve the vomiting, pain and distension.

Fluid and electrolytes are given intravenously to replace the losses; as much as 5–6 litres may be administered daily. An accurate record of all fluid output and intake is necessary. The doctor bases the electrolyte replacement as well as the amount of intravenous fluid on the volume of intestinal fluid lost in vomiting and aspiration.

If there is evidence of interference with the blood supply to the obstructed intestine, emergency surgery is undertaken.

The surgical procedure used in intestinal obstruction depends upon the cause of obstruction and the patient's general condition. If the obstruction is due to adhesions, they are severed. It may involve resection of the affected area of intestine and anastomosis to restore continuity of the tract or a bypass of the lesion by anastomosing a part above the obstruction to a lower part (usually the colon). In the case of an incarcerated hernia, volvulus or intussusception, the obstruction is relieved and the intestine examined for viability. If the blood supply has been interrupted for some time or is not re-established, a segment of the bowel may be gangrenous, necessitating resection and anastomosis. The surgery may entail an ileostomy, caecostomy, or colostomy, which may be a temporary measure while an anastomosis heals or it may be done to establish drainage above the obstruction, making it possible to delay more extensive surgery until the patient's condition improves. In some instances, the enterocutaneous fistula (colostomy or ileostomy) is permanent. (*Ileostomy* is an opening from the ileum onto the external surface of the abdomen. Intestinal content is eliminated through this opening. *Caecostomy* is an opening through the abdominal wall into the caecum to provide elimination of the intestinal contents. *Colostomy* is an opening through the abdominal wall into the colon. Faeces are diverted through this opening onto the external surface of the abdomen.)

For nursing care of the surgically treated patient, see Chapter 11.

Intestinal obstruction due to paralytic ileus is treated symptomatically. A nasogastric or intestinal tube is passed to drain gas and fluid and reduce distension. Fluid and electrolyte deficiencies are corrected; the serum potassium level receives special attention because hypokalaemia favours peristaltic dysfunction. Paralytic ileus is most frequently a secondary condition; as the primary disorder improves and decompression occurs, peristalsis is usually re-established gradually.

CANCER OF THE INTESTINE

The most common site is the rectum; the sigmoid, caecum and ascending colon are next in order of frequency. Colorectal tumours are the second most common form of cancer in the United Kingdom and account for 12% of all deaths from malignant disease. They are fairly equally distributed between the sexes. Small bowel cancers are uncommon and account for 2% of all gastrointestinal tumours. Cancer of the colon or rectum may occur at any age but has its highest incidence in the fifth and sixth decades. The incidence is high in Western countries and low in underdeveloped countries.

CONTRIBUTING FACTORS

The cause of colerectal cancer is believed to be multifactorial. Studies show a relationship between high-fat, low-fibre diets and colorectal cancer. Specific substances in the mucous membrane lining the intestine may be the cause. The fat and fibre content of the diet, transit time of bowel contents and intestinal bacteria alter the microenvironment of the intestine.

A number of conditions carry an increased risk of developing large bowel and rectal cancer. These include: prolonged history of inflammatory bowel disease, familial polypsis, neurofibromatosis (von Recklinghausen's disease) and juvenile polyposis. As there is a considerable familial tendancy with a number of these conditions there is a major place for screening and surveillance programmes.

TYPES

The malignant growth may be papillary, soft and friable, or a firm nodular mass projecting into the lumen; it may be a ring-shaped (annular) mass of firm fibrous tissue, causing a constriction of the bowel, or it may be ulcerative and necrotic, leading to bleeding and perforation.

METASTASES

The malignant cells from bowel cancer may be spread by blood and lymph and by direct extension to neighbouring tissue and structures. Frequent sites of secondary growths are the liver, stomach, bones, and peritoneal cavity. Direct extension may involve the bladder and reproductive organs.

CLINICAL CHARACTERISTICS

Manifestations vary with the location of the lesion in the intestine. If the neoplasm is in the *small intestine*, the symptoms develop insidiously and are vague and less noticeable. They include anorexia, nausea and vomiting, anaemia, loss of weight and strength, and occult blood in the stool. Obstructive symptoms appear gradually and the patient develops abdominal pain. If the tumour is in the duodenum, the manifestations may be similar to those of a peptic ulcer.

If the site of the neoplasm is in the *colon* or *rectum*, the most common early signs are a change in bowel habit and blood in the stool. Any person manifesting either of these signs is urged to seek *prompt medical attention*.

There may be increasing constipation or perhaps alternating bouts of constipation and diarrhoea. The stool may gradually become smaller and ribbon-like in form and may be streaked with blood, mucus and pus. A continuous defecation urge and the feeling that evacuation is incomplete after passing a stool may be experienced. The patient presents a general picture of ill health with a loss of weight and progressive anaemia. Laboratory examination of the stool will probably reveal occult blood. In cancer of the large bowel, abdominal pain is usually a late symptom; at first the patient may have a vague discomfort, and later he may experience a colicky pain which gradually becomes more severe. Unfortunately, if the cancer is in the caecum or ascending (right) colon, the early symptoms are more insidious and difficult to detect until the mass is large enough to be observed by palpation. Occasionally, the first symptoms recognized are those associated with complications, such as obstruction or perforation of the bowel.

SCREENING AND EARLY DETECTION

The 5-year survival rate for colerectal cancer remains under 50%; early detection therefore provides the best chances for survival. If the cancer is detected early, before lymph nodes become involved, the 5-year survival rate increases to 70–80%. The goal is to detect the malignant lesion before symptoms occur.

Screening for colorectal cancer at present is dependent upon occult blood estimation in stool samples. This test is estimated to produce a 25% false-positive result. However in one study (Clark et al, 1987) of an asymptomatic population over 40 years, using occult blood tests 1:1000 were diagnosed as having cancer. Another study (Mitchell and Silman, 1983) describing a screening programme found that people were frightened to participate in case cancer was found, and despite health education initiatives only achieved a slightly greater than 50% participation. It is suggested that the development of a more acceptable test, such as 'magic toilet paper', may help in increasing participation in screening programmes.

DIAGNOSIS

A neoplasm in the *small intestine* may be recognized when barium sulphate is taken by mouth and the passage of the barium through the small intestine followed. Any delay at a given section may indicate narrowing of the lumen by a mass. The intraluminal contour of the small intestine is also recorded by X-rays.

Investigation of the large intestine involves a colonoscopy, sigmoidoscopy or proctoscopy. A biopsy of the lesion, if it is located, is done at the time of the endoscopic examination. X-ray is done with a barium enema providing a contrast medium. The patient's haematocrit and haemoglobin are checked for possible anaemia, and stool specimens are examined for blood, parasites and pus. Liver function tests may be done, especially if the neoplasm is in the small intestine, to determine if the malignancy has metastasized to the liver.

A carcinoembryonic antigen (CEA) test may be done. This antigen is produced within *some* malignant growths and released into the blood. The test is not a reliable diagnostic measure since not all tumours produce the antigen. A normal level does not rule out carcinoma but a high level points to a problem. The test is of greater value in assessing the patient's progress following treatment; increasing levels indicate a progressive growth and spread of the disease (normal level, 2.5–3.0 ng/ml).

TREATMENT

Surgery is the treatment of choice and usually includes removal of the tumour, a section of bowel and the regional lymph nodes. If the disease is more extensive, a partial or complete colectomy may be required. A temporary or permanent colostomy, may be formed to permit elimination of body wastes. The development of the end to end anastomosis (EEA) stapling device has meant that fewer individuals require the formation of a temporary or permanent stoma.

Chemotherapy, either as a single agent or a combination of agents, is used to manage recurrent disease and metastatic disease. The agent 5-fluorouracil (5-FU) has been shown as the most effective to date, producing short-term response in some patients. Radiotherapy is increasingly being used to control local recurrence of cancer. In some centres, radiotherapy is being used either preoperatively or postoperatively as part of the overall treatment approach for those individuals most likely to develop recurrent disease.

Other drugs are being tested for the prevention and treatment of colorectal cancer. Ascorbic acid (vitamin C) has been shown to retard carcinogenesis and is being tested on persons with familial polyposis following colectomy.

NURSING INTERVENTION

Prevention

Evidence is accumulating in support of high dietary fibre as a protection against the development of colonic cancer. A low-fat diet is also recommended. Other dietary constituents affect the metabolism of chemical carcinogens by the microsomal mixed-function oxidase enzyme system of the gastrointestinal tract. Antioxidants that have been shown to have these anticarcinogenic effects include the trace element selenium, vitamins C and E, and butylated hydroxytoluene (BHA).

A major nursing issue is the promotion of colorectal cancer screening. The nurse is in a key position to teach individuals about the risk factors, to inform them about screening recommendations and encourage participation in screening programmes. Nurses in primary health care, occupational settings and out-patient departments may have greater opportunities for initiating intensive health education programmes. An informed public recognizes the importance of early detection and treatment. Misconceptions exist that bowel cancer equates with a colostomy. The nurse can stress the positive outcomes of early detection and impress on patients that a colostomy may not be necessary. It depends on the location, extent and stage of the tumour. The examination of stools for occult blood, although far from ideal, is a simple non-invasive procedure that all persons over 40 should take advantage of on a regular basis.

THE PERSON WITH ALTERED BOWEL ELIMINATION: FAECAL DIVERSION

Ileostomy and Colostomy

The treatment of some intestinal disorders may necessitate surgery that establishes an opening into the bowel through which the intestinal content is discharged on to the surface of the abdomen. The opening may be temporary or permanent. A temporary diversion of the bowel content may be necessary while some abnormal condition below the level of the stoma is corrected or for quick decompression and drainage in obstruction. Later, the normal continuity of the tract is restored and the stoma is eliminated. If the opening is permanent, the portion of the bowel below is generally removed.

The operations performed are ileostomy, caecostomy and colostomy.

ILEOSTOMY

An ileostomy involves transection of the ileum and bringing the proximal end out to the abdominal surface to form a stoma. An ileal stoma usually protrudes 2–3 cm which makes the management easier than with a stoma that is level with the abdominal surface. The latter predisposes to seepage around the ileostomy appliance and excoriation of the skin. The removal of the distal severed portion of the bowel may be done at the same operation or may be postponed until the patient's condition is improved. If the lower part of the intestine is to be retained for a period of time, it is closed or, in some instances, the severed end may also be brought out to the abdominal surface.

An ileostomy is most frequently performed for Crohn's disease, or for ulcerative colitis that does not respond to medical treatment and is incapacitating. It may also be necessary for patients with multiple polyposis of the colon or an intestinal obstruction in the upper portion of the colon.

A reservoir referred to as a pouch ileostomy or continent ileostomy, may be created by the surgeon to improve the quality of life for the patient (Figure 16.8). Continent ileostomies are not usually performed on patients with regional enteritis (Crohn's disease) since the pouch may become affected.

The surgical procedure involves the formation of an internal pouch in the distal segment of the ileum. The pouch serves as a reservoir for the intestinal content. The pouch is drained at regular intervals by the insertion of a catheter through the stoma. The capacity of the reservoir gradually increases, and may reach 500–1000 ml over several months to a year. As the capacity increases, there is a corresponding decrease in the frequency of drainage required. Continuous discharge and leakage of the fluid or semifluid between evacuations of the pouch is prevented by the formation of a valve-like structure at the internal end of the ileum that leads from the stoma to the ileal pouch. Pressure of the contents of the pouch closes the valve, but it is

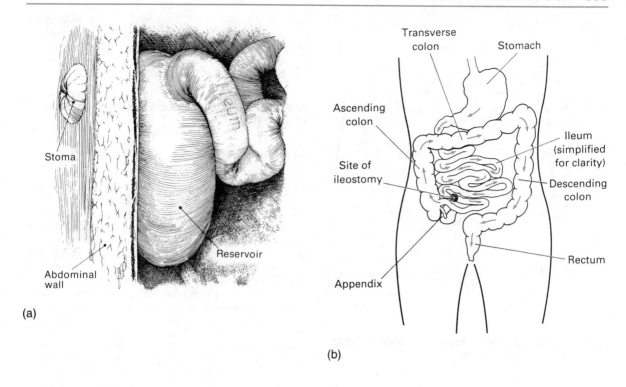

(a)

(b)

Figure 16.8 (a) Pouch (continent) ileostomy. (b) Diagram showing the location of the ileostomy. Arrows show direction of movement of bowel contents.

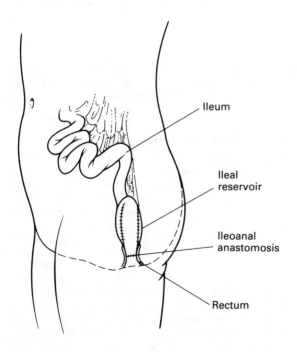

Figure 16.9 Ileoanal reservoir.

structured so that it opens when the gentle pressure of a catheter is exerted against it on the stomal side.

An alternative approach involves the surgeon constructing an ileal pouch and connecting it to the anus (Figure 16.9). In over 75% of patients this gives rise to a continent bowel elimination process. The operation is in two stages, with bowel resection and construction of the ileoanal pouch being accompanied by an ileostomy, but only on a temporary basis. At the second stage the ileostomy is closed and the pouch is activated to permit anal elimination.

The postoperative period for the pouch ileostomy is longer than that for the patient who has had the conventional ileostomy. It involves gastrointestinal drainage via a nasogastric tube, intravenous fluids and continuous catheter drainage of the pouch for several days while the pouch heals. In addition, the patient will probably have had a colectomy or an abdominoperineal resection of colon, rectum and anal canal. However, the advantages associated with an ileal pouch, such as the elimination of continuous drainage and the wearing of a bag, make the more involved procedure acceptable to the patient.

COLOSTOMY

A colostomy is an opening of the colon on to the surface of the abdomen. It may be in the ascending, transverse,

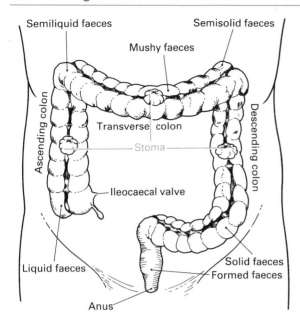

Semiliquid faeces · Semisolid faeces · Mushy faeces · Ascending colon · Transverse colon · Descending colon · Stoma · Ileocaecal valve · Liquid faeces · Solid faeces · Formed faeces · Anus

Figure 16.10 Colostomy sites and variation in faecal consistency within the colon.

descending, or sigmoid colon. The types of stoma include:

- *Permanent, end or terminal colostomy*, usually formed after resection of part of the colon, rectum and anal canal or following a Hartmann's procedure where the rectal stump is oversewn and the proximal colon is brought on to the abdominal wall to form the stoma.
- *Temporary colostomies*, fashioned using any part of the colon, but the transverse colon is the usual segment.

Various techniques can be used to fashion these types of stoma such as:

- *Loop colostomy* where a section of the colon is brought out on to the abdomen, supported on the surface by a rod or bridge, opened longitudinally and the mucosal edges sutured to the skin.
- *Spur colostomy (Mikulicz)* where the two ends of the colon are sutured together to make a spur and brought out on to the abdomen. Ultimately an enterotome is placed into the two openings of the spur, which produces continuity without further major surgery.
- *Double-barrelled colostomy* where the proximal and distal ends of the stoma are brought out on to the abdomen to form two separate openings.

CAECOSTOMY

Rarely, in large bowel obstruction, decompression of the distended bowel is achieved by a caecostomy. A small opening is made in the caecum through a small lower right abdominal incision and a fairly large tube is inserted through which the bowel content escapes to the exterior. The tube is attached to a drainage receptacle and remains in place until the patient's condition is such that he can withstand the more extensive surgery necessary to relieve the obstruction.

NURSING CONSIDERATIONS IN ILEOSTOMY AND COLOSTOMY

Differences between ileostomy and colostomy

Certain differences exist between an ileostomy and colostomy that result in different problems and necessitate different types of care. For example, control of the discharge is determined by the location of the stoma; drainage from the ileum is of liquid consistency and is rich in enzymes that cause excoriation and erosion of the skin. It flows almost continuously, requiring the constant wearing of a receptive appliance unless an ileal pouch is constructed. There may be quiescent periods but they are not predictable and cannot be controlled. Complications are a more common occurrence with an ileostomy than with a colostomy, and odour presents a greater problem if there is continuous drainage. Irrigations are not used with the conventional ileostomy; the introduction of anything into the ileal stoma is discouraged for fear of injury to the intestine.

Colostomy drainage is usually more manageable and less irritating to the skin unless the opening is into the ascending colon; the drainage then is similar to that from an ileostomy. The colostomy is more often in the transverse or descending colon and much of the fluid and electrolytes have been absorbed from the faecal content, leaving it semisolid or solid by the time it reaches the stoma (Figure 16.10). Irrigations may be necessary but, in some instances, the sigmoid colostomy may be so well controlled that it resembles normal bowel movement, and the patient does not have to wear an appliance continuously.

Intestinal activity in the individual with a colostomy or ileostomy may be influenced by diet, fluid intake and emotions, just as in the normal person.

Psychological preoperative preparation

When the doctor advises the patient preoperatively that a colostomy or ileostomy may or will be necessary, the patient is often emotionally disturbed. If the colostomy is a temporary measure it may be accepted more readily but, if it is likely to be permanent, the patient may be more concerned about this than about the operation or the primary condition. The immediate response may be 'it would be better to die than have that'. The patient may become resentful or show marked depression, withdrawal and despair, perceiving this change to the body as making him unclean and unacceptable to society. There are fears because of odour and soiling. It is best to let the patient, family and partner express their feelings before attempting explanations. The nurse can help by being a willing listener, answering their questions and using every opportunity available to assure the patient that the 'ostomy' can be cared for

Table 16.11 Sites to be avoided when positioning a stoma.

- Areas affected by skin conditions
- Bony prominences
- Fatty bulges or skin folds or creases (present on lying, standing or sitting)
- Groin creases
- Old scars
- Pubic area
- Site of surgical incision
- Site which cannot be seen
- Umbilicus
- Under large breasts
- Waistline

without interfering with his work and social life. When the patient recovers from the initial blow, discussions may then be held as to how to care for the ileostomy or colostomy.

The stoma care nurse should be notified and meet with the patient and family preoperatively. If no stoma care nurse is available, the nurse can encourage the patient and partner to handle the appliances, ask questions and look at literature or audiovisual resources on care and management of ostomies. It is important to reinforce that support and teaching will be available postoperatively.

Some individuals, their families and significant others may welcome a visit from someone who has experienced a similar operation. Local branches of self-help groups such as The Ileostomy Association of Great Britain and Ireland or the Colostomy Welfare Group have a list of suitable visitors. Some centres develop their own group of ex-patients who can fulfil this function.

Physical preoperative preparation

Physical preparation for the formation of a stoma is important. This will include siting of the stoma and bowel preparation. Correct siting of the stoma will ensure ease of mastery of the techniques of management and ultimately speedier adaptation to altered bowel elimination. Although the site may be chosen by the stoma care nurse or surgeon, the nurse may be involved in assessing the patient and identifying physical disabilities (i.e. poor eyesight, poor dexterity, etc.) which will influence where the stoma is sited. Table 16.11 outlines the sites which should be avoided. The nurse may also be involved in applying test patches (patch testing) of appliances, skin protective wafers and adhesives to prevent later problems with skin sensitivity.

Bowel preparation should be carried out according to local policy as methods vary. Whatever method is used the nurse should prepare the person by explaining the procedure and the reason why it is necessary. This will increase co-operation. Adequate privacy and hygiene needs should be provided, and monitoring of the patient for signs of dehydration, electrolyte disturbance,

discomfort and exhaustion must be carried out. Bowel preparation can be psychologically traumatic, particularly if the individual experiences episodes of incontinence, as it may bring with it feelings of loss of control and realization of the impact of the planned surgery and future ramifications. The nurse should be supportive and encourage expression of anxieties about the future.

NURSING ASSESSMENT

Initial and continuous assessment of the following is necessary:

- The patient's perception of the ileostomy or colostomy.
- The volume, colour, composition and consistency of the effluent (drainage).
- The patient's nutritional and hydrational status. The fluid intake and the quantity and composition of meals are noted. The patient's weight is recorded.
- The condition of the stoma and surrounding skin surface.
- The reaction to self-care.
- The family's perception and reaction to the ileostomy or colostomy.
- The patient's ability to manage stoma care.

PATIENT PROBLEMS

Health problems common to the person with a stoma during the postoperative and early rehabilitation periods include:

- *Altered bowel elimination* due to the faecal diversion.
- *Potential for impairment of skin integrity* related to leakage of intestinal/bowel contents on peristomal skin.
- *Altered nutrition* related to differences in consistency of faeces at the level of the stoma and changes in control of elimination of abdominal contents.
- *Disturbances in body image* due to the abdominal stoma, the surgical incision, changes in faecal elimination and control of odours.
- *Altered sexuality pattern* related to altered self-image, stoma, ostomy appliance, altered sexual responses and lack of knowledge.
- *Deficit of knowledge* related to self-management of the stoma.

GOALS

The patient will demonstrate:

- A healthy stoma with clean, intact peristomal skin.
- Ability to look at and touch the stoma.
- Active participation in care.
- Ability to empty, clean, change, prepare and dispose of appliances.
- Absence of diarrhoea, constipation, excessive gas and abdominal distention.
- Awareness of how diet and fluid intake affect bowel function.
- Recognition of signs of complication and actions to take.

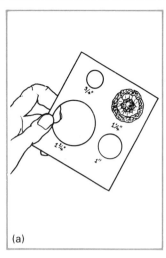

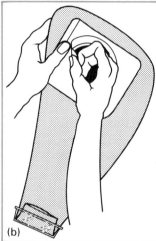

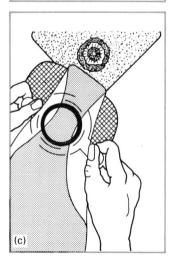

Figure 16.11 Procedure for the application of a one-piece ostomy pouching system. (a) Check size of stoma and select appropriate appliance. (b) Remove backing paper from skin barrier. (c) Apply pouch smoothing barrier against skin preventing creases. Modified from Erickson (1987).

- Verbalization of feelings, concerns, questions and perceptions of self as a stoma patient.
- Awareness of community resources.
- Understanding of how to obtain further supplies of appliances and accessories.

NURSING INTERVENTION

Physical Management of the Stoma

The ileostomy site is usually located through the rectus muscle in the lower right quadrant of the abdomen, about 5 cm below the waist and high enough to permit normal leg movement without dislodging the pouch.

Postoperative Assessment
The patient will usually return from the theatre with a clear pouch in place to allow for observation of the stoma. Initially the stoma is swollen and oedematous, pink to bright red in colour and shiny in appearance. A deep red or dusky colour and coolness to touch indicate ischaemia. The volume of drainage is small. The baseline assessment data includes the colour, temperature, size, type and location of the stoma. It is important to note if the stoma is flush, retracted or prolapsed and to document the condition of the skin. The stoma is assessed at least every 8 hours for the first 24 hours postoperatively, and at least daily during the remainder of the hospitalization. The pouch is usually removed in 24 hours to allow for thorough observation of the stoma and stutures. The peristomal skin is inspected each time the appliance is changed. If a loop ostomy has been created, note the type of support system (e.g. rod, bridge, drain). It is important to label the pouch to alert others to remove the pouch gently if a rod is in place.

Selection of the drainage appliance
Appliance selection is important for the person to be able to resume usual physical and social activities. The selected system should; (1) be odour proof, (2) protect the peristomal skin, (3) stay secure, (4) be readily available in the community, (5) be acceptable to the patient, and (6) be invisible under ordinary clothing (Table 16.12). Pouches come as one-piece or two-piece systems. The one-piece appliances are most commonly used. The skin barrier is incorporated into the pouch, eliminating the possibility of separation. Two-piece systems require that the drainage bag be snapped on over the solid skin barrier which is fitted around the stoma against the skin. The pressure of snapping the pouch in place can be uncomfortable against a newly-operated area. There are two-piece systems available that avoid this pressure. Postoperatively all ostomy patients will require a system with a drainable bag. An ostomy belt may be attached to the appliance to hold it secure during activities and to prevent undue pull on the seal, but is usually unnecessary. The skin barriers often come in precut sizes and the pouches are available in different shapes and sizes, clear or opaque, odour-proof and drainable. Some can be cut to fit, decreasing the need for hospitals to stock all options. Figure 16.11 illustrates the application of a one-piece ostomy appliance.

Table 16.12 Types of drainage appliance and indications for selection.

Type of pouch	Consideration for use
One-piece closed pouch	Suitable for solid effluent Discarded after use once emptied Changed once/twice daily Patient may need to use a peristomal wafer if skin sensitivity occurs Discrete appearance
Two-piece system	Skin sparing, because the baseplate or flange stays in place for 3–7 days Interchangeable sizes of pouch: • Activity pouch • Closed pouch • Drainable pouch Can be used with a belt for extra security
One-piece drainable pouch	Suitable for liquid effluent Wear times of 3–5 days can be achieved Can be washed via emptying portal Clip or clamp used to empty device Can be used with a belt for extra security
Colostomy plug (Bucharth et al, 1986)	Suitable for solid effluent, where stoma acts three or less times daily Stoma should be < 45 mm in diameter Stoma should not protrude > 6 mm from skin Manufacturer suggests that a 12-day training period is necessary Patient may experience initial discomfort Patient needs to be motivated and dextrous Can be used with colostomy irrigation techniques Discrete appearance

From Borley (1989)

The size of the stoma is determined by a stoma-measuring card and bags of corresponding size are used. Too large an opening in the adhesive that attaches the bag exposes the skin to irritating drainage; too small an opening may traumatize or constrict the stoma.

The disposable bag is emptied when it is one-third to one-half full; if allowed to fill it becomes too heavy and the pull on the bag may break the seal of the stoma and cause leakage. The lower end of the bag is opened and the contents allowed to drain into a receptable. Using a syringe or small jug the bag is then rinsed with lukewarm water. The volume and characteristics (colour, consistency and composition) of the drainage are noted and recorded. The appliance is changed as regularly as necessary but at least twice weekly to permit inspection and cleansing of the peristomal skin.

The stoma care nurse will help the individual choose the system most suited to the individual's needs and to make any adjustments required because of variations in the size, characteristics or placement of the stoma. Persons with diversions of the large bowel may not require skin barriers because the stool is usually formed. A small stoma pouch or cap can be worn by persons who have achieved continency of a sigmoid colostomy. Persons with an internal continent pouch usually require only a stoma cap or a gauze square with vaseline ointment over the stoma.

Colostomy irrigation

A colostomy can in some circumstances be controlled entirely by diet, especially if the colostomy is in the descending colon or sigmoid. Irrigation can be used to achieve control when the colostomy exudes solid faecal material. The technique can be time consuming and requires motivation and dexterity to master. The purposes of irrigating the colostomy are to remove faeces, gas and mucus from the intestine and establish a regular time of emptying the lower tract so that spontaneous, irregular drainage is less likely to occur and interfere with the person's activities and usual life-style. The technique usually takes approximately 30–40 minutes to perform and is usually done every 24 to 48 hours. It involves lavaging the terminal colon with 1 litre of warm tap water. The individual wears a long drainable pouch for the procedure but usually only wears a mini-pouch or cap to collect mucus or minimal faecal discharge at other times.

If the patient is constipated it may be necessary to irrigate the colostomy. An irrigation set can be used or alternatively a funnel is attached to one end of a catheter; the other end is lubricated and placed about 10 cm into the colon. Warm water is placed in the funnel which is held above the level of the colostomy, and the water is allowed to run into the patient. The catheter is then removed and the outflow runs into the toilet. All the water that was instilled into the colostomy must be returned before the process is complete. When evacuation is complete, the patient cleans the skin and applies a new drainage bag.

The irrigation is most effective early in the morning, since this approximates the normal time of defecation. If bowel regularity is maintained, irrigation should be unnecessary unless the person decides they wish to use irrigation as means of stoma control.

Care of a pouch ileostomy

The procedure of tube drainage of the ileal pouch, the nasogastric drainage and the withholding of food and fluids by mouth that follow the operation are discussed with the patient and family preoperatively and opportunities are provided for them to ask questions.

The patient is returned from the operation with a catheter inserted through the stoma and valve into the pouch. The catheter is connected to a closed drainage system. It is important to maintain continuous drainage and prevent an accumulation of secretions, gas and faecal matter in the pouch in order to promote healing and prevent complications. If the pouch becomes distended, ileal contents may seep through the suture lines and cause peritonitis. Regular, frequent irrigation of the tube may be required to promote drainage. Sterile normal saline or water may be used, and a directive is received regarding the exact volume that is to be introduced very gently with a syringe. Suction is not applied to withdraw the fluid; the return flow should drain by gravity through the catheter. If it is retained, the doctor is notified.

The colour of the drainage is checked frequently; it may be coloured by blood at first but the blood content progressively decreases over the first 2 days. If it does not, it is reported. The volume of the ileal discharge is also recorded. The faecal drainage eventually may become semiliquid as the diet is increased and the capacity and retention of the pouch increase. Thicker pouch content may cause a drainage problem since 'solid' particles may obstruct the drainage tube, necessitating irrigation, increased fluid intake and adjustment in the diet.

A lightweight dressing with a slit for the catheter covers the stoma and surgical wound. This is changed daily and the stoma inspected for colour, swelling and oedema.

The nasogastric tube is attached to a drainage bag to prevent the possibility of gastric secretions and gas accumulating and distending the gastrointestinal tract. The patient is not allowed anything by mouth until the tube is removed, hydration being maintained intravenously. The fluid balance and serum electrolyte levels should be accurately recorded as they will determine the i.v. fluid regimen prescribed for the patient.

The catheter into the pouch is disconnected from the closed drainage system in approximately 10–12 days and is clamped. The clamp is removed hourly for drainage of the pouch. During the night the catheter is reconnected to the drainage system. The period between the drainages is gradually increased by 15-minute intervals and eventually, when the interval has been lengthened to approximately 3 hours, the catheter is removed. The pouch is then drained every 3 hours by reinsertion of the catheter.

The capacity of the pouch gradually increases and, in 6 months to a year, a capacity of 500–1000 ml is achieved. As the pouch progressively accommodates more and more, the frequency of the catheter insertion for drainage decreases, the objective being three or four times daily. Twenty-four-hour drainage is measured and recorded for many weeks. If the pouch does not drain freely when the tube is introduced, gentle irrigation with a prescribed volume is used.

When the nasogastric tube is removed, the patient receives small amounts of clear fluid exclusive of carbonated drinks. If these are tolerated without distension or vomiting the amounts are increased, followed by a progressive increase from more nourishing fluids through soft to a light normal diet. Food tolerance tends to be an individual matter; the introduction of 'new' foods one at a time makes it possible to identify those that are troublesome. Gas-forming foods, raw fruits and vegetables, foods with a high cellulose or fibre content, corn, celery, lettuce, beans, peas and cabbage are frequently among those not tolerated.

Maintenance of skin integrity
Each time the appliance is changed, the condition of the skin and stoma are noted. The latter should be bright red and moist; if it is bluish or grey or dry the doctor is notified, as the change may indicate impaired circulation. The skin is examined carefully for possible excoriation or any break. Skin irritation is treated promptly and a more effective protective barrier is provided. Fewer skin problems are encountered by the colostomy patient than the ileostomy patient.

The peristomal skin is washed with warm water and patted dry. Skin preparations that provide an effective barrier include karaya which comes in the form of washers, powder and paste. The actual preparation used will vary with the hospital.

Factors affecting the integrity of the peristomal skin include allergic responses, trauma, chemical irritants and infections. The individual may develop sensitivities to any of the products or appliances used to manage the ostomy. These include the skin barrier preparations, the adhesive agents, the pastes, the pouches, clamps and belts. Known irritants are avoided and the method of use of each product is assessed and proper techniques taught. For example, skin barriers should be applied dry, not wet, to avoid moisture under the pouch and against the skin. The use of adhesive tape should be kept to a minimum.

Mechanical trauma most often occurs as a result of frequent, repeated changes of the pouching system. The pouch should be changed every 3 to 7 days and whenever leaking occurs. If the person is changing it more frequently, the nurse should assess the technique being used and consult with the stoma care nurse regarding other actions the person might use to overcome the identified problem. Perhaps a different pouch system would be more appropriate for the person and the individual's particular activity pattern, or there may be another type of adhesive that will hold better. Use of a belt may provide the support needed to prevent pull on the pouch. Tapes are avoided and if necessary are used sparingly. The belt and loops are checked regularly for indications of pressure.

The location of the stoma affects the composition, consistency and quantity of the faecal discharge. The drainage from an ileostomy contains more proteolytic digestive enzymes which quickly erode the skin. Skin barriers are sized or cut to fit snugly around the stoma to protect the skin from faecal drainage but should not cut into the stoma itself as this will cause local trauma. The pouch should be changed regularly and the underlying skin cleansed and inspected to guard against hidden leakage. Soaps are avoided on the peristomal skin as they leave a residue. If solvents are used, care must be taken to ensure that the skin is well cleaned. Adhesive preparations should be applied sparingly.

Infections of the intact peristomal skin are not

common. *Candida albicans* (Monilia) is the most common infection. It is usually treated with nystatin in the form of a powder. If infection is suspected, a swab is taken and sent to the laboratory and the surgeon is notified.

Alterations in nutrition

The ileostomy or colostomy patient usually starts out on a light, low-residue diet to which foods of a regular, normal diet are added gradually. Tolerance varies with patients but, by careful personal experimentation with foods, each person will recognize what can and cannot be taken. The foods that most often have to be excluded are those with a high-fibre or high-cellulose content. Nuts, prunes, celery, corn, pineapple, turnips, beans, cabbage and onions tend to be troublesome.

A well-balanced diet is encouraged and the person's weight followed. Patients are advised to eat slowly and to chew their foods well, which reduces the risk of a faecal bolus blocking the stoma.

Considerable water and salts are lost in ileostomy drainage, especially during the first 2 or 3 months. Gradually, the small intestine adapts to the lack of colonic function and absorbs more water and salts. Until then extra water and food rich in sodium and potassium should be taken. The patient may erroneously think that limiting fluid intake will cause the intestinal drainage to be less fluid. Fluid intake should be more than 1.5 litres/day.

Coping with the change in body function

As soon as practicable after the operation, the nurse concentrates on helping the patient to accept the 'ostomy' and on teaching the necessary care and management. Although there may have been considerable dicussion of the modified method of elimination preoperatively, when the patient is actually faced with it, revulsion, discouragement and depression may still occur. The patient with a temporary ostomy experiences the same feelings as the individual with a life-long diversion. The emotional responses to illness, discussed in Chapter 5, all come into play when a person is faced with the reality of a change in body image and a loss of function that conflict with the social norm for a healthy, well-functioning body. The patient is again concerned about future social acceptance. Acceptance comes first from the nurse, who willingly makes every effort to keep the patient clean and comfortable without any hesitation or aversion. Personal contact by touch, when bathing the patient and positioning and cleansing around the stoma for example, in a perfectly natural and matter-of-fact manner helps the patient to feel that the stoma is acceptable. The nurse should encourage the patient and gradually introduce self-care with an understanding of the patient's reactions to the adjustments that are required. Competence in self-care of the ostomy promotes psychological adjustment. The patient may find it helpful to be visited by someone who has a stoma and is coping well. A visit by a stoma therapist should also be arranged.

Sexuality
Opportunities are created for the patient to interact and socialize with other patients on the ward. Return to normal activities and work are encouraged and may be achieved within 3 months.

The patient and partner are encouraged to ask questions about resuming normal sexual functioning, particularly as the partner may have more anxiety than the patient. Literature and pamphlets are available that may be given to the patient and partner regarding sex. Further opportunity for discussion should be arranged after they have read the information and formulated their personal questions and concerns.

Satisfactory sexual function improves the quality of life of the patient and promotes the closeness and sharing that the individual may perceive as lost or unattainable as a result of the alterations in body image and function. Identification of the patient's and partner's perceptions of the impact of the surgery on their sexuality patterns and relationship should be assessed on an ongoing basis as they begin to cope with the realities of their situation. Table 16.13 lists the physical and psychological effects of ostomy surgery on sexual function. The patient and partner need help in understanding the meaning of these changes to their relationship. Misconceptions need to be identified, discussed and solutions explored. Responses to common misbeliefs about ostomy surgery and sexuality include:

- A stiff penis does not make a solid relationship nor does a wet vagina.
- Absence of sensation doesn't mean absence of feeling.
- The presence of deformities doesn't mean absence of desire.
- Inability to perform doesn't mean inability to enjoy.
- Loss of genitals doesn't mean loss of sexuality.

The nurse plays an important role in helping the patient and partner adjust to the surgery and the effects of ongoing treatment and in the identification of problems related to altered sexuality patterns. If problems persist and interfere with the achievement of a satisfactory quality of life, the nurse should ensure that the patient and partner are referred appropriately and encouraged to utilize professional services.

As outlined in Table 16.3, a number of physical problems can occur following stoma surgery, especially when the rectum is excised. Impotence can be treated and options such as intracavernosal self-injection, penile prostheses and vacuum devices should be discussed. Careful counselling of both partner and individual is important to ensure a satisfactory outcome. It should be remembered that impotence can resolve up to 2 years after surgery. Women can experience dyspareunia, and careful assessment of the nature of the problem and appropriate advice can promote return to the desired level of sexual activity. Painful intercourse can be helped by strategies such as adopting different positions during intercourse, extended foreplay to encourage relaxation, use of water-soluble lubricants or saliva, or use of vaginal dilators. Some women respond to replacement oestrogen therapy.

Nurses can have a major role in encouraging

discussion of issues related to sexuality and sexual functioning but it should be noted that it is an issue that is highly charged and requires sensitivity and understanding. Disclosure by the patient and the partner may threaten the attitudes and beliefs of the nurse, and, similarly, suggested strategies may frighten or disgust the individual's or partner's value system. If the nurse is unable to deal personally with this area it should not be ignored. Encouragement to utilize other services eg. counselling or to discuss problems with the stoma care nurse or general practitioner may be more advantageous in some circumstances in order to achieve a satisfactory outcome.

Self-care

A plan of education is developed to prepare the patient for assuming care of the ileostomy or colostomy and for living a healthy, active life. During the first few days after the operation, the patient's experience with pain and discomfort generally precludes concern about the stoma and future care and activity. Gradually an awareness of the situation develops and the patient's reaction must be assessed. There may be a brief period of depression and withdrawal. Obviously, while reacting in this way, the patient is not receptive to any formal teaching. The nurse encourages expression of concern by being a good listener and accepting the patient's reactions and anxiety.

The preparation for the patient's discharge from the hospital should include a member of the family. Participation of a person with an ileostomy or colostomy who may have already visited the patient may be very helpful in reinforcing the information. Teaching includes explanations, discussions and demonstrations related to the following factors:

Management of the ileostomy and colostomy
Active patient participation in stomal and appliance care is introduced gradually but as early as possible. On discharge, the patient should be engaged in self-care and be confident in the fact that support and assistance are available in the hospital and at home.

At first, as the nurse cares for the ileostomy or colostomy, each step of the procedure is clearly described without minute details. Then, gradually, the patient participates in the care until eventually self-care is achieved. This progressive, step-by-step approach takes time and patience but is less frustrating and discouraging for the patient. As self-care progresses, the community nurse should discuss any problems of self-care after discharge.

More formalized and detailed instruction includes directions for and demonstrations of:

1. *The necessary equipment and supplies.* In addition to discussing and demonstrating the various parts of the appliance, a written list is provided and information given as to how and where the products may be obtained. Information regarding obtaining exemption from prescription charges, if not already exempt, should be provided.

2. *Emptying the pouch, care of the stoma and changing of the appliance.* Planned discussions reinforce the learning that took place as the patient undertook, step-by-step, the daily care. It also gives the patient and the members of the family an opportunity to ask questions.

   Additional directions for care and use usually accompany the appliance and should be read by the patient. Several useful booklets about ileostomy and colostomy care are usually available from the Colostomy Welfare Group or the Ileostomy Association of Great Britain and Ireland.

   The hospital may also issue printed directions which serve as a guide for the patient. The importance of establishing a regular schedule for care is emphasized.

3. *Irrigation of the colostomy* (only if required by the patient). In addition to demonstrating and explaining the procedure and having the patient do it himself, written directions may be given. Assistance may be necessary in deciding how the irrigation can be fitted in with daily routine.

4. *Care of the skin.* The need for thorough but gentle cleansing of the skin is stressed, as is the use of a protective skin barrier because of the irritating effect of the enzyme-containing discharge. Inspection for redness and excoriation is described and advice given as to what should be done if either is present.

5. *Emptying the bag.* The role of regular emptying, changing and thorough cleansing of the appliance in controlling odour is discussed.

6. *Problems or complications.* Problems such as excessive drainage, blockage of the stoma, excoriation, burning sensation or itching of the skin are discussed as to possible causes, how they are recognized and the appropriate action.

Nutrition and fluids
The patient is advised that foods high in cellulose and fibre and some raw vegetables and fruits may be troublesome. A list of foods known to lead to a problem, and therefore to be avoided is provided. The import-

Table 16.13 Sexual problems related to ostomy surgery

Direct effect	Indirect effect
1. Damage to sympathetic and parasympathetic nerves: (a) Erectile difficulty (b) Retrograde/no ejaculation (c) Change in ejaculatory amount or force (d) Orgasmic problems 2. Penetration problems related to shortening or removal of vagina	1. Altered expression related to: (a) Altered body image (b) Physical change (c) Lack of knowledge 2. Fears: (a) Stomal/pouch appearance (b) Noise/odour (c) Leaking (d) Rejection (d) Pain

From Shipes (1987).

ance of a well-balanced diet and the taking of additional amounts of sodium, potassium and water is explained. It is suggested that one new food be added at a time so those that cannot be tolerated may be identified.

Bathing

The patient may take a shower or bath with the appliance in place. Showering without the appliance is good for the skin and for cleansing the stoma. The patient must be sure that no soap is used on the peristomal skin. Bathing is usually done before applying a fresh appliance because the moisture is likely to loosen the adhesive disc.

Some people with stomas may have sufficient confidence to go swimming, since the appliance is concealed by a bathing suit.

Activity

Activity for the ileostomy and colostomy patient is normal except for heavy lifting, which predisposes to prolapse of the stoma and hernia, and body contact sports, which could result in injury to the stoma. The patient is encouraged to return to his occupation and recreational activities. Many people find that their general health is so much better than previously that they enjoy being able to participate in new activities.

The patient may be concerned about sexual relationships and is advised that the change in body image need not be a deterrent to satisfactory sex relations. If an abdominoperineal resection has been done, injury to parasympathetic nerves may very occasionally result in impotency. A woman may experience some discomfort during intercourse for a period of time because of the perineal wound. This matter of sexual relationships is something the individual may wish to discuss freely with the stoma therapist. Further help may be available from SPOD (Association to Promote the Sexual and Personal Relationships of People with Disabilities).

Medications

Laxatives or other drugs should not be taken unless prescribed. If a medicine is ordered by a doctor other than the gastroenterologist, the patient should remind the doctor of the ileostomy. Some preparations should be only in powder or liquid form to ensure absorption.

Sources of assistance

The patient is likely to be very apprehensive about leaving the protective hospital environment. A list of persons or associations from whom advice or assistance may be sought is provided with their telephone numbers. This list may include the stoma therapist, general practitioner or community nurse, and the relevant associations.

Care of the ileal pouch

As soon as the tube is removed, plans are made to teach the patient how to insert the catheter to empty the pouch. The catheter is passed every 2 hours at first, and then the interval is gradually lengthened over the next 4–6 months. The patient is advised that if discomfort or a full sensation in the pouch is experienced the pouch should be intubated to avoid distension and excessive

pressure on the valve. The nurse may demonstrate pouch catheterization to the patient, who is then encouraged to undertake self-catheterization. The nurse remains during the procedure until assured that the patient is competent and sufficiently confident. If the ileal flow is slow, the patient is advised to bear down. Instructions are given as to the frequency and volume of drainage that would be considered inadequate, and what to do if this occurs.

Cleansing of the stoma and the skin and covering it with a small dressing (e.g. 5 cm² Band-Aid or a piece of gauze) are reviewed in preparation for discharge.

The necessary supplies are obtained for the patient and include a small case with two catheters, water-soluble lubricant for the catheter, a syringe, dressings and non-allergenic tape. The sources for supplies are given and instructions supplied as to their care. The patient is instructed to wash the catheter in detergent solution thoroughly and rinse well.

It is important for the person with an ileal pouch to carry a card or to wear a Medic Alert bracelet or pendant indicating the need for drainage of the pouch and giving medical details of the surgery should the patient lose consciousness or be injured; this would be necessary to avoid excessive and dangerous distension of the pouch.

Complications

Potential complications of an ileostomy or colostomy include prolapse or retraction of the stoma, obstruction of the stoma, fluid and electrolyte imbalance, renal calculus and fistula.

In *prolapse of the stoma*, the mesentery of the remaining intestine is not secured sufficiently to the abdominal wall and/or opening in the abdominal wall is too large. Increased intra-abdominal pressure results in a segment of the ileum or colon being forced out onto the abdomen. If several inches of the bowel is extruded, the patient should be placed in the dorsal recumbent position with the head and shoulders slightly raised and the knees flexed. A dressing moistened in sterile water or normal saline is placed over the area. The doctor may attempt manual replacement of the extruded segment or recommend surgical repair.

Retraction of the stoma occurs as the result of shrinking scar tissue in the supporting tissues of the abdominal wall. The opening becomes flush with the abdominal surface, making it difficult to protect the skin from the irritating effluent. Correction is by surgery.

Obstruction of the stoma may be caused by a faecal bolus formed as a result of insufficient mastication of food or the ingestion of fibrous or cellulose foods that are too bulky to pass through the stoma. Examples of such foods are corn, celery, bran, coconut and nuts. The blockage may be relieved by an irrigation. An obstruction may also be caused by a volvulus of the ileum near the stoma. If there is no ileal or colostomy discharge, the doctor is notified. Unless the obstruction is relieved, the patient will develop nausea, vomiting, crampy pain and abdominal distension.

Ileostomy dysfunction sometimes occurs, and is characterized by sporadic free liquid drainage with a very offensive odour. It is associated with peristomal scarring and stenosis which causes trapping of the intestinal contents until pressure and irritation result in the discharge. Dilatation of the stoma may be necessary.

Normally, much of the water and electrolytes contained in the small intestine content is reabsorbed in the colon. The person with an ileostomy loses considerable water, sodium and potassium in the ileal drainage and may develop *fluid and electrolyte imbalance*. The patient is encouraged to drink a minimum of 1500–2000 ml of fluid daily, add salt to foods and include potassium-containing foods (e.g. orange juice, banana, meat) in the diet. If the ileal drainage becomes excessive, fluids containing potassium and sodium, such as fruit juice, are increased to compensate for the loss. If the excessive drainage cannot be controlled, the doctor should be notified. An antidiarrhoeal drug may be prescribed, serum electrolyte levels determined and intravenous fluids administered to correct dehydration and electrolyte imbalance.

The ileostomy patient is predisposed to the formation of a *renal calculus* (kidney stone) because of the water and sodium loss in drainage. This further emphasizes the importance of a greater fluid and electrolyte intake for the person with an ileostomy or colostomy, especially if the latter is on the right-hand side.

Rarely, an ileostomy or colostomy is complicated by a *fistula*. An opening develops in the ileum and the drainage forms a tract to the surface. This may be the result of a poorly fitting appliance or the recurrence of the primary disease. The drainage causes tissue irritation and erosion. Surgical intervention may be used to resect the tract and may include reconstruction of the stoma. Healing may necessitate complete rest of the intestine; the patient may receive total parenteral nutrition until the area is healed.

Herniation of the intestine due to a weakness of the muscular tissue at the site of the stoma may occur. It is recognized as a bulging area. Support may be provided by the ileostomy or colostomy appliance.

Evaluation

Physical management of the stoma is an important step in the person's adjustment to the change in body image and altered control of an important body function. Ostomy surgery impacts on the person's total well-being and family and social relationships. Adjustment is slow

and requires support from the nurse, other health care providers and the patient's spouse and family.

A variety of products and appliances are available for ostomy care. The stoma therapist and/or nurse should assist the patient in selecting a drainage system most suited to his or her individual needs. Achievement of self-management and an acceptable quality of life are realistic goals for most persons following bowel diversion surgery.

SUMMARY

The gastrointestinal tract serves to supply the body cells with a constant supply of nutrients, electrolytes and water. It does this through the mechanisms of motility, secretion, digestion and absorption. Disorders in one mechanism anywhere along the tract affect the other activities above and below the area. Function of the gastrointestinal tract is influenced by external and internal environmental factors. Physical and life stresses have been shown to affect gastrointestinal motility and secretion.

Discussion in this chapter focuses on the person with disorders of the various functions and parts of the gastrointestinal system: Disorders of swallowing and absorption of foods are discussed. Diarrhoea and constipation are health problems that we all experience at sometime in our lives. Constipation is a common, yet largely preventable problem in the elderly. Research findings are presented on the impact of chronic inflammatory bowel disease on the person's quality of life. Implications for nursing are discussed. The creation of a surgical faecal diversion also has a tremendous impact on the quality of life of the patient and family. Adjustment is slow and requires teaching and support from nurses and other health professionals. Cancer of the gastrointestinal tract effects both men and women of all ages and carries a poor prognosis. Early diagnosis and treatment are important for a positive outcome. Screening programmes for all persons over 50 are recommended. Preventive measures include the adoption of a diet high in fibre, fruits and vegetables, with adequate vitamins C and D and micronutrients such as selenium, and low in fat, nitrate-preserved foods, salt and alcohol.

LEARNING ACTIVITIES

1. Explore how your gastrointestinal tract usually responds to your life stresses. What gastrointestinal responses (e.g. nausea, vomiting, anorexia, constipation or diarrhoea) have you experienced with: (a) happy events such as an engagement, wedding, birthday or graduation; (b) losses such as death of a family member or friends, a move to another community by yourself or best friend, or termination of a romantic relationship; (c) accidental trauma to yourself or others.
2. Find between two and five patients in your clinical setting who are experiencing problems with constipation.
   (a) What contributory factors are identified on each patient's records?

    (b) How often has each patient received a laxative in the past 2 weeks?

    (c) Is there documentation of the reason for the administration of each laxative dose and evaluation of the effectiveness of each dose?

    (d) What other nursing measures to prevent/manage the constipation are identified on each patient's care plan and nursing documentation?

    (e) Review and discuss critically the nursing literature for evidence of the effectiveness of the identified practice measures in alleviating/preventing constipation.

3. Explore the resources in your community for people with ostomies and for obtaining supplies for ostomy management.

4. Sexual functioning can be affected by surgery in the lower gastrointestinal tract.

    (a) Do you feel able to discuss sexual issues with patients and their partners?

    (b) If not, can you identify why you feel unable to discuss sexual issues?

    (c) If lack of knowledge is an area you have identified, review the nursing literature and develop resources which can increase your knowledge and understanding of the subject.

    (d) Identify a patient in your clinical area who may encounter or has difficulties relating to sexuality. From the nursing records or, if you feel able and prepared, from the patient, assess the nature of the problem and interventions that have been explored and evaluate the outcome.

REFERENCES AND FURTHER READING

Alderman C (1988) Colorectal cancer. *Nursing Times* **2(36):** 33–34.

Borley D (ed.) (1989) *Oncology for Nurses and Health Care Professionals. Vol. 33: Cancer Nursing*, p. 294. Beaconsfield: Harper and Row.

Breckman B (ed.) (1981) *Stoma Care*. Beaconsfield: Beaconsfield Publishers.

Bridges J (1987) Restorative proctocolectomy to avoid a stoma. *Nursing Times* **83(4):** 63–66.

Brown MK & Everett I (1990) Gentler bowel fitness with fibre. *Geriatric Nursing* **1:** 26–27.

Brunt PW (1988) *Gastro-enterology*. London: Heinemann.

Bucharth F et al (1986) The colostomy plug: a new disposable device for a continent colostomy *Lancet* **i:** 1062–1063.

Clark ML et al (1987) Tumours of the gastrointestinal tract. In Weatherall DJ et al (eds) *Oxford Textbook of Medicine*. Oxford: Oxford Medical Publications.

Clarke B (1989) Bowel preparation for operative procedures. *Nursing Times* **85(5):** 46–47.

Coloplast (1987) *Ostomy and Ostomy Patients: An Introductory Guide for Nurses*. Oxford: The Medicine Group (UK) Ltd.

Davenport HW (1982) *Physiology of the Digestive Tract* 5th edn. Chicago: Year Book Medical.

Davis K (1990) Impotence after surgery. *Nursing* **4(18):** 23–25.

Dewer BJ (1986) Total parenteral nutrition at home. *Nursing Times* **82(28):** 35–38.

Dunwoody CJ (1987) Patient-controlled analgesia: rationale, attributes, and essential factors. *Orthopaedic Nursing* **6(5):** 31–36.

Erickson BJ (1987) Ostomies: The art of pouching. *Nursing Clinics of North America* **22:** 316–317.

Finch M (1989) Continuous pain relief. *Nursing Times* **85(26):** 30–31.

Fox JET & Monna K (1980) How to relieve your dysphagic patient's pain with a double swallow. In MacKay RC & Silm G (eds) *Research for Practice*. Halifax, Nova Scotia: Dalhousie University.

Ganong WF (1989) *Review of Medical Physiology* 14th edn, p. 399. Norwalk CT: Appleton & Lange.

Gingell JC & Desai KM (1988) Treatment of erectile failure. *Practical Diabetes* **5(1):** 7–9.

Guyatt G, Mitchell A, Irvine EJ et al (1989) A new measure of health status for clinical trials in inflammatory bowel disease. *Gastroenterology* **96:** 804–810.

Harvey RF & Bradshaw JM (1980) A simple index of Crohn's disease activity. *Lancet* **i:** 514.

Haverty S, MacLeod Clark J & Kendall S (1986) Nurses and smoking education: a literature review. *Nurse Education Today* **6:** 237–243.

Hendriksen C & Binder V (1980) Social prognosis in patients with ulcerative colitis. *British Medical Journal* **281:** 581–583.

Hinchcliff S & Montague S (1988) *Physiology for Nursing Practice*, pp. 395–440. London: Baillière Tindall.

Holmes S (1986) Nutritional needs of surgical patients. *Nursing Times* **82(13):** 30–32.

Joachim G (1989) Sad times can be growing times. *The J.—A Quarterly Publication of the Canadian Foundation for Ileitis and Colitis* **December:** 5–6.

Joachim G & Milne B (1985) The effects of inflammatory bowel disease on lifestyle. *Canadian Nurse* **81(10):** 39–40.

Kane NE, Lehman, ME, Dugger R, Hansen L & Jackson D (1988) Use of patient controlled analgesia in surgical oncology patients. *Oncology Nursing Forum* **15(1):** 29–32.

Kelly M (1985) Loss and grief responses to surgery. *Journal of Advanced Nursing* **10:** 517–525.

Kelly M (1986) The subjective experience of chronic disease: some implications for the management of ulcerative colitis. *Journal of Chronic Disease* **39(8):** 653–666.

Kelly M (1987) Managing radical surgery: notes from the patients viewpoint. **GUT 28:** 81–87.

Krause MV & Mahan LK (1984) *Food, Nutrition and Diet Therapy* 7th edn, Chapter 6. Philadelphia: Saunders.

Lepczyk M, Raleigh EH & Rowley C (1990) Timing of preoperative teaching. *Journal of Advanced Nursing* **15(3):** 300–306.

MacLeod Clark J & Webb P (1985) Health Education—a basis for professional nursing practice. *Nurse Education Today* **5:** 216–214.

MacLeod Clark J, Haverty S & Kendall S (1990) Helping people to stop smoking: a study of the nurse's role. *Journal of Advanced Nursing* **15(3):** 357–363.

Mallett SJ, Lennard-Jones JE, Bingley J et al (1978) Colitis. *Lancet* **ii:** 619–621.

Metheny N (1988) Measures to test placement of nasogastric and nasointestinal feeding tubes: a review. *Nursing Research* **37(6):** 324–329.

Michie B (1988) Making sense of TPN. *Nursing Times* **84(20):** 46–47.

Mitchell A, Guyatt G, Singer J et al (1988) Quality of life in patients with inflammatory bowel disease. *Journal of Clinical Gastroenterology* **10:** 306–310.

Mitchell A, Guyatt G, Singer J, Irvine EJ, Tompkins C & Goodacre R (1989) A method to measure quality of life in patients with inflammatory bowel disease. In *Current Topics in Inflammatory Bowel Disease: Symposium Proceedings,* pp. 3–7. New York: McGraw-Hill.

Mitchell P & Silman (1983) Screening for colorectal cancer. *Nursing Times* **79:** 58–61.

Myer SA (1984) Overview of inflammatory bowel disease. *Nursing Clinics of North America* **19(1):** 3–9.

Pritchard AP & David JA (1988) *The Royal Marsden Manual of Clinical Nursing Procedures* 2nd Edn, pp. 78–96, 234–239, 240–251, 344–354.

Rolstad BS (1987) Innovative surgical procedures and stoma care in the future. *Nursing Clinics of North America* **22(2):** 353.

Roth PT & Creason NS (1986) Nurse-administered oral hygiene: is there a scientific rationale? *Journal of Advanced Nursing* **11:** 321–331.

Salter M (ed.) (1988) *Altered Body Image.* Harrow: Scutari.

Shipes E (1987a) Psychosocial issues: the person with an ostomy. *Nursing Clinics of North America* **22(2):** 291–302.

Shipes E (1987b) Sexual function following ostomy surgery. *Nursing Clinics of North America* **22(2):** 305.

Smith DB & Johnson DE (1986) *Ostomy Care and the Cancer Patient.* Orlando: Grune & Stratton.

Topping AE (1989) Nursing patients with tumours of the gastrointestinal tract. In Borley D (ed.) *Oncology for Nurses and Health Care Professionals: Vol. 3 Cancer Nursing* pp. 261–308. Beaconsfield: Harper & Row.

Topping AE (1990) Sexual activity and the stoma patient. *Nursing Standard* **4(41):** 24–26.

Tschudin V (ed.) (1988) *Nursing the Patient with Cancer,* pp. 203–266, 227–244. Hemel Hempstead: Prentice Hall.

Truelove SC (1984) *Ulcerative Colitis.* London: Update Publications.

Wade B (1989) *A Stoma is for Life.* Harrow: Scutari.

Williams G, Mulcahy MJ & Kiely EA (1987) Impotence: treatment by autoinjection of vasoactive drugs. *British Medical Journal* **295:** 595–596.

Wilson-Barnett J (1978) Patients' emotional responses to barium X-rays. *Journal of Advanced Nursing* **3:** 37–46.

Wilson-Barnet J & Bateup L (1988) *Patient Problems,* pp. 86–99. Harrow: Scutari.

Caring for the Patient with Disorders of the Liver, Biliary Tract and Exocrine Pancreas

17

OBJECTIVES

On completion of this chapter, the reader will be able to:

- Describe the structure and function of the liver, biliary tract and exocrine pancreas
- Assess the individual for alteration in function of the liver, biliary tract and exocrine pancreas
- Appreciate the role of the nurse in the early detection and treatment of persons with alcohol abuse problems
- Explore personal attitudes towards persons with alcohol abuse problems
- Discuss measures to prevent the transmission of hepatitis to health professionals and the public
- Discuss the nursing management of persons with disorders of the liver, biliary tract and exocrine pancreas

PHYSIOLOGY

The biliary system consists of the liver, gallbladder and bile ducts.

Liver

The liver is the largest organ of the body and is situated in the upper abdominal cavity immediately below the diaphragm. It is divided into four lobes and is highly vascular, receiving its blood supply from two sources. The portal vein carries blood from the stomach, intestines, spleen and pancreas into the liver. The hepatic artery delivers blood from the aorta. The blood from both sources leaves the liver by a common pathway, the hepatic vein, which joins the inferior vena cava.

The liver tissue is organized in functional units called lobules. Each lobule consists of rows of cells radiating out from a central vein. Subdivisions of the hepatic artery and portal vein deliver blood into small spaces called sinusoids between the rows of cells, bringing the blood in direct contact with the hepatic cells. From the sinusoids it enters the central vein (Figure 17.1). Large phagocytic, reticuloendothelial cells called Kupffer cells lie scattered within the sinusoids to ingest and destroy organisms and other foreign material within the blood. The central veins from the lobules empty into sub-lobular collecting veins, which unite to form the hepatic vein. Minute ducts into which bile is discharged are also formed between the rows of hepatic cells. The small lobular bile ducts are directed toward the surface of the lobules where they unite to form larger ducts. Eventually, the bile from the lobules is transmitted in one main channel, the hepatic duct, which joins the bile duct from the gallbladder (cystic duct) to form the common bile duct (see Figure 17.2).

FUNCTIONS OF THE LIVER

The liver performs a variety of very important complex functions. It is a vital organ, performing a major role in total body metabolism. The liver synthesizes, processes and/or stores many of the substances that are essential to normal body functioning. It also processes and excretes some substances that would be harmful if left in their original form or retained.

Bile production and excretion

The liver cells secrete 500–1000 ml of bile daily into the hepatic ducts. It is a yellow-green or brownish fluid that is strongly alkaline and bitter to the taste. The

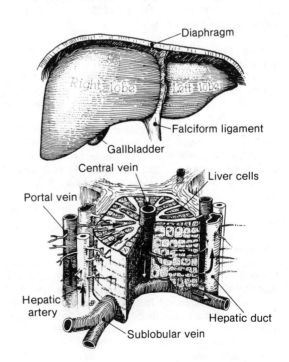

Figure 17.1 The liver and an enlarged section of a lobule.

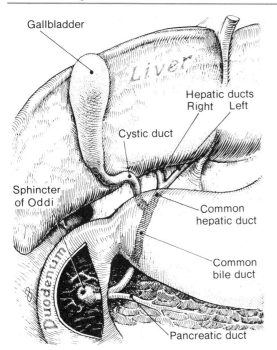

Gallbladder

Liver

Hepatic ducts
Right   Left

Cystic duct

Sphincter
of Oddi

Common
hepatic duct

Common
bile duct

Duodenum

Pancreatic duct

Figure 17.2 The gallbladder and extrahepatic biliary tract.

constituents of bile include water, bile pigments and bile salts.

Water (90–97%). The water content is reduced when the bile is stored in the gallbladder where it is concentrated six to ten times.

Bile pigments. The pigments resulting from the breakdown of red blood cells and from foods are excreted as the bile pigments *bilirubin* and *biliverdin*. Bilirubin is orange-red and is in greater concentration in man; biliverdin is green and predominates in those persons or species whose diet is mainly vegetable.

In the intestine, bile pigments are acted upon by bacteria and reduced to urobilinogen. Part of the urobilinogen is excreted in the faeces, giving them the normal brown colour. The remainder is re-absorbed through the intestinal mucosa into the blood. A small amount is excreted in the urine and the rest is returned to the liver, where it is reconverted to bilirubin and again is secreted in the bile.

Bile salts. These are sodium and potassium salts of certain amino acids that function in digestion and absorption. The bile salts emulsify fats, increase the digestive action of the fat-splitting enzyme, and promote absorption of fats, fat-soluble vitamins and calcium salts. The bile salts are reclaimed from the intestine and returned to the liver by the portal circulation where they stimulate the hepatic cells to secrete bile. They are reused in the secretion.

Other constituents. Sodium and calcium salts, choles-

terol, fatty acids and lecithin are other substances in bile.

Bile is discharged by the common bile duct into the duodenum through the sphincter of Oddi. The functions of bile may be summarized as follows:

Bile promotes the digestion and absorption of fats in the small intestine. Because it is alkaline, it neutralizes the acidic chyme when it moves into the small intestine. It stimulates peristalsis of the large intestine, which was the basis of the use of bile salts in preparations of laxatives. The reabsorbed bile salts stimulate hepatic cells to secrete bile. Bile is an excretory medium for some drugs, toxins, excess minerals (e.g. copper and zinc), pigments and cholesterol.

Metabolic functions

The liver has a role in the metabolism of *carbohydrates, proteins and fats*. Briefly, it converts glucose to glycogen and stores it (glycogenesis), reconverting it to glucose and releasing it into the blood when required in order to maintain an adequate blood sugar concentration. Glucose in excess of what can be converted to glycogen is converted to fat (lipogenesis) in the liver. The simple sugars, or monosaccharides, fructose and galactose cannot be utilized by the cells, so the liver changes the molecules to glucose.

Fats may be both synthesized and catabolized by the liver. Cholesterol, lecithin, phospholipids and lipoproteins are examples of substances that may be formed by the liver. Fats are desaturated or may be broken down into ketone acids or acetate.

Protein may be deaminized, a process in which the amine radical is removed and the remaining elements are used to form glycogen or other compounds to meet tissue needs. The amine radical is converted to urea and released into the blood for elimination by the kidneys. Amino acids are also used in the liver to form blood proteins, enzymes and structural compounds. Amino acids may be converted to carbohydrates to provide a source of energy.

Storage

The liver stores glycogen, vitamins A, D, E, K and B_{12}, iron, phospholipids, cholesterol, and a small amount of protein and fat.

Formation of certain blood components

In the fetus, the liver produces the erythrocytes. This activity gradually diminishes after midterm when erythropoiesis in the bone marrow increases. After birth, the liver stores vitamin B_{12} and releases it as necessary to promote the production of erythrocytes.

Heparin, and the blood proteins serum albumin, fibrinogen and α and β globulins are formed by the hepatic cells. The liver also synthesizes most of the blood-clotting factors; it is the primary source of prothrombin, fibrinogen and Factors V, VII, VIII, IX, XI and XII.

Destruction of erythrocytes

The Kupffer cells break down the worn-out erythrocytes. The haemoglobin is released, the iron and globin are split off, and bilirubin is formed from the waste products and is excreted in bile. The iron is reclaimed, combined with a protein to form ferritin and stored until it is needed for the formation of haemoglobin.

Detoxification of harmful substances

Certain drugs and chemicals that could be harmful to tissue cells are changed by the liver and rendered harmless before being circulated and excreted by the kidneys. The liver detoxifies by conjugation, oxidation or hydrolysis. In conjugation, it combines the toxic substance with some other material to produce an inoffensive compound (e.g. benzoic acid is changed to hippuric acid). Barbiturates, nicotine and strychnine are drugs that are oxidized and completely destroyed by the liver. Laxative drugs and some nutrients such as vitamin D are neutralized in the liver.

The body itself produces certain chemicals (hormones) that, unless destroyed, would reach too high a concentration. Examples of physiological products that are destroyed in the liver are the antidiuretic hormone (ADH), progesterone and adrenocorticoid secretions. Some hormones such as insulin and glucagon undergo deamination (removal of amino acids) in the liver, which renders them inactive.

The Kupffer cells also protect the body by destroying organisms that may have been absorbed from the intestine.

Heat production

The liver is second only to muscle tissue in the production of heat by its continuous cell activity. Under basal (resting) conditions, the liver is responsible for most of the body heat.

Gallbladder and Bile Ducts

The gallbladder is a sac on the undersurface of the liver with an average capacity of 40–50 ml. The cystic duct leading from the gallbladder merges with the hepatic duct to form the common bile duct. The latter unites with the pancreatic duct to form the ampulla of Vater, which opens into the duodenum. This opening is controlled by the sphincter of Oddi (Figure 17.2).

Smooth muscle, connective tissue and a mucous membranous lining compose the walls of the gallbladder and ducts.

The functions of the gallbladder are to concentrate and store the bile. When the stomach and duodenum are empty of food, the sphincter of Oddi remains contracted. During this period, the bile that is continuously secreted accumulates in the gallbladder. Contraction of the sac to eject the bile is dependent upon hormonal stimulation. When food containing fat and partially digested protein enters the duodenum, a hormone called cholecystokinin-pancreozymin (CCK-PZ or CCK) is secreted by cells of the duodenal mucosa. It is carried in the blood and, on reaching the gallbladder, stimulates the smooth muscle tissue to contract and eject bile. CCK also produces relaxation of the sphincter

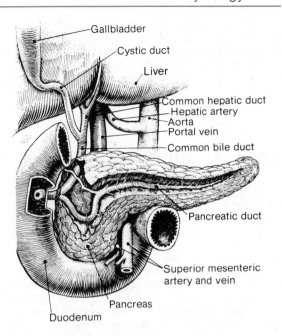

Figure 17.3 Diagram of the pancreas and central pancreatic duct in relationship to the duodenum and common bile duct.

of Oddi which allows the flow of bile into the duodenum.

Pancreas

The pancreas is a fish-shaped gland; the thicker portion, referred to as the head, lies in the curve of the duodenum, and the remainder extends to the left directly behind the stomach (Figure 17.3). It has two distinct types of essential functional cells. Groups of one type secrete into small ducts which drain into a main channel running the length of the gland. This collecting channel is called the *pancreatic duct*, or the duct of Wirsung, and passes out of the head of the pancreas to unite with the common bile duct to form the ampulla of Vater. In a few people, the duct may have a direct entrance to the duodenum via the duct of Santorini. Because the secretion of this type of cell flows through ducts, it is classified as an *external* or *exocrine secretion*.

The other type of parenchymal cell is scattered in insular groups, forming what are known as the islets of Langerhans. These cells produce secretions which are classified as *internal* or *endocrine secretions* because they are absorbed into the blood and are not secreted into ducts.

EXOCRINE FUNCTIONS

The external secretion passes through the ampulla of Vater and sphincter of Oddi into the duodenum. It is strongly alkaline, owing to a high bicarbonate content. Several important digestive enzymes (see Table 16.1) (trypsinogen, chymotrypsin, procarboxypeptidase, amylopsin, lipase, ribonuclease and deoxyribonuclease) involved in the breakdown of proteins, carbohydrates and fats are contained in the exocrine secretion. Regulation of the secretion of these enzymes and their role in digestion is discussed under Digestion in the Small Intestine on page 442.

ENDOCRINE FUNCTIONS

The endocrine functions of the pancreas are the production of insulin, glucagon, somatostatin and pancreatic polypeptide hormones.

Insulin is secreted by the β cells of the islets of Langerhans in response to a rise in blood glucose concentration. It has a major role in the metabolism of glucose and regulation of the blood sugar level. The transfer of glucose from the blood into most body cells is facilitated by insulin, but neurones and erythrocytes are not dependent upon it for the uptake of glucose. Insulin promotes utilization of glucose by the cells and the storage of glucose as glycogen in the liver. It also influences fatty acid synthesis (esterification) in fatty tissue and the uptake and conversion of amino acids into body proteins. It is rapidly removed from the blood and degraded by the liver.

Glucagon is formed by the α cells of the islets of Langerhans and by similar cells in the walls of the stomach and duodenum. Glucagon functions to increase the blood glucose concentration by breaking down liver glycogen (glycogenolysis) and increasing the synthesis of glucose (gluconeogenesis) by the liver. It also promotes the breakdown of fats to fatty acids and glycerol and the release of potassium from the liver. Physical exercise, stress and the sympathetic nervous system also stimulate glucagon secretion thus mobilizing the body's energy stores.

The two main hormones, insulin and glucagon, secreted by the islets of Langerhans are opposite in effect. Insulin secretion increases during absorption of a meal high in carbohydrate in response to the increase in plasma glucose concentration. Absorption of a meal low in carbohydrate and high in protein increases plasma amino acid concentration which stimulates the release of glucagon as well as insulin, thus maintaining the plasma glucose level. Following absorption of a usual meal, the increase in plasma glucose and amino acid concentrations counteract each other and the result is an increase in insulin secretion with only a minimal change in glucagon. During the postabsorptive period following a meal and during fasting, glucagon secretion increases and insulin secretion decreases as the plasma glucose concentration falls.

Somatostatin, secreted by the cells of the islets of Langerhans, functions to maintain a relatively constant blood glucose level by inhibiting the secretion of insulin and glucagon.

Pancreatic polypeptide hormone is secreted by cells of the islets of Langerhans. Its function is not clear. Secretion increases following ingestion of protein, fats or glucose.

ASSESSMENT

Disorders of the liver, biliary tract and pancreas affect overall body functioning. The body's energy balance is affected when the supply and storage of nutrients is altered, fluid and electrolyte balance is disrupted, bowel and bladder elimination is altered, blood clotting mechanisms are affected, and heat production diminishes. Patient assessment includes the collection of data on life-style, behaviour patterns, dietary habits and changes in physiological functioning of most body systems. Also, the nurse should have some understanding of the various examinations and tests carried out, and the implications of the results of these for the patient. Knowledge of the manifestations of disorders of the liver, biliary tract and pancreas will also help her to assess the patient and to plan nursing care.

Subsequent sections of this chapter will address specific disease processes and the clinical manifestations that they produce. This information is important for the nurse in assessing the patient as it gives guidance to the areas deserving particularly careful enquiry. Equally important however is the effect of a symptom on the patient, how the patient and family interpret that symptom and how they feel about it.

It is not enough therefore to note that a patient appears jaundiced. The alteration in skin colour may make the patient embarrassed or ashamed and be a cause of great concern to the family. The person may have heard 'old wives' tales about jaundice, or associate the condition with a fatal outcome, consequently patient education is required to relieve a great deal of possible anxiety and fear. Jaundice represents a significant alteration in body image which requires the patient to adapt to this change. The nurse therefore needs to assess how effectively the patient is coping, as maladaptive behaviour, if present, suggests the need for nursing intervention.

It is important therefore that the nurse considers the effects of the various clinical manifestations of biliary, hepatic and pancreatic disease on the whole patient, besides the obvious physical changes that are present. This consideration should be borne in mind while studying the rest of this chapter. The question 'What does the patient make of this?' should therefore be to the forefront throughout the assessment stage.

HISTORY

1. *Activity and life-style*. Data are collected on: the type and extent of daily activities; how the person feels following activity; how leisure time is used and the usual pattern and amount of sleep received.
2. *Nutritional history* includes identification of daily food intake, eating habits, and factors affecting eating. Daily food intake is analysed for adequacy of essential nutrients, vitamins, fluid volume and kilocalories. How the individual responds to food is elicited as well as symptoms that occur following ingestion of food. The presence of nausea, vomiting, anorexia, excessive thirst and changes in body weight are determined. Use of alcohol and drugs is carefully recorded.

3. *Elimination*. The person's usual bowel habits are determined and questions related to the nature, formation, colour and odour of stools are asked. The presence of steatorrhoea, melaena and clay-coloured stools is noted.

   The volume and colour of urine and frequency of voiding are determined as well as the presence of nocturia.
4. *Changes in blood clotting* may be identified by questioning the person about the presence of blood in urine or stools, petechiae in the skin, bruises, or cuts that bleed for an unusual length of time.
5. *Environmental and occupational history* includes the identification of factors in the person's work and home environment that might be toxic to the individual.
6. *Pain and discomfort* are identified by questioning the patient about the location and duration of abdominal or epigastric pain or discomfort and factors which precipitate discomfort.
7. *The patient's psychological and social status* should also be assessed, including the patient's own perceptions of his or her health.

PHYSICAL EXAMINATION

1. *General appearance*. Changes in posture or weight distribution as seen with abdominal ascites are observed, as well as the general colour of the skin and the sclera of the eyes.
2. *Height and weight* are measured and recorded. Changes in body weight are noted.
3. *Skin-fold thickness and body circumferences* may be measured to determine the amount of subcutaneous body fat.
4. *Temperature, pulse, respirations and blood pressure* are recorded. Body temperature reflects both liver function and cellular metabolism.
5. *The skin* is inspected for signs of petechiae or bruises, open lesions that have not healed, and jaundice as evidenced by a yellowish colour to the skin and sclera and itching of the skin. Skin turgor is assessed by lifting a fold of skin and observing for mobility of the tissue and the rate at which it returns to its previous position. Peripheral oedema is determined by pressing firmly for about 5 seconds with the thumb over a bony prominence such as the dorsum of the foot; on release of the pressure, the skin is observed and palpated for pitting or indentations and the rate at which it returns to normal.
6. *Abdominal ascites*. Inspection of the abdomen containing ascites will show distension, protrusion of the umbilicus and asymmetry when the patient shifts position.

DIAGNOSTIC TESTS

LABORATORY TESTS FOR LIVER, BILIARY AND PANCREATIC FUNCTION (TABLE 17.1)

Blood tests

Plasma protein electrophoresis (serum albumin and globulin concentrations). Serum albumin is produced by the liver and, normally, is of greater concentration than globulin, most of which is produced by the lymphoid tissues. In disease of the liver cells, the amount of albumin decreases, and the ratio of albumin to globulin is reversed.

Serum bilirubin. This test gives an estimation of the concentration of bilirubin in the blood and indicates whether it is conjugated or unconjugated. Normally, the liver cells extract the pigment from the blood and convert it to a water-soluble compound (bilirubin diglucuronide) before excreting it in bile. Unconjugated bilirubin is usually reported as 'indirect bilirubin' and the conjugated form as 'direct bilirubin'. In obstructive jaundice, the conjugate (direct) bilirubin level is increased. In haemolytic jaundice, unconjugated (indirect) bilirubin is the predominant pigment in the blood.

Serum alkaline phosphatase. Normally this enzyme is excreted in the bile by the hepatic cells. The blood concentration may be increased when there is liver disease or obstruction in the bile ducts.

Serum enzymes (liver and pancreatic).

1. *Liver enzyme tests*. The liver cells contain the enzymes serum alanine aminotransferase (ALT), formerly referred to as serum glutamic-pyruvic transaminase (SGPT), and serum aspartate aminotransferase (AST), previously called serum glutamic oxaloacetic transaminase (SGOT). Since they are released into the blood when the cells are damaged, their concentration may be used to estimate liver damage. Opiates can cause a rise in ALT and AST.

   Gamma-glutamyl transferase (GGT) is an enzyme found in greatest concentration in the liver and kidneys; it indicates liver cell dysfunction and alcohol-induced liver disease.
2. *Concentration of pancreatic enzymes*. Some of the enzymes secreted by the pancreas are normally absorbed into the blood and eventually are excreted in the urine. An elevation of the serum amylase and lipase levels occurs when there is an obstruction of pancreatic ducts and necrosis of cells.

Serum calcium. Pancreatitis causes a decrease in the blood calcium level.

Prothrombin time. The liver is responsible for the synthesis of several clotting factors. The prothrombin time or activity reflects the effects of liver dysfunction on blood coagulation.

Bromsulphalein (BSP) test. Bromsulphalein is a dye normally excreted by the liver cells in the bile. The test is used to detect liver cell damage and impaired function. It is not used if obstruction in the bile ducts is suspected, because the dye would be retained in the body. Five milligrams of bromsulphalein for each kilogram of the patient's body weight is given intravenously, and a venous blood specimen is collected from another vein in 45 minutes. Normally, only 5% or less of the dye given remains in the blood.

Table 17.1 Tests used to assess liver, biliary and exocrine pancreatic function.

Diagnostic test	Normal values	Description/discussion
Blood tests		
Plasma protein electrophoresis (serum albumin, and globulin concentrations)	Total serum proteins: 60–80 g/l Albumin: 40–50 g/l Globulin: 5–15 g/l A/G Ratio 3:1	Serum albumin produced in the liver is normally found in greater concentration than globulin which is produced by the lymphoid tissues With liver disease, serum albumin levels decrease and globulin levels increase
Serum bilirubin: conjugated (direct), unconjugated (indirect), and total	Direct bilirubin: 2.0–8.0 μmol/l Indirect bilirubin: 0–12 μmol/l Total bilirubin: 3.5–20.5 μmol/l	Bilirubin is normally extracted from the blood and converted to a water-soluble compound in the liver before being excreted in bile In obstructive jaundice, the conjugated (direct) bilirubin level is increased In haemolytic jaundice, unconjugated or indirect bilirubin is increased
Serum alkaline phosphatase	35–105 iu/l at 37°C or 5.0–13.0 King-Armstrong units	Alkaline phosphatase is an enzyme excreted in the bile by hepatic cells. Serum concentrations increase with liver disease or obstruction of the bile ducts
Prothrombin time (PT)	11–15 s	Prothrombin time is prolonged in liver diseases as the liver cells cannot synthesize prothrombin
Liver enzyme tests Serum alanine aminotransferase (ALT)	ALT (SGPT): 1–12 iu/l (or 4–24 iu/l at 30°C)	These enzymes are released when cells are damaged. Elevated levels provide an estimate of liver damage
Serum aspartate aminotransferase (AST)	AST (SGOT): 0–40 iu/l	
Gamma glutamyl transferase (GGT) (gamma glutamyl transpeptidase; GGTP)	GGT: female, 4–18 iu/l male, 6–28 iu/l	
Pancreatic enzyme tests Serum amylase	0–130 u/l (or 50–150 Somogyi units/dl)	Elevated serum amylase and lipase levels occur when there is an obstruction of the pancreatic ducts and necrosis of cells
Serum lipase	0–160 u/l	
Serum calcium	2.2–2.6 mmol/l	Serum calcium increases with pancreatitis
Bromsulphalein (BSP) test	5% or less of the injected dye remains in the blood 45 minutes later	Used to detect liver cell damage and impaired function. Bromsulphalein is a dye normally excreted by the liver cells in the bile. Retention of the dye increases with liver cell damage or decreased hepatic blood flow
Blood lipids Serum cholesterol	3.6–6.0 mmol/l	The cholesterol level in the blood falls in liver disease when cell function is impaired and rises in obstructive jaundice
Cholesterol esters	50–70% of total cholesterol	
Blood ammonia	47–65 μmol/l	Blood ammonia concentrations increase in severe liver impairment and may lead to hepatic coma
Hepatitis viral studies	Negative	These tests are used to identify the known antigens and antibodies associated with hepatitis virus A, hepatitis virus B, and non-A, non-B hepatitis viruses
Blood glucose	Fasting 3.9–6.1 mmol/l	An elevated blood glucose may result from a decrease in insulin secretion if the cells of the islets of Langerhans are damaged

Table 17.1   *Continued*

Diagnostic test	Normal values	Description/discussion
Leucocyte count	$4.0–11.0 \times 10^9$ per litre or 5000–10000 per mm^3	Elevated white blood counts occur with pancreatitis
Urine tests		
Urinary bilirubin	0	This bile pigment, normally absent in the urine, may be present in obstructive jaundice and hepatocellular jaundice
Urinary urobilinogen	0–6.8 µmol/dl (0–4.0 mg) in 24 hours or less than 1.0 Ehrlich unit per dl	In obstructive jaundice, when bile does not reach the intestine, conjugated bilirubin is not changed into urobilinogen and so urinary levels are decreased, as it is when oral antibiotics are administered When liver cells are damaged urinary urobilinogen concentrations increase
Urinary amylase excretion	260–950 King-Armstrong units/24 hours or up to 5000 Somogyi units in 24 hours	Elevations occur in pancreatitis with increases in the excretion of the enzyme amylase
Glycosuria	0	Glucose may be present in the urine with pancreatic dysfunction and decreased insulin production producing hyperglycaemia and glycosuria
Stool tests		
Faecal fat test	3–5 g in 24 hours	Elevated levels occur with obstruction of bile ducts

The normal values presented are a general guide as they vary from laboratory to laboratory. It is advisable to refer to local values.

Blood lipids. The concentration of cholesterol and cholesterol esters in the blood falls in liver disease, when cell function is impaired, and rises in obstructive jaundice.

Blood ammonia. In severe impairment of liver function, the ammonia concentration in the blood is elevated and may lead to hepatic coma.

Hepatitis tests. Viral hepatitis is caused by hepatitis virus A, hepatitis virus B, and non-A, non-B hepatitis viruses. Tests are available to identify the known antigens and antibodies associated with these viruses.

Blood glucose concentration. Damage to the islets of Langerhans may cause a reduction in insulin secretion and hyperglycaemia.

Leucocyte count. The white blood count is elevated in pancreatitis with a marked increase in the polymorphonuclear leucocytes in necrotizing and haemorrhagic pancreatitis.

Urine tests

Urinary bilirubin. A urinalysis may be requested for bilirubin. Normally, this bile pigment is not present in urine. Conjugated, or direct bilirubin, is water soluble and is present in the urine in obstructive jaundice and hepatocellular jaundice but is absent in haemolytic

jaundice. Phenazopyridine (Pyridium) can produce a false-positive bilirubin result.

Urinary urobilinogen. Conjugated bilirubin is changed to urobilinogen by bacterial action when the bile reaches the small intestine. Most of the urobilinogen is then excreted in the faeces, and the remainder is absorbed. A small amount of the absorbed urobilinogen is excreted in the urine, but the larger portion is claimed by the liver to be excreted in the bile. If the liver cells are damaged they may not perform this latter function, and the amount of urobilinogen excreted by the kidneys is increased. The amount of the pigment in the urine may be decreased below the normal amount of obstructive jaundice when bile is not reaching the intestine or if the bacterial content of the intestine is reduced, as it is in oral administration of antibiotics. If the individual is taking antibiotics this information should be noted on the laboratory form.

Urinary amylase excretion. Urinalysis may indicate an increase in the excretion of the enzyme amylase in pancreatitis.

Glycosuria. Dysfunction of the pancreas may incur a deficiency of insulin, resulting in hyperglycaemia and the excretion of excess glucose in the urine.

Stool test

Faecal fat test. Analysis of stool specimens made over a

specified number of hours may be done to determine the fat content. Failure of the pancreatic lipase to reach the intestine results in undigested and unabsorbed fat.

X-RAY

A radiological examination is made of the abdomen. It may reveal gallstones, accumulation of gas in the duodenum or calcification in the pancreas.

PANCREAS SCAN

A scan may be done if tumours of the pancreas are suspected or to assess the extent of fibrosed, non-functional tissue. The patient receives selenium-75 (^{75}Se) tagged with methionine by intravenous injection. The radioactive substance is taken up by the pancreas; methionine is used in the formation of enzymes. The pancreas is then scanned with a scintillation counter; a graph is produced which indicates the *amount* of the radioactive tracer taken up by the different areas of the pancreas. Abnormal areas of tissue do not take up the radioactive selenium and so leave voids in the scan.

ULTRASOUND EXAMINATION

Ultrasound is a quick, cheap and non-invasive method of assessing the pancreas. While it is less reliable in obese individuals or those with an excess of bowel gas, it can frequently detect enlargement of the gland due to inflammation or neoplasm. It is particularly useful in the follow-up of patients with acute pancreatitis to identify either pseudocyst or abscess formation.

Ultrasound is the initial investigation for patients with jaundice because it is very sensitive in the diagnosis of bile duct dilatation. This is important because the management (surgical versus medical) of patients with jaundice secondary to bile duct obstruction is very different to those with normal bile ducts. Ultrasound accurately detects gallbladder pathology, notably gallstones; focal hepatic lesions, e.g. metastases are also well demonstrated as an alteration in echo character.

In suspected cases of portal vein thrombosis, real-time ultrasound combined with Doppler (duplex scanning) can identify both thrombus within the vessel and flow disturbances.

COMPUTERIZED TOMOGRAPHY

Computerized tomography (CT) detects most liver lesions; information about their density and enhancement characteristics often allows a specific diagnosis to be made, e.g. in haemangioma. As with all radiological examinations, the images must be interpreted within the clinical context. CT is a useful means of evaluating the pancreas; factors degrading the quality of ultrasound (adipose tissue and intestinal gas) enhance the quality of CT. So when ultrasound fails, for example in the confident exclusion of pancreatic pseudocyst or abscess, CT is the next investigation of choice.

ENDOSCOPIC RETROGRADE CHOLANGIOPANCREATOGRAPHY (ECRP)

A fibreoptic endoscope can be used to cannulate the papilla of Vater in the duodenum. This gives access to both the bile and pancreatic ducts. Pancreatography is done to detect the presence of pancreatic disease, to delineate the pancreatic duct when a precise knowledge of its anatomy is needed for surgery, and to obtain histological or cytological evidence of disease. Retrograde cholangiography is performed to determine the cause of biliary problems, to diagnose cholestatic jaundice, and to remove gallstones which are obstructing the common bile duct. X-ray films are taken during the procedure. A catheter (stent) or T-tube may be inserted endoscopically to bypass the obstructive lesion and relieve the jaundice in some patients with malignant biliary obstruction.

When gallstones are removed by an ERCP and sphincterotomy, the patient will need blood coagulation levels measured, and blood typed and crossmatched. An antibiotic and intravenous fluid are usually administered prior to the procedure. The major problems that may occur are haemorrhage and infection, and the patient is assessed for any signs of these following investigation.

Cholangiography may be used to aid diagnosis of the cause of jaundice, the location of stones within the biliary tract, in diagnosing cancer of the biliary system, and when investigating recurrent symptoms in individuals who have already had cholecystectomy. Contrast medium (e.g. Cholografin sodium) is injected either intravenously or directly into the common bile duct. Direct injection can be performed during operation, percutaneously (via a tube or cannula) or retrogradely during ERCP.

CHOLECYSTOGRAPHY

Radiography is also used in the diagnosis of gallbladder disease and the procedure may be referred to as cholecystography. A radiopaque organic iodine compound (e.g. Telepaque or Cholografin) that is eliminated in the bile is given orally or intravenously. The patient receives a fat-free evening meal which is followed by the administration of the contrast medium the night before the X-ray examination. Then the patient must not take anything by mouth until after the first X-ray. The iodine compound is absorbed, excreted by the liver cells in the bile and, normally is concentrated in the gallbladder, since there was no fat in the meal to stimulate the emptying of the gallbladder. An X-ray film is taken in the morning (approximately 12 hours after the contrast medium was given) to determine if the gallbladder has filled. Calculi are observed if present.

Following this first film, the patient is given a meal containing fat. After one hour, a final X-ray is taken. Normally, after a fatty meal, the gallbladder contracts and empties bile into the small intestine via the common bile duct.

To summarize, cholecystography provides information as to whether the gallbladder fills and empties and whether it contains gallstones.

PERCUTANEOUS LIVER BIOPSY

A small specimen of liver tissue may be examined microscopically to assist in the diagnosis of liver disease. The specimen is obtained by aspiration with a special liver biopsy needle. Using a lateral approach, the needle is passed through the right eighth, ninth or tenth intercostal space, or may be introduced below the costal margin if the liver is enlarged.

Previous to the procedure, the patient's blood coagulation is evaluated by performing a partial thromboplastin time and platelet count. Blood is typed and crossmatched so that blood is available for transfusion if required. An explanation is made to the patient of the purpose of the biopsy and what will happen during and after the procedure. Pulse, respirations and blood pressure are noted by the nurse as a baseline for comparison following the biopsy.

The patient is placed in the supine position close to the right side of the bed. The area is cleansed, and an antiseptic and sterile drape are applied. A local anaesthetic is then injected at the puncture site. The patient is instructed to take two or three deep breaths, and then to stop breathing following exhalation. The doctor should quickly introduce the biopsy needle, aspirate and withdraw, taking only a few seconds.

Following the biopsy, absolute bed rest is necessary until the next morning. The patient is required to lie on the right side with a small pillow under the costal margin. This position places pressure against the biopsy site, preventing the escape of blood and bile. Close observation is made of the patient for haemorrhage for 24 hours. The pulse, respirations, blood pressure, colour, puncture site and general condition are noted and recorded every 15 minutes for 2 hours, then every 30 minutes for 2 hours. The interval is then gradually increased if there are no significant changes. Abdominal pain, tenderness and any rigidity are reported, since they may indicate irritation and inflammation of the peritoneum due to the leakage of bile from the liver. Severe pain and breathlessness are reported promptly as they may indicate that the lung or colon is perforated.

RADIOISOTOPE LIVER SCAN

The Kupffer cells of the liver phagocytose small particles in the blood such as technetium-99m sulphur colloid. When injected intravenously this accumulates in the liver (and spleen). Any lesion in the liver does not take up the radiocolloid and appears as a cold area in the gamma camera image.

BILIARY SCINTIGRAPHY

Technetium-99m labelled derivatives of iminodiacetic acid (e.g. [^{99m}Tc]HIDA) injected intravenously are extracted by the liver, rapidly excreted in bile and accumulate in the gallbladder. Failure to accumulate in the gallbladder indicates an obstructed cystic duct and is typical of cholecystitis. Failure to pass into the bowel indicates an obstructed common bile duct.

Clinical Characteristics of Disorders of the Liver and Biliary Tract

Liver function is essential to life and, fortunately, this large organ has exceptional functional ability and regenerative capacity. If liver disease is limited and tissue damage is localized to one area of the organ, the body is not likely to suffer serious impairment of function. If there is diffuse disease and parenchymal damage, dysfunction is more marked. Liver disease may be acute or chronic, and disturbed function may be reversible or irreversible, depending on the amount of tissue involved and the nature of the cause.

Disorders of the gallbladder and bile ducts interfere with the flow of bile into the duodenum. They may be acute or chronic and the intensity of the signs and symptoms parallels the severity of the condition. Like the liver, the pancreas has a large reserve capacity; a portion of the gland may be destroyed or become nonfunctional and the remainder will compensate sufficiently to maintain normal physiology.

Jaundice (icterus)

This is an indication of an excess of bilirubin in the blood, resulting in a yellowish staining of the tissues that may be seen in the sclerae, mucous membranes and skin. The cause may be intrahepatic or extrahepatic disease, and according to the cause, the jaundice may be classified as hepatocellular, obstructive or haemolytic (Table 17.2).

The *hepatocellular type of jaundice* is associated with intrinsic liver disease and is due to failure of the hepatic cells to take up the bilirubin resulting from the breakdown of red blood cells and excrete it as bile. Jaundice may not be present in chronic liver disease (e.g. cirrhosis), especially in the early stages, since regeneration of the hepatic cells may parallel the damage.

Obstructive jaundice is caused by an interference with the flow of bile in the extrahepatic ducts. It is most often due to the impaction of gallstones in the common bile duct, but may occur as the result of a stricture in the duct or neoplastic disease in neighbouring structures (e.g. pancreas) compressing the duct. *Haemolytic jaundice* occurs when there is an inordinate destruction of red blood cells, resulting in excessive bilirubin formation.

The jaundiced patient's urine is likely to be dark because of the bilirubin or urobilinogen content. Urobilinogen is not present in obstructive jaundice, since it is formed in the intestine. The stools are pale grey in obstructive and severe hepatocellular jaundice.

Pruritus

The itching of the skin experienced by many patients with jaundice is attributed to irritation of the cutaneous sensory nerves by the retained bile salts.

Table 17.2   The characteristics of different types of jaundice.

	Haemolytic	Hepatocellular		Obstructive	
Abnormality	Increased bilirubin load	Deficiency of transferase	Cellular damage	Intrahepatic fibrous obstruction	Extrahepatic obstruction
Example	Hereditary spherocytosis	Gilbert's disease	Infective hepatitis	Biliary cirrhosis	Carcinoma of head of pancreas
Urine					
Colour	Normal	Normal	Dark	Dark	Dark
Urobilinogen	Increased	Variable	Variable	Absent	Absent
Bilirubin	Absent	Absent	Increased	Increased	Increased
Faeces					
Colour	Dark	Normal	Paler than normal	Pale	Pale
Stercobilinogen	Increased	Normal	Low	Absent	Absent
Plasma					
Unconjugated bilirubin	Increased	Increased	Decreased	Increased	Increased
Conjugated bilirubin	Normal	Decreased	Increased	Increased	Increased

From Storer (1988).

General constitutional symptoms

The patient complains of a poor appetite, vague digestive discomfort and flatulence, and loses weight. Lassitude, weakness and muscle wasting develop as a result of the impaired storage of carbohydrates and protein metabolism. A low-grade fever may be present.

Pain

Dull, aching pain in the right upper abdominal quadrant is a common symptom, especially in acute liver disease. Tenderness is manifested on palpation.

The pain associated with gallbladder or biliary duct disease may be felt in the right upper abdomen or midepigastric region, or is referred to the right scapular area. It may be a persistent, dull ache or very severe and disabling. The onset may follow a meal containing fatty foods. When it is very severe, causing the patient to writhe about, the pain is described as biliary colic.

Bleeding tendency

Inadequate production of prothrombin and other blood-clotting factors results in failure of the normal clotting process. Spontaneous bleeding may occur, manifested by purpura, epistaxis, bleeding of the oral mucous membrane, and/or melaena.

Ascites and oedema

An accumulation of fluid in the peritoneal cavity develops with progressive liver disease, such as cirrhosis. The hepatic tissue damage, obliteration of blood vessels, and compression by the fibrous tissue (scar) replacement produce a resistance to the inflow and outflow of blood from the portal vein. The resulting increase in the blood pressure within the portal vein and its contributaries promotes the escape of fluid into the peritoneal cavity.

Some individuals also develop a generalized oedema because of the failure of the liver to produce sufficient serum albumin to maintain the normal colloidal osmotic pressure of the blood (see Chapter 7). Some blood protein is also lost in the transudate in ascites. Reduced liver activity results in increased concentrations of antidiuretic hormone and aldosterone (an adrenocorticoid secretion), further contributing to oedema. These secretions, normally destroyed by the liver, promote reabsorption of water and sodium by the kidneys.

Dilated veins and varicosities

The portal hypertension associated with liver disease is reflected in changes within the veins that drain into the portal vein. They become dilated and varicosities develop. The oesophageal and gastric veins are commonly affected and, because they are close to the surface, one may rupture, resulting in massive haemorrhage manifested by haematemesis or melaena or both. Haemorrhoids develop because of the pressure and resistance to blood flow within the rectal veins.

Splenomegaly

The spleen enlarges because of the hyperplasia of the reticuloendothelial tissue and congestion, causing considerable discomfort for the patient.

Skin changes

In progressive chronic liver failure, several changes are

likely to appear in the skin. Arterial spiders (spider angiomas or naevi) may develop in which a superficial arteriole gives rise to a series of fine, radiating branches readily visible on the surface. These lesions are seen predominantly on the face, neck, arms and chest, and are attributed to high oestrogen levels in the blood. Gynaecomastia and atrophy of the testicles may occur in males for the same reason. Normally, oestrogen is destroyed in the liver.

The palms of the hands are frequently mottled, bright red and warm because of capillary dilatation (palmar erythema). There is a loss of axillary and pubic hair in both sexes, and facial hair grows more slowly than usual in the male.

Neurological disturbances

Severe hepatic insufficiency leads to various mental changes. The patient may manifest irritability and behaviour not previously characteristic such as becoming inactive, apathetic and forgetful. These symptoms may progress to confusion, lack of co-operation, stupor and eventually coma.

Twitching and a peculiar coarse tremor, referred to as flapping tremor, develop. Flapping tremor consists of a series of rapid, irregular alternating flexion and extension movements at the wrist and finger joints. The tremor may be referred to as *asterixis*. It occurs when the arms and hands are extended.

Ammonia toxicity is considered to be an important factor in producing the mental changes, coma and other abnormal central nervous system responses. The liver is unable to convert the ammonia that results from the breakdown of amino acids to urea.

Fetor hepaticus

In advanced liver disease, the breath has a faecal odour and the patient complains of a bad taste in the mouth. It is attributed to disturbed amino acid metabolism and abnormal bacterial action in the intestine.

Digestive disturbances

The patient with impaired bile transport may experience flatulence and an uncomfortable full feeling or nausea, especially after the ingestion of fatty or fried foods. Vomiting is usual if the patient has biliary colic or develops obstructive jaundice.

Fever

Chills and an elevation of temperature frequently accompany infection and inflammation within the gallbladder or bile ducts.

THE PERSON AT RISK OF DISORDERS OF THE LIVER AND EXOCRINE PANCREAS

Alcohol and Alcohol Abuse

Alcohol consumption is closely associated with liver and pancreatic disorders. The current recommendations by the Health Education Authority are that women should not drink more than 13 units of alcohol per week, and men no more than 20 units per week. One unit of alcohol is equivalent to half a pint of beer, one measure of spirits or one glass of wine.

Nurses are reported (Sullivan and Hale, 1987) to hold negative attitudes towards individuals with drinking problems. This may be due to experiences of frequent casualty attenders, and in-patients with alcohol-related conditions who resume drinking despite advice to the contrary. These experiences can lead to stereotyping the problem drinker as potentially violent, hopeless, or unable to maintain relationships, employment or 'normal' social activity, whereas the reality in the United Kingdom is that regular moderate drinking or occasional intoxication results in a range of alcohol-related health problems. Recurrent stomach disorders, hypertension and stroke, damage to brain, liver and heart, domestic, occupational and road traffic accidents and injury, can result from quite light or moderate drinking. It is estimated that 20% of all acute hospital beds in general hospitals are occupied by men whose drinking habits put their health at risk (Catalan et al, 1985) and that, after cardiovascular disease and cancer, alcohol is a major cause of morbidity and mortality.

Early identification and education may be effective with 'at risk' drinkers in reducing serious health problems and dependence. Nurses, as the largest group of health care professionals with the greatest patient contact, may be ideally placed to re-educate and promote healthy drinking behaviour. Recent evidence suggests (Rowland and Maynard, 1989) that educational initiatives to increase nurses' knowledge of the effects of alcohol and consequences for health produces a more positive attitude.

ALCOHOLISM

Alcoholism, like abuse of other substances, is a complex illness. Theoretical explanations of the causes all attempt to explain the unique relationship between the alcoholic and his or her environment. Many myths about this major health problem and its treatment exist. It has been labelled as a hopeless, untreatable, progressive illness. There is a myth that the person must reach 'rock bottom' and 'want' treatment before there can be any benefit from a therapeutic programme. The opposite is true. When alcoholism is identified and treated in the early stages, before individuals lose their jobs and family, there is a 68–85% recovery rate (Tweed, 1989).

Nurses encounter persons with alcohol abuse problems in their daily practice, both in hospitals and the community. The informed nurse who recognizes that alcoholism is an illness and that treatment can be beneficial, is more likely to assess the problem and refer the patient to a treatment programme.

The numerous physiological, psychological and sociological health problems experienced by the alcoholic person present complex challenges for nurses. A survey of nurses working in medical–surgical hospital settings (Fitzgerald et al, 1987) identified *potential for injury* related to neurological changes and *fluid volume deficit* as the most difficult physiological problems. *Alteration in coping* was the most frequently cited difficult patient problem overall. Other psychosocial problems included *alterations in relationships with family or significant others* and *non-compliance* in self-management of health.

CLINICAL SITUATION: MR COLIN BEARDSLEY, A PERSON WITH ALCOHOLISM

Colin Beardsley is a 31-year-old salesman who is married with two children. He was admitted via the emergency department with an acute case of pancreatitis. He appeared to smell of alcohol but explained that he had just come from a family celebration. Blood tests revealed his liver enzymes were generally at the high end of the normal range; his GGT results were elevated by a factor of four.

The nurse was aware that Mr Beardsley might have a drinking problem and that the nursing assessment would need to explore this possibility. The nurse therefore not only asked about alcohol consumption patterns, but asked broad questions about legal, employment, social and family difficulties related to alcohol use. (For example: Have you ever had any difficulties at work related to the use of alcohol?) Mr Beardsley seemed annoyed with these questions. He explained he usually had a few drinks on a daily basis in order to entertain customers. 'I certainly can't ever get drunk or I'd lose customers. I'm very careful about how much I drink.' He denied any alcohol-related problems, except for two impaired driving charges. One charge was after an office Christmas party and the other after taking a client out to lunch to seal an important business transaction. Mr Beardsley explained he was just in the wrong place at the wrong time; such charges are an 'occupational hazard' for salespersons who are expected to do a lot of entertaining.

The nurse's awareness of a likely alcohol problem allowed anticipation of the potential problems of alcohol withdrawal. The symptoms of withdrawal include *nausea, vomiting, agitation, heavy perspiration.* As withdrawal progresses, symptoms such as *confusion, hallucinations* and *convulsions* may develop. The risk of convulsion was noted on the care plan (see Chapter 21 for nursing care during and following convulsions). When Mr Beardsley became confused and appeared to be having visual and tactile hallucinations, the nurse recognized these as symptoms of alcohol withdrawal rather than a psychotic episode. Hallucinations and other psychotic symptoms (delusions, thought disorder) are frequently treated with antipsychotic medication. However, in the case of alcohol withdrawal this would

not be done, since antipsychotics would generally further lower the seizure threshold and therefore further increase the risk of convulsions.

In the period of detoxification and following detoxification, the fluid balance frequently needs monitoring. The patient is often prone to dehydration and will therefore generally need frequent fluids. In addition, from a behavioural point of view, the patient has become accustomed when drinking alcohol to consuming large quantities of fluid and may attempt to drink large quantities of other fluids to replace this loss. The writer had one patient who, even after several months of sobriety, would drink 24 cans of ginger ale an evening. It is quite common for large quantities of coffee to be consumed as a readily available substitute. This can create difficulties since coffee can have a further diuretic effect, and the caffeine is also addictive. The patient could experience further withdrawal symptoms when later attempting to cut back coffee consumption.

The nurse was also aware of the potential for cross addiction: almost all people with an addiction have more than one. Mr Beardsley was also a heavy smoker and frequently drank coffee. The nurse, being aware of the high incidence of depression that accompanies substance abuse, monitored Mr Beardsley for signs of depression and suicidal risk (see emotional responses to illness in Chapter 5).

Once the immediate physical problems related to withdrawal had passed, Mr Beardsley's nurse recognized his need to have specific treatment for his alcoholism. Options include self-help groups such as Alcoholics Anonymous (AA) or more formal treatment programmes. Assessment and referral programmes may be community or hospital based. Similarly, treatment programmes may operate on an out-patient, day-patient or in-patient basis. It is therefore important to be aware of community resources.

In the case of Mr Beardsley, the nurse made a referral to a social worker who further assessed the drinking problem and then discussed treatment options. Mr Beardsley was able to take advantage of an employee assistance programme through his place of work to arrange for a four-week day hospital programme, followed by a year of weekly out patient follow-up.

The issue of denial frequently interferes with the identification of alcoholism and the acceptance of treatment. It is difficult for people with alcoholism to accept both their alcoholism and a positive self-concept if they held a negative stereotype of alcoholics. People with alcoholism who reject society's negative stereotype of alcoholics, are able to accept their own alcoholism and still maintain a positive self-concept. Discussing what alcoholism is, and dispelling myths associated with the alcoholic stereotype, can be an important nursing intervention in assisting the individual to accept the alcoholism and the treatment for it.

It is important for the nurse caring for a patient with alcoholism to examine his or her own feelings, beliefs and attitudes towards alcohol, alcoholism and alcoholics. Stereotypes not only make it difficult for the patient to accept their alcoholism, but also can prevent the nurse from being supportive and emotionally available to assist the patient.

At times, the individual with alcoholism (or other substance abuse disorders) will continue to deny the problem and/or refuse assistance. It is important to recognize that there is still likely to be a need for family support (e.g. Al-Anon treatment programme). Family members and significant others may require information about programmes and support even if the family member with alcoholism refuses treatment.

THE PERSON WITH DISORDERS OF THE LIVER

Viral Hepatitis

The most common inflammatory disease of the liver is due to viruses. Viral hepatitis is transmitted by human blood and body fluids and therefore is an occupational risk for nurses and other health care workers. Three types of hepatitis are currently recognized and they are referred to as hepatitis A (HA), hepatitis B (HB), and non-A, non-B hepatitis. Hepatitis due to the A virus (HAV) may be referred to as infectious (or epidemic) hepatitis; that caused by hepatitis B virus (HBV) was formerly referred to as homologous serum hepatitis. One or more additional hepatotropic viruses are known to exist and are referred to as non-A, non-B viruses (NANBV). The principal differences in the three types of hepatitis are in their mode of infection, incubation period, severity and chronicity.

Hepatitis A

This type of hepatitis accounts for the greater number of cases. The disease may be epidemic and has a higher incidence in children and young adults. It has an incubation period of 10–50 days and is included in the list of *reportable* diseases. It is an acute, self-limited disease which does not usually lead to chronic hepatitis or a carrier state.

Large amounts of the virus are eliminated in the faeces in the week preceding the onset of jaundice. The stools therefore constitute a low infection hazard once symptoms appear. Transmission is by the faecal–oral route and is therefore facilitated by poor hygiene. This disease may spread rapidly, especially in overcrowded and poor sanitary conditions.

Hepatitis B

Hepatitis B is caused by the virus B, which consists of an inner DNA core enclosed in a protein coat. Both the inner core and the large surface mass contain distinctive antigens. The principal mode of transmission is by the injection of infected blood and blood products. Because of this, hepatitis B is a common problem among drug addicts who are sharing injection equipment. Needle-stick injuries may result in transmission of the virus to health care workers. The same mechanism is also apparent in HIV infection. Hepatitis B can be transmitted like HIV, by intimate contact with carriers or those with acute disease. The virus can be found in saliva, semen, vaginal secretions, as well as blood. The incubation period for hepatitis B ranges from 6 weeks to 6 months. It is more common in adults than children, while hepatitis A tends to have a higher frequency in children and young adults. Hepatitis B has an insidious onset; it may persist or become chronic, or produce a carrier state in which the individual may be asymptomatic but harbour the virus.

Non-A, non-B hepatitis

This term is applied to viruses causing syndromes similar to hepatitis A and B, but which have not yet been characterized in the laboratory; they can at present be diagnosed only by excluding the presence of HAV and HBV. One form of non-A, non-B hepatitis is spread in water supplies contaminated by sewage; this type resembles hepatitis A; another, more like hepatitis B, is transmitted by blood products such as Factors VIII and IX, thus putting haemophiliacs at special risk. The virus appears to be bloodborne but sexual contact can be a mode of transmission. The incubation period is 2 to 5 months.

PREVENTION AND SCREENING

Prevention of the transmission of viral hepatitis focuses on two areas: education of carriers to prevent transmission to others, and protection of at-risk groups against contamination of the virus. Nurses have an important contribution to make in giving advice to carriers and their significant others to allay fears, reduce anxiety, provide education regarding potential routes of contamination, and abating misconceptions. However, this information should be relayed in such a way as to ensure reduction of risk to others but without promoting unnecessary restrictions or precautions which could cause distress. In a study (Ho-Yen et al, 1985) of nurses' knowledge about hepatitis B it was found that nurses had considerable gaps in their knowledge, particularly about transmission routes and mortality rates associated with the disease.

At-risk groups include: drug addicts, male homosexuals, prostitutes, in-patients in institutional care, and individuals who have received multiple transfusions of blood and blood products. Education for drug addicts should focus on safe use and disposal of needles and syringes. Information regarding safe sexual practice, the use of condoms, etc. should be given and reinforced at every opportunity to homosexuals, prostitutes and drug addicts. Leaflets and other education material can be useful for spreading sound information and can be easily displayed in many health settings to which the public have access. The parallels with the prevention of the spread of HIV are obvious.

Screening for hepatitis in hospital settings is usually targeted on the following: all admissions to renal dialysis and transplant units; individuals who have recently travelled to countries with high levels of hepatitis, such as developing countries; drug addicts; in-patients of institutions for the mentally handicapped; individuals who have received blood or blood products; the acutely or recently jaundiced; and sometimes individuals with tattoos.

CLINICAL CHARACTERISTICS

The virus attacks the hepatic cells, and inflammation and necrosis follow. The swelling and congestion interfere with normal bile formation and flow, resulting in intrahepatic obstructive jaundice and elevated blood bilirubin levels. Serum enzyme levels (alanine amino-transferase (ALT) and aspartate amino transferase (AST)) rise sharply because of the necrosis, and the protein electrophoresis and serum albumin:globulin ratio may indicate a reduced formation of albumin and an increase in the gamma globulin. The latter points to the acute infectious nature of the disorder. Urinalysis reveals an excess of urobilinogen, especially in the initial stage. The blood is examined for the presence of hepatitis virus antigens and antibodies that have been identified (hepatitis A virus (HAV), hepatitis A antigen and hepatitis A virus antibodies (anti-HAV) and hepatitis B virus (HBV), hepatitis B surface antigen (HBsAg), hepatitis B surface antibody (HBsAb), hepatitis core antigen (HBcAg), hepatitis core antibody (HBcAb), hepatitis B e-antigen (HBeAg), hepatitis B e-antibody (HBeAb)). Antibodies to the core antigen can be detected when symptoms develop. Antibodies to the 'e' and surface antigens may develop within a month of onset of symptoms. Fortunately, in most cases complete regeneration of the liver cells occurs on recovery with a minimum of fibrous tissue formation and scarring. Very few persons experience residual impairment of liver function.

The signs and symptoms may vary in intensity from one individual to another. The onset is usually manifested by vague symptoms such as fatigue, loss of appetite, nausea, vomiting, headache, fleeting abdominal and joint pains, and fever. After several days, abdominal tenderness and pain in the right upper quadrant are more predominant, the urine becomes dark, either constipation or diarrhoea may be troublesome, the stools may be abnormally light in colour and jaundice becomes evident. Hepatitis B is usually more prolonged and debilitating. Table 17.3 lists the clinical characteristics of viral hepatitis.

DIAGNOSTIC PROCEDURES

Urine specimens are submitted for assessment of urobilinogen content. In viral hepatitis there is an excess of this substance in the initial stage of the disease. If the inflammatory process is widespread, intrahepatic biliary obstruction may result in the appearance of bilirubin in the urine and the disappearance of the urobilinogen.

The serum bilirubin level is elevated, serum flocculation tests are positive and the serum enzymes ALT (SGPT) and AST (SGOT) are elevated. Blood specimens are examined for the hepatitis A and B virus antigens and their associated antibodies. Specimens of faeces are examined for the hepatitis A virus.

Table 17.3 Assessment of the person with viral hepatitis.

Pathophysiological alterations	Clinical characteristics
Liver structure and function Hepatomegaly	The liver is tender and enlarged on palpation Abdominal discomfort
Altered bile production, excretion and reabsorption	Pruritus Jaundice of skin and sclerae Urine, dark orange in colour Stools, clay-coloured Diarrhoea or constipation
Altered metabolism of carbohydrates, proteins and fats	Nausea and vomiting Anorexia Flatulence Malaise, weakness and fatigue Irritability Weight loss Muscle wasting Fever
Altered production and destruction of blood components	Spontaneous bleeding Purpura Melaena Haematuria
Extrahepatic	Skin rashes Arthralgia Headache Sore throat, cough, coryza Depression

TREATMENT

Since there is no specific treatment for viral hepatitis, supportive therapy and attention to the patient's discomforts constitute the principal care. Most patients are managed at home.

Interferon α-2b injections have been effective in inducing a sustained loss of hepatitis B replication, producing remission of the disease in one-third of patients with chronic hepatitis B infection (Perrillo et al, 1990). Since hepatitis B remains chronic in 10% of infected persons, this finding is significant in terms of their longevity, decreasing their risk for liver cancer and decreasing the potential for transmission to others.

ASSESSMENT

Health history. The person is questioned regarding exposure to hepatitis viruses from blood transfusions, the use of contaminated needles, or contact with infected individuals. Emphasis is placed on identification of the clinical symptoms the person is experiencing. Since the course of the disease varies from asymptomatic and mild to acute, fulminating and life-threatening, symptoms vary considerably as to frequency and severity. The patient is asked specific questions related to gastrointestinal disturbance, and changes in the colour of the skin and mucous membranes, sclera, stools and urine. Changes in the tendency to bleed are also noted.

Physical examination includes the measurement of the person's temperature; observation of the skin, mucous membranes and sclera for changes in colour; observation of urine and faeces; observation of the skin and gums for signs of bruising and bleeding; and palpation of the abdomen for distention, discomfort and liver enlargement.

NURSING INTERVENTION

The *goals* of care are that the person will demonstrate:

- Alleviation of symptoms.
- Fluid balance.
- Maintenance of desired body weight.
- Return of appetite.
- Knowledge of self-management.
- Resumption of usual daily activities.

It is also important that there should be no evidence of transmission to others.

Rest. The person is encouraged and helped to get adequate rest and relaxation. Both at home and in the hospital, plans should be developed to provide uninterrupted periods of rest throughout the day as well as at night. Activity is resumed slowly, and the person is observed for reactions. Liver function is monitored by repeated tests to detect any adverse effects of increased activity.

Medications. Many drugs (such as barbiturates, oral contraceptives and morphine) which are normally inactivated by the liver are not prescribed. The patient is advised against taking any drug that has not been prescribed by the doctor during this illness. Alternative barrier methods of contraception and issues relating to safe sexual practices should be discussed.

Nutrition and fluids. In the acute stage, it is difficult for the person to take sufficient fluids and food because of the nausea, vomiting and aversion to food. An increased fluid intake of at least 3000 ml is necessary because of the fever and to promote urinary elimination of the serum bilirubin. If the patient cannot tolerate fluids orally, intravenous fluids may be given. The patient is observed closely for signs of overhydration manifested by sudden weight gain, oedema and respiratory distress. Fluid intake and output are recorded. Parenteral administration of vitamin K may be recommended if blood coagulation is impaired as a result of impaired absorption of vitamin K when bile salts are decreased.

A high-calorie diet of 3000 kcal is recommended; nutritional deficiency retards the liver's ability to overcome the infection and regenerate functional tissue. As soon as the nausea and vomiting are controlled, the patient is offered small amounts of high-calorie foods

frequently. These are gradually increased until the ultimate goal of 3000 kcal is achieved.. The diet consists principally of protein and carbohydrate. The fat content may be restricted while there is jaundice but is increased, as tolerated, by the addition of dairy products, which make the diet more palatable. Fried foods, fat meat and rich foods, such as pastries, usually are avoided for several weeks or months after recovery. The person is advised not to take alcohol for at least 6 months.

The individual's weight is checked at regular intervals, since there may have been a considerable loss in the early phase of the disease.

Skin care. Frequent bathing and changes of linen during the period of fever are necessary. The use of soap is avoided; emollients may be added to the bathwater to relieve the itching. Calamine lotion may be used and fingernails are cut short and kept clean.

Prevention of the spread of infection. All patients with viral hepatitis are treated as potentially infectious. Universal and body substance precautions are used with all patients, therefore no additional measures are required. Needle-stick injuries pose the greatest threat to health care workers as HBV is transmitted through the blood. As with all patients, needles should never be recapped and only disposable needles and syringes should be used for persons with hepatitis. Invasive procedures should be avoided whenever possible. Gowns and gloves should be worn whenever direct contact with blood or faeces is possible. Personnel caring for the patient are informed of the possible sources of the infective organisms (faeces, vomitus, urine and blood) and of the fact that they are usually resistant to heat, antiseptics, and prolonged exposure to cold and freezing.

The hands are scrubbed under running water with liquid soap after each contact. Bed linen contaminated with faeces or blood is placed in a clean bag at the bedside which is identified as an isolation bag. No special precautions are necessary regarding dishes or glasses. The use of disposable equipment for procedures involving penetration of the skin (e.g. needles and syringes) is recommended, and gloves should be worn by those handling them. Used needles and syringes are placed in a puncture-resistant container used for all such supplies. Blood, urine, faeces and sputum specimens should be clearly labelled 'Biohazard' to protect laboratory personnel.

If it is necessary to take the temperature by rectum, the nurse wears gloves while handling the thermometer, which is thoroughly disinfected after use. Disposable supplies are preferred.

The person is advised of the importance of thorough hand washing after going to the toilet. Gloves are worn when handling the patient's bedpan; excreta should be flushed promptly down the toilet. If the patient is being cared for at home, the patient and family are taught simple precautions and the importance of good hand washing.

Contacts. Known contacts of infectious hepatitis A are

advised to consult a doctor as soon as possible. An intramuscular injection of human immune serum globulin may be given to provide protection. It is effective against the virus A organism. Hepatitis B immune globulin is available for contacts of hepatitis B virus. Its use is usually reserved for individuals exposed to hepatitis B virus through needle pricks or other accidental injection. The γ globulin may not always provide immunity, but is found to lessen the severity of the disease should the person develop it.

Vaccines for active immunization against hepatitis are recommended for high-risk groups, especially health professionals at risk of contamination with patient's blood. Hepatitis B vaccine is available to nurses in the high-risk groups and to all who wish it through most employee occupational health services. Immunization involves three intramuscular injections, with the second and third doses being given at 1 and 6 months respectively. Antibodies persist for at least 3 years. Booster doses are given at regular intervals. HBV vaccine is also available in the community for individuals who are at risk for contacting the infection. High-risk groups include those with illness-related factors requiring repeated transfusions of blood or blood products, and those with life-style related factors such as homosexual practices, intravenous drug use and prostitution.

Follow-up. The person is encouraged to attend outpatient appointments; laboratory and physical examinations are done to detect possible progressive or residual impairment of liver function. Supervision is usually continued for 1 year. The intervals between visits to clinics or doctor are gradually increased if the findings are favourable. The person who has had hepatitis B, or non-A, non-B hepatitis is advised not to serve as a blood donor.

Evaluation

Achievement of the established goals for the individual with hepatitis is determined by on-going assessment showing alleviation of the person's symptoms. The individual's body weight should be maintained at a desirable level. The patient and family should be able to describe plans for meeting nutritional needs and needs for increased rest, as well as precautionary measures to prevent transmission of the virus to others. They should be familiar with plans for follow-up care.

Toxic Hepatitis

Rarely, inflammation and degenerative changes in the liver occur as a result of a chemical. Carbon tetrachloride, phosphorus, sulphonamides, arsenical preparations and chloroform are examples of suggested offenders. The patient is treated by prompt withdrawal of the causative chemical, rest and supportive care.

Cirrhosis of the Liver

The term cirrhosis denotes chronic diffuse degenerative tissue changes occurring in the liver. There is destruction of parenchymal cells and formation of excessive dense fibrous scar tissue. Blood, lymph and bile channels within the liver become distorted, compressed and effaced, with subsequent intrahepatic congestion, portal hypertension and impaired liver function. (For functions, see p. 515.) The fibrous tissue changes result in the liver becoming firmer. The surface is usually rough because of small projecting nodules of regenerated hepatic cells, and is frequently described as a 'hobnail surface'.

CAUSES

The mechanisms responsible for cirrhosis of the liver are not clearly defined.

Alcoholism. Cirrhosis of the liver is a common sequel to chronic alcoholism. Ingestion of moderate to large quantities of ethanol (ethyl alcohol) over several years can produce fatty infiltration of the liver and liver dysfunction. The toxic effects of ethanol on the liver develop more readily in the presence of malnutrition. Many persons show a marked improvement in the earlier stages of cirrhosis when alcohol ingestion is discontinued.

Hepatitis. Severe type B viral hepatitis in which there has been extensive necrosis followed by considerable scarring may lead to cirrhosis.

Chronic cholestasis. Degenerative changes characteristic of cirrhosis may also occur with prolonged cholestasis (obstruction to the flow of bile). The cause is usually partial obstruction by a stone or stricture within the extrahepatic bile ducts, but may be intrahepatic as a result of infection or inflammation and subsequent stricture of the small ducts within the liver.

Hepatic infiltration. Fibrotic changes in the liver may be associated with the infiltration of certain substances. Examples include excessive glycogen which accumulates in the liver in the individual with von Gierke's disease, enlargement and fibrosis develop. Similarly, Gaucher's disease results from an abnormal reticuloendothelial cell content that incurs liver fibrosis and dysfunction.

CLASSIFICATION

Certain terms may be used to classify cirrhosis according to the cause and changes that occur. Cirrhosis associated with alcohol abuse accounts for 60–70% of the cases. When cirrhotic changes are a result of massive hepatic necrosis and subsequent fibrous scarring, the condition is known as *postnecrotic cirrhosis*. The term *biliary cirrhosis* is used to denote cirrhosis associated with cholestasis. Other forms include pigment cirrhosis (haemochromatosis), cardiac or congestive and rare forms of uncertain aetiology.

Cirrhosis may also be classified as micronodular, macronodular or mixed, according to the size and thickness of the nodules. Since it is generally a progressive disease, the size of the nodules progressively changes.

CLINICAL CHARACTERISTICS

The liver has considerable reserve; early cirrhotic changes generally go unrecognized without apparent manifestations. With the characteristic insidious progress, signs and symptoms of impaired liver function appear gradually over a period of years. In the early stages the symptoms are vague digestive disturbances: the person experiences anorexia, flatulence, nausea and loss of weight. Later, jaundice, dependent oedema, spider angiomas, anaemia and increased abdominal girth develop. Splenomegaly, neurological involvement (hepatic coma) and haemorrhage from oesophageal varices are characteristic of advanced cirrhosis and serious liver dysfunction.

The severity of liver dysfunction is determined by various liver function tests (see earlier) as well as by history, symptoms and physical examination. Palpation of the liver and spleen provides significant information. The liver is enlarged and firm and may have a rough surface; the spleen is enlarged owing to the resistance by the liver to flow of blood from the portal vein.

TREATMENT

The care required by the patient with cirrhosis depends upon the extent of the liver damage.

Medications. Multivitamin preparations are prescribed. Parenteral vitamin K may be given if the prothrombin level is below normal and if a tendency to bleeding is manifested by petechiae, ecchymosis, epistaxis, melaena or haematemesis. Vitamin B_{12} injections may be necessary to correct anaemia.

Although the patient with cirrhosis usually develops oedema and ascites due to portal hypertension and decreased plasma oncotic pressure because of reduced liver production of blood proteins, the doctor may be reluctant to prescribe a diuretic because of the possible electrolyte imbalance and excessive reduction of intravascular volume. Diuretics that are given initially are potassium-sparing diuretics (e.g. spironolactone), as hypokalaemia may precipitate hepatic encephalopathy. Cirrhotic ascites is often refractory and requires the use of a combination of diuretics. Rapid acting diuretics waste potassium and necessitate frequent determinations of electrolyte and fluid balance.

Potentially toxic drugs normally inactivated by the liver are avoided. Examples of these are paracetamol, diazepam, oral contraceptives and opiates.

Abdominal paracentesis. An abdominal paracentesis may be necessary if the fluid in the peritoneal cavity reaches a volume that is causing respiratory distress, compression of abdominal viscera and blood vessels and considerable pain and discomfort. The nurse explains the aspiration procedure to the patient, and makes sure the bladder is empty. The head of the bed is elevated and the patient is supported with pillows. The doctor may wish to have the patient sitting on the side of the bed with a support for the back and feet. A sphygmomanometer is placed in readiness on one arm so that the blood pressure may be monitored during and after the paracentesis. The necessary sterile equipment and fluid receptacle are brought to the bedside. Following the application of an antiseptic and sterile towels, the doctor injects the site with a local anaesthetic before introducing the trocar and cannula. A tube is attached to the cannula to drain the fluid into the receptacle.

During the procedure, the nurse checks the patient's pulse, colour and blood pressure and provides necessary psychological support. The doctor should be alerted promptly if the pulse becomes rapid and weak, pallor is noted, or there is a fall in blood pressure. No more than 1 or 2 litres is withdrawn at one time. Removal of the fluid results in the loss of considerable plasma protein, especially serum albumin. Also, the sudden reduction of intra-abdominal pressure results in a dilatation of the abdominal blood vessels and a pooling of a large volume of blood that may lead to circulatory collapse and shock.

A sterile dressing is applied to the site of the paracentesis when the cannula is withdrawn. The patient is returned to the dorsal recumbent position, and the head of the bed is lowered. The amount and character of the fluid are recorded and a specimen of the fluid is labelled and sent to the laboratory for examination. The abdominal site is kept clean and dry to prevent infection and discomfort. The pulse, colour and blood pressure are checked at frequent intervals for several hours. A plasma or whole blood infusion may follow the paracentesis to replace the lost protein. Increased diuresis may be observed with the decreased pressure on the renal blood vessels.

Peritoneovenous shunt. When ascites is consistent or recurring, a shunt may be surgically performed to relieve portal hypertension and ascites (see Figure 17.6). The mortality rate from these procedures is high because the patients are such poor surgical candidates. A peritoneovenous shunt may be performed, which avoids the necessity of major surgical intervention. A tube is inserted into the superior vena cava and is connected by a one-way valve to a perforated collecting tube in the peritoneal cavity. The valve opens in response to pressure in the peritoneal cavity; ascitic fluid flows into the venous circulation and is transported by the venous tube from the peritoneal cavity into the superior vena cava. Infection is a major complication associated with this procedure.

COMPLICATIONS OF CIRRHOSIS AND THEIR MANAGEMENT

Hepatic encephalopathy and coma, and oesophagogastric varices are common complications.

Hepatic coma

Before the patient with cirrhosis of the liver develops coma, neurological disturbances are manifested. These include mental dullness, slow responses, forgetfulness and disorientation. Muscle reflexes are exaggerated, and muscular rigidity and asterixis (flapping tremor) are also present. The cause of the neurological involvement is failure of the liver to metabolize and detoxify nitrogenous substances; the toxic materials such as ammonia remain in the blood and are carried into the cerebral circulation. The failure may be due to hepatocellular necrosis or because portal blood bypasses the liver and reaches the central nervous system by being shunted directly into the systemic circulation.

Nursing measures used in the care of any unconscious person are applicable to the patient in hepatic coma (see Chapter 21). The condition is managed by reducing the level of nitrogenous substances. This is achieved by cleansing the gastrointestinal tract by administering lactulose orally and giving enemas (disposable magnesium sulphate). Sometimes a non-absorbable antibiotic (neomycin) is prescribed to suppress urea-splitting bacterial gut flora. Protein intake is restricted.

Portal hypertension

The flow of blood from the portal vein through the liver may meet with resistance due to disease and cirrhotic changes in the liver. Pressure rises within the portal venous system, causing portal hypertension. The latter is defined as a portal pressure in excess of 30 cm of saline. The increased pressure in the portal vein produces a back-up in the veins that normally empty into the portal system. Collateral circulatory channels develop between the portal vein and the systemic circulatory system to bypass the liver.

The veins most seriously affected by portal hypertension are those in the gastric cardia region and the lower part of the oesophagus. The veins become engorged and tortuous; the walls are weakened, predisposing them to rupture. These varicosed veins appear as large bulbous protrusions under the mucosa. The congestion in the mesenteric veins causes haemorrhoids and is also reflected in the apparent congested cutaneous veins around the umbilicus (caput medusae). In addition to varices, problems associated with portal hypertension include congestive splenomegaly and ascites.

The severity of portal hypertension may be assessed indirectly by evidence of oesophageal varices, which may be visualized using fibreoptic endoscopy or by liver scan. Direct measurement of portal hypertension requires surgical intervention and is rarely performed.

Bleeding oesophagogastric varices

The oesophagogastric varices are frequently the site of rupture of the vascular wall and severe haemorrhage. The perforation and bleeding may be caused by mechanical trauma from 'rough' food passing over a varicosity, erosion and ulceration of the mucosa and venous wall by gastric acid secretion, or sudden increased intra-abdominal pressure associated with coughing, vomiting, straining at stool or physical exertion. Severe haematemesis occurs; some blood will enter the intestine and eventually the person passes tarry stools.

Prompt emergency treatment and care of bleeding oesophagogastric varices are necessary; the excessive loss of blood is life-threatening.

Control of bleeding. Various measures are used to control bleeding and include the following:

- *Balloon tamponade.* A Sengstaken–Blakemore tube, a nasogastric tube with three or four lumens, may be inserted. One lumen ends in an elongated balloon that is inflated to exert pressure against the oesophageal wall; another ends in a small balloon that is positioned just within the stomach and, when inflated, compresses varices in the cardia and anchors the tube in place (Figure 17.4); and the third lumen opens into the stomach, extending well beyond the balloon in the cardia. The third lumen permits drainage or aspiration of the gastric content; its proximal end may be attached to suction. Removal of gastric contents reduces the amount of blood entering the intestine. Digestion of blood in the intestine produces nitrogenous wastes that, when absorbed, predispose the patient to hepatic coma. Some Sengstaken–Blakemore tubes have a fourth lumen which permits suction above the oesophageal balloon. Continuous suction is applied so as to aspirate any blood or secretions above the oesophageal balloon. Before the tube is inserted, the tube and balloons are tested for leaks. Before insertion the tube is usually chilled, which makes it firmer and easier to manipulate, and is lubricated to ease insertion. The nurse makes sure that the proximal end of each lumen is identified and clearly labelled to prevent possible error in inflation or deflation of tubes after insertion. The pressures to be maintained within the balloons are indicated by the doctor and are usually 25–30 mmHg; excessive pressure can cause tissue ulceration (Figure 17.5). Inadequate inflation is ineffective in checking bleeding and may also permit shifting of the tube. The gastric drainage is checked frequently for blood content which should progressively decrease following the insertion of the tube. In some instances, when the tube is in place and the balloons inflated, the doctor may lavage the stomach with ice water until the return flow is clear.

  A nurse remains in constant attendance; the patient is observed closely for any indication of respiratory distress. Saliva or blood escaping around the tube into the oropharynx may be aspirated. The patient is unable to swallow saliva, so provision is made for suction or for expectoration into tissues or a basin.

  The tube is positioned within the nostrils to exert a minimum of pull and pressure, and then secured. Frequent moistening and a very light application of a lubricant to the nasal mucosa may reduce the irritation. Some doctors position the tube via the mouth.

  Compression by the inflated balloons is not usually continued longer than 48 hours. Pressure for a longer period could cause oedema, ulceration and

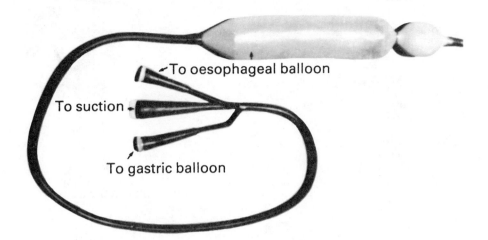

Figure 17.4 A Sengstaken–Blakemore tube which is used in the treatment of bleeding oesophageal varices. The tube has three lumens. One leads to the longer inflatable balloon that is positioned in the oesophagus to provide pressure. A second lumen ends in the smaller balloon that lies just within the stomach. The third lumen opens into the stomach to permit gastric drainage.

perforation. The tube is left in position for continued gastric drainage and for the balloons to be reinflated readily if bleeding resumes. In some instances, the doctor may order deflation of the balloons for 5 minutes at regular intervals to reduce the risk of tissue damage. Vomiting with the tube in place can lead to aspiration of the fluid and in some instances another nasogastric tube is inserted to drain fluid above the oesophageal balloon.

● *Vasopressin infusion.* Vasopressin (Pitressin) may be administered by an intravenous route or, with the assistance of angiography, may be given directly into the superior mesenteric artery. The vasopressin produces arterial vasoconstriction which reduces portal venous pressure by decreasing the volume of blood entering the portal system. The patient may experience crampy abdominal pain and be incontinent of stool.

● *Sclerotherapy.* This is the primary method of treatment. A coagulating substance is injected into the oesophageal varices. Visualization of the varices is achieved using fibreoptic endoscopy and a coagulating substance is injected. The patient is closely monitored following the injection. The patient will be required to have this procedure repeated at regular intervals for 1–2 years.

● *Percutaneous transhepatic portal vein embolization.* This procedure is performed by the radiologist under X-ray guidance. It involves the selective catheterization of the portal vein in patients with bleeding varices. Embolic material (steel coils, gel-foam), is passed down the catheter to occlude the vessels leading to the site of bleeding.

● *Surgical treatment.* If the measures cited above are not effective in checking the haemorrhage, emergency surgery may be performed to relieve portal

hypertension. Different surgical procedures are used. A portacaval shunt in which an anastomosis is made between the portal vein and the inferior vena cava (Figure 17.6b), a splenorenal venous shunt (Figure 17.6c), an anastomosis between the superior mesenteric vein and the inferior vena cava (mesocaval shunt, Figure 17.6d) or a transoesophageal ligation of the varices may be done. As an emergency measure, there is considerable risk. It is preferable if the patient's condition can be stabilized and surgery undertaken when bleeding is arrested.

Care following a surgical shunt is similar to that of patients undergoing any abdominal surgery. Close

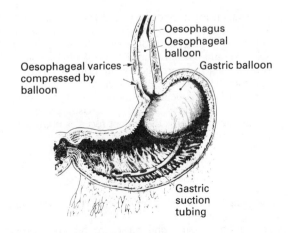

Figure 17.5 A Sengstaken–Blakemore tube in position with the oesophageal and gastric balloons inflated.

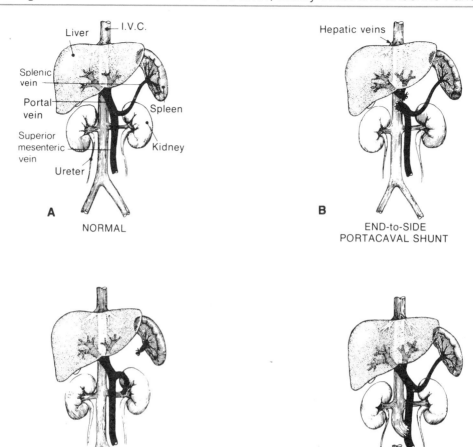

Figure 17.6 Portal shunts used to relieve portal hypertension: (A) normal portal system; (B) end-to-side portacaval shunt: anastomosis of the portal vein and the inferior vena cava; (C) end-to-side splenorenal shunt: anastomosis of the splenic vein and the renal vein; (D) mesocaval shunt: anastomosis of the superior mesenteric vein and the inferior vena cava.

observation for haemorrhage and abdominal distension is important. If a nasogastric tube is passed to control vomiting and distension, a soft tube is selected and is introduced very gently to avoid precipitating haemorrhage by rupturing a varicosity. Specific orders are received from the surgeon as to how much the patient may move and whether deep breathing, coughing, and leg exercises are to be carried out. Similarly, the patient receives nothing by mouth until specifically ordered.

Vitamin K. Parenteral injections of vitamin K are prescribed to increase the patient's blood-clotting power.

Assessment. The patient requires continuous attention and on-going assessment.

The blood pressure and pulse are recorded every 15–30 minutes until the bleeding is controlled. The intervals are gradually increased as the patient's condition shows improvement and stabilization. The patient's respirations, colour and responses are noted; persisting grey pallor, rapid shallow respirations and dulling of awareness and responses are unfavourable signs.

The pressures in the balloons are checked at frequent intervals and corrected if necessary to the prescribed pressure. The gastric drainage is observed for amount and blood content. Persisting bright blood in the drainage is brought to the doctor's attention. The fluid intake and output are recorded, and the balance determined daily. Stools are examined for blood content.

Supportive measures. The patient with bleeding oesophagogastric varices is critically ill and needs physical and psychological support.

- *Blood transfusion.* Replacement of the blood lost is imperative. Fresh blood rather than stored is preferable in order to replace the thrombocytes lost.
- *Nutrition and fluids.* An intravenous line is maintained until the patient is able to take fluids by mouth.

Fluids may be introduced via the tube in the stomach before it is removed. When the tube is removed, small amounts of nutritious fluids are given. The diet is progressively increased to a light diet as tolerated. Roughage and raw fruits and vegetables are avoided. The patient is advised to chew food well, and in small amounts so that the bolus is small and less likely to cause trauma to a vulnerable area in the oesophagus or cardia of the stomach.

- *Rest and positioning.* The patient is kept absolutely at rest to avoid displacing the balloons. Passive movements of the lower limbs and deep breathing are usually carried out to prevent circulatory stasis and to promote airway clearance. The head of the bed is elevated, unless contraindicated by shock. This position may reduce the flow of blood into the portal system.
- *Psychological support.* The haematemesis, emergency measures and rapid loss of strength are very frightening to the patient. Fears and concerns should be acknowledged, and reassurance provided that everything possible is being done. Explanations are calmly made as to what is happening and what is going to be done. Sedation may be necessary to allay the patient's tension and anxiety and provide rest. The patient may be less apprehensive and more relaxed if a family member is present. The family should be kept informed about the patient's progress and what is being done.
- *Mouth care.* The inability to swallow saliva and to receive anything by mouth necessitates special mouth care. Suction may be necessary to remove secretions. Tissues or a basin should be provided into which the patient may expectorate. The mouth is cleansed with moist applicators and petroleum jelly or cold cream is applied to the lips to prevent irritation that may develop with the repeated use of tissues.

NURSING MANAGEMENT

Assessment

Health history. The person's perceptions of symptoms and cause of the illness are obtained. Data is collected about changes in body weight and the appearance of ascites; nausea and vomiting and any loss of appetite; skin colour and itching; changes in mental status; changes in bowel habits; changes in energy level and feelings of tiredness.

Ongoing assessment includes recording of the person's fluid intake and output and accurate assessment of nutritional intake. A mental status examination is performed frequently if there is indication of confusion, lethargy or altered level of consciousness.

Physical examination. The person is weighed daily as short-term changes will reflect changes in body fluid. The abdomen is examined daily for signs of ascites and the presence of oedema should be monitored. The skin is inspected for changes in colour associated with jaundice and for petechiae and bruising which indicate bleeding.

Nursing intervention

The *goals* of care are that the person with cirrhosis of the liver will demonstrate:

- Adequate nutritional intake.
- Absence of pain and discomfort.
- Regular, rhythmic respirations.
- Loss of weight associated with a decrease in the ascites.
- Absence of signs of infection.
- Verbalization of feelings and concerns.
- Understanding of the treatment regimen.

Nutrition. Since the progress of the disease is influenced by nutrition, a diet of 2500–3000 kcal, high in carbohydrates and vitamins is recommended. Protein may be high (110–150 g), but can be restricted to 40 g, or eliminated according to the severity of the disease. Sufficient fat to make the diet palatable is added if the patient can tolerate it and is not jaundiced. Three small meals with in-between snacks will probably be more acceptable than three large meals. Sodium intake is restricted because of the tendency to develop oedema and ascites. Low-sodium protein concentrate and low-sodium milk are available and may be used to assist with the protein intake. Total abstinence from alcohol is very important.

If the liver insufficiency is serious, and the patient is exhibiting neurological disturbances (e.g. depressed awareness, dulled mentation, confusion, asterixis and hyperreflexia) and an elevation in blood ammonia, protein is eliminated from the diet. The patient is sustained with carbohydrates. The disturbance of the nervous system is attributed to failure of the liver to metabolize the nitrogenous wastes; the ammonia level rises because it is not deaminized to form urea. If coma develops, intravenous infusions are used to support the patient.

Control of pain and discomfort. The person's skin should be kept clean and dry. Soaps and perfumed skin products are avoided. The skin is inspected for areas of redness or breakdown. Moisturizers are used to treat dryness and antipruritic lotions may be applied to alleviate itching. The person's nails are kept short and they are encouraged not to scratch. Diversional therapy may be useful. The person will be more comfortable in a cool environment and should be cautioned to avoid heat and heavy clothing which will increase itching.

The person will probably be more comfortable in a sitting position to alleviate discomfort from abdominal distention due to the ascites. The sitting position also alleviates respiratory distress. The person's respirations are monitored regularly as indicated and the patient encouraged to carry out deep breathing and coughing exercises if respirations are impaired.

Prevention of infection. Resistance to infection is lowered in the patient with cirrhosis of the liver. Precautions should therefore be taken to prevent possible exposure to any source of infection.

Patient and family teaching. Significant changes in life-style are required after discharge and these should be carefully discussed with the patient and family. Strict adherence to diet, total abstinence from alcohol, and the avoidance of infection and physical strain are stressed when interpreting the regimen to the patient and family. (If cirrhosis has been caused by alcoholism the nurse should encourage participation and commitment to therapy and provide information and contact numbers and addresses of self-help groups such as Alcoholics Anonymous for the individual and significant others.)

The increased bleeding tendency associated with liver disorders makes it important to stress the need to avoid injuries and abrasions to the skin.

A referral to the community nursing service, community psychiatric nurse or the primary health-care team may be necessary so that consistent support and supervision is ensured.

The prognosis for patients with cirrhosis depends on the degree of liver insufficiency. If treatment is instituted in the early stages and the patient is sufficiently motivated to adhere to the suggested care, a normal life span is still possible. If portal hypertension has developed with resultant ascites and oesophageal varices, the prognosis is grave.

Evaluation
The person with cirrhosis of the liver is assessed on an on-going basis for relief from symptoms and absence of discomfort. The skin is inspected for signs of irritation, scratches, breaks and signs of bleeding. The client and family should understand dietary and comfort measures and recognize when to seek professional help. The patient and family should be comfortable verbalizing their concerns and anxieties and be aware of the prognosis for the patient. They should be aware of support groups related to alcoholism and palliative care in the hospital and the community.

Accidental Injury to the Liver

Rupture of the liver in accidents is not uncommon. Any interruption of the capsule enclosing the hepatic tissue carries the risk of severe internal haemorrhage that may prove fatal before surgical intervention is possible. A blood transfusion is given, and surgical repair undertaken. Control of the bleeding is of prime importance. The area may be sutured or packed, or oxidized cellulose (Oxcel) gauze may be applied. The latter supplies fibres on which the clot may form more easily. In addition to the loss of blood incurred in injury, peritonitis may develop as a result of the chemical irritation caused by the bile that may escape from the liver. Destruction of liver cells may also follow the injury, resulting in impaired liver function.

Neoplastic Disease

Benign and primary malignant neoplasms are rare in the liver, but it is a frequent site of metastasis, especially if the primary malignant neoplasm is in the abdominal

cavity. The malignant cells may be transported to the liver via the portal venous or hepatic arterial blood or via the lymph. In many instances, secondaries in the liver are discovered before the primary source. The liver enlarges and signs of liver insufficiency develop. The patient experiences pain, food intolerance, anaemia, emaciation and ascites.

If a primary neoplasm is confined to one lobe of the liver, a hepatic lobectomy may be done. Following the operation, the patient is observed closely for possible haemorrhage and biliary peritonitis. More often, chemotherapy is used (see Chapter 10). Drugs may be administered by direct hepatic arterial infusion.

Liver Abscess

Infection with subsequent abscess formation occurs rarely and is most often associated with amoebic dysentery. The causative organisms (*Entamoeba histolytica*) are carried by the portal bloodstream from the bowel. The pyogenic infection may also be caused by staphylococcus, streptococcus, or *Escherichia coli*. Along with manifestations of impaired liver function, the patient has chills and a high fever. There may be one or multiple small abscesses which frequently coalesce, forming one large cavity.

The patient is treated with antibiotics and also receives chloroquine or emetine hydrochloride (antiamoebic drugs) if the abscess is a complication of amoebiasis. The abscess is drained by aspiration followed by the injection of an antibiotic into the cavity. Open surgical drainage is avoided if possible because of the danger of dissemination of the infection within the peritoneal cavity and resultant peritonitis.

Liver Transplantation

Human liver transplants have been carried out since 1963. With improved surgical techniques, better means of preserving the donor liver and advances in immunosuppressive therapy, patients receiving liver transplants are surviving longer. The number of liver transplants being performed is increasing each year, although the procedure remains limited to a few centres. Persons with end-stage liver disease should have the opportunity to be evaluated at a transplant centre. If the person is accepted as a possible transplant candidate, both he or she and the family need support during the stressful wait for a suitable donor. The complex problems that are present preoperatively affect the patient's post-transplant recovery. Donor organs are generally matched to the recipient according to body size and blood type, as the liver is not as immunologically active as other organs. The recipient's immune system is suppressed usually with cyclosporine in combination with low dose corticosteroids.

Nursing intervention is directed at management of the side-effects of immunosuppressive therapy which include control of the resulting stomatitis and prevention of infection. The patient is instructed as to the act side-effects and prescribed regimen for maintenance immunotherapy as well as measures to prevent infection and actions to take if infection or signs of rejection occur. Patients and families require a great deal of emotional support and therapeutic intervention to help them deal with the transplant and the implications for the patient's life and the quality of life that can be anticipated. A team of nurses, doctors, social workers and possibly pastoral counsellors usually work collaboratively to help the patient and family through the decision-making period prior to transplantation, the wait for a donor liver, and the adjustment that occurs following the procedure.

THE PERSON WITH DISORDERS OF THE GALLBLADDER AND BILE DUCTS

Cholelithiasis

Cholelithiasis is the term used for stones in the gallbladder (Table 17.4). They vary in shape and size and consist mainly of cholesterol and bile pigments. There may be one stone or many and, although they may develop in both sexes, they occur more often in middle-aged females. The incidence is high in individuals with regional enteritis.

CLINICAL CHARACTERISTICS

Cholelithiasis may not give rise to any disturbance in many persons; in others, the stones cause signs and symptoms ranging from mild digestive disturbances following fat ingestion to all those previously cited under manifestations. Gallstones may cause acute or chronic inflammation of the gallbladder (cholecystitis), or cholestasis (stasis of the bile) within the liver leading to impaired function of that organ. Small stones tend to cause more acute problems, since they may escape into the ducts. They may pass into the duodenum, or may lodge in the cystic or common bile duct or the ampulla of Vater. Impaction of a stone in the common bile duct leads to obstructive jaundice and intense, incapacitating pain.

TREATMENT AND NURSING INTERVENTION

Cholelithiasis is treated surgically by removal of the gallbladder (*cholecystectomy*) and exploration of the common bile duct for a stone or stricture. When impaction of a stone in the common bile duct occurs, leading to obstructive jaundice, the stone may be removed endoscopically (see p. 522).

During an episode of biliary colic, an antispasmodic drug such as propantheline (Pro-Banthine) may be ordered to relieve the painful reflex spasm that occurs in response to the stone in a duct. Morphine or pethidine may also be prescribed in conjunction with an

Table 17.4 Nomenclature in disorders of the extra-hepatic biliary system.

Cholelithiasis	Gallstones or calculi in the gallbladder
Cholecystitis	Inflammation of the gallbladder
Cholecystectomy	Surgical removal of the gallbladder
Cholestasis	Stoppage or suppression of the flow of bile
Cholecystostomy	Incision into the gallbladder and the insertion of a tube for drainage
Choledocholithiasis	Gallstone(s) in the common bile duct
Choledochitis	Inflammation of the common bile duct
Choledocholithotomy	Surgical removal of stone from the common bile duct
Choledochotomy	Incision and exploration of the common bile duct
Choledochoduodenostomy	Anastomosis of the common bile duct to the duodenum

antispasmodic drug, but some doctors avoid their use because they oppose relaxation of the sphincter of Oddi.

Food and fluids by mouth are withheld, and the patient is given intravenous fluids. If vomiting and abdominal distension occur, a nasogastric tube is passed and regular aspiration is performed.

Following the acute episode and removal of the nasogastric tube, clear fluids are given and gradually increased to a light, low-fat diet as tolerated.

The patient is observed for signs of jaundice, and the colour of all stools is noted. The stools may be saved for examination for the presence of the stone that may have passed from the biliary tract into the intestine.

If the patient is jaundiced, and the stools are a pale grey, indicating an absence of bile in the intestine, a daily dose of vitamin K is given parenterally to maintain prothrombin formation and prevent bleeding.

Cholecystitis

Inflammation of the gallbladder may be acute or chronic. Acute cholecystitis is most often associated with gallstones but may occur as a result of infection. The patient manifests pain and tenderness in the right upper abdominal quadrant or mid-epigastrium, fever, nausea and vomiting and leucocytosis. The severity of the symptoms varies with the degree of inflammation. Jaundice may develop if the inflammation involves the biliary ducts.

MANAGEMENT

The treatment includes rest, intravenous fluids, analgesics and antibiotics. If the condition persists or worsens, it may indicate suppuration (empyema of the gallbladder), necessitating prompt surgery. A *cholecystostomy* (drainage of the gallbladder) or a *cholecystectomy* (removal of the gallbladder) may be done.

Chronic cholecystitis is characterized by a long history of vague digestive complaints. The person experiences abdominal discomfort and flatulence after a large rich meal or one high in fats. A dull, aching pain and nausea and vomiting may occur at times. The intensity and probably the frequency of the symptoms insidiously increase over months or years.

The chronic inflammation results in scarring and thickening of the wall of the gallbladder and cholestasis. If calculi are present, they progressively increase in size or number. The person may have subacute or acute exacerbations leading to nausea and vomiting, moderate fever and probably colic. The condition is usually treated surgically by removal of the gallbladder.

Bile Duct Disorders

Obstruction of the common bile duct may occur as a result of a gallstone that has escaped from the gallbladder (*choledocholithiasis*), inflammation (*choledochitis* or *cholangitis*), neoplasm or a stricture formed by scar tissue following trauma and inflammation. The duct above the obstruction dilates and obstructive jaundice develops.

In the case of an impacted stone, retrograde cholangiography may be done and the gallstone removed during the cannulation of the common bile duct. Surgery may be undertaken to open the duct and remove the calculus. When a stricture is present and the area is sufficiently small, it is resected and an end-to-end anastomosis performed. If the obstruction is due to primary carcinoma, excision may be undertaken and the duct stump anastomosed to the duodenum (*choledochoduodenostomy*) or the jejenum (*choledochojejunostomy*).

Extrinsic pressure on the bile ducts obstructing the flow of bile may occur with cancer of the pancreas or duodenum.

When surgery involves an extrahepatic bile duct, a T-tube is inserted at the site of entry into the duct to maintain bile drainage during recovery of the tissues (*choledochostomy*). The stem portion of the tube is brought out on the abdominal surface through a stab wound or the incision and is attached to a drainage receptable. Surgery on a bile duct is usually accompanied by a cholecystectomy, since the gallbladder is frequently the origin of the problem.

NURSING CARE OF PATIENTS WITH EXTRAHEPATIC DISORDERS

The patient is kept at rest, and food is withheld as the patient is usually nauseous and vomiting. If there is vomiting, a nasogastric tube is passed and regular aspiration is performed (see Chapter 16). The temperature, pulse and respirations are recorded regularly. The patient should be checked for signs of obstructive jaundice and abdominal distension.

When the vomiting is controlled and the nasogastric tube removed, oral fluids are given and graduated, as tolerated, to a light, low-fat diet. If the patient is obese, the caloric intake is limited to approximately 1000 kcal daily.

PREOPERATIVE CARE

Preoperative preparation (see Chapter 11) for surgery on the extrahepatic biliary system includes close observation for jaundice and the administration of vitamin K to raise the prothrombin level. Special attention is given to having the patient understand the importance of the frequent coughing and deep breathing that will be required after the operation. Because of the site of the surgery, the patient tends to take very shallow breaths to prevent pain and discomfort, predisposing to respiratory complications as insufficient lung expansion occurs, which may lead to an accumulation of secretions and atelectasis. A nasogastric tube may be passed before the patient is taken to the operating theatre.

POSTOPERATIVE CARE

General postoperative care as outlined in Chapter 11 is applicable. Close observation for bleeding is necessary, since low prothrombin levels may still exist.

The drainage tube (T-tube) that is inserted in the common bile duct is generally clamped during the transfer from the operating room; after the patient is transferred, it is immediately attached to a drainage receptacle. The tubing leading to the receptacle is secured to the dressing and lower bed linen and should have sufficient slack to prevent traction and dislodgement. The patient is advised as to how to turn to avoid a pull on the tube and of the need to be sure that it is not kinked or compressed. The drainage is observed frequently during the first 24 hours in case of haemorrhage. There may be a small amount of blood mixed with bile in the first few hours, but persistent bleeding is reported to the surgeon. The character and daily amount of bile drainage are recorded. If there is a prolonged loss of bile, it may be given back to the patient through a nasogastric tube for the purpose of promoting more normal digestion and absorption in the intestine.

The dressing is checked frequently for possible bleeding or bile leakage. After a few days, the T-tube is clamped for stated intervals and is removed when oedema of the common bile duct subsides. This is usually established by administration of a radio-opaque substance into the tube and the subsequent X-rays will show the outline of the biliary tract. Alternatively, the tube is clamped for 24 hours and if the individual remains pain free the tube is removed. Following removal of the tube, the dressing is observed for bile seepage. If the dressing is soiled with bile, it is changed frequently; the skin and wound are cleansed. Should excoriation of the skin occur due to chemical irritation caused by strongly alkaline bile, a protective dressing such as a hydrocolloid wafer should be applied to the skin. If the drainage is heavy, application of a drainage bag may reduce soiling of clothing and reduce embarrassment or distress. The patient should be reassured that it will cease. The patient is also observed for signs of peritonitis, such as an elevation of temperature, abdominal pain, distension and rigidity.

Until the procedures become less painful and the patient is less fearful, the nurse's assistance and support are required during the frequent, regular coughing, deep breathing and changes of position that are required.

Early ambulation is encouraged, and provision is made for a small drainage receptacle that may be attached to the patient's dressing gown if there is a T-tube in the common bile duct.

The urine, stools, sclerae and skin are checked for any indication of obstructive jaundice.

The patient receives intravenous fluids until the nasogastric tube is removed and oral fluids and food are tolerated. The fat content of the diet is limited.

In preparation for discharge, the patient's diet is discussed. The individual can usually gradually include fat as tolerated in the diet but the health advantages of a low-fat diet should be discussed.

THE PERSON WITH DISORDERS OF THE PANCREAS

Inflammation and neoplastic disease are the pathological conditions seen most frequently in the pancreas.

Pancreatitis

Inflammation of the pancreas may be acute or chronic with recurrent acute episodes.

ACUTE PANCREATITIS

Acute pancreatitis is a potentially serious and life threatening disorder; the severity of the inflammation varies. In the mild form the pancreas becomes swollen and oedematous and, with treatment, the patient is likely to recover within a few days. If the process is severe and persists, necrosis and haemorrhage ensue. Necrosis results from intrapancreatic activation of the proteinases and lipase, initiating autodigestion of the pancreatic tissue and blood vessels. Enzymes and blood may escape into the surrounding tissue and peritoneal cavity; peritonitis, paralytic ileus or ascites may develop.

CAUSE

Pancreatitis is considered to be the result of some factor or change within the pancreas that effects activation of the proteinases and lipase of the exocrine secretion, with subsequent breakdown of the ducts, parenchymal tissue and blood vessels. The causative factor may be an obstruction to the flow of the pancreatic secretion

within the ducts. Continued secretion produces dilatation and back pressure, resulting in duct disruption and the escape of enzymes into the parenchyma. The obstruction may be due to a calculus in the pancreatic duct, a neoplasm, or fibrosis following some irritation within the pancreas.

A gallstone in the ampulla of Vater, compression of the ampulla by an extrinsic neoplasm, or spasm or oedema of the sphincter of Oddi may be the initiating factor. It is suggested that such an obstruction causes a reflux of bile into the pancreas, promoting activation of the enzymes and ensuing autodigestion.

Other possible aetiological factors are considered to be infection and injury of the pancreas. Pancreatitis is most frequently associated with biliary tract disease and alcoholism and has a higher incidence in middle-aged individuals.

CLINICAL CHARACTERISTICS

Acute pancreatitis has a sudden onset, being preceded usually by only mild, vague digestive disturbances. The principal signs and symptoms are pain, gastrointestinal disturbances, obstructive jaundice, shock and hyperglycaemia.

Pain. At first, constant severe incapacitating pain occurs in the upper abdomen, penetrating through to the back. It may be described as burning or boring. Later, with progression of the disease, the pain becomes more generalized in the abdomen.

Gastrointestinal disturbances. Nausea and vomiting occur and persist. Constipation may be a problem. Abdominal distension and rigidity appear as a result of the development of peritonitis. The latter is caused by chemical irritation of the viscera and peritoneum by the enzymes that escape from the pancreas. Peristalsis diminishes, and eventually paralytic ileus and intestinal obstruction may complicate the patient's condition further.

Shock. Shock is attributed to the severity of the constant pain, the exudation of plasma into the peritoneal cavity that occurs with the peritonitis, and the loss of blood resulting from the erosion of vessels within the pancreas associated with necrotizing and haemorrhagic pancreatitis.

Vital signs. The temperature may be elevated in the early stage but may become subnormal if peritonitis and shock develop. The pulse is rapid, and the blood pressure falls with the decrease in the intravascular volume. The patient is flushed at first, and then usually becomes pale. If peritonitis develops, a dusky or cyanotic colour is possible.

Obstructive jaundice. If the head of the pancreas is involved, it may compress the common bile duct and cause obstructive jaundice.

Blood changes. With the escape of enzymes into the pancreatic parenchyma and peritoneal cavity, fatty tissue is broken down into glycerol and fatty acids. The latter combine with calcium to form insoluble calcium compounds. The serum calcium level falls and may be severe enough to produce tetany and affect heart action (prolonged diastole). The serum bilirubin level may be elevated after 2–3 days.

Haemoconcentration develops as a result of the loss of plasma. The prothrombin level falls because of the lack of absorption of vitamin K. Serum amylase and lipase levels are elevated.

Disturbance in glucose metabolism. A deficiency of insulin may develop when the islets of Langerhans are involved in the pathological process, and hyperglycaemia and glycosuria (sugar in the urine) may be present.

TREATMENT

The patient with acute pancreatitis is critically ill. Care is directed toward the reduction of pancreatic secretion to a minimum, relief of pain, prevention of shock or correction if it has developed, of electrolyte and fluid imbalances and prevention of infection.

Medications. Analgesia should be given regularly to relieve pain and discomfort and promote rest. Pethidine is usually prescribed as it depresses the central nervous system and relaxes smooth muscle. Opiates can induce spasm of the pancreatic and biliary ducts, thereby increasing pain. The patient may receive an anticholinergic drug such as propantheline bromide (Pro-Banthine) by intramuscular injection, which will inhibit vagal nerve stimulation of pancreatic enzymes and promote relaxation of the sphincter of Oddi. If an anticholinergic drug is prescribed, the patient will experience a very dry mouth and close observations are made for the possible side-effects of urinary retention and paralytic ileus.

An antibiotic is often prescribed as a prophylactic measure since inflammation and necrosis make the pancreas very vulnerable to infection.

When gastric drainage is discontinued, an antacid such as aluminium hydroxide gel or a combination of aluminium hydroxide and magnesium hydroxide may be given orally at frequent intervals to reduce the acidity of the chyme entering the duodenum.

Parenteral administration of vitamin K may be necessary to maintain normal prothrombin production and prevent bleeding.

Complications. If *paralytic ileus* and intestinal obstruction develop, a nasogastric tube may be passed into the stomach and decompression suction established (see Chapter 16). *Obstruction of the duodenum* may develop because of the swollen oedematous pancreas. Escaping pancreatic enzymes may digest an area of the gastric or duodenal wall, causing *severe haemorrhage* as well as perforation of the eroded organ.

Renal failure may develop within 24 hours of the onset of acute pancreatitis, necessitating dialysis.

Another complication that rarely develops in pancreatitis is the formation of one or more *pseudocysts.*

Accumulations of inflammatory exudate, liquefied necrotic tissue and secretions become walled off by a capsule of fibrous tissue. The cyst is atypical in that there is no epithelial lining characteristic of true cysts. This accounts for the term pseudocyst. A pseudocyst may form within or on the surface of the pancreas or in a neighbouring area into which pancreatic secretions have escaped. It may enlarge and impose on surrounding structures. The common bile duct may be blocked, the duodenum or stomach may be displaced, or the diaphragm may be elevated. The deviation and location are usually recognized in an X-ray.

The symptoms depend on the size and location of the cyst(s). In some instances resolution takes place spontaneously, or the cysts may produce persisting pain, digestive disturbances, anorexia, loss of weight and mechanical interference with other organs. Surgical drainage may be necessary and may be internal or external, depending on the location of the cyst. Internal drainage is achieved by anastomosing the cyst to the small intestine. Surgical drainage through the skin is occasionally but rarely performed as it can lead to the development of pancreatic fistulae. Meticulous skin care and protection is essential to prevent excoriation. Use of skin protective wafers or drainage bags with integral skin-saving adhesive plates may prevent problems. Early consultation with the stoma care nurse, (if available) concerning skin care and appropriate appliances may prevent problems with skin integrity.

Surgical intervention. Surgery is not usually undertaken during an acute attack of pancreatitis unless there is increasing obstructive jaundice due to an impacted stone. The various operative procedures that may be used to treat the patient may be performed on the biliary tract or directly on the pancreas. They include exploration of the common bile duct and ampulla of Vater and the insertion of a T-tube for drainage, cholecystostomy, cholecystectomy, sphincterotomy to relieve obstruction caused by spasm of the sphincter of Oddi, anastomosis between the common bile duct and duodenum, or anastomosis between the gallbladder and the jejunum. Surgery on the pancreas may involve the removal of calculi in the pancreatic duct, drainage of a pseudocyst, or partial or complete pancreatectomy. Rarely, in severe chronic pancreatitis, sensory nerves (splanchnic nerves) which transmit pain impulses from the pancreas may be interrupted to relieve intractable pain.

The nursing care of patients having surgical treatment is similar to that required by patients having gastric surgery (see Chapter 11).

NURSING MANAGEMENT

Assessment

The person's condition may change rapidly with progressive necrosis and resulting haemorrhage. The *vital signs* and the *general response and appearance of the patient* are observed frequently. A rapid weak pulse, a fall in blood pressure, pallor and increasing weakness may manifest haemorrhage or shock and are immediately brought to the doctor's attention. Frequent *haemoglobin* and *haematocrit estimations* may be requested by the doctor to detect haemoconcentration which would indicate the loss of plasma into the peritoneal cavity. An accurate record is kept of the *fluid intake* and *output*.

The *intensity and location of the pain* are noted, and the abdomen is examined for distension and rigidity. All *stools* are examined and, if they are bulky, greasy and foul-smelling or show other abnormalities, they may be saved for medical examination.

The *sclerae and skin* are observed for any yellow tinge that would indicate the development of jaundice.

Nursing intervention

The *goals* of care are that the person with acute pancreatitis will demonstrate:

- Fluid and electrolyte balance.
- Blood glucose levels within normal range.
- Absence of pain and discomfort.
- Absence of respiratory complications.
- Gradual increase in self-care activities.
- Knowledge of prescribed dietary and life-style measures.
- Plans for follow-up care.

Gastric drainage. A nasogastric tube is passed and regular aspiration is performed. This relieves vomiting and distension and prevents the acid gastric secretion from entering the duodenum, which would stimulate the release of the hormones secretin and cholecystokinin-pancreozymin. The colour, consistency and 24-hour volume of the drainage are recorded.

Fluids and nutrition. The patient receives nothing by mouth to avoid stimulating the secretion of the pancreatic enzymes. The restoration and maintenance of normal blood volume is very important to prevent or correct shock. Plasma or whole blood may be given intravenously, in addition to electrolyte and glucose solutions. A close check is kept on the blood chemistry, volume of gastrointestinal drainage, urinary output and amount of perspiration to determine the specific electrolyte and fluid needs. Total parenteral nutrition may be prescribed during the acute and convalescent phases of the illness. Regular (4–6 hourly) monitoring of blood glucose levels should be performed using a reagent strip (see care of the patient with hyperglycaemia). Insulin may be prescribed and titred according to blood glucose levels.

When oral intake is permitted, fluids are introduced in small amounts. The principal nutrient given at first is carbohydrate; protein is added gradually, according to the patient's tolerance. Fats are avoided. The diet is progressively increased to a high-protein, high-carbohydrate, low-fat, light diet. Four or five small meals are recommended. A preparation of extract of pancreas (pancreatin) may be prescribed orally with meals to assist in digestion. Large meals are avoided, and total abstinence from alcohol is stressed.

Mouth and nasal care. Frequent cleansing and rinsing of the mouth are necessary during the period in which oral intake is restricted because the anticholinergic drug which the patient may be receiving suppresses salivary secretion. Oil, petroleum jelly or a cream is used on the lips to prevent cracking. The nostrils are cleansed with an applicator which has been slightly moistened with normal saline, and a light application of petroleum jelly or water-soluble lubricant is made to the nostril through which the tube passes to prevent irritation and excoriation.

Pulmonary care. The person with acute pancreatitis can develop respiratory difficulties due to acid–base abnormalities, distended abdomen preventing full expansion of the lungs, or experience of pain on respiration causing reduced effort. Anticholinergic drugs can reduce normal secretions of the respiratory tract. The person should be nursed in a semi-upright position to reduce pressure on the diaphragm and promote full lung expansion. Deep breathing exercises and coughing should be taught and the patient should be encouraged to perform them regularly. Should oxygen therapy be prescribed, humidification may prevent further drying of the respiratory tract, and the use of nasal cannulae rather than a face mask may improve tolerance.

Psychological support will be necessary throughout the illness as it is clearly a very stressful experience for the patient and family. This will only be compounded by worries and anxieties over social factors such as loss of earnings, or even job, while a history of alcohol abuse brings with it a whole sequence of psychological and social problems.

Follow-up care. A long convalescence follows recovery from an acute episode of pancreatitis. The necessary care to avert an exacerbation is discussed with the patient and family. The importance of strict adherence to the prescribed diet, total abstinence from alcohol and the avoidance of large meals are explained. Verbal and written instructions are given about the content and preparation of the recommended low-fat, high-protein, high-carbohydrate diet.

If anticholinergic drugs or antacids are to be continued, verbal and written directions are given which include advice as to early side-effects that should be reported to the doctor. To assist with digestion, the patient with chronic pancreatitis may need to continue to take extract of pancreas (pancreatin) orally with each meal.

Activities are gradually resumed and the individual may return to work in 1–3 months if the person's job has been kept available.

Evaluation
Evaluation of the outcomes of nursing intervention for the person with acute pancreatitis includes assessment of the person's symptoms and evidence that they have been alleviated; particularly important is the absence of pain. Vital signs and fluid and electrolyte balance should be returning to the person's usual levels. The patient

should increasingly assume self-care activities. The patient and family should be able to describe the prescribed dietary measures, understand the need for rest, state plans to alter life-style factors such as alcohol consumption, and verbalize plans for follow-up health care.

CHRONIC PANCREATITIS

Chronic pancreatitis may develop following an initial acute episode or may develop insidiously. Recurrent acute exacerbations are likely to occur. It is frequently associated with alcoholism, chronic biliary tract disease, or hypercalcaemia due to hyperparathyroidism.

The chronic form of the disease is characterized by progressive fibrosing and calcification of areas in the pancreas following inflammation and necrosis. The degree of impaired function and the intensity of its signs and symptoms are proportionate to the amount of continuing inflammation or frequency of acute episodes and ensuing tissue damage.

CLINICAL CHARACTERISTICS

The person with chronic pancreatitis experiences recurrent attacks of pain in the epigastric region and right upper quadrant which progressively becomes persistent. Anorexia, nausea, flatulence and constipation are common problems. Episodes are frequently precipitated by the ingestion of alcohol or a large meal with considerable fatty content.

As more and more of the pancreatic parenchyma becomes non-functional, a deficiency of enzyme secretion occurs in the intestine. Less fat and protein are digested; the person's stools become bulky, greasy and offensive (steatorrhoea) and there is a progressive weight loss. A deficiency of insulin secretion may result in diabetes mellitus.

TREATMENT AND NURSING INTERVENTION

In some instances, slight impairment by chronic pancreatitis may be controlled by dietary adjustments and the avoidance of emotional stress, fatigue and infection.

A low-fat diet and four or five small meals rather than the usual three larger ones are recommended. The person's fear of precipitating more severe pain may lead to a reluctance to eat and a resulting serious weight loss; consequently encouragement to take nourishing foods that can be tolerated is needed. Impaired digestion due to insufficient quantities of enzymes in the intestine may be corrected by the administration of pancreatic enzyme supplements (preparation of pancreatic extract). Vitamin supplements, including vitamins A, D, K, folic acid and B_{12} may be required. Total alcohol abstinence must be respected to avoid precipitation of an acute episode.

Decreased insulin secretion may necessitate the giving of insulin to control glucose metabolism.

As the disease becomes more advanced, the pain experienced by the patient may indicate frequent doses of an analgesic. Not infrequently, this becomes complicated by the person's development of a tolerance for the

drug, necessitating progressively larger doses or a change in the prescribed medication regimen.

Rarely, surgical intervention may be used to drain pseudocysts or to relieve intractable pain. Partial pancreatectomy or anastomosis of the pancreatic duct with the jejunum may be undertaken.

Neoplasms of the Pancreas

CARCINOMA

Cancer of the pancreas usually arises from the ducts and, although it may occur in any part of the organ, it is most commonly seen in the head. It is usually fatal.

The patient experiences pain, progressive weakness and loss of weight. Obstructive jaundice develops if the neoplasm encroaches on the ampulla of Vater or common bile duct. The cancer may spread by direct invasion to adjacent structures or by metastasis to the liver.

TREATMENT

The condition is treated surgically if recognized sufficiently early and if it is the head of the pancreas that is involved. Neoplasms in the body and tail have usually metastasized by the time they are identified. Rarely, a pancreatoduodenal resection may be done. This procedure involves resection of the head of the pancreas, ampulla of Vater, duodenum and pylorus with anastomosis between the common bile duct and jejunum, anastomosis between the pancreas and jejunum, and a gastrojejunostomy. Palliative operations that may be used include a cholecystojejunostomy to relieve obstructive jaundice and a side-to-side anastomosis of the main pancreatic duct (duct of Wirsung) to the jejunum. Radiation therapy and/or chemotherapy may be used but have not been found to be very effective.

Preparation for surgery includes a high-calorie, low-fat diet if tolerated by the patient, intravenous rehydration, blood transfusions, and parenteral vitamin K if there is jaundice. Postoperative care includes gastrointestinal decompression to prevent distension of the jejunum and pressure on the sites of the anastomoses. The patient is supported by blood transfusions and intravenous fluids. Vitamin K administration may be continued.

TUMOURS OF ISLET CELLS

A benign tumour may develop in non-β islet cells and may become malignant. The tumour cells secrete gastrin freely, causing the Zollinger-Ellison syndrome, which is characterized by gastric hypersecretion and persisting peptic ulceration. The treatment is surgical removal of the tumours or total gastrectomy. Nursing care of the patient is similar to that cited under gastric surgery, see Chapter 11.

Occasionally an adenoma develops from β cells of the islets of Langerhans, causing an excessive secretion of insulin (hyperinsulinism) and hypoglycaemia. The adenoma is usually benign but, rarely, may be adenocarcinoma.

The symptoms presented by the patient are mainly due to the effect of the abnormally low blood sugar on the brain cells. Brain cells are more sensitive to glucose deficiency than other body cells. The initial symptoms are hunger, restlessness and apprehension. These progress to weakness, loss of co-ordination, tremors, diaphoresis, disorientation, convulsions and coma. The manifestations appear during a fasting period (early morning) or following extreme exertion. Prompt administration of some form of glucose is necessary to raise the blood sugar. If the hypoglycaemia remains untreated, the glucose deficiency may result in permanent brain cell damage or death. When early signs are recognized, the patient is given sugar or orange juice with sugar. In the more advanced stage of hypoglycaemia, glucose 50% is given intravenously.

Surgical treatment may consist of excision of the adenoma or subtotal or total pancreatectomy. Preparation for the surgery includes a high-carbohydrate, high-protein diet and intravenous infusions of glucose solution to restore glycogen reserves. The glucose infusion is continued during the operation. Following surgery, close observation is made for a recurrence of hypoglycaemia. If a total pancreatectomy is done, the patient will receive supplemental insulin and pancreatic extract for the remainder of his life.

Diabetes mellitus is discussed in Chapter 19.

SUMMARY

This chapter provides an overview of the structures and functions of the liver, biliary tract and exocrine pancreas. The clinical characteristics and the nursing assessment of alterations in function demonstrated by the person with disorders of the liver, biliary tract and exocrine pancreas are discussed. Emphasis is placed on the role of the nurse in the early detection and treatment of persons with alcohol abuse problems and the potential for preventing serious disorders of the liver and pancreas.

The assessment and nursing management of persons with the more common acute and chronic disorders of the liver, biliary tract and exocrine pancreas are described. Discussion focuses on the occupational risk for hepatitis and measures to prevent the transmission of hepatitis B virus to nurses and the public.

LEARNING ACTIVITIES

1. (a) Write a list of your personal attitudes toward people with alcohol-related problems.
   (b) Write a second list describing how you believe the nursing profession may help people with alcohol problems.
   (c) Identify similarities and differences between the two lists you have formulated. Discuss reasons for these differences.
2. Develop a resource pack of health education material for use in teaching patients about healthy drinking.
3. Hepatitis B can be transmitted by sexual intercourse.
   (a) Write down what you consider to be safe sexual practice.
   (b) Refer to p. 24 (HIV/AIDS and safe sex); does the information compare with what you have noted as safe sexual practice?
   (c) Develop resources which will assist you in health education activities regarding safe sexual practices.
4. A small overdose of about 10–15 paracetamol tablets may cause life-threatening damage to the liver. Discuss whether paracetamol should be withdrawn from use or what steps may be taken to prevent deaths from paracetamol overdose.
5. 'Cirrhosis of the liver in alcoholics is a self-inflicted injury.' Discuss the merits and implications of this statement.

REFERENCES AND FURTHER READING

Bergman B, Larsson G, Brismar B & Klang M (1989) Battered wives and female alcoholics: a comparative social and psychiatric study. *Journal of Advanced Nursing* **14**: 727–734.

Catalan J, Batten R & Litvinoff S (1985) Alcohol abuse in patients admitted to a general hospital: a continuing detection failure. *British Journal of Clinical and Social Psychiatry* **3**: 56–59.

Close D (1989) Training for alcohol education in the south west. *Health Education Journal* **48(2)**: 74–76.

Cotton G (1989) A little of what you fancy.... *Nursing Times* **85(40)**: 37.

Fitzgerald AP, Bartek, JK, Lindeman MG, Newton M & Hawks JH (1987) Nurse reported patient problems in alcoholism. In McLane AM (ed.) *Classification of Nursing Diagnoses: Proceedings of the Seventh Conference: North American Nursing Diagnosis Association*, p. 296. St Louis: Mosby.

Health Education Council (1985) *That's the Limit*. London: HEC.

Ho-Yen DO, Crossan MN & Walker E (1985) Nursing knowledge of hepatitis B infection. *Journal of Advanced Nursing* **10**: 169–172.

Kedzierski M (1991) Managing liver disease in adults. *Nursing Standard* **5(41)**: 25–28.

Kedzierski M (1991) Management of viral hepatitis. *Nursing Standard* **5(42)**: 29–32.

Knowles R (1990) Clearing your head. *Nursing Times* **86(27)**: 65–67.

Neuberger JM (1989) Transplantation for alcoholic liver disease. *British Medical Journal* **299**: 693.

Pearson M (1990) Small steps to progress. *Nursing Times* **86(42)**: 28–30.

Perrillo RP, Schiff ER, Davis GL et al (1990) A randomized, controlled trial of interferon alfa-2b alone and after prednisone withdrawal for the treatment of chronic hepatitis B. *New England Journal of Medicine* **323(5)**: 295–301.

Quaghebeur G & Richards P (1989) Comotose patients smelling of alcohol. *British Medical Journal* **299**: 410.

Reed MT (1986) Descriptive study of chemically dependent nurses. In Brooking J (ed.) *Psychiatric Nursing Research*, pp. 157–173. Chichester: Wiley.

Robinson BG & Gaskell K (1989) Prevalence and characteristics of at-risk drinkers among a health visitor's caseload. *Health Visitor* **62**: 242–243.

Rowland N & Maynard AK (1989) Alcohol education for patients: some nurses need persuading. *Nurse Education Today* **9**: 100–104.

Royal College of General Practitioners (1986) *Alcohol — a balanced view*. London: RCPG.

Royal College of Physicians (1987) *The Medical Consequences of Alcohol Abuse: A Great and Growing Evil*. London: Tavistock.

Smith C, Roberts JL & Pendleton LL (1988) Booze on the box. The portrayal of alcohol on British television: a content analysis. *Health Education Research* **3(3)**: 267–272.

Storer J (1988) In Hinchcliff S & Montague S (eds) *Physiology for Nursing Practice*, pp. 441–464. London: Baillière Tindall.

Sullivan EJ & Hale RE (1987) Nurses' beliefs about the aetiology and treatment of alcohol abuse: a national study. *Journal of Studies on Alcohol* **48**: 456–460.

Tedder RS (1980) Hepatitis B in hospital. *Journal of Hospital Medicine* **23(3)**: 274–279.

Tweed SH (1989) Identifying the alcoholic client. *Nursing Clinics of North America* **24(1)**: pp 13–32.

Wood D (1986) *Beliefs about alcohol*. London: Health Education Council.

Caring for the Patient with a Nutritional Disorder

18

OBJECTIVES

By the end of this chapter, the reader will be able to:

- Assess a person's nutritional status through interview and physical examination
- Recognize (1) normal values of laboratory tests, and (2) how they would be altered in a disorder of nutrition or metabolism
- Describe current guidelines for nutritional intake related to: (1) food groups, (2) proportion of intake as carbohydrate, protein or fat, and (3) recommendations for fibre, alcohol and salt
- Understand the metabolism of carbohydrates, protein and fat
- Relate a variety of factors to the causation and maintenance of over or undernutrition using the examples of obesity and eating disorders
- Implement an educational and supportive role with patients who have a problem of over or undernutrition
- Discuss ethical issues related to the provision of nutrition and hydration

NUTRITION

Nutrition refers to the process of ingesting, assimilating and utilizing food. All living cells require a continuous supply of nutrients for survival. Body cells utilize the molecules from ingested food to provide the energy and materials necessary to maintain their structure and function. The cells, particularly those of the liver, are capable of converting the wide range of molecules from different foods to another type of molecule for use.

Nutritional Requirements

Certain nutrients are considered to be *essential* and must be ingested in adequate amounts to meet body needs. These include: protein (8 of the 20 amino acids that cannot be produced in the body), some fatty acids, vitamins and minerals. To obtain essential nutrients, the individual must consume a daily diet composed of a variety of foods as no one food provides all essential elements. Tables of recommended daily allowances of essential nutrients have been developed to meet the nutritonal needs of healthy individuals (DHSS, 1979; Howe, 1981).

A balanced diet consists of foods from each of the basic food groups of milk, meats, fruits, vegetables, and grains. An adequate daily diet for an adult includes:

- Two servings of milk or milk products such as cheese or yogurt.
- Two servings of meat, fish, poultry or lentils.
- Four servings of fruits and vegetables, including a citrus fruit, a dark green and a root vegetable.
- Four servings of grain in the form of bread, or whole grain cereals.

If variety of intake from each of these food groups is consumed, vitamin supplementation should not be necessary.

Basic food group guides are useful in planning diets for healthy individuals and for adjusting diet to meet specific needs such as altered energy intake or increased or decreased intake of specific nutrients. Energy requirements are met primarily by carbohydrates (50%) and fats (35%), with about 15% provided by protein. For kilocalorie-reduced diets, it is recommended that fats (mainly) and carbohydrates be reduced and protein content remain the same (12% of the dietary kilocalories). Use of non-nutritive sweeteners is questionable as there is some evidence that they may increase one's appetite for sweet tastes.

Energy requirement for an individual is determined by:

1. The amount of energy needed to maintain involuntary body functions at rest (basal metabolic rate, BMR).
2. The amount of energy required to metabolize food.
3. Physical activity.

When kilocalorie intake equals kilocalorie use, body weight is maintained.

The use of food additives is a highly controversial area directing much current research. Additives are important to preserve freshness, to increase nutritional value, to improve flavour and to ease preparation. However, there is concern about potential carcinogenicity and toxicity. In absence of 'facts' about the effects of additives, it is recommended that one eat predominately food which is unprocessed (e.g. oatmeal instead of commercial sweetened and coloured cereal).

Factors Which Influence Dietary Patterns

Dietary behaviour is influenced by physiological, psychological, sociocultural and environmental factors, as well as knowledge of food and food requirements. The consumption of food is usually a social activity; eating habits are very complex and are resistant to change as they become an integral part of the individual and family life-style.

Physiological factors influencing nutritional needs and eating behaviour include the individual's metabolic rate, growth phase, body excretions, reproductive functions and level of daily physical activity. Increased energy and nutrients are required by the individual during periods of rapid physical growth, pregnancy and lactation, increased basal metabolic rate (e.g. hyperthyroidism) and increased physical activity. Fewer kilocalories are needed by elderly individuals because of their lower basal metabolic rate and decreased activity and by those with sedentary life-styles.

The hypothalamus, the limbic system of the brain and gut hormones regulate food intake by influencing appetite, hunger and satiety. *Hunger* is a physiological phenomenon involving unpleasant sensations of abdominal discomfort and irritability which prompt the individual to search for food. *Appetite* involves the conscious desire to eat. *Satiation* is the pleasant feeling of being fully satisfied after a meal. *Anorexia* is the abnormal loss of the desire to eat which may be influenced by both physiological and psychological factors.

Emotions are important in determining eating behaviour. Food has different meanings for each individual, and responses to stress or happiness are often expressed as changes in eating habits. Some individuals respond to stress and decreased self-esteem by overeating, while others have loss of appetite and decrease their food consumption. It is possible that some people may experience both increases and decreases in consumption depending on the degree of stress perceived. Eating habits are believed to be formed early in life and become fixed responses.

Sociocultural factors influencing eating behaviour include religious and ethnic practices and the use of foods which have special meaning for the individual and family. The media also play an important role in influencing food consumption: advertisements relating to specific foods have a great impact on individuals and families; the portrayal of an 'ideal' body appearance greatly influences dietary intake and patterns of food consumption in girls and young adult females (Orbach, 1986). Sociocultural factors also influence the proportion of meals eaten in restaurants as opposed to the home, and the quality of restaurant chosen. Advertising is heavy for the 'fast food' chains which tend to have foods of higher saturated fat and salt than one might consume in a meal prepared at home. Social class may affect diet, with knowledge about what constitutes a healthy diet being greater in higher social class families.

Environmental factors include the availability, cost and convenience of foods. The individual's income may be inadequate to meet the cost of the essential foodstuffs or disability may limit a person's ability to prepare food or shop for food. The environment in which food is prepared and eaten also influences eating behaviour. Appetite is usually stimulated when eating takes place in a pleasant and relaxed social milieu.

Knowledge of dietary requirements and food values is an important factor in the individual's or family's eating patterns. In some instances, persons may not understand that in planning a balanced diet, expensive food elements can usually be substituted by less expensive items that will meet the essential dietary requirements.

These non-biological influences on the use of food may contribute to the development of nutritional disorders and are important restraining factors when attempting to change eating habits.

METABOLISM

When food is absorbed, it is taken from the blood by tissue cells. Some of it is used by the cells to meet material requirements for the construction of tissue, for growth and maintenance or for the production of substances such as hormones and enzymes. Much of the food is broken down to produce the energy required by the body to carry out its many functions. All cells require substances that provide energy, but since those of different tissues vary in composition and function, the cells select materials to meet their special needs in respect to such differences. Glucose and fat are used mainly to supply energy, while requirements for cellular structure and chemical products are met principally by the amino acids and minerals.

When the foods are taken into the cells, they undergo physical and chemical changes which comprise *metabolism*. When the cellular activity results in the synthesis of tissue substance, the process is referred to as *anabolism*, or anabolic metabolism. The processes that break down the materials into simpler forms and release energy are called *catabolism*, or catabolic metabolism.

Anabolism exceeds catabolism during the absorptive phase, following ingestion and digestion after a meal. Monosaccharides and amino acids are absorbed from the intestinal tract into the blood and are transported to the liver where the monosaccharides are immediately converted into glucose to supply the body's major source of energy during this absorptive period. Excess calories are stored in the liver and adipose tissue, mostly as fats.

During the postabsorptive period, which occurs about four hours following ingestion of a meal, during the night and during periods of fasting, energy is supplied by the stores of glycogen in the liver and muscles and by the breakdown of neutral fat stored in adipose tissue. When fasting is prolonged, body protein is catabolized to provide energy.

Fate of Carbohydrates in the Body

Carbohydrates are absorbed as glucose, fructose and galactose and are the main energy source. Fructose and most of the galactose are converted to glucose by the liver. Some galactose remains as such and is one of the components of the myelin sheath found around many nerve fibres. The sheath is a fatty, insulating membrane that prevents the loss of the nerve impulse.

Glucose may be oxidized by the cells to provide energy; it is temporarily stored as glycogen in the liver or muscles or converted to fat and stored as such. It is also used in small amounts in the synthesis of tissue substances and secretions and is circulated in the blood for a period of time, providing what is known as the blood glucose. If it is in excess, some may be excreted in the urine.

OXIDATION OF GLUCOSE

The oxidation of glucose by the cells to acquire energy is a complex process involving a series of many chemical reactions. Each reaction is catalysed by a specific enzyme, with the final end-products being energy, water and carbon dioxide.

It is not the intent to give the details here of the biochemical reactions that take place in the oxidation of glucose. If such detailed information is desired, the reader should consult a textbook of biochemistry or medical physiology. In principle the catabolism of glucose involves two main processes, glycolysis and the citric acid cycle (Krebs cycle or tricarboxylic acid cycle).

Glycolysis splits the glucose molecule into two pyruvic acid molecules, at the same time releasing some energy. Ten successive chemical reactions are necessary to achieve glycolysis. The pyruvic acid molecules then embark on a series of chemical reactions which compose the citric acid cycle. Each of the ten chemical changes occurring in the citric acid cycle also requires a specific enzyme. The net result of the metabolism of one molecule of glucose is energy (E) plus six molecules of carbon dioxide plus six molecules of water:

$$C_6H_{12}O_6 + 6O_2 \rightarrow E + 6CO_2 + 6H_2O.$$

Some of the energy that is released by the chemical reactions forms heat energy, and the remainder is stored in the cell as adenosine triphosphate (ATP). ATP is a compound with three phosphoric acid radicals; two of these radicals are connected to the compound by high-energy bonds which can be split off readily when energy is needed by the cell to promote other chemical changes. If one phosphate radical is released, the compound is changed to adenosine diphosphate (ADP). As energy is released by other chemical reactions, the energy is used to bond the free phosphate radical to ADP and regenerate ATP. These energy changes go on continually with the chemical processes that constitute metabolism.

The glucose that is not needed to maintain a normal concentration in the blood or for immediate oxidation is converted by several chemical reactions and enzymes to glycogen and stored as such. Most of the glycogen is found in the muscle and liver cells. The muscle cells store it for their own use for contraction. The liver stores it and, as the blood concentration falls, converts the glycogen back to glucose and releases it into the blood. The process by which the glucose is converted to glycogen is known as *glycogenesis; the reconversion of the glycogen to glucose is called glycogenolysis.*

BLOOD GLUCOSE

The blood glucose concentration is relatively constant, the normal being 3.9–6.1 mmol/l of blood. It may rise to 7.2–8.0 mmol/l after a meal, but falls to normal within 2–3 hours. Maintenance of the blood glucose level within normal limits is especially important for normal functioning and survival of the brain cells. A concentration of at least 3.9 mmol/l of glucose in the blood is necessary in order to meet the needs of the cells.

A deficiency in the blood glucose concentration is quickly manifested by central nervous system disturbances. The person may become confused and lose muscle co-ordination and strength. If the deficiency is severe, loss of consciousness may occur and, unless corrected, death may ensue. If the brain cells are deprived of glucose for even a very few hours, they may suffer permanent damage.

Hypoglycaemia is the term given to a blood sugar concentration below the normal. If the concentration is above the normal, the condition is known as *hyperglycaemia.*

REGULATION OF BLOOD GLUCOSE CONCENTRATION

Maintenance of blood glucose within normal limits is achieved mainly by hormones. When the blood glucose concentration falls, the liver cells may be activated by two hormones, glucagon and adrenaline, to convert glycogen to glucose and release it into the blood. Glucagon is secreted by the pancreas when the blood glucose falls below the normal level. Adrenaline is secreted by the medulla of the adrenal glands. Sympathetic innervation to the adrenal glands is excited by a low blood glucose concentration, resulting in release of adrenaline into the blood. Adrenaline also stimulates the breakdown of muscle glycogen to lactate, which must return to the liver for gluconeogensis to occur.

Insulin, a hormone secreted by cells in the islets of Langerhans of the pancreas, brings about a decrease in the blood glucose concentration by promoting the transport of glucose into the tissue cells. If the blood glucose level decreases towards or below the lower normal limits, there is a corresponding decrease in the secretion of insulin.

The adrenal cortex also secretes the hormones known as glucocorticoids that increase the blood glucose concentration. A decrease in the blood glucose stimulates the adenohypophysis (anterior pituitary gland) to release the adrenocorticotropic hormone (ACTH) which brings about the release of glucocorticoids. The increase in blood sugar is brought about by the glucocorticoids stimulating the liver cells to form glucose from noncarbohydrate substances. Protein and fats may be broken down and glycogen or glucose formed. This process may be referred to as glyconeogenesis or, if glucose is produced, as *gluconeogenesis.*

Similarly, the lowered blood glucose may cause the release of thyroid-stimulating hormone (TSH) by the adenohypophysis and a resulting increase in the output of thyroxin, which promotes gluconeogenesis.

LIPOGENESIS

When the absorbed glucose exceeds what the cells use and what can be stored as glycogen, it may be converted to fat and stored in the fat depots of the body. Insulin plays an important role in stimulating the deposition of fat.

EXCRETION OF GLUCOSE BY THE KIDNEYS

As the blood flows through the kidney, about one-tenth of the water in the blood and its associated solutes with a molecular weight of less than 67 000 are filtered by the glomeruli of the kidneys. Normally, all of the filtered glucose is reabsorbed by the tubules and the urine is sugar-free. If the blood glucose becomes abnormally high, not all the glucose is reabsorbed from the kidney tubule back into the blood; that which is not reabsorbed by the tubules passes out into the urine. The level of blood sugar at which glucose is excreted in the urine is referred to as the *renal glucose threshold* and is approximately 10 mmol/l, but this may vary with individuals. This excretion of the glucose, rather than its usual reabsorption, does reduce blood sugar to some extent and is considered as a mechanism active in the regulation of blood glucose.

Fate of the Fats in the Body

Fatty acids and glycerol are absorbed into the microvilli of the intestinal cells. There they are combined to form triglycerides which are coated with phospholipids to become chylomicrons. The absorbed fat is carried into the major lymph channels and reaches the blood through the thoracic lymphatic duct. Fats may be used by the body cells to provide energy, synthesize fat compounds or be stored as fatty tissue.

In the use of fats to provide energy, the triglycerides are first broken down by the liver into glycerol and fatty acids. The glycerol is converted to glycogen, which is then converted to glucose.

The fatty acids are split by a series of chemical changes, mainly occurring in the liver. In each reaction, two carbon atoms and energy are freed in an oxidation process, finally ending up with acetoacetic acid and smaller amounts of β-hydroxybutyric acid and acetone. These acids, because of their chemical structure, may be referred to as ketone acids or ketone bodies and the process by which they are formed is called *ketogenesis*. The ketones move out of the liver into the blood and are transported to the cells in need of energy, where they are metabolized via the citric acid cycle, releasing energy and ending up as waste carbon dioxide and water. Although one gram of fat has more than twice as much energy value (9.3 kcal or 38 kJ; 1 kcal = 4.184 kJ) as does one gram of glucose (4.1 kcal or 17 kJ), as long as glucose is available to the cells it is used in preference to fats.

The amount of ketones in the blood is normally very low and depends on a balance between the production by the liver and the assimilation by the tissue cells. Occasionally, the rate of ketogenesis may exceed the rate at which the cells complete the metabolism, resulting in an accumulation of ketone acids in the blood and ketonuria. The condition is called ketosis and may occur when there is an increased use of endogenous fat for energy, as in starvation, or if there is a deficiency of glucose or a disturbance in the metabolism of glucose, as in diabetes mellitus. Ketosis may also develop with a diet high in fats (ketogenic diet).

Fat in the body is necessary for the formation of some essential fatty compounds such as phospholipids, lecithin, steroids and cholesterol. These compounds are built into other tissues: for example, phospholipids and cholesterol are necessary components of cell membranes.

The fat that is not used for energy or for the synthesis of certain tissue substances is stored as fatty tissue in areas of the body called the fat depots. Most of the fat is deposited in the subcutaneous tissue, in the abdomen, especially on the mesentery and omentum, around the kidneys and between the muscle fibres.

A certain amount of stored fat is of value. The subcutaneous fatty tissue insulates the body against excessive heat loss and against the cold of the external environment. Fatty tissue also provides a protective cushion for the body against trauma.

Not all the absorbed fat may enter the liver after a meal. Some of it moves directly into the fat depots so that the concentration of fat in the blood is quickly lowered. The fat in the tissues is mobilized when it is needed for energy. There is a constant movement of fat in and out of the fatty tissue (Figure 18.1).

As with carbohydrate metabolism, certain hormones produced in the body may influence fat metabolism. Most of them increase fat mobilization and fat utilization by the cells. These hormones include the growth (somatotropic) hormone secreted by the anterior pituitary gland, thyroxine, cortisone secreted by the adrenal cortices, and adrenaline released by the medulla of the adrenals. Insulin increases lipid synthesis and utilization. Oestrogen secreted by the ovaries increases the deposition of fats in the tissues.

Fate of Protein in the Body

The absorbed amino acids may be built into body tissue or used in the synthesis of cell products, such as enzymes and hormones, or the formation of protein compounds, such as plasma proteins. They may be converted to non-nitrogenous substances, such as carbohydrate or fat, which may be stored or oxidized to produce energy. From the large number of different amino acids, the cells select only those that they need to produce their particular type of protoplasm and cell products. Amino acids are very important to the growing child, whose protein requirement is more than twice that of the adult.

The amino acids that are not used by the cells for structure or cell products are taken into the liver where they may be stored or converted to a non-nitrogenous compound; the liver thus prevents an excessive concentration of amino acids in the blood. Only a small

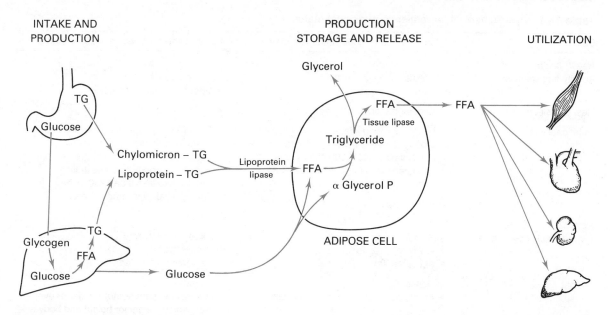

Figure 18.1 Fat homeostasis in normal man. The liver is a major site of the synthesis of fat, which is released as the triglyceride (TG) moiety of lipoproteins. The adipose cell is the major storage reserve of fat. Release of fatty acids from the adipose cell depends on the activity of a hormone-sensitive tissue lipase. The free fatty acids (FFA) released to the circulation are largely oxidized by skeletal and cardiac muscle, and to a smaller extent by kidney and liver.

amount can be stored, but when the blood concentration of amino acids falls, the liver releases the reserve.

Amino acids may be converted to glucose by the liver cells by a process called *deamination*. The amino radical is removed from the amino acid, forming ammonia. Since the ammonia would be toxic to tissue cells, it is combined with carbon dioxide to form urea. The urea is released from the liver into the general circulation and excreted by the kidneys.

The residual molecular elements of the amino acid are converted to glucose or fat and are oxidized to meet energy requirements. Normally, carbohydrate and fat provide the energy required by the cells. If these become deficient, protein is moved into the liver and is deaminated to meet the cells' energy needs. In starvation, this involves the use of blood proteins and tissue protein and deprives the cells of structural and functional amino acids. The cells' normal activities are disrupted and survival is threatened.

Some amino acids may be synthesized by the liver cells. The amino radical is removed from one amino acid and is attached to the molecule of a carbohydrate or a fatty acid. This process is called *transamination*.

Protein metabolism is influenced by certain hormones. The growth hormone, thryoxine and testosterone (male sex hormone) stimulate the use of protein in the synthesis of tissue and cell products. The glucocorticoids promote mobilization of amino acids into the blood from the cells and their conversion to glucose.

THE PERSON WITH POTENTIAL OR ACTUAL ALTERED NUTRITION AND METABOLISM

ASSESSMENT

The body's energy balance and body functions are affected when the supply of nutrients is altered. Assessment of the patient with an actual or potential disorder of nutrition and metabolism includes the collection and analysis of information regarding lifestyle, behaviour patterns, dietary habits and changes in physiological functioning of most body systems (Table 18.1).

In community or hospital settings, the nurse may initially assess the patient. If the result of that assessment is that the patient has an actual alteration in nutrition and metabolism, the nurse would usually refer the person for more indepth assessment (including laboratory assessment) by a dietician and/or physician.

Health history

1. *Age and sex.* The patient's age and sex are noted as these influence basal metabolic rate as well as lifestyle, activity and nutritional needs.
2. *Activity and life-style.* The amount of energy the patient expends daily is determined by finding out the type of occupation and extent of daily activities.

Table 18.1   Assessment of the patient's nutritional status.

Data	Characteristics of good nutritional status	Characteristics of poor nutritional status
Health history		
Activity and life-style	● Consistent daily activity	● Sedentary life-style ● Sporadic excessive activity
Rest and sleep	● Regular pattern	● Inconsistent
Nutritional intake	● Usual daily food intake contains basic food groups and all essential nutrients ● Fluid intake 1500–2000 ml/day ● Balanced calorie intake for size and activity	● Some food groups and essential nutrients missing from diet ● Calorie intake less than or greater than required for body size and activity ● Fluid intake less than 1200 ml/day ● Abuse of laxatives and diuretics
Physical examination		
General body appearance	● Stands erect ● Alert ● Abdomen flat	● Drooped shoulders ● Inattentive ● Abdomen protruded
Weight	● Constant ● In proportion to height and body size	● Variable ● Twenty per cent or more under or over suggested weight for height and body type
Skinfold thickness	● Within 80% of standard value for age and sex	● Twenty per cent or more above or below standard value for age and sex
Circumference measurement	● Body muscle stores are within 90% of standard value for age and sex	● Body muscle stores are 80% or less of standard value for age and sex
Skin	● Clean, dry and intact	● Dry, transparent, scaly with petechiae
Oral mucous membrane	● Clean, moist and intact	● Gums swollen and bleeding
Teeth	● Clean, smooth, regular edges, straight and symmetrical and intact	● Dental caries ● Discoloration ● Irregular edges ● Malpositioned and absent teeth
Lips	● Smooth, intact	● Red and swollen with fissures
Hair	● Shiny and clean	● Dull, listless and brittle
Nails	● Smooth, shaped and intact	● Brittle, ridged, irregular edges
Eyes	● Clean, focused ● Conjunctiva pink and moist	● Sunken ● Conjunctiva pale ● Discharge

How the patient feels following activity and the perception of activities that can or cannot be performed is also assessed.

3. *Rest and sleep* are assessed in relation to the patient's usual pattern.

4. *Nutritional history* includes identification of past weight loss or gain, or attempts at either, daily food intake, eating habits and factors affecting these. The patient may be asked to record total food and fluid intake over a 24-hour period and include information about the time and circumstances under which the food was consumed, the method of preparing the food and the consumption of dietary supplements and snacks between meals. How the individual responds to food (has or has not an appetite for it, has strong likes or dislikes) is elicited, as well as

symptoms that occur following ingestion of foods. The patient's daily food intake is analysed for adequacy of the essential nutrients, vitamins and minerals, energy intake and fluid volume. The presence of nausea, vomiting, anorexia, excessive thirst and changes in body fat may be indicative of metabolic and/or eating disorders. Food preferences, dislikes, food allergies and sociocultural factors which may influence eating habits are documented.

5. *Elimination.* Bowel habits are determined, and information related to the nature, formation, colour, odour and frequency of stools, and use of laxatives, stool softeners or supplemental fibre is obtained. The volume, frequency and colour of urine output is determined, as well as the presence of nocturia and the use of diuretics. The urine should be tested for

any abnormalities with a chemical reagent strip test.
6. *Socioeconomic factors* affecting the availability, storage and preparation of foods are identified.

Physical examination

1. *General body appearance* is observed. The patient's general stature and posture, distribution of body fat and general state of alertness reflect the state of health.
2. *Height and weight* are measured and recorded, and changes in body weight over given periods are identified (e.g. weight loss or gain over so many weeks or months).
3. *Skin-fold thickness* is measured to determine the amount of subcutaneous body fat. Callipers are used to measure the skin-fold thickness over the triceps, scapular region and upper abdomen (Goodinson, 1986). Results are compared with a table of normal values for the individual's age and sex. (Skin-fold thickness and circumference measurements are not routine observations, but are sometimes used with some emaciated, obese or debilitated patients.)
4. *Circumference measurements* are taken bilaterally at mid-arm and mid-thigh level. The arm muscle circumference is determined by subtracting the triceps skin-fold measurement from the arm circumference measurement. Results are compared with a table of normal values for the individual's age and sex. These calculations provide information on the body's muscle stores.
5. *The skin* is inspected for rashes, lesions, petechiae, bruises and changes in colour. The presence of infections and lesions that fail to heal may indicate increased blood glucose levels, while indications of prolonged bleeding may reflect a vitamin K deficiency.

Diagnostic tests

Blood and urine studies may be undertaken. These will reflect changes in the metabolism of carbohydrates, proteins and fats, and may be used to determine the level of vitamins and minerals. The tests and normal values are summarized in Table 18.2.

DIET AND HEALTH

Over the last 10 years, many reports have been produced linking our way of eating with health problems. These reports make recommendations on food and health in terms of prevention of diseases attributed to inappropriate food intake. Two recent reports should influence the advice given by nurses (Table 18.3): these are the reports of the National Advisory Committee on Nutrition Education (NACNE) (1983) and the report of the DHSS Committee on Medical Aspects of Food Policy (the COMA Report) (1984). A summary of their recommendations follows.

Guidelines for healthy eating

1. *Maintain a desirable weight.* A body mass index (BMI) (which is weight (kg) divided by height (metres)^3 of between 20 and 25 is associated with an appropriate weight for most people and is associated with the lowest occurrence of morbidity and mortality (Gregory et al, 1990).
2. *Fat is implicated in heart disease and some cancers.* The reports recommend a reduction in the total amount of fat consumed to 30–35% of total energy intake, and a reduction in diary fat and meat fat to between 5 and 10%, that is, to less than a third of total fat. (This is not, however, recommended for infants and children under 5 years.) This means less fried foods, eating more fish and poultry and less red meats and using skimmed or semi-skimmed milk.
3. *Reduce sugar intake by half.* Currently, the average person in the United Kingdom eats about 115 g (4 oz) of sugar per day and this should be reduced by cutting down on sweets, snacks and sugary drinks and increasing the intake of complex carbohydrates (Royal College of Physicians, 1983).
4. *High blood pressure is a major risk factor in heart disease.* Some individuals seem unable to cope with excess salt and it is recommended that salt is reduced from the present average of 2.5 teaspoons a day to less than 2 teaspoons. This means less salt in cooking and adding less at the table. Continue a diet rich in potassium.
5. *'Energy values should be maintained because more exercise is to be encouraged.'* Exercise reduces cardiac risk factors and promotes positive feelings about one's self and body. Reduction in energy as a result of cutting down fat and sugar should be balanced by more bread, potatoes, fruit and other vegetables.
6. *Lack of dietary fibre* has been associated with a variety of bowel disorders and with certain types of cancer, particularly bowel cancers. Fibre intake should be increased to an average of 25–30 g per person per day. This means increasing wholemeal bread, whole grain cereals, fruit, vegetables and pulses.

Health education programmes have had some impact on the awareness of the general public, but a recent national survey commissioned by the Department of Health suggests that dietary habits may not have changed significantly among British adults (Gregory et al, 1990). The survey of the diet of people between the ages of 16 and 64 revealed an increase in the recorded prevalence of obesity and higher than recommended intakes of carbohydrate, protein and fat.

1. The average BMI in men was 24.9 and in women 24.6. The prevalence of obesity, as defined by a BMI of 30 or more, was 12% in women and 8% in men. (This compares with an estimated 8% and 6% in women and men respectively in 1980); (Knight, 1984.)
2. Fat intake: only 12% of men and 15% of women had intakes which met with COMA target of deriving 35% or less of food energy from fat.
3. Sugar continues to provide an average of 45% of carbohydrate intake and should be substituted with more complex carbohydrate sources.
4. Protein contributes an average of 15.2% of energy intake in women and 14.1% in men. These are significantly higher than the recommended daily average of 10% (DHSS, 1979).

Table 18.2 Diagnostic tests used to assess nutritional status.

Test	Normal values	Discussion
Carbohydrate metabolism		
Blood glucose	3.9–6.1 mmol/l (70–110 mg/dl)	Serum osmolality increases as the amount of glucose in the serum increases Serum glucose and serum osmolality may increase with obesity in relation to the decrease in insulin receptors
Serum glucagon	50–100 mg/l	
Serum osmolality	280–300 mmol/kg	
Urine: glucose	Negative	The presence of glucose and ketone bodies in the urine
ketone	Negative	indicates hyperglycaemia and fatty acid metabolism
Fat metabolism		
Total blood lipids	4.0–8.5 g/l	Low levels of lipids in debilitating stages of malnutrition
Cholesterol	3.9–7.2 mmol/l	Elevated levels of lipids may indicate excessive intake of
HDL cholesterol	0.8–2.35 mmol/l	foods high in cholesterol and saturated fats, or diabetes
LDL cholesterol	1.30–4.90 mmol/l	mellitus
Triglycerides	< 1.8 mmol/l	
Phospholipids	1.6–3.9 mmol/l	
Protein metabolism		
Total serum proteins	60–80 g/l	Serum protein levels decrease with undernutrition
Albumin (A)	40–60 g/l	Haemoglobin levels decrease with iron and protein
Globulin (G)	20–30 g/l	deficiencies
A/G ratio	3:1	Plasma amino acid fractionation may be undertaken to
Urine protein	< 0.15 g/dl	diagnose protein deficiencies
Haemoglobin	Male: 13–18 g/dl Female: 12–15 g/dl	
Vitamins		
Serum vitamin levels		Decreased levels of fat-soluble vitamins A, D, E and K results from impaired fat absorption
Prothrombin time (PT)	11–15 seconds (75–100% activity)	Absorption of vitamin K is reflected by the prothrombin time. With a vitamin K deficiency, the prothrombin time is prolonged
Minerals		
Serum mineral levels	See Chapter 7	Decreased levels of minerals occur with specific dietary deficiencies

HDL, high density lipoprotein; LDL, low density lipoprotein.

Table 18.3 Nutritional guidelines for health education in Britain.

Dietary component	Estimated average intake	NACNE 1983 Recommended average intakes		COMA 1984
		Long term	Short term	Individual recommendation
Energy intake	—	Recommended adjustments of types of food eaten and an increase in exercise output so that adult body weight is maintained within the optimal limits of weight for height.		Obesity should be avoided
Total fat intake	38% of total energy (128 g)	30% of total energy (101 g)	34% of total energy (115 g) 10% reduction	35% of total energy

Table 18.3 *continued*

Dietary component	Estimated average intake	NACNE 1983 Recommended average intakes		COMA 1984
		Long term	Short term	Individual recommendation
Saturated (S) fatty acid intake	18% of total energy (59 g)	10% of total energy (33 g)	15% of total energy (50 g)	15%
Polyunsaturated (P) fatty acid intake	—	No specific recommendations; if total fat intake is reduced to 30% then this will automatically tend to increase the P:S ratio		3.5–6.8%
Cholesterol	—	No recommendations		No recommendations
Sucrose intake	38 kg/head per year	20 kg/head per year (approx. 50% reduction)	34 kg/head per year (approx. 10% reduction)	No further increase
Fibre intake	20 g/head per day	30 g/head per day (50% increase)	25 g/head per day (25% increase)	No recommendation
Salt intake	8.1–12 g/head per day	Recommended reduction by 3 g/head per day	Recommended reduction by 1 g/head per day	No further increase Ways to decrease should be considered
Alcohol intake	4.9% of total energy	4% of total energy	5% of total energy	Excessive alcohol to be avoided
Protein intake	11% of total energy	No recommendations		No recommendations

From Janes (1986).

5. Intake of dietary fibre appears to have increased, although only 25% of men and 6% of women consumed the NACNE recommended intake of 30 g per day; 45% of men and 16% of women had an average daily intake of 25 g.

Nurses clearly have a continued role in health education.

HEALTH PROBLEMS RELATED TO POTENTIAL AND ACTUAL ALTERATIONS OF NUTRITION AND METABOLISM

Nutritional and metabolic changes affect all body systems and produce a variety of manifestations which vary according to the specific nutritional problems, extent of the deficit or excess and the duration of the change. Nutritional status is also reflected in the individual's physical appearance, energy level and behaviour. Dietary deficits and excesses in nutritional requirements may be the result of specific disorders and are discussed in the relevant topics of other chapters.

THE PERSON WITH ALTERED NUTRITION ASSOCIATED WITH OBESITY

Obesity is a condition characterized by an excess of adipose tissue. Many different definitions exist but an individual is commonly classed as overweight when 10% over some standard (usually the national mean for individuals of the same sex, age and height), and obese when 20% over the standard.

RELATED FACTORS

Today, most people adhere to a model of obesity which emphasizes its heterogeneous and multidimensional nature. There are environmental, behavioural, genetic, physiological and socioeconomic variables influencing the development and/or maintenance of obesity. Simplistically, obesity is caused by the ingestion of too many calories, and/or the utilization of too little energy. An excess of 3500 kcal (14644 kJ) would accumulate 0.5 kg of fat (Howe, 1981). Figure 18.1 summarizes the process of storage and release of fat in the body. Only a small amount of excess is stored as carbohydrate and there is only a slight increase in the protein mass; the excess is stored as triglycerides in the form of adipose tissue. However, there are many different potential causes of this energy imbalance. Sclafani (1984) has classified 50 different animal models of obesity into neural, endocrinal, pharmacological, nutritional, environmental, seasonal, genetic, viral and idiopathic categories. The many different types of animal obesities indicate that no single type can serve as a general model of human obesity.

CONSEQUENCES

The model of complex and multiple aetiologies for obesity explains the variability in physical and laboratory findings for obese people. Some obese people are actually undernourished in one or more essential food factors. Not all obese individuals overeat and there is no characteristic eating style in the obese. Some obese people have metabolic changes including hyperinsulinaemia, impaired glucose tolerance, hyperlipidaemia, and hyperuricaemia. Where overeating does occur, it may result in a chronic increase in insulin production. This might eventually lead to a reduction in the number of insulin receptors in the target cells, thereby reducing insulin responsiveness and resulting in increased glucose concentration in the blood. Serum levels of free fatty acids are elevated with movement of fats in and out of the fatty tissue. Therefore, some types of obesity increase the risk of the individual developing cardiovascular disease, hypertension and diabetes mellitus. Repeated unsuccessful attempts at weight loss may exacerbate these risk factors. Furthermore, distribution of fat (abdominal versus gluteal-femoral) may be more important in determining risk than overall weight. For this reason, waist: hip ratio is sometimes calculated. Higher risks of heart disease and diabetes mellitus are associated with abdominal fat distribution.

Probably more widespread than the metabolic changes and their associated increase in health risk factors is the psychologically stressful effect of being overweight. Given the social pressures to be thin and the discrimination against those who deviate from the ideal, it 'is remarkable that the obese show no greater psychopathology than the non-obese in the general population (Wadden and Stunkard, 1985). However, those who are sensitive to the pressure to conform to the ideal may suffer from a poor body image and low self-esteem.

LABORATORY INVESTIGATION

Medical assessment should particularly include thyroid function, glucose tolerance, triglyceride, total and low density lipoprotein/high density lipoprotein and cholesterol levels. Diagnosis and treatment of any medical disorders is essential before any actual treatment of obesity.

ASSESSMENT

1. *Health history.* In addition to a general history, the patient should be questioned specifically about the history of weight fluctuations, past attempts at weight control, binge–purge symptoms or periods of restrained eating, depression, drug and alcohol abuse or dependency. Any family history of weight problems, hypertension, diabetes mellitus and heart disease should also be identified. The nurse should probe for dissatisfaction regarding body weight and shape. It is important to discern daily pattern and amount of food intake (proportion of intake in complex versus simple carbohydrates, fat and protein) and exercise pattern.
2. *Physical assessment* should include measurement of height and weight, calculation of BMI, measurement of blood pressure and possible measurement of waist and hips for calculation of ratio (waist (cm) divided by hips (cm)).

IDENTIFICATION OF PATIENT PROBLEMS

The following are examples of health problems which may be found in people with obesity. Not all will be evident in every patient but those relevant will be identified as a result of findings from careful history taking.

1. Actual or potential nutritional intake of more than body requirements. The patient's overall goals are to:
   - Acquire knowledge of the food requirements of the body, the relationship between food intake and energy expenditure, and the effects of excessive body fat and obesity on the body.
   - Reduce body weight and body fat by decreasing calorie intake and increasing energy expenditure.
   - Maintain weight at a desirable level.
   - Acquire knowledge about a normal pattern of intake.
   - Acquire the skills to achieve a normal pattern of intake.
   - Acquire knowledge about the cyclical nature of restricted eating/bingeing.
2. Actual or potential disturbance in self-concept and body image due to deviance from culturally prescribed norm. The overall goals are to:
   - Acquire knowledge of the many factors which could cause or maintain obesity.
   - Acquire knowledge about the 'ideal' body as a sociocultural phenomenon which has changed over time.
   - Gain self-acceptance by valuing functional aspects of the physical self, by reducing the importance that body image plays in determining overall self-esteem, and by valuing non-physical attributes of the self.

GOALS

The goals may be said to have been achieved if the patient is able to:
- State the components of a nutritionally balanced diet.
- Describe the potential effects of excessive weight and body fat on health.
- Describe and implement a plan to increase physical activity.
- Eat a diet containing essential food groups.
- Space intake of food over the day.
- Recognize feelings of hunger (as opposed to appetite) and satiety.
- State positive attributes of the body and self.
- Resist weight preoccupation.
- State the dangers of severe food restriction.

NURSING INTERVENTION

Prevention of overweight and control of obesity are important nursing responsibilities. However, given the many complex and multiple causing and maintaining factors in obesity, the effectiveness of interventions will vary.

If obesity is life threatening, the treatment of choice may be hospitalization for gastric-stapling surgery, calorie restriction and/or appetite-suppressant drug therapy. In this case, the role of the nurse is daily measurement of weight, and the monitoring of emotional reactions, food intake, drug effectiveness, and side-effects. There is little reported about the long-term maintenance of weight lost after gastric stapling. However, the use of anorectic drugs produces only short-term results. Out-patient clinical programmes all produce short-term weight loss, with few people maintaining weight loss at the end of one year. Because of the poor results from weight loss strategies, and the possible negative effects of dieting such as impaired glucose tolerance, increased blood lipid levels, increased risk for eating disorders, and lower self-esteeem, it may be better for some people to stop repeated weight loss programmes, stabilize their eating and increase their activity level (Wooley and Wooley, 1984).

The majority of people with a weight problem will be treated in the community. Community nurses have a vital role in assessing patients and supporting them in their attempts to reduce or stabilize their weight.

Health education should begin with parents during the prenatal period, and focus on the development of healthy eating habits during infancy and childhood. Parents need help in assessing the food requirements of developing infants. Education can be given by the health visitor regarding when and how to introduce solids, and how to comfort a crying infant without always relying on food.

Changing life-long overeating patterns in adults is a difficult process. When a careful patient history reveals that the weight problem is probably due to overeating or lack of activity, the nurse can have an impact through education, support and behaviour modification (see Chapter 2 for details regarding interventions for promoting behaviour change). The knowledge required by the individual relates to:

1. Basic nutritional requirements of the body (energy, nutrients and fibre).
2. The relationship between food intake and energy input.
3. The potential effects of obesity on health.
4. The role of activity and exercise in reducing health risks.

Maintenance of weight control is a life-long process and depends largely on the establishment of healthy eating and activity patterns. Family members and friends can do much to reinforce the habits initiated during a weight management programme. Individual and group counselling sessions are useful in initiating and supporting changes in attitude and behaviour.

Community nurses can also help the individual who suffers from a poor body image and low self-esteem as a result of having a body which is larger than society dictates is the norm. Needs of this individual include:

- Skills to reduce the importance of body weight in determining self-esteem.
- Knowledge about the cultural imperative for thinness in women and how to resist this message.

- Skills in the use of clothes and cosmetics to enhance appearance.

If a person has a family history of weight problems, and/or a history of several weight losses which were not maintained, and/or a current food intake which appears to be of normal quantities (or below normal), it may be that the individual has a strong genetic predisposition to overweight, and will be put at greater risk, healthwise, to continue the 'yo-yo' pattern of weight loss and regain. The knowledge required by this individual relates to:

- The biological controls over weight.
- Difference in health risks associated with obesity depending on distribution of fat (abdominal versus femoral-gluteal).
- Ineffectiveness and dangers of severe food restriction.
- Benefits of mild exercise.
- Strategies to retrain oneself to respond to hunger and satiety.

Because of the social pressures, the individual needs to feel accepted by significant others regardless of weight. The nurse can assist others to be supportive of the individual in adopting a healthy eating and activity pattern which will maintain weight and not necessarily result in weight loss.

Evaluation

Prevention of obesity is of primary importance in preventing the usual accompanying risk factors. People with an established weight problem can be helped, but success becomes less likely as the degree of excess weight increases. Frequent evaluation of progress towards goals needs to be carried out by the patient and nurse, in order to monitor progress continuously and change the plan as necessary.

THE PERSON WITH ALTERED NUTRITION: LESS THAN BODY REQUIREMENTS

Humans normally ingest food intermittently throughout each day, with the period of fasting varying from a few hours to 12–14 hours. A typical daily Western European or North American diet consists of 2000–3000 kcal (8368–12552 kJ) in the form of 40–45% carbohydrate, 40% fat and 15–20% protein. (See Table 18.3 for the NACNE and COMA recommendations on healthy eating.) Daily requirements vary with body size, physical activity and growth. Fat storage in adipose tissue provides the largest fuel reserves, consisting of 15–25% of body weight in an adult male. Protein, consisting of 12–17% of body weight in men, is found primarily in muscle tissue. Carbohydrate reserves consist of glycogen stored in the liver, muscle glycogen and circulating blood glucose. These reserves are adequate to meet the needs of the brain and physiological processes during the usual intervals between meals and during short periods of exercise. If fasting extends beyond 18–24 hours, these reserves are rapidly depleted (Hinchcliffe and Montague, 1988).

Undernutrition occurs when the energy intake is less than the energy expenditure. Body fat is depleted for energy, and protein, mineral and vitamin deficiencies develop. The individual is underweight compared to ideal-weight charts.

Smith describes starvation as a continuum that can be divided into three phases: 'the postabsorptive state (9–15 hours after food intake); short-term starvation (lasting to 7 days); and prolonged starvation (2 weeks or longer) (Smith and Thier, 1985). During the postabsorptive state, three-quarters of the glucose used to supply the energy needs of the brain, muscles and vital organs is provided from the carbohydrate stored in the liver and muscle and from circulating blood glucose. The remainder is formed from the mobilization and breakdown of fat. The blood glucose level is maintained, but the catabolic processes are initiated during the first 24 hours of fasting. Short-term starvation is characterized by the breakdown of fat deposits, since the glycogen stores are already depleted. Plasma insulin levels decrease and glucagon levels rise, stimulating glyconeogenesis and ketogenesis. Blood glucose levels drop and ketones function as fuel for the brain. The ability of the brain to utilize ketone bodies as well as glucose for its energy needs prolongs survival by decreasing the need for body protein to be utilized for glucose production.

Prolonged starvation is characterized by continued fat breakdown and mobilization, gluconeogenesis and proteolysis. The rate of protein breakdown decreases as fasting continues and ketones are utilized for energy; analysis of urine samples show that less urea is eliminated and more ammonia is excreted. The blood glucose level stabilizes at a low level. The liver produces less glucose, but some additional glucose is produced by the kidney. Insulin levels remain low and glucagon levels remain normal.

RELATED FACTORS

Undernutrition may result from inadequate food intake or a pathophysiological condition. The cause of inadequate food intake may be:

- Famine, unavailability of food.
- Poverty, which prevents the individual from obtaining sufficient food.
- Inability to shop for or prepare food, such as may occur in the elderly, disabled or housebound individual.
- The lack of knowledge of essential nutritional needs.
- The influence of the mass media in promoting nutritonally unbalanced 'junk foods'.
- Emotional disturbance (such as eating disorder, extreme fear of fat or desire to be thin).
- Pathophysiological conditions. These include those which: interfere with ingestion, digestion, absorption and/or metabolism of food; increase the body's requirements for energy; or result in loss of body fluids and their constituents.

IDENTIFICATION OF PATIENT PROBLEMS

The problem is a nutritonal intake of less than body requirements.

The overall goal for the individual is to achieve a state of optimal nutrition.

GOALS

The individual will be able to:

- Demonstrate understanding of basic nutritional needs of the body.
- Gain weight progressively towards the normal range.
- Express awareness of underlying emotional disturbances.
- Comply with the prescribed dietary regimen and, if indicated, with a counselling or psychotherapy programme.

NURSING INTERVENTION

Malnutrition from inadequate food intake due to socioeconomic factors is a world-wide problem, existing in industrialized countries as well as in developing nations. Alleviation of this problem requires increasing the world's food supply and its distribution, as well as providing economic assistance to those in need. Individuals and families require knowledge of basic nutritional needs as well as assistance in the selection and preparation of foods to ensure an adequate diet within the limits imposed by their sociocultural and economic situations.

For the individual who is underweight because of inadequate intake of food although it is available, nursing interventions include:

1. Providing information about basic nutritional needs of the body. This may be by discussion and the provision of pamphlets which outline a dietary plan containing the essential food groups (see Table 18.3).
2. Identifying the causes of inadequate nutrition.
3. Assisting the individual to develop a diet regimen that will promote the development of body tissue.

Being thin may be currently fashionable and peer pressure tends to reinforce the idea. Simply increasing calorie intake may serve only to increase body fat; the diet should be balanced and contain extra protein as well as carbohydrates and fats. Meals should be regular and between-meal snacks of protein and complex carbohydrates encouraged. Moderate activity serves to build body tissue, but adequate and regular rest is essential to conserve energy and promote weight gain.

When emotional disturbances are the primary factor of malnutrition as, for example, in the patient with anorexia nervosa or bulimia nervosa, intervention is focused on identifying the underlying emotional cause. This is a long-term process that requires counselling and psychotherapy for the patient and usually the family as well. The person needs help to acquire a realistic appraisal of self and body which may be distorted. Harmful and bizarre behaviours need to be identified and attitudes changed. The patient may have to be admitted to hospital initially. Environmental change may also be helpful to initiate changes in eating patterns and attitudes toward food. Maintenance of changes in eating patterns and self-image takes time and continuous therapy.

Undernutrition in the hospital patient is now being recognized as a major problem. Hinson (1985) states that there is convincing evidence that many patients in hospital are malnourished, yet the condition frequently goes unrecognized and untreated. Malnutrition is believed to contribute to the frequency of complications experienced by patients and to increase their stay in hospital. The illnesses leading to admission serve to reduce further the nutritional status of patients. A nutritional assessment should be made on admission and at regular intervals throughout the hospital stay. Measures are required to improve the nutritional status of many patients, especially in intensive care and during the post-surgery period.

Undernutrition in certain groups in the community may also be prevalent. The elderly may be at particular risk of nutritional deficiencies. This may be related to physiological changes, such as diminished appetite, taste sensation and salivary secretion; dental problems, impaired digestion and absorption, and physical or mental disability. In addition to these factors, social isolation and poverty and a lack of knowledge regarding essential nutrients may make the elderly particularly vulnerable (Holmes, 1989a). Calorific requirements in the elderly may fall with advancing age as the basal metabolic rate decreases and energy expenditure lessens due to reduced physical activity. This may lead to overweight if the intake of calories is not reduced. However, their general nutritional requirements differ little from the general population, although surveys suggest that the intake of certain nutrients is considerably lower than is desirable. This is particularly true of vitamins C, B and D, potassium, certain trace elements and dietary fibre (DHSS, 1979). Since nutritional deficiency may be both the cause and effect of illness, it is important that those at risk are identified and nutritional support and education provided.

Evaluation

Achieving a state of optimal nutrition is often a slow and variable process. The undernourished individual needs to be frequently reassessed and compared with the stated outcome criteria so that progress can be monitored and the plan of care altered as necessary. Often knowledge and understanding are relatively easy for the patient to accomplish; however, weight gain, awareness of underlying emotional disturbance and compliance with prescribed diet are much more difficult to achieve.

THE PERSON WITH ALTERED NUTRITION: LESS THAN BODY REQUIREMENTS DUE TO WITHHOLDING/WITHDRAWAL OF NUTRITIONAL SUPPORT

ETHICAL ISSUES

The withdrawal or withholding of nutritional support from a patient is one of the more controversial ethical dilemmas faced by patients, families, surrogates and health professionals. Is it ever ethically justifiable to withdraw food and fluids? Conversely, are there circumstances in which it would not be justifiable to institute nutritional support? The provision of food and water holds moral and emotional significance. The symbolic value of providing nourishment may be greater than any resulting therapeutic benefit. In certain clinical circumstances it may be necessary to determine if the provision of nutrition and fluids is for the purpose of sustaining life, a therapeutic measure, or a part of basic nursing care. What is the desirable goal for the individual? What are the social and legal implications of withholding nutrition and hydration? What are the implications for the nurse as a participant in the ethical decision-making process and in the implementation of the outcomes?

Clinical/therapeutic factors

Many persons in hospitals, nursing homes and the community are unable or unwilling to take food orally. Advanced technology provides the means to nourish and hydrate patients who would otherwise die. Is the provision of nutritional support through nasogastric and gastrostomy tubes or peripheral and central venous lines medical therapy or routine care? If, as many believe, nutrition provided through mechanical means is a therapeutic measure, what are the implications for the administration or withholding of the therapy? Campbell-Taylor and Fisher (1987), in their assessment of tube feedings for the terminally-ill elderly, identified risk factors and hazards associated with the procedure. They recommend against tube feedings for this patient group, stating that the probability of the patient developing aspiration pneumonia is as great or greater than with careful spoon feeding. Patients experience some degree of discomfort from the continuous use of invasive tubes and lines. Diarrhoea is also a common side-effect of tube feedings. For many terminally ill patients, the provision of nutritional support will not change the overall outcome of their illness. Clinical evidence indicates that the thirst and dry mouth experienced as a result of dehydration in dying patients can be effectively relieved by moistening the lips and mouth with ice chips or lubricant without rehydrating the patient (Billings, 1985). In the last days before death, patients may spontaneously reduce their intake of food and water without experiencing hunger or thirst. The provision of nutritional support results in benefits and burdens which must be assessed and balanced.

Human factors

Recognition must be given to the significance of nutritional support to the patient and family. Actual and perceived psychological benefits are, in many circumstances, equally as important as the physiological effects. Every effort should be made to determine and fulfil the patient's wishes. The intent of a patient's behaviour when refusing food by turning the head away, or not opening the mouth, or by pulling out tubes and lines, is often difficult to assess, especially if the patient is cognitively impaired. Living wills or statements made by patients expressing wishes to forgo life support systems which will prolong life rarely specify the person's wishes in relation to nutritional support.

Implications for the nurse

The provision of nourishment to patients may be viewed as symbolic of the caring and nurturing nature of nursing. The withholding or termination of nutritional support to patients may provoke strong feelings in the nurse and may be morally offensive. In certain clinical situations, nurses may feel that by providing food and fluids by technical means, they are prolonging a person's dying rather than supporting life. In other situations, they may feel that the lack of adequate nourishment is contributing to the patient's death.

Ethical decisions about a patient's care should be made by the health care team in collaboration with the patient or family. Decisions relating to the provision of food and fluids fall within the scope of nursing. The nurse not only has a vested interest in the decision-making process, she also has a responsible role to play in implementing the decisions and in evaluating the consequences. The nurse, therefore, must be an active participant in the decision of the health care team.

Nurses have obligations to themselves, their professional colleagues and their patients to be informed about the beneficial and detrimental effects of procedures they implement, even apparently basic activities such as the provision of food and water. They should work together to become informed, active participants in the identification and analysis of clinical ethical dilemmas and to ensure that the employing agency develops policies and guidelines to facilitate and monitor decisions.

IDENTIFICATION OF THE PATIENT PROBLEM

The health problem faced by the individual is an intake of food and water less than body requirements due to an inability to ingest adequate nourishment.

The objective for the individual might be that if the patient is sufficiently aware, he or she would appreciate that his or her wishes be honoured in the resolution of ethical dilemmas related to the provision of nutritional support.

GOAL

There will be written, verbal and/or behavioural evidence that the provision of or the withholding/withdrawal of nutritional and hydrational support benefited the person in relation to the defined goals of care.

ASSESSMENT

Whenever a nurse suspects that an individual's state of nutrition and hydration are not adequate to meet physiological and psychological needs, a nutritional assessment should be performed. Reassessment should occur regularly, as factors which affect nutritional intake,

such as swallowing and level of consciousness, change.

Every effort should be made to identify the person's perspective and wishes related to the provision of nutritional support. Behavioural indicators of refusal of food and water should be identified and interpreted in relation to the total patient situation.

Information should be documented by the multidisciplinary team regarding the person's medical diagnosis and prognosis, and whether any associated dysphagia, confusion or vegetative state are temporary in nature or expected to be permanent.

INTERVENTION

Ethical decision-making process

Under certain circumstances, it may be ethically justifiable to withhold or withdraw nutritional support (Knox, 1989). The possibility of abuse demands that such decisions be made with caution and on an individual basis, as situations occur.

When it is identified that an individual's nutritional state is inadequate or deteriorating, the nurse should discuss this with the dietician and doctor. If an ethical conflict arises regarding the provision of nutritional support, all responsible individuals should participate in determining its resolution.

Patients and their families may be unaware of the options available for the provision of nutritional support. The nurse, as a health professional in frequent contact with the patient and family and one who may have established a receptive and therapeutic relationship with them, should initiate discussion and facilitate inquiries. Opportunities for discussion should be ongoing as the patient's status changes. Patient and family meetings, with all relevant health care providers present, facilitate dialogue and promote participative decision-making. All health professionals caring for the patient should be informed of decisions to forgo nutrition and hydrational support and be aware of the process used to arrive at the decision.

Implementation of the decision

Time-limited trials are recommended to permit evaluation of the outcomes and to allow all responsible participants to come to terms with the decision. During this period, the nurse assumes a role in evaluating the patient's response and in identifying changes in the patient's situation that impact on the outcome and may warrant further discussion. When an ethically appropriate decision has been made to forgo nutritional support, symptomatic and supportive care continues. Moistening the lips and mouth and frequent cleansing of the mouth are necessary to prevent and alleviate any feelings of thirst or discomfort. Oral fluids and food are given as requested or tolerated. The decision-making process and the decision reached must be documented. Consent from the patient or family should be obtained before any action is taken.

Evaluation

In a situation where an individual is unable to take food orally, resolution of the resulting ethical dilemma should follow an appropriate decision-making process. Documentation should demonstrate that consideration was given to the perspective of the individual, relevant therapeutic factors and the expected benefit for the individual.

EATING DISORDERS: ANOREXIA NERVOSA AND BULIMIA NERVOSA

ANOREXIA NERVOSA

Anorexia Nervosa (AN) is characterized by dissatisfaction with body weight and shape and a relentless pursuit of a thinner body size. There is severe weight loss achieved by strict dieting, excessive exercise, laxative abuse or vomiting. Patients become emaciated, with a weight of only 85% of expected body weight, and menstruation ceases.

Bulimia nervosa is characterized by similar concerns about body weight and shape, and the pursuit of a thinner body shape or fear of fatness. Individuals experience episodes when they consume large quantities of food in short periods of time, accompanied by a sense of loss of control. Foods chosen for these binges usually involve those the individual forbids themselves to eat while dieting. Binge episodes are usually followed by vigorous exercise, strict dieting or purging (by vomiting, use of diuretics or laxatives). Individuals with bulimia nervosa may be thin, of normal weight or obese.

The most common age for anorexia nervosa and bulimia nervosa to develop is between 13 and 18, but it is not unusual for it to arise in the late 20s. The conditions are far more common in females, with about one anorectic male for every 20 female cases, and about one bulimic male for every 10 female cases.

CAUSES

The development and maintenance of eating disorders are related to a variety of risk factors. Cultural factors (such as the ideal of thinness, perceived pressure to this ideal from family and peers, or involvement in a sport or occupation which requires a thin body such as modelling or dance; Orbach, 1986), family and individual factors are all implicated. Individual factors include:

- Weight preoccupation, history of weight loss attempts and fear of fat
- Poor hunger awareness and control
- Poor self-esteem, sense of ineffectiveness
- Autonomy, identity and separation concerns
- Body image disturbances
- Chronic medical illness (insulin-dependent diabetes)
- Obesity.

Family risk factors include:

- Inherited biological predisposition (family history of eating disorders, alcholism, affective disorders)
- Lack of conflict resolution
- Overprotectiveness
- Rigidity
- Enmeshment.

Usually one of these factors is insufficient to cause an eating disorder, but they may work in combination to start or maintain the problem. In addition, the syndrome is often maintained by symptoms of semistarvation.

LABORATORY INVESTIGATION

Medical assessment includes electrocardiography (ECG), full blood count, urea nitrogen, electrolytes, urinalysis and serum creatinine.

ASSESSMENT

The nurse should use the guidelines of the assessment provided in this chapter related to obesity because the same assessment applies with patients with eating disorders. the physical assessment should particularly include weight, height, and assessment for presence of dehydration, swollen salivary glands, muscle weakness, emaciation, bradycardia and hypotension.

The patient's overall goal is to resolve the eating disorder and its underlying maintaining factors.

GOALS

The patient will be able to:

- Demonstrate understanding of food requirements of the body.
- Maintain BMI between 20 and 27.
- Space food intake at two meals a day and one or two snacks.
- Seek and comply with counselling or psychotherapy programme.
- State positive attributes of the body and self.

TREATMENT OF EATING DISORDERS

In-patient care is indicated where weight loss is extreme, potassium levels are low, there are ECG or cardiac enzyme changes, severe dehydration, acute abdominal symptoms, presence of convulsions, or suicidal behaviour. Bulimia nervosa patients may be admitted to stabilize chaotic eating behaviour. In-patient, out-patient, or day hospital therapy (group, individual and family) may be given, usually by a multidisciplinary team. Cognitive-behavioural and psychodynamic approaches have been effectively used. Nursing care includes emotional support around meal times and monitoring of weight changes and the effectiveness and side-effects of drug treatment. In out-patient treatment, nurses are involved in patient education. Individuals with eating disorders require knowledge about:

- Skills to resist social pressures
- Assertiveness
- Meal planning

- Relaxation skills
- Quantity, quality and pattern of intake which might be described as normal eating
- Physical and emotional effects of starvation
- Ineffectiveness of the binge–purge cycle for maintaining low weight
- Physical consequences of eating disorder
- Dangers of dieting.

Evaluation

Anorexia nervosa is considered a chronic disease, with estimates as high as 50% non-recovered 5 years after diagnosis. Less evidence is available regarding bulimia nervosa but the disease is considered similar in its chronicity. Early identification and treatment improves prognosis, but sufferers are reluctant to seek and accept treatment in the early stages. The nurse may be instrumental in early identification, particularly if working in schools. There is also a valuable role for nurses to establish and lead community support groups for sufferers and/or their families.

DISORDERS OF CARBOHYDRATE METABOLISM

Diabetes mellitus is a common disorder of carbohydrate metabolism that affects a large number of persons and is characterized by hyperglycaemia. The reader is referred to Chapter 19 for a detailed discussion of the disorder and the care of patients with diabetes mellitus.

Hypoglycaemia may result from inadequate food intake. It may also occur in response to endocrine disorders of the pancreas, disorders of ingestion or liver dysfunction.

DISORDERS OF FAT METABOLISM

Diabetes mellitus, obesity and underweight are examples of disorders involving fat metabolism. Atherosclerosis is a chronic degenerative disease of the blood vessels characterized by the development of fatty plaques in the intima of the vessel walls. Diabetes mellitus, obesity, diet, smoking and genetic factors may predispose the individual to the development of the disease.

DISORDERS OF PROTEIN METABOLISM

Protein deficiency results primarily from inadequate intake of the essential amino acids which cannot be synthesized in the body. Anaemia, underweight, fatigue and retarded growth are signs of protein deficiency. Kwashiorkor results from a diet deficient in the quality and quantity of protein in infancy and childhood despite an adequate total energy intake. Protein–calorie mal-

nutrition (PCM) occurs when the diet lacks both protein and calories. Protein deficiencies may occur with disorders of the digestive system and with serious illnesses when excessive protein is lost, for example, burns, draining wounds, pressure sores and some renal diseases in which there is a loss of protein in the urine. Immobility is a further cause of protein loss and occurs in debilitated patients on bed rest.

SUMMARY

Current scientific knowledge is able to tell us far more about levels of nutrient intake needed to prevent deficiency diseases than levels needed for optimum health. There is much ongoing research activity around the world to discover the qualities, amounts and patterns of nutrient intake which will provide the individual with a feeling of energy and well-being, as well as reducing health risk factors. The current recommendations consist of maintaining a protein intake of about 15% of total, lowering fat intake to about 35% of total, reducing simple carbohydrates and increasing complex carbohydrates to 60% of total intake. They also suggest increasing fibre, and reducing salt and alcohol consumption.

It is an important skill to be able to assess a person's nutritional status, as nutrition is such a key component of growth, general health and well-being, and a potential cause or complicating factor in illness. Observation of the individual and the ability to take a complete diet history are essential to problem identification.

In addition to issues of assessment and problem identification, this chapter includes the physiology and pathophysiology related to the metabolism of protein, carbohydrates and fats. Also, the role of the nurse in health education, and supportive interventions are explored.

Obesity and eating disorders are reviewed in more depth as they are more common in industrialized countries than deficiency diseases. However, the nurse must keep malnutrition in mind as a potential problem. Issues and principles guiding ethical decision making related to the use of nutrition and hydration to sustain life are presented.

REFERENCES AND FURTHER READING

Billings JA (1985) Comfort measures for the terminally ill: is dehydration painful? *Journal of the American Geriatric Society* **33(11):** 808–810.

Campbell-Taylor I & Fisher RH (1987) The clinical case against tube feeding in palliative care of the elderly. *Journal of the American Geriatric Society* **35(12):** 1100–1104.

Coates VE (1985) *Are They Being Served?* London: RCN.

Davidson S, Passmore R, Brock JF & Trusswell AS (1986) *Human Nutrition and Dietetics.* Edinburgh: Churchill Livingstone.

Department of Health and Social Security (DHSS) (1979) *Recommended Daily Amounts of Food Energy and Nutrients for Groups of People in the United Kingdom.* London: HMSO.

LEARNING ACTIVITIES

1. Keep a diary of your own food intake for 3 days. Include what you ate, quantity, and the time. Did the exercise of keeping a diary alter your usual pattern of intake? Analyse how your own intake compares with the current recommendations for inclusion of food groups, lowering of fats, simple carbohydrates, salt and alcohol. Are there any areas you need to change? If so, use the strategies in Chapter 2 to make a behaviour modification plan.

2. Mrs Smith, a 77-year-old woman has a leg ulcer which has been healing slowly for the past month. Her general practitioner has asked you to visit her to dress her ulcer. You are concerned that she appears to be rather thin; she weighs 43 kg and is about 1.65 m tall. Her skin is very thin and fragile. Describe the factors you would wish to consider and the problems you would look for when assessing her nutritional status.

3. Identify situations in which you might consider withholding nutritional and/or hydrational support to be ethically justifiable. In what circumstances would you consider it to be unacceptable?

Department of Health and Social Security (DHSS) (1979) *A Nutrition Survey of the Elderly*. Report on Health and Social Subjects No. 3. London: HMSO.

Department of Health and Social Security (DHSS) (1984) *Committee on Medical Aspects of Food Policy 'Diet and Cardiovascular Disease'*. Report on Health and Social Subjects No. 28 ('The COMA Report'). London: HMSO.

Dickerson JWT & Booth EM (1985) *Clinical Nutrition for Nurses, Dietitians and Other Health Care Professionals*. London: Faber & Faber.

Exton-Smith AN (1988) Nutrition in the elderly. In Dickerson JWT & Lee HA (eds) *Nutrition in the Clinical Management of Disease*. London: Edward Arnold.

Goodinson SM (1986) Assessment of nutritional status. *Nursing* **3(7):** 252–258.

Gregory J, Foster K, Tyler H et al (1990) *The Dietary and Nutritional Survey of British Adults*. OPCS Social Survey Division. London: HMSO.

Hinchliffe S & Montague S (1988) *Physiology for Nursing Practice*, p. 170. London: Baillière Tindall.

Hinson LR (1985) Nutritional assessment and management of the hospitalized patient. *Critical Care Nurse* **5(2):** 53–60.

Holmes S (1987) Nutrition in the critically ill. *Nursing* **3(15):** 561–566.

Holmes S (1989a) Nutrition and the elderly. *Nursing* **3(37):** 18–21.

Holmes S (1989b) Diet and heart disease. *Nursing* **3(36):** 9–11.

Howe PS (1981) *Basic Nutrition in Health and Disease* 7th edn. Philadelphia: Saunders.

Huskisson J (1985) *Applied Nutrition and Dietetics*. Eastbourne: Baillière Tindall.

Janes EMH (1986) Changing our eating habits. *Nursing* **3(7):** 269.

Jones DC (1975) *Food for Thought*. London: RCN.

Knight I (1984) *The Heights and Weights of Adults in Great Britain*. London: HMSO.

Knox LS (1989) Ethical issues in nutritional support nursing. *Nursing Clinics of North America* **24(2):** 427–436.

Lask S (1986) The nurses' role in nutritional education. *Nursing* **3(8):** 296–300.

Macleod S (1981) *The Art of Starvation*. London: Virago.

Moghissi K & Boore J (1983) *Parenteral and Enteral Nutrition for Nurses*. London: Heinemann.

National Advisory Committee on Nutrition Education (NACNE) (1983) *Guidelines for Health Education in Britain*. London: Health Education Council.

Orbach S (1986) *Hunger Strike: The Anorectic's struggle as a Metaphor for our Age*. London: Faber & Faber.

Orr J (1985) Obesity. *Journal of Advanced Nursing* **10(1):** 71–78.

Potts NL (1984) Eating disorders: the secret pattern of binge/purge. *American Journal of Nursing* **84(1):** 32–35.

Royal College of Physicians (1983) *Report on Obesity*. London: HMSO.

Sanger E & Cassino T (1984) Eating disorders: avoiding the power struggle. *American Journal of Nursing* **84(1):** 31–33.

Sclafani A (1984) Animal models of obesity: classification and characterization. *International Journal of Obesity* **8:** 491–508.

Smith LH & Thier SO (1985) *Pathophysiology* 2nd edn, sect. 6 & 7. Philadelphia: Saunders.

Wadden TA & Stunkard AJ (1985) Social and physiological consequences of obesity. *Annals of Internal Medicine* **103:** 1062–1067.

Winkler ER (1987) The morality of withholding food and fluids. *Journal of Palliative Care* **3(2):** 26–30.

Wooley SC & Wooley OW (1984) Should obesity be treated at all? In Stunkard & Stellar (eds) *Eating and Its Disorders*. New York: Raven Press.

Caring for the Patient with a Disorder of the Endocrine System

19

OBJECTIVES

On completion of this chapter the reader will be able to:

- Describe the endocrine functions of different tissues and organs
- Discuss how hormones function to regulate growth, maturation, metabolism and reproduction
- Identify and describe health problems experienced by persons with hypersecretion and hyposecretion of hormones of the pituitary, thyroid and adrenal glands and the endocrine pancreas
- Describe nursing assessment, planning, intervention and evaluation of patients with acute episodic complications of hormone imbalance
- Recognize the lifelong implications for hormone replacement therapy
- Describe nursing responsibilities and guidelines for patient/family teaching for hormone replacement therapies
- Describe nursing responsibilities related to teaching patients and families self-management of the endocrine imbalance
- Acknowledge the rights and responsibilities of the patient and family for self-management of the endocrine disorder

THE ENDOCRINE SYSTEM

A gland is an organ which extracts substances from the blood and produces one or more new chemical substances, referred to as secretions. Glands may be classified as exocrine or endocrine. The secretion of an *exocrine gland* is carried along a duct into a body cavity or to the external surface of the body. Examples of such glands are the salivary, gastric, mammary and sweat glands. *Endocrine glands* do not have ducts; their secretions, which are called *hormones*, pass directly into the blood and act on remote tissues.

The glands usually cited as composing the *endocrine system* are the anterior and posterior pituitary glands, thyroid gland, four parathyroid glands, two adrenal (suprarenal) glands, islets of Langerhans and two gonads (ovaries or testes) (Figure 19.1). Unlike other body systems in which the component organs are located close together and are connected, the glands are situated in various parts of the body. There are other organs which are known to demonstrate endocrine action through their liberation of chemical agents into the blood. They are not considered to be part of the endocrine system since they are a more integral part of other major systems. These include the gastrointestinal glands, which secrete gastrin, secretin and cholecysto-kinin-pancreozymin (see Chapter 16), and the kidneys, which secrete renin and the renal erythropoietic factor into the blood (see Chapter 20). The placenta, formed in pregnancy, also serves as an endocrine gland because of its production of progesterone, oestrogen and chorionic gonadotrophin.

Co-ordination and integration of the development and functions of the body that maintain homeostasis are dependent upon the nervous system and the endocrine system. The endocrine system is concerned mainly with growth, maturation, metabolic processes and

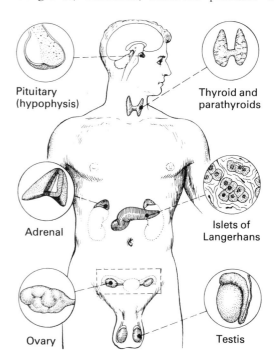

Figure 19.1 Endocrine glands in the body.

reproduction. The action of each hormone is specific. One hormone may modify the activity of all body cells (e.g. thyroxine); other affect the activity of only one particular organ (e.g. adrenocorticotrophin). The site of action of any hormone is referred to as the *target organ or tissue*.

Target cells contain *receptors* for which specific hormones have an affinity. Some hormones are necessary for survival (e.g. adrenocorticoid); others are not essential to life (e.g. gonadal secretions).

TYPES OF HORMONES

There are three chemical classes of hormones:

1. *Amine hormones* are derived from the amino acid tyrosine and include the hormones produced by the adrenal medulla and the thyroid gland.
2. *Peptide and protein hormones* comprise the majority of hormones and include most of the hormones secreted by the hypothalamus, the pituitary, parathyroid, pancreas and gastrointestinal system.
3. *Steroid hormones* are produced by the adrenal cortex and the gonads (testes and ovaries) as well as the placenta during pregnancy. These hormones affect carbohydrate metabolism, fluid balance and reproductive functions.

MECHANISM OF HORMONE ACTION

Hormones are transported in the blood either freely in solution or in combination with a carrier protein. The water-soluble hormones, including the polypeptide and protein hormones, bind with the receptors on the surface of the target cells. the steroids and thyroid hormones require a carrier for transportation to the target cells and bind with intracellular receptors.

Hormones (the first messengers) which bind with surface receptors on the target cells act by altering a membrane-bound enzyme which stimulates the production of a 'second' messenger in the cell; the second messenger then activates enzymes within the cell to produce the specific cellular functions. The second messenger is believed in most instances to be cyclic adenosine monophosphate (cAMP).

Steroid hormones cross the membrane of cells containing their specific receptors and bind with the intracellular receptors. The receptor is altered by the hormone, allowing it to enter the cell nucleus and combine with the chromatin of certain genes. The messenger RNA is formed which migrates to the cell cytoplasm where it influences the synthesis of specific peptides and proteins. These peptides and proteins carry out the metabolic functions of the cells that were in the past attributed to the steroid hormones.

The precise mechanisms for other hormone actions, such as the alteration of cell permeability to specific substances by insulin, the catecholamines and acetylcholine, are not known.

REGULATION OF SECRETION

The production of endocrine secretions is generally controlled according to the need for their action; that is, production and release into the bloodstream are stimulated when their action is needed and are inhibited when the effect is achieved. Secretions by the pituitary gland are regulated by either hormonal or nervous signals originating in the hypothalamus. The control mechanism may be influenced by the blood concentration of the target organ, or by physicochemical processes. For example, regulation of secretion by the thyroid, adrenal cortices and the gonads is maintained by hormones which are produced by the anterior pituitary gland and are liberated in response to the blood concentration of the hormones of those glands. To illustrate, the anterior pituitary gland secretes a thyroid-stimulating hormone (TSH or thyrotropin), and the output of TSH is controlled by the level of thyroid hormones in the blood. This reciprocal arrangement is referred to as a *negative feedback mechanism*, in that the higher the level of thyroxine, the lower the level of TSH and vice versa. A hormone which stimulates the secretion of another hormone is referred to as a *trophic hormone*. An example of control by a *physicochemical process* is the influence of the osmotic pressure of the blood on the output of the antidiuretic hormone (see p. 566).

DYSFUNCTION

Disorders of an endocrine gland may incur an excess or deficiency of its hormone(s). Signs and symptoms of the disorder are predominantly manifestations of dysfunction in the target organ or tissues. Enlargement or outgrowths of a gland may also impose on neighbouring structures, interfering with their function(s).

Pituitary Gland (Hypophysis)

The pituitary gland is a very small gland located at the base of the brain in the sella turcica, a depression in the sphenoid bone. It lies just below the anterior part of the third ventricle and adjacent to the optic chiasm. It is attached to the hypothalamus by a stalk, the *infundibulum*, which contains nerve fibres and blood vessels. The gland has two distinct parts: the anterior lobe, or anterior pituitary, and the posterior or neural lobe (posterior pituitary). The anterior pituitary is an embryological outgrowth of the roof of the mouth and is completely separated from its origin. The posterior pituitary develops from the base of the brain, remaining connected to the hypothalamus by many nerve fibres (Figure 19.2).

The cells of the anterior pituitary are truly glandular in that they extract substances from the blood and secrete new chemicals (hormones). The posterior pituitary consists mainly of many terminal nerve fibres which originate with nerve cells (neurones) in the hypothalamus. The fibres are supported by non-secreting cells called *pituicytes*. The hormones released by the posterior pituitary are secreted by the neurones of the hypothalamus and are released at the nerve endings in the posterior pituitary.

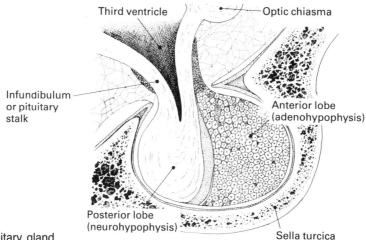

Third ventricle

Optic chiasma

Infundibulum or pituitary stalk

Anterior lobe (adenohypophysis)

Posterior lobe (neurohypophysis)

Sella turcica

Figure 19.2 The pituitary gland.

ANTERIOR PITUITARY LOBE (ADENOHYPOPHYSIS)

The anterior pituitary secretes the following hormones:
- Thyroid-stimulating hormone (TSH).
- Growth hormone (GH).
- Prolactin (PRL), which affects lactation.
- Adrenocorticotrophic hormone (ACTH), which stimulates the adrenal cortex and related peptides: β-lipotrophin (β-LPH), α-melanocyte stimulating hormone (MSH), which increases pigmentation of the skin and mucous membranes, and β-endorphin (a substance with morphine-like actions).
- Follicle-stimulating hormone (FSH), which stimulates the development of mature Graafian follicles in women and stimulates spermatogenesis in men.
- Luteinizing hormone (LH) which stimulates the development and maintenance of the corpus luteum in women; in men, where it is called interstitial cell-stimulating hormone (ICSH), it affects secretion of testosterone.

The cells of the pituitary are classified as:
1. Somatotrophs (secrete GH)
2. Corticotrophs (secrete ACTH, β-LPH)
3. Thyrotrophs (secrete TSH)
4. Lactotrophs (secrete PRL)
5. Gonadotrophs (secrete LH and FSH).

The hormones TSH, ACTH, FSH and LH stimulate other glands; GH, PRL and MSH act directly on tissues of the body.

A branch of the internal carotid artery supplies the anterior pituitary, but the blood is circulated through the lower hypothalamic tissue before entering the gland. It is carried from the hypothalamus in hypothalamic-hypophyseal portal vessels in the infundibulum (pituitary stalk) to the sinusoids of the anterior pituitary. Control of the various secretions is mediated by the hypothalamic releasing factors which are liberated by special hypothalamic neurones into the hypothalamic-hypophyseal portal system. On reaching the sinusoids, these substances influence the secretory activity of the respective glandular cells.

REGULATION OF ANTERIOR PITUITARY GLAND SECRETIONS BY HYPOTHALMIC HORMONES

Hypothalamic hormones control, by stimulation or inhibition, the release of hormones from the pituitary gland.

The hypothalamic hormones comprise:
- Growth hormone releasing hormone (or factor) (GHRF)
- Growth hormone release inhibiting hormone (somatostatin; GHRIH)
- Thyrotrophin-releasing hormone (or factor) (TRH)
- Corticotrophin-releasing hormone (CRF)
- Gonadotrophin-releasing hormone (GnRH)
- Prolactin release inhibiting hormone (PIH).

FUNCTIONS OF THE ANTERIOR PITUITARY HORMONES

Figure 19.3 depicts the metabolic functions of anterior pituitary hormones. The *growth hormone* is concerned with the growth of the body and plays an important role in determining a person's size. The most striking effect of the hormone is evidenced in the skeleton. Bones increase in length and thickness until late adolescence, the muscles enlarge and there is a corresponding growth of the viscera. Many metabolic processes are influenced by GH, and a positive nitrogen balance develops because of the increased use of proteins in tissue synthesis (i.e. fatty acids are mobilized from adipose tissue and used for energy). Growth is also dependent upon the secretion of normal amounts of other hormones. The thyroid hormones are necessary to maintain an adequate metabolic rate, and insulin must be available to promote glucose metabolism for the provision of energy. The growth hormone is diabetogenic; it increases the breakdown of glycogen in the liver, promotes the release of glucose into the blood and also produces an anti-insulin effect in muscles. This promotes the synthesis and conservation of protein, conservation of glucose and utilization of fat.

The secretion of GH is controlled by the hypothalamus which produces two regulating hormones; one

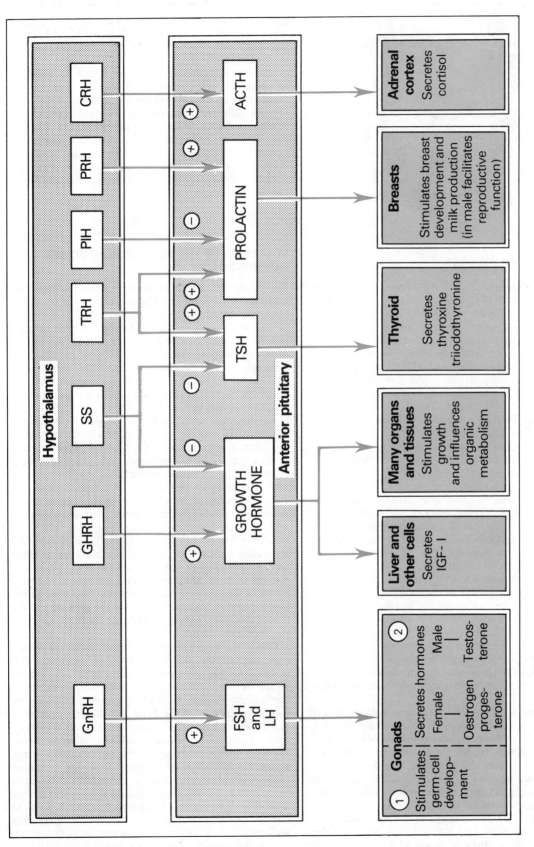

Figure 19.3 Summary of the hypothalamic–anterior pituitary system. GnRH, gonadotrohpin-releasing hormone; GHRH, growth hormone-releasing hormone; SS, somatostatin; TRH, thyrotrophin-releasing hormone; PIH, prolactin release-inhibiting hormone; PRH, prolactin-releasing hormone; CRH, corticotrophin-releasing hormone; FSH, follicle-stimulating hormone; LH, luteinizing hormone; TSH, thyroid-stimulating hormone; ACTH, adrenocorticotrophic hormone; IGF-1, insulin-like growth factor 1. Modified from Vander et al (1990).

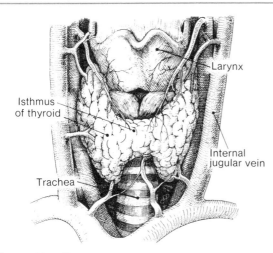

Larynx

Isthmus of thyroid

Internal jugular vein

Trachea

Figure 19.4 The thyroid gland.

stimulates the release of GH and the other, somatostatin, inhibits the release of GH by the anterior pituitary. The secretion of GH is influenced by the state of nutrition; hypoglycaemia, fasting, exercise, stress and trauma increase its production. Hyperglycaemia and high concentrations of cortisol decrease the secretion.

Thyroid-stimulating hormone (TSH) promotes the growth and secretory activity of the thyroid gland, the function of which is the production of hormones which regulate the metabolic rate of all tissues. The production of TSH is regulated by a negative feedback mechanism. A decrease in the blood concentration of thyroid hormones increases the secretory output of thyrotropin; conversely, when the thyroid hormones reach a normal or above normal level, there is a reciprocal decrease in the release of thyrotropin.

Adrenocorticotrophic hormone (ACTH) has as its target organ the adrenal cortices, influencing their secretory output of several cortical secretions. ACTH secretion is regulated by an ACTH releasing factor produced in the hypothalamus in response to a decreased blood level of cortisone, or to nerve impulses initiated by biological stress (e.g. trauma, pain).

The *follicle-stimulating hormone (FSH)* causes the development of the ovarian follicle and the secretion of oestrogen. The secretion of FSH is reciprocally related to the blood level of oestrogen; FSH production is increased as the oestrogen level declines (see Chapter 22 for details of its role in the female menstrual cycle). In the male, FSH promotes the production of spermatozoa in conjunction with the male hormone testosterone.

Luteinizing hormone (LH) promotes ovulation and is necessary for the formation of the corpus luteum in the ruptured follicle. When the corpus luteum develops and secretes progesterone, the production of LH is suppressed. In the male, this hormone may be called the interstitial cell-stimulating hormone (ICSH) because it stimulates the production of the male hormone testosterone by the interstitial cells of the testes.

Prolactin (PRL) stimulates the corpus luteum to secrete progesterone and initiates and stimulates the secretion of the mammary glands which have under-

gone preparatory changes in response to the oestrogen and progesterone blood levels. It is similar to luteinizing hormone. Its action in the male, if any, is undetermined.

An anterior pituitary hormone which is normally secreted in very small amounts in man is the *melanocyte-stimulating hormone (MSH)*, which increases skin pigmentation. Its chemical structure is similar to that of ACTH, and pigmentation of the skin may occur in the human with a high blood concentration of ACTH. Pigmented areas of the skin are frequently seen in persons with a deficiency of adrenocortical secretion which results in an increased, compensatory output of ACTH.

POSTERIOR PITUITARY LOBE

FUNCTIONS OF THE POSTERIOR PITUITARY HORMONES

Two hormones, the antidiuretic hormone (ADH) and oxytocin, are released by the posterior pituitary gland. ADH, also called vasopressin, increases the permeability of the distal and collecting tubules of the kidneys, resulting in increased reabsorption of water. Release of ADH by the posterior pituitary lobe is regulated by osmoreceptors in the hypothalamus. When the osmotic pressure of the blood is elevated (for example, because of dehydration or increased salt ingestion) the neurones sensitive to changes in the osmotic pressure of the blood transmit impulses to the posterior pituitary to release ADH into the circulating blood. Conversely, if the solute concentration of the blood is below normal, nerve impulses are not produced and release of ADH is inhibited. The reduction in the blood concentration of ADH decreases the permeability of the renal tubules to water. A decrease in effective intravascular volume, regardless of osmolality, also results in a decrease in the secretion of vasopressin. This hormone plays an important role in maintaining normal fluid balance, and influences sodium ion concentration through its effect on the osmolality of the extracellular fluid. When it is present in large amounts, ADH stimulates a relatively transient, generalized vasoconstriction and thus affects blood pressure. ADH released into the general circulation is destroyed rapidly by enzymatic action, mainly in the liver and kidneys.

Oxytocin excites contractions of the pregnant uterus, especially during the latter part of gestation. The mechanism that prompts the release of oxytocin to initiate labour contractions is not known. Sensitivity of the uterine muscle to the hormone is thought to increase gradually throughout pregnancy, reaching a maximum at term. This hormone plays an important role in lactation; suckling initiates afferent nerve impulses which on reaching the hypothalamus bring about the liberation of oxytocin from the posterior pituitary gland. The hormone is carried by the blood to the mammary glands, stimulating the release and flow of milk. It is also suggested that oxytocin which is secreted during sexual stimulation of the female, promotes fertilization of the ovum by stimulating uterine contractions which propel the sperm towards the uterine tubes.

Thyroid Gland

The thyroid is situated in the neck and consists of two lateral lobes, one on each side of the trachea immediately below the larynx. These lobes are connected by a band of tissue, the thyroid isthmus, lying across the anterior surface of the trachea (Figure 19.4). The lobes contain numerous vesicles or follicles, and the walls of the follicles are composed of a layer of secreting cells. The follicles contain a clear, colloidal protein–iodine compound called thyroglobulin. The gland has an abundant blood supply; paired superior and inferior thyroid arteries arise from the external carotid and subclavian arteries.

Three hormones are produced and released into the blood. These are *tri-iodothyronine* (T_3) and *thyroxine* (T_4) which are produced by the follicular cells, and *calcitonin* (thyrocalcitonin, TCT) which is secreted by the parafollicular (C) cells. Thyroxine (T_4) occurs in greater amounts than (T_3). The thyroid hormones are formed by the combination of the amino acid tyrosine and iodine. The tyrosine molecule first combines with one or two iodine atoms to form monoiodotyrosine (MIT) and diiodotyrosine (DIT), respectively. Oxidative reactions, promoted by enzymes, combine these compounds to form T_3 and T_4 (MIT + DIT → T_3; DIT + DIT → T_4). T_3 and T4 are stored in the thyroglobulin in the follicles. They are freed from the thyroglobulin and released into the blood as needed. In the blood most of the thyroid hormone combines loosely with a globulin fraction of the blood proteins from which it readily separates at cellular level.

The thyroid hormones (T_3 and T_4) increase the metabolic rate in most of the cells by stimulating oxidative processes. There is a notable increase in cellular activity, oxygen consumption and heat production. The hormones are essential for normal physical growth, maturation and mental development. The production and release of the thyroid hormones are controlled by TSH secreted by the anterior pituitary. It is also influenced indirectly by the nervous system through the hypothalamus, which is closely linked with the anterior pituitary via the hypothalamic-hypophyseal portal vessels. TSH promotes the uptake of available tyrosine and iodine as well as the release of the hormones from the thyroglobulin into the blood. A reciprocal or negative feedback relationship exists between TSH and the thyroid hormones. When the blood concentration of the thyroid hormones decreases, the hypothalamus produces a releasing factor (TRH) which alerts the anterior pituitary to release TSH. Production of TRH is influenced also by emotional factors and environmental temperatures. Conversely, with an increase in the thyroidal hormone concentration of the blood, a corresponding decrease of the TSH output occurs.

Calcitonin is secreted in response to an above-normal elevation in the blood calcium or an excess of glucagon in the blood. It lowers the serum calcium and phosphate levels by promoting their excretion in urine and movement into the bones.

Parathyroid Glands

The parathyroid glands are small oval bodies attached to the posterior surface of the lateral lobes of the thyroid (Figure 19.5). The number may vary but is usually four. The principal secretion of the parathyroid glands is parathyroid hormone (PTH), which regulates the concentration of calcium and inorganic phosphorus in the blood through its action on the intestine, bone tissue and kidneys. It promotes absorption of calcium in the intestine and demineralization of bone and the movement of the calcium into the extracellular fluid. In the kidneys, the hormone increases the excretion of phosphorus by decreasing its reabsorption from the glomerular filtrate and conversely, the reabsorption of calcium is increased, decreasing its excretion in urine.

The parathyroid hormone, through its regulation of blood calcium and phosphorus levels, plays an important role in normal physiology. A normal concentration of calcium is essential for the normal structure of bones and teeth, coagulation of blood, maintenance of normal cardiac rhythmicity, normal neuromuscular excitability and cellular membrane permeability. The greater part of the absorbed calcium is deposited in bones. The optimal blood calcium level for meeting these functions is 2.2–2.55 mmol/l. Phosphorus functions in cellular metabolism, bone structure and the maintenance of a normal pH of body fluids. The normal blood concentration of serum phosphorus in adults is between 0.6 and 1.3 mmol/l.

The rate of secretion of the parathyroid hormone is controlled by the concentration of calcium in the blood. When the calcium level rises above normal, the glands are inhibited and less hormone is produced. A fall in the blood calcium level stimulates the glands, resulting in an increased output of PTH.

Calcitonin is secreted by the C cells of the thyroid and has the opposite effect on blood calcium as that of PTH. Output is stimulated by an elevation in the calcium

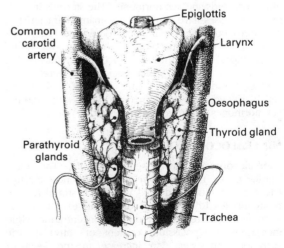

Figure 19.5 Posterior surface of the thyroid gland, showing the parathyroid glands.

of the blood. It inhibits bone resorption and promotes the excretion of calcium and phosphorus in urine and the movement of calcium into the bones.

In summary, a feedback system exists between the parathyroid glands and the circulating blood calcium level. Following a decrease in calcium concentration there is an increased secretion of the parathyroid hormone. The hormone thus acts to: (1) raise the serum calcium level; (2) lower the serum phosphorus level; (3) decrease the urinary output of calcium; (4) increase the renal excretion of phosphate; and (5) promote the movement of calcium from the bones and the absorption of calcium from the intestine. A feedback mechanism also operates to regulate the secretion of calcitonin; hypercalcaemia stimulates its production.

Adrenal Glands

The two adrenal or suprarenal glands are situated immediately above the kidneys. Each one is enclosed within a capsule and consists of two distinct parts, the cortex and medulla, which are functionally unrelated and are of different embryological origin. The cortex develops from germinal mesodermal cells. The medulla is derived from the ectoderm in close association with the sympathetic division of the autonomic nervous system with which it is functionally related. The adrenal glands have an abundant blood supply through branches of the aorta and the inferior phrenic and renal arteries.

ADRENAL CORTEX

The cortex forms the outer part as well as the greater portion of the gland and produces hormones essential to life. These are steroids and collectively are called the *adrenocorticoids*, corticosteroids or corticoids. Cells of the cortex have a high cholesterol and vitamin C content which is used in the production of many steroid substances. Those secreted in physiologically significant amounts fall into three classes: mineralocorticoids, glucocorticoids and sex hormones. The steroids in each of these classes have some predominant characteristics or actions, but may overlap into another class. There are three zones or groups of cells: the outer one (zona glomerulosa) secretes the mineralocorticoids; the middle, thicker area of cells (zona fasciculata) secretes the glucocorticoids; and the inner layer of cells (zona reticularis) adjacent to the medulla secretes the adrenal sex hormones (androgens and oestrogen).

MINERALOCORTICOIDS

Mineralocorticoids are essential to life. The most significant one is *aldosterone*, which influences electrolyte concentrations and fluid volume. It stimulates the renal tubules to reabsorb sodium and excrete potassium, and it decreases the sodium concentration while increasing the potassium content of saliva, gastric secretion and sweat. An increase in the level of circulating aldosterone causes an increase in the serum sodium level, and that in interstitial fluid. The consequent elevation in their osmotic pressure causes an increased release of the ADH and a resultant retention of water. Conversely, a decreased output of aldosterone reverses these reactions.

The secretion of aldosterone is regulated in the interest of maintaining a normal sodium concentration and normal fluid volume. Factors which influence the amount of aldosterone released are the blood sodium and potassium levels and the blood volume. A decrease in the sodium concentration stimulates an increased output of aldosterone and, conversely, a rise in sodium to above the normal level decreases the output of the hormone. The effect of potassium is the reverse of that of sodium; that is, the adrenal cortices respond to an elevated potassium concentration by an increased secretion of aldosterone and vice versa. Decreases in renal arterial blood pressure such as occur in shock, physical trauma and haemorrhage increase renin secretion by the kidneys. The production of angiotensin II that results from the release of renin (see Fig. 20.5) stimulates the adrenal cortex to secrete aldosterone. The adrenocorticotrophic hormone (ACTH) also stimulates the secretion of aldosterone as well as glucocorticoids, but more is required than that necessary to initiate an output of glucocorticoids.

GLUCOCORTICOIDS

Several glucocorticoids have been recognized, but *cortisol* (hydrocortisone) is considered to be the most important, since it is more potent and is produced in much greater amounts than the other cortical hormones. Cortisol influences the metabolism of glucose, protein and fat, and is involved in the body's responses to physical and mental stress. Its actions are complex and not clearly understood; for example, it enables a person to deal more effectively with stress, but how this is achieved is not known. Cortisol elevates the blood sugar level and the liver glycogen stores are increased. Tissue protein is broken down and the amino acids are converted to glycogen or glucose in the liver (gluconeogenesis). Fat is also mobilized, some of which is also converted to glucose.

Glucocorticoids are secreted in response to circulating ACTH. In turn, the production and release of ACTH by the anterior pituitary depends upon the release of corticotrophin-releasing hormone (CRH) which is secreted by the hypothalamus and delivered to the corticotrophs of the anterior pituitary. The production of CRH is influenced by a negative feedback mechanism; that is, a low concentration of adrenocorticoid secretions in the blood initiates the hypothalamic responses. With an elevation of blood glucocorticoids, the output of ACTH is depressed. Physical and psychological stress and hypoglycaemia also stimulate the release of CRH through impulses delivered from the cerebral cortex or midbrain to the hypothalamus. ACTH is secreted in diurnal rhythm; the secretory output is highest in the morning and lowest in the evening.

A concentration of cortisol in excess of the normal is of clinical significance because it suppresses local inflammatory responses to irritating substances (anti-inflammatory effect), delays healing through depressed fibroplasia and reduces tissue sensitivity reactions to antigens (antiallergic reaction). Glucocorticoids have a tissue-wasting effect; they promote the breakdown of body proteins and tend to inhibit amino acid uptake and tissue synthesis. Other effects also associated with an excess of cortisol are atrophy of the lymphoid tissues, a decreased production of antibodies, an increased secretion of gastric hydrochloric acid and pepsinogen which predisposes to the development of ulcers, and increased cerebral excitability manifested by restlessness and euphoria. The glucocorticoids, as well as the mineralocorticoids, may also cause some sodium retention, resulting in a positive fluid balance.

ADRENAL SEX HORMONES

The adrenal cortices of both sexes secrete both male and female hormones: namely, *androgens, oestrogen* and *progesterone*. Oestrogen and progesterone are produced in lesser amounts than the androgens but, normally, the quantity of any of these hormones is considered to be physiologically insignificant compared with the amounts produced by the gonads.

ADRENAL MEDULLA

The medulla forms the central portion of each adrenal gland and is composed of specialized neurones (nerve cells) which secrete two hormones, *adrenaline* and *noradrenaline*. Because of their chemical composition, they are frequently referred to as catecholamines. During any stress or threat to the organism, the hormones are released and serve with the autonomic nervous system to produce defensive reactions throughout the body. Their production is controlled by nerve impulses transmitted to the medullae by sympathetic nerve fibres, and their effects are similar to those produced by sympathetic innervation. Approximately 80% of the secretion is adrenaline and the remainder is noradrenaline.

Adrenaline causes constriction of the peripheral and renal blood vessels and dilatation of the coronary and skeletal muscle vessels. The rate and force of contraction of the heart and skeletal muscle is increased. The smooth muscle of the bronchioles, gastrointestinal tract and urinary bladder relaxes. The dilator muscle fibres of the irises contract, resulting in dilatation of the pupils. The blood sugar is elevated by increased glycogenolysis (conversion of glycogen to glucose) in both the liver and skeletal muscles. The metabolic rate is accelerated, and there is an increased alertness and awareness due to stimulation of the brain. Adrenaline also promotes the release of ACTH, which in turn increases the secretion of glucocorticoids.

Noradrenaline causes a more generalized vasoconstriction and does not cause dilatation of any vessels. Because of this action, it is more effective in raising the blood pressure; both systolic and diastolic blood pressures rise.

Pancreas (Islets of Langerhans)

The pancreas is both an exocrine and endocrine gland. Its exocrine secretions are carried by a system of ducts

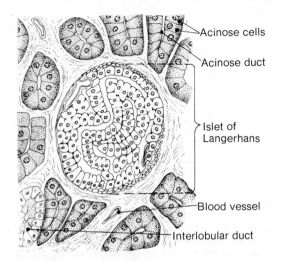

Figure 19.6 Location of cells of the islets of Langerhans between lobules of the pancreas.

to the duodenum and contain enzymes which play an important role in digestion. The islets of Langerhans form the endocrine component of the pancreas and consist of irregularly scattered groups of cells which are totally independent of the pancreatic system of ducts (Figure 19.6). The islets are highly vascularized and consist of four types of cells: α cells, which secrete the hormone glucagon; β cells, which produce insulin; δ cells, which may secrete small amounts of gastrin and somatostatin (growth hormone-releasing inhibiting hormone) (GHRIH); and F cells which secrete pancreatic polypeptide. Insulin and glucagon are proteins and are rendered inactive in the gastrointestinal tract by the proteolytic enzymes: when prescribed, they must be administered parenterally.

SECRETIONS AND FUNCTIONS

Insulin

This hormone plays a dominant role in carbohydrate, fat and protein metabolism, especially in the liver and muscular and adipose tissues. Figure 19.7 depicts the production, release, transport and action of insulin on cells of peripheral tissues. Knowledge of the ways in which insulin promotes specific metabolic cellular activities is incomplete, but it has been established that it binds to receptors in cell membranes and stimulates the following actions: (1) the transfer of glucose into most cells and its metabolism by those cells (not all cells are *insulin-dependent* for the transfer of glucose; notable in this respect are the brain cells, erythrocytes, kidney tubules and intestinal mucosa); (2) the formation of glycogen by the liver and muscle cells; (3) the synthesis of fatty acids and storage of fat in adipose tissue; (4) the uptake and incorporation of amino acids into cell proteins; and (5) an increased uptake of potassium by cells. These activities result in a lower concentration of glucose in the blood.

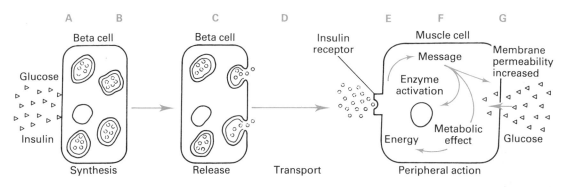

Figure 19.7 Action of insulin. The rise in blood glucose associated with a carbohydrate meal induces the beta (β) cells in the islets of Langerhans to secrete insulin into the circulation. The insulin is then carried in the bloodstream to target cells throughout the body, where it binds to receptor molecules on the cell surface. This interaction triggers a series of events inside the cells that enhance the uptake of glucose from the blood and its subsequent breakdown for metabolic energy or storage as glycogen (animal starch) and fat. A defect anywhere along this pathway could result in diabetes. Possible causes include destruction of β cells (A), abnormal synthesis of insulin (B), retarded release of insulin (C), inactivation of insulin in the bloodstream by antibodies or other blocking agents (D), altered insulin receptors or a decreased number of receptors on peripheral cells (E), defective processing of the insulin message within the target cells (F), and abnormal metabolism of glucose (G). Current evidence points to the β cells as the site of primary defect in type I diabetes.

The chemical structure and composition of the insulin that is initially secreted by the beta cells is called preproinsulin. This is rapidly broken down to form a large molecule called proinsulin. Proinsulin undergoes chemical changes which are activated by proteolytic enzymes within the cells to form insulin.

The secretion of insulin is regulated by a variety of stimulatory and inhibiting factors most of which are related to glucose metabolism or the cyclic AMP system. The concentration of blood glucose is the major controlling factor. An elevation increases the production of insulin and, conversely, a decrease below the normal blood level of glucose suppresses its secretion. Thus, a positive feedback mechanism is established which controls the output of insulin in order to maintain the blood sugar level within a normal range. Some amino acids have a similar effect on insulin secretion. Their action is enhanced when glucose levels are elevated. The synthesis of insulin is also stimulated by an excess of growth hormone and glucocorticoids but somatostatin is an inhibitor of both insulin and glucagon secretion. The glucocorticoid hormones act by decreasing intracellular adenosine monophosphate (AMP). The amount of insulin circulated in the blood increases when carbohydrate foods are ingested; this is attributed to the effect of the gastrointestinal hormones (e.g. gastrin, secretin, cholecystokinin-pancreozymin) on the beta cells. Glucose given intravenously does not produce the same effect as when it is taken orally.

Calcium ions are necessary for the release of insulin by the β cells. Other factors that result in an increased insulin level include vagal nerve stimulation and oral hypoglycaemic agents.

Glucagon

This hormone may also be referred to as the hyperglycaemic factor, since its primary effect is stimulation of glycogenolysis (the conversion of glycogen to glucose) and its release into the blood by the liver to increase the blood glucose concentration. It also promotes gluconeogenesis, lipolysis, and secretion of the growth hormone and insulin. Its secretion by the α cells is stimulated by a low blood sugar level. An oral intake of proteins initiates an increased secretion of glucagon, greater than that seen in response to intravenous administration of amino acids. This suggests a gastrointestinal hormone that stimulates the secretion of glucagon. Sympathetic nervous stimulation of the pancreas also increases the glucagon output.

Somatostatin (growth hormone release-inhibiting hormone, GHRIH)

This hormone is found in cells of the hypothalamus, where it passes down the portal vessels to the anterior pituitary, gastrointestinal tract and islets of Langerhans. It inhibits the secretion of insulin, glucagon, pancreatic polypeptide, GH and various gastrointestinal hormones. It interferes with carbohydrate absorption and possibly with the absorption of protein and fat.

Pancreatic polypeptide

This hormone is known to decrease glycogen in the liver and to slow the absorption of food. Release of the hormone is stimulated by protein ingestion, fasting, exercise and hypoglycaemia.

BLOOD SUGAR LEVEL

The normal blood sugar (glucose) level 3–4 hours after a meal varies from approximately 6.5–7.5 mmol/l. Fluctuations occur as a result of energy expenditure and the ingestion of foods. The types of food taken also influence the degree of change; obviously, a meal high in carbohydrate produces a greater concentration of glucose for a period of time than a meal with a low carbohydrate content. An elevation of the blood sugar level above the normal is known as *hyperglycaemia*. A level below normal is referred to as *hypoglycaemia*.

As cited previously, the blood sugar level is regulated by the hormones of the islets of Langerhans (insulin, glucagon and somatostatin). It may, however, be influenced by several other endocrine secretions. An excess of GH produces a tendency toward hyperglycaemia by decreasing the utilization of glucose and stimulating the production of glucagon. The release of glucocorticoids (cortisol) by the adrenal cortices promotes gluconeogenesis (formation of glucose from amino acids and the glycerol portion of fat), resulting in an elevation of the blood sugar. Adrenaline and noradrenaline stimulate liver glycogenolysis and the metabolism of muscle glycogen to lactic acid, which is then converted to glucose by the liver. The thyroid hormones also increase the blood sugar level by an acceleration of gluconeogenesis.

Clinical Characteristics of Disorders of the Endocrine System

Signs and symptoms of endocrine dysfunction may be non-specific, resulting from changes in the wide-spread target tissues and are common to many disorders. They include the following:

- *Alterations in growth.* Growth may be delayed or excessive. *Delayed growth* can occur from endocrine and metabolic disorders as well as genetic factors. Delayed growth from endocrine disorders usually occurs during a specific period of development. *Excessive growth* may result from endocrine disorders in which an excess of adrenal, ovarian or testicular or pituitary hormones is produced. Excessive pituitary secretion of growth hormone causes gigantism.
- *Obesity.* Obesity can be associated with hormonal disorders and may be a causative factor (as in diabetes) as well as a result of a disorder.
- *Appetite changes* include anorexia and polyphagia. Excessive eating (polyphagia) is most often seen with uncontrolled diabetes, hyperthyroidism and occasionally with a hypothalamic disorder.
- *Polyuria and polydypsia.* Excessive urinary output and abnormal thirst are frequently the result of uncontrolled diabetes mellitus or diabetes insipidus.
- *Weakness and exhaustion.* Excessive weight loss, muscle wasting, weakness and exhaustion may be seen in patients with uncontrolled disorders of the pancreas, thyroid or adrenal glands.
- *Skin pigmentation.* Changes in skin pigmentation may develop in patients with disorders of the pituitary, parathyroid and adrenal glands.
- *Hirsutism.* Changes in the distribution and texture of body hair occur with several endocrine disorders. Facial hair in the female may occur with adrenal or ovarian disorders.

- *Sexual disturbances.* Impotence, menstrual disorders and infertility may be associated with endocrine disturbances. Impotence may occur in men who have had diabetes mellitus for several years. The onset of puberty and delay in the development of secondary sex characteristics may occur with deficiency of the growth hormone and gonadal dysfunction.
- *Bone and joint disorders* accompany changes in the secretion of the growth and thyroid hormones and adrenocorticoids.
- *Renal colic and stones* may be associated with bone disorders in patients with disorders of secretion of the thyroid and adrenal gland.
- *Hypertension* occurs as a result of hyperactivity of the adrenal cortex.
- *Personality changes* including lethargy, confusion, nervousness, restlessness, convulsions and coma may result from acute metabolic disorders associated with uncontrolled diabetes mellitus as well as with disorders of secretions of the pituitary gland, adrenal gland and thyroid.

THE PERSON WITH DISORDERS OF THE PITUITARY GLAND (HYPOPHYSIS)

ASSESSMENT

Assessment of the person with disorders of the pituitary gland, as with other endocrine disorders, requires analysis of data and recognition of the underlying pattern of the pituitary disorder. The signs and symptoms of pituitary dysfunction are varied and reflect not only the increase or decrease in the production of one or more of the pituitary hormones, but also the resultant changes in the target tissues. Pituitary hormones, their functions and associated disorders are listed in Table 19.1.

Health history

The health history should include questions related to:

- *Growth and development.* Questions relate to changes in growth pattern, general rate of growth and perceived changes in appearance or clothing size. The development of secondary sex charactersitics and abnormalities of secondary sex characteristics may be explored, but only with sensitivity, given the delicate nature of the topics involved. For the female, questions are asked about changes in the menstrual cycle and, if relevant, problems with pregnancies and lactation. For the male, questions relate to sexual dysfunctions, in particular difficulties in attaining and maintaining an erection and any changes in body hair growth and distribution.
- *Appetite and body weight.* Recent changes in appetite and the pattern of weight gain or loss are determined. It is important to ask questions about the volume of fluid intake, any cravings for salt, preferences for cold liquids and whether thirst is

Table 19.1 Pituitary gland hormones.

Gland	Hormones	Functions	Disorders
Anterior pituitary	Growth hormone (GH)	Growth; aids in determining size; accelerates metabolism; diabetogenic	Panhypopituitarism Gigantism—increase in GH in childhood Acromegaly—increase in GH in adulthood Short stature—decrease of GH in childhood
	Thyroid-stimulating hormone (TSH)	Promotes secretory activity of thyroid	Hyperthyroidism secondary to increase of TSH Hypothyroidism secondary to decrease of TSH
	Adrenocorticotrophic hormone (ACTH)	Stimulates secretion of adrenal cortices	Cushing's syndrome and excess TSH Addison's disease secondary to pituitary disorder
	Gonadotrophins —Follicle-stimulating hormone (FSH)	In women: development of ovarian follicle and secretion of oestrogen In men: promotes production of spermatozoa	Tumours Amenorrhoea Infertility
	—Luteinizing hormone (LH)	In women: induces ovulation, stimulates secretion of progesterone In men: stimulates production of androgens	
	—Prolactin	Initiates and sustains lactation	Galactorrhoea Infertility
	Melanocyte stimulating hormone (MSH)	Pigmentation of skin cells	Increase in pigmented areas
Posterior pituitary	Antidiuretic hormone (ADH)	Increases permeability of distal and collecting tubules of kidneys (i.e. increases reabsorption of water)	Tumour
	Oxytocin	Contracts pregnant uterus; stimulates release and flow of milk	

relieved. Alteration in heat tolerance may also be present with metabolic changes.
- *Elimination patterns.* Changes in the volume, frequency and pattern of urinary elimination are determined. The person is asked specifically about getting up at night to void. Changes in bowel habits, constipation and/or diarrhoea are identified.
- *Skin and hair.* Alteration in skin colour, texture, dryness, bruising and ability to heal may be caused by pituitary dysfunction. The patient can validate the nurse's observations as he or she is in the best position to recognize changes.
- *Activity tolerance.* Questions are asked about feelings of tiredness or exhaustion related to usual daily activities and on exertion. Knowledge of the person's usual pattern of daily activity provides a basis for comparison.

- *Cognitive/perceptual function.* Changes in memory, ability to concentrate, decreased attention span and visual losses may result from pituitary disorders or altered function of the target tissues. How the person usually responds to stressful physical and emotional events is elicited in detail and recent changes in these responses are also recorded.

Physical examination

The pituitary gland is not palpable, therefore the presence of pituitary disorders generally requires an assessment of most body systems.

- *General appearance.* The patient's general appearance, body build and fat distribution provide valuable information about pituitary abnormalities and overall growth and development of the individual.

- *Body weight and vital signs.* The patient's weight and vital signs (temperature, pulse rate and rhythm, respirations and blood pressure) are recorded.
- *Skin, hair and nails.* The skin is observed and palpated for pigmentation, dryness, oiliness, elasticity, hydration, temperature and breaks in the integrity and any resulting discharge. The pattern of distribution and amount of body hair are observed and the texture and dryness noted. Nails are observed for thickness and changes in growth.
- *Genitalia and breasts.* The genitalia of the male and female are observed for size and shape and the breasts are examined to assess development and maturation.
- *Neurological examination* may be done in detail if degenerative changes are noted in the examination or history. Changes in sensation, pain, discomfort, reflexes and muscle tone are noted. The patient's speech is carefully listened to for huskiness, slurring, hoarseness, volume and pitch and rationality.
- *Visual fields.* Assessment is carried out if there is any indication of a pituitary tumour.

Diagnostic measurements

Hormone levels are measured by *radioimmunoassay*.

- *Serum growth hormone (GH).* Fasting levels of serum GH may be determined by radioimmunoassay.
  Normal: adult male, 0–238 pmol/l (0–5 ng/ml); adult female, <380 pmol/l (<8 ng/ml); prepubertal child, <238 pmol/l (<5 ng/ml).
- *Somatomedin-C* is a growth hormone dependent polypeptide that is increased with acromegaly and decreased in persons with hypopituitarism.
- *Thyroid-stimulating hormone* promotes the secretory function of the thyroid gland. Changes in levels of this hormone are reflected in thyroid function.
- *Gonadotrophins: follicle stimulating hormone; luteinizing hormone* and *prolactin* levels are indicative of pituitary gland function as well as functioning of ovarian and breast tissues.
- *Melanocyte-stimulating hormone* levels are reflected in the pigmentation of the skin.
- *Adrenocorticotrophic hormone* levels are increased with decreased adrenal function. Decreased levels may be caused by a pituitary disorder.
- *Antidiuretic hormone* levels are used to diagnose diabetes insipidus and the syndrome of inappropriate antidiuretic hormone secretion.

Challenge tests are used to determine the reserve function of the pituitary gland when other tests show low or borderline levels of specific hormones.

- *Growth hormone stimulation tests* are used to detect a deficiency of growth hormone. Base-line fasting blood levels of serum GH, glucose, cortisol and insulin are determined. The test consists of the intravenous administration of insulin followed by the determination of GH levels at 0, 15, 30 and 60 minutes. Other stimulation tests may be used, such as levadopa and glucagon.

Normally, GH levels increase in response to insulin stimulation.

- *Thyrotropin-releasing hormone challenge* is used to stimulate the release of thyroid stimulating hormone in order to differentiate pituitary and thyroid causes of hypothyroidism or hyperthyroidism. Measurements are made before, immediately and at regular intervals after intravenous administration of TRH.

Water deprivation tests (Mosenthal test). ADH secretion is normally stimulated when water is withheld and the urine output decreases. The test involves withholding fluids for up to 8 hours and measuring the urinary output and osmolality of each voiding. Plasma osmolality tests are made also, and the patient's weight loss is recorded. Failure to increase urine osmolality and the presence of increased plasma osmolality are characteristic of diabetes insipidus.

Suppression tests are used to confirm hyposecretion of specific pituitary hormones by suppressing a known stimulus.

- *Growth hormone suppression test* is used to assess hypersecretion of growth hormone. Glucose is administered orally or intravenously as in a glucose tolerance test. Normally, the level of GH will decrease.

Urine and serum osmolality tests. These tests are used to evaluate ADH regulation. Normally, urine osmolality is higher than serum osmolality. With an ADH deficiency, the urinary output increases and plasma concentrations of sodium increase.
  Normal: serum osmolality, 275–295 mosmol/kg; Urine osmolality, maximum dilution 50 mosmol/kg, maximum concentration 800–1500 mosmol/kg.

Radiological studies. These include X-rays of the sella turcica and computerized axial tomography (CT) scan. Radiological examination of the sella turcica demonstrates changes in its size, shape and density. Tumours may be identified by a CT scan.

PATIENT PROBLEMS

Problems associated with disorders of the pituitary vary greatly, depending on which lobe is involved, the nature of the disease (hyperplasia, neoplasm or destruction of tissue) and the particular type of cell of the anterior pituitary that is involved. Dysfunction may be manifested in one or more of the gland's target organs, reflecting either an excessive or deficient output of one or more pituitary hormones. Secondary neurological disturbances may also occur as a result of pressure on neighbouring brain tissue by a pituitary neoplasm. For example, early manifestations may include altered perceptual/visual function. The visual disturbances frequently occur because of the proximity of the visual tract. Conversely, primary pathological lesions in the brain, especially in the hypothalamic region, may cause secondary involvement of the pituitary.

The more commonly recognized disease entities associated with the anterior pituitary include: gigantism, the result of an excessive secretion of GH in childhood; acromegaly, due to an excessive secretion of GH commencing in adulthood; dwarfism, resulting from a deficiency of GH in childhood; Cushing's disease, the result of a hypersecretion of adrenocorticotrophic hormone and Simmonds' disease (panhypopituitarism), which occurs with a deficiency of all the anterior pituitary hormones. Hyperthyroidism (Graves' disease) may also be secondary to an excessive production of TSH or an abnormal form of the hormone and is discussed in the section on disorders of the thyroid.

The most common disorder associated with the posterior pituitary is diabetes insipidus, which is a result of a deficiency of ADH.

Hypersecretion of Growth Hormone: Acromegaly

An overproduction of GH before closure of the epiphyses causes a rapid overgrowth of the bones, producing the condition known as *gigantism*. *Acromegaly* results from an excess of growth hormone after puberty.

CLINICAL CHARACTERISTICS

A person with gigantism may attain a height of 7–8 feet (2.1–2.4 metres). Most cases are attributed to an adenoma of the somatotrophs or acidophilic cells (α cells). When the person passes adolescence, acromegaly is superimposed on the gigantism.

If the adenoma develops after the epiphyses have closed, longitudinal growth cannot occur, but marked thickening of the bones occurs and acromegaly develops. Enlargement of the head, jaws, hands and feet becomes apparent. Increased growth of cartilage produces an increase in the size of the nose, ears, costal cartilages and larynx. Hypertrophy of the larynx may be accompanied by a deepening of the voice, and the change in the costal cartilages results in an increase in the thoracic circumference. The skin, subcutaneous tissues and lips thicken, the chin lengthens and the lower teeth separate because of the overgrowth of the mandible. Viscera enlarge and may become overactive, leading to disturbances.

As well as the evident skeletal changes and alteration in appearance, the patient experiences lethargy, weakness, increased metabolic rate and excessive sweating due to hypertrophy of the thyroid. Common complaints are joint pains, stiffness in the limbs, and tingling or numbness in the hands. Impaired carbohydrate metabolism and hyperglycaemia develop owing to the diabetogenic effect of GH. Pressure from the causative expanding neoplasm may cause headache, insomnia and loss of visual acuity and fields. Increased gonadal function may be associated with the early stage of acromegaly but, later, loss of libido and amenorrhoea are common. Osteoporosis, rarefaction of bones due to loss of calcium, may develop, especially in the vertebrae, and kyphosis (forward curvature of the spine) may be seen in the advanced stage. Hypertension is a common complication. The course of the disease varies con-

siderably from one patient to another; it may develop slowly over many years in some, but in others it may prove fatal in 3 or 4 years. Destruction of pituitary tissue by progressive growth and spread of the tumour may cause a general hypopituitarism.

Diagnostic investigation involves X-rays of the skull in which the sella turcica is checked for widening. Laboratory studies include: serum inorganic phosphorus, which may be elevated; blood glucose level, which may be increased; and measurement of plasma GH concentration, which is elevated and remains elevated when glucose is administered.

TREATMENT

Acromegaly may be treated by external or internal irradiation of the pituitary or by a hypophysectomy or transphenoidal microsurgery to remove the hyperfunctioning tissue. Internal radiation may be achieved by the implantation of radioactive gold (^{198}Au) or yttrium (^{90}Y) seeds in the pituitary. The gland is approached through the nasal cavity and sphenoid bone. Synthesized somatostatin (growth hormone release inhibiting factor) may be used to treat acromegaly. Bromocriptine has also been administered orally when other forms of treatment have been ineffective. Substitution hormal preparations are prescribed if a hypophysectomy is done or if the patient manifests insulin, thyroid, adrenal or gonadal insufficiency in the advanced stage of the disease. Treatment arrests further changes but the changes in bony structures are irreversible.

NURSING INTERVENTION

Health problems experienced by the person with acromegaly and his or her family vary with the stage and type of therapy, the impact of the disorder and treatment on the individual's life-style and the person's ability to meet developmental tasks. Common health problems include: (1) *anxiety* related to the surgery and treatment; (2) *altered self-esteem* related to changes in physical appearance; (3) *sexual dysfunction* related to possible amenorrhoea, decreased libido or impotence; (4) *altered nutrition* related to increased physical growth and metabolic rate; (5) *perceptual deficits* related to visual impairment; and (6) *knowledge deficit* related to surgery or radiation therapy and possible long-term hormone replacement therapy.

The nurse supplies support and counselling to the patient and family to help them verbalize and deal with their concerns and anxieties. The reasons for the physiological changes are explained and they are helped to understand the expectations of acute and long-term therapy. The nurse helps the patient and family to develop a self-care plan that includes a diet that is well-balanced but high in calories, and plans for long-term hormone replacement therapy.

Panhypopituitarism (Simmonds' Disease)

This disease denotes a deficiency of all the anterior pituitary hormones. The condition may be the result of a primary lesion, such as a tumour or cyst, within the anterior lobe itself, or it may be secondary to a space-occupying lesion in neighbouring structures or to interference with the blood supply to the gland. The latter may occur with thrombosis of the hypophyseal vessels rarely associated with postpartum shock (Sheehan's syndrome). Frequently the causative lesion is a craniopharyngioma which is derived from vestigial cells of Rathke's pouch. This tumour occurs most often in children but may not give rise to symptoms until adulthood because it grows slowly. A second neoplasm that may be responsible for panhypopituitarism is an adenoma of the chromophobe cells. The cells of both these tumours are non-secreting and, as they enlarge, they compress and destroy the secreting cells. Surgical excision or irradiation of the gland for the purpose of suppressing the secretion of certain hormones in the treatment of carcinoma of the breast (see Chapter 23) or acromegaly may incur hyposecretion of all the adeno-hypophyseal hormones.

CLINICAL CHARACTERISTICS

The multiple hormone deficiency results in a lack of stimulation to the thyroid, adrenal cortices and gonads. Secondary atrophy and a hyposecretion of their hormones ensue. If the condition occurs in childhood, failure of the secretion of GH along with the others produces dwarfism. Growth and development are arrested, the skin becomes wrinkled and the child develops an appearance characteristic of a 'wizened old person'.

In the adult, there is also a general wasting of all body tissues and the person exhibits emaciation and severe weight loss. The skin is dry and wrinkled and may assume a yellowish cast. The body hair becomes sparse. Decreased thyroid activity causes a reduction in the metabolic rate, leading to a subnormal temperature and extreme weakness. Arrested function of the gonads results in failure of ovulation and amenorrhoea in the female and an absence of spermatogenesis and impotence in the male. Concomitant hypoglycaemia and hypotension are seen and may lead to shock and coma. The low blood sugar is attributed to the decreased GH and adrenocorticoid secretions. If the panhypopituitarism is due to an expanding neoplasm, the posterior pituitary and the infundibulum (neural stalk) may become involved, manifested by polyuria and extreme thirst, which is characteristic of a deficiency of ADH. An expanding lesion may impose itself on the optic tract, impairing vision. The hypothalamus may also be affected and varied neurological disturbances become evident; for example, the patient may experience severe anorexia.

TREATMENT

Treatment includes the administration of substitution hormones of the target glands. The patient receives corticosteroids and thyroid hormone in dosages adjusted to individual needs. Thyroid hormone is prescribed only when the patient is receiving corticosteroids. Gonadal hormones may be prescribed, depending on the patient's age. Testosterone (male hormone) may be administered to both sexes for its anabolic effect. Oestrogen may be used with the female to preserve female secondary sex characteristics. Human GH, if available, may be given to children to increase height.

If the cause is a tumour, it is removed by transphenoidal microsurgery and/or treated by irradiation.

NURSING INTERVENTION

The nurse assists the patient and family in setting realistic long-term goals to promote adjustment to the chronic endocrine dysfunction. Patient and family concerns are identified and explored in depth, since the disorder has profound effects on both the individual and family.

The nurse plays an important role in encouraging patients to take a high-calorie, high-vitamin diet. Since anorexia is a frequent problem, resourcefulness is necessary to gain the patient's co-operation and ensure adequate nourishment. Various methods and approaches must be tried. It is usually helpful to provide small servings of high-calorie foods at frequent intervals rather than the usual three or four regular meals. Varying the foods, adding concentrates to fluids, determining the patient's preferences, having favourite 'dishes' prepared at home, eating with others and a change of environment are just a few suggestions that may prove beneficial.

The lethargy and apathy generally associated with Simmonds' disease predisposes to the patient's immobility. Prompting the patient to change position and exercise is necessary to stimulate circulation and prevent complications.

The nurse provides instruction about the long-term hormone replacement therapy.

ADH Hyposecretion: Diabetes Insipidus

CAUSATIVE FACTORS

The causative factor in this disorder maybe a deficiency of ADH (arginine vasopressin, AVP) or failure of the renal tubules to respond to ADH. In the latter case, the disorder may be referred to as nephrogenic diabetes insipidus and is a rare sex-linked, recessive hereditary condition present at birth but may be acquired in adults secondary to renal disorders. A deficiency of ADH is most commonly due to hypoactivity or destruction of a part of the hypothalamic–posterior pituitary system resulting from primary or metastatic neoplasms or infection, such as encephalitis, meningitis or brain injury. In some instances, no apparent cause can be identified.

CLINICAL CHARACTERISTICS

Diabetes insipidus is characterized by a very large urinary output (polyuria) and extreme thirst (polydipsia). The daily output may range from 5 to 20 litres and the patient may experience anorexia, headache, muscular pains, loss of weight and strength and electrolyte imbalance. The urine has an abnormally low specific gravity and does not contain any abnormal constituents. If fluid is withheld or does not keep pace with the output, an excessive loss of urine continues, leading to severe dehydration and shock. The persisting symptoms of polyuria and polydipsia day and night interfere with rest and normal activities.

DIAGNOSIS

Investigation of the disorder usually involves water deprivation tests. Failure to increase the specific gravity of the urine and an elevation of plasma osmolality are characteristic of diabetes insipidus. Stimulation of ADH may also be achieved by parenteral administration of a hypertonic solution. If these studies are positive for diabetes insipidus, a trial dose of vasopressin (Pitressin) is given; if the polyuria and thirst are not relieved, nephrogenic diabetes insipidus is suspected and kidney function studies may be done.

Investigative procedures may also include neurological examination, X-rays of the skull, visual field tests and a CT scan.

TREATMENT

The patient is treated by replacement therapy with hypotonic parenteral fluids and unlimited oral fluids; a preparation of posterior pituitary extract or vasopressin is prescribed. The preparations used include an aqueous solution of vasopressin (Pitressin) every 3–6 h s.c. or i.v. during the acute phase, and vasopressin tannate (Pitressin Tannate) in oil, given intramuscularly every 2 or 3 days. The latter preparation is absorbed more slowly and is usually administered in the evening. If the patient is allergic to the above animal vasopressin preparations, a synthetic substitute is available in the form of a nasal spray, lypressin (Syntopressin). One spray (or two may be necessary) is generally used on each nostril four times daily. The use of the nasal spray is more convenient but irritation of the nasopharyngeal mucosa may develop. Desmopressin (DDAVP) is a longer acting synthetic ADH substitute that may be inhaled intranasally. Chlorothiazide, an oral diuretic, has been found to be effective in some cases, possibly by causing sodium loss. Chlorpropamide and clofibrate have also been found to be effective in some cases.

The patient is usually hospitalized during diagnostic investigation and regulation of medication.

NURSING INTERVENTION

Nursing care focuses on the two major health problems demonstrated by individuals with diabetes insipidus: (1) fluid volume deficit due to polyuria; and (2) knowledge deficit concerning hormone replacement therapy.

Fluid volume deficit.   The nurse is responsible for the ongoing assessment of the person's fluid balance and for teaching the patient and family to recognize signs of dehydration and hypovolaemia. Vital signs, mental status, intake and output, urine specific gravity and skin integrity are assessed and recorded regularly. Daily

weights are determined. The person with fluid volume deficit will have a rapid, thready pulse, decreased blood pressure, poor skin turgor, dry mucous membranes and decreased mental alertness.

Provision of adequate fluid intake is achieved by the intravenous administration of hypotonic fluids, which serve to reduce the existing hypertonic state, and unlimited oral fluids. When the thirst mechanism is intact, the person will seek fluids which should be readily available. If the person lacks the desire to drink, the nurse must be creative to ensure that the oral intake is maintained and/or supplemented with parenteral fluids.

Patient and family teaching.   Lifelong dependence upon medication is not an easy fact for the patient to accept. The nurse can help the patient to plan for necessary readjustments, while giving reassurance that a normal pattern of life can be resumed.

The patient and a family member are taught the details of how to administer the drug, including care of the equipment. The instructions are also given in writing. They may require further explanation of the disorder to appreciate the importance of regular administration of the drug, and should be advised that in the case of vasopressin, it is ineffective if taken orally because it is inactivated by the digestive enzymes. The patient is advised to record the weight every 2 or 3 days and note the urinary volume. Water retention indicated by weight increase and scanty urine may necessitate a decrease in vasopressin dosage.

ADH Hypersecretion: Syndrome of Inappropriate Antidiuretic Hormone (SIADH)

CAUSES

Inappropriate production of antidiuretic hormone (ADH or AVP) may be caused by malignant tumours, respiratory and central nervous system infections, head trauma or positive pressure ventilation. The exact mechanisms producing the excessive ADH secretion are not fully understood.

CLINICAL CHARACTERISTICS

The clinical characteristics of SIADH are those of water intoxication. The blood volume increases, haemodilution results and serum sodium and osmolality are decreased. Oedema is absent as a result of the hyponatraemia. The person's urine is concentrated and the volume is diminished. Weight gain, nausea and vomiting, a decreased level of consciousness and seizures may be present.

TREATMENT

Treatment depends on the severity and duration of the water intoxication. In an emergency situation, intravenous hypertonic saline solutions are administered along with diuretic drugs such as frusemide. In less acute situations, the restriction of fluids to 500 ml daily may be sufficient. Demeclocycline or lithium chloride may be prescribed because they inhibit the renal response to ADH. The underlying cause of the increased ADH secretion must be treated.

NURSING INTERVENTION

Nursing care is directed toward: (1) management of the fluid volume excess; (2) assessment and control of the altered thought processes which occur as water moves into the cerebral cells; and (3) patient teaching for the person with chronic SIADH.

Fluid volume excess. Assessment of the person's fluid balance includes monitoring vital signs, serum electrolytes, urine osmolality, fluid intake and output, body weight and mental status. Oral fluids are restricted to about 500 ml a day. The nurse helps the patient develop a daily plan for distribution of the limited fluid intake and for the types of fluids to be taken. Intravenous infusions are closely monitored and administered slowly to prevent further fluid overload and aggravation of the neurological manifestations.

Mental status. The patient's level of consciousness and mental alertness are assessed regularly and changes documented. If the patient's level of consciousness is decreased or if seizures are likely, safety precautions are implemented. The side-rails should be up on the bed and someone should be with the patient if ambulant.

Patient/family teaching. The patient and family are helped to understand the disease and to recognize signs and symptoms of water toxicity. Specific instruction is provided about the administration and side-effects of prescribed medications. The nurse assists the patient and family to plan and implement safety precautions in the home to protect the patient from injury until the disorder is controlled. Safety measures may include the use of night lights and the removal of mats. Information is provided about Medic Alert identification. The patient is instructed to monitor body weight and changes in the amount of urine output.

Pituitary Ablation

The anterior and posterior pituitary gland may be removed or destroyed because of hyperfunction or a neoplasm of the gland. Hypophysectomy is also employed in the treatment of diabetic retinopathy and cancer of the breast and prostate. Malignant disease of the latter organs in many instances is supported by the sex hormones oestrogens and androgens, respectively. Removal of the source of gonadotrophic hormones reduces support for the primary neoplasm and its metastasis. Withdrawal of the hormones does not cure the disease, but usually produces a remission for a period of several months.

Pituitary ablation may be carried out by radiation therapy, surgical excision or destruction by stereotactic radiofrequency or cryosurgery (freezing). Irradiation may be from an external source or radioactive yttrium-90 may be implanted. Access to the gland is usually by a nasal–trans-sphenoidal approach but a transfrontal approach may be used if the tumour is large and has spread. Trans-sphenoidal surgery involves the use of televised radiofluoroscope and a binocular microscope. Hypophysectomy results in the withdrawal of ACTH, TSH, and probably ADH as well as the gonadotrophins. In some instances, the neural stalk, which transmits the nerve fibres from the hypothalamus to the posterior pituitary gland, may be preserved at operation, thus preventing diabetes insipidus. The patient requires cortisone, thyroxine and possibly ADH replacement for the remainder of his life. Gonadal function ceases, and the patient becomes infertile. If the surgery was done because of disease of the pituitary gland, the male patient may be given testosterone to prevent impotence.

PREOPERATIVE PREPARATION

The patient and family are likely to be very apprehensive. The nurse should therefore encourage them to talk about their fears and ask questions and provide necessary emotional support. The permanent results of the surgery will have been explained by the doctor but the nurse, knowing what the patient has been told, should be prepared to answer their questions and explain the hormonal replacement. •

The patient is advised that there will be frequent recording of blood pressure, temperature, pulse and respirations following the operation. Nasal packing will be inserted if a trans-sphenoidal approach is used. The patient is taught deep breathing techniques, encouraged to practice mouth breathing preoperatively and is cautioned against nose-blowing, sneezing and coughing postoperatively. A corticosteroid preparation is usually given the day before operation and again before going to the operating theatre.

POSTOPERATIVE CARE

The care following a hypophysectomy is similar to that of any patient who has had intracranial surgery. The patient is placed in a semi-Fowler's position to decrease swelling and promote drainage. Close observation is made for early signs of acute adrenal insufficiency (see p. 591) or fluid imbalance. An adrenocorticoid steroid is given intravenously until the patient can tolerate it orally. The dose is gradually decreased until the maintenance dose is established. Vasopressin (Pitressin) may be necessary to control the fluid loss; the dosage is adjusted to the urinary volume. Thyroid extract may be started orally on the second or third postoperative day.

The intravenous infusion is usually discontinued the morning following surgery. Oral fluids may be started the evening of surgery or the next morning. If a trans-sphenoidal approach was used, the incision will be above the front teeth. The patient is instructed not to brush the teeth until the incision is healed and the sutures are removed. Dental floss and mouth-washes are used to maintain dental and oral hygiene. The patient is taught to carry out meticulous oral hygiene regularly until healing has taken place in about 4–6 weeks. The

Table 19.2 Assessment of the person with altered thyroid function.

Patient problems	Clinical characteristics of hypothyroidism	Clinical characteristics of hyperthyroidism
1. Altered nutrition and metabolism	• Pulse rate decreased • Blood pressure low • Respirations decreased • Appetite poor • Weight gain • Serum cholesterol elevated	• Pulse rapid and bounding • Palpitations • Increased blood pressure • Respiratory rate increased • Appetite increased • Weight loss • Serum cholesterol decreased
2. Altered activity tolerance	• Weakness and fatigue • Slow movements • Dyspnoea • Decreased muscle tone and reflexes	• Weakness and fatigue • Weakness of eyelid muscles • Shortness of breath on exertion • Tremor of hands • Increased muscle tone and reflexes
3. Altered skin integrity	• Skin dry, thick and pale • Eyelids oedematous • Lips and tongue enlarged • Hair coarse and sparse • Interstitial oedema	• Increased sweating • Skin warm and moist • Eyelids retracted • Hair loss
4. Altered thought processes and emotional responses	• Slow mental processes • Increased sleep and lethargy • Speech hoarse, slow and monotonous • Depression • Mental disturbance	• Anxiety, apprehension • Restlessness • Irritability • Emotional instability • Insomnia
5. Altered bowel elimination	• Decreased gastrointestinal motility • Constipation	• Increased gastrointestinal motility • Diarrhoea
6. Altered thermoregulation	• Sensitivity to cold • Decreased body temperature	• Sensitivity to heat • Increased body temperature
7. Altered sexuality patterns	• Metrorrhagia • Amenorrhoea • Low sex drive • Infertility	• Oligomenorrhoea or amenorrhoea • Low sex drive • Impotence

period of hospitalization is relatively short; instruction about the taking of the necessary hormones (cortisone, vasopressin and thyroxin) is carried out throughout the postoperative period and, if necessary, a referral is made for follow-up instruction and supervision by a community nurse.

THE PERSON WITH DISORDERS OF THE THYROID GLAND

Disease of the thyroid may cause a hyposecretion or hypersecretion of the thyroid hormones and a change in the size of the gland. A deficiency in the secretion is called *hypothyroism*; an excessive secretion is referred to as *hyperthyroidism*. The normally functioning gland is referred to as *euthyroid*.

ASSESSMENT OF THYROID FUNCTION

Assessment of the person with disorders of the thyroid gland begins with a comprehensive health history. The health problems experienced by the individual usually develop gradually and are vague and general in nature. Knowledge of the clinical characteristics of altered thyroid function assists the nurse to organize data collection, to formulate specific questions for the health history and to identify patterns of responses demonstrated by the patient. Table 19.2 lists the common health problems experienced by persons with thyroid disorders and the clinical characteristics of hypothyroidism and hyperthyroidism.

Health history

The patient is asked about changes in physical appearance, activity tolerance and energy level, skin moisture, muscle tone, body weight, diet, menstrual cycle and thought processes. Specific questions related to usual and current daily routine and activity patterns and how the individual organizes the day may provide clues to subtle changes and how the person is compensating. With questioning, the person may recognize that they have become more forgetful and have compensated for the changes by instituting reminders for themselves to keep appointments and fulfil commitments. They may also recognize insidious changes in physical activity and usual exercise patterns. Other specific information includes any difficulty swallowing, episodes of palpitations, prescription and non-prescription medications taken and any family history of thyroid disease. It is important to identify the onset and duration of the symptoms.

Physical examination

Physical examination begins with observation of the person's *general appearance*. Changes which may indicate decreased thyroid function are paleness, facial puffiness and a non-expressive appearance. The person with increased thyroid function may appear anxious and agitated and their eyeballs may protrude.

The *skin* and *hair* are inspected for dryness, brittleness and texture. The density and pattern of hair distribution are noted.

Vital signs are measured as changes in respiratory rate and depth, blood pressure and cardiac rate and rhythm may be present.

The *thyroid gland* is observed by facing the patient and asking the person to extend the neck slightly and

Table 19.3 Diagnostic measurements of thyroid function.

Diagnostic tests	Normal value	Description
Serum thyroxine (T_4)	50–150 mmol/l	The total amount of thyroid hormone in the blood
Thyroid stimulating hormone (TSH) radioimmunoassay	0–7 µu/ml	The serum level of TSH
Serum tri-iodothyronine test (T_3)	1.2–3.1 nmol/l	Radioimmunoassay to determine the serum level of T_3
Thyrotrophin-releasing hormone (TRH) test	Increased levels of TSH	The thyrotropic cells are normally stimulated by the intravenous administration of synthetic TRH to release TSH
Radioactive iodine thyroid uptake (RAIU)	At 24 hours: 7–25% absorbed	Determines the rate at which the thyroid removes iodine from the blood and uses it
T_3 suppression test	25% decrease in radioiodine uptake in the second test	A 24–hour radioiodine uptake is followed by daily administration of thyroid hormone for 7 days. The radioiodine uptake test is then repeated
T_3 resin uptake test	25–35%	T_3 tagged with radioiodine is added to a specimen of the patient's blood. The amount of binding by the erythrocytes is noted
Thyroid scan	Symmetrical with no areas of increased density	A scan is made of the thyroid following administration of a tracer dose of ^{99m}Tc
Achilles tendon reflex time	240–380 ms	The relaxation time is prolonged in hypothyroidism and more rapid and greater in hyperthyroidism
Thyroid stimulation test	A normal radioiodine uptake and normal protein-bound iodine indicate the problem is related to secretion of TSH and not thyroid function	The response of the thyroid to an injection of TSH is measured by a radioactive uptake or a serum protein-bound iodine estimation
Thyroid antibody test	Increased levels demonstrate involvement of immune system	Antibodies commonly measured are thyroglobin, thyroid microsomes, thyroid colloidal proteins and antinuclear antibodies

swallow a sip of water. The neck is observed for movement of cartilages and muscles and the shape and contour of any mass. Normally the thyroid gland is not observed and is not palpable. The gland is palpated using either a posterior or anterior approach by placing the fingers of both hands on the sides of the patient's neck with the finger tips meeting in the centre. The patient is asked to swallow to facilitate palpation during movement. If the gland is felt, the degree of firmness of the tissue and the presence of any nodules are noted.

Diagnostic measurements

The various medical tests that may be performed are summarized in Table 19.3.

Hypothyroidism

Hypothyroidism is a common disorder characterized by a hypometabolic state. It is more common in females and can occur at any age but the incidence is higher in the elderly.

CAUSES AND CONTRIBUTING FACTORS

The deficiency of thyroid hormones may be primary, due to a disorder in the thyroid itself, or may be secondary as a result of a pituitary or hypothalamic disturbance. If the dysfunction is congenital or develops in infancy or early childhood, it gives rise to cretinism which is characterized by a failure to achieve normal physical growth and mental development. In the adult it produces myxoedema.

Primary hypothyroidism accounts for about 95% of the cases of hypothyroidism in adults. It is due to destruction of thyroid tissue by disease or surgery. Autoimmune thyroid disease (Hashimoto's thyroiditis) is the most common cause of hypothyroidism.

A less common cause is iodine deficiency, which produces an enlargement of the thyroid gland or a goitre. The enlargement of the thyroid in iodine deficiency occurs because of stimulation by an increased release of TSH by the anterior pituitary in response to the low thyroxine concentration of the blood. The follicles increase in number and size and the thyroid becomes more vascular. If the iodine deficiency and excessive TSH stimulation are prolonged, the gland tends to develop nodules which contain greatly distended follicles that may eventually undergo degeneration.

A deficiency in the natural supply of iodine in the water and soil occurs in inland areas distant from the sea (e.g. Derbyshire). The addition of iodine to the salt used in food has largely eliminated this once endemic cause of hypothyroidism.

Other factors which contribute to the development of hypothyroidism include the use of antithyroid drugs such as the thiocarbamides, sulphonylureas, lithium and iodine. Excessive and regular use of substances found in goitrogenic foods such as cabbage, broccoli, turnips, cauliflower, Brussels sprouts, carrots, soyabeans, spinach, peaches and pears inhibits hormone synthesis.

CLINICAL CHARACTERISTICS

A decreased production of T_3 and T_4 influences most metabolic processes of the body, resulting in many and varied manifestations.

The symptoms and the rate at which they develop correspond to the degree of thyroid inactivity (see Table 19.2). An abnormal decrease in thyroid hormone causes a general reduction in cellular metabolism, producing mental and physical sluggishness. The person gradually exhibits apathy and slowness in responses. An abnormal deposition of a mucopolysaccharide, which tends to hold water, occurs in the subcutaneous tissues, giving the person an oedematous appearance. The skin becomes dry and thick, the face (particularly the eyelids) appears puffy and the lips and tongue enlarge. The person experiences weakness, fatigue and an increased sensitivity to cold, and appetite is poor although there may be a gain in weight. The temperature, pulse and blood pressure may be abnormally low. Mental processes are slow and the patient sleeps a great deal. Impaired function of the reproductive system is manifested by menstrual disorders, such as metrorrhagia and amenorrhoea, and loss of sexual drive. Hoarseness and slow, monotonous speech may be noted. Because of complacency and dull mental processes, the condition may appear to be of much less concern to the patient than to the family or friends witnessing the changes. Allowed to progress, the disorder may lead to arteriosclerotic changes, cardiac insufficiency, depression and psychosis with hallucinations and delusions ('myxoedema madness'), or the patient may pass into a comatose state.

Severe hypothyroidism may be complicated by coma, which may be precipitated by exposure to cold, infection, trauma or the taking of medications which depress the central nervous system. Older persons with hypothyroidism are more predisposed to develop coma. Their temperature falls to hypothermic levels and respiratory insufficiency may develop.

With a goitre, the enlarged gland may cause disfigurement which creates embarrassment for the person. More serious symptoms are pressure on the larynx and trachea, manifested by a chronic cough and respiratory difficulty, interference with swallowing, and compression of nerves in the area.

TREATMENT

Hypothyroidism is treated favourably in uncomplicated cases with thyroxine. In cases where there are complications, such as ischaemic heart disease, tri-iodothyronine (T_3) may be given. T_3 acts very rapidly, but the effect is sustained for a shorter period than thyroxine which is not fully effective before 7–10 days. The dosage is usually small to start with and is gradually increased to guard against a too sudden and excessive demand on the heart by rapid acceleration of metabolism. The pulse is checked and recorded frequently until the maintenance dose is established. Drug therapy is essentially replacement of naturally occurring hormones. Adverse effects are almost entirely related to underreplacement with the symptoms of hypothyroidism remaining, or overreplacement, producing symptoms of hyperthyroidism. Allergic reactions are rare. It takes several months to achieve metabolic equilibrium. The maintenance dose is individualized on the basis of the person's responses and on levels of TSH and T_4 and T_3. Elderly persons usually require smaller doses. Drug replacement is life-long.

NURSING INTERVENTION

It may be necessary for the nurse to explain the condition to the patient and family and emphasize that replacement therapy must be continued indefinitely. The patient may neglect to take the medication if feeling better. During the myxoedematous state, it is important that the family appreciate that the patient's lethargy and dullness are a part of the disease. The nurse, the patient and the family must be tolerant of this slowness, and encouragement and time should be given to complete responses and activities. Early indications of improvement and response to the drug therapy may be pointed out as reassurance that the physical condition is reversible although depression does not always resolve.

Much of the nursing care is symptomatic. For example, extra warmth is provided because of the patient's lower heat production and consequent decreased tolerance to cold. Without extra clothing and bedding, the person may be uncomfortable in an environmental temperature that is comfortable to others. A minimum of soap is used on the patient's skin, and oily lotions or creams are applied to relieve the dryness. The diet should be low in calories to decrease and/or maintain body weight; low in fat and cholesterol because of the accompanying increase in serum cholesterol; and high in fibre with increased fluid intake to promote bowel function. Laxatives or enemas may be necessary to maintain adequate bowel elimination. The hypothyroid patient is seen at the outpatient clinic or by the general practitioner at regular intervals; adjustment of the drug dosage is necessary from time to time.

The patient with hypothyroidism must learn self-management in relation to the drug therapy and symptom control. Teaching is individualized and planned according to the identified needs of the individual, the severity of symptoms, the impact the disorder is having on the person's life and daily functioning, and the ability of the family to adjust to the changes in the patient prior to achieving control and during episodes when readjustment of the treatment plan is necessary.

CLINICAL SITUATION: MRS JANE GREEN WHO HAS HYPOTHYROIDISM

Mrs Green is a 34-year-old wife, mother and office manager. She and her husband Robert, an engineer, usually share household tasks and child care activities and like to participate in outings which include their 4-year-old and 8-month-old sons.

Jane makes an appointment to see you as practice nurse. She tells you that she is having difficulty balancing her job and her family life since returning to full-time work after the birth of her last child. She is constantly tired and falls asleep each evening while reading bedtime stories to the children. She feels pressured by the demands of her job and is concerned that she is becoming forgetful and disorganized.

You question Jane about any physical and emotional changes she has experienced since the birth of the baby and discover that: Jane has not been able to lose the extra weight she had gained; her menstrual periods are still not regular; her hair and skin have become very dry; she feels cold and wears an extra sweater, socks or other clothing to keep warm; she is frequently constipated; and she feels she is pushing herself to get through the day. She states that her husband complains about her disinterest and feels that she is not fulfilling her share of household tasks. Following discussion with her general practitioner (GP) you take blood, and arrange for Jane to see her GP.

On Jane's next visit to the surgery, her GP, on reviewing the health history and the results of Jane's laboratory tests concludes that Jane has primary hypothyroidism. The test results are: TSH 16 µu/ml; T_4 55 mmol/l; T_3 1.5 mmol/l. Jane is to begin thyroid replacement treatment with thyroxine 0.025 mg daily. The dose is to be adjusted in 3–4 weeks according to her serum TSH level and response to drug therapy.

You meet with Jane and mutually set the following learning objectives. Jane will be able to:

- Understand the reasons for the physical and behavioural changes she has been experiencing.
- Take her prescribed hormone replacement regularly, safely and knowledgeably.
- Recognize the clinical signs and symptoms of hypothyroidism.
- Discuss actions to take to alleviate the health problems she is experiencing related to changes in *activity tolerance, temperature regulation, nutrition, constipation, skin integrity, sexual pattern* and *thought processes*.

Jane's lethargy, decreased attention span and distress at her diagnosis are impeding her ability to comprehend instructions at this time. It was agreed that you review her medication plan and answer immediate concerns.

Thyroid hormone replacement. The medication is taken daily on an empty stomach. Jane decides that she will take her tablet as soon as she wakes up each morning. You tell her not to exceed the prescribed dose and explain the importance of continuing with drug therapy. You review the signs of under replacement which are the same symptoms that Jane is presently experiencing. The half-life of thyroxine is 6–7 days therefore Jane should not expect immediate relief from her symptoms. You explain to Jane that her blood pressure and pulse rate will be monitored on each visit. She is currently hypotensive and her pulse is slow at 60 per minute. As her hormone levels rise, her pulse and blood pressure should return to her usual levels. Since Jane is not taking any other prescription or non-prescription medications she does not need to be cautioned about the fact that thyroxine potentiates the effects of anticoagulants, insulin and oral hypoglycaemic agents.

It is agreed that on a later visit you will discuss the symptoms of overreplacement and any concerns Jane has after starting her hormone replacement.

Evaluation. Jane returns to the surgery in 3 weeks with her husband. At this time her symptoms are beginning to abate. She is still extremely tired and sensitive to cold but is taking more interest in family and work activities. You discuss the function of the thyroid gland and its hormones and help Jane and her husband to understand the cause of her symptoms. You emphasize that although she will require hormone replacement for life her symptoms can be controlled and she should return to her previous level of functioning. She requires regular medical supervision to monitor her control and to make periodic adjustments in her hormone replacement. Jane's husband is encouraged to learn about her responses to decreased thyroid hormone levels and the symptoms of hyperthyroidism so he can help Jane to recognize changes and to seek further medical evaluation. An appointment is made for Jane to meet the dietician to discuss her dietary needs. She is taking her medication regularly. The increase in the dose prescribed by her GP is explained to her. Her blood pressure is 115/80 and her pulse rate is 72 per minute. Arrangements are made to review Jane's learning needs on her next visit.

Hyperthyroidism

Hyperthroidism implies an excessive secretion of the thyroid hormones and may be called *thyrotoxicosis, toxic goitre, exophthalmic goitre* or *Graves' disease*. The terms exophthalmic goitre, or Graves' disease are reserved for hyperthyrodism that is accompanied by exophthalmos and extreme nervousness.

CAUSES

The exact cause of hyperactivity of the thyroid in most patients is not clear. In many cases it is thought to be due to autoimmunity. Thyroid-stimulating immunoglobulins (TSI) are found in almost all people with Graves' disease. Excessive secretion of TSH by the pituitary gland may also cause enlargement of the thyroid gland and thyroiditis. Overreplacement of thyroid hormones is the most common iatrogenic cause of hyperthyroidism. Hyperthyroidism affects females more often than males, and is rare in childhood. Frequently, the onset is closely related to an emotional crisis in the person's life.

CLINICAL CHARACTERISTICS

Some enlargement of the gland may be evident owing to a diffuse hyperplasia of the gland or the development of one or more adenomas. It may be readily seen to move upward with the larynx in swallowing.

The increased blood level of thyroid hormones accelerates the metabolic rate. The patient's appetite increases and, unless the food intake keeps pace with the rapid metabolic rate, there is a marked loss of weight. Lowered heat tolerance and excessive sweating are manifested. The hyperthyroid patient is uncomfortably warm in an environmental temperature quite acceptable to others.

Nervousness, apprehension, emotional instability and restlessness are evident, and the hands are warm and moist in contrast to the cold, moist extremities associated with anxiety. Despite eating more, the patient may complain of weakness and quick fatigue. The pulse is rapid and exhibits a sharp rise on exertion. The increased pulse rate is due to the increased metabolic demands and the effect of thyroxine on the sympathetic nervous system. Shortness of breath on exertion and palpitation are experienced as a result of the increased metabolic rate. The diastolic blood pressure is usually lower than normal because of widespread vasodilation. A fine, rapid tremor develops in the hands and is accentuated when they are outstretched. Diarrhoea, resulting from increased gastrointestinal activity, may be troublesome. Menstrual disorders, such as oligomenorrhoea (scant flow) or amenorrhoea, are common (see Table 19.2).

Eye changes may appear in hyperthyroidism. Exophthalmus may be evident when the upper eyelids are retracted, showing the upper sclerae, and the eyes appear to be protruding. The lids fail to follow the movement of the eyes when the person looks down (lid lag).

TREATMENT

Hyperthyroidism may be treated by antithyroid drugs, radioactive iodine (^{131}I) or surgery.

Drug therapy

The drugs most commonly used suppress the formation of the thyroid hormones. They may be used alone or as an interim treatment prior to surgery; they include carbimazole and propylthiouracil. The drug is generally taken over a prolonged period of 1–2 years if the patient remains free of side-effects. These antithyroid drugs are potentially toxic. Side-effects which may develop are dermatitis, agranulocytosis and fever. Rarely, hepatitis, joint and muscle pain and neuritis have been reported. The patient is advised to report promptly a sore throat, swollen tender 'neck glands', fever, rash or jaundice. It is important that the patient understand the necessity for taking the drugs regularly and at the hours suggested in order to obtain the desired effect and prevent a remission. Some compensatory enlargement of the gland may occur and the patient is reassured that this is not serious.

The patient is followed closely; weekly visits to the general practitioner or clinic are usually required for 4–6 weeks and the interval is gradually lengthened. A blood specimen is taken for determination of serum levels of T_4, T_3 and TSH, and a leucocyte count is made on each visit. The reports may indicate a need for an adjustment in the dosage of the anti-thyroid drug.

Drug therapy may be given to reduce the hyperthyroid patient's nervousness and agitation; for example, propranolol a β-adrenergic blocking agent may be prescribed to treat some of the toxic manifestations of hyperthyroidism. It decreases the heart rate and rapidly abates the fever of thyrotoxicosis.

Radiation treatment

Iodine-131 therapy of hyperthyroidism is being used in many patients as an alternative to antithyroid drugs. This is particularly useful in patients who fail to respond to the usual doses of antithyroid drugs or who are unable to tolerate these drugs. Treatment by radioiodine is very simple. It is given orally and is trapped in the thyroid, where its radiations destroy tissue, reducing the functioning mass. Improvement is usually evident in 3 weeks and the metabolic rate is expected to reach a normal level in 2–3 months. Radioiodine is not generally given for therapeutic purposes to persons who are likely to want to have children, and is never given during pregnancy. The therapeutic dose is not considered large enough to constitute a radiation hazard to those in the person's environment.

The patient is observed closely for signs of aggravation of the disease and thyroiditis, manifested by tenderness and soreness in the area of the gland. Rarely, a thyroid crisis may develop (see p. 587). After receiving the ^{131}I, regular visits to the clinic or the doctor are necessary. The patient is examined for remission of the disease and for possible hypothyroidism. The serum T_3, T_4 and TSH levels are determined. If hypothyroidism is indicated, a replacement preparation (e.g. a thyroxine preparation) is prescribed.

Surgical therapy

A partial thyroidectomy may be done if radioactive iodine is contraindicated: for example if the patient is young, if antithyroid drug therapy has failed, if sensitivity precludes its prolonged administration, or if the gland is very large, causing disfigurement or pressure on the respiratory tract or on the oesophagus. In hyperthyroidism, approximately three-quarters of the gland is removed; in the case of cancer of the thyroid, a complete thyroidectomy is done, which necessitates continuous replacement drug therapy during the remainder of the patient's life.

NURSING ASSESSMENT

An accurate record of the person's temperature, pulse and respirations is made at least every 4 hours, and the responses and degree of restlessness and agitation are noted frequently. This is necessary so that an early indication of increasing thyrotoxicosis and cardiac insufficiency may be recognized and receive prompt attention. The patient is told that the vital signs will be checked at regular intervals, to avoid undue apprehension associated with such frequent checking. The doctor may request the recording of a sleeping pulse; in hyperthyroidism, the elevated rate persists during sleep. The patient is weighed daily or every second day to determine if calorie intake is keeping pace with metabolic rate. Reactions to visitors are noted; an elevation in pulse rate and increased agitation and excitement may indicate the need for additional limitations on visitors.

PATIENT PROBLEMS

The patient with hyperthyroidism is expending energy in excess of the body's ability to produce energy. Metabolic processes are increased, requiring more calories to prevent excessive weight loss. Environmental stimuli increase energy demands further. Health problems which are experienced by the person with hyperthyroidism are listed in Table 19.2.

GOALS

The patient and family will be able to:

- Understand the reasons for the physical and behavioural changes.
- Recognize the clinical signs and symptoms of hyperthyroidism.
- Describe the prescribed medication and/or treatment plan.
- Describe the expected and possible adverse responses to therapy.
- Discuss actions to take to alleviate the health problems experienced in relation to changes in *thought processes and emotional responses, nutrition, activity tolerance, thermoregulation, skin and eye integrity, sexual pattern and body image.*
- Describe plans for ongoing therapy and health supervision.

NURSING INTERVENTION

1. *Altered thought processes and emotional responses.* The *goal* is that the patient will appear less anxious.

- *Environment.* Because of the patient's nervousness and hyperexcitability, quietness is very important. An established routine may prevent unnecessary disturbance which only aggravates the condition. If the patient is being cared for at home, the family is made fully aware of these needs. They are advised that irritability, restlessness and emotional lability are characteristic of the illness and are helped to develop strategies to cope with the situation and to avoid upsetting the individual.
  In the hospital careful consideration should be given to placement on the ward. Exposure to very ill, talkative or otherwise disturbing patients should be avoided.
- *Information.* The nurse explains all procedures and medical treatment to the patient and family and answers questions regarding care. They receive an explanation of the disease, the cause of symptoms, what to expect from treatment and are taught measures to relieve symptoms. The nurse works in a calm, quiet, competent manner and, whenever possible, the same nurse cares for the patient, since adjusting to strange personnel may be stressful.
- *Identification of additional stresses.* The nurse works with the patient and family to identify additional stresses that may have resulted from the patient's illness or existed previously. Referrals to community resources are made if relevant.
- *Visitors.* Visitors and family members require information on the need for limiting visitors and

suggestions as to how they can best contribute to the patient's well-being and avoid aggravating the condition.

2. *Altered nutrition.* The *goal* is that the patient will maintain or increase body weight.

- *Diet.* The patient requires a high-protein, high-carbohydrate, high-calorie diet (4000–5000 kcal) to prevent tissue breakdown by the high metabolic demand and to satisfy the patient's increased appetite. A snack between meals and at bedtime is provided. Tea and coffee are usually restricted to eliminate caffeine stimulation. Decaffeinated coffee may be used as a substitute.
- *Fluids.* The patient's excessive heat production and resulting perspiration increases fluid loss, necessitating extra fluids. Also, there is an increased production of metabolic wastes, requiring dilution for elimination by the kidneys. A minimum intake of 3000–4000 ml daily is recommended, unless contraindicated by cardiac or renal dysfunction. An explanation of the importance of this amount of fluid is made to the patient to gain co-operation, and a variety of fluids are provided.

3. *Hyperactivity and fatigue.* The *goal* is that the patient will decrease energy expenditure.

- *Rest and activity.* Activity is restricted because it increases the metabolic rate, but the patient's nervous excitability makes it difficult to rest. Efforts are made to provide some quiet activity such as reading that expends little energy. The patient is helped to plan activities and daily routines to obtain sufficient rest.

  Activities requiring fine motor movements are kept to a minimum. When necessary, assistance is provided by the family or nurse.

4. *Altered thermoregulation.* The *goal* is that the patient will state that he or she feels comfortably cool.

  Since the patient is producing more than the normal amount of body heat, comfort will only be achieved in an environment of lower temperature than normal. Scant, lightweight clothing is used and the room is kept well-ventilated and cool.

5. *Altered skin and eye integrity.* The *goals* are that the patient will maintain skin integrity and avoid injury to the eyes.

- *Skin care.* A daily bath is necessary because of the profuse perspiration. If the patient is extremely restless, has lost weight and has decreased mobility, special attention is given to the pressure areas.
- *Eye care.* If the patient has exophthalmos, the eyes should be protected from irritation by sunglasses. Methylcellulose (a conjunctival lubricant) drops (0.5–1%) may be recommended to prevent drying of the conjunctiva and cornea. The patient's vision is tested frequently, especially if the exophthalmos is progressive; compression of the optic nerve and artery may occur, with ensuing visual impairment.

6. *Altered sexual patterns and self-image.* The *goal* is that the patient will express concerns regarding alterations in body image and changes in sexual patterns.

  The patient and partner are helped to understand that the changes in menstrual cycle, low sex drive and/or impotence are a result of the hyperthyroidism and that they will abate or disappear once thyroid hormonal balance is achieved.

  Repeated explanations of the causes of the physical changes and assurance should be given. There is a prolonged phase of gradual improvement of the eyes once the hormone imbalance is corrected. It should be said, however, that the eyes may not return to the normal state. Good grooming and attractive dress promote self-confidence and the feeling of wellness.

7. *Knowledge deficit* related to the disease process, therapeutic plan and self management. The *goal* is that the patient will achieve self-management of the therapeutic regimen and self-care.

  The patient and family are given information about hyperthyroidism, causes, manifestations and treatment. Learning needs are assessed and they are assisted in developing a plan for home care of the patient. The dietitian may be consulted about diet and meal planning.

Evaluation

The physical and behavioral changes that the person is experiencing should begin to diminish with treatment. With drug therapy, clinical improvement should be apparent after several weeks. The dose of the medication will then be decreased by the doctor according to symptomatic changes and decreases in the T_4 level. The person should begin to regain weight. As weight approaches the person's desirable level, and energy expenditure is consistent and within usual parameters, the diet is adjusted and caloric intake decreased.

The patient and family should demonstrate understanding of the hyperthyroidism, the treatment plan and medication regimen. They should be able to describe and implement measures to alleviate symptoms by: (1) the provision of a quiet, cool environment; (2) the avoidance of undue stress; (3) provision for sufficient rest and sleep and decreased physical activity; (4) adequate caloric and fluid intake; (5) maintenance of dry clean skin; and (6) protection of the eyes. The person should verbalize a decrease in anxiety and begin to take responsibility for self-care.

The Person Having Thyroid Surgery

In caring for the patient who has had a thyroidectomy, pertinent factors to be kept in mind are: the *location of the gland in relation to the trachea and larynx*; its *proximity to the recurrent laryngeal nerve*, which controls the vocal cords; its *abundant blood supply*; and that the *parathyroid glands*, which influence neuromuscular irritability through their control of the blood calcium level, lie on the posterior surface of the thyroid. The nurse must be constantly alert for manifestations of disturbances due to these factors.

PREOPERATIVE PREPARATION

The hyperthyroid patient who is to have surgery is given an antithyroid drug for several weeks prior to operation to reduce the metabolic rate, and return the gland to as near the euthyroid state as possible; alternatively propranolol in increasing dosage is given, until effective β-blockade has been achieved. During this period, whether at home or in the hospital, the care cited in the preceding section is applicable. The antithyroid drugs produce some compensatory enlargement of the gland and an increased blood supply. When the metabolic rate has been reduced to a satisfactory level, the drug is discontinued. Then, in a few days, a course of potassium iodide (Lugol's iodine) is commenced and continued for approximately 10 days. This reduces the size and vascularity of the gland, facilitating surgery and lessening the problem of bleeding. Since potassium iodide has a disagreeable taste and may also irritate the mucous membrane, it is well diluted in fruit juice or milk.

Preparation includes an electrocardiogram to obtain further information about the patient's cardiac status and blood typing and cross matching for transfusion. The female patient may have some concern for the cosmetic effect of the operation. She is assured that consideration is given to this and that the scar becomes barely perceptible in a few months. During the interval, it may be concealed by a scarf or necklace. Remembering that the hyperthyroid patient may be hyperexcitable and apprehensive, judicious explanations are made of what may be expected after the operation. Demonstration and practice in supporting the head with the hands while turning in bed is carried out to decrease stress on the neck.

PREPARATION TO RECEIVE THE PATIENT AFTER OPERATION

Special equipment to be assembled and ready for use when preparing to receive a patient following a thyroidectomy includes: (1) sandbags or small firm pillows to immobilize the head; (2) suction equipment and catheters for clearing mucus from the throat; (3) sterile clip removers or stitch cutters in case of a haematoma at the site of surgery obstructing the trachea by compression; (4) a humidifier to relieve tracheal and laryngeal irritation and facilitate the removal of mucus; (5) intravenous infusion equipment; (6) a sterile emergency intubation and tracheostomy tray in the event of respiratory obstruction; (7) equipment for obtaining a blood specimen quickly for blood calcium determination; and (8) ampoules of calcium chloride or calcium gluconate, with the necessary equipment for intravenous administration in the event of the complication of tetany (hypocalcaemia).

POSTOPERATIVE CARE

The patient is usually very apprehensive, and serious complications may *develop rapidly*. Table 19.4 lists potential problems and their causative factors relevant to the patient following thyroid surgery.

Assessment

The blood pressure, pulse and respirations are recorded every 15 minutes; the frequency is gradually reduced if they remain stable. The body temperature is recorded every 4 hours. The degree of restlessness and apprehension is noted and, if not relieved by the prescribed sedation, is brought to the surgeon's attention. Particular attention is paid to the patient's respirations; any complaint or sign of respiratory distress and cyanosis is reported promptly, since it may indicate laryngeal paralysis or compression of the trachea by accumulating blood. Some hoarseness is common and is due to irritation of the larynx by the surgery and the endotracheal tube used in administering the anaesthetic. The doctor is advised if the horseness and weakness of the voice persist beyond 3 or 4 days.

Potential patient problems (see Table 19.4)

1. Obstructed airway, because of:
   (a) Oedema, decreased head and neck mobility and

Table 19.4 Identification of patients' problems following thyroid surgery.

Patient problem	Causes
1. Ineffective airway clearance	• Haematoma pressing on trachea • Tracheobronchial irritation from anaesthesia • Difficulty in coughing up bronchial secretions because of oedema, pressure and pain at operation site, decreased head and neck mobility
2. Alteration in comfort: pain	• Surgical intervention
3. Wound healing	• Surgical intervention • Pain and discomfort
4. Altered nutrition: intake of less than body requirements	• Difficulty in swallowing
5. Potential complications (haemorrhage, respiratory distress, loss of voice or tetany)	• Surgical intervention to neck
6. Knowledge deficit related to follow-up care	• Lack of information, experience and resources

tracheal-bronchial secretions from the anaesthetic, which all contribute to a difficulty in expectorating secretions.
(b) Haematoma formation behind the wound site pressing on the trachea.
2. Pain related to surgical intervention.
3. Impaired mobility of head, neck and shoulders related to surgical intervention, pain and discomfort.
4. Inadequate nutrition because of difficulty in swallowing.
5. Potential for injury (complications) as a result of the surgical intervention.
6. Inadequate knowledge about follow-up care.

Goals

Following thyroid surgery, the patient will be able to:

- Maintain a patent airway.
- State that pain is absent.
- Assume self-care activities.
- Achieve and maintain desirable body weight.
- Demonstrate ability to safely perform neck exercises.
- Describe a plan for follow-up care.

Nursing intervention

1. *Ineffective airway clearance.* The *goal* is that the patient will maintain a patent airway.

- The patient is assisted to a sitting position with support given to the head and neck in order to help the patient to cough and expectorate. Suction of the oropharynx is carried out if the accumulation of secretions is severe. Deep breathing and coughing should be encouraged several times each hour.
- The nurse should observe the wound and ensure free drainage from the wound drains is maintained (see below under Complications) to prevent the formation of a haematoma.

2. *Pain.* The *goal* is that the patient will state that pain is absent. Pethidine or morphine may be ordered to keep the patient comfortable and less apprehensive during the first 48 hours. Narcotics should be administered regularly and consistently to control pain. Respirations are assessed for evidence of a decrease in rate or depth.

3. *Wound healing.* The *goal* is that the wound will heal and the patient will maintain range of movement of the neck.

After recovery from the anaesthetic, the patient is placed on his back and the head of the bed is moderately elevated to facilitate breathing. The head and neck are supported by a pillow and are positioned in good alignment, preventing flexion and hyperextension. When the patient's position is changed, the nurse lifts and supports the head, preserving good alignment. The patient is taught to lift and support the head by placing the hands at the back of the head when wishing to move.

The patient often returns from the operating theatre with surgical drains inserted. These should be checked at intervals to ensure free drainage and, if a closed system, that the mechanism is functioning. While large accumulation of blood behind the wound site can cause respiratory obstruction, smaller haematomas can increase vulnerability to infection and delayed wound healing.

If the vital signs are stabilized and normal, the patient is assisted out of bed on the first post-operative day.

Following removal of the drains, the sutures or skin clips and firm healing of the incision, head exercises, which include flexion (forward and lateral), hyperextension and turning, are gradually introduced with the surgeon's approval. To prevent contraction of the scar, the patient may be taught to massage the neck gently twice daily, using lanolin, cold cream or an oily lotion.

4. *Altered nutrition.* The *goal* is that the patient will maintain adequate food intake.

Some difficulty in swallowing is usually experienced for a day or two, but fluids by mouth are encouraged as soon as tolerated. Intravenous fluids are given until an adequate amount can be taken orally. The patient progresses through a soft diet to a full diet in 2–3 days.

5. *Potential complications.* The *goal* is that complications will be promptly identified and corrected.

- The nurse must be aware that haemorrhage, respiratory difficulty, loss of voice and tetany are serious complications which may occur following thyroid surgery. The first three may develop with startling rapidity and are usually seen within 48 hours of operation.
- *Haemorrhage* may be manifested by a rapid pulse, fall in blood pressure and evident bleeding. The bleeding may only be discovered by frequent checking of the dressing and by sliding the hands under the shoulders and behind the neck. Blood may collect quickly within the tissues and cause pressure on the trachea. The patient may complain of a choking sensation and shortness of breath; cyanosis and dyspnoea develop and, unless the pressure is relieved quickly, asphyxia may occur. The surgeon is notified immediately at the earliest sign of change. The dressing is loosened to promote freer, outward drainage. Instruments for removing the sutures or skin clips should already be at the bedside and the emergency tracheostomy tray is made ready, since the surgeon may consider an immediate tracheostomy necessary. On reporting the situation, the nurse may be instructed to remove the skin clips to allow the escape of blood. A thick sterile dressing is then applied until the surgeon arrives. The patient will probably be returned to the operating theatre to bring the bleeding under control. Blood replacement may be necessary.
- Occasionally, *injury to one or both recurrent laryngeal nerves* may occur during thyroid surgery. These nerves control laryngeal muscles, the opening of the glottis and voice production. Injury to one nerve produces hoarseness and weakness of the voice but no serious respiratory disturbance. Bilateral nerve injury causes paralysis of muscles on both sides of the larynx, resulting in closure of the glottis and

respiratory obstruction. The patient is unable to speak and stridor occurs (i.e. respirations become shrill and crowing), cyanosis develops and loss of consciousness ensues unless respirations are quickly re-established. Prompt endotracheal intubation or emergency tracheostomy is done, and oxygen is administered via either tube. The injury and paralysis are rarely permanent; function is usually gradually restored, and the tracheostomy tube is removed.

- During surgery, interference with the blood supply to the parathyroid glands or injury or removal of parathyroid tissue may occur which depresses secretion by the glands. Decreased parathyroid hormone concentration leads to *hypocalcaemia*, resulting in increased neuromuscular irritability and the condition known as *tetany*. Early signs of this complication include complaints of numbness and tingling in the hands or feet, muscle twitching and spasms, and gastrointestinal cramps. A change may be evident in the voice; it may become high-pitched and shrill because of spasm of the vocal cords. To confirm increased neuromuscular irritability due to hypocalcaemia, the patient is examined for a positive Chvostek's or Trousseau's sign. Chvostek's sign is demonstrated by twitching of the upper lip and contraction of the facial muscles in response to tapping of the facial nerve in front of the ear. Trousseau's sign is elicited by the inflation of a blood pressure cuff around an arm; if the blood calcium level is low, spasmodic contraction of the forearm muscles occurs, producing a claw-like flexure of the hand and fingers. A blood specimen is obtained for serum calcium determination with the appearance of early symptoms. Calcium gluconate 10% may be slowly administered intravenously by the doctor; then, an oral preparation is given until normal parathyroid function resumes. The patient is encouraged to take milk and calcium-containing foods.
- *Thyrotoxicosis* or thyroid crisis rarely complicates the postoperative period following a thyroidectomy. This emergency situation is attributed to (1) the release of a large amount of thyroid hormone into the circulation to produce a hypermetabolic state; (2) adrenergic hyperactivity which may potentiate the hypersecretion of thyroid hormone; and (3) excessive lipolysis and fatty acid production which cause an increase in oxygen consumption and thermogenesis (Evangelisti and Thorpe, 1983). The patient's symptoms develop abruptly and change quickly, requiring constant monitoring and intensive nursing intervention.

6. *Knowledge deficit related to follow-up care.* The goal is that the patient will verbalize understanding of a plan for post-hospital care and follow-up.

The patient's hospitalization is usually brief if no complications develop. Information as to the amount of activity that may be resumed is discussed with the patient. Extra rest will still be necessary, and the patient is advised to continue neck exercises until there is freedom of movement without any feeling of pulling. Follow-up is usually at the out-patient clinic for about a year, checking for any residual laryngeal damage,

hypoparathyroidism, recurring hyperthyroidism, or developing hypothyroidism. If no problems develop during that year, an annual checkup is then recommended. Information is provided on the administration and effects of prescribed thyroid hormone replacement. Following a total thyroidectomy, hormone replacement will be life long.

Evaluation

Following a thyroidectomy the patient will show absence of complications: the serum calcium level will be within normal range, Chvostek's and Trousseau's signs will be negative and there will be no muscle twitching, hoarseness or breathing difficulties. The patient and family will describe plans for follow-up care and demonstrate understanding of the prescribed neck exercises, medication schedule and other self-care activities.

THE PERSON WITH DISORDERS OF THE PARATHYROID GLANDS

Primary disease of the parathyroid glands is rare; the disturbances seen are most often secondary to thyroid disease.

ASSESSMENT OF PARATHYROID FUNCTION

The *health history* begins with the collection of information related to the health problems experienced by the individual. Table 19.5 lists health problems common to individuals with increased and decreased parathyroid function. The nurse asks specific questions to determine: the presence, duration and severity of the associated signs and symptoms; vitamin D and calcium intake; the use of drugs such as thiazide diuretics; and any history of renal calculi. The person is asked about any family history of metabolic bone disease, endocrine tumours, renal calculi, hypercalcaemia or intractable peptic ulcer disease.

Physical examination of the gland is not possible. The nurse inspects the person's skin, hair and nails for specific changes. Muscle tone, spasms, increase or slowness of reflexes and bone tenderness are assessed. The person's blood pressure is measured as elevations occur with hyperparathyroidism.

Hypoparathyroidism

CAUSES

Parathyroid insufficiency may be the result of idiopathic atrophy of the glands or surgery on the thyroid. In the case of surgery, there may have been interference with the blood supply to the glands, injury which inhibits secretion or, rarely, inadvertent removal of them.

·CLINICAL CHARACTERISTICS

The deficiency of PTH causes hypocalcaemia. Symptoms of increased neuromuscular excitability and tetany are

Table 19.5 Assessment of the person with altered parathyroid function.

Patient problems	Clinical characteristics of hypoparathyroidism	Clinical characteristics of hyperparathyroidism
1. Altered activity tolerance	• Muscular cramps and spasms • Numbness and tingling of extremities • Tetany	• Muscle weakness and fatigue • Decreased muscle tone • Bone tenderness and pain on weightbearing • Pathological fractures
2. Altered thought process and emotional response	• Irritability, agitation • Depression • Psychosis • Slow mental processes • Anxiety	• Lethargy • Drowsiness • Impaired memory • Disorientation
3. Altered nutrition	• Nausea and vomiting • Abdominal cramping	• Loss of appetite • Nausea and vomiting • Abdominal discomfort • Weight loss
4. Altered elimination	• Constipation or diarrhoea	• Constipation • Increased urinary output
5. Impaired skin integrity	• Skin coarse, scaly and dry • Alopecia • Loss of eyebrows • Nails brittle with horizontal ridges	
6. Ineffective breathing pattern	• Laryngeal spasm • Wheezing	

usually the first manifestations (muscle cramps, carpopedal spasms, laryngeal spasm affecting the voice, dysphagia, convulsions). Wheezy respirations may be heard due to bronchospasm. Less calcium than normal is excreted in the urine because of the low blood calcium level, and the bones tend to become more dense. Renal excretion of phosphorus is reduced and the serum phosphate level is elevated, which predisposes the patient to acidosis. If the hormone deficiency is prolonged, calcium deposition may develop in the lens and conjunctiva of the eyes, the brain, lungs or gastric mucosa. The hair becomes thin and grey; areas of alopecia and loss of eyebrows are common. The skin becomes coarse and scaly and the nails are brittle and have horizontal ridges. Mental changes include depression, fatigue, psychosis, mental retardation and deficiency.

TREATMENT

The hypocalcaemia is corrected initially by the intravenous administration of calcium gluconate 10%. The patient is then given regular oral doses of a calcium salt, such as gluconate or lactate, along with a preparation of vitamin D to promote the absorption of the calcium. The patient is followed closely; frequent determinations of blood phosphorus and calcium levels are made in order to adjust vitamin D dosage. Overdosage may cause renal damage. Phosphorus-containing foods may have to be limited to avoid complications; these are principally

dairy products. An alternative may be the prescription of aluminium hydroxide gel which binds the phosphorus in the intestine, preventing its absorption. The patient is encouraged to take extra fluids to promote renal excretion of phosphorus.

The need for long-term calcium replacement therapy should decrease with the move toward autotransplantation of parathyroid tissue.

Hyperparathyroidism

CAUSES

The cause of an excessive secretion of PTH is usually an adenoma but may rarely be hyperplasia or carcinoma of the glands.

CLINICAL CHARACTERISTICS

The high PTH concentration in the blood causes decalcification of the bones, and hypercalcaemia occurs. The blood level of inorganic phosphorus falls as its renal excretion increases, and the concentration of calcium in the glomerular filtrate is higher than normal, predisposing to the formation of renal calculi. Neuromuscular excitability is depressed and loss of muscle tone is evident. Demineralization of the bones may be so marked that fibrous cystic areas develop which frequently lead to deformities and pathological

Table 19.6 Adrenal gland hormones.

Tissue	Hormones	Functions	Disorders
Adrenal cortex	Adrenocorticoids (corticosteroids, corticoids)		Addison's disease (hypofunction of cortices Cushing's syndrome (hyperfunction of cortices)
	—Mineralocorticoids (aldosterone) —Glucocorticoids, cortisol (hydrocortisone) —Sex hormones (androgens, oestrogen and progesterone)	Influences electrolyte concentration, fluid volume, blood pressure Influences metabolism of glucose, protein and fat; concerned with body's responses to physical and mental stress.	Primary aldosteronism (increase of aldosterone)
Adrenal medulla	Adrenaline	Constricts peripheral and renal blood vessels; dilates coronary and skeletal muscle vessels; relaxes smooth muscle of bronchioles, gastrointestinal tract, urinary bladder; dilates pupils; elevates blood sugar; promotes release of ACTH; accelerates metabolic rate	Phaeochromocytoma (increase of production of both hormones)
	Noradrenaline	Generalized vasoconstriction	

fractures. In some instances bone tumours consisting of an overgrowth of osteoclasts develop. When bone changes occur, the disorder may be referred to as *von Recklinghausen's disease* or *osteitis fibrosa cystica*, and the patient may experience tenderness and pain in the bones, especially with weight bearing.

The patient with hyperparathyroidism may develop acute pancreatitis. Muscular weakness, loss of appetite, nausea, vomiting and constipation may also develop. The urinary volume is usually increased because of the excessive amounts of calcium and phosphorus to be excreted. Renal function may become impaired; the tubular epithelium may be damaged by the excessive excretion of calcium or the formation of renal calculi. Frequently, the disease is only recognized when some deformity develops or a pathological fracture occurs.

TREATMENT

The patient with hyperparathyroidism should receive 3–4 litres of fluid daily followed by the administration of a diuretic such as frusemide (Lasix) to increase urinary excretion. If anorexia, nausea and vomiting are problems, intravenous infusions may be necessary to ensure an adequate intake. Fluid intake and output are carefully monitored. Foods containing calcium are restricted in the diet.

Hyperparathyroidism is treated by surgical excision of the gland with the adenoma or, in the case of hyperplasia, removal of all the glands but one. Normal residual parathyroid tissue may be allografted into a muscle to preserve as much of the patient's parathyroid function as possible. Following surgery, the patient is observed closely for the early signs of possible hypocalcaemia (tetany). Frequent serum calcium and

phosphorus determinations are made. A diet high in calcium and phosphorus may be necessary to restore normal bone structure.

THE PERSON WITH DISORDER OF THE ADRENAL CORTICES

As with other endocrine glands, dysfunction of the adrenal cortices may involve hyposecretion or hypersecretion of their hormones (Table 19.6). Adrenocortical hypofunction produces Addison's disease. Hyperfunction may cause Cushing's syndrome or primary aldosteronism.

ASSESSMENT OF ADRENOCORTICAL FUNCTION

Assessment of the person with altered adrenocortical function includes the identification of health problems common to persons with increased or decreased production of the adrenocortical hormones (Table 19.7).

Common characteristics identified during the *health history* include progressive fatigue and weakness and changes in appetite and weight. The patient and family are questioned regarding changes in emotional responses including irritability, lability or depression. Questions are posed to identify changes in sexuality patterns in both males and females.

The *physical examination* focuses on observation of the skin and secondary sex characteristics.

The *skin* is inspected for signs of oedema or dehydration; increased bruising and pigmentation may be present on the palms and exposed body surfaces,

Table 19.7 Assessment of the person with altered adrenocortical function.

Patient problems	Clinical characteristics of adrenocortical insufficiency (Addison's disease)	Clinical characteristics of adrenocortical hyperfunction (Cushing's disease)
1. Altered nutrition and metabolism	• Hypoglycaemia • Anorexia, nausea • Abdominal pain • Weight loss	• Hyperglycaemia • Abdominal discomfort • Weight gain
2. Altered fluid and electrolyte balance	• Dehydration • Increased serum potassium • Decreased serum sodium • Hypotension	• Oedema • Decreased serum potassium • Increased serum sodium • Hypertension
3. Altered skin and hair integrity	• Skin dusky, bronze • Increased pigmentation	• Purple striae • Bruising • Thinning of skin and hair • Hirsutism
4. Altered activity tolerance emotional responses	• Weakness • Constant fatigue	• Weakness, fatigue • Muscle atrophy
5. Increased potential for infection		• Delayed wound healing • Suppression of usual signs of infection
6. Altered sexuality patterns	• Decreased pubic and axillary hair in females	• Secondary male sex characteristics in females • Amenorrhoea • Development of breasts in males
7. Ineffective individual coping	• Depression • Irritability • Restlessness	• Depression • Apathy • Mood changes

joints, genitalia and oral mucosa. The abdomen is observed for the presence of purple striae. The development of a 'moon face' or the existence of fat deposits, particularly a 'Buffalo hump' (cervicodorsal fat), are characteristic signs that may be observed.

Changes and deviations in the structure of the breasts and in the distribution and amount of body hair, particularly scant pubic and axillary hair and excessive facial hair in the female, are noted.

Body height and weight are measured and alterations in normal growth and development are assessed.

Adrenocortical Insufficiency (Addison's Disease)

CAUSES

Primary failure of the adrenal cortices to produce corticosteriods is most often the result of atrophy of the glands but may also be caused by congenital adrenal hyperplasia, tubercular infection, adrenal haemorrhage or a neoplasm. Atrophy of the glands is attributed to an autoimmune reaction; specific antibodies to the adrenal glands are present in up to 60% of patients with primary

adrenal insufficiency (Dillon, 1980). Secondary hypofunction of the adrenal cortices occurs with hypopituitarism and the concomitant deficiency of ACTH and with excessive administration of steriods. The patient undergoes various diagnostic procedures to distinguish between primary and secondary adrenocortical insufficiency. This is important since, in secondary insufficiency, the secretion of aldosterone usually remains normal and mineralocorticoids should not be administered.

CLINICAL CHARACTERISTICS

In Addison's disease there is a deficiency of cortisol which interferes with the maintenance of a normal blood sugar level; the body cannot compensate by gluconeogenesis, liver glycogen is depleted and hypoglycaemia develops, especially between meals. There is a general depression of metabolic activity and energy production. The ability to cope with even mild stress is greatly diminished and minor infections, slight injuries, exposure to extremes of temperature, or emotional problems that are relatively insignificant to the normal person may prove very serious to these individuals.

The patient complains of weakness and constant

fatigue which becomes progressively more severe and incapacitating unless treatment is instituted. Listlessness, irritability and impaired mental ability may be manifested. Anorexia, nausea, abdominal pain and constipation alternating with diarrhoea are common complaints. Increased sensitivity to cold develops. The patient loses weight. The skin takes on a dusky, bronze hue and brown pigmented areas appear, especially in sites normally exposed to light, pressure or friction such as the backs of the hands (particularly over the knuckles), face, neck, axillae and 'belt' areas. Patchy areas of pigmentation may also be observed in the oral mucosa and conjunctivae.

The adrenocortical insufficiency causes an outpouring of the hormone ACTH, which is similar in chemical structure to the melanocyte-stimulating hormone (MSH) and, in high concentration, may produce similar effects. As a result, pigmented areas of the skin are common to the patient with Addison's disease.

The aldosterone deficiency incurs decreased reabsorption of sodium by the renal tubules with a consequent excessive loss of water as well as sodium in the urine. Severe dehydration may develop, leading to a depletion of the intravascular volume and ensuing reduced cardiac output, hypotension and shock. There is not the normal exchange of hydrogen ions for reabsorbed sodium ions in the kidneys, and acidosis may develop. Increased reabsorption of potassium by the tubules produces an elevated blood level, and hyperkalaemia may develop (see Chapter 7) and cause cardiac arrhythmias. Hypotension is invariable and it would be unlikely that someone with a systolic blood pressure above 110 mmHg would have the disease. An infection or trauma may precipitate a slowly progressive disorder.

TREATMENT AND NURSING INTERVENTION

Addison's disease is treated by maintenance doses of corticosteroid preparations. The glucocorticoids are replaced by the oral administration of a cortisol preparation (hydrocortisone) two or three times daily. The deficiency of mineralocorticoid (aldosterone) associated with primary adrenocortical insufficiency is met by giving fludrocortisone (synthetic aldosterone) orally once daily. The patient with secondary adrenocortical insufficiency does not require the aldosterone replacement.

The nurse caring for a patient receiving corticoid preparations must be familiar with the potential adverse effects of these drugs. If the patient receives corticoids in doses even slightly in excess of the amounts normally secreted, certain changes are likely to occur, especially with prolonged administration. Constant observation is necessary for early signs of side-effects. Restlessness, insomnia, euphoria and swings in mood may be manifested. The patient's susceptibility to infection may be markedly increased by the drug's suppression of lymphocyte and antibody production and local inflammatory responses. Muscle wasting and weakness may occur as a result of an excessive protein breakdown and increased loss of potassium in the urine. Sodium and water retention may be evidenced by oedema. Increased fat deposition on the trunk and face may develop,

changing the patient's general appearance. Increased fullness and rounding of the face produces the characteristic change referred to as the 'moon face'. Females may develop secondary male characteristics accompanied by growth of hair on the face, and growth of the breasts in males is occasionally seen. Prolonged administration of corticoids in excess of normal secretion may produce hyperglycaemia and glycosuria. The patient also becomes predisposed to the development of gastrointestinal lesions, such as peptic ulcers.

The patient with Addison's disease is encouraged to take a high-carbohydrate, high-protein diet. The danger of hypoglycaemia which may occur with glucocorticoid deficiency may be offset by the patient taking nourishment between meals and at bedtime. In primary adrenal insufficiency the patient may require additional sodium chloride. A directive as to the amount of salt to be included in the diet should be received from the doctor; the average amount served with meals may be sufficient. The patient with secondary adrenocortical insufficiency will not require additional salt.

Acute corticoid insufficiency, which is also referred to as *Addisonian crisis*, may develop when corticoid replacement is inadequate or omitted, or it may be what brings the patient for medical attention before the disease is diagnosed. Frequently a crisis is precipitated by some physical or psychological stress such as infection, exposure to extremes of temperature, gastrointestinal upset (e.g. vomiting and diarrhoea), fever, profuse perspiration, strenuous activity, anxiety or grief. Acute insufficiency is serious and, unless treated promptly, can rapidly lead to death. Early symptoms are nausea, vomiting, diarrhoea, abdominal pain, fever and extreme weakness. Severe hypoglycaemia and dehydration develop rapidly; the blood pressure falls, and shock and coma may follow. Blood glucose, sodium and cortisol levels are low and the potassium and urea concentrations are markedly elevated.

Addisonian crisis is treated by continuous intravenous infusion of dextrose in normal saline to which hydrocortisone (cortisol) is added for at least the first 24 hours. Hydrocortisone is also given orally or intramuscularly. The large doses of hydrocortisone which the patient receives usually exert a sufficient sodium-retaining effect, eliminating the need for supplementary administration of a mineralocorticoid preparation.

Frequent recordings of the blood pressure, temperature, pulse respirations and level of response are made. The patient is kept at absolute rest to avoid expenditure of energy and is turned, bathed and fed by the nurse. He or she is kept flat and any change of position is made slowly because of the hypotension. Frequent, high-carbohydrate feedings are given as soon as they can be tolerated. When the patient's blood pressure and other vital signs have returned to normal and are sustained, and the condition which precipitated the crisis has been controlled, the corticoid dosage is gradually reduced to maintenance level.

Patient and family teaching

The overall goals are to learn self-regulation of the disease and to maintain a satisfactory level of functioning.

Goals

The patient and family will be able to:

- State the purpose of life-long steroid replacement therapy.
- Describe a plan for taking medications daily.
- State the names, dosage, frequency, actions and side–effects of each prescribed medication.
- State the effects of stress on his disease.
- Describe a plan to minimize stress.
- Describe actions to take to minimize the effects of stress when it occurs.
- Discuss plans to minimize exposure to infection.
- Describe symptoms that indicate Addisonian crisis and actions to take if symptoms develop.
- Wear a Medic Alert tag and/or carry a steroid card identifying the disorder and medication plan.
- Describe a plan for continuing health care.

Nursing intervention

Since primary adrenal insufficiency requires life-long replacement therapy, an important nursing function is teaching the patient and family about the disease and necessary care. A simple explanation is given of the nature of the condition with reassurance that, although hormone replacement will be necessary for life, if the prescribed therapeutic regimen is followed, a relatively normal life can be expected.

Activity tolerance The importance of regular and adequate hours of rest, stopping activities short of fatigue and avoiding exposure to cold are stressed, indicating the effect of exposure and overexertion on cellular activity and the blood sugar level.

Medication therapy No medications, including laxatives, except those ordered by the doctor should be taken. Explicit instructions are given regarding the taking of the prescribed corticoid preparations; directions are written clearly, and the importance of taking the exact amounts at the prescribed times is emphasized. The patient is warned of the dangers of being without medication. Increased doses of medication may be recommended during periods of stress.

Nutrition The high-carbohydrate, high-protein diet with the amount of sodium recommended by the doctor is discussed in detail, explaining the need for nourishment between meals and at bedtime to maintain a normal blood sugar level.

Prevention of infection The patient and family are advised of the need for avoiding contact with those with an infection as much as possible, and suggestions are made as to how this may be achieved.

Individual coping They should understand that a stressful situation or illness demands more corticoids. To prevent a serious crisis or acute corticoid insufficiency, prompt medical attention is necessary with any disorder such as a respiratory infection, vomiting, diarrhoea, fainting or sudden weakness. The role of worry and emotional situations in precipitating a crisis is emphasized.

Safety measures The patient with Addison's disease should always carry a steroid card or wear a Medic Alert bracelet or pendant which clearly indicates the presence of corticoid insufficiency and what should be done in the event of injury or sudden collapse.

In teaching, the nurse does not attempt to provide all the necessary information at one time. The instruction is planned to cover several sessions; salient points are clarified and reinforced by repetition, and opportunities are provided for the patient and family members to ask questions. and to participate actively in the learning process.

Evaluation

The patient and family should be able to administer the prescribed corticosteroid replacement therapy safely and to recognize side-effects of over- or underreplacement. The patient should be able to describe plans to receive adequate rest, to decrease exposure to infection, to minimize the effects of added physical and emotional stress and for ongoing health care and supervision.

The patient should maintain a desirable body weight and quickly identify fluctuations in weight pattern.

The nurse is responsible for the evaluation of patient and family teaching and for validating the effectiveness of teaching with the patient and family. Reassessment of learning needs should be done on each nurse–patient encounter.

Adrenocortical Hyperfunction (Cushing's Syndrome)

CAUSES

This is a rare disorder which is more common in females and results from an excessive secretion of adrenal corticoids. It may be due to primary hyperfunction of one or both of the adrenal cortices or may be secondary to a pathological hypersecretion of ACTH by the anterior pituitary gland. Primary hyperactivity of the adrenal cortex is usually caused by a neoplasm, most frequently an adenoma, but may also occur as a result of unexplained hyperplasia. A common cause is excessive administration of ACTH.

CLINICAL CHARACTERICISTICS

These will vary in individuals according to age and the amount of corticoid being produced in excess of the normal. The increased output of cortisol causes excessive protein catabolism, gluconeogenesis, an abnormal distribution of fat and atrophy of lymphoid tissue. The person manifests a decreased glucose tolerance, hyperglycaemia, and muscle wasting and weakness. The appearance changes because of the increased deposition of fat on the trunk, thin wasted limbs, and a round, bloated-looking face ('moon' face). Purple striae may appear, notably on the abdomen, buttocks and thighs, and are due to increased fragility of the blood vessels and atrophy of the skin. Ecchymoses are common. The production of lymphocytes is suppressed, increasing the patient's susceptibility to infection. Osteoporosis may occur, usually in the vertebrae, because of calcium mobilization; the patient frequently complains of backache.

The excessive secretion of mineralocorticoids results in electrolyte, fluid and acid–base imbalances. Hypernatraemia, water retention and hypokalaemia develop. The increased reabsorption by the renal tubules of sodium ions in exchange for hydyrogen ions (see Chapter 7) depletes the acid ions, producing alkalosis. The low blood level of potassium may cause extreme weakness and cardiac dysfunction. Hypertension due to the sodium and water retention is common.

As a consequence of the increased production of androgens, the female patient develops secondary male characteristics. There is a marked growth of hair on the face, the voice deepens, breasts atrophy, amenorrhoea occurs and the clitoris may enlarge.

If the disease is secondary to a hypersecretion of ACTH, the disturbances are associated principally with an excessive production of the glucocorticoids only.

TREATMENT AND NURSING INTERVENTION

The treatment of Cushing's syndrome depends upon whether the hypersecretion of corticoids is due to primary dysfunction of the adrenal cortices or is the result of a hypersecretion of ACTH. In the case of an adrenocortical neoplasm, the affected gland is removed. If the cause is hyperplasia, a bilateral adrenalectomy is usually done. The patient then receives hormonal replacement therapy as outlined under Addison's disease. If the condition is secondary to a pituitary tumour the tumour is usually treated by irradiation or surgical removal.

Nursing case of the patient with Cushing's syndrome is mainly symptomatic (Table 19.7). Precautions are necessary to prevent accidental falls which may occur because of weakness. The fluid intake and output are recorded to determine the amount of water retention, and sodium intake is restricted. The blood pressure and pulse are taken at regular intervals so that early changes may be detected. Changes in mood and behaviour are common and should be recorded. Exposure to persons with infection is avoided because of the patient's lowered resistance.

Hyperaldosteronism

An excessive production of aldosterone occurs rarely and is usually caused by an adenoma or hyperplasia of the particular adrenocortical cells which secrete the hormone. The most striking features of the disease are the excessive renal loss of potassium, retention of sodium and hypertension. The person experiences severe generalized muscular weakness due to the hypokalaemia. Depletion of the body potassium reduces the kidneys' ability to concentrate the urine, and polyuria occurs. Despite an increased retention of salt, there is no corresponding retention of water or oedema. This is attributed to an increased glomerular filtration rate and the polyuria. As a result of the

hypernatraemia and polyuria, the person usually experiences severe thirst. An elevation of arterial blood pressure is characteristic. In addition to hypernatraemia and hypokalaemia, laboratory investigation reveals elevated urinary and plasma aldosterone levels and normal renin concentration. Treatment consists of surgical removal of the adenoma or affected gland preceded by administration of potassium salts.

Secondary hyperaldosteronism due to an excessive secretion of renin by the kidneys may occur. It may be treated with spironolactone, an aldosterone antagonist, or renal surgery.

THE PERSON WITH DISORDERS OF THE ADRENAL MEDULLAE

ASSESSMENT OF ADRENAL MEDULLARY FUNCTION

The *health history* focuses on identification of the person's usual responses to stress and documentation of episodes of excessive stress reactions (flight or fight reaction).

Physical examination involves the documentation of fluctuations in and excessively high blood pressure readings.

Excess of Adrenaline and Noradrenaline (Phaeochromocytoma)

Disease of the adrenal medullae is rare and most commonly occurs in the form of a neoplasm known as a phaeochromocytoma, which produces an excessive amount of adrenaline and noradrenaline. The tumour is usually unilateral and benign and causes hypertension, hyperglycaemia and hypermetabolism. The increased liberation of large amounts of the hormones is usually paroxysmal at first, lasting from a few minutes to hours, but is likely to eventually become persistent. The patient frequently complains of a pounding headache, nausea, vomiting, palpitation, air hunger, nervousness, tremor and weakness. Sweating, pallor, dilatation of the pupils, tachycardia and a sharp rise in the blood pressure are also manifested. The increased glucogenolysis and subsequent elevated blood sugar may result in glucosuria.

Tests used to establish the diagnosis of phaeochromocytoma include the estimation of the blood and urinary content of the hormones or their major metabolite, vanillylmandelic acid (VMA). Computerized axial tomographic (CT) scanning and ultrasonography are more favoured because they are noninvasive.

The patient with phaeochromocytoma is treated by surgical removal of the tumour of the affected gland. Sympathetic blocking agents are administered preoperatively to decrease blood pressure and reduce other symptoms.

Nursing in Adrenal Surgery

Surgery of the adrenal glands may be done on patients with hypersecretions of hormones due to hyperplasia or tumours of one or both glands. The procedure may involve the removal of both adrenal glands (bilateral or total adrenalectomy), the removal of one gland (unilateral adrenalectomy) or resection of a part of a gland (subtotal adrenalectomy). Bilateral adrenalectomy is occasionally undertaken in patients with cancer of the breast and occasionally in those with cancer of the prostate. Malignant disease of these organs is dependent to some extent on sex hormones, and, since the adrenal cortices produce both oestrogens and androgens, their removal eliminates a source of the supporting hormones. In the case of cancer of the breast, adrenalectomy is preceded by oophorectomy (removal of the ovaries). Occasionally the patient with cancer of the prostate undergoes orchidectomy (removal of the testicles) before adrenalectomy is considered.

PREOPERATIVE PREPARATION

Preparation of the patient for adrenal surgery includes the general preparation cited in Chapter 11. Blood studies are done to determine electrolyte concentrations, and corrections are made as indicated. Because of an excessive potassium excretion, a solution of potassium chloride may be ordered to restore the normal level of potassium in the blood. The blood sugar level and glucose tolerance are investigated. The patient is given a high-protein diet because of the protein depletion due to excessive glucocorticoid secretion. The fluid intake and output are measured, and the balance is noted. The blood pressure is recorded at least once daily to serve as a postoperative comparative baseline. The patient with hyperfunction of the adrenal cortices frequently has experienced hypertension for some time. Phentolamine (Rogitine) and/or phenoxybenzamine hydrochloride may be prescribed preoperatively to reduce vasomotor tone and hypertension because the anaesthetic and actual surgery may precipitate severe hypertension.

If both adrenal glands are to be removed, the patient and the family must understand that constant hormone replacement will be necessary for the remainder of the patient's life.

After operation, the patient's respirations tend to be shallow because the incision is close to the diaphragm. Careful teaching about postoperative breathing and coughing exercises are therefore essential.

The surgeon's approach to the adrenal gland is usually through a high flank incision or occasionally through the abdomen. When a bilateral adrenalectomy is done, two incisions are made unless the transabdominal approach is used.

Hydrocortisone may be administered before and during as well as following the operation to prevent adrenal insufficiency in the immediate postoperative period. An intravenous solution is run slowly and continuously. This is in preparation for prompt administration of corticosteroids or a vasopressor, as indicated.

POSTOPERATIVE CARE

Assessment and management of medication and fluid therapy

During the first few postoperative days, and until the maintenance dosages of hydrocortisone and fludrocortisone are established in the case of adrenalectomy, special attention is paid to the patient's blood pressure, fluid balance and blood chemistry. Constant nursing care is necessary until the vital signs and the corticoid, sodium and potassium concentrations are stabilized. The blood pressure, respirations and pulse are recorded every 15 minutes for several hours and the interval gradually lengthened if they remain satisfactory. Any rapid or significant fall in the blood pressure, dyspnoea, or tachycardia is reported promptly. The fluid intake and output are accurately measured, and any imbalance is brought to the doctor's attention. Frequent checks are made of the blood sodium, potassium and glucose levels which influence the amount of corticoids given. Vomiting, increased weakness, dehydration, hypotension and an elevated temperature may indicate acute corticoid insufficiency.

Intravenous corticoids are given continuously for a day or two with the dosage and rate of flow adjusted to the patient's clinical condition and the electrolyte and fluid balances. Oral doses of hydrocortisone and fludrocortisone are started as soon as tolerated by the patient. The dosage of both corticoid preparations is gradually tapered off until maintenance amounts are established. When the intravenous corticoids are withdrawn, an intravenous infusion of glucose in water or normal saline is continued slowly even though the patient may be tolerating fluids by mouth. The purpose of this is to keep the route available for quick administration of corticoids or a vasopressor (e.g. metaraminol (Aramine) or noradrenaline acid tartrate (Levophed)) if needed. The patient's condition tends to be labile and may change quickly. The nurse must be constantly alert for signs of corticoid insufficiency or indications of excessive corticoid administration.

When surgery is performed to remove a phaeochromocytoma, monitoring of the blood pressure is necessary every ½–1 hour for at least 36–48 hours; severe fluctuations may occur. A marked rise may occur during or immediately following surgery because of an excessive liberation of catecholamines from the tumour during removal. An adrenergic blocking agent such as phentolamine (Rogitine) is kept available for quick intravenous administration to neutralize the medullary hormones.

More often the problem following surgery is severe hypotension and concomitant shock. The blood pressure is maintained by giving a vasopressor such as noradrenaline acid tartrate or metaraminol in an intravenous solution. The rate of flow must be carefully controlled and adjusted according to frequent blood pressure recordings and the doctor's directives. The patient is kept flat, and any change in position achieved slowly.

When unilateral adrenalectomy or a subtotal resection of one or both glands is done, the patient may receive some hydrocortisone following operation. Less will be required than in total adrenalectomy and it is gradually withdrawn.

Following adrenal surgery, the patient usually remains in bed until the blood pressure remains at a satisfactory level. Before commencing ambulation, the head of the bed is elevated and the blood pressure checked. The patient should not be left unattended during mobilization and frequent blood pressure checks should be carried out. If a significant decrease in blood pressure occurs, the patient is returned to bed and kept flat.

Patient teaching

In preparation for discharge, the patient who has had a bilateral adrenalectomy receives the same instruction as the patient with Addison's disease (see p. 591). If one gland has been removed or a subtotal resection done, the patient is cautioned to avoid overfatigue, exposure to extremes of temperature (especially cold), infections, and emotional disturbances as much as possible. It is possible that stress may precipitate an acute adrenal insufficiency or crisis because the remaining adrenal tissue cannot meet the increased hormonal demand. If the patient experiences weakness, fainting, fever, or nausea and vomiting, the general practitioner should be contacted immediately and a corticoid supplement will be required.

Following any adrenal surgery, the patient should resume activity very gradually and is followed closely as an out-patient. Usually several months are required to adjust the hormonal replacement satisfactorily. The patient who has had hypertension due to phaeochromocytoma may not regain a stable blood pressure level for 3–4 months.

THE PERSON WITH DISORDERS OF THE ISLETS OF LANGERHANS

Diabetes Mellitus

Diabetes mellitus is a heterogeneous group of disorders of carbohydrate, fat and protein metabolism characterized by chronic hyperglycaemia, degenerative vascular changes and neuropathy. It tends to accelerate degenerative changes throughout the body by widespread vascular changes in the large blood vessels and the microvessels.

CHARACTERISTICS

As a result of a deficiency of insulin or inadequate insulin function there is an inadequate transfer of glucose into the cells; the utilization of glucose for energy and cellular products and its conversion to glycogen or fat and storage as such are depressed. Glucose accumulates in the blood, causing hyperglycaemia.

Fat may be mobilized from adipose tissue and broken down to provide a source of energy. The mobilized fat is withdrawn from the blood by the liver and broken down to glycerol and fatty acids. The fatty acids are oxidized by the hepatic cells to ketone bodies (acetoacetic acid, β-hydroxybutyric acid and acetone), which are then circulated and may be metabolized by cells to produce energy, carbon dioxide and water. Only a limited amount of ketone acids can be utilized by the cells. If ketogenesis proceeds rapidly, exceeding the rate at which they can be metabolized, the ketone acids accumulate in the blood, causing ketosis or ketone acidosis.

Tissue protein may also be broken down to amino acids which are used in gluconeogenesis, contributing to the hyperglycaemia. Both the uptake of amino acids by the cells and body protein synthesis are decreased.

Insulin-dependent diabetes mellitus (IDDM) usually has a sudden onset in a severe, acute form. In non-insulin-dependent diabetes mellitus (NIDDM) the onset is most often insidious, going undetected and untreated for a considerable period of time (see Clinical situations type I and type II). The diabetes may be recognized in a routine examination in which glucosuria is discovered, or eventually a distressing symptom presents which prompts the patient to consult a doctor.

The patient excretes an excessive volume of urine (polyuria) as a result of the increased concentration of glucose in the glomerular filtrate. The glucose increases the osmotic pressure of the filtrate, preventing the reabsorption of water. As a result of the excessive water loss, the patient experiences a persisting thirst (polydipsia), and dehydration and electrolyte imbalance may develop. The blood glucose concentration exceeds the capacity of the renal tubules to reabsorb it from the glomerular filtrate, and glucose is excreted in the urine (glycosuria). The maximum capacity of the renal tubules to reabsorb glucose represents what is referred to as the glucose renal threshold. The normal is 10–12 mmol/l.

Weakness and fatigue are common complaints because the glucose cannot be utilized to produce energy. There is a loss of weight which is attributed to the mobilization of fat from adipose tissue and the breakdown of protein. Some patients also experience an increased appetite (polyphagia).

Female patients may develop pruritus of the vulva, usually due to infection by fungi which thrive on the glucose deposit from the urine. The vulva becomes swollen and inflamed.

Table 19.8 lists the clinical characteristics of persons with the two major types of diabetes mellitus.

CHRONIC COMPLICATIONS OF DIABETES

The blood vessels of practically all diabetics undergo degenerative changes to some extent. These changes may be both microvascular and macrovascular. *Microvascular degenerative changes* are specific to diabetes; the basement membrane in the capillaries and arterioles thickens. The retinae, kidneys and skin are the areas most affected by *microvascular changes*.

Diabetic retinopathy occurs in the form of minute aneurysms in the retinal vessels. These dilatations are prone to rupture and cause a haemorrhage into the eye. The resultant visual loss varies with the location and proliferation of the lesions. Poor diabetic control, increased diastolic blood pressure, impaired renal function, deterioration in motor nerve conduction and increased triglyceride levels increase the risk for diabetic retinopathy.

Renal function may be slowly impaired by changes in the glomerular capillaries (intercapillary glomerulo-sclerosis or Kimmelstiel–Wilson syndrome) and by sclerotic changes in the larger renal vessels. The patient may manifest albuminuria and some degree of hypertension.

Macrovascular degeneration involves the development of atherosclerosis (deposits of the fatty substance cholesterol) in the arteries, narrowing their lumen. Atherosclerosis of the coronary arteries of the diabetic frequently leads to angina pectoris and myocardial infarction, especially in older persons.

Defective circulation due to vascular changes in the lower limbs may lead to gangrene. A small superficial injury may be a precipitating factor and the ensuing gangrene may necessitate the amputation of a toe, foot or leg. Restricted circulation may produce abnormal coldness of the extremities, numbness, discoloration, muscular cramps, weakness, burning pain or a small ulcer that does not heal.

Diabetic neuropathy. Neuropathy may be defined as a non-inflammatory, non-specific pathological or functional disorder of the peripheral nervous system. This complication affects all parts of the nervous system except the brain. Peripheral neuropathy is usually bilateral and worsens at night. The patient may experience muscular cramps, tingling and burning sensation as well as pain. Deep tendon reflexes are absent and the patient's vibratory and position senses may be impaired. Changes occur in the shape of the hands and feet; muscle atrophy and demineralization of bone occur. Joints deteriorate (Charcot's joints) and foot drop may develop. Autonomic neuropathy usually causes changes in gastrointestinal and oesophageal functioning. Impotence and retrograde ejaculation may occur in the male.

INCIDENCE

Type I or *insulin-dependent diabetes mellitus (IDDM)* has its peak onset between 11 and 12 years of age. Studies of the incidence of IDDM lack standardization showing variability between countries and individual studies. Ranges vary from 0.07–3.5 per 1000 population (Office of Health Economics, 1989). Seasonal variations occur in the onset of the disorder; the highest onset occurs in the autumn and winter and the lowest frequency in the summer.

Type II or *non-insulin dependent diabetes mellitus (NIDDM)* is one of the most common chronic disorders and is seen most often in middle-aged and older persons. While prevalence rates show variations in different studies, there is evidence of an increase of diabetes. The incidence is higher in persons who are obese, among relatives of diabetics, and in persons of middle to upper socioeconomic groups.

CAUSES AND RISK FACTORS

The exact causes of the major types of diabetes mellitus are not known. A common factor in all types is hyperglycaemia.

Glucose metabolism. Diabetes mellitus can be caused by a variety of pathological processes that interfere with the metabolism of glucose. Such changes may occur anywhere along the insulin pathway depicted in Figure 19.7. The dysfunction may occur in the pancreas and interfere with the production or secretion of insulin, in the bloodstream, or at the level of target tissue cells disrupting glucose uptake or utilization by the cells. Possible causes of diabetes include: (1) destruction of the β cells; (2) abnormal synthesis of insulin; (3) retarded release of insulin; (4) inactivation of insulin in the bloodstream by antibodies or other agents; (5) altered insulin receptors or a decreased number of receptors on peripheral cells; (6) defective processing of the insulin message within the target cells; and (7) abnormal metabolism of glucose (Norkins, 1979). Defects in the β cells appear to be the primary cause of insulin-dependent diabetes.

Genetic and autoimmune mechanisms. It is now generally accepted that certain histocompatability antigens (e.g. HLA-B8, HLA-BW15 and HLA-BW18) occur more often in insulin-dependent diabetics than in healthy people. In NIDDM there is often a family history but this does not seem to be linked to HLA markers (Hassan, 1985).

As many as 85% of newly diagnosed patients with IDDM have been found to possess an antibody which reacts with the α, β and δ cells of the islets of Langerhans, suggesting an autoimmune factor is present. Islet cell antibodies have not been shown to be of any significance in patients with NIDDM. It is also suggested that a relationship exists between the HLA types and the development of microvascular disease and neuropathy in patients with IDDM (Albin and Rifkin, 1982). The interaction between an individual's genetic make-up and environmental or life-style factors is complex and unclear. As a result the risk of development of type I or type II diabetes cannot be accurately predicted.

Obesity. The majority of diabetics who develop their disease after the age of 40 years are obese or have a history of obesity. It is believed that the number of insulin receptors on tissue cells is decreased with obesity and that the level of serum insulin increases. With weight loss and exercise, the number of cellular insulin receptors increase, insulin binding is more effective and the serum insulin level drops to a normal range. The association of diabetes with obesity is a very significant factor in considering prevention.

Infectious agents. There is increasing evidence that viral infections, especially in genetically predisposed individuals, may cause insulin-dependent diabetes. Indirect evidence of this association includes the seasonal variations found in the onset of the disease. Onset of IDDM also increases following childhood viral infections.

CLASSIFICATION OF DIABETES

Diabetes mellitus is classified as:

- *Insulin-dependent diabetes mellitus (IDDM), type I.* Individuals in this group are usually but not necessarily, non-obese, develop diabetes suddenly, usually in youth, are likely to be linked to certain HLA types, and have a family history of the disease in only about 10% of cases. They are ketosis prone if insulin is withdrawn and therefore are usually insulin dependent.

- *Non-insulin-dependent diabetes mellitus (NIDDM), type II.* Individuals with type II are generally obese, have a family history of NIDDM, develop the disease insidiously as adults, are non-ketosis prone and may demonstrate hyperinsulinism as well as hyperglycaemia.

- *Other types (type III).* This class includes people with diabetes mellitus associated with other identifiable causes. Causes include: pancreatic disease, hormonal disorders (e.g. Cushing's disease), drug or chemical causes, insulin receptor abnormalities and certain genetic syndromes.

Additional subgroups included in the international classification are:

- *Impaired glucose tolerance (IGT).* This group may be further divided into obese and non-obese. The prognosis can be improved if the individual stops smoking and loses weight.

- *Gestational diabetes (GDM).* Glucose intolerance may have its onset during pregnancy.

- *Statistical risk groups.* Included in this category are individuals at greater risk than the general population of developing diabetes. Risk factors may include: immediate family members with the disease, the presence of islet cell antibodies, and obesity.

Table 19.8 outlines the clinical characteristics presented by patients with IDDM (type I) and NIDDM (type II).

PREVENTION OF DIABETES MELLITUS

Primary prevention

Diabetes mellitus is not a single entity but a group of heterogeneous disorders caused by a combination of genetic, environmental and viral factors. With the knowledge now available, primary preventive measures are limited but measures can be taken to prevent and/or correct obesity and stop smoking. This is especially important for those with a family history of diabetes or a suggestive obstetric history. As indicated previously, the majority of non-insulin-dependent diabetics are either obese at the time their disease is manifested or have a history of obesity. The incidence of diabetes among women who have previously given birth to an infant of 4.5 kg (10 lb) or more is sufficiently significant to recommend that they maintain their ideal weight and be checked annually for diabetes mellitus. Hospital and community nurses have a responsibility to advise people who are overweight of the many adverse effects of obesity and that they are possible candidates for diabetes mellitus. Progress in defining genetic markers may soon lead to the ability to identify individuals at risk of developing insulin-dependent diabetes and the possibility of immunization or other measures to prevent the disease.

Secondary prevention: detection

Programmes for screening and education of the general public about diabetes mellitus are organized by national diabetic associations in some countries. Routine blood glucose testing at the time of health checks for job applicants, and when people are attending a hospital clinic for any reason, may unexpectedly uncover hyperglycaemia. Women with a history of having had a large baby should be alert to the possibility of being a latent diabetic.

Detection of impaired glucose tolerance in the elderly is important to alert patients and health professionals to the increased risk for diabetes and to the need for preventive measures. Routine screening, using 2-hour post-glucose blood glucose levels, of all individuals admitted to homes for the elderly or nursing homes will detect those at risk for type II diabetes. Measures can then be instituted to correct obesity, alter diet to limit

Table 19.8 Classification of diabetes mellitus.

	IDDM (type I)	NIDDM (type II)
Synonyms	Juvenile onset	Maturity onset
Age of onset	Usually before 30 years	Usually after 40 years
Type of onset	Frequently sudden	Usually gradual
Presentation	Polydipsia, polyuria	Often asymptomatic
Body weight	Thin	Usually (80%) obese
Ketoacidosis	Ketosis-prone	Ketosis-resistant
Control of diabetes	Difficult; brittle	Generally easy
Control by diet alone	Not possible	Frequent
Control by oral agents	Not possible	Frequent
Long-term complications	Frequent	Frequent

simple sugars and calories, and to promote physical and mental activities.

Informing the public as to the characteristics of diabetes mellitus, susceptibility factors (obesity and family history) possible consequences of undetected and uncontrolled diabetes by, for example, occupational health departments associated with the workplace is important.

MANAGEMENT AND EDUCATION OF THE DIABETIC PATIENT AND FAMILY

Although inroads are being made in the prevention of diabetes, to date no cure exists. Individuals must therefore live with this chronic disorder and the potential complications. The diabetic patient may be dependent on health professionals for restoration of health when the disease is first diagnosed and during episodes of acute illness. As the individual acquires knowledge and skill to make alterations in life-style to regulate the hyperglycaemia, greater independence may be achieved (see Figure 2.1). All persons with diabetes mellitus must alter their life-styles and health behaviours to regulate their blood glucose levels. Most adults are able to achieve self-regulation of their diabetes and move to higher levels of independence.

MANAGEMENT OF DIABETES MELLITUS

Management of diabetes mellitus is directed towards establishing and maintaining metabolic control by correcting the hyperglycaemia. The plan of treatment for each person is determined on an individual basis; the therapeutic requirements for control in the case of one diabetic patient may be quite different from that of another.

General principles of treatment includes (Toews, 1987):

1. *Decrease body insulin resistance.* In the early stages of type II diabetes, the person may produce adequate amounts of insulin which the cells are not able to utilize. Insulin resistance can be decreased by weight reduction in the obese person with type II diabetes and by an aerobic training programme. This approach is less effective in persons with Type I diabetes and in the advanced stages of type II, when insulin secretion is diminished.
2. *Control the dietary carbohydrate load.* The level of blood glucose following a meal depends on the amount of carbohydrate in the diet. Most of the dietary carbohydrate should be from complex carbohydrate found in starchy foods, while the use of simple sugars from fruit and milk should be limited.
3. *Delay intestinal absorption of carbohydrate.* Decreased absorption rates of ingested carbohydrate will deliver the total glucose load over a longer period of time, resulting in lower blood glucose levels. Unrefined or high-fibre foods are slower to hydrolyse in the gut and therefore produce a decreased glycaemic response, while refined carbohydrates and simple sugars are rapidly absorbed. Dietary fibre should be gradually increased to 40 g daily. Soluble fibre found in oat and rice brans, barley and legumes works best to slow the absorption of glucose as well as to reduce serum lipid levels (Tredger, 1989).
4. *Increase endogenous insulin production.* Drugs such as thiazides, diazoxide and phenytoin, may inhibit insulin secretion and should be discontinued. Sulphonylurea drugs increase insulin secretion and potentiate the metabolic actions of insulin. These oral hypoglycaemic drugs may be prescribed for persons with type II diabetes. Transplantation of the pancreas or of the insulin-producing islet tissue is feasible but is not currently realistic for the large number of people with diabetes.
5. *Administer exogenous insulin.* Subcutaneous insulin administration is the standard method of maintaining therapeutic serum glucose levels for individuals with type I diabetes. Insulin may also be administered intravenously or intramuscularly to treat hyperglycaemic reactions. Persons with type II diabetes may require insulin administration at times of increased stress.

Blood glucose levels are controlled by balancing the person's energy intake with energy utilization or output. *Dietary measures*, *medication* and *physical activity* are adjusted to achieve the best possible glycaemic control for the individual.

Diet

The patient's *goals* are: to restore and maintain blood glucose and lipid levels to normal; to prevent wide fluctuations in blood glucose levels throughout the day; to attain and maintain a desirable body weight; and to prevent or delay the development of cardiovascular, renal and neurological complications.

Diet is a major factor in the control of diabetes. The prescribed 'diabetic diet' has been replaced by an individualized diet regimen with the patient assuming responsibility for planning, implementing and adjusting the diet to needs and life-style. The diet should be quite similar to that advocated for the nondiabetic and must provide sufficient variety to make it appetizing and palatable (British Diabetic Association, 1984).

The *dietary plan* indicates the number of calories required each day and the proportions of these calories to be allocated to carbohydrate, protein and fat. The number of calories is determined by the person's ideal and present weight, age, sex, activity and previous dietary intake. Initially, if the non-insulin-dependent patient is overweight, the number of calories must be lower than the figure indicated as needed for his ideal weight. The objective is to bring about a gradual and steady loss of weight until the normal weight is achieved. Appropriate increases in the food plan are usually made as the weight approaches normal. The insulin-dependent diabetic who is losing energy through glycosuria, has impaired protein and fat synthesis as well as inefficient use of glucose and so an overall increase in calorie intake is required until better control achieves weight gain.

Generally, the proportion of prescribed calories allocated to each food type is approximately 55–60% carbohydrate, 12–20% protein and less than 30% fat. In providing the necessary carbohydrates, concentrated forms of simple sugars, such as sugar, sweets, jam, jelly, preserves, honey, ice cream, pastries, cake and sweetened beverages are strictly limited and then only permitted as part of a meal to prevent rapid increases in blood sugar levels. Unrefined carbohydrates with fibre, such as whole grain breads and cereals, fruit and vegetables, should be substituted for the refined carbohydrates. It is believed that foods with a high soluble fibre content improve glucose tolerance, lower insulin-secretion, reduce glycaemia and glucosuria and lower lipoprotein levels. The mechanism of action of fibre in achieving these results is not entirely understood, but improvement in glycaemia and lipid regulation is widely reported (British Diabetic Assocation, 1984). Foods high in soluble fibre include oat, rice and corn brans, legumes and lentils. Carbohydrate intake is distributed over the day to avoid abnormal fluctuations in blood glucose concentrations. In the selection of fat, the substitution of unsaturated for saturated fats is recommended because of the diabetic's predisposition to the development of atherosclerosis and vascular lesions. As public awareness of the benefits of soluble fibre and low fat diets increases, recipes and products using soluble fibre and less fat are becoming readily accessible to consumers.

It is currently believed that the amount of protein in the diet of persons in most Western countries should be decreased. Evidence suggests that individuals with diabetic complications such as neuropathy should limit their protein intake.

Food exchange information provides help for patients and their families to select a varied diet. Food intake is usually best divided into at least three main meals. If an oral hypoglycaemic drug or insulin is used, the carbohydrate intake is usually divided across meals and snacks distributed throughout the day and evening.

Careful education and the availability of good eating guides or exchange lists permit the diet to be varied and takes into account the availability of foods as well as the person's preferences. Cookery books, extensive information about food values, and general dietary guidelines are available from the British Diabetic Association. This material can be useful in supplementing the basic but individualized food plan that will be given to each person on diagnosis by the local dietetic team.

It must be impressed upon the person that all of the daily food allowance should be eaten, especially if insulin or a hypoglycaemic drug is being taken. If the insulin-taking patient is unable to take his usual diet, the carbohydrate requirement is made up in some way (e.g. orange juice, milk). Meals should be taken regularly; the delay or missing of a meal may upset the blood glucose level and promote the breakdown of fat. Foods of no significant nutrient value or 'extra' foods which the person may have as desired include clear broths and consommé, clear tea and coffee, and artificially sweetened carbonated beverage. Non-caloric sweeteners such as aspartame and saccharin may be safely used by diabetics. These sweeteners are found in many low-caloric beverages and prepared foods.

Sorbitol (a sugar alcohol) has been used as a sweetening agent, as has fructose (crystalline fruit sugar). Both are virtually all absorbed and metabolized but the rate of absorption from the gut is slow and it has less effect on blood sugar than glucose. Both are often used in the manufacture of 'diabetic' jams, boiled sweets, biscuits and chocolate. Because they do not offer any energy savings they should not be used for slimming purposes, or by diabetics whose main therapeutic aim is to reduce weight.

The use of artificial non-nutritive sweeteners and the bulk nutritive sugar substitutes are not necessary in the management of diabetes, but many people find their use improves the quality of their life and helps make dietary restrictions more acceptable.

The diabetic diet is very much an individual factor. Following the initial dietary plan, the patient is followed closely to determine if it is satisfactory; the blood glucose levels are checked several times a day, or urine may be checked for glucose, weight is recorded daily, and general reactions (physical and psychological) are noted. Adjustments in the total calorie intake and distribution of food throughout the day are often necessary. Diabetics interviewed by Daschner (1986) identified the following problems, in order of frequency, in adhering to their prescribed diets: self-discipline; the influence of other people; impact of events especially eating out; control of emotions; lack of material resources; self-image and time constraints. To increase compliance with dietary regimens patients need assistance with self-management techniques and require psychosocial support during the adjustment period.

To summarize, the following are important points for individuals with diabetes mellitus to note:

1. The diet provides approximately 55–60% of calories as carbohydrate, 12–20% as protein and less than 30% as fat.
2. Total calorie intake will be adjusted as necessary, for the individual to achieve and maintain a desirable weight.
3. Calorie intake is adequate to provide for optimal growth and development (childhood, pregnancy and lactation).
4. Carbohydrate intake is evenly distributed throughout the day and consistent from day to day.
5. The diet should consist of normal foods with a preference for foods which contain unrefined carbohydrates and are high in soluble fibre.
6. Food intake is adjusted to accommodate changes in life-style (e.g. illness, physical activity, emotional stress, eating-out and travel).
7. Meal plans are individualized and consider social, cultural and ethnic values of the patient and family.

Medication

The *goal* of drug therapy is that the patient will maintain therapeutic glucose levels by increasing endogenous insulin production and utilization; or by maintaining serum insulin levels through the administration of exogenous insulin.

Insulin

Insulin is prescribed for all insulin-dependent diabetics. Non-insulin-dependent diabetics may require insulin

Table 19.9   Examples of commonly used insulins.

Category	Preparation	Source*	Action (hours)†		
			Onset	Peak	Duration
Rapid-acting	Human Actrapid	Human	0.5	2–5	8–10
	Humulin S	Human	0.5	1–3	5–7
	Velosulin	Pork	0.5	1–3	8–10
	Human Velosulin	Human	0.5	1–3	8–10
	Hypurin Neutral	Beef	0.5	2–5	8–10
Intermediate-acting	Semitard MC	Pork	2	4–10	18
	Humulin I	Human	1	2–8	18–20
	Hypurin Isophane	Beef	1	4–10	16–24
	Insulatard	Pork	1.5	4–10	16–24
	Human Insulatard	Human	1.5	4–10	16–24
Long-acting	Human Monotard	Human	2.5	6–16	24
	Humulin Zn	Human	3	6–16	24
	Lentard MC	Pork and Beef	3	8–18	24
	Human Ultratard	Human	4	8–30	36
Mixture of rapid-acting and intermediate-acting insulins	Humulin M2 (20/80)	Human	0.5	1–9	14–16
	Initard 50/50	Pork	0.5	3–8	16–24
	Human Initard 50/50	Human	0.5	3–8	16–24
	Mixtard 30/70	Pork	0.5	3–8	16–24
	Human Mixtard 30/70	Human	0.5	3–8	16–24
	Rapitard MC	Pork and Beef	0.5	3–12	22

* All pork and beef insulins are highly purified.
† Times of action vary in different patients and according to the source of insulin. Human insulin may have a more rapid onset than pork or beef insulin.

during periods of stress (e.g. infection, surgery, pregnancy or emotional crisis). Insulin is prescribed for the individual whose plasma glucose cannot be controlled at acceptable levels despite weight control and adherence to dietary regulation, and for the treatment of ketoacidosis and non-ketotic hyperglycaemia.

Insulin. (a protein) can be prepared from natural sources (i.e. pancreas of cattle and pigs) or synthetically by genetic engineering. Because it is a protein, insulin is destroyed in the gastrointestinal tract by proteinases; therefore, it must be given parenterally. Several types are available and may be classified as rapid-acting with shorter period of action, intermediate-acting with longer period of action, and long-acting with prolonged period of action. The *rapid-acting* preparations include unmodified, clear solutions such as soluble insulin. The *intermediate-acting* insulins include isophane insulins and *medium-acting* insulin zinc suspension (lente) insulins. *Long-acting* insulins, having an extended effect on lowering blood glucose are mostly prolonged-action insulin zinc suspension (ultralente) insulins; protamine zinc insulin is used less frequently. See Table 19.9 for the onset and duration of action of each type of insulin. These figures are approximate, since individual differences in responses do occur.

It is important that the nurse caring for or counselling

diabetics be familiar with the action characteristics of the various types of insulin so that appropriate instruction can be given and the patients assisted in monitoring their medication.

Administration of insulin. Insulin is measured in units. Each patient's regimen is determined individually in relation to a particular schedule and diet plan in an attempt to achieve a normal physiological level of glucose throughout a 24-hour period. The regimen is organized so that insulin action coincides with major meals and also provides action overnight. Diet and activity may have to be readjusted with the insulin routine to facilitate physiological control. Blood glucose levels are normally lowest during the night and begin to rise in the early morning hours. Most insulin regimens consist of combinations of rapid-acting and intermediate-acting insulin. A mixture of two insulins may be administered twice daily (morning and evening), which the patient may mix himself or which may be premixed (e.g. Initard 50/50, Mixtard 30/70). Alternatively, patients may use a multi-injection regimen with an intermediate-acting insulin given at bedtime and a rapid-acting insulin administered immediately before meals. Most patients can be taught to adjust or supplement their insulin regimen in response to changes in their blood glucose levels, changes in activity, eating patterns, stress or illness.

Insulin is given by subcutaneous injection below the subcutaneous fat to prevent lipodystrophy. The arms, thighs and abdomen are the areas used, (Figure 19.8). Injections should be at least 2.5 cm (1 in) apart until the full site is completely used. The site is then rotated. Too frequent use of one site causes fibrosing and scarring which delay absorption as well as make the injection more difficult. Disposable syringes with non-detachable needles of finer gauge are less traumatizing to tissue and decrease the air bubbles in the syringe. With these shorter needles, the needle is inserted at a 90° angle. The use of an injection 'pen' makes the process of injecting more convenient and discreet (Manning, 1989). The device, similar to an ordinary cartridge pen, is loaded with a prefilled cartridge of insulin. The 'nib' of the pen is a disposable needle. The dose of insulin required is selected on the dial on the body of the pen, or clicks are counted and the insulin injected at the usual site. Individual regimens are planned with the patient according to needs and abilities. Cleaning the skin with alcohol prior to injection is contraindicated. If the skin is not clean, then soap and water will suffice. Alcohol may be a contributory factor to hardening of the injection areas.

All insulin other than the soluble clear insulin must be thoroughly mixed before use to ensure uniform suspension and concentration throughout. This is done by rotating the bottle and inverting it slowly from end to end; vigorous shaking is avoided to prevent the formation of froth.

Some patients require a combination of extended-acting insulin (lente, isophane) with soluble insulin. If soluble and extended-acting insulin are to be mixed in the same syringe before injection, the following procedure should be adopted:

- Inject air into cloudy insulin (lente, isophane).
- Inject air into clear insulin (soluble).
- Draw up correct dose of clear insulin and remove all bubbles of air.
- Draw up correct dose of cloudy insulin.

If too much extended-acting (cloudy) insulin is drawn up into the syringe, do *not* inject it back into the vial, since the syringe contains a mixture of insulins, but dispose of the contents of the syringe and start again.

If soluble insulin and insulin zinc suspension (lente, ultralente) are mixed in the syringe, they must be given immediately. This is because excess zinc in the lente and ultralente preparations can delay the effect of the soluble insulin after mixing.

Soluble insulin and isophane (NPH) insulin can be mixed in the syringe and then stored in a refrigerator for up to 5 days, but it is normal practice to use them the same day. Before injecting the insulin it is important that the syringe is rotated between the hands for 10–15 seconds to ensure that the insulin is well mixed.

Each bottle of insulin bears an expiry date beyond which the content should not be used. Insulin should be kept in a cool place, preferably a refrigerator; freezing is avoided. Extremes of temperature and exposure to sunlight are likely to cause deterioration.

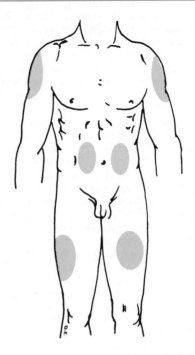

Figure 19.8 Suitable locations for insulin injections.

Insulin pumps. A portable insulin infusion pump provides continuous, subcutaneous delivery of regular insulin to maintain a basal insulin level. Predetermined or self-regulated amounts of insulin to correspond with meals, unusual activity or illness are released (see Figure 19.9). Some machines can be adjusted to decrease the rate of insulin delivery in the early morning hours. The goal of continuous insulin infusion therapy is to maintain blood glucose levels as close to normal physiological levels as possible; they fluctuate over a 24-hour period. Individuals using these devices must be willing to be active participants in their disease management, follow dietary and activity regimens and monitor their blood glucose levels several times a day. Insulin pumps provide the person with greater flexibility in travelling, the timing of meals and in participation in unusual activities. The pump may also be disconnected for 1–2 hours for swimming or bathing. Patient satisfaction is generally high although some individuals find the wearing of a pump is a constant reminder of having diabetes. Difficulties related to insulin pumps include battery failure, blocked needles and occasionally infection at injection sites.

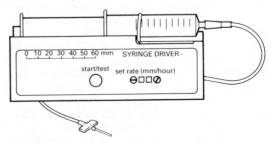

Figure 19.9 Example of an insulin pump.

Complications of insulin therapy. Various local and general reactions to insulin may occur. The *local reactions* are minor in nature and include local sensitivity, lipodystrophy and fibrosis. Frequently, when insulin therapy is first started, sensitivity may be manifested at the site of injection because the insulin is a foreign protein and antigenic. The area becomes red, swollen and itchy but the response is generally temporary and disappears as the patient becomes desensitized by the repeated doses of insulin.

The local action of insulin on the adipose tissue cells may incur a swelling of the fatty tissue followed by atrophy which leaves a hollow space in the area. These atrophic areas are not serious but present an undesirable cosmetic effect. Management may consist of switching the patient to a more purified pork insulin. Frequent and repeated injections into one area of tissue may result in hypertrophy of tissue and eventual fibrosing. Fibrous tissue has poor vascularization which decreases the rate of absorption of insulin. This complication may be prevented by systematic rotation of the injection sites and avoiding the use of any one spot more often than once every 4 weeks. The nurse should also recommend that the injection site is not wiped with alcohol.

General insulin reactions include insulin resistance and hypoglycaemia. *Insulin resistance* is said to be present when diabetes cannot be controlled with less than 200 units of insulin per day (Metz and Benson, 1988). It may occur secondarily to some other diseases, such as severe adrenocortical hyperfunction, acromegaly and thyrotoxicosis. As a primary condition, it is attributed to an antigen–antibody reaction. Antibodies are developed in response to the foreign protein (insulin). It is more likely to occur with insulin extracted from cattle than with that prepared from the pancreas of the pig. Insulin resistance usually develops insidiously several months after insulin treatment has begun. Treatment includes the use of highly-purified porcine insulin, or human insulins.

Hypoglycaemia is discussed on p. 614.

Oral hypoglycaemic drugs.
There are two groups of drugs which lower blood glucose: sulphonylurea compounds and biguanides (Table 19.10). The fact that they may be taken orally provides a distinct advantage. Their use is limited mainly to non-insulin-dependant diabetics.

The *sulphonylurea compounds* lower the blood glucose by stimulating the secretion of insulin and are usually used for non-obese type II diabetes. These preparations include tolbutamide, chlorpropamide and glibenclamide. The principal difference between these preparations is in the duration of their action; tolbutamide has a half-life in lowering the blood glucose for 5–10 hours, chlorpropamide 24–40 hours, and glibenclamide for 10–15 hours. The biguanide preparation available is metformin which has a half-life of 2 hours. The action of the biguanide preparation is not clearly understood, but it is thought to improve glucose assimilation and insulin efficiency.

It must be remembered that it is still important for the person receiving oral hypoglycaemic agents to

Table 19.10 Oral hypoglycaemic drugs.

Group	Half-life (hours)	Action
Sulphonylurea compounds		Stimulate the β islet cells of the pancreas to produce insulin
—Tolbutamide	5–10	
—Chlorpropamide	24–40	
—Glibenclamide	10–15	
Biguanide preparations		May increase uptake of glucose in peripheral tissues
—Metformin	2	

adhere to the prescribed diet and other therapeutic measures. Although the risk of hypoglycaemia is less than with insulin therapy, it may occur, and the patient must be made aware of the early manifestations. Hypoglycaemia is more likely to occur in elderly persons and patients with renal or liver dysfunction, and with the concurrent taking of certain drugs. Examples of the latter are alcohol, aspirin, phenylbutazone, suphonamides and methyldopa (Aldomet). Occasionally, oral hypoglycaemic agents produce some side-effects, such as gastrointestinal disturbances (heartburn, nausea, vomiting, diarrhoea), headache, skin rash and itching. Long term responses to these drugs (over 5 years) is unclear.

Activity

The *goals* of activity and exercise for the person with diabetes mellitus are to: (1) establish a daily activity and exercise pattern to promote metabolic control; (2) reduce the risk for cardiovascular and peripheral vascular complications; and (3) assist in weight control.

Diabetes should not interfere with everyday life. Physical activity promotes health and should be encouraged in moderation and at a consistent level for everyone. It promotes the use of glucose and may diminish the amount of insulin or oral hypoglycaemic needed to control the blood glucose level. It also stimulates and improves the circulation, helps to maintain muscle tone, prevents obesity and promotes a sense of well-being. Some diabetics have sufficient exercise in their occupation, but those in sedentary jobs or who are retired should have a planned programme which is introduced gradually. Since the prescription for diet and a hypoglycaemic agent is based on the patient's physical activity, the regimen should be approximately the same each day to minimize fluctuations in the blood glucose concentration. When variations in daily energy expenditure are necessary, adjustments in the diet may be needed. Extra carbohydrate in the form of fruit, milk or bread may be added if activity is increased, or even more concentrated carbohydrate forms may be required if activity is strenuous or prolonged. When the usual amount of activity is decreased for some reason (other than illness or infection), some decrease in the calorific and carbohydrate intake is usually indicated.

Active exercise at regular intervals is encouraged

during hospitalization if at least a moderate degree of glycaemic control has been achieved. With an anticipated increase of activity on discharge from the hospital, the insulin dosage may be decreased and the food plan amended accordingly. For the older diabetic a daily routine of walking and light home chores (house and garden) is recommended.

The aim is to maintain a balance between energy expenditure and the prescribed treatment (diet with or without insulin or oral hypoglycaemic). More than the usual amount of excercise lowers the blood glucose; less than the usual amount will raise it. Patients must be cautioned that exercise may aggravate the glycaemic state, causing hyperglycaemia and hyperketonaemia, when the person's glycaemic control is poor (if the blood glucose level is greater than 10 mmol/l (Hunter, 1990)).

The diabetic participating in strenuous activity, particularly if on insulin therapy, should advise a colleague or, in the case of sports, a friend or sports supervisor that he is a diabetic in case of a hypoglycaemic reaction. The person is instructed to increase carbohydrate intake and/or decrease insulin dose before undertaking the increased energy expenditure. The diabetic person should also carry sugar cubes or sweets which can be taken at the first signs of weakness and hypoglycaemic reaction. Blood glucose levels should be monitored before and after exercise to allow for appropriate adjustments to food and insulin intakes. When making a change in occupation that involves either a decrease or increase in activity, the diabetic should review the plan of treatment with the doctor.

PATIENT AND FAMILY EDUCATION

The overall goals of diabetic education are to:

- Impart the knowledge and skills necessary to maintain optimal glycaemic control.
- Develop and foster the attitudes, beliefs and behaviours which are conducive to metabolic control.
- Promote a quality of life whereby the individual's disease and lifestyle are harmoniously balanced.

The person with diabetes mellitus has a chronic lifelong disease. To achieve a state of health and an acceptable level of functioning, the person must learn to coordinate the treatment regimen of diet, activity and medication into a daily routine of work or school and recreation to achieve and maintain normal physiological blood glucose levels. The diabetic is ultimately responsible for the self-management of health care. To do this, adequate knowledge and skill to be able to make informed decisions about current health problems and an understanding of the implications of present actions on future health status are required.

Nursing intervention

The nurse, with the doctor, dietitian and pharmacist, is responsible for assessing learning needs, helping the patient to set realistic goals, providing knowledge, teaching necessary skills, identifying relevant learning resources and evaluating the outcomes of teaching. Successful diabetic education programmes have been developed using a team of health professionals working together to teach groups of diabetic patients and their families (British Diabetic Association, 1988).

All nurses should possess the knowledge and skill necessary to teach diabetic patients and their families what they need to know about diabetes and its management to enable them to function safely on discharge. Nurses are responsible for reinforcing learning with the patient and family, for identifying ongoing learning needs and for ensuring that individuals and their families are aware of available resources. More advanced knowledge of diabetes care and skills as an educator and counsellor are required to assist patients to achieve greater levels of self-management. Teaching plans must be individualized to meet the unique needs of each patient and family.

Assessment of learning needs
Assessment of what the patient already knows, learning capability and life-style factors which will influence learning and compliance with the therapeutic plan is important before a learning plan can be developed. For a previously diagnosed diabetic, information is required about the usual diabetic routine at home, work or school, how usual activities have changed, community resources used and what further information and skills are needed. Guidelines for assessing patients' learning needs are discussed in Chapter 3.

The patient's responses to diagnosis and treatment influence readiness to learn. Initial responses to the diagnosis may include fear, withdrawal, or anger. Assessment of learning needs continues as patients work through their immediate reactions reaching a phase in which they may talk about their feelings and are prepared to listen and accept the reassurance that their disease can be controlled and that the necessary treatment and care can soon become a routine part of their life without seriously altering it.

Development of a teaching plan
Once learning needs are identified, the nurse, with the patient and family, sets priorities. These may be dictated by the fact that the patient will be discharged in a few days and will be responsible for preparing meals and/or administering insulin. The knowledge and skill necessary for safe functioning assumes priority and must be adjusted according to the readiness of the patient to learn. Information available from the British Diabetic Association may provide further support after discharge home.

In planning the instruction, it is necessary to know the patient's background so that care can be adapted as much as possible to normal living patterns. The amount of information given at one time depends on the patient's ability and willingness to receive it. Generally, brief periods of discussion are more effective than the presentation of a large amount of information at one time. Group instruction may be used in the hospital or clinic for some topics, but it must be remembered that each diabetic's treatment and life-style are unique. A large part of the discussion must be on an individual basis. Patient negotiation and learning contracts (see Figure 2.3) are useful strategies to assist individuals with the development of self-management skills.

Teaching is begun as soon as possible to avoid giving too much at one time, leading to confusion and discouragement, and to allow time for the patient to practise self-care, read and ask questions.

Explanations are made in simple lay terms; and demonstrations are broken into steps, made slowly, repeated as often as necessary, and sufficient opportunity is provided for the patient to practise. Follow-up discussion of signs and symptoms experienced during episodes of hypoglycaemia and hyperglycaemia and responses to interventions, helps the patient to develop the problem-solving skills needed for self management. Illustrations, films and written explanations and directions may be used for clarification. Reading material (books, pamphlets) written for diabetics are available from The British Diabetic Association.

An instruction programme should cover the following: (1) an explanation of diabetes; (2) diet; (3) insulin therapy or oral hypoglycaemic agents, if appropriate; (4) activity; (5) assessment of glycaemic control; (6) metabolic emergencies; (7) diabetic identification card; (8) special personal care; (9) regular health supervision; and (10) sources of information and assistance.

Goals

Following completion of the learning plan the diabetic patient and relevant family members will be able to undertake the following:

Knowledge of diabetes mellitus.

- Define diabetes mellitus.
- Describe particular type of diabetes mellitus in relation to other types.
- Describe how diabetes affects usual daily activities.

Diet.

- Describe a meal plan appropriate for the disease and usual life-style of the patient.
- Describe how the meal plan can be adjusted to accommodate illness and changes in activity.
- List foods which should be limited or avoided.
- Describe a plan to achieve or maintain desired body weight.

Medication (if applicable).

- State the name of the prescribed oral hypoglycaemic agent and its purpose.
- Describe a plan to take medication daily.
- Describe side-effects of the prescribed oral agent.
- Describe the action of insulin and its interrelationship with blood glucose and exercise.
- State the name, dosage and time of administration of prescribed insulin(s).
- Demonstrate the correct technique of preparing insulin for injection, rotation of injection sites, injection of the insulin and care and disposal of equipment.
- State the prescribed medication routine for periods of illness and/or when the doctor should be notified during illness.

Activity.

- State the reasons for maintaining regular exercise.
- Describe how diet and insulin may be adjusted as activity levels change.

Skin integrity.

- State the need for regular skin care.
- Demonstrate how feet are cared for.
- Describe situations (infection, skin breakdown) requiring health supervision.

Assessment of glycaemic control.

- Demonstrate the technique of blood glucose monitoring.
- Demonstrate a technique of testing urine for glucose and ketones (if applicable).
- Describe a plan for regular testing of blood glucose.
- Discuss the significance of blood glucose results in relation to time of day, associated food intake, recent activity and medication.
- Suggest appropriate action for adjustment of diet, activity and/or medication plans in response to the test results.

Acute metabolic emergencies.

- Define hypoglycaemia and hyperglycaemia.
- Discuss causes of hypoglycaemia and hyperglycaemia that might apply to his personal situation.
- Describe the symptoms experienced with (a) hypoglycaemia and (b) hyperglycaemia.
- Describe a plan of action should symptoms of (a) hypoglycaemia and (b) hyperglycaemia occur.

Health management.

- List community resources available for diabetic patients and families.
- Describe plans for attaining regular medical, dental and eye care.
- Describe information to be provided to various health professionals.
- State the importance of wearing an identification tag and/or carrying a card to identify the type of diabetes and medication plan.

Implementation of the Teaching Plan.

How the learning plan is implemented depends upon the immediate patient situation and the agreed goals and plan. Rarely does one nurse have the opportunity to work with a patient and family throughout the learning process. Teaching carried out in hospital, whether with the newly diagnosed diabetic or with an established diabetic patient and family, requires evaluation and supplementation in the community as the person has opportunity to apply knowledge and skill and learning needs continue to evolve.

The following is presented as an example from which the nurse can select the content relevant to an individual patient in a given situation.

1. *What is diabetes mellitus?* A simple basic explanation is made of the nature of diabetes, relating it to the

symptoms experienced by the patient. To illustrate, the patient may be told that sugar and starches (such as bread and cereal) are converted by digestion to a simple form of sugar called glucose, which is the body's chief source of energy. In order for the cells to extract it from the blood and use it, the chemical insulin is necessary. There are two types of diabetes. In Type I or insulin-dependent diabetes, there is not sufficient insulin being produced to use the amount of sugar and starches being taken, so glucose accumulates in the blood in excess of the normal. The kidneys remove some of the excess, which is why the diabetic voids a lot of urine which contains sugar. The loss of large amounts of urine results in thirst. Weakness, fatigue and hunger occur because the sugar is not being 'burned' to produce energy. The body, in an effort to provide energy, may break down body tissue, causing a loss of weight. Daily insulin injections and dietary measures are necessary to control this disorder.

With type II or non-insulin-dependent diabetes enough insulin to handle the amount of sugar may be produced but the cells cannot effectively utilize the glucose. This type of diabetes can usually be controlled by diet and activity to achieve a desirable body weight. Some patients may require an oral hypoglycaemic agent.

2. *Diet.* The prescribed diet must be clearly and carefully interpreted to the patient and family. The initial instruction is usually given by a dietitian, but con-siderable clarification and reinforcement by the nurse, who is with the patient more often and for longer periods, is usually necessary. The dietitian explains the prescribed diet and reviews the foods allowed each day and how these may be distributed into meals and snacks. It is helpful for the patient to plan meals for several days. The purchase and preparation of food and how it may be worked in with the family meals are discussed. The general principles which apply to the diabetic diet are discussed (see p. 598).

The patient and health professional discuss and agree on a target or ideal body weight for the person. A plan to achieve and/or maintain the desirable weight is mutually developed and should include plans for regular weight checks.

Adjustment of diet and medications in relation to increased stress and changes in life-style is important. Diabetic patients can be taught to adjust their diet and medication in relation to change in demand for glucose and insulin. Blood glucose monitoring by patients has made it possible for them to achieve good glycaemic control during illness and to be more flexible in their eating patterns, activity and travel.

Eating out and delayed meals may also necessitate changes in food intake. Whenever possible, diabetics should maintain their usual eating pattern, including the time of meals and the content of each meal. They quickly learn to select appropriate meals from menus or from the selection offered by friends and relatives. When eating out, the diabetic should be prepared for delays and the possibility of hypoglycaemia by carrying sugar lumps or other sources of quickly absorbable carbohydrate. When aware that meals will be delayed the patient is instructed to have a small snack before

leaving home. Insulin-dependent diabetics with good understanding of their disease and its management, may be provided with guidelines from their doctor on the use of compensatory insulin supplements prior to large meals. Patients using insulin pumps and blood glucose monitoring quickly learn to take an extra bolus of insulin with an unusually large meal.

The patient is encouraged to read and obtain for personal use books and pamphlets which contain considerable detail on diabetic dietary plans. The dietitian will give more detailed advice and the British Diabetic Association literature can reinforce and extend the basic dietary education.

3. *Drug therapy.* If the patient is on *insulin* therapy advice is required on equipment and where it may be obtained. An explanation is made of what insulin is, types available and the name and nature of the insulin prescribed, and how it is identified. Unit dosage is explained and measurement by units is demonstrated. The patient is encouraged to practice handling the syringe and needle and the measurement of the prescribed dose. Instruction and demonstrations are then given to facilitate aseptic handling of the syringe and needle, rotating of the vial to equalize the suspension of insulin, withdrawal of the required amount of insulin, the necessary rotation and prepara-tion of sites for injection, the actual injection and the safe disposal of the equipment. Storage and main-tenance of an adequate supply of insulin are discussed. Insulin is only available on prescription. Automatic injectors are available which may be of assistance to those patients who find the injection of the needle difficult. The injector has a mechanically controlled spring which, when released, pushes the needle quickly through the skin. The need to plan and break down all this information into small logical teaching units or blocks is again emphasized. If discouragement and frustration are evident, further instruction is delayed and another approach considered.

If an *oral hypoglycaemic* agent is prescribed, the importance of taking the drug in the exact dosage at the times ordered is stressed. Written directions are given, and the patient is advised that if headache, nausea, vomiting or other disturbances are experienced, the general practitioner should be contacted. The patient is reminded not to experiment with the dosage of the drug and that adherence to the prescribed diet is most important even though medication is also being re-ceived.

Illness will affect drug medication. Diabetics are instructed on how to manage their disease during illness. If nausea and vomiting are present, the diet plan may be converted to liquids. A balanced diet may still be obtained. Vegetables and fruit may be ingested in the form of juices or soups. If oral intake is not possible, parenteral fluids are administered. The insulin-depend-ent diabetic and patients on oral hypoglycaemics should continue to take their medication during an illness. Larger doses of insulin with more frequent supplement-ary doses may be required. Insulin dosage should be adjusted according to prescribed guidelines in relation to blood glucose determinations. Insulin may be switched to soluble, short-acting insulin for the duration of illness.

Travel may also necessitate changes in drug therapy. The insulin-dependent diabetic needs to take precautions to avoid hypoglycaemia while travelling. If travelling by car, snacks or juices are kept available. On planes and trains while meals may be obtained if delays occur, it is still important to carry some food in the handbaggage in case there are problems. Travelling through several time zones should not pose any difficulties, providing that a plan is developed ahead of time. The insulin-dependent diabetic must remember to carry insulin and syringes and be prepared to inject insulin wherever required. It is important for the patient to take a sufficient quantity of insulin and supplies for insulin administration and blood glucose monitoring or urine testing for the duration of any stay, as products may vary or be difficult to obtain in different countries. Insulin should be refrigerated whenever possible but will be quite safe if kept in a small insulated container to prevent exposure to high temperatures and bright light.

4. *Activity.* Regular activity is beneficial and an integral component of the person's diabetic control. The nurse and patient should review usual activity patterns and develop plans for the person to receive consistent exercise. The person who participated in extended exercise activities prior to diagnosis is helped to develop a modified routine until glycaemic control is achieved and the skill of balancing diet and insulin in relation to activity has been learnt.

Precautions to avoid exercise induced hyperglycaemia and hyperketonaemia include:

- Regulation of food and insulin intakes in conjunction with excercise.
- Regular monitoring of blood glucose levels.
- A readily available source of carbohydrate.
- A decrease in insulin dosage prior to extended exercise.
- Use of an injection site that is not active during excercise (e.g. the abdomen).

Precautions to avoid exercise induced hyperglycaemia and hyperketonaemia include:

- Regular monitoring of blood glucose levels.
- Avoiding exercise when glycaemic control is poor.

5. *Skin integrity.* Diabetes increases the individual's risk for infection and skin breakdown. The person is taught to keep the skin clean, warm and free of irritation and pressure as much as possible. Precautions are taken to prevent cracks and breaks in the skin. Scratches, cuts and abrasions are cleaned and protected by a dressing. The use of strong antiseptics (such as iodine) and adhesive is avoided. Prolonged exposure to sunlight and the use of local heat applications (electric heating pad, hot water bottle) are discouraged.

The adult diabetic's feet require regular special attention because of the increased susceptibility to circulatory disorders and loss of sensation. The patient is directed to bathe the feet daily with warm (not hot) water, using a mild antibacterial soap and a small amount of bath oil, and to dry them thoroughly, especially the areas between the toes, using gentle

pressure rather than vigorous rubbing. Talcum powder may be used sparingly if the feet tend to be moist and perspire; if they are dry and scaly, a light application of lanolin or prescribed lotion is rubbed into the skin. The toenails are cut straight across with scissors. If calluses and corns cannot be controlled by rubbing them lightly with a pumice stone, they should be treated by a state registered chiropodist who is advised of the person's diabetes. The patient is cautioned against attempting to remove them by cutting or applying commercial preparations. Stockings or socks should fit well to avoid any constriction or wrinkles that might cause irritation or pressure and are changed daily. To prevent possible interference with the circulation, garters are not worn. Shoes should be well-fitting so there is no irritation or pressure on any part of the foot, and new shoes are worn only for brief periods until 'broken in'. Walking barefoot and the application of heating appliances are discouraged. The feet should be examined daily for breaks in the skin, discoloration, dryness and drainage. Numbness, persisting coldness, discoloration, a burning feeling, pain or any unusual condition of the lower limbs should be reported to the doctor.

6. *Assessment of glycaemic control.* Assessment of metabolic control of glucose can be achieved by the person on a continuous or intermittent basis by monitoring of blood glucose and/or the testing of urine for glucose and ketones.

Urine glucose monitoring is not adequate to enable good control of glycaemia. It does not identify hypoglycaemia and may not reveal hyperglycaemia; the latter is detected only when the blood glucose levels exceed the renal threshold, which is variable and may change in older diabetics and those with renal complications.

Blood glucose monitoring is easily mastered by most patients once they adjust to the invasive aspect of pricking their finger to obtain a drop of blood. Self-monitoring of blood glucose levels facilitates understanding of diabetes and gives the patient an active role in the management of the disorder. Satisfaction is generally high; infections and other complications due to self-monitoring are negligible.

The accuracy of glucose monitoring by diabetic individuals in their homes has been found to be approximately 80%. Inaccuracies were found to be unrelated to training programme, type of monitor used, age, sex, duration of diabetes, frequency of monitoring, educational level or knowledge of the monitoring technique (Most et al, 1986).

Self-monitoring of blood glucose is recommended for all persons going home on insulin, pregnant women with diabetes and during episodes of illness and hypoglycaemia.

Monitoring of blood glucose levels may be done: (1) continually, with diet, activity and insulin adjusted as indicated; (2) intermittently, with the person using a blood glucose profile of a 'typical day' to assess glycaemic control; or (3) only during episodes of illness or when problems occur. The monitoring schedule will vary for each person. A stable, non-insulin-dependent diabetic may take three to seven fasting tests per week while insulin-dependent diabetics continue to monitor glucose levels about 2–4 times daily.

Self-monitoring of blood glucose may be done with a reagent strip, with or without a machine. Both methods are sufficiently accurate for self-monitoring but the machines are best used when meticulous control of glycaemia is desired. It is important to follow the manufacturer's instructions precisely, particularly as regards accuracy and timing. It is a common mistake to use the test strips after the recommended expiry date or to fail to store the strips in the airtight container.

The finger is cleansed and pricked with a single-prong lancet, either manually or using an automated device. A drop of blood large enough to cover the reagent pads is placed on a reagent strip and left for the period of time recommended by the manufacturer; it is then washed or wiped off and the results interpreted either by comparing the strip with a chart or placing the strip into a machine which provides a digital read-out of the results. Most meters available today are small, portable and simple to use. Differences between machines include the method of calibration prior to use. The person who chooses to use a monitor is told about the sources where information may be acquired on the various types of equipment and also receives instruction on their use. Pamphlets, audiovisual presentations and individualized instruction are usually available from the supplier. The person should begin to keep a record of the results of the blood glucose tests while in hospital. The nurse and doctor discuss these with the patient each day, comparing results to the previous day and exploring factors which influenced any changes. The newly diagnosed diabetic patient may not grasp the significance of the results initially, however involvement in the decision making process about disease management will promote responsibility for self-care.

The individual can discuss daily records, actions taken and results obtained with the community health nurse, doctor and/or out-patient clinic staff.

Specific written instructions are provided to help the patient adjust insulin dosage according to the results of blood glucose tests when this is relevant.

Urine testing. This provides a simple and convenient measurement of the concentration of blood glucose over the renal threshold level. Non-insulin-dependent diabetics are less likely to have glycosuria except occasionally following a large meal. Insulin-dependent diabetics who use this method to monitor their diabetes control usually test their urine for glucose four times a day (i.e. before meals and at bedtime or perhaps only once daily). Testing the urine for ketones is done:

- When the blood glucose test result is greater than 13.3 mmol/l.
- During periods of illness.
- When the person experiences signs and symptoms of hyperglycaemia or ketoacidosis.
- During episodes of vomiting or diarrhoea.
- During episodes of emotional stress.
- During pregnancy.
- During vigorous and extended exercise.
- When oral hypoglycaemic agents are started.
- When insulin dosage is being adjusted.

Urine should be tested on a 'double-voided' specimen. The first specimen, consisting of urine contained in the bladder for a period of time is discarded.

A second specimen for testing is obtained 30 minutes later. This fresh specimen more accurately reflects the urine glucose level at that time.

A variety of agents in the form of dip sticks and tablets are available for urine testing by the patient. Specific instructions are packaged with each product. Choice of product will depend on the person's manual dexterity, the ease with which the product can be used while travelling and the colour scales of the product (many elderly patients with impaired vision have difficulty differentiating certain colours).

7. *Knowledge of metabolic emergencies* (hypoglycaemia and hyperglycaemia). The diabetic who is receiving insulin or an oral hypoglycaemic agent should know that under certain circumstances the blood glucose level may fall below normal, resulting in what is called an insulin or *hypoglycaemic* reaction. The patient and family should be familiar with the symptoms which usually begin to appear when the blood glucose level falls below 3.3 mmol/l. A hypoglycaemic reaction in a person receiving rapid-acting insulin usually occurs approximately 2–6 hours after the injection. In a person receiving intermediate-acting insulin, the reaction happens more commonly in the afternoon or evening. Hypoglycaemic reactions to slow-acting insulin generally occur during the night or the following morning. It is possible for persons receiving oral hypoglycaemic drugs to develop hypoglycaemia. Symptoms vary from one person to another but are usually similar with each reaction for the same person. The early signs and symptoms include sweating, tremor, apprehension, hunger, weakness, rapid pulse and palpitations. More advanced symptoms are faintness or dizzyness, blurring of vision or diplopia, headache, slow reactions, uncoordinated movements, twitching, disorientation and confusion. The possible causes of hypoglycaemia are the delay or omission of a meal following administration of insulin or oral medication, excessive energy expenditure with prolonged and/or strenuous exercise, an overdose of insulin, anorexia, vomiting or diarrhoea, increased utilization of glucose and weight loss without readjustment of insulin dosage.

The person is instructed that on experiencing early symptoms carbohydrate should be taken immediately. With more pronounced symptoms, a quick acting form of carbohydrate will be required, for example two or three cubes of sugar, tea or coffee with 2 or 3 teaspoonsful of sugar, two or three small sweets, orange juice or grape juice (112 g or 4 oz) or 2 teaspoonfuls of honey or syrup may be used. If the symptoms do not disappear in 10 minutes, the administration is repeated. The patient on insulin is advised to always carry lump sugar or boiled sweets or glucose tablets.

The family should know that if the diabetic cannot swallow or retain sugar, glucagon should be administered or a doctor summoned at once. Alternatively the person should be taken as quickly as possible to a hospital accident and emergency department. Friends and associates as well as the family should know that the diabetic receives insulin and may experience a reaction. The patient is advised that insulin reactions should be reported to the doctor as the insulin dosage or diet may require adjustment.

The patient should also be able to recognize early symptoms of uncontrolled diabetes, which cause *hyperglycaemia*. If it is not corrected in the early stage it may lead to the serious complications of diabetic ketoacidosis or hyperosmolar non-ketotic coma. Hyperglycaemia and dehydration with or without ketosis, develop more slowly than hypoglycaemia, usually over several days. The disturbance is usually manifested by loss of appetite, nausea, vomiting, thirst, weakness, drowsiness and general malaise. Glucose will be present in the urine and blood levels are greatly increased. They are frequently associated with infection or stress or may be due to prolonged dietary indiscretion or omission of insulin or oral hypoglycaemic agent. The patient is advised that the general practitioner should be contacted as soon as symptoms are experienced. Until medical attention is obtained the patient should remain in bed, keep warm, and try to drink clear fluids *without sugar*, to avoid dehydration and electrolyte imbalance, even if this causes vomiting; if possible, someone should remain with the patient.

8. *Health management*. The newly diagnosed diabetic will be required to make more frequent visits to the general pracittioner or the diabetic clinic. These will become fewer as the disease and treatment are stabilized. The nurse in either situation checks how the patient is managing and gives the patient the opportunity to ask questions. Some aspects of care may require repetition and reinforcement. Before leaving the hospital, the importance of keeping appointments is stressed. In the case of older persons, assistance may be necessary in making some arrangements for transport to the clinic.

It is advisable for the diabetic to have an annual *eye examination* because of the predisposition to visual change which can only be detected by an ophthalmologist. There is an increased tendency for retinal haemorrhage in diabetes which must be identified promptly and treated with laser beam.

Diabetic identification card. Every diabetic should carry a diabetic identification card at all times so that his condition will be made known quickly in the event of a reaction, illness or accident. Cards which carry appropriate information are available from the hospital, doctors, the diabetic clinic and the British Diabetic Association or its local branches; a written one may be carried temporarily.

Sources of assistance. The patient and family are made aware of the available sources of help and information. These include the national and local diabetic associations. The services provided by the various organizations and recommended publications are cited. Patients are encouraged to join. This entitles them to the regular periodical and additional literature published by the association.

Evaluation of patient and family teaching.
It is recognized that patient and family education positively influences metabolic control and prevents or delays the onset of chronic complications. Results of a meta–analysis of 47 studies on the effects of patient teaching on knowledge, self-care behaviours and metabolic control supported the assumption that teaching has positive outcomes for diabetic adults (Brown, 1988). Less is known about the factors that contribute to learning.

Studies of diabetic education use a variety of outcome measures to evaluate the effectiveness of education programmes and individual teaching.

Knowledge of the disease and its management can be evaluated using tested tools and by documenting the frequency of hospital admissions or clinic visits related to diabetes control. It has been demonstrated that patients taking insulin scored higher on knowledge tests than diabetics not taking insulin. Diabetic education leads to improved knowledge but learning is an ongoing process requiring reassessment of learning needs and further input in relation to identified deficits or changes in personal goals and objectives.

Glycaemic control can be evaluated using blood glucose and glycosylated haemoglobin levels. Blood glucose levels are useful for daily monitoring by the patient as well as by health professionals. The determination of glycosylated haemoglobin levels gives an indication of glucose control over a period of time. This test measures the amount of glucose that adheres to haemoglobin during the life span of the red blood cell (about 2–3 months).

Hospital admissions and visits to diabetic clinics give an indirect measure of the person's self-management skills and ability to identify potential problems and use resources appropriately. Comparative studies generally indicate fewer admissions to hospital following educational interventions. Quality assurance programmes in the health care agencies provide useful data on the freqency and reason for admissions and some programmes provide measurements of patient outcomes.

Complications. Documentation of the frequency of episodic acute metabolic complications and the development of chronic complications, provides further evidence of the effectiveness of diabetic education.

Personal meaning of diabetes. Attention must be given to the patient's attitudes to diabetes and what it means to them. Patient education should help diabetics achieve the highest standards of glycaemic control, but this should be accompanied by satisfactory emotional adjustment and social fulfilment. Diabetes educators need to address the affective or attitudinal aspects of coping with this life-long condition (British Diabetic Association, 1987).

The nurse in any clinical setting should always use the best source available to evaluate the effectiveness of teaching *the patient and family*. Only the patient and those close to him or her can determine if the knowledge and skills taught met their needs and if the teaching contributed to their psychological and social adjustment to diabetes.

PATIENT EDUCATION: THE PERSON WITH TYPE II DIABETES MELLITUS

Clinical situation: *Mrs Grace Cook who has type II diabetes mellitus.*

Mrs Cook is a relatively inactive 60-year-old lady who enjoys baking and gardening. She is 10 kg over-weight. She has been having a problem with a cut on her right middle finger that 'just won't heal'. She has also been experiencing blurring of her vision, has less energy than usual and when questioned thinks that she has been urinating more frequently. Her fasting blood glucose level was 13 mmol/l and negative for ketones when tested by her general practioner.

Mrs Cook's doctor referred her to a dietitian for dietary assessment and a diet for type II diabetes. The dietitian found that Mrs Cook was drinking a lot of fruit juices. She skipped breakfast but ate a very large evening meal with her husband and continued to eat snacks throughout the evening while watching television.

Discussion. Grace is typical of many persons with type II diabetes mellitus. Her symptoms developed slowly, she has the major risk factor of obesity and she is within the age group of 40–65 when over 50% of non-insulin-dependent diabetics are diagnosed. Symptoms of hyperglycaemia experienced by Grace included decreased energy, urinary frequency, blurred vision and impaired healing. Her fasting blood glucose level was elevated.

The patient's overall goals were to return to a normal body weight for her age and height and to have blood glucose within normal limits.

Goals. Grace will:

- Decrease her body weight by 10 kg over the next 6–8 months.
- Establish a regular pattern of exercise.
- Alter her eating habits to decrease calorie intake, increase dietary carbohydrate and fibre and eat three meals a day.
- Have a blood glucose of <9 mmol/l.

Intervention and Evaluation. The dietitian prescribed a weight reducing diet which included 3 meals a day. She helped Grace to select foods which were high in complex carbohydrate and fibre. She told Grace to drink water or diet fizzy drinks rather than fruit juices for thirst. Grace was able to lose 1 kg in the first month of her diet and her fasting blood glucose level dropped to 10 mmol/l.

Exercise recommendations for type II diabetics include low intensity exercise over 40–60 minutes at least 5 days each week. Grace began taking a walk after breakfast. She did this for 30 minutes almost every day and was able to lose an additional 0.5 kg in the second month. Her fasting blood glucose dropped to 8.7 mmol/l.

THE PERSON WITH TYPE I DIABETES MELLITUS

Clinical situation: *Mr Tom Tolly who has type I diabetes mellitus and ketoacidosis*

Mr Tolly, who is 22-years-old, was married 2 weeks ago. He is a construction worker.

Mr Tolly experienced a weight loss of 9 kg in the past 2 weeks. He has been very thirsty and has been urinating large amounts. He has been getting up at night to urinate and to drink fluids. He states that his vision is blurred and that he is tired and lacks energy. His appetite has been very poor for the past few days and he has experienced nausea and stomach pain.

The patient went to his general practitioner who tested his urine for glucose with a reagent stick and found large amounts of glucose and ketones. Mr Tolly was sent to hospital for blood glucose tests. The results were: blood glucose 36 mmol/l, positive ketones; pH 7.0; and bicarbonate level 17 mmol/l.

Mr Tolly was admitted to hospital with a medical diagnosis of severe *diabetic ketoacidosis*. The medical goals of care are to rehydrate him and to treat his diabetes with insulin.

The priorities for nursing care relate to the patient's hyperglycaemic state. Although diabetic ketoacidosis can be resolved in 24 hours, it can be life threatening. Nursing actions include immediate and continuous assessment of Mr Tolly's metabolic state and the identification of associated health problems, as well as collaborative activities related to implementation and evaluation of medically directed care. The long-term goal of Mr Tolly and his wife is to control and achieve self-regulation of his diabetes.

ACUTE METABOLIC EMERGENCIES: TYPE I DIABETES MELLITUS

Diabetic ketoacidosis

Diabetic ketoacidosis is a serious metabolic complication which develops when there is too little insulin and an excess of glucose.

The cause of insulin deficiency may be due to inadequate production of insulin in the undiagnosed diabetic, inadequate administration of insulin or an increased need for insulin resulting from emotional or physical stresses such as infection. Excess glucose may result from increased hepatic production of glucose, decreased utilization of glucose by peripheral tissue and increased ingestion of glucose in the diet.

The production of *ketone bodies* involves processes occurring in adipose tissue, liver and muscle. The glucose in the blood cannot be utilized by the cells, and fat is broken down to provide energy. Fat is mobilized and broken down rapidly, producing ketone bodies (acetoacetic acid, β-hydroxybutyric acid and acetone) in excess of the tissue cells' ability to metabolize them. Alterations in liver metabolism lead to further ketone production. This process is accelerated when glucagon levels rise. An associated decrease in the ability of muscle tissue to utilize these organic acids further contribute to ketoacidosis. The acids and acetone accumulate in the blood. At first the normal pH is maintained by the buffer systems, but eventually the alkali reserve becomes depleted and the pH of the body fluids falls, resulting in acidosis. At the same time, the increased concentration of glucose causes an increased output of urine (osmotic diuresis), and dehydration develops. The increased osmotic pressures of the extracellular fluid result in the movement of fluid out of the cells accompanied by electrolytes. Serious sodium, potassium and phosphate deficiencies develop.

Ketoacidosis has an insidious onset over several days, being preceded by *symptoms* characteristic of uncontrolled diabetes (polyuria, thirst, glycosuria, weakness). The symptoms related to the accumulation of ketones and reduced alkalinity of body fluids include anorexia, nausea, vomiting, deep and rapid respirations, drowsiness, weakness which progresses to prostration, and abdominal pain or muscular cramps. The skin and mouth are dry, and the eyeballs are soft because of dehydration. The patient may appear flushed in the early stages but later becomes pale owing to hypotension. The pulse is rapid and may be weak because of severe dehydration and the reduced intravascular volume. Unless the condition is recognized and treated promptly, the blood pressure falls, the patient becomes comatose, and brain damage will occur unless the situation is quickly reversed. (Coma is uncommon in patients with known diabetes because of greater awareness through patient and family education leading to early adjustment of insulin therapy and prompt medical referrals.)

The patient's urine shows a high concentration of glucose and ketones. The blood glucose is elevated and the sodium and chloride blood levels are lower. The potassium level may be low at first owing to polyuria and vomiting; then it may become normal or elevated as the electrolyte moves out of the cells. The blood urea level is usually higher, and the leucocyte count is generally elevated. The carbon dioxide concentration and combining power are lowered as well as the pH. Plasma concentrations of blood ketones: β-hydroxybutyrate, acetoacetate and acetone are elevated.

The *treatment and nursing intervention* for the patient with diabetic ketoacidosis requires emergency care which is directed toward stimulating the utilization of glucose by the cells and decreasing the production of ketone bodies by the administration of insulin, and correction of dehydration and the electrolyte imbalance. Any causative disorder is also treated.

Immediate blood determinations are made of the glucose, carbon dioxide, potassium, sodium, chloride, phosphate, and urea concentrations. The haematocrit is also checked to determine haemoconcentration. An indwelling catheter may be inserted if the patient is comatose, to enable monitoring of urinary output. If the patient is stuporous or comatose, a nasogastric tube is passed to avoid risk of aspiration of vomitus. The patient receives repeated doses of soluble (rapid-acting) insulin intravenously and/or a continuous intravenous infusion. The solution for the infusion and the dosage of insulin are based on the laboratory blood findings. Continuous cardiac monitoring is done to detect changes in heart action characteristic of an abnormal potassium blood level. Intravenous fluids are given to correct electrolyte deficits as well as dehydration. The initial solution used is usually normal saline; potassium phosphate may be added to the solution. As cited previously, potassium moves out of

the cells and at first the serum concentration may be normal or even elevated. With the administration of the intravenous insulin and solutions, plasma potassium moves into the cells and hypokalaemia may develop which may then necessitate the administration of a potassium solution. Repeated blood electrolyte, glucose and ketone determinations are necessary. When the blood glucose level approaches normal, the frequency of administration and the dosage of insulin are decreased, and an intravenous glucose solution (5% in water or saline) may be ordered. If the patient's blood pressure is low and shock is present, plasma or plasma expanders may be given. Unless the cause of the ketoacidosis was evident at the onset, efforts are made to determine why it occurred.

Clinical Situation (continued)

Mr Tolly's hyperglycaemia is related to diabetic keto-acidosis and is due to inadequate production of insulin associated with his undiagnosed type I diabetes mellitus. He demonstrates the characteristic clinical picture of a person with diabetic ketoacidosis. His symptoms, which developed over a 2-week period, include thirst, polyuria, blurring of vision, weakness, loss of appetite, nausea and gastrointestinal discomfort. The results of diagnostic tests show that Tom has glycosuria, as evidenced by the presence of glucose and ketones in his urine, and that he is hyperglycaemic; his blood glucose level is elevated and ketones are present. His bicarbonate level is decreased (normal 24–32 mmol/1) and his pH is below normal (normal 7.35–7.45). As the nurse, you expect to observe changes in respirations. *Kussmaul breathing* (rapid, deep respirations) is usually present in diabetic ketoacidosis when the pH is below 7.2. When the bicarbonate level decreases, hyperventilation occurs in order to drive off excess carbon dioxide in an attempt to maintain the pH at a physiological level. When the pH is less than 7.0, the compensatory mechanisms change and slower respirations result. Tom is in a very vulnerable state with a pH of 7.0.

The nurse must also be alert for the development of drowsiness and confusion as Tom's metabolic state is no longer compensated and increases in PCO_2 will have a depressing effect on his central nervous system.

The actual and potential *patient problems* on admission to hospital are listed in Table 19.11.

The *goals* for Tom on admission to hospital are that: (1) he will achieve fluid, electrolyte, acid–base and metabolic balance; and (2) he and his wife will develop a basic understanding of his diabetes and resulting ketoacidosis.

Table 19.11 presents the care plan developed for a patient with ketoacidosis.

Evaluation. On admission to hospital Mr Tolly was acutely ill and required skilled care from knowledgeable, experienced nurses. The nurses worked in collaboration with the doctors to manage the acute medical problems presented by Tom. Many of the patient problems discussed in Table 19.11 fall primarily into the realm of nursing. The patient usually makes a good recovery with prompt care and will normally be

Table 19.11   Care plan for the patient with ketoacidosis

Patient problem	Goals	Nursing intervention	Rationale
1. *Fluid volume deficit* due to polyuria and glycosuria	• Fluid intake and urine output will be in physiological balance • Mucous membranes will be moist • Blood glucose levels will decrease towards normal	• Administer 0.9% saline at 650 ml/h for the first 2 hours as ordered. Adjust rate as indicated • Accurately record fluid intake and output hourly • Assess for signs of fluid overload: dyspnoea, pulmonary crackles and wheezes, increased central venous pressure • Assess blood pressure, pulse and respirations hourly • Record patient's temperature 2–3 hourly • Provide mouth care regularly	• The severe dehydration is life-threatening. Isotonic fluids are administered rapidly to restore the intravascular volume and increase cardiac output • Hypotension and tachycardia occur in response to hypovolaemia and decreased tissue perfusion • Dehydration produces a rise in body temperature
2. *Metabolic imbalance: ketoacidosis* related to decreased production of insulin	• Serum glucose level will be 5.6–7.8 mmol/l • Serum acetone level will be 51.6–344.0 mmol/l • Urine will be negative for glucose and ketones	• Administer regular insulin by continuous i.v. infusion (8 u/h) and adjust rate as ordered • Monitor blood glucose and acetone levels, urine glucose and ketones and urinary output hourly • Assess hourly for signs of hypoglycaemia	• Low dose infusions of insulin are effective in decreasing the catabolic process and promoting glucose uptake by the cells • The rate of flow (dosage) is determined by blood glucose levels and decreased ketosis • Sudden reduction in blood glucose levels can cause tachycardia and symptoms of hypoglycaemia
3. *Ineffective breathing pattern* related to hyperventiliation in response to metabolic acidosis	• Respirations will be 20–24/minute and regular • Blood gases, pH and bicarbonate levels will return to normal range	• Assess respiratory rate, depth and rhythm hourly • Change position 2-hourly and assess response to position change • Administer oxygen by nasal cannulae as ordered • Evaluate blood gas level	• Hyperventilation occurs with acidosis. Respirations decrease with pH less than 7.0 • To increase tissue perfusion
4. *Sensory/perceptual deficits* due to ketoacidosis, central nervous system depression, and blurring of vision	• pH will be within normal limits • Serum glucose levels will be within normal limits • Patient will respond appropriately to the environment and to verbal commands	• Assess level of consciousness and pupillary responses, reflexes and behavioural responses 2-hourly and record • Call by name • Explain all procedures and activities and describe what is happening	• Cognitive and perceptual changes are multifactorial in origin and can develop in response to aggressive rehydration and treatment of acidosis • Awareness that blurring of vision is transient helps to decrease fear

Table 19.11 *Continued*

Patient problem	Goals	Nursing intervention	Rationale
		• Explain that vision will clear when diabetes is controlled	
		• Keep cot sides in place on bed	
5. *Alteration in nutrition: intake of less than body requirement* due to inability to utilize glucose as a result of insulin deficit, loss of appetite, nausea and gastrointestinal discomfort	• Abdominal distension and discomfort will be absent • Gastrointestinal sounds will be present on auscultation • Patient will take oral fluids with no discomfort	• Assess for abdominal distension and signs of increased abdominal discomfort • Assist with nasogastric intubation • Document amount and colour of aspirated gastric content • Following removal of nasogastric tube, administer small amounts of clear fluid and assess for distension and discomfort • Answer questions regarding diabetic diet and explain that the dietitian will see the patient prior to discharge	• Gastric mobility is impaired with ketoacidosis • To decompress gastrointestinal tract and reduce discomfort
7. *Impaired physical mobility* related to weakness, fatigue and restrictions of treatment	• Peripheral pulses will remain palpable • Peripheral skin will be normal and warm to touch • Patient will move to bedside chair within 24 hours • Rehydration will be evident by urine output of >1.5 l/day and normal vital signs	• Assess peripheral skin colour and peripheral pulses 2-hourly • Provide antiembolic stockings if prescribed • Perform passive leg exercises 2-hourly while awake until fully mobile • Mobilize patient as soon as possible	• Patient is at risk for developing vascular thrombi due to decreased intravascular volume with dehydration, and acidosis, increased blood viscosity, decreased tissue perfusion, decreased cardiac output and increased adhesiveness of platelets
8. *Knowledge deficit* related to diabetes mellitus, ketoacidosis and their management	• Patient and family will be able to describe the causes of ketoacidosis, and signs of hyperglycaemia • Patient and family will verbalize plans to begin learning about diabetes and its management	• Assess level of understanding of diabetes and ketoacidosis • Provide explanations of all procedures and activities • Answer questions from patient and family • Develop an initial learning plan with the patient and family as soon as they are able to participate	• If the patient and family are knowledgeable about the signs and symptoms of hyperglycaemia and appropriate interventions, future episodes of ketoacidosis are largely preventable

awake, self-caring and mobile within 48 hours of admission.

Teaching Plan. A teaching plan is developed with Tom and his wife. Teaching will be carried out in short intervals throughout the day to accommodate his limited physical tolerance and shortened attention span. Teaching sessions with the dietitian, pharmacist and nurse are arranged for late afternoons when Mrs Tolly will be present. Because of the overwhelming quantity of new knowledge and skills faced by Mr Tolly and his wife, care is taken to limit teaching to that which they need to know to function safely on discharge. The following expectations are agreed to.

Goals. The reader is referred to the list on p. 603. Additional goals which might be incorporated in a teaching package include the ability for Mr and Mrs Tolly to:

- Experience a gradual increase in weight for Mr Tolly from his present 65.5 kg to his ideal body weight of 72 kg.
- Understand how insulin works.
- Describe the role of exercise in diabetes management.
- Discuss with health professionals the adjustments to insulin dose as a result of changes in blood glucose levels.
- Verbalize awareness of complications of diabetes.
- Describe the relationship between diabetes control and the development of complications.
- Talk about the meaning of the diabetes to themselves, their new relationship and their future life-styles.
- Confirm that their major concerns have been addressed.
- Describe an agreed plan for continuing education and medical supervision on discharge.

Mr Tolly's major expressed difficulties are: (1) how he can continue his current job, which often does not have regular coffee and lunch breaks and is very physically demanding; and (2) acceptance of the fact that he has diabetes when he is a young, healthy man, recently married and enjoys sports and drinking alcohol with friends.

The nurse should discuss Tom's concerns with him and arrange for the dietitian to talk with him about possible solutions to the irregular meals and snacks he will experience at work. It will be possible for him to learn to adjust his insulin administration when he knows meals will be delayed. He can also carry snacks with him to take when meals are delayed. Although his present insulin dosage is being regulated according to his restricted activity in hospital, this will be increased and regulated according to the demands of his usual work activity. He should be referred to the occupational health department in his place of work. He should be told that he will still be able to participate in active sports. It is important that he participate in regular, consistent exercise. When exercise is extended or excessive he will have to take glucose supplements such as fruit and sweets and adjust his insulin. He is assured that he will have opportunity to learn these skills once metabolic control is re-established and after he learns

the basics of diet, insulin and exercise management. The doctor will help him with the regulation of the insulin and a referral will be made for the diabetic nurse specialist to work with Tom and his wife when he returns home.

Another area to explore with Tom concerns sex, as he may have experienced difficulty in maintaining an erection due to his diabetes. It should be explained that the severely high blood glucose levels he experienced with the uncontrolled diabetes may cause impotence and that this will resolve when metabolic control is re-established. The diabetes will not affect his sexual desire but when the diabetes is uncontrolled he may be unable to achieve or maintain an erection. Since this problem may impede progress, alter self-concept and affect his new role as a husband, the nurse should encourage him to discuss this with his wife. The initial and later changes in sexual function associated with diabetes can represent the most difficult adjustments faced by persons with diabetes. The reality of impotence, concerns about infertility and the stress these place on the marriage relationship are major concerns for any patient and family. The nurse may give Tom a pamphlet on sexual health and diabetes and plan to reassess his concerns and discuss them further prior to his discharge.

ACUTE METABOLIC COMPLICATIONS: TYPE II DIABETES MELLITUS

Hyperglycaemic, hyperosmolar, non-ketotic diabetic coma

This serious metabolic complication is characterized by severe hyperglycaemia with no significant ketosis. Serum osmolarity is elevated; insulin is deficient but not absent; and severe dehydration and hypovolaemia exist.

Hyperglycaemic, hyperosmolar non-ketotic coma is most likely to occur in non-insulin-dependent diabetics who are controlled by diet and hypoglycaemic agents and who are elderly, institutionalized, physically or mentally incapacitated, or experience a precipitating stress such as infection. Renal insufficiency is frequently an underlying cause, with the kidneys failing to regulate glucose levels. When renal compensatory mechanisms are inadequate and dehydration also is present as may occur in the elderly who are infirm or ill, non-ketotic coma may develop.

The lack of ketosis in patients with this disorder has been attributed to the extreme dehydration which is believed to suppress the release of free fatty acids from the adipose tissue and inhibit the pancreatic insulin response to glucose.

The onset of hyperglycaemic, hyperosmolar non-ketotic coma is insidious, occurring over several days. The patient demonstrates weakness, polyuria and polydipsia. As intracellular dehydration progresses and fluid shifts to the extracellular spaces, symptoms of neurological involvement, lethargy, confusion, convulsions and eventually coma develop.

Treatment is directed toward reversing the hyperosmolar state with fluid replacement and correcting underlying causes. The prognosis for patients with this condition is generally poor but is improved with prompt treatment. Treatment differs in three ways from that of ketoacidosis: (1) large volumes of hypotonic solutions are given intravenously instead of the isotonic solutions used to treat ketoacidosis; as many as 4–6 litres of hypotonic saline may be given during the first 10 hours. When the blood glucose is lower than 14.4 mmol/l, 5% dextrose may be given. (2) Insulin is administered intravenously, but lower doses are required than for ketoacidosis. (3) Less potassium replacement is required. Other electrolytes are replaced as indicated by determination of blood levels. A nasogastric tube may be inserted to control gastric distension and prevent aspiration.

Nursing intervention is similar to that outlined in Table 19.11 for the patient with diabetic ketoacidosis. Careful monitoring and recording of the large volumes of hypotonic parenteral solutions that are administered is important. The patient is assessed for signs of fluid overload which include dyspnoea, pulmonary crackles and wheezes, and increased central venous pressure. The low doses of insulin prescribed are administered using an infusion controller to carefully regulate the dosage. Observations should be made for signs of hypoglycaemia as a precaution.

Care of the patient with altered levels of consciousness is discussed in Chapter 21. Nursing intervention includes measures to maintain a patent airway and personal safety.

The patient and family's level of understanding of diabetes, the causes of metabolic complications, general disease management and actions to take when complications occur are assessed. An individualized teaching plan is developed, implemented and evaluated; referrals are made to the community nurse where appropriate. Attempts are made to determine the factors precipitating the episode and to institute measures to prevent future episodes of hyperosmolar, non-ketotic coma.

Hypoglycaemia

Hypoglycaemia implies an abnormally low blood glucose concentration. The onset of symptoms varies with individuals; some may develop symptoms at a higher level of blood glucose, while others may not manifest the disturbance until a lower level is reached. Adults tend to have symptoms earlier than child diabetics.

The *causes* of hypoglycaemia are overproduction or over-replacement of insulin. Hypoglycaemia may be caused by the delay or omission of a meal after having taken insulin or an oral hypoglycaemic agent, an undue amount of energy expenditure, an overdosage of insulin, a gastrointestinal disorder which produces anorexia, vomiting or diarrhoea, improvement in the diabetic's ability to utilize glucose, failure to adjust insulin dosage when significant loss of weight occurs, or it may occur following a gastrectomy.

The *manifestations* of hypoglycaemia are as follows: A hypoglycaemic reaction in a patient receiving rapid-acting (soluble) insulin usually occurs approximately 2–6 hours after the injection. In the patient receiving an intermediate-acting insulin given in the morning, it happens more commonly in the afternoon or evening. Hypoglycaemic reaction to a slow-acting insulin generally occurs during the night or early in the morning of the following day.

It should be kept in mind that it is possible also for the patient receiving an oral hypoglycaemic agent to develop hypoglycaemia. It develops insidiously and may occasionally go unrecognized.

The signs and symptoms manifested by an abnormally low blood glucose are a reflection of its effect on the central nervous system. The brain is very dependent on a constant, adequate supply of glucose. Any deprivation, even for a relatively brief period, may seriously impair cerebral activity and result in permanent damage. Similarly, repeated occurrences of hypoglycaemia, even of short duration, especially in children, may incur some permanent cerebral impairment. The manifestations of hypoglycaemia vary from one patient to another but tend to be the same with each reaction for the same person, which makes it more easily recognizable by the individual. The earlier signs and symptoms include sweating, tremor, apprehension, hunger, weakness, tachycardia and palpitation. Symptoms usually do not appear until the blood glucose level is 2.8–3.3 mmol/l. More advanced symptoms are faintness or dizziness, blurring of vision or diplopia, headache, slow reactions, uncoordinated movement which occasionally leads to mistaking the patient's condition for alcohol intoxication, muscular twitching that may progress to convulsions especially in children, disorientation and confusion, stupor and eventual loss of consciousness. The urine is usually negative for glucose although occasionally, a trace may be found if the bladder has not been emptied for a few hours. All diabetics, their immediate family and close associates should be familiar with the early signs and symptoms of hypoglycaemia and should know what to do.

If the patient can still swallow, some form of rapidly absorbable concentrated sugar should be given. Ten to 20 g of carbohydrate are usually sufficient to restore the blood glucose level. Orange juice (120 ml) or other sweetened fruit juice or 2 teaspoonfuls of syrup, honey or sugar with a glass of water may be used. Fifteen to 20 minutes after eating, the person should measure the blood glucose level. If there is no improvement the administration is repeated. If the patient is unconscious or uncooperative, 30–50 ml of 50% glucose are given intravenously. Glucagon (1–2 mg) subcutaneously may be ordered to promote glycogenolysis and subsequent increase in blood glucose. Family members may be taught to administer the glucagon. A venous or capillary blood specimen is collected as soon as possible and is repeated at frequent intervals for blood glucose determinations until the patient is stabilized.

Following a reaction, the patient is encouraged to rest for several hours in order to decrease the utilization of blood glucose. Carbohydrate administration may be repeated and some form of protein (cheese or milk) should be given to the patient to provide additional glucose which is produced gradually as a result of protein metabolism. The nurse should check with the doctor before giving the next scheduled dose of insulin. If the patient is at home, instructions should be given not to take more insulin or hypoglycaemic agents at that time. Adjustments are usually made in the carbohydrate content of the diet and in the insulin dosage.

Most diabetic patients and their families are taught

which symptoms signal hypoglycaemia or hyperglycaemia. Evidence suggests that people miss hypoglycaemia or hyperglycaemia symptoms and erroneously believe that their blood glucose levels are within normal range or feel they are hypoglycaemic or hyperglycaemic when they are not. Self-monitoring of blood glucose, while readily available and used by many diabetic patients, is not necessarily used appropriately to confirm subjective symptoms. A survey of 79 IDDM patients found that the majority reported not using self-measurement to confirm low blood glucose levels before taking action to raise the levels (Gonder-Frederick and Cox, 1986). It is suggested that the individual's ability to distinguish good predictors of blood glucose levels can be improved through systematic training. The person may be helped to review documented daily blood glucose levels and associated symptoms and to identify which cues are predictive of the actual blood glucose levels. This problem-solving approach requires that the patient and a family member or close associate be knowledgeable of the symptoms, the measurement of blood glucose levels, the associated risk factors and the treatment of hypoglycaemia. The patient and family member will learn from the experience if encouraged to examine the reaction in retrospect. A discussion of the possible cause and the early symptoms may be helpful in preventing further reactions and in having the patient recognize hypoglycaemia at the onset.

The *Somogyi effect* occurs in insulin-dependent diabetics who are treated too aggressively in an attempt to normalize blood glucose levels. The hypoglycaemia resulting from administration releases counter-regulatory hormones, producing a rebound hyperglycaemia. The insulin produces a decrease in blood glucose which triggers the sympathetic nervous system to release ACTH. The liver releases glycogen and the blood glucose rises. Further administration of insulin causes a repeat of the cycle. Sudden falls in blood glucose levels followed by rebound hyperglycaemia are characteristic of the Somogyi effect. Treatment consists of gradually decreasing the insulin dosage. The phenomenon is less frequent in patients whose diabetes is controlled by insulin infusion pumps.

SUMMARY

The endocrine system contributes to the homeostatic control of many body functions. Disorders of the endocrine system and its interrelated components are of three major types: (1) increased production of one or more hormone(s); (2) decreased production of one or more hormone(s); and (3) failure of the target organ or tissue to respond to the hormone.

Clinical characteristics of endocrine disorders are varied, subtle and slowly progressive. The patient and family are the best source of assessment information as they are usually aware that something is wrong before a pattern of characteristic signs and symptoms can be recognized. The health problems common to most persons with endocrine disorders include: altered nutrition and metabolism, changes in activity tolerance, altered thought processes and emotional responses, altered sexuality patterns, altered fluid balance, impaired skin integrity and impaired thermoregulation.

The person with a hormone imbalance is at risk for the development of life-threatening as well as chronic complications. The nurse provides intensive care during acute episodes and assists the patient and family to recognize the early warnings of endocrine imbalances and actions to take to prevent complications.

The discussions in this chapter focus on the more common endocrine disorders of type I and type II diabetes mellitus and hypothyroidism and hyperthyroidism. Individuals with disorders of the pituitary gland, parathyroid and adrenal glands, experience similar and equally devastating problems. Many persons with endocrine disorders require life-long hormone replacement therapy as a result of decreased production of hormones with disease and/or therapeutic destruction of the involved gland. All are faced with the need to make major adjustments in their lives. The patient ultimately becomes responsible for self-management of the endocrine disorder.

The growing body of nursing knowledge available to resolve patient health problems is useless if it is not transmitted to patients and their families to enable them

LEARNING ACTIVITIES

1. Sit down with a colleague. Imagine he or she has just been diagnosed as suffering from type I IDDM. Explore the changes this would mean in life-style and the feelings these changes would generate. Reverse roles.
2. List the complications of diabetes. Devise a teaching package to use about the complications for:
   (a) A 17-year-old type I diabetic male.
   (b) A 70-year-old type II diabetic male.
3. Imagine you suffer from type I IDDM and you are refusing to co-operate with treatment. Justify your non-compliance to a colleague. What is the response? What steps might reduce your non-compliance?

to assume control of their own care. Throughout this chapter the importance of patient and family teaching is stressed. Emphasis is placed on the provision of information about the survival skills or the basic knowledge and skill the person requires to function safely. Nurses are also responsible for evaluating the effectiveness of health teaching and for determining whether the patient and family understand the need for continuing therapy.

Advanced teaching and counselling skills are needed to help people change their habits and life-styles. Although all nurses do not have the opportunity to follow individuals for an extended period of time to enable them to provide this level of teaching, they can ensure that all persons with long term endocrine disorders are aware of the many resources available in the community.

REFERENCES AND FURTHER READING

Albin J & Rifkin H (1982) Etiologies of diabetes mellitus. *Medical Clinics of North America* **66(6):** 1209–1226.

Almond J (1986) Measuring blood glucose levels. *Nursing Times* **Oct. 8:** 51–54.

British Diabetic Association (1982) Dietary recommendations for diabetes in the United Kingdom. *Human Nutrition: Applied Nutrition* **36a(5):** 378–394.

British Diabetic Association (1984) *Dietary Fibre in the Management of the Diabetic.* London: British Diabetic Association.

British Diabetic Association (1987) *Minimal Education Requirements for the Care of the Diabetic in the United Kingdom.* London: British Diabetic Association.

British Diabetic Association (1988) *What Professional Supervision Should Adults with Diabetes Expect?.* London: British Diabetic Association.

Brown SA (1988) Effects of educational interventions in diabetes care: a meta-analysis of findings. *Nursing Research* **37(4):** 223–230.

Burton B (1989) Corticosteroid therapy. *Nursing* **3(4):** 17–19.

Cagno JM (1989) Diabetes Insipidus. *Critical Care Nurse* **9(6):** 86–93.

Daly H (1988) *Diabetes Care: A Problem Solving Approach.* London: Heinemann.

Daschner BK (1986) Problems perceived by adults in adhering to a prescribed diet. *Diabetic Education* **12(2):** 113–115.

Dillon RS (1980) *Handbook of Endocrinology* 2nd edn. p. 510. Philadelphia: Lea & Febiger.

Evangelisti JT & Thorpe CJ (1983) Thyroid storm: a nursing crisis. *Heart and Lung* **12(2):** 184–193.

Ganong WF (1989) *Review of Medical Physiology* 14th edn. sect. IV. Norwalk CT: Appleton & Lange.

German K (1987) Fluid and electrolyte problems associated with diabetes insipidus and syndrome of inappropriate antidiuretic hormone. *Nursing Clinics of North America* **22(4):** 785–796.

Gonder-Frederick LA & Cox DJ (1986) Behavioural responses to perceived hypoglycaemic symptoms. *Diabetes Education* **12(2):** 105–109.

Guyton WF (1986) *Textbook of Medical Physiology* 7th edn. chapters 74–79. Philadelphia: Saunders.

Hamara E, Cassmeyer V, O'Connel KA et al (1988) Self-regulation in individuals with type II diabetes. *Nursing Research* **37(6):** 363–367.

Hardcastle W (1989) Management of Addison's Disease. *Nursing* **3(4):** 7–9.

Hassan T (1985) *A Guide to Medical Endocrinology.* London: Macmillan.

Hunter B (1990) The benefits of exercise. *Nursing* **4(6):** 23–24.

Jowett N & Thompson D (1986) Diabetic heart disease. *Nursing Times* **Oct. 29:** 33–34.

Keele CA, Neil E & Joels N (eds) (1982) *Samson Wright's Applied Physiology* 13th edn. Oxford: Oxford Medical.

Knight B & Watkinson S (1987) Nursing care of the patient with diabetic retinopathy. *Senior Nurse* **7(5):** 23–25.

MacKinnon M, Wilson RM, Hardisty CA & Ward JD (1989) Novel role for specialist nurses in managing diabetes in the community. *British Medical Journal* **299:** 552–554.

Manning V (1989) No more watching the clock. *Nursing Times* **85(26):** 39–40.

Metz R & Benson JW (1988) *Management and Education of the Diabetic Patient,* p. 75. Philadelphia: Saunders.

Morrison H (1988) Diabetic impotence. *Nursing Times* **84(32):** 35–37.

Most RS, Gross AM, Davidson PC & Richardson P (1986) The accuracy of glucose monitoring by diabetic individuals in their home setting. *Diabetic Education* **12(1):** 24–27.

Moyer A (1989) Caring for a child with diabetes: the effect of specialist nurse care on parents needs and concerns. *Journal of Advanced Nursing* **14:** 536–545.

Norkins AL (1979) The cause of diabetes. *Scientific American* **241(5):** 62–73.

Office of Health Economics (1989) *Diabetes: A Model for Health Care Management.* London: Office of Health Economics.

Nyhlin KT (1990) Diabetic patients facing long term complications: coping with uncertainty. *Journal of Advanced Nursing* **15:** 1021–1029.

O'Riordan JLH, Malan PG & Gould RP (1988) *Essentials of Endocrinology* 2nd edn. Oxford: Blackwell.

Rosenberg C (1990) Wound healing in the patient with diabetes mellitus. *Nursing Clinics of North America* **25(1):** 247–261.

Smith LH & Thier SO (1985) *Pathophysiology,* sect. 8 Philadelphia: Saunders.

Toews CJ (1987) *Guidelines for the Management of Diabetes Mellitus,* pp. 7–9. Hamilton, Ont.: McMaster University.

Tredger J (1989) Diet in the treatment of diabetes mellitus. *Nursing* **3(41):** 20–21.

Tucker SM, Cannobbio MM, Paquette EV & Wells MF (1989) Hyperthyroidism: thyroid crisis. *Journal of Emergency Nursing* **15(4):** 352–355.

Vander AJ, Sherman JH & Luciano DS (1990) *Human Physiology: The Mechanism of Body Function* 5th edn, pp. 255–282. New York: McGraw-Hill.

Caring for the Patient with a Disorder of the Renal System

OBJECTIVES

On completion of this chapter, the reader will be able to:

- Identify normal kidney structure and function and the abnormalities that can occur
- Describe the mechanisms of urinary elimination
- Describe the characteristics and composition of urine
- Identify how aberrations in kidney function can manifest themselves in the person with acute or chronic disease
- State the nursing issues involving comprehensive and holistic care of the individual with acute or chronic renal dysfunction and his or her family
- Discuss the contributing factors and clinical characteristics of functional, stress, reflex, urge and total urinary incontinence, and urinary retention
- Discuss a systematic approach for the assessment of individuals with urinary incontinence and with retention of urine
- Value the role of the nurse in the identification and management of individuals with urinary incontinence and urinary retention
- Discuss the nursing measures to prevent the development of urinary tract infections
- Discuss self-care for an individual with a urinary diversion

INTRODUCTION

Understanding the renal and urinary systems is complex and challenging. Renal and urinary tract anatomy and physiology is intricate, yet delivery of expert, comprehensive care to the person with a disorder in either system involves understanding the full impact of that disorder on the individual's quality of life. The purpose of this chapter is to give the practitioner an overview of the normal kidney and urinary tract and how disorders affect the rest of the body. This will assist the nurse to understand the impact of disease and how to deliver care to the person within a holistic framework.

To facilitate this understanding, the chapter will be organized with discussion of the structure and function of the renal system and urinary tract followed by a discussion of how disorders of the renal system affect the person and a discussion of the care needed by persons with disorders of urinary elimination.

THE RENAL SYSTEM AND URINARY TRACT

STRUCTURE OF THE KIDNEYS

The kidneys are paired organs that lie retro-peritoneally against the dorsal abdominal wall. Each kidney is enclosed in a fibrous capsule and is embedded in fatty tissue. It consists of approximately 1 000 000 nephrons, collecting tubules, and a pelvis. The kidney is anatomically divided into an outer, dark red portion called the *cortex* and an inner, lighter-coloured section lying between the cortex and the pelvis called the *medulla* (Figure 20.1). The medullary tissue is arranged in *conical* or *pyramidal masses* separated by *renal columns* formed by projections of cortical tissue. The blood vessels, nerves and ureter enter or leave the kidney at the hilum, the indentation on the medial surface.

NEPHRON

The nephron is the functional unit of the kidney. It consists of a narrow, convoluted tubule and a tuft of capillaries referred to as a *glomerulus*. The upper end of the tubule is dilated and invaginated to envelop the glomerulus and is called *Bowman's capsule*. According to their position, the nephrons may be classified as superficial cortical or juxtamedullary nephrons. The latter lie deep in the cortex with their glomeruli and capsules close to the medulla and their tubules extending deep into the medulla.

The tubule is divided into three segments: the *proximal convoluted tubule*, the hairpin-like *loop of Henle* and the *distal convoluted tubule* (Figure 20.2). A major function of the tubules is to convey water and solutes in either direction across the tubular cells between the interstitial fluid and the tubular content.

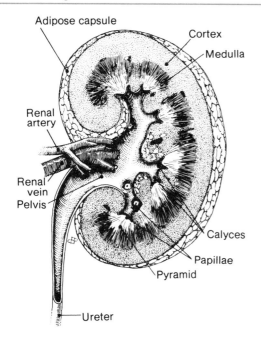

Figure 20.1 Cross-section of the kidney.

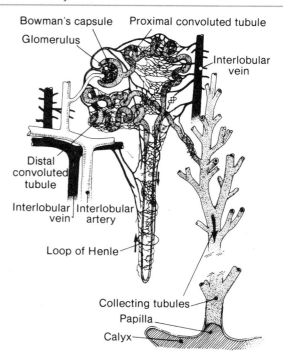

Figure 20.2 A renal unit or nephron of the cortex of the kidney is shown with its blood supply and a collecting tubule.

The thickness and structure of the walls differ from one segment to another: this arrangement accounts for different substances being reabsorbed and secreted in different sections of the tubule. (In relation to kidney function, *reabsorbed* means the movement of substances from the tubular content to the interstitial fluid. *Secreted* implies the transport of substances from the interstitial fluid to the tubular lumen. *Endocrine secretion* indicates the cellular production of a substance and its release directly into the bloodstream.) Movement across the tubular membrane may be active (using cellular energy) or passive.

The proximal convoluted tubule is the longest portion of the nephron and has thin walls consisting of a single layer of cells. The intraluminal surface of the cells has minute finger-like extensions known as *microvilli*, forming what is called a brush border layer. The villi play an important role in reabsorption of glucose and amino acids. These absorptive cells rest on a basement membrane. At the brush border, the cells are joined by *tight junctions* which block communication between the intercellular channels and the tubular lumen (Figure 20.3).

The loops of Henle vary in length and lie mainly in the medulla. The walls in the descending limb become thinner as they approach the loop. Modifications in the cells result in the walls of the ascending limb of the loop being thicker. Its terminal portion approximates the glomerulus of the nephron, of which it is a part, and its afferent arteriole.

The distal convoluted tubule is shorter than the other portions of the tubule. In the area of the tubule where the distal tubule commences, the epithelial cells differ and form an area referred to as the *macula densa*. The

cells in the remainder of the tubule are sensitive to the concentration of antidiuretic hormone (ADH) and adrenocortical steriods which influence reabsorption of substances by the distal tubule.

COLLECTING TUBULES

The distal tubules coalesce to form straight collecting tubules which unite to form progressively larger collecting tubules. Groups of the larger tubules come together to form a pyramid-like structure in the medulla. The apex of each pyramid is known as the *papilla* and contains the terminations of collecting tubules through which the urine passes into a cup-like pouch (calyx) of the renal pelvis.

RENAL PELVIS

When the ureter joins the kidney, it expands to form a funnel-shaped receiving basin for the urine delivered by the collecting tubules. It has numerous projecting pouches (calyces), each of which encases a renal papilla and is called a *calyx*.

BLOOD SUPPLY

The renal artery to each kidney arises from the abdominal aorta. When the artery enters the kidney, it

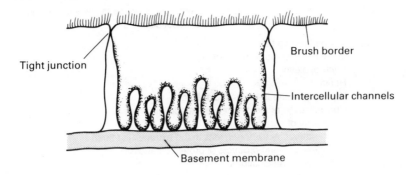

Tubular lumen

Tight junction

Brush border

Intercellular channels

Basement membrane

Peritubular Interstitial Space
(ECF)

Figure 20.3 Structure of the proximal tubular cells concerned with the reabsorptive process.

progressively subdivides to become afferent arterioles. Each *afferent arteriole* enters a nephron to form a glomerulus. The glomerular capillaries unite to form the *efferent arteriole*, which terminates in a second capillary network in which the tubule is invested. The blood pressure in this second set of capillaries is much lower than that in the glomerulus. The blood is then collected into venules and eventually into a renal vein that carries it to the inferior vena cava.

A large volume of blood is continuously circulated through the kidneys. It is estimated that the renal blood flow averages about 1000–1200 ml per minute in an adult, approximately 23–24% of the cardiac output. Receiving an adequate blood supply under the appropriate driving pressure is critical to maintaining kidney function.

Just before the afferent arteriole becomes the glomerulus, the cells change and increase in the middle tissue layer of the vascular wall. These special cells are known as *juxtaglomerular cells*. They are responsible for the production of the chemical *renin*.

NERVE SUPPLY

Sympathetic nerve fibres from the thoracolumbar autonomic nervous system transmit impulses to the afferent and efferent arterioles, causing vasoconstriction.

RENAL FUNCTION

Normal functioning of the body cells is greatly dependent upon a relative constancy of the internal environment. The kidneys play a major role in maintaining this constancy by regulating the water and electrolyte content and the acid-base balance of the body; they *conserve* appropriate amounts of essential substances vital to normal cellular function (e.g. glucose) and

excrete excesses, the waste products of metabolism, toxic substances and drugs in the urine. The kidneys also have an important *endocrine role*: the production of renin and erythropoietin, and their release into the blood when needed. In addition, the kidney is the major organ responsible for the production of the most active vitamin D metabolite, 1,25-dihydroxycholecalciferol (calcitriol). Its major effect is to stimulate calcium absorption from the gut, thereby assisting to maintain development of healthy bone. The processes involved in these functions performed by the kidneys are filtration, selective reabsorption, the transport of substances from the interstitial fluid to the tubule and endocrine secretion (Table 20.1).

FILTRATION

The permeability of the glomerular capillaries is greater than that of capillaries elsewhere in the body as a result of the unique three layer structure which permits most dissolved substances in the plasma to pass through into the Bowman's capsules. The same principles that govern the movement of fluid out of the arteriolar ends of the capillaries throughout the body are applicable to the filtration process in the glomeruli. The hydrostatic pressure of the blood in the glomerular capillaries is approximately 60 mmHg, which is considerably higher than that in the other capillaries of the body. This hydrostatic pressure is opposed by the osmotic pressure of the blood proteins (approximately 28 mmHg) plus the hydrostatic pressure in Bowman's capsule (about 18 mmHg). The net filtration force is 14 mmHg (hydrostatic blood pressure [60] – colloidal osmotic pressure [28] – capsular hydrostatic pressure [18] = 14 mmHg).

The average volume of filtrate in both kidneys is estimated to be about 180 litres each day. The glomerular filtration rate (GFR) is directly proportional to the filtration force; the normal rate is approximately

Table 20.1 Renal functions.

Overall function: Homeostasis—the maintenance of a suitable environment for optimum cellular function
Principal function: To regulate the volume and composition of the extracellular fluid

The kidney maintains homeostasis by performing the following roles:
1. *Production:* Vitamin D metabolite (Calcitriol)
   Erythropoietin
   Renin
2. *Regulation:* Volume of water in extracellular fluid
   Concentration of electrolytes in extracellular fluid
   Osmolality of extracellular fluid
   Concentration of hydrogen ions in the extracellular fluid
3. *Excretion:* Endogenous—end-products of protein catabolism
   Exogenous—medications

125 ml per minute. Factors which may alter the glomerular filtration rate are:

1. Change in glomerular capillary hydrostatic pressure, which may be incurred by an increase or decrease in systemic blood pressure or by constriction or dilatation of the afferent and efferent arterioles.
2. Increase or decrease in renal artery blood volume.
3. Increase or decrease in the hydrostatic pressure within Bowman's capsule due to compression by ureteral obstruction or disease within the kidney, causing swelling confined within the renal capsule.
4. Decrease or increase in the oncotic pressure (concentration of plasma proteins).
5. Increased glomerular permeability due to disease, such as nephrotic syndrome.
6. Decrease in glomeruli incurred by pathological destruction.

The glomerular filtration rate can be measured by determining the excretion volume and plasma concentration of a substance (e.g. creatinine) which is readily filtered through the glomeruli but not secreted or reabsorbed by the renal tubules.

Many solutes escape from the blood in the glomerular filtrate, but small amounts of only a few of them appear in urine. The formed elements and plasma proteins of the blood do not normally pass out of the glomeruli; the composition of the filtrate is the same as plasma minus the plasma proteins.

TUBULAR REABSORPTION

Reabsorption and secretion are complex renal activities. The composition and volume of the filtrate which enters Bowman's capsule differ markedly from those of urine. Of the 180 litres of filtrate produced in 24 hours, only about 1.5 litres are excreted as urine. Most of the water and many of the solid constituents of the filtrate are needed by the body to maintain homeostasis and normal cell metabolism. Other substances, such as urea,

creatinine, uric acid, sulphates and phosphates are waste products of metabolism and are excreted in the urine. The tubule cells selectively reabsorb according to the body's needs. Certain substances, such as glucose and amino acids, are completely reabsorbed when their plasma concentrations are within normal range but appear in the urine when the normal is exceeded. About 99% of the water in the filtrate is reclaimed. Reabsorption of the inorganic salts (e.g. sodium, chloride, calcium, potassium, bicarbonate) is variable, depending mainly on their plasma levels. Reabsorption and secretion are carried out selectively, based on the preceding factors.

Some constituents of the filtrate are passively reabsorbed by diffusion or carrier-mediated transport through the tubular membrane. Others are reabsorbed by active cellular transport, which entails energy expenditure on the part of the tubular cells and the presence of certain enzymes. Active reabsorption of substances in the proximal tubule is believed to be in cotransport with sodium. The location of reabsorption and secretion in the tubules varies with different filtrate constituents. The *proximal convoluted tubule* is responsible for the greatest amount of reabsorption. All of the glucose and amino acids and a large proportion of the water and other essential substances are reabsorbed here. Only about 35% of the total volume of filtrate enters the loop of Henle.

In the medulla there are branches of the efferent arterioles of juxtamedullary nephrons that form hairpin loops which approximate the loops of Henle. Each vascular loop of capillaries is called a *vasa recta*. The flow in the ascending limb of the vascular loop is sluggish, so ions diffuse out of the blood readily.

The vasa recta and the loop of Henle play an important role in concentrating the urine and conserving water by means of the countercurrent mechanism and determination of the peritubular osmolality. The countercurrent mechanism implies a U arrangement in which the fluid flows in opposite directions in the two limbs (ascending and descending) and there are interactions between them that alter the osmolality of the fluid along its course in the tube, with the

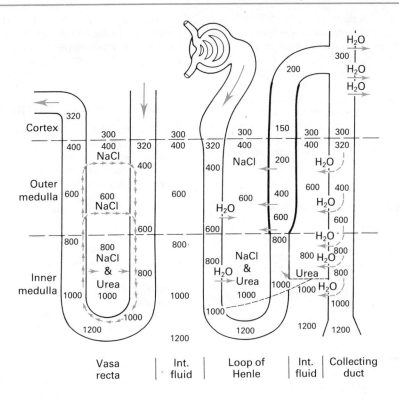

Figure 20.4 The countercurrent mechanism for concentrating the urine.

modification being greatest at the base of the loop (Figure 20.4).

The *loop of Henle* seems to be concerned principally with the transport of sodium chloride ions and water. The ascending limb (the thicker segment) is impermeable to water. It actively transports sodium and chloride ions out into the interstitial fluid, and the tubular fluid becomes hypotonic. The descending limb of the loop of Henle is permeable to water; water moves out to the interstitial fluid which has become hypertonic. At the same time sodium and chloride ions diffuse into the descending limb. The osmolality of the fluid within the descending limb progressively becomes more hypertonic as it approaches the base of the loop. The osmolality of the medullary interstitial fluid is increased, and sodium chloride diffuses into the blood in the descending limb of the vasa recta. But, as the blood flows in the opposite direction in the ascending limb, sodium chloride readily diffuses out again into the medullary interstitium; the osmolality of the blood as it leaves the medulla is only slightly higher than when it entered the vasa recta.

The maintenance of the volume and concentration of body fluids within a narrow range is largely controlled by the ability of the kidney tubules to concentrate or dilute the urine. When body fluids are diluted by an excess of water or diminished solute intake (especially sodium), the urine becomes dilute and the volume is increased. Conversely, if the concentration of body fluids is raised to above the normal level by an excessive intake of solutes or an extrarenal loss of water, water reabsorption from the filtrate is increased, concentrating the urine and decreasing the output volume.

The dilution and concentration of urine depend principally on two factors: first, the osmotic pressure of the peritubular fluid, which in turn is mainly dependent on the normal functioning of the loop of Henle and the distal convoluted tubules; and secondly, on the concentration of ADH in the blood.

The fluid entering the distal tubule is hypotonic, but the volume and osmolality are modified selectively as it proceeds through the distal and collecting tubules.

Reabsorption of water from the hypotonic filtrate in the distal convoluted and collecting tubules is regulated by ADH, which increases the permeability of their membranous walls. It is produced by the hypothalamus in the brain, and is stored and released into the blood by the posterior pituitary gland (neurohypophysis). Receptors in the hypothalmus are sensitive to changes in the osmotic pressure of the blood. When the pressure is increased to above normal (for example, by additional sodium), impulses are delivered to the posterior pituitary, resulting in the release of ADH which increases water reabsorption in the tubules. Conversely, if the osmotic pressure falls below the homeostatic level, the release of ADH is inhibited. The tubular membrane becomes relatively impermeable, restricting the reabsorption of water, and the urine is dilute.

The reabsorption of sodium by active cellular transport in the distal and collecting tubules is influenced by the adrenocortical hormone *aldosterone*. A high concentration of aldosterone stimulates the distal tubular cells to reabsorb increasing amounts of sodium. A deficiency of the hormone, such as occurs in Addison's disease, reduces the amount of sodium reclaimed, resulting in an excessive loss of urine. Aldosterone also affects the amount of potassium reclaimed and excreted. Increased concentrations of the hormone promote excretion of potassium, and a deficient amount of aldosterone produces excessive retention of potassium.

TUBULAR SECRETION AND EXCRETION

Tubular cells are capable of actively transporting some substances from the blood into the filtrate—a reverse process to that of reabsorption. The potassium concentration of plasma is regulated by this process. Practically all of the potassium that escapes from the plasma into the filtrate is reabsorbed in the proximal tubule. Any excess in the blood is then actively secreted by the distal tubules and is excreted in exchange for sodium ions.

Cells of the distal tubules play an important role in maintaining a normal *acid–base balance* in the blood and extracellular fluid. In association with the respiratory system (p. 371) the kidneys regulate the body's systemic arterial pH within a narrow range of 7.35–7.45.

The first lines of defence against alteration in body pH are the extracellular and intracellular buffers. The major extracellular buffer is bicarbonate and the buffering capacity of the HCO_3–CO_2 system is greatly extended by the regulation of CO_2 gas tension by the respiratory system.

The kidney's role in acid–base homeostasis is to stabilize the balance between H^+ and HCO_3^- in the blood. This is accomplished by four processes:

1. Secretion of hydrogen ions.
2. Reabsorption of sodium and bicarbonate ions.
3. Acidification of phosphate salts.
4. Synthesis and secretion of ammonia.

When the levels of the bicarbonate ion in the blood are elevated, the kidney decreases the quantity of bicarbonate that is reabsorbed. The quantity of bicarbonate in the urine is therefore increased. The kidney also excretes monosodium phosphate and the hydrogen ion, and conserves sodium by eliminating the phosphate ion in the monsodium form and excreting the anions as ammonium salts. All these mechanisms serve to restore the hydrogen ion concentration so that the pH of the blood is maintained within normal limits.

Of critical importance to the maintenance of acid–base homeostasis is the kidney's role in stabilizing bicarbonate concentration. This can be summarized in the following two processes:

1. Reabsorption of virtually all of the filtered bicarbonate.
2. Regeneration of the sodium bicarbonate lost by the buffering of metabolic acids (products of breakdown of food stuffs, sulphuric acid and phosphoric acids).

Some drugs are also excreted by active tubular removal from the blood into the tubules. These include diodone, amminohippuric acid and phenolsulphonphthalein, which may be used to investigate renal function.

ENDOCRINE RENAL SECRETIONS

The kidney produces two endocrine secretions, renin and erythropoietin.

Renin is a proteolytic enzyme that reacts with an inactive precursor fraction of the plasma globulin (angiotensinogen), producing a substance called angiotensin I which is converted to angiotensin II by another enzyme in the lungs. As angiotensin II circulates it causes vasoconstriction of the systemic arterioles and stimulates the secretion of aldosterone and, to a lesser degree, glucocorticoids (Figure 20.5). Angiotensin II is changed to angiotensin III by an aminopeptidase in the red blood cells and many other tissues, including the adrenal gland. It is believed to stimulate aldosterone secretion.

Five mechanisms are suggested as influencing the production and release of renin. (1) The juxtaglomerular cells release renin in response to decreased arteriolar blood volume and pressure. (2) The macula densa is sensitive to sodium and chloride concentrations; a decrease in the sodium and chloride content of the tubular fluid entering the distal tubule brings about the release of renin. The release of renin and the ensuing formation of angiotensin II and III stimulates the release of aldosterone which promotes the retention of sodium ions. (3) Sympathetic stimulation of the juxtaglomerular cells may be associated with the production of renin. The stimulation may be mediated by the release of catecholamines (e.g. adrenaline) by the adrenal medulla or by renal sympathetic innervation. (4) Prostaglandins act on the juxtaglomerular cells to stimulate renin secretion. (5) Potassium concentrations also influence renin release by influencing sodium and chloride levels in the macula densa.

A second hormone produced by the kidneys is the *renal erythropoietic factor* (REF, erythrogenin). It is produced and secreted into the blood in response to hypoxia, cobalt salts and androgens, and functions in the maintenance of normal erythrocyte production by the bone marrow. REF reacts with a plasma globulin to produce erythropoietin which stimulates the bone marrow to produce and release blood cells.

CHARACTERISTICS AND COMPOSITION OF URINE

When the filtrate flows into the main collecting tubules and renal pelvis, it becomes urine. The average volume excreted in 24 hours is approximately 1.5 litres but varies with fluid losses through other channels (e.g. sweat) and fluid intake. The reaction of urine is usually acid, with a pH of about 6.0, but may range from 4.5–8.5 with a varied dietary intake. The acidity increases with high protein ingestion and tissue catabolism, while a vegetable diet produces an alkaline urine.

The specific gravity, which gives a rough estimate of

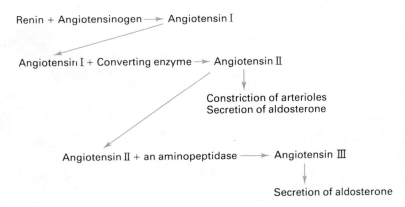

Figure 20.5 Effects of renin secretion.

the concentration of solids, ranges from 1.003–1.040. The composition of urine varies with dietary intake and metabolic wastes produced. Normally, about 90–95% of urine is water. An average of 50 g of organic and inorganic solid wastes are eliminated daily. The chief solutes are urea, creatinine, uric acid and the chlorides, phosphates and sulphates of sodium, potassium, calcium, magnesium and ammonia.

URETERS, BLADDER AND URETHRA

URETERS

Each of the two ureters is a tube 25–30 cm (10–12 in) in length, extending from a kidney to the bladder. They are situated behind the parietal peritoneum and enter the posterior wall of the lower half of the bladder obliquely. The slanted entrance forms a flap in the bladder wall that serves as a valve to prevent a reflux of urine as the bladder fills or contracts. Each ureter consists of an outer fibrous covering, a middle layer of muscle tissue, and a mucous membrane lining which is continuous with that of the bladder and the renal pelvis.

The function of these tubes is simply to convey urine from the kidneys to the bladder. Contraction of the ureteral muscular tissue produces peristaltic waves which move the urine along the tube and into the bladder in spurts.

BLADDER

The urinary bladder serves as a temporary reservoir for the urine, which it expels at intervals from the body. It is a collapsible muscular sac that lies behind the symphysis pubis. Three layers of plain muscle tissue form the bladder walls. The fibres are arranged in longitudinal, circular and spiral layers. Collectively, these layers are referred to as the *detrusor muscle*. The ureteral orifices in the posterior wall and the urethral opening outline a triangular area called the *trigone*. When the bladder is empty, the mucous membrane lining falls into folds (rugae) except in the area of the trigone (Figure 20.6).

URETHRA

The urethra is a slender tube that conveys urine from the bladder to the exterior. It has a thin layer of smooth muscle tissue and is lined with a mucous membrane which is continuous with that of the bladder. The opening from the bladder is controlled by two sphincters: an internal one which is under autonomic (involuntary) nervous system control, and an external one which is voluntarily controlled by the cerebral cortex. The external urethral orifice is known as the urinary meatus.

In the female, the urethra is about 4 cm (1.5 in) long and lies anterior to the vagina. The male urethra is approximately 20 cm (8 in) in length and, on leaving the bladder, passes through the prostate gland. As well as conveying the urine, the male urethra receives the semen from the ejaculatory ducts of the reproductive system, transmitting it through the meatus (see Figure 20.6).

MICTURITION

This is a term used for the elimination of urine from the bladder. The process involves both autonomic (involuntary) and voluntary nervous impulses. When 300–400 ml of urine collect in the bladder, receptors that are sensitive to stretching initiate impulses which are transmitted by afferent nerve fibres into the lower part of the spinal cord (Figure 20.7). A reflex response via parasympathetic nerves to the bladder results in contractions of the detrusor muscle and relaxation of the internal sphincter.

The initial impulses from the stretch receptors are also relayed via a spinocortical tract to the cerebral cortex, producing an awareness of the need to void. When a person is prepared to empty the bladder, voluntary impulses are initiated which descend the cord and are carried out to the external sphincter, causing it to relax. With both sphincters relaxed, the detrusor muscle contracts and urine flows from the bladder through the urethra. Voluntary micturition may also be accompanied by relaxation of the perineal muscles and

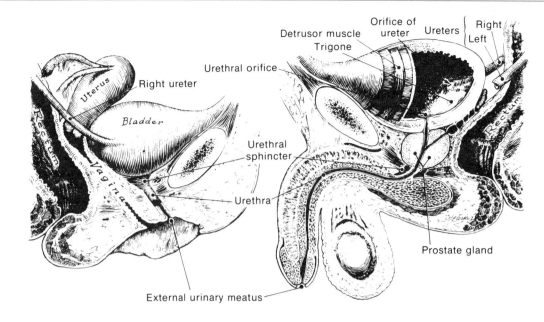

Figure 20.6 The bladder, ureters, urethra and prostate. Left, female; right, male.

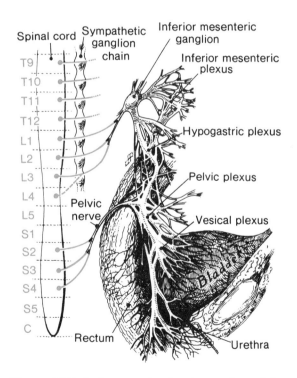

Figure 20.7 A diagram showing innervation of the bladder.

contraction of abdominal muscles. Infants and very young children empty their bladder whenever the micturition reflex is initiated, as they have not yet developed voluntary control over the external sphincter.

Obviously, any interruption of the spinocortical impulse pathway interferes with control of the external sphincter, resulting in involuntary voiding or retention.

THE PERSON WITH ALTERED RENAL FUNCTION

ASSESSMENT OF RENAL FUNCTION

The investigation of renal dysfunction may include examination of urine specimens (which may be voided or obtained by bladder or urethral catheterization), blood chemistry determinations, renal function tests, X-ray studies and ultrasound procedures.

Urine output

Perhaps one of the most crucial nursing functions in the care of the person with renal dysfunction is the accurate measurement of urine output and fluid balance.

Urine colour

It is important that the nurse be aware of the colour of the urine being eliminated. Changes from the normal amber, clear urine can be an indication of many things, such as urinary tract infection (cloudy urine), bleeding into the urinary tract (blood-stained urine) or dehydration (darker, more concentrated urine).

Routine urinalysis

Routine urinalysis is usually a nursing responsibility; it is relatively fast, simple and accurate because of the wide availability of reagent strip tests which allow the nurse to test for protein, glucose, ketones, acetone, blood and bilirubin, as well as to measure pH.

Urine for bacteriological examination

This is achieved by culturing the urine; the organism is identified using a microscope. Sensitivity to microbial agents (antibiotics) is determined by placing impregnated discs of specific agents upon the culture plate and observing the colonization pattern. Areas where colonies of micro-organisms fail to grow indicate sensitivity to the specific antibiotic.

Urine specimens for bacteriological examination should be fresh, or refrigerated following collection. The first morning specimen is the most concentrated and therefore most likely to reveal abnormalities. A clean catch mid-stream specimen (MSU) is the most effective method of obtaining urine for bacteriological examination. The patient should be given clear instructions on how to prepare himself or herself and which part of the urine stream should be collected. The external genitalia should be cleaned with water, antiseptic solution or sterile saline solution (depending on local policy). The individual should start passing urine and, once the urine is being voided, a sterile container should be used to collect it. The last part of the stream should be avoided. In the catheterized patient the specimen should be obtained, using a syringe and needle, from the rubber portal on the collecting tube, not from the reservoir or collecting bag.

24-hour urine collection

A 24-hour urine specimen means collection of all the urine that a person produces in a 24-hour period. Collection is begun first thing in the morning, with the urine of the first void being discarded. For the next 24 hours all the urine must be saved and collected in a container, including the first void of the next day. The urine can be examined to determine the amounts of specific substances that the person's kidney is capable of excreting, based on calculations that include height, weight and total volume excreted during the 24-hour period. By making a quantitative determination of the total solid content of such substances as urea, creatinine, protein, urinary electrolytes and glucose, a statement can be made about the glomerular filtration capacity of the kidney. The container should be refrigerated during the period of collection. Some 24-hour collections may be needed for specific tests and a stabilizer or preservative may be added to the receptacle prior to collection.

Blood chemistry determinations

Impaired glomerular filtration and loss of the tubular ability to reabsorb and excrete discriminately lead to alterations in plasma composition. Blood specimens may be requested to determine the concentration of a number of substances. The nurse is often the first health care provider to be informed of results, and therefore should have an understanding of normal serum concentrations so that abnormal levels can be promptly reported. The following normal values are of particular importance for patients with renal disorder:

- Urea nitrogen. Normal: 2.9–8.9 mmol/l
- Creatinine. Normal: 60–120 μmol/l
- Uric acid. Normal: 0.22–0.48 mmol/l

Haematological tests

The haemoglobin concentration and haematocrit are determined, since anaemia is a common problem. If infection is suspected a leucocyte count is done, and a platelet count and prothrombin time may be needed in advanced chronic renal failure.

Renal function tests

Renal function tests may be classified according to the kidney function being evaluated. In renal function, the removal or clearance of substances from the blood is achieved by glomerular filtration and tubular cell activity. If a substance passes freely through the glomeruli, and is neither reabsorbed or secreted by the tubules, the quantity appearing in the urine is the same as that filtered by the glomeruli. By measuring the amount excreted in the urine in a specified period of time, information is obtained about the efficiency of glomerular filtration. The substances used for this evaluation may be creatinine or urea, which are naturally occurring metabolites, or inulin.

The nurse needs to understand what is involved in these tests for two reasons: firstly to ensure the patient is properly prepared and cared for prior to and after any procedure. The second aspect concerns the nurse's role in reducing anxiety and fear by answering questions and giving explanations to the patient.

Glomerular filtration rate. For determining the glomerular filtration rate, creatinine or [51Cr] EDTA clearance tests are used most frequently.

In the *creatinine clearance test*, the patient maintains normal but not excessive activity, since endogenous creatinine is produced in muscular activity. No special diet is necessary but excessive intake of tea, coffee and meat is avoided for a 24-hour period before the test. A 24-hour specimen of urine and a venous blood specimen are collected for creatinine concentration determinations. The rate of urinary excretion per minute is calculated. The normal amount of creatinine excreted in 24 hours varies with age: in an adult the normal is about 1.2–1.7 g, and in a child it is approximately 0.36 g. Calculations are made to determine the volume of plasma cleared of creatinine per minute, which is the glomerular filtration rate.

[51Cr] EDTA, a radioactive isotope, is given intravenously into one arm. Blood tests from the other arm are taken hourly for 3 hours and from the rate of clearance from the plasma, the GFR is calculated.

Tubular function. Assessment of tubular function involves testing the kidneys' ability to concentrate solid wastes, excrete phenolsulphonphthalein (PSP) and excrete acids in the urine.

In order to maintain homeostasis, normal kidneys are able to vary the concentration of solid wastes and the volume of urine according to the volume of body fluids. When there is an excessive loss of body fluid by other channels or a restricted intake, more water is reabsorbed by the renal tubules; the solid wastes are excreted in a smaller volume of urine and the specific gravity is high. Conversely, with a large fluid intake: less water is reabsorbed by the tubules, the volume of urine is greater and the specific gravity and osmolality are lower than usual. This ability to vary the volume and concentration of the urine appropriately is impaired in tubular damage and may be tested by a concentration test.

The *concentration test* is designed to determine the kidney's ability to concentrate urine when the fluid intake is restricted. Fluids are restricted over a specified period. Then, two or three urine specimens are collected, and the osmolality and specific gravity of each are determined. If the kidneys are normal, the specific gravity is not less than 1.024 and the osmolality is greater than 8000 mosmol/kg of water and greater than the serum osmolality which should be unchanged. The procedure regarding the period of fluid restriction and the number of specimens collected varies in different institutions. The commonly used Fishberg concentration test involves restricted fluids with the evening meal (approximately 200 ml) and then no food or fluid until the test is completed the next morning. Three hourly urine specimens are collected in the morning (e.g. at 6, 7 and 8 a.m.). The time of voiding each specimen is indicated on the labels. *All urine voided each time must be submitted to the laboratory.* Before the test is begun, the reasons for the fluid restriction and collection of specimens should be fully explained to the patient. This test must not be performed on patients with known renal impairment as dehydration may precipitate an acute deterioration in renal function.

Renal scanning

The use of radioisotope scanning techniques may demonstrate areas of renal dysfunction and is becoming increasingly widespread as an investigative procedure.

Ultrasound

There is no preparation for an ultrasound and there are no X-rays or injections needed, although if the person is not anuric a full bladder may be requested as it provides a good 'landmark' for the technician. The examination is used to look at the size and structure of the kidneys and other organs. Renal lesions seen in polycystic kidney disease and hydronephrosis can be distinguished. Ultrasound is also widely used in determining the position of a kidney for renal biopsy.

Intravenous pyelography (IVP) or intravenous urography (IVU)

This procedure involves the intravenous administration of a radio-opaque contrast medium. This fluid concentrates in urine and, as it is excreted through the kidney (pyelogram) and the ureters and bladder (urogram), X-rays are taken. Patient preparation varies, but fluids are usually restricted 4 hours prior to the procedure; sometimes a laxative is administered the night before the examination. This avoids bowel content or gas obscuring the outline of the urinary tract. It is important to ascertain if the individual has a history of allergies, particularly to iodine preparations, as severe reactions to the contrast medium can occur.

Cystoscopy and retrograde pyelography

Cystoscopy involves the passage of a cystocope through the urethra into the bladder. The instrument is equipped with a light which permits direct visualization of the internal surface of the bladder. A long, fine catheter may also be introduced into each renal pelvis through the cystoscope (ureteric catherization), and a urine specimen collected from each kidney. Ureteric catheterization may be used to obtain specimens from one or both kidneys for microscopic examination and culture, or in renal function tests when the function of each kidney is to be determined. For example, during cystoscopy and ureteric catheterization, phenosulphonphthalein may be given intravenously and its appearance in the urine from each kidney noted and timed. Normally it appears within 4–6 minutes of administration. The specimens must be labelled as to right or left ureter.

A radiopaque iodide preparation may then be introduced into the catheters, and X-rays which outline the renal pelvioes and ureters are taken. This procedure is referred to as retrograde pyelography. The examination is used to exclude or delineate a ureteral obstruction when excretion of contrast by the kidney during an IVP is poor.

Preparation of the patient for a cystoscopy includes an explanation of the procedure. The patient's signature indicating consent for the examination is required. The procedure may be performed under local epidural or general anaesthetic; food and fluid therefore are restricted for 6–8 hours preceding the examination and intravenous fluid is administered to ensure hydration and hence urinary flow.

If a general anaesthetic is contraindicated, the procedure may be performed under sedation. Increasingly, it is possible to perform cystoscopy with a flexible cystoscope under sedation without discomfort.

Upon completion of the examination, the person rests in bed for a few hours. Additional fluids are encouraged. It is important that the nurse examine the urinary output for haematuria, and any severe pain or persisting bright blood in the urine is reported to the doctor. Should the individual report inability to pass urine it may be necessary for an indwelling catheter to be inserted. Severe haematuria may necessitate catherization and irrigation of the bladder with fluid to control bleeding and flush debris and blood clots.

Computerized tomography

Computerized tomography (CT) is used in the detection of renal tumours and cysts. The patient is given an oral contrast medium before the scan to opacify the bowel; food is not allowed for 4 hours prior to the procedure.

Renal angiography

Renal blood vessels may be outlined on an X-ray film following the administration of a radio-opaque substance into the vascular system. The procedure is performed under local anaesthesia by a radiologist; it is used to explore the blood supply to the kidneys. The main indication for a renal angiogram is for a diagnosis of renal artery stenosis or to differentiate renal masses, e.g. tumours or cysts. As the person may be sensitive to the radio-opaque iodide preparation, the same precautions as cited for intravenous urography should be followed. Preparation of the patient is similar to that for intravenous urography. After the procedure, the site of catheter introduction into the femoral artery has a firm dressing applied and frequent inspections are made for bleeding. The person may be on bed rest for several hours after the procedure to reduce the risk of bleeding. The site is also observed for local swelling, redness and tenderness. The temperature of the lower limbs is noted and the popliteal and pedal pulses are checked so that any indication of impaired circulation may be reported promptly.

Magnetic resonance imaging

This technique is also being developed to permit investigation of the kidneys and has been shown to have an important role in the detection of abnormalities of renal tissue.

Percutaneous renal biopsy

A biopsy is a valuable test in diagnosis and assessment of the effects of treatment but carries with it the risk of haemorrhage. It is frequently used to determine the underlying pathology of renal dysfunction so that appropriate treatments may be selected. Renal biopsy is also performed in selected cases in renal transplant patients in order to diagnose rejection. It is contraindicated if the person has hypertension, a bleeding tendency, only one kidney, or suspected perirenal abscess. Before a person is booked for renal biopsy, coagulation, bleeding and prothrombin times are determined. If these are satisfactory, the person's blood is grouped and crossmatched, and compatible blood is kept available in the event of haemorrhage. An explanation is given to the person of what to expect and that he or she will be put in the prone position over a firm pillow (kidney elevator) for a brief period.

The exact location of the kidney is identified by X-ray, which may include an intravenous urogram or an ultrasound scan, and the position indicated on the skin surface. The skin is cleansed and local anaesthesia is infiltrated. The person is instructed to hold the breath during the insertion of the needle and the actual taking of the specimen. Following the removal of the biopsy needle, pressure is applied to the site for a few minutes.

The blood pressure and pulse are recorded every 15 minutes for 1 hour, then every 30 minutes for a period of 1–2 hours, and then every 4 hours for 24 hours. The risk of heavy bleeding after the procedure is very real, therefore the nurse must carefully observe the person for signs of shock, and assess the urine for prolonged haematuria. Any undue pain, haematuria or change in vital signs should be immediately reported. The person is kept on bed rest in the dorsal recumbent position for 18–24 hours or until the urine is cleared of blood.

CLINICAL CHARACTERISTICS OF RENAL DYSFUNCTION

In impaired kidney function, the constancy of the internal environment (homeostasis), which is essential for the normal functioning of all body cells, is disrupted. The normal volume, composition and reaction of the body fluids may be altered by the inability of the kidneys to conserve essential substances and excrete excesses, metabolic wastes and toxic substances; disturbances in the functioning of other organs readily develop. Consequently, the signs and symptoms of renal insufficiency are varied, and many are not directly referable to the urinary system. Whether the disease is acute or chronic and whether it affects the glomeruli or the tubules will also affect the manifestations.

As the nurse assesses the patient the following physical signs must be borne in mind as evidence of significant renal dysfunction. The nurse should be alert to the possible psychological sequelae of these clinicial signs as such effects may be a cause of great distress requiring urgent nursing intervention, for example, a change in the colour of a person's urine.

Abnormal urinary volume

Oliguria or anuria may develop, especially in acute and advanced renal failure. *Oliguria* means that less than 500 ml of urine is formed in 24 hours. *Anuria* implies a urinary output of less than 250 ml in 24 hours and is sometimes referred to as a renal shutdown. The diminished urine formation may be associated with decreased glomerular filtration due to renal disease (e.g. glomerulonephritis), hypotension as in shock and dehydration, decreased renal blood flow or an obstruction within the tubules.

Polyuria, a volume of urine in excess of the normal (over 2000 ml in 24 hours), may also indicate renal disturbance in which the ability of the tubules to reabsorb water and concentrate the solid wastes is limited. It is most often seen in chronic kidney disease or it may be secondary to diabetes insipidus as a result of a deficiency in the secretion of vasopressin (antidiuretic hormone). Polyuria may not be a manifestation of renal disease but may indicate a disorder elsewhere. Frequently, polyuria is the symptom that may cause an individual to go to a doctor where, on investigation, diabetes mellitus is diagnosed.

Nocturia (voiding during the night) usually accompanies polyuria and the person becomes desperate for undisturbed sleep. Inability of the kidneys to reabsorb the normal amount of water and to concentrate the wastes may be referred to as *hyposthenuria*. As well as the excessive volume, a low specific gravity of the urine persists because the impaired tubules cannot concentrate or vary the amount of solids.

Abnormal constituents in the urine

Abnormal constituents revealed in urinalysis vary with the underlying renal disease. They include protein (usually albumin), blood, casts, pus and organisms.

The large molecular structure of serum albumin inhibits its filtration through normal glomeruli. *Albuminuria* usually indicates inflammation and almost always indicates damage to the glomeruli. *Haematuria* denotes blood in the urine and may be macroscopic or recognized only by microscopic examination. It indicates some pathological process within the kidneys or postrenal structures.

Urinary casts are microscopic cylindrical structures formed in the distal and collecting tubes by the agglutination of cells and cellular debris in a protein matrix. They are moulded or cast in the shape of the tubule. Depending on their composition, casts are usually classified as red blood cell, epithelial, hyaline, granular or fatty. They point to the presence of some inflammatory or degenerative process within the tubules. Obviously, *pus and bacteria* in the urine indicate infection in the kidneys or urinary tract.

Abnormal urine colour

Abnormal discolouration of urine may be associated with infection within the urinary tract, but more often occurs with a disorder extrinsic to the kidneys and urinary tract. Examples of disorders in which the urine is discoloured are: obstructive jaundice, where the urine appears a dark colour due to the presence of bilirubin haemoglobinuria, which may develop following a blood transfusion reaction in which there is a breakdown of erythrocytes and the release of haemoglobin; porphyria, a genetic disorder in which normal use of porphyrin in the formation of haemoglobin does not occur, resulting in porphyrins being eliminated in the urine; and melanoma, a skin neoplasm characterized by excessive pigmentation.

It should be remembered that urine can sometimes be discoloured by the contrast media used in intravenous X-ray examination, or by the eating of beetroot.

Uraemia

Metabolic wastes accumulate in the blood. Urea, creatinine and uric acid levels are elevated. In acute failure and anuria, the levels rise rapidly. In chronic kidney disease, even though there may be polyuria, the blood urea progressively rises.

Fluid, electrolyte and pH imbalances

Generalized *oedema* may be one of the early symptoms of renal insufficiency and usually becomes apparent first around the eyes. It may be due to decreased glomerular filtration and the retention of water and sodium, or to an abnormal permeability of the glomeruli to plasma proteins, especially serum albumin. The latter defect is associated with a condition known as nephrosis that occurs more often in children. The loss of plasma protein causes a decrease in the colloidal osmotic pressure of the blood, and an excess of water remains in the interstitial spaces. The urine is high in albumin, and the plasma protein is abnormally low.

In some instances of chronic renal failure due to impaired tubular function, the excessive volume of urine excreted (polyuria) may lead to *dehydration* unless there is a corresponding increase in the water intake.

Deficiencies or excesses of electrolytes may occur, depending on the nature of the renal disturbance and the degree of tissue damage. Failure of impaired tubules to secrete potassium ions is a serious development in renal insufficiency. Abnormal concentrations of sodium and calcium as well as hyperkalaemia may develop, and may seriously affect cardiac function and threaten the patient's life.

Failure of the kidneys' capacity to excrete hydrogen ions by the formation and excretion of acid sodium phosphate and ammonia results in their accumulation in the blood causing *acidosis* (see Chapter 7).

Vital signs

An elevation of blood pressure occurs in most patients with renal insufficiency associated with parenchymal disease of the kidneys. It is attributed to an increase in the blood volume as a result of the retention of sodium and water or a decrease in the renal blood flow and consequent secretion of renin by the juxtaglomerular cells. The renin results in the formation of angiotensin II and III which cause vasoconstriction of the arterioles and increased aldosterone release.

The pulse may become weak because of heart failure which may result from hypertension, excessive fluid load or electrolyte imbalance. Of the electrolyte disturbances, hyperkalaemia (elevated serum potassium) is the most serious (see Chapter 7).

The patient may experience dyspnoea due to pulmonary oedema. Kussmaul's breathing (deep rapid respirations), characteristic of acidosis, may be manifested. In advanced renal failure, the breath has an ammoniacal or 'uraemic' odour.

Pyrexia is associated with infection in the kidneys or secondary infection, such as pneumonia, that may develop readily if pulmonary oedema is present.

Gastrointestinal disturbances

The patient experiences anorexia and, in the later stages of renal dysfunction, nausea and vomiting. Diarrhoea may also be troublesome in the acute stage. Hiccups may develop in advanced failure, and the oral mucosa may become sore and ulcerated.

Headache and pain

Headache is an early complaint as a result of the hypertension and cerebral oedema. Pain and tenderness in the back between the lower ribs and iliac crest occur in acute kidney disease because of the stretching of the renal capsule.

Visual disturbances

The patient may complain of 'spots before the eyes' or blurred vision which are attributed to oedema of the optic papillae (papilloedema). Loss of vision may actually occur as a result of a retinal haemorrhage.

Neurological manifestations

Signs of both irritation and depression of the nervous system appear in renal failure. The patient becomes irritable, lethargic and drowsy. Family members may be distressed at perceived personality changes in the person. Short-term memory may also be affected, hence clear explanations and repetition will be necessary. It is important to assess the level of consciousness as the person may become disorientated and progress to a comatose state. Muscular twitching may be noticeable and, in advanced kidney disease, may be an indication of ensuing convulsions.

Skin changes

In progressive renal insufficiency, the skin may take on a yellowish-brown appearance. Dryness and scaliness, known as xerosis, are common with chronic disease and polyuria. The patient may complain of pruritus, and excoriated lesions may appear from scratching. Pruritus is often persistent and there is no treatment that appears to have a lasting effect. Consequently, pruritus can be a debilitating and depressing experience.

In advanced failure, urea frost may be manifested, although this will only be seen in those persons for whom dialysis intervention is not possible. As the individual becomes progressively uraemic, deposits of small white crystals of urea are excreted by the sweat glands. The frost is usually first seen around the mouth.

Haemtological changes

Most patients with prolonged renal disease show a reduction in the production of red blood cells, a shortened red cell survival time with a resultant anaemia. Normal kidneys, as well as the liver, contribute erythropoietin which stimulates erythropoiesis. In renal dysfunction, this activity may be decreased.

With uraemia, the patient develops a bleeding tendency; the platelets are defective and the bleeding time increases. Petechiae, purpura or bleeding from mucous membranes, particularly the gums, may be present. The person with renal dysfunction is most likely to notice an increased propensity to bruising.

THE PERSON WITH IMPAIRED RENAL FUNCTION

Renal dysfunction may be due to a primary disease within the kidneys or may be secondary to a disorder elsewhere in the body. When kidney function is impaired, dysfunction of extrarenal systems ultimately develops. Similarly, primary dysfunction in other systems may readily affect renal function.

The Person with Renal Failure

When the kidneys are unable to excrete metabolic wastes and perform their role in fluid, electrolyte and acid-base balance, renal failure exists. Homeostasis of the internal environment is no longer maintained. The retention of the waste and excess products normally excreted in the urine may be referred to as *uraemia*. The latter is not a disease but rather a syndrome or complex of symptoms reflecting failure of the kidneys to carry out their role in regulation of the fluid volume, acid-base and electrolyte balances and excretion of metabolic wastes. Renal production of renin, erythropoietin and vitamin D_3 is also disturbed. With failure of fluid volume regulation the patient becomes either oedematous or dehydrated and the acid-base imbalance leads to metabolic acidosis. Electrolyte imbalances occur and an accumulation of nitrogenous wastes produces elevated blood levels of non-protein nitrogenous substances such as urea, creatinine and uric acid. The disturbance in the secretion of hormones leads to alterations in blood pressure, erythrocyte production and calcium absorption by bone tissue. As renal efficiency diminishes, symptoms develop reflecting impairment of function in other body systems. Figure 20.8 illustrates the systemic effects of renal failure. Renal failure may be acute or chronic.

The nursing care of the person with renal failure, whether acute or chronic, is complex. The working relationship between patient and nurse must begin with an assessment and baseline physical examination to establish appropriate, individualized health care needs.

HEALTH HISTORY

When exploring health history it is essential to consider symptoms that pertain to the renal system as well as the psychological and social impact the disease process and hospitalization are having on the patient and family. It is especially important to realize that patients with chronic renal failure will often be initially diagnosed as 'acute' because they have no previous symptoms or knowledge of renal disease. Admission to hospital and initiation of invasive investigation and treatment will often be sudden, unexpected and frightening for the patient. The nurse must be sensitive to the fact that the patient and family may well be overwhelmed by technical procedures that are difficult to understand.

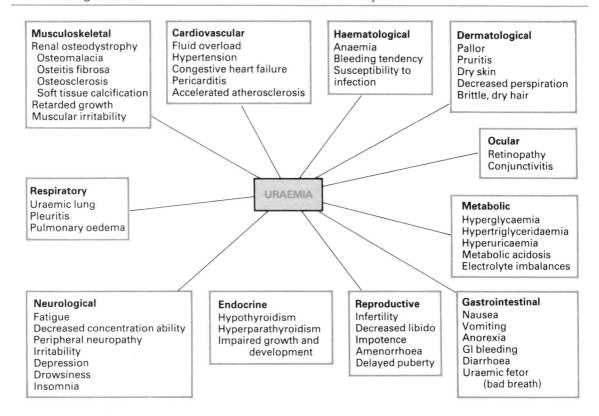

Musculoskeletal
Renal osteodystrophy
 Osteomalacia
 Osteitis fibrosa
 Osteosclerosis
 Soft tissue calcification
Retarded growth
Muscular irritability

Cardiovascular
Fluid overload
Hypertension
Congestive heart failure
Pericarditis
Accelerated atherosclerosis

Haematological
Anaemia
Bleeding tendency
Susceptibility to
 infection

Dermatological
Pallor
Pruritis
Dry skin
Decreased perspiration
Brittle, dry hair

Ocular
Retinopathy
Conjunctivitis

Respiratory
Uraemic lung
Pleuritis
Pulmonary oedema

URAEMIA

Metabolic
Hyperglycaemia
Hypertriglyceridaemia
Hyperuricaemia
Metabolic acidosis
Electrolyte imbalances

Neurological
Fatigue
Decreased concentration ability
Peripheral neuropathy
Irritability
Depression
Drowsiness
Insomnia

Endocrine
Hypothyroidism
Hyperparathyroidism
Impaired growth and
 development

Reproductive
Infertility
Decreased libido
Impotence
Amenorrhoea
Delayed puberty

Gastrointestinal
Nausea
Vomiting
Anorexia
GI bleeding
Diarrhoea
Uraemic fetor
 (bad breath)

Figure 20.8 Systemic effects of uraemia (Lewis, 1981).

HEALTH ASSESSMENT

In assessing the patient the nurse needs to explore the physical, psychological and social effects of the illness on the person's normal functioning. Not only should the patient's self-caring or adaptive abilities and family resources be examined, but it is also important to discover the patient's own perceptions and understanding of the illness and health status.

PHYSICAL ASSESSMENT

The physical assessment of the patient with acute or chronic renal failure will focus upon collecting information on the effects of renal impairment on extracellular fluid volume and the body systems. The nurse should begin by making careful observation of the person's overall appearance, noting the skin's colour, turgor, intactness and texture. The nurse should observe for signs of circulatory overload, such as periorbital oedema, peripheral oedema, increased respirations, agitation and anxiety. General activity and comfort level should be assessed by noting posture, movement, gait, stength and restlessness. Mental status is assessed by noting the level of consciousness, orientation, appropriateness of verbal responses, and motor responses to stimuli.

Since fluid volume assessment is critical in acute and chronic renal failure, the nurse looks for distinctive changes that might suggest circulatory overload or dehydration. Records of fluid intake, urine output and daily weights might show trends that indicate gains or losses. The nurse then assesses the pulse and blood pressure for hypertension. Circulatory overload may manifest as breathing difficulties such as dyspnoea and orthopnoea. Pulmonary congestion and oedema can result from renal disease. The nurse should observe the individual for breathlessness, alteration in respiratory effort, restlessness, sounds accompanying breathing, and engorgement of jugular veins.

The skin at the base of the spine should be inspected for oedema, particularly in the patient who is critically ill and is in a dependent position in bed: extracellular fluid expansion may manifest itself in oedema at the base of the spine rather than at the periphery. It is crucial for the nurse working with the hospitalized renal patient to perform a fluid volume assessment on at least a daily basis.

ACUTE RENAL FAILURE

Acute renal failure is a sudden, severe interruption of kidney function that in most instances is a complication of another disorder and is reversible. It is important to understand, however, that persons with progressive chronic renal disease may experience an event that results in an acute episode of renal dysfunction. After treatment, the renal function may or may not return to the preillness capacity. What is critical here is that some persons may have an acute episode that results in hastening end-stage renal failure in the face of slowly progressing renal disease.

CAUSES

The primary or initiating causes of acute renal failure are many but the basic mechanisms causing the failure, in most instances, are tubular necrosis due to inadequate tissue perfusion and hypoxia, or acute inflammation of glomeruli. Causes may be classified as prerenal, intrarenal or postrenal.

Prerenal refers to extrarenal disorders *which cause inadequate renal perfusion* as a result of a decrease in vascular volume or cardiac output or obstruction of a renal artery. The renal insufficiency is secondary to a condition which reduces the blood supply to the kidneys. The condition may be haemorrhage, dehydration, shock, cardiac failure, burns or renal artery occlusion by thrombosis or an abdominal mass.

Intrarenal refers to disorders in which there is actual renal tissue irritation and destruction which impairs renal functions; for example, acute inflammation of the glomeruli (glomerulonephritis), acute tubular necrosis and acute inflammation of the kidney tissue and renal pelvis (pyelonephritis). The primary renal tissue damage may be induced by a chemical or biological product or an infectious agent.

Renal failure may be the result of glomerulonephritis which is secondary to an *extrarenal Streptococcus haemolyticus* infection. The antigen complexes formed in response to the infection are trapped in the glomeruli and initiate the inflammatory process.

Nephrotoxic agents that are possible causes of a renal shutdown may be endogenous or exogenous in origin. Epithelial cells are destroyed; the tubular lumens are obliterated by swelling and oedema of the tissues as well as by casts formed from the sloughed cells. Examples of endogenous nephrotoxins are haemoglobin, released in haemolysis of erythrocytes following incompatible blood transfusion, and myoglobin, released from muscle cells in crushing injuries. The molecules of haemoglobin pass through the glomeruli and become concentrated in the tubules, obstructing the flow of filtrate. Similarly, the tubular necrosis that follows a crushing injury is attributed to the myoglobin accumulating in the tubules and causing an obstruction, as well as to shock. The individual who has been 'pinned down under a weight' for a period of time or who has been subjected to limb ischaemia may appear in satisfactory condition when released, but should be put to bed under close observation. Severe shock, acute renal failure and gross oedema of the injured part may develop hours later.

Exogenous nephrotoxins may be poisonous chemicals or drugs. Poisons, which may be taken accidentally or with suicidal intent, include carbon tetrachloride, ethylene glycol (a constituent of antifreeze), bichloride of mercury, chloroform and lead. Common pharmaceuticals which may prove toxic and damaging to the tubules include sulphonamide preparations (e.g. sulphadiazine), salicylates, phenacetin, paracetamol, vancomycin, amphotericin B, cyclosporin, non-steroidal anti-inflammatory agents, a cephalosporin and frusemide combination, and aminoglycoside antibiotics (kanamycin, gentamicin, tobramycin, etc.). Interstitial nephritis may be produced by methicillin and some analgesics. Obstructive disorders may result from cytotoxic drugs.

Postrenal causes of acute renal failure are conditions which result in an obstruction to the outflow of urine. Calculi, a neoplasm or prostatic hypertrophy may obstruct collecting tubules, the pelvis, a ureter or the bladder; the accumulation of fluid within the kidney compresses blood vessels and nephrons, seriously reducing kidney function.

CLINICAL CHARACTERISTICS

Patients with acute renal failure fall into two distinct categories: those who are oliguric, passing less than 500 ml of urine per day, and those who are never oliguric but who continue to pass 1000–1500 ml of dilute urine per day. The effects of a decreased urinary output are retention of an excess of certain biochemical substances in the blood and a decrease in the pH of body fluids. Blood urea and serum creatinine, potassium and sodium chloride concentrations are elevated; the pH is decreased and hydrogen carbonate, haematocrit and haemoglobin levels are below normal.

The first sign of acute renal failure may be oliguria, which may progress rapidly to anuria. The oliguric phase may last for 7–10 days and the urine contains blood and protein. An output of less than 30 ml per hour is an indication for concern and should be reported immediately. If oliguria and anuria persist for a few days, manifestations of water retention and disturbances of blood chemistry are likely to develop. Sodium and water retention cause oedema and, unless the fluid intake is controlled, overhydration may lead to cardiac failure and pulmonary oedema. The serum sodium levels may suggest hyponatraemia because of the diluting effect of the retained fluid in the vascular compartment.

The elevation of serum potassium becomes a serious threat to cardiac muscle. In addition to the fact that potassium is not being eliminated by the kidneys, haemolysis and the breakdown of tissue cells by the primary condition (trauma, burns, sepsis, etc.) increase the concentration of potassium ions in the blood. Metabolic acidosis which also develops in acute renal failure promotes the movement of potassium out of the cells. Cardiac arthythmias are common, and cardiac arrest may occur.

The rate of the accumulation of nitrogenous wastes (urea and creatinine) in the blood varies with the cause of the renal insufficiency. If there is rapid catabolism, as in infection, fever, and pathological destruction of tissue, the blood concentration of nitrogenous wastes may rise more quickly. The onset of the uraemic state is usually marked by mental changes, nausea and vomiting, and probably hiccups. The patient may complain of pruritus.

Metabolic acidosis develops because the hydrogen ions produced in metabolism are not being eliminated by the renal tubules. Respirations are increased in rate and depth, and an acidotic odour of the breath becomes noticeable.

Leucocytosis may be present; anaemia is likely to develop fairly quickly, and is manifested by a decrease in the haematocrit and haemoglobin. If the renal failure persists, the patient may develop a bleeding tendency. Ulcerated areas in the mouth are common and may bleed. Vomit and stools may contain blood, and petechiae and ecchymoses may appear. As the condition worsens, disseminated intravascular coagulation (DIC) may develop (see p. 276).

The patient becomes drowsy and may progress to a comatose state. Muscle twitching and convulsions may also develop.

The outcome in acute renal failure is unpredictable. Many patients do recover; tubular healing and repair occur within 2–6 weeks and there is no serious functional impairment. Those who do not recover do not necessarily die from renal failure alone; frequently, the cause of death is the seriousness of the underlying cause or the combination of several associated disorders and complications. The patient with renal insufficiency is very susceptible to infection, especially pulmonary. Fluid in the alveoli (pulmonary oedema) and the retention of secretions due to inability to cough because of weakness predispose to pneumonia. Early recognition of renal insufficiency and prompt treatment are important. The nurse may play an important role in early recognition by being familiar with the possible causes of renal failure and by being alert to any significant decrease in a patient's urinary output.

Diuretic phase

If the renal failure is reversible, the patient experiences a period of diuresis following the oliguric period; large volumes of urine are excreted. The tubules are unable to concentrate urine and serum creatinine and blood urea remain elevated. A diuretic phase may not be observed if the patient has been treated by dialysis.

Recovery phase

Improvement in renal function continues over 3–12 months. As it returns, the urine becomes more concentrated but some residual impairment often remains.

COMPLICATIONS

Complications which commonly develop in renal failure include hyperkalaemia, cardiac insufficiency, convulsions and coma.

Hyperkalaemia. Normal serum potassium levels of 3.5–5.0 mmol/l can be maintained until the 24-hour urine output falls below 500 ml with a decreased glomerular filtration rate. There are a few visible signs of hyperkalaemia that the nurse may observe until the serum reaches 7–8 mmol/l. At this elevated level severe electrocardiographic changes may rapidly occur. Cardiac function becomes impaired, and failure or sudden cardiac arrest may occur.

The nurse should be aware of the possible clinical symptoms of potassium intoxication which include generalized muscular weakness, shallow respirations, complaints of a tingling sensation or numbness in the limbs and around the mouth, a slow irregular pulse and a fall in blood pressure. ECG changes are the single most important indication of potassium intoxication. The critical aberrations include tall, tented T waves, ST segment depression, prolonged P–R interval and broadening of the QRS complex, with eventual ventricular fibrillation and cardiac standstill.

Since the outcome of hyperkalaemia can be life threatening, its management focuses on prevention, early detection and treatment of emergencies.

As well as ensuring that no potassium is ingested in fluid or food, preventive measures may include the oral or rectal administration of a cation exchange resin, such as calcium resonium. The resin preparation combines with the potassium in the gastrointestinal secretions, preventing its absorption. Care must be taken to give a stool softener with it, as constipation and occasionally bowel obstruction are complications. Potassium loss via the gastrointestinal tract is only effective if a regular and effective bowel habit is established. If hyperkalaemia develops, an intravenous infusion of glucose with a dose of human soluble insulin may be given. This is to promote the deposition of the glucose as glycogen, a process which utilizes potassium. A solution of sodium bicarbonate or sodium lactate and probably calcium may be administered to counteract the effect of the excess potassium on the heart. An antiarrhythmic drug may also be prescribed. The only permanent and effective way for potassium to be removed from the body is by dialysis.

Cardiac insufficiency. Heart failure may occur as a result of the retention of sodium and water. The pulse may become weak and pulmonary oedema may develop, causing dyspnoea and moist respirations. If hypertension is associated with the renal failure, it may also be a factor in heart failure. Urgent fluid removal by ultrafiltration is required to ensure the safety of the patient. Only when this facility is not available should prescription of a vasodilating agent such as isosorbide dinitrate or reduction of intravascular volume by venesection be considered as a temporary measure until the patient can be transfered urgently to a dialysis unit.

Convulsions. Convulsions may occur and are usually preceded by muscular twitching, persisting severe headache, severe hypertension, increasing oedema and rising blood urea level. Benzodiazepines and diazepam (Valium) may be prescribed to control the seizures.

Coma. Increasing drowsiness may indicate increasing uraemia and may progress to disorientation and coma. The delirious patient requires constant attendance, and a sedative such as diazepam (Valium) may be prescribed. If the patient becomes comatose, the care appropriate for any unconscious patient is applicable (see Chapter 21). At this stage an urgent decision needs to be made either to refer the patient for dialysis or to institute palliative care.

MANAGEMENT

Medical management of acute renal failure is aimed at regulating fluid and electrolyte balance, controlling nitrogen imbalance, maintenance of nutrition and treatment of the underlying cause. Dialysis is initiated before the uraemic state develops to reestablish a normal homeostatic environment for tissue repair and restoration of renal function. Haemodialysis is considered preferable for the patient with acute renal failure. (See discussion of haemodialysis pp. 640–644 and peritoneal dialysis pp. 638–640). Daily dialysis is usually required but the frequency will vary according to the rate of catabolism and the fluid imbalance. Excess fluid may be removed by haemofiltration using continuous, slow ultrafiltration. The use of ultrafiltration filters permits continuous fluid removal from the patient's intravascular content without the side-effects of sudden fluid loss, and without altering serum osmolality as occurs with diffusion dialysis. *Ultrafiltration* can be monitored by the nursing staff in an intensive care unit and has the advantage of allowing intravenous fluids and medications to be given to treat the cause of the patient's acute renal failure while controlling the fluid balance.

Conservative treatment includes the administration of diuretics to increase urine output. Frusemide (Lasix) may be given intravenously. If the urinary output is not satisfactory after 1 or 2 doses, the drug is not usually repeated. Fluid intake is restricted to 500 ml plus the previous day's output. The dietary protein should not be limited to decrease the production of nitrogenous wastes but maintained to provide adequate resources for tissue repair and the patient should be dialysed as often as necessary to keep nitrogenous wastes at an acceptable level. In other words; dialysis is performed as often as needed to 'make room for' a healthy protein intake. This will often mean daily dialysis. The calorie intake is maintained by the administration of glucose. The electrolyte balance is closely monitored, sodium and potassium are restricted and dialysis is used to lower the potassium level.

PATIENT PROBLEMS

The nursing management of persons with acute renal failure is challenging and complex. Virtually every body system will be affected and the nurse must be able to assess how the disease process is affecting the patient as a whole. Table 20.2 lists actual and potential health problems and outcome criteria for care relevant to most persons with acute renal failure.

NURSING INTERVENTION

Assessment. The patient with acute renal failure is seriously ill and requires constant nursing care and *close observation* for changes which may occur suddenly. An accurate record of the *fluid intake and output* is essential as an output of less than 30 ml hourly or 500 ml daily is ominous. Any evident sweating as well as vomiting is recorded and taken into consideration when estimating the volume of fluid the patient should be given.

The *pulse, respirations* and *blood pressure* are checked frequently. Cardiac function may be impaired by the retention of potassium and fluid or by hypertension which may accompany renal parenchymal disease. Blood tests are carried out at least every 4 hours to detect changes in the serum potassium level (hyperkalaemia). Continuous electrocardiographic monitoring may be established if the plasma potassium remains elevated.

Any oedema is noted, and the patient's weight is recorded daily as a gain usually indicates fluid retention. Breathing is observed for signs of developing pulmonary oedema, which may result from overhydration and cardiac failure. A noticeable increase in the volume and depth of respirations may point to acidosis.

The blood pressure is recorded at frequent regular intervals to provide information on the patient's progress. A progressive rise in excess of normal levels is reported to the doctor; it may point to increasing fluid volume. The temperature is taken every 4 hours, even if normal, since a sudden elevation may occur and indicate complicating infection.

Muscular twitching, increasing drowsiness and disorientation are recorded, since they may be manifestations of uraemia, cerebral oedema and approaching convulsions and coma.

Frequent laboratory determinations of blood urea and serum creatinine and electrolytes are followed closely. The sodium and potassium levels are especially important in decisions relating to the types of solutions to be administered, and the patient's fluid balance and weight are used in determining the daily volume of fluid to be given.

Patient responses to medications are carefully assessed. Administering a drug to a patient in renal failure requires knowledge of the metabolic and excretory course of the drug, that is, what happens to it within the body. Those drugs with which renal cells normally react or which are excreted by the kidneys are not given or, if used, are administered in smaller dosage than usually prescribed and levels monitored. Drugs containing potassium or sodium are not given.

Fluid volume excess. The daily fluid intake is limited to 500 ml plus an amount equal to the urinary output of the preceding 24 hours. The 500 ml replaces the obligatory loss through the skin and lungs. The fluid that may be given will depend on the laboratory findings. An explanation of the fluid restriction is essential if the patient is to understand the reasons for such severe limits on fluid intake.

Nutrition. A minimum of 100–200 g of potassium-free carbohydrate is given daily to reduce the amount of tissue protein and fat broken down for energy. Protein is not restricted to avoid a further rise in blood urea. Often patients initially do not tolerate large amounts of food and so are fed nasogastrically or intravenously until they have a desire to eat. If hyperkalaemia is present, 50 ml glucose 50 % may be given intravenously with a dose of soluble insulin. This promotes the movement of

Table 20.2 Actual and potential health problems of persons with acute renal failure.

Patient problem	Goals	Outcome criteria
1. Excess circulating fluid volume due to inability of kidneys to excrete water	• The patient will achieve a state of fluid balance with intake and output within normal limits	• The patient's weight will be stable and within 2 kg of usual weight • Fluid intake and output are balanced and within normal volumes
2. Alteration in electrolyte levels, particularly life-threatening hyperkalaemia, due to inability of kidneys to maintain normal serum electrolyte levels	• Electrolyte levels will be within normal limits	• Serum electrolyte concentrations, pH and osmolality will be within normal range
3. Loss of lean body mass due to malnourishment	• No loss of lean body mass will occur	• The patient experiences no true weight loss • Serum creatinine and blood urea nitrogen are within an acceptable range for the patient
4. Potential impairment of oral mucosa and skin integrity due to oedema and increased excretion of waste through the skin	• Patient's skin and oral mucosa will be clean and intact	• The oral mucosa will have a normal healthy appearance
5. Potential for infection and bleeding due to effects of uraemia on patient's resistance to infection and clotting mechanism	• Infection and bleeding will not occur	• Temperature < 37°C; respiration < 20/minute • No evidence of petechiace, haematuria or melaena
6. Anxiety due to lack of knowledge and loss of control over events	• Patient will be able to talk about anxieties and ask questions	• The patient states that he or she is less anxious and shows some understanding of the disease process and its implications
7. Potential for injury due to confusion	• No injury will occur	• The patient does not injure self despite altered cognition or level of consciousness
8. Dehydration due to excessive fluid loss associated with diuresis or diuretic therapy	• The patient will not become dehydrated	• The patient will be in fluid balance • Signs of dehydration, e.g. dry mouth, loss of skin elasticity, will be absent
9. Knowledge deficit regarding plans for future management	• Patient will be aware of long-term implications of the illness for future life	• The patient and family understand how to manage convalescence • The patient is aware of support services within the community and how to use them to promote recovery

potassium into the cells as well as providing calories.

Essential amino acids as well as hypertonic glucose may be provided by the administration of total parenteral nutrition (TPN) (see pp 496–497). Adequate protein is necessary for synthesis of body tissues, enzymes and antibody production. The delivery of these nutrients requires the administration of a considerable volume of fluid, so parenteral administration of nutrients is used if the patient is treated by ultrafiltration to remove the excess fluid and prevent overloading the heart.

Activity. Activity is not restricted but most patients are initially very ill and therefore need help with all activities. Early involvement of the physiotherapist and

occupational therapist is important so that a co-ordinated excercise regimen, including active and passive exercises and use of appropriate devices and aids, is used to support and assist activities so that independence is enhanced. The family should be consulted to determine the usual level of pre-illness function. Preparations for rehabilitation and discharge should be initiated early, involving other appropriate health care professionals and referral to community services so that recovery is supported both in hospital and at home.

Skin and oral mucosa. In renal failure, the mouth requires special care. The tongue becomes coated, salivary excretion is reduced, and the mucosa and lips are dry and frequently encrusted. Ulcerative lesions may develop, and the patient may be distressed by the disagreeable taste frequently associated with uraemia. Mouth lesions predispose to respiratory infection, local mouth infections and parotitis. Frequent cleansing of the mouth with hydrogen peroxide and rinsing with a mouthwash are necessary. Petroleum jelly or cold cream is applied to the lips. The limited fluid intake and dry mouth are frequently a great source of distress to the patient. Resourcefulness on the part of the nurse may reduce the discomfort. Rinsing the mouth with ice-cold mouthwash or water is more acceptable than using lukewarm solutions. Occasional rinsing of the mouth with ice-cold fruit juice or ginger ale provides a change. Tart fruit or boiled sweets such as fresh pineapple or 'lemon drops' are helpful to stimulate secretions, reduce thirst and, at the same time, supply a little sugar.

The patient is bathed daily to remove the increased wastes that may be excreted in sweat and to provide comfort. Regular assessment of pressure risk should be carried out, with inspection of at risk areas at frequent intervals. Meticulous pressure area care is essential (see Chapter 26).

Anxiety. Acute renal failure that is secondary to some serious disorder heightens the patient's fear and anxiety. Giving information to the patient and creating time in which the patient can ask questions or just talk about feelings are essential aspects of care. Relatives are kept informed of the patient's progress and encouraged to visit. They require support in understanding changes observed in the patient's behaviour and level of awareness.

Potential for injury. Cot-sides may be kept in position since the uraemic patient may become drowsy and disorientated. Uraemia frequently leads to convulsions and coma, but regular dialysis will prevent this.

Fluid volume deficit (diuretic phase). Improvement in renal function is manifested by a steady increase in the volume of urine. The latter may rise rapidly to as much as 6000–8000 ml in 24 hours. The diuresis is accompanied by marked losses of potassium, sodium and water because the tubules have not yet regained their ability to regulate the volume and composition of urine. Frequent serum electrolyte determinations continue, and necessary replacements are made either orally or intravenously. The fluid intake is increased to cover the volume lost. The nitrogenous waste concentration (urea) decreases more slowly.

The patient is offered a soft diet and then a light diet. The nurse continues to record the intake and output, and renal concentration tests may be done to determine if there is some residual insufficiency due to tubular necrosis.

Patient education. Preparation for discharge requires a multi-disciplinary approach in order for the anticipated needs of the individual, family and significant others to be met. The patient and family should be actively involved in discharge preparation to promote a sense of personal control and to ensure adaptation and compliance with ongoing management. The nurse may be a key member of the team ensuring co-ordination and reinforcing information so it is fully understood. Early involvement of the dietitian is important so that dietary restrictions can be discussed against a background of the individual's food preferences, usual eating patterns and food preparation practices at home.

Education should include information concerning recognition of the signs and symptoms of volume overload and hyperkalaemia, and monitoring of dialysis access sites for bleeding and infection. Written and verbal information and contact addresses and telephone numbers should be provided. Community services such as district nursing should be discussed and organized. Again, written and verbal communication with the community services will assist in ensuring continued and appropriate support. Discharge planning should also include outpatient follow-up plans so that the person clearly understands when the doctor will need to review progress and plan further care.

The prolonged convalescence frequently causes socioeconomic problems for the person and family. The nurse may be able to assist by a referral to a medical social worker. It is important to understand the uncertainty of this period because many patients may be discharged before renal function is fully recovered. Consequently, the nurse who is working with the individual, planning the discharge, must be sensitive to the need for continued emotional support of the patient within the community.

CHRONIC RENAL FAILURE

Chronic renal insufficiency is due to progressive disease of both kidneys. Irreversible damage to nephrons occurs which eventually leads to the retention of many waste and toxic products of metabolism, fluid and electrolyte imbalances, metabolic acidosis, anaemia, hypertension and decalcification of bone tissue (renal osteodystrophy).

CAUSES

The most frequent causes of progressive renal failure are the following:

- *Glomerulonephritis.* This involves a variety of immuno-logically-induced diseases which cause inflammation, fibrosis and destruction of glomeruli, with tubular degeneration.
- *Renal vascular disease.* This involves a nephro-sclerosis secondary to hypertension, renal artery stenosis or atherosclerosis.
- *Diabetes mellitus.* Diabetic nephropathy involves extensive glomerular and arteriolar impairment. The glomeruli lose their structure and no longer act as filters.
- *Polycystic kidney disease.* Progressive enlargement of the cysts compresses functional renal parenchyma, increasing renal insufficiency in this inherited disease.

- *Drug-induced nephropathy.* Drug and analgesic abuse may lead to chronic interstitial nephritis and gold therapy can cause nephrotic syndrome.
- *Miscellaneous.* Other diseases which may cause chronic renal failure include chronic pyelonephritis, systemic lupus erythematosus, obstructive postrenal disease (e.g. calculi and neoplasms), and hyperparathyroidism. The aetiology of some individuals' renal disease often remains unknown.

CLINICAL CHARACTERISTICS

Regardless of the cause of the chronic renal failure, the disease progresses through three stages: (1) *diminished renal reserve* which is characterized by an asymptomatic decrease in renal function, (2) *renal insufficiency* demonstrating slightly elevated serum creatinine and blood urea nitrogen levels, and a glomerular filtration rate of about 25% of normal, and (3) *end-stage renal failure or uraemia* which occurs when the glomerular filtration rate is less than 10% of normal, and functional disturbances are apparent.

The patient may pass through the early stage of chronic kidney impairment without the renal disease being recognized. It may first be discovered in a routine physical examination, revealed by an elevation in blood pressure and by albuminuria. The rate of destruction of functional tissue varies among individuals and with the primary causative factor. Some persons live a normal active life for many years because the functioning nephrons compensate to some extent for those destroyed. Others, whose disease progresses rapidly, may enter the advanced uraemic phase in a matter of a few months. In compensation the glomerular filtration rate per nephron is increased as are the reabsorption and secretory functions of the tubules. However, a deficit still exists which progressively increases.

Gradually, with increasing nephron destruction, the patient enters the phase in which renal compensation can no longer maintain homeostasis, and symptoms become apparent. Filtration is impaired, and there is a loss of tubular ability to vary the composition and volume of urine according to the need to conserve or eliminate urinary solutes and water.

The signs and symptoms vary considerably in individuals in the early stages of uncompensated insufficiency but tend to become similar in the more advanced stage (Table 20.3). An elevation in blood pressure, lassitude, headache and loss of weight may be the earliest manifestations. Urinalysis reveals albumin due to increased permeability of glomeruli. The loss of plasma protein as the disease progresses may be severe enough to produce the nephrotic syndrome (see p. 656). As more and more nephrons are destroyed, decreased filtration results in the retention of metabolic wastes. The blood urea and serum creatinine levels rise. Creatinine and urea clearance tests show a decrease in ml per minute, and the severity of failure may be categorized as mild, moderate, severe, end-stage, or anuria on the basis of the clearance test findings. For example, if the creatinine clearance test is used,

Table 20.3 Physiological alterations related to chronic renal failure.

Fluid and electrolyte alterations
  Volume overload or depletion
  Hyperkalaemia or hypokalaemia
  Metabolic acidosis
  Hypercalcaemia and hypocalcaemia
  Raised serum phosphorus

Cardiovascular and pulmonary alterations
  Arterial hypertension
  Heart failure
  Pericarditis
  Pulmonary oedema

Neurological alterations
  Fatigue, lassitude
  Headache, irritability
  Impaired cognition
  Seizures
  Peripheral neuropathy

Gastrointestinal alterations
  Anorexia, nausea and vomiting
  Weight loss
  Peptic ulcer
  Gastrointestinal bleeding

Haematological alterations
  Anaemia
  Bleeding tendency
  Increased potential for infection

Musculoskeletal alterations
  Muscular twitching and weakness
  Renal osteodystrophy
  Calcium deposition in muscle tissue

Skin alterations
  Pruritus associated with xerosis
  Thinning, loss of elasticity
  Increased potential for bruising
  Increased potential for skin breakdown and infection
  Calcium deposition in the skin

Metabolic and endocrine alterations
  Hyperlipidaemia
  Sex hormone disturbances
  Secondary hyperparathyroidism
  Hyperglycaemia

50–84 ml per minute may be interpreted as mild failure, 10–40 ml per minute as moderate failure, less than 10 ml per minute as severe failure, and 0 ml per minute as anuria or end-stage failure.

With a progressive decrease in glomerular filtration and the development of hypertension, the patient experiences increasing fatigue and lassitude, more severe headaches and loss of weight. Nausea, especially in the mornings, and anorexia become troublesome. Fat and glucose metabolism are impaired, as well as protein metabolism. Serum triglycerides increase and a moderate hyperglycaemia occurs as a result of increased sensitivity to insulin.

Initially, in chronic renal failure the 24-hour urinary volume is increased and the patient experiences nocturia as a result of tubular inability to concentrate the glomerular filtrate. The concentration of solutes in the urine is invariable, producing a fixed specific gravity. If the fluid intake does not cover the increased fluid loss, the patient develops a negative fluid balance and the retention of solid wastes is increased.

Tubular destruction causes electrolyte imbalances. There is usually an excessive loss of sodium which may produce hyponatraemia unless there is adequate replacement. Potassium retention is not usually a problem until the terminal oliguric phase. In moderately severe failure, metabolic acidosis develops and hypocalcaemia may also be a problem, contributing to muscular twitching and general weakness.

Eventually, the urinary output is reduced, hypertension becomes severe, and the nitrogenous waste and potassium blood concentrations rise sharply. The patient is pale, and the haematocrit and haemoglobin determinations indicate anaemia which accounts in part for the fatigue and reduced activity. In chronic renal failure a bleeding tendency is also manifested; the thrombocyte count is low and the prothrombin time is abnormal. Petechiae, ecchymoses and bleeding of mucous membanes may be observed.

The central nervous system is affected by the retained wastes; the person is irritable; memory, reasoning and judgement are impaired and the attention span is shortened. In the advanced uraemic stage, the patient manifests confusion, disorientation, drowsiness and stupor. Restlessness and twitching may be observed and frequently precede convulsive seizures. Retention of phosphate and decreased synthesis of the active metabolite of vitamin D by the kidney alter bone metabolism, producing renal osteodystrophy (osteomalacia, osteitis fibrosa, soft tissue calcification and osteosclerosis).

Pruritis can be a severe problem for the person with renal failure; it is attributed to the precipitation of retained phosphates into the skin.

Alterations in ovulatory and menstrual patterns occur in women experiencing renal failure. Although pregnancy has been reported, few women can successfully continue a pregnancy to term because of the overwhelming physiological changes in the body. Both women and men often experience changes in sexual desire and expression. This is for a variety of reasons but fatigue, lowered self-esteem and changed perceptions of attractiveness to their partners appear to play a great part.

Late symptoms are anuria, generalized oedema, persistent headache of increasing severity, nausea and vomiting, hiccups, diarrhoea, muscular twitching, convulsions, ulceration of the mouth, fetid breath, rapid deep respirations indicating acidosis, drowsiness, disorientation and coma. As a result of the severe hypertension and water retention, a cerebrovascular accident or cardiac failure and pulmonary oedema may supervene.

MANAGEMENT

The nurse works with the person to identify patient-centred goals so that the individual will experience life as productively, comfortably, and satisfyingly as possible within the limitations imposed by the disease. It is necessary to create a positive relationship so that the nurse and patient can work together to meet patient-centred goals effectively. The notion that patients with chronic renal failure want to participate in their care is well supported by the work of Stapleton (1983) and Lubkin (1986).

The primary cause of renal failure is treated to retard progression of the disease (e.g. hypertension, pyelonephritis). The therapeutic plan includes measures to correct the body biochemistry and modify symptoms.

Conservative treatment is reserved for those patients who can be maintained without dialysis or kidney transplantation. The dietary and fluid intake are adjusted to maintain water and electrolyte balance and to reduce the retention of nitrogenous waste. Dietary protein may be decreased and limited to proteins high in essential amino acids (i.e. eggs, meat, fish and poultry) and to proteins from vegetables and grains. Carbohydrate intake is increased to provide adequate calories and to prevent the catabolism of body protein. Polyunsaturated fats are recommended and cooking with fats is avoided. A normal sodium intake is maintained if the patient has no signs of oedema or hypertension, but is restricted if these symptoms develop. Dietary potassium is usually restricted and potassium exchange resins are prescribed if hyperkalaemia persists. *Serum phosphate levels are controlled by the use of phosphate binders such as aluminium hydroxide gel.* Multivitamin tablets are prescribed daily to prevent deficiences of water-soluble vitamins which may develop when the diet is low in protein and potassium. Serum calcium is monitored closely and if generalized bone pain, muscle weakness or radiological evidence of bone changes are present, vitamin D in the form of 1α-hydroxycholecalciferol is given and calcium supplements may be prescribed if the phosphate level has been lowered.

The patient is closely monitored for symptoms of complications, and treatment is initiated promptly to control hypertension, fluid and electrolyte imbalances, metabolic acidosis, anaemia and altered bone metabolism.

When conservative treatment will no longer adequately control the blood concentration of wastes and the fluid and electrolyte balance within limits compatible with life, regular *dialysis* may be employed to maintain the patient and a kidney transplant is considered.

THE PERSON UNDERGOING DIALYSIS

When the person with renal failure is being cared for on a conservative therapeutic regimen, he or she will be monitored closely for manifestations that suggest that dialysis needs to be initiated. When the serum creatinine level reaches 800–1200 µmol/l, dialysis will probably need to be instituted. However, blood concentrations alone do not indicate clinical need for dialysis. The signs and symptoms that the nurse must be aware of and that should be reported are progressive hypertension, fluid retention, anorexia, nausea, vomiting, twitching and/or pruritus. These symptoms are often experienced to a degree of debilitation that indicates that dialysis needs to be initiated.

Dialysis is a therapeutic procedure used in acute and chronic renal failure to lower the blood level of metabolic waste products (urea, creatinine, uric acid) and toxic substances and to correct abnormal electrolyte and fluid balances. Two methods currently in use are *peritoneal dialysis* and *extracorporeal haemodialysis*. The latter dialysis takes place outside of the body using a dialysis machine to which an artificial kidney is attached. Although the procedures in the two types of dialysis differ, the purposes and principles are basically the same. In haemodialysis a semipermeable membrane separates the patient's circulating blood from a specially prepared solution known as the *dialysate*. In peritoneal dialysis, the peritoneum is the membrane which separates the dialysate from the person's interstitial fluid, the dialysate being introduced into the peritoneal cavity. By using the principles of osmosis and diffusion, the dialysis procedure can partially replace some of the excretory and regulatory functions of the nephrons of the kidney. It is important to understand that the endocrine function of the normal kidney cannot be replaced by either haemodialysis or peritoneal dialysis.

Peritoneal dialysis

Peritoneal dialysis may be used for most people with symptomatic renal failure and a healthy peritoneal surface area. It is most suitable as a treatment for persons who are independent, live alone, or have limited living space.

In this method of dialysis, the dialysate is introduced into the peritoneal cavity, which is lined by a membrane, the peritoneum. The potential space between the two layers of the peritoneum forms the peritoneal cavity and normally contains only a small amount of serous fluid. For substances to pass from the blood vessels into the peritoneal cavity they must pass through the mesothelium, or outer layer, and five thin layers of fibrous and elastic tissue that comprise the visceral peritoneum. Water is removed across the peritoneal membrane as the result of the osmotic difference between blood and the dialysate.

Continuous ambulatory peritoneal dialysis (CAPD) was developed for use in individuals with renal failure in 1978. This technique involves instilling a dialysis solution in the peritoneal cavity. The dialysate is replaced 3–6 times a day. Scheduling of exchanges is very flexible and the equipment is portable to permit travel, work and schooling and as a consequence this method is increasingly replacing extra-corporeal dialysis in the U.K.

Peritoneal catheters. A permanent peritoneal catheter is required for CAPD. A catheter with several openings in the tip, such as the Tenckhoff catheter or a modification of it is inserted into the peritoneal cavity (see Figure 20.10).

Tissue cells (fibroblasts) grow into the two Dacron cuffs on the subcutaneous section of the catheter in 2–3 weeks, stabilizing the catheter position and decreasing the incidence of infection and escape of fluid. The procedure is usually carried out in the operating theatre under either a local or a general anaesthetic.

Dialysates. Dialysates are commercially available in 1, 2 or 3 litre plastic bags and provide various options of dextrose concentration and osmolarity. Dextrose concentrations above 1.5% increase the osmolarity of the dialysate above that of the plasma and promote water removal. Additional electrolytes and medications are added to the dialysate according to the needs and serum electrolyte concentrations of the individual patient.

Dialysis cycles. Each exchange of dialysate is divided into three stages; the instillation time, dwell time and drainage time. The solution is warmed to body temperature and infuses fairly rapidly into the peritoneal cavity by the force of gravity. The *instillation time* for the 2 litres of solution usually used for an adult requires approximately 10 minutes. *Dwell time* is the period of time the dialysate remains in the peritoneal cavity. For CAPD this varies from 4 to 8 hours and exchanges are carried out continuously, 7 days a week. Smaller molecules such as blood urea nitrogen equalize in 2–3 hours; larger molecules take longer to equalize. The osmolarity of the solution influences the dwell time required to remove water. Higher concentrations of dextrose (4.25%) remove larger volumes of water in less time than solutions of 1.5% dextrose. *Drainage time* is the third phase of the cycle which is the period in which the solution drains from the cavity and takes up to 20 minutes.

Continuous ambulatory peritoneal dialysis is currently the treatment of choice for most patients because it permits independence from machines, a more varied diet and a more flexible life-style. It has proven to be effective in removing small and middle-sized molecules, sodium, potassium and water and in controlling hypertension and anaemia. The procedure involves: (1) connection of the catheter to tubing from a plastic bag containing the dialysate solution; (2) instillation of the dialysate; (3) folding of the plastic bag into a waist, leg or pocket pouch worn under the clothing; (4) drainage of the peritoneal cavity by gravity into the plastic bag about 6 hours later; (5) disposal of the filled bag; (6) connection and instillation of a fresh bag of dialysate (Figure 20.9). Bags containing 2 litres of dialysate are exchanged approximately four times a day, 7 days a week. The exchange schedule may be adjusted allowing 6 hours between two exchanges, 4 hours between the next exchange and an 8-hour interval at night to permit uninterrupted sleep.

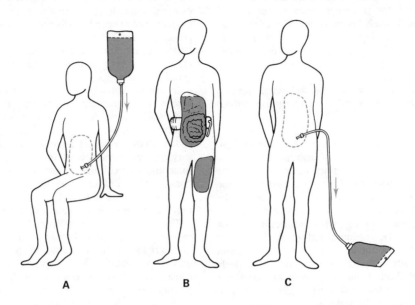

Figure 20.9 Continuous ambulatory peritoneal dialysis. (A) Fluid flows from bag into peritoneal cavity through permanent access tube. (B) Patient wears bag around waist or leg and resumes normal activity. (C) Bag is lowered and fluid drains out. Bag is then discarded and procedure is repeated with fresh fluid.

Complications of peritoneal dialysis

Peritonitis. This is the major complication of peritoneal dialysis. The causative organisms have been shown to colonize all catheters and peritonitis may be due to a sudden increase of organisms by contamination of equipment, or dialysate fluid, or a decrease in the patient's ability to clear the organisms. Reasons for this are not yet known. Symptoms include abdominal pain and tenderness, cloudy effluent, fever, and occasionally vomiting and paralytic ileus. The peritoneal effluent is cultured for identification of organisms and white blood cell count. Treatment may consist of peritoneal lavage; this may be performed by continuously flushing with dialysis solution, without dwell time, for a brief period or for up to 48 hours. This may be followed by repeated exchanges with dwell times from 1–6 hours. Antibiotics are infused into the peritoneal cavity in the dialysate.

Catheter complications. Leakage around the catheter, obstruction of the catheter, retention of fluid and infection of the exit site are the most common complications associated with the catheter. Leakage occurs most often in the first 2 weeks following insertion of the catheter. Occlusion of the catheter may require the use of heparin in the dialysate to prevent or dislodge fibrin clots. Maintenance of regular bowel elimination helps to prevent problems with the flow of solution into the peritoneal cavity. Infection of the catheter site should be identified and treated promptly. Systemic antibiotics are given if positive cultures are

obtained. Tunnel infections along the path of the catheter may necessitate replacement of the catheter.

Dehydration may result from use of large volumes of 4.25% dextrose dialysate. The patient will be hypotensive manifesting pallor, weakness, fainting and a rapid, weak pulse and will experience muscle cramps and may also be hyperglycaemic.

Pain. This may be due to the tip of the catheter pressing on viscera or overheating of the dialysate.

Protein catabolism and anorexia. The breakdown of tissue protein may occur because of loss of protein in the dialysate. Maintenance of adequate protein intake is necessary to prevent this complication.

Anorexia may occur initially, accompanied by a feeling of fullness when the dialysate is held in the peritoneal cavity. This problem usually disappears in a few months. When anorexia is present, the patient is assessed for signs of dehydration from excessive fluid loss.

Nursing care of the person undergoing long-term peritoneal dialysis
Because of its relative simplicity, nurses often make the assumption that the person undergoing long-term peritoneal dialysis should adjust quickly and easily. It is also expected that the patient should learn CAPD rapidly. However, it is wrong to imply that peritoneal dialysis is 'easy' since it involves skill, problem-solving ability and fine motor co-ordination that some patients

may not possess. By careful assessment the nurse can begin to work with the patient to promote self-care as independently and safely as possible. The nurse can assist patients to develop new methods of self-care which are unique to their particular needs and situation. At all times the nurse must be aware of the patient's perspective of the illness.

Nurses should be aware of the following general issues when giving care to patients undergoing dialysis in hospital.

Predialysis. Preparation of the patient involves evaluating the person's understanding of dialysis. An explanation of the procedure and its purpose is given to the patient and family. Assessing their continued education needs is very crucial, since the effects of uraemia, by interfering with cerebral function, may prevent the patient from understanding what is being taught. Information should be repeated and given clearly and simply. While the patient is learning CAPD, frequent assessment is very important and should include recording of BP (both lying and sitting or standing), pulse, respirations, temperature and weight in order to establish a baseline for physical signs. Signs of oedema, respiratory distress and dehydration should also be noted. The abdomen is examined for distention and tenderness that might indicate peritonitis, and the area around the exit of the catheter is observed for redness, drainage and infection. It is important to assess how the patient is feeling and how the forthcoming dialysis is viewed. When outflow is completed, the volume of fluid drained should be measured and recorded in order to ensure all dialysate is drained.

The person may be more comfortable in an easy chair rather than in bed; being occupied by watching television, listening to the radio, reading, or talking with the nurse usually helps the patient through the cycle. Activity is encouraaged as much as possible; equipment may be attached to movable poles, permitting a greater degree of mobility.

If CAPD is to be established, the patient and family require detailed, individualized education and training before the patient is ready to begin to dialyse independently. The nurse working with individuals learning to undertake their own dialysis should assess their knowledge and needs to provide a baseline from which to plan and implement a step-by-step programme. This will assist the development of confidence and autonomy and encourage adaptation and normalization.

Haemodialysis

Haemodialysis can remove water and catabolic wastes at a faster rate than peritoneal dialysis. Because of this efficiency, it may not always be used for patients who are haemodynamically unstable, as can be the case in certain cardiac diseases. It is a complex procedure that requires expensive and sophisticated equipment.

In haemodialysis an extracorporeal dialysing system is used to remove toxic wastes. During haemodialysis the person's uraemic blood is purified by drawing it from an artery, passing it through a sterile extracorporeal circulation, through a dialyser in which dialysis takes place, and returning it to the venous system in its purified state. It is within the dialyser that the actual exchange of material across the dialysis membrane takes place. Figure 20.10 illustrates the relationship of the patient to the equipment. During routine haemodialysis, clearance of body toxins and filtration of water occur simultaneously.

In haemodialysis, both solute and solvent transfer across the membrane under the force generated by hydrostatic pressure, in addition to that created by osmotic pressure.

The dialysate is an aqueous solution that contains varying concentrations of the body's normal extracellular and intracellular cations and anions. The cations commonly found in dialysate are sodium, potassium, calcium and magnesium. The anions found in dialysate may be acetate, bicarbonate and glucose.

The concentrations within the dialysate solution promote the removal of toxic substances, such as excess urea, creatinine and uric acid, from the body, as well as excess potassium, sodium, phosphate and water. Because of the semipermeable nature of the dialysis membrane it readily allows the passage of small molecules such as urea, potassium and sodium, while retaining such large molecules as proteins, glucose and red blood cells. The small molecules that can pass through the pores of the membrane will always travel from the area of greater to lesser concentration so that there is equal composition and concentration on both sides of the membrane. Because of the hydrostatic pressure across the membrane, excess water can be removed as the water flows toward the dialysate solution, which is of greater osmolality.

Vascular Access

Maintenance haemodialysis requires direct access to the circulating blood by the extracorporeal dialysing system. The requirement for vascular access in persons with renal failure can be either permanent or temporary. Patients using long-term haemodialysis will need a permanent access because the duration of the treatment will be months or many years. The types of access are the arteriovenous fistula, the arteriovenous graft and the arteriovenous shunt. Each access requires specialized nursing care, the focus of which should include assessing the access for patency, pain, signs of infection, tissue trauma or oedema, and bleeding. The nurse will also work with the patient to ensure that he or she can monitor the vascular access thoroughly and independently.

The *arteriovenous (AV) fistula* is most frequently used and is surgically constructed by a side-to-side or end-to-end anastomosis between an artery and a vein in the forearm. The anastomosis may be between the cephalic vein and the radial artery, or between the cephalic vein and brachial artery (Figure 20.11). This redirects arterial blood through the vein, thereby causing enlargement of the vein in response to the increased rate of blood flow and the higher pressure of arterial blood now passing through it. This engorgement of the arterialized vein requires 6–12 weeks to 'mature' before it is able to withstand the changing pressures against its vessel wall and the repeated insertion of dialysis needles.

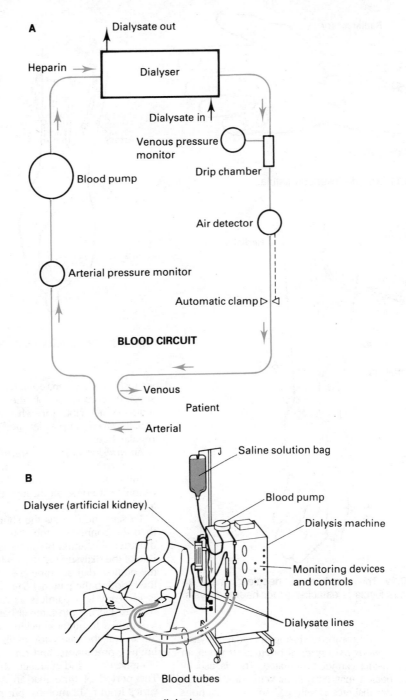

Figure 20.10 Diagrammatic representation of haemodialysis.

Haemodialysis with an AV fistula involves the insertion of two needles into the vein. One needle is inserted at least 2 cm above the anastamosis and is connected to the arterial line of the dialyser. The second needle is inserted 3–4 cm above the outflow needle and is connected to the tube that returns the blood from the dialyser. Blood flows out from the distal needle through the dialyser and back via the proximal needle (Figure 20.12). The limb in which an arteriovenous fistula is developed should not normally be used for taking blood pressure or blood samples, as either may jeopardize the patency of the fistula.

The AV fistula is often the preferred access for long-term haemodialysis because it has several distinct advantages. It is completely subcutaneous, thus lessening the possibility of infection and reducing the risk of

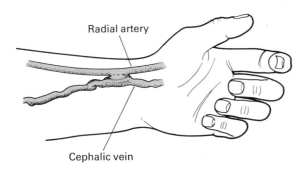

Figure 20.11 An arteriovenous fistula.

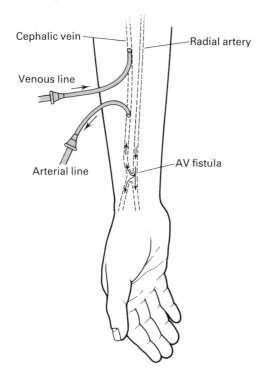

Figure 20.12 The position of needles when an arteriovenous fistula is established for haemodialysis.

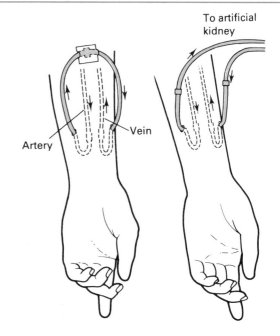

Figure 20.13 Arteriovenous shunt.

haemorrhage and thrombosis during everyday activity.

The *arteriovenous (AV) graft* is often used when an adequate AV fistula cannot be created. This is usually because the person may have poor veins due to small vasculature or diabetes mellitus. An arteriovenous connection is then made via a tube graft made from polytetrafluoroethylene (PTFE; Teflon).

The graft does have a drawback in comparison to the fistula in that the graft has a higher rate of infection and thrombosis. Some graft infections may occur without local signs as the infecting organism may become embedded in the weave of the graft material itself. Prompt therapy with antibiotics is essential. If the infection is unresponsive to medication, the graft will have to be removed.

Thrombosis of an AV graft is usually caused by stenosis at the anastomotic sites. This necessitates surgical correction of the defect. To reduce the tendency to clot, for whatever reason, patients are usually given antiplatelet medications to be taken on a regular basis.

An *arteriovenous (AV) shunt* is established by exposing an artery and an adjacent vein and implanting a cannula in each (Figure 20.13). The ends of the cannulae are brought through the skin and are joined by a short connecting tube.

To start the dialysis the shunt-tubing is clamped and then the connecting tube on the AV shunt is removed; the arterial cannula is connected to the inflow (arterial) line of the dialyser and the venous cannula is attached to the outflow dialyser tube (i.e. to the tube which returns the blood to the patient). The advantage of the AV shunt is its ready and painless accessibility for commencing dialysis. During the interval between dialyses, however, it requires frequent checking, dressing and protection. Since available sites for establishing an AV shunt are limited, precautions and care are necessary to prevent complications and maintain the patency of the shunt. The period of time that an AV shunt remains patent varies from 6–12 months, but may be several years.

The loop of the tube is checked frequently for blood flow. Clotting in the shunt system and obstruction of the flow may occur with kinking or malalignment of the tubes or pressure being exerted on them. *The blood becomes dark red, and the bruit that is normally heard with a stethoscope over the venous side is absent.* If clotting is suspected, no attempt is made to clear the tube by 'milking'. The problem is reported immediately to the doctor or dialysis unit. Efforts will be made to remove the clots by aspiration and the use of heparinized saline and declotting catheters.

The site is also checked for bleeding. If the tubing becomes disconnected, free bleeding is quickly recognized and the clamps previously mentioned are applied promptly to the tubing. Subcutaneous bleeding may result from the displacement of a cannula or erosion of the artery or vein. This is reported promptly; pressure is applied over the site to control bleeding.

The limb in which there is an AV shunt must not be used to determine blood pressure or administer intravenous infusions.

There are two temporary types of vascular access that can be used in a variety of clinical situations. For example, a patient may have a clotted AV shunt that cannot be used but needs urgent dialysis before a permanent access can be re-established. In these cases, the patient may undergo haemodialysis with a *subclavian catheter* or a *femoral catheter*. In either case, access is gained to the circulation by percutaneous insertion of a cannula.

The subclavian catheter can be inserted quickly and easily at the bedside. Blood flows are lower and therefore clearances of body toxins and water are not as efficient as they would be using a permanently established fistula or graft. The subclavian access can be used for a period of from 1 to 6 months.

The femoral catheter is most often used in the clinical management of the person with acute renal failure. The technique is simple and safe and can be easily performed at the bedside. The disadvantage is that the catheter is in an area where it is difficult to maintain adequate hygiene. Consequently, there is a high risk of infection. Patients must also stay on bed rest while the catheter is in place to avoid groin or retroperitoneal haematomas. To avoid the possibility of infection and haematoma formation, a cannula in the femoral vein is usually removed within 72 hours.

Table 20.4 outlines issues for the immediate postoperative care of the patient with a newly created AV fistula, graft or shunt or temporary access.

Nursing intervention in haemodialysis
Nurses responsible for the care of patients receiving dialysis require specialized preparation. Dialysis is a complex therapeutic procedure used to correct a life-threatening body dysfunction. Staff on general medical and surgical units and in the community should also have an appreciation of the implications for and the concerns of the renal patient and family. Personnel working in dialysis units usually assume responsibility for the specialized needs of dialysis patients being cared for in other areas of the hospital.

Factors to be considered in the nursing care plan for the haemodialysis patient include the following:

Emotional and socioeconomic concerns. When the person's chronic renal failure necessitates haemodialysis, it is natural that the patient and family will be concerned. It is likely to have many implications; knowing that the disease has progressed to this stage and that life becomes dependent upon the procedure is extremely threatening. Severe anxiety may be manifested due to concern for the future and life expectancy. Acceptance may be very difficult for some patients and they may manifest resentment and anger at first, followed by a period of depression. A regular schedule of dialysis two or three times weekly imposes modifications on the patient's and family's life pattern. Treatment may mean changing occupation or giving up employment or, at best, working only part-time unless home dialysis can be provided. The adjustments that have to be made may cause both social and economic changes for family members. The patient may be the main source of income or the mother or combine both roles. Special diet requirements and transport to and from the dialysis unit or the need to accommodate dialysis equipment in the home may incur worrisome additional expense. A referral to a social worker may be helpful.

It is important for the nurse to be a willing listener and encourage the patient and family to reveal their concerns and problems; these vary from person to person and family to family. An understanding of their situation and recognition of their reactions are essential to providing the appropriate support and care, and in assisting them to accept necessary modifications in lifestyle. A positive attitude on the part of the health care team promotes realistic patient and family acceptance and adaptation. Many people obtain support and pleasure through socialization and the establishment of close relationships with other dialysis patients.

Gradually, as the uraemic toxicity is reduced, the person experiences physical and emotional improvement and, by degrees, becomes more active and interested in living and may lead a relatively normal productive life.

Table 20.4 Guidelines for nursing care of the patient with a permanent or temporary vascular access for haemodialysis.

1. Elevate affected arm or leg on pillow to minimize tissue swelling
2. Check dressing for any bleeding; document and report to the doctor
3. Check warmth, colour and mobility of fingers or toes for circulation
4. Oedema is expected postoperatively but excessive oedema should be reported to the doctor
5. Access insertion is a painful procedure, therefore analgesia should be given as required during the postoperative period
6. Teach the patient to monitor own access for bleeding and swelling, and to report pain. If it is an AV shunt, teach the patient how to use bulldog clamps and ensure that the patient understands that clamp must be present on shunt dressing at all times
7. No blood specimens, intravenous infusions, blood pressure monitoring, etc. to be performed on access arm
8. Psychological support should be given to the patient at all times

Predialysis responsibilities. The patient and family should receive a simple explanation of the purpose of dialysis and what to expect during the procedure. Many units have prepared brochures and audiovisual programmes to provide information and reinforce verbal explanations and instruction. If the patient is to be dialysed at home, an extensive home training programme is planned. Prior to the initial treatment, if the patient's condition permits, he or she should visit the dialysis unit, meet the dialysis staff and may have the opportunity to chat with a patient on a regular dialysis programme. Such preparation is helpful in reducing the person's fear.

For dialysis, the patient is positioned comfortably in a bed or a reclining chair with the limb with the AV fistula or shunt exposed and supported. Temperature, pulse, respirations, lying and standing blood pressure and weight are recorded before the dialysis is commenced to provide a baseline. Blood specimens are obtained when the needles are introduced (or cannulae are opened) for laboratory determination of the haematocrit, electrolyte (K^+, Na^+), blood urea, and creatinine levels and clotting time. Anxiety is often greatly reduced if the patient and a relative are actively included even for the first dialysis. This might mean helping to set up the machine or preparation of the patient's dialysis access. A working knowledge of the equipment often greatly reduces fear.

The vascular access site is examined for signs of a haematoma or infection. Observations are made of the person's colour and the condition of the skin (dryness, turgor, abrasions) and for oedema. Weight is compared with that recorded following the last dialysis to check fluid accumulation. Weight changes, as well as blood chemistry and physical findings determine the desired fluid loss and the appropriate dialyser, dialysate and flow-rate.

Responsibilities during dialysis. During dialysis the patient is monitored continuously for indications of the effectiveness of treatment and signs of complications. Each unit or home programme will have a schedule for observing and recording vital signs, equipment used, rate of flow, composition and temperature of dialysate, heparinization and blood clotting times, as well as ongoing monitoring of the functioning of the equipment. The person is closely observed for signs of dehydration or overhydration. Changes in blood pressure and respirations are recorded and the flow rate through the dialyser is regulated accordingly. If there is a rapid, excessive loss of water into the dialysate, the ensuing reduction in the intravascular volume causes a sharp fall in the blood pressure. Overhydration may be indicated by respiratory distress, moist sounds and an increase in the blood pressure.

Blood analysis for potassium and sodium levels may be repeated at intervals during dialysis. Adjustments may be necessary in the dialysate in accordance with the electrolyte values.

The clotting time is usually checked hourly by a simple ward-based test.

Headache, vomiting and twitching may develop if the patient becomes dehydrated and should be brought to the doctor's attention. The first dialysis should be short (i.e. 2–3 hours) to allow a gentle clearance of nitrogenous waste. This prevents the complication of cerebral oedema associated with disequilibrium syndrome which may be present as disorientation or a convulsion.

If the individual is on regular medication, the administration of these during dialysis is considered. Those which are dialysed out are often given post dialysis, especially if taken in once-daily doses. Antihypertensive preparations are not given, since they may cause hypotension.

The length of time the patient is kept on the dialyser varies with the patient's condition and type of machine used. The average range is 4–6 hours. The frequency also varies with patients. In acute renal failure, daily dialysis may be necessary until renal function is reestablished. Persons with chronic renal insufficiency are dialysed two or three times weekly and may lead a relatively normal productive life the remainder of the week. The dialysis programme may be long-term, extending over years, or may be a temporary measure for the individual who is awaiting a kidney transplant.

Postdialysis care. Upon completion of the dialysis the arterial line is clamped and as much blood as possible in the dialysing circuit lines is returned to the patient. The needles are removed or, in the case of a shunt, the dialysing lines disconnected and the cannulae reconnected. Dressings are applied and the area observed until there is no evidence of bleeding; it may be necessary to apply some pressure for a brief period. The patient's weight, blood pressure, lying and standing, pulse and temperature are recorded for comparison with the original baseline observations.

Patient education. When a regular dialysis programme is recommended, the person and a relative receive detailed instruction concerning diet and fluid intake, care of the fistula site or cannulae, activity, and recognition of disturbances that should prompt immediate notification of the doctor or dialysis unit. The brochure given out by the dialysis unit that explains dialysis also discusses these factors.

The diet prescribed varies from person to person and with doctors. The food intake must be balanced with the renal capacity to eliminate protein waste and prevent excesses of electrolytes (K^+, Na^+) and water. The protein content may be 60–80 g per day, allowing 0.75–1 g per kg of body if dialysis facilities are limited, otherwise a normal diet or a high protein diet is encouraged and dialysis hours adjusted to control nitrogenous waste.

NURSING THE PERSON WITH CHRONIC RENAL FAILURE

Patient problems

Health care providers have long since acknowledged that patients with chronic renal failure have much to overcome. They are particularly vulnerable to reactive

Table 20.5 Actual and potential health problems of the person with chronic renal failure.

1. Altered fluid and electrolyte balance (deficit or excess)
2. Altered nutrition: nutritional intake lower than body requirements
3. Potential for infection and bleeding
4. Activity intolerance
5. Impaired skin integrity and altered oral mucosa
6. Altered thought processes
7. Ineffective individual and family coping patterns
8. Knowledge deficit related to:
   (a) Kidney function
   (b) Methods of treatment (dialysis or transplant)
   (c) Self-care measures
   (d) Necessary alterations to life style.

depression, social isolation and a whole host of physiological complications (Stapleton 1983). In an attempt to capture the full impact of chronic renal failure on the individual, research has focused on quality of life measures (Janes, 1990a, 1990b), compliance (Eddins, 1985) and control (Poll and Kaplan De-Nour, 1980). The experiences of individuals undergoing long-term dialysis are beginning to be investigated by exploring the subjective experiences of patients undergoing different treatment approaches (Buck et al, 1986). This approach allows the practitioner to gain insight into patients' experiences and interpretations. Feelings of powerlessness are frequently reported in relation to long-term dialysis and by those awaiting transplantation. The nurse is in a unique position to explore with patients the impact of the disease and management on them and their relationships, and to help individuals develop skills and strategies to cope (Lubkin, 1986; Weems and Patterson, 1989). All practitioners need to be aware of the unique health care needs of the person with chronic renal disease because of the prevalence of the condition in the general population.

Table 20.5 lists actual and potential health problems common to most patients with chronic renal failure, however care should be individualized to meet the needs of each patient. The needs of patients and their families will also vary as the disease progresses.

Nursing intervention

1. Altered fluid and electrolyte balance. Assessment of fluid and electrolyte balance is continuous. The patient and family should be taught to identify signs and symptoms of fluid excess or dehydration and to adjust fluid intake accordingly. The patient is also taught to recognize the signs of hyperkalaemia and other electrolyte imbalances and to adjust diet as necessary.

In the early stages of chronic renal failure, tubular reabsorption of water is decreased so the intake must be increased accordingly to avoid dehydration. Generally a minimum of 2000 ml is required to prevent dehydration. When oliguria is present the fluid intake is limited

to 400–500 ml plus the measurable loss (e.g. urine and vomit). Fluid restriction may be minimal for the person on CAPD because fluid is continuously removed; however fluid restrictions may be introduced in the individual on CAPD who exhibits signs of fluid volume expansion that could jeopardize cardiovascular integrity.

2. Nutrition. The prescribed diet varies with the severity of the disease and the type of maintenance treatment used. In the early stages, protein restrictions may be based on the glomerular filtration rate (GFR), but when the GFR decreases to 4–5 ml/min, protein restrictions are no longer effective in reducing the retention of nitrogenous wastes and dialysis is required. Protein is lost during peritoneal dialysis and the loss is greater if peritonitis develops. Less protein is lost during haemodialysis, but some free amino acids escape with this treatment. The protein intake must be adjusted to compensate for the loss and prevent catabolism of body protein. Calorie intake must be sufficient to permit activity without breakdown of tissue protein. The person on CAPD absorbs some glucose from the dialysate and so carbohydrate intake is adjusted accordingly to individual requirements to maintain a healthy body weight and blood glucose concentrations.

Electrolyte balance is maintained by adjusting the dietary intake according to serum electrolyte levels. Since impaired tubular reabsorption results in an excessive loss of sodium, salt is not restricted in the diet unless there is oedema or hypertension. Dietary sodium is restricted following a transplant as corticosteriod therapy leads to sodium and water retention. Foods high in potassium are restricted for most renal patients because potassium is not effectively removed by impaired kidneys. Transplant recipients receiving diuretic therapy may require potassium supplements. The serum phosphate level is usually controlled by the use of phosphate binders, such as an aluminium hydroxide antacid, and avoidance of foods high in phosphorus.

Nutritional management in chronic renal failure is complex. Because of the multiplicity of factors to be considered in determining dietary modifications for each individual, patients experience some difficulty in understanding restrictions and in following the prescribed diet. Since diet is such an important part of disease management, the individual and family require considerable teaching and prolonged support from the nurse as well as the dietitian. It is essential that a person's previous meal patterns and food preferences be incorporated into any management plan.

Dietary management becomes more complex for the person with chronic renal failure who experiences sudden stress such as infection, surgery or trauma. Food and fluid intake must be closely monitored and adjusted to body needs. Total parenteral nutrition may also be used to maintain adequate nutrition for the critically ill patient.

3. Preventing infection and bleeding. Immunosuppressive drugs or uraemia affect white cell activity, making the person prone to infection. Preventive measures and prompt treatment of infection are essential. Uraemic blood also has altered clotting ability and the patient therefore needs to be monitored for signs of bleeding from the dialysis access, mucous membranes or surgical sites.

4. Activity intolerance. The individual with chronic renal failure experiences considerable fatigue and lethargy; anaemia may contribute to the decreased energy. The anaemia may be due to decreased erythropoeitin production, depression of the bone marrow associated with uraemia, or to blood loss due to increased tendency to bleed and through dialysis. It develops gradually and may not be symptomatic at first.

In the early stages of the disease, kidney function may be adequate as long as the prescribed diet and fluid intake are followed and metabolic extremes are avoided. The patient should be encouraged to remain as active as possible, as the ability to continue to be a useful, independent member of society bolsters self-esteem and emotional well-being.

If the person develops severe anaemia that manifests itself in fatigue, shortness of breath or angina, periodic transfusions of whole blood or packed cells may be given. The nurse working with haemodialysis patients should therefore take precautions to minimize blood loss during dialysis. The taking of blood for laboratory tests is reviewed to limit the amount of blood being taken. Promising research results suggest that the monitored administration of a manufactured form of erythropoietin, recombinant human erythropoietin, may be instrumental in increasing haemoglobin concentrations. This will improve the person's energy level and quality of life dramatically. However, the cost of this drug may mean that it is used selectively or prohibits generalized use within the National Health Service.

Enquiry should be made concerning joint and muscle pain and any changes in range of motion or mobility. Signs of hypocalcaemia, tetany, carpopedal spasm, seizures, numbness and tingling of extremities or confusion should be noted and reported to medical staff. When signs and symptoms of altered serum calcium and phosphorus develop, the patient's compliance with medication therapy and dialysis is assessed and changes made as necessary. An activity and exercise plan is developed to maintain muscle tone and mobility.

5. Skin and oral mucosa. Assessment of the skin of the patient with chronic renal failure may show pallor, a yellow-grey colour, dryness, bruising and decreased sweating. The patient complains of itching. The hair is dry, becomes brittle and the nails are rigid and dry. Uraemic frost on the skin from crystallization of urea deposits is rare except in terminally ill patients. The mouth should be inspected regularly for signs of inflammation and bleeding.

The patient is taught to care for skin, mouth, hair and nails; This includes following the dietary regimen to control serum calcium and phosphorus levels and avoiding tissue trauma.

6. Altered thought processes. Changes in the patient's level of awareness usually develop gradually as uraemia increases. Rapid progression of the disease produces severe disturbances in behaviour and cognition. Dialysis should be started before the progression of these neurological complications.

Early symptoms may include headache, lethargy, dizziness, euphoria, depression, apathy, sleeplessness or drowsiness. Recent and remote memory and attention span are decreased and decision making is impaired. In the late stages of renal failure, confusion, slurred speech, stupor, coma and convulsions may develop.

The patient is assessed for orientation to time, place and person. Changes in behaviour as perceived by the patient and family are noted and relatives are helped to understand that the patient cannot always control behaviour.

Cognitive abilities should be evaluated before patient teaching is started. Explanations of procedures should be simple, broken down into steps and repeated frequently. It is possible that the patient's home environment may need modification to promote safety.

Many of the behavioural and cognitive changes are reversible with dialysis. The importance of following the dialysis schedule is stressed and additional dialysis time may be planned when neurological symptoms indicate more severe renal insufficiency.

7. Coping patterns. Adaptation to chronic renal failure is a complex process and varies with each patient, the degree of loss of renal function, the type of treatment selected and support available.

Assessment of the patient's coping includes learning about pre-illness personality and the degree of dependence and independence assumed in daily life. The number and type of losses and changes required in the patient's life-style such as: loss of job and financial security; loss of position in the family; loss of freedom because of actual or perceived dependence on a machine; loss of stamina and sense of well-being; loss of self-esteem and self-worth; and reduced life expectancy. Further changes in family roles and relationships are increased by decreased sexual function. The previously independent person has the most difficulty adjusting initially, but measures to prevent feelings of helplessness and dependence can be effective. Selection of home dialysis or continuous ambulatory peritoneal dialysis forces the patient to become an active participant in care, while hospital dialysis may reinforce dependence and emphasize losses.

Information about how the patient coped with stress in the past helps the nurse in assessing the patient's present coping responses and in assisting in developing new coping strategies. Some coping mechanisms used every day are dangerous when employed by the person with chronic renal failure. For example, a period of denial or non-adherence to the management plan is often seen in persons with chronic illness as they strive to deal with the staggering life changes necessary. The nurse should accept this as the patient works through the denial period, and should work with the person in exploring thoughts and feelings about the impact of chronic illness on life-style.

Changes in cognitive ability and behaviour affect the patient's perceptions of the illness, ability to comprehend what is happening, to understand and adhere with treatment and make informed, rational judgements about care; dependency on others is increased. Chronic fatigue and lethargy further impair the patient's ability to cope.

The presence of family and other support groups enhances positive coping. The responses of family members and friends and their influence on the patient are evaluated. They require knowledge of the disease, understanding of the patient's responses and behavioural changes and understanding of the treatment plan so they can be informed participants. They will need help in developing new patterns of interacting with each other and new coping strategies.

Decisions about care are made with the patient and family as active participants and should be directed to achieving the goals of the patient. Doctors and nurses should avoid giving ambiguous messages to the patient and family by first expressing the desire for patient participation in decision-making and then imposing their own expectations of patient behaviour. Patient responses change as each new phase of treatment is encountered. The patient starting dialysis must acknowledge dependence on machines to sustain life. Transplantation usually results in an initial state of euphoria which is followed by reactions to living with a foreign body, before eventual acceptance of the graft occurs. These patients live with a life-long need for medication and constant fear of graft rejection. Even with a successful transplantation the patient needs help adjusting to the changes imposed by this life-long process.

8. *Lack of knowledge.* Since the patient and family must assume the responsibility for following the prescribed regimen, formal and informal instruction is planned. Patient education is started at the time of diagnosis and the teaching is adjusted as the patient's needs change with progression of the disease and revision of the treatment plan. The decision about home or institutional dialysis influences the degree of responsibility the patient and family assume for self-care and the resources needed to help them. Some patients and families learn to follow the treatment programme, make necessary observations, recognize significant changes, adjust care according to predetermined guidelines and seek help when needed. Other patients require a referral to community services because a regular support person is unavailable. Medical supervision is provided by the dialysis unit or treatment centre. If the patient is returning to work, the occupational health nurse at the place of employment should be advised of the situation so that he or she may provide the necessary assistance and follow the patient's progress if desired.

When a patient with chronic renal failure is admitted to hospital it is important that the nursing staff assess the patient's understanding of care and support the individual's achievements by encouraging active patient participation in care. Taking away the patient's control on each hospital admission retards progress already made and contributes to feelings of dependency.

Goals for education should be established for each patient and teaching methods varied with available resources. Many pamphlets are available for patient use. Renal centres will have instruction sheets, guidelines and audiovisual programmes which are useful to teach skills and reinforce demonstrations and practice sessions. Written instructions are given to each patient regarding specific dietary modifications, medications, care of the fistula, shunt or catheter, and treatment schedule. Group teaching may be useful to impart general content and to allow patients and families to share experiences and to learn alternative coping strategies from each other.

A patient and family teaching programme includes: the function of the kidneys, types of treatment (dialysis or transplant), self-care measures and life-style adaptations.

The function of the kidney. The healthy kidney regulates body fluid volume, excretion of waste and secretion of hormones to control blood pressure, red blood cell production and calcium absorption. When kidney insufficiency occurs, waste products and fluid are retained, blood pressure rises, anaemia develops and weakness of the bone structure occurs.

Types of treatment. When end-stage renal failure develops the patient becomes dependent on dialysis or receives a kidney transplant. Information is provided about: intermittent and continuous peritoneal dialysis; haemodialysis; types of vascular accesses available and the options of treatment at home or in a dialysis centre. The suitability, availability and implications of transplant are discussed.

A home peritoneal dialysis teaching plan includes knowledge and practice of the principles of asepsis, the techniques of changing dialysate bags, the catheter dressing procedure, the taking and recording of blood pressure and weight. It is necessary for the patient to have an understanding of the role of dialysis, the significance of weight changes and recognition of the signs of fluid overload, dehydration and peritonitis. Active patient participation and supervised practice sessions are essential.

A teaching programme for home haemodialysis includes knowledge of and practice in the principles of asepsis and care and assessment of the shunt or fistula. The patient learns to palpate the AV shunt, feeling a 'thrill' and to use a stethoscope to listen for a bruit proximal to the venous insertion site resulting from the turbulence created by the high arterial pressure flowing into the vein. Safety measures to prevent haemorrhage are employed. The patient practises the dialysis procedure under supervision and learns to care for the equipment. Assessment of complications of fluid and electrolyte imbalance, infection and clotting of the vascular access are taught and actions to take when problems occur are discussed.

Following transplantation the patient has a life-long need for immunosuppressive drugs. Instruction includes the name, dosage, method of administration, action and side-effects of the medications. Sodium and fluid restrictions may be necessary with corticosteroid therapy.

Self-care measures.

- *Nutrition and fluid.* Basic nutrition and the role of proteins, carbohydrates, fats and fluids in the body are discussed. The patient's diet plan is reviewed and foods that contain protein of high caloric value which should be included are discussed and lists of foods that provide necessary calories without excessive protein, electrolytes and fluid are provided. The measurement and distribution of the required fluid intake over 24 hours are planned. The patient is instructed to record weight daily and to do this at the same time each day with the same amount of clothing.

  The dietitian helps the patient and family plan a meal schedule that includes foods the patient prefers, supplies recipes to allow for variety in meals and instructions on the preparation of foods. Reinforcement of compliance with dietary restrictions is provided by discussing and relating weight changes, the results of blood tests and blood pressure readings with the patient.
- *Medications.* The pharmacist or nurse provides instruction regarding medications. Participation in a self-administration of medications programme in hospital, provides opportunity for the patient to assume responsibility for his medication regimen, to adjust the schedule to his daily routine, and to begin to identify side-effects of the medications.
- *Monitoring of signs and symptoms of uraemia.* The patient is taught to identify signs of fluid overload and retention of nitrogenous wastes and to accurately measure and record weight, temperature and blood pressure as well as to understand the signficance of changes and what to do when they occur.
- *Use of resources.* The patient is introduced to the multidisciplinary team and is provided with information on who to call when specific needs arise. As the patient's knowledge and confidence increase, so too should the patient involvement in decision making. Referrals are made to nursing services in the community as necessary.

  Patients are taught the importance of interpreting their treatment plan to other health professionals, especially when travelling or on admission to hospital for reasons other than for the renal programme. Medic-Alert tags and bracelets may be worn and include identification of a vascular access or peritoneal catheter.

Necessary alterations to life-style. Helping the person adjust his or her life-style is an individual process. The teaching programme includes consideration of the following:

- *Work.* The person's treatment plan, chronic fatigue and lethargy may limit the ability to retain gainful employment. Liaison with the individual's employer and occupational health service, if available, or employment counselling may assist the person to continue working. Referral to the Employment Services Agency, particularly the local disablement resettlement officer, may prove useful to some individuals, particularly if currently unemployed.

- *Sexuality.* Counselling of the patient and partner helps them to understand the reasons for changes in sexual desire and expression. Many persons do not ask about the effects of renal disease on this aspect of their life-style. The nurse therefore needs to be sensitive to the couple's need to discuss this issue. Birth control information is necessary since pregnancy is possible, although there is a high likelihood of spontaneous abortion in the second trimester.

  Many couples affected by renal disease are able to have a satisfying sexual relationship by exploring alternative ways of expressing affection. The nurse should encourage the couple to participate in decision making and care and assist them to establish and maintain open communication, thereby fostering the solidarity of the emotional and sexual relationships.
- *Holidays.* The person and family are helped to plan holidays and are informed of resources available. These include portable machines which may be borrowed, a directory of renal units in other cities nationally and internationally, and trips and camping facilities available through the local or national Kidney Foundation.
- *Exercise.* The patient is helped to plan an activity schedule that includes moderate exercise and is taught that regular exercise improves circulation and appetite and promotes rest and a sense of well-being.
- *Social activities.* Alterations in social activities, such as eating and drinking, that are required by the treatment regimen need to be fully discussed. Support and encouragement from staff and families are needed for the person to initiate and increase social interaction.

KIDNEY TRANSPLANTATION

The development of donor selection by tissue typing and the steady progress that has been made in managing the rejection process, have resulted in an increase in the number of kidney transplants.

An advantage of a kidney transplant for the person who has severe renal failure is the discontinuance of the demanding dialysis schedule; considerable time is saved, and the individual's employment is uninterrupted and more productive. Dietary restrictions are lifted and constraint of activity is slight. The patient must be aware of the possible adverse effects as well as the benefits of transplantation prior to deciding on this mode of treatment. Some experience few complications and their quality of life is greatly improved. Others experience side-effects from the drugs used to control the rejection process and graft rejection. Transplantation requires major surgery and a life-long dependency on immunosuppressive drugs. Rejection of the transplant necessitates return to dialysis and consideration for retransplantation.

Transplant recipients

The patient and family should be informed of the available types of treatment of chronic renal failure and the risks and benefits of each, as well as the implications for their well-being and quality of life. Given such understanding, the person makes the final decision whether to have the transplant or not.

The criteria for the selection of transplant candidates have become more liberal in the past few years. Uncontrolled infection and malignancy are the only firm contraindications at present. Treatment of the malignancy followed by a year without recurrence and an absence of infection for several months would make the person for reconsideration as a candidate. The selection of candidates for kidney transplant is based on factors which will influence the outcome of the organ transplantation. These factors include: biological and physiological age, psychological status and the patient's primary disease process. If the renal failure is associated with diabetes mellitus, systemic lupus erythematosus, amyloidosis or scleroderma, the chances for success are decreased.

Immunological factors

The greatest hazard associated with any organ or tissue transplant from another person is the incompatibility of the recipient's tissue with that of the donor, and the ensuing rejection process. Secondary to this are the effects of the immunosuppressive drugs used to depress the rejection process; the most formidable is the recipient's increased susceptibility to infection.

The rejection process is an antigen-antibody reaction or immune response; the recipient's immune system recognizes the graft as a foreign substance, and specific antibodies and sensitized lymphocytes attack the foreign tissue.

The antigenicity and compatibility of the donor and recipient in tissue and organ transplants are determined by heredity. The antigens of concern, being determined by genes, are specific for each individual and are located on the surfaces of nucleated cells and red blood cells. Erythrocyte antigens compose the ABO antigen system used in blood typing and matching in blood transfusions, and may be present in vascular endothelium of the graft. Blood groups must be compatible in organ transplant.

The donor-recipient relationship is an important factor in influencing acceptance or rejection of a graft. The closer the relationship, the greater is the possibility of compatibility. Because cellular proteins and antigens are specific for each individual, donor tissue is rejected by the recipient's body unless it is taken from an identical twin. In this case, the transplant is compatible because the antigens of both the host and donor are identical, having been determined by the same genetic blue-print of a single fertilized ovum. Such a graft (with identical cellular proteins and antigens) is referred to as an *isograft*. A graft between two genetically dissimilar persons is known as an *allograft* or *homograft*.

The antigens located on the nucleated cells belong to the system designated HLA (human leucocyte antigen). These antigens, present on cell membranes of most tissues, are easily detected on leucocytes which are readily accessible for tissue typing and clinical tests for histocompatibility of potential donor tissue. Histocompatibility may be understood as the ability of cells to be accepted and to function in a new situation.

The HLA complex is located on the sixth chromosome in man. Four major HLA loci (A, B, C, D) have been identified in this region with each locus having multiple alleles. Although over 77 antigens have been identified, each person possesses two antigens for each locus, one inherited from each parent. Locus D antigens which are subdived into D and DR (D-related) are believed to be of particular significance in graft survival.

The principal methods used to determine the recipient's immunological response to potential donor tissue are: (1) tissue or HLA typing to identify the antigens at each HLA locus; (2) ABO blood-typing to identify compatability of red blood cells; (3) white blood cell cross-matching to detect the presence of preformed antibodies from previous exposure to an antigen; and (4) mixed lymphocyte culture to assess the degree of incompatibility between donor and recipient cells.

Tissue typing is the typing of antigens of the recipient and each potential donor. Antigens are identified by mixing lymphocytes with a series of standard sera which contain HLA antibodies. The reaction of the donor's and patient's cells to each serum is observed; lysis of the cells indicates that the antigen is specific to the known antibody. The patient's HLA typing is then compared to that of the donor.

ABO blood typing identifies the red blood cell antigens present in the recipient and donor. Antigens are identified when agglutination occurs on exposure of red blood cells to serum containing identified antibodies.

White blood cell cross-matching is performed by mixing blood from the recipient and donor and observing the reactions of the cells. Cell agglutination or lysis indicates a positive response; compatibility is indicated by a negative response.

The *mixed lymphocytes culture* involves making a culture of a mixture of the recipient's and potential donor's lymphocytes. The response of the recipient's lymphocytes to donor antigens is observed; reaction is demonstrated by the degree of change in the recipient lymphocytes in response to the other lymphocytes' antigens. The donor cells are treated before culturing to inhibit their response to the recipient's antigens. This test takes 5–7 days and can only be used with living donors.

Donor

In early transplants, the kidney was always obtained from a live blood relative. Now, cadavers serve as the principal donor source. The cadaver is frequently an accident victim or someone who has had a sudden death and who is known to have been in good health.

If a living donor is used, he or she is usually related to the patient. The donation is more likely to be successful if the relative is close (e.g. sibling, parent) than if the donor is a genetically non-related person (e.g. cousin, uncle by marriage).

Obviously, the living donor must be in good health. A thorough investigation is required and includes an intravenous urogram and a renal angiogram to ensure normal kidneys with a normal vascular supply. The donor must have volunteered willingly and made the decision without pressure from others. The decision is a major one; it requires a mature, stable person. The immunological and other investigations preceding the operation to remove the kidney, the nature of the surgery, the inherent risk in being left with one kidney and the possibility of rejection of the graft by the recipient are explained and discussed freely with the prospective donor. A consent form is signed for the removal of the kidney following the investigation period.

Immediate preoperative preparation and postoperative care of the donor is similar to that cited in the section on nursing in renal surgery. The function of the remaining kidney is monitored closely. Blood urea and serum creatinine levels are followed for 2–3 weeks to assess compensatory efficiency. The donor's psychological state should be carefully observed as realization of the risks involved may produce significant disturbance.

The demand for kidneys is much greater than the supply, and locally available kidneys may not be immunologically compatibile. An established central service or register is maintained; persons with end-stage renal failure are registered with their tissue and blood types. When a locally available kidney is not compatible, one that matches may become available in another part of the country and is obtained through the United Kingdom transplant centre based in Bristol. Because of the demand for kidney transplants, various educational programmes have been organized to alert the public to the need for donors.

Legal and ethical considerations include the need for donation consent and the determination of death. Organ donation cards, making a gift of any organ for the purpose of transplantation in the event of death can be completed and carried at all times. These cards are available from surgeries, most health care settings, and public buildings, and are sometimes displayed in shops and public houses. Nurses can play a significant role in encouraging the general public to participate in this programme. The next of kin may also provide written authorization for the donation of organs if death is imminent. Laws in most countries define brain death and policies are established to ensure independence of the doctors treating the donor patient from the transplant team. Most regions now have a transplant co-ordinator who is responsible for co-ordination of organ transfer. This person will often meet the potential donor, next of kin and ward staff and is responsible for feedback of information to them after the transplant. The co-ordinator also has a very important role in the education, not only of the medical and nursing staff, but also the general public to encourage greater referral of potential donors.

When death occurs, the kidneys are removed with their arteries, veins and ureters. The blood vessels are flushed out with an 'extracellular' electrolyte solution such as Ringer's lactate.

The organs are kept cool during transport and storage, until implantation. Transplantation should be done within 72 hours of obtaining the kidney from the

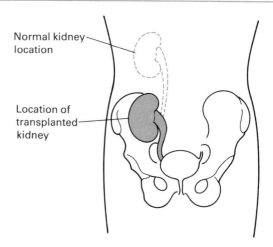

Figure 20.14 Location of transplanted kidney.

donor. Storage up to 2–3 days requires pump oxygenator perfusion. When a cadaver kidney is used in transplant, the source remains anonymous to the recipient and the family.

Transplant procedure

The donor kidney is placed in the recipient's iliac fossa, usually on the side opposite to that from which it was taken: that is, a left donor kidney is placed in the recipient's right iliac fossa. Its renal artery may be anastomosed to the host's hypogastric artery, and the renal vein of the graft is anastomosed to the common or external iliac vein (Figure 20.14). The ureter is implanted in the recipient's bladder via a submucosal tunnel; the latter prevents urinary reflux. A J-stent may be inserted into the transplanted kidney's ureter to prevent obstruction. It will normally be removed by cystoscopy after 3 months.

The patient's own kidneys are removed if there is recurrent infection or uncontrolled hypertension. Polycystic kidneys may need to be removed to provide room for the graft. Usually this will have been performed while the patient awaits transplantation.

In the case of a living donor, the removal of the kidney and the surgical implantation in the recipient are synchronized in adjacent operating theatres; this greatly reduces the period of ischaemia and the risk of tissue damage.

When a person is selected as a candidate for a renal transplant a full and detailed discussion with the surgeon is necessary. The patient and family are informed of what is entailed in the surgery: that the kidney graft may be rejected, necessitating the resumption of a maintenance haemodialysis programme; that continuous drug therapy and close supervision will be needed; and that precautions against infections will be necessary. The patient is encouraged to be as fit as possible whilst awaiting a transplant. This may involve taking calorie supplements to improve nutritional status.

During the period before the operation, the blood pressure, which is likely to be elevated, is monitored closely. If an antihypertensive drug is being administered, the nurse is alert for side effects and sharp pressure swings up or down. An accurate record is made of the fluid intake and output; the intake is regulated daily according to the output of the previous day to avoid overloading the cardiovascular system and promoting electrolyte imbalances. Efforts are made to improve the person's nutritional status and to meet caloric requirements.

Histocompatibility tests will have been completed prior to the scheduling of surgery. A detailed medical history and examination are done as well as a chest X-ray, electrocardiogram and other tests recommended as a result of the medical examination. Blood tests are extensive and include a full blood picture, serum electrolytes, creatinine, blood urea and blood coagulation determinations. Blood is cross-matched for the operation. If the serum potassium and creatinine and blood urea are elevated, the patient is dialysed prior to surgery.

If the patient's anaemia is severe, blood transfusions may be given. Controversy exists as to whether blood should be given; transfusions are believed to increase graft survival but may also cause pre-sensitization.

The patient's family's level of anxiety is assessed. The patient receiving a cadaver graft will have little notice prior to the actual surgery. Preparations must be made quickly but opportunity is provided for the person to review the decision and to ask questions and share feelings. A consent form will be completed.

Deep breathing and coughing are taught and practised and the patient is informed about what to expect postoperatively. If the person is known to have respiratory problems, baseline blood gases will be measured preoperatively. Immunosuppressive drug therapy is commenced preoperatively. The following drugs may be used in combination: azathioprine, prednisolone and cyclosporin. A central venous pressure line will be established under anaesthetic so the intravascular fluid volume can be monitored intra- and postoperatively. A retention (Foley) catheter is introduced into the bladder in the theatre under strict aseptic conditions for accurate monitoring of urine output.

Nursing intervention

The nursing care of the patient who has received a kidney transplant includes measures to maintain fluid balance, kidney function, prevention of infection and assessment for possible graft rejection and other complications. The immediate care is the same as that for any patient recovering from anaesthetic.

Assessment. Vital signs, urinary output, fluid intake and electrolyte concentrations are monitored, and frequent observations are made for bleeding from the wound and early signs of infection and rejection. A renal scan is performed the day following surgery to provide a baseline for graft function.

Maintenance of fluid balance and kidney function. The retention catheter is connected to a sterile closed-drainage system; the urinary output is recorded hourly.

Frequent urinalyses and cultures are made and 24-hour urine specimens may be obtained for measurement of creatinine clearance. Blood-stained urine may be expected at first but should progressively clear over a few days. Bleeding is due to the bladder incision made to implant the ureter in the bladder wall and the high vascularity of the bladder.

The transplanted kidney usually begins to excrete urine soon after the surgery. The volume may increase rapidly, resulting in profuse diuresis. Unless there is adequate replacement during this diuretic phase, dehydration, shock and electrolyte imbalance may develop. The patient may experience bladder spasm and pain with the large urine volume, because the bladder has not been used to receiving urine for some time preoperatively. If the transplant fails to excrete sufficient urine for several days, haemodialysis or peritoneal dialysis may be used until kidney function improves. If peritoneal dialysis is considered the surgeon must be consulted to ensure that the peritoneum was not damaged during the operation. Fluid and electrolyte restrictions are required until adequate urine volume is achieved. Once kidney function appears to be stabilized the hourly measurement can be discontinued. The catheter is removed, normally at about 4–5 days. The person is encouraged to void frequently to avoid overdistension of the bladder and pressure on the ureteral implantation area. If the patient's own kidneys have been retained, consideration must be given to their usual output when assessing the function of the graft kidney. The patient's weight is recorded daily and changes noted.

The central venous pressure is recorded at least hourly initially. A regime of fluid replacement is normally prescribed to maintain the central venous pressure as 0–5 cmH$_2$O measured at the sternal notch. This allows accurate assessment of fluid status and prevents dehydration or fluid overload. An increased intravascular volume places an increased demand on the pulmonary circulation, while dehydration may cause poor perfusion to the transplanted kidney and jeopardize its survival.

The fluid balance is determined every hour by comparing the total intake with total fluid loss and is assessed with other observations. The electrolyte composition of the intravenous fluids is based upon the laboratory reports.

Prevention of infection. The person is receiving immunosuppressive medications and is at greater risk of infection. The application of good asepsis is stressed; thorough handwashing is important before each contact with the patient. The patient is usually cared for in a transplant unit or area with consistent and specially prepared nursing staff. Extensive protective isolation techniques used in the past are no longer believed necessary.

Because the patient's immune system is suppressed, normal inflammatory responses to infection may not occur. The patient's skin and oral mucosa are examined frequently for redness, swelling, drainage, warmth and tenderness. The temperature is taken every 4 hours and the patient is asked to report any pain or discomfort.

The white blood cell count is monitored frequently and if severely depressed, protective measures may be instituted and immunosuppressive therapy decreased for a brief period.

The patient is required to carry out regular frequent periods of deep breathing and coughing and ambulation is encouraged. Recipients are treated prophylactically with antimicrobial agents (e.g. co-trimoxazole) to prevent opportunistic lung infections and pneumocystis. Early removal of central venous lines and the urethral catheter eliminates potential sources of infection and facilitates ambulation. Mouth care should be carried out regularly, particularly following meals. The use of a soft toothbrush will reduce trauma to gums. Oral mouthwashes with antifungal agents (e.g.nystatin) help prevent mucosal fungal colonization. These individuals are especially prone to this as a side-effect of steroid and antibiotic therapy.

Any invasive investigation must be covered with antibiotic treatment and any sign of infection investigated and broad-spectrum antibiotics given immediately. The appropriate antibiotic is identified quickly and given as the patient may develop septicaemia rapidly.

Rejection. The nurse must be constantly alert for early manifestations of the rejection process, which may occur as early as the second or third day. There may be swelling and increasing tenderness over the kidney, fever, general malaise, headache, an elevation in the leucocyte count, anorexia, decreased urinary output, hypertension, oedema and elevated levels of serum creatinine, sodium and potassium and blood urea.

The patient may become anxious at first and then appears gradually apathetic and lethargic. The kidney becomes swollen, oedematous and congested; thrombosis occurs in the renal blood vessels and tissue necrosis follows due to ischaemia.

The intensity of the rejection process and the rapidity with which it develops correspond to the degree of difference between the recipient's and donor's cellular antigens; the greater the difference, the more severe and rapid is the rejection. *Hyperacute rejection* occurs within minutes or hours of the transplant, due to preformed antibodies attacking the homograft. This severe type of reaction may be attributed to presentization to donor antigens as a result of previous transfusions or several pregnancies. Widespread intravascular coagulation occurs in the transplanted kidney, and failure develops.

Acute or early rejection may develop in the postoperative or convalescent period or it may occur 1–4 months following the transplantation. Oliguria and increasing blood urea and creatinine levels are manifested. Rejection can usually be reversed by increased dosage of immunosuppressive drugs.

Chronic or late rejection develops insidiously after 3 or 4 months, or it may occur several years after the homograft was received. This type of rejection is characterized by arterial impairment due to intimal hyperplasia. It is attributed to chronic reaction between circulating antibodies and the antigens of the vascular endothelial cells. This process cannot be reversed with medication.

Prevention of rejection

The administration of immunosuppressive drugs is resumed in the immediate postoperative period and continued. These drugs depress the body's responses to the donor kidney's antigens. The drugs which may be used are azathioprine (Imuran) and a corticosteroid preparation (prednisolone) (Table 20.6) but cyclosporin A is currently the preferred immunosuppressive drug and is used with lower doses of steroids. Antilymphocytic globulin (ALG) may be given intravenously as an infusion in a progressively decreasing daily dose for 10 days if rejection is suspected.

The dosage of azathioprine and prednisolone are adjusted according to the leucocyte count and the patient's reactions to these drugs. It is necessary for the nurse to be familiar with their side-effects. Azathioprine may depress the bone marrow production of leucocytes and produce leucopenia. Reactions to prolonged administration of prednisolone may include the retention of sodium and water, an elevation of blood pressure, hirsutism, development of a round puffy face ('moon face'), euphoria, gastrointestinal ulceration, impaired liver and pancreatic function, and arrested growth in a child.

Cyclosporin A is severely nephrotoxic and so blood levels are closely monitored. It may also produce hepatic impairment and lymphomas. Patients often become hirsute and have tremors, especially in the early stages. This tends to disappear as the dosage is reduced. Since ALG is a serum, one must be alert for an anaphylactic reaction; an intracutaneous sensitivity test is done before the initial dose.

The signs and symptoms of rejection are cited above. When rejection is suspected the patient is given higher doses of prednisone; it may be given intravenously as well as orally. Plasma exchange may be carried out to remove antibodies and immune complexes and thus reduce the rejection response. This will depend on the patient's original disease. If the reaction is severe and there is marked fluid retention and the elevation of serum potassium and creatinine and blood urea, dialysis may have to be resumed. Fluid intake and dietary restrictions may also be necessary.

If the rejection process is irreversible, the immunosuppressive drugs are discontinued and the graft may be removed. The patient may well become discouraged and the nurse should be prepared to offer support and reassure the patient that a second graft may be considered.

Other medications. Since most medications are eliminated through the kidneys, as few drugs as possible are given following a renal transplantation. Small doses of an analgesic may be prescribed, if necessary, for the relief of pain and discomfort when nursing measures do not provide adequate palliation.

Patient education for health management

The patient may become apprehensive about leaving the hospital and becoming independent. The need to follow a prescribed pattern of living indefinitely and be con-

Table 20.6 Immunosuppressive drugs.

Drug	Dosage	Action	Side-effects
Azathioprine (Imuran)	2–3 mg per kg body weight per day orally. Regulated by leucocyte count	Inhibits the synthesis of nucleic acids in cell production. Depresses the production of leucocytes (especially lymphocytes) and antibodies	Bone marrow depression; mouth ulcers; alopecia; and, rarely, hepatitis
Adrenocorticosteroid (e.g. prednisone, oral; methyl prednisolone, intravenous)	0.2–0.4 mg per kg body weight per day, orally. Rejection normally treated with 1 g intravenously for 3 days	Suppresses the inflammatory response. Suppresses lymphocyte and antibody formation	Lowered resistance to infection; gastrointestinal ulceration; bleeding; oedema and hypertension due to sodium retention; mood swings; weight gain; moon face and cataracts
Antilymphoctye globulin (ALG) and Antilymphocyte serum (ALS)	20–60 mg per kg body weight per day, 10 daily doses intravenously as an infusion. Dose decreases over the 10 day period. May be given prophylactically to patients with known antibodies to prevent rejection	Suppresses lymphocyte action	Anaphylaxis (patient requires very close observation); Alopecia; bone marrow suppression and haemorrhagic cystitis
Antithymocyte globulin (ATC)	Given intravenously as an infusion 2 mg per kg per day. Daily for 10 days. May be given prophylactically to patients with antibodies.	Suppresses thymocyte action	Anaphylaxis; alopecia; bone marrow suppression and haemorrhagic cystitis
Cyclophosphamide (Endoxana)	1–5 mg per kg body weight, oral or intravenously (rarely used)	Suppresses cell reproduction	Bone marrow depression; alopecia and haemorrhagic cystitis
Cyclosporin	5–16 µg per kg body weight orally or intravenously regulated by blood levels	Depresses humoral and cellular immunity	Nephrotoxicity, hepatic impairment, lymphomas, hirsutism and tremors

stantly alert for early signs of rejection and complications may provoke considerable anxiety. Consequently a good teaching programme for both patient and family is essential.

A social worker can be of considerable assistance to the patient and family in planning for the future. The social worker may provide assistance in finding suitable employment or, if work is not possible, may help in obtaining financial assistance. Suitable forms of recreation and sports should also be discussed.

The patient should fully understand the drug regimen that will be required after discharge. It is helpful if a sample of each is attached to a card on which the name of the drug, its strength, and directions for taking are clearly printed. The nurse stresses the importance of these drugs, and that if they cannot be taken or retained because of illness, the person must contact a general practitioner or the renal unit promptly. The cards are taken to the outpatient clinic or the general practitioner when visits are made so that if the dosage is changed the directions on the cards may be changed.

The person is instructed to keep a daily record of weight, fluid output and medications taken. Verbal and written explanations are made of the content and preparation of the diet. Since the prednisolone may increase appetite and promote sodium retention, the person is advised to guard against exceeding his or her normal weight. Dietary restrictions are few and are individualized. Sodium intake may be restricted, and as cyclosporin may cause acidosis and hyperkalaemia in some patients, especially in the early days, potassium intake may need to be restricted.

Suggestions are made as to how infections may be prevented. Close contact with persons with a cold or other types of infections should be avoided. Good hygienic practices in food handling and the frequent washing of the hands are stressed. Good personal hygiene is essential.

The early signs of rejection are reviewed with the patient and family. By this time the patient is usually quite familiar with them and realizes that prompt action is necessary. The patient and family are cautioned to report immediately a cold, sore throat, fever, dysuria, frequency or other disturbances which may indicate infection. The patient is also urged to contact the unit promptly if there is a sudden gain in weight (for example, 1kg in a day), swelling of the ankles or puffiness of the face, pain, tenderness and/or swelling in the area of the graft, decrease in urinary output, headache, unaccounted for fatigue, or elevation in temperature.

Following discharge, the patient is followed closely by visits to the outpatient department at least once a week, since constant surveillance plays an important role in progress and the development of acceptance of the situation with less fear. If progress is satisfactory, and understanding and efficient management of care are demonstrated, the intervals between visits are gradually lengthened. The patient and family may appreciate information regarding self-help organizations such as British Kidney Patient Association.

Complications

In addition to infection and the rejection process, complications which may develop in the recipient after a kidney transplantation include the following:

Tubular necrosis. This is attributed to the ischaemia of the kidney during the period between its removal and grafting. It is manifested by oliguria and the effects of the retained metabolic wastes and excess fluid.

Gastrointestinal ulceration and bleeding. These may be caused by the corticosteroid preparation which the patient receives to suppress the immune response to the graft. Any vomitus or faeces containing blood is reported to the doctor. An H_2 antagonist (cimetidine or ranitidine) may be prescribed as prophylaxis. Dyspepsia is investigated promptly by endoscopy to detect erosions.

Cataracts. These are also a side-effect of the prednisolone. Patients are advised to have their eyes examined annually.

Urinary fistula. This may be due to failure of healing of the ureter at the site of anastomosis with the bladder.

Lack of wound healing. This may be caused by the steroid medication or urine leakage.

Bone marrow depression. This is due to the immunosuppressive drugs. Leucopenia develops, which predisposes the individual to serious infections; erythrocyte production is depressed, and the signs and symptoms of anaemia develop; normal coagulation may be impaired when the platelets are decreased, and bleeding from mucous membranes, petechiae and ecchymoses may become evident.

Other Disorders of Renal Function

GLOMERULONEPHRITIS

This disease is usually characterized by a diffuse, non-infectious inflammation of the glomeruli of both kidneys. Since the blood supply that supports the tubules normally passes through glomerular capillaries before reaching them, fibrous scarring and obliteration of some glomeruli lead to secondary degenerative changes in the associated tubules, blood vessels and interstitial tissues. Glomerulonephritis is more common in children and young adults and has a higher incidence in males. It may be acute or chronic.

CAUSES

The glomerular injury is usually caused by immunological processes. Three major immunological mechanisms are recognized. In one, antigen–antibody complexes formed extrarenally are trapped in glomeruli and initiate the inflammatory process; this is a common reaction responsible for glomerulonephritis. The second immune reaction involves antibodies that are formed against an antigen in or produced by the glomerular basement membrane, initiating glomerular inflammmation. The third mechanism involves activation of the alternate complement pathway.

A common cause of glomerulonephritis is the β-haemolytic streptococcus (group A, types 12, 4 and 1). The patient's history usually reveals that the renal disturbance follows an infection, such as a sore throat or respiratory infection of some form, by a latent period of 2–4 weeks. In some instances, the infection may have been so mild that little or no attention was given to it at the time. Post streptococcal glomerulonephritis is produced by immunological processes probably involving one or more of the above causative mechanisms.

Glomerulonephritis may also be associated with other diseases such as systemic lupus erythematosus, polyarteritis nodosa, scleroderma, diabetes mellitus, amyloidosis and bacterial endocarditis.

CLINICAL CHARACTERISTICS

The onset is generally abrupt but in some instances may be insidious. The affected glomeruli are partially or completely obstructed, resulting in reduced filtration. Some glomeruli rupture, permitting the escape of blood into the tubules. The permeability of the glomeruli that remain patent is increased. The scant output of urine is cloudy and contains albumin, blood cells and casts.

Oedema develops and is usually seen first in the periorbital areas and ankles. The patient complains of pain and tenderness in the back, headache, and weakness. Visual disturbances may also be manifested. The blood pressure is elevated, and decreased filtration results in a gradual accumulation of nitrogenous wastes in the blood; the blood urea and serum creatinine levels may be elevated.

Nasal and throat swabs may be taken to determine if streptococci are still present. Examination of the blood may reveal an elevation in antistreptolysin O titre (ASO titre).

Neurological signs and symptoms corresponding to the degree of hypertension may be present (see Chapter 21). Unless the renal insufficiency is reversed, uraemia, pulmonary oedema and cardiac failure may ensue.

MANAGEMENT

The treatment of patients with acute glomerulonephritis consists mainly of rest, fluid and diet regulation, and chemotherapy to eliminate possible residual streptococcal infection. The daily fluid intake is restricted to 400–500 ml in excess of the urinary output of the previous 24 hours. The blood chemistry is followed closely and the sodium, potassium, and chloride intake regulated according to the findings. The patient receives a high carbohydrate diet to reduce the breakdown of tissue protein. Protein may be provided in the form of essential amino acid or keto analogues to achieve nitrogen balance. Similarly, salt restriction in the diet is regulated according to the degree of oedema and hypertension.

If the low output of urine is prolonged and the blood potassium and nitrogenous waste levels are progressively increasing, diuretic therapy is initiated or peritoneal dialysis or haemodialysis may be instituted (see pp 638–644).

Plasma exchange may be carried out to remove antibodies and immune complexes since the disorder is usually caused by immunological processes. Precautions are necessary to protect the patient from exposure to infection. A superimposed infection could aggravate the disease or cause pneumonia that could prove fatal.

The frequent association of glomerulonephritis with respiratory infections emphasizes their potential danger and the importance of prevention and prompt, adequate treatment of such infections. Too often they are ignored, considered as unavoidably seasonal and treated very lightly. Women who have a history of acute glomerulonephritis are advised to consult a doctor before planning a pregnancy, since they are more likely to develop toxaemia and eclampsia.

According to the literature, the majority of patients with acute glomerulonephritis associated with infection (e.g. streptococcal) recover with no residual kidney disease. These patients generally show an increase in the volume of urine and a decrease in the blood pressure and serum urea levels within 1 week. The albuminuria and microscopic haematuria may persist for much longer. A few patients progress through a subacute phase to chronic glomerulonephritis. Others may be asymptomatic for a period of months or years and then experience an insidious development of the chronic disease which may progress to chronic renal failure.

PYELONEPHRITIS

This is an inflammation of the pelvis and parenchymal tissue of the kidney due to infection. The predominant causative organisms are the gram-negative enteric bacilli which have invaded the lower urinary tract and ascended to the kidney via the ureters. In rare instances,

the pathogen, such as the staphylococcus or streptococcus, may be bloodborne.

Significant predisposing factors are defective urinary drainage and reflux of urine from the bladder into the ureters. Obstructions to the flow of urine from the kidney may be the result of a renal calculus, neoplasm, stricture of a ureter due to pressure, scarring or congenital anomaly. Stasis of urine in the lower urinary tract due to bladder or urethral dysfunction may increase the intravesical pressure sufficiently to produce a reflux into the ureters.

Pyelonephritis is more common in females than males. The incidence is relatively high in female infants and children, due perhaps to faecal soiling and *Escherichia coli* contamination of the urethral meatus. Its frequent occurrence in pregnant women is attributed to stasis of urine incurred by pressure from the enlarging uterus and atonia of the ureters due to the effect of progesterone. It may also occur following urethral catheterization; infection introduced into the bladder may ascend through the ureters to the kidney. Pyelonephritis in males in the later years of life is generally associated with defective urinary drainage as a result of an enlarged prostrate.

CLINICAL CHARACTERISTICS

The onset is usually sudden. In children it may be accompanied by a convulsion. Manifestations include chills, fever, headache, nausea and vomiting, pain and tenderness in the loins, leucocytosis, and frequent and painful micturition (dysuria). The urine is cloudy and contains bacteria, pus, blood and epithelial cells.

TREATMENT

The patient is encouraged to take liberal amounts of fluid unless there is complete obstruction of urinary drainage. An accurate record of the fluid intake and output is necessary. A culture will be made of the urine and the causative organism antibiotic sensitivity determined. Antibiotic therapy is prescribed. If nitrofurantoin (Furadantin) or a sulphonamide preparation is used, the patient is observed for possible reactions which usually appear in the form of nausea and vomiting and a skin rash.

Unless there is complete eradication of the infection, pyelonephritis may become chronic with insidious destruction of nephrons, leading to chronic renal failure and uraemia. Following the initial episode of acute pyelonephritis, the patient generally undergoes a thorough investigation for a predisposing obstructive lesion. Antimicrobial therapy and a high fluid intake are needed beyond the disappearance of acute signs and symptoms in order to ensure complete eradication of the infective organism. Specimens of urine are examined and cultured at regular intervals after the antimicrobial drug is discontinued.

TUBERCULOSIS OF THE KIDNEY

Tubercular infection in the kidney is usually secondary to tuberculosis elsewhere in the body; most often the primary site is a lung or lymph node. The tubercle bacilli are carried by the blood to the kidneys. Scattered characteristic granulomatous lesions (tubercles) develop, eroding renal tissue and leaving cavitations. The infection may involve pyramids and calyces, interfering with tubular drainage and leading to hydronephrosis. The infection may spread to involve the bladder.

The systemic symptoms characteristic of any tubercular infection are usually present: low-grade fever, night sweats, loss of weight, fatigue and a positive tuberculin skin test. The urine contains pus and blood; smears and a culture reveal the presence of tubercle bacilli. The patient complains of back pain, which may become quite severe in advanced disease. An intravenous urogram is done to determine whether the disease is unilateral or bilateral.

The patient receives a prolonged, intensive course of antituberculous drugs and should be observed for possible reactions to the drugs which may take the form of dermatitis, fever, dizziness and impaired hearing. A nutritious full diet is encouraged without restrictions if there is adequate renal function to prevent oedema, hypertension and the accumulation of wastes in the blood. Frequent urine smears and cultures are made to determine the progress of the patient's disease. Treatment is continued for a period of 12–18 months even if the cultures become negative for tubercle bacilli.

THE NEPHROTIC SYNDROME (NEPHROSIS)

The characteristic symptoms of the nephrotic syndrome are proteinuria (greater than 3.5 g of protein in 24 hours), hypoproteinaemia, generalized oedema and usually hyperlipidaemia. It may develop in a patient with primary renal disease, or it may be associated with other conditions in which kidney involvement is secondary. Systemic disorders (e.g. diabetes mellitus, systemic lupus erythematosus and amyloidosis), circulatory disturbances and infections are some of the causes.

The proteinuria, which is chiefly albumin, is the result of some change in the glomeruli that causes an increase in their permeability to the plasma proteins. Obviously, the loss of the proteins reduces the colloidal osmotic pressure of the blood, contributing to increased movement of fluid into the interstitial spaces as well as to its decreased reabsorption into the capillaries. The resulting decrease in intravascular volume leads to retention of sodium and water by the kidneys. The excessive concentration of serum lipids, which is determined by estimation of the cholesterol level, is not understood.

The urine is reduced in volume and usually contains casts as well as large amounts of albumin. In contrast with other forms of impaired renal function, the blood pressure and nitrogenous waste levels of patients usually remain within a normal range in the absence of advanced damage to glomeruli.

The severity of the nephrotic syndrome is variable. In some, the oedema may cause only slight puffiness in the periorbital areas and ankles, yet in others it may be so extreme that ascites (accumulation of fluid in the peritoneal cavity) and pleural effusion develop. The oedematous areas are generally soft and readily pit on pressure. The patient is usually pale, may be breathless,

complains of fatigue and may experience anorexia, which further complicates the problem of hypoproteinaemia. Susceptibility to infection increases and the incidence of venous thrombosis is greater as anticoagulant substances are lost in the urine. The onset may be insidious or abrupt.

TREATMENT

When the nephrotic syndrome is secondary, the treatment is directed toward inducing diuresis, reducing oedema, producing and maintaining a normal serum albumin level and reducing the lipid level in the blood.

The patient receives a low-sodium, high-protein full diet. The recommended daily protein is usually 1 g per kg of body weight plus an amount equivalent to the daily loss in urine. This implies that 24-hour collections of urine are made for estimation of the amount of protein excreted. Intravenous infusions of plasma or albumin may be given and infection is treated promptly with an antibiotic when it occurs. The patient may require anticoagulation with subcutaneous or intravenous heparin to cover the acute period.

The patient is particularly susceptible to infection because of the lowered resistance of oedematous tissues and reduced plasma gammaglobulin which is essential in the formation of antibodies. Precautions are necessary to avoid exposure to infection.

An adrenocorticosteroid preparation such as prednisone may be prescribed. It is usually given for a period of 3–4 weeks, with the dosage gradually being reduced until the minimum maintenance level is reached. It is then continued in that dosage. Immunosuppressive drugs such as azathioprine or cyclophosphamide may be given in combination with corticosteroid preparations to induce a remission when nephrosis is due to underlying autoimmune disease.

A diuretic such as frusemide may be used in some instances if there is not a satisfactory response to the corticoid preparation and a reduction of the oedema.

The patient is not usually hospitalized after a satisfactory therapeutic regimen is established, nor confined to bed; activity is encouraged. Treatment is generally required over a long period, and frequent medical check-ups are necessary.

NEPHROLITHIASIS (RENAL CALCULI)

Stones or small concretions may develop in the collecting tubules, calyces or the pelvis of a kidney. They are formed by the precipitation of various substances in the urine; if retained, the initial precipitation forms a nucleus or matrix which promotes further precipitation and calculus enlargement. The substances commonly involved in calculus formation are calcium, oxalate, phosphate, uric acid, cystine, xanthine and ammonia, but most often the stones are of mixed composition (e.g. mixed phosphates and oxalates). They vary in size from tiny particles to large smooth or irregular masses. The irregular stone that forms in the pelvis and has projections into the calyces is referred to as a *staghorn calculus*. The usual composition of the latter type of calculus is phosphate.

CAUSES

The constituents of renal calculi are present in normal urine; any condition which increases their concentration, reduces their solubility or promotes retention of the urinary salts, favours their precipitation, calculus formation and possible obstruction to urinary flow. Conditions favourable to their formation include hypercalcaemia, as occurs with hyperparathyroidism, excessive vitamin D, an excessive ingestion of milk or an alkali and prolonged immobilization. Other causes are hyperuricaemia associated with gout (an error in uric acid metabolism), cystinuria, resulting from a genetic metabolic disorder in which cystine and other amino acids are excreted in excess by the kidneys, dehydration, a highly acid urine and infection by *Proteus* (Gram-negative bacteria usually associated with faeces). *Proteus* infection changes the urine to alkaline; this results in the precipitation of phosphates, forming what may be referred to as a struvite calculus.

SYMPTOMS

The manifestations of renal calculus depend upon the size of the stone and whether it remains stationary. It may remain latent over a long period, producing no symptoms. Small, gravel-like stones may be passed without any disturbance.

The majority cause some pain, haematuria, infection and, if large, kidney damage and renal insufficiency. Renal calculi may obstruct renal drainage by impaction of the tubules, by completely filling calyces and the pelvis, or by lodging in a ureter. The urine accumulates in the pelvis and tubules, dilating them and creating a back pressure; this condition is known as *hydronephrosis*. Compression of the blood vessels and nephrons by the mass of fluid leads to their destruction and obliteration and to renal insufficiency.

The patient may complain of pain in the back which may be caused by irritation of tissues by movement of the stone or the back pressure and accumulation of fluid if the stone is obstructing renal or ureteral outflow. A small stone may enter the ureter and initiate *ureteric colic*. The patient complains of excruciating pain radiating from the back to the front along the groin into the genitalia; this may be associated with pallor, sweating, restlessness and vomiting.

Haematuria results from injury to the membranous lining of the pelvis or ureter. Infection is frequently associated with a calculus and, if present, chills, fever, leucocytosis and pyuria are likely to be manifested.

Complete obstruction of the kidney outflow is eventually reflected in renal insufficiency and a palpable mass in the renal area as a result of the hydronephrosis. The total volume of urine is less than normal, and blood investigations indicate reduced elimination of waste products.

Investigation of the patient for nephrolithiasis includes: midstream specimen of urine for culture and sensitivity, abdominal X-ray, intravenous urography or pyelography, and sometimes cystoscopy with retrograde pyelography. Serum calcium and uric acid levels are determined and renal function tests may be done (for the latter, see p. 625). Investigation includes examination of the urine for crystals, 24- or 48-hour serial pH analysis in which the pH of each voiding is recorded, and 24-hour urine studies for calcium, phosphorus, uric acid, creatinine and sodium oxalate.

TREATMENT AND NURSING INTERVENTION

If the urogram indicates that the calculus is small and may be passed by the patient, activity and large amounts of fluids are encouraged. All urine is strained through several layers of gauze or a filter paper and is observed. All sediment or solid particles passed are saved and submitted for identification of their composition.

During an attack of ureteric colic, the patient usually receives an analgesic, such as pethidine, to relieve the pain, and an antiemetic. When the pain subsides fluids should be encouraged once nausea is no longer a problem.

If the calculus is in the lower third of the ureter, a special ureteric catheter with a looped or corkscrew tip may be passed and an attempt made to withdraw the stone. This procedure is referred to as 'removal by instrumentation'.

When a stone in the kidney or ureter is too large to be passed, open surgery may be undertaken. Removal of a stone through the renal parenchyma is called a *nephrolithotomy*. Removal of a stone directly from the renal pelvis is known as a *pyelolithotomy*. The operation for extracting a stone from the ureter is a *ureterolithotomy*. If the calculus is in the lower part of the ureter, it is approached through an abdominal incision. When it is lodged in the upper part of the ureter, the approach is through an incision in the flank. Some stones in the renal collecting system are amenable to percutaneous extraction under radiological guidance.

More recently, renal calculi have been treated by lithotripsy (extracorporeal shock-wave lithotripsy, ESWL). After placing the patient in a special tank of water, shock waves are propelled by a machine, the lithotripser, directly at the stone(s) to cause it to disintegrate. The patient is then required to ingest a large quantity of fluid for several days to wash out the stone particles. Renal colic may be experienced intermittently for several days while the stone fragments are passed.

Calculi are prone to recur in patients with a history of previous episodes. In an effort to prevent the formation of new stones or the enlargement of existing stones, the pH of the urine is controlled according to the type of stone involved by a special diet and medication, and measures are used to eliminate any known or suspected infection. For the latter, an antibiotic or sulphonamide preparation is prescribed.

The patient is advised that a high fluid intake of at least 3000 ml daily is essential to maintain a dilute urine. A portion of this should be taken at bedtime and during the night to prevent the concentration of urine that normally occurs at night. If the climate or patient's occupation are such that there is an excessive loss of fluid in sweat, the intake should be increased by 1000 ml.

If the principal calculus component is calcium the prescribed diet is low in calcium and vitamin D. If the stone is of calcium phosphate, acidification of the urine with three to four glasses of cranberry juice daily is recommended. If uric acid is involved, alkalinization of the urine is important. Solubility is promoted by the administration of sodium bicarbonate or a citrate mixture. The pH of the urine is monitored and an effort made to maintain it at a level above 6.5. Allopurinol is prescribed to lower the serum uric acid level.

The formation of cystine stones is usually seen in children. Alkalinization of the urine and a diet low in methionine are recommended. For details as to the foods which are high and low in the different substances involved in calculus formation, the reader is referred to a diet therapy or urology text. A problem in relation to dietary restriction is that most stones are of mixed composition.

If the patient should become ill, prolonged immobility should be avoided as the effects of immobility on calcium metabolism increase the probability of stone formation.

NEOPLASMS IN THE KIDNEYS

Neoplasms in the adult kidney are of lower incidence than those in many other areas of the body. When they occur, they are usually malignant and are seen more often in males than in females. Tumours may arise in parenchyma or the collecting system of the kidney. The most common form of parenchymal tumours in adults is adenocarcinoma (also called Grawitz, hypernephroma or renal cell carcinoma). It readily invades the blood vessels, causing early metastases to bones, lungs or liver, which may be the lesion that brings the person to the doctor. Wilms' tumour is a highly malignant adenosarcoma which occurs in young children and may grow very large before being discovered. Tumours that arise in the renal pelvis and ureter are the same histologially as bladder cancers; 85% are transitional cell in origin, the remainder being squamous cell or adenocarcinoma-type cancers. Tumours of the renal pelvis and ureter are ten times less common than those developing in the bladder.

CLINICAL CHARACTERISTICS

In the adult, the first symptom is usually haematuria. As the neoplasm enlarges, the kidney becomes a palpable mass and the patient experiences pain, abdominal discomfort from pressure, anorexia and loss of weight. Ureteric colic may occur as a result of a blood clot entering the ureter. Polycythaemia develops in some patients due to an overproduction of erythropoietin by the affected kidney. Others may have marked anaemia. In children, the neoplasm is frequently noted first as an abdominal mass or swelling by the mother.

A cystoscopy with ureteric catheterization is done to determine if the source of the bleeding is unilateral or bilateral. Radiological studies are made, using an intravenous or retrograde pyelogram to determine filling defects and the location of the neoplasm. A renal angiogram may also be done to assess the extent of blood vessel involvement. Renal ultrasound may be performed to assess the nature of the lesion and allow visualization of the lesion to facilitate aspiration.

TREATMENT

Nephrectomy is the usual treatment for parenchymal tumours; treatment may also involve local lymph node dissection. Embolization of the kidney may be used to prevent or relieve symptoms of metastatic disease when nephrectomy is not performed. Radiotherapy may be used but its effectiveness with these tumours is debatable, except for prophylaxis of metastatic symptoms. Chemotherapy, immunotherapy, hormone manipulation and the use of interferon are currently being investigated to determine their value in treating these cancers.

POLYCYSTIC DISEASE OF THE KIDNEYS

This disorder is characterized by the widespread distribution of cysts of varying sizes throughout both kidneys. The disease is congenital and familial and affects both sexes. It is predominant in infants and adults over 40 years of age. In infants and young children, other abnormalities may be present. The disease is often found in more than one member of the family and in successive generations. Because of the distinct difference in the age of the groups in which the disease is manifested, it is suggested that there are two different genetic types. When it occurs in infants and young children, it is considered to be autosomal recessive, but the polycystic disease which becomes manifest in adults is autosomal dominant.

THE PERSON WITH DISORDERS OF THE URINARY SYSTEM

CLINICAL CHARACTERISTICS OF POSTRENAL/ URINARY DISORDERS

Clinical characteristics of impaired bladder function and urinary elimination include abnormal constituents in the urine and altered patterns of urinary elimination (functional, reflex, stress, total and urge incontinence, and urinary retention). Alterations in voiding may be related to infection in the urinary tract, emotional stress, a neurological disorder, bladder calculi, obstructive disease of the bladder or urethra and rarely, chemicals excreted in the urine.

Abnormal constituents in urine

Blood, pus, micro-organisms and mucus may be present in the urine as a result of inflammation, tissue necrosis or a malignancy in the lower urinary tract. The urine may be cloudy or blood-coloured and have an ammoniacal odour.

Alteration in patterns of urinary elimination

Symptomatic changes in voiding include *frequency, urgency, dysuria, residual urine, alterations in the urinary stream, retention* and *incontinence.*

Frequency, urgency and dysuria. Irritation of the bladder or urethral mucosa may give rise to an abnormally frequent desire to void, urgency and painful micturition. Frequency due to a urological disturbance is generally accompanied by an *urgency* which implies that there is an intense desire to void immediately. The normally voluntary control to retain the urine cannot be maintained, and some urine may escape before the person can reach the toilet or use a bedpan. *Dysuria* refers to the abnormal discomfort, pain, burning or smarting sensation that may accompany voiding. *Strangury* is a term used occasionally when the dysuria is unusually severe and there is increasing frequency of decreasing amounts of urine.

Residual urine. Micturition may not completely empty the bladder, leaving a residue of urine. This problem is diagnosed, and the amount determined, by catheterizing the patient immediately after voiding. Residual urine is usually the result of an obstruction to the bladder outlet and causes a stagnation that predisposes to bladder and kidney infection and calculus formation.

Alterations in the urinary stream. The person may have difficulty in initiating the urinary flow. This symptom of hesitancy is usually due to some obstruction in the bladder–urethral orifice or the urethra. Pressure within the bladder must be increased beyond the normal to force the urine past the obstructing lesion. Because of resistance to the urinary outflow, the muscle tires before the bladder is empty; after a few moments, it contracts again and voiding is resumed.

Retention of urine. The inability of a person to void is a relatively common problem. The distension of the bladder and stasis of urine predispose to the development of ureteric back pressure, reflux of urine into the ureters, and infection of the bladder and kidneys. The reaction of the bladder to progressive obstruction of the outflow is hypertrophy of the detrusor muscle. Diverticulae may develop; these are saccular protusions of the mucosa between the muscle fibres. The sacs fill with urine which becomes stagnant and readily infected. Calculi may also form within the diverticula.

Retention of urine is suspected if the person has had a normal fluid intake and has not voided within a period of 8–10 hours or if there is a distension of the lower part of the abdomen. A distended bladder may also be present with frequent voiding of small amounts (30–50 ml), which is termed *retention with overflow.* The person may experience a constant desire to void but efforts to do so are ineffective.

URINARY INCONTINENCE

This is an embarrassing, isolating and debilitating problem. It is estimated that over 3 million people in the UK suffer from incontinence. It is not a problem only effecting the elderly. Approximately 1 million adults between 15 and 65, and half a million children cope with incontinence. Incontinence probably goes untreated or unassessed because of associations with sexuality and social interaction and can exert severe stress both on the individual, partner and carers. Urinary incontinence presents a real challenge to nurses to assist in improving the quality of life of a significant number of the population.

The classification of types of urinary incontinence can be confusing. The following is one classification system (North American Nursing Diagnosis Association, 1989) and will be used in this text:

- *Stress incontinence* is the state in which an individual experiences a loss of urine (less than 50 ml) which occurs with increased abdominal pressure.
- *Reflex incontinence* is the state in which an individual experiences involuntary loss of urine at somewhat predictable intervals when a specific bladder volume is reached.
- *Urge incontinence* is the state in which an individual experiences involuntary passage of urine occuring soon after a strong sense of urgency to void.
- *Functional incontinence* is the state in which an individual experiences an involuntary, unpredictable passage of urine.
- *Total incontinence* is the state in which an individual experiences a continuous and unpredictable loss of urine.

Other terms used to describe characteristics of urinary incontinence include:

- *Overflow incontinence* which occurs with retention and is characterized by the voiding of small amounts (25–50 ml) of urine at frequent intervals.
- *Enuresis* usually implies nocturnal urinary incontinence or bed-wetting. It most often occurs in children but may continue into adulthood in a few instances.
- *Dribbling* or continuous urinary incontinence in conscious, alert persons usually results from damage to or degeneration of the urethral sphincter. Unawareness of dribbling is usually associated with a neurological condition.
- *Postmicturition dribbling* causes soiling of clothing which is embarrassing for the person and those around him. It is more common in men of all age groups and may develop following urinary infection, an invasive procedure of the urinary tract or prostatectomy.

The Person with Urinary Incontinence

Urinary incontinence is a major health problem. Studies (Thomas et al, 1980; Egan et al, 1983) have shown that incontinence is not just a problem of the elderly, although its prevalence increases with age. Incontinence brings with it many hardships, not only is there the cost, but also the effort involved in maintaining hygiene and containing the problem, together with the emotional

Table 20.7 Comparison of characteristics of five types of incontinence.

Characteristic	Functional	Stress	Reflex	Urge	Total
Character of voiding urge	Usually strong	Sudden and associated with increased abdominal pressure	None	Very strong	None
Amount voided	Moderate to large	Small	Moderate	Small, moderate to large	Constant leakage
Nocturia	May be present	Possible, not usual	Always	Common	Always
Precipitating factors	Inability to reach receptacle	Increased intra-abdominal pressure	Full bladder, uninhibited bladder contraction/spasm	Sensation of full bladder, inability to reach toilet on time	Unpredicatable
Awareness of incontinence	Aware	Aware	Unaware	Aware	Unaware
Frequency of urination	Variable	Increased	Regular intervals related to volume	Increased	Unpredictable and constant
Anatomical problem	Not urinary, but sensory, cognitive, mobility, or environmental defects	Increased urethrovesicular angle, sagging support structures, weak sphincter tone	Nerve pathway problems	Stretch receptor changes, reduced bladder capacity, detrusor over-activity	Sensorimotor nerve damage, no neurone control, fistulas
Related factors/ causes	Altered environ-ment, sensory deficits, mobility, deficits, drug use, stool impaction, closed head injury, emotional illness	Obesity, gravid uterus, increased age, incompetent bladder outlet, weak pelvic muscles, over-distension between voiding, jolting exercise (for instance jogging)	Spinal cord injury, multiple sclerosis, spinal cord tumours, spondylosis, cerebral lesions	Abdominal surgery, catheter use, bladder infections, alcohol intake, caffeine use, increased fluid intake, increased urine concentration, overdistension of bladder, neuro-logical disorders (cerebrovascular accident, incom-plete supraspinal cord injury, multiple sclerosis, Parkinson's disease, brain tumours, trauma), Alzheimer's disease, cancer of bladder, urethritis	Neuropathy, neurological misfiring, surgery, trauma, spinal cord diseases, anatomical problems (fistula), severe neuro-logical diseases

Compiled from Irrgang SJ: *J Enterostom Ther* 13: 62, 1986: McLane AM: Classification of nursing diagnoses: proceedings of the seventh conference, St Louis, 1987, The CV Mosby Co; Orzeck S and Ouslander JG: *J Enterostom Ther* 14: 20, 1987; Resnick NM and Yalla SV: *N Eng J Med* 313: 800, 1985; and Voith AM: *Rehabil Nurse* 11: 18, 1986.

From: GK McFarland & EA McFarlane (1989) *Nursing Diagnosis & Intervention: Planning for Patient Care*. St. Louis: CV Mosby, pp. 282 & 283.

hardships in relation to the isolating and demeaning aspects of the problem. A survey of hospital in-patients showed that 5–7% of patients aged between 5 and 64 years and 18–21% of those over 65 are incontinent. The average prevalence on general wards was 9–10%. A conservative estimate of the cost of coping with incontinence within the National Health Service in 1984 was £72 million per annum. The burden posed by urinary incontinence on the individual and care-givers is substantial. The reported prevalence in long-term care institutions has been consistently high and is estimated to range from 38 to 55%. The incidence of incontinence increases with age but for some types of incontinence it may be more closely related to functional disability than age.

It is generally acknowledged that most people with urinary incontinence can benefit from treatment, yet many receive only palliative remedies of protective pads and urinary appliances while the basic problem remains unidentified and untreated. One study found that 5% of the incontinent group in the home care population surveyed had undergone urodynamic assessment in the previous year, despite the fact that incontinence had persisted for at least 6 months in 72% of the patients.

CONTRIBUTING FACTORS

Established urinary incontinence may be due to: degenerative tissue changes, as seen in the elderly; neurological disease or injury which results in loss of bladder sensation or interruption of innervation to the detrusor muscle and sphincters; loss of cerebral awareness that may occur in any illness and in shock; relaxation of the pelvic floor muscles; infection or irritation of the bladder; or a congenital anomaly (e.g. hypospadias).

About one-third of episodes of incontinence are transient, resulting from treatable or preventable causes. These include faecal impaction, impaired mobility, urinary tract infections or the use of drugs such as diuretics and sedatives.

Risk factors for urinary incontinence include age, female sex, immobility, confusion, hospitalization and the use of indwelling catheters. Oestrogen deficiency in postmenopausal women may contribute to the development of stress incontinence.

CLINICAL CHARACTERISTICS

Table 20.7 provides a comparison of the clinical characteristics of each of the five types of established incontinence. Differences related to the urge to void, the amount voided, nocturia, predisposing factors, awareness, frequency, anatomical problems and related factors are described.

ASSESSMENT

Urinary elimination is a personal and private activity; social norms and personal habits influence how individuals respond when problems develop with urinary emission. Patients may be uncomfortable and embarrassed discussing their problems and delay seeking assistance. When obtaining a health history and examining a patient with a urinary system disorder the nurse should assess each individual's level of anxiety, allow the patient to express feelings of discomfort or embarrassment, acknowledge awareness of these feelings and reassure the patient that everything possible will be done to ease any embarrassment and provide privacy. It is also important to establish the terms and expressions used by the patient to describe the act of voiding and to ensure that the terminology used by the nurse is understood.

Health history

The person should be asked about any *family or personal history* of: (1) urinary system disorders or infections; (2) diseases affecting the urinary system such as diabetes mellitus or hypertension; and (3) past use of drugs (either prescribed or bought over the counter).

Female patients should be asked about their obstetric history due to the effects of pregnancy on the pelvic floor muscles.

Specific information about the person's usual and present *pattern of urinary elimination* is obtained. Information includes frequency of voiding, volume of urine excreted at each voiding and in a 24-hour period and usual times of voiding. Any changes in the usual pattern of elimination such as nocturia or frequency are identified. The person is asked about the colour, odour and clarity of urine and if there is any discomfort or pain associated with voiding. It is important to determine how long the incontinence has been present.

Incontinence
Figure 20.15 provides an overall approach to the assessment of incontinence. Data should be determined from the health history.

Factors influencing urinary elimination
1. *Past experiences and attitudes.* Urinary habits vary with each individual. The nurse should discuss the person's usual habits, attitudes to urinary elimination and experiences with toilet training which may have influenced present attitudes. The person may associate urinary incontinence with loss of control of body function, and see the problem as regression towards infancy; sensitivity on the nurse's part is therefore of paramount importance.
2. *Diet and fluid intake.* The volume of fluid intake has a direct effect on the urinary output. The person who suffers from incontinence may well restrict fluid intake in order to try and reduce the problem. Unfortunately, this may lead to dehydration and in increased risk of urinary tract infection (UTI). For patients with renal disorders it is important to identify usual eating habits and the relative amounts of protein and sodium in the daily diet.
3. *Life-style factors* that influence elimination include accessibility of toilet facilities, privacy and any unusual stresses associated with voiding.
4. *Activity, mobility and dexterity.* Physical activity is necessary to maintain muscle tone and normal

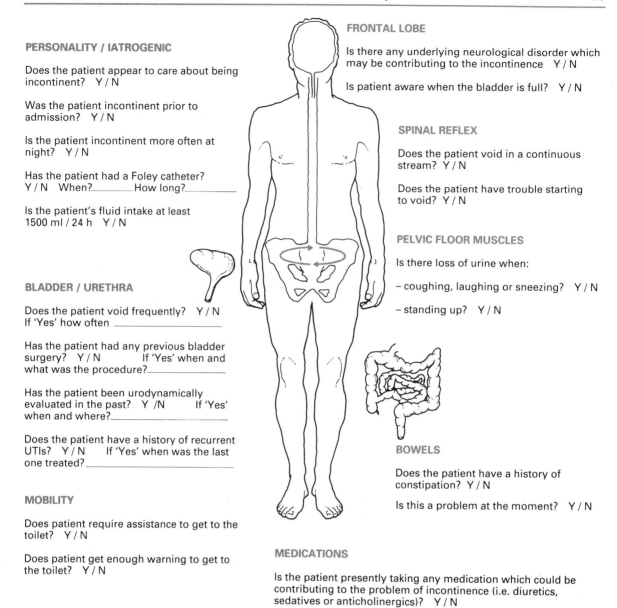

PERSONALITY / IATROGENIC

Does the patient appear to care about being incontinent? Y / N

Was the patient incontinent prior to admission? Y / N

Is the patient incontinent more often at night? Y / N

Has the patient had a Foley catheter? Y / N When?_____ How long?_____

Is the patient's fluid intake at least 1500 ml / 24 h Y / N

BLADDER / URETHRA

Does the patient void frequently? Y / N If 'Yes' how often _____

Has the patient had any previous bladder surgery? Y / N If 'Yes' when and what was the procedure?_____

Has the patient been urodynamically evaluated in the past? Y / N If 'Yes' when and where?_____

Does the patient have a history of recurrent UTIs? Y / N If 'Yes' when was the last one treated?_____

MOBILITY

Does patient require assistance to get to the toilet? Y / N

Does patient get enough warning to get to the toilet? Y / N

FRONTAL LOBE

Is there any underlying neurological disorder which may be contributing to the incontinence Y / N

Is patient aware when the bladder is full? Y / N

SPINAL REFLEX

Does the patient void in a continuous stream? Y / N

Does the patient have trouble starting to void? Y / N

PELVIC FLOOR MUSCLES

Is there loss of urine when:

– coughing, laughing or sneezing? Y / N

– standing up? Y / N

BOWELS

Does the patient have a history of constipation? Y / N

Is this a problem at the moment? Y / N

MEDICATIONS

Is the patient presently taking any medication which could be contributing to the problem of incontinence (i.e. diuretics, sedatives or anticholinergics)? Y / N

Figure 20.15 Assessment of urinary incontinence. Modified from Turpie & Skelly (1989) with permission.

amounts of calcium in the bones. Bed rest and immobility predispose to the formation of calculi. Impaired mobility and dexterity may interfere with the individual's ability to get to the toilet quickly enough to use it effectively.

5. *Level of awareness and orientation.* Confusion, disorientation and difficulty following directions may interfere with the individual's ability to respond appropriately to the urge to void as well as to meet fluid and nutritional needs.

6. *Medications.* The name, dosage, frequency and duration of use of any medications being taken is recorded. Diuretics have a direct effect on urine production, while sedatives may alter cognition.

Assessment

General appearance. The patient is observed for general state of health, lethargy, fatigue and degree of alertness.

Urinary meatus and perineum. The urethral orifice is observed for signs of drainage, oedema, redness or ulceration and underclothing is examined for urine or other stains. A vaginal examination may be done by the doctor on a female patient to identify possible uterine prolapse or cystocele; the prostate gland is palpated by rectal examination to assess its size (see p. 667).

Table 20.8 Basic skills required to achieve urinary continence

- The ability to initiate micturition voluntarily at an appropriate time
- The ability to delay, temporarily, the onset of micturition
- Perception of the urge to urinate well in advance of reflex voiding
- Awareness of socially acceptable places and/or circumstances to urinate
- The ability to communicate needs and interpret oral directions and written signs to get necessary assistance or locate the toilet
- The physical mobility and manual dexterity to reach the toilet, to assume and maintain body posture during micturition, adjust clothing, deal with doors, locks, flushing systems, seats and washing facilities

Bladder. The bladder is not normally palpated but may be felt if it is overdistended. With the person supine, gently palpate and percuss the area just above the symphysis pubis; the distended bladder feels smooth and firm. The degree of elevation above the symphysis pubis is measured. Palpation of a distended bladder causes increased discomfort for the patient.

Neurological examination. A complete neurological examination is done (see Chapter 21) in patients with neurological impairment and sensory losses such as absence of the sensation or urge to void.

Assessment of functional status. The person's mobility, manual dexterity and communication skills are determined. Figure 20.15 describes the basic skills which should be identified for the individual to control urinary elimination.

Table 20.8 lists the basic skills required by an individual to achieve control of micturition. The nurse and patient collectively identify which of these basic skills the patient possesses, where difficulties are encountered in the course of daily activities, and what measures and techniques the patient uses to compensate for these deficits and their effectiveness.

Analysis of medical and nursing assessments may demonstrate the need for further evaluation by members of the multidisciplinary team such as continence nurse advisor, occupational therapist, physiotherapist or speech therapist. Early referral to the continence nurse advisor may assist in the appropriate management of the incontinence, the supply of appliances or aids, and liaison with community services in anticipation of discharge to ensure continuity of care. The occupational therapist will evaluate the home environment and toilet facilities in relation to the patient's mobility, dexterity and awareness. Difficulties manipulating clothing are also identified. The speech therapist will assess communication skills and recommend means by which the patient can communicate needs. The role of nursing staff and relatives in contributing to the patient's incontinence is also assessed, especially in the in-

stitutionalized, elderly and the disabled. Assistance to allow a schedule of regular voiding may be lacking, resulting in incontinence. Staff and family attitudes and relationships with the patient can be changed by helping them define expectations, set goals and develop strategies for dealing with the individual problem.

Clinical Diagnostic Measurements

Urine tests. A random or midstream urine specimen may be sent to the laboratory for routine and microscopic analysis.

Residual urine determination. To identify overflow incontinence associated with urinary retention, an in-and-out catheterization is performed immediately following voiding. The amount of urine that remained in the bladder after the person voided is measured and recorded.

Urodynamic investigations. These studies provide information on bladder sensation and detrusor muscle and urethral sphincter function. The tests consist of: (1) urine flow studies, (2) filling and voiding cystometrography, (3) urethral pressure profile, and (4) synchronous pressure-flow cystourethrography and video recording.

Urine flow studies measure the time and amount voided and usually include determination of the amount of residual urine in the bladder following voiding.

The cystometrogram is a method of recording the bladder's responses to increasing distension. A two-way catheter is inserted; the bladder is filled with fluid through one lumen while pressures are recorded via the second lumen. By this simple procedure, measurements are made of the volume of residual urine, resting intravesicular pressure, bladder capacity, intravesicular pressures during filling and at the point of emptying, the point at which sensation to void is felt, and the pressure and timing of any uninhibited contractions.

The synchronous video pressure flow cystourethrography is a newer, more sophisticated and expensive method of evaluating bladder and urethral function; it provides information on the appearance of the bladder during the micturition cycle.

Incontinence voiding record or diary

Documentation of the person's ability to void and episodes of incontinence may be obtained in the form of a patient log book or diary or a record by the individual, carers or nurse. The data is collected for several days to two weeks to enable analyses of the frequency of the incontinence and its relationship to fluid intake and physical and social activities and events. This record is useful in helping the patient, family and health care professionals to develop a management programme appropriate to the needs of the individual.

MANAGEMENT

Interventions to reduce or manage urinary incontinence include: (1) drug therapy, (2) pelvic floor exercises, (3) behavioural interventions, (4) protective pads and appliances, and (5) surgery. In some instances, the doctor can treat the cause directly and alleviate the disorder. In other cases, a multidisciplinary approach is required, using a variety of techniques to control the symptoms and help the individual to adjust and acquire socially and personally acceptable means to control the problem.

General measures directed to the alleviation of contributing factors include:

1. Weight reduction if the person is overweight.
2. Maintaining a fluid intake of at least 2000 ml per day.
3. Decreasing fluid intake if it has been excessive.
4. Review of medication for possible contributing factors and adjustment of these medications if necessary.
5. Adjustment of any diuretic therapy so that the action of the drugs occurs during the day.
6. Decrease in alcohol intake.
7. Institution of measures to suppress a chronic cough.
8. Treatment of any underlying urinary tract infections.
9. Increase in daily physical activity.
10. Prevention or treatment of constipation.

1. *Medication* is also used in the control of incontinence. Many drugs are available which influence the activity of the detrusor muscle and urethral sphincter but their use is limited because of the other generalized effects of these drugs and the unpleasant side-effects produced. Drugs which may be prescribed include:

- Cholinergic agents such as bethanechol chloride which stimulates detrusor contractions. These agents are used when the bladder is atonic or hypotonic.
- Anticholinergic agents, which include propantheline, empronium, oxybutynin and trodiline, decrease smooth muscle activity of a hypertonic bladder and may be used to treat urge incontinence related to neurogenic impairment and detrusor muscle instability.
- α-adrenergic agents such as adrenaline, phenylpropanolamine and imipramine (Tofranil) may be used to treat stress incontinence as they increase urethral sphincter resistance.
- α-drenergic blocking agents e.g. phenoxybenzamine decrease urethral sphincter resistance in patients with overflow incontinence.
- β-Adrenergic blocking agents (e.g. propranolol (Inderal)) increase sphincter resistance and may be used to treat stress incontinence.
- Calcium antagonists (e.g. flunarizine), antispastic agents (e.g. baclofen) and prostaglandin synthetase inhibitors (e.g. indomethacin) can all be used to manage detrusor instability, with varying results.
- Oestrogen therapy is used either topically, orally or by transdermal patch to manage atrophic vaginitis in postmenopausal women with incontinence.

2. *Pelvic floor exercises.* Kegel exercises increase the tone of muscles involved in micturition. They may be taught to control stress incontinence in women. The person sits with the feet on the floor and knees apart and is instructed to tighten the perineal muscles, as if stopping the flow of urine, and to hold the muscle contraction and then relax. This excercise is repeated several times every 2–4 hours throughout the day. During voiding, the patient is instructed to stop and start the urinary stream by contracting the perineal muscles. A feedback device may be used for patients who lack sensory input as it provides them with pressure readings, demonstrating the effectiveness of the muscle contractions.

3. *Behavioural interventions. A bladder training programme* is developed whenever possible with the active participation of the patient and family. A detailed chart or diary of urine frequency and volume, fluid intake, the times of fluid intake and voiding and the circumstances surrounding incidents of incontinence is kept for several days. From this information, the nurse and patient can develop a voiding schedule and a plan that considers the person's needs and daily activities. Voiding normally occurs on arising in the morning, before or after meals and before retiring in the evening. The voiding schedule may begin by having the person void every 1 or 2 hours, with the intervals increased gradually as control is acquired. The person's level of awareness and perception of the urge to void influence the degree of personal control that can be expected. When a patient is confused and disorientated, it is necessary for others to prompt the patient to follow the schedule and to provide assistance in tasks such as getting to the toilet and manipulating clothing.

Fluid intake of at least 2000 ml daily is maintained throughout the programme to avoid the risks of dehydration and urinary tract infection. Physical activity is increased.

Toilet facilities, a commode chair, bedpan or urinal should be within reach of the person and privacy provided. An assessment of the home environment is done and recommendations made if necessary for modifications to the home or the purchase or loan of a commode chair or bedpan. A night light should be provided. Voiding should always take place in the usual sitting posture for females and standing posture for males, with the nurse or a relative providing the necessary assistance.

For those with flaccid, hypotonic bladders, Credé's manoeuvre is taught. The hands are placed flat over the abdomen below the umbilicus. Manual pressure is exerted over the bladder to initiate flow of urine. Suprapubic tapping or stroking of the thighs may also be used to stimulate reflex voiding when incontinence is the result of neurogenic dysfunction (reflex incontinence).

Suggestions are provided for adapting clothing for the person with impaired manual dexterity or the individual who has minimal time between the sensation or urge to void and the act of voiding (urge incontinence). The person may need instruction and practice with the manipulation of zippers, buttons or other aspects of clothing.

Positive reinforcement or contingency management is a behavioural approach using positive verbal and social reinforcement to establish continent behaviours.

McCormick and Burgio reported on a study which demonstrated a 45% increase in the frequency of correct toileting when used with a small group of nursing home residents who were cognitively impaired (McCormick and Burgio, 1984). They cautioned that staff and patient rights must be considered and patient consent obtained for such a programme.

Prompted voiding and socialization are behavioural techniques that have been used effectively with female nursing home residents to decrease episodes of incontinence (Creason et al, 1989). The technique used involved asking residents if they needed to void and if so, assisting them with toileting. The schedule for prompting must be established for each individual in relation to their voiding pattern and activities.

Biofeedback used alone or in combination with bladder training and positive reinforcement has been shown to be effective in the treatment of stress and urge incontinence. This procedure provides the person with information about bladder and abdominal pressures which is useful in learning to voluntarily inhibit bladder contractions. This method is most effective when used with cognitively aware individuals.

4. *Protective pads and appliances.* Various aids are used in the management of incontinence. Self-control of continence cannot be achieved for every patient. Some may continuously require protective measures. Others may require protective measures during assessment and treatment or during periods of illness. Many protective devices and aids are available and include the following:

- *Protective pants and pads.* Underpads may be used on bed linen or furniture or pads are available to be worn by the person. Various types of waterproof pants and pads are also available. Each type is designed to meet a specific need and the absorbancy of the various pads vary. The marsupial pants (Kanga pants) are designed with a waterproof pouch to hold the pad in place. Most products are available in a variety of sizes and styles and some are disposable while others are washable. Use and selection of pants and pads must be individualized and requires the individual's interest and co-operation. Protection of clothing allows the patient to dress normally and participate in social functions. The use of pads or plastic or rubber pants for adults may be demeaning and serve to promote feelings of dependence and withdrawal if their use is not discussed and agreed with the person. Sanitary towels are not designed to contain urine and are inappropriate, ineffective and an expensive means of containing incontinence.
- *External urinary drainage devices.* A condom with an attached drainage bag is useful for male patients. It may be worn only at night or during the day under clothing; care must be taken to select an appropriately sized condom. The penis is checked frequently for oedema, redness or excoriation. A female external urine collecting device is available. It has an adhesive plate similar to a stoma wafer with an integral pouch which can be attached to a collecting bag. Wear times achieved by this device vary and mobility can be restricted. In order to achieve

adherence the skin around the external genitalia is shaved and a skin protective gel is applied.
- *Catheter.* Catheterization as a means of controlling incontinence is not considered until other alternatives have been tried. An indwelling catheter may be used in some instances to permit increased independence for the patient. Intermittent catheterization is preferred to an indwelling catheter; the person or carer is taught to perform the procedure. The risk of infection is reduced with intermittent catheterization as opposed to an indwelling catheter. It is performed on a regular schedule which is determined in a similar manner to the bladder training schedule.
- *Electrical devices.* Electrical stimulators are receiving moderate attention as a means of increasing the tone of pelvic muscles. They create continuous contraction of the pelvic muscles which is relieved by releasing the electrical stimulation to facilitate voiding when desired.
- *Occlusive devices* are not satisfactory for long-term use. Penile clamps and an inflatable pad which applies pressure against the perineum to close the penile urethra are available for men.

  Occlusive devices for females are vaginal tampons and an inflatable vaginal balloon which elevate the bladder neck and apply pressure on the urethra through the vagina and may be useful for minor stress incontinence or during periods of physical activity.

5. *Surgery.* Surgical intervention for incontinence is directed to the correction of anatomical defects that contribute to the incontinence (for example: correction of obstructions in the urinary tract, repair of a cystocele, or uterine prolapse, or prostatic hypertrophy). Urethrovesical resuspension may be done in women with severe stress incontinence. This procedure increases the support for the bladder and restores the closure of the bladder outlet. Sometimes urinary diversion is performed for uncontrollable incontinence. This is occasionally necessary following radiotherapy for bladder cancer, where the bladder becomes atrophied with a small capacity, or for congenital malformations of the bladder, e.g. ectopic vesicae, or in spina bifida.

Artificial urethral sphincters can be implanted in men and women. Various types of devices are available but they generally consist of a cuff filled with fluid and a mechanism for diversion of the fluid when voiding is desired.

NURSING INTERVENTION

Effective management of urinary incontinence usually involves the collaborative efforts of a multidisciplinary team and the active participation of the individual and carers. The nurse is an important member of this team and is often in the best position to initiate and co-ordinate activities.

Assessment. Assessment is the key to the identification of the problem and to determining accurately the type of incontinence and the contributing factors. The nurse plays a vital role in the assessment process in identifying individuals at risk for or with incontinence and in promoting verbalization and recognition that a problem exists. The nurse is able to document the person's patterns of urinary elimination over a period of time and to identify factors associated with the incontinent episodes. The nurse assumes responsibility for ongoing patient assessment and thus reassesses the need for indwelling catheters and ensures that they are removed as early as possible once the reason for their insertion is resolved.

Development of the patient plan of care. The nurse should collaborate with the person and family to develop an effective plan to manage the person's urinary incontinence. Patient and family input is necessary to establish realistic goals and to develop a plan to meet the needs, activities and life-style of the patient and family members.

There is a need for nursing research to evaluate the effectiveness of the many incontinence pads and urinary devices available. Currently there are few, if any, standards for absorbency of pads. Urinary appliances vary in design and complexity. Studies of these products have had small samples and have lacked scientific rigor in their methodologies. The nurse needs to identify and document the need for each product used and to evaluate its effectiveness in controlling the incontinence of the individual patient. Patient co-operation is essential before any protective pads or appliances are introduced.

Self-concept. Urinary incontinence has a negative impact on the individual's self-esteem and self-concept. Studies of the prevalence of incontinence recognize that many cases are hidden. They are not identified because the person is reluctant to disclose the information. One of the more constructive interventions the nurse can perform is to get the person and family to verbalize the problem and to recognize that incontinence is not a normal consequence of ageing or childbirth and that something can be done to help them. Plans for managing the incontinence should consider the impact of the problem on the person's social activities and include strategies for increased socialization.

In a study of 43 elderly women in a retirement community, Simons (1985) found that 51% identified themselves as being incontinent and that 50% of this group had reported their incontinence to their doctors. Comments of the doctors who responded included: 'Don't worry about it' and 'It's normal for your age'. Over 40% of the incontinent group had not previously disclosed their problem to a health care provider. The nurse has a responsibility to open the lines of communication with individuals who may be experiencing undetected incontinence and to help them deal with the problem constructively.

Patient and family teaching. Patients and families generally lack information about the nature of urinary incontinence and its management. Patients and families need help to develop self-care skills related to the numerous products and appliances used to control the incontinence. Roe (1990b) found that patients lacked basic knowledge of their indwelling catheters and that teaching by nurses about catheter care was not comprehensive or consistent. She recommended the use of information booklets to enable learning to take place over time. Not all patients want to learn or are capable of learning about their incontinence and its management. Assessment of learning needs should be ongoing to identify when and if the patient is ready for further information.

Clinical Situation: Mrs Jarvis, an elderly woman with urge incontinence

Mrs Jarvis is a 76-year-old woman who was admitted to hospital for a total knee replacement. Following her surgery the nursing staff noted that she was requesting the bedpan frequently and was often incontinent by the time they got to her.

Mrs Jarvis had a 10-year history of problems with urgency, frequency and incontinence of urine. She had bladder surgery 8 years ago but this was only effective for the first year. When her symptoms returned she consulted her doctor who told her there was nothing further to be done and she would have to learn to live with it.

Assessment
Bladder. A postvoiding residual was requested to determine how well Mrs Jarvis was emptying her bladder. A toileting routine was instituted for the next 48 hours to assess the amount and frequency of her voiding. Mrs Jarvis voided 50–75 ml every 2 hours and the frequency increased in direct relation to her intake. In the initial postoperative phase she had an intravenous infusion at 100 ml per hour and was voiding every half hour, once the infusion was stopped this decreased to every 2 hours.

Bowel. Mrs Jarvis stated that her bowels had not moved since before her surgery 5 days previously. An abdominal assessment and rectal examination were done. Her abdomen was distended, with bowel sounds present, and was firm on palpation. The rectum was full of very hard, constipated stool.

Once the assessment was complete it was determined that Mrs Jarvis was voiding small amounts frequently with a normal postvoiding residual and was felt to have detrusor instability. The instability was being further exacerbated by her faecal impaction.

Intervention.
Mrs Jarvis was put on a bowel programme to resolve her constipation. She was also started on an anticholinergic medication to reduce the irritability of her bladder, thus allowing an increase in voided volumes and the time between voiding. A postvoid residual was repeated at 5 and 10 days following the start of the anticholinergic treatment to ensure that she was not in retention.

Evaluation. Mrs Jarvis was discharged home 3 weeks after surgery and was delighted to have regained her continence after so many years.

Table 20.9 Causes and characteristics of urinary retention

Causes	Clinical Characteristics
• Obstructive disease of the bladder or urethra • Surgical intervention • Neurological disease • Embarrassment or fear • Constipation	• Frequent voiding of small amounts • Absence of voiding in 8–10 hours with adequate fluid intake • Bladder distension • Urgency and persistent desire to void • Restlessness • Pain and discomfort in the region of the bladder and/or kidney

The Person with Urinary Retention

Urinary retention is *the state in which the individual experiences incomplete emptying of the bladder* (North American Nursing Diagnosis Association, 1989). It is characterized by a distended bladder and a sensation of bladder fullness. The person may be unable to void when fluid intake has been adequate, may experience difficulty with starting a stream of urine, or bladder emptying may be incomplete. The person may void frequent small amounts of urine and may experience dribbling. It may be described as a type of incontinence (urinary incontinence with overflow).

Retention may be related to obstructive disease of the bladder or urethra (usually due to enlargement of the prostate gland with ageing in male patient, see below), surgical intervention or neurogenic disease (Table 20.9).

BENIGN PROSTATIC HYPERTROPHY

Obstructive disease of the bladder is caused by benign prostatic hypertrophy (BPH), a common condition in later life which affects a high proportion of men. As the prostate gland enlarges it interferes with normal urinary outflow from the bladder. The condition is insidious in onset with the person becoming aware of increasing difficulty in passing urine, dribbling and frequency may develop. In time chronic retention may develop where the person has a large residual volume of urine in the bladder which then becomes very prone to infection. Alternatively acute retention may develop; in this situation the patient will have a distended lower abdomen and be in acute pain and distress as he is unable to pass any urine. (See also pp. 815–817.)

It is important therefore in assessing any male patient aged over 50 to enquire carefully about any changes in micturition, remembering the possible embarrassment this may cause the patient. It is interesting to note that a national survey by the British Market Research Bureau (Nursing Standard 1991) found that although the symptoms of BPH were widespread, knowledge of what the condition involved and its treatment were poor. Only 28% of persons with symptoms had consulted a GP while only 2% stated that they had consulted a nurse about the problem. This is an area where the nurse has a vital role in the early detection of symptoms and referral for medical treatment in addition to having a strong health education role.

The surgical treatment of BPH involves transurethral resection of the prostate (TURP), whereby a cutting diathermy instrument is introduced via a cystoscope and under direct vision the hypertrophied prostate is tunnelled through to enlarge the opening from the bladder and allow normal urinary drainage. Postoperative care is concerned with ensuring that drainage from the catheter is kept free and not blocked by any clots which may form and lead to clot retention. Bladder irrigation using a two way catheter is therefore required and care must be given to ensuring that the patient regains normal bladder control when the catheter is removed.

ASSESSMENT

The time of last voiding, the volume of fluid intake and the volume of urinary output are determined. Fluid loss by channels other than urinary is also considered. The patient's lower abdomen is examined for distension of the bladder. The patient may complain of low abdominal pain or the distress of feeling the need to void but being unable to initiate voiding. The comprehensive assessment approach described in Figure 20.15 is applicable to the person with urinary retention.

NURSING INTERVENTION

The *goal* is that the patient will establish and maintain a flow of urine from the bladder.

Promotion of spontaneous voiding. Nursing measures used to induce voiding include increasing the fluid intake (unless contraindicated), providing privacy, pouring of warm water over the perineum, letting the patient hear running water, stroking of the inner portions of the thighs, and, unless contraindicated, assisting the patient to assume the normal position for voiding. Females are encouraged to use a commode at the bedside; male patients may stand beside the bed. A warm bath may prove effective with some patients.

Urinary retention in a postoperative patient may result from incisional pain and discomfort or be associated with embarrassment at the lack of privacy. Analgesics are administered prior to offering the patient a bedpan or urinal or assisting them to a sitting position, commode chair or to the bathroom. Privacy should be maintained at all times. Bethanechol chloride or neostigmine (Prostigmin), which are parasympathomimetic agents, may be prescribed to stimulate voiding. These drugs increase the tone of the detrusor muscle stimulating bladder contractions.

Urethral catheterization. Emptying of the bladder by the insertion of a catheter into the urethra and bladder may be done on an intermittent or continuous basis. Urinary catheterization may be performed for reasons other than urinary retention; it may be necessary to assess urinary output accurately in a critically ill patient, to promote healing following surgery in the perineal region, to administer medications directly into the bladder or to measure the volume of residual urine remaining in the bladder following micturition. Before inserting a Foley catheter, the need for it should be thoroughly assessed and documented. Because of the increased risk for infection, as well as the patient's discomfort and loss of dignity, the catheter should be removed as soon as possible.

The procedure and the purpose for it are explained to the patient and privacy is provided throughout the procedure. Precautions are taken to avoid the introduction of organisms and trauma of the mucosa; sterile gloves are worn, and strict aseptic technique is observed throughout the procedure. The catheter is handled with great care in order to minimize trauma. If the retention has been acute and severe, not more than 1000 ml of urine are removed initially. The sudden, complete emptying of an overdistended bladder may result in an atonic bladder wall. The sudden release of pressure on the blood vessels in the bladder region causes a sudden inflow of blood and sometimes capillary bleeding may occur. Rarely, the patient may experience faintness. The catheter is removed or may be clamped after 1000–1500 ml is drained and then reopened to allow further drainage at a later time.

Management of an indwelling urethral catheter. A closed drainage system is used to maintain a continuous urinary flow and decrease the potential for the entry of organisms into the system. The catheter is attached to tubing and a collecting bag with a drainage valve or to a leg bag which contains a valve to prevent backflow of urine into the bladder. The leg bag or regular drainage bag is kept below the level of the bladder and attached to a hanger or hook on the side of the patient's bed or chair. A leg bag is used for the patient who is mobile since it is less cumbersome and can be worn under clothing. The drainage system should not be disconnected unnecessarily for fear of introducing infection to what should be a closed, sterile system.

The drainage system is assessed frequently for patency; kinks in the tubing and tension on the catheter and tubing are avoided. In the female patient, the catheter is taped to the inner thigh; in the male patient the catheter is taped laterally to the upper thigh or abdomen to prevent pressure on the penile–scrotal angle. The latter is an important preventive measure since erosion of tissue at the penile–scrotal angle may develop if tension is applied to the catheter and the resulting fistula can only be corrected by plastic surgery.

Indwelling urethral catheters are changed at varying intervals and may be left in place for 4–6 weeks depending on the type of material used in the catheter; information is usually available on the catheter package. Collecting tubing and drainage bags are changed every 2–7 days. Urethral catheters are inconvenient for the patient, but should not interfere with the performance of usual daily activities. Showers are generally permitted.

Measures to prevent the development of urinary tract infections from catheter use are discussed on p. 670.

Patient teaching. Individuals requiring retention catheters during periods of hospitalization require information about the purpose of the catheter and general principles of care and the importance of preventing infections. Individuals are taught to keep the drainage bag below the level of the bladder, to prevent tension on the catheter and to maintain a closed system.

The person requiring intermittent or continuous catheterization at home requires detailed instruction about the supply and care of equipment, and the performance of the procedure if necessary. Horsley (1982), in reviewing the current literature on catheterization procedures, concludes that the use of clean intermittent catheterizations promotes improvement in urinary incontinence, urinary infections, renal function and bladder emptying and this is therefore the procedure of choice. Frequency of catheterization is determined by the volume of urine. Referrals are made to the community nurse or continence adviser to assist the person and family in managing the catheter. At home, the drainage tubing and bag required for night use may be cleaned with soap and water and stored dry during the day before reconnection at night. With intermittent self-catheterization it is also possible to wash through the catheter and store in a clean dry place until required again. Good clean technique is necessary whatever system is adopted.

Management of the person following removal of the catheter. An indwelling catheter is removed as soon as possible to lessen the trauma to urethral sphincters and the loss of muscle tone that ensues. After the catheter is removed, the person is encouraged to pass urine hourly for a few hours and the time and amount of each voiding are recorded as well as the fluid intake. The patient is assessed for any discomfort, dribbling of urine due to dilatation of the sphincter by the catheter, sensation of urgency or stress incontinence. If the person is unable to void in 6–8 hours and has had an adequate fluid intake, intermittent catheterization may be necessary. If only small amounts of urine are voided, catheterization may be done to measure the amount of residual urine. A bladder training programme may be instituted if difficulties persist after a few days (see p. 664).

Suprapubic catheterization. The insertion of a catheter into the bladder through the suprapubic area is a surgical procedure and requires local or general anaesthetic. Nursing care of the patient with a suprapubic catheter and closed drainage system is similar to that of the patient with an indwelling urethral catheter. The suprapubic catheter is sutured in place and is then taped to the abdomen to prevent tension on the catheter. The exit site is cared for as a surgical incision. Stomahesive can be used to protect the skin around the insertion site or a transparent, sealed dressing (e.g. Opsite) is used.

Clinical Situation: Mrs Lee, a woman with urinary retention

Mrs Lee is an 80-year old woman who was admitted to hospital in a diabetic crisis in an effort to stabilize her blood sugar. She was incontinent of large amounts of urine over the first 24 hours and the nursing staff requested an indwelling catheter. They were concerned that prolonged incontinence would put her at risk for skin breakdown and increase the number of linen changes which would be required.

Mrs Lee complained of an ongoing problem with incontinence that started several years before but had worsened in the past few months.

Assessment
Bladder. Inserting an indwelling catheter at this point would simply postpone the problem of determining the cause of her incontinence and the appropriate treatment. Instead, a postvoiding residual was done to determine the extent to which she was able to empty her bladder completely.

Mrs Lee voided 100 ml and was catheterized for a residual volume of 1000 ml. She did not even seem to be aware that she had to void or that her bladder was so overdistended.

Bowel. An abdominal assessment and rectal examination determined that she was having difficulty emptying her bowels and was in fact constipated.

Mrs Lee was in urinary retention secondary to three factors: diabetic neuropathy which reduced her sensation of filling; faecal impaction which was partially obstructing her urethra; and immobility which made it very difficult for her to get to the bathroom so she often lost the urge to void or ignored. it.

Intervention
Mrs Lee was started on a programme of intermittent catheterization four times a day until her residual volumes reduced to 350 ml, when catheterization was reduced to three times a day. As her bladder tone returned she began voiding again and her residuals were reduced to twice daily.

Her faecal impaction was initially treated with a series of enemas and, once resolved, she continued on a regular bowel programme.

Evaluation. Mrs Lee's condition stabilized over the next few days and she was then transferred to a rehabilitation setting to improve her mobility and evaluate her ability to look after herself. Her urinary retention slowly resolved and she was still on daily residuals when discharged. These were done by the district nurse for another 2 weeks before they were low enough to be discontinued.

The Person with a Lower Urinary Tract Infection

Lower urinary tract infection (UTI) refers to an acute or chronic infection and inflammation of the bladder (*cystitis*) and the urethra (*urethritis*). It is a common health problem affecting at least 20% of women during their lifetime, with about 3% experiencing recurrent infections. The incidence is less in men but increases after 65 years of age, probably as a result of obstructive disorders and the loss of bactericidal activity of prostatic secretions.

CAUSES

Lower urinary tract infection is most often due to infection caused by the ascent of organisms by way of the urethra, but it may also be associated with the administration of certain drugs (e.g. cyclophosphamide) and radiation therapy of the lower abdomen. Predisposing factors are the use of indwelling catheters, trauma of the tissues, stagnation of the urine, and distortion or compression of the bladder by an enlarged neighbouring organ. The latter condition is a factor in cystitis that not infrequently develops in the pregnant woman, especially in the last trimester; the enlarging uterus compresses the bladder. The higher incidence in females is attributed to the shorter urethra of a relatively wide calibre. Sexual intercourse and the type of contraception, particularly diaphragm use, are precipitating factors. Poor bladder emptying is a precipitating factor in older women. Organisms from rectal and vaginal discharge can enter readily. In the male, it is usually secondary to prostatic hyperplasia or infection or to congenital malformation (e.g. hypospadias).

CLINICAL CHARACTERISTICS

Frequency, urgency, dysuria and abnormal urine constituents are the primary characteristics of a UTI. The inflammation is generally confined to the mucosa and submucosa which are hyperaemic and oedematous. Scattered haemorrhagic areas are present, and small ulcerative lesions may develop as a result of sloughing of the lining tissue of the bladder. The urine contains blood cells, pus, bacteria and mucus. If the urinary tract infection becomes chronic, the inflammation may extend into the detrusor muscle. Fibrosis of the tissues occurs with persisting inflammation, which reduces the bladder capacity and increases the problem of frequency.

TREATMENT

In some instances, a UTI is of brief duration, being resolved spontaneously. There is always the danger that the infection may ascend via the ureters and cause pyelonephritis. The infection is treated by the administration of an antibiotic or urinary antiseptic such as co-trimoxazole or amoxycillin. A urine specimen obtained before any antimicrobial drug is given may be cultured to determine the infective organism and its drug sensitivity. A specific antibiotic may then be ordered. Sodium bicarbonate or sodium citrate may also be prescribed for the purpose of making the urine alkaline to decrease the bladder irritation and dysuria. Warm baths may reduce bladder spasm and provide considerable relief. The person is encouraged to drink liberal amounts of fluids which should include citrus fruit juices.

If the condition persists, the UTI is suspected of being secondary. The patient is then investigated for a primary condition which might be pyelonephritis, a bladder calculus, urethral stricture or, in the case of the male, an enlarged prostate.

Since a UTI is frequently the result of an ascending infection and occurs readily in females, good personal hygiene and efficient cleansing of the perineum, especially after defecation, are extremely important and require emphasis in health teaching. Adequate cleansing is often very difficult for the ill person who is weak or handicapped and confined to bed. It becomes the nurse's responsibility to see that the patient is thoroughly cleansed.

PREVENTION OF URINARY TRACT INFECTIONS

The nurse has responsibilities for health promotion and patient teaching to decrease the development or recurrence of urinary tract infections in individuals at risk and to prevent and/or decrease episodes of catheter or therapy induced UTIs.

Patient Teaching

Hand washing and personal hygiene. Since most urinary tract infections result from bacteria that originate in the gastrointestinal tract, frequent handwashing, especially after defecation, is an important preventive measure. Women should be taught to wipe their perineal areas from the front to the back and then dispose of the tissue. This avoids contamination from the rectal area and should be practised after each bowel movement.

Sexual intercourse is a contributing factor in the development of UTIs in women. For women who experience repeated UTIs associated with sexual intercourse, both partners should wash their genitals prior to intercourse and the female should empty her bladder just before and again after intercourse. She should be taught to drink lots of fluids to keep the urine dilute. The use of condoms should be discussed.

Treatment of altered patterns of urinary elimination. Elimination disorders that result in retention and stasis of urine predispose the individual to urinary tract infections. If complete emptying of the bladder is not possible a programme of intermittent catheterization may be indicated. It is important to identify and treat persons with urinary incontinence and retention.

Catheter-induced urinary tract infections

Use of urinary catheters
Catheters are a major cause of urinary tract infections. They allow entry of micro-organisms to the bladder, they offer a surface for the organisms to grow, they are a foreign body and therefore interfere with the body's immune responses, and they may cause chemically-induced inflammation of the urethral and bladder mucosa. Catheters also stretch the urethral orifice and injure the tissues. Obstruction of a catheter produces increased intravesicular pressure, promoting the spread of organisms across the mucosa and up into the ureters.

- Evidence indicates that urinary catheters contribute to urinary tract infection, their use should therefore be limited. The need for a catheterization, either intermittent or indwelling, should be assessed and documented prior to the procedure.
- Indwelling urinary catheters should be removed as soon as possible because of the risk of infection.
- External urinary devices, such as condom catheters for men, should be used in place of urinary catheters whenever feasible.
- Intermittent catheterization should be used in preference to indwelling catheters. The incidence of infection is decreased with intermittent catheterization. In hospitals or other institutions, strict aseptic technique is required when inserting any catheter. Patients can be taught intermittent self-catheterization, to be performed at home using clean, non-sterile technique.

Care and management of urinary catheters

- When an indwelling catheter is in place, a closed system should be maintained to decrease infection.
- Urine specimens should be obtained from the designated port of a closed catheter system using a syringe with a small-bore needle. The system should not be opened to obtain a specimen.
- Wash hands and wear gloves prior to handling the catheter system and teach the patient to wash the hands before touching the catheter and attached drainage receptacles.
- When emptying the drainage bag ensure that the tap does not come into contact with other surfaces thereby reducing the risk of infection.
- The site of the catheter insertion at the urethral opening provides a port for entry of organism. Many topical antiseptic agents and cleansing procedures have been tested to decrease contamination of the urinary meatus. There is no evidence to warrant adoption of any of these protocols in clinical practice (Conti and Eutropius, 1987).
- The addition of bactericidal agents to urine drainage bags has been frequently tested. Most well-designed studies have failed to show any benefits from this practice.
- Bladder irrigations are recommended only to prevent or alleviate obstruction of the catheter. Neither intermittent nor continuous irrigations have been shown to prevent UTIs and may actually increase the risk of infection. Intermittent bladder irrigations require entry into the closed drainage system, which should be avoided whenever possible.

Bladder Injury

Accidental injury of the urinary bladder, causing perforation and ensuing extravasation of the urine (escape of urine from the bladder), is not uncommon. It may occur when the pelvis is fractured or as a result of direct blows to the lower abdomen. If the bladder is full and distended at the time of accident, it is more vulnerable.

If the laceration occurs in the upper portion, the rupture is intraperitoneal. Urine escapes into the peritoneal cavity and produces peritonitis. The patient becomes shocked (see Chapter 12) and experiences abdominal pain and tenderness, with a rigid distended abdomen and usually a paralytic ileus (see Chapter 16).

Rupture of the lower part of the bladder is usually extraperitoneal; urine escapes into the surrounding tissues, and infection, cellulitis and necrosis of tissue may ensue. Occasionally an abdominal or perineal fistula develops.

When there is a history of an injury or blow to the lower abdomen followed by pain and tenderness, injury to the bladder is suspected. A urine specimen is obtained promptly, either by having the patient void or passing a catheter, to determine if there is haematuria. If blood is present in the urine, a cystogram may be done to confirm the diagnosis and locate the laceration.

TREATMENT

The injury is a serious threat to life and requires prompt treatment. The shock and haemorrhage are treated with a blood transfusion and intravenous infusions. An indwelling catheter is inserted into the bladder, and the patient is prepared for abdominal surgery. The site of injury is repaired and a temporary cystostomy (incision of the bladder and introduction of a suprapubic catheter) is done to establish urinary drainage and prevent the possibility of pressure on the repair suture line. If the rupture was intraperitoneal, the extravasated fluid is aspirated before closure.

Following surgery, the patient is observed closely for signs of infection. Antibiotics may be administered immediately. An accurate record of the fluid intake and all drainage is very important. (See section on nursing care of the patient having had a cystostomy, pp. 673. For the care of the patient with peritonitis and paralytic ileus, see Chapter 16.

The Person with a Tumour of the Bladder

Tumours in the bladder may develop at any age but occur more frequently after the age of 50 and have a high incidence in males. The majority arise from the epithelial lining (transitional cell) as papillomas and may be benign or malignant. Those that are benign and recur tend to become malignant eventually. Others appear as ulcers which are usually malignant and are more invasive of deeper tissue layers.

RISK FACTORS

Prolonged occupational exposure to aniline dyes is recognized as a predisposing factor. It is recommended that the period of working with these chemicals should be limited to 3 years and that during this period such persons should have urinary examinations for malignant cells. Workers are also advised of the importance of prompt reporting of any blood in the urine or slight bladder irritation. Smoking has also been cited as a predisposing cause of bladder cancer.

CLINICAL CHARACTERISTICS

The first symptom is usually intermittent painless haematuria, or cystitis may be the initial factor that brings the person to a general practitioner. The lesion may encroach on the urethral orifice, giving rise to hesitancy and a decreased force and calibre of the urinary stream. Suprapubic pain and a palpable mass generally indicate that the condition is in an advanced stage. The person may experience pain in the flank region if the growth obstructs a ureteral orifice which causes hydronephrosis. The lesion ulcerates, which accounts for the haematuria, and readily becomes infected. If the infection is severe and anaemia has developed, the patient manifests weakness and loss of weight.

DIAGNOSTIC TESTS

Diagnostic procedures include a cystoscopy and biopsy; urine specimen for cytology and midstream specimen of urine for culture and sensitivity; intravenous urogram to identify obstruction or defects of the urinary system; and a CT scan may be performed to identify invasion of other organs by tumour.

TREATMENT

The treatment used depends upon whether the neoplasm is benign or malignant and, in the case of malignancy, upon the stage and the depth of the tissue involved. Surgery, radiation, chemotherapy, or a combination of these may be used. Small papillomatous growths may be treated by transurethral resection followed by electrocoagulation of the base tissue. An indwelling catheter may or may not be inserted in the bladder on completion of the operation. The urinary drainage is observed frequently for possible bleeding. Bladder spasm and irritability may cause considerable discomfort which may be reduced by a warm bath. The patient is encouraged to take a minimum of 2000 ml of fluids daily.

Since papillomas, benign as well as malignant, tend to recur, these patients are followed closely for 5–6 years. They are advised to report any bleeding or bladder irritability promptly. A cystoscopic examination is usually done every 3 months during the first year following the resection, every 6 months during the second year, and then annually for 3 or 4 years.

If the neoplasm is malignant, a partial resection of the bladder or total cystectomy (removal of the bladder) may be done.

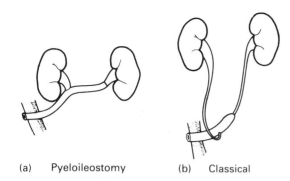

(a) Pyeloileostomy (b) Classical

Figure 20.16 Methods of permanent urinary diversion: the ileal conduit. (a) Pyeloileostomy. (b) Classical.

Partial cystectomy

A partial cystectomy is only used if the cancer is in the upper part of the bladder well above the urethral orifices. At operation, a tube or catheter is placed in the bladder and brought out through the incision, and an indwelling catheter is also introduced through the urethra. Removal of a part of the bladder obviously reduces its capacity. Adequate drainage in the postoperative period is necessary to prevent distension and possible disruption of the suture line. The tube in the incision may be connected to gentle intermittent suction. The length of time it remains in the bladder will depend on the rate of healing.

The urethral catheter usually remains in place for approximately 2–4 weeks. On its removal, frequency becomes a problem for the patient because of the reduced bladder capacity. Thus may lead to discouragement and depression, consequently understanding support from the nurse is essential. Any attempt to reduce the frequency by cutting down fluid intake must be guarded against. The importance of a minimum fluid intake of 2000 ml to prevent dehydration and the spacing of the fluids so the intervals between voiding may be increased during certain periods (e.g. at night) should be discussed with the patient. The traumatized bladder gradually becomes less irritable and increases its capacity.

Cystectomy

A total cystectomy with ureteric transplantation for permanent urinary diversion is used when the cancer is situated in the lower part of the bladder or is quite extensive. Permanent urinary diversion may be achieved by cutaneous ureterostomy, continent ileal urinary pouch or the formation of an ileal conduit (Figure 20.16).

In *cutaneous ureterostomy*, the detached ends of the ureters are brought through the abdominal wall and secured at skin level. This is rarely the procedure of choice. Maintaining the patency of the ureters is difficult because strictures tend to develop. If catheters are placed in the ureters to maintain drainage, they readily block and are difficult to keep in place. Chronic kidney infection is a frequent complication with subsequent renal failure.

Continent ileal urinary pouch. Several surgical procedures (e.g. Koch, Camay, Mitroffonoff, Indiana) are being done to create a continent ileal or internal reservoir from an isolated segment of ileum which is then connected to the abdominal wall. A nipple-like valve is created to allow insertion of a catheter to drain urine. The internal pouch replaces the external urine collecting bags worn by persons without the built-in reservoir.

The *ileal conduit (ureteroileostomy)* involves removal of a segment of the ileum with its mesentery and blood supply. The open ends of the ileum left by the resection are anastomosed to re-establish intestinal continuity. One end of the resected ileal section is closed. The open end is brought through the abdominal wall to the skin surface and secured. The detached ends of the ureters are implanted in the ileal segment near its closed end.

Radiation

Internal or external radiation may be used in treating cancer of the bladder. It may be used alone, as an adjunct to surgery, or with chemotherapy. External radiotherapy may be used to treat the tumour as an adjunct to surgery, or prophylactically to reduce pressure symptoms or tumour mass. During treatment the individual is likely to experience gastrointestinal disturbance (nausea, vomiting and diarrhoea) and cystitis. This should be discussed with the person prior to commencing therapy. Information booklets may be useful in reinforcing verbal information. Long-term side-effects of radiotherapy include chronic urinary disturbance, telangiectasia of the bladder mucosa with chronic haematuria, and usually loss of erectile function in men and decreased orgasmic sensation in women. Intracavity radiation may be achieved by the enclosure of a radiosotope (e.g. ^{60}Co, ^{198}Au) in a catheter balloon which is placed within the bladder. The catheter is connected to a drainage receptacle, and all urine is saved and sent to the radioisotope department. In some instances, radon seeds or radiotantalum (^{182}Ta) needles may be implanted around the lesion. Safety precautions are necessary in the handling of these radioactive materials and are cited in Chapter 10. Internal radiation causes cystitis, and the patient usually experiences considerable bladder spasm and discomfort. Fluids are given freely and analgesics may be necessary. The application of heat over the bladder region may provide some relief.

For care of the patient receiving external radiation therapy, the reader is referred to Chapter 10.

In advanced carcinoma of the bladder and when metastases are suspected, chemotherapy may be used as well as surgery and irradiation (see Chapter 10). Local or intravesical chemotherapy can be used for the control of some bladder cancers. This can be performed on an in-patient or out-patient basis. The management of this procedure is often performed by nurses and safety precautions in relation to the handling of cytotoxic drugs should be observed (see Chapter 10).

Bladder Surgery

Operative procedures used in the treatment of bladder disease may be transurethral or by open surgery. Open surgery involves an incision through the abdominal wall. Transurethral operative procedures may be performed to obtain a biopsy, remove a neoplasm or calculus, or resect the prostate gland. The resectoscope, which is used to resect tissue, is similar to a cystoscope but has insulated walls and is equipped with a wire loop which is activated by a high frequency current to cut tissue and contol haemorrhage by electrocoagulation (diathermy). The procedure is referred to as a transurethral resection of the prostate (TURP). A lithotrite, which is a special crushing instrument, is used to remove a stone, and the procedure is called litholapaxy.

Open surgery on the bladder may be undertaken for repair of a perforation or laceration, the removal of a neoplasm, calculus, or the prostate gland, or a segmental resection or removal of the bladder. The open operative procedures include *cystotomy* (an incision into the bladder and closure without a drainage tube), *cystostomy* (an incision into the bladder and the insertion of a drainage tube which is brought out on to the abdominal surface), *segmental resection* (the removal of a section of the bladder) and *total cystectomy* (the removal of the bladder, involving ureteral transplantation and urinary diversion). A suprapubic approach is most commonly used in open bladder surgery, with the bladder being opened below the peritoneum.

NURSING CARE OF THE PATIENT HAVING BLADDER SURGERY

Preopreative preparation

Unless the bladder is injured or there is acute retention that cannot be relieved by urethral catheterization, the patient who is to have bladder surgery usually undergoes investigation and preparation. Kidney function is assessed and certain blood chemistry levels are determined (e.g. urea, creatinine, potassium, sodium, chloride, calcium). The urine is examined microscopically and, if infection is present, a urinary antiseptic or an antibiotic is prescribed. The patient is encouraged to take 2500–3000 ml of fluid daily unless a large amount of fluid is contraindicated by cardiac or renal insufficiency. The fluid intake and output are recorded and the balance noted. The patient's nutritional status frequently requires attention. Many of these patients are elderly and the existing condition may have contributed to their lack of interest in food, resulting in deficiencies. In encouraging the patient to take nourishment, its importance in recovery is explained. Dietary adjustments and supplements may be necessary to meet nutritional needs.

During the preparatory period, an indwelling catheter may be used to provide adequate drainage and reduce

Table 20.10 Identification of problems relevant to the patient who has just had a cystotomy, cystostomy or segmental bladder resection.

Patient problem	Goals
1. Altered pattern of urinary elimination related to bladder incision, urethral catheter and cystostomy tube	● Patient will achieve fluid balance
2. Ineffective airway clearance related to anaesthesia and decreased mobility	● Patient will show normal respiratory function
3. Impairment of skin integrity related to surgery and possible leakage of urine	● Wound will heal without complications
4. Alteration in comfort: pain related to surgical intervention and bladder spasms	● Patient will be free of pain
5. Alteration in nutritional and fluid balance related to surgery and discomfort	● Patient will maintain nutritional status
6. Altered bowel elimination related to surgery and discomfort	● Patient will have normal bowel actions
7. Knowledge deficit related to fluid intake, catheter care and health supervision	● Patient will show understanding of condition and requirements after discharge

the residual urine. The patient is usually encouraged to remain ambulatory.

Psychological support in the preoperative phase is equally as important as physical care. Opportunities should be provided for the discussion of feelings and concerns and for the patient to ask questions. The patient and family are advised as to what may be expected following the operation. If the patient is to have a partial cystectomy, this explanation will include a discussion of the frequency of voiding that will be experienced when the tubes are removed because of the reduced capacity of the bladder. Reassurance is given that this gradually becomes less troublesome.

The immediate preparation for open bladder surgery is similar to that for any patient having abdominal surgery (see Chapter 11).

Postoperative nursing intervention

Preparation to receive the patient after operation includes the assembling of sterile tubing and drainage receptacles ready for prompt connection to an indwelling urethral catheter and a cystostomy tube. A tray of sterile equipment and solution for irrigating the catheters in the event of obstruction by clots should be readily available. Goals for the patient following a cystotomy, cystostomy or segmental bladder resection are listed in Table 20.10.

1. Maintenance of urinary elimination. The patient returns from the operating theatre with an indwelling urethral catheter which is secured to the upper thigh to prevent traction. It is connected to sterile tubing leading to a closed sterile drainage receptacle. The length of the tube should allow for turning and moving the patient without tension being exerted on the catheter.

If there is a cystostomy as well, a tube is anchored in the bladder by a suture at the time of operation. The cystostomy tube is attached to a sterile tube and receptacle.

Both drainage systems are checked frequently (at least hourly for the first 36–48 hours) for patency. The characteristics (colour, consistency, and content or sediment) of the drainage are noted at the same time. The urine will be blood-stained for the first 2–3 hours, gradually becoming lighter. The drainage is best examined in the plastic connecting tubes before it becomes mixed with what is already in the receptacles.

The cystostomy tube, urethral catheter or tubing may become obstructed by a blood clot. The drainage system is checked for patency. If blockage of the tubing is indicated, it may be 'milked' or changed. If the obstruction is within the catheter tube in the bladder, an order may be given to irrigate with sterile normal saline. Fifty to 75 ml of the fluid are introduced; if the initial fluid does not return, no more fluid is instilled and the surgeon is consulted. Adequate postoperative drainage is very important to prevent bladder distension and pressure on the suture line.

Bladder irrigation systems are available that may be used to prevent clots blocking the catheter. Specially made-up sterile bags of sterile irrigation fluid may be run into the bladder under gravity and then allowed to drain. It is important to ensure that fluid instilled is drained off before any further fluid is run into the bladder, for reasons discussed above. This procedure is particularly important after TURP (see p. 816).

The drainage from each system is measured and recorded every 4 hours. Care of the tubing and drainage bag varies with local policy. It may be replaced daily with a fresh sterile set or changed every second day or twice weekly.

The cystostomy tube usually remains in place from 4–7 days, depending on the patient's healing. The urethral catheter is generally left for a few days longer or until the incisional opening in the bladder heals. When the cystostomy tube is removed, some urine will escape onto the dressing for a few days until the fistula heals over.

Following the removal of the urethral catheter, a close check is made of the patient's frequency of voiding and the volume of the daily output for several days. The ambulant patient should be encouraged to record the necessary information. When a urethral catheter that has been in place for several days is removed, dribbling is a frequent problem because of the bladder-urethral

sphincters have been continuously dilated for a period of time. Frequent perineal exercises, which consist of contracting the abdominal, gluteal and perineal muscles while continuing to breathe normally, may help the sphincters recover their tone and control. Occasionally, a patient may not be able to void and catheterization may be performed if voiding has not occurred within 8 hours.

A permanent cystostomy is sometimes done as a palliative measure for a patient who has an inoperable obstruction of the urethra (e.g. advanced carcinoma of the urethra, bladder neck or prostate). A urethral catheter is not inserted in this patient; bladder drainage is entirely dependent upon the cystostomy tube.

Assessment. As well as frequent checking of the drainage system(s), the patient's blood pressure, pulse, colour and level of consciousness are noted and recorded at frequent intervals, which are gradually lengthened if the vital signs are satisfactory. Haemorrhage and shock are possible complications following either transurethral resection or open bladder surgery. Bleeding may be evident in the drainage, but the dressing, surrounding skin areas and groins are also examined.

The daily fluid intake and output are recorded for a longer period than with most surgical patients. The ratio of the intake to the output is examined by the nurse so that he or she is alert to possible renal insufficiency or retention of urine. The characteristics of the urine are noted for a period of 10–14 days. The appearance of sediment, blood, shreds of mucus-like material, cloudiness or the presence of an unusual odour is reported. Sloughing and ensuing bleeding may occur 8–10 days following the removal of a lesion.

2. Maintenance of airway clearance. The reader is referred to Chapter 11 for a discussion of the importance of avoiding respiratory and cardiovascular complications in the postoperative period.

3. Impairment of skin integrity. Compared with other abdominal surgery, the dressing is changed earlier and more frequently for patients who have had open bladder surgery. There is almost certain to be some leakage of urine through the incision and around the tube. The skin is cleansed of urine frequently and is kept as dry as possible to prevent excoriation and infection. Application of a skin protection preparation may aid in preventing excoriation. If excoriation occurs the use of stoma or hydrocolloid dressing wafers may help in preventing further skin breakdown and encourage healing. Early referral to the stoma care nurse or wound care specialist nurse (if available) may help obviate problems. The lower back, buttocks, groin, inner thighs and perineum are examined each time the dressing is changed. If any areas are moist with urine drainage, they are washed and thoroughly dried to prevent excoriation. The bedding is changed as often as is necessary to ensure dryness and comfort.

4. Control of pain. Bladder trauma and irritation cause bladder spasms which are very painful, and the patient may also experience the desire to void frequently, even though the bladder is emptied by tube drainage. In the case of the sensation of frequency, it may be necessary to explain to the patient that the bladder is empty and that trying to void only increases bladder spasms and pain. An analgesic such as pethidine is usually necessary at regular intervals during the first 48 hours. If the pain and discomfort are not relieved, the surgeon is consulted. Either the catheter or cystostomy tube may require adjusting to relieve the pressure of its tip on the bladder wall.

5. *Maintenance of fluid balance and nutrition*. A daily fluid intake of at least 2500–3000 ml (unless contraindicated by other coexisting disease) is necessary to ensure adequate irrigation of the bladder as well as to maintain satisfactory hydration. Most of it usually has to be administered by intravenous infusion during the first day or two. A soft diet is given and is progressively increased to a regular diet as tolerated.

6. *Maintenance of bowel elimination*. The patient may be given a mild laxative after 2 days, or an enema may be given. Constipation and straining at stool should be avoided since they tend to increase the patient's pain.

7. *Patient education*. Most patients who have had a cystotomy or cystostomy remain in the hospital until the wound is healed and normal micturition is re-established. The nurse should discuss the resumption of their previous activities with them and explain any restrictions indicated by the doctor. They are advised to continue taking a minimum of 2000–2500 ml of fluid daily. Some may require reassurance that no special care of the wound is necessary and that they may resume baths.

If the cystostomy is permanent or a urethral catheter is to remain in place, the patient and a family member are given detailed instruction about the necessary care. This instruction is given over several days and should be completed soon enough for the patient to demonstrate satisfactory self-care before going home. This gives confidence and provides the opportunity to clarify certain points. Verbal and written instructions will include an explanation of the necessary equipment, its use and maintenance, how it may be acquired, and any precautions to be observed in its use. An inconspicous plastic leg bag which can be strapped to the thigh may be required by the patient if an indwelling catheter is to be used. The lower end of the bag has a valve which permits emptying of the bag into the toilet at necessary intervals. The importance of thorough washing of the hands with soap and running water before connecting or disconnecting the equipment is stressed to reduce the possibility of ascending infection. The patient and a relative are also taught how to anchor the tube that is in the patient to the abdomen or thigh to prevent traction on it.

The patient is reminded of the need to continue taking at least 2000–2500 ml of fluid daily to provide adequate bladder irrigation. Odour is likely to be less of a problem with more dilute urine, and there is less danger of infection with constant washing out of the bladder.

A referral may be made to the district nurse for assistance and supervision when the patient goes home. This is likely to be needed when the patient is elderly and finds it difficult to cope with the necessary care. The patient and family are advised how often the catheter needs to be changed and should be referred to the community continence advisor where possible.

Evaluation

On discharge from hospital, the patient should be able to perform usual daily activities with minimal discomfort and only temporary changes in activity tolerance. The patient and family should be aware of expectations for self-care and community resources available. They should be able to describe plans for follow-up health supervision.

The Person with a Urinary Diversion

Complete removal of the bladder necessitates establishing a new urinary outlet; this may be achieved by cutaneous ureterostomy, ileal conduit (ureteroileostomy) or an internal continent ileal pouch. For a description of these procedures, see p. 672.

Following operation, the patient who undergoes a cystectomy and ureteral transplant is seriously ill. The amount of surgery usually involved predisposes the patient to shock. Frequently, considerable surrounding tissue is resected with the bladder (e.g. lymphatics, prostate gland), and if the ileal conduit procedure or internal ileal pouch is used, an intestinal resection and anastomosis are done. The patient will have a large vertical or transverse incision through which the bladder is removed, the ureters are freed for transplant, and the intestine is resected. The stoma through which the urine will drain is made separately in the right abdominal wall and an internal pouch may be created. Care of the patient requires consideration of the needs incurred by the cystectomy, the intestinal surgery, the ureteric transplantation and urinary diversion as well as the individual patient's psychological and physiological responses to such radical surgery.

PREOPERATIVE PREPARATION

The operative procedure and the permanent change in urinary drainage that will ensue should be explained to the patient and his family by the surgeon and the stoma therapist. This is likely to produce considerable anxiety and despair and will prompt many questions. The nurse needs to show acceptance of these understandable concerns and provide opportunities for the patient and family to express their feelings and ask questions and, when they are ready, the necessary adjustments and care associated with urinary diversion are outlined in simple terms. They are told that a relatively normal, active life is possible. This may be reinforced by having a person who has had a permanent urinary diversion and has made a successful adjustment talk with them. If such a person is not available, someone with an ileostomy may prove helpful. The nurse who is willing to take time to talk freely with the patient, discussing future plans, and is patient in repeating answers and reinforcing what has probably already been said can provide immeasurable support. A rapport can be developed that contributes to acceptance of the situation and the development of positive attitudes on the part of the patient and family.

The sexual implications of the surgery should be discussed with the individual and partner, together with the treatment options available should difficulties arise postoperatively. Whenever sexual issues are discussed sensitivity and tact are of the utmost importance because of the personal nature of this subject and the potential threat to self-image and self-esteem. Many men and women who undergo surgery of this type fear rejection and abandonment by their partners, or if single, believe they will never have a physical relationship again. The following changes can result from radical bladder surgery: in men, sexual desire and genital sensation is often normal, orgasm intensity may be reduced, ejaculation dry, and erectile dysfunction may be present; women may experience dyspareunia and reduced vaginal secretion but orgasm normally remains the same. Treatment options for men include intercavernosal self-injection technique, penile prosthesis, or use of vacuum devices. Women who experience painful intercourse may wish to adopt the following strategies: different positions for lovemaking, extended foreplay, or the use of lubricants (e.g. water soluble gel or saliva). Vaginal dilators may be useful to dilate the vagina. Some women respond to replacement hormone therapy.

As part of the physical preparation for surgery, kidney function is assessed and the blood levels of nitrogenous wastes, potassium, sodium and chloride are determined. The patient usually receives a blood transfusion during and probably following the surgery, so typing and cross matching are necessary. At least 2500 ml of fluid daily are given unless contraindicated by cardiac insufficiency or urinary obstruction.

If the intestine is to be entered, the patient may receive a low-residue diet for 3 or 4 days, then clear fluids only for 2 days before operation to reduce the faecal content. The reasons for these restrictions are explained in order to gain the patient's co-operation and acceptance. Laxatives and enemas are also used for cleansing purposes, and a course of an antimicrobial drug that is poorly absorbed from the gastrointestinal tract is given orally to destroy intestinal organisms (e.g. silver sulphadiazine, neomycin). A nasogastric tube is passed at the operation to provide drainage of secretions and prevent intestinal distension after the surgery. The remainder of the preparation is similar to that for any major abdominal surgery (see Chapter 11).

The operation is a lengthy procedure; relatives should be informed when they may call to enquire about the person's condition and/or visit.

MANAGEMENT OF THE PATIENT WITH A URINARY DIVERSION

A large part of the required care is essentially the same as that for any patient having an intestinal resection (see Chapter 16). Table 20.11 lists goals relevant to the patient with a urinary diversion.

Table 20.11 Identification of problems relevant to the patient with a urinary diversion

Patient problem	Goals
1. Altered pattern of urinary elimination related to formation of a ureteroileal conduit	● The patient will maintain urinary elimination
2. Potential impairment of skin integrity (stoma and peristomal skin) due to surgical intervention and irritation	● The integrity of stoma and peristomal skin will be preserved ● Infection will not occur
3. Alteration in mobility related to surgical intervention and pain	● The patient will be pain free ● Normal mobility will be regained
4. Alteration in nutrition and fluid balance related to surgery on intestine, bladder and ureters	● The patient will maintain nutritional status and fluid balance
5. Disturbance in body image related to the urinary diversion and creation of the abdominal stoma	● The patient will demonstrate a healthy body image
6. Disturbance in sexual functioning related to damage to nerves, surgical excision of tissue, and trauma to reproductive system	● The patient will demonstrate understanding of potential alterations in sexual functioning
7. Knowledge deficit related to self-care of the urinary diversion and follow-up care	● The patient will show knowledge, skills and resources to manage health care regimen

1. Maintenance of urinary elimination. On completion of the operation a disposable clean plastic ileostomy bag is secured to the skin around the stoma. This allows for vizualization of the stoma and drainage. A cessation of drainage may indicate occlusion of the stoma by mucus or by swelling and oedema of the tissues, and the surgeon is notified immediately. A sterile catheter may be inserted periodically to determine if there is residual urine.

2. Maintenance of integrity of stoma and peristomal skin. The appliance should be removed gently to prevent trauma to the peristomal skin. A tissue or wipe can be used to cover the stoma to collect urine. The skin is gently washed with mild soap and water and dried. Barrier creams, adhesive preparations and skin sealants may be used on intact skin. A new appliance is applied carefully, ensuring correct fit around the stoma. Transient erythema is usual on appliance removal but this should rapidly resolve. Any persistent redness, broken skin, complaints of discomfort or allergic reactions should be investigated and rapidly treated. The stoma should be monitored for signs of oedema, bleeding, excoriation, ulceration, unusual drainage or discoloration. (See care of the individual with a fecal diversion, Chapter 16.)

Odour control may be a problem for some individuals. Advice should be given concerning avoidance of foods which produce strong odours in urine. Introduction of a few drops of vinegar or commercial deodorizer into the appliance via the outlet spout may reduce stale urine odours.

Abdominal pain, distension or rigidity, nausea, vomiting or fever is reported promptly. Any of these symptoms may indicate peritonitis, resulting from the escape of intestinal content from the site of the intestinal anastomosis or from a leakage of urine from the ileal conduit or ureters into the peritoneal cavity.

3. Maintenance of mobility and physical function. Since the ileal conduit opens on to the right side of the abdomen, more complete drainage occurs when the patient is on the right side or back with the trunk elevated. With each change of position, the bag and tubing are checked for any kinks or compression.

Early amubulation is encouraged to foster adequate drainage and prevent complications.

Good pain relief is essential and the nurse carries the main responsibility for ensuring the patient is pain free in this postoperative period.

4. Maintenance of nutritional status and fluid balance. The nasogastric tube remains in place for 3–4 days and the patient is given intravenous fluids. The patient is observed for any signs of distension. Once bowel sounds indicate the re-establishment of peristalsis, and there is no distension, the nasogastric tube is removed. The intake of clear fluids is gradually increased and the diet progresses through soft foods to a light solid diet. Gas-forming foods are avoided for 4 to 6 weeks and then added gradually as tolerated.

5. Promotion of a healthy body image. The person with a urinary diversion must deal with the altered body structure of an abdominal stoma that is initially red, swollen and tender, the loss of control of urine and the perceived effects on social interactions and sexual activity. Acceptance of body image changes takes place slowly. It is important that the nurse encourages the patient to verbalize concerns and to talk about them with both partner and family.

Initially patients are often uncomfortable looking at the stoma. The nurse can support them in looking and talking about it as care procedures are being performed. The person will need support to touch the stoma and to gradually assume self-care activities. Some patients benefit from talking with others who have learned to manage their urinary diversions and sharing experiences related to care and the resumption of social activities. Information regarding self-help groups should be offered. Prior to discharge, patient concerns related to sexual function should be assessed and addressed. If the actual or perceived concerns are beyond the scope of the nurse, plans may be made for further assistance from specialists or resources in the community or hospital.

6. Patient and family education. The patient and a family member are taught the care of the stoma, skin and appliance following the same plan as that outlined for the ileostomy patient in Chapter 16. Emphasis is placed on the precautionary measures necessary to prevent infection. Once the oedema subsides and the stoma shrinks, the stoma is measured for a permanent appliance (approximately 7 days). The patient is taught to measure the stoma in order to adjust the size of the appliance as healing continues to take place.

If a continent internal pouch has been constructed, the individual is taught to insert a catheter through the valve to drain the urine. The nurse helps the person to develop a schedule and to adapt it to usual daily activities as control is established. During this period, the importance of continuing a daily intake of 2500 to 3000 ml to keep the ureters and ileal conduit patent should be emphasized. The patient and family are cautioned that the doctor is to be consulted immediately if there is a decrease in urinary drainage, abnormal constituents such as blood in urine, fever, pain in the back or abdomen, severe skin excoriation or general malaise. Mucus from an ileal conduit or internal pouch is normally present in the urine. This should be explained to avoid distress or concern. The patient is followed closely after hospital discharge. A referral may be made to the district nurse and community stoma care nurse, and the patient is seen at regular intervals at the clinic or by the general practitioner. These visits may be frequent at first, and the intervals are gradually increased to 3 to 6 months if the patient's progress is satisfactory.

URINARY DIVERSION: SUMMARY

Factors to be considered in caring for a patient who undergoes permanent urinary diversion, regardless of the method used, include the following:

- The individual's psychological reaction to a change in body image and normal pattern of function requires thoughtful understanding on the part of the nurse, with sincere efforts to reduce the patient's despair and promote acceptance and adaptation.
- Preoperative cleansing and 'sterilization' of the bowel are necessary if the operative procedure involves resection of or entry into the intestine.
- Maintenance of continuous, adequate urinary drainage from the ureters postoperatively is essential to prevent renal complications.
- Drainage of urine through an opening on to the skin necessitates special skin care to prevent excoriation and maceration.
- A daily fluid intake of 2500 to 3000 ml of fluid is important to provide good internal irrigation of the renal pelvis and ureters.
- A planned programme of teaching the care of the stoma, skin and appliance or drainage of the pouch is given to the patient and a relative. It should take

place over a period of time that will allow them to acquire a satisfactory understanding and competence by the time the patient leaves the hospital. The instruction includes an explanation of the need for ample fluids and prompt reporting of decreased urinary drainage and significant symptoms.

- Information about the person's previous employment is obtained, and consideration is given as to whether it is possible for previous employment to be resumed or whether a referral to a social worker would be of assistance in finding other employment.
- The person requires close follow-up. Frequent home visits by a district nurse, especially during the first few weeks after leaving the hospital, can provide assistance and considerable support to the patient and family. Regular visits to a clinic or the general practitioner are necessary.

SUMMARY

This chapter provides an overview of the structure and function of the kidneys, the formation and composition of urine and the mechanisms of urinary elimination. The nursing management of persons with acute and chronic disorders of renal function are discussed.

Urinary incontinence is a prevalent health problem, especially in elderly women. Clinical situations are included to illustrate the experiences of two women, one with urinary incontinence and one with retention of urine. Comprehensive assessment of the person with urinary incontinence is essential to accurately define the type of incontinence and the contributing factors. The nurse plays an important role in the assessment process and in promoting effective patient management. Participation of the patient and family in the care process enables the development of a relevant and realistic management programme and facilitates acceptance of the plan of care. Urinary catheters are identified as the major cause of nosocomial infections. The nurse has a responsibility to prevent urinary tract infections from being acquired as a result of catheter use. Permanent urinary diversions cause a disturbance in self-image and necessitate skilled patient and family teaching by the nurse.

Throughout this chapter, emphasis is placed on the impact of renal disorders and altered urinary function on the quality of life of the person and the resulting effects on the family. The nurse plays a vital role in identifying the impact of the disorder on the patient and family, in teaching them self-management skills and in helping them to develop appropriate coping patterns.

LEARNING ACTIVITIES

1. Arrange to visit a local dialysis unit and observe how nurses and patients interact. Discuss how nurses can encourage patients to participate in their care.
2. Arrange to meet and talk to a patient undergoing long-term dialysis. Interview the person to find out what impact having renal failure has had on his or her life-style and family.
3. Evaluate the care plan and other records of a patient who is incontinent of urine.
   (a) Using Figure 20.15 as a guide, review the assessment data available related to the person's urinary incontinence. Is the documented data comprehensive?
   (b) Is there documentation of a plan of care for this patient related to the incontinence?
   (c) Is there documentation of patient and family involvement in the development and implementation of the plan?
   (d) Is there documentation that evaluation of the effectiveness of the nursing interventions has been carried out?
   (e) Would you recommend that the documented plan of care be continued? If yes, what is your rationale for continuing the plan? If no, describe a revised approach/plan to manage the patient's urinary incontinence.
4. Develop a resource file related to sexuality and sexual dysfunction associated with renal disorders and altered urinary function. Identify information concerning:
   (a) The nature and extent of problems experienced by this patient group.
   (b) Agencies or support available to assist individuals with difficulties.
   (c) Approaches which can be used to assist patients with difficulties associated with altered sexual functioning.
   (d) Strategies which you and others can use when discussing sexuality with patients.

REFERENCES AND FURTHER READING

Alderman C (1989) Catheter care. *Nursing Standard* **4(3)** (Supplement): 1–15.

Barnes KE & Malone-Lee J (1986) Long term catheter management: minimizing the problem of premature replacement due to ballon deflation. *Journal of Advanced Nursing* **11**: 303–307.

Brown SM (1990) Perioperative anxiety in patients undergoing extracorporeal piezolithotripsy *Journal of Advanced Nursing* **15(9)**: 1078–1082.

Brown J, et al (1991) Campaigning for Continence. *Nursing Times* **87(14)**: 66–68.

Buck N, Roy C & Atcherson E (1986) Life with dialysis: structured interviews provide feedback. *Journal of Nephrology Nursing* **15(2)**: 78–81.

Churchill DN, Morgan J & Torrance GW (1984a) Quality of life in end-stage renal disease. *Peritoneal Dialysis Bulletin* **2(1)**: 20–22.

Churchill DN, Bear JC, Morgan J, Payne RH, McManamon PJ & Gault MH (1984b) Prognosis of adult onset polycystic kidney disease re-evaluated. *Kidney International* **26**: 190–193.

Conti MT & Eutropius L (1987) Preventing UTIs: what works? *American Journal of Nursing* **87(3)**: 307–309.

Creason NS, Grybowski JA, Burgener S, Whippo C, Yeo SA & Richardson B (1989) Promoted voiding therapy for urinary incontinence in aged female nursing home residents. *Journal of Advanced Nursing* **14(2)**: 120–126.

Crow RA, Chapman RC, Roe BH & Wilson JA (1986) *A Study of Patients with Indwelling Urinary Catheters and Related Nursing Practice*. Guildford: University of Surrey Nursing Practice Research Unit.

Eddins BR (1985) Chronic self-destructiveness as manifested by noncompliance behaviour in the haemodialysis patient. *Journal of Nephrology Nursing* **14(4)**: 194–196.

Egan M, Plymat K, Thomas T & Mead T (1983) Incontinence in patients in two district general hospitals. *Nursing Times* Feb.2: 22–23.

Getliffe K (1990) Catheter blockage in community patients. *Nursing Standard* **5(9)**: 33–36.

Goodison S & Holmes S (1985) Acute renal failure: aetiology and treatment. *Nursing* **42**: 1254–1257.

Hagan T (1990) Nurses take the lead in continence work. *Nursing Standard* **4(40)**: 24–28.

Havard C (1989) Nursing patients with urinary tract cancers. In Borley D (ed.) *Oncology for Nurses and Health Care Professionals, Vol. 3 Cancer Nursing* 2nd end, pp 389–421. Beaconsfield: Harper & Row.

Hinchliff SM & Montague SM (1988) *Physiology for Nursing Practice*, pp 512–545. London: Baillière Tindall.

Horsely J, Crane J & Reynolds MA (1982) *Clean Intermittent Catheterization (CURN Project)*. New York: Grune & Stratton.

Janes G (1990a) A better life than before: quality of life in people with renal failure. *Professional Nurse* **6(1)**: 26–28.

Janes G (1990b) An open approach to minimize the effect sexuality and renal patients. *Professional Nurse.* **6(2)**: 69–71.

Jeter K, Falter N & Norton C (1990) *Nursing for Continence*. London: WB Saunders

Lubkin I (1986) Illness roles. In Lubkin I (ed.) *Chronic Illness: Impact and Interventions*, pp 42–62. Boston: Jones & Bartley.

Luker KA & Box D (1986) The response of nurses towards the management and teaching of patients on continuous ambulatory peritoneal dialysis (CAPD). *Journal of Advanced Nursing* **23(1)**: 51–59.

McCormick KA & Burgio KL (1984) Incontinence: an update on nursing measures. *Journal of Gerontological Nursing* **10(10)**: 16–23.

McFarland GK & McFarlane EA (1989) *Nursing Diagnosis and Intervention: Planning for Patient Care*, pp 272–331. St Louis: Mosby.

MacIver C (1989) Polycystic kidney disease. *Nursing Times* **85(6)**: 52–54.

McKeever MP (1990) An investigation of recognized incontinence within a health authority. *Journal of Advanced Nursing* **15(10)**: 1197–1207.

Moody M (1990) *Incontinence—Patient Problems and Nursing Care*, Oxford: Heineman.

Mulhall A (1991) Biofilms and urethral catheter infections. *Nursing Standard* **5(18)**: 26–28.

North American Nursing Diagnosis Association (1989) *Taxonomy 1: Revised 1989: With Official Diagnostic Categories* pp 24–30. St Louis: NANDA.

Norton C (1986) Nursing for Continence, Beaconfield Publishers. UK.

Nursing Standard Clinical News (1991) *Nursing Standard*, **5:** 10, 15.

Poll IB & Kaplan De-Nour A (1980) Locus of control and adjustment to chronic haemodialysis. *Psychological Medicine* **10**: 153–157.

Roe B (1990) Do we need to clamp catheters? *Nursing Times* **86(43)**: 66–67.

Roe BH (1989a) Study of information given by nurses for catheter care to patients. *Journal of Advanced Nursing* **14**: 203–211.

Roe BH (1989b) Use of bladder washouts: a study of nurses' recommendations. *Journal of Advanced Nursing* **14**: 494–500.

Roe BH (1990a) The basis of sound practice. *Nursing Standard* **4(51)**: 25–27.

Roe BH (1990b) Study of the effects of education on patients' knowledge and acceptance of their indwelling urethral catheters. *Journal of Advanced Nursing* **15(2)**: 223–231.

Roe BH & Brocklehurst JC (1987) Study of patients with indwelling catheters. *Journal of Advanced Nursing* **12**: 713–718.

Simons J (1985) Does incontinence affect your client's self-concept? *Journal of Gerontological Nursing* **11(6)**: 37–43.

Skelly J & Turpie ID (1989) Management strategies for urinary incontinence. *Geriatrics* **44(6)**: 17–22.

Stapleton S (1983) Recognizing powerlessness: causes and indicators in patients with chronic renal failure. In Miller JF (ed.) *Coping with Chronic Illness*, pp 135–148. Philadelphia: Davis.

Thomas TM, Plymar KM, Blannin J & Meade TW (1980) Prevalence of urinary incontinence. *British Medical Journal* **281**: 1243–1245.

Thompson J (1991) The significance of urine testing. *Nursing Standard* **5(25)**: 39–40.

Toppng AE (1990) Sexual activity and the stoma patient. *Nursing Standard* **4(41)**: 24–26.

Turpie ID & Skelly J (1989) Urinary incontinence: current overview of a prevalent problem. *Geriatrics* **44(9)**: 32–36, 38.

Uldall R (1988) *Renal Nursing* 3rd edn. London: Blackwell.

Watson R & Kuhn M (1990) The influence of component parts on the performance of urinary sheath systems. *Journal of Advanced Nursing* **15(4)**: 417–422.

Weems J & Patterson ET (1989) Coping with uncertainty and ambivalence while awaiting a cadaveric renal transplant. *American Nephrology Nursing Association Journal* **16(1):** 27–31.

Wheeler V (1990) A new kind of loving? The effect of continence problems on sexuality. *Professional Nurse* **5(9):** 492–494.

Winder A (1990) Intermittent self-catheterization. *Nursing Times* **86(43):** 63–64.

Wright K (1988) Male reproductive system cancers. In Tscudin V (ed.) *Nursing the Patient with Cancer*, pp 229–307. Hemel Hempstead: Prentice Hall.

OBJECTIVES

On completion of this chapter, the reader will:

- Have knowledge of the basic anatomy and physiology of the nervous system
- Have knowledge of the pathophysiology of the various disorders affecting the nervous system
- Be able to identify the major concepts relevant to the care of a neurological patient and family
- Have an overview of the nursing care required by patients with neurological disorders

THE NERVOUS SYSTEM

The nervous system is an integrated, multipurpose system made up of many parts. It contains the higher human functions such as memory and reasoning, controls and co-ordinates all parts of the body and provides a complex communication system between the body's internal and external environments.

Structurally, the nervous system is composed of two parts: the *central nervous system* (CNS) and the *peripheral nervous system*. The CNS consists of the brain and the spinal cord, while the peripheral system consists of the spinal and cranial nerves.

The two functional divisions of the nervous system are the *somatic* or *voluntary nervous system* and the *autonomic* or *involuntary nervous system*. The somatic system is primarily concerned with the transmission of impulses to and from the non-visceral parts of the body such as the skeletal muscles, bones, joints, ligaments, skin, eyes and ears. Its activities are usually conscious and willed responses. The autonomic system is concerned with regulation of the activities of visceral muscles and glands.

Division of the nervous system into discrete parts is useful for discussion purposes in the abstract. However, in the body, the activities of each division are *interrelated*, and the nervous system and the endocrine system work in concert to harmonize the many complex functions of the total system.

This section focuses on some of the major structural and functional components of the nervous system which have implications for nursing. Muscle tissue is also considered, because disturbances in movement such as paralysis and spasticity due to nervous system dysfunction are relatively common. Few primary disorders of muscle activity are encountered in nursing practice. With the exception of cardiac and intestinal muscle, the nervous system initiates and co-ordinates contraction of muscle tissue to produce body movements, including visceral activity.

NEURONE

The neurone or nerve cell, is the structural and functional unit of the nervous system (Figure 21.1). Each neurone consists of a cell body and cytoplasmic processes. The cell body contains a nucleus and other structures and masses concerned with cell maintenance and activity. The cytoplasmic processes include a single axon and one or more dendrites.

The *axon* is a tubular process which conducts nerve impulses away from the cell body, out to the dendrites of other neurones or to muscles and glands. Near its end, the axon divides into numerous fine branches, each of which has a specialized ending called the presynaptic terminal. *Dendrites* are short, thin projections which branch profusely as they extend from the cell body. They receive stimuli and carry impulses generated by the stimuli toward the nerve cell body. Most stimuli affecting nerve cells are chemical messengers (neurotransmitters) that are secreted from one neurone to an adjacent neurone. The profuse branches of dendrites increase the surface area over which impulses may be picked up.

The processes (axons and dendrites) may be referred to as *tracts* if they are inside the CNS or as a nerve if outside the CNS. The latter is formed by a bundle of neuronal processes. The term *ganglion* refers to a collection of cell bodies outside the brain and spinal cord. Within the brain and spinal cord, such a collection may be referred to as a nucleus.

Neurones may be classified according to their function: *motor* (efferent or effector) neurones, *sensory* (afferent or receptor) neurones, and *connecting* (internuncial) neurones. The axons of motor neurones transmit impulses from the CNS to stimulate muscle or glandular tissue. Axons of sensory neurones transmit impulses to areas of the brain or spinal cord from the periphery. Connecting neurones, which occur only in the grey matter of the brain and spinal cord, convey

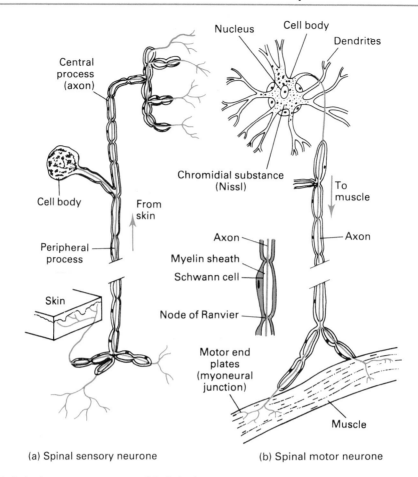

(a) Spinal sensory neurone   (b) Spinal motor neurone

Figure 21.1 (a) Spinal sensory neurone. (b) Spinal motor neurone.

incoming stimuli to neurones of various integrating centres of the CNS. The connecting neurones form the association areas in the cerebral cortex. They have an important role in the CNS because they 'decide' the responses to the incoming (sensory) impulses and promote the initiation of the appropriate motor neurone response.

Neurones are designed to initiate, receive and react to stimuli, transmit impulses, process and store information. Neuronal activity results in a wide variety of responses ranging from a simple reflex to complex behaviour requiring central co-ordination.

Unlike most body cells, neurones lose their ability to undergo mitosis early in life. They lose their viability if denied a supply of oxygen or glucose for more than a few minutes. When neurones are destroyed in the peripheral system, neuronal processes may be replaced under favourable conditions. However in the CNS neurones are not replaced. These unique properties of nerve tissue have important implications for the nursing care of patients with neurological dysfunction.

NERVE IMPULSE

The functions of the nerve cells are to receive, initiate and conduct 'messages' known as nerve impulses. An impulse is a combination of physical and chemical processes which are initiated at the point of stimulation. It occurs as the result of a mechanical, chemical or electrical change at some point in the immediate environment of the neurone. This change temporarily alters the permeability of the cell membrane at that point and is referred to as the stimulus. The series of events that result from the change in the membrane permeability produces an electrical current (Figure 21.2).

When a normal neurone is in a resting state, the outer surface of its membrane is electropositive, but the inner surface is electronegative. As a result, it is said to be polarized. This electrical polarity is attributed to the selective action of the cell membrane by which a higher concentration of sodium ions is maintained outside the cell. The positive sodium ions, which are normally attracted to the negative ions within the cell, are not

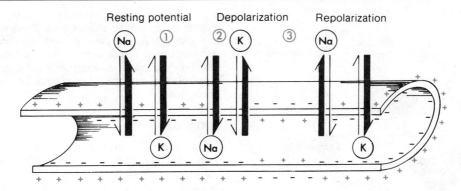

Figure 21.2 Transmission of a nerve impulse—depolarization and repolarization.

allowed to cross the membrane; if they do so, they are ejected by the cell membrane. The electronegativity within the cell is mainly due to the non-diffusible protein anions and retained chlorine anions. When the stimulus occurs, the membrane becomes permeable to sodium. The influx of cations depolarizes the membrane; a reversal of the electrical potential develops as the outer surface of the membrane becomes electronegative and the inner surface becomes electropositive. This change alters the electrical relationship of the excited area to the adjacent portions; the shift of ions acts as a stimulus, and a wave of depolarization passes along the length of the neuronal process. In a fraction of a second, following depolarization, the membrane recovers its normal permeability and the resting electrical polarity is restored. The electrical currents that are generated as impulses sweep over the fibres and may be recorded and used in assessing function (e.g. electroencephalogram).

During the conduction of impulses, the neurones consume oxygen and glucose and produce heat and carbon dioxide. The velocity of impulse transmission is determined by the diameter of the neuronal process (nerve fibre) and the presence or absence of a *myelin sheath*, a white lipid and protein insulating cover. Nerve fibres enclosed in a myelin sheath are referred to as myelinated. Larger, myelinated fibres conduct more quickly than smaller, unmyelinated ones. Neural impulses move at a maximum of 100 metres per second in large fibres.

Synapse

A synapse is the junction, or discontinuity, between the axon of one neurone and the dendrite of another. A release of chemicals at the synapse provides for the transmission of impulses from neurone to neurone. The termination of a nerve fibre in a muscle cell is called a *neuromuscular junction*. This is basically similar to the synapse between two neurones. The synapse of each axon terminal of a motor neurone on a voluntary muscle cell is referred to as a *motor endplate*.

Chemicals released from the terminal portion of the axon can have an excitatory or inhibitory effect on the transmission of impulses across a synapse. There is evidence that about 30 different neurotransmitter substances exist. The chief excitatory transmitter is acetylcholine. Glutamic acid, secreted in some of the sensory pathways is also an important excitatory transmitter. Noradrenaline and adrenaline cause excitation in some areas but inhibition in others. The chief inhibitory substances are γ-aminobutyric acid (GABA), glycine, dopamine and serotonin (5-hydroxytryptamine). The transmitter acetylcholine is destroyed by the enzyme cholinesterase within about one millisecond of its release, and others transmitters are similarly destroyed or reabsorbed into the axon. In this way, rapid, repetitive, discrete stimulation (or inhibition) of neurones is possible; this is an essential factor in the function of the nervous system.

Reflex arc, receptor, effector

A large amount of body activity occurs at an unconscious, involuntary level in response to particular types of stimuli. Reflex arcs are the involuntary, fixed motor responses to sensory stimuli. The reflex arc includes a sensory or receptor neurone (afferent), an integrating centre within the CNS at any level below the cerebral cortex and a motor neurone (efferent). A reflex is often a defence mechanism that permits quick, automatic responses to painful potentially harmful situations. Its basic purpose is to maintain total body integrity.

A receptor consists of bare nerve endings or specialized structures sensitive to specific stimuli. An effector is muscular or glandular tissue. When a receptor is stimulated by a change in its environment (e.g. pressure, temperature, chemical, stretching), it evokes an impulse in the nerve fibres. The impulse is carried through the cell body of the sensory neurone and along its axon into the CNS. Here, it may pass through one, several or many connecting neurones before it excites a motor neurone whose axon (efferent or motor fibre) carries the impulse out of the CNS to the effector tissue or organ. The terminal portion of the efferent fibre releases a chemical at its junction with the effector, initiating its response. For example, this response is contraction in the case of muscle, and is secretion if it is a gland that is innervated (see reflexes).

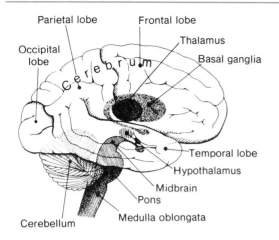

Figure 21.3 Diagram of the brain and its major parts.

NEUROGLIA

The nervous system is composed of two types of cells, namely, neurones and neuroglia (glia). The *neurones* are the essential units of the conduction system of the nervous system while *neuroglial* cells provide structural support for the neurones.

Neuroglial cells lack axons. They are generally divided into five major classes:

1. *Astrocytes* (astroglia) are star-shaped and are implicated in providing essential nutrients for neurones, in the blood–brain barrier concept, in information storage processes, and in the maintenance of bioelectrical potentials of neurones.
2. *Oligodendroctyes* form and maintain the myelin sheaths of axons in the CNS.
3. *Microglia* are phagocytic cells which are related to the macrophages of the connective tissues. They remove disintegration products of the neurones.
4. *Ependymal cells* line the ventricular system and the choroid plexuses (see p. 690). They are involved in the production of cerebrospinal fluid.
5. *Schwann cells* form the myelin sheath around the axons of the peripheral neurones.

Neuroglial cells comprise about 40% of the total volume of the brain and spinal cord. Since strong intracellular substances such as collagen and elastin are lacking in neuroglial cells, fresh brain and spinal cord tissue appears soft and jelly-like. In contrast to neurones, neuroglial cells retain their mitotic abilities throughout the life span of the individual. From a clinical viewpoint, neuroglial cells are important because they are the most common source of primary tumours in the nervous system.

Central Nervous System

BRAIN

The human brain is the organ concerned with thought, memory and consciousness. It is also concerned with a range of sensory experiences, with motor activity, the regulation of visceral, endocrine and somatic functions and with the use of symbols and signs that underlie communication. For descriptive purposes the brain may be subdivided into the cerebrum, basal ganglia, thalami, hypothalamus, midbrain, pons, medulla oblongata and cerebellum.

CEREBRUM

The cerebrum is an important part of the nervous system. It accounts for 80% of the total weight of the brain. It is divided into two hemispheres by the *longitudinal fissure*. The two hemispheres are joined at their bases by bands of neuronal fibres collectively forming the *corpus callosum*. It is believed that the corpus callosum transfers information from one hemisphere to the other. A fold of dura (see p. 691) called *falx cerebri* lies between the two hemispheres.

In selected higher functions, one cerebral hemisphere appears to be the 'leading' one and is referred to as the *dominant hemisphere*. Cerebral dominance tends to be most complete in relation to the complex aspects of language. Handedness also is related to cerebral dominance although its relationship is less clearcut than previously believed. In true right-handed persons it is nearly always the left hemisphere which is dominant and governs language; but the converse of this is not necessarily true. The degree of cerebral dominance appears to vary among individuals and with respect to different functions. Recent research indicates that each hemisphere, independently, contains the ability to learn but that the right hemisphere has a superior role in intuitive and creative responses and in spatial perception. The concept of cerebral dominance has implications for nursing care of patients with stroke or head injury in which there is damage in one hemisphere.

Each cerebral hemisphere is subdivided into four anatomically distinct regions called lobes: the frontal, parietal, temporal and occipital (Figure 21.3). The frontal lobe is separated from the parietal lobe by the central fissure. The temporal lobe is separated from the parietal and frontal lobes by the lateral fissure of Sylvius and the occipital lobe is separated from the parietal and temporal lobes by the parieto-occipital fissure. These four regions underlie the skull bones which have the corresponding names. Some texts refer also to insular and limbic lobes but neither are true lobes. The insular cortex lies in the depth of the lateral cerebral fissure. The limbic lobe is based largely upon a physiological concept.

The brain contains areas of grey and white matter. The *grey matter* is a collection of neuronal bodies and unmyelinated processes. *White matter* consists primarily of myelinated fibres coming off cell bodies. Grey matter, which forms the surface of the cerebrum, is called the *cerebral cortex*. The cortex is believed to contain about 100 billion neurones. It is 2–5 mm thick and is arranged in a series of convolutions or coil-like elevations called gyri. Shallow crevices between the gyri are called sulci (Figure 21.4). The folding into gyri and sulci appears to be a means of increasing the surface area of the brain. Sulci that are particularly deep are called fissures.

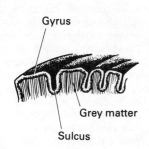

Figure 21.4 The surface of the cerebrum.

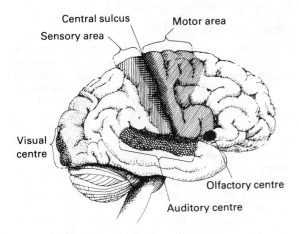

Figure 21.5 Major centres of the cerebrum.

The cerebral cortex is a highly specialized area whose functions are not precisely understood at present. It is known to have an essential role in consciousness, mental ability, and memory. Some texts refer to the cerebral cortex as the neocortex in the belief that it appeared fairly late in vertebrate evolution.

The cerebral cortex of each hemisphere is made up of primary sensory areas or centres, primary motor areas or centres and association areas. Primary *sensory areas* are receptive areas for incoming impulses. Primary *motor areas* are concerned with dispatching outgoing impulses to prompt action responses in peripheral structures (Figure 21.5).

Association areas, which are areas that do not perform primary functions, lie around the sensory and motor areas. They occupy the greater portion of the cortex and have multiple connections with the sensory and motor centres. The functions of the association areas are somewhat general but nevertheless are very important. Functional loss of sensory association areas greatly diminishes the ability of the brain to analyse characteristics of sensory experience, to give them meaning and make decisions as to appropriate responses. Responses involving storage of perception in memory or stimulation of motor centres to bring about body movement or speech could be adversely affected.

The primary sensory and motor centres occupy certain areas of the cerebral cortex and perform highly specialized functions. The motor area that initiates all

voluntary movements of the body occupies the strip of the frontal lobe immediately anterior to the central fissure. In general, the motor area in one hemisphere controls the movements on the opposite side of the body. The various muscles are spatially represented on the motor strip so that the feet are located in the area of the longitudinal fissure and the muscles of chewing are located at the opposite end of the motor strip. The size of the cortical area representing the body parts is proportional to the complexity and functional importance of the part. This is shown diagramatically in Figure 21.6. The area anterior to the primary motor area is known as the *premotor* or *secondary motor* area. It is believed to be concerned with control and co-ordination of skilled movements of a complex nature. It has direct connections with the primary motor area and lower levels of the brain.

The sensory impulses that enter the cerebral cortex are transmitted to specific areas of the cortex, depending on their origin. Impulses concerned with the *somataesthetic senses* such as touch, pressure, temperature, pain and the sense of body position and its parts are transmitted to the parietal lobe immediately posterior to the central fissure. As with the motor areas, sensations from the lower part of the body are received at the medial portion lying within the longitudinal fissure. Impulses from the head are received at the lower part of the strip. Sensations originating in the right side of the body are transmitted to the left hemisphere and those originating in the left side are received in the right hemisphere.

The primary receptive area for vision is located in the posterior part of the occipital lobe. The *visual centre* in the right occipital lobe receives impulses from the right half of the retina of each eye and, conversely, the left cerebral visual centre receives impulses from the left half of each eye. Visual association areas are immediately anterior to the primary receptive area for vision. With destruction of the visual association area, the person can clearly see objects but will be unable to recognize or identify them. This disability is known as *visual agnosia*.

The *primary auditory receptive areas* or *centres for hearing* are located in the superior parts of the temporal lobes. Impulses from both ears are received in both the right and left auditory centres. The auditory association area occupies a part of the temporal lobe immediately below the primary areas. It is known as Wernicke's area. Damage to Wernicke's area results in receptive *aphasia*. This means that the person hears words but they are not meaningful. The person would be able to speak but because of comprehension failure would make errors in speech content. The *olfactory sense* or *sense of smell* is also represented in the temporal lobes.

At the junction of the lateral fissure where temporal, parietal, and occipital lobes meet is a very important area called the *interpretive area*. This area provides an integration of the somatic, auditory, and visual association areas, and plays the greatest role of any area of the cerebral cortex. Any destruction of tissue in this area will result in impaired intellectual ability.

The frontal lobes contain the motor area described above. Other areas in the frontal lobes are the premotor

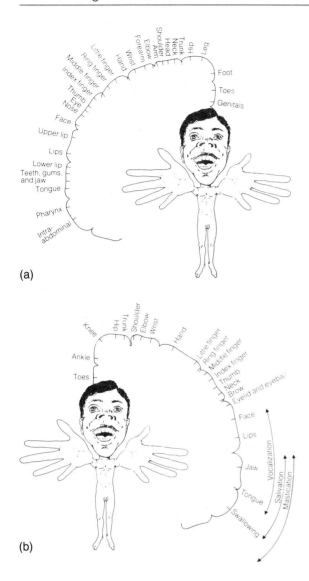

(a)

(b)

Figure 21.6 (a) Sensory homunculus. (b) Motor homunculus. Reproduced from Penfield W & Rasmussen T (1950) *The Cerebral Cortex of Man.* New York: Macmillan, with permission.

cortex, the prefrontal areas, and Broca's area. The premotor cortex is also known as the motor association or secondary motor area. It plays a role in the activities of several cranial nerves. The prefrontal areas of the frontal lobe provide additional cortical area for cerebral function. They are concerned with memory and ability to concentrate, and ability to think in abstract terms. They are also concerned with personality, emotional reactions, initiative and sense of responsibility for socially acceptable standards. *Broca's area* is categorized as an association area because it aids in the formulation of words. Injury to this area results in the inability of the person to speak in sentences; the vocabulary is limited to 'yes' and 'no'.

Beneath the grey cerebral cortex, the cerebrum is mainly composed of white matter. Myelinated neuronal processes are arranged in functionally related bundles called tracts. These are classified as commissural, asociation, and projection tracts. The *commissural tracts* transmit impulses between the two hemispheres. The *association tracts* carry impulses from one area of the cortex to another in the same hemisphere. *Projection tracts* are ascending and descending pathways from one level of the central nervous system to another. One of the most important of these is the internal capsule. The *internal capsule* is a massive bundle of efferent and afferent nerve fibres that connect the various subdivisions of the brain and spinal cord.

BASAL GANGLIA (NUCLEI)

Basal ganglia are groups of nerve cell bodies deeply embedded within the white matter of each cerebral hemisphere. Anatomically, they are very complex. Physiologically, the parts include four main nuclei. These are the *lenticular nucleus* (composed of the globus pallidus and putamen), the *caudate nucleus*, the *amygdaloid body*, and the *claustrum*. The lenticular nucleus and the caudate nuclei are collectively called the *corpus striatum* (striate body). Major portions of the thalamus, reticular formation, and red nuclei (pigmented grey matter) operate in close association with these and are part of the basal ganglia system for motor control.

The functions of the basal ganglia are complex and not clearly understood. The system actually operates, along with the motor cortex and cerebellum, as a total unit, and individual functions cannot be ascribed solely to the various parts of the system. One of the general functions of the basal ganglia is inhibition of muscle tone throughout the body. With widespread destruction of this system, muscle rigidity occurs throughout the body. The resultant phenomenon is known as *decerebrate rigidity* (also termed *spastic extension*). The corpus striatum helps to control gross intentional movements which are normally performed unconsciously. It is believed that the principal function of the globus pallidus (see above) is to provide background muscle tone for intended movements.

THALAMI

The thalami are a pair of egg-shaped masses of grey matter at the base of each hemisphere. Each mass is referred to as a thalamus and forms part of the lateral walls of the third ventricle. The thalami form the main relay centre for sensory impulses and cerebellar and basal ganglia projections to the cerebral cortex. Impulses are 'sorted' in the thalami and forwarded to appropriate cerebral cortical areas. *Encephalins and endorphins* (compounds with morphine-like action) have been found in some nuclei of the thalami. It is believed that these substances have a role in pain relief (see Chapter 9).

HYPOTHALAMUS

This is an important grey mass which lies beneath the

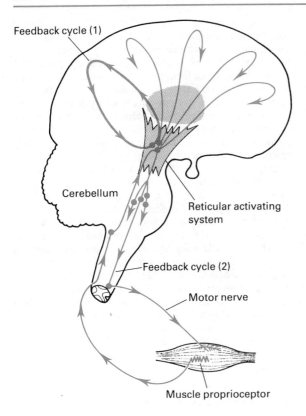

Feedback cycle (1)

Cerebellum

Reticular activating system

Feedback cycle (2)

Motor nerve

Muscle proprioceptor

Figure 21.7 Feedback mechanisms of the reticular activating system (RAS). 1, Impulses carried to the cerebral cortex and back to the RAS; 2, impulses to peripheral muscles and back to the RAS.

thalamus. It forms the floor and part of the wall of the third ventricle. It contains nuclei of the autonomic nervous system for the control of most of the body's involuntary functions as well as many aspects of emotional behaviour. There are neuronal links between the hypothalamus and the posterior pituitary gland. The hypothalamus exerts a control on vasomotor tone and heart rate. It is concerned with regulation of body temperature, and it regulates body water. Body water regulation is achieved by creating the sensation of thirst and by controlling the excretion of water in the urine. Neurones in the hypothalamus serve as osmoreceptors (cells sensitive to changes in osmotic pressure of body fluid) and regulate the production and release of the antidiuretic hormone (ADH), which plays an important role in maintaining or restoring body fluid balance. ADH causes reabsorption of water in the kidneys, thereby decreasing water loss in the urine. The hypothalamus is also concerned with gastrointestinal and feeding regulation. Hunger centres and a satiety centre have been identified in this grey mass. In addition, it activates feeding reflexes such as licking the lips and swallowing. The cells of certain hypothalamic nuclei secrete the hormone oxytocin which is concerned with uterine contraction and with the expulsion of breast milk for infant feeding. The hypothalamus also plays an important role in the secretion of hormones by the anterior

pituitary gland. It is also known to affect responses such as pleasure and fear. Endorphins, which are believed to function as excitatory transmitters that activate portions of the brain's analgesic system, have been found in abundance in the hypothalamus.

BRAIN STEM

The brain stem is composed of the pons varolii and the medulla oblongata, although the midbrain may be considered as the upper part. The *pons varolii* is located between the midbrain and medulla. It consists of numerous tracts which link various parts of the brain and serve as conduction pathways. The pons also contains portions of the reticular formation and groups of neurones (nuclei) which give rise to cranial nerves V–VIII (inclusive).

The *medulla oblongata* lies between the pons and the spinal cord. It is composed of ascending and descending conduction pathways. Autonomic centres that regulate such vital functions as breathing, cardiac rate and vasomotor tone as well as centres for vomiting, gagging, coughing and sneezing reflex behaviours are located in the medulla. Cranial nerves IX–XII have their cell bodies in this area.

Reticular formation (reticular activating system, RAS)

This is a diffuse system of motor and sensory fibres and nerve cells which forms the central core of the brain stem (Figure 21.7). It has widespread afferent connections, receiving sensory impulses from all over the body. The cerebral cortex can stimulate this system. The actual function of the RAS continues to be the subject of research and speculation. However, it is known to be associated with initiation and maintenance of wakefulness and alertness which make perception possible. The neurones of this area learn to be selective, making judgements as to whether the cortex should be alerted or not. For example, a mother may sleep through hearing traffic noise but she is aroused by the slightest whimper from her infant. When specific areas of the reticular formation are damaged severely, as occurs in diseases such as encephalitis lethargica (sleeping sickness), or when a brain tumour develops in this region or serious haemorrhage occurs, the person becomes comatose and is resistant to normal awakening stimuli.

Consciousness

Consciousness may be defined as the complete awareness of self and environment, with appropriate responsiveness to stimuli. It is a dynamic experience involving a series of different elements whose relationship changes incessantly. The precise limits are hard to define as consciousness is inferred from a person's appearance and behaviour.

Two physiological components affect conscious behaviour. These are *content* and *arousal*. Mental activities involve the contents of sensation, perception, attention, memory and volition. Analysis and synthesis of information, along with emotional implications, also occur. The *content* aspects generally refer to those mental functions carried out in the cerebral cortex. The *arousal* aspects are reflected in the person's appearance of wakefulness. Cognitive functions are not possible without some degree of arousal. Arousal can exist without the emotional and thinking components of content.

The system of consciousness is driven by an arousal mechanism. Full consciousness depends upon the interaction between the cerebral cortex and the reticular activating system. This is a mesh-like network of undifferentiated neurones located throughout the central portion of the brain stem. These neurones receive collateral nerve fibres from all sensory pathways that enter the brain via the upper spinal cord or cranial nerves. It has been demonstrated that if the sensory pathways are blocked impulses travel by the collaterals to the reticular activating system then to the thalamus and on to innervate the cortex. This activation of the cortex produces a state of alertness. Further, it has been postulated that impulses are conducted via a feedback loop back to the reticular activating system, which in turn stimulates the cortex. This continuous circuitry of arousal maintains the state of readiness of the cortex to receive and interpret incoming sensory impulses. A further function of the reticular activating system is to screen and modulate incoming messages so that the cortex is able to process significant information.

Sleep

Normal sleep is a periodic depression of the physiological function of the parts of the brain concerned with consciousness from which a person can be aroused to awareness. Sleep occurs in two ways: first, as a result of decreased activity in the reticular activating system, which produces slow-wave or normal sleep. This is a restful type of sleep during which the respiratory and pulse rates and blood pressure fall, the pupils constrict and react more slowly to light, the eyes deviate upwards and tendon reflexes are abolished.

The second way by which sleep occurs results from the abnormal channelling of brain signals and is referred to as paradoxical or desynchronized sleep. Short episodes of paradoxical sleep usually occur about every 90 minutes throughout a night. Heart and respiratory rates and blood pressure alter; cerebral blood flow increases, clonic jerks may occur and rapid eye movements (REM) take place. Most dreams occur during paradoxical sleep.

During normal sleep, activity of the reticular activating system is decreased, while in paradoxical sleep some cerebral areas are active while others are suppressed.

During sleep a person may be easily aroused to wakefulness or consciousness by cerebral arousal through stimuli such as pain or unaccustomed noise. The return to wakefulness shows that the reticular activating system is still functioning and capable of screening and discrimination.

CEREBELLUM

This part of the brain lies beneath the posterior portion of the cerebrum, posterior to the pons and medulla. It is separated from the cerebrum by a fold of meningeal membrane (dura mater) called the tentorium cerebelli. Three pairs of cerebellar peduncles attach the cerebellum to the midbrain, pons and medulla. These peduncles receive direct input from the spinal cord and brain stem and convey it to the deep cerebellar nuclei and cerebral cortex. The result is both an excitatory and inhibitory influence on the cerebellar nuclei, with a predominance of excitatory influences. An excitatory effect on the brain stem and on the thalamic nuclei maintains a tonic discharge to the motor system.

The cerebellum is integrated into many connective pathways throughout the brain for the provision of muscle co-ordination in the body. All sensations are relayed through the cerebellum, thus providing information about muscle activity. For example, afferent impulses are delivered to the cerebellum from the labyrinth of each internal ear. These impulses prompt reflex muscle responses to maintain balance of position or postural equilibrium. The functions of the cerebellum are essentially to control fine movements and balance, to control co-ordination of movement, and maintain feedback loops to correct movement, and to co-ordinate the action of muscle groups. Dysfunction of the cerebellum can result in gait disturbance, equilibrium ataxia (overstability or understability), and tremors.

BLOOD SUPPLY TO THE BRAIN

The ever-active brain receives about one fifth of the blood pumped by the heart and it consumes about 20% of the oxygen utilized by the body. Approximately 800 ml of blood flows through the brain each minute, with 75 ml present in the brain at any given time. The brain requires a continuous flow of blood since it can store only minute quantities of glucose and oxygen and derives its energy almost exclusively from the metabolism of glucose delivered by the blood. Its blood requirement is the same whether one is mentally active or sleeping.

Brain cells are extremely sensitive to hypoxia, particularly those of the cerebral cortex. Interruption of blood supply to the brain produces loss of consciousness in seconds. Irreversible brain damage occurs if the blood supply is interrupted for 2–4 minutes. Brain stem neurones are less sensitive to hypoxia than cortical cells; individuals experiencing prolonged hypoxia may survive because the vital centres in the medulla are more resistant and recover, but irreversible cortical damage persists, resulting in mental deficiency.

Various built-in protective mechanisms of the brain act to increase blood flow and nutrient supply when the need arises. These mechanisms include arterial anastomoses and autoregulatory mechanisms which: (1) increase cerebral blood flow even in profound hypotension; and (2) help to extract greater amounts of glucose and oxygen from perfusing blood. Even after other organs are deprived of blood and can no longer function, blood flow within the brain may remain near normal levels. Factors which affect cerebral blood flow include arterial and venous blood pressure at brain level, conditions of the vessels (e.g. atherosclerosis),

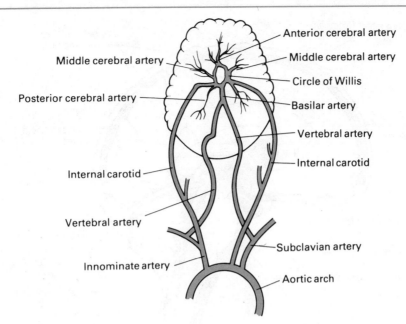

Figure 21.8 Blood supply to the brain.

intracranial pressure, viscosity of the blood, and, to a lesser extent, constriction and dilatation of cerebral vessels.

The arterial blood supply to the brain is derived from *two internal carotid arteries* and *two vertebral arteries* (Figure 21.8). The vertebral arteries originate from the subclavian arteries and unite at the junction of the pons and medulla to form the *basilar artery*. The basilar artery continues to the midbrain level where it divides to form the paired posterior cerebral arteries. In general, the vertebral arteries and their branches (posterior cerebral arteries) supply blood to the lower third of the diencephalon (thalamus and hypothalamus), the cerebellum, and the occipital region of the cerebral hemispheres. The internal carotid arteries arise from two different vessels. The left common carotid artery originates in the aorta directly while the right common carotid artery arises from the innominate artery which originates in the aorta. The common carotid arteries branch to form the external and internal carotid arteries. The internal carotid arteries supply blood, via the anterior and middle cerebral arteries, to most of the hemispheres excluding the occipital lobes, the basal ganglia, and the upper two thirds of the diencephalon.

Although the vertebral basilar arterial tree and the internal carotid arterial tree are essentially independent, some anastomotic connections between the two systems exist. Small posterior communicating arteries connect the two systems to form an arterial crown known as the cerebral arterial *circle of Willis*. The anterior communicating artery which connects the two anterior cerebral arteries completes the circle. It allows an adequate blood supply to reach all parts of the brain even after one or more of the four supplying vessels is obstructed.

The veins draining the brain stem and cerebellum follow the arteries to these structures. Veins draining the cerebrum have short, stocky branches which come off at angles and drain into superficial venous plexuses and the *dural sinuses*. Dural (venous) sinuses are valveless channels located between two layers of dura mater. Most venous blood drains into the internal jugular veins at the base of the skull.

Blood–brain barrier

This is a unique relationship between the capillary walls in the brain and the glial cells. It is believed that the blood–brain barrier limits entry of substances, which may be harmful, into the extracellular space of the brain around the neurones. This barrier phenomenon effectively keeps micro-organisms out of the brain. However, it is equally effective in keeping most antibiotics out, thus complicating therapy for intracranial infections. The brain cells of infants, particularly if premature, are readily permeable to some substances (e.g. bilirubin, radioactive phosphorus) that are prevented from reaching the neurones when the glial cells are mature or fully developed. Techniques for reversibly opening the blood–brain barrier and the synthesis of therapeutic agents that can cross the barrier are areas that are currently under study.

VENTRICLES AND CEREBROSPINAL FLUID

The ventricular system is a series of cavities within the brain (Figure 21.9). Each cerebral hemisphere contains a *lateral ventricle*, each of which communicates with the *third ventricle* by means of an intraventricular foramen (foramen of Monro). The third ventricle is a slit-like space between the thalami and it is continuous with the fourth ventricle through a narrow channel called the

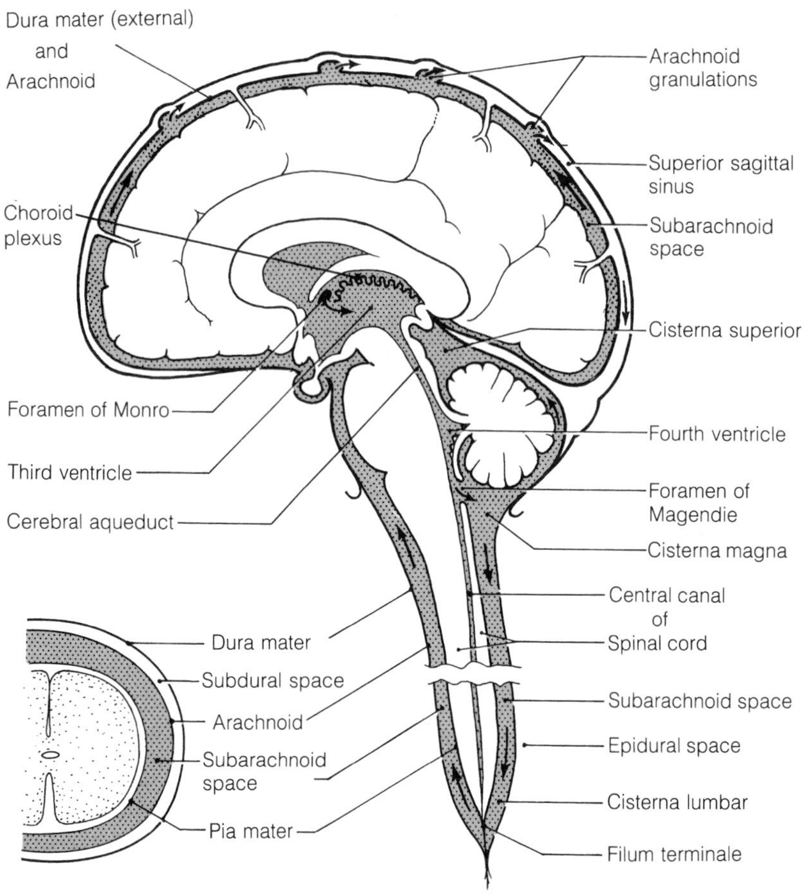

Figure 21.9 Path of flow of cerebrospinal fluid. Based on an illustration by R.J. Demarest in Noback CR (1967) *The Human Nervous System.* New York: McGraw-Hill.

cerebral aqueduct (aqueduct of Sylvius). The *fourth ventricle* is located between the pons and the cerebellum and is continuous with the subarachnoid space (see Meninges) and with the central canal of the medulla and the spinal cord. The medial opening of the fourth ventricle, allows cerebrospinal fluid (CSF) to circulate around the cord. Two lateral openings channel fluid around the brain. This distribution of CSF provides a protective cushion for the brain and cord.

The ventricular system is lined by ependyma (see p. 684) and is filled with CSF. Each ventricle contains a *choroid plexus* which is a rich network of blood vessels covered by a layer of ependymal cells which constantly secrete CSF. The CSF is a clear, colourless, water-like fluid with a specific gravity of 1.007. It contains occasional lymphocytes and traces of the minerals and organic materials found in blood. The glucose concentration is normally 2.8–4.5 mmol/l and protein concentration is 0.1–0.4 g/l at the lumbar level. The total volume of CSF in the adult ranges from 125 to 150 ml. Normal pressure is 40–180 mmH$_2$O.

The CSF circulates through the ventricular system and around the brain and cord in the subarachnoid space. It is steadily reabsorbed into the *arachnoid villi*, which are projections from the subarachnoid space into the venous sinuses of the brain. Any interruption within the CSF circuit, such as occurs with a congenital absence of openings between the fourth ventricle and subarachnoid space, results in an excessive accumulation of fluid within the ventricles. The condition is referred to as hydrocephalus. The brain tissue becomes compressed between the skull and the expanding volume of fluid.

MENINGES

The soft brain and spinal cord are surrounded by three layers of connective tissue membranes known as the meninges. The three meninges from the outermost layer inward, are the dura mater, the arachnoid mater, and the pia mater. The *dura mater* is a thick, tough, inelastic, collagenous double membrane. One layer of the dura is attached to the skull while another is adjacent to the arachnoid. Two potential spaces associated with the dura are the epidural (or extradural space) and the

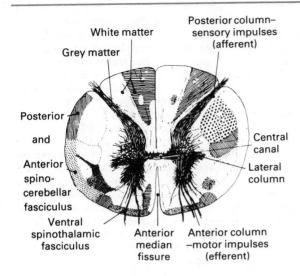

Figure 21.10 Cross-section of the spinal cord.

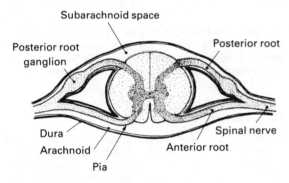

Figure 21.11 The spinal nerve: its posterior root ganglion, posterior root and anterior root.

subdural space. *Epidural space* refers to the potential space between the cranium and the periosteal layer of the dura. *Subdural space* describes the potential space between the dura and the arachnoid, and is said to contain a thin film of fluid. However, recent electron-microscopic findings indicate that when the dura and arachnoid appear to separate, the separation actually occurs within the innermost cellular layer of the dura. In several places the inner dural layer is reflected as sheet-like protrusions into the cranial cavity. These are called dural septa. The principal dural septa are the *falx cerebri* between the two hemispheres, and the *tentorium cerebelli* between the cerebral hemispheres and the cerebellum. The tentorium cerebelli separates the superior surface of the cerebellum from the occipital lobes, defining the *supratentorial* and *infratentorial cranial compartments*. The opening in the tentorium through which the brain stem passes is known as the *tentorial notch* or *tentorial incisura*. This notch is of clinical significance when intracranial pressure increases.

The *arachnoid* ('spider-web-like') is a thin, avascular, delicate membrane. It conforms to the general shape of

the brain. A subarachnoid space, filled with CSF, is located between the arachnoid and pia mater. Several large spaces referred to as cisterns occur in the subarachnoid space and can be useful radiological landmarks. The *pia mater* ('gentle mother') is a thin, vascular, elastic membrane which adheres closely to the brain and spinal cord, following every sulcus and gyrus. The choroid plexuses arise from the vascular structure of the pia mater. The arachnoid and pia mater are sometimes collectively referred to as the *leptomeninges*.

SPINAL CORD

The spinal cord is long, cylindrical structure of grey and white matter within the vertebral column. It is continuous with the medulla oblongata, originating at the foramen magnum of the skull and extending to the first or second lumbar vertebrae. It tapers off into a fine, non-neural cord called the *canda iguina* which continues inferiorly (caudally) to its attachments in the coccyx. A small canal (central canal) extends the full length of the cord. It contains CSF, and the upper end opens into the fourth ventricle. The cord is surrounded by the three meninges which are continuous with those encapsulating the brain. The meninges extend to the level of the fifth lumbar vertebra.

The grey matter (cell bodies) in the spinal cord is concentrated in its interior, roughly in the form of an H. White matter, composed of nerve tracts and fibres, surrounds the H-shaped grey matter (Figure 21.10). Afferent impulses are received by neurones in the posterior columns or horns of grey matter. Efferent impulses are discharged by neurones in the anterior columns or horns of the grey matter. The grey matter also contains neurones which may transmit impulses from one lateral half of the cord to the other, from posterior to anterior and to other levels of the CNS.

Nerve fibres emerge from the spinal cord in uninterrupted series of posterior (sensory or afferent) and anterior (motor or efferent) rootlets which unite to form 31 pairs of posterior and anterior roots. In the area of an intervertebral foramen, a posterior and an anterior root meet to form a *spinal nerve* (Figure 21.11) which supplies innervation to a segment of the body. The cord has two enlargements: cervical and lumbar. The cervical enlargement (plexus) is associated with nerve roots which innervate the upper limbs, and the lumbar enlargement (plexus) innervates the lower limbs.

The spinal cord has three major functions: (1) It carries impulses via sensory nerves through ascending tracts up to the brain. (2) It carries impulses from the brain via motor nerves through descending tracts to nerves supplying effector organs (muscle and glands). (3) It functions as a centre for reflex actions (see p. 700).

NERVES AND TRACTS

Nerves are bundles of neuronal processes which extend beyond the CNS, while tracts are bundles of processes within the CNS. Nerves consisting only of afferent fibres, which transmit impulses from the periphery to the CNS, are called *sensory nerves*. *Motor nerves* are composed entirely of efferent fibres, which transmit impulses from the CNS out into the periphery. Many nerves, for example, all spinal nerves, contain both efferent and afferent fibres and are known as *mixed nerves*.

Structurally, three types of nerve fibres or processes occur. One type known as a medullated or myelinated fibre is enclosed in a lipoprotein sheath (myelin) and an outer membranous sheath called the *neurilemma* (sheath of Schwann). Another type has no myelin sheath but does have a neurilemma and is referred to as a non-myelinated or non-medullated fibre. Most non-myelinated fibres belong to the autonomic nervous system, which is concerned with visceral activity. A third type of neuronal process has a myelin sheath but lacks the neurilemma. All fibres within the CNS, as well as the optic and auditory nerves, are of this type. Neuronal processes lacking the neurilemma cannot regenerate following injury.

Nerve tracts transmit impulses that are usually similar in origin, termination and function. The origin and destination may be determined from the name of the tract. For example, the corticospinal tract carries impulses originating in the cerebral cortex to the spinal cord; the spinothalamic tract transmits sensory impulses from the spinal cord to the thalamus.

NERVE REGENERATION

Unlike most cells in the body, the adult nerve cells cannot reproduce by mitosis to replace any that are destroyed. Some, however, can respond to injury by reconstitution. If a nerve fibre's connection with its cell body is interrupted, the fragment distal to the cell body ceases to function and degenerates. If a neurilemma sheath is present however, the fibre may regenerate and restore function. Nerve fibres within the CNS have no neurilemma and cannot regenerate to re-establish function. If research could solve this problem many tragic effects of stroke or trauma of the CNS could be relieved. Spinal cord reconstruction has been attempted in recent years.

When a fibre with a neurilemma is damaged, the fragment distal to the nerve cell body disintegrates and the debris is removed by phagocytic glial cells. The neurilemma (Schwann cells in the proximal end near the interruption and in the distal stump, divide mitotically to form continuous cords of neurilemma cells. The distal ends of the proximal axons branch into numerous sprouts which grow into the interruption and distal stump along neurilemmal cords which guide them to the sites of the nerve endings. This is a slow process. Non-myelinated fibres regenerate more rapidly than those that must form a myelin sheath.

Interruption of a peripheral nerve is followed by loss of sensation and movement in the part served by the affected nerve. If the two cut ends of the nerve are approximated and sutured, less scar tissue forms, favouring the regeneration process. Occasionally, because of fibrous scar tissue, a branch or bud of viable fibre stump may not find its way into the 'tube' of Schwann cells which is essential to the growing fibres. In such an instance, multiple growing tips may be produced by the fibre stump and may form a small mass referred to as a neuroma.

Peripheral Nervous System

The peripheral nervous system is composed of nerves and ganglia. The nerves may be divided into two main groups, *cranial* and *spinal* nerves, according to whether they emerge from the central nervous system at the cranial or spinal level.

CRANIAL NERVES

There are 12 pairs of cranial nerves that are considered to be part of the peripheral nervous system. They emerge from the undersurface of the brain and are numbered according to the sequence in which they arise from the front to back. For example, the first cranial nerve is located most anteriorly in the frontal lobe, and the twelfth is located most posteriorly in the medulla. Cranial nerves are also named according to their function or distribution. Some of the cranial nerves consist mainly of afferent (motor fibres), three are comprised of afferent (sensory) fibres, and others are made up of both motor and sensory fibres and are

Table 21.1   Origin and functions of the cranial nerves (12 pairs).

Number	Name	Origin of main nerve fibres	Function
I	Olfactory	Sensory fibres: neurones in nasal mucosa	Olfactory sense (sense of smell)
II	Optic	Sensory fibres: neurones of retina	Vision
III	Oculomotor	Motor fibres:* nucleus in midbrain	Movements of the eyeball and upper eyelid: size of the pupil of iris (i.e. constriction and dilatation of pupil to regulate amount of light admitted): control of ciliary muscle to regulate degree of refraction by the lens

Table 21.1 *Continued*

Number	Name	Origin of main nerve fibres	Function
IV	Trochlear	Motor fibres: nucleus in midbrain	Movement of eyeball by superior oblique muscles
V	Trigeminal	Motor fibres: nucleus in pons	Motor function: mastication
	Largest cranial nerve has three sensory divisions: ophthalmic, maxillary, mandibular	Sensory fibres: gasserian or semilunar ganglion in temporal bone	Sensory function: sensations (pain, touch, temperature) of the face, nose, teeth and mouth
VI	Abducens	Motor fibres: nucleus in pons	Movement of the eyeball by lateral rectus muscle
VII	Facial	Motor fibres: nucleus in pons	Motor function: contraction of facial and scalp muscles (facial expression); secretion of saliva by submaxillary and sublingual glands
		Sensory fibres: geniculate ganglion in temporal bone	Sensory function: taste (from anterior two-thirds of tongue)
VIII	Auditory (acoustic) Has two divisions: vestibular cochlear	Sensory fibres: vesticular branch: vestibular ganglion in internal ear cochlear branch: spiral ganglion in internal ear	Sensory function: vestibular branch: equilibrium (position, balance) cochlear division: sense of hearing
IX	Glossopharyngeal	Motor fibres: nucleus in medulla	Motor function: swallowing reflex, control of blood pressure through connection with carotid baroreceptors: salivary secretion by parotid glands
		Sensory fibres: jugular and petrous ganglia	Sensory functions: taste and oral and pharyngeal sensations
X	Vagus Has very wide distribution	Motor fibres: nuclei in medulla	Motor function: muscles of pharynx, larynx, thoracic and abdominal viscera (e.g. regulates gastrointestinal motility of peristalsis; influences cardiac rate); secretion by gastric, intestinal and pancreatic glands
		Sensory fibres: jugular and nodosa ganglia	Sensory function: sensations in pharynx, larynx, and thoracic and abdominal viscera
XI	Accessory	Motor fibres: nucleus in medulla and the spinal cord	Movement of shoulder and head by trapezius and sternocleidomastoid muscles
XII	Hypoglossal	Motor fibres: nucleus in medulla	Movements of the tongue

* Most motor nerves are considered to also contain some sensory fibres by which information as to the existing conditions in the muscles concerned (proprioceptive data) is transmitted into the central nervous system. The proprioceptive impulses result in appropriate motor responses to facilitate the required pattern of movement.

referred to as mixed nerves. Cell bodies of the motor fibres form nuclei within the brain stem. With the exception of the olfactory nerves and the optic nerve, sensory fibres originate in ganglia (groups of cell bodies outside the CNS). Olfactory fibres originate in the nasal mucosa and optic fibres arise from the retina of the eyeball. The origin and functions of cranial nerves are described in Table 21.1.

SPINAL NERVES

Thirty-one pairs of nerves arise from the spinal cord. The are numbered and named according to the order in which they arise and the vertebral level at which they emerge. There are *eight cervical, twelve thoracic, five lumbar, five sacral pairs* and *one coccygeal pair.*

All spinal nerves are mixed (sensory and motor) and

each one has two origins which are referred to as anterior and posterior roots (Figure 21.11). The anterior roots carry two types of motor fibres: (1) the *general somatic efferent fibres* which have axons originating from lower motor neurones (anterior horn cells in the spinal cord) and which innervate voluntary striated muscles; and (2) the *general visceral efferent fibres* (autonomic nerves) which innervate visceral and cardiac muscle, and regulate glandular secretions. The posterior roots convey sensory input via two types of sensory fibres: (1) the *general somatic afferent* fibres which carry impulses for pain, temperature, touch, and proprioception from the body wall, tendons, and joints into the central nervous system; and (2) *general visceral afferent fibres* which carry sensory impulses from the viscera into the central nervous system.

After emerging from the vertebral canal, each spinal nerve divides into two major branches: the anterior and posterior rami. The *posterior rami* divide into smaller branches which go directly to the muscles and skin of the posterior portions of the head, neck and trunk. The *anterior rami* supply all the structures of the extremities and lateral and anterior portions of the trunk.

The branches of the anterior rami tend to form intricate networks of interlacing nerve branches before proceding to the structures they innervate. These networks are referred to as *plexuses*. Spinal nerves lose their individuality after passing through a plexus and they emerge as peripheral nerves. Four major plexuses are formed by the anterior rami of spinal nerves: the cervical, brachial, lumbar and sacral plexuses. The *cervical plexus* gives rise to peripheral nerve branches that innervate muscles of the neck and shoulders. It also gives rise to the phrenic nerve which supplies the diaphragm. Important peripheral nerves which arise from the *brachial plexus* are the musculocutaneous, median, radial and ulnar nerves, all of which supply the upper limbs. The *lumbar plexus* generates the femoral, saphenous and obturator nerves which innervate the lower abdominal wall, external genitalia, and parts of the thigh and leg. The nerves leaving the *sacral plexus* supply the buttocks, perineum and lower extremities. The most important nerve derived from this plexus is the sciatic, the longest and largest nerve in the body.

GANGLIA

A ganglion is a group of nerve cell bodies located outside the CNS. Many important drugs known as ganglion blocking agents exert their effects by inhibiting impulse transmission in this area.

The ganglia which form the posterior or sensory roots of the spinal nerves lie just outside the spinal cord within the vertebral column. These are the spinal or posterior root ganglia.

The ganglia associated with the autonomic (visceral) nervous system may be divided into three groups according to their location. The vertebral, sympathetic, or lateral ganglia occur in two chains. One chain of 22 ganglia lies on each side of the vertebral column. A second group of autonomic ganglia is called the collateral or paravertebral ganglia. These lie in front of the vertebral column and close to large arteries from

which they are named (e.g. iliac, mesenteric). A third group is referred to as the terminal ganglia. They lie close to or within the viscera which the nerve fibres supply.

AUTONOMIC NERVOUS SYSTEM

The autonomic nervous system controls the visceral functions of the body. This system helps to control such phenomena as arterial blood pressure, gastrointestinal motility and secretion, urinary bladder emptying, sweating and body temperature. It carries only efferent impulses and the responses are involuntary.

The autonomic system is largely activated by centres located in the spinal cord, brain stem and hypothalamus. In addition, parts of the cerebral cortex can transmit impulses to the lower centres and in this way influence the autonomic system. For example, chronic emotional stress can result in excessive stimulation of the autonomic system, which in turn may contribute to the development of gastric or duodenal ulcers or other stress-related problems. Often, the autonomic system operates by means of visceral reflexes. That is, sensory signals enter the centres in the CNS and these in turn transmit appropriate reflex responses back to the organs via the autonomic system to control their activities.

The autonomic nervous system is divided into the *parasympathetic* and *sympathetic* systems. Most viscera have a nerve supply from each division; impulses delivered from one system excite visceral activity, and those originating with the other division inhibit activity (Table 21.2).

PARASYMPATHETIC NERVOUS SYSTEM

The parasympathetic fibres leave the CNS through several cranial nerves (75% are in the vagus nerve) and through the pelvic nerves. For this reason, the system may also be referred to as the craniosacral division. This system has both preganglionic and postganglionic fibres. With only a few exceptions, the preganglionic fibres pass uninterrupted to the ganglia which are located within or close to the viscera they innervate. Postganglionic fibres of this division are short and are located within the respective organs (Figure 21.12).

The responses to parasympathetic stimulation are localized and specific for parts of the body.

Generally, parasympathetic innervation promotes a normal state; it is concerned with the restoration and conservation of body energy and elimination of body wastes (Table 21.2).

SYMPATHETIC NERVOUS SYSTEM

The sympathetic nerves originate in the thoracic and lumbar regions of the spinal cord. The sympathetic nerves leave the spinal cord via the anterior roots and form the white communicating rami of the thoracic and lumbar nerves. Through these, nerves reach the trunk ganglia of the sympathetic chain. Upon entering the chain, these preganglionic fibres may synapse with a host of ganglion cells, pass up or down the sympathetic

Table 21.2 Autonomic effects on various organs of the body.

Organ	Effect of sympathetic stimulation	Effect of parasympathetic stimulation
Eye: Pupil	Dilated	Constricted
Ciliary muscle	Slight relaxation	Contracted
Glands: Nasal	Vasoconstriction and slight secretion	Stimulation of thin, copious secretion (containing many enzymes for enzyme-secreting glands)
Lacrimal		
Parotid		
Submaxillary		
Gastric		
Pancreatic		
Sweat glands	Copious sweating (cholinergic)	None
Apocrine glands	Thick, odoriferous secretion	None
Heart: Muscle	Increased rate	Slowed rate
	Increased force of contraction	Decreased force of atrial contraction
Coronary arteries	Dilated (β_2): constricted (α)	Dilated
Lungs: Bronchi	Dilated	Constricted
Blood vessels	Mildly constricted	Dilated
Gut: Lumen	Decreased peristalsis and tone	Increased peristalsis and tone
Sphincter	Increased tone	Relaxed
Liver	Glucose released	slight glycogen synthesis
Gallbladder and bile ducts	Relaxed	Constricted
Kidney	Decreased output	None
Bladder: Detrusor muscle	Relaxed	Excited
Trigone	Excited	Relaxed
Penis	Ejaculation	Erection
Systemic blood vessels:		
Abdominal	Constricted	None
Muscle	Constricted (adrenergic α)	None
	Dilated (adrenergic β)	
	Dilated (cholinergic)	
Skin	Constricted	None
Blood: Coagulation	Increased	None
Glucose	Increased	None
Basal metabolism	Increased up to 100%	None
Adrenal cortical secretion	Increased	None
Mental activity	Increased	None
Piloerector muscles	Excited	None
Skeletal muscle	Increased glycogenolysis	None
	Increased strength	

chain to synapse with ganglion cells at a higher or lower level, or pass through the trunk ganglia and out to the tissues and organs that are innervated by these nerves (Figure 21.13).

The sympathetic system produces generalized physiological responses rather than specific, localized ones. It responds to stress, strong emotions, severe pain, cold, or any threat. The purpose of the responses induced is to mobilize the body's resources for defensive action ('fight or flight') (Table 21.2).

Stimulation of the sympathetic nervous system results in stimulation of the adrenal medullae. Increase in secretion of adrenaline and noradrenaline results, and this augments the body defence responses mediated by the sympathetic nervous system.

Chemical mediators

In both the sympathetic and parasympathetic nervous systems the transmission of impulses from the preganglionic fibres to the ganglia is dependent upon the release of *acetylcholine* by the preganglionic axon terminals. Acetylcholine is rapidly deactivated by *cholinesterase*. The postganglionic fibres of the parasympathetic system also release acetylcholine at their junction with the effector organs to facilitate the transmission of their impulses. The neurotransmitter that is released by the postganglionic nerve terminals in the sympathetic system is *noradrenaline* which is deactivated by enzymes (e.g. monoamine oxidase,) or taken up again by the nerve terminals.

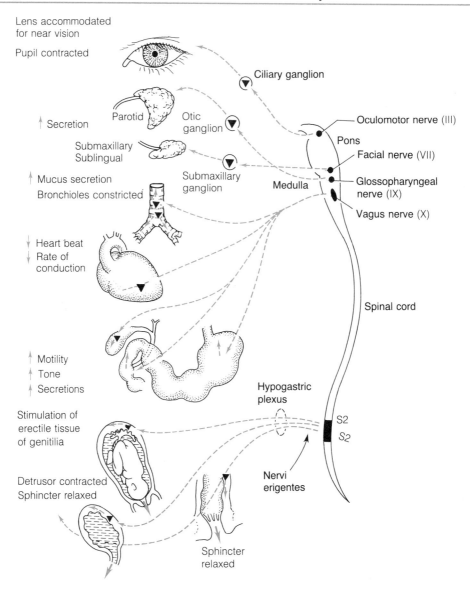

Figure 21.12 Diagram of the parasympathetic division and innervation of some key organs.

Muscle Tissue and Activity

Muscle tissue comprises up to 50% of the total body weight. This tissue performs activities which are critical to survival such as respiration, circulation of the blood, and peristaltic movement of food through the gastrointestinal tract. It is also responsible for movements of body parts as well as the mobility of the body as a whole. The capacity of the body to carry out its vital activities is dependent upon the specialized physiological properties that are unique to muscle tissue (Table 21.3).

During muscle contraction, the chemical reactions which occur liberate both mechanical and heat energy.

The heat energy contributes to the maintenance of body temperature. At rest, most of the body heat is produced by metabolic activities such as occur in the liver.

Muscle cells, because of their elongated shape, may be referred to as muscle fibres. In most muscles, the fibres extend the entire length of the muscle. The cell membrane of the muscle fibre is called *sarcolemma*. Three types of muscle tissue with different types of control are present in the body to meet its need for varying degrees of muscular activity. These are *cardiac*, *smooth (visceral or involuntary)*, and *striated (skeletal or voluntary)* muscle tissue. Cardiac muscle tissue is discussed in Chapter 14.

Smooth muscle tissue is present in walls of blood

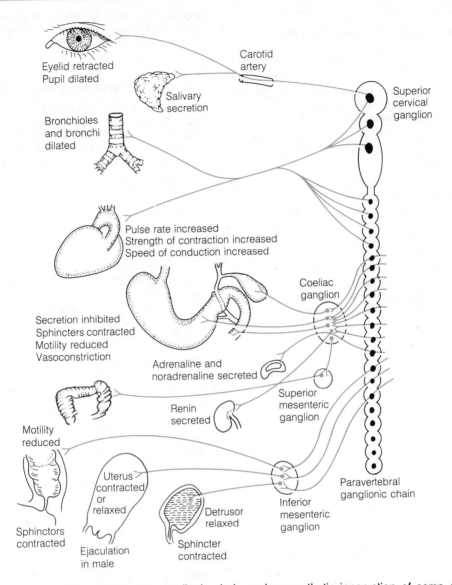

Figure 21.13 Diagram of the sympathetic ganglionic chain and sympathetic innervation of some of the key organs.

vessels and most hollow viscera. The cells are smaller and are arranged in sheets or layers and their sarcolemmae are not as well defined as in skeletal muscle. Smooth muscle has inherent, rhythmic contractile activity and is under autonomic control.

Skeletal muscle tissue forms the muscles which are attached to bones and is responsible for external body movements and the maintenance of position against gravity. It is called striated because of variations in protein concentration which are evident with light microscopy. Its cytoplasm, which may be called *sarcoplasm*, contains hundreds or thousands of myofibrils and its sarcolemma is well defined. Unlike most body cells, each skeletal muscle fibre has several nuclei. A skeletal muscle is composed of both muscle and

connective tissue. Groups of muscle fibres are arranged in bundles (fasciculi) and are held together by connective tissue. Groups of these bundles are bound together and the entire muscle is encased in a tough sheath of connective tissue (epimysium) and may also have a tough fibrous coating, called *fascia*. The muscle sheath contains blood and lymph vessels and nerve fibres. Prolongations of the connective tissues extending beyond the actual muscle fibres form the tendonous attachments to bones. Each skeletal muscle has an *origin*, which is the stationary attachment of muscle to skeleton, and an *insertion*, which is the attachment to the moveable part. When the muscle contracts, the insertion is pulled toward the origin. The thick part of the muscle consisting of the bundles of fibres may be

Table 21.3 Physiological properties of muscle tissue.

Property	Description
Contractility	The shortening and thickening of muscle cells as a result of their ability to convert chemical energy to mechanical energy
Elasticity	The capacity to stretch. The ability to resume original length after a stretching force is removed
Excitability Sensitivity	The capability to respond by contraction to a change in the environment which may be initiated by a nerve impulse, pressure, stretching, chemical changes (e.g. calcium concentration) or temperature changes (e.g. cold stimulates contraction)
Clonus	The sustained partial contraction maintained by groups of muscle cells contracting in relays in response to nerve impulses from the spinal cord. This is a state of readiness for action

referred to as the *body* of the muscle. Individual skeletal muscles are usually named according to action (e.g. flexor or extensor), location or origin.

MOTOR AND SENSORY INNERVATION OF SKELETAL MUSCLES

Contraction of skeletal muscles normally only results from impulses discharged by motor neurones within the CNS and transmitted along peripheral nerve fibres to the muscle. Since the motor centres lie within the cerebral cortex, contractions are usually voluntarily produced. Involuntary contractions occur in the form of reflex responses (see p. 700).

The process whereby a nerve impulse is converted into a muscle action current is referred to as *neuromuscular transmission*. Each nerve fibre terminates at a specialized region of the muscle fibre, called *myoneural* or *neuromuscular function* or *motor end-plate*. The end-plate is a localized specialization of the sarcolemma. Essentially, the release of acetylcholine at the end-plate and its rapid destruction by the enzyme cholinesterase is at the basis of electrical and chemical reactions and the release of mechanical and heat energy in the contraction of muscle fibres.

It has been estimated that at least 40% of nerve fibres innervating a given muscle are sensory rather than motor end-organs. Three major types of end-organs (receptors) that are sensitive to changes in muscle fibres and that initiate impulses which are transmitted by afferent nerve fibres from skeletal muscles to the CNS are known to exist. These are muscle spindles, Golgi bodies and free nerve endings. *Muscle spindles* lie between muscle fibres. They are excited by stretching and are associated with the stretch reflex. *Golgi bodies* are proprioceptors located in tendons and are sensitive to tension; when the tension becomes excessive,

impulses are initiated which result in inhibition of muscle contraction. *Free nerve endings*, which are mainly associated with blood vessels in muscle tissue, give rise to pain impulses.

CHEMICAL COMPOSITION AND CONTRACTION

Skeletal muscle is composed of 75% water, 20% protein, and 5% inorganic material, organic 'extractives' and carbohydrates (glycogen and its derivatives). The proteins myosin, actin, tropomyosin, troponin and myoglobin give muscle fibres their elasticity and contractile power. The major inorganic constituents of muscle include potassium, sodium, magnesium, and calcium. Phosphate chloride and small amounts of sulphate are also present. Compounds which can be extracted from muscle include creatine and phosphocreatine, adenine, guanine, uric acid and adenylic acid (from adenosine triphosphate or ATP).

Almost everything discussed regarding initiation and conduction of action potential in nerve fibres applies equally well to skeletal muscle fibres (see p. 682). Energy for muscle contraction is generated by a series of chemical reactions within the fibres. Briefly, these include the following: the motor nerve impulse causes depolarization of the sarcolemma, leading to the sudden breakdown of adenosine triphosphate (ATP) to adenosine diphosphate (ADP) and the release of phosphate and energy; the energy promotes the interaction of actin and myosin filaments which produces the actual shortening and thickening of the muscle (contraction); phosphocreatine is hydrolyzed and gives up phosphate, which combines with ADP to quickly restore the ATP so that a constant source of energy for contraction is maintained; glycogen is then broken down, releasing phosphate and lactic acid; the phosphate molecules combine with creatine to replenish the phosphocreatine; about one-fifth of the lactic acid is oxidized to energy, carbon dioxide and water; and the remainder of the lactic acid is reconverted to glycogen. The initial reactions which provide instantaneous energy for contraction do not utilize oxygen (anaerobic). The oxidation of lactic acid requires oxygen and the energy released is utilized in the resynthesis of the basic compounds used during contraction. In hypoxaemia or in strenuous exercise, the oxygen supply is generally inadequate to oxidize lactic acid and provide the required energy for resynthesis. Lactic acid accumulates and the condition is said to have incurred an oxygen debt; that is, the oxygen provided was not sufficient to keep pace with the production of lactic acid.

The initial source of energy for muscle contraction is oxygen and the basic food substances, particularly the metabolism of carbohydrates and fats. Therefore, interruption of blood flow through a contracting muscle quickly leads to muscle fatigue.

The *strength of the contraction* of a muscle depends on the number of fibres excited, the length of the fibre, and the size of the muscle. When stimulated, each fibre contracts to its fullest capacity (all-or-none law) and when the stimulus is maximal or intense, all fibres are involved. The force of contraction of a fibre increases proportionately with its length up to a certain point,

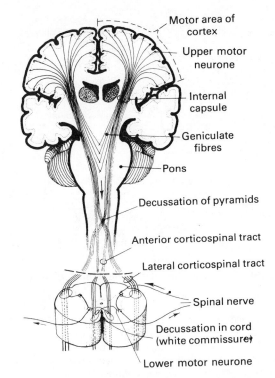

Motor area of
cortex

Upper motor
neurone

Internal
capsule

Geniculate
fibres

Pons

Decussation of pyramids

Anterior corticospinal tract

Lateral corticospinal tract

Spinal nerve

Decussation in cord
(white commissure)

Lower motor neurone

Figure 21.14 The pyramidal tract (corticospinal tract).

after which it decreases. The larger the muscle mass, the greater amount of energy produced. A muscle responds to repeated, increased demands by hypertrophy of individual fibres, and to decreased demands by atrophy.

Muscle contractions are referred to as twitch, tetanic, isotonic, and isometric. A single stimulus to a muscle produces a quick, brief contraction referred to as a *twitch*. *Tetanic contraction* occurs when a muscle is stimulated at progressively greater frequency and a sustained contraction results due to a fusion of successive contractions. Muscle contraction is said to be *isometric* when the muscle length does not change during contraction but its tension is increased. It is said to be *isotonic* when muscle shortens and produces movement but the tension in the muscle remains constant.

Muscles are arranged to function in pairs; the contraction of one of the pair is accompanied by relaxation of the other (reciprocal inhibition). For example, if the biceps is to contract to flex the forearm, the triceps must relax. The muscle which contracts is called the agonist, and the one which relaxes at the same time is known as the *antagonist*. Other muscles may be necessary in certain patterns of movement and may be classified as *synergists* or *stabilizers*. They facilitate the work of the agonist.

VOLUNTARY MOVEMENT

Normal voluntary movements are the result of controlled contraction and relaxation of groups of muscles. All willed movements depend upon excitation of

neurones within the cerebral cortex (upper motor neurones) as well as at a lower level (lower motor neurones). Those at a lower level may be the motor components of cranial nerve nuclei in the brain stem or they may be in the spinal cord. Two major neuronal pathways in the CNS are involved in voluntary muscle activity. These are referred to as the pyramidal tract and the extrapyramidal system.

PYRAMIDAL TRACT (CORTICOSPINAL TRACT)

The pyramidal tract arises in the sensorimotor cortex of the cerebrum and is one of the major pathways whereby motor signals are transmitted from all the motor areas of the cortex to the anterior motor neurones of the spinal cord.

Voluntary movement begins with the stimulation of a discrete area of neurones in the motor area of the cerebral cortex. If the movement applies to only muscles on one side of the body, only the motor area of the cerebral hemisphere on the opposite side will be involved. As the axons of the motor neurones of each hemisphere descend, they converge to form a compact mass referred to as the *internal capsule*. The fibres continue downward through the brain stem and in the lower medulla approximately 90% decussate (cross over) to form the pyramids of the medulla (Figure 21.14). These fibres descend in the lateral corticospinal tract of the cord and terminate in posterior horns of cord grey matter. Fibres which did not decussate earlier, continue ipsilaterally in the anterior corticospinal tracts and cross over further down the cord.

At various levels in the cord, the fibres synapse with neurones in the anterior horns of grey matter. The axons of these neurones form the motor fibres of the peripheral nerves whereby the impulses are delivered to muscle fibres. Some fibres in the tract may synapse in the brain stem with nuclei of cranial nerves. The impulses are then carried out to a muscle by motor fibres of a peripheral cranial nerve.

The neurones of the cerebral cortical motor area are referred to as the upper motor neurones. Those with which the axons of upper motor neurones synapse are called *lower motor neurones*. The cell bodies of lower motor neurones reside within the CNS and their axons carry the impulses to skeletal muscles in the periphery.

Interruption of the pyramidal tract at any level produces muscle paralysis. Spastic paralysis occurs with damage of an area above the lower motor neurones. The muscles controlled by the affected upper motor neurones resist passive movement and exhibit increased tone and exaggerated reflexes, because the inhibiting influence of higher centres is interrupted. Injury to lower motor neurones or their axons results in flaccid paralysis in the respective muscles, loss of tone and reflexes and wasting (atrophy) of the muscles.

EXTRAPYRAMIDAL SYSTEM (EXTRAPYRAMIDAL TRACTS)

This system includes all the tracts exclusive of the pyramidal tract, that transmit motor signals from the brain to the spinal cord (Figure 21.15). Unlike the

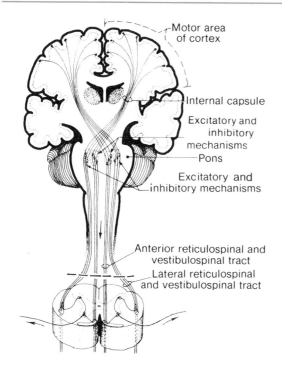

Figure 21.15 The extrapyramidal tract.

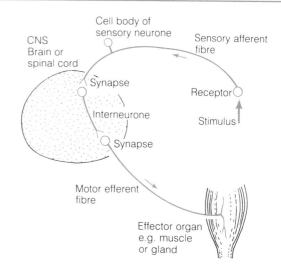

Figure 21.16 The component structures of a reflex arc.

pyramidal tract, which is a direct link from the cerebral cortex to the spinal cord, the extrapyramidal system conveys its influences to the cord via multineuronal and multisynaptic linkages involving the cortex, basal ganglia, thalami, cerebellum, brain stem and related structures. Extrapyramidal impulses are initiated in several areas of the brain below conscious level and all are transmitted by reticulospinal tracts to lower motor neurones. The lower motor neurones provide the final common pathway for all the afferent impulses (both pyramidal and extrapyramidal) to skeletal muscles. Inhibition, facilitation, and co-ordination, essential for smooth, precise muscle activity is normally provided by the extrapyramidal system.

An imbalance in the interactions within the complex circuitry of the extrapyramidal system occurs with malfunction of various nuclear complexes. The motor disorders resulting from the improper functioning of the extrapyramidal system and associated nuclei include various abnormal movements such as paralysis agitans, athetosis and choreas.

Voluntary muscle activity involves the pyramidal and extrapyramidal tracts in concert. The pyramidal tract transmits the impulses which are consciously initiated to produce a given movement. The other essential components of the movement such as reciprocal relaxation of certain muscles, correlation, stabilization and adjustment in posture are automatically contributed by the extrapyramidal system.

The following activity illustrates the role of the pyramidal and extrapyramidal tracts in voluntary movement. If a person who is standing reaches out to pick up a pen from a table, he or she consciously concentrates on the action of the fingers and thumb necessary to grasp the object. Several muscle responses are involved as well as the flexion of fingers and thumb. The forearm is extended to reach the pen (the biceps relaxes and the triceps contracts); muscles contract to stabilize the shoulder and wrist; leaning forward to reach the pen may be necessary, so the trunk flexes and shifts the centre of gravity, necessitating muscle action in the trunk and lower extremities to ensure maintenance of the upright position.

REFLEXES

A reflex is an involuntary, stereotypic response mediated by the nervous system. It serves as a defence mechanism and it may involve the contraction of muscle tissue or the secretion of a gland. Although reflexes occur without voluntary or willed initiation, the person usually becomes conscious of the reflex activity because the impulses reach the cerebral cortex and are interpreted as sensation. The pathway over which nerve impulses pass is called a reflex arc (Figure 21.16). The arc is comprised of receptors, an afferent pathway (sensory nerve fibres), CNS connections, motor neurones, efferent pathway (motor nerve fibres) and effector organ (muscle fibres or glandular cells). The simplest reflex arc consists of two neurones: a sensory and a motor neurone. The patellar reflex ('knee-jerk') which is elicited by tapping the tendon of the quadriceps femoris muscle is an example of this type of reflex.

Reflex responses are either protective or postural. *Protective reflexes* are produced in response to irritating or painful stimuli. Examples include: the closing of the eyelid when the cornea is lightly touched (blink reflex); rapid withdrawal of a hand from a hot stove (withdrawal reflex); and contraction of superficial abdominal muscles and movement of the umbilicus in the direction of the skin area stimulated in response to light, rapid stroking of the cutaneous surface of the abdomen (abdominal reflex).

Postural reflexes maintain an appropriate degree of muscle tone which is essential in supporting the body against gravity and maintaining an upright position. The body can stay upright because muscles exert a continual pull on bones in the opposite direction to ever-present gravitational forces. Reflex mechanisms which regulate the muscle contraction necessary to provide the antigravity force are the stretch reflex and impulses originating in the internal ear. With a change in position, movement of the fluid in the semicircular canals in the ears elicits sensory impulses which are conveyed by the vestibular fibres of the eighth cranial (auditory) nerve to nuclei in the brain stem. From here, impulses are transmitted via vestibulospinal tracts to motor neurones which discharge impulses to appropriate muscles, producing an increase in their tone in support of the body's upright position.

Reflexes which are clinically important may be organized into four groups: (1) superficial (or skin and mucous membrane) reflexes, (2) deep (or myotatic) reflexes, (3) visceral (or organic), and (4) pathological (or abnormal). The nasal (or sneeze) reflex and the pharyngeal (or gag) reflex are examples of *mucous membrane reflexes*. The abdominal reflex and the plantar reflex are *skin reflexes. Deep reflexes* include those in which receptors are located in deeper tissue such as tendons. The biceps reflex, which is flexion at the elbow when the biceps tendon is struck, is a deep reflex. *Visceral reflexes* include pupillary reflexes such as constriction in response to light stimulus, the oculocardiac reflex (slowing of the heart rate in response to pressure over the eyeballs), and the carotid sinus reflex (decrease in heart rate and blood pressure in response to pressure over the carotid sinus in the neck).

Pathological reflexes are usually elicited only when neurological disease is present. Primitive defence responses, normally suppressed by cerebral inhibitory influences, are frequently present in these reflexes.

ASSESSMENT OF THE PERSON WITH ALTERED NEUROLOGICAL FUNCTION

Neurological assessment provides the base from which both medical and nursing problems will be identified and decisions about intervention will be made. Baseline neurological assessment may be performed in an initial visit to a doctor's surgery, in a casualty department or once the patient has been hospitalized. There can be the formal step-by-step assessment which will include assessment of cognitive status (a mental status examination), cranial nerve assessment, motor and reflex testing, sensation and cerebral function. Neurological assessment (evaluation) may include: a neurological history or interview, the neurological examination, assessment of the effect of neurological dysfunction on daily living, emergency assessment—craniocerebral and spinal testing, continuous intracranial monitoring observations, and diagnostic studies.

NEUROLOGICAL HEALTH HISTORY (INTERVIEW)

The neurological history is part of the general health history. It usually includes demographic data, a description of the patient, the history of the present disorder, past history, a review of systems and family and social history. Since neurological illness frequently affects mental status, the patient's mental condition and perception of the problem are evaluated. If the patient is unable to provide reliable information, the history may be obtained from a relative or friend who is familiar with the patient. The source of the data is included in the history.

Many aspects of assessment may be carried out by the nurse at the bedside while observing the patient on a day to day basis or assisting the patient to complete basic hygienic functions. The data ascertained by the nurse provides direction both for the identification of patient problems and for decisions about nursing interventions.

CEREBRAL ASSESSMENT OF COGNITIVE STATUS

The neurological examination is that part of the physical examination which evaluates the function of the cerebrum and the cranial nerves as well as the motor and sensory status, reflex status and the status of the autonomic nervous system.

Cerebral function

Evaluation of cerebral function includes information obtained from observing the patient, evoking responses and from family and friends. It relates to the appropriateness of the individual's appearance, behaviour, level of consciousness (Glasgow coma scale, see p. 706), mood, attitude and flow of speech. Cognitive functions such as orientation, speech comprehension, general intelligence, attention and concentration, memory retention and immediate recall, vocabulary, judgement and abstract reasoning are also evaluated. Deterioration in one or more of these functions commonly occurs with cerebral dysfunction.

Disease involving the CNS may affect the patient in many ways. The patient's family may report a change in his appearance, particularly facial expression, posture and personal grooming. Disordered emotional reactions may be evident in the patient's fluctuating attitudes. There may be inappropriate laughing, crying, irritability or unprovoked expressions of anger. Sharp mood swings may occur; the patient who is withdrawn and depressed or anxious may suddenly become excited or euphoric. Impaired reasoning, unjustified fears, distortion in perception and loss of memory may occur. The attention span may be abnormally short and there may be inability to do very simple calculations or to identify normally familiar objects or sounds. Confusion or disorientation as to time, place or person may occur with a cerebral lesion. The patient's response to stimuli may vary from a coherent verbal response to no response of any sort, even to painful stimuli.

Speech dysfunctions which occur with cerebral lesions vary with the location, size, and nature of the lesion. Aphasia, dysphasia, agnosia and apraxia are examples of speech disorders which may occur.

Aphasia refers to the loss of ability to understand words or to use them to communicate. Difficulty in using words to communicate due to lack of co-ordination and ability to put words in order occurs more commonly and is referred to as *dysphasia*. Aphasia may be classified as *motor* (*expressive*, *Broca's*) or *sensory* (*receptive*). Motor aphasia implies the person understands spoken and written words and knows what he or she wants to say but cannot speak the words. Motor aphasias include any loss of communication by writing, speaking or making signs. Sensory aphasia implies that the comprehension of written and spoken words is affected. A patient may suffer auditory aphasia (word deafness) which is the inability to make sense of sound because of an inability to comprehend symbolic communication associated with sound. Some may experience visual aphasia ('word blindness') which means loss of ability to understand the symbolic content of written words or figures and even though they can see them they cannot read them. In many instances of aphasia, elements of both expressive and receptive communication are lost.

Certain areas of the cerebral cortex are essential to the recognition of objects by sight, sound, feeling, smell and taste. Cerebral dysfunction may result in the inability to recognize objects through any of the senses and is referred to as *agnosia*. Agnosia may be visual, auditory or tactile. A cerebral lesion may also result in *apraxia* which is the inability to carry out purposeful, useful, or skilled acts in the absence of paralysis, or use objects correctly. *Dyslexia* means inability to comprehend written words.

Cranial nerves

Cranial nerves are referred to by specific name or number (see Table 21.1). Most arise from the brain stem, and much information can be obtained by testing cranial nerve function. Evaluation of cranial nerve function involves the following:

Olfactory (I). The patient is asked to close the eyes and to identify a series of odorous substances such as coffee, peppermint, oil of cloves. Each nostril is tested separately. Inability to identify the substances (in the absence of a cold or allergy) may suggest a lesion in the frontal lobe such as a basal skull fracture or a tumour of the olfactory groove.

Optic (II). This test includes ophthalmoscopic examination and evaluation of visual acuity and visual fields. Visual acuity may be grossly evaluated by asking the person to read from a printed page or distant sign both with and without corrective lenses if such are used. See assessment in Chapter 28.

Ophthalmoscopic examination may reveal papilloedema which is oedema of the area where the optic nerve and blood vessels enter and leave the eyeball, and is a classical sign of increased intracranial pressure.

Oculomotor (III), trochlear (IV) and abducens (VI). These nerves are usually tested together since they are all involved in the muscles that rotate the eyeball, constrict the pupils and elevate' the eyelids. On examination, pupils should be round and equal in size and shape. Each pupil is tested, in a darkened room, for the direct light reflex. A light is directed into each pupil and the response is observed. The normal pupil constricts briskly in response to light stimulus. The consensual light reflex is also tested. This is a slightly weaker constriction of one pupil when the other is stimulated by light. Accommodation is tested by asking the person to look at a distant spot and then to follow the examiner's finger to within 15 cm (6 in) of the person's nose. Visualization of a distant object causes pupillary dilatation while viewing a near object produces constriction and convergence. Abnormal pupillary responses suggest neurological dysfunction. The range of ocular movements is evaluated by asking the person to follow the examiner's finger as it moves up, down, medially and laterally. Inability to move the eyeball in a particular direction may result in *diplopia* (double vision). Normal eyes move conjugately (track together). Disconjugate movement implies failure of function of one or more of the eye muscles. Abnormal eye movements can result from injury to the nerves themselves or their nuclei in the midbrain and pons. During examination of ocular movements, observations for *nystagmus* are made. This is an involuntary rhythmic movement of one or both eyes in a lateral or vertical direction. It may occur in normal persons with severe myopia or fatigue or it may occur with neurological disease. *Ptosis* (drooping) of the eyelid may occur with paralysis of the levator palpebrae muscle due to damage of cranial nerve III.

Trigeminal (V). The trigeminal nerve has *sensory* and *motor* components. The sensory function is assessed by testing both sides of the face and mouth for touch, temperature and pain sensations while the person's eyes are closed. The motor function is evaluated by having the person make chewing and biting movements. The ophthalmic branch of the trigeminal nerve controls the corneal reflex. If this reflex is intact, the person blinks briskly when the cornea of each eye is lightly touched with a wisp of cotton wool. The corneal reflex is one of the last to disappear when the patient's condition is deteriorating.

Facial (VII). The facial nerve has a sensory and motor component. The sensory component is tested by seeing if the person can recognize the taste of sweet and salty substances respectively when applied to the anterior part of the tongue. The motor divisions are tested by asking the person to use the facial muscles in such expressions as smiling, frowning, closing the eyes tightly and puckering the lips.

Acoustic (auditory, VIII). This nerve has two divisions, the cochlear nerve and the vestibular nerve. The cochlear nerve is tested for hearing acuity by whispering in one ear, using a ticking watch and a tuning fork (see Chapter 27). Loss of hearing or reports by the patient of constant or abnormal recurring sounds described as roaring, ringing, buzzing or swishing should be recorded and reported to the doctor. The vestibular nerve, concerned with equilibrium reflexes, is tested by rotating the patient and performing the caloric test (see p. 711). Dizziness and loss of position balance (equilibrium) may occur with disturbance in the semicircular canals of the internal ear, of the vestibular part of the auditory nerve, or pathway within the brain.

Glossopharyngeal (IX) and vagus (X). These nerves are usually examined simultaneously because of their overlapping innervation of the pharynx. In response to touching of the pharynx with a tongue depressor, a brisk gag reaction should be elicited. Ability to swallow water is assessed and the posterior third of the tongue may be tested for taste. Absence of the gag or swallowing reflex occurs in neurological damage and it renders the person vulnerable to aspiration. To assess the vagus nerve, the ability to speak and to cough is evaluated. Ineffectual cough and a weak, hoarse voice suggest possible vagal involvement.

Accessory (XI). This nerve is tested by inspecting the sternocleidomastoid muscle and the upper portion of the trapezius muscle for symmetry, atrophy and strength. The person is asked to elevate the shoulders with and without resistance from the examiner's hand, and to rotate the head to each side against the pull of the chin to the midline by the examiner's hand.

Hypoglossal (XII). This nerve is assessed by observing various movements of the tongue and examining it for symmetry, atrophy and tremor when protruded.

Motor function

This is evaluated by examining muscle symmetry, size, shape, tone and movement. Muscle function, balance accuracy, and muscle strength are assessed. Inspection and comparison of muscles on both sides of the body, palpation and measuring the circumferences of areas with a tape measure provides information about size and shape and can reveal abnormalities such as atrophy or hypertrophy. Muscle tone is assessed by palpating muscles at rest and noting the resistance to passive movement. Excessive resistance (*spasticity*), a constant state of resistance (*rigidity*) and decreased muscle tone (*flaccidity or hypotonia*) are examples of abnormal muscle tone.

Movements are examined for 'fine' and 'gross' abnormalities. Fine muscle abnormalities are *fasiculations* which are involuntary ripples, or twitches, which occur when the person is relaxed. They suggest lower motor neurone disease. Gross abnormal movements may indicate extrapyramidal disease and include athetoid, choreiform and dystonic movements, spasms, myoclonus, tics, and tremors.

Athetoid movements are involuntary, repetitive, slow and writhing. They may be unilateral or bilateral and follow a definite pattern in the individual patient, ceasing only during sleep. Athetosis is commonly seen in persons with cerebral palsy.

Choreiform movements are involuntary, rapid, rhythmic and jerky. They begin abruptly, are variable in pattern and distribution and may occur during sleep. The limbs, face and tongue are most often involved, and difficulty in speaking, chewing and swallowing may be present. The forcefulness of the movements may lead to injury unless protection is provided. *Spasms or cramps* are sudden, violent, involuntary contractions of a muscle or muscle groups which result in pain, interference with function and voluntary movement. Muscles of the limbs and neck are most frequently affected. The cause may be a lesion within the CNS (e.g. degenerative changes in the extrapyramidal system, a deficient blood supply to the muscle(s), overstretching and injury of the muscle fibres or, a blood calcium or sodium deficiency). *Dystonic movements* involve spasms in portions of the limbs as well as the trunk. The result is usually slow, grotesque, twisting movements and abnormal posture. *Myoclonus* is shock-like contractions of a portion of a muscle, an entire muscle or group of muscles restricted to one area of the body or appearing synchronously or asynchronously in several areas (seen most commonly in epilepsy). Tics are frequently of psychogenic origin. They are stereotyped, repetitious, purposeless movements which vary from individual to individual. Twitching of a cheek is an example of a tic. *Tremors* are involuntary shaky movements, particularly of the limbs, which may have a physical or psychological aetiology. A fine, rapid tremor, particularly of the hands, may be associated with anxiety, fatigue or toxic conditions such as thyrotoxicosis, uraemia and alcoholism. *Intention tremor* occurs when a voluntary movement is initiated and progressively intensifies especially with precision movements. A *resting tremor* is one that diminishes with voluntary movement and disappears during sleep.

Muscles are further evaluated by putting all the joints through a full range of passive movement. Pain, contractures and muscle resistance are abnormal findings.

Muscle strength may be assessed by flexion and extension and other movements, first without resistance and then with the examiner offering resistance. In addition, the person may be asked to hold the arms straight in front with the palms up and the eyes closed for 20–30 seconds. If one arm moves downward or one hand begins to pronate, a *drift* is said to be present, suggesting muscle weakness in that arm. Drift can be tested in the lower limbs by asking the person to raise both legs off the bed while in a supine position.

Co-ordination, balance and *accuracy* of muscle function is largely mediated by the cerebellum. These attributes may be assessed by point-to-point tests (e.g. with the eyes open, then repeated with the eyes closed, the person repeatedly touches the examiner's finger and then his or her own nose). Co-ordination and balance may also be assessed by observing the person's gait while the eyes are open and again when closed. Locomotion depends upon a normal degree of tone, close integration and co-ordination of the involved muscles of the lower limbs and trunk. These factors are primarily dependent upon normal innervation.

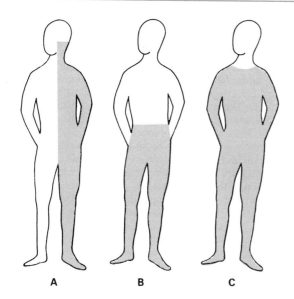

Figure 21.17 (A) Hemiplegia. (B) Paraplegia. (C) Quadriplegia.

Various abnormal gaits may be observed in the presence of neurological dysfunction. The *ataxic gait* is an unsteady, uncoordinated walk. With the feet placed far apart to provide a wide base for support, each foot is lifted abnormally high and slapped down with each step. The steps are unsure, unevenly spaced and may deviate to one side. Ataxic gait is associated with a loss of proprioceptive sense and a lack of co-ordination of muscle action. It tends to be more pronounced in the dark, as visual influences diminish. The *stepping gait* (foot drop gait) is characterized by foot drop due to paralysis of the anterior tibial muscles, usually secondary to lower motor neurone disease. The person looks as though he or she is walking upstairs, because the advancing leg is lifted abnormally high to avoid dragging the foot and stumbling. *Cerebellar ataxia* is staggering, unsteady and wide based. Turns are made with difficulty. The person is unable to stand steadily with the feet together, whether the eyes are open or closed. It is associated with damage in the cerebellum or related tracts. *Parkinson's gait* is characteristic of patients with the basal ganglia defects of Parkinson's disease (see pp. 751–753). With this gait, the trunk is stooped forward, the knees are slightly flexed, steps are short and often shuffling and the speed of walking progressively accelerates. Turning occurs stiffly and as if 'all in one piece'.

Paralysis or loss of motor function is a common occurrence in neurological disease or injury. Paralysis may be partial and exhibited by weakness (*paresis*) or complete and may be classified according to the extent of the involvement. *Monoplegia* refers to paralysis of one limb. *Hemiplegia* means paralysis of one side of the body. There is loss of muscle power in the limbs and the muscles of the face on the same side. If the side of the face opposite to that of the paralyzed limbs is affected, the term *alternate hemiplegia* may be used

(Figure 21.17a). *Paraplegia* denotes paralysis of the legs or the lower half of the body (Figure 21.17b). *Quadriplegia* or *tetraplegia* refers to paralysis of the trunk and all four extremities (Figure 21.17c). Isolated paralysis indicates the loss of the contractile ability of one muscle of a group. It is frequently associated with peripheral nerve damage and is usually accompanied by loss of sensation in the area supplied by the injured nerve.

Paralysis may also be classified as that due to an upper or lower motor neurone lesion. Damage to the motor areas of the cerebral cortex or their projection pathways (corticospinal or pyramidal tracts) produces paralysis due to an upper motor neurone lesion or what may also be termed *spastic paralysis*. Since the lower motor neurones and reflex arc are intact, the affected muscles are still capable of reflex movements and exhibit hypertonicity (spasticity) as well as exaggerated reflexes. There is increased activity of postural (stretch) and protective reflexes. Paralysis resulting from injury of the motor neurones in the nuclei of cranial nerves or in the anterior horns or columns of grey matter in the spinal cord or damage to their axons in the periphery may be referred to as that due to a *lower motor neurone lesion* or as *flaccid paralysis*. Flaccidity occurs because the reflex arc is interrupted: there is a lack of reflex innervation and responses.

Serious abnormal postures which may develop with some cerebral and brain stem disorders are *decerebrate rigidity* and *decorticate rigidity* (see p. 730). Normally, primitive reflex spinal mechanisms which initiate involuntary muscular responses are kept inactive by cerebral control. These primitive involuntary responses may be referred to as spinal automatisms. When control from the higher centres is abolished, sustained rigid posturing develops.

Sensory function

This includes assessment of the visual, auditory, olfactory, gustatory, touch, proprioceptive, pain and temperature senses. Most of these have been discussed in conjunction with assessment of the cranial nerves. The body areas usually tested for touch, pain and temperature are the face, hands, arms, trunk, thighs, feet, perineal and perianal regions. The patient is asked to close the eyes, and each side of the body is compared to the other. Sensitivity to touch (a wisp of cotton wool), superficial pain (a pin prick), deep pressure pain, heat and cold, vibration and position is tested. In addition, the patient is asked to differentiate among various textures.

Sensory tests are often difficult to evaluate and a great deal depends upon the co-operation of the patient. Neurological lesions more often result in a diminution of sensation than in total anaesthesia. A sensory disturbance may be localized in one particular area of the body because of the different sensory pathways being associated with different parts. Hyposensitivity or hypersensitivity in the area may provide information about the location of a lesion.

NORMAL
CONSCIOUSNESS

1   Eyes open, oculomotor activity
    is normal
    Spontaneous interaction with
    environment; oriented normal
    speech

    **Normal voluntary motor and
    reflex function**

2   Eyes open to speech
    Talks but is disoriented about
    time and/or place and person
    May still obey commands slowly
    with repeated requests

3   Opens eyes to painful stimulus
    Conversation is not initiated or
    sustained; words are inappropriate
    Tries to remove painful stimulus
    or flexes to pain

4   Eyes generally closed
    Moans and groans but no recognizable
    words

COMA   Flexes or extends to painful
        stimuli

5   No response

Figure 21.18 Signs of altered consciousness.

Reflex status

Evaluation of reflexes provides valuable information about the nature, location and progression of neurological disorders in both the conscious and unconscious patient. Exaggeration or diminished responses of normal reflexes and the presence of pathological reflexes are frequently among the earliest indications of neurological disturbance. Reflexes most commonly tested are the deep tendon or muscle-stretch reflexes, superficial reflexes and pathological reflexes. The part of the body tested should be relaxed and the stimulus applied with the same intensity to each side of the body. Rapidity and strength of the muscle contractions are noted.

The *deep reflexes* are tested by tapping briskly on a tendon over a bony prominence, evoking an instantaneous stretching of certain muscles and their resulting contraction. The maxillary, biceps, brachioradialis, triceps, patellar and Achilles reflexes are the most common tested. *Superficial reflexes* are elicited by light, rapid stroking of a particular area of the skin or mucous membrane with an object. The corneal and pupillary reflexes, the pharyngeal or gag reflex, abdominal and plantar reflexes are the common superficial reflexes tested. Diminished superficial reflex responses occur on

the opposite side of the body when lesions are present above the decussation of the corticospinal tract. Loss of these reflexes occurs on the same side as the lesion when the lesion is below the corticospinal tract decussation.

The *Babinski reflex* is a useful *pathological reflex* suggestive of neurological disease, particularly of the pyramidal tract. In response to light stroking of the lateral aspect of the sole of the foot, an extension or dorsiflexion of the big toe and fanning of the other toes occurs.

UNCONSCIOUSNESS

Interruption of impulses from the reticular activating system, or failure of the cerebral cortical neurones to respond to incoming impulses, produces a loss of consciousness. Other than destruction of the cortical or cortical activating cells (reticular formation) by trauma, the basic factors contributing to unconsciousness are considered to be oxygen and glucose deprivation. Neurones require a constant supply of both of these substances for cellular activity. A deficiency of oxygen for even a few seconds decreases neuronal metabolism to a point at which unconsciousness ensues. Figure 21.18 describes the effects of alterations in level of consciousness from a state of normal awareness to coma or unconsciousness.

CAUSES OF ALTERATIONS IN CONSCIOUSNESS

The patient's level of consciousness may be depressed due to the effects of abnormal metabolic processes or disease, including trauma, involving the brain or brain stem.

1. Processes which may interfere with the metabolism of the brain stem and cerebral cortex include: hypoglycaemia or diabetic ketoacidosis which produces a deficiency of glucose that is essential for cerebral neuronal functioning; respiratory failure which produces cerebral hypoxia; renal and hepatic failure which cause an accumulation of metabolic wastes; electrolyte imbalance; infections and autoimmune disorders; and drug overdose. Patients' manifestations resulting from altered metabolism show symmetrical changes in motor function.
2. Space-occupying lesions affecting the brain may alter the level of consciousness and include: cerebral haemorrhage from vascular diseases and trauma, tumours, abscess and haematoma from skull injuries. Manifestations are usually unequal on each side and may include hemiplegia and small reactive pupils which later become fixed.
3. Brain stem lesions that may cause unconsciousness include: cerebral haemorrhage and brain stem infarction, tumours, and abscesses, as well as trauma which produces direct pressure on the reticular formation tissue in the brain stem. Symptoms include loss of reflexes and pupillary reactions. Patients with trauma or metabolic disturbance will show signs of generalized brain dysfunction rather than focal signs; it is important to assess overall brain function and vital signs frequently.

Assessment of Level of Consciousness

Decrease in responsiveness to stimuli indicates progressive deterioration in brain function. The chance of complete recovery decreases with increase in the duration of impaired consciousness; decrease in responsiveness to stimuli must be reported immediately in order that measures can be implemented to reduce the risk of irreversible neurological dysfunction or death. The patient whose level of consciousness is decreasing may become progressively lethargic, irritable or restless, disinterested in the environment and eventually disorientated. Orientation to time is usually lost first; loss of orientation to place occurs next and lastly, orientation to person.

Health History

The patient with an altered level of consciousness is unable to relate a history. Therefore, information must be obtained from the family members, friends, witnesses, police or rescue workers.

The health history should include:

1. A description of the onset of injury. What events, behaviour changes or other unusual factors preceded the incident? When did the injury occur? What type of accident was it and where did it occur? What position was the patient in when found?
2. Whether there is evidence of an infection or a history of a recent infection.
3. History of previous seizures.
4. Information about associated health problems such as diabetes mellitus, cardiovascular or renal disease, respiratory disorder or psychiatric disturbance, which may have affected consciousness or will influence treatment.
5. Recurring headaches, nausea and vomiting, changes in attention span or irritability.
6. The use of prescription and non-prescription drugs. Drug containers in the patient's home, bag or other personal effects or in the area of the incident should be collected and examined in relation to the possible toxic effects of their contents. The nurse should also look for a Medic-Alert bracelet and items such as a diabetic card.

Once information relevant to the initiation of treatment has been obtained and necessary life support procedures have been instituted, further information is obtained about the patient. This may include identification of the patient and the family or friends who should be notified, past medical history, allergies, sensory deficits and corrective measures (e.g. use of hearing aid, contact lenses, glasses), work experiences, life-style, usual health habits, social and recreational interests, language spoken and relevant cultural and religious beliefs and practices. Knowledge of the patient's daily routine may be useful to the nurse in planning and structuring care that is relevant and meaningful and which may stimulate further awareness on the part of the patient.

Physical assessment

It is difficult to define consciousness and to differentiate between levels or degrees of impairment. Terms such as confusion, drowsiness, stupor, semicomatose and deep coma have obscure meanings and are subject to varying interpretations by different observers. The Glasgow coma scale is a simple assessment tool for consciousness which standardizes observations. It provides for accurate graphical recording of three aspects of behavioural response and the assessor is not required to interpret the observations. Changes in the patient's level of consciousness can be made by comparing current observations with previous results. The scale provides an assessment of overall brain functioning.

Glasgow coma scale
The Glasgow coma scale provides for evaluation of eye opening and the best verbal and motor responses. Within each of these three parameters, there are a variety of responses which are arranged in scales of increasing dysfunction, as outlined in Figure 21.19. Each aspect is assessed independently of the others.

1. Eye opening.
- *Spontaneous opening* (4). The nurse approaches the patient's bedside and notes whether the eyes are open or closed. Spontaneous opening of the eyes indicates that the arousal mechanism in the reticular activating system of the brain stem is functioning.
- *Opening to speech* (3). If the patient's eyes are closed, the observer speaks, addressing the patient by name. If there is no response to a normal speaking voice, the volume should be increased.
- *Opening to pain* (2). Physical stimulation, usually in the form of pressure on the fingernail bed using a pencil or pen is applied. It is important that observers use the same method of applying physical stimulation to ensure consistent, accurate findings.
- *No eye opening* (1). If no response is demonstrated in either eye to increased pain stimuli, there is depression of the arousal system.

The patient may be sufficiently alert to respond by opening his eyes, but is restricted by swelling of the eyelids. If the eyelids are swollen shut, the observer records this as a 'C'.

2. Best verbal response. The patient's ability to speak and to understand the language spoken are determined. If the patient is intubated or has a tracheostomy, verbal response cannot be observed and 'T' is recorded. Speech is first used to stimulate a verbal response by askin the patient simple, direct questions. If there is no response a light touch is used or, if necessary, painful physical stimulation. Patient responses are rated as being: *orientated* (5) if able to respond as to who he or she is, where he or she is and give the year, month and day; *confused* (4) if not fully orientated to time, place and person; *inappropriate* (3) if the patient utters words in a disorganized way, swears or does not engage in meaningful conversation; *incomprehensible* (2) when responses are limited to moaning, groaning or mum-

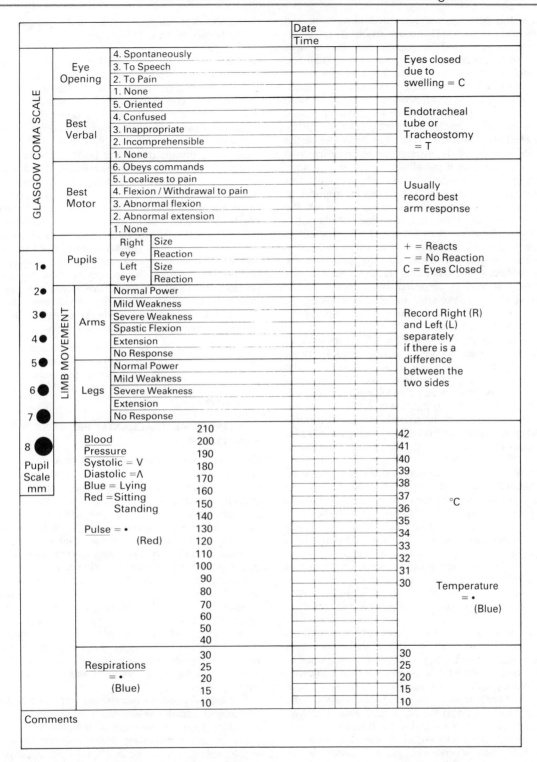

Figure 21.19 Assessment: level of consciousness.

bling sounds with no recognizable words; and *no response* (1) when no sounds are made in response to noxious stimuli.

3. Best motor response. The best possible motor

response in either arm is usually observed. The patient is asked to raise the arms and hold them outstretched for 10 seconds. The ratings in order of decreasing levels of function include: *obeys commands* (6) when the patient understands verbal, written instructions or gestures and performs the requested movement, and *localization to pain* (5) occurs when there is no response to command. A painful stimulus is then applied such as pressure on the patient's fingernail bed or stimulation to an area of the head or trunk. The patient moves a limb in an attempt to locate and remove the stimulus. (*Flexion* and *Extension* are the terms used in this assessment as opposed to *decorticate* and *decerebrate* which involve more subjective interpretation.) *Flexion withdrawal to pain* (4) occurs when the arm bends at the elbow in response to fingernail bed pressure or other local stimulation. Leg flexion is not a reliable gauge because with brain death, a spinal reflex may be present causing the legs to flex in response to localized pain. *Abnormal flexion* (3) occurs when the arm flexes at the elbow and pronates, making a fist. *Abnormal extension to pain* (2) occurs when the elbow straightens and the arm abducts (usually with internal rotation) in response to localized pain applied to the fingernail bed. If one arm flexes and the other extends, the best response is recorded. *No response* (1) is recorded when no detectable movement or change in the tone of the limbs is observed in response to repeated and varied stimuli.

Assessment of pupil responses and limb movements provides information and assists in localizing lesions; for example, if the pupil starts to dilate, pressure on the third cranial nerve is present, and neighbouring parasympathetic fibres which control pupillary constriction are affected. This may indicate coning or herniation of brain tissue through the tentorial hiatus. The nurse should check that the eye is real and functioning; it may be a 'glass eye'.

4. Pupils. Each pupil is examined for size and reaction. Normally, the pupils are round in shape, equal in size and constrict in response to direct light. The *size* of each pupil is measured by comparing it with the pupil scale as illustrated in Figure 21.19. Pupil *reaction* is measured in response to light; the beam of a pentorch is brought in from the patient's side and directed on one eye at a time. Constriction of the pupil is recorded as '+', or '−' when no reaction is obtained.

The surroundings should be dimly lit and the light beam of adequate intensity to obtain accurate results.

5. Limb movement. Verbal commands are used to elicit movement in each limb. When the patient does not respond to commands, painful stimuli are applied to the nail bed of a finger or great toe. Responses in order of decreasing function are recorded as: *normal power* when the limb movements are appropriate to the normal muscle strength for the patient; *mild weakness* when one limb shows normal strength but its opposite is weaker; *severe weakness* when the difference between two limbs is very much marked; *spastic flexion* when there is slow, stiff movement of the arm with the flexed forearm and hand held against the body; *extension* when the elbow or knee are straightened in response to painful stimulation; and *no response* when painful stimulation produces no movement and the limb remains limp.

It is important to compare each side and to record differences between right and left limbs and changes in the responses of an individual limb.

6. Vital signs. The vital signs (i.e. temperature, pulse, respiration and blood pressure) should be recorded frequently when the patient's level of consciousness is changing or severely impaired. The comatose patient is not able to communicate whether he or she feels too cold or too warm. With head trauma and certain medical problems, the heat-regulating centre in the hypothalamus is disturbed and the body temperature may fluctuate rapidly. Continuous monitoring of temperature is instituted or individual readings taken every 15–30 minutes. Body temperature may be recorded every 2–4 hours when the patient is in a stable but unconscious condition. Changes in the pulse rate and rhythm and blood pressure provide information about possible increased intracranial pressure, internal bleeding or shock. In addition to observing the rate, rhythm and depth of respirations, the equality of chest movements on both sides and any sounds associated with inspiration or expiration are noted. The chest is auscultated by the doctor for possible retention of secretions and inadequate ventilation of some lung areas.

It should be remembered that any changes in the patient's cerebral condition will manifest first as changes in level of consciousness, hence the importance of frequent and accurate observation, using the Glasgow coma scale.

CONTINUOUS INTRACRANIAL PRESSURE MONITORING

Continuous or direct intracranial pressure monitoring is an invasive procedure which is used in selected situations. It can provide reliable information indicating changes in intracranial pressure before such changes are clinically evident. It does not replace non-invasive clinical monitoring of neurological signs. It is valuable in patients whose 'neuro-signs' cannot be readily assessed because they have been given muscle-relaxant drugs so they can be mechanically ventilated.

Several different intracranial monitoring devices are available. They may be intraventricular, subarachnoid, subdural or epidural. Each device is complex, works differently, has a different set of advantages and disadvantages and requires different nursing considerations. Since the pressure in one compartment of the brain is normally not necessarily the same as that in another one, the values obtained with each device will vary.

Intracranial pressure monitoring involves a pressure sensor and transducer implanted inside the skull. The transducer converts mechanical impulses to electrical impulses and a recording device converts these into visible tracings on an oscilloscope or on graph paper. *Nursing care* includes maintenance of sterility, observing the dry sterile dressing around the insertion site for drainage, positioning the patient and the equipment properly, keeping the system intact and operational, and interpreting intracranial pressure waves.

Intracranial *pressure waves* are defined as abnormal spontaneous alterations in intracranial pressure. Three wave patterns have been identified but only the plateau, or A waves, are considered to have clinical significance because of the cerebral ischaemia and brain damage which they incur. Plateau waves are sudden, transient waves lasting 5–20 minutes. They usually begin from a baseline of already elevated intracranial pressure. They increase ventricular fluid pressure and intracranial pressure by 50–100 mmHg (normal intracranial pressure is 4–15 mmHg or 60–160 mmH$_2$O).

Transient, observable clinical symptoms of plateau waves are called pressure wave symptoms. These symptoms may be associated with deterioration in consciousness, abnormal respiratory patterns and pupillary reactions, altered motor function such as paresis, characteristic changes in vital signs, headache, nausea and vomiting, dysphasia, and other symptoms of cerebral dysfunction. Early recognition of any of these changes and early intervention to control the pressure can prevent permanent brain damage or even death.

Identification and control of factors which initiate these plateau waves are important considerations. These factors include: hypercapnia, hypoxaemia, cerebral vasodilating agents, Valsalva's manoeuvre, prone position, neck and hip flexion, isometric muscle contractions, coughing, sneezing, rapid eye movement, arousal from sleep, and emotional upset.

OBSERVATIONS

The patient responses which may suggest neurological changes and which need to be observed, recorded and reported are discussed below.

Focal signs
These are signs of neurological dysfunction which are related and limited to a specific cortical area of origin. They may be motor, sensory or psychological. For example, a lesion or pressure on the motor strip or the visual pathway will produce signs of motor or visual deficits which reflect interference in these areas. Focal signs may include such phenomena as paralysis of one limb, facial paralysis and loss of sensation, loss of hearing or vision, aphasia, ataxia, seizures, changes in personality and disorientation.

Lateralizing signs
These are signs of neurological dysfunction which are confined to one side of the body. For example, paralysis of one side of the body as occurs in stroke.

Restlessness
This may range from slight increase in activity with decreased level of consciousness to severe agitation in the alert individual. The cause needs to be identified and the patient protected from injury. Restlessness in the neurological patient may be the first sign of increasing intracranial pressure. It may be due to irritation or injury of brain tissue, airway obstruction and respiratory insufficiency, returning consciousness, pain, malposition, full bladder or rectum, tight dressings or other restraints. Restlessness may precede a seizure.

Fits or convulsions
These are common in patients with discrete lesions involving the frontal or parietal lobes and in patients with increased intracranial pressure. Seizures are sudden episodes of disturbances in consciousness which may be accompanied by uncoordinated, purposeless muscle contractions and changes in sensations or behaviour. Those which place the patient at risk of injury and require immediate intervention are those which involve the entire body in tonic and clonic movements and when there is loss of consciousness. *Tonic* refers to sustained muscle spasm while *clonic* means alternate contraction and relaxation of muscle. Seizures are due to excessive, neuronal discharges within the brain. They should be prevented if possible since they may worsen the patient's condition and/or cause injury.

Specific information about the patient's fits may help to identify the cause and to localize a brain lesion. The patient's level of consciousness and his activity before, during and after the seizure are recorded. In addition, answers to the following questions are sought and documented: Where did the fit begin and what was the initial activity? Did the patient cry out? What was the progression of the seizure activity? What body parts were involved? Was the activity tonic, clonic, localized or generalized and did the movements change in character during the fit? Was there deviation of the head or eyes and to which side? Were the eyes open or closed? Did the pupils change in size? Were the pupils equal and did they react to light? Was there incontinence of urine or faeces? Was there thick salivation of mucus (frothing at the mouth)? What was the patient's colour? What was the respiratory status throughout the seizure? What was the duration of the seizure activity? Did the patient experience a warning prior to the seizure? Was it auditory, visual, olfactory, tactile or other? Was there any weakness or paralysis of the extremities after the episode?

Headache
This may be due to inflammation or traction on pain-sensitive structures such as blood vessels, cranial nerves and dural attachments and it is an important symptom of increasing intracranial pressure. The location of the headache, its duration and severity are recorded as well as the position the patient assumes for maximum comfort. The headache of neurological origin is usually intermittent, deep, aching and pressure-like and it is intensified by coughing, straining and change in posture. Other characteristics will depend upon the location of the lesion.

Nuchal rigidity
This is an involuntary stiffness of the neck muscles and is assessed by asking the patient to flex his head. Pain in the neck and rigidity may indicate cervical spine injury, meningeal irritation, or subarachnoid bleeding.

Posturing
Decerebrate or decorticate posturing (see p. 730) may suggest worsening of the patient's neurological status.

Vomiting
This occurs particularly during the night or early morning. It may be due to direct pressure on the vomiting centre in the medulla. Nausea is usually absent and the vomitus is precipitous and forcefully ejected (projectile vomiting).

Cerebrospinal fluid leakage
This may occur from a head wound, from the posterior pharynx, the nose, or the ear. CSF leakage is potentially serious since micro-organisms may enter the subarachnoid space and give rise to meningitis or brain abscess. To determine whether drainage from the nose is CSF or mucus, a glucose indicator may be used. CSF is a dialysate of blood and is positive for glucose. Another method to test for CSF is the 'halo ring' method. A gauze pad is held under the dripping fluid and if blood and CSF are both present the two will separate on the pad, a red drop will form in the centre with a serous ring around it indicating the presence of CSF.

Incontinence of urine and faeces
This is common in disease of the brain and spinal cord.

DIAGNOSTIC TESTS: PATIENT EDUCATION AND SUPPORT

Neurodiagnostic procedures supplement and add precision to clinical data. As with any procedure, the patient needs both *physical and psychological preparation* to promote confidence in unfamiliar personnel and procedures. During procedures the patient needs privacy, support and encouragement. Following completion of the procedure, the patient needs observation for complications and protection from injury or complications. Neurodiagnostic procedures may be classed as invasive or non-invasive.

Non-invasive neurodiagnostic procedures

Non-invasive procedures pose minimal risks to the patient but may still provoke a high level of anxiety. This level of anxiety can be decreased by clear explanations that can be supplemented by charts, diagrams, pamphlets as well as audio visual supplements, if these are available. Once the material is reviewed, patients should be encouraged to ask questions in order to clarify any misconceptions. A signed consent is not usually required prior to the test, but if a contrast medium is injected intravenously during the procedure, a signed consent will be required.

Neuroradiography. Conventional X-rays of the skull and spine are frequently the first investigation in neurological disease. A wide spectrum of abnormalities may be demonstrated, including fractures, bone destruction, calcification and congenital lesions. In fact, they may give specific clues to the nature of the underlying problem. *Tomography* involves layered radiological exposures at measured depths which permits examination of single layers of tissues and provides some idea of the two-dimensional shape of the defects. However, in most centres, conventional tomography has been replaced by computerized tomography.

Computerized tomography (CT) of the head provides valuable information about the skull and its contents as it may diagnose a spectrum of lesions, e.g. tumour, abscess or haematoma. In patients who have suffered head injury, CT accurately locates the site(s) of intracranial haemorrhage, providing the surgeon with prognostic information on which he can base a decision about surgery.

Magnetic resonance imaging (MRI) gives unique information about the brain and spinal cord. The physics of MRI is very complex; the basic principle is that a powerful magnet aligns hydrogen nuclei. Their orientation is then changed by a radio frequency pulse; during realignment, the nuclei emit a signal which can be recorded. Computerized interpretation of this signal results in an image. During scanning, the patients should not have any metal objects on them as this will interfere with the procedure. MRI has several advantages over CT, notably in investigating the posterior cranial fossa and the spinal cord. It also more clearly demonstrates certain brain lesions, such as the demyelinating plaques of multiple sclerosis. Disadvantages include its high cost and the time required to obtain the images. The test requires patients to be enclosed in a long cylindrical tube, often giving a sensation of claustrophobia.

Cerebral angiograms are used to diagnose vascular lesions, particularly aneurysms, arteriovenous malformations (AVM) and tumours. These patients have often had a prior CT scan showing blood in the subarachnoid space or abnormal enhancing foci, close to the circle of Willis in the case of aneurysms or deeper within the substance of the brain in the case of AVMs.

Brain scan (radioisotope uptake). This technique detects regions of increased or decreased blood flow in the brain, and breakdown in the blood–brain barrier. A radioactive isotope is injected rapidly intravenously. Images are taken of the arrival and washout of isotope in the brain. These initial blood flow images are useful in detecting relative changes in regional blood flow in the brain. The brain images obtained 1–2 hours later reflect changes in the integrity of the blood–brain barrier. For example, the blood vessels in brain tumours and in the area of a brain infarction are much more porous than normal. The isotope will therefore accumulate in these regions and produce an abnormal region of uptake on the scan.

Carotid Doppler study. This non-invasive diagnostic study is used to assess the blood flow through the carotid arteries and the extent of sclerotic vascular change that may be partially or completely obstructing the normal flow of blood to the brain. The study may be done on persons who are considered at risk of stroke because of attendant signs and symptoms (e.g. transient ischaemic attacks).

The study involves the placing of a probe over the carotid area. The probe gives off ultrasound waves and receives them back as they rebound from erythrocytes flowing through the carotid arteries. The probe is connected to an oscilloscope which indicates the difference between the frequency of the waves given off by the probe and those that rebound. The difference is known as the Doppler shift and may be interpreted to yield information about blood flow in the artery under examination.

Positron emission (transaxial) tomography (PET scan or PETT). This new technique is similar to the CT scan but has other advantages. Minute doses of radioactive tracers prepared in a cyclotron are inhaled or injected into a vein. The radioactive emissions (positrons) of the tracer are picked up by sensitive detectors around the head as it distributes in the brain. The PET scan provides safe, rapid scanning of blood flow in the brain as well as biochemical mapping. It can be used to study diseases related to chemical changes in the brain and to localize the area of action in the brain.

Electroencephalography (EEG). The EEG is a recording of the brain's electrical activity. Several small electrodes are superficially placed on the scalp in standard positions. The electrodes are attached to an amplifier and recorder. It is believed that the electrical activity of neuronal dendrites of the superficial layers of the brain are responsible for the low-voltage electrical waves. If the patient has been prescribed an anticonvulsant drug it is usually withheld for 24 hours or more prior to the test. The patient needs assurance that an electric shock will not occur during the test and that the machine cannot 'read the mind'. The technician cleans the scalp and applies the electrodes with collodion. In some instances needle electrodes are inserted into the scalp, which necessitates cleansing the scalp before the needles are inserted. The patient lies or sits in a quiet dimly lit room. In order to evoke or accentuate certain abnormal wave patterns the patient may be asked to hyperventilate or the technician may flash bright lights before the eyes. Some abnormalities only become evident during sleep; therefore, a sedative may be prescribed and recordings made before, during, and after sleep.

The EEG may take up to an hour to complete. Following the test the patient may need assistance in using acetone to remove the collodion from the hair and scalp. The EEG is particularly useful in evaluating seizure disorders and it may help to localize tumours.

An ambulatory EEG may be performed over a 24-hour period, using a portable recorder attached to the patient's waist. This is used to diagnose petit mal, temporal lobe epilepsy or seizures of unknown origin.

EEG telimetery is frequently used as with this method the patient can be observed by using a video camera, whilst at the same time the EEG tracing can be seen and recorded. This method gives essential information on seizure type and patients' behaviour.

Electromyography (EMG). This is a record of the electrical currents produced by skeletal muscles. Small needle electrodes are inserted into a muscle and the electrical currents are recorded with the muscle at rest and during activity. The test is useful to monitor changes in peripheral nerve dysfunction, to determine types of primary muscle disease and to identify defective transmission at the myoneural junction. The patient usually experiences some discomfort when the needle electrodes are inserted and if many muscles are tested some discomfort may persist.

Nerve conduction study. This is frequently done with the EMG (above). It studies the excitability and conduction velocities of motor and sensory nerves to help diagnose disease of peripheral nerves. During the procedure the patient may experience a mild electrical shock.

Caloric test. This test evaluates the function of the vestibular portion of the eighth cranial nerve. It helps to differentiate lesions of the brain stem and the cerebellum. Normally, stimulation of the auditory canal with hot water produces a rotary nystagmus toward the side of the irrigated ear. The nystagmus is away from the irrigated ear when ice-cold water is used. Nystagmus does not occur if pathology is present. The patient needs to know that he may experience vertigo, nausea, and vomiting but that a nurse will be available to assist him.

Neuropsychological tests. These tests are done when deficits in adaptive abilities are suspected. Motor, perceptual, language, visual–spatial, cognitive and other abilities can be assessed to determine the extent of impairment in brain functions. The tests measure deficits in coping skills by evaluating these skills directly rather than indirectly. They require several hours to complete and they may result in recommendations concerning educational and vocational placement.

Invasive neurodiagnostic procedures

Invasive procedures may be very complex and the patient may experience pain and discomfort. Invasive procedures carry a risk of morbidity and mortality. The degree of risk should be communicated to the patient and/or family so that the decision to undertake the test is an informed one. Prior to each of these procedures, craniocerebral testing is done in order to provide baseline information for comparison during and after the test. A signed consent form must be obtained prior to many of these procedures.

Lumbar puncture (LP). A lumbar puncture *is not performed* on a patient when increased intracranial pressure is suspected. Removal of cerebrospinal fluid may cause coning or herniation of the brain leading to damage affecting the brain stem as medial brain structures are forced through the tentorial notch in response to the increased pressure gradient. A lumbar puncture involves the insertion of a spinal needle into the lumbar subarachnoid space of the spinal canal by the doctor. The needle is passed through the intervertebral space between the third and fourth or fourth and fifth lumbar vertebrae, stopping at a safe distance from the cord.

The puncture may be performed to determine the pressure of CSF, to obtain specimens of the fluid for examination, or to inject drugs for anaesthesia or other purposes.

Lumbar pucture is performed in cases of suspected benign intracranial hypertension (pseudo tumour cerebri), having first excluded space occupying lesions by means of a CT scan. The pressure, which may be greater than 400 mm H_2O, can be safely reduced to 120 mm H_2O and the procedure is often repeated at weekly intervals over several months.

The patient assumes the lateral recumbent position, with the back on the edge of the bed, and flexes the knees to the chest so that they touch the chin, in order to widen the interspinous spaces. The nurse may need to support the patient behind the neck and knees. Asepsis is emphasized to prevent infection in the spinal canal which could be serious and even fatal. The skin is prepared, local anaesthetic injected and a spinal needle inserted. If the needle contacts one of the dorsal nerve roots, pain down one leg occurs. Needle removal rectifies this and the patient is assured that no damage has occurred. The fluid pressure is measured with a manometer and several samples of CSF are collected in sterile tubes for examination. Following needle removal a small sterile dressing is applied to the site.

Normal CSF pressure in the recumbent position is 40–180 mm H_2O. Abnormally low pressure may indicate an obstruction in the spinal subarachnoid space above the puncture site. Elevated pressure may signify infection or a space-occupying lesion such as a brain tumour or blood clot. Generally, LP is contraindicated in the presence of a space-occupying lesion because the rapid reduction in pressure caused by the removal of CSF can cause the brain to shift downward and herniate in the foramen magnum ('coning'). This, in turn, compresses the vital centres in the medulla and could cause sudden death. Should sudden collapse occur, airway establishment and resuscitation are necessary. Removal of CSF from the lateral ventricles may also be required.

Nursing care following LP includes keeping the patient flat in bed for 6–24 hours (depending on policy and presence of headache), monitoring neurological signs and encouraging fluids (unless contraindicated). When increased intracranial pressure is present, herniation of the brain does not necessarily occur during or immediately after LP but rarely may occur several hours later. The patient should have frequent neurological checks for several hours post-LP and adverse changes should be reported to the doctor.

Post-LP problems may be transient difficulty in voiding, temperature elevation due to meningeal irritation, pain, oedema, or haematoma at the puncture site and pain radiating to the thigh due to nerve root irritation. Post-LP headache may also occur. This is normally attributed to the removal of CSF during the test or to later leakage of the fluid into the tissues. The headache is typically frontal and suboccipital and is relieved when a horizontal position is assumed. The patient lies flat, a cold compress or ice-bag may be applied to the head, and a mild analgesic may be prescribed.

Cisternal puncture. This is done if an LP is contraindicated or if there is a block in the spinal subarachnoid space. A short needle is inserted into the cisterna magna (a small sac of CSF between the cerebellum and medulla) just beneath the occiptal bone. Because this puncture is close to the brain and the patient's co-operation is necessary, anxiety-reducing and supportive measures are essential. The nape of the neck is shaved, the patient is positioned on the side and the head is flexed forward and held firmly by the nurse, or the patient may be sat upright, resting the arms on pillows on a bed-table. Observation is necessary for signs of respiration difficulty which may suggest that the needle has made contact with the medulla. Usually the patient resumes normal activity soon after the procedure.

Cerebral angiography. This is performed by injecting radio-opaque material into the carotid and vertebral arteries. While this can be done by a direct puncture of the vessel, the method of choice is by a catheter, manipulated into the origin of the vessel via the femoral artery. Under local anaesthetic, sterile technique and with the patient sedated, a suitably-shaped catheter is passed retrogradely up to the aorta over a guide wire. Selective catheterization of the carotid and vertebral arteries can be undertaken as indicated. During the injection, X-ray images are obtained in rapid sequence. following removal of the needle, a sterile gauze pad is applied over the injection site and firm pressure is applied for 5–10 minutes to prevent haemorrhage and haematoma formation.

Following the angiogram the patient remains on bed rest for at least 8 hours. Neurological observations are carried out frequently and the pressure dressing is checked for bleeding. A cold compress or ice-bag may be applied to the injection site to control oedema and discomfort and to reduce the possibility of bleeding. If a limb was used for the puncture site (e.g. femoral artery), the distal part is checked for colour, temperature, and presence of a pulse. It is important to assess the adjacent extremity because vasospasm, thrombosis or formation of a haematoma can occur, obstructing the blood supply to the distant part.

Rarely, cerebral angiography may precipitate a stroke, seizure, allergic reaction to the contrast substance, or other serious complications. Any signs of deterioration in the patient's condition must be reported to the doctor immediately.

Myelography. This is an X-ray examination of the spinal cord and vertebral canal following injection of a radiopaque contrast substance into the spinal subarachnoid space. It is used to detect and localize lesions which may be compressing the spinal cord or nerves. Water soluble, non-ionic contrast medium is injected into the cerebral spinal fluid surrounding the spinal cord and emerging nerve roots. The most common access site is the lumbar region (as for lumbar puncture), but when pathology is suspected in the cervical region, a lateral puncture of the dura may be made, between the spinous processes of C1 and C2.

As with all procedures, an explanation is given so that the patient will know what to expect and can co-operate more fully. A history of any allergy is recorded and brought to the doctor's attention. Food and fluid are withheld up to 6 hours prior to the test and sedation may be prescribed 1 hour prior to the procedure. The lumbosacral area of the back is shaved if necessary.

Following the procedure, the patient rests supine in bed, with the head and trunk at 45°. This position will minimize the volume of contrast that enters the CSF surrounding the brain. Serious complications of myelography are fortunately rare, particularly with the use of the new non-ionic contrast media. However, the neurological status of the patient should be kept under review following the procedure; persistent headache, pain and/or the development of neck stiffness should be reported.

THE PERSON WITH NEUROLOGICAL DISORDERS OR ALTERED NEUROLOGICAL FUNCTION

The highly complex nature of the nervous system is revealed through its numerous and diverse disorders. The dysfunctions which result depend primarily on the area(s) of the nervous system affected the extent of the lesion, and, to a lesser degree, the nature of the pathological process. For this reason, it is difficult for health care professionals to predict outcomes and thereby develop outcome criteria. The focus of nursing activity includes disease stabilization, health promotion and prevention. The family is an integral part of patient care and members are encouraged to participate in all aspects of care, including decision making, to the degree that they are able. Pathology of the central nervous system often compromises intellectual and reasoning process, hence the added importance of family involvement and the need for nurses to be aware of concepts such as maintenance of dignity and need for advocacy. There are recurrent legal and ethical issues inherent in the care of patients with neurological dysfunction. Issues such as brain death, persistent vegetative state, and surrogate decision making are only some examples where nurses face ethical dilemmas.

The following sections present a discussion of common disorders which are most often encountered in nursing practice; a review of nursing interventions is also included.

THE PERSON WITH ALTERED LEVEL OF CONSCIOUSNESS

PATIENT PROBLEMS

Problems relevant to the patient with an altered level of consciousness are:

1. Alteration in sensation: visual, auditory, kinaesthesic, gustatory, tactile and olfactory.
2. Alteration in thought processes.
3. Ineffective airway clearance.
4. Impaired physical mobility.
5. Potential for injury.
6. Potential impairment of skin integrity.
7. Alteration in nutrition (less than body requirements).
8. Alteration in patterns of urinary elimination: incontinence.
9. Alteration in bowel elimination: incontinence.
10. Inability to maintain self care: feeding, bathing/hygiene, dressing, grooming and toileting.

GOALS

These principal problems lead to a set of patient goals which involve the patient avoiding harmful complications, maximizing independence and adapting to altered functioning in the above areas.

NURSING INTERVENTION

Identification of changes in neurological function

Monitoring of the patient's level of consciousness, pupillary responses, limb movements and vital signs is done continuously. If the patient's condition is changing, data are recorded every 15 minutes. When the patient's neurological status stabilizes, recordings are gradually made less often. Early signs of increasing intracranial pressure should be reported promptly to ensure immediate action to prevent cerebral coning. The first sign of increasing intracranial pressure is a decrease in level of consciousness, as measured on the Glasgow coma scale; hence the importance of these observations.

Maintenance of body functions and prevention of complications

1. Maintenance of a patent airway. The first priority in caring for an unconscious patient is the establishment of a patent airway. As the patient's level of consciousness decreases, the ability to maintain a clear airway is limited. The cause may be obstruction of the airway by the tongue when the jaw and tongue relax, vomit, blood or other inhaled foreign material such as dentures. Ineffective ventilation may occur due to depression of the respiratory centre, accumulation of secretions and foreign material, as a result of depression of the cough reflex and immobility and weakness of respiratory muscles.

The unconscious patient is placed in a lateral or semiprone position (unless contraindicated by a chest or spinal injury), with the neck aligned with the spine. If the patient is unconscious as a result of a head injury, a spinal injury should be assumed to be present until proven otherwise. See p. 737 and Chapter 24 for movement of spinally injured patients. Either position facilitates the drainage of mucus and vomit and prevents obstruction of the airway by the relaxed tongue and jaw. If mucus collects in the oropharyngeal cavity, frequent suctioning with a flexible catheter will be necessary. The suction catheter should have several holes at its tip for adequate collection of the mucus during the procedure. The catheter is moistened with water prior to its insertion and is handled gently during insertion and on withdrawal to avoid trauma to the delicate tracheal mucous membranes.

If the patient has lost the gag reflex an artificial airway will be needed. An oropharyngeal airway or an endotracheal tube may be inserted to maintain the airway and facilitate the removal of secretions by suctioning.

Oxygen may be administered by nasal cannulae or mask, or mechanical ventilation may be instituted. If the patient is able to follow instructions, deep breathing is practised hourly. Hard, sustained coughing is contraindicated as it causes an increase in intracranial pressure. If coughing is necessary to remove secretions and the patient is able to do so, staged coughing is taught. This involves the patient taking a deep breath while relaxing the abdominal muscles, holding the breath, and then exhaling in short, staged intervals involving 4–5 expirations. Postural drainage and chest percussion and vibration are carried out several times a day by the physiotherapist to promote drainage of respiratory secretions.

The patient's position should be changed every two hours to prevent pressure sore formation and facilitate the removal of secretions from the lungs. Observations are made following each change of position to determine the effect on respirations. Chest expansion is observed and the rate and rhythm of respirations are noted as well as the patient's colour and general status.

2. Care of the eyes. Loss of the corneal reflex and depression of lacrimal secretion may result in prolonged exposure, drying and injury to the cornea which may lead to ulceration. The eyes should be examined regularly for signs of inflammation or injury. Contact lenses are removed. Ophthalmic solutions may be prescribed to irrigate the eyes three or four times a day. The eyes may be covered with dressings to protect them.

3. Care of the mouth. Dentures should be removed if the patient is unconscious. The mouth is cleansed several times a day and teeth are cleaned by brushing when possible. The lips are moistened with a water-soluble ointment or cream. The mouth should be inspected daily for signs of crusting or ulceration of the mucosa.

4. Positioning. When the patient is placed in the lateral or semiprone position (as cited above), attention is given to good body alignment and to the prevention of contractures, foot and wrist drop, muscle strain, joint injury, and interference with circulation and chest expansion. The head should be positioned so that the neck is aligned with the spine. The arm that is uppermost is flexed at the elbow and rested on a pillow to prevent a drag on the shoulder and wrist drop. The arm that is down is drawn slightly forward, flexed at the elbow, and lies on the bed parallel with the neck and head. The lower limb that is uppermost is flexed at the hip and knee, and supported on a firm pillow; the other lower limb is slightly flexed. The feet are positioned at a

90° angle to the leg and care is taken that *no* pressure is applied by firm objects placed against the feet.

5. Joint movement. The extremities are passively moved through their normal range of motion at least twice daily to preserve joint function and prevent circulatory stasis. Active exercises are initiated as soon as the patient is able to follow instructions.

6. Protection from injury. The cot-sides of the bed are always maintained in the up position when the patient is unconscious unless someone is in constant attendance on the patient. It may be necessary to pad the sides of the bed if the patient is restless and thrashing about. Alternatively, the patient may be nursed on a mattress on the floor. A very agitated patient may climb over cot sides and suffer serious injury from the ensuing fall. Placing mittens on the hands may be necessary if the patient is restless, scratches, or pulls on the nasogastric or intravenous tube or the urethral catheter. The mittens are removed at least twice daily; the hands are bathed, the nails are kept clean and short, and the fingers put through their normal range of motion by passive exercise.

The nurse should not attempt to force resisting extremities (such as in spastic flexion or extension) to assume a different position. Forcing a rigid extremity into a different position could result in a fracture of that limb. The use of depressant drugs to control agitation is contraindicated as they may further depress the arousal system.

When the patient is ambulatory but has some impairment of awareness, a safe environment should be provided. Scatter rugs and objects are removed from the patient's path to prevent falling. Sharp objects are removed from the immediate environment.

7. Fluids and nutrition. The patient is assessed for a gag reflex; as soon as it is present, and the patient is conscious, oral feeds are initiated. When the patient is unconscious or the gag reflex is absent the patient's nutrition may be sustained by intravenous infusion or feeds given via a nasogastric feeding tube. The liquid feed given by tube contains the essential food elements and the amount is individually calculated to provide adequate caloric intake for the patient's size and metabolic activity. The dietitian should be consulted for advice. Frequency of feeding varies from slow continuous to every 4 hours. If there is any regurgitation (fluid welling up around the tube into the mouth), the volume given at one time is decreased and the frequency of the feeds is increased. If the patient's condition permits, it is helpful to elevate the head of the bed slightly during the feeding and for a brief period following. The tube is rinsed with 30–45 ml of water after each feeding.

The presence of the tube in a nostril tends to irritate the mucous membrane and stimulate mucus secretion. The area is cleansed twice daily with applicators which have been moistened with normal saline, and is then also lubricated lightly. The tube should be secured loosely enough so that it does not continuously press on any one area of the nostril.

8. Elimination. The unconscious patient has urinary incontinence. An indwelling catheter is inserted initially only if it is necessary to facilitate accurate monitoring of output or if retention of urine occurs. The catheter is removed as soon as possible to prevent complications and promote the return of normal bladder functioning. Condom drainage is established with the male patient as soon as his condition is stable. While the catheter is in place it is taped to the thigh to prevent undue traction. The complete set of tubes and drainage receptacle constitutes a closed sterile system. The urethral meatus and surrounding area may be cleansed with an antiseptic solution two or three times daily, but as discussed in Chapter 20, there is no evidence to show this reduces infection risk.

If a catheter is not used, frequent attention is necessary to protect the skin. Incontinence pads are used to absorb the urine and are changed promptly after voiding. The skin is washed after each voiding and dried thoroughly. A barrier cream may be applied to the skin. The bed linen is changed as necessary.

The patient may be incontinent of faeces, particularly if receiving tube feedings. Prompt cleansing and changing of soiled pads and bedding are necessary. If the bowels do not move regularly, the doctor will prescribe an aperient, suppositories or an enema.

9. Skin care. The unconscious patient is predisposed to the rapid development of pressure sores. Precautions should be taken to keep the skin clean and dry and the bedding free of wrinkles. Pressure areas are bathed and gently dried. Sheepskins may be used to prevent friction damaging the patient's skin while a Spenco mattress or an alternating air pressure (ripple) mattress may be used to relieve pressure; particular attention should be paid to the heels and ankles. The patient's position is changed at least every 2 hours. If a pressure sore develops it is treated aseptically, just as any wound, and the patient is positioned to avoid pressure on the area.

Care should be taken to maintain daily personal hygiene. This includes hair and face washing and shaving. Families should be encouraged to help in these activities if they feel comfortable about it. It is important for families to be included as part of the caring team.

Maintenance or restoration of sensation, perception and awareness

Fluctuations in consciousness affect the patient's ability to receive a stimulus, interpret its meaning and respond with appropriate behaviour. The arousal mechanism may be affected so that repeated stimulation may be required to elicit a response. Sensory stimulation is an important aspect of the care of every patient experiencing alterations in the level of consciousness. The type of stimulation, how it is structured and presented and its complexity must be planned for each individual according to his level of consciousness, the cause of the decreased consciousness and the relevance and meaning of the stimulus to this particular individual.

Types of stimuli include the following (*Stimulation Program for Cognitive Deficits in Traumatic Head*

Injured Adults. Unpublished, Hamilton General Hospital, Hamilton, Ontario):

- *Auditory* stimulation is provided by the nurse who regularly addresses the patient by name, explains where he or she is and states the date and time and what is happening at any given time. Family members and friends are encouraged to talk to the patient. Radio, tape recordings of music or conversations from friends and family or talking books may also be used to provide auditory stimulation. Environmental noises are interpreted by the nurse to prevent misunderstanding; bedside curtains and room doors are left open to allow for visualization of the source of sounds.
- *Olfactory* stimulation by noxious odours such as sulphur or ammonia may be used to evoke a response. The patient is also exposed to familiar, accustomed pleasant odours; these may include perfumes, coffee, tea or flowers.
- *Visual* stimuli may be provided by a stimulation board placed at the foot or side of the bed; cards, posters and photographs of family members may be pinned to the board. Mobiles can be made to serve the same purpose. Personal possessions, favourite toys and pictures are placed in the patient's line of vision. Television also provides visual and auditory stimulation.
- *Tactile* stimulation may be provided by the nurse and family members; the latter are encouraged to use touch and to have the patient touch them in return. Tactile stimuli may take the form of massage, gentle touching or brisk rubbing.
- *Kinaesthesic* sensations may be promoted by 'range of motion' exercises of the extremities and by changes in body position. A programme of mat activities may be provided by the physiotherapist.
- *Vestibular* stimulation may be provided by tilt tables.
- *Oral* stimulation may be produced by cotton swabs or flavours may be used on swabs, or ice chips may be given for sucking if the gag reflex is present. Foods of varying textures are provided if the patient is able to swallow, when consciousness returns.

The nurse should always speak to the patient, by name and explain what is being done, and the patient should be informed before procedures such as feeding and turning occur. Touch is used as much as possible. Environmental noise is decreased and night orientation is practised to provide rest. Multisensory stimuli sessions may be carried out three or four times a day. Each method of stimulation is introduced one at a time in a form that is meaningful to the patient.

THE PERSON WITH CEREBROVASCULAR DISORDERS

Cerebrovascular disorders are among the most common of all neurological disorders. The greater number may be classified as ischaemic or haemorrhagic. *Either may cause a cerebrovascular infarction which is commonly known as a stroke* or may also be referred to as cerebrovascular accident (CVA).

Stroke (Cerebrovascular Accident)

INCIDENCE

Strokes are a leading cause of death and disability. They have their highest incidence in those over 60 years of age.

A stroke or CVA involves an interruption of the blood supply to a part of the brain and the development of neurological deficits. If the ischaemia persists, necrosis of the deprived area follows, the infarcted area eventually liquefies and is absorbed and the neurological deficits remain. The cause of the stroke may be atherosclerosis, cerebral thrombosis or embolism, or intracranial haemorrhage. The artery that ruptures is usually vulnerable due to degenerative vascular changes (atherosclerosis) or the presence of an aneurysm. A haemorrhagic stroke may be precipitated by an elevation of blood pressure and is usually associated with some physical or emotional stress.

According to the rate of development and permanence of the neurological effects, a stroke may be categorized as a transient ischaemic attack, stroke in evolution or completed stroke. Gradual development of stroke symptoms over a period of several hours or days is usually associated with a cerebral thrombosis or slow leak in a cerebral artery. This type of stroke is referred to as a stroke in evolution. A stroke is classified as a completed stroke when the neurological deficits remain longer than 3 or 4 days.

CEREBRAL ATHEROSCLEROSIS

This is a chronic degenerative process of the cerebral arteries in which the intimal layer gradually develops atheromas (fibrous fatty plaques). These narrow the vascular lumen, damage the underlying layer of tissue media and tend to undergo calcification, ulceration with overlying thrombosis and intraplaque haemorrhage which worsen the luminal narrowing or cause total occlusion. These degenerative changes result in interference with cerebral perfusion. Although the brain represents only about 2% of the body's weight, it consumes 20% of its oxygen. Since the brain cannot store energy nor temporarily exist by anaerobic metabolism, deprivation of oxygenated blood for even a very few minutes leads to neuronal death.

Atherosclerosis affects the larger vessels at the base of the brain first, particularly at the points of vessel branching and tends to develop silently. The incidence increases with increasing age. Its presence is manifested when it is well advanced by: (1) the development of ischaemia of vital organs (e.g. deterioration of mental faculties); (2) episodes of local neurological dysfunction, which are referred to as transient ischaemic attacks; (3) predisposition to thrombosis which may give rise to emboli; (4) weakening of an arterial wall resulting in an aneurysm. Occasionally, on routine physical examination, a noise or bruit may be heard through a stethoscope placed over the eye or carotid artery when there is turbulent blood flow due to irregularities in the vessel wall.

Since the cause of atherosclerosis continues to elude scientists, interventions are directed to reducing the risk factors. This diagnosis can promote much anxiety and uncertainty in the patient and family, who will consequently require information about risk factors such as smoking, cholesterol (LDL), obesity, etc., and a discussion about possible changes in life-style that will decrease the level of risk. Risk factors that are the target of educational interventions include: (1) diets high in cholesterol and saturated fat, (2) hypercholesterolaemia, (3) hypertension, (4) cigarette smoking, and (5) diabetes. Controversy continues with regard to the control of atherosclerosis by modification of diet and blood lipid values. In addition, some defend and others deny a role for control of blood sugar in the progression of atherosclerosis, but the desirability of controlling hypertension and cigarette smoking is unquestioned. An anticoagulant (e.g. aspirin, warfarin) may be prescribed.

Surgical therapy for atherosclerosis causing cerebral ischaemia involves a carotid endarterectomy or cerebral artery bypass (see Chapter 14).

CEREBRAL THROMBOSIS AND EMBOLISM

This is the most common cause of stroke and is usually due to atherosclerosis of the carotid, vertebral or larger cerebral arteries. The narrowing of the lumen of the vessel by atherosclerotic plaques leads to thrombus formation, occlusion of the artery and ischaemia of the respective brain area. Inadequate delivery of blood to the brain and subsequent thrombosis may be secondary to cardiac insufficiency, shock or to reduced intravascular volume as occurs in haemorrhage and severe dehydration.

Embolic material, which may be a thrombus or atherosclerotic plaque, which becomes free in the bloodstream, lodges in a cerebral artery, occluding the vessel and resulting in a cerebral infarction (stroke). The middle cerebral artery is the most frequent location. The occlusion occurs suddenly; there is no warning or time for the development of collateral circulation. Anticoagulant therapy may be prescribed to prevent a second stroke.

TRANSIENT ISCHAEMIC ATTACKS

A large percentage of patients with an atherothrombic stroke have a history of transient ischaemic attacks. These episodes of local neurological dysfunction may last a few seconds to several hours; most last 5–10 minutes. There may be only a few attacks or as many as several hundred before an actual stroke. These transient attacks are due to focal ischaemia incurred by temporary occlusion of an artery by vasospasm microemboli or insufficient blood supply. They are usually associated with atherosclerosis.

Transient attacks are warning signs of impending complete stroke. Manifestations include transient paresis or hemiplegia, visual deficits (decreased vision in one eye), difficulty in or loss of speech, difficulty in comprehension, dizziness, unsteadiness and sudden falls.

Lack of knowledge in the patient experiencing transient ischaemic attacks is a major concern. It is a nursing responsibility to assess the patient's understand-

Table 21.4 Organization of a functionally orientated nursing neurological evaluation.

General category	Functional category	Examples of specific function which may be tested
Consciousness	Arousing (reticular activating system)	Arousability, response to verbal and tactile stimuli
Mentation	Thinking (general cortical function plus specific regional functions)	Educational level Content of conversation Orientation Fund of information Insight, judgement, planning
	Feeling (affective)	Mood and affect Perception and reaction to ability, disability
	Language	Content and quantity of speech Ability to name objects Ability to repeat phrases Ability to read, write, copy
	Remembering	Attention span Recent and remote memory
Motor function	Seeing (cranial nerves, II, III, IV, VI)	Acuity Visual fields Extraocular movement Pupil size, shape, reactivity Presence or absence of diplopia, nystagmus
	Eating (cranial nerves V, IX, X, XII)	Chewing Swallowing Gag (if swallowing impaired)
	Expressing (facially) (cranial nerve VII)	Symmetry of smile, frown
	Speaking (cranial nerves VII, IX, X, XII)	Clarity, presence or absence of nasality
	Moving (Motor and cerebellar systems)	Muscle tone, mass, strength Presence or absence of involuntary movements Coordination: heel-to-toe walk, observing during dressing Posture, gait, position
Sensory function	Smelling (cranial nerve I)	Ability to detect odours
	Blinking (cranial nerve V)	Corneal reflex
	Hearing (cranial nerve VII)	Acuity, presence or absence of unusual sounds
	Feeling (sensory pathways)	Pain-pinprick Touch, stereognosis Temperature—warm, cold

Note: Examples of specific functions that may be tested in each functional category are shown. The structures involved in each of the functions categorized are indicated in parentheses.

ing of the episodes and urge prompt, medical attention. Timely and appropriate therapy can reduce the number of these attacks and may reduce the risk of a disastrous stroke in the near future.

The therapeutic regimen may involve a low fat diet, control of hypertension, no smoking and an anticoagulant such as warfarin or aspirin. Selected patients are treated surgically by a carotid endarterectomy or cerebral artery bypass.

ENDARTERECTOMY

Endarterectomy of the internal carotid involves the removal of the atheroma from the intima. A venous graft or dacron prosthesis may be necessary to reinforce the vascular area from which the plaques are removed.

Not all patients with atherosclerosis or experiencing transient ischaemic attacks are candidates for surgery; those who are very elderly and have extensive vascular disease or who have serious heart or renal problems are a high risk.

Nursing intervention

Preoperative preparation of the patient for an endarterectomy includes an explanation of the procedure and what may be expected immediately after the operation. The patient receives an anticoagulant such as heparin. Baseline neurological information is recorded for postoperative comparison. The care is the same as for a general preoperative preparation (see Chapter 11) except that a specific directive may be received

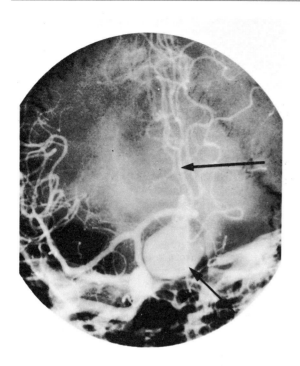

Figure 21.20 Cerebral aneurysm (arrowed).

concerning skin preparation.

Postoperative nursing care as with any patient who might develop neurological complications, involves frequent craniocerebral testing which is necessary to detect early evidence of neurological deficit (see Table 21.4). Frequent monitoring of the blood pressure is essential: an elevation may place stress on the operative site and cause severe haemorrhage. Hypotension predisposes to thrombus formation within the artery at the surgical site. Frequent observation of the operative site for evidence of bleeding or oedema in the area is necessary. The neck circumference is observed frequently for swelling due to internal bleeding. Respiratory distress is reported promptly; swelling due to oedema or clot formation may compress the trachea and interfere with respirations. Observations are also made for signs of any intracranial functional changes.

The patient is kept at rest and quiet with a minimum of stimuli during the first 24 hours; all exertion on his part is avoided. After this period, the patient is gradually mobilized if his vital signs are satisfactory and stable.

An anticoagulant is prescribed and is usually continued for about 6 months following the surgery. Regular checking of prothrombin time is necessary. On discharge from the hospital, the patient is advised to report any blood in the urine or stool, bleeding of gums or discoloured bruised areas (ecchymoses). Former activities are resumed very gradually.

CEREBRAL ARTERY BYPASS

Cerebral artery bypass surgery may be performed on patients who have lesions in the smaller arteries inside the skull which cannot be corrected by endarterectomy. Using microsurgical techniques and a craniotomy just above the ear, a large scalp artery (e.g. superficial temporal) is anastamosed to a blocked artery in order to supply blood beyond the stenosis.

Nursing intervention

Nursing care postoperatively is similar to postendarterectomy. Frequent craniocerebral testing allows for early detection of neurological changes suggestive of compromised cerebral blood flow or increased intracranial pressure.

The major complications following bypass surgery include interruption of blood flow through the graft, stroke and subdural haematoma due to bleeding at the surgical site. The patient is positoned off the operative side with the head of the bed elevated 30°. Anticoagulant therapy may be continued for several months following surgery. Long-term benefits and indications for cerebral bypass have not been firmly established but there is some evidence of decreased stroke rate and improvement in the quality of life of those patients who have had a bypass.

CEREBRAL ANEURYSM

An aneurysm is a saccular dilatation of an arterial wall, thought to be caused most often by the congenital absence of muscular and elastic tissue in the wall of that area of the vessel. It may also develop as a result of degenerative vascular changes. The most common cerebral aneurysm is referred to as a *berry aneurysm* because it is a rounded, outpouching on a stem (Figure 21.20). The majority occur at the base of the brain in the circle of Willis at points of bifurcation. The lesion does not always produce symptoms and may be single or there may be several.

Aneurysms are the cause of death in over 50% of all fatal cerebrovascular lesions in persons under the age of 45 years. Although the weakness in the arterial wall is congenital, actual distension of the vessel occurs much later in life. The distension may produce localizing symptoms by pressure on adjacent strucures (e.g. paralysis due to pressure on cranial nerves). Rupture of the artery is the most serious consequence. It may be preceded by a series of small leaks over several weeks manifested by headache and stiffness of the neck but more often the rupture occurs without any warning. The most vulnerable persons are those who are 35–60 years of age and those with hypertension or polycystic disease of the kidneys. Rupture may be precipitated by physical or emotional exertion and the bleeding may occur into the subarachnoid space, cerebral substance or both those areas.

Assessment

Clinical characteristics
Rupture of a cerebral aneurysm forces blood under arterial pressure into the brain tissue and subarachnoid space giving rise to an explosive headache, nausea,

Table 21.5 Classification of cerebral aneurysms.

Classification	Patient response
I. Minimal bleed	Alert, minimal headache, neurological deficits absent
II. Mild bleed	Alert, mild to severe headache, neck rigidity, minimal neurological deficits (e.g. oculo-motor palsy)
III. Moderate bleed	Drowsy or confused, neck rigidity, may have mild focal deficit such as limb weakness
IV. Moderate to severe bleed	Responds only to painful stimuli; neck rigidity, major neurological deficits (e.g. hemiparesis), possible early decerebration
V. Severe bleed	Unresponsive, decerebrate rigidity, moribund appearance

vomiting and in some, rapid loss of consciousness. Symptoms of meningeal irritation will also be present, which include pain and neck rigidity, positive Kernig's sign (inability to extend the knees without pain while in supine position with hips flexed), positive Brudzinski's sign (person in supine position bends the knees to avoid pain when the neck is flexed), photophobia, blurred vision, irritability, restlessness and possible temperature elevation. The presence and severity of symptoms are determined by the location and extent of the bleeding.

Investigation

When an aneurysm is suspected on the basis of the presenting symptoms a CT scan of the head will be done to detect the presence of blood in the ventricular system or any intracerebral clot. This may then be followed by a lumbar puncture, which will reveal blood in the cerebrospinal fluid. The next investigation will be the cerebral angiogram to look for aneurysms of the circle of Willis. This is performed in the neurological X-ray department by passing a catheter into the patient's femoral artery and feeding it into the subclavian artery. An injection of radio-opaque contrast medium will outline the blood vessels. When the diagnosis is confirmed, the clinical data are used to grade the aneurysm; the classification is used as a guide to therapy and to establish the prognosis (Table 21.5). The nurse's role is one of monitoring, supporting and preventing complications. An important role is to support the family during this difficult time.

Prognosis

The prognosis following the initial bleed of a cerebral aneurysm is grave; many patients succumb at this time. Of those who survive the initial onset, a large number (approximately 42%) die of a recurrence of bleeding within a few days or weeks. Others may die as a result of cerebral infarction due to severe vasospasm. Survivors of a cerebral aneurysm haemorrhage may recover with few neurological deficits but many are partially or totally disabled due to paralysis, mental deterioration and/or seizures.

Medical management

The patient with a cerebral aneurysm requires prompt treatment. Those categorized as grade III, IV or V are managed conservatively until they progress to grade I or II. Only those classified as grade I or II are considered to be candidates for surgery.

Conservative treatment includes a hypotensive agent to lower the blood pressure, a mild sedative to reduce agitation and anxiety, a mild analgesic (usually codeine) to relieve pain, and a steroid preparation, for example dexamethasone, to control cerebral oedema and intracranial pressure. Analgesics and sedatives are used cautiously since they tend to mask neurological changes and symptoms. To reduce the risk of a rebleed, an antifibrinolytic agent may be administered orally or parenterally.

Surgical treatment involves microsurgical technique because of the critical location, size and fragility of some aneurysms. If the aneurysm can be clipped, a metal, self-closing, spring clip or ligature is applied to the neck of it to occlude the aneurysm. Those which cannot be occluded may be wrapped in a special gauze-like material and coated with an acrylic substance to reinforce the vascular walls to prevent another leak or rupture. Another procedure may involve proximal and distal ligation of the aneurysm which embolizes it. If the lesion is surgically inaccessible, gradual occlusion of the common carotid artery on the affected side by the application of a Selverstone clamp may be done; the blood supply to the affected side of the brain is gradually reduced. This latter procedure places the patient at risk of hemiplegia and is rarely undertaken these days.

Nursing care

Assessment

Vital signs and neurological status are assessed at frequent intervals (15 or 30 minutes) during the acute stage: a decrease in the level of consciousness, disorientation or other neurological changes are recorded and reported promptly to the doctor. The blood pressure is followed very closely since an elevation may increase the bleeding or precipitate rebleeding. If receiving a hypotensive drug, there is the risk of the pressure falling to a level that incurs ischaemia of the brain tissue; in addition there is the risk of rebleeding, vasospasm and secondary hydrocephalus. The latter may develop as a result of interference with the normal absorption process of the CSF by the accumulation of blood in the subarachnoid space into the venous sinuses. Hydrocephalus compresses the brain, giving rise to signs of increased intracranial pressure.

Patient problems
The problems of the patient treated *conservatively* include:

1. Potential for continued intracranial bleeding or for recurrence of bleeding.
2. Loss of self-care abilities.
3. Headache.
4. Anxiety and ineffective coping. Fear of the circumstances and concern for the outcome.
5. Potential for injury secondary to altered level of awareness, disorientation and immobility.
6. Alteration in food and fluid intake due to nausea, vomiting and restricted fluid intake.
7. Alteration in urinary and bowel elimination secondary to reduced level of awareness, decreased intake and enforced immobility.
8. Potential for complications: rebleeding, hydrocephalus and vasospasm.
9. Potential for residual mental and/or physical impairment resulting in need for rehabilitation.

Goals
The patient goals are to avoid the complications associated with the above problems and to achieve maximum independence and self-care.

Nursing intervention
Those treated conservatively are usually patients categorized as grade III, IV or V (Table 21.4). If the patient is unconscious, nursing measures will include those which apply to any unconscious patient (see pp. 713–715).

1. Observe for bleeding or a rebleed.   The patient is kept on complete bed rest with one pillow under the head or the head of the bed elevated about 30° to promote venous drainage and prevent increased intracranial pressure. The blood pressure is monitored frequently; it is important that it remain within the extreme low range of normal. Visitors are limited; family members are informed that they may sit quietly with the patient.

Because self-care requires exertion which increases the blood pressure predisposing to rebleeding, bathing, feeding and change of position are done by the nurse. In change of position and when getting on and off the bedpan, the patient is cautioned against physical effort and also against straining at stool.

If the patient is unable to rest, a mild sedative may be prescribed but only used with caution because it may mask neurological changes. The essential immobility predisposes to venous stasis and thrombophlebitis; the application of antiembolic stockings to the lower limbs may be recommended. They are removed and reapplied according to manufacturers instructions.

Vomiting and coughing are controlled because they increase the intracranial pressure. If the patient is nauseated and vomiting, oral fluids and food are withheld and an antiemetic prescribed. Deep breathing is encouraged at regular intervals to promote pulmonary ventilation.

2. Alteration in comfort.   The severe headache which the patient experiences causes restlessness, nausea and vomiting. Nursing measures include keeping the patient at rest and as quiet as possible. Cold applications to the head may help and a mild analgesic (e.g. codeine) is usually prescribed.

3. Anxiety and ineffective coping.   The patient will probably be very fearful and concerned for the future. It is important therefore to allow and encourage the patient to talk about these fears and answer questions openly. It will help if the serial assessments, procedures, enforced immobility and restrictions are explained if the patient is alert. A calm, reassuring approach can be therapeutic.

The family's perception of the illness, their expectations and coping patterns are assessed. Their role in keeping the patient quiet and at rest is explained to them. They are kept informed as to the patient's progress, and opportunities are provided for expression of feelings and for questions. Tests and procedures are explained to them.

4. Potential for injury.   Impairment of awareness may occur resulting in disorientation. Cot sides are kept up and frequent close observation made for confusion and restlessness: a mild sedative may be necessary. It may be necessary to have someone remain constantly with the patient to avoid personal injury.

When the comatose patient regains consciousness, frequent orientation to place and circumstances is necessary as well as reassurance as to care and progress.

5. Potential pressure sores.   The regular assessment of pressure areas and a 2-hourly turning regimen are essential, together with the use of equipment such as a ripple mattress, if pressure sores are to be prevented.

6. Fluid and food intake.   When tolerated, the patient receives a soft diet initially. The fluid intake may be limited to a specific volume per 24 hours to promote a reduction in cerebral oedema and in the intracranial pressure. This varies from unit to unit. Some units have a policy of a 3-litre minimum intake in 24 hours. An accurate record of the fluid intake and output is maintained.

7. Urinary and bowel elimination.   Rarely, the patient has difficulty voiding in the supine position and requires catheterization. In some instances an indwelling catheter may be used in the acute phase to prevent the exertion in using a bedpan, to protect the skin if the patient is incontinent or to closely monitor the urinary output.

A mild laxative or stool softener may be prescribed

after 3 or 4 days to prevent constipation and straining at stool. Enemas are contraindicated.

8. Potential complications. As well as the danger of a recurrence of bleeding by the aneurysm, the patient is at risk of developing vasospasm of cerebral vessels. Initially the spasm occurs in vessels in the region of the aneurysm, then spasms may become more extensive through the brain. The patient manifests symptoms of cerebral ischaemia. The nurse should be alert for changes in level of consciousness and vital signs, together with the symptoms of paresis, paralysis or speech impairment. If the spasm persists, infarction of the brain tissue occurs, causing serious neurological deficits.

Secondary hydrocephalus may develop as a result of interruption of the normal drainage of CSF into the general circulation system, by the residue of blood in the fluid blocking absorption by the arachnoid villi. The accumulation of CSF causes increased intracranial pressure (ICP) and compresses the brain.

Treatment may involve a cranial burr hole and the placing of a tube in a ventricle (ventriculostomy) for external drainage of the CSF. If the hydrocephalus persists, a permanent ventriculoatrial or ventriculoperitoneal shunt may be done to drain the CSF.

9. Residual impairment. The patient may recover and be left with brain damage that results in reduced physical and/or mental capacity. This clearly has long-term social and psychological implications for the patient and family which must be addressed realistically and with the support of a wide range of agencies.

The patient treated by surgery
Generally, only patients classified as grade I or II are considered as surgical candidates.

Most surgeons wait several days before operating to allow time for the postrupture oedema of the brain to reduce. The greatest challenge to the nurse may be the patient in grade I or II category during this waiting period. He or she may be a young person who is worried about being away from work and family, may not feel particularly ill and finds it very difficult to understand why it is necessary to be kept immobile and treated as though helpless. The nurse spends time talking quietly, explaining and reassuring, and making every effort to prevent incidents that are likely to increase the blood pressure and initiate rebleeding.

A specific directive is usually received from the surgeon as to the preoperative preparation: otherwise it is similar to that cited for intracranial surgery (see p. 733).

Postoperative care is that outlined for the patient having intracranial surgery. If no complications arise, ambulation is started within 2 or 3 days after operation. Progression from lying to the sitting position and then to standing is made very slowly as the patient will have been on complete bed rest for a period before the surgery.

The integrity of the surgical procedure may be checked by a postoperative cerebral angiogram.

EFFECTS OF A CVA ON THE PATIENT

Whether the CVA was due to atherosclerosis, thrombosis, embolism or a ruptured cerebral artery, it may produce a wide range of severe effects, leading to the following range of problems.

- *Alteration in level of consciousness.* The patient may experience only a decrease in responsiveness to stimuli, confusion or clouding of consciousness while others may suddenly or gradually become unconscious. The coma may last a few hours to days; the gravity of prognosis tends to increase if the coma extends beyond 36 hours.
- *Headache and vomiting.* If remaining conscious, the patient may complain of severe headache as a result of increased intracranial pressure. Vomiting frequently occurs with the initial onset and may be recurring in the conscious patient.
- *Neuromuscular deficits.* The immediate onset may be accompanied by convulsive movements which may be local or general. The effects of the impairment of neuromuscular control by stroke vary from only a muscular weakness to complete paralysis. Hemiplegia (paralysis of one side of the body) is one of the most common effects of a stroke and indicates interruption of motor pathways. The interference with impulses usually involves the internal capsule in the affected hemisphere. The axons of motor neurones which initiate willed movements in each hemisphere converge into the internal capsule (see p. 699). The motor fibres from each hemisphere cross over in the medulla; as a result, paralysis of one side of the body indicates that the cerebral lesion is on the other side; that is, a stroke in the right side of the brain causes paralysis of the left arm and leg. For a few days, there is a marked loss of tone in the affected muscles and an absence of normal reflexes. Even though the patient is in coma, a greater loss of tone in the affected limbs is recognizable (when flexed the limb falls more quickly in a limp, lifeless manner). Later this flaccidity is replaced by spasticity.

  One side of the face may be paralysed, which causes the alternating abnormal distension and retraction with each respiration. The mouth is also drawn to one side.

  When conscious, the patient may experience difficulty in swallowing (dysphagia) indicating some paralysis of the swallowing muscles.
- *Incontinence.* Urinary and bowel incontinence are common in the early stage. The bladder is atonic and the patient does not experience the desire to void. Later, tone returns and the bladder may become spastic and the patient experiences frequency and urgency. Unless the cerebral damage is extensive, involving both hemispheres, bladder control may be re-established with training. The patient may be insensitive to the defecation reflex, resulting in incontinence.
- *Eye changes.* The pupils may be unequal in size; the larger of the two is on the side of the lesion. The eyes as well as the head tend to turn to the side of the lesion in the early stage; later the deviations may be reversed. Hemianopia (loss of vision in half of the

Table 21.6 Common types of aphasia.

Auditory aphasia	Inability to comprehend spoken word. May be referred to as *word deafness*
Expressive aphasia	Individual understands spoken and written words and knows what he or she wants to say but cannot speak the words. Also referred to as *motor or Broca's aphasia*
Global aphasia	Complete aphasia involves both the sensory and motor functions that provide all forms of communication
Receptive aphasia	Inability to comprehend spoken, written or tactile symbols. Also referred to as *sensory aphasia*

visual field) occurs and may be temporary. In the unconscious patient, the corneal and pupillary reflexes may be absent and the fundus may reveal papilloedema due to increased intracranial pressure or hypertension.

● *Impairment of speech.* There may be complete or partial loss of the ability to communicate. The speech centre is in the dominant cerebral hemisphere; if the stroke occurs on that side, aphasia is likely to occur. The left hemisphere is dominant in the majority of persons. The patient may not only be unable to communicate verbally but may manifest some impairment of comprehension of either or both written or verbal communication.

The aphasia may take various forms (Table 21.6). In motor or expressive aphasia, the person understands and knows what he or she wants to say but cannot utter the words. In receptive aphasia the person does not comprehend either written or spoken words. If there is total loss of speech and communication it is referred to as global aphasia and indicates a serious, massive lesion.

● *Mental impairment.* A stroke may impair the patient's memory, comprehension and the ability to reason and make judgements. There may be inability to recognize previously familiar objects or sensory impressions (agnosia) and to use objects correctly (apraxia).

Emotional lability is common; the patient may cry or laugh inappropriately.

● *Vital signs.* The respirations are usually slow and stertorous or may be Cheyne–Stokes. The pulse is usually slow, full and bounding in the initial phase. The temperature may be normal during the first few hours and then becomes elevated. Hyperpyrexia is an unfavourable sign.

DIAGNOSTIC PROCEDURES

When a stroke occurs, procedures may be carried out to identify the underlying cause because the therapy for an ischaemic stroke differs from that of a haemorrhagic stroke. Diagnostic procedures also may reveal the extent and location of involvement. They may include the following:

1. A CT scan may be done; a collection of blood, cerebral oedema or an infarcted area will show up

because of a change in density. It will also demonstrate the displacement of tissue.
2. An EEG may be used to determine the amount of brain wave activity and differentiate a thrombotic or haemorrhagic stroke. High-voltage slow waves are characteristic of a haemorrhagic stroke; if the cause is thrombosis, the tracing usually shows low-voltage slow waves.
3. Rarely, a lumbar puncture is done, and in the case of a stroke and infarction there is an elevation in the leucocyte count in the CSF; the presence of blood in the CSF indicates haemorrhage.

ONGOING ASSESSMENT

An initial assessment of the vital signs and neurological status establishes a base for on-going evaluations and prompt recognition of changes. During the acute phase, vital signs, level of consciousness and motor and sensory functions are monitored at frequent intervals.

Following the acute stage, the patient's motor functions and level of awareness are assessed daily. Some improvement may occur day to day as the cerebral oedema and pressure are reduced and collateral circulation is established. The regaining of function tends to follow a pattern in which the facial and swallowing muscles recover first, then those of the lower limbs. Usually, speech and arm function return more slowly and less completely. Observations are made frequently for early signs of complications such as contractures and pressure sores.

PATIENT PROBLEMS

1. Altered level of consciousness: coma.
2. Alteration in respiratory process:
   (a) Ineffective breathing pattern.
   (b) Ineffective airway clearance.
   (c) Impaired gas exchange.
3. Potential increased intracranial pressure secondary to cerebral oedema and haemorrhage.
4. Headache and vomiting due to increased intracranial pressure.
5. Alteration in elimination processes:
   (a) Possible urinary retention with overflow.
   (b) Incontinence.
   (c) Potential constipation, faecal impaction and bowel incontinence.

6. Alteration in fluid and food intake: deficit due to coma, vomiting and/or dysphagia. The taking of food may also be influenced by difficulty with mastication as well as swallowing.

7. Potential for injury secondary to neurological deficits, confusion or fits.

8. Potential pressure sores related to immobility and incontinence.

9. Self-care deficits due to coma, paralysis, impaired cognition and awareness.

10. Impaired verbal communication: aphasia.

11. Impairment of mobility: occurs in varying degrees ranging from weakness to complete paralysis.

12. Cognitive dysfunction: impaired awareness, confusion, loss of memory, reasoning and judgement.

13. Emotional lability: inappropriate responses, for example inappropriate outbursts of anger, crying and laughing. If awareness is not impaired, the patient is usually manifests the characteristics of the grieving process (denial, anger, depression, gradual acceptance and resolution).

14. Lack of knowledge about rehabilitation and home management.

GOALS

In the acute phase the goals are that the patient will not develop complications related to the problems stated above, while in the convalescent and rehabilitative phase additional goals involve the recovery of maximum independence and adaptation to reduced function.

NURSING INTERVENTION

A great deal of patience is needed to support both family and patient in striving to meet these goals.

The degree of recovery following a stroke is determined by the size of the haemorrhage and infarction and is influenced by the patient's age, available rehabilitation programmes and the individual's personality and behavioural responses. Improvement can occur but deficits which are present after 6 months are usually permanent. Early, sustained and intensive therapy for the highly motivated patient with strong professional and family support frequently results in independence and a very satisfying recovery and quality of life.

Treatment and nursing care of a patient with a thrombotic stroke will differ somewhat with that of a haemorrhagic stroke and of course it varies with the degree of cerebral damage and ensuing neurological deficits. In the case of a thrombotic stroke, in evolution, an anticoagulant such as heparin may be administered and efforts are directed to maintaining a normal level of blood pressure. The patient is kept on bed rest with a minimal of disturbance and environmental stimuli to reduce the potential for haemorrhage. Surgical removal of the thrombus may be undertaken. When the stroke is due to a cerebral haemorrhage, therapy and nursing involve efforts directed towards relief of the increased intracranial pressure, life-support measures, relief of hypertension to prevent further bleeding and the prevention of complications.

The care required by the stroke patient during the acute phase following the initial onset differs from that required during the convalescent and rehabilitative phase. The care will also vary with the severity of the cerebrovascular accident and extent of brain damage. During the acute phase, intervention is principally directed towards maintaining life and preventing increased neurological deficits and complications.

Much of the nursing care surrounding problems such as diminished level of consciousness, altered respiratory processes, headache, elimination, personal hygiene and pressure care has already been discussed. Care must be taken with nutrition.

When consciousness is regained, the gag reflex is tested before giving any fluids orally. If the patient can swallow, a soft diet is given and progressively increased to a full balanced diet as tolerated. The hemiplegic patient may have to be fed at first if the dominant arm is affected, but with the necessary assistance, is encouraged to feed unaided as soon as possible to establish independence.

If one side of the face is paralysed, food is placed in the opposite side of the mouth. Mouth care is then given following each meal to remove retained food particles from the affected side to prevent aspiration and the development of ulcers.

Protection from injury is necessary due to the motor deficits and possible seizures. Contractures and deformities may develop because flexor muscles take over and loss of range of joint movement occurs. Limbs are supported in a natural position. Passive movements of all joints are carried out at regular intervals, for example when changing the patient's position.

Sensory function may also be impaired; as well as a reduced sensitivity to pressure, pain and temperature, there may be loss of the ability to know the location of parts of his body in space (impaired spatial perception). Cot sides are kept up; the patient may be disorientated and also if turning in bed, may not have the normal reflexive muscular responses that would maintain balance and prevent the patient falling from the bed. When allowed up, precautions are taken to prevent falls and accidents (sufficient assistance, hand-rails, walking frames or sticks).

As soon as the condition has stabilized, opportunity is provided for the patient to regain as much independence as possible as active assistance is gradually withdrawn while giving support and encouragement. The call light or buzzer, water, toilet articles and other needed items are placed within the patient's reach. The nurse should encourage the patient to be aware of and to use the affected side if possible.

Heparin or warfarin may be prescribed. The INR (international ratio) blood estimation will be necessary at frequent intervals, initially on alternate days until the correct level of anticoagulation is achieved (normal = 1; controlled needs to be 2.5–3). Care should be taken to ensure that the patient is not taking other drugs which could prolong the clotting time, e.g. aspirin or one of the non-steroidal anti-inflammatory drugs. If the blood pressure is elevated, an antihypertensive drug or diuretic may be prescribed. The blood pressure is monitored at frequent, regular intervals; a low normal blood pressure is desirable.

If there is a confirmed diagnosis of cerebral thrombosis or embolism, an anticoagulant such as heparin may be prescribed.

Family assessment. Once a family assessment has been carried out and problems or concerns are identified, the family will require some assistance in developing both short-term and long-term plans. Questions may arise about community resources, self-help groups, rehabiliative facilities, home adaptations, social security payments and possibly employment prospects, to name but a few of the areas of long-term concern for the patient and family.

Rehabilitative phase following stroke

Rehabilitation really commences with the initial onset and acute phase: certain aspects of the care received in the early stage of the illness play an important role in the patient's rehabilitation. As soon as the patient is well enough, an assessment is made of residual disabilities and remaining capacities. A multidisciplinary team then becomes involved in plans to assist the patient to develop maximum potential, independence and to assist the family with the necessary adjustments. Both patient and family should participate in setting achievable goals. Attainment of the goals usually requires months of perseverance and patience. The patient and family naturally experience periods of frustration, depression and pessimism. Activities are taken in steps so that achievement is experienced. Complete restoration to previous functional ability may not be possible but much can be done to restore the patient to a degree of independence that makes life more tolerable for him and his family.

Impaired communication. The *aphasia* associated with a stroke most often is expressive in type although variants do occur (Table 21.5). The sudden loss of the ability to communicate creates fear and frustration in the patient; feelings of isolation, insecurity and loneliness develop. The nurse endeavours to allay some of the anxiety by anticipating the patient's needs as much as possible, acknowledging the difficulty and concern and indicating time and willingness to work through the problem. The patient is likely to benefit psychologically from knowing that someone understands and will help. Many aphasic patients can recover the ability to communicate to some degree. It is not possible to predict this at the onset; speech is usually recovered very gradually and slowly and requires the assistance of those around the patient. The nurse avoids conveying what may be false optimism at first but reassures the patient and family that special assistance will be given to minimize speech and other neurological deficits. In the early stage, gestures to indicate needs and wishes may be encouraged but should not be accepted indefinitely since established use of them inhibit efforts to speak.

If the services of a speech therapist are available, a retraining programme is planned. In many situations, the nurse will be mainly responsible for helping the patient recover the ability to communicate. It is necessary, as soon as possible, to determine whether the patient can express ideas verbally or by written work and whether the spoken and written word is understood. Comprehension may be limited to short simple phrases or single words. Rarely, intellectual impairment occurs (e.g. receptive aphasia) which precludes speech rehabilitation. It is important to talk normally and with ease to the patient; auditory stimulation and socialization can play important roles and are considered as valuable as structured remedial drills. It must be remembered that the fact that speech has been lost is no indication that intelligence, comprehension and hearing are impaired. The patient should be included in the conversation taking place in his presence. Short simple sentences, kept at functional level relating to present and immediate needs and environment are used if there is evidence of difficulty in comprehension. When encouraging the patient to try, emphasis is placed on nouns and simple responses such as 'yes' and 'no' at first; then progression through verbs and adjectives to short sentences is made. The necessary retraining in many instances is much the same as the process used with the young child learning to communicate. The use of several sensory avenues is usually more effective than the use of just one at a time. Hearing words in direct association with the objects and the printed words that represent them contributes to recovery.

During speech therapy; the patient should be rested and relaxed and in a quiet undistracting setting. The periods of instruction are kept brief as the patient may tire easily and have a short attention span. Emphasis on exact pronunciation is unnecessary and may lead only to frustration and discouragement.

Early in the illness, the family members and others are helped in understanding the patient's communication problems and their role in the recovery of speech. The importance of conversing normally with the patient, expecting a response, making every effort to understand and giving plenty of time to respond should be emphasized to the family who should be fully involved in speech therapy. At least one member should be given the opportunity to observe a teaching session carried out in the hospital or rehabilitation unit. The need for patience and the need for providing opportunities for the patient to practise and use what speech he or she has are stressed. The family is advised that progress may be slow and are cautioned against making excessive demands on the patient. Progress should be acknowledged because it encourages and prompts motivation for continued effort.

Impaired mobility. The muscles of affected limbs are flaccid for a few days after CVA, then became spastic. The paralysed arm becomes adducted and flexion occurs at the elbow, wrist, fingers and thumb joints. The lower limb assumes a position of external rotation at the hip, flexion of the thigh and leg and plantar flexion of the foot (Figure 21.21). With immobility, muscles atrophy and the collagen fibres of the connective tissue of the tendons, ligaments and joint capsules tend to shorten and become dense and firm. The process may be hastened by circulatory stasis, oedema and trauma. As a result, if the affected limbs are permitted to remain

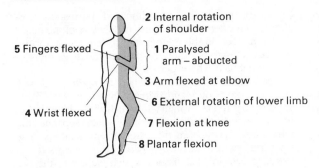

2 Internal rotation of shoulder

5 Fingers flexed

1 Paralysed arm – abducted

3 Arm flexed at elbow

4 Wrist flexed

6 External rotation of lower limb

7 Flexion at knee

8 Plantar flexion

Figure 21.21 Contractures which develop with hemiplegia.

immobile in the positions they automatically assume, contractures and reduced range of joint motion may become permanent. Deformities are created which actually increase the person's disability and make rehabilitation difficult. Liaison with the physiotherapist is essential when caring for the stroke patient.

Maintenance of joint motion, support to prevent the pull of gravity on joints and subsequent subluxation, and positioning to prevent contractures and maintain good alignment are essential from the onset of the stroke.

When lying on the unaffected side, the patient's unaffected shoulder is brought slightly forward and the arm should lie straight, in line with the trunk. The unaffected leg should be straight. A pillow is placed under the affected arm, which is straightened at the elbow; the hand is straightened, with the fingers spread over the upper part of the pillow. The affected leg is flexed at the knee and hip, with a pillow underneath for support. A pillow is placed along the back of the patient for support.

When the patient is lying on the affected side, a reverse, similar position is adopted, except that the unaffected arm is flexed at the elbow, with the hand towards the edge of the bed. The affected leg is flexed slightly at the knee. Pillows are this time placed under the unaffected, not the affected, limbs for support and to prevent friction and pressure. A pillow at the back should support the patient.

Marked spasticity of the affected hand may necessitate the application of a padded splint, especially at night, to prevent flexure contractures of the wrist and fingers. A support may be provided to prevent foot drop.

The limbs are passively moved through a full range of movements 2 or 3 times daily. While the patient is dependent and confined to bed, the position is changed and passive movements carried out every 2 hours.

The stroke patient is usually assisted out of bed for progressively increasing periods as soon as the condition has stabilized. Balance should be assessed and improved (if possible) before walking is commenced. Being up reduces the possibility of complications and may help promote a more positive attitude on the part of the patient towards the future. When the patient is up, support of the affected arm in a sling may sometimes be necessary to prevent subluxation of the shoulder joint. A pillow may be used to support the arm when sitting in a chair. Most hemiplegic patients fortunately experience extensor spasm of the affected knee and hip muscles with weight-bearing, which stabilizes the leg as the unaffected leg is carried through a forward step. Some patients do experience spasm of flexor rather than extensor muscle in the affected leg and as a result when the patient attempts to walk, the knee and hip flex and do not support him. This necessitates the application of a leg brace for stabilization. When assisting the patient who is walking, the nurse or family member provides support from the affected side. An aid, such as a walking frame, may be required to help regain independence. If plantar flexion and toe-dragging interfere with walking, a drop-foot splint may be used. A few hemiplegic patients suffer ataxia and loss of balance which may prevent walking and confine the patient to a wheelchair.

As soon as possible the retraining for self-care is begun. Retraining carried out by the occupational therapist and the nurse includes the simple useful functions on which every person is dependent in normal living. Examples are dressing and undressing, opening doors, using the telephone, writing and the handling of various articles (e.g. cutlery). The hemiplegic patient is taught how to change position in bed (turn, sit up, transfer to a chair, stand up). The bed is lowered and made stationary when transfer techniques are carried out. A schedule of exercises is established to strengthen the trunk and unaffected limb muscles. The programme includes the affected limbs; if the muscles are weak, active assistive and active exercises are used. If the muscles are unresponsive, passive movements are carried out to prevent contractures and ankylosis.

Sensory deficits. The patient is assessed for possible impairment of sensory functions such as pain, pressure and temperature. There may also be loss of the ability to know the location of parts of the body in space (proprioception deficit) making the judging of distances and movements more difficult. The patient's vision may also be impaired by the loss of function in the corresponding halves of the visual fields (homonymous hemianopia) in both eyes. The inability to recognize objects by touch, sight or hearing may be manifested. The necessary precautions are established to prevent accidents such as falls and burns and become an important part of the rehabilitation programme.

Health education. The patient may be required to continue taking an anticoagulant, therefore it is important to teach both patient and family its purpose and the importance of prompt reporting of signs of bleeding. A balanced diet with less fat content may be recommended and a dietary plan reviewed with the patient and family that will meet caloric needs according to weight and energy expenditure. The patient is strongly advised against smoking. It is recommended that younger female patients should not take contraceptive pills.

Predischarge planning. The total care and rehabilitation programme should be fully discussed with a member of the family. The importance of encouraging and permitting the patient to do things unaided is emphasized. Family and friends find it difficult to stand back while the patient struggles and perseveres with activities. Prior to discharge, the patient may be encouraged to spend 1 or 2 days at home, e.g. at the weekend, and a home assessment may be carried out by appropriate personnel. Following discharge from hospital, both patient and family still require considerable support and assistance; referrals should be made to appropriate support and community services. Modifications of the environment may be necessary to facilitate the development of independence and prevent accidents. Handrails in the bathroom, placement of articles for ready accessibility, making the bed stationary and the removal of scatter rugs and wax from floors are a few examples of adjustments that may be made in the environment.

The assistance of social services may be necessary to help solve the problems imposed by the illness and residual disabilities. The family should be taught to recognize the signs of resentment at loss of independence by the patient. By listening to their points of view, by explaining the patient's condition and unusual patterns of behaviour and by helping the family organize themselves so that all share in the increased responsibility, complete rejection of the patient may be prevented.

Social contact. The patient is encouraged to develop interests and worthwhile hobbies and to gradually assume responsibility for domestic tasks as far as possible. The performance of some useful tasks promotes the patient's morale and greater harmony within the family.

Friends are encouraged to visit and the patient should be included in the social activities of the family. Domestic arrangements may however be less than ideal. The patient may live alone in a large house with no close family or live in a small flat in considerable poverty. Elderly patients may have several concurrent medical problems as well as social problems to contend with. Whatever the difficulties, nurses should not be judgemental about families who refuse to have an elderly relative to live with them after a CVA; this will serve no useful purpose for the patient, and antagonism between family and hospital staff is in nobody's interests. The patient may now have to face leaving a home they have lived in for many decades, losing their independence in the process, although this is to be avoided if at all possible; hence the importance of community care.

THE PERSON WITH TRAUMA OF THE NERVOUS SYSTEM

Head Injuries

Accidents on the roads, in industry and sports, and violence on the streets and in the home are the major causes of head injury, which ranks high on the list of causes of morbidity, mortality and permanent disabilities. Frequently, head injury is only one of the major problems seen in the traumatized patient and priorities of care are established on the basis of the assessment of the patient as a whole person.

Head injuries may be classified as open or closed, coup or contrecoup, and primary or secondary. *Closed head injury* refers to injury in which there is no break in the tissues (scalp and skull) which separate the intracranial cavity from the external environment (e.g. subdural haematoma). *Open head injury* means that a break exists in the tissues which separate the intracranial contents from the external environment (e.g. compound or perforating skull fracture).

Coup and contrecoup injuries result from direct trauma to the head in which the sequence of intracranial events resembles an acceleration–deceleration phenomenon. *Coup* refers to bruising of the brain tissue which directly underlies the site of impact and which rebounds against that portion of the cranium. *Contrecoup* is brain injury on the side opposite to the site of impact. It is due to the wave of pressure created by the impact, compressing the brain substance against the bony ridges and opposite wall of the cranium. For example, a fall on the back of the head may cause injury to the frontal and temporal cerebral lobes. Injury to the nerve fibres, and blood vessels in the brain stem results from the stress of shearing forces.

PRIMARY HEAD INJURIES

FRACTURE OF THE SKULL

A skull fracture is particularly significant if there is communication between the intracranial contents and the outside (open head injury), or there is depression of a piece of skull, compressing the brain below. If the fracture involves the base of the skull, CSF leakage occurs and there is potential communication between the oropharynx and the meninges, leading to the risk of infection entering the meninges. This is known as meningitis.

No specific treatment is used for a simple linear or comminuted skull fracture but the patient is kept at rest and under close observation because of potential bleeding and haematoma. Meningeal blood vessels may have been torn and incur extradural, subdural or subarachnoid haemorrhage. Concussion or contusion of the brain is a frequent result.

Early surgical exploration is indicated when a depressed fracture occurs. Skull fragments are elevated and splinters and debris removed. Severe fragmentation and depression may necessitate removal of that area of the skull. Later, a cranioplasty may be done; a plate of inert material (e.g. titanium) is inserted to protect the brain and improve the patient's appearance.

BRAIN INJURY

Injury to the brain may result from a blow to the head and may or may not be associated with a fracture of the skull. A head injury may cause concussion, cerebral contusion or laceration, haemorrhage and/or compression.

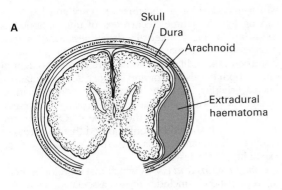

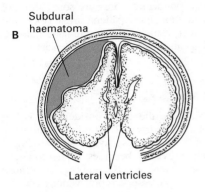

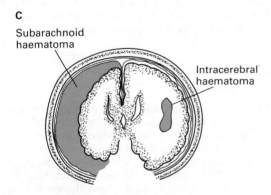

Figure 21.22 Cranial haematomas.

A brain injury may be mild and reversible or may be severe and irreversible, leaving residual neurological deficits if the patient survives. Oedema of the brain and intracranial haemorrhage increase intracranial pressure which, if severe, may compress the brain stem and its vital centres (supratentorial herniation). Initially, *every head injury is considered serious*; it must be emphasized that regardless of outward appearance, the person requires close observation for evidence of developing secondary brain damage which could result in permanent disability or death.

Concussion may be described as a temporary cerebral paralysis as a result of a blow to the head. It is characterized by a brief period of unconsciousness due to jarring of the brain and its sudden forceful contact with the rigid skull. The period of unconsciousness is usually at most only a few minutes, depending on the severity of the injury. When the patient regains consciousness, he or she may be confused, dazed and restless and be unable to recall events which preceded the accident. Headache is a common complaint. If there is no haemorrhage or brain tissue damage, no abnormal neurological findings are present: normal reflexes and muscle tone return.

Nursing intervention for concussion includes observation for evidence of neurological deterioration if the patient is admitted, and, if discharged, ensuring that a reliable person is available. The responsible person is instructed to remain with the patient. If the patient becomes increasingly drowsy or difficult to rouse or, if he or she experiences headache, vomiting, visual disturbances, seizures or a reduction in limb strength, the patient should be brought back to hospital by ambulance immediately. It is advisable to provide instructions in writing for the responsible person since anxiety may affect the ability to recall what has been said. Recovery following an uncomplicated concussion occurs within a short period of time, although some side-effects may persist for weeks (Walsh, 1990).

Cerebral contusion and laceration refers to bruising and tearing of superficial brain tissue. The multiple areas of tissue damage may give rise to a wide variety of patient responses. It must be emphasized that a patient with a head injury can have significant trauma and still be alert. Loss of consciousness is not a requirement for a diagnosis of severe head injury. Aphasia may result with a frontal–temporal contusion. A temporal lobe contusion may give rise to agitation, confusion and 'foul-mouthed' responses. Lesions of the brain stem are usually of the more serious type. Level of consciousness may be altered for several hours or weeks. A variety of other neurological abnormalities are usually present on both sides of the body. If neurological signs are present on one side of the body, it is probable that a secondary event such as the development of a haematoma has occurred. The tissue injury is usually accompanied by brain swelling and oedema. Recovery may be a lengthy process; permanent tissue damage and scarring may result in permanent disability if the patient survives.

SECONDARY EVENTS FOLLOWING HEAD INJURY

INTRACRANIAL HAEMORRHAGE

Haemorrhage within the cranium and the formation of a haematoma following a head injury frequently leads to rapid deterioration in the patient's condition. The bleeding may be extradural, subdural, subarachnoid or intracerebral. The clinical characteristics presented are due to increased intracranial pressure and compression of areas of the brain (see p. 729).

An *extradural haematoma* is an accumulation of blood between the dura and skull (Figure 21.22A) and is a serious complication. Since the meningeal artery is frequently torn, extradural bleeding is at arterial pressure. The brain is compressed and displaced and the intracranial pressure rises rapidly. The patient may be comatose for a brief period, regain consciousness, then gradually develop serious neurological symptoms (disturbed vision, dilated pupil and loss of reflex to light in the eye on the affected side, severe headache, confusion, decreased motor and sensory function, seizure, vomiting) and loss of consciousness. Prompt treatment is essential. If an extradural haemorrhage is not recognized and promptly treated, the rapidly increasing intracranial pressure may cause tentorial herniation, pressure on vital centres and death within a few hours.

Subdural haemorrhage is another possible complication of head injury. Blood accumulates in the subdural space (Figure 21.22B), gradually forming a haematoma which compresses the brain and increases intracranial pressure. The bleeding may occur following a seemingly minor head injury. Since the bleeding is usually at venous pressure, the development of symptoms may be delayed and vague but progressively worsen and eventually, increasing intracranial pressure and brain compression lead to coma.

As cited previously, all head injuries should be treated initially as serious and a potential threat to life.

Subdural haemorrhage may be subacute or chronic in patients of advanced age or with cortical atrophy. In these patients, evidence of increased intracranial pressure usually appears very gradually and intermittently.

Subarachnoid haemorrhage is bleeding of cerebral vessels into the space between the arachnoid and pia mater. The clinical characteristics are similar to those presented by the patient with a subdural haemorrhage and depend on the area of the brain involved. This is rarely seen in trauma and is much more likely to be due to a cerebral aneurysm.

Intracerebral haemorrhage is bleeding resulting from a torn or diseased vessel within the cerebrum, it may occur as a result of contrecoup injury, a penetrating wound such as a gun-shot or stabbing or a CVA (stroke). The symptoms depend on the particular vessel and cerebral area (Figure 21.22C).

BRAIN SWELLING AND OEDEMA

Infection, brain injury and cerebral haemorrhage and infarction cause brain swelling and oedema and consequent increased intracranial pressure which may lead to tentorial herniation. Oedema develops as a result of an inflammatory response; the swelling occurs when there is oedema or an accumulation of blood in the brain tissue. Infection such as meningitis or brain abscess develops most commonly with an open head injury or basilar skull fracture.

SUMMARY

To summarize, the clinical characteristics associated with a head injury depend on the area of the brain involved and the nature and severity of the tissue damage. They may appear immediately following the injury or several hours afterward as a result of intracranial haemorrhage, cerebral oedema and swelling of the brain and the ensuing compression and elevation of intracranial pressure.

The symptoms may include: loss of consciousness which may develop at the time of injury and last for a varying length of time; recurrence of unconsciousness following a lucid interval; drowsiness and stupor progressing to coma; severe headache or dizziness; disturbed vision; dilatation and failure to react to light of one or both pupils; motor and sensory deficits, seizures, nuchal rigidity, speech impairment, disorientation, changes in vital signs indicative of increasing intracranial pressure (see p. 730); and the escape of CSF from the ear or nose. It should be remembered that a decreased level of consciousness is the first warning of an expanding brain lesion.

Complications and events which may develop in head injured patients include those associated with immobilization (e.g. contractures, pressure sores, thrombi and emboli). In addition, these patients are at risk of the development of such problems as post-traumatic epilepsy, intellectual deficits and marked memory deficits.

EMERGENCY CARE

As in all emergencies, the first consideration is the establishment of a clear airway. The brain cells are very dependent upon a continuous oxygen supply and, if injured, adequate provision becomes even more imperative. A clear airway is also important because obstruction tends to increase cerebral venous congestion and intracranial pressure. It should be kept in mind that serious intracranial damage can occur without external signs of head trauma. An assessment is made of:

- Vital signs
- Level of consciousness (Glasgow coma scale)
- Pupil size, equality and reaction
- Motor function in limbs.

If signs of shock are observed in the patient with a head injury, an examination is made for the presence of other injuries, which may be the cause. If unconscious, the victim is turned to a lateral or semiprone position and a Guedal airway inserted, if tolerated, to minimize the danger of obstruction of the airway and aspiration. The spine is kept straight and the head aligned; flexion and hyperextension of the head must be avoided as a spinal injury should be assumed until otherwise proven.

An open scalp wound is covered with available clean material and direct pressure used to control bleeding.

ASSESSMENT

On admission to hospital, further consideration is given to supporting respiratory function and the patient's physical status and neurological status are assessed. A record of the initial findings serve as a base for ongoing comparative assessment so that even slight changes may be readily recognized.

The neurological observations are repeated at half-hour to hourly intervals for at least 24 hours. The doctor should be promptly notified of any decrease in level of consciousness, increased blood pressure, inequality of pupils, change in respiratory pattern and loss of strength in one or more limbs; a change may indicate an increase in intracranial pressure. The interval between assessments is gradually lengthened depending on the basis of the patient's progress. Hourly recordings are made of the temperature if hyperthermia develops.

The escape of blood and CSF from an ear or nasal passage may occur with a fracture of the base of the skull and tearing of the dura mater between the brain and the ear or nasal passage. It is therefore a key observation. The drainage may be confirmed as CSF by a simple test (see p. 710). Such injury creates a potential for intracranial infection such as meningitis or brain abscess. The drainage is allowed to flow freely; the patient is positioned on the affected side. A dry sterile towel is placed under the head or a dry sterile dressing placed loosely over the orifice and changed frequently since moisture provides a most favourable environment for growth of organisms. Those caring for the patient should wash their hands well before working in the area of the drainage. The patient is cautioned not to blow the nose and not to suppress a sneeze. Under no circumstances should the drainage passages be packed, and suction to the nasal passages is never performed if CSF leakage is suspected. The patient is observed closely for signs of infection; and a prophylactic antibiotic may be prescribed.

PATIENT PROBLEMS

The following is a list of some of the main problems encountered in the early stages of recovery from brain injury.

1. Respiratory dysfunction secondary to:
   (a) Loss of patency of airway.
   (b) Injury to or compression of the respiratory centre in the brain stem.
2. Alteration in level of consciousness.
3. Alteration in comfort when conscious: mild to severe headache.
4. Motor and sensory deficits due to brain compression and damage.
5. Alteration in level of awareness of self and environment.
6. Potential for injury related to reduced level of consciousness, confusion, motor and sensory deficits or seizures.
7. Impairment of skin integrity secondary to scalp wound or immobility (pressure sores).
8. Alteration in fluid and food intake secondary to comatose state, fluid intake restrictions per 24 hours, or anxiety.
9. Alteration in elimination patterns:
   (a) Urinary (incontinence, retention).
   (b) Bowel (constipation and potential impaction).
10. Self-care deficits affecting personal hygiene secondary to unconsciousness, enforced immobility or motor deficits.
11. Anxiety related to confusion and loss of memory of previous events.
12. Lack of knowledge about diagnostic and therapeutic procedures, condition, hospitalization and post-hospital care.

GOALS

The fundamental goal is that the patient will regain consciousness with no long-term deficits. This involves a series of short-term goals, such as a normal breathing pattern and patent airway, avoiding further injury and the complications of having a decreased level of consciousness leading to confusion and immobility. Goals relating to normal body function such as fluid intake and output should also be set.

NURSING INTERVENTION

If the patient is comatose, the care is the same as that described for the unconscious patient. The patient is also at risk of increased intracranial pressure.

The head-injured patient is at risk of infection if an open scalp wound is present; the wound is cleansed, debrided if necessary, and sutured. A reinforcing dose of tetanus toxoid may be prescribed as a prophylactic measure, or human tetanus immunoglobulin may be given.

Loss of the corneal reflexes, periorbital oedema and ecchymoses are common problems with a head injury. If the corneal reflex is absent, the eyelid may be taped shut with non-allergic tape to protect the cornea from drying and abrasions. The tape is removed every two hours and the eye irrigated with normal saline and artificial tears instilled before retaping. If the eyelids are swollen, it may be necessary for a second nurse to hold the lids open while pupillary reflexes are assessed. If the lids cannot be opened, the doctor is notified; it is important that pupillary changes be detected in sufficient time to institute treatment.

Hyperthermia may develop following head injury due to a disturbance of the temperature control centre in the hypothalamus leading to temperatures of 40°C or more. Vigorous interventions are required to reduce such extremely high temperatures.

Increased Intracranial Pressure

The cranium, which, in the adult is a rigid vault allowing practically no expansion of the content, contains the brain, CSF and blood. An increase in the volume of any one (brain, blood or CSF) causes an increase in the intracranial pressure and a comparable decrease in the volume of one or both of the other contents. The response may be:

1. Displacement of CSF.
2. A compromise in cerebral blood supply which causes cerebral ischaemia. The latter leads to hypoxia, hypercapnoea and acidosis at cellular level, resulting in interruption of cell metabolism.
3. Displacement of brain tissue (*herniation* of brain tissue). This occurs when the other compensatory mechanisms fail. Brain displacement may occur in the supratentorial compartment or infratentorial compartment. The tentorium is a fold of the dura mater which lies below the cerebrum, separating it from the cerebellum and brain stem. As the brain

Table 21.7 Effects of increased intracranial pressure.

Headache
Restlessness, disorientation
Changes in responsiveness (decreased level of
   consciousness)
Changes in vital signs:
   ↑ systolic blood pressure
      widening pulse pressure
   ↓ pulse rate
      altered respiration rate and rhythm
      may develop periods of apnoea
   ↑ temperature (later sign)
Vomiting—usually projectile
Changes in pupillary size, equality and reflex responses
Change in posture—rigidity may develop
Loss of motor function
Loss of sensory function

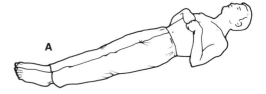

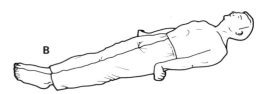

Figure 21.23 Posture in (A) decorticate rigidity, and (B) decerebrate rigidity. (Also termed spastic flexion and spastic extension respectively.)

stem ascends to join the cerebrum, it passes through a small space referred to as the tentorial hiatus or notch. Increasing intracranial pressure may cause a downward displacement of the cerebrum through the hiatus, causing a supratentorial herniation or coning. It causes compression of the brain stem; the patient becomes comatose and respiratory and circulatory failure may develop rapidly. A lesion in the temporal lobe compresses the mid-brain and third cranial nerve, first causing dilatation of the pupil.

Infratentorial herniation involves displacement of brain stem or cerebellar tissue through the foramen magnum. Coma, motor dysfunction and respiratory depression develop.

4. An increase in BP as more powerful cardiac contractions are required to force blood into the cranium. A reflex slowing of the pulse also occurs.

CAUSES OF INCREASED INTRACRANIAL PRESSURE

The causes of increased intracranial pressure are swelling of the brain, increased CSF volume and increased blood volume.

Swelling of the brain may be due to a tumour (increased mass of tissue cells), abscess, inflammatory exudate, or cerebral oedema. An increase in the cranial volume of CSF is usually associated with a disturbance in the absorption or the outflow of the fluid; it accumulates in the ventricles, compressing brain tissue and blood vessels. An increase in the intracranial blood volume may be due to compression of the venous sinuses or jugular veins, vasodilatation of the cerebral vessels or be associated with trauma.

NURSING THE PATIENT WITH POTENTIAL OR ACTUAL INCREASED INTRACRANIAL PRESSURE

Treatment may be medical, surgical or a combination of both. Surgical intervention usually deals with the specific cause and may involve ventricular drainage.

Medical treatment includes the intravenous administration of osmotic diuretics (e.g. mannitol) and the corticosteroid, dexamethasone to try and reduce cerebral oedema.

Assessment

The effects of rising intracranial pressure on the patient will vary with the speed at which pressure is rising and hence the nature of the lesion itself. The pressure may increase very rapidly, as with an extradural haemorrhage, or it may increase very gradually, as with a slow-growing tumour.

Early symptoms include headache which progressively becomes more severe, drowsiness, slowing of responses and vomiting, which may not be preceded by nausea. It is important that the nurse obtain information from the family about the patient's normal behaviour as a baseline against which to compare current functioning. With further development there is decreasing consciousness, an increase in the systolic blood pressure with a widening pulse pressure, change in respiratory pattern, eye changes (pupillary dilatation, loss of reflex to light stimulus), papilloedema and bradycardia (Table 21.6).

The patient's vital signs and neurological status are assessed to provide a baseline against which any signs of deterioration may be detected. Assessment of the patient's neurological status also includes observations for involuntary movements (twitching, tremors or convulsion), restlessness, rigidity and posturing (decerebrate or decorticate rigidity) (Figure 21.23).

It is important to assess the patient's level of understanding of the current situation and communication skills, and how the family are reacting to the situation.

The physical assessment should include a careful check on the patient's skin to assess for signs of dehydration and pressure area breakdown. One of the standard risk assessment scales such as Norton or Waterlow should be used.

Patient problems

The following is a list of potential problems frequently encountered by patients suffering raised intracranial pressure.

1. Alteration in respiratory function related to:
   (a) Ineffective clearance of airway.
   (b) Injury or compression of the respiratory centre.
   (c) Obstruction of the airway by the tongue or aspirate, if unconscious.
2. Potential for injury due to disorientation and impaired awareness, restlessness, seizures.
3. Severe headache.
4. Potential hyperthermia.
5. Alteration in cardiac function secondary to compression and ischaemia of vital centres in the medulla.
6. Potential for skin breakdown due to immobility and possible restlessness and hyperthermia.
7. Potential fluid imbalance due to osmotic diuretic, inadequate intake and vomiting.
8. Nutritional deficit due to inadequate intake and increased metabolic rate with hyperthermia and injury.
9. Alteration in elmination; bowel and urinary.
10. Self-care deficit in personal hygiene due to reduced level of consciousness and motor and sensory changes.

Goals

The goals for the patient revolve around being free from any of the complications outlined in the above list of problems, having the maximum possible insight into the situation and a satisfactory standard of personal hygiene and comfort.

Nursing intervention

1. Ineffective respiration

The standard measures, already outlined, to maintain a patent airway and promote adequate ventilation should be carried out.

If sufficiently alert, the patient is cautioned not to cough and sneeze if possible, due to the effect this may have on intracranial pressure, and is prompted to take several deep breaths at regular intervals (every 2 hours). Chest physiotherapy may be used to help mobilize secretions.

If respiratory insufficiency develops due to weak ventilatory function, endotracheal intubation or a tracheotomy may be done and the patient supported by a mechanial ventilator. Hyperventilation and a lowered P_{CO_2} level is desirable to reduce cerebral vasodilatation and promote cerebral venous return, reducing cerebral blood volume and intracranial pressure.

When oral fluids are permitted, only a very small amount is given at first to test the swallowing reflex to prevent choking, coughing and aspiration.

2. Potential for injury

Increased intracranial pressure. Planning and implementation of care must take into consideration the prevention of *further increase* in the intracranial pressure as well as the reduction of the existing increased intracranial pressure.

Positions and activities which raise the intracranial pressure are avoided. The head of the bed is usually elevated about 30°; the patient with potential or actual increased intracranial pressure is never placed in a head-low position but is positioned to prevent any impediment of cerebral venous return. The head is aligned with the spine; flexion and twisting of the head, anything tight around the neck that might compress the jugular veins and extreme hip flexion are avoided. When moving or changing position, the conscious patient is instructed not to push with the feet or push or pull with the arms and to breathe out through the mouth. The latter prevents the Valsalva manoeuvre, which quickly raises the intracranial pressure.

The corticosteroid dexamethasone (Decadron) is commonly used to help reduce the intracranial pressure; the exact mechanism of the action is unclear. The patient receiving dexamethasone is observed for possible side-effects and complications since corticosteroids suppress the immune response, making the patient more susceptible to infection and also may cause gastrointestinal bleeding. An antacid or an antisecretory agent such as the H_2 receptor antagonist cimetidine (Tagamet) may be prescribed to protect the stomach and intestine.

Disorientation and impaired cognitive function. The patient's orientation, judgement, level of consciousness and mobility may change quickly. Protection from injury is necessary. Cot sides are kept in position unless someone stays at the bedside with the patient. This applies for a considerable period of time even though the patient is conscious and orientated. Following an intracranial disorder and increased intracranial pressure, patients are frequently subject to spells of dizziness or lapses of orientation, or may be slow in regaining their postural reflexes.

Restlessness. This may be due to cerebral hypoxia or increasing elevation of the intracranial pressure but it should be kept in mind that restlessness may also be associated with retention of urine, pain, an uncomfortable position, the regaining of consciousness, or fear and concern about the situation. The cot sides are padded for protection. Efforts are made to determine the cause if the patient is restless and to eliminate it if possible. If there are neurological symptoms and changes in vital signs that indicate a further increase in the intracranial pressure, they are reported promptly so that further treatment may be undertaken. If the restlessness occurs with the regaining of consciousness, the patient is reorientated to the situation: if the cause of the restlessness is thought to be the patient's anxiety, he or she is encouraged to express concerns and receives explanations and reassurance.

Narcotics and strong sedation are not given to a

patient with increased intracranial pressure; they mask neurological signs and depress respirations. Nursing measures such as position change and staying with the patient and encouraging expression of concerns may promote comfort and reduce restlessness. The environment should be quiet and the lighting subdued. In extreme restlessness a mild sedative may be prescribed to prevent exhaustion.

It should be remembered that the patient with reduced consciousness may be able to hear and comprehend although not able to respond; hearing is the last sensation to be lost. It is important that those caring for the patient continue to communicate with the patient and the guard against inappropriate conversation. Verbal communication provides cerebral stimulation and information; it can be comforting and reassuring to the patient. Non-verbal communication by touch and presence is also reassuring to both patient and family. Family members are advised of the possibility of the patient hearing and are encouraged to communicate with the patient even though unresponsive.

3. Headache

The patient usually experiences headache with the onset of increased intracranial pressure which progressively becomes more severe as the intracranial pressure rises. A mild *non-narcotic* analgesic such as paracetamol may be prescribed. The patient may find that cold applications provide some relief. As the intracranial pressure increases and the patient loses consciousness, pain perception diminishes. A quiet room, subdued lighting and a minimum of environmental stimuli are important while sudden movements should be avoided.

4. Alteration in body temperature

Compression of the temperature regulating centre by increased intracranial pressure may result in a marked elevation of the temperature and, at the same time, the normal physiological heat dissipating mechanisms are suppressed (dilatation of superficial blood vessels and perspiration). The metabolic rate is increased in proportion to the fever: with a temperature of $40.5°C$, there is an increase in metabolism of approximately 50%. Oxygen demands are increased and carbon dioxide production increases.

The room is kept at $18–20°C$ and a light cotton sheet used to cover the patient. If the temperature is elevated, the sheet is arranged to cover only the lower half of the body. Tepid sponging may be ordered and an electric fan directed on the patient to help cool the body surface. An antipyretic such as aspirin, administered by rectal suppository, may be prescribed. The patient should not be cooled too quickly; shivering must be prevented since it increases metabolism, oxygen consumption and the production of carbon dioxide and other metabolites which increase intracranial pressure.

5. Alteration in cardiac function

The compression and ischaemia caused by increased intracranial pressure may seriously affect the cardiac and vasomotor centres. Close monitoring of the pulse for irregularity and changes in the rate and volume is necessary. A decrease in cardiac output reduces cerebral perfusion to a greater degree, resulting in ischaemia, increased Pco_2 and vasodilatation and an ensuing increase in the intracranial pressure. Changes in the pulse are brought promptly to the doctor's attention; continuous cardiac monitoring may be established and an antiarrhythmic drug prescribed if necessary. The excessive loss of body fluid as a result of osmotic diuretic therapy may cause a reduction in intravascular volume and a corresponding reduction in cardiac output. Cardiac failure is more likely to occur if the patient has a pre-existing cardiac problem.

6. Potential for skin breakdown

Maintenance of skin integrity requires special attention because of the patient's immobility and possible restlessness and hyperthermia. The patient's position is changed from side to back (only if conscious) to side every 2 hours unless contraindicated by the location of the patient's intracranial lesion or surgery. For example, if a relatively large space-occupying lesion has been removed, the patient is not permitted to lie on the operative side to prevent a shifting of the brain into the remaining space.

When repositioned, the patient is turned slowly and gently. Bony prominences and pressure areas receive special attention to maintain skin integrity. The bedding must be kept dry and free of wrinkles. An alternating air pressure (ripple) or Spenco mattress may be used to relieve pressure, and pieces of soft resilient material (synthetic sheepskin) are placed under vulnerable areas to reduce friction.

7. Potential fluid imbalance

The fluid intake is usually restricted to a stated volume distributed over 24 hours to maintain slight dehydration which reduces the extracellular volume and intracranial pressure. Intravenous fluids are infused slowly and must be closely monitored; rapid infusion could cause a serious, rapid rise in the intracranial pressure. A sign placed in a conspicuous place on the patient's bed alerts personnel and family to the fluid restriction.

An osmotic diuretic may be prescribed to dehydrate the brain; the drugs administered for this purpose are principally hyperosmolar solutions which are given intravenously (e.g. mannitol). They promote the transfer of fluid from the brain tissue into the vascular compartment by osmosis and increase the urinary output.

Fluid intake is usually calculated each 8–12 hours according to the output; 400–500 ml are added to the output volume to cover insensible loss. Intravenous infusion is usually necessary owing to an inability to take sufficient fluid orally because of nausea, vomiting or coma.

8. Nutritional deficit

The headache, nausea, vomiting or loss of consciousness results in the patient's inability to take adequate food, which is reflected in changes in his strength and muscle mass. Nasogastric feeding may be given every 4 hours to provide necessary fluid and calories. If the patient is febrile, the increased metabolic rate requires more calories; if the caloric requirement is not met, the patient becomes seriously debilitated.

9. Alteration in elimination

Bowel elimination. The patient is discouraged from straining to defecate since the effort involved raises intracranial pressure. A mild bulk laxative or stool softener may be given or a bisacodyl (Dulcolax) suppository may be used as faecal impaction must be avoided.

Urinary elimination. If the patient is unresponsive, incontinence is a problem, making a retention catheter necessary so that an accurate assessment can be made of the output, as well as to maintain skin integrity. The output is noted every 1–2 hours to evaluate the effectiveness of the osmotic diuretic.

The fluid intake and output are monitored for oliguria and water retention or an excessive volume of urine with a low specific gravity. The excessive output may develop as a result of a disturbance in the secretion of ADH by the posterior pituitary lobe. An increase in ADH causes decreased urine formation, while a deficiency of ADH causes large volumes of urine to be excreted, necessitating the administration of vasopressin (Pitressin).

The catheter is removed as soon as possible due to the risk of urinary tract infection. For this reason the use of a condom-type catheter is preferable.

10. Self-care deficit in personal hygiene

The nurse provides the personal care that the patient would normally carry out unaided, such as bathing, cleaning of teeth and mouth, combing of the hair and feeding. Nursing care should be carried out with undisturbed intervals between to permit adequate rest. If the eye reflexes are absent, the eyes may be irrigated with sterile normal saline and hypromellose drops (artificial tears) instilled 3 or 4 times daily to keep the surface of the eye clean and moist. If one or both eyes remain open a protective shield is applied.

If permitted, the limbs are moved slowly and gently through their range of motion to preserve joint movements.

Ventricular drainage in increased intracranial pressure

A ventricular puncture may be done via a burr hole in the skull and a tube inserted into a ventricle to establish drainage of CSF to lower the intracranial pressure. Externally, the tube is attached to a sterile closed system. The level at which the tubing and bag are placed is prescribed by the doctor. The bed is usually kept flat unless otherwise indicated by the doctor. The rate of drainage is monitored very closely; too rapid drainage is to be avoided and blockage of the tube is to be reported promptly. Strict asepsis must be observed in handling the tubes and the dressing at the burr hole. The patient may be given an antibiotic as a prophylactic measure. If the patient complains of severe headache or a neurological disturbance (e.g. disturbed vision) develops that was not experienced before the ventricular puncture, the doctor is notified.

THE PATIENT TREATED BY INTRACRANIAL SURGERY

PREOPERATIVE NURSING CARE

Assessment

If the preoperative period extends over several days, the patient is observed for possible neurological changes from day to day which may indicate a worsening of his condition. The vital signs are followed closely; pupils are checked regularly for size, equality and reaction to light, and the patient's alertness, orientation, sensory perception, motor ability and strength of limbs are noted.

Vital signs and neurological observations are recorded to provide a base-line for measuring progress in the postoperative period.

Patient problems

The patient faces all the usual problems associated with surgery, plus the following problems which are unique to intracranial surgery:

1. Anxiety related to the intracranial surgery and the outcome.
2. Potential for intracranial infection due to surgery.
3. Fluid deficit due to the administration of an osmotic diuretic because of increased intracranial pressure.
4. Potential increased intracranial pressure.
5. Potential for respiratory depression and thrombophlebitis.
6. Embarrassment and concern related to the shaving of the head.

Goals

The patient goals involve avoiding the potential problems outlined above and being able to talk freely about fears and anxieties, including appearance after head shaving.

Nursing intervention

1. Anxiety. Any impending surgery is perceived as a threat to the person and generates anxiety, but that involving the brain is even more threatening. The alert patient and the family are usually very fearful of a fatal outcome or permanent changes, disability and a loss of intellect and competence. Expression of doubts and concerns is encouraged; time and opportunities for questions and answers are provided. The patient is not left alone for long periods; contact with others interrupts concentration on the operation and provides the opportunity to express fears. Visits are limited to family members and friends who can control their anxiety and show a quiet, reassuring presence with the patient.

It is necessary to explain to the patient and family the need for the surgery, the nature of the procedure, the risks and possible outcome. The nurse should be able to answer questions, clarify misconceptions and refer, if appropriate, any special problems to the doctor. The sort of information the family requires is that the patient may have temporary oedema and discoloration of the face and eyes and possible neurological deficits such as facial paralysis and aphasia after the operation. The fact these signs are common after surgery will help reduce the anxiety they generate. Particular sensitivity must be shown over the issue of head shaving. The patient should be advised that a wig of choice will be supplied free once the head dressings and sutures have been removed. It is advisable to ask the appliance officer to visit the patient prior to surgery so that a wig may be chosen and ordered in readiness. The psychological trauma of having the head shaved cannot be overemphasised.

2. Potential for infection. Because of surgical interruption of the integrity of the scalp and cranium, the head must be cleansed and prepared to minimize the possibility of infection. Unless it is an emergency, the hair is washed the day before the operation and the required area of the head shaved, usually after anaesthesia has been induced, leaving, if possible, some hair to cover the scar. In some instances, the entire head is shaved to provide adequate and safe exposure. Any rash, infection or abrasion of the scalp is brought to the surgeon's attention.

3. Fluid deficit. Usually, there is concern if a preoperative patient manifests dehydration and efforts are made to re-establish normal hydration. A fluid deficit in the patient who is to have intracranial surgery may be an important therapeutic measure. A restricted fluid intake may be necessary to control intracranial pressure or an osmotic diuretic such as mannitol to reduce increased intracranial pressure may be given.

No attempt is made to increase the fluid intake without a specific directive. The patient may have water up to 4 or 5 hours before the operation unless otherwise indicated.

4. Potential for increased intracranial pressure. Frequent assessment of neurological and vital signs is made during the preoperative period to detect early signs of increasing intracranial pressure. The patient does not receive the usual preoperative cleansing enema. (An enema is contraindicated because of the risk of increased intracranial pressure with straining at stool.) A mild laxative may be prescribed 2 days before the surgery if necessary. The patient is cautioned not to strain when defecating.

COMMON INTRACRANIAL SURGICAL PROCEDURES

Intracranial surgery necessitates an opening in the skull. The size and location of the opening depend upon the nature and site of the lesion and the amount of exposure needed for the operation. If the lesion is in the cerebrum, it is referred to as being *supratentorial* and the incision is well above the hairline. If it is in the cerebellar or brain stem regions, it is designated as *infratentorial* and the incision is usually in the occipital region.

The surgical procedures include:

- *Burr hole.* This is a small circular opening into the cranium made with a bone drill. The purpose may be to obtain tissue for a biopsy, aspirate CSF from a ventricle, or relieve pressure caused by swelling and oedema of the brain or a tumour.
- *Craniotomy.* In this procedure a scalp incision and two or more burr holes are made over the area to be explored. The bone between the burr holes is incised allowing elevation of a *bone flap* to provide access to the brain. The opening is curved so the scalp and bone flap can be folded back to expose the affected brain area.
- *Craniectomy.* This involves excision of a portion of the skull and may vary from a small burr hole to a sizeable area of several square centimetres. The craniectomy may be done to remove shattered bone or to relieve pressure by expanding cranial contents.
- *Cranioplasty.* This is a replacement of a section of the cranium with a synthetic material such as titanium to re-establish the contour and integrity of the skull. In some instances, the bone flap that was initially separated from the skull is replaced; this is referred to as an *osteoplastic craniotomy.*

POSTOPERATIVE NURSING CARE

Since all patients suffer some elevation of pressure inside the cranium following brain surgery, the nursing care described for increased intracranial pressure as well as the care of the unconscious patient are applicable in the postoperative phase.

Assessment

Vital signs and neurological status are determined when the patient is returned from the operating theatre as a baseline against which progress can be assessed. If the patient is conscious, alertness, orientation, speech and ability to move limbs are checked. The required frequency of these observations may be indicated by the neurosurgeon but usually begins with 15–30 minute intervals which are gradually lengthened to 1 hour then 4 hours if the evaluations indicate stability. Care should be taken to assess for pain, headache or other discomfort, as well as for signs of fear and anxiety.

Assessment of the patient's status includes observations for involuntary movements (twitching, tremor, seizure, restlessness, rigidity and posturing (decerebrate rigidity or decorticate rigidity).

The head dressing is examined for security, for moistness suggesting leakage of CSF and for evidence of bleeding. There may be a drain attached to a gentle negative-pressure system; if so, the amount and type of drainage should be noted as a baseline.

Patient problems

Following intracranial surgery, much of the care cited for the patient with increased intracranial pressure and for the unconscious patient is applicable, together with care applicable to any patient after surgery. Consideration is also given to the following problems:

1. The potential for further increased intracranial pressure due to the reaction to the trauma imposed by the surgery.
2. Potential for injury (risk of injury due to malpositioning or disorientation).
3. Potential for infection due to open wound and lowered resistance.
4. Hyperthermia secondary to the disturbance of the temperature-regulating centre.
5. Knowledge deficit. The patient and family require assistance in making necessary adjustments and planning home management.

Goals

The principal patient goal is a safe recovery from surgery, avoiding the potential problems outlined above and the other general problems related to any postoperative patient or person with reduced consciousness.

Nursing intervention

1. Potential for increased intracranial pressure. All patients experience some elevation of intracranial pressure following brain surgery due to the oedema and swelling resulting from the trauma and inflammation incurred by surgery. Frequent vital signs and neurological evaluations are necessary to recognize significant changes indicating increased intracranial pressure.

The head of the bed may be elevated about 30° to promote cerebral venous return unless contraindicated by shock or a specific directive from the surgeon. A small pillow may be necessary under the head to maintain good neck alignment which promotes cerebral venous return. Following infratentorial surgery (cerebellum or brain stem) the bed is generally kept flat for 2–3 days to prevent pressure on the brain stem and its vital centres.

The fluid intake is usually restricted to a stated volume distributed over 24 hours to maintain slight dehydration which reduces extracellular fluid and intracranial pressure. Intravenous fluids are infused slowly and closely monitored; rapid infusion could cause a rapid rise in intracranial pressure. An osmotic diuretic may be prescribed to dehydrate the brain.

2. Potential for injury. Following intracranial surgery, the patient is at risk of injury from malpositioning. The required position depends on the patient's level of consciousness and the location and nature of the surgery.

While unconscious, the patient is positioned to promote cerebral venous return as well as to prevent obstruction of the airway and aspiration of secretions. The limbs are positioned and supported in the normal way for an unconscious patient. The head of the bed may be elevated 25–30° and the head aligned with the spine. The patient with potential or actual increase in intracranial pressure is never placed in a head-low or prone position. Flexion or twisting of the head and extreme hip flexion are voided because this may increase intracranial pressure.

If a relatively large space-occupying lesion has been removed, the patient is not permitted to lie on the operative side in order to prevent a shifting of the brain into the remaining space. Following infratentorial surgery, the patient lies on either side using a small pillow under the head to maintain alignment. Keeping the patient off the back for 2–3 days prevents pressure on the incision, as well as possible forward flexion on the incision. A specific directive as to positioning may be given by the surgeon.

The position is changed at regular intervals (e.g. every 2 hours) from side to side to back to side unless contraindicated. When repositioned, the patient is turned slowly with adequate support for the head, so that it and the trunk are turned as if they were one unit. Sudden movement and jarring are avoided at all times.

Trauma to the brain stem may depress the gag and swallowing reflexes predisposing to aspiration. When oral fluids are permitted, only a very small amount is given at first to test the swallowing reflex.

3. Potential for infection. Following intracranial surgery the risk of infection arises from the open wound, from the patient's lowered resistance as a result of the illness and its related stresses and from the possible administration of a steroid preparation (e.g. dexamethasone). Since infectious processes increase metabolism, waste products such as carbon dioxide and lactic acid are produced in greater amounts. Waste products in increased amounts cause cerebral vasodilatation which increases intracranial blood volume and pressure. Strict asepsis is essential when the head dressing is changed. The wound is inspected for redness, swelling, offensive odour and drainage; signs of infection are reported promptly and a swab of the wound drainage is taken for culture purposes. Immediate treatment to prevent meningitis, encephalitis or brain abscess is essential; an antibiotic is prescribed.

4. Hyperthermia. The patient may develop an elevation of temperature. To counteract this tendency, the room temperature is kept at 18–20°C and only a cotton sheet and bedspread are used as covers. If hyperthermia develops, a sheet is arranged to cover only the lower half of the body. An antipyretic (e.g. acetyisalicylic acid) is prescribed and administered by rectum. If the temperature continues to rise, tepid sponging is given and an electric fan is directed on the patient.

5. Decreased intellectual function. In some instances, there may be some residual neurological deficit following some intracranial surgical procedures. A rehabilitation programme is planned and instituted as soon as possible with the goal of restoring the patient to independent useful living within his or her potential. This may involve the physiotherapist, speech therapist, occupational therapist and social worker as well as the doctor and nurse. The patient may have to relearn the performance of ordinary daily activities and progress from the simple to the more complex much as a child learns. It is frequently a slow process and both the patient and family are likely to have periods of depression and discouragement. The nurse assists them in making their plans for home management and the necessary activities and exercises. A referral is made to appropriate support services so that support and guidance are continued.

Spine and Spinal Cord Injury

Spinal cord injury is a major cause of serious disability, particularly in males between the ages of 15 and 30 years. Motor vehicle accidents continue to be a major cause of spinal injuries and frequently alcohol and drugs are involved. Other causes are falls, diving accidents and sports injuries, particularly horse riding and rugby.

TYPES OF INJURY

A spinal injury may or may not involve injury to the spinal cord. Fracture of one or more vertebrae may occur with no displacement of fragments resulting in the cord escaping injury. However, rupture of the ligaments holding the vertebrae in alignment may allow displacement of the vertebral column, leading to serious cord injury, even if no fracture occurs. Injury may be the result of: (1) sudden forceful angulation of the spine (hyperextension, hyperflexion, or hyperextension–hyperflexion) with or without rotational forces; (2) excessive force applied along the axis of the spine causing burst fractures and vertical compression (e.g. landing on the feet or buttocks from a height); (3) a direct blow to the area of the spine.

EFFECTS OF SPINAL INJURIES

Injuries to the vertebrae may result in spinal cord contusion, laceration and compression. Bleeding into the tissues and oedema occur, causing swelling and compression of nerve tracts. The damage may be slight and completely reversible or it may leave a minor degree of residual impairment. Oedema and bleeding in the cervical cord area is very serious; compression may interrupt innervation of the diaphragm incurring respiratory failure. A laceration which transects the cord or causes severe compression may result in complete, irreversible interruption of ascending or descending tracts. Destruction of the cord resulting in interruption of its tracts is not always due to transection. Injury may incur haemorrhage, circulatory stasis, extravasation of fluid and blood cells, ischaemia and necrosis of the tissue. Interruption of ascending tracts causes loss of sensation below the site of injury. This means that pain, pressure and temperature sensation may be dulled or lost and the patient may be unable to appreciate the position of affected limbs due to interference with proprioception impulse pathways. Interruption of descending tracts results in paralysis of the parts deriving their innervation from the cord below the level of the lesion. Flaccid paralysis and an absence of reflexes occur first and are usually followed by spastic paralysis and exaggerated tendon reflexes. Bladder, bowel and autonomic nervous functions are disturbed.

When the spinal cord is suddenly transected, a phenomenon known as *spinal shock* develops in which all cord functions including involuntary reflex responses are depressed; there is the sudden loss of all motor, sensory, reflex and autonomic responses below the site of cord injury. This occurs due to the sudden interruption of the initiating and regulatory impulses between the higher centres and the cord below the site of injury; that is, impulses are no longer being passed to or from neurones below the lesion. The result is loss of muscular tone (flaccid paralysis), an absence of reflexes and loss of sensation below the lesion. Cord reflexes for voiding and defecation are suppressed and retention and overflow incontinence occur. Vasomotor tone is lost and the blood pressure falls. Body temperature control is affected since there is no perspiration below the lesion; hyperthermia may develop. Spinal shock may subside in a few days or may persist for a much longer period. The loss of autonomic impulses and tone in the intestine may cause distension and paralytic ileus (see Chapter 16). Occasionally, recovery of reflex activity following spinal shock is characterized by hypersensitivity of the spinal neurones; for example, spasticity of the muscles develops and the bladder becomes hypertonic, resulting in diminished capacity and frequent reflex voiding.

The victim with injury to the spine without cord involvement retains motor and sensory functions and complains of pain at the site of the trauma and in parts innervated by that area. Later this may change; bleeding into the tissue and oedema may occur causing swelling and compression of the cord. *Initial management of spine-injured patients is on the basis of preventing potential cord damage.*

The spinal cord and its tracts are not capable of regeneration but regeneration of the nerve roots (outside the cord) can occur if the neurilemma is not severely damaged (see p. 692). Some recovery of function may occur in the first few weeks as oedema subsides and neurones, which were compressed but not destroyed, resume activity.

The paralysis which occurs with spinal cord injury may be complete or partial (paresis) and may be paraplegia or quadriplegia. If quadriplegia is complete there may be no voluntary control of function below the neck and very little potential for independence in self-care. With incomplete quadriplegia, voluntary control of selected muscles in the upper limbs may be restored and independence in many areas of self-care may be possible. Respiratory insufficiency or failure is a major concern in quadriplegia since there is usually some involvement of the nerve supply to the diaphragm and intercostal muscles.

CARE OF PATIENT WITH SPINAL INJURY

Care of the spine-injured patient involves three phases: the emergency, acute and rehabilitative phases.

EMERGENCY CARE AT THE SCENE OF AN ACCIDENT

The principal *problem* is the potential for further cord damage to occur and the *goal* is therefore that the patient will suffer no further cord damage.

Intervention

Spinal cord injury and permanent disability may be minimized with accurate assessment and appropriate care immediately following the accident. Injury to the spinal cord is suspected if the victim is unable to move his limbs, if numbness or peculiar sensations are present, if there is unexplained shock or if the person is unconscious after a head injury. The victim may also be having difficulty breathing if the injury is cervical. Wounds about the head or shoulders, pain, tenderness or deformity adjacent to the vertebral column also suggest spinal cord injury. If there is doubt regarding the presence of cord injury, the patient should be managed as if one were present.

Usually the spinal cord injured victim is conscious. The patient should be kept flat to permit free diaphragmatic breathing and should be advised to keep the head still; neck flexion or side to side rotation could seriously aggravate an injured cervical spine. A quick assessment is made for other injuries using the ABC checklist (Airway, Breathing, Circulation). Airway obstruction and inadequate ventilation have first priority but in establishing an airway or in providing assistance, extension of the neck must be avoided. If the patient is unconscious, the modified jaw thrust may be used to open the airway; two fingers are placed at the angle of the lower jaw to lift it forward. With cervical cord injury, the chest wall muscles may be paralysed and entire respiratory function is dependent on the diaphragm; respiratory assistance and suctioning may be necessary.

The patient should not be moved, except for life saving purposes, until the Ambulance Service are present. Ambulances carry a special 'scoop stretcher' for moving such patients with the minimum disturbance. All movements should be smooth and well co-ordinated. Immobilization of the head and neck are essential before the victim is moved. A firm cervical collar or sand bags taped to each side of the head may be used if available.

CARE DURING THE ACUTE PHASE (HOSPITAL)

Assessment

1. A brief history of the accident is obtained from the victim or person who was at the site.
2. An immediate assessment is made of the vital signs and continuous monitoring established if necessary.
3. If the patient's condition permits, or a family member is available, a brief review is made of the health history so that significant factors such as allergies, pre-existing disorders and medications being taken are identified.
4. The patient is examined for other injuries and a neurological evaluation is made to identify spinal cord damage. An assessment is made of:
   (a) Level of consciousness.
   (b) Orientation.
   (c) Motor and sensory functions (e.g. movement of the limbs; levels of sensation).
   (d) Reflexes (e.g. patellar, abdominal).
   (e) Condition of the skin: cold or warm, moist or dry all over or above or below a certain level.
5. The patient's understanding of the situation should be ascertained together with his or her feelings.

Patient problems

1. Potential for further cord injury.
2. Anxiety due to fear of paralysis.
3. Complications of actual cord injury e.g. spinal shock, respiratory failure, urinary retention/incontinence, pressure sores.

Goals

The goals are that no further injury will occur, complications of actual injury will be avoided and that the patient will verbalize fears and anxieties freely.

Intervention

The treatment of the spine-injured patient depends on:

- Whether there is cord injury and neurological deficits or not.
- The level of the injury.
- The nature of the injury (e.g. fracture fragments compressing the cord, laceration of the cord).

Immediate efforts are directed towards sustaining life and preventing cord damage or, where it has occurred, preventing further injury. The spinal lesion is treated by immobilization of the spine. Realignment of vertebrae and relief of pressure on the cord or spinal roots may be achieved by traction. In some instances surgery (decompression laminectomy) is undertaken to relieve pressure on the cord, remove vertebral fragments which are hazardous to the cord or to realign dislocated vertebrae which do not respond to traction of hyperextension. The surgery may include spinal fusion (see Table 21.8) or wiring of the spinous processes to stabilize the spine.

Cervical spine injury

A cervical collar may be applied as a first aid measure and should be left in place. When there is a fracture–dislocation with or without neurological deficit, skeletal traction is applied by means of Crutchfield tongs, a halo traction device or a halter.

Tongs are inserted into the skull at approximately the midlateral line, a short distance above the ears. The areas are prepared for the insertion by shaving, cleansing and the injection of a local anaesthetic. A very small incision is made in the scalp and small holes made in the skull with a drill to accommodate the tongs. The scalp may require sutures before a dressing is applied. The sites of insertion of the tongs are inspected daily for signs of infection, the areas are cleansed with an

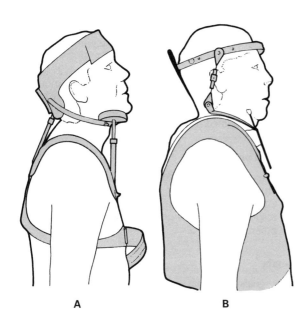

Figure 21.24 Halo traction (used in cervical vertebral fracture). (A) Four poster brace; (B) halo jacket.

antiseptic and fresh sterile dressings are applied. Traction of 4.5–13.2 kg (10–40 lb) may be applied and is achieved by a rope that overlies a pulley; one end is affixed to the tongs and the other hangs free with the prescribed weight attached. The prescribed weight depends on the size of the patient and the amount of displacement. It is usually heavy at first and altered as indicated by X-ray or clinical progress; that is reduced as realignment of the vertebrae or fragments occurs.

The patient may be placed on a turning bed (e.g. Egerton electrical turning and tilting bed) which is fitted with a pivoting device; this permits turning without interference to the traction. An ordinary bed with a fracture board, if necessary, beneath the mattress and the head board removed to allow clearance for traction may be used. The head of the bed is elevated to enable the body to act as counteraction for the weights and prevent the patient sliding toward the head of the bed. When realignment of the vertebrae or fragments and sufficient healing are achieved, the patient is fitted with a plastic collar or neck brace to provide cervical immobilization and support and is gradually ambulated.

The *halo traction device* involves the application of a metal ring to the head which is secured to the skull by the insertion of four pins (similar to the application of tongs). The sites of insertion into the skull are anterior, posterior and lateral. The ring is firmly anchored to a body cast or special vest by metal rods. This form of cervical immobilization and traction allows the patient to be ambulatory (Figure 21.24).

If only slight traction is required, a halter-like arrangement may be used in place of the tongs. The halter is arranged to place traction under the chin and

occipital area. Prolonged continuous application usually causes considerable discomfort and skin irritation for the patient by the pressure and pull, especially under the chin. Careful monitoring of neurological status and breathing are essential, together with meticulous pressure care. The patient's personal hygiene is also crucial.

A great deal of psychological support is needed. It is not possible to say in the first few days after injury how much recovery will occur. The nurse should therefore be honest in talking to the patient and family and say it is just too soon to know the extent of possible recovery. A truthful answer is better than avoiding the question or giving false hope to the patient.

Thoracic or lumbar spinal fracture
Where there is a fracture of the spine in the thoracic or lumbar region without dislocation and compression of the spinal cord the patient may be placed flat on a firm mattress on a bed with a firm base, or on a fracture board on an ordinary bed, or on a turning bed for several weeks. If the ordinary bed is used, specific directions are received as to whether the patient must remain on his back at all times. If turning is permitted, precautions are taken to ensure good alignment and avoidance of movement and displacement of the fragments ('log-rolling'). When there is sufficient healing, the patient is gradually ambulated. A brace, plaster jacket or firm corset may be necessary for several months to provide support and immobility of the spine.

A *fracture dislocation* of thoracic or lumbar vertebrae may be treated by hyperextension of the spine which may be achieved by various methods. One method is the placing of a firm roll or sandbag across the bed under the mattress to provide the required angulation. Fracture boards are placed on the bed if it has a sprung base, and a very firm mattress is used on which a sponge rubber mattress is placed, since the patient must remain in the supine position.

LONG-TERM CARE OF THE PATIENT WITH SPINAL CORD INJURY

After the initial stage of admission and stabilization, the patient faces a long road to recovery with the possibility of severe residual disability. Continuous assessment of progress is essential to monitor the effectiveness of care and to detect any of the potential complications of cord injury and immobility. Psychological care is of paramount importance in this period, together with an awareness of how the family might be affected.

Patient problems

1. Alteration in breathing pattern; respiratory insufficiency due to interruption of normal innervation of the diaphragm and/or intercostal muscles.
2. Potential for pressure sores as a result of immobility and impaired tissue perfusion.
3. Alteration in urinary elimination: retention with overflow or incontinence, due to disturbed innervation.
4. Alteration in bowel elimination: distension, constipation, incontinence secondary to spinal shock and immobility.

5. Alteration in food and fluid intake secondary to gastrointestinal distension, anxiety and difficulty in eating caused by immobility and position.
6. Self-care hygiene deficits due to paralysis and enforced immobility.
7. Alteration in comfort: pain and spasticity.
8. Potential for infection.
9. Potential for muscle contractures, deformities, osteoporosis and thrombophlebitis.
10. Inability to control body temperature due to dysfunction of the autonomic nervous system.
11. Disturbance in sleep pattern due to impact of accident, dependency and permanent disability.
12. Patient and family reactions to change in patient's role, loss of mobility and independence.
13. Potential for injury due to paralysis, immobility, muscle spasm, loss of sensation.
14. Sexual dysfunction.
15. Lack of knowledge and depression due to loss of mobility, independence and roles.

Goals

The patient's goals are to avoid the potential problems listed above and to adapt to altered levels of functioning whilst regaining maximum independence.

Nursing intervention

1. Respiratory dysfunction. In the *acute phase*, the patient with cervical or high thoracic cord injury is at risk of respiratory failure, reduced gas exchange and ineffective airway clearance. Initially, diaphragmatic function may appear to be adequate, but during the first 48 hours, oedema develops in the area of the injury. Its progress in the patient with a cervical injury may compromise vital centres in the medulla; respiratory failure develops as well as hypotension and weakening of the pulse. Chest trauma or pre-existing respiratory disease seriously complicates respiratory function.

Endotracheal intubation or a tracheostomy and oxygen administration may be necessary. If ventilatory muscle function is not adequate to maintain blood-gas levels, mechanical respiratory assistance is provided. Chest physiotherapy and increased humidity of inspired air and oxygen are provided to mobilize the secretions.

When the patient recovers sufficiently and the blood-gas analyses indicate satisfactory levels, mechanical respiratory assistance is discontinued and a regimen of deep breathing and coughing is established.

The patient continues to be at risk of respiratory insufficiency and complications in the post-acute phase. Abdominal muscle function may be weak or lacking, and, as a result, the cough is weak in the paraplegic and absent in the quadriplegic patient. Suction equipment should be readily available and intensive physiotherapy provided to help the patient develop an effective cough if possible, as well as to mobilize secretions. During the period that they must remain flat while the spine heals and stabilizes, spinal cord-injured patients are predisposed to bronchopneumonia and atelectasis.

2. Potential for pressure sores. The changes in vasomotor tone and the resulting impairment of tissue perfusion, the enforced immobility and the loss of cutaneous sensation contribute to tissue breakdown. If a decubitis ulcer occurs, healing is difficult in patients with spinal cord injury and rehabilitation is delayed.

The patient needs to understand the importance of keeping the skin intact and his or her role in maintaining its integrity. Following the period of immobilization to stabilize the spine, as the patient begins to assume the self-care within his or her potential, the importance of shifting of pressure is explained and the patient is taught how to change position at frequent regular intervals in bed and in a wheelchair. The patient is taught to inspect the vulnerable areas at least once daily using a mirror.

Most patients with paraplegia or quadriplegia are eventually mobilized by light-weight wheelchairs. The patient is taught transfer from bed to chair and from chair to toilet and that at regular intervals the body weight must be shifted. The patient learns to lift the trunk by pushing with the arms and hands on the chair arms or seat in order to relieve constant pressure on the buttocks and sacral region. Aids such as sheepskins and cushions filled with polyester granules may be provided.

3. Alteration in urinary elimination. During the spinal shock, the bladder is atonic and there is retention of urine with overflow. The statsis of urine predisposes to infection and the distension may cause fissures or areas of pressure necrosis in the bladder wall. Ureteral openings are dilated allowing reflux of urine into the kidneys. An indwelling catheter or intermittent catheterization is introduced soon after admission to prevent overdistension of the atonic bladder. The prevention of incontinence also assists in protecting the skin from irritation and breakdown. If continuous catheter drainage is required, a sterile closed drainage system is used; precautions must be strictly observed to prevent infection. Renal complications (e.g. pyelonephritis) leading to renal failure are the major cause of mortality in cord-injured persons. The atony of the bladder remains for a varying length of time before hyperreflexia takes over and the bladder becomes hypertonic, resulting in frequent automatic emptying of small volumes. To counteract the hypertonicity and diminished bladder capacity, an indwelling catheter is used, or if intermittent catheterization is used the intervals are gradually increased. Catheter use is discontinued as soon as possible because of the risk of infection and a bladder training programme is initiated. The reflex emptying of the bladder and incontinence are very distressing to the patient, who may resist an adequate fluid intake with the thought that it may at least lessen the frequency of involuntary voiding. This is dangerous since it predisposes to infection and the formation of calculi. Some patients become dependent on catheter use on a permanent basis, and may have to be taught intermittent self-catheterization.

Ideally a bladder training programme should be introduced as soon as possible to avoid dependency on a catheter. The patient is taught to initiate the reflexive emptying of the bladder by the Credé manoeuvre or the Valsalva manoeuvre. With some patients, stretching of the anal sphincter by the insertion of a gloved finger into the anal canal in combination with the Valsalva manoeuvre is more effective. The bladder may not completely empty and stasis of urine predisposes to infection. Periodic catheterization may be done to determine residual volume; less than 75–100 ml is usually acceptable. A specimen of urine is submitted for analysis at regular intervals and also if the urine has an offensive odour, is cloudy or there is blood or sediment.

4. Alteration in bowel elimination. With spinal shock the gastrointestinal tract becomes atonic; severe distension and vomiting without effort may develop. Gastrointestinal aspiration via a nasogastric tube may become necessary until peristalsis is re-established; abdominal distension causes respiratory embarrassment by pressure on the diaphragm.

The spinal cord injury interrupts impulses from the higher centres of awareness and control. The sensation of the need to defecate is lost and the rectal and anal sphincters function reflexly (automatic spinal cord response). Because of the immobility and dietary changes the patient experiences constipation, and impaction develops readily. When bowel sounds are present, a mild laxative or suppository (glycerin or bisacodyl) may be used to evacuate the bowel at first then, as the patient's condition improves and a more normal diet is taken, involuntary defecation occurs. A diet high in fibre is usually necessary to prevent constipation. The diet is adjusted to the stool consistency and frequency. As soon as the patient is able to sit in a chair, training for bowel elimination by conditioned reflex begins. A regular hour for bowel elimination may be established; morning is the normal time for most patients. The procedure involves a warm beverage, followed in one-half hour by the insertion of a glycerin or bisacodyl (Dulcolax) suppository and stimulation by inserting a lubricated gloved finger every 10–15 minutes until defecation occurs. Once a pattern of regular reflex evacuation has been established the patient may find that digital stimulation alone or the use of a device to massage the anal canal may be effective.

The patient is assisted to a commode or toilet at the same time each day or every other day. Privacy should be provided. A member of the patient's family should be involved in the bowel training programme as part of the preparation for home management.

5. Alteration in food and fluid intake. During the initial phase oral food and fluid are withheld. Some degree of paralytic ileus develops in most spinal cord-injured patients due to spinal shock. Fluids are administered by intravenous infusion to maintain hydration. A nasogastric tube may be inserted and aspiration established to relieve gastric and intestinal dilatation. When peristalsis is re-established, fluids are administered orally and, if tolerated, solid foods are added. A high calorie, high protein diet is important to combat the tendency toward a negative nigrogen balance which is commonly associated with immobility. An adequate nutritional intake also plays a role in promoting tissue healing and resistance to breakdown (e.g. pressure sores) and provides energy for exercises and the rehabilitative programme. Adequate dietary intake is made more difficult by the patient's positioning. Dietary supplements between meals may be necessary. Later, calorie intake may have to be reduced to prevent obesity, which complicates rehabilitation and increases the risk of complications. Bulk and roughage are necessary in the diet to promote bowel elimination.

Calcium intake (milk and milk products) may be restricted to prevent urinary calculi which may develop as calcium moves out of immobilized bones. A fluid intake of at least 3000 ml a day is encouraged to prevent concentration and stasis of urine. Grape and apple juices are preferable to citrus fruit juices; they produce an acid urine which reduces the precipitation of calcium and the formation of calculi as well as reducing the risk of infection. Organisms are less likely to grow in an acid environment.

Some cord-injured patients develop stress ulcers (gastric or duodenal). The aetiology has yet to be fully determined; hyperacidity due to histamine release following the trauma, or mucosal ischaemia, are among the leading theories at present. Ranitidine may be prescribed as a prophylactic measure. Dietary adjustments may be necessary to meet these patients' tolerance.

Food must be placed readily within reach and the patient encouraged to feed unaided as soon as the condition permits. Initially those with quadriplegia will require assistance with feeding until appropriate assistive devices are available. Swallowing may be difficult in the recumbent position and inhalation may occur. The patient is encouraged to take only small amounts at a time and swallow frequently. Suction equipment should be readily available in the event of inhalation.

If the partial quadriplegic patient has motor function in the triceps and biceps muscles, self-feeding may be accomplished. With flexion at the elbow and the fitting over the hand of a wide elastic band with a pocket, self-feeding may be achieved. Special utensils such as a spoon fit into the pocket.

6. Self-care hygiene deficits. The patient will become increasingly aware of limitations and dependency; personal care must be provided with sensitivity to the patient's feelings. It is difficult to convince the patient in the early stages that eventually it is possible that considerable independence will be regained.

In order to regain even minimal independence in self-care, the individual must be able to move about and be able to have some grasp in at least one hand. Paraplegic persons do have the distinct advantage of having the use of both hands and are capable of achieving self-care. The quadriplegic is dependent on head movements, assistive devices and care provided by others.

7. Alteration in comfort. The patient with a spinal cord injury may experience pain which radiates along the spinal nerves that originate at the level of injury. Spasticity of the muscles below the level of the cord injury is also a source of severe discomfort in paraplegia and quadriplegia and may lead to contractures and deformities. The pain is severe and fatiguing and may be embarrassing at times for the patient. It may retard rehabilitation. The muscle spasms are hypersensitive reflexes which develop after spinal shock subsides. The stimulus may not even be obvious. Examples of stimuli which may initiate the spastic response include light touching of the skin, jarring of the bed, turning, cold, fatigue, a distended bladder and emotional reactions. Regular passive moving of the limbs through their range of motion is beneficial especially when done under water. Rarely, severe painful spasticity is treated by surgery; various procedures have been done and include severing of tendons, transection of a nerve root (rhizotomy) and neurotomy (cutting of nerves).

Narcotics and strong analgesics are not used with the patient with high cervical injury because of the depressing effect on respiration.

8. Potential for infection. The risk of urinary and respiratory tract infections has already been discussed.

9. Potential for complications: muscle contractures, deformities, osteoporosis and thrombophlebitis. Patients with spinal cord injury and the resulting paralysis develop muscle and tendon contractures and ankylosis of the joints unless preventive measures are observed. The shortening of the muscles and tendons may cause serious deformities which restrict rehabilitation. For example a flexure contracture of the thigh at the hip joint may inhibit the patient's use of a wheelchair. Wrist drop and foot drop develop readily in paralysed limbs unless preventive measures are instituted. Immobility, muscle spasticity and poor alignment in positioning the patient are contributing factors. Preventive measures include frequent change of position and maintenance of good body alignment using sand bags, and pillows if necessary, regular passive range-of-movement exercises and a physiotherapy programme as soon as the patient's condition permits.

The health of bones normally depends on stress due to muscle pull and weight bearing. When these are lacking, as with paralysis and prolonged immobilization, bone demineralization and osteoporosis occurs. Therefore, weight bearing is started as soon as possible to stimulate osteoblastic activity and prevent demineralization. The head of the bed is gradually elevated as tolerated, and, when safe, the patient is positioned upright on a tilt table. Weight bearing for at least a few minutes each day may also help to prevent contractures, particularly in the hips.

Regardless of intervention, eventually atrophy of paralysed muscles does occur to some degree. This is primarily due to absence of nerve impulses to the muscle.

Thrombophlebitis is a common problem in a paralysed patient, particularly in the first 3 months following injury. Absence of the pumping action of contracting muscle and poor skeletal muscle tone which results from paralysis and immobility, leads to pooling of blood in the lower viscera and extremities and a reduced venous return. This predisposes to thrombophlebitis. Localized oedema, redness, warmth, tenderness and red streaks of an extremity suggest thrombophlebitis. Deep venous thrombosis may also occur. Because of loss of sensation, pain and tenderness are not perceived. Assessment for venous thrombosis, done daily, includes calf observation, gentle palpation for calf firmness and measurement of the circumference of the thigh and calf. The tape measure is placed at the same level above and below the knee each time. Management to prevent thrombosis includes a regular schedule of range of movement and exercises (these activities act as a mechanical pump to increase circulation), frequent change of position, elevation of the legs 15° for stated periods and the wearing of antiembolic stockings while in bed. Anticoagulant therapy (e.g. acetylsalicylic acid) may be prescribed as a prophylactic measure. Subcutaneous Heparin 5000 units twice daily is often prescribed for the first 3 months following paraplegia.

10. Inability to control body temperature. This is a common problem for patients with a spinal cord injury. Dysfunction of the autonomic nervous system occurs and there is decreased ability to lose or conserve heat in the paralysed parts of the body. Room temperature is controlled to meet the patient's need since he or she is mainly dependent on environmental temperature for the avoidance of hypothermia.

11. Disturbance in sleep pattern. This is a common problem as a result of the psychological impact of the traumatic event and enforced immobility and dependency. The cord-injured patient may experience frightening dreams in which the accident is relived. Discomfort and the necessary frequent repositioning as well as a high level of anxiety may disrupt the patient's sleep.

Lack of adequate rest and sleep depletes the person's energy and endurance which are essential for healing and rehabilitation.

Nursing care involves the provision of a quiet environment, comfort measures such as position change, warm drinks and remaining with the patient, encouraging the discussion of anxieties and feelings and to provide reassurance that he or she is not alone. Regular rest periods are scheduled to prevent exhaustion.

12. Sexual dysfunction. The potential for sexual fulfilment is a major concern of the patient with permanent disability. Some patients may express this concern directly but more often concern is present long before it is expressed. One paraplegic reported: 'It is such a personal thing. If someone else had brought up the subject I might have felt more comfortable about asking the questions I had.' If the patient brings up the topic of sexuality, a free and open discussion should be encouraged.

The cord-injured patient needs to know that meaningful and satisfying relationships are still attainable and that even though he or she may no longer be able to function sexually in the same ways as before the injury, new ways of giving and receiving sexual satisfaction can be learned. The patient needs to understand that the sexuality of an individual involves the total person and that self-image is an important dimension in the resocialization process in disability.

The question of fertility and ability to procreate may also be raised by patients with a spinal cord injury. Male infertility is not uncommon following a cord injury because of testicular atrophy, decreased production of sperm and infrequency of ejaculation. The female with cord injury is usually able to conceive and deliver a child with few adaptations being necessary. Since there exists a vast body of knowledge specific to sexuality in disability, it is appropriate to discuss other resources of information with the patient. Referral to a qualified counsellor or agency may be advisable. Issues such as parenting, adoption, contraception and artificial insemination as they relate to the physically disabled are currently receiving attention and are being studied.

13. Patient and family reactions. It is understandable that a spinal injury which results in paralysis is a very traumatic psychological experience. Suddenly, the victim is changed from an independent person to one who is dependent on others for even very personal care. Responses and adjustment to the loss of body functions usually parallel the grief reaction with feelings of anger and despair mixing with frustration and depression.

Initially, shock and denial of reality help the victim to maintain self-control and survive. Consistent, high-quality nursing care is supportive in this phase. Gradually, a beginning awareness develops and the patient responds with anger and resentment that this has happened to him. The nurse needs to listen and try to understand the patient's responses; support at this time may help to strengthen the patient's tenuous grasp of reality. Anger may be followed by a period of despair and depression in which the patient may eat or drink very little and does not manifest any interest in rehabilitation, family or others. Close observation of reactions and comments indicate to the nurse when to encourage conversation or when presence alone is preferable to the patient. At the appropriate time, the nurse verbally acknowledges recognition of how the situation looks to the patient. The patient may raise questions that relate to concerns such as independence, financial support and sexuality in the future. Anxiety may escalate in proportion to the unknown; anxiety depletes energy and tends to distort reality. The patient should be assured that everything possible will be done to help regain the ability to do some things unaided. Reassurance should be realistic; offering false hope must be avoided. The quadriplegic patient poses the greater challenge to the nurse.

It will be some time before the patient begins to see things realistically and explore possibilities for the future. In this reorganization phase, learning to cope with body changes predominates. Assimilation of the changes in body image and pattern of life takes considerable time; periods of withdrawal and depression are to be expected from time to time. Such reactions are accepted but with expectation that efforts will be resumed. Thinking is directed to the positive and as soon as possible, the patient is encouraged and expected to do the things that the functional motor

capacity allows. The acknowledgement of improvement and achievement helps to sustain motivation. The development of a sense of worthiness and self-esteem essential for resocialization greatly depend on the positive attitude, appreciation and reliance conveyed by professionals and significant others.

The victim's injury and the possible implications of disability are difficult for family members to accept. As well as concern for the patient, the situation may involve a complete change of life-style for them. They may be faced with financial hardships and a disruption of home management. Role functions change, responsibilities are shifted and plans and goals may be shattered.

Family bonds may become greater as they face the situation together; new strengths, capabilities and determination to cope with their problems may be revealed. In other instances, the reaction of some family members after the patient's acute phase may be resentment for the individual whose accident has altered their life. The patient is rejected and feelings of loneliness, fear and depression are increased. There may also be profound feelings of guilt if a family member was in some way responsible for the original accident.

The nurse takes time to talk with the family; they are kept informed of the patient's progress and of the therapeutic and rehabilitative programmes. Their role in supporting the patient is discussed. Time is given to discussing family problems and suggestions made that assist them in planning and resolution.

Family and friends are encouraged to spend time with the patient to provide support and reinforce the impression that they are not rejecting the patient as useless. Encouraging and letting the patient do things unaided are emphasized. A major multidisciplinary effort will be needed to provide the long-term community care the patient needs.

14. Potential for injury. Limited sensation in the paralysed parts, limited mobility, muscle spasm and dependency place the paralysed patient at risk of injury and complications. It is necessary for the patient to develop the necessary strength in the unaffected parts to mobilize and control the affected parts in order to prevent complications incurred by immobilization and falls. The bones in paralysed limbs are easily fractured due to osteoporosis. A waist strap is used while the patient is in a chair until he or she is strong enough to control the trunk. Consistent use of wheelchair brakes during transfers is essential for safety.

Any local heat application is used judiciously; loss of cutaneous sensation predisposes to burns. The skin is inspected daily for abrasions, bruises, pressure ischaemia and irritated areas.

15. Rehabilitation. As soon as the patient is well enough, an active rehabilitation programme is planned and instituted. The patient and family participate in the planning and scheduling of the programme to meet their knowledge deficits and adjustments. Family members should be involved in order to support the patient and maintain consistent care. Rehabilitation begins with simple self-care activities, progressing to more complex as skill is achieved. With increasing independence, the

Table 21.8 Spinal surgical procedures.

	Procedure	Conditions in which used
Laminectomy	Partial or complete removal of the vertebral arch by the two laminae. It precedes other spinal operations to provide access to the canal	Chronic low back pain (disc problems) Spinal fracture (to remove fragments) Cord decompression Removal of a neoplasm
Discectomy	Excision of an intervertebral disc	Ruptured or herniated disc Chronic low back pain
Spinal fusion	Application of bone grafts to two or more adjoining vertebrae to ankylose them	Ruptured or herniated disc Relief of nerve or cord compression
Rhizotomy	Division of transection of a nerve root either outside or within the spinal cord	Chronic pain
Cordotomy	Division of the pain-conducting pathways (spinothalamic antero-lateral tracts) in the spinal cord Percutaneous cordotomy involves the insertion of a needle (under X-ray) into the spinal cord	Intractable pain (usually associated with malignant disease)

paraplegic patient learns to turn, transfer from bed to chair and chair to toilet. Progress is slow and requires persistent effort and repeated encouragement; recognition of even the slightest gain prompts motivation. Planned periods of rest and diversion are necessary to offset intensive exercises and prevent exhaustion. The family are cautioned against fostering dependence by doing things that the patient has the capacity to do or learn to do alone.

A major component of rehabilitation concerns work. Some patients may be able to manage to return to their previous employment but many will not. Retraining may be possible and every effort should be made to allow the patient to regain meaningful employment as this will be beneficial to morale, self-concept, and also the patient's finances.

NURSING THE PATIENT TREATED BY SPINAL SURGERY

Spinal surgery may be performed to: remove a neoplasm, a herniated or ruptured disc or bony fragments following an injury; reduce a fractured vertebra; decompress the spinal cord following an injury; relieve intractable pain or spasticity; or suppress involuntary movements. For common spinal surgical procedures see Table 21.8.

The care following spinal surgery varies with the surgery, the patient's response to it and the surgeon's preferences. For example some patients are immobilized for weeks while others are ambulated a day or two following the procedure. An understanding of what was done and specific directives are necessary in planning care, especially in relation to positioning and movement. The major principles to be observed with all patients in moving and positioning are the maintenance of proper spinal alignment, the avoidance of any twisting, angulation and jerky movements of the spine and the prevention of strain on the back muscles.

Assessment

The patient's vital signs and responses are recorded as a baseline against which any changes in condition will become apparent.

When the surgery is below the thoracic region, assessment includes an evaluation of sensation and motor ability in the lower limbs. The colour and temperature of the limbs and leg and foot pulses may be checked since vascular problems may develop. If the surgery was cervical or high thoracic, close observation of the person's respiratory pattern is necessary as well as sensorimotor responses of the arms. Hoarseness of the voice and ineffective cough may develop due to injury of the recurrent laryngeal nerve.

Wound area(s) are checked for possible haemorrhage, leakage of CSF and contamination. The patient's sensation of pain should be carefully assessed, together with the standard postoperative parameters of urine output, wound drainage, skin condition, etc.

Patient problems

1. Potential for spinal injury. Even slight angulation or tension or jerky movements may injure the spine and cause nerve or cord damage.
2. Potential for respiratory insufficiency due to cord and nerve compression in cervical spinal surgery, immobility and shallow respirations because of the pain.
3. Pain due to oedema in the operative area, irritation and trauma of nerves at the time of surgery and muscle spasm.
4. Alteration in elimination pattern: retention of urine, paralytic ileus, constipation.
5. Potential for wound haemorrhage or infection.
6. Alteration in food and fluid intake.
7. Potential impairment of skin integrity due to immobility and later due to the wearing of a brace or corset.

Table 21.9 Intracranial tumours.

Name of neoplasm	Origin	Most frequent sites	Comments
Gliomas	Neuroglial tissue		Most common type of intracranial neoplasm; rate of growth varies with type of glioma
Astrocytoma	Astrocytes	Adults—cerebrum Children—cerebellum	Most common glioma grows very slowly; infiltrates surrounding tissue
Glioblastoma	Undifferentiated glial cells	Frontal, parietal and temporal lobes	Highly malignant
Medulloblastoma	Undifferentiated glial cells	Cerebellum	Rapid extension: highly malignant
Ependymoma	Ependymal cells of the lining of the ventricle and aqueducts	Fourth ventricle	Rare; frequently papillomatous; may obstruct flow of CSF
Oligodendroglioma	Oligodendrocytes	Cerebral hemispheres	Rare; grows very slowly; tends to calcify
Meningioma	Meninges	Along the course of the intracranial venous sinuses	Are extracerebral, causing compression of brain tissue; usually encapsulated; grow slowly
Haemangiomas Angioma	Blood vessel wall	Middle cerebral artery	(Not a true neoplasm) Congenital mass of tortuous, enlarged vessels; benign, but may interfere with adjacent tissues
Angioblastoma	Blood vessel wall	Cerebellum	Tendency to form cysts
Pituitary adenomas			
Chromophobe adenoma	Adenohypophyseal glandular tissue	Anterior pituitary lobe (adenohypophysis)	Encapsulated; compresses pituitary gland tissue and optic nerves, leading to hypopituitarism and impaired vision
Chromophil adenoma (acidophilic adenoma)	Adenohypophyseal glandular tissue	Anterior pituitary lobe (adenohypophysis)	Seen less often than chromophobe adenoma; causes hyperpituitarism (gigantism or acromegaly)
Craniopharyngioma	Embryological defect in craniopharyngeal duct	Anterior to the pituitary stalk	Produces pressure on surrounding structures, interfering with function
Acoustic neuroma	Eighth cranial (acoustic) nerve		Encapsulated

8. Impairment of mobility: enforced immobility and maintenance of spinal alignment.
9. Lack of knowledge. Information is required to prevent recurrence of the back problem and assistance is needed in planning the necessary adjustments in the resumption of activity and management at home.

Goals

Patient goals are similar to those set in the postoperative care of any general surgical patient. In addition, the patient should not suffer any complications related specifically to the spinal surgery.

Nursing intervention

The patient should be nursed in accordance with the same principles as a general surgical patient but also taking into account the nursing interventions specifically designed to deal with spinal problems that have been discussed earlier in this section.

THE PERSON WITH A NEOPLASM OF THE NERVOUS SYSTEM

Intracranial Neoplasms

Intracranial tumours may be primary or secondary (metastatic), may occur at any age and in any part of the brain. *Primary* neoplasms may be benign or malignant and commonly arise from the neuroglial tissue, meninges, cerebral blood vessels, hypophysis and nerve fibres are named according to their tissue origin (Table 21.9). Most primary intracranial tumours are gliomas. Unlike neoplasms elsewhere in the body, primary neoplasms of the brain rarely metastasize. *Secondary* intracranial tumours commonly originate in the lungs or breast.

Brain tumours vary in size, location and pattern of growth. The glioblastomas are highly malignant and invasive while others like the meningiomas are benign and compressive. This accounts for the great variability in the development of symptoms and in the prognosis following surgery. Most brain tumours in the adult tend to occur in the supratentorial compartment (above the brain stem and cerebellum).

EFFECTS ON THE PATIENT

Any intracranial neoplasm is a space-occupying lesion; as it grows, intracranial content and pressure increase within the rigid cranium. The effects of rising intracranial pressure have already been discussed. The manifestations reflect the location; neurological deficits (sensory and/or motor) and behavioural changes appear as the tumour involves specific cerebral areas, some deficiency in mental capacity may develop and seizures may occur due to alterations in the electrical potential of cells. Hydrocephalus may develop if there is interference of the normal flow and absorption of CSF, and endocrine imbalances may occur associated with the compression or invasion of the pituitary gland.

MEDICAL MANAGEMENT

The treatment used for a brain tumour depends on the location and type of neoplasm and the condition of the patient. It may involve surgery, radiation and/or chemotherapy. Whenever possible, surgical excision of the neoplasm is the method of choice but in some instances it may be inaccessible or involve vital areas (e.g. brain stem) making removal impossible. Non-encapsulated neoplasms infiltrate surrounding tissue, making surgery less effective. In some instances, surgical decompression is indicated to relieve compression symptoms by a craniotomy (see p. 734). If the lesion is obstructing the CSF and is inoperable a palliative shunt may be done involving the placement of a tube between the lateral ventricle and the subarachnoid space in the posterior fossa below the brain (cistern magna) or between the ventricle and the superior vena cava or the peritoneal cavity. Radiotherapy is employed with tumours which are surgically inaccessible or which cannot be entirely excised. It is effective in slowing the progress of some primary neoplasms (e.g. gliomas) and metastases, improving the quality of the patient's life as well as lengthening it. Radiation may cause temporary cerebral oedema and an increased intracranial pressure; a corticosteroid preparation may be administered to lessen these side-effects. Hair loss may result from irradiation to the head.

Certain chemotherapeutic drugs, for example vincristine, may be used alone or in combination with surgery or radiation. However, many of the cytotoxic drugs are unable to penetrate the blood–brain barrier, if it remains intact.

NURSING THE PATIENT WITH A BRAIN TUMOUR

Assessment

An initial evaluation is made and recorded of the patient's motor and sensory functions, speech ability, orientation, behavioural responses, pupillary reactions and any complaints of headache, dizziness and tingling or numbness. It is important to obtain information about the patient's normal behaviour before the development of the tumour. Assessment is an ongoing process through successive contacts so that changes and newly developed symptoms may be recognized promptly. The nurse's recognition and recording of physical and behavioural changes may play an important role in the diagnosis and localization of the intracranial tumour. Knowing that a space-occupying lesion is suspect, the nurse is especially alert for signs of increasing intracranial pressure. It is crucial to discuss the patient's and family's understanding of the condition in order to plan how they may be assisted and supported. Anxieties and fears, together with the patient's level of knowledge and any coping mechanisms being employed, should all be ascertained.

Patient problems

The patient faces the whole range of potential problems associated with immobility and raised intracranial pressure (see preceding sections). In addition there is the very real fear of death itself, understandably leading to severe anxiety and depression as well as seriously stressing family networks.

Goals

Patient goals revolve around avoiding the complications of immobility and raised intracranial pressure in general, and specifically in adapting to the fact that the illness may prove fatal.

Nursing intervention

The nursing care discussed in preceding sections will be required, adapted to the individual, in addition to care needed to help the patient deal with the fear and anxiety produced by the knowledge that this may be a fatal disease. No single intervention can entirely relieve these concerns but an understanding and supportive approach helps. Acknowledging the fear as understandable, encouraging the patient to talk about concerns, express feelings and ask questions may ease the situation somewhat. Information is provided to prepare the patient for investigative procedures and treatment and the patient should be involved in making decisions.

The family's anxiety is understandable. Their strengths and weaknesses that may have implications for the patient's progress are identified. They are kept informed about the patient, what is being done and how they may provide support. Opportunities are provided for them to ask questions and express their concerns. In some instances, it may be necessary to suggest to the family that they avoid conveying their emotions to the patient. Information about the hospital chaplaincy service may be useful to the patient and family, as will contact with a social worker, who can advise about social security assistance, etc.

Relief of pain is very important in helping the patient deal with this situation. The assessment and management of pain associated with cancer is discussed in depth on pp. 176–181.

THE PERSON WITH A DEGENERATIVE DISORDER

Commonly occurring degenerative disorders of the nervous system include Alzheimer's disease, multiple sclerosis, Parkinson's disease, myasthenia gravis and motor neurone disease. In addition, patients with AIDS will also suffer chronic neurological disease.

AIDS

Thirty to 70% of all individuals with HIV infection will at some time during their illness develop neurological manifestations of the disease. The brain, spinal cord and peripheral nerves can all be involved in HIV infection, with the symptoms being very similar to those seen in depressive or anxiety syndromes, or may imitate those of manic depression and schizophrenia. Opportunistic infections of the brain include viral infections such as cytomegalovirus, herpes simplex, adenovirus, varicella zoster virus and papovavirus. The most common bacterial infections include cryptococcasis and toxoplasmosis, which respond well to drug therapy but this must be continued for the patient's life-time.

The most frequent problem affecting the spinal cord is a condition known as vascular myelopathy, a degenerative condition which presents as difficulty walking, numbness in the feet and paraplegia. There is currently no treatment for this condition.

HIV can also directly invade brain tissue resulting in a condition known as AIDS dementia complex (ADC) or AIDS encephalopathy. ADC has an insidious onset, with impairment in memory and concentration and subtle changes in personality being early signs. The condition may advance to motor difficulties, with ataxia being present, or to psychiatric manifestations such as psychosis or hallucinations. The patient often becomes depressed, resulting in social withdrawal and apathy. It is often difficult to differentiate between psychological symptoms of the illness and neurological changes.

Early and ongoing nursing assessment of neurological change is crucial. Questions relating to memory, concentration, orientation and judgement need to be asked in a safe, non-threatening environment. Safety issues must be continually examined, with the patients often requiring orientation cues and written instruction. Eyesight may be hindered by cytomegalovirus retinitis, eliminating the use of this modality. Family and significant others are crucial resources at this time and may provide helpful information in relation to the patient's behaviour.

The diagnosis of a chronic neurological problem can affect a patient's self-esteem and feeling of confidence, as well as generating fear for the future. These feelings can be manifested as symptoms of anger, denial, powerlessness and depression. The nurse, in caring for the family and the patient, has to be aware of the difficulties in adaptation the patient may have at any given time. There are periods of stability, both emotional and physical, together with periods of increased stress when the illness exacerbates.

An explanation of the disorder and the prescribed therapy is made to the patient and family. Opportunities are provided for discussions in which they can ask questions and express their feelings and concerns. They are assisted in planning how to maintain a satisfactory life-style, role functions and socialization. The patient is encouraged to be independent and carry out self-care activities. Those around are advised that the patient's intellectual ability is unimpaired; it should be emphasized that he or she needs to be treated normally, to socialize and to do things unaided even though it may take much longer. The environment should be cheerful and free of haste and confusion.

The general *goals* of the patient and family in cases of degenerative neurological disorder are that they will:

1. Have knowledge of the disease process and potential complications.
2. Have knowledge of the health care system and available support systems.
3. Be aware of interventions that maintain optimal functioning.

Alzheimer's Disease

Alzheimer's disease is a *presenile dementia* of unknown aetiology and is the most common degenerative brain disorder. A history of familial incidence is considered to play a role in the development of the disease, which is incurable at present. The age of onset is between 45 and 65 years of age. Both males and females are equally affected. The frontal and temporal lobes are most affected but gradual progressive atrophy of the entire brain occurs. Microscopically, there is wide-spread loss of nerve cells.

EFFECTS ON THE PATIENT

In the progress of the disease three stages may be identified. The first stage lasts 2–4 years and is characterized by subtle changes which may be dismissed as inattention or carelessness. Eventually, there are recognizable changes in personality, loss of memory for recent and remote events, apathy, loss of spontaneity and initiative, neglect of personal hygiene and appearance, and a suspiciousness of other's motives with a tendency to blame them for one's incapacities. Loss of spatial orientation is seen in the inability to put on a garment without confusion as to top and bottom and sleeve and neck. Weakness, muscular twitching or seizures may occur, and motor aphasia (the person cannot recall words he or she wishes to say) and speech slurring may become evident. Indifference to social customs and graces develops.

In the second stage of the disease, the changes of the first stage intensify. Disorientation is complete; emotional lability increases and there may be restlessness at night. Memory loss becomes so severe that even close friends and relatives are not recognized and the patient may not recognize himself or herself in the mirror. Movements are slow, and simple writing, reading, mathematical skills and reasoning deteriorate seriously. Other deficiencies such as inability to recognize objects by way of the senses become obvious. Motor dysfunction may progress from unsteady gait to inability to stand or walk. The person loses weight due to poor nutrition and shows no interest in meals.

In the final stage of the disease, movements become stereotyped, there is inability to use language, urinary and bowel incontinence, abnormal reflexes and muscular rigidity develop and eventually, there is flexion of the lower extremities and the individual becomes bedridden and totally helpless. There is a marked tendency to grasp objects and put them to the mouth. The disease may last for several years. Death usually results from bronchopneumonia or infected pressure sores.

NURSING CARE

Assessment

The patient assessment involves a detailed physical assessment, paying particular attention to nutritional and fluid balance status, skin condition, general personal hygiene and appearance and elimination patterns. The patient's level of understanding, memory and orientation are key parts of the psychological assessment, whilst social and family circumstances must also be explored.

Patient problems

The patient's carers may be the focal point of nursing interventions. The age, the health and support systems of the care-givers are important considerations when a patient remains at home. The following is a list of core problems, many more individual problems are possible:

1. Ineffective coping because of altered cognitive functioning.
2. Potential for injury due to loss of memory, impaired motor and cognitive functioning.
3. Self-care deficits in relation to adequate rest, nutrition and personal hygiene.
4. Alteration in elimination patterns: urinary and bowel incontinence.
5. Potential for social isolation due to loss of interest, initiative and memory (friends and relatives not recognized).
6. Potential for complications:
   (a) Respiratory dysfunction due to inactivity and lowered resistance to infection.
   (b) Impairment of skin integrity due to immobility, incontinence, malnutrition and injury.
7. Inadequate knowledge.

Nursing intervention

1. Ineffective coping. In the early stage, the patient and particularly the family require considerable counselling. Expectations of the patient's abilities should be lowered. The patient needs to be understood and accepted as he or she is, because memory cannot be restored nor behaviour changed. A written outline of daily routines to be carried out may prove helpful. For example, if the person is to carry out a job away from home, it may be useful to refer to a written note.

Each day, the patient identifies a few essential tasks on which to focus, since coping with more than these is too difficult.

2. Potential for injury. The environment is kept free of hazards and stress as much as possible. As disorientation develops and as body movements become increasingly more awkward the risk of falls increases. The patient may forget that a cigarette is burning or that a gas stove has been turned on. With progressive loss of memory, the person requires close supervision. It is important that he or she carries identification in case of wandering off and becoming lost and exposed to the elements. It should be remembered that restlessness and disorientation are likely to be worse at night when sensory stimuli are minimal and there is some decrease in cerebral perfusion.

The patient can usually manage for a longer period and be capable of doing more if in the familiar surroundings of home where an automatic routine is established.

3. Self-care deficits. Regular periods of rest are planned for the person: fatigue tends to aggravate the manifestations of deterioration. Some patients respond to relaxation therapy tapes. The daily food and fluid intake are noted and the patient is weighed at regular intervals. In the early stage of Alzheimer's disease, the patient gradually loses the appreciation of nutritional needs. The person becomes unable to shop and prepare food and eventually skips meals. Prompting and assistance with meals and in between snacks are necessary to ensure that the patient gets sufficient nutrition. High calorie foods and supplements are used when necessary. Plans are made to provide hygienic care as neglect becomes obvious. Provision is made for bathing, grooming, dressing and frequent change of washable clothing.

4. Alteration in elimination pattern. With progression of Alzheimer's disease, the patient develops urinary and bowel incontinence. A schedule for prompting the patient to go to the toilet at intervals determined by customary elimination frequency may help in avoiding incontinence. When the patient is incontinent, the perineum and surrounding area are cleansed and dried promptly to prevent excoriation. Constipation may be a problem due to the immobility and reduced food intake. The roughage content of the diet may be increased and a mild laxative (bulk producing or stool softener) administered. If the constipation is not recognized and corrected, faecal impaction develops readily.

5. Potential for social isolation. The patient tends to avoid social situations as cognitive and communicative skills diminish. Efforts should be made for exposure to human interaction and for socialization just as long as they have even the slightest meaning. Including the person in short social events and in small-group affairs could be helpful. If a day care centre is available, the patient will be able to get out of the home and participate in structured social activity.

6. Potential for complications. Because of inactivity and malnutrition, the patient is predisposed to respiratory infection. An exercise programme, walking, deep breathing and coughing, adequate nutrition as well as protection from exposure to those with an infection contribute to the prevention of respiratory infection.

As the immobility, helplessness and malnutrition worsen, the patient becomes more and more predisposed to pressure sores. Regular bathing, careful observation and protection of vulnerable areas, repositioning at regular intervals and prompt changing of clothing or bedding following incontinence are necessary.

7. Inadequate knowledge. Some major adjustments in the life-style and relationships of the family, as well as the patient, are necessary as the disease advances. Planning for these at an early stage of the disorder facilitates the change process as it becomes necessary. A major effort involving social workers and various members of the community care team is needed to support the family in caring for the patient at home. Although the life span of the person with Alzheimer's disease cannot be protracted, the quality of the life of all those concerned can be enhanced through early professional intervention, counselling and effective planning. It is helpful to introduce the family to the local branch of the Alzheimer's Society. The association provides family support through meetings, pamphlets and community referrals. The Society also provides education for the general public.

In the early stages, the family is advised of ways to help the patient maintain independence and carry on at home. The family is informed of signs of progression of the disorder and how members can best cope with increasing dependency of the patient. They are alerted to the hazards that may develop with the increasing dementia. When the affected person is no longer productive, roles and relationships must change. It is particularly difficult when a formerly responsible and productive person becomes dependent upon others for decision-making and personal care. The process of adjustment is slow and requires understanding and acceptance of the patient's condition. The family's reactions may indicate the need for a referral for professional counselling.

In the later stages of the disorder, management focuses on helping the family cope with extremely difficult situations. The family may consist of one person or several people. Anticipatory planning for institutional care has to be encouraged so that, when it becomes necessary, it is part of a rational decision-making process. The family may need considerable persuasion and support in making this decision.

Multiple Sclerosis (MS, Disseminated Sclerosis)

Multiple sclerosis is a chronic, progressive, degenerative disease that is characterized by patches of demyelination throughout the brain and spinal cord. Myelin is the lipoprotein sheath surrounding the axons of the neurones and enables impulses to travel much faster along the fibre than is possible in unmyelinated fibres. The destruction of areas of myelin is followed by a proliferation of neuroglial cells. Scar tissue forms as hardened (sclerotic) white elevations known as plaque. Nerve fibres (axons) eventually degenerate; there is loss of impulse transmission and focal deficits occur which in some instances may be permanent. The optic nerves and the cervical spinal cord tend to be most vulnerable to this degenerative demyelinating process in the initial episodes.

INCIDENCE AND POPULATION AT RISK

Multiple sclerosis has a worldwide distribution and affects 40–60 people per 100 000 of the population. People are twice as likely to be stricken if they live in cold damp climates. The United Kingdom has been recognized as a high risk zone; in north-east Scotland and Ulster, the incidence is 100 per 100 000 population, and in the Shetlands and Orkney, 300 per 100 000. The onset of the disease is highest amongst persons aged 17–30 years with a slightly higher incidence among women. A familial tendency has been recognized but a definite genetic pattern has not been identified.

AETIOLOGY

The specific cause of multiple sclerosis continues to elude scientists; current evidence suggests that genetic factors, environmental factors, viruses and the individual's immune system may be collectively implicated. The view that viral infection and an immunological abnormality interact to induce the central nervous system damage is particularly favoured.

EFFECTS ON THE PATIENT

Multiple sclerosis is characterized by remissions and relapses. The course and the effects vary widely from one person to another and are unpredictable. Spontaneous remissions of varying lengths are common particularly in the early years of the disease, and in some instances appear to be permanent. Rarely multiple sclerosis takes a fulminating, malignant course in which a combination of cerebral brain stem and cord manifestations develop suddenly; the patient becomes comatose; there is no remission and death may occur within a few weeks.

Most patients survive more than 20 years after the initial onset and lead active productive lives for many of those years. A lesser number experience a steady progression of their disease with frequently recurring relapses leading to a chronic incapacitated state, dependency and complications.

The initial onset of symptoms of multiple sclerosis usually develops suddenly (within a day or two) but with some, may develop slowly over several weeks. The initial onset of exacerbation usually coincides with a stressful experience such as anxiety, trauma, infection, excessive fatigue, exposure to an extreme of temperature and pregnancy.

Since the location and extent of the demyelination are so variable, the clinical characteristics are also highly variable from one patient to another. They may include the following:

- Extreme fatigue
- Visual dysfunction (e.g. diplopia, blurring of vision, nystagmus)
- Transient tingling sensations or numbness (paraesthesia) or loss of sensation
- Intention tremor
- Ataxia
- Muscular weakness in one or both arms and legs
- Paraparesis
- Bladder and bowel dysfunction
- Impairment of speech (scanning)
- Emotional lability: alternating periods of euphoria, depression and irritability
- Personality changes
- Cognitive dysfunction: loss of memory and confusion

Deficits which persist beyond 3 months are usually permanent. Weakness of the respiratory muscles and cough reflex may develop, predisposing the patient to pulmonary complications.

There is no cure for multiple sclerosis; the treatment is symptomatic and supportive and increases in amount and complexity as the patient's disease progresses. Corticosteroids are now used for severe relapses and a dose of 500 mg methylprednisolone daily for 5 days is the accepted regimen. There is no consensus on the role of any specific dietary measures. Physiotherapy is prescribed for most patients to promote activity and independence as long as possible.

Assessment

Assessment should focus on the current neurological problems being experienced by the patient, together with the degree of insight the patient has into the illness. Fears, anxieties and other feelings such as frustration should be gently explored together with the social and family circumstances of the patient.

PATIENT PROBLEMS

The following is a list of the more commonly found problems associated with multiple sclerosis; it should be remembered that many other individual problems are also possible.

1. Inadequate or inaccurate knowledge about the disorder, health maintenance and management of a remission.
2. Alteration in self-image and fear due to the potential change in life-style, disability and dependence.
3. Potential remissions; adjustments in activities to maintain health.
4. Impaired mobility secondary to muscular weakness, fatigue, ataxia and/or paralysis.
5. Potential for injury because of difficulty in walking.

6. Potential sensory deficits: abnormal vision and diminished cutaneous sensation may occur.
7. Alteration in pattern of elimination:
   (a) Urinary frequency, urgency or incontinence.
   (b) Constipation.
8. Alteration in nutritional status due to loss of appetite secondary to anxiety and depression, weakened mastication and swallowing muscles and/or inability to prepare meals.
9. Self-care deficits due to muscular weakness or paralysis, immobility and depression.
10. Impairment of verbal communication secondary to weakness or paralysis of the muscles involved in producing speech.
11. Potential for complications:
    (a) Impairment of skin integrity.
    (b) Respiratory insufficiency and infection.

GOALS

The patient's *goals* can be summarized as avoiding the complications listed in the above problems and as adapting life-style to the progressive deterioration in function that occurs. A key goal is to maintain maximum independence for as long as possible.

NURSING INTERVENTION

Good counselling and care may contribute to the prevention of relapses as well as help in keeping the patient active and independent for as long as possible. Hospital care usually becomes necessary during acute exacerbations or when complete dependence has been reached.

1. Inadequate knowledge.   The patient and family are informed about multiple sclerosis, the nature of the disease, effects, the fact that relapses of varying length occur and the potential precipitating factors in relapses. They are advised that it is not possible to predict the course of the disorder. Management is discussed in detail with emphasis on continuing former activities and gainful employment and the necessary modifications in life-style to avoid those factors known to contribute to a recurrence of symptoms. Important factors in the prevention of potential injuries and complications are outlined.

Community resources for assistance are made known to the patient and family. These include the Multiple Sclerosis Society, social services and community nurses. During relapses, or as the disorder progresses leaving residual disability, assistive devices (e.g. wheelchair), assistance with physical care and/or home management, financial assistance and support and encouragement may become necessary. The local branch of the Multiple Sclerosis Society is an excellent source of information and assistance. For example, it helps in securing assistive devices, transporting patients to the physiotherapy department or clinic and contacting other resources for assistance (e.g. Social Service Department) if necessary. The society also has voluntary workers who make home visits and arrange occupational and recreational programmes for multiple sclerosis patients. If the patient's former occupation is too strenuous or stressful, vocational retraining may be appropriate so that the person can return to gainful employment during remissions.

2. Alteration in self-image and fears. The changes in body function and capacity and increasing loss of independence alter the patient's image of self. Feelings of uncertainty may arise because the outcomes are unclear and planning may be difficult. Roles and relationships change, counselling around sexuality may be helpful, and responsibilities shift. Sensory and motor deficits which occur with multiple sclerosis frequently lead to impaired sexual functioning which may affect relationships. Fear of the long-term consequences of the disease, increasing dependency and the reactions of others are threatening. Both patient and family are likely to experience the stages of grief reaction as they come to grips with the realities of the situation. Nursing care involves acceptance of their reactions, supportive understanding and open discussion of concerns. Providing information about the illness, the symptoms and the potential therapy helps to decrease the uncertainty and promote realistic expectations. Anxiety and depression on the part of the patient and family may delay the process of acceptance of the diagnosis with the result that counselling may be helpful. The patient and family should be allowed to make decisions and be part of the planning for the future.

3. Maintenance of health. In early remissions when the residual effects are likely to be minimal, the patient is encouraged to resume their usual pattern of life, modifying it as necessary to avoid overfatigue, emotional stress and infections since these may precipitate a relapse. Regular and adequate rest, a well-balanced diet and learning to accept what cannot be readily changed to avoid emotional stress, reduce the risk of an exacerbation.

In the case of the female patient, menstruation and fertility are unaffected but she is advised of the increased risk of a relapse incurred by pregnancy. In addition, delivery may be complicated by spasms of the hip adductor muscles. Contraceptive pills may aggravate symptoms of multiple sclerosis.

4. Impaired mobility. Muscle spasticity and weakness, especially in the lower limbs, is a common disabling factor in multiple sclerosis. A carefully controlled physiotherapy programme is instituted within the patient's tolerance to keep the patient active and prevent muscle contractures and atrophy. Exercises in a warm pool reduce the spasticity. Close observation is made for signs of excessive fatigue and a rest period should follow the exercise period.

A walking stick or crutches may be necessary to assist the patient in maintaining mobility. Walking between parallel bars may be helpful. When walking becomes impossible, a wheelchair is provided and the patient is taught to transfer from the bed to chair and from chair to toilet unaided if there is sufficient strength in the arms.

Family members require instructions on how to transfer the patient from the wheelchair to the bed and vice versa if the patient is experiencing weakness or motor deficit in the upper limbs.

Spasticity may become a painful problem in the disabled limbs. Passive movements of the affected limbs may reduce the spasticity and prevent contractures.

5. Potential for injury. The patient is at risk of injury especially as walking becomes increasingly more difficult. In order to prevent falls, floors are kept clear of scatter rugs, stools, electric flexes and other articles over which the patient might trip. Hand-rails in appropriate places facilitate safer mobility. Shoes that provide firm support and have non-slip soles are worn.

6. Potential sensory deficits. Sensory deficits such as impaired vision and diminished temperature and pressure sensations increase the patient's potential for injury. If a portion of the visual field is affected, the patient learns to turn the head in order to bring objects into the range of vision. Diplopia may be relieved by the wearing of an eye patch on one eye and then periodically placing it on the other eye. The patient and family are taught safety measures to prevent burns; for example control of the temperature of food and beverages as well as bath water. Areas of diminished sensation are inspected daily for irritation and injury.

7. Alteration in pattern of elimination. Urinary frequency and urgency are common problems for the patient with multiple sclerosis. Later, as the disease progresses, loss of sphincter control and incontinence develops. The patient is advised to set up a regular schedule for going to the toilet to avoid the distress caused by urgency and dribbling or incontinence. If the patient's mobility is impaired, a prompt response to the patient's request for assistance is necessary.

Some patients experience urinary retention or may not completely empty their bladder when voiding. The use of catheterization is avoided if possible because of the risk of ascending urinary tract infection. If catheterization becomes necessary, strict asepsis is observed, a high fluid intake is encouraged (3000 ml daily) and regular assessment is made for infection (temperature, culture of urine).

Constipation is a frequent problem as a result of the reduced mobility and should be dealt with by standard methods (high-fibre diet, etc.).

8. Alteration in nutritional status. The patient's weight is recorded at regular intervals since the food intake is frequently reduced due to a poor appetite which develops due to the patient's anxiety, immobility, weakness in mastication and swallowing, or the patient's inability to shop and prepare meals.

Well-balanced meals that are easily digested are necessary; the food intake is monitored. High-calorie drinks may be necessary in order to meet the patient's requirements for energy and tissue maintenance. If the patient is overweight, a decreased caloric intake is prescribed to reduce the burden on weakened muscles.

9. Self-care deficits in hygiene. Nursing care includes repeated assessments of the patient's ability to complete self-care, which may become increasingly difficult as the disease progresses and the provision of the care needed increases. For example, muscular weakness or paralysis of the arms may prevent the patient from cleaning the teeth and combing the hair. Food particles and mucus may accumulate in the mouth if swallowing is difficult, necessitating mouth care after each meal.

10. Impairment of verbal communication. The speech may progressively become slower and more difficult as muscular weakness increases, creating frustration for both the patient and carers. Referral to a speech therapist may be helpful. Nursing care includes support and reinforcement of the therapy, talking with the patient, encouraging verbal responses and acknowledging even slight achievement without, however, being patronizing.

11. Potential for complications. As mobility and sensory perception deteriorate, the potential for skin breakdown increases; meticulous pressure care is therefore required.

Parkinson's Disease (Paralysis Agitans)

Parkinson's disease is a complex clinical syndrome associated with a decreased concentration of the chemical dopamine and its major metabolite. Dopamine is essential for normal neurotransmission and functioning of the basal ganglia. It is produced by the substantia nigra (black substance), a nucleus of highly pigmented cells in the midbrain which function as a part of the extrapyramidal system. Dopamine exerts an inhibitory effect on movements by opposing or lessening the stimulating effect of acetylcholine. When a deficiency of dopamine occurs, tremors, rigidity, slowness and limited voluntary movement become evident.

TYPES, AETIOLOGY AND INCIDENCE

The cause of the illness is usually unknown, although it may occasionally appear as a side-effect of some drugs (e.g. the phenothiazines).

Parkinson's disease affects one person out of 1000 in the United Kingdom, with 1 person in every 100 affected in the 60–70 year age group. Men and women are affected equally. There is no evidence of familial influence nor is the disorder more prevalent in any part of the world.

EFFECTS ON THE PATIENT

The disease produces increasing physical disability as it progresses. At first, tremor and muscular rigidity develop insidiously and disappear with voluntary movement and sleep, though becoming more pronounced with fatigue and stress. The tremor initially usually develops in the fingers and thumb producing the characteristic pill-rolling movement. The arms are adducted and semiflexed and the normal arm swing associated with walking is absent. Movements are slowed and a monotone becomes evident in the speech.

As the disease progresses the trunk and head are flexed forward, the patient may have difficulty in starting to walk and in turning and the gait is slow and shuffling. Rigidity of the facial muscles and unblinking eyes produces a mask-like inexpressive appearance.

With further deterioration the patient becomes more stooped and when walking there is a progressive acceleration of steps, producing what is known as a festination gait, making stopping difficult and predisposing to falls. There is difficulty in changing postion and the patient has difficulty with tasks involving finger movements.

Drooling occurs due to the decrease in automatic swallowing of saliva. Disturbances in autonomic innervation may develop; there may be excessive, or an absence of perspiration, and disordered temperature regulation. Excessive lacrimation, ptosis and/or pupillary constriction may develop. Gastrointestinal activity may be slowed, causing constipation.

Pain and fatigue are experienced due to the continuous increased traction of muscles on their attachments. Speech becomes weak, slurred and devoid of any inflections as the muscles concerned with articulation become more involved.

In the final stages the patient becomes disabled to a greater degree because of the inability to initiate voluntary movement. Speech becomes incoherent and difficulty in mastication and swallowing develops. The respiratory volumes are reduced and the ability to cough is diminished, predisposing to respiratory complications.

Up to now, the patient's intellectual functioning is unaffected, but at this later stage dementia may become evident in some patients.

ASSESSMENT

Assessment of the patient should focus on the degree of disability and any techniques the patient may use to help cope with such disability. The effects on family and the social circumstances should be investigated, together with the patient's feelings about the condition.

PATIENT PROBLEMS

1. Inadequate or inaccurate knowledge about the Parkinsonian syndrome, its characteristics, prescribed treatment and management.
2. Muscular dysfunction due to impairment of extrapyramidal control: tremor, rigidity, slowness and lack of co-ordination.
3. Potential for injury due to muscular dysfunction.
4. Altered body image and loss of self-esteem secondary to incapacity, change in role, appearance and dependency.
5. Nutritional deficit due to difficulty in eating, mastication and swallowing, anorexia and nausea caused by the prescribed medication.

6. Impairment in communication. Speech difficulty secondary to the rigidity of the muscles involved in speech and reduced pulmonary volumes.
7. Potential for complications:
   (a) Respiratory complications due to respiratory muscle dysfunction, causing reduced pulmonary volumes and the inability to cough to remove secretions.
   (b) Break in skin due to immobility and falls.
   (c) Impairment of eye function due to diplopia or due to drying and injury of the cornea caused by a reduction in blinking and moistening of the surface of the eye.
   (d) Medication reaction (see side-effects, above); medication withdrawal.

The *goals* are that the patient and family will accept and adjust to the situation and the patient will maintain independence, accustomed role and a relatively normal life-style for as long as the condition permits.

NURSING INTERVENTION

The patient with Parkinson's disease is managed at home on a drug programme until the advanced stage of the disorder causes marked disability and dependency. The clinic or community nurse assumes the major role in assessing the patient's needs and providing the necessary counselling and guidance for the patient and family at the onset and through successive months and years. It is important that the nurse recognizes the emotional, physical and socioeconomic problems incurred by the disease. The fact that the *patient's intellect is unimpaired* must be kept in mind as well as a tendency to become very self-conscious, depressed and withdrawn because of the appearance and limitations enforced on the patient by the disease.

The patient is advised to contact the national Parkinson's Disease Society. Socialization in structured groups of persons with similar problems is helpful.

Difficulty in movement requires care to be taken to avoid hazards which may cause falls and also emphasizes the need for teaching about pressure care. Encouragement with a physiotherapy programme is essential to promote inability for as long as possible.

Loss of normal smooth, co-ordinated mobility, change in appearance, loss of the capacity for gainful employment and self-care and loss of accustomed social interaction result in the patient's altered self-image, loss of self-esteem and depression. The patient is encouraged to express his feelings, to take an active role in setting realistic goals and planning management. The patient may develop an acute sense of humiliation leading to withdrawal and isolation.

The patient's strengths and potential capacity should be emphasized and independence encouraged in order that socialization and group activities may be promoted. Every effort should be made to try and encourage the patient's self-esteem.

The expertise of other professionals may be required to provide counselling, motivation, guidance and support. Involvement in the local branch of the Parkinson's Disease Society may promote acceptance and adjustment.

The quality and quantity of food taken by the patient and body weight are followed closely. Only a small amount of food may be taken because of fatigue and depression. The patient should be encouraged to be as independent as possible in feeding. The patient may be less self-conscious and eat more if privacy is ensured and ample time is allocated for each meal. Sensitive provision of protection for clothing at meal times is essential to preserve the patient's fragile self-esteem.

Constipation is a common occurrence because of the decreased activity, decreased food (bulk) intake and decreased fluid in the gastrointestinal tract due to an inadequate intake and the loss of saliva (drooling). The drug therapy may also contribute to the problem.

The fluid, roughage and bulk intake are increased. A stool softener or bulk-producing laxative (e.g. bisacodyl) may be necessary to prevent faecal impaction. The patient is encouraged to establish a regular time for defecation and a raised toilet seat will make it easier.

Urinary dribbling and incontinence may occur; the cause may be the inability of the patient to reach the toilet soon enough. A regular toileting schedule is arranged and the patient prompted and assisted if necessary. A commode or urinal is kept readily available for use at night.

The patient experiences the discomfort of continually contracted muscles and readily becomes fatigued. Physiotherapy, avoidance of prolonged periods in one position and planned rest periods contribute to comfort.

As a result of disturbed autonomic nervous system control, excessive perspiration may occur. Daily bathing and frequent change of clothing may be needed to promote comfort and control body odour.

The rigidity of the muscles involved in speech and the reduced pulmonary volumes which may develop interfere with the patient's enunciation and volume of speech. Deep breathing with slow exhalation, singing and speech classes in groups help to improve speech. Facial exercises such as smiling, blowing out, grimacing, eye movements and neck extension performed before a mirror may lessen facial rigidity.

The patient may experience prolonged exposure and drying of the surface of the eye due to a reduction in the normal frequency of blinking. This may lead to corneal irritation. The instillation of artificial tears may be prescribed and the patient and/or a family member is taught how to instil the solution. Diplopia may become a problem. A patch on one eye may help.

The patient is observed for any reaction to prescribed medication. Carbidopa (Sinemet) is commonly given to promote the entrance of levodopa, the precursor of dopamine, into the brain. Long-term side-effects include memory loss, mood swings and behaviour change. Anticholinergic drugs such as benzhexol (Artane) may be used to try and reduce muscle tone, but they too have side-effects such as blurring of vision, retention of urine and palpitations. An assessment is made for positive responses as well as for undesirable side-effects. For example: Is the tremor less? Has the patient's gait improved? If side-effects develop, the doctor is notified; an adjustment in dosage may be necessary or another drug prescribed.

Sudden withdrawal of an antiparkinsonian drug or

severe emotional disturbance may precipitate a reaction referred to as a parkinsonian crisis. It is characterized by a marked aggravation of tremors, rigidity and akinesia. Tachycardia, increased respirations, acute anxiety and diaphoresis also occur.

The reaction is a medical emergency requiring prompt treatment. Treatment includes respiratory and cardiac support, the administration of an antiparkinsonian preparation and the parenteral administration of a sedative such as phenobarbitone may be necessary.

Huntington's Chorea (Corticostriatonigral Degeneration)

First described by George Huntington, a New York physician, in 1872 as an inherited condition of chorea and dementia in a group of families on Long Island. Early in the seventeenth century many Englishmen migrated to America for religious and political reasons. Three men from the Suffolk village of Bures landed in Boston in 1630. Three hundred years later a researcher was able to trace the transmission of many cases of Huntington's chorea, via 1000 affected descendants, back to these men.

INHERITANCE

The patient is transmitted by a dominant gene which, when present, will always produce Huntington's chorea. As the gene is carried on an autosome it is an autosomal dominant disease. Both sexes are equally affected and each child of an affected parent has a 50% chance of developing the disease in later life.

PATHOLOGY

It has been shown biochemically that GABA, an inhibitory neurotransmitter, is greatly reduced in the substantia nigra, with a resultant fall in the activity of the enzyme, glutamic acid decarboxylase (GAD). It therefore appears that there is death of the nerve cells producing GABA. Experiments suggest that GABA pathways exist between the basal ganglia and the substantia nigra.

About 7 people per 100 000 population in the UK suffer from the disease, making a total of about 5000. It occurs in all racial groups. For every affected individual there are about two more who carry the abnormal gene and will later develop the disease.

Huntington's chorea appearing before the age of 20 years is passed from the father in 80% of cases; in cases of very late onset the abnormal gene is more commonly transmitted by the mother. The nature, course and prognosis of the disease should be very carefully explained to the family and they should be offered genetic counselling and encouraged to join the Association to Combat Huntington's Chorea.

Motor Neurone Disease (Amyotrophic Lateral Sclerosis)

This is a progressive chronic disease in which there is a degeneration of motor neurones in the spine (anterior horn cells), brain stem and/or cortical motor areas.

The cause of motor neurone disease is unknown. The onset of the disorder occurs most often between the ages of 40 and 60 years. The muscles innervated by the affected neurones lose their ability to contract, and atrophy.

EFFECTS ON THE PATIENT

The first symptom is usually weakness of the hands and arms; finer movements are lost and articles are dropped. Twitching and hyperreflexia develop along with the spasticity and weakness of the lower limbs. As the disorder progresses, speech, swallowing and respiration are impaired as motor neurones at higher levels are involved. The diagnosis is made on the patient's symptoms and their progressive nature. Electromyographic studies are done to confirm the loss of innervation to the muscles. The course is usually progressively retrograde; rarely is there a remission.

TREATMENT AND NURSING CARE

There is no specific treatment for motor neurone disease. When the disease is diagnosed, the patient and family are advised by the doctor of the expected progression and fatal outcome of the disorder. They require support, opportunities to express their feelings and ask questions, explanations and assistance in planning home management. The nurse can advise them to contact the Motor Neurone Disease Society. The patient is encouraged to remain active within the potential muscular ability and every effort should be made to encourage independence despite increasing disability. It should be kept in mind that in motor neurone disease, the cognitive ability remains unaffected. Obviously home management must be individualized because of the variability of symptoms and stages of the disease in patients. Progression of the disease and increasing dependency eventually necessitates the use of a wheelchair.

The speech therapist has a vital role to play in the management of swallowing and speech. He or she should be introduced to the patient early on in the illness and will monitor progression and introduce communication aids at the appropriate stages.

Dysarthria and dysphagia are very distressing features in the later stages of the illness. The patient may become very embarrassed by the speech and the constant drooling of secretions. Privacy at meal times is very important, with the patient given small meals and nourishing drinks frequently. A portable tracheal suction machine can be supplied for home use and it is important that the patient and family are taught the correct way to use it. It may become necessary in the later stages to feed the patient via a nasogastric tube, or a gastrotomy tube may be inserted under X-ray control.

These are very distressing procedures to both patient and family and much time must be taken with them to explain and teach them how to use the tubes.

Myasthenia Gravis

Myasthenia gravis is not a degenerative condition but is included here because of its chronic, progressive nature. It is a neuromuscular disorder characterized by weakness and easy fatigability of voluntary muscles due to interference with impulse conduction at the neuromuscular junction.

The *cause* is unknown. It has been suggested that there is a deficiency of either acetylcholine or the enzyme cholinesterase. In addition, a deficiency in the number of acetylcholine-sensitive receptors in the motor end-plate has been identified. There is some evidence that autoimmune and genetic factors are implicated in the disease. Abnormalities of the thymus gland and increased antibodies that react against muscle tissue elements have been identified in some patients with myasthenia gravis.

INCIDENCE

It is not a common disorder. The incidence is highest between 20 and 30 years of age, and women are affected more frequently than men at this age. In later years, men and women are equally affected.

EFFECTS ON THE PATIENT

The onset of myasthenia gravis may be insidious with the symptoms of fatigue and weakness being associated with muscular activity. Initially, only the extrinsic ocular and levator palpebrae muscles may be involved resulting in ptosis of the eyelids and diplopia. This may be referred to as ocular myasthenia. More generalized muscle involvement (generalized myasthenia) with progression of the disease produces the following manifestations: an expressionless appearance due to weakness of facial muscles; difficulty with mastication and swallowing; nasal voice tone that loses volume as the patient talks; limb weakness, which becomes evident with the patient experiencing difficulty with self-care management (e.g. bathing, brushing the teeth, combing the hair); respiratory difficulty; and loss of control of bladder and rectal sphincters.

Muscle weakness is most noticeable at the end of the day and following exercise. Some recovery of strength is evident upon rising in the morning or following a period of rest. Mild atrophy may occur in the affected muscles and some aching may be present. Usually, sensation is unchanged.

There is great variability in the course of the disease; spontaneous remissions may occur. Factors which may aggravate symptoms include infection, temperature extreme, exposure to sunlight, emotional stress and physical exertion. Weakness of the diaphragm and intercostal muscles is serious; respiratory insufficiency and complications may be fatal.

MEDICAL MANAGEMENT

There is no known cure for myasthenia gravis. Treatment includes the administration of drugs, plasmaphaeresis and surgery. The drug most commonly used is a cholinesterase antagonist preparation such as neostigmine (Prostigmin) or pyridostigmine (Mestinon). Response to such a drug is used as a diagnostic test during medical investigations for myasthenia gravis. The patient is usually hospitalized and observed for reactions to the drug. If the patient does not respond to the anticholinesterase, the corticosteroid prednisone may be given for its antibody suppressant effect, on the basis that the disorder is an abnormal immune response.

Surgical therapy involves thymectomy (the removal of the thymus gland). Hyperplasia occurs in many of the patients, or a thymic tumour may be present, and removal of the gland results in a marked improvement in some and complete remission in others. Surgery is used mainly in younger patients in the early stages of the disease.

PROBLEMS AND GOALS

The patient faces lengthy periods of remission and progressively deteriorating exacerbations of the illness. The familiar problems of progressive disability have to be faced (see preceding sections), with most of the patient's care taking place in the community.

NURSING INTERVENTION

Most patients with myasthenia gravis are managed in the home. Hospitalization may be necessary for evaluation, establishing the required medication dosage, exacerbation of symptoms, respiratory failure or myasthenic crisis. Nursing management is primarily concerned with maintenance of muscle strength and the prevention of complications especially the potentially fatal respiratory failure and muscle atrophy.

The reader is referred to preceding pages in this chapter for a discussion of the general care required.

A major potential problem unique to myasthenia gravis which may occur involves a crisis reaction to drugs. The patient who requires high doses of an anticholinesterase drug is at risk of developing a *cholinergic crisis*. This is a life-threatening reaction resulting from overmedication necessitating prompt emergency treatment. A dramatic increase in myasthenic symptoms occurs in about one hour, the patient experiences extreme weakness, blurred vision, nausea, vomiting, intestinal cramping, diarrhoea, increased salivation and bronchial secretions, respiratory insufficiency, bradycardia, constricted pupils and increased perspiration.

Treatment involves withholding the anticholinesterase. Endotracheal intubation, mechanical respiratory assistance and frequent suction are necessary to prevent severe respiratory failure, hypoxia and death. Atropine sulphate may be prescribed to lessen the secretions. Following the cholinergic crisis, regular dosage of the anticholinesterase is decreased.

A crisis may also develop due to *undermedication*

which is referred to as *myasthenic crisis*. The symptoms are similar to those that occur in a cholinergic crisis but develop three or more hours after taking the anticholinesterase drug. An anticholinesterase preparation is given as well as supportive treatment as indicated (e.g. respiratory assistance). Regular dosage of the anticholinesterase is increased.

In order to determine whether the crisis is cholinergic or myasthenic, edrophonium chloride may be administered, intravenously by the doctor. If the crisis is myasthenic the patient's muscle weakness is reversed and regular. If the muscle weakness is increased, cholinergic crisis is indicated and anticholinesterase drug preparations are withheld and atropine sulphate may be prescribed as an antidote for anticholinesterase.

THE PERSON WITH A PAROXYSMAL DISORDER

Epilepsy (Seizures)

A seizure is the manifestation of abnormal, rapid and uncontrolled neuronal electrical discharges within the brain. It is characterized by sensory, motor, and autonomic disturbances and changes in level of consciousness. The term *epilepsy* refers to a chronic disorder characterized by recurring seizures of unknown cause. In the normal brain, a certain stability exists between excitation and inhibition. When a seizure occurs, the ability to suppress abnormal neural activity may be impaired or lost, or there may be increased excitation within the neurones. The abnormal activity may occur in a small group of neurones and remain relatively localized or may spread to involve extensive areas of neurones. In some seizures, no focal origin of abnormal electrical discharges can be identified; large areas of the brain appear to be involved simultaneously.

INCIDENCE AND CAUSE

The disorder characterized by recurring seizures and commonly referred to as epilepsy represents one of the most common neurological problems affecting individuals irrespective of geographical location, sex and race. About one person in 20 has a seizure of some type during life, and in the population at large about one in 200 has epilepsy (recurrent seizures). Most of those who develop idiopathic epilepsy do so before the age of 20 years.

Epilepsy may be *idiopathic* (without known cause) or *symptomatic*. The latter type of seizures are secondary and may be caused by almost any intracranial pathological condition and by many general systemic disorders. Symptomatic seizures may occur with increased intracranial pressure or brain damage associated with a head injury, cerebral oedema, or an intracranial space-occupying lesion, haemorrhage or infection. They may be a sequel to brain injury or infection that has resulted in brain damage and scar tissue formation. General systemic conditions in which seizures most commonly occur include hypoglycaemia, hypocalcaemia (tetany), renal insufficiency (uraemia), hypoxia, high fever (especially in children), toxaemia of pregnancy and chemical poisoning (e.g. alcohol, strychnine, amphetamine, lead, some insecticides).

There is no known specific cause of primary (idiopathic) epilepsy but an inherited predisposition to hypersensitivity and dysrhythmia of the neurones is considered to play a role.

EFFECTS ON THE PATIENT

The type of seizure that a nurse is most likely to encounter is known as a *generalized* seizure. Other types may be localized to one part of the brain, only producing their effect in one localized area of the body (*Jacksonian* seizure).

During a generalized fit abnormal neuronal discharges spread throughout the brain, producing grand mal (major) or absence (petit mal) seizures.

Absence (petit mal) seizures are characterized by sudden cessation of activity with a momentary absence of consciousness (5–30 seconds). The person stares blankly into space and the eyes usually roll upward. Objects being held may be dropped. Occasionally a few involuntary movements and falling may occur. More often, the episodes are unnoticed and the person resumes activity, unaware that there has been an interruption.

Absence seizures may occur as often as a hundred times in a day. Attention and learning are affected with frequent occurrence. They usually have their onset in infancy or early childhood and either cease during adolescence or develop into grand mal seizures.

Grand mal seizures are now referred to as major motor or tonic–clonic seizures. The seizure may develop with or without warning to the patient. Some patients experience irritability, tension or headache for a period before the episode. A brief sensory or perceptual aberration, referred to as an aura, may immediately precede the impending seizure. The aura may be auditory, visual, gustatory, olfactory or numbness or tingling in an area of the body. The aura is related to the focus of origin of the seizure and is specific for each patient.

The seizure begins with sudden loss of consciousness and the tonic phase of the seizure. The person falls to the floor; the tonic spasm of the muscles causes rigidity and distortion of the body. An involuntary cry is heard. The latter is caused by the sudden contraction of the thoracic and abdominal muscles forcing air through the spastic glottis. Respirations are arrested temporarily and cyanosis may develop. The jaws are fixed, hands clenched, the eyes opened widely and the pupils dilated. The initial tonic phase may last up to 60 seconds and is followed by a clonic phase of irregular jerky movements. Breathing is re-established and is stertorous, blowing out frothy saliva which cannot be swallowed due to spasms. There may be some bleeding caused by biting of the tongue, lips and oral mucosa. Urinary incontinence is common and rarely, faecal incontinence occurs.

The clonic movements gradually subside and consciousness is regained soon after. The patient may be confused, dazed or respond normally, falling into a deep sleep for several hours and awakening with no memory of the seizure. During the postseizure (postictal) period, the patient may be disorientated or may complain of headache, fatigue and muscular soreness. (*Ictus* means seizure or sudden attack.) In rare cases, the patient may become aggressive or violent.

Status epilepticus is a serious form of epilepsy in which seizures occur in such rapid succession that recovery of consciousness between the episodes does not occur. Hyperpyrexia develops, coma deepens and permanent brain damage occurs due to anoxia. Complete exhaustion and death occur, if the patient is not treated.

The most common cause of status epilepticus is considered to be abrupt discontinuation of an anticonvulsant drug. Untreated or inadequately treated seizures may also lead to this emergency condition.

In status epilepticus, the seizures must be controlled by firstly the use of intravenous diazepam. If this and other anticonvulsant drugs fail the patient is given muscle relaxants, intubated and ventilated.

ASSESSMENT

A grand mal seizure is a sudden emergency that will be over very quickly. It is important that the nurse can give a clear account of the fit to medical personnel when required, so close observation is essential.

PATIENT PROBLEMS

1. Potential for injury due to the loss of consciousness and uncontrolled strong muscular contractures.
2. Lack of knowledge about the disorder, the treatment and necessary modications in life-style which may be necessary.
3. Alteration in self-image due to anxiety, and the stigma which a segment of society attaches to epilepsy.

GOALS

The goals are that the patient will suffer no harm as a result of the seizure and also be aware of the needs for long-term self-care in avoiding further fits.

NURSING INTERVENTION

1. Potential for injury. When a patient has a seizure, the most important function is to protect the patient from injury. When a patient is known to be subject to seizures or is suspect because of the condition, precautions include: having the patient near the nursing station, or where he can be readily observed; keeping the bed low; taking the temperature by axilla; having padded sides in place on the bed; and staying with the patient during a bath or shower.

During a seizure, the nurse stays with the patient; safety and the observations and recording of events are paramount. A seizure cannot be stopped once it has begun; it is self-limiting and no immediate treatment will shorten it. If the patient is in bed, the pillow is removed and the top bedding turned down so that the patient's responses can be observed. If the patient is up, and has not already fallen, he or she is eased to a semiprone position and a folded blanket or towel placed under the head to prevent injury during the clonic phase. Restrictive clothing at the neck is loosened and the immediate area cleared of anything that might contribute to injury (e.g. furniture, electric fan, lamp). No attempt is made to insert anything between the teeth as the teeth are clenched and there would be a risk of pushing the tongue into the oropharynx, obstructing the airway. In addition, injury to the teeth and soft tissue may occur; aspiration of blood or a broken tooth may become a possibility. As soon as the clonic phase begins to subside, the patient is turned on the side to promote drainage of secretions and prevent aspiration. Suction may be necessary. The patient is protected as much as possible from exposure to others.

During the seizure, the following *observations* are made:

- The mode of onset; did the patient indicate an aura? Was there a cry? Is there deviation of the head and eyes—if so, to what side? In what part of the body did the initial phase start?
- Are the seizure movements localized or generalized? If generalized, are they symmetrical or asymmetrical?
- Is the patient cyanosed?
- Are the teeth clenched and is there frothing at the mouth?
- Is there incontinence of urine or faeces?
- How long did the seizure last?

Following the seizure the patient will be drowsy and disorientated for some time; close observation is therefore essential for the patient's safety. When the patient wakens, reorientation may be necessary as well as an explanation of the event.

In the interest of safety and the prevention of injury for self and others, the person with epilepsy may not be allowed to drive a motor vehicle, operate certain machines or work at heights or where there is loud noise or flashing lights. The doctor may also advise the patient against swimming, climbing, riding, cycling and participation in contact sports. Decisions regarding activities are based on the type, frequency and severity of seizures and the patient's response to the prescribed drug.

Family members are taught what to do when a seizure occurs so that they can respond effectively.

2. Knowledge deficit. Information about the prescribed anticonvulsant drug is provided. The client and family shouild be alerted to the potential side-effects and are advised to get in touch with the doctor if they occur (Table 21.10). They should know that if the drug is not tolerated that there are others that will be prescribed until optimal control of fits with minimal side-effects is achieved. It is emphasized that the drugs must be taken at the prescribed frequency even though there are no seizures; effective blood levels of the drug must be maintained by compliance with the prescribed dosage

Table 21.10 Anticonvulsant drugs.

Drug	Side-effects and comments
Phenytoin (Epanutin)	Nausea, ataxia, diplopia or nystagmus, slurring of speech, gingival hyperplasia, rash and hirsutism. Drug should be taken with meals. Good oral hygiene, gum massage and regular dental supervision are necessary
Carbamazepine (Tegretol)	Bone marrow depression, nausea, vomiting, headache, urinary retention, oedema, rash and drowsiness. Blood cell counts and haematocrit should be done at least monthly
Phenobarbitone (Luminal)	Incapacitating drowsiness, rashes
Primidone (Mysoline)	Depression, irritability, dizziness, ataxia and, rarely, impotence. If used with symptomatic seizures, dosage decreased gradually before withdrawal
Ethusuximide (Zarontin)	Gastrointestinal irritation, drowsiness and headache. Should be taken at meal-time with a large amount of fluid. Primarily for use in petit mal epilepsy
Sodium Valproate (Epilim)	Gastrointestinal irritation, bleeding tendency and liver dysfunction. Drug should be taken with meals. Frequent blood cell counts and bleeding times should be performed

and frequency and alcohol should not be consumed. Drug doses must not be altered except with the doctor's approval; the drug is prescribed on an individual basis according to the type, severity and frequency of the seizures and the individual's response. The patient is cautioned against the taking of any non-prescription drug.

The importance of regular visits to the doctor is emphasized. Blood serum levels of the anticonvulsant drug are determined and dosage adjustment made it indicated. Since a blood dyscrasia is a potential side-effect of many of the drugs used, blood cell counts, haematocrit and bleeding time are evaluated regularly.

The patient and family are requested to keep a record of seizures which includes antecedent events or any known or suspected precipitating factor(s). Information about the British Epilepsy Association may be very useful. The mutual support offered to the patient and family by groups such as this can be invaluable. A Medic Alert identification bracelet or pendant should be worn so that appropriate care can be given during a fit or an emergency. The patient should always carry the names, addresses and telephone numbers of persons to be contacted.

3. Alteration in self-image. Patients express anxiety and embarrassment and see themselves as being different and inferior, having to adjust to potentially disruptive seizures and dependency on medication. Acceptance of the diagnosis is difficult for the patient who may respond with denial, anger, resentment and despair before acceptance and adaptation. Fears and anxieties which are unexpressed and unrelieved may result in ineffective coping. A thorough evaluation of the patient's attitude toward epilepsy and expectations concerning health maintenance is essential. The at-

titudes and expectations of family members should also be evaluated since their understanding and support is crucial to the patient's ability to adjust to his condition.

Epilepsy is not yet clearly understood and there is no known cure. Because of this, and the historical context, fear of the disorder is widespread. At one time the disorder was thought to be caused by the possession of a person by devils, and even today, myths, misunderstandings and social stigma still exist. As a result, the patient may fear rejection by peers and employers and refuse to disclose the health problem even though it would be wiser to do so. Concerns about the person's intellectual abilities psychological stability and ability to perform efficiently on the job have been expressed by educators and employers. It is important for the nurse to be aware of potential prejudices which may be encountered by the patient and his family. The fact that mental capacity and abilities are as varied among people with epilepsy as in any cross-section of society and that epilepsy is not synonymous with mental handicap or psychosis requires emphasis.

Some controversy exists concerning genetic predisposition to epilepsy. It is considered by some authorities to be greatest when epilepsy develops early in childhood and when both parents suffer epilepsy. Genetic counselling may therefore be advisable for a person with epilepsy who is contemplating having children.

THE PERSON WITH AN INFECTION OF THE NERVOUS SYSTEM

There are a range of infective conditions which may affect the nervous system, for example encephalitis (infection of the brain), cerebral abscess, poliomyelitis and rabies. Fortunately these conditions are very rare, as also is tetanus which is a condition in which the nervous system is attacked by the exotoxins of the *Clostridium tetani* organism. Tetanus may be fatal due to effects of the exotoxin on the nerves controlling respiration, hence the importance of tetanus prophylaxis.

Meningitis

Meningitis is an acute inflammation of the pia and arachnoid meningeal membranes (leptomeninges) of the brain or spinal cord. The cause is usually bacterial or a virus. Almost any bacteria can cause meningitis but the most common are the meningococcus, the pneumococcus and *Haemophilus influenzae*. Meningitis is frequently secondary to infection of the sinuses, ears or respiratory tract. A less common form is tuberculosis meningitis.

EFFECTS ON THE PATIENT

The onset of meningitis tends to be insidious when caused by a virus. The bacterial type is more sudden and acute, manifested by headache, irritability, nausea, vomiting, back pain, chills and fever and symptoms of meningeal irritation. Photophobia is a common complaint. The classic signs of meningeal irritation include neck rigidity (stiffness of the neck and severe pain with forceful flexion), positive Kernig's sign (inability to straighten the knee when the hip is flexed), and positive Brudzinski's sign (hip and knee flexion in response to forward flexion of the neck). Signs of increased intracranial pressure such as blood pressure elevation, pupillary changes, changes in respiratory patterns, seizures, bradycardia, confusion, drowsiness and coma may develop. Focal neurological signs rarely occur.

The medical diagnosis of meningitis is made on the basis of clinical signs and symptoms and is confirmed by isolating the organism from the CSF. The CSF is under increased pressure, is cloudy or purulent, and has an increased leucocyte count, a high protein content and a reduced concentration of glucose. Blood, nose and throat cultures are done to assist in identifying the organism and X-rays may be done of the chest, skull and sinuses to detect areas of inflammation.

Meningitis requires emergency treatment, since delay may result in cerebral damage and disability or death. It includes elimination of the source of infection, massive doses of an appropriate antibiotic and an anticonvulsant drug if seizures occur. The antibiotic may be administered intrathecally as well as parenterally. There is no specific treatment for viral meningitis.

ASSESSMENT

A full assessment of the patient along the lines discussed earlier in the chapter is essential, paying particular attention to the level of consciousness and other neurological parameters.

PATIENT PROBLEMS

A wide range of problems associated with immobility, a severe infection and a diminished level of consciousness may be encountered by the patient. They are summarized below; other individual problems may also coexist.

1. Alteration in comfort due to the headache, back pain and fever.
2. Potential for increased intracranial pressure secondary to the intracranial inflammatory process.
3. Fluid and nutritional deficit due to nausea, vomiting, headache, fever, confusion and decreased awareness.
4. Potential for injury due to seizures, disorientation or coma.
5. Potential spread of infection to others, particularly if the causative organism is meningococcus.
6. Self-care deficits secondary to discomfort, reduced awareness, weakness or coma.
7. Inadequate knowledge about management of the convalescent period and residual disabilities.

GOALS

Patient goals will be the avoidance of complications and potential problems as outlined above while making a full recovery without any long term deficits.

NURSING INTERVENTION

Much of the care required has already been discussed in this chapter; the following special points should however be noted.

A major problem of the patient with meningitis is *discomfort* due to headache, back pain, fever, photophobia and anxiety. Nursing care includes provision of emotional support, reassurance that help is available and an explanation of all nursing activities. Irritability due to increased reaction to sensory stimuli is minimized by maintaining a cool, quiet, darkened environment, by approaching the patient gently with a soft, calm voice and by keeping communication simple and direct.

The possible spread of the patient's infection to others must be considered. The hospital infection control department is consulted; it may be necessary to use isolation procedures.

Following meningitis the patient is usually debilitated and readily fatigued and may have some residual neurological deficits. Several weeks or months may be needed for the patient's convalescence and rehabilitation. The family and patient should be forewarned of this and given support and encouragement throughout this difficult period. Following the initial acute phase, a highly nutritious diet is encouraged and a regimen of range-of-movement exercises is established to prevent weakness, contractures and joint ankylosis, and to promote circulation.

Minor disabilities may reverse with time while others may be residual and require detailed evaluation and an intensive rehabilitation programme. The nurse plays a role in supporting the patient and interpreting the rehabilitation programme to the family and in assisting them in making plans for adjustments and home management.

THE PERSON WITH PERIPHERAL NERVE DISORDER

Disorders of the cranial nerves may be secondary to other diseases but a few are primary to specific nerves. The more common of these are trigeminal neuralgia and Bell's palsy. Peripheral nerve dysfunction may be incurred by direct local trauma (pressure, severance, infection and inflammation) or may be secondary to a variety of general conditions such as malnutrition, alcoholism and chemical poisoning.

Trigeminal Neuralgia (Tic Douloureux)

Trigeminal neuralgia is a very painful disorder of the sensory fibres of the trigeminal (fifth cranial) nerve. It is characterized by recurring episodes of excruciating pain along the distribution of one or more divisions of the nerve. The attack is brief, lasting from seconds to 2 or 3 minutes. The episodes recur frequently, day or night for several weeks at a time. The onset of an episode may occur spontaneously or may coincide with touching or movement of the face or exposure to cold or a draught. The patient may relate the precipitation of pain to eating, talking, cleaning the teeth, or washing or shaving the face. The recurring incapacitating pain has been known to cause severe depression and even suicide. The cause of the neuralgia is unknown.

The patient may be treated by medication or surgery. There is no specific drug for the disorder. Anticonvulsant agents such as phenytoin (Epanutin) or carbamazepine (Tegretol) may suppress or shorten the painful episodes. These drugs may produce side-effects (Table 21.10). An analgesic may be prescribed; if a narcotic is used, there is the risk of addiction. Drug therapy may provide relief at first but, usually, gradually loses its effectiveness.

Injection of alcohol into the affected nerve branch may be performed to interrupt the sensory impulses and usually provides relief for several months. During this period of effectiveness, the patient has loss of sensation in the areas of distribution of the injected nerve branch.

A popular surgical measure is percutaneous radiofrequency thermocoagulation. This procedure, with the patient conscious, permits destruction of the pain sensory fibres by use of an electrode and leaves the neurones and fibres concerned with other areas and the corneal reflex intact.

Bell's Palsy (Peripheral Facial Paralysis)

Bell's palsy is a disorder of the motor component of one of the facial (seventh cranial) nerves and is characterized by loss of the ability to move the muscles on one side of the face.

The condition is most common in persons between 20 and 40 years of age. The patient may experience pain behind the ear or in the face for a day or two prior to the onset of paralysis. When paralysis occurs, a drawing sensation on the affected side is experienced. There is flaccidity, drooping of the mouth, drooling, flattening of the nasolabial fold, widening of the palpebral fissure and inability to completely close the eye on the affected side. There may be watering of the eye. The individual is unable to smile, whistle or grimace. The taste sensation is lost over the anterior two-thirds of the tongue on the respective side. Herpes lesions may appear on or in the corresponding ear. In 80% of the victims, muscle tone begins to return in a few weeks and movement is usually restored over a period of months.

Treatment is usually provided on an outpatient basis. It may include analgesics for discomfort due to herpes, or application of acyclovir (Zovirax) cream, a corticosteroid preparation to relieve oedema and inflammation, application of moist heat and gentle facial massage and electrical stimulation of the facial nerve to maintain muscle tone.

Polyneuritis (Multiple Peripheral Neuritis)

Although the term neuritis implies inflammation, it is more often applied to any neuropathy where there is dysfunction and pain of peripheral nerves from any cause. Polyneuritis is a disorder in which there is pain and impaired function along the distribution of many peripheral nerves. It is usually symmetrical and both motor and sensory disturbances occur.

EFFECTS ON THE PATIENT

The symptoms generally start in the parts innervated by the distal portions of the nerves and spread proximally. The patient first experiences pain, pins and needles, tingling and weakness in hands and feet ('glove and stocking' effect) then, a progressive loss of sensation, diminished tendon reflexes and inability to perform finer movements. The areas are tender and sore when subjected to even light pressure.

The causes include toxicity, nutritional deficiencies (especially vitamin B complex), metabolic disorder and cell-mediated immunological response. In some instances the cause is not identified.

Some of the more common polyneuropathies are diabetic polyneuritis, vitamin deficiency polyneuritis associated with alcoholism, arsenic or lead polyneuritis, malnutrition polyneuritis and acute idiopathic polyneuritis (Guillain–Barré syndrome).

Guillain–Barré Syndrome (Acute Infective Polyneuropathy)

The Guillain–Barré syndrome is an inflammatory disease of the spinal nerve roots within the dural sheath, peripheral nerves and may also involve the cranial nerves. The loss of nerve impulse conduction that occurs is due to compression, demyelination and nerve degeneration as a result of the inflammation and oedema.

INCIDENCE AND AETIOLOGY

It may occur at any age but the incidence is greater in persons 30–40 years of age. Men and women are equally affected. The cause of the disorder is unknown but viral infection and immunological reaction are both suspect. Frequently, the patients give a history of having 'just had' an upper respiratory infection or a gastrointestinal disturbance.

EFFECTS ON THE PATIENT

The onset of Guillain–Barré syndrome is usually abrupt. Bilateral muscle weakness, beginning in the legs, may ascend to involve the trunk, arms and cranial nerves. Paraesthesia may precede the weakness. Within a few days, the weakness is followed by flaccid motor paralysis with weakness of the respiratory muscles. If the cranial nerves become involved, inability to swallow, talk, or even close the eyes develop. Muscle tenderness or sensitivity of the nerves to pressure may be experienced. Autonomic changes include sinus tachycardia and hypertension in the acute phase followed by hypotension.

Guillain–Barré syndrome is life-threatening due to potential respiratory and vasomotor failure if mechanical ventilation and vasopressor drugs are not promptly available. The mortality rate is estimated at 10–20%; death may result from a superimposed infection. Complete spontaneous recovery within weeks or months in usually anticipated in the survivors.

In some instances steroids may be used to counteract the inflammation. Treatment is mainly supportive and intensive nursing care along the lines discussed in this chapter is needed to help the patient survive the acute episode.

SUMMARY

The critical importance to human functioning of the nervous system cannot be over-emphasized and the features unique to this system must be borne in mind at all times. Health problems may affect a person at any age and be potentially devastating in impact leaving major long term deficits. The nurse's role in health education is a key one in preventing head injuries for example, while the nurse as teacher features prominently in the rehabilitation of patients after brain trauma or cerebrovascular accident. The nursing care of patients whose central nervous system has been impaired by trauma or disease is a challenging and long term commitment in many cases, with a major contribution being made by informal carers in the home setting. There is unfortunately little evidence to suggest a reduction in the numbers of patients requiring care in the fields of neurosurgical and neuromedical nursing in the immediate future.

LEARNING ACTIVITIES

1. Investigate the number of pedal cyclists who die or are seriously injured as a result of head injury. Carry out a census to determine the proportion of cyclists who are wearing helmets. Should helmets be compulsory for pedal cyclists in the same way they are for motorcyclists?
2. How many students in your group carry organ donor cards? Should the law be changed in such a way that consent for organ donation in cases of brain death be assumed to have been given unless a person carries a card to say they specifically refuse consent? Organize a debate on this topic in class.
3. Investigate the self help and support groups that are available in your area for patients and their families in cases of illness such as multiple sclerosis, Alzheimer's disease or brain injury.
4. An elderly lady has suffered a right sided cerebrovascular accident which has left her with significant functional deficits. She is to be discharged home to her daughter's care. Plan out the topics you would cover in discussing the patient's needs with her daughter, role play the interview with a colleague.

REFERENCES AND FURTHER READING

Agee BL (1985) Helping your patient survive the perils of CNS infection. *Nursing 85* **15(5):** 11–13.

Agee BL & Herman C (1984) Cervical logrolling on a standard hospital bed. *American Journal of Nursing* **34(3):** 314–318.

Allan D (1984) Glasgow coma scale. *Nursing Mirror* **158(23):** 32.

Allan D (1988) *Nursing and the Neurosciences.* Edinburgh: Churchill Livingstone.

Association to Combat Huntington's Chorea (1984) *Facing Huntington's Chorea.* Hinkley, Leicestershire: ACHC.

Baumann A & Joseph L (1985) Acute stroke: early recognition is the key to successful treatment. *Canadian Nurse* **81(10):** 22–28.

Beatty R (1982) Cerebral haemorrhage: 'A patient's view'. *Nursing Times* **78(46):** 1956.

Beckingham A & Baumann A (1990) The aging family in crisis: assessment and decision making. *Journal of Advanced Nursing* **15(7):** 782–787.

Bingham E (1990) Motor neurone disease. *Nursing Times* **86(19):** 28–31.

Chung Ho (1982) Infective polyneuritis (Guillain–Barré syndrome). *Nursing Times* **78(8):** 315–319.

Clough CG (1990) Neurosurgical treatment of Parkinson's disease. *Care of the Elderly* **2(8):** 306–307.

Csesko P (1988) Sexuality and multiple sclerosis. *Journal of Neuroscience Nursing* **20(6):** 353–355.

Cummings JL & Benson DP (1983) *Dementia: A Clinical Approach*. London: Butterworth.

Dening F (1987) Nuclear magnetic resonance. *Professional Nurse* **3(2):** 5.

Harrison MJ (1987) *Neurological Skills*. London: Butterworth.

Hickey J (1979) *The Clinical Practice of Neurological and Neurosurgical Nursing*. Philadelphia: Lippincott.

Illis LA, Glanville HH & Sedgwick EM (1982) *Rehabilitation of the Neurological Patient*. Oxford: Blackwell.

Milne C (1989) Motor neurone disease. *Nursing Standard* **3(26):** 20–21.

Parkinson's Disease Society (1982) *Living with Parkinson's Disease*. London: PDS.

Purchese G & Allen D (1984) *Neuromedical and Neurosurgical Nursing* 2nd edn. London: Baillière Tindall.

Roberts A (1989) Systems of life: cerebrovascular disease I. *Nursing Times* **85(28):** 51–54.

Stevens SA & Becker KL (1988a) A simple step-by-step approach to neurologic assessment. Part I. *Nursing 88* **18(9):** 53–61.

Stevens SA & Becker KL (1998b) A simple step-by-step approach to neurologic assessment. Part II. *Nursing 88* **18(10):** 51–58.

Teasdale G & Mendelow AD (1986) Management of head injuries. *Nursing Times* **82(20):** 59.

Gray-Vickrey (1988) Evaluating Alzheimer patients. *Nursing 88* **18(12):** 34–40.

Walsh M (1990) *A & E Nursing: A New Approach* 2nd edn. Oxford: Heinemann.

OBJECTIVES

At the end of this chapter the reader will be able to:

- Describe the structure and functioning of the male and female reproductive systems
- Demonstrate an awareness of issues involving sexuality
- Discuss methods of contraception and be aware of issues connected with infertility
- Show understanding of the principal forms of pathology that effect the reproductive system of both males and females
- Discuss the assessment and planning of care for patients with disorders of the reproductive system
- Be aware of the nurse's role in helping patients faced with difficult ethical decisions related to reproductive physiology

EMBRYOLOGY

The reproductive system is unique in mammals in that it differs markedly between sexes. Sex is determined at the time of fertilization by the inclusion of the XX chromosomal pair of the female or the XY genotype of the male. In this early period of human development, sex differentiation can be determined microscopically by the presence or absence of Barr bodies in a cell nucleus which has been taken from the embryo. These Barr bodies, which are always one less than the number of X chromosomes, indicate the genotype of the embryo.

As the embryo grows, an internal genital ridge develops but remains undifferentiated in either sex until the seventh week of intrauterine life. At that time, under the regulation of the Y chromosome seminiferous tubules and Sertoli cells differentiate. The Sertoli cells produce H-Y antigen which promotes masculine development and the Müllerian inhibition factor. At this time sex differentiation can be made morphologically because the genital ridges of the embryo, accompanied by the primordial germ cells, have grown and differentiated into a rudimentary testis or ovary, depending on the sex of the cell (Figures 22.1 and 22.2).

An elaborate bilateral duct system also develops. In the male much of this duct system degenerates, and the remaining portion forms the epididymis and vas deferens, which then join the male urethra. In the female the duct systems develop bilaterally and, as growth continues, the two ducts meet and fuse in the midline. The portion which fuses becomes the uterus, cervix and vagina. This process of fusion takes some weeks to complete and, indeed, may never occur, giving rise to paired uteri and vaginas. Fusion may be incomplete, causing some abnormalities of the uterus (Figure 22.3).

While internal development proceeds the external genitalia are also becoming differentiated. In the 'neuter' phase of development three small protuberances appear caudally on the external surface of the embryo. These protuberances consist of the 'genital tubercle' and, on either side of this tubercle, the genital swellings. In the male the tubercle becomes elongated and develops into the male phallus while the genital swellings become the scrotal tissue. These two swellings must develop, descend and fuse, closing the urethra in the male penis and forming the pendulant scrotum. Should fusion not be complete on the dorsal surface, a condition known as hypospadias occurs (Figure 22.4). Epispadias, a rarer malformation, may also occur. Here the failure of the urethra to fuse completely occurs on the ventral side of the penis. From these swellings, the prepuce, or foreskin, of the penis also arises. The foreskin is attached to the penile shaft at the base of the glans. The foreskin then drops down like a hood over the glans and remains partially fixed until sometime between birth and 3 years of age. During this time the congenital adhesions break down and the prepuce is then easily retractable over the glans penis.

The female genitalia arise from the same three ridges. The tubercle becomes the clitoris, and the genital swellings develop into the labia majora and minora. As the labia meet anteriorly, they form a loose-fitting, hood-like fold over the clitoris. This fold is similar to the prepuce of the male penis. Posteriorly, the labial folds fuse just before the anus. Thus, male and female reproductive systems have homologous counterparts.

By the sixteenth week of embryologic life the sex of the infant can be determined externally. At this time the testes of the male, which normally reside in the scrotum, are not there. In early development the testis and ovary are abdominal organs. As further growth takes place, they descend over the pelvic brim in the case of the ovaries or into the scrotum in the case of the testes. The descent of the testes appears to be in response to

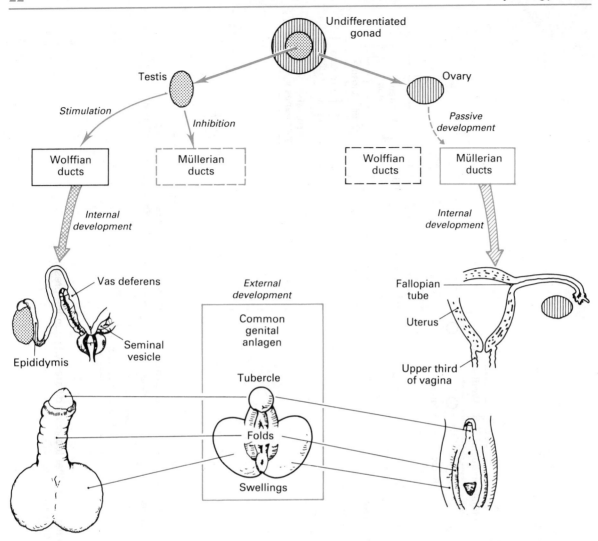

Figure 22.1 Normal sexual development in the male and female.

hormonal and mechanical control. As the fetal testes begin to produce testosterone, in about the seventh month of fetal life, descent occurs, and they pass through the inguinal canal and the external inguinal ring to enter the scrotum by the ninth month. During descent the testis is surrounded by a tube of peritoneum known as the processus vaginalis. After descent has occurred, this tissue generally becomes obliterated, leaving the testis covered by the tunica vaginalis. Following descent, the testis shows a decline in its production of testosterone until puberty. As in all processes, descent may not occur or may occur imperfectly. This may result in undescended testes. Other genetic and exogenous influences may disrupt the process of differentiation either internally or externally, producing a variety of rare sexual malformations.

PHYSIOLOGY

Male Reproductive System

The system consists of the paired testes, epididymis, vas deferens, common ejaculatory ducts, urethra, penis and the scrotum. The accessory organs are the seminal vesicles, prostate gland and the bulbourethral glands (Figure 22.5). A cross section of the testis (Figure 22.6) demonstrates the relationships between the seminiferous tubule, rete testis, efferent ductules, epididymis and vas deferens.

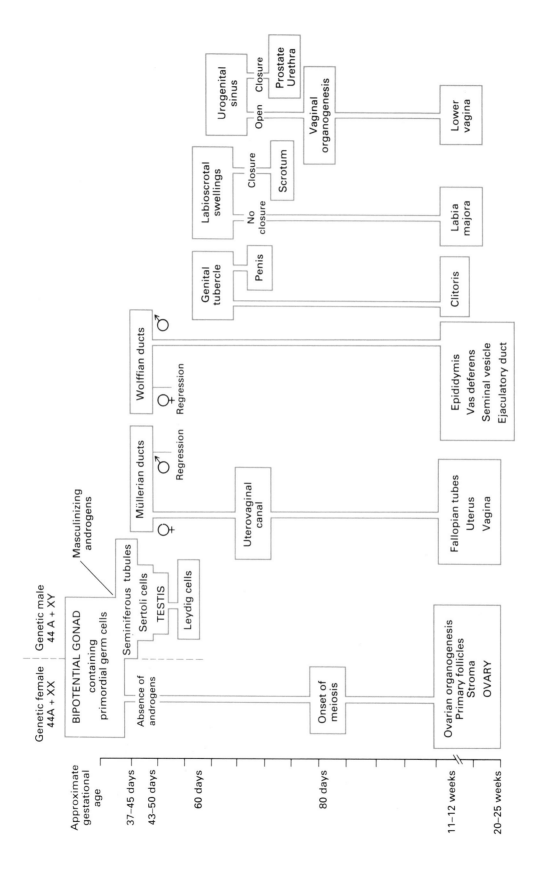

Figure 22.2 Sequence of sexual differentiation in the human. Note that testicular differentiation in the presence of masculinizing androgens precedes all other forms of differentiation.

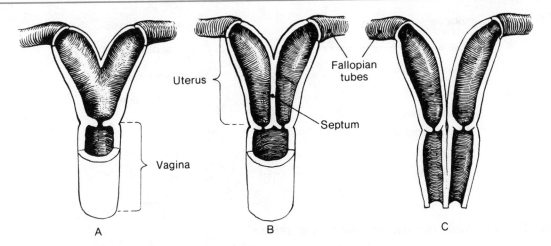

Figure 22.3 Some abnormalities of the uterus resulting from incomplete fusion of the ducts. (**A**) Bicornu-ate uterus; (**B**) uterus septus and a double cervix; (**C**) double uterus, cervix and vagina.

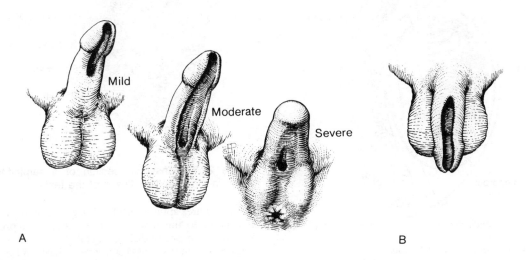

Figure 22.4 (**A**) Hypospadias: mild, moderate and severe. In severe hypospadias note the similarity to the female (see Figure 22.10). (**B**) Epispadias.

THE TESTES

Each lobe of the testis contains a seminiferous tubule surrounded by tissue. In this tissue are interstitial (Leydig) cells, which are endocrine in action, producing the male hormones of which testosterone is the most prominent. These cells become activated to produce some androgens in the fetal period but remain nearly dormant until puberty. At puberty, under the complex control of the hypothalamus and pituitary glands, the testes are stimulated to produce male hormones. Under the influence of these androgens, the body begins the process of puberty. The external organs of reproduction grow and develop. The distribution of body hair

changes to that of the adult male. The larynx and musculoskeletal systems develop and change. Concurrently, the testes begin to produce sperm. Puberty ends with the sexual and reproductive maturity of the individual.

Spermatogenesis

Spermatogenesis begins in the seminiferous tubule (Figure 22.7). Here a basilar membrane around the lumen of the tubule is lined with two major cell types which project into the lumen of the tube. The first of these, the germ cells, are called spermatogonia. These

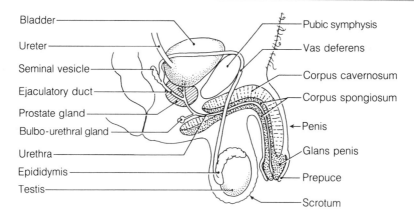

Figure 22.5 The male reproductive system and pelvis.

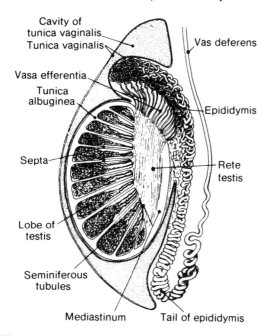

Figure 22.6 Section of the testis.

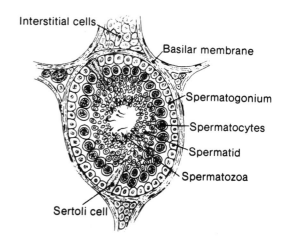

Figure 22.7 Transverse section of a seminiferous tubule in the interstitial tissue of the testis.

cells undergo growth and multiplication to become primary and secondary spermatocytes and then spermatids. Until this phase is complete the cell appears to have sufficient nutrients in itself. Now, however, the second type of cell, the Sertoli or sustentacular cell, is apparently necessary to provide nutrition for the spermatid. The spermatid is engulfed by the Sertoli cell and begins a metamorphosis which produces viable spermatozoa.

When growth is complete, the sperm is released into the lumen of the seminiferous tubule and is rapidly transported to the epididymis and thence through the duct system. Although sperm may appear to be mature at the time of release into the tubule, they do undergo further maturation, increasing in fertility and vigour as they progress through the ducts. Sperm removed from the tail of the epididymis rather than the head are more fertile. If sperm are not ejaculated, they degenerate and are absorbed. Spermatogenesis is continuous and a

sperm requires approximately 75 days to mature. This is in contrast to the female, whose mature ova present from her own primordial germ cells.

Spermatogenesis is also sensitive to heat, and occurs at a temperature a few degrees lower than body temperature. It is for this reason that the testes are suspended in the scrotum, allowing the temperature of the testes to be regulated by the body. The dartos muscle within the scrotum contracts or relaxes in response to varying temperatures. Coldness causes it to contract, bringing the testes closer to the body for extra warmth. The reverse is true in heat. It is also known that men with uncorrected cryptorchism remain sterile, because body temperature intra-abdominally is incompatible with successful spermatogenesis.

A feedback mechanism controls the production of sperm and testosterone (Figure 22.8). The anterior pituitary gland, when stimulated by the gonadotrophin releasing hormone (GRH) of the hypothalamus, releases two hormones: the follicle-stimulating hormone (FSH) and luteinizing hormone (LH). FSH stimulates the seminiferous tubule to begin spermatogenesis and the Sertoli cells to produce nutrients for the sperm. The Sertoli cells also release a hormone named inhibin

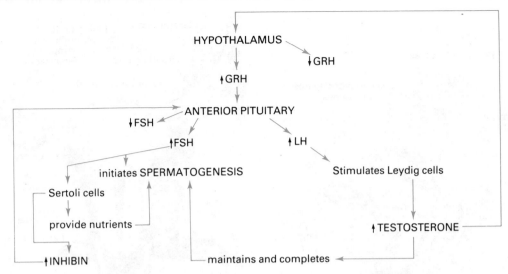

Figure 22.8 Feedback mechanism for spermato-genesis and production of testosterone.

which signals the anterior pituitary to reduce production of FSH.

The luteinizing hormone stimulates the interstitial cells of the testes to produce testosterone which maintains and completes spermatogenesis. Spermatogonia will proceed to the spermatocyte stage under the influence of FSH but testosterone is necessary to complete the step from spermatocyte to fertile spermatozoa.

High levels of testosterone exert an inhibitory effect on the hypothalamus. When testosterone reaches a low level it no longer exerts this inhibitory effect and more GRH is released, repeating the cycle.

DUCT SYSTEM AND ACCESSORY GLANDS

The viable sperm must be transported from the testis to the penis and thence to the female reproductive tract so that fertilization may take place. Here the duct system and the accessory glands play a major role. As the vas deferens ascends into the pelvic cavity, it widens into a broad ampulla. The duct of each seminal vesicle and the ampulla of the adjacent vas deferens meet to form the common ejaculatory duct. As a secretory organ, the seminal vesicle does not store sperm but rather produces a fluid which is rich in nutrients and prostaglandins. These nutrients provide for the sperm until fertilization. The prostaglandins are believed to aid fertilization by reacting with cervical mucus to make it more penetrable by sperm and to induce contractions in the uterus and tubes which help sperm to reach the ovum.

The prostate gland, which is fused to the neck of the bladder, is divided into three lobes which surround the urethra. The prostate develops in puberty and is easily palpable on rectal examination. During the years of sexual maturity the prostate secretes a thin, milky-looking fluid which contains among other substances a clotting enzyme and a profibrinolysin. The fluid is alkaline and reduces the acidity of seminal fluid and vaginal secretions. This is an important reproductive function, as the motility and viability of sperm are greatly reduced in an acid solution. Sperm are more motile in a neutral or slightly alkaline solution.

Further fluid is added to the semen by the bulbourethral glands. These paired glands lie posterior to the urethra and discharge their fluid into it when they contract at ejaculation. This fluid seems to function merely as a lubricant and fluid medium for the sperm.

Deposition of the semen in the vagina of the female is one function of the penis. The penis also serves as an excretory organ. In order to obtain intromission, the penis must move from its normally flaccid state to one of erection. Such a change is due to engorgement with blood of the corpora cavernosa and the corpus spongiosum.

Semen is a milky, viscous fluid varying at one ejaculation from 2–7 ml in quantity and containing about 60 000 000 to 100 000 000 sperm per millilitre. The alkaline fluid is rich in nutrients and minerals to support the sperm. It coagulates a few minutes after ejaculation and then reliquefies later. The clotting enzyme of the prostatic fluid acts on the fibrinogen of seminal vesicle fluid to form a coagulate. This coagulate spontaneously dissolves some 15–20 minutes later under the influence of the fibrinolysin formed from the prostatic profibrinolysin. During this time the sperm are immobile; following reliquefaction they are highly motile. The sperm, which are now actively motile by lashing their tails, move rapidly up through the uterus into the outer third of the fallopian tube where fertilization usually takes place. It is believed that the acrosome or projection on the head of the sperm releases hyaluronidase, an enzyme which dissolves the outer wall of the ovum. This allows a sperm to enter the ovum and fertilization to take place.

Female Reproductive System

The female reproductive tract consists of paired ovaries, uterine tubes, a uterus and vagina (Figure 22.9).

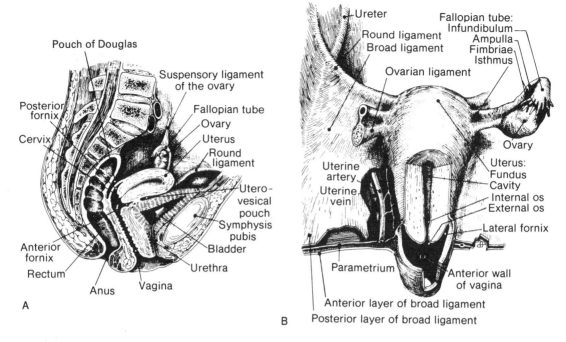

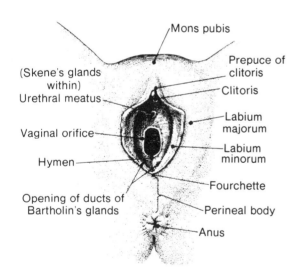

Figure 22.9 (**A**) Median sagittal section of the female pelvis. (**B**) Uterus and adnexa, posterior view (uterus, cervix and vagina wedge sectioned).

Figure 22.10 Female external genitalia.

Externally, the labia, clitoris, and Skene's and Bartholin's glands are part of the reproductive system (Figure 22.10). The external area may be collectively referred to as the vulva, perineum or pudenda. Generally, perineum refers to the area stretching from the symphysis pubis laterally to the thighs and posteriorly to the tip of the coccyx. This is arbitrarily divided into the anterior and posterior perineum by an imaginary line drawn between the ischial tuberosities. Anteriorly, this contains

the urogenital triangle and posteriorly the rectal triangle, including the perineal body. The area between the labia majora is referred to as the pudendal cleft. That area which lies between the labia minora and extends from the clitoris to the fourchette is referred to as the vestibule. Bartholin's glands, whose ducts open into the vestibule, may be referred to as the greater vestibular glands, Skene's being the lesser.

The female reproductive system functions to produce the female hormones (oestrogen and progesterone), to ripen ova for fertilization, and for intercourse which permits fertilization of ova and the release of sexual tension. In addition, the organs of reproduction incubate the human conceptus, providing it with safety and nourishment until the fetus is expelled from the uterus to continue its growth and development externally.

THE OVARY

The ovary is a small, almond-shaped organ lying posterior to the broad ligament of the uterus and attached to it by the mesovarium. Cross-sections of the ovary show a cortex and a medulla. The cortex, or outer layer, is composed of connective tissue and cells, among which are scattered the ova and developing follicles. Over this outer layer of the cortex is a thin layer of germinal epithelium. The medulla is composed of connective tissue containing blood vessels and smooth muscle fibres.

The fetal ovary is recognizable very early. By the fourth month of intrauterine life some cells in the ovary

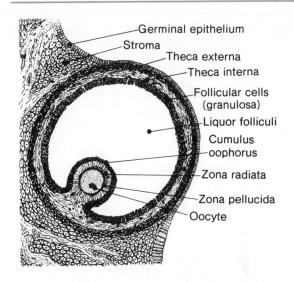

Germinal epithelium
Stroma
Theca externa
Theca interna
Follicular cells (granulosa)
Liquor folliculi
Cumulus oophorus
Zona radiata
Zona pellucida
Oocyte

Figure 22.11 Mature graafian follicle.

have differentiated enough to be recognizable as primary oocytes. Initially these oocytes number in the millions but most degenerate. At birth less than two million are present; at puberty there are about 300 000, and of these only 400–500 will develop to ovulation. By the menopause few primordial follicles remain and they soon degenerate. Throughout childhood certain of these oocytes develop but never reach maturity and ovulate. Then, under the influence of the maturing hypothalamus, which stimulates the anterior lobe of the pituitary to produce hormones, puberty begins.

The secondary sex characteristics begin to develop. First there is growth and development of the breast tissue. Pubic hair appears and the internal and external organs of reproduction become fully developed and functional. The vagina, under the influence of oestrogens, thickens and develops several layers of squamous epithelium. This makes it more resistant to infection. Previously, the vaginal pH had been neutral or alkaline; now it becomes acidic. This is largely due to Döderlein's bacillus which oxidizes the glycogen which has been deposited in the vagina to form lactic acid. Concurrently, the ovaries are developing and menarche, or the beginning of menstruation, occurs.

As in the male, GRH stimulates the anterior pituitary gland to release two hormones: FSH and LH. FSH and LH are not secreted continuously but in a pulsating manner with the amplitude and frequency of the pulses varying with the phase of the cycle. Under this hormonal influence, primordial follicles in the ovary begin to develop. Each primordial follicle is composed of an oocyte and surrounding granulosa cells. As growth occurs the oocyte or ovum enlarges and there is an increase in the number of granulosa cells. Growth is eccentric and the ovum comes to lie at one side of the group of granulosa cells. Fluid, rich in oestrogens and inhibin collects between these cells and the ovum. Inhibin is produced by the granulosa cells under the stimulation of FSH. As more inhibin is produced, it

exerts an inhibiting effect on the production of FSH, causing the levels to fall. High inhibin levels are associated with several follicles developing simultaneously. A clear membrane, the zona pellucida, develops and surrounds the ovum. As the follicle grows, cells begin to form around it and are called thecal cells. These thecal cells, stimulated by the FSH and LH, produce oestrogens.

Many follicles in both ovaries start to ripen but usually only one follicle continues on to ovulation. The others undergo degeneration. The mechanism of this atresia is still unknown. The thecal cells surrounding these degenerated (atretic) follicles continue to produce oestrogens. The mature follicle may now be termed a graafian follicle, after de Graaf who first described it in 1672 (Figure 22.11).

As the graafian follicle approaches ovulation, it comes to lie close to the surface of the ovary. The tissue over it becomes thin and taut. Soon the follicle wall ruptures and the ovum, surrounded by the zona pellucida and attached cells, is expelled into the abdominal cavity. The time of rupture is designated as ovulation and marks the end of the preovulatory (proliferative or follicular) phase.

The ovary now embarks on the luteal (secretory) phase of its cycle. Immediately following ovulation, the wall of the follicle collapses inward and some haemorrhage may occur into this cavity. In a few hours the remaining granulosa cells hypertrophy and begin to show the characteristic yellow of the corpus luteum. These yellowy granulosa cells are now called luteal cells. The luteal cells are stimulated by LH to become the corpus luteum and to begin producing progesterone. Oestrogen continues to be produced as well. The corpus luteum reaches full maturity by about the ninth day following ovulation. At this time it is easily recognizable on the surface of the ovary as a raised yellowy area and may constitute nearly half the volume of the ovary. Near this time the corpus luteum may receive a message that the ovum has been fertilized. If it does so, the corpus luteum is maintained and becomes known as the corpus luteum of pregnancy. If fertilization does not occur, the luteal site begins to degenerate, and progesterone production drops. As the site degenerates, so do the thecal cells. Oestrogen production from this source declines. The luteal site shrinks to form a small mass of whitish scar tissue on the surface of the ovary which is known as the corpus albicans.

Hormones and the ovarian cycle

In response to the falling oestrogen and progesterone levels, the hypothalamus signals the anterior pituitary gland to release FSH and LH. Under this stimulus the follicles begin to develop and the thecal cells produce oestrogen. The rising levels of oestrogen exert a negative feedback effect on the hypothalamus to reduce the amount of GRH released and hence the amount of FSH and LH, for the levels of FSH and LH fall slightly following the initial rise in oestrogen levels (Figure 22.12). As oestrogen peaks, it is thought to exert a positive feedback effect on the hypothalamic–pituitary axis that results in a surge of LH and, to a lesser extent, FSH. This surge of LH

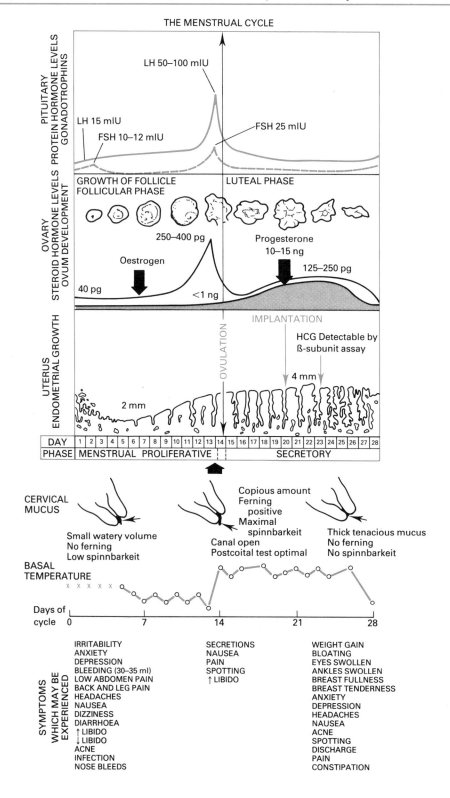

Figure 22.12 Summary of menstrual cycle events. HCG: human chorionic gonadotrophin.

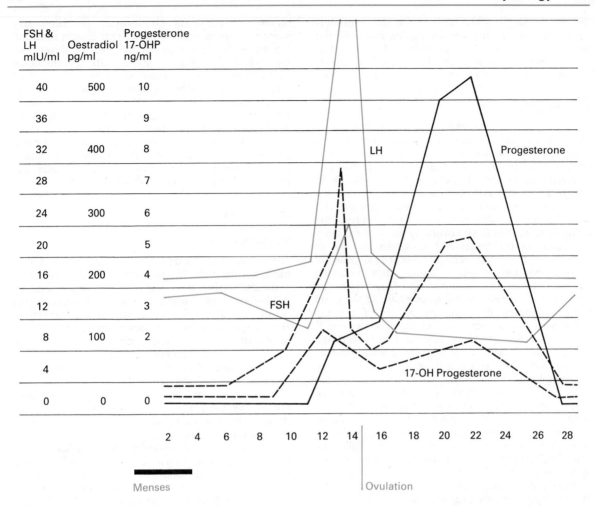

FSH & LH mIU/ml	Oestradiol pg/ml	Progesterone 17-OHP ng/ml
40	500	10
36		9
32	400	8
28		7
24	300	6
20		5
16	200	4
12		3
8	100	2
4		
0	0	0

Figure 22.13 Plasma concentrations of gonadotrophins and ovarian hormones during one ovarian cycle.

occurs about 24 hours before ovulation (Figure 22.13).

In cycles where the LH surge does not occur or is of insufficient magnitude, ovulation fails to occur. Exactly how the LH surge affects ovulation is unclear except that it is necessary for completion of the cycle. Follicles will grow and develop under FSH stimulation but will fail to ovulate without the surge of LH.

Ovulation occurs in a climate of falling oestrogen, LH and FSH levels and a rising progesterone level, as LH stimulates the follicular site to begin production of progesterone. As the preovulatory cycle is one of high oestrogen level, the postovulatory phase is one of high progesterone level. The other hormones continue to be produced but at lower levels. These levels of FSH and LH are too low to stimulate development of new follicles.

The cells of the corpus luteum are organized to enlarge, proliferate, secrete and then degenerate. The surge of LH seems to be the main organizing factor for this. This stabilizes the corpus luteum and the length of the postovulatory phase of the cycle. As the 12-day-old corpus luteum degenerates and becomes a corpus albicans the levels of progesterone and oestrogen drop,

signalling the hypothalamus to begin releasing GRH again, thereby repeating the cycle.

In response to this cycle, the endometrium of the uterus also undergoes cyclic phenomena. These phenomena are known as the uterine cycle. The two cycles, uterine and ovarian, are intimately related and occur simultaneously.

THE UTERUS

The uterus is a thick-walled, muscular, pear-shaped organ about 7.5 cm (3 in) in length in the adult virgin. It is held in position by its ligaments and by the pelvic floor. The uterus is composed of three layers: (1) an inner mucous layer, or endometrium; (2) a middle muscular layer, or myometrium; and (3) an outer serous layer which covers the entire body of the uterus except where it is reflected up and over the bladder. The uterus is divided into two distinct parts, the body and the cervix.

The cervix projects into the vagina. It appears to be mainly connective tissue, and only 10% is muscle. The endometrial lining of the body of the uterus extends downward, undergoing certain modifications in the cervical canal and terminating just above the external os of the cervix where it meets the stratifed squamous epithelium of the vaginal wall.

Uterine cycle

In the uterine cycle the endometrium plays a major role. The endometrium is a thin, pink membrane which is attached directly to the underlying muscle layer. It is composed of surface epithelium, uterine glands and connective tissue, and is richly supplied with blood vessels and tissue spaces. The thickness 'of the endometrium varies with the cycle. At the beginning of a new cycle it is probably about 0.5 mm thick. In response to the oestrogens of the preovulatory phase of the ovary it begins to proliferate and continues to do so throughout the cycle until it reaches a peak of proliferation and secretion several days following ovulation. In addition to the effect of oestrogen, the progesterone released in the luteal phase of the ovary further promotes the secretory activity of the endometrium. In this secretory stage the endometrium is oedematous, the glands are large and sacculated, the arteries have developed their typical coiled, tortuous pattern and some connective tissue has undergone hypertrophic stages. The rich, succulent endometrium now contains much glycogen. At this time the endometrium may be 5–6 mm in depth. In short, all is ready for the implantation of the fertilized ovum, should it appear. In perfect timing the endometrium reaches its peak development approximately 7–8 days following ovulation, or just when the fertilized ovum should appear in the uterine cavity ready for implantation.

If the ovum has been fertilized and the corpus luteum is continuing to secrete progesterone, the endometrium is maintained and implantation may occur successfully. However, should the corpus luteum not receive this message, it begins to degenerate. Oestrogen and progesterone production decline. This decline in hormone level causes the endometrium to retract and degenerate. Vasoconstriction of blood vessels occurs and the uterus becomes ischaemic. Shortly thereafter the endometrium begins to slough away and menstruation begins. The process of sloughing takes from 3–7 days, with each woman usually establishing her own pattern. Menstrual flow is composed of endometrial tissue, mucus and some blood. As the tiny arterioles constrict and relax, bleeding occurs. Usually not more than 50–60 ml of blood per menstrual period is lost. This blood does not clot because of the action of fibrinolytic enzymes released into the uterine cavity during menstruation. Occasionally, a heavy menstrual loss neutralizes the available fibrinolysins and clots occur. At the completion of menstruation the endometrium has returned to its unproliferative state. It is now ready to respond again to the rising oestrogen levels.

Myometrial muscle tone and contractility varies throughout the menstrual cycle. Prostaglandins produced in the uterus act on smooth muscle to produce contractions. The contractions are of insufficient mag-

nitude to be felt by the woman except perimenstrually when they are at peak levels. Uterine muscle tone and the amplitude of these contractions increase throughout the cycle from a relaxed uterus with low amplitude contractions in the follicular phase to a less relaxed uterus with contractions of increasing amplitude in the luteal phase. At the onset of menstruation the uterus may be tense and having contractions of sufficient amplitude to be felt as cramps by many women. These cyclical changes are controlled by hormones because anovulatory cycles are not associated with cramping at menstruation. The contractions increase circulation and empty the uterus of menstrual debris.

OVULATION

Menstrual cycle

The uterine and ovarian cycles are often referred to as the menstrual cycle. This cycle begins on day one, which is the day menstruation begins, and continues until the day before menstruation begins again. Ovulation occurs on or around the fourteenth day of a 28–day cycle. However, this is subject to many factors, and the timing of ovulation in any one woman is a matter of considerable variation (Figure 22.14).

The menstrual cycle is divided into two independent sections: the pre- and postovulatory phases. The two phases are independent because the length of one does not control the length of the other. Ovulation· is the dividing factor signalling the end of one phase and the beginning of the next.

Not all cycles are ovulatory and it is known that women can have an anovulatory cycle and still menstruate. The precise mechanism for this phenomenon is not clearly understood. The most common explanation is that a follicle develops, there is a failure of the LH surge and the follicle degenerates. Anovulatory cycles are most common in adolescent girls in whom the first menstrual periods may be anovulatory and in women at the menopause.

Follicles do not mature at the same rate each month. This produces a month to month variation in the timing of ovulation and the length of the preovulatory phase in any one woman. This variation in timing is evident by variation in the onset of menstruation.

The onset of menstrual flow is controlled by the corpus luteum of the ovary. Once ovulation occurs, menstruation follows 14 (±1) days after and this time relationship is constant. Fluctuations in the length of the cycle arise in the preovulatory phase.

These events produce a natural variation in cycle length from month to month. Each woman establishes her own rhythm and this may differ from other women. When expressed as an average, one woman will have an average cycle length of 22 days and another of 32 days. Each is normal for that individual and is the result of physical differences between women as well as the influence of environmental factors.

Age is an important physical influence on cycle length in women. The menstrual pattern throughout life is divided into three zones: two of transition and a central period of increasing stability. The two transition periods

Table 22.1 Mean cycle interval in days of successive 5-year age groups from three studies.

Age (years)	Gunn, 1937			Chiazze, 1968			Shields-Poë, 1981		
	Mean	SD	n	Mean	SD	n	Mean	SD	n
15–19	32.1	3.64	3	30.8	3.38	436	—	—	—
20–24	30.1	3.84	59	30.5	3.99	257	29.6	2.56	5
25–29	29.9	5.71	63	29.6	2.68	266	29.4	2.46	17
30–34	27.6	2.74	34	29.0	2.92	505	29.4	2.51	17
35–39	27.4	2.44	25	28.5	2.58	550	27.9	3.02	13
40–44	27.0	2.55	24	28.3	2.77	302	26.2	4.55	11

n, Numbers of women recording menstrual cycles; SD, standard deviation.
From Shields-Poë DA (1981).

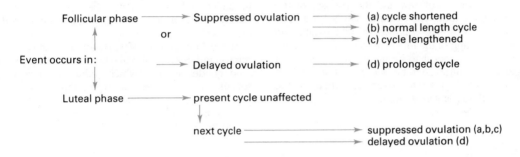

Figure 22.14 Effects of life events on menstrual cycle length and ovulation.

(postmenarche lasting about 5–7 years, and premenopause lasting about 6–8 years) are characterized by variation in cycle length.

As a girl ages, her average cycle length shortens and variation in cycle length reduces. The younger the girl experiences menarche the sooner she begins to develop a more 'regular' cycle.

The central period, from age 20–40 years, shows a continued reduction in variation and a shortening cycle interval. The average cycle length shortens between 0.1 and 0.18 of a day per year. Maximum stability is reached from age 35–39 years (Table 22.1).

As ageing continues there is a decrease in the number of follicles which begin to develop. This results in a gradual reduction in hormone levels, particularly inhibin, with corresponding increases in circulating FSH throughout the cycle. Documentation of these high FSH levels is the first laboratory indication of the perimenopausal period.

These high FSH levels induce rapid follicular development and a correspondingly shorter preovulatory phase. As the process continues there is a failure of the LH surge and anovulation follows, contributing to increasing irregularity in the cycle length. Eventually the ovary ceases to respond and menopause occurs.

Transitory variation in cycle length occurs in response to significant life events. Events associated with excitement, stress, a change of environment or anxiety can delay the ripening of a follicle and, consequently,

ovulation. An area of the posterior hypothalamus seems to allow psychological impressions to enhance or decrease the secretion of GRH. Without GRH, FSH and, particularly, LH are not released by the pituitary. This delays the ripening of a follicle or prevents a sufficient surge of LH to take place. Figure 22.14 demonstrates the effects observed in the cycle in response to these life events. If the event occurs in the follicular phase of the cycle it may either inhibit (anovulatory cycle) or delay ovulation. If ovulation is inhibited, the cycle in which the event occurred could be shorter in length, normal in length or prolonged in length. If ovulation is delayed, the cycle is prolonged in length. If the event occurs in the luteal phase of the cycle that cycle is unaffected but the succeeding cycle may show the expected effects.

Cervical, vaginal and tubal cycles

Changes also occur in the cervix, vagina, and fallopian tubes in response to stimuli from the ovary. Oestrogen prompts the endocervical glands to respond by increasing their secretions and becoming longer and more tortuous. This is accompanied by increased vascularity and tumescence of the cervix. From about the seventh day of the menstrual cycle to about the twenty-first the cervical mucus gradually increases in amount. The mucus contains an increasing concentration of sodium chloride, which causes it to show a typical ferning pattern when allowed to dry on a slide. During the other periods of the cycle and during pregnancy the dried cervical mucus shows a beaded pattern. The mucus reaches its peak of production at ovulation. The consistency changes at ovulation and becomes thinner and can be drawn out into long, thin threads; this is called spinnbarkeit. These changes demonstrate the timing of the body as the mucus will permit easy entry of the sperm at ovulation, the most logical time. Indeed, it appears that the cervical mucus permits passage of sperm through the cervix only at this particular time.

Changes in the vagina and fallopian tube are minimal compared to the changes in the ovary, uterus and cervix. The vaginal epithelium proliferates and reaches a peak at ovulation time. The fallopian tube becomes swollen. Its secretory cells enlarge and project beyond the ciliated cells. Maximum development is timed to occur simultaneously with ovulation and the passage of the ovum through the tube. The ovum is also assisted in its passage by the wave-like contractions of the fallopian tube and the beating of the tubal cilia toward the uterus. These contractions appear to be under the influence of oestrogens. The fallopian tube secretes fluids, which provide nutrients first for the ovum and then for the conceptus until implantation occurs.

SEXUALITY

Sexuality is broadly defined as the becoming and being of a man or a woman. As such, adult sexuality has four major divisions (Figure 22.15).

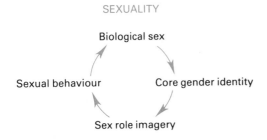

Figure 22.15 Divisions of adult sexuality.

Biological sex refers to the individual's physical attributes. This is based in the genotype (XX, XY or other combinations) and includes internal and external genitalia with the corresponding underlying hormonal, neural, vascular and physical components.

Core gender identity refers to one's inner sense of being a man or a woman and is established early in life, usually by 3 years of age. At this age, the child knows he is a boy or a girl. In most cases the core gender identity corresponds to the physical attributes of the individual.

Sex role imagery refers to the learned behaviour that the particular society subscribes to their men and women. Sex or gender role imagery is complex because it includes the myriad beliefs about what is labelled feminine or masculine in a society. It also conveys the image of appropriate sexual conduct for particular social groups. Some examples of these beliefs are: trousers are worn by men, skirts by women; women are passive, men are active. Sex role imagery is of great interest because it represents much of the learned behaviour which influences human choice and life-style. Much stereotyping of human behaviour has resulted from the need for society to set up expectations by which to guide and judge sex role behaviour. The learning of sex role imagery begins in infancy and continues throughout most of life. This learned behaviour, combined with personal experience, is internalized and becomes the individual's personal belief about sexuality.

Sexual behaviour refers to sexual expression and is the acting out of sexual feelings and beliefs. It includes a broad spectrum of human behaviour and varies from how one walks, to how and with whom one performs the sex act. For example, is the individual heterosexual in outlet and object? Does the person indulge in a variety of sexual practices, for example masturbation or oral sex?

These four aspects of sexuality are interrelated and reinforcing. Biological make-up and learning promote a core gender identity which influences acceptance of specific sex roles. Sexual expression reflects biology, gender identity, sex role and behaviour. For further discussion on sexuality see the appropriate references in the list at the end of the chapter.

Physiological Aspects of Sexual Response

Human sexual response occurs as a result of stimulation. The ability to respond physiologically to this stimulation exists in all healthy persons. The stimulation which elicits a response varies from purely mental images such as fantasy, dreams or remembered events to stimulation received through the senses. Touch is probably the most important source of stimulation and certain areas of the body appear to be more sensitive as stimulators of sexual arousal than are others. These sensitive areas vary for each individual but the sexual organs (penis in the man and clitoris, labia and vagina in the woman) are usually the most sensitive of the areas.

Learning modifies the emotional and physiological responses of people to sexual stimuli. As a result of prior learning or past experience similar sexual stimuli may elicit a wide range of response. However in all situations the appropriate psychological stimuli for that individual will increase pleasure in and ability to perform the sex act.

The response of the body to sexual stimulation is a total one, but the most noticeable changes are seen in the primary sexual organs. Tables 22.2 and 22.3 outline these responses. The sexual response cycle has been divided into four progressive phases. The phases do not differ between the sexes and depend in each sex on the same physiological mechanisms. The first is the excitement phase, in which the person becomes sexually aroused. It occurs in response to any source of stimulation, somatogenic or psychogenic or any combination of these. This phase is quite sensitive to outside

Table 22.2 General body reactions during the sexual response cycle.

Phase	Male	Female
1. Excitement	Nipple erection (30%)	Nipple erection (consistent) Sex-tension flush (25%)
2. Plateau	Sex-tension flush (25%) Carpopedal spasm Generalized skeletal muscle tension Hyperventilation Tachycardia (100–160 beats per minute)	Sex-tension flush (75%) Carpopedal spasm Generalized skeletal muscle tension Hyperventilation Tachycardia (100–160 beats per minute)
3. Orgasmic	Specific skeletal muscle contractions Hyperventilation Tachycardia (100–180 beats per minute)	Specific skeletal muscle contractions Hyperventilation Tachycardia (110–180 beats per minute)
4. Resolution	Sweating reaction (30–40%) Hyperventilation Tachycardia (150–180 beats per minute)	Sweating reaction (30–40%) Hyperventilation Tachycardia (150–180 beats per minute)

From Katchadourian and Lunde (1987).

Table 22.3 Reactions of sex organs during the sexual response cycle.

Phase	Male	Female

1. Excitement	Penile erection (within 3–8 seconds)
	
	As phase is prolonged:
	  Thickening, flattening and elevation of scrotal sac
	As phase is prolonged:
	  Partial testicular elevation and size increase
		Vaginal lubrication (within 10–30 seconds)
		As phase is prolonged:
		  Thickening of vaginal walls and labia
		
		As phase is prolonged:
		  Expansion of inner two-thirds of vagina and elevation of cervix and corpus
		As phase is prolonged:
		  Tumescence of clitoris

2. Plateau	Increase in penile coronal circumference and testicular tumescence (50–100% enlarged) Full testicular elevation and rotation (orgasm inevitable) Purple hue on corona of penis (inconsistent, even if orgasm is to ensue) Mucoid secretion from bulbourethral gland	Orgasmic platform in outer third of vagina Full expansion of two-thirds of vagina, uterine and cervical elevation 'Sex-skin': discolouration of minor labia (constant, if orgasm is to ensue) Mucoid secretion from Bartholin's gland Withdrawal of clitoris
3. Orgasmic	*Ejaculation* Contractions of accessory organs of reproduction: vas deferens, seminal vesicles, ejaculatory duct, prostate Relaxation of external bladder sphincter Contractions of penile urethra at 0.8 second intervals for 3–4 contractions (slowing thereafter for 2–4 more contractions) Anal sphincter contractions (2–4 contractions at 0.8 second intervals)	*Pelvic response (no ejaculation)* Contractions of uterus from fundus toward lower uterine segment Minimal relaxation of external cervical opening Contractions of orgasmic platform at 0.8 second intervals for 5–12 contractions (slowing thereafter for 3–6 more contractions) External anal sphincter contractions (3–4 contractions at 0.8 second intervals)

Table 22.2 Continued

Phase	Male	Female
		External urethral sphincter contractions (2–3 contractions at irregular intervals, 10–15% of subjects)
4. Resolution	Refractory period with rapid loss of pelvic vasocongestion Loss of penile erection in primary (rapid) and secondary (slow stages)	Ready return to orgasm with retarded loss of pelvic vasocongestion Loss of 'sex-skin' colour and orgasmic platform in primary (rapid) stage Remainder of pelvic vasocongestion as secondary (slow) stage Loss of clitoral tumescence and return to postion

From Katchadourian and Lunde (1987).

influences and if the stimuli are interrupted or not intense enough the excitement phase may be prolonged or aborted.

As sexual arousal continues to mount, the individual enters the plateau phase. Sexual tension is intensified and reaches the preorgasmic level. Alteration in stimuli may also cause this phase to be prolonged or to revert to the pre-plateau level of sexual arousal.

Orgasm is the phase of release of sexual tension and is accompanied by ejaculation in the male. It is experienced as an involuntary subjective feeling of pleasure or relief. This feeling is concentrated in the clitoris, vagina and uterus of the woman and in the penis, prostate and seminal vesicles of the male. There is much individual variation in the intensity and duration of orgasm; generally this relates directly to the degree of sexual arousal which preceded the orgasm.

Following orgasm the individual enters the resolution phase or period during which the body returns to its pre-excitement state. Within this resolution phase the male passes through the refractory period, a time during which the male cannot be restimulated to orgasm. The length of the refractory period varies with sexual episodes and may vary from a few minutes to several hours in the same individual.

Most of the observed responses during sexual excitement and resolution are due to two physiological mechanisms: vasocongestion and myotonia. Vasocongestion occurs as the muscular walls of the arterioles relax and expand allowing blood to rush in. This marked influx of blood into the area exceeds the ability of the veins to remove it and a period of vasocongestion occurs. Myotonia is increased muscle tension. During sexual activity, both smooth and skeletal muscles are affected.

Vasocongestion is a vascular phenomenon triggered by a nervous impulse. Effective stimulation activates the parasympathetic nervous system and inhibits the sympathetic fibres. The parasympathetic nerve fibres cause the arterioles to relax and expand allowing blood to rush in. Vasocongestion and penile erection result. At orgasm the sympathetic fibres are stimulated causing the arterioles to constrict, reducing blood flow to the area,

and the muscles to contract rhythmically. These impulses are transmitted through the spinal cord to the brain where they are experienced as pleasure.

A simple reflex arc also exists in the spinal cord. With genital stimulation, erection and ejaculation will occur after the spinal cord has been severed if the area of spinal nerve damage was above the sacral and lumbar areas governing erection and ejaculation. Because pleasure is experienced via sensory input to the brain, the sexual response is not felt by the individual if the spinal cord is transected.

The influence of sexual hormones on sexual response in humans cannot be clearly separated from learned responses. High circulating levels of hormones are important in stimulating the adolescent to overcome the latency period of childhood and become sexually orientated. Surgical removal of ovaries or testes later in life is not associated with a marked decrease in sexual interest in most adults. Adrenal hormones seem to be important to the continued sex drive or libido.

MALE SEXUAL RESPONSE

The most dramatic change in the male during sexual excitement is the erection of the penis. This is due to engorgement with blood of the corpora cavernosa and the corpus spongiosum. Erection of the penis may be partial but it is considered to be functionally erect if vaginal penetration can be achieved. Following full erection, further engorgement of the corona of the glans penis occurs just before orgasm. Concurrent with penile erection, the scrotum becomes contracted and thickened. This tightening of the scrotal sac assists in the elevation of the testes. The testes increase in size and are elevated until they are pressed against the body. Under parasympathetic nervous control, the bulbourethral glands secrete a few drops of fluid which is seen at the urethral orifice (Figure 22.16).

Ejaculation occurs in two phases: the first phase or emission involves the upper part of the male reproductive tract; the second expels sperm and semen from the body. At ejaculation the seminal vesicles contract and seminal fluid is forced into the common ejaculatory

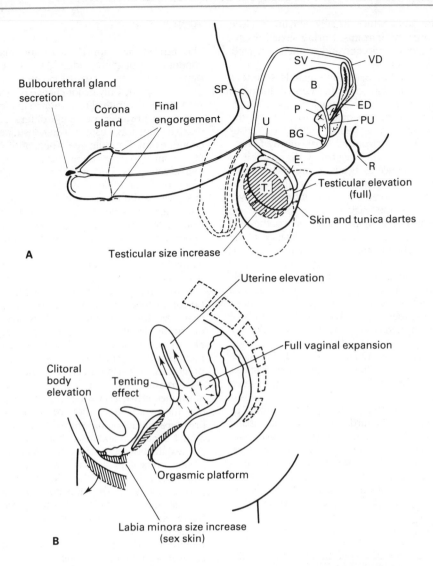

Figure 22.16 Sexual response. **(A)** Male pelvis: plateau phase. **(B)** Female pelvis: plateau phase. SP, symphysis pubis; SV, seminal vesicle; VD, vas deferens; B, bladder; ED, ejaculatory duct; P, prostate; PU, prostatic urethra; BG, bulbourethral gland; U, urethra; E, epididymis; T, testis; R, rectum.

ducts and into the urethra. The muscular layers of the prostate gland contract rhythmically forcing prostatic fluid into that portion of the urethra near the prostate. Simultaneously with these contractions of prostatic muscle, the fibres at the neck of the bladder continuous with muscle fibres in the prostate gland also contract, closing the internal urethral orifice. The contracting ampulla of the vas deferens discharges its contents into the prostatic urethra. When all fluids are pooled in the prostatic portion of the urethra the first phase of ejaculation has been completed. The man is aware of ejaculation coming and he can no longer control or delay the process.

The second phase is accomplished by rhythmic contractions that force the semen along the length of the urethra and expel it from the urinary meatus under pressure. The man responds with pleasure to the contractions of the penis and accessory organs and the feeling of fluid volume escaping. Generally, the first few expulsive contractions and a greater volume of ejaculate are associated with greater pleasure.

FEMALE SEXUAL RESPONSE

The vagina, a fibromuscular tube from 7.5–10 cm (3–4 in) long, is the female organ of intercourse. Here sperm is deposited. It also serves as a passage for the fetus from intrauterine to extrauterine life. The vagina is protected by the labia, which usually remain in close approximation over the introitus. During sexual excitement the labia become engorged and swollen and gape, thus exposing the vestibule.

Under neural stimulus, Bartholin's glands secrete a fluid which serves to lubricate the vaginal introitus. However, the mucus these vulvovaginal glands secrete is minimal and not of sufficient quantity to lubricate the entire vagina. Hence, most vaginal lubrication arises from the vaginal walls themselves. Very quickly following sexual stimulation the vaginal walls exhibit a 'sweating'-like appearance as beads of mucoid material appear throughout the rugal folds. Soon the droplets run together to form a complete coat of lubrication over the inner surface of the vagina. Since there are no glandular elements in the vaginal wall, it is hypothesized that the exudation is a result of marked dilatation of the venous system which surrounds the vagina. The cervix, once thought to be the source of much of the lubrication of the vagina, also appears to play a relatively minor role. This seems to be confirmed by the fact that little or no secretory activity of the cervix has been observed during sexual activity. Also, women who have undergone total hysterectomy and bilateral salpingo-oophorectomy produce reasonable vaginal lubrication in response to sexual stimulation. Indeed, the same response will develop in artificially constructed vaginas, and the source of the lubricating material is presumed to be the same.

The vagina also responds to sexual stimuli by enlarging. The inner two-thirds of the vagina expand and lengthen, forming a basin for the seminal pool which will form in the posterior fornix of the vagina just below the cervical os. The outer third of the vagina becomes engorged and constricted, serving to assist the vagina to form a reservoir for the semen. Engorgement of pelvic organs also results in a slight elevation of the uterus and cervix.

An orgasm may occur as a generalized systemic feeling, with sensation localized in the clitoris, and rhythmic muscular contractions of the outer third of the vagina and the uterus. With orgasm, pelvic engorgement of blood vessels is rapidly resolved. This causes the uterus to return to its normal position, placing the cervix very near to or in the seminal pool, thus facilitating movement of sperm through the cervix.

The clitoris seems to be a unique organ in human anatomy. As the primary focus of sensual response, it appears to serve no other function. Made of fibrous tissue with two corpora cavernosa and richly innervated, it undergoes engorgement and enlargement when the female is sexually stimulated either physically or mentally. The tumescent clitoris then retracts against the symphysis pubis and becomes difficult to see or feel.

The subjective experience of orgasm is synchronous with orgasmic platform contractions and the pleasure associated with orgasm is related to their number and intensity.

Following orgasm the woman enters the resolution phase. Unlike the male, a woman, if provided during this phase with sufficient further stimulation, may return to the orgasmic level.

MENOPAUSE

The reproductive functions of the male and female continue throughout adult life. Given health and opportunity, the male's sexual and reproductive capabilities are life-long; the only major change is a slowing of sexual response and a gradual reduction in libido (sexual drive).

Women, however, present a different picture. Reproductive function, usually demonstrated by menses, continues until middle age. Then, at the average age of 50, women cease menstruating. The cessation of menstruation is perhaps the most obvious sign of menopause, or 'change of life'. This transitional period is known as the climacteric. The climacteric may take a few months to several years and is the result of altered ovarian function. Ovarian follicles cease to ripen. The endometrium does not respond as richly, and menstruation becomes scantier and shorter in duration. The woman may have several anovulatory cycles, just as she may have had in puberty. Eventually the menses may become irregular and finally cease. Menopause is said to be complete when the woman has had no menses for 1 year. As the perimenopausal woman may ovulate erratically, family planning advice is important to her. She cannot assume she will not become pregnant until menopause is complete, after which the risks of pregnancy occurring are very slight.

Decreasing oestrogen levels stimulate gonadotrophic hormones (FSH, LH) which show a proportionate rise, but the ovary does not respond fully. The body, previously functioning smoothly under balanced hormonal control, responds to these imbalances with 'hot flushes' in about 85% of women. A hot flush is a sudden feeling of heat in the face, neck and chest associated with patchy flushing of the skin. There is usually profuse perspiration, perhaps palpitations, a generalized feeling of heat and a sensation of acute physical discomfort. Some are accompanied by nausea, dizziness and headache. A hot flush lasts about three minutes. The monitoring of women having hot flushes confirms that an average temperature shift of about 4°F (2°C) from core to skin occurs. The hot flush is followed by vasoconstriction and shivering as the body attempts to correct the shift in temperature from skin to core. Hot flushes begin gradually, reach a plateau by 6–8 weeks following the last period and can occur for several years after the menopause. There is no difference in the severity between the natural menopause and a surgical one. Hot flushes occur in parallel with LH pulses and are not co-ordinated with oestrogen levels. The exact mechanism is not understood but the same factor(s) that triggers a rise in LH is also thought to trigger a hot flush. Low circulating levels of oestrogen contribute as in double blind trials it has been found that the only symptoms controlled by oestrogen are hot flushes. Additionally, obese women report fewer hot flushes, presumably because of higher circulating levels due to conversion of some androgens to oestradiol. However, these symptoms are unpredictable, hence uncontrollable, and can be embarrassing, anxiety producing and sleep disturbing. Much of this may be unsettling to the woman, especially when accompanied by cessation of reproductive function and fears of advancing age and of loss of usefulness, sexual function and love of her husband.

Many women accept these changes with only some minor disturbance. It would seem that education and reassurance will help most women. Only about 25% of women require hormone replacement treatment. This is in the form of short-term therapy with oestrogens, usually by the transdermal patch route. The dosage is individualized to relieve the symptoms (the patient is instructed to keep a chart of her symptoms) and is continued for 2–3 months, at which time a reassessment is made. An oral progestational agent may be added after the initial oestrogen treatment because of the effects of long periods of unopposed oestrogen on the endometrium. Usually the dosage of oestrogen and progesterone will be reduced and the woman gradually weaned off drugs by about 9 months to 1 year. Because the prolonged use of unopposed oestrogens is associated with an increased risk of cancer of the endometrium, women should be alerted to the risks of long-term therapy.

It should be understood that all oestrogen production does not cease at menopause. The ovaries do not appear to be inert postmenopausally, and it is thought that they continue to excrete small amounts of hormones. This is in addition to oestrogens from the adrenal gland. Over the years oestrogen production declines further and the development of other organ changes occurs. The vulva becomes atrophic and thin from a reabsorption of fatty tissue. The uterus decreases in size; the endometrium becomes thin and atrophic. The vaginal epithelium thins out and is more susceptible to injury and infection. Lubrication of the vagina may require supplementation so that dyspareunia (painful sexual intercourse) need not occur.

Sexual function can continue with little change in the vast majority of postmenopausal women. The most important factors in the continuance of sexual function appear to be the opportunity for and the frequency of intercourse, so that the changes of menopause themselves do not mean this phase of a woman's life must cease. Indeed, relief from fear of pregnancy may make the experience a more enjoyable one.

DISORDERS OF THE REPRODUCTIVE SYSTEM

ASSESSMENT

Assessment of a patient with a disorder of the reproductive system includes a tactful and sensitive history. Information is obtained about the following:

1. History of any disorders, illnesses, injuries, surgery and diagnostic investigations of the reproductive system.
2. History and character of menstruation (including menarche, last menstrual period, length of cycle, duration of flow, amount of flow, menopause and last cervical smear test).

3. History of reproductive events including number of pregnancies and the outcome of these (abortion, premature, full-term), delivery (types), children (any stillbirth or neonatal death and cause if known), present health status, complications of pregnancy, history of infertility and cause if known, and present and past use of contraception.
4. Review of function. In reviewing a system questioning should elicit:
   (a) Any changes or disturbances in function (for example, dysmenorrhoea, dissatisfaction with sexual functioning or birth control).
   (b) The presence of any symptoms of disease. If symptoms are present they are explored in order to determine their location, character, duration and severity. The common manifestations of disorders are: pain, lesions, discharges, itching, non-cyclical bleeding, swellings and masses.
5. The patient's sexual roles and how the presenting health problem may affect self-concept and relationships with significant others.

The medical examination includes a general physical examination, with inspection and palpation of internal and external genitalia (Figures 22.17 and 22.18). The examination is personal and invades body boundaries and there is a sense of exposure, particularly during vaginal examination. For these reasons the woman having her first vaginal examination should be prepared in advance for what is involved. The examination procedure is described and she is shown the equipment. The patient undergoing a vaginal examination may have a sense of physical and emotional exposure; the nurse can help to reduce these feelings by a sensitive and supportive approach. This includes such measures during the examination as maintaining privacy by correct draping, restricting access to the room, introducing and explaining the role of those present, including the patient in conversations taking place around her, and accepting her reaction to and fears surrounding the examination.

PATIENT PROBLEMS

The patient with a disorder of the reproductive system presents some special concerns for the nurse. Knowing he or she is a man or a woman gives the person a set of behaviours, culturally and physiologically determined, which help to guide his or her actions. The normal functioning of the reproductive system gives constant reassurance of a person's essential maleness or femaleness. The distortion or interruption of these processes may prove very disturbing to the individual and family.

The person may experience problems in relation to self-image and have fears about future sexual performance and attractiveness. Body parts that contribute to self-esteem and identity have a high psychological investment. The threat posed by loss of these body parts depends on:

* Their meaning to the individual.
* His or her stage of development of body image and self.

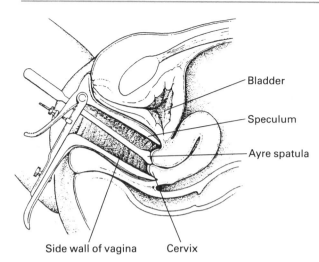

Figure 22.17 Internal vaginal examination demonstrating the position of the speculum and Ayre spatula used to obtain cervical cells for a smear test.

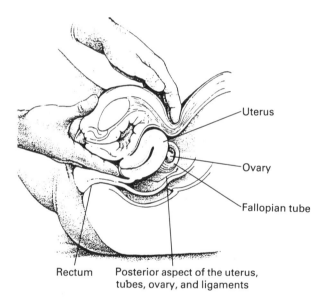

Figure 22.18 Bimanual vaginal examination.

• The reactions of the social group including the spouse, to which the patient belongs.

The person may fear loss of reproductive function. The ability to reproduce is seen by many as a criterion of usefulness and sexuality. The loss of function may be followed by feelings of uselessness or of being only half a person. These feelings can be particularly distressing to the woman who has defined herself in terms of her reproductive and sexual function. To her the removal of her uterus or ovaries may be tantamount to removing her femaleness. Because she may feel less a woman, she fears her husband will see her as less a woman. Indeed, in some unfortunate situations, he may. Thus, to the fear

of loss of reproductive function may be added the fear of loss of a loved one. For some the fear of loss of libido as well as sexual function may be very frightening and can cause the patient much anguish.

Also, most patients have been culturally conditioned to the idea that these areas of the body should not be discussed, much less exposed, in examination or discussion. Such experiences may disturb the individual and produce shame that may be enhanced by lack of privacy and exposure of the body in examinations or during care. Other patients may feel guilt over their illness. Sexually transmitted disease, abortion and cancer arouse guilt feelings in certain individuals which may be expressed as a feeling of 'being punished for past deeds'.

The nurse may be dealing with patients who experience anxiety and fear, shame, guilt, diminished self-esteem or re-awakened anxieties over personal identity. In addition, the long shadow of AIDS may be a particular, unspoken fear for many patients.

GOALS

Patient goals may include:

1. Resolving dysfunctional sexual problems.
2. Achieving a sense of self-worth.
3. Being able to verbalize fears and anxieties.
4. Showing understanding of health problems and what medical intervention involves.
5. Adapting to a change in sexual role and/or function.
6. Being aware of and avoiding risk factors in sexual activity.

NURSING INTERVENTION

These goals may be achieved by the following nursing interventions. The nurse should:

1. Assess the degree of threat posed by loss of function or body parts to the individual and plan, give and evaluate nursing care for that individual based on the assessment.
2. Give physical nursing care which:
   (a) Promotes feelings of dignity, self-worth and attractiveness by attention to personal hygiene and grooming.
   (b) Promotes the return of health, control over body functions and independence.
3. Reduce fear and guilt by:
   (a) Acknowledging and discussing feelings.
   (b) Anticipating the need for explanations and interpretations.
   (c) Clarifying and correcting misinformation about causes of illness, physiology and the consequences, if any, of treatment on present function.
   (d) Maintaining a confident, non-judgemental approach to the patient.
   (e) Assisting in acknowledging the loss, if any.
   (f) Obtaining appropriate additional sources of spiritual or emotional help for the patient.

EVALUATION

Interventions are successful if behavioural changes have occurred, although behavioural changes may be difficult to document in areas such as self-concept, anxiety and guilt. The patient may, for example:

1. State that he or she feels better, less frightened or happier.
2. Take an interest in personal appearance and renew interests in social life, which may also indicate a return to a more positive outlook toward the future.
3. Demonstrate an understanding of the illness, treatments and any residual changes in function to the level of ability or willingness.
4. Demonstrate a knowledge of the risk factors which may lead to a recurrence of the problem and the actions which may reduce or eliminate the risk factors, if appropriate.
5. Discuss alterations in body function and structure with the nurse and so indicate a willingness to begin to deal with the problem or to accept it with appropriate adjustments.

Adjustment to many of these changes requires some time and complete resolution is rarely seen in hospital. Expectations of resolution and effectiveness of intervention must be realistic.

SEXUAL ISSUES ASSOCIATED WITH GIVING NURSING CARE

Several issues involving sexuality may arise in the course of nurse–patient interactions. They reflect the changing role of the patient and involve confusion over the meaning of nursing or patient actions. The most common arise from the intimate level of care involved in nursing and acting out sexual behaviour by the patient.

Touch

The nurse may feel uncomfortable at having to touch the genitals or breasts of patients. The patient may also experience discomfort at being cared for so intimately by the nurse. It reinforces for many adults the dependent child-like role associated with nursing care. On the other hand, touch may be a source of great comfort to patients. Touch should be used with discrimination and its purpose should be understood by both patient and nurse.

Prior to giving nursing care the nurse gives an explanation of what will be done so that the patient is not surprised and has time to adjust. The nurse's movements should be firm, purposeful and reflect a knowledge of the procedure.

Touch for the purpose of comfort is offered as seems appropriate to the situation and patient. Many patients are grateful for a hand to hold during frightening or stressful procedures or times. Other patients would be uncomfortable offered that form of comfort. A knowledge of and sensitivity to the patient assists the nurse in judging what forms of comfort are helpful to which patients.

Male erection

The erections which occur during the delivery of nursing care are most often the result of the stimulation of the spinal reflex arc. The stimulus from a full bladder or perineal care may produce this non-sexual or non-psychological erection. Should this occur during care it is important for the nurse to remain calm, acknowledge the situation and finish care. A flustered nurse who 'runs away' from the patient may increase his confusion, shame and guilt. The patient also needs to understand the nature of reflex, non-sexual erections.

Sexual acting out

A patient may act out sexually to test sexual image, to gain control of the situation, or to attract attention. Examples of sexual acting out in this context include touching the nurse inappropriately, improper suggestions or gestures toward the nurse or self-exposure. The nurse should address the situation directly and unambiguously. The nurse–patient relationship should be defined and any misconceptions about role and function clarified. Limits are set, clearly defined and enforced. Sexual harassment from *any* source, patient or staff is unacceptable.

Meanwhile the patient is helped to explore anxiety and fears. As these are identified and appropriately dealt with, the sexual acting out usually ceases.

Disorders of Sexuality

Disorders of sexuality can occur in each of the four areas of sexuality (see Figure 22.15) but most disorders are psychosexual in origin. Only a few arise from physical illness and trauma or congenital error. Most become obvious through difficulties in sexual expression.

Variations in sexual expression are classified by object choice and sexual aim. Object choice refers to problems such as paedophilia, incest, animal contacts or fetishism (inanimate objects). Variations in sexual aim refers to problems such as voyeurism, exhibitionism and sado-masochism.

Transsexuality is a problem in which the individual appears to have a gender identity at odds with his or her physical self. This results in cross-dressing. The person may seek out sex change therapy because of a deep need to have a body similar to the gender identity.

Occasionally a child reaches puberty and is then discovered to be genetically and internally different from the external genitalia. Because the child has been socialized in the sex role defined by the external genitalia, continuation in the sex assigned at birth is usually advised. It is usually more successful to alter the physical state than to attempt to reverse gender identity and several years of gender role learning. Parents of a child born with ambiguous genitalia should understand the necessity to delay sex assignment until careful physical and genetic screening indicates the true sex of the infant.

SEXUAL CONCERNS

Many persons experience doubts over their inner feelings of being a man or a woman. This may be more prominent in adolescence when the final development of gender identity takes place, but may recur throughout the individual's life. Since sexual identity is considered to be an important component of overall identity, this may stimulate concerns over self-identity.

Concerns over performance are also prevalent. The individual may doubt whether he or she has the necessary physical attributes, experience or appeal to attract, satisfy and keep a sexual partner.

SEXUAL DYSFUNCTION

Sexual dysfunction in the male is most frequently associated with the inability to achieve an erection (impotence) and to delay ejaculation until both partners achieve a sense of satisfaction (premature ejaculation).

In the female, sexual dysfunction may be associated with inhibition of or lack of response (frigidity). Some women may not become sexually excited or, if aroused, do not experience orgasm with intercourse. Women may also complain of painful intercourse (dyspareunia) or a strong contraction of the outer one-third of the vagina (vaginismus) which makes insertion of the penis extremely difficult.

Sexual dysfunction can be the result of psychological, interpersonal or physical factors. Psychological causes may be anger, depression, anxiety, ignorance, or deeper psychosexual conflicts. Interpersonal factors involve conflicts with the partner or an inability to establish interpersonal relationships. Physical causes include illness, injury or drugs.

Diagnosis and treatment involve a history, physical examination and laboratory tests to ascertain the most likely cause. Nurses may be involved in all stages of assessment but are most frequently involved in history taking and case finding.

During history taking the patient is asked if there are any sexual complaints. This makes sexuality an acceptable topic to discuss should the patient have a problem or develop one in the future. If the patient does present with a sexual problem, it is discussed in a frank, open manner, maintaining a broad, objective attitude toward the patient's sexual beliefs and practices. The patient is not urged to disclose more information during a session than he or she is comfortable in revealing. The patient's sexual concerns are assessed in the context of other problems and in the context of value systems.

Once the nature of the problem has been identified, treatment commences. Sexual counselling operates at four levels: (1) permission, (2) limited information, (3) specific suggestions, and (4) intensive therapy. Permission involves reassurance that the patient is normal and may continue doing what he or she has been doing. Limited information involves providing information specific to the patient's concern or problem. This frequently allows the patient to make appropriate changes in behaviour. These changes in behaviour usually involve the patient following a suggested course of action. This may vary from the treatment of organic

disorders to the relearning of sexual behaviours through more in-depth education and sexual exercises. The fourth level, intensive therapy, is highly individualized, in-depth therapy provided by professionals who have advanced experience and knowledge in the sex therapy field.

It is the responsibility of the nurse to create an atmosphere conducive to the identification of sexual problems; if unable to provide the appropriate intervention the nurse should refer the patient to another professional. Nurses with the requisite knowledge and skills and who are comfortable with the subject function in levels one and two, providing reassurance and knowledge of human sexual response and practice in health and illness. Nurses with additional and advanced preparation and experience in sexual therapies may function at higher levels.

Rape Trauma Syndrome

The legal definitions of rape and sexual assault vary between legal jurisdictions. In the United Kingdom rape is legally defined in the 1976 Sexual Offences (Amendment) Act as when a man 'has unlawful sexual intercourse with a woman without her consent and at the time he knows that she does not consent to the intercourse or is reckless as to whether or not she consented to it.' By defining rape as a form of assault the primary motivating factors of anger, aggression and need for power are acknowledged.

Sexual assault is considered a crisis in the life of the victim. It contains the elements of suddenness, arbitrariness and unpredictability: three factors associated with crisis and with rape. A crisis demands psychological and physical adaptation or response from the individual. Crisis is recognizable by the disruption of regular patterns of behaviour and thought which occur in the individuals involved. The degree and nature of the response will vary from one individual to another. Several key factors should be kept in mind in assessing both an individual's initial response to crisis and eventual resolution of crisis. They are:

1. How the individual perceives and understands the incident and feelings about the incident.
2. The emotional stability of the individual prior to the crisis.
3. The coping skills possessed by the individual.
4. The presence or absence of support systems such as family, friends, and colleagues who will be available to assist the individual in the next few days and weeks.

The person in crisis is acutely sensitive to the responses of the individuals around them. The type of intervention a person experiences immediately after sexual assault may either aggravate the crisis or ameliorate it. As the effects of sexual assault may be long-lasting if the crisis is not resolved in a positive manner, it is important for the professionals in contact with the victim to attempt to alleviate the situation. The victims of such assaults have the right to expect to be treated with dignity and respect in a manner that does not take away personal control and to receive prompt physical and emotional support.

In order to provide such services many areas have established rape crisis centres. These centres ensure that the victims are treated in a knowledgeable, caring manner. Some rape crisis centres are independent clinics; others are designated as a part of the emergency department of a hospital. All personnel associated with them should understand and be experienced in dealing with the social, emotional, legal and medical issues surrounding rape and sexual assault.

REACTION TO SEXUAL ASSAULT

Three phases of response to this form of physical and psychological trauma have been identified by Burgess and Holmstrom (1974). They identified a model encompassing the elements of the possible reactions to rape. These are an acute or impact phase, a recoil or adjustment phase and finally a post-traumatic or re-integration phase.

Acute phase

In the acute phase the victim presents a variety of reactions. Initially many will appear very upset; others will appear calm and controlled. The state of seeming control and calm may be an indication of the state of shock the person is in rather than the intensity of their eventual reaction. The individual may express disbelief, fear, anxiety, guilt, shame, helplessness, anger, or rage. Some may be highly irritable and moody; all seem to share a fear of death, fear the attacker will return and fear that it will happen again. Some women fear becoming pregnant and, in the present climate there is also the added fear of having contracted AIDS. They are concerned over why it happened. Some will see their behaviour as contributing to the event; they feel guilty and worry that somehow they encouraged the attack. Occasionally society, with its biases, may support this view. The victim expresses anger toward the assailant and some may convert their anger and helplessness into depression and further guilt.

Physically these women complain of disturbances in eating and sleep patterns, increased headaches, fatigue and gynaecological symptoms and general body pain. Socially, they are fearful and may shun going out. They have increased dependency needs and may find decision-making difficult. Much anxiety may centre around the decision to press charges against the individual or to tell family, friends, and colleagues beccause of fear of misunderstanding by family members and others of their role in the event. Sexually they may retreat from encounters and be unable to enjoy or even tolerate sexual contact for a period of time. This is further aggravated by any physical trauma they have suffered. This phase lasts from a few days to a few weeks.

Adjustment phase

As the victims progress from the initial shock of the acute phase, defence mechanisms emerge and most of the disturbances of that phase decrease. They return to

their normal activities of work, school or home and appear outwardly composed. Most will now attribute the rape to chance or some other societal cause but not to self. They see little need to continue professional counselling or to continue talking about the situation. This is healthy and to be expected and should be encouraged. Most women will pass into this phase. Others will show a maladaptive response such as excessive self-blame, severely altered self-image or agitation and depression. The adjustment phase can last a few weeks to years.

Integration phase

Following the adjustment phase most individuals will feel a need to discuss their experiences. This need is usually triggered by some event, such as an anniversary of the rape. The person may feel emotionally upset, depressed, fearful, angry and may need to talk about the experience.

During this phase the person resolves feelings about the rapist and her role in the rape. She develops a new self-image which allows for the episode of rape. Following this period of sorting-out, the individual is free to take control of her life, accepting the feelings surrounding the assault in a more dispassionate manner. Some patients may never reach this stage.

ASSESSMENT

An accurate and precise history of the event and a physical examination are the first steps in care. Before proceeding, the doctor must obtain a signed consent form from the woman or guardian. The consent, which must be witnessed, obtains permission to do a complete physical and pelvic examination, and to collect the necessary specimens.

The history and physical examinations are used to assess the extent of trauma but are also used to collect evidence that may be used for forensic purposes. Because of the need to collect legal evidence there is usually a well-defined protocol to follow which outlines the information to be obtained and the specimens that are to be collected. Nurses involved in emergency departments must be familiar with the protocol for the assessment of rape victims applicable in their setting.

Most protocols include: a detailed history and description of the assault and the assailant; a recent sexual and menstrual history; a precise description of the physical findings; laboratory tests for infections, sperm, pregnancy and any identifying markers, for example hair which the attacker may have left. The woman's emotional state is also assessed and described.

TREATMENT

The patient receives immediate treatment appropriate to the injuries identified during examination. Follow-up care is equally important in order to prevent un-desirable sequelae.

Extragenital and genital bruising and lacerations are the most common injuries suffered. Bruises are usually not evident at initial examination but will be identified at a follow-up visit. A few patients will be more severely injured and require immediate and extensive medical and nursing care. Occasionally a patient may require a pelvic examination under anaesthesia, with suturing and repair of injury. Most patients, however, will receive treatment for trauma in the emergency department.

The possibility of infection must not be overlooked. A referral to the sexually transmitted disease (STD) clinic (or department of genitourinary medicine as it is officially known) is essential for investigation and follow-up care.

Pregnancy is a potential sequela of rape. Prophylactic treatment is instituted at the discretion of the doctor. A careful sexual, menstrual and birth control history is mandatory in assessing risk. If there is a possibility of pregnancy the patient may receive hormone therapy ('morning-after pill') to prevent it. A combined oestrogen–progestogen preparation is used, for example two tablets of Eugynon or Ovran (equivalent to 100 mg ethinyloestradiol plus 500 mg levonorgestrel). It is given within 72 hours of unprotected intercourse and repeated once 12 hours later. The use of combined oestrogen and progestogen has fewer side-effects when compared with the use of oestrogen alone. The patient is also requested to return in 6 weeks for a pregnancy test so that she may be offered an abortion or pregnancy counselling if it is required. HIV and STD screening is also done at this time.

PSYCHOLOGICAL SUPPORT

Intervention and assessment go hand in hand in the treatment of sexual assault patients. Although separated in this format, the integration of emotional support with assessment and treatment is imperative in the care of these patients. Immediate interventions should include the following:

1. Assume the patient is telling the truth.
2. Go out of your way to demonstrate concern.
3. Advise the patient not to bathe, douche, or clean up in any way as this may destroy vital forensic evidence, and to seek medical attention immediately.
4. In the emergency room, give the patient as much privacy and priority as is possible.
5. Allow a supportive person to remain with the patient.
6. Do not take away personal control.
7. Be gentle in word and deed.
8. Explain clearly the reasons for all examinations and collection of specimens.
9. Assess the extent of the emotional crisis for the individual. For example: What is her manifest emotional state? Is she able to make decisions? What evidence of coping is there? What personal supports does the person have?
10. Allow the expression of feelings.
11. Listen supportively.
12. Explain follow-up and counselling services.
13. Give teaching about tests and follow-up care.

The spouse and family may have a variety of emotions about the assault. Some will be supportive to the victim; others may not. Most families require help in understanding the processes of the examination and emotional reaction of the patient. They should be included in the care by the nurse.

Congenital Anomalies of the Reproductive System

MALDESCENT OF TESTES

Approximately 4% of newborn males will exhibit some form of maldescent of the testes. Unilateral maldescent of testis is about four times as prevalent as bilateral maldescent. The condition is usually the result of hormonal deficiency or mechanical malfunction. The majority of testes descend during the first 3 months of extrauterine life. Many more descend at puberty under the influence of rising testosterone levels. Probably less than 1% of men remain with undescended testes following puberty. The principal sign is an inability to palpate one or both testes in the scrotal sac.

It is important to distinguish between three possible types of maldescent. Retractile testes are those which, under the influence of a strong muscular reflex, are drawn up to the external inguinal ring. This gives a false impression on palpation that the testes are not in the scrotum. No treatment is required. Ectopic testes are those which have descended to an abnormal site. Commonly this is the superficial inguinal pouch but may be almost anywhere near the normal path of descent. Cryptorchidism is a condition in which the descent of the testis is interrupted anywhere along the normal path of descent.

Because histological changes are observed in the undescended testes as early as 4 years of age, treatment is initiated early to ensure maximum functioning of the testes. Orchidopexy (surgical placement and fixation of the testes in the scrotal sac) is the primary method of treatment and should be completed by the age of 1 year. Hernioplasty may also be done to repair the inguinal hernia which is often present in these cases. Hormone therapy in the form of GRH alone or followed by human chorionic gonadotrophins may be given to stimulate production of testosterone in cases of bilateral undescended testes. Successful descent may occur and no other treatment is required, or partial descent may occur, frequently placing the testes in a more favourable position for surgery. Hormone therapy is less successful with unilateral conditions.

Should the condition not be diagnosed until after puberty, orchidopexy is indicated even though the man may be sterile. First, the Leydig cells of the testes continue to produce male hormones which will sustain the secondary sex characteristics. Secondly, such testes have a higher incidence of malignancy than do normally positioned testes and can be more easily examined yearly for malignancy in the scrotum than in the abdomen. In unilateral conditions, the extrascrotal testis will be removed to reduce the possibility of malignancy further. This leaves the man with one functioning testis as a source of sperm and male hormones.

ABSENCE OR DUPLICATION OF ORGANS (MALE)

Congenital absence of the penis, scrotum and vas deferens is very rare. However, in certain genetically determined syndromes, the testicular tissue may be absent or non-functioning. One such example is Klinefelter's syndrome. The person with this syndrome has an XXY genotype; this produces atrophic testes and sterility. The person may also have eunuchoid development, and mental retardation may or may not be present. Androgens are administered to prevent feminization. Other examples are hermaphrodites, or persons who have some characteristics of both sexes. This could be genetically determined as true hermaphroditism or could be due to a feminizing lesion, producing pseudohermaphroditism.

HYPOSPADIAS

Hypospadias arises from a failure of the folds to fuse (see Figure 22.4). Chordee, a curvature of the penis, usually accompanies hypospadias and epispadias. Since the sex of the child may be doubtful, chromosome and endocrine studies will be carried out and treatment based on the results of these findings. In mild cases of hypospadias, no treatment is necessary, as function is usually not impaired. In more severe cases, surgical repair will be necessary. This repair will straighten the penile shaft so that normal intercourse is possible. In addition a urethra will be formed which extends as near as possible to the tip of the glans so that semen is deposited deep in the vagina.

EPISPADIAS

Epispadias is much rarer than hypospadias and is often associated with exstrophy of the bladder (see Figure 22.4). Because of the possible bladder involvement, the patient may be incontinent as a result of imperfect or absent urethral sphincters. Surgical repair provides the child with a functioning penis and urethra.

ABSENCE OR DUPLICATION OF ORGANS (FEMALE)

The uterus, cervix and vagina can undergo duplication or incomplete fusion (see Figure 22.3). The exact incidence of such anomalies is unknown, since they are largely asymptomatic. Some may cause sterility in women or an increased risk of abortion. Rarely an organ is completely absent. Also, as in the male, some absence (agenesis) or maldevelopment of tissue (dysgenesis) is genetically determined. Ovarian agenesis may be the result of an XO genotype (Turner's syndrome). The patient with this genotype may present a characteristic appearance from birth with a webbed neck, multiple anomalies, small birth weight or irregularities of the hairline. However, in others, the patient may present in adolescence because of the failure of the menarche to appear. Treatment may be oestrogen replacement therapy, with 20 µg being given every day for 3 weeks, followed by withdrawal combined with norethisterone, 5 mg daily on days 12–21. Withdrawal of oestrogen permits the endometrium to slough away, thus simulating a menstrual period. The addition of progesterone prevents endometrial hyperplasia due to oestrogen stimulation. Because the ovaries do not exist, the patient remains sterile.

IMPERFORATE HYMEN

Normally the hymen is patent. Rarely, it may not be. Usually the condition is not discovered until adolescence when the girl may present herself because of absence of menstrual flow. Menstruation occurs but the menstrual blood is retained behind the closed hymen. The patient may complain of crampy, lower abdominal pain occurring monthly. She may also notice dysuria, frequency, and urinary retention as the growing mass of retained menstrual blood accumulates in the vagina, putting increasing pressure on the bladder and urethra. Treatment consists of a cross-shaped incision of the hymen which allows drainage of the debris. This debris is often a thick, chocolate-like material. Because of this old blood, the risk of postoperative infection is greatly increased. Antibiotics are usually ordered. The nurse must pay careful attention to good aseptic technique postoperatively to reduce the risk of infection further. The nurse must see that adequate drainage is maintained, frequent cleansing of the perineum occurs, and perineal dressings are changed frequently.

The hymen may also be rigid. This is usually discovered when the patient presents with a complaint of dyspareunia. In mild cases the patient will be instructed to dilate the hymen digitally, usually while sitting in a bath of warm water. If this does not succeed, vaginal dilators may be inserted by the doctor or nurse and later by the patient. In difficult cases, hymenotomy is performed.

Fertility and Infertility

CONTROL OF FERTILITY

Perhaps one of the greatest problems facing the world today is the control of fertility. The implications of overpopulation have usually been stated in terms of the developing nations, but have taken on a global context. In addition, contraception is considered a matter of personal decision—it can exercise an important liberalizing potential for the family or the single person. In the light of these discussions the health professional has a responsibility to extend the knowledge and availability of contraception to anyone who requests it. With more birth control clinics available the nurse has a major role in the control of fertility.

NURSING RESPONSIBILITIES

Generally, the nursing responsibilities include referral of the patient to the appropriate clinic or doctor and education and interpretation. Depending on the nurse's situation and knowledge, these may be taken care of in an initial interview (or group discussion) with a patient (or a group of patients) seeking birth control advice.

The nurse can assist the patient or couple in making a decision by presenting concise, factual information about the methods available. The couple should choose a method which will be most compatible with their personal circumstances. Most certainly this should be the one they will use and feel comfortable in using. No method of birth control is effective unless it is used constantly. This final decision is usually made with medical counsel. As the doctor reviews the patient's history, he or she may make other recommendations which will affect the person's or couple's choice. The patient or couple will need counselling in the proper use of the method they have chosen and what to expect in the period of initial adjustment. The nurse should validate the patient's real understanding of the method chosen and provide explanations and interpretations if necessary. In a simple fashion the knowledge of an alternative emergency method should be provided as well, for it is this which may prevent a pregnancy. The patient should leave the clinic or hospital with knowledge of an alternative method. Usually, the use of spermicidal foam or the use of a condom by the male will overcome these situations and has the added advantage of safety in terms of risk reduction with regard to sexually transmitted disease (e.g. AIDS). The nurse is responsible for gaining sufficient knowledge of the complex subject of contraception to be able to present factual knowledge to couples and to discuss the advantages and disadvantages of each method. In addition, the nurse will need to understand much of the emotional, social and religious aspects of contraception. A detailed presentation of family planning is beyond the scope of this work, but a brief outline of methods follows.

METHODS OF CONTRACEPTION

Coitus interruptus

This method consists of the male withdrawing his penis from the vagina before ejaculation occurs and ejaculating outside the vagina. Coitus interruptus, or withdrawal, is better than no attempt at birth control but is still very unreliable. Care must be taken not to ejaculate on or near the vulva, as the sperm may make their way into the vagina and pregnancy can result. The method requires the man to have advance awareness of ejaculation. This control and knowledge may be difficult to establish and may require more sexual experience than the man or couple possesses. Also, some sperm may escape before ejaculation occurs. The method has also come under considerable criticism for its psychological effects. These have been associated principally with frustration as a result of unresolved sexual tensions on the part of one or both partners. However, if the method is accepted by the couple and orgasm and ejaculation do occur, the resulting psychological stresses are probably minimal.

Condom

The condom is a thin rubber sheath which is placed over the penis before intromission. It prevents pregnancy by acting as a mechanical barrier to the sperm. Proper use includes application before intromission to avoid the possibility of a pre-ejaculatory emission of semen into the vagina and careful withdrawal of the penis and condom following intercourse to be sure that some semen is not lost into the vagina or over the vulva (see Table 3.2). Some doctors advise the use of a spermicidal jelly as a lubricating agent over the condom. This is a method of additional safety, particularly if the condom should be defective. However, newer methods of manufacture have greatly reduced this hazard. The condom is reasonably priced and is available without prescription. This greatly increases its availability and makes it one of the most widely used methods in the world.

Some couples find it objectionable as a method of birth control because it may interrupt sexual foreplay, it can lessen sensation, and its effective use relies heavily on the motivation of the male. These objections can be overcome if it is used by a man who is taking mature responsibility for his behaviour, especially in view of the hazards of contracting AIDS (see Table 3.3).

Diaphragm

The diaphragm is a thin rubber cap which is inserted into the vagina by the woman and placed over the cervical os. The cap provides a mechanical barrier to the sperm. In addition a spermicidal jelly is placed on both sides of the cap. When the diaphragm is in place the spermicidal jelly will be in touch with the cervix and vagina.

The diaphragm is not dispensed without a prescription and requires individual fittings by a doctor initially, after a few months of use and following pregnancy or miscarriage. The woman also requires careful teaching in the proper insertion and care of the diaphragm. The diaphragm is inserted manually or with an inserter which is provided. The position of a diaphragm should be checked following each insertion. The woman stands with one foot elevated or squats. The diaphragm is squeezed between two fingers, thus narrowing it, and the woman slips the diaphragm into her vagina. In its proper position, the diaphragm cups the cervix with its anterior side behind the pubic bone and its posterior side in the posterior fornix of the vagina. Following insertion, the woman must be taught to check the position of the diaphragm to see that it is properly situated. Properly positioned, it is not felt by either partner. It can be left in place for 24 hours but should then be removed and cleansed with soap and water. Removal should not take place until at least 6 hours postcoitus to ensure death of all sperm present in the vagina.

Used by well instructed, highly motivated, women it is a highly effective method of birth control. Some women find it distasteful to insert the diaphragm and to check its position; for these women it is probably a poor method of birth control.

Spermicidal preparations

In more recent years chemicals with a spermicidal

action have been placed in gels, creams, aerosol foams, suppositories and foam tablets. These are inserted into the vagina about 30 minutes before intercourse. The foam or jelly coats the cervix and inner vaginal walls. It should remain in the vagina for at least 6 hours to be sure that all sperm are dead. Used consistently, the method can be effective, particularly for the older woman approaching the menopause. Objections to the method revolve around the messiness which can result after coitus. Some men may complain of a slight urethral irritation when some foaming types of preparations are used.

Douche

The vaginal douche or irrigation may be used for cleanliness following coitus or may be considered to be a method of birth control by those who are under the impression that it 'washes the sperm away'. In fact, it may force the sperm into the uterine cavity and merely speed them on their way. It is not a method of contraception.

Breast-feeding

Under the stimulus of breast-feeding many women remain anovulatory for several months. Others quickly regain their fertility. Hence, breast-feeding should not be considered a method of birth control.

Rhythm method

This method requires temporary abstinence from coitus during the possible ovulation time of the woman. It is the only method of birth control officially sanctioned by all religions. The rationale of the method is based on several assumptions. First, a woman is only fertile at the time of ovulation, which occurs once monthly at a predictable time, and the ovum lives for approximately 24 hours. Secondly, sperm will survive in the genital tract for only 3 days. Placing these facts together, and allowing 3 days before and after ovulation for the life span of the sperm, we arrive at 6 days. Since we know that the time of ovulation varies in any one woman we must allow 1 or 2 days for extra safety on either side. This now gives us a fertile period of approximately 8 days' duration, falling near the middle of the menstrual cycle.

The crux of the problem is the timing of ovulation. Since no anticipatory method of timing ovulation has been discovered, we must rely on a retrospective view of the time of ovulation in any one woman. Under the influence of the rising progesterone levels following ovulation, the basal body temperature in women shows a rise. This rise should be noticeable within the first 24 hours following ovulation. The temperature remains slightly elevated for the remainder of the cycle. Also, at the time of ovulation, the cervical mucus changes. There is an increase in amount and a reduction in viscosity. Women can be taught to recognize and record these changes. Most doctors will attempt to predict the time of ovulation for any one woman after she has carefully recorded the dates of her menstrual periods, the mucus

changes, and her temperatures taken daily at a uniform time. Depending on the woman, doctor or clinic, this may be done for 3–6 months. An average is then calculated from these dates and her individual period of likely fertility is plotted. The calculated fertile period should be reviewed at specified intervals. At periods of her life when ovulation is being established or re-established, during post partum and lactation or menopause and during periods of emotional stress the method is highly unreliable. In women of very regular periods and with high motivation the method has had success. However, until a foolproof method of anticipating ovulation is achieved, this method is unreliable.

Intrauterine device

An intrauterine device (IUD) is an object placed inside the uterus which remains in the uterus and prevents pregnancy. The action is not completely understood. Some doctors believe that an IUD creates a hostile intrauterine environment either for sperm or for the fertilized ovum. Others feel that it is implantation which is prevented.

The IUD ranks as a very effective method of birth control in about 80% of the women who try it. Most IUDs used today are made of a flexible plastic and are in several shapes. The addition of copper or progesterone to the IUD produces a more effective device.

The device must be inserted by a doctor or other suitably trained person. It is a sterile procedure. First, the doctor will sound the uterus, confirming its depth and position. Then, having threaded the IUD into the inserter, he or she will insert this through the cervix, push down the plunger and retract the inserter. The use of the uterine sound and the skill of the person greatly reduce the risk of perforating the uterus. Uterine perforation during insertion remains a rare complication. Insertion of an IUD may be painful in the nullipara because of the tightness of the cervical os. Insertion is tolerated well by a majority of women.

Many devices are equipped with strings which hang into the vagina just below the cervix. The woman is taught to check for the presence of these strings monthly after her menstrual period. The IUD can be expelled from the uterus, and this is most likely to occur during the menstrual period. Women who have never been pregnant have an increased tendency to expel the device, as have women who have previously expelled it. If the woman notices that the IUD appears to have been expelled, she should report this to the doctor so that this can be confirmed. The use of an alternative form of birth control would be advisable in the interim.

Removal of the device is carried out by a doctor. A woman should be discouraged from removing her own IUD. Some are difficult to remove because of their shape.

Complications and contraindications of the use of an IUD include increased menstrual loss and cramping. These are the most common side-effects and approximately 15% of women will require removal of the IUD for these reasons.

Pregnancy does occur in about 3% of women using an intrauterine device. If the patient wishes to continue with the pregnancy, the IUD is removed if possible. The risk of spontaneous abortion is about 50% with the IUD in place and there is an increased risk of infection. These risks vary with the type of IUD and its location in the uterine cavity.

The IUD contributes to the development of pelvic inflammatory disease (PID) in about 2% of women. If neglected, PID contributes to sterility. The only sign of this infection may be irregular intramenstrual bleeding and complaints of pain. If an infection is suspected, the IUD is removed and the infection treated. The IUD is contraindicated in women with a pelvic infection or those at high risk of one.

Rarely an IUD can pass silently through the uterine wall into the abdominal cavity. This may be discovered when the woman cannot locate the strings, gets pregnant, or experiences abdominal or pelvic symptoms. It is removed during laparotomy.

Oral contraceptives

Birth control pills are synthetic chemical hormones which resemble the female hormones of the ovary. In suppressing ovulation they mimic the action of pregnancy. The high hormone levels depress the hypothalamus, which in turn inhibits the release of pituitary gonadotrophins which stimulate ovulation. Thus, the woman is anovulatory. Protection is established as soon as the woman begins taking the pills, if she starts taking them on day 1 of the menstrual cycle.

The pills are divided into two types, the combined pill and progestogen pill. The combined pill contains synthetic oestrogen and progesterone hormones in each pill. This pill is more effective in preventing pregnancy because it induces changes in the cervix, making the mucus thicker and more impenetrable by sperm. Also, changes occur in the endometrium which would discourage implantation should fertilization occur.

The progestogen or 'mini-pill', contains a progestational agent and no oestrogen. It should not be confused with the low-dose (30 µg oestrogen) combined pill. Many of a woman's menstrual cycles while on the progestogen pill may be ovulatory. This pill depends on the effects of progestogen to produce changes in cervical mucus, the endometrium and hormonal levels to inhibit fertilization. Because of the reduced oestrogenicity of the pill it has fewer major side-effects than the combined pill but is slightly less effective in

preventing pregnancy. This makes the low-dose combined pill the pill of choice initially. The risk of pregnancy in both types of pills is minimal if taken as prescribed.

The combined pill is taken once a day for 21 days (sometimes 20) and no pill for the next 7 days, regardless of the woman's period. Initially, the first pill is taken on the first or fifth day of the woman's menstrual period. Now the pill will regulate her menstrual cycle and she takes them as prescribed. It is wise for her to cross them off on a calendar or devise a method of knowing when to start again because each succeeding 21-day series of pills is begun on the basis of when she took the last pill, not on her subsequent menstrual period. She begins again regardless of the state of her menstrual period. Progestogen pills are taken every day without omission. This does make it easier for women to follow, for no timing, counting or remembering other than to take the pill is required. Also, to maintain consistently high hormonal levels in the body, the pill should be taken at approximately the same time each day.

Withdrawal bleeding is regulated by the pill and occurs regularly at some time during the 7 pill-free days. This withdrawal bleeding simulates true menstruation. With the withdrawal of the high hormone levels, the endometrium sloughs away. However, menstruation is usually scantier and shorter, since the endometrium is thinner. A woman may miss one period but, should she miss two, this should be reported to the doctor immediately.

Much discussion has occurred over the possible side-effects or complications attendant on the use of oral contraceptives. For many women, adjustment to oral contraceptives may take some months (Table 22.4). During that time she may experience nausea, fullness and tingling in her breasts, headache, some spotting between menstrual periods, weight gain, chloasma or masking of pregnancy, acne, loss of libido or changes in vaginal discharge. On the other hand she may feel better, have relief from menstrual cramps and have an increased libido. Sometimes changes in dosages or in the timing of taking the pill helps. If she takes the pill with supper or lunch, she may feel less nauseated later.

The missed pill is cause for concern in many women. The woman should take the pill when she remembers it and take the next pill as she is accustomed to do. This may mean taking two pills in one day. Should more than

Table 22.4   Side-effects of oral contraceptives.

Oestrogen	Progestogen	Oestrogen and progestogen
Breakthrough bleeding	Acne	Weight gain
Nausea	Depression	Post pill amenorrhoea
Headaches	Dry vagina	Increased breast size
Chloasma	Loss of	Breast tenderness
Increased vaginal discharge	libido	
Cervical erosion		
Cystic breast changes		

one pill be missed, then the couple should use an alternative form of birth control for the remainder of that cycle. If several pills are missed, the doctor should be consulted, as the cycles may be sufficiently interrupted as to require some further regulating under medical supervision.

The major complications of the pill are rare but serious. For some women the hazards of the pill are still less than the hazards of a pregnancy or an abortion. Major concern revolves around the increased incidence of diseases of the circulatory system in women using the pill. The major circulatory diseases include thromboembolic disease, coronary artery disease, cerebrovascular accidents and hypertension. The risks rise with age, cigarette smoking, and duration (over 5 years) of pill use. Thus the smoking woman who has been using oral contraceptives for 5 years or more and is over 35 is placing herself at considerable risk if she continues use of the pill. Such women should be counselled to give up smoking and if unable to do so, to consider another method of birth control.

The long-term taking of pills (5–7 years) with high oestrogen content is associated with an increased risk of developing a rare, benign tumour of the liver. These tumours may cause rupture of the liver capsule with subsequent haemorrhage.

These complications have brought prolonged use of oral contraceptives into question. However, medical opinion still supports widespread use of the pill for carefully chosen women. The role of the family planning doctor and nurse is of great importance. The factors of past health, age, and smoking history are important, as is the duration of use.

Some benefits may accrue for a woman who has taken oral contraceptives. The risk of PID is lower, and women who have taken the pill for longer than 1 year have lower risks of developing cancer of the uterus and ovary. No association between cancer of the breast and the pill has been demonstrated.

Women on a contraceptive pill should see a doctor every 6 months to have their blood pressure and weight monitored and for an assessment of their general health. Pelvic examination is carried out annually and a cervical smear test is performed at least every 3 years. They are taught to seek prompt medical care if they experience severe or recurrent abdominal pain, chest pain and shortness of breath, severe headaches, eye problems such as blurred vision, flashing lights or tenderness and warmth over veins in the legs.

Safe birth control, compatible with the woman's lifestyle, will demand the use of several different methods of birth control throughout her life. The pill is best during periods of high risk for pregnancy and a strong desire to avoid pregnancy; the IUD, diaphragm, or condom for periods of higher risk but less desire to avoid pregnancy or to space children; finally, sterilization for those who wish no more worries in this direction.

Long-acting injectable steroids are used in some countries. Most are in depot form but some are in capsules inserted surgically under the skin. Capsules avoid the depot's disadvantage of not being able to immediately to stop the action of the drug. Both types produce highly effective long-term suppression of ovulation producing amenorrhoea. They have the same side-effects as the pill but, in addition, return of ovulation may be delayed for 5 months after removing the capsule or after the depot has ceased to release steroids. These problems have delayed their universal acceptance.

Sterilization

Sterilization means the termination of reproductive capacity. As the social and emotional barriers to sterilization have altered, it has increased in popularity. When family size is complete, many couples choose sterilization as the method of birth control. In other cases, when the hazards of pregnancy are lifethreatening, it may be strongly indicated.

Removal of any or all of the major organs of reproduction in either male or female results in sterility. Generally that is considered too extreme. A simple method of mechanically barring sperm and egg from meeting is required which will neither reduce natural hormone levels nor affect sexual capacity.

Vasectomy

In men vasectomy will accomplish this purpose. This simple operation can be done on an out-patient basis or at a clinic. On the surface of the scrotum the ascending spermatic cord is palpated and identified. Under local anaesthetic a small incision is made slightly to one side of each cord. The vas deferens is exposed, severed and electrocoagulated. Thus, new sperm are barred from reaching the vagina. Other sperm are still present in the tract above the ligation. For this reason a man is not considered sterile until he has had two negative sperm counts postoperatively.

The first sperm count is done after 10 ejaculations and is repeated following a further series of ejaculations until a negative sperm count is obtained.

In the immediate postoperative period the man may expect some minor bruising and discomfort for 24–72 hours. The discomfort is relieved by a simple analgesic, rest and wearing a scrotal support. Protected intercourse is resumed when he feels comfortable to do so. Few major side-effects, either physical or emotional, are reported following the procedure. Some cases are recorded of reconstructing the vas deferens. However, the rate of successful reconstruction is low. This is partly due to extravasation of sperm which causes the development of sperm antibodies following vasectomy. Even though physical reconstruction of the vas deferens might be possible, the antibodies continue to destroy the sperm. Vasovasostomy (repair of the separated vas deferens) produces fertility in only 22% of men. Thus, the patient should regard a vasectomy as irreversible.

Tubal ligation

Tubal ligation is the comparable operation in women. It can be done vaginally but is usually done abdominally. Under a general anaesthetic two small incisions are made in the abdomen. The fallopian tube is dissected, a loop of tube is lifted up, ligated, and above the ligation is either crushed with a clamp or severed. In some operations the uterine end of the tube may be turned back and embedded in the posterior wall of the uterus. Various names for these techniques include Madlener, Pomeroy and Irving. Tubal coagulations, in conjunction with a laparoscopy, may also be done. The surgeon identifies the tubes through the laparoscope and then applies the heat source which coagulates the tube. In the hands of a skilled operator the procedure is safe and associated with few side-effects. As in the male, the tubes can be reconstructed, but the success rate is not high. Thus, the patient should see the operation as irreversible. The operation is not entirely harmless. Rare major complications postoperatively can be pulmonary embolism and later tubal pregnancy. These make the operation a more hazardous procedure than a vasectomy.

Nursing responsibilities in both operations include regular preoperative and postoperative care. However, in addition to the consent for operation, there is a separate consent form for sterilization which must be signed before the operation.

INFERTILITY

Infertility is defined as the failure to conceive after 12 months of adequate exposure without the use of contraceptives. Primary infertility refers to a couple who have never conceived. Secondary infertility refers to a couple who have had a previous pregnancy but now cannot conceive. Approximately 10% of couples prove infertile. Of this 10%, about 40% of the problem rests with the man, 40% with the woman and from 5–10% with the couple as a unit.

CAUSES OF INFERTILITY

The possible causes of infertility are too numerous to list. However, the major causes can be grouped under several headings. Any impairment of ovarian function which interrupts ovulation creates infertility. This may be caused by hormonal imbalances or may be due to some intrinsic defect in the ovaries themselves. The same is true of the testes. The conducting system may not be patent. Infections leading to adhesions are a major cause in both men and women. Malformations or displacements of the organs of the reproductive tract may contribute to infertility. The problem may arise because of unique factors particular to the union. Vaginal secretions may not be compatible with the seminal fluid, causing the sperm to die.

ASSESSMENT AND DIAGNOSIS

The investigation usually begins when the woman presents herself to the gynaecologist with a complaint of failure to conceive. By this time the problem may have become a nagging fear for both her and her husband. Often reassurance and ventilation of the anxiety seem to help the patient, for many patients are reported as returning shortly thereafter as pregnant. A persistent infertility case will require thorough investigation. Many gynaecologists prefer to see the couple together so that both partners may receive an outline and discussion of the approach which will be used. The doctor's assessment of the possible cause of the infertility will guide the direction of the investigation. Some techniques which are used in investigating infertility are described.

Medical history and physical examination

A detailed medical history and physical examination are done for both partners. Particular attention will be paid to the development of the secondary sex characteristics and any evidence of virilizing or feminizing effects. Any history of infections, and injuries involving the genitourinary tract will be carefully noted. In addition the doctor will take a marital history to gain an adequate picture of the couple's sexual pattern. The woman will be asked to give a detailed menstrual history. At this point some education in human reproduction may help the couple.

Before other tests are begun, infections, particularly cervicitis and prostatitis, are likely to be treated, as they may contribute to infertility. Anaemia, poor health, exhaustion, overwork, stress and other psychological situations all may be causative factors, and the doctor often tries to relieve these first if they seem of sufficient magnitude to be affecting the sexual adjustment of the couple.

Ovulation

Whether or not ovulation occurs monthly may have to be established. The patient is asked to keep a basal body temperature chart. This also helps the doctor to estimate hormonal levels. The woman is asked to come to the surgery or clinic near ovulation time. Cervical smears will be taken and tested for spinnbarkeit and ferning. Respectively, these tests help to time ovulation and indicate how receptive the cervical mucus is to sperm. If ferning appears to be unsatisfactory, the patient may be requested to return for serial vaginal smears, which give indications of ovulation.

Plasma assay will be done to assess the levels of FSH and LH. Plasma progesterone levels are sampled one week after the biphasic shift in the basal body temperature graph, or day 21 in the 28-day cycle. These results, together with the graphs and other tests, permit an outline of the events of the menstrual cycle that are occurring in the woman.

Urinalysis

Urine tests may be done to measure urinary oestriols and, if the doctor feels it is warranted, the presence and amount of 17-ketosteroids.

Endometrial biopsy

This is done to indicate whether or not a healthy endometrium is present. If it is not, then the problem may be one of failure of the fertilized ovum to achieve successful implantation. Occasionally tuberculosis, hitherto unsuspected, is discovered, and may be the cause of the infertility.

Laparoscopy

Laparoscopy allows the direct visualization of pelvic contents and an opportunity to perform ovarian biopsies if necessary. It may also be combined with a hysterosal-pingogram.

Hysterosalpingogram

A hysterosalpingogram is the injection of a radiopaque contrast medium into the genital tract. It serves to outline the uterine cavity and uterine tubes. The patient may not be anaesthetized. The test is done in the X-ray department under sterile technique. The patient is usually asked to move from side to side after the injection in order to promote spilling of the contrast medium into the abdominal cavity. This test provides information about the exact location of any abnormality.

Possible complications of tubal patency tests. Pain, collapse and vomiting may be experienced shortly after the test is done, especially in women who were not anaesthetized. The patient should be observed for these signs for approximately 3 hours following a test. Helping the patient to assume a knee–chest position for a few minutes before standing up may prevent further discomfort. Cramps and vomiting may be more prevalent following cervical dilatation.

Other complications may include exacerbation of pelvic infections, air embolism or sensitivity reactions to the contrast medium and inadvertent abortion.

On the other hand, either of the tests may be therapeutic because they may have opened the tract. This is supported by many patients who conceive with no further treatment.

Sims–Huhner postcoital test

Postcoitally, a specimen of seminal fluid from the posterior fornix of the vagina and the cervical canal is aspirated. The specimen is examined for motility of the sperm and their ability to survive in the cervix or vagina. The test is best performed at the time of ovulation. The patient will be instructed not to douche or use lubricants for 2 days before the test. Following inter-course she will remain supine, hips elevated on a pillow for 30 minutes. Within the next 2–4 hours she will come to the doctor's surgery or the fertility clinic, at which time the specimen will be taken. A reading will assess how many live, motile sperm are in the specimen. Should the sperm not be present, the investigation may be directed toward the male. Does he have sperm? If he does, why is he not capable of depositing them near the cervix? If they are dead or non-motile, the vaginal environment may be hostile to them. One such reaction is due to the stimulus a foreign protein (sperm) evokes in the woman's body. Consequently, antibodies develop. The antibodies in the female inactivate the sperm before fertilization can take place. Following a 3–6-month period of abstinence or the use of a condom by the male, circulating antibodies may be sufficiently reduced to permit sperm to live long enough to fertilize.

Cross hostility

This test is carried out when the postcoital test is negative. A drop of ejaculate is placed on a slide with a drop of cervical mucus. Sperms should be seen actively invading the mucus. If not, the mucus may be impenetrable for several reasons or the sperm may have low motility. If the problem is with the mucus, any infection which is present is treated and oestrogen may be given from day 1 to day 10 of the menstrual cycle to produce a more watery penetrable mucus.

Semen analysis

A specimen of seminal fluid will be examined for volume and the number, morphology and motility of sperm. Ideally, 2–5 ml of fluid should be present. The fluid should gel and then reliquefy after 15–20 minutes. The sperm should number above 60 million per millilitre of ejaculate, and 60% should still show vigorous activity when examined at room temperature 2 hours after ejaculation. Not more than 20% of the sperm should show abnormal forms.

The specimen is collected after a 3-day period of abstinence from coitus. It is collected in a dry, sterile jar by masturbation or coitus interruptus and is brought to the clinic for examination within 2 hours of collection.

If no sperm are present in the ejaculate, the patency of the duct system may be assessed by a vasogram. Testicular biopsy may be indicated. If the biopsy shows living sperm, then the failure of the sperm to arrive in the seminal fluid may be due to a blockage in the tube. If the semen is acidic, it may result from a failure of seminal vesicle fluid to reach the prostatic fluid and neutralize the semen. Hormone assays of FSH, LH and testosterone will also be done.

Sperm penetration assay

This test assesses whether or not sperm can penetrate a hamster egg. The sperm are washed with a buffer solution and transported to the laboratory where the test is done. Whether the sperm washed in the buffer solution have improved penetrating capacity, both in vivo and in vitro, is determined. Some sperm which cannot penetrate an ovum before being washed can do so afterwards. Even if the washed sperm do not penetrate a hamster egg, there have been cases where they have penetrated the wife's ovum. However, a penetration of 0% of the hamster egg is a poor prognosis for fertility.

The test is a useful and rapid way to test male fertility, particularly in oligospermic men. It can be a method of treatment if washed sperm are used to fertilize the wife's ovum.

TREATMENT

Surgery

In both male and female, surgery is aimed at restoring function. Adhesions may be released; the ducts are reconstructed. Cysts and tumours are removed as indicated. The nursing care is the same as that for any pelvic operative procedure.

Hormone therapy

Clomiphene. Hormones may be administered to in-duce ovulation. Clomiphene (Clomid) is an antioestrogenic substance which stimulates the hypothalamus to stimulate the pituitary to increase the output of FSH and LH. By displacing the circulating oestrogens, the hypothalamus is released from the inhibiting effects of high levels of oestrogen. In addition, clomiphene may increase ovarian sensitivity to FSH and LH.

Treatment consists of administering 50–200 mg pills daily for 5 days. These tablets may be started on the fifth day of the cycle or at any time if no cycles are occurring. Ovulation is expected 7–12 days following treatment. The patient must be instructed to monitor her basal body temperature carefully, as a rise in temperature is expected with ovulation. Coitus should occur close to ovulation. Treatment may be repeated several times until pregnancy occurs or the treatment is judged ineffective. Good rates of success are recorded. Clomiphene is more successful when used in situations of altered function, such as amenorrhoea following the oral contraceptives or anovulation in Stein–Leventhal syndrome.

The drug does stimulate the growth of benign ovarian cysts which usually disappear after its use. The incidence of multiple births is increased in couples using this medication. There do not appear to be any long-term effects.

Gonadotrophins. The gonadotrophins may be supplied artificially. Hypothalamic-releasing factors may be given to stimulate the pituitary. Human pituitary gonadotrophins made from freeze-dried human pituitaries may be administered. These are, in effect, the FSH and LH hormones. The patient receives injections of FSH to ripen a follicle and then LH to stimulate ovulation. The process is complex, necessitating close monitoring of the patient for ovulation and for overstimulation of the ovaries. Ovarian cysts follow its use, as do multiple pregnancies. Like clomiphene, good pregnancy rates have been achieved. Because of abortions and high fetal wastage associated with prematurity and multiple births, the overall success rate in terms of live children is lower.

Bromocriptine. Occasionally, a woman experiences amenorrhoea due to elevated prolactin levels secondary to pregnancy, steroid contraceptives, pituitary tumours or other drugs and treatments. High prolactin levels inhibit the effect of FSH and LH on the ovary. Bromocriptine is an ergot derivative which inhibits release of prolactin from the pituitary. As the prolactin levels fall FSH and LH stimulate the ovary to ovulate. About two-thirds of patients treated become ovulatory. The major side-effects are nausea and dizziness.

Hormone therapy may also be instituted in the man. Gonadotrophins may be prescribed and have achieved some success in raising the sperm counts of men with low counts. Sometimes vitamin B will be prescribed to ensure the normal inactivation of oestrogens by the liver. Varying doses of testosterone may be tried with varying rates of success.

NURSING RESPONSIBILITIES

Most infertility investigations and treatments are done on an out-patient basis or during short hospitalization. Some nurses may be involved in infertility clinics; others may see the patient only during a brief visit to hospital to have an investigative test. Depending on the involvement, the nurse may be expected to:

1. Provide education in human reproduction and sex education.
2. Teach the patient how to perform certain tests or treatments accurately, using clear detailed instructions.
3. Prepare the patient physically and emotionally for the procedure.
4. Assist the patient and doctor during investigative procedures.
5. Monitor the patient's physical and emotional status post-treatment for the development of complications.
6. Respond appropriately to changes in patient condition, for example if the patient experiences vomiting, nursing measures for dealing with vomiting are used.
7. Realize that the patient may come to the investigation with a sense of failure and decreased self-esteem and respond in ways which do not increase the sense of failure or further decrease self-esteem.
8. Be sensitive to the possible grief over loss of reproductive function and feelings of inadequacy.

Disorders of the Menstrual Cycle and Menstruation

MITTELSCHMERZ

Mittelschmerz is a feeling of lower abdominal pain on one side on or near ovulation day. It is thought to be caused by fluid or blood escaping from the ruptured follicle site and causing peritoneal irritation. It occurs in about 25% of women. Occasionally when the right side is involved, fear of appendicitis may bring the woman to the doctor.

PREMENSTRUAL TENSION

This syndrome (PMS) is probably experienced by most women in mild forms. However, extreme cases are seen. The symptomatology includes a feeling of fullness or heaviness in the lower abdomen, backache, painful breasts, irritability, headache, weight gain premenstrually, nervousness, depression and insomnia.

The absence of normative data on the physical and emotional changes in the menstrual cycle mean that the syndrome has not been clearly defined. No single aetiology has been identified and several theories of aetiology exist. Diuretics are now considered to have been over-used and the theory relating all symptoms to fluid retention has not been supported.

What seems clear is that somatic and psychological symptoms exist; they occur cyclically but in varying degrees with each cycle. There is usually an abrupt onset and departure of the symptoms and the woman tends to be 35 years of age or older.

Among the treatments that are usually tried are birth control pills, pyridoxine (vitamin B_6), progesterone and bromocriptine. Any of these treatments may help some women. For patients suffering severe psychological symptoms, psychotherapy may be recommended both to provide support and to distinguish between other emotional disturbances which may be present and masking as premenstrual tension.

Treatment consists in taking a sympathetic and understanding approach, as the patient may be very upset by the changes of mood and behaviour which she experiences. Women are taught to chart their symptoms to reduce the unexpectedness of them, to talk about these changes with husband and family in order to increase family understanding, to eat nutritious, regular meals, and to reduce stress during the latter half of the menstrual cycle.

Further research into the complex neuroendocrinological relationships of the menstrual cycle is needed before all the symptoms associated with the menstrual cycle can be fully understood and effectively treated.

DYSMENORRHOEA

Dysmenorrhoea is defined as pain with menstruation. Two types, primary and secondary dysmenorrhoea, are commonly distinguished.

PRIMARY DYSMENORRHOEA

Primary dysmenorrhoea is a spasmodic type of pain, occurring at the onset of the menstrual period and lasting from 1–24 hours. It is most common among young girls, rarely beginning with the menarche and fading away spontaneously around 24 years of age or following the delivery of a full-term infant. No pathology in pelvic structures is associated with this type of dysmenorrhoea. In addition to the cramps, there may be shivering, a feeling of tension, nausea, vomiting, pallor and fainting.

Prostaglandins are considered the cause of the increased myometrial activity and subsequent pain experienced. Excessive quantities of prostaglandins are synthesized during the breakdown of the secretory endometrium in some women. They cause increased muscular contractions, uterine ischaemia and are also responsible for the symptoms of nausea, vomiting and pallor by their influence on smooth muscle. Other cramps are caused by clots stretching the internal os of the cervix.

Dysmenorrhoea is also associated with ovulation, as anovulatory cycles are rarely accompanied by dysmenorrhoea. This probably explains why the first cycles are pain-free and dysmenorrhoea in some girls is synchronous with ovulation. Also, the daughters of women who have suffered dysmenorrhoea are more frequently dysmenorrhoeic. Whether this is learned or inherited is unclear. In any case the psyche can play a role in aggravating the symptoms but is very rarely the sole explanation. A woman's personal tolerance for discomfort undoubtedly affects her response to any pain, dysmenorrhoea being no exception.

Treatment includes a kind and sympathetic approach by all members of the health team. Prostaglandin inhibitors such as acetylsalicylic acid (aspirin) and mefenamic acid (Ponstan) may be prescribed. The addition of analgesics is useful for some women and the doctor may prescribe a course of oral contraceptives. This induces anovulatory periods and may be followed by very good results. It may also be diagnostic. Should dysmenorrhoea continue, the doctor may look for other causes.

Nursing intervention

The school and occupational health nurses commonly deal with the girl or young woman suffering from dysmenorrhoea. She may present herself in their office, or the nurse may be asked to interview the girl or woman who frequently misses school or work because of dysmenorrhoea. Frequent, severe dysmenorrhoea should always be investigated by the gynaecologist, and it is the nurse's responsibility to suggest this to the patient and assist her in obtaining this care.

In regard to general care, the patient may need instruction in the normal anatomy and physiology of menstruation. This serves to eradicate misconceptions and lessen the fear and anxiety which may be associated with her periods. She may need some instruction in menstrual hygiene so that her period does not seem distasteful and restricting. This may simply mean a switch from sanitary pads to tampons and frequent bathing.

Immediate care involves providing a sympathetic, understanding approach, a place to lie down, a blanket for warmth, application of heat to the lower abdomen and a mild analgesic. When the symptoms are relieved, the girl often continues with her work. If the patient requires medication for relief, she should be instructed to take the tablet before dysmenorrhoea becomes acute. This will prevent the symptoms and the girl or woman feels that she has some control over the events which are happening to her rather than being totally subject to them.

SECONDARY DYSMENORRHOEA

Secondary dysmenorrhoea is a constant type of pain which often starts 2–3 days before the period and persists well past the first day. It may continue for a day or two following the period. Pain may radiate through the abdomen into the back and down the thighs. It occurs after several years of normal painless menses and is frequently associated with pelvic pathology. The most frequent causes are tumours, inflammatory diseases, endometriosis and fixed malpositions of the uterus. It is essentially a symptom of disease. Should the nurse be consulted by a woman describing these symptoms, the woman should be referred to a gynaecologist immediately.

AMENORRHOEA

Amenorrhoea, or absence of menstruation, may be primary or secondary. Secondary amenorrhoea is that which occurs after several months or years of normal menses.

MENORRHAGIA

Menorrhagia is excessive bleeding at the time of normal menses.

POLYMENORRHOEA

Polymenorrhoea refers to cyclic bleeding which is normal in amount but occurs too frequently.

EPIMENORRHAGIA

Epimenorrhagia is cyclic bleeding which is both excessive and too frequent.

METRORRHAGIA

Metrorrhagia refers to any bleeding which occurs between menstrual periods. Any bleeding per vaginam at any time other than normal menses is included, even if it amounts only to slight staining.

DYSFUNCTIONAL UTERINE BLEEDING

True dysfunctional uterine bleeding refers to that which occurs in the presence of endocrine dysfunction rather than organic disease. It may be seen as chronic epimenorrhagia or as an episode of acute bleeding. Some episodes of haemorrhage are caused by high levels of oestrogen in the proliferative phase of the cycle. These high levels depress the hypothalamus–pituitary complex and no ovulation occurs. Because there is no ovulation, no progesterone is produced and the endometrium remains proliferative and becomes cystic. As oestrogen levels fall, usually after a 6–8-week period of amenorrhoea, bleeding occurs. This disorder is associated with the older woman.

Other episodes of bleeding are related to fluctuating oestrogen levels produced by an imperfectly functioning hypothalamus–pituitary–ovary feedback mechanism. Follicles are stimulated to partial maturation; some oestrogen is produced but then the level falls, producing intermittent irregular and possibly prolonged bleeding. The causes are related to immaturity or ageing of the feedback mechanism and to imbalance induced in the system from physical or psychological factors.

In most cases treatment consists of administering the combined oral contraceptives. They exert a regulating and inhibiting effect on the endometrium and feedback mechanism. Three to six cycles of hormonal therapy are usually required to re-establish the normal menstrual pattern. A dilatation and curettage may be done initially. The endometrium is scraped, a biopsy done and then hormone therapy is initiated. If required, adjunctive therapy such as iron replacement is also started. More severe cases are treated with higher and more complex doses of oestrogens and progestins, in combination or sequence. In some cases when hormone therapy does not succeed, a hysterectomy may be necessary.

ENDOMETRIOSIS

Endometriosis is the location of endometrial tissue outside the uterine cavity. Although the location may be varied, the most frequent locations are in or near the ovaries, the uterosacral ligaments and the uterovesical peritoneum. Extrapelvic sites may be as varied as the umbilicus, an old laparotomy scar, vulva or even lungs. The tissue responds to the hormones of the ovarian cycle and undergoes a small menstruation just like the uterine endometrium. Statistics vary, but perhaps 5% of all patients seen by the gynaecologist suffer from endometriosis.

AETIOLOGY

Causes may be varied. Two major theories are prevalent. One concludes that small bits of endometrial tissue are forced or regurgitated back up the fallopian tube and escape into the abdomen during menstruation. The other theory points out that the peritoneum and reproductive tract derive from the same early embryological tissues. Some of the tissues may be misplanted from that early time. Under sufficient stimulation, these cells respond and differentiate into a fuctioning endometrial tag. Rare cases seem to be caused by small pieces of endometrium being transported to other parts of the body through the lymphatics or by the blood. This seems to be true of endometrial tissue in the limbs or in lung tissue. As the ectopic endometrium menstruates, the blood collects in little cyst-like nodules which have a characteristic bluish-black look. Usually they are pea-sized but may be much larger. Those in the ovary and uterosacral area often attain a size of 3–6 cm. These ovarian cysts are sometimes termed 'chocolate cysts' because of the thick, chocolate-coloured material which they contain. The cysts become surrounded by fibrous tissue which makes them easy to palpate, as they feel firm and well defined. Frequently the cyst perforates and spills its sticky contents into the abdomen. The resulting irritation promotes the formation of adhesions which readily fix the ovary or the affected area to the broad ligament or other pelvic structures.

The disease is seen most frequently in the nulliparous woman, aged 30–40. It occurs more commonly in the upper economic and social groups, presumably because of less frequent and later childbearing.

EFFECTS ON THE PATIENT

The patient may have no symptomatology, and the disease may only be discovered incidental to abdominal surgery. More commonly, the patient complains of pain. Secondary dysmenorrhoea may appear, with pain becoming severe 1–2 days before menstruation. The pain gradually becomes worse and may be described as 'boring'. This is due to the distension and pain of the swollen, shedding areas contained within the fibrous capsule of the cysts. The patient may also complain of backache, dyspareunia of a deep nature localized in the posterior fornix of the vagina or persistent lower abdominal pain occurring throughout the cycle. Pain may be of an acute nature, localized in the abdomen when a cyst ruptures. The gynaecologist may suspect endometriosis when a patient is infertile, since this is a common symptom of this group. Sometimes the adhesions become severe enough to cause a bowel obstruction or painful micturition.

Diagnosis is frequently confirmed on bimanual examination when firm nodular lumps are felt in the adnexa. Visualizing the typical bluish nodules may be done by culdoscopy, laparoscopy or during a laparotomy. Diagnosis is confirmed by biopsy when endometrial glands and stroma are seen microscopically.

Laparoscopy. The gynaecologist may feel that direct viewing of the pelvic organs is necessary. Examination under anaesthesia involving colpotomy, culdoscopy and culdocentesis may be used but these procedures are now being replaced by laparoscopy. It provides better lighted, direct visualization of the anterior aspect of the tubes and ovaries. The procedure is done under a general anaesthetic and aseptic conditions.

To avoid damage and to obtain better visualization of the abdominal and pelvic contents, the cavity is distended by the introduction of carbon dioxide. The abdominal wall is lifted by the gas above the underlying organs. The patient is tilted head downwards to about a 45° angle, shifting the abdominal contents up and away from the site of insertion of the laparoscope and from the pelvis. Through a small incision in the lower rim of the umbilicus a trocar and cannula are inserted on an angle; the trocar is then withdrawn and the endoscope inserted. It enters the peritoneal cavity approximately half-way between the umbilicus and the symphysis pubis. The contents of the abdomen and pelvis are observed and the uterus may be manipulated from below by a clamp in the cervix: this changes angles and brings the organs into better view. At the end of the procedure the endoscope is withdrawn, the gas expressed from the abdomen through the cannula and the incision closed with a clip or stitch which is removed in 24–48 hours.

There are few complications, but cardiac arrhythmias, collapse and death have been recorded. The patient may complain of some mild abdominal or shoulder pain following the procedure. This is usually abdominal gas which collects beneath the diaphragm and is not intestinal colic. The gas is absorbed gradually over a few days, but a change of position may help. Severe pain or signs of abdominal tenderness or tightness should be reported.

The patient receives preoperative and postoperative care, but does not require a shave preparation. She is ambulatory on return from the recovery room and generally returns to a full diet immediately.

TREATMENT

This is based on the age of the patient, her desire for more children and the severity of the disease. Pregnancy relieves the symptoms and may be advised if the couple want children. Pseudopregnancy may be achieved by the administration of progesterone for varying periods of time, or danazol 200–800 mg daily for 6 months. Danazol is a synthetic androgen which suppresses ovulatory function and inhibits LH and FSH synthesis and release. This produces amenorrhoea and an atrophic endometrium, usually for the duration of therapy. Some women will have intermittent spotting during therapy. The patient is usually on Danazol for 6 months, or possibly 9 months. When therapy is discontinued the patient usually remains symptom free for a period.

Treatment may be surgical and is directed at preserving reproductive function. Affected areas are removed, and fixed organs released. Infertility often ceases following surgery. In severe cases a hysterectomy may be done. Depending on the extent of the cystic involvement, oophorectomy may also be performed. The symptoms usually disappear at menopause as ovarian atrophy begins and hormonal stimulation declines.

ADENOMYOSIS UTERI

This condition is similar to endometriosis in that it is characterized by endometrium within the muscular wall of the uterus or the fallopian tube. The cause is unknown. In any case, the uterine endometrium appears to grow downward between the muscle bundles of the myometrium. This produces a uniform, moderate enlargement of the uterus. The patient may complain of menorrhagia and dysmenorrhoea. Often pelvic endometriosis is also present. Then the uterus may be fixed (frozen) in the pelvis, and pelvic nodules may be palpated. The patient may complain of pain in the sacral or coccygeal area as well.

Interruptions of Pregnancy

ABORTION

An abortion is the cessation of a pregnancy before the 28th week of pregnancy. It may either be induced or occur spontaneously, the lay term for a spontaneous abortion being a 'miscarriage'.

The incidence of abortion is difficult to state accurately but between 10 and 20% of all conceptions are thought to abort. See Figure 22.19 for classification of abortions.

CAUSES

Most known causes can be separated into three major groups: fetal, maternal and faulty environment. Fetal causes are often associated with chromosomal or other abnormalities which are incompatible with life. This has been considered to be as high as 40% of all causes of abortion. Maternal and faulty environment causes are more varied. Endotoxins, as a result of severe infections in the mother, may invade the fetus, usually causing its death and later expulsion. Drugs ingested by the mother may damage the fetus directly or may damage the placenta and hence the nutrition of the fetus. Hormonal imbalances may be the cause of some abortions, especially in cases in which the thyroid gland is involved. Lack of progesterone may result in a poorly developed endometrium. As a result, implantation of the fertilized ovum in the endometrium (nidation) does not occur or does so ineffectively. Anatomical uterine defects or uterine pathology cause some abortions.

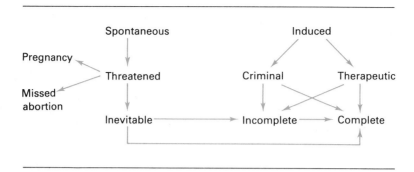

Figure 22.19 Classification of abortion.

Nutritional factors are linked to abortion and premature labour, for adequate nutrition of the woman bears an important part in her reproductive capacity. The emotional state of the woman is also considered a possible contributing factor. This often centres on fear, grief or emotional trauma in susceptible women. Physical trauma can also induce an abortion. This may be true of surgery performed during pregnancy.

A threatened abortion is one in which the threat to the pregnancy is slight. With care, the woman may carry the pregnancy to term. Since any bleeding, however minor, per vaginam is abnormal in the pregnant woman, any evidence of such bleeding is taken as a sign of threatened abortion until proven otherwise. In addition, some backache or mild intermittent lower abdominal pain may be present. If the abortion is not to be immediate, cramping and bleeding continues, cramps become stronger and regular, the cervix dilates and the membranes rupture. The inevitable abortion becomes the complete abortion when all products of conception are expelled. This usually occurs before the twelfth week of gestation. The abortion is incomplete when some of the products of conception are retained. This is usually the placenta and membranes and is more frequent following the twelfth week, when the placenta is more firmly embedded. The umbilical cord breaks, leaving the placenta and membranes in utero. A missed abortion is one in which the fetus dies; symptoms of abortion cease and the products of conception are retained in the uterus for 2 or more months. Following this, the uterus is not observed to increase in size. Indeed, it begins to regress slightly as the amniotic fluid is absorbed. No fetal heart is heard. The patient remains amenorrhoeic, and the breasts regress. The abortus is usually expelled spontaneously but may be retained for many months or years. In such cases it becomes a shrivelled sac with areas of dense calcification.

A woman is considered to be an habitual aborter when she aborts three or more consecutive pregnancies. The causes can be any of the causes of a single abortion but persist through several pregnancies. In addition, an incompetent cervix is frequently sited as a cause of habitual abortion. Possibly because of inherent problems in the cervix or trauma to the cervix, the cervix dilates easily and will not retain the pregnancy. Loss of the pregnancy usually occurs later at about 16–20 weeks. Dilatation of the cervix is rapid, with little pain and bleeding. Rupture of the membranes occurs, followed by the expulsion of the fetus.

TREATMENT AND NURSING CARE

Threatened abortion

The treatment of threatened abortion is aimed at preserving the pregnancy. Every pregnant woman should be told the danger signs of pregnancy. Often this instruction is the responsibility of the nurse in either the clinic or the surgery. Thus, the woman should recognize bleeding as abnormal and be aware that she should notify her doctor immediately. She should then go to bed and rest unless otherwise instructed by her doctor. If the bleeding is slight, the patient is managed at home and advised to get extra rest for a few days. For some patients this may be impossible, and admission to hospital is necessary.

On admission to the hospital, the patient is placed on bed rest. Temperature, pulse and blood pressure are noted as frequently as the patient's condition warrants. All the pads, linen and clothing stained with blood are kept in order to estimate blood loss. In addition, the patient is observed for any increased bleeding or cramping which would indicate a change in status. A diet low in roughage is ordered. Purgatives and enemas are not given in order to avoid stimulation of the uterus. Rectal and vaginal examinations are contraindicated. Bleeding usually ceases within 24–48 hours if the pregnancy is going to continue. At this time the doctor will probably perform a careful speculum and bimanual examination, since other possible causes of bleeding must be ruled out. These causes could be carcinoma or other complications of pregnancy.

On discharge home the patient is instructed to get extra rest and to avoid strenuous exercise, heavy lifting, excitement or fatigue. Coitus may be restricted for a period of 2 weeks or longer. Should bleeding recur, the patient is advised to notify her doctor and remain in bed.

Missed abortion

The patient will be followed by her obstetrician to see that the pregnancy progresses normally. If it does not and a persistent brownish discharge recurs, missed abortion may be suspected. A positive pregnancy test may only indicate that placental tissue still remains living. An ultrasound examination of the fetus usually confirms the diagnosis. The obstetrician is faced with the choice of interfering to evacuate the uterus or waiting until it is done spontaneously. Physically, there is usually no pressing need. Emotionally it is very distressing to the woman and her family to know that she is carrying a dead fetus. The danger from disseminated intravascular coagulation (DIC) as a complicating factor to intervention by the obstetrician increases as the dead fetus is retained. Presumably this occurs as some of the degenerating products of the fetus enter the maternal bloodstream. This danger appears to be most serious about 4–6 weeks after fetal death. Coagulation studies may be done before intervention is attempted.

For these reasons the obstetrician usually intervenes approximately 2 weeks after death of the fetus. The dead fetus may be aborted by means of suction evacuation if death occurs before 12 weeks of gestation or by prostaglandin administration if it occurs during the second trimester. The procedure is emotionally and physically exhausting for the patient. She requires much supportive nursing care. Also, the contractions are painful, and some analgesic should be administered. Since no danger can result to the fetus, the mother need not suffer unduly. Close observation of the patient's condition for overyhydration is necessary because of the danger of administering large amounts of fluid containing synthetic oxytocin, which has an antidiuretic action. An intake and output record should be kept.

Inevitable abortion

The treatment of an inevitable abortion is similar to that of a threatened abortion. The patient is placed on bed rest. Blood will be taken for haemoglobin, typing and cross-matching. The amount and character of the bleeding is observed carefully. Blood pressure and pulse may need to be taken every 10 minutes if bleeding is profuse, and the patient must be observed for other signs of shock. Any tissue or suspicious clots are saved to be examined for traces of fetus and placenta. Good perineal care is maintained by frequent cleansing of the vulva to reduce the risk of infection and to promote the patient's comfort. Procedures for perineal care will vary. Generally, soap and water are sufficient. The perineum is swabbed from the pubes to the perineal body (front to back) and from the vulva out to the thigh. The rectal area is washed last. This is to prevent the spread of bacteria from the rectum upward into the vagina and thence to the endometrium. If the abortion seems to be approaching a conclusion, it is not assisted. However, with the membranes ruptured, the cervix dilated and contractions tapering off, the process may be hastened by the administration of intravenous oxytocin.

If the abortion has been complete and the obstetrician is satisfied of this, the woman is treated similarly to the postpartum patient. If the patient is Rh negative blood group, she receives Rh_0 (anti-D immunoglobulin) to prevent the formation of antibodies in further pregnancies. A slight lochial discharge is expected and the woman must be taught perineal care. She will be discharged home in 1–2 days, depending on the state of her health. To reduce the risk of infection, coitus is contraindicated until lochial discharge has ceased. This usually occurs within 2 weeks.

When the products of conception are retained, the uterus must be emptied. Two of the major causes of bleeding associated with pregnancy result from the partially separated placenta and retained fragments of conception. The uterus cannot contract effectively; the torn blood vessels remain open and bleed. Also, the risk of infection is much increased by the debris lying in the uterus. If the bleeding is acute, the patient is usually taken to the operating theatre and an emergency evacuation of retained products of conception (ERPC) is done. Under a general anaesthesia, the cervix is gently dilated until the passage of a curette is possible. Dilatation is accomplished by using the dilators or by the use of a special vibrating dilator. The curette is used to scrape the tissue from the walls of the uterus.

Following this operation the patient receives perineal care and is observed for signs of haemorrhage and infection. She may receive an intravenous oxytocic solution to help involution of the uterus. Because of the danger of accidental perforation of the uterus with the instruments, the patient is observed postoperatively for signs of peritoneal irritation or abdominal (concealed) haemorrhage. Packing may or may not have been inserted in the vagina to help control or prevent haemorrhage. This should be carefully noted on the chart. If packing was inserted, the nurse observes the patient even more carefully for signs of shock, since any bleeding may be concealed by the packing. If there is packing, it is removed within several hours to allow free drainage of lochia and thus help prevent infection. By altering urethrovesical relationships, vaginal packing increases a woman's inability to void postoperatively. Inability to void with subsequent bladder distension should be avoided, either by removing the packing or inserting a urethral catheter.

Incompetent cervical os

The patient who has had several abortions will probably receive a thorough assessment between pregnancies in an attempt to ascertain her problem. Should the cause be considered an incompetent cervical os, the obstetrician may attempt to tighten the cervix with a suture. This is usually done during the twelfth to sixteenth week of pregnancy. The Shirodkar technique consists of running a non-dissolving suture around the cervix like a drawstring or purse string.

On return from the operating theatre, the pregnant patient is observed for signs of labour and imminent abortion. Should the abortion appear inevitable, the suture must be removed or serious tearing of the cervix might occur. At 38 weeks, the suture is removed and vaginal delivery follows, or the suture is retained and delivery is by caesarean section.

Emotional response to spontaneous abortion

Response to early abortion. Early pregnancy is characterized by feelings of unreality while the mother strives to confirm that the pregnancy is real. The first trimester is also a stage of ambivalence toward the pregnancy and its timing. Emotional energy appears to be invested in accepting and acknowledging the pregnancy and this is true both of planned and unplanned, wanted and unwanted pregnancies. The fetus is rarely described at this time as a baby. Consequently most women do not appear to be deeply attached to the fetus. About a third of women in the first trimester exhibit attachment and relate to the fetus as a baby. Most women respond to a spontaneous abortion with a sense of loss. To some, it will be the loss of a pregnancy but to others the loss of a baby.

The response to the loss may be surprise, disappointment, grief, guilt and anger in differing proportions depending on the meaning of the loss at that time. The woman who has had several abortions may be experiencing this loss and also the threat of the loss of ability to ever bear a live child.

Most women express surprise at the abortion. They are unprepared for the pain, loss of blood and if recognizable or noticed, the sight of the fetus. It seems that the concept of a baby is so vague in their minds at this time that such real evidence of a fetus is unexpected. Because of the ambivalence of the first trimester many feel guilt associated with the negative thoughts they may have had about the pregnancy or its timing.

Response to late abortion. By mid-gestation, the pregnancy usually has been accepted as real and the fetus becomes a baby to the majority of women. Most couples have begun to establish a relationship with the baby and loss at this stage is usually perceived as the loss of a baby. There may be more desire to see the fetus, to know the sex and weight and to identify the baby by name even though it may legally be an abortion. Emotional response may be more intense and appear more painful if there is no 'object' to attach the pain to. Seeing the infant or keeping a picture of the baby may assist with grieving and the resolution of the loss for some parents. Others will not choose or require such a method of relating to the fetus.

Parents will exhibit immediate responses similar to those with an early spontaneous abortion. Questions of 'Why me?' and 'What did I do?' will also surface as they search for an explanation for the event. The associated physical discomforts seem to make the stress worse for the mother. The father, who usually becomes the supporter and planner at this stage, may feel overlooked and his grief unacknowledged. The couple may mourn unequally and in different ways, making it difficult for them to support one another.

The reactions of parents who have chosen therapeutic abortion for genetic reasons are similar to these parents. Guilt may be increased in some. Others are fearful of the censure and disapproval of hospital staff. Immediate nursing interventions are aimed at acknowledging the loss, accepting the feelings and wishes of the parents and reinforcing reality. This assists in promoting the long-term goal of resolution of normal grieving, which takes a few months.

The patient experiencing the loss of a desired child derives little consolation from being told that she can have other children or that she has children at home. It is the loss of this child which she feels; she needs sympathy, understanding and someone to listen. She requires factual information about the events, the baby and future childbearing. If the couple wish to see the baby, they are prepared verbally for what they will see. For example, the baby is shown to them wrapped in a blanket. If deformed, it is wrapped to cover all but the face. After preparation, the baby may be unwrapped to reveal the body if they wish. This is an area where the nurse must use judgement and discretion. Some parents like a short time alone with the baby. If the parents do not wish to see the baby, their decision is respected. It is not a positive or necessary step for all parents.

A brief review of the grieving process with the parents is helpful so that they will understand the feelings of grief, irritability and fatigue which may come. The value of rest, sleep and exercise in coping with grieving is stressed. Unequal patterns of grieving and ways of obtaining support are discussed.

Religious rites

If the patient who aborts is Roman Catholic, the fetus can be baptized. In addition, some Protestants may feel strongly that the fetus should be baptized. The nurse may ascertain this by tactfully inquiring what the patient's wishes are. Baptism may be performed by any person, regardless of his religious beliefs. If available, a member of the clergy should be asked to perform this rite; if not, the nurse may have to baptize the fetus. Clear water must be poured over the head of the fetus while the nurse pronounces the words 'I baptize you in the name of the Father and of the Son and of the Holy Spirit'. The water must come into direct contact with the fetus. Therefore, if the fetus is still in the amniotic sac, the sac must be broken before the baptism is performed. The procedure is similar for all religions. If the fetus is very small, it may have to be immersed in water to ensure that water reaches the head. Sometimes a conditional baptism is given with the words, 'If thou art living, I baptize thee ...' This is done in cases in which the fetus may have died before delivery, but the exact state is unknown.

Other religious groups may have special rites which they wish to perform. The nurse assesses this with the parents and provides support and help.

Some late abortions may require burial. The parents may need practical assistance on how to go about this, for example referral to the appropriate chaplaincy or social work services.

Therapeutic abortion

The past few years have seen a large increase in the number of therapeutic or induced abortions performed throughout the world, in response to the liberalization of abortion laws. It is estimated that legal abortion for social and medical reasons is now available to over half the world's population, making the therapeutic abortion

Table 22.5 Indications for therapeutic abortion under the Abortion Act (1967).

1. The continuance of the pregnancy would involve risk to the pregnant woman greater than if the pregnancy were terminated
2. The continuance of the pregnancy would involve risk of injury to the physical or mental health of the pregnant woman greater than if the pregnancy were terminated
3. The continuance of the pregnancy would involve risk of injury to the physical or mental health of the existing child(ren) of the family of the pregnant woman greater than if the pregnancy were terminated
4. There is a substantial risk that if the child were born it would suffer from such physical or mental abnormalities as to be seriously handicapped

The restrictions
1. That one or more of the above conditions are believed to be present in the opinion of two doctors, who are acting together in good faith and in full knowledge of the facts
2. That this opinion be notified to the DHSS
3. That the operation be carried out in a NHS hospital or an approved establishment
4. That the doctor carrying out the operation notify the DHSS
5. That the consent of the woman be obtained. If the patient is under the age of 16 the consent of the parents is also necessary

one of the most common medical procedures performed.

Because an abortion concerns the life and death of at least two people, it is governed by religious and legal codes. Complex issues surround the topic of induced abortions and a discussion of all of them is beyond the scope of this work. Only a brief discussion of the law and medical and nursing management is presented here.

The laws governing abortions vary from country to country. In all nations legal codes exist defining the conditions under which an abortion may be done. They outline who may do an abortion, where it may be done (in or outside the hospital), and when it may be done in relationship to the length of gestation. The law also defines the social and medical conditions which constitute cause for an abortion. In the United Kingdom, the Abortion Act (1967) gives indications and restrictions for therapeutic abortion (Table 22.5). All abortions performed outside the limits of the legal condition are illegal. In many countries, assisting a patient to procure an abortion outside the law is also punishable by law. For these reasons the nurse should be acquainted with the law pertaining to the area in which he or she practises.

Abortions can be divided into two groups on the basis of risk to the woman and her future childbearing potential. Low-risk or early abortions are those done before 12 weeks of gestation. Late or high-risk abortions are done from the thirteenth week of gestation onward. As the upper limits of abortion are defined by the law

they will vary from 20–28 weeks of gestation, depending upon the jurisdiction. An abortion may carry greater risk if the patient has a serious accompanying medical condition.

Early abortions
Most abortions performed before 12–14 weeks of gestation are done by suction dilatation and curettage (D and C). If done before 8 weeks of gestation the cervix usually does not require dilatation but it is more difficult to ensure complete evacuation of the products of conception. The procedure is most commonly done on an out-patient basis. A general anaesthetic may be given but many abortions, particularly those not requiring cervical dilatation, may be done without anaesthesia or with a local anaesthetic such as a paracervical block. Some surgeons administer intravenous oxytocin (Syntocinon) before suctioning to ensure a strong firm contraction of the uterus; others do not feel this is necessary.

Following these initial steps the doctor determines the size, shape and position of the uterus by bimanual examination. The cervix is then visualized and immobilized by forceps and the cervical canal sounded for direction and the uterus for depth. Should the cervix require further dilatation, it will now be done to the size of the cannula required to perform the D and C. The size of the cannula is determined by the length of gestation. A flexible plastic suction tip is then slipped through the cervix. It is attached to a vacuum source which sucks out the uterine contents. The pressure of the pump is carefully regulated to achieve evacuation while avoiding damage to the walls of the uterine cavity. The doctor judges when the uterus is empty by the grating feel of the denuded uterine walls, the contractions of the uterus and the content and character of the aspirated fluid. The aspirated tissue is caught in a gauze trap to facilitate recovery for immediate inspection and for examination by the pathologist. Immediate identification of fetal tissue is important to confirm the diagnosis of an intrauterine pregnancy which has been completely evacuated. As the operator becomes more experienced, the need for postsuction curettage of the uterus declines but may still be performed in cases of doubtful complete emptying of the uterus. It is necessary to confirm the intrauterine pregnancy to avoid an ectopic pregnancy continuing unnoticed. Immediate inspection and, later, pathology reports may confirm a molar pregnancy which, if left undetected, would deprive the patient of important follow-up care.

Following the procedure the patient recovers as determined by the anaesthetic she received. Many patients experience some cramping postabortion, which is normal. The cramps are frequently gone by the time the effects of the anaesthetic, either general or paracervical, are over, but may persist for longer. A mild analgesic may be required. The patient is then observed for a few hours more or allowed to go home with instructions, depending upon her condition.

Late abortions
When the pregnancy is more than 12–14 weeks a D and C becomes more difficult. Other methods must be

selected by the gynaecologist, who may decide to induce labour by the use of an intra-amniotic injection. The technique and preparation are similar to a paracentesis, but an amniocentesis is done. With strict sterile technique the patient's abdomen is prepared and draped. A skin wheal is made with a local anaesthetic agent. Then a needle is inserted through the abdomen, and into the amniotic cavity. One of several agents is injected into the uterine cavity: urea, glucose, hypertonic saline and prostaglandins have all been used. Hypertonic saline and prostaglandins seem to be the most commonly used. If the drug chosen is saline, some amniotic fluid is withdrawn and replaced by an equal amount of 20% saline solution. The fetus dies, and the uterus is apparently irritated and begins to contract. The contractions may need to be assisted with an oxytocic medication given intravenously.

Later pregnancies of 16–20 weeks' gestation may be terminated by the performance of a hysterotomy. This means that an incision is made into the uterus and the contents removed. It is a miniature caesarean section. The preoperative and postoperative care is similar to abdominal surgery. Postoperatively, the fundus must be checked for firmness and position. Lochia is observed for colour, amount and odour, since haemorrhage or infection may occur postoperatively. Vulval care is carried out.

Prostaglandins. Prostaglandins are naturally-occurring fatty acids which were first isolated in semen and thought to arise in the prostate gland. Since then they have been found in all tissues. One of their actions is the ability to make smooth muscle contract. This ability is pronounced in relation to uterine muscle. Two forms of prostaglandins, E_2 and $F_{2\alpha}$ are used therapeutically. E_2 is several times stronger than $F_{2\alpha}$. The most common side-effects described are nausea, diarrhoea, pyrexia and local tissue reactions at the site of injection. Synthetic analogues of both F and E groups are now made. They produce fewer side-effects and still stimulate uterine contractions. One of their major uses is to induce abortion and to stimulate labour in full-term pregnancies.

Prostaglandins may be given in an intravenous drip which is carefully regulated by an infusion pump. The dosage is started at very low levels; the responses of the patient, fetus and uterus are carefully monitored. The dose is gradually increased until the uterus is contracting satisfactorily. Labour and delivery or abortion will follow for most patients in 12–24 hours. If the stimulation is not sufficient, additional stimulation with oxytocin may be given. This is associated with an increased risk of rupture of the cervix and uterus, so the response of the contracting uterus must be carefully monitored. The patient's complaints of discomfort or pain should be carefully heeded.

Intra-amniotic injections of prostaglandins may also be given. The procedure is similar to the injection of saline. The prostaglandins are absorbed and the uterus begins to contract. Delivery usually occurs about 20 hours after the injection. Occasionally additional stimulation with an oxytocin (Syntocinon) drip is required. The use of oxytocin reduces the time to abortion by 6–8 hours.

Side-effects include nausea, vomiting and diarrhoea. Because the action is directly on smooth muscle, antiemetic drugs which act on the central nervous system are only partially successful. Diphenoxylate (Lomotil) does reduce the diarrhoea and is usually given. Prostaglandins may produce bronchospasm in asthmatics.

Extra-amniotic injection with prostaglandins is another common method of inducing abortion. A polyethylene tubing or a Foley catheter is passed under aseptic conditions through the cervix, and is directed between the uterine wall and the membranes. The bag of the Foley catheter is inflated to help retain the catheter in the uterus. The tube is attached to further tubing attached to a syringe containing the solution. The rate of infusion is controlled by an infusion pump. Small amounts are injected and the uterine response observed. The dose is gradually increased. Abortion occurs in anywhere from 12–24 hours.

Nursing intervention
The therapeutic abortion is not a totally benign procedure. Physical and mental complications can arise. Thus, the decision to perform an abortion is a weighty one for the gynaecologist as well as for the woman. She and her family will need support and acceptance. Some patients will benefit from counselling beforehand, especially those for whom the abortion involves conflict. All patients require an explanation of the procedure. Unfortunately, many patients are so driven by the overriding need to have the pregnancy terminated that detailed explanation or teaching is not absorbed. Most patients appear less tense, more relaxed and less hostile once they know that the pregnancy is terminated. They are then more receptive to teaching and explanations about follow-up. Anxiety, loneliness and fear are the problems expressed by patients waiting for their contractions to start. Some have told no one, and have no friends or family to support them through the procedure. The nurse can be an important factor in their experience of the event.

Postoperatively the patient is nursed similarly to the patient who has had a spontaneous abortion and a D and C to complete the process. In late abortions the patient requires more intensive nursing care. While the intra-amniotic injections are being given the patient must be observed for reactions to the drug injected. Hypertonic saline may be absorbed into the circulatory system. To avoid this a small amount is injected, the patient's response assessed, and then the remainder injected. If saline is being absorbed intravascularly she may complain of confusion, heat sensations, headache, tinnitus, a dry mouth and tachycardia. In this event the saline is stopped and the injection site altered. When the injection is completed, the patient then awaits the beginning of contractions. To reduce the risk of infection, oxytocin is usually begun within 12 hours if uterine contractions are not adequate. The patient may express some thirst during this period of waiting. All patients who have been given saline absorb a portion of it, thus producing some electrolyte imbalance. Fluid is required and she should be allowed to drink. The patient experiences labour and requires the support and nursing care which is given to a labouring patient. The contractions are distressing, especially since they appear to be for a negative purpose. Analgesia is required by some patients and should not be withheld. Bed rest is usually maintained after active labour begins or after administration of a sedative. In extra-amniotic injection of prostaglandins the catheter may be expelled as the uterus contracts and the cervix dilates. Oxytocin stimulation may be required to maintain labour.

As progress is difficult to assess, the patient frequently aborts in bed alone or with the nurse in attendance. If previously warned she may call the nurse when she feels pressure. However, the patient herself frequently receives little warning.

All products of conception are retained for examination by the doctor and the pathologist. Often the placenta is retained and only the fetus expelled. The nurse should clamp and cut the cord and remove the fetus. Now the patient enters one of the hazardous periods during an abortion, and requires close observation by the nursing staff. Severe haemorrhage may result from the partially separated placenta or the retained products of conception. Haemorrhage may take several forms: the sudden gush, a steady trickle, or small gushes interspersed with periods of minor loss. In all cases the nurse must assess the cumulative loss as well as the immediate one. Individual episodes of bleeding might not alert the nurse to haemorrhage but she must assess the loss over the period of time from the beginning of bleeding to the present. In this way morbidity is reduced, since evacuation of the uterus is begun before the patient has suffered loss. If the placenta is not expelled spontaneously within 2 hours and bleeding does not indicate immediate removal, the patient will be scheduled for a D and C for a convenient time within a few hours. Meanwhile, frequent observations of the lochia must be maintained, as the patient's status may change at any time. Following the D and C she is nursed as other patients postabortion who have had a D and C.

Infection may develop, and the patient is monitored for signs of pelvic infection every 4 hours during the hours when she is aborting. Regular daily checks of temperature, general well-being and the character of the lochia follow.

Most abortion patients are discharged within hours of being aborted or within 1 or 2 days. They need clear discharge instructions so that they may take care of themselves in the days that follow. Each patient should be told:

1. To resume normal activities, except for hysterotomy patients who as postoperative patients may do so more gradually.
2. To expect intermittent menstrual-like discharge for the next week or two, but no heavy, bright-red bleeding.
3. To use sanitary pads as long as bleeding occurs. The use of tampons is inadvisable.
4. Some cramping may occur but should not persist or be severe.
5. To report any fever or unusual discomfort.
6. To expect her menstrual period within 4–5 weeks after the procedure. If it does not occur, it may indicate a continuing intrauterine or extrauterine pregnancy or a new pregnancy. Ovulation occurs as

early as 18 days following an abortion and pregnancy is possible immediately. Birth control advice and teaching should be given to the patient as necessary.
7. It is wise to limit coitus while the menstrual-like flow continues, to reduce the risk of infection.
8. To contact her doctor or clinic immediately if any of the unusual signs should occur.
9. When she is to return for a follow-up visit.

While the therapeutic abortion is now associated with low maternal morbidity and mortality statistics (lower than pregnancy in many countries), it does carry some serious risks which need to be considered. Psychiatric sequelae are rare but do occur. The main concern appears to be an increased incidence of spontaneous abortion and premature labour in those women who have had a prior abortion. The risk is greatest with the older methods of dilatation and curettage, and is greater still when damage to the cervix has been documented. It is important to educate women to seek abortion as early as possible so that the need for dilating the cervix will be reduced. Prevention is better than cure, and birth control should be seen as the first line of defence. Nursing has an important role to play by providing knowledge of and access to birth control to those who need it.

Criminal abortion

The criminal abortion is a dangerous procedure. Often women attempt to abort themselves by the use of strong douches or instruments which they insert into the uterus. Frequently, the instrument used punctures the posterior fornix of the vagina, the cervix or perforates the uterus. The bowel may be involved should the instrument be inserted far enough. Conditions are furtive, untrained people frequently officiate, and sterility is not maintained. These patients frequently contract an infection and present a grave situation. The situation is known as a septic abortion. Infection is essentially an endometritis, which may spread to peritonitis or to septicaemia.

ECTOPIC PREGNANCY

Implantation of the fertilized ovum anywhere outside the uterine cavity is considered an ectopic pregnancy. Most frequently this occurs in the ampullary portion of the fallopian tube, but it may be ovarian, abdominal or cervical. Women with a history of one ectopic pregnancy have an increased risk of having a second one.

An ectopic pregnancy results when the passage of the zygote to the uterine cavity is impeded or slowed. Any blocking of the tube or reduction in tubal peristalsis will achieve this. Former salpingitis, tumours and hormonal imbalances may all play a part.

As implantation occurs, the chorionic villi burrow into the thin tubal wall. Eventually, they burrow into a blood vessel, and bleeding occurs. If the bleeding is sufficient, the fetus dies. This is the fate of most. The abortus may be retained in the tube as a tubal mole or may be extruded through the end of the fallopian tube as a tubal abortion. Occasionally, the trophoblast burrows through the wall of the tube and out into the peritoneal cavity. This is known as a ruptured tubal pregnancy and often occurs as the result of a pregnancy in the narrow isthmus of the tube. A secondary abdominal pregnancy may follow if the chorionic villi settle elsewhere in the abdominal cavity and begin to grow. This is rare.

The incidence of ectopic pregnancies has been increasing throughout the Western world in the last 10–15 years. The increase seems to be due to many factors such as an increase in pelvic infections, widespread IUD use, fertility induced by ovulatory agents, reconstructive surgery of fallopian tubes or better and earlier diagnosis. The condition is a serious one and ectopic pregnancy still contributes significantly to maternal mortality statistics.

EFFECTS ON THE PATIENT

The woman has a history of the early signs of pregnancy, including amenorrhoea usually of 6–10 weeks' duration. Soon after her first missed period she may have complaints of a localized pain on one side, due probably to the distension of the tube. Following that she may have sharper intermittent pain in the same area. This may be due to strong peristaltic waves of the tube attempting to pass the embryo or abortus along the tube. At some point the patient may experience a sharp, severe pain. This is probably synchronous with separation of the embryo and some haemorrhage. The sharp pain may be followed by generalized abdominal discomfort as blood spills into the abdomen. Referred shoulder pain may occur. At this point many women present for treatment. It is wise to remember that pain may not be a reliable guide to the extent of haemorrhage and that in young healthy women blood pressure and pulse are slow to respond to blood loss. If she does not present, then 4–5 days following this episode there is bleeding per vaginam due to falling hormone levels, which occur following the death of the fetus and cause the endometrium to regress and menstruation to occur.

Diagnosis will usually include a single radioimmunoassay pregnancy test, or serial ones, ultrasound and, if necessary, culdocentesis or laparoscopy, depending on the urgency of the presenting symptoms. Examinations of patients with suspected ectopic pregnancy should be gentle as too vigorous an examination may precipitate an acute rupture before surgery can prevent it.

Acute ruptured tubal pregnancy

Sometimes the patient reports no early symptoms but experiences one episode of acute abdominal pain shortly after her missed period. This acute pain is often accompanied by vomiting and fainting. Some vaginal bleeding may be present but appears too minimal to warrant the reaction of the patient. The patient may rapidly go into shock with a drop in blood pressure, rapid weak pulse, pallor, sweating, low temperature and cold extremities. The abdomen is distended with blood and may be tight and tender to the touch. A pelvic examination of the patient may be difficult because of the exquisite tenderness. The patient presents as an emergency situation.

When the diagnosis of a tubal pregnancy is confirmed, a salpingectomy (removal of the fallopian tube) with the

Table 22.6   Trophoblastic tumours.

Benign $\longrightarrow$	Intermediate $\longrightarrow$	Malignant
Hydatidiform mole	Metastasizing mole Chorioadenoma destruens	Choriocarcinoma (chorioepithelioma malignum)

removal of the fetus is performed. This is usually done within 24–48 hours of diagnosis unless the situation is acute, in which case it is done immediately.

Ectopic pregnancies in other locations will be investigated in a similar fashion. Treatment is usually surgical removal of the fetus. However, abdominal pregnancies have carried to term and been delivered by laparotomies.

Because ectopic pregnancy involves the loss of a pregnancy and possibly the loss of reproductive ability, these patients require the same emotional support a patient requires after a spontaneous abortion (see p. 798).

TUMOURS OF THE TROPHOBLAST

Trophoblastic tumours are a group of neoplasms which arise in the chorionic villi of the fertilized ovum during the trophoblast stage. The condition is rare in Europe and North America, occurring about once in every 2500 pregnancies. It is more prevalent in the Far East. The reason for this is not known. The tumours range from benign to malignant (Table 22.6). Not all benign tumours become malignant, nor are all malignant tumours preceded by a benign stage.

HYDATIDIFORM MOLE

Hydatidiform mole is an abnormal development of the chorionic villi of the conceptus. A true mole is now known to occur when the chromosomal pattern is 45,XX and the source of the chromatin material is paternal. No maternal chromatin exists. This is the result of a normal sperm fertilizing an ovum with no genome. The maternal chromatin has been lost or inactivated. The haploid sperm (23) then undergoes endoreplication. Some moles are 46,XY and these are the result of two sperms fertilizing one empty ovum. The conceptus is really an abnormal development of the placenta, which begins to develop the characteristic mole pattern about the fifth week of life. Fluid accumulates and the chorionic villi distend into small, clear vesicles clinging to thin threads of connective tissue in a grape-like mass. Partial moles also exist. They have a fetus or an amniotic sac and some normal-appearing placental tissue associated with the mole tissue. These result from a conceptus with the chromosomal pattern 69,XXY or 69,XYY and contain one maternal and two paternal haploid elements.

Why these events occur is unknown. Age seems to play a role as moles are more common in women over the age of 40.

The condition is the most common of all the tumours. Thus, the majority of women who have a molar pregnancy do not need to fear malignancy. Only 3–7% of benign moles will proceed to malignancy.

The intermediate stages are characterized by an increased ability to invade uterine musculature and to send bloodborne deposits of trophoblast cells throughout the body. However, in some cases, the host, or pregnant woman, seems able to contain the spread of the tumour and it disappears. The intermediate stage is frequently not identified clinically, but is obvious only on pathological examinations of specimens of tissue. This means that all moles must be treated as potentially malignant until demonstrated otherwise.

Effects on the patient

The patient exhibits the signs and symptoms of early pregnancy. Vomiting may be more frequent. The uterus is often much larger than expected for the weeks of gestation. About the twelfth week, some vaginal bleeding may occur, and this is often the first sign of some abnormality. No fetal movements are reported by the mother, and no fetal parts can be palpated. On palpation the uterus may have an elastic consistency. There is an increased incidence of pre-eclampsia. Urine tests for the quantity of chorionic gonadotrophins excreted show very high titres which persist and do not fall as is usual in a normal pregnancy. These high levels also stimulate the formation of theca lutein cysts in the ovary. The cysts regress following the abortion of the mole.

Treatment and nursing responsibilities

The patient is usually admitted to the hospital and nursed as a threatened abortion until proven otherwise. All perineal pads are carefully inspected for pieces of the mole, as this would be diagnostic. Thyroid function tests may be ordered, for high levels of chorionic gonadotrophins may exert a thyroid-stimulating effect.

An ultrasonic scan of the abdomen is done. The scan plots a 'snowflake' pattern, which is typical of a mole and is considered diagnostic. In preparation for an ultrasound scan the patient is instructed to drink 6–8 large glasses of water in quick succession. The bladder fills within 15–20 minutes, after which the scan is performed. The full bladder pushes the bowel away from the uterus and tubes, permitting better penetration of sound waves. At the same time the uterus is pushed up and away from the symphysis pubis, allowing better visualization. The full bladder provides a water path or window through which to look, a landmark in the abdomen, for it is clearly outlined, and an internal reference standard for density comparisons.

In scanning soft tissue, two types of measurements are done; one outlines tissue and the other estimates density of the tissue outlined. The snowflake pattern of a mole reflects an irregular shaped mass with areas of alternating density. Because sound waves can be dispersed or lost, a contact gel is used between the transducer and the skin of the patient. This keeps the sound waves on track, as it were. The area is carefully mapped out as the transducer is moved in lines 1 cm apart up and down and across the area. The findings are displayed on a monitor screen. Print-outs can be obtained for permanent record.

Ultrasound is being used increasingly in gynaecology for the localization of foreign objects in the uterus, the diagnosis of tumours of the uterus, ovary and tubes, ectopic pregnancy, and as a device to outline precise areas for irradiation. The patient suffers no discomfort save that of a full bladder during the procedure.

Often the mole is partially aborted spontaneously. Haemorrhage may be acute. Oxytocics will be given to control the bleeding, and a careful and complete evacuation of the uterus will be done. Because of the danger of perforating the uterus in areas weakened by the erosion of the mole, a curette is not used. Instead, the cervix is dilated and suction equipment used to evacuate the uterine contents. Postoperatively the patient is observed for signs of haemorrhage.

Because of the possibility of a malignancy occurring, the patient receives close follow-up care during the next 12–18 months. The first signs of the recurrence of the mole or the development of a malignancy is a rising chorionic gonadotrophin level. Therefore, the urinary levels of gonadotrophin will be monitored at regular intervals. Amenorrhoea, metrorrhagia or persistent cystic ovaries may alert the gynaecologist to look for rising hormone levels. The patient is advised against pregnancy during this period, as early pregnancy also produces high chorionic gonadotrophin levels which could mask the signs. Cytotoxic drugs (such as methotrexate) are given in all intermediate cases, and may be given as prophylaxis to all women who have had a molar pregnancy.

CHORIOEPITHELIOMA MALIGNUM

Chorioepithelioma is a malignant tumour of the embryonic chorion and is marked by invasion of the uterine musculature by malignant trophoblastic cells which have lost their original villous pattern. Destruction of uterine tissues with accompanying necrosis and haemorrhage is the result. The growth quickly metastasizes, and the most frequent site is the lung. The condition is extremely rare but because of its rapid advancement is considered to be one of the most malignant of all pelvic neoplasms. Death usually occurs within 12 months unless the patient receives early treatment. Fifty per cent of all cases of chorioepithelioma are preceded by a mole. The others are preceded by a normal pregnancy or abortion. Because of careful follow-up of patients who have had a molar pregnancy, the number of deaths from this disease have been reduced.

The chemotherapeutic agent methotrexate is the treatment of choice but may be combined with surgery. The drug is a folic acid antagonist and may be administered orally or parenterally for 5 consecutive days and then withdrawn for a week. The course may need to be repeated several times if chorionic gonadotrophin titres do not regress. Actinomycin D may also be used alone or in combination with methotrexate (see Chapter 10).

Infections of the Reproductive Tract

INFECTIONS IN THE MALE

BALANITIS

Balanitis is an infection of the glans penis. Many different organisms may be causative. It is generally associated with poor personal hygiene in the uncircumcised male, but it may be associated with sexually transmitted diseases. Symptoms include redness, swelling, pain and a purulent discharge. The disease may be chronic and may cause the formation of adhesions and scarring.

Treatment

The infection is treated with the appropriate antibiotic following culture and sensitivity tests. Once the inflammatory process is controlled, circumcision, the excision of the prepuce, is advised.

On return from the operating theatre, the patient has a small petroleum jelly gauze dressing which is changed following each voiding. The patient may be taught to do this and how to care for the dressing at home.

Should bleeding occur, a pressure dressing is applied. The dressing may make voiding impossible or difficult. Usually the dressing can be removed within a short period of time.

PHIMOSIS

Phimosis is a condition in which the preputial orifice is too small to permit retraction over the glans. It may be congenital but is most frequently a sequel to infection or trauma. Circumcision is advised.

PARAPHIMOSIS

Paraphimosis occurs when a narrowed prepuce is either forced back over the glans or is gradually retracted over it. It then forms a tight, constricting band around the glans; venous return is impaired, and swelling and pain follow. Usually pain is too severe to permit manipulation, so a general anaesthetic is given, and the foreskin is pulled forward. Occasionally the foreskin may have to be incised, and a slit is made up the dorsal surface. This is usually followed by circumcision after the treatment of any infection which may have been present.

PROSTATITIS

Prostatitis is usually an ascending infection of the genitourinary tract, but it may also be the result of the haematogenous spread of the organism. It is often secondary to urethritis or instrumentation of the urethra, as occurs in the use of an indwelling catheter.

In the acute stage, fever and chills are accompanied by haematuria, frequency and dysuria. A urethral discharge may be noted. Rectal examination usually reveals an enlarged, tender, 'hot' prostate. Since infection of the seminal vesicles almost invariably accom-

panies prostatitis, the seminal vesicles can be palpated as well. Prostatic massage and instrumentation of the urethra are avoided to prevent possible spread of the infection to the epididymis, bladder and kidney. Exceptions are made only to relieve acute urinary retention, which may be a sequel to the enlarged prostate. A small urethral catheter will be used. In severe cases, drainage may be by suprapubic cystostomy rather than by catheterization. Prostatic abscesses may develop and usually drain through the urethra. Occasionally, excision and drainage are required.

The patient is placed on bed rest. Hydration, analgesics and stool softeners are useful as supportive therapy. Appropriate drug therapy is prescribed; this is usually cotrimoxazole (Bactrim). The patient is in considerable pain. The nurse often sees a tense, anxious and frightened patient who needs reassurance and support. Analgesics and warm baths help to relieve the pain and bladder spasms. The irritable bladder may require special attention, and antispasmodics and bladder sedatives are frequently ordered.

In cases in which treatment is early, excellent results usually follow. However, the acute picture may become chronic. The symptoms are mild and include a low-grade fever and some bacteria and pus in the urine. Fertility and potency are not affected unless complications ensue. The chronic infection may stubbornly resist treatment. Prostatic massage every 7–14 days is done by the doctor and helps by draining the bacteria away. Sexual intercourse or masturbation accomplishes the same purpose. Daily baths also help resolve the infection.

EPIDIDYMITIS

Epididymitis may be caused by any pyogenic organism. It frequently follows prostatitis and may be a complication of prostatectomy. Fever, malaise and chills accompany swelling and pain in the scrotum. The patient may be so uncomfortable that he may walk in a waddling fashion. Symptoms of cystitis may be present, and a hydrocele often develops. The swelling and irritation cause congestion of the testes which impedes the circulation of blood. Sterility follows from necrosis of the tubular epithelium and fibrosis which occludes the ducts.

The patient is placed on bed rest. The scrotum is elevated on towel rolls. Local applications of heat or cold may be ordered. After the patient is ambulant, a roomy scrotal support is worn.

Antibiotics are given but are not usually curative. If the disease is diagnosed early, a local anaesthetic agent is injected into the spermatic cord above the testes. Symptoms are usually absent in a day or two following this treatment. Chronic epididymitis may follow an acute episode. If the involvement is bilateral, sterility follows.

ORCHITIS

Inflammation of the testes may follow any infectious disease or may be acquired as an ascending infection from the genital tract. Most commonly it follows mumps parotitis. The mumps virus is excreted in the urine;

therefore, the spread to the testes in this case appears to be by descent. The onset is sudden, manifested by pain and swelling of the scrotum followed by fever and prostration. Urinary symptoms are usually not present. A hydrocele may develop, and the involvement may be unilateral or bilateral. Sterility probably follows death of the spermatogenic cells from ischaemia. Bed rest, scrotal support and local applications of heat or cold are ordered. A padded athletic support may be worn continuously.

Antibiotics are used in some situations but are not of value against the mumps virus. Local infiltration of the spermatic cord with a local anaesthetic may relieve the symptoms. The prevention of mumps in the postpubertal male has some value. If a man who has not been immunized as a child against mumps or who has not previously had mumps has been in contact with the virus, γ-globulin is usually administered.

INFECTIONS IN THE FEMALE

BARTHOLINITIS

Bartholinitis is an infection of the greater vestibular gland and may or may not be gonorrhoeal in origin. The infection is an ascending one, progressing up the ducts to the gland. Symptoms are usually those of an acute infection: pain, swelling, inflammation and a purulent discharge. Cellulitis of the surrounding tissues aggravates the situation, but the infection may localize and become an abscess. This is usually excised and drained. Sometimes the infection subsides, leaving the duct scarred and occluded. This may be followed by a cyst filled with the secretions of the gland which now cannot escape. The cyst is usually a painless swelling in the lower third of the labium minus. Treatment is to excise the cyst and gland. Alternatively, a marsupialization (conversion of the duct into a pouch) of the cystic duct may be done. This leaves the functioning gland in place.

Hot baths, saline soaks and/or the use of a bidet may be ordered following surgery. The patient should be advised on frequency of bathing and how to perform adequate vulval toilet before she is discharged.

VAGINITIS

Physiological leucorrhoea

Physiological leucorrhoea is a normal whitish discharge which helps to keep the vagina moist. It is composed of endocervical secretions, leucocytes, desquamated epithelial cells and other normal flora of the vaginal tract. The pH is normally 4–5 but varies during the life-cycle of the woman. At birth, it may be as low as 5 under the hormonal stimulus of the mother. As a child it is 6–7. At menarche the pH becomes acidic again, and assumes the adult pH of 4–5. Postmenopausally, oestrogen is withdrawn, and the pH rises to 6–7 again. The quantity of the discharge also varies among women, during stages of the menstrual cycle and during pregnancy. An increase is usually noticed at ovulation, during sexual stimulation and during pregnancy. The most characteris-

tic symptom of a vaginitis is a change in the normal vaginal discharge.

Trichomoniasis

The most common cause of vaginitis is a flagellated protozoon, known as a trichomonad. Trichomonads may be found in the large bowel and occasionally in the bladder and vestibular glands. They can be sexually transmitted and in men trichomonads may be harboured in the urethra, bladder or prostate.

The woman presents with symptoms of a heavy, greenish-yellow, frothy discharge which has a slight odour. This heavy discharge may be irritating to the vulva, causing pruritis and excoriation. The vaginal mucosa is reddened and is slightly oedematous. The patient may complain of dyspareunia and, if the bladder is involved, of dysuria and frequency. As the condition becomes chronic, the woman has fewer symptoms. Diagnosis is confirmed when trichomonads are seen microscopically in a vaginal smear.

Men frequently have few symptoms. There may be some urethral itching and a slight discharge. Invasion of the bladder may produce frequency and burning on micturition. Wet smears are made of the urethral discharge, and the protozoa seen microscopically confirm the diagnosis.

Treatment is usually the oral administration of metronidazole (Flagyl) 250 mg three times a day for 10 days. Repeat smears will then be done, and a repeat course of therapy may be necessary. During the treatment, a condom should be worn until both partners are considered cured. The woman may be given vaginal pessaries instead of oral therapy. A pessary is inserted morning and night daily for 4–8 weeks. This is continued through the menstrual period, for the menstrual flow is alkaline and provides an excellent medium for the protozoa. Insertion is like that of a vaginal tampon. The patient is instructed to remain flat for about 10 minutes following insertion.

Monilial vaginitis

Monilial vaginitis occurs when the vagina is invaded by the fungus *Candida albicans*. The vaginal pH is usually 5–7. Pregnant women and diabetics are predisposed because of glycosuria and the increased glycogen present in the vagina during pregnancy. Contamination may be from the rectum. A thick, white, curdy vaginal discharge is present which frequently causes pruritus and irritation of the vulva. The vaginal walls are reddened and covered with typical white patches. When the patches are swabbed off, bleeding may occur. Diagnosis is confirmed microscopically from a vaginal smear.

The patient is instructed in careful perineal care and hand washing to avoid reinfection and spread of the fungus to others, especially children. Nystatin vaginally or in the form of pessaries achieves good results. It may be given to pregnant women.

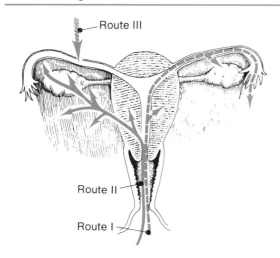

Figure 22.20 Common routes of the spread of pelvic inflammatory disease. Route I, commonly gonococcus and staphylococcus; route II, frequently streptococcus; route III, tuberculosis, usually a descending infection from another source.

Atrophic vaginitis (senile)

Because of hormonal changes following the menopause, the pH rises and the glycogen stores are reduced in the vagina. The vagina loses its rugae and becomes smooth and shiny. It is now more susceptible to invasion by organisms. A sticky, mucoid discharge may appear. The patient complains of a burning in the vagina, dyspareunia and pruritus of the vagina. Occasionally, the discharge is blood flecked, as areas of the vagina ulcerate and adhesions develop and tear. Severe infection is controlled by the use of systemic antibiotics or sulpha drugs. Oestrogens are prescribed.

TOXIC SHOCK SYNDROME

Toxic shock syndrome is a rare systemic disease occurring as the result of circulating toxins produced by *Staphylococcus aureus (S. aureus)* bacteria. The organisms produce two toxins; enterotoxin F, which affects intestinal mucosa causing gastroenteritis, and exotoxin C, which is pyrogenic. Signs and symptoms occur following the introduction of toxins into the bloodstream. The disease varies from a subclinical form to a severe septicaemia.

Clinical characteristics commonly include a high fever, rash, vomiting, diarrhoea, headache, sore throat and muscle pain. Hypotension progressing to shock occurs within 48 hours in severe cases. Laboratory results indicate renal, hepatic and haematological involvement. Diagnosis is confirmed by swabs positive for *S. aureus* taken from the patient's nose, throat, vaginal discharge and tampon, where applicable.

The disease is associated with intravaginal tampon use but is not caused by them. A significant number of women in the severe state are menstruating and using tampons. It is related to the fact that women have *Staphylococcus aureus* present in the vagina. Tampons act as a dam to vaginal flow providing ideal conditions for bacterial growth. Some tampons were found to carry the organisms and have now been withdrawn from the market. The new synthetic material tampons aggravate the situation by their greater drying effect. They may create microulcerations in the vaginal mucosa, allowing micro-organisms to escape into the bloodstream.

Treatment is supportive, aimed at relieving the symptoms and curative by eradicating the source of toxin production. If associated with tampon use, the tampons are removed and the vagina cleansed with a disinfecting solution and daily saline douches. The patient receives systemic medication to which the organisms are sensitive. These measures prevent further development of the bacteria but are ineffective against the already-circulating toxins.

Patient teaching is aimed at prevention of a recurrence. The patient with toxic shock syndrome associated with tampon use is advised to discontinue the use of tampons entirely or until she has three negative vaginal cultures for *S. aureus*, each culture a month apart. The patient then follows general instructions for the use of tampons.

1. Use only one tampon at a time.
2. Use the tampon of the absorbency that will control the flow; that is, never use one of super absorbency when a regular one would do. This reduces the chance of vaginal drying with subsequent trauma and ulceration.
3. Change the tampon frequently (every 4–6 hours).
4. Do not forget a tampon; always check by finger insertion in the vagina if you think you may have forgotten one.
5. If you suspect an infection, immediately remove the tampon and consult your doctor.

CERVICITIS

The cervix is the main barrier against ascending infections of the genital tract. As such it is exposed to many insults. The majority of these are small lacerations which occur during childbirth or injuries associated with surgery, instrumentation or sexually transmitted disease. When the cervical epithelium is damaged, infection may easily spread to the endocervix. Congestion and oedema follow. An increase in cervical mucus results in an elevation in vaginal pH. The cells of the endocervix begin growing out around the external os. This outgrowth of cells produces a red, granular raised lesion. As the cervix is exposed to further trauma, the eroded areas become infected again and again. Chronic cervicitis results.

The symptoms vary. Usually a heavy vaginal discharge exists. The patient may notice deep dyspareunia or some bloodstained discharge following intercourse.

The diagnosis depends on the characteristic appearance of the lesion. Cytological studies are usually done to distinguish cervicitis from early carcinoma. When carcinoma is ruled out, the condition is generally treated by cautery of the endocervix. After cautery the old tissue sloughs away, followed by the regeneration of the new from the outside edges of the lesion. The patient should expect a brownish discharge for 1–2 weeks as the old tissue sloughs away.

Often patients with cervicitis need to be taught proper perineal care.

PELVIC INFLAMMATORY DISEASE (PID)

Pelvic inflammatory disease has come to mean all ascending pelvic infections once they are beyond the cervix. Many organisms may be responsible for the symptoms. However, among the most frequent are the gonococcus and *Staphylococcus aureus*. On occasion, tuberculosis and anaerobic bacteria can be causative. Symptoms may follow labour and delivery, a criminally induced abortion, surgical procedures, or a contact with gonorrhoea or cervicitis. The condition may be acute or chronic.

Effects on the patient

The typical picture is one of a systemic infection with fever, chills, malaise, anorexia, nausea and vomiting. This is usually accompanied by lower abdominal pain which is either unilateral or bilateral. In more chronic cases, this pain is increased before and during menstruation. Pain is experienced on movement of the cervix. Leucorrhoea is present. With gonorrhoeal or staphylococcal infections the discharge is usually heavy and purulent; streptococcal infections cause a thinner, more mucoid discharge.

Spread of the infection occurs by two typical routes, which are demonstrated in Figure 22.20. Symptoms depend on which route the infection follows. In route I the bacteria spread along the surface of the endometrium to the fallopian tubes and into the peritoneum. The consequences of this route may be adhesions or cysts of the tube, with consequent infertility. In more advanced cases abscesses develop about the ovary or in the cul-de-sac. Infection following route II is spread mainly through the lymphatics and produces a pelvic cellulitis in contrast to the more localized endometritis or salpingitis (infection of the fallopian tube) of route I. Thrombophlebitis may follow this cellulitis. Advanced and virulent infections admitted by either route may become systemic and may show all the signs of septicaemia.

Treatment and nursing care

The patient with an acute episode is usually admitted to the hospital. She may or may not be isolated, depending on the cause of her infection. The patient is placed on bed rest in semi-recumbent position to promote drainage of pus into the vagina and the cul-de-sac. Vulval toilet should be done as needed to keep the patient clean and comfortable. Heat to the lower back and abdomen may be soothing. Analgesics and sedation may be ordered. The patient will receive antibiotics following culture and sensitivity studies. In some cases blood cultures may be obtained. Surgical treatment is deferred, if possible, until the infection is controlled. A culdocen-

tesis or colpotomy may be done to drain a pelvic abscess. Tubo-ovarian abscesses may require an abdominal approach. In cases of prolonged, debilitating infections which are resistant to conservative treatment, salpingectomy or hysterectomy may be done.

Sexually Transmitted Diseases

The health problem of greatest concern is AIDS. This produces a range of effects on the person and has been dealt with as appropriate elsewhere in this text. Other sexually transmitted diseases will be considered in this section. Table 3.1 lists the degree of risk for specific sexual practices.

GONORRHOEA

The specific organism causing gonorrhoea is *Neisseria gonorrhoeae*, and it is transmitted almost exclusively by sexual intercourse. The organism dies quickly when not harboured in the human body.

EFFECTS ON THE PATIENT

Symptoms appear 2–10 days after the initial contact. In the male urethritis occurs, heralded by a purulent urethral discharge. Some itching and burning about the meatus are also present. The urethral meatus is red and oedematous. The infection may remain localized and in about 2% of men is asymptomatic. An ascending infection involving the prostate, seminal vesicles, bladder and epididymis may result. If adhesions develop, they may damage the urethra and duct system with consequent urethral stricture and infertility.

Diagnosis is confirmed when the gonococcus is seen microscopically in smears or cultures taken from the site of infection. If urethral discharge is slight, the first urethral washings may be used. These are obtained by collecting the first portion of a voided urine specimen. The penis is not swabbed off before collecting the specimen.

In the adult female the vagina with its layers of squamous epithelium is resistant to the gonococcus. Therefore, the vulnerable areas are the vestibular glands, the urethra and the endocervix. The glands become red, swollen and sore. A purulent discharge may drain from the urethra and the ducts of the glands. Leucorrhoea is present in cases in which cervicitis accompanies the picture. Dysuria and frequency often occur. In about 50% of women the symptoms may be mild and vague. The infection may ascend above the cervix and may form the characteristic picture described in pelvic inflammatory disease.

Diagnosis is made on the basis of organisms seen in smears or cultures. To obtain these specimens the patient is instructed not to void or douche for approximately 2 hours before the cultures are taken. The vulva is not cleansed first. With the patient in a lithotomy position, smears are taken from the urethra, cervix and the ducts of the vestibular glands.

TREATMENT

In 1976 a drug-resistant strain of *Neisseria gonorrhoeae* was identified; this strain of the organism produces an enzyme (penicillinase) that inactivates penicillin. Patients infected with this resistant strain are treated with spectinomycin or a cephalosporin. Treatment is successful in cases in which repeated cultures are judged to be negative. Ceftriaxone, an injectable third generation cephalosporin, is presently used in the treatment of gonorrhoea.

NON-SPECIFIC URETHRITIS

Non-specific urethritis is far more common than gonorrhoea in the UK. The man complains of mild gonorrhoea-like symptoms which may become severe. It is important to rule out gonorrhoea as a cause. The onset of the symptoms is frequently related to coitus, often during menstruation when vaginal bacteria are increased, but in other cases no obvious link exists.

The infection may be due to one of several agents, but in 40% of cases is the result of a chlamydial infection. Chlamydia are a group of organisms which multiply like bacteria but do so only in the host cell, like viruses.

The infection frequently coexists with gonorrhoea but may persist as a postgonococcal urethritis following successful treatment of the gonorrhoea. This can be anxiety producing for the patient. Reassurance and teaching about the complaints are helpful in relieving anxiety.

Cultures for *Chlamydia trachomatis* are made from swabs of the anterior urethra and from first urethral washings. Tetracycline is the treatment of choice. Those unable to take tetracycline, including pregnant women and children, are treated with erythromycin. Sexual intercourse is contraindicated during the acute stage as it prolongs the symptoms. Repeat cultures are made to confirm the effects of treatment.

The infection may progress to a chronic state or to epididymitis, prostatitis and rarely Reiter's syndrome. In women the organism contributes to non-specific cervicitis, vaginitis and pelvic inflammatory disease. The newborn may acquire the infection during delivery through the vagina. For these reasons many doctors treat the female partners of infected men. It is hoped this will prevent later development of chlamydial-related pelvic disease in these women and reduce the incidence of newborn eye and chest infections.

HUMAN PAPILLOMAVIRUS INFECTION

Human papillomavirus (HPV) is the causative organism in condylomata acuminata or genital warts. These warts can be confused with those of syphilis but are different. They are less flat and more cauliflower like. Some attain a large size. This viral infection was previously thought to be benign but recently HPV has been associated with several genital cancers in both men and women.

The infection can be silent. No visible warts are present, but a type of HPV-induced cervical dysplasia exists which is seen during colposcopy or as a result of a smear test. In a number of those cases the dysplasia

may progress to a cervical neoplasia or, if on the vulva or vagina, to vulvar intraepithelial neoplasia (VIN). Some forty or more types of the virus exist but only HPV types 16 and 18 are associated with malignant changes. The virus is not thought to be carcinogenic. Some other agent may trigger it to induce malignant changes or it may simply coexist with the oncogenic agent. It is more common in women and during pregnancy but many men also have the infection. A number of babies develop laryngeal papilloma and the route of transmission is thought to be vaginal, during birth. The infection appears to go through stages from infection with visible warts to a spontaneous regression of the warts in a significant number of women. It may then enter a latent phase.

The risk factors for acquiring the virus are early age at first intercourse (less than 17 years old), multiple sex partners, a history of sexually transmitted diseases, poor personal and sexual hygiene, a sexual partner with a similar history, a history of anal intercourse, and immunosuppression or immunodeficiency for any reason. Sexual intercourse is the major method of transmission.

Patients presenting with external warts will be screened for other sexually transmitted diseases, and if present they will be treated. A colposcopy examination and smear tests will be done. The partners of infected patients should also be examined and treated if necessary. External warts are treated with podophyllin 10–25% in tincture of benzoin. This caustic agent is applied with a cotton applicator and washed off in 4 hours. The surrounding skin is coated with vaseline before application of the podophyllin. It is not used on internal warts. Cervical and vaginal warts may be bathed in an 85% solution of trichloroacetic acid. This produces a stinging sensation; a vaginal discharge follows for about 1 week as the tissue sloughs away.

Non-visible warts (small flat warts on the cervix or areas of dysplasia associated with the HPV on vulva or penis) are frequently vaporized with a carbon dioxide laser. Because the virus tends to recur, treatment during pregnancy is delayed until the third trimester. The virus is a stable one and can be transmitted from specula to other patients if instruments are not properly cleaned and sterilized.

SYPHILIS

Syphilis is a serious disease and, fortunately, is much less common than gonorrhoea. The causative organism is the spirochaete *Treponema pallidum*.

EFFECTS ON THE PATIENT

Incubation varies between 10 and 90 days. In most cases the disease is spread by sexual intercourse. As with the gonococcus, the spirochaete does not survive outside the host. In the untreated condition, three stages are distinguished. The stages may overlap or be widely separated. The primary lesion is a small, painless chancre or ulcer. It is deep and has indurated edges. Usually, this chancre heals spontaneously, giving the false impression that the disease is cured. This primary lesion appears most commonly on the penis of the male. In the female, it may appear on the labia, vagina or cervix. The secondary stage is usually characterized by a rash appearing over the body. This rash may be accompanied by condylomata lata on the female vulva. This is a cauliflower-appearing collection of flat, grey vulvar warts. As are all lesions of syphilis, these are teeming with spirochaetes and are highly infectious. The rash is usually accompanied by malaise and fever. In a short period the rash regresses and the patient enters the latent stages. Latency refers to the absence of symptoms in the infected individual. Pregnant women can still infect their fetus in utero, thus demonstrating the infectiousness of the blood. However, progress of the disease in the individual seems arrested and only rarely can others be infected in this stage. Three outcomes are now possible: (1) the patient proceeds immediately or after a delay of 10–30 years to the third stage; (2) the disease remains latent for the rest of the person's life; or (3) a spontaneous cure occurs. In the tertiary stage the bones, heart and central nervous system, including the brain, can be affected. Personality disorders arise and the typical ataxic gait of the tertiary syphilitic appears. A large, ulcerating necrotic lesion known as a gumma now occurs. Rarely is it seen in the genital tract, but it may occur on the vulva or in the testes. At this stage the disease may be arrested but not reversed.

Diagnosis is made by a careful history, clinical findings, and cultures or biopsies from the lesions. Blood serology is also assessed. Since blood serology is not positive for about 4 weeks after the onset of the disease, the early diagnosis is made from scrapings of the lesions. They can be seen on dark-field examination. These scrapings are made before antibiotic therapy is initiated so that the diagnosis can be confirmed.

TREATMENT

Treatment is by antibiotic, and penicillin is the drug of choice. A series of injections is necessary; oral medication is not effective. The Jarisch–Herxheimer reaction is a local and systemic reaction which may occur after beginning antisyphilitic therapy. Fever, sweating and headache appear 2–12 hours after treatment. The reaction should be differentiated from a penicillin reaction.

NURSING INTERVENTION

Most cases of sexually transmitted disease are treated on an out-patient basis, and patients must be taught how to protect themselves and others. First, the nature and transmission of the disease should be understood. No immunity develops and reinfection can occur easily. Strict personal and perineal hygiene should be observed. Hand washing following any handling of the genitalia is imperative, as the gonococcus can be readily carried to the eye, which quickly becomes infected. Blindness may ensue if treatment is not received. Women who are handling small children need to be especially careful. The vagina of a pre-pubertal girl is sensitive to the gonococcus because it lacks the protective layers of squamous epithelium. A form of vulvovaginitis may occur as a result of contamination from a family member. Sexual abuse is the cause of some cases in children. Sexual intercourse is to be avoided until the doctor notifies the patient he or she is cured. All equipment must be sterilized following use, and dressings or swabs are disposed of in a safe way. Syphilis may be transmitted by direct contamination with living spirochaetes of a laceration. For this reason, the routine use of universal body substance precautions will also control inadvertent transmission of this disease to health professionals. Once therapy has been initiated, the patient is usually non-infectious within 48 hours.

The disease may be very distressing to the patient. The patient may experience guilt feelings, and marital difficulties may arise when one partner infects the other. The disease carries a social stigma. For these reasons, confidentiality must be maintained by the nurse at all times; the issue is protected by law and the disease is reportable. Contacts must be identified and discreetly followed by the contact tracer. The contact tracer, by explaining the nature of the disease, usually obtains the patient's co-operation in identifying contacts.

The contact tracer will have to take a sexual history to identify sexual practices and contacts so that appropriate follow-up and health teaching can be done. Table 22.7 outlines a series of questions which a contact tracer might go through to obtain the necessary information. The interview requires privacy, reassurance of confidentiality, and is done while the patient is dressed, before the physical examination. The contact tracer should explain clearly to the patient the purpose of the

Table 22.7 Questions that might be asked of a patient when taking a sexual history.

1. Are you currently sexually active?
   If not, when was your last sexual contact?

2. When you engage in sexual activity is it with men, women or both?

3. Are you currently active with more than one partner?
   If yes, trace each partner in the last three months.
   If no, have you had any other sexual partner in the last three months?

4. Can you describe the kinds of sexual practices you do; for example, oral, anal, genital sex? This is important because it helps us decide what tests we need to do and what risks of other diseases you may have.

5. What kinds of protection do you or your partner(s) use during sexual activity?

6. How have your symptoms affected your sexual activity and relationships?

7. Have you any questions about your sexual activity?

8. Have you thought about how to tell your partner(s) about the problem?

Modified from Andrist (1988).

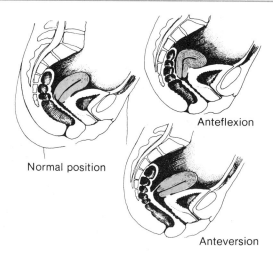

Figure 22.21 Normal position of the uterus; anteflexion and anteversion.

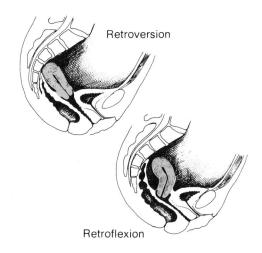

Figure 22.22 Retroversion and retroflexion of the uterus.

questions and why they are necessary. In addition, the nurse should include sexually transmitted diseases in any lectures prepared on general health education in schools so that the population may become more aware of the signs and symptoms, the modes of transmission, and the safe sex practices needed to prevent spread of these diseases (see p. 25).

Responsible sexual conduct, based on a healthy understanding of human sexuality, should be taught. The definition of responsible sexual conduct varies considerably. For some it means complete abstinence from sexual intercourse or activity until permitted by religious or cultural laws. For others, a wide range of sexual practices are accepted and practised. However low-risk sex practices should be known to all (see Table 3.1), and some safe sex guidelines follow.

1. Reducing the number of sexual partners is very important. Abstinence is safe. Adolescents and adults should be encouraged to avoid casual sexual encounters. Longer term monogamous relationships with known sexual partners reduce the risks by reducing the opportunity for exposure. Within such a long-term relationship, the latitude available for sexual practices can be broader and still be considered safe from the threat of disease.
2. Avoid the exchange of body fluids by:
   (a) Using a condom during vaginal, anal and oral intercourse. Condoms have been shown to be effective barriers to bacterial and viral agents. Use each condom only once.
   (b) Never using saliva as a lubricant. Use spermicides or water soluble jelly.
   (c) Not following or preceding anal intercourse with vaginal penetration without a change of condom.
   (d) Using gentle sexual practices which avoid trauma to mucous membrane or skin.
   (e) Avoiding other sexual practices such as oral–anal, oral–genital sex as it is difficult to avoid the ingestion or exchange of body fluids or or-

ganisms. Gonorrhoea, hepatitis, HIV and other viruses can be transmitted in these ways.
   (f) Avoiding prolonged wet (French) kissing unless with a partner whom you consider to be safe.

Displacements and Relaxations of the Female Genital Organs

RETROVERSION AND RETROFLEXION OF THE UTERUS

The normal position of the uterus is one of some anteversion and anteflexion (Figure 22.21). It is not a fixed organ. The filling of the bladder or bowel may cause a change in uterine position. On occasion, the uterus assumes a retroverted or retroflexed position. When retroverted, the fundus points toward the sacrum and the cervix toward the anterior vaginal wall. Retroflexion refers to the position of the fundus of the uterus in relation to the cervix. In retroflexion the fundus bends back over the cervix (Figure 22.22). Degrees of retroversion and retroflexion are possible so that the case may be mild or extreme.

The aetiology appears to lie in a weakness of the supporting structures which may be either congenital or acquired. The acquired weakness is frequently due to injuries during the maternity cycle. Adhesions and tumours may pull or push the uterus into this position.

The patient may complain of backache, infertility, dyspareunia or dysmenorrhoea, but she is frequently symptomless unless the situation is extreme. Backache and dysmenorrhoea are probably associated with pelvic congestion. Infertility may arise because the cervix does not reach the seminal pool. Frequently, the ovaries prolapse into the cul-de-sac and become congested and enlarged. Because of this, intercourse may be painful.

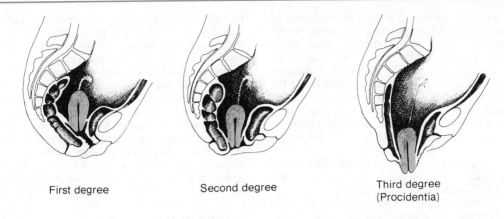

First degree   Second degree   Third degree (Procidentia)

Figure 22.23 Uterine prolapse: showing first-degree; second-degree; and third-degree (procidentia) pro-lapse.

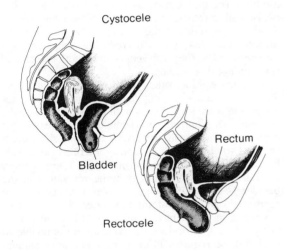

Cystocele

Bladder

Rectum

Rectocele

Figure 22.24 Cystocele and rectocele.

TREATMENT

Usually the uterus is manually replaced, and a vaginal pessary is inserted to hold the uterus in place. The pessary functions by holding the cervix in a posterior position. This in turn rotates the uterus forward. When the pessary is properly in position, the patient is unaware of its presence and no difficulty is experienced on voiding or during intercourse. The patient will return in about 4–6 weeks to have the pessary checked and removed for cleaning. The gynaecologist may then give the patient a 6-week trial period without the pessary to see if she remains free of symptoms. If not, a further trial with the pessary may be given.

All pessaries are irritating, especially those which are rubber and have some degree of movement. An offensive-smelling leucorrhoea usually develops, and chronic ulceration may occur.

In other cases the uterus will be surgically suspended by shortening the round ligaments. This is done when the pessary does not correct the situation.

PROLAPSE, CYSTOCELE AND RECTOCELE

Uterine prolapse refers to the downward displacement of the entire organ. Prolapse (Figure 22.23) may occur in varying degrees. First-degree prolapse describes the condition existing when the uterus descends within the vagina. Second-degree prolapse occurs when the cervix protrudes through the introitus. Procidentia, or third-degree prolapse, refers to the entire uterus protruding through the introitus with total inversion of the vagina.

Cystocele, urethrocele, rectocele and enterocele refer to herniations or relaxations of the bladder, urethra, rectum and small bowel into the vagina (Figure 22.24). They may occur singly or in combinations with some degree of uterine prolapse.

The single most important aetiological factor in the development of these conditions is thought to be injury at childbirth. The pelvic floor and supporting structures may be stretched and torn during the process of delivery and are thereby weakened. Further relaxation results after menopause as the tissues atrophy following oestrogen withdrawal. Large intra-abdominal tumours may also place an added strain on already weakened tissue. In some rare cases, the structures seem to be congenitally weak.

The patient with a prolapse often complains of a feeling of 'something coming down'. She may have a dragging or a heavy feeling in the pelvis, accompanied by backache and bladder symptoms of either retaining or losing urine. She may have recurrent cystitis. When the cervix protrudes through the introitus, it may become ulcerated from constant friction. This may produce pain and bleeding. The patient with a cystocele frequently has symptoms of stress incontinence.

Diagnosis is usually confirmed by bimanual and rectal examinations. The patient will be asked to bear down, cough or strain while the doctor estimates the degree of prolapse or herniation.

TREATMENT AND NURSING RESPONSIBILITIES

The best treatment is prevention. Better care during the

maternity cycle has helped to reduce the incidence of these complications. Exercises should be taught by the physiotherapist and encouraged by the nurse to all patients in the postpartum period and the same exercises may be taught to help relieve mild prolapse. These consist of alternately tightening and relaxing the gluteal and perineal floor muscles. Practising starting and stopping the stream of urine also helps the patient regain good perineal muscle tone. She should continue to practise these exercises several times a day for several weeks.

In situations in which surgery is contraindicated, the use of pessaries may be employed. A variety are available for different degrees of prolapse.

Surgical intervention is frequently necessary to correct the situation. An anterior and posterior colporrhaphy and perineorrhaphy repair a cystocele and rectocele, respectively.

In some women where prolapse of the uterus is present and future childbearing is not an issue, a Manchester repair may be done. This combines the amputation of an elongated cervix and shortening of the cardinal ligaments with an anterior and posterior repair. Although childbearing is not precluded by an anterior and posterior repair, delivery by caesarean section is usually recommended in order to retain this repair. Vaginal hysterectomy with an anterior and posterior repair is usually performed for more severe uterine prolapse. The fallopian tubes and the uterus with all or part of the cervix will be removed. The ligaments and blood vessels are ligated, and a cuff is made in the upper portion of the vagina.

The nursing care of these patients is similar to that given to any patient undergoing surgery. The nurse assists the patient in understanding the limitations, if any, surgery will impose on sexual and reproductive capacity, since misunderstandings frequently occur. The nurse should assess the psychosocial impact the surgery may have on the patient.

During surgery the patient may receive an intravenous vasoconstrictor to reduce the danger of haemorrhage. Blood loss during vaginal surgery tends to be heavy and is heavier still in premenopausal women.

In theatre the patient's legs are carefully lifted together to be placed into and removed from the stirrups. No one should lean or apply pressure on the anaesthetized leg to avoid thrombus formation. These measures reduce postoperative discomfort, avoid strain on the repaired perineal muscles and help reduce the incidence of postoperative emboli. These same measures should be used whenever a patient's legs are placed in stirrups.

Following vaginal surgery, the nurse observes the patient for signs and symptoms of haemorrhage, urinary tract infection, thromboemboli and infections at the surgical site. Haemorrhage may be frank, oozing or in the form of a large haematoma. The oozing of blood may not be readily noticed by the patient or the staff; therefore, the nurse must be careful to observe the estimated blood loss over a period of time, not just each time she checks the patient. A haematoma is a form of concealed haemorrhage; the blood vessels bleed into the tissue of the vagina or perineum. The patient complains of discomfort or pain over the site. The tissue bulges and may be so taut as to glisten. The nurse should notify the doctor immediately and be prepared to assist with treatment and the possible return of the patient to the operating theatre. Blood transfusions may be required. The clot may be evacuated, the bleeding vessels ligated or the site firmly packed. An antibiotic may be ordered to lessen the chance of infection.

Postoperatively the patient returns with a suprapubic drain. This is a small polyethylene tube which has been threaded through a needle into the bladder. The abdomen is surgically prepared, the bladder filled with sterile saline solution, and the needle inserted. The tube is taped or caught with a stitch to the skin to avoid accidental removal and attached to a sterile drainage system. It drains freely for 3–4 days and the patient voids as she can. Seventy per cent of women void spontaneously before the tube is clamped, starting on the fourth day. If the tube leaks, tape may be placed around the base. The tube can be used to obtain residuals, but occasionally a catheter may have to be used. Suprapubic drainage has reduced the incidence of postoperative urinary tract infections by reducing the need for catheterizations. They also reduce the emotional tension surrounding first voiding.

In some cases the patient may have catheter drainage. She is catheterized preoperatively, and the catheter remains in place for 7–9 days until the oedema has been resolved. The catheter is clamped and released for periods of time, finally removed, and then the patient attempts voiding. She is usually catheterized twice daily for residual urine during the first 24–36 hours without the catheter. If the amount or urine remaining in the bladder is above 75–100 ml, a Foley catheter may be reinserted or the cystostomy tube opened.

Voiding in sufficient quantities should occur at least every 6 hours. To induce the patient who is unable to void to do so requires all the nurse's skill in an attempt to avoid catheterization. Patients are usually encouraged to move about early and getting up to void helps. If the use of a bidet or vulval toilet is allowed, it usually helps if these are encouraged immediately before the patient attempts to void. When catheterization is necessary, the strictest aseptic technique should be followed.

Perineal care is important to the prevention of infection. Depending on the extent of the surgery, sterile technique may be required. It should be as frequent as necessary to keep the perineal area clean and dry. General principles of working from front to back are followed. In addition, sterile pads are applied. Vulval toilet may be ordered with sterile or plain water or some solutions. The nurse or patient runs the solution from a bag and tubing over the perineum into a basin. If the patient is well enough, she is taught how to do these procedures.

Straining at stool is avoided by a low residue diet and the avoidance of constipation.

On discharge the patient may receive further instructions; some doctors definitely restrict heavy lifting and prolonged standing, walking and sitting. Intercourse is contraindicated for approximately 6 weeks.

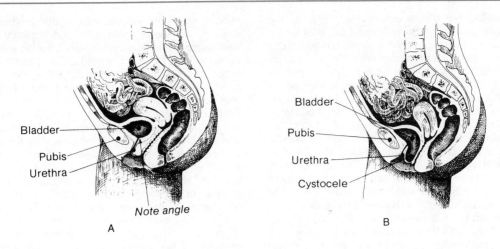

Figure 22.25 (A) The bladder at ease; no stress incontinence. **(B)** Cystocele without stress incontinence.

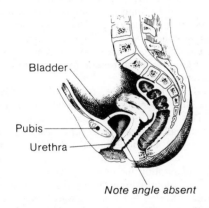

Figure 22.26 The bladder during micturition.

STRESS INCONTINENCE

Stress incontinence is the involuntary loss of small amounts of urine when a woman coughs, sneezes or otherwise suddenly increases the intra-abdominal pressure and, therefore, the intravesical pressure. It should be distinguished from urge incontinence and frequency related to abnormal detrusor function. See Chapter 20 for further discussion.

The urge to void and the ability of the bladder to contract are controlled by the detrusor muscle which lines the bladder wall. As the bladder fills, the detrusor muscle is stretched and nerve endings send a message of the need to void to the brain via the spinal cord. In some people, more commonly women, an irritable detrusor muscle overreacts sending a message before the bladder is really full and contracting quite vigorously, sometimes involuntarily. The patient complains of an urgent desire to void and not always reaching the lavatory on time.

Continence is maintained at the junction of the urethra and bladder by continuous spiral muscles from the base of the bladder to the upper urethra. Assistance is also received from the muscles surrounding the urethra, as well as a tight supporting perineal floor. In the continent woman these relationships can be demonstrated radiologically by observing that the angle between the urethra and posterior wall of the bladder is approximately 90° (Figure 22.25). Normally, this angle is only obliterated at micturition (Figure 22.26) when an increased intra-abdominal pressure combines with a relaxed urethrovesical muscle and perineal floor to lower the base of the bladder. However, in stress incontinence, the slight effort of straining, coughing or sneezing is sufficient to reduce this angle, and an involuntary loss of urine occurs. This explanation is thought to describe about 90% of cases of stress incontinence. A woman may have a cystocele (see Figure 22.25) and still be continent if the relationships demonstrated by the angle are maintained. However, many women with a cystocele also have accompanying stress incontinence.

Occasionally, stress incontinence follows a cystocele repair. This is probably due to elevation of the bladder to a position which obliterates the angle. For this reason many surgeons check the angle following repair to be sure it will be adequate.

The symptoms may become distressing to the woman. Frequent small dribbles of urine cause wetness, irritation and an offensive odour. The woman may have to wear protective pads and gradually she may become shy of social contacts and confine herself to home.

Diagnosis is made following a physical examination and a urodynamic evaluation. A pelvic and modified neurological examination is done to diagnose any underlying pelvic or neurological disease. The urodynamic evaluation, which includes a series of tests, helps to distinguish true stress incontinence from other conditions. The series of tests usually requires a day at the hospital and is done on an out-patient basis. In preparation the patient is instructed not to void or take self-medication for 6–8 hours before going to the urodynamic laboratory. This provides a full bladder for testing and avoids drug effects on nerve conduction.

Initially uroflowmeter readings are done. The patient is instructed to void into a funnel connected to a flowmeter. This meter is an electronic device which calculates the rate at which urine flows, the time taken to void and the volume voided. The results are printed on a graph. An abnormally high rate of flow is associated with stress incontinence. Immediately following this the patient is catheterized for residual urine. This test may be followed by a cystometrogram. During this latter procedure a catheter is passed, attached to a transducer and the bladder is filled with fluid, usually water. The patient is asked to tell the doctor when she feels a sense of fullness and when her bladder actually feels full. She is told to void and then asked to stop voiding. The transducer meanwhile records on a graph the changes in bladder pressure associated with these events. The doctor can assess how the patient perceives and responds to these sensations and requests. Normally bladder pressure increases when voiding as the bladder is contracting and drops when voiding ceases and the bladder relaxes. This may be combined with a urethral pressure profile. Urethral pressure is recorded as the catheter is slowly withdrawn at a constant rate through the urethra.

More elaborate tests may be done such as electromyograms to measure response and strength of bladder muscle, videorecordings and measurements of intra-abdominal pressure by rectal electrodes. They are used less often in stress incontinence.

These procedures, with the exception of the uroflowmeter, require sterile equipment, appropriate preparation of the patient and sterile gowning and gloving of the staff. A few patients may require an anaesthetic.

TREATMENT

Treatment begins with prevention of injury and ensuing incontinence by good maternity care and the practise of postpartum exercises in the immediate postpartum period.

Stress incontinence is aggravated by chronic urinary tract infections, obesity and chronic coughing. Prevention includes the education of women about stress incontinence and the aggravating factors. Any urinary and vaginal tract infections are treated; the obese patient is advised to lose weight and an appropriate diet is discussed to assist her with this. The heavy smoker is advised to reduce or stop smoking as a means of reducing coughing, and is also instructed about stop-smoking programmes designed to help in this. Mild stress incontinence and abnormal detrusor activity are treated similarly. They also frequently coexist. The patient is assisted to re-establish a normal voiding pattern and bladder control. She is usually provided with a bladder drill and exercise regimen.

Bladder drill involves routines related to voiding. The patient is instructed to void each hour by the clock whether she feels the need to or not. When she has kept herself dry this way for three or four days she increases the time interval between voidings by one-half hour every 3 days until she can comfortably hold urine for three hours. She is instructed to drink plenty of non-stimulating fluids (e.g. caffeine-free) during the day, to drink nothing for 2 hours before going to bed and to empty her bladder completely before going to sleep. She is also instructed to empty her bladder before and after sexual intercourse.

The exercises consist of always giving an extra push at the end of voiding to make sure all urine is expelled. She also is instructed to practise tightening the buttocks and pelvic floor muscles and stopping and starting the stream of urine during micturition. The exercises are practised several times a day. If the patient is unsure whether or not she is practising them correctly, she can be taught to insert two fingers into the vagina and contract the vaginal muscles to grip the fingers as tightly as possible. This provides the patient with a direct measure of her progress. Once she has learned the technique, it can be practised without inserting her fingers.

Various smooth muscle relaxants which inhibit detrusor activity and increase bladder capacity may be prescribed while the patient is practising the bladder drill and re-establishing a voiding pattern. This regimen is successful for detrusor problems and for correcting mild stress incontinence. In incontinence of a more severe nature, surgery may be necessary in order to support the urethra and restore the proper urethrovesical relationship.

Several operations are commonly used. In the Aldridge sling operation the surgeon makes a sling of fascia. This sling is then attached to the anterior abdominal wall. This serves to support the urethra. The approach may be abdominal, vaginal or both. Occasionally, the sling is too tight and the patient has difficulty micturating and emptying the bladder properly. Cystitis and other complications may occur. Teaching the patient to bend her body forward when attempting to void postoperatively helps. This relaxes the muscles of the abdomen, thereby loosening the sling and lowering the base of the bladder.

The Marshall–Marchetti–Krantz operation supports the urethra by suturing the anterior vaginal wall on each side to the periosteum of the pubic bone and the anterior wall of the bladder to the pubic bone.

In the Burch colposuspension operation the procedure is carried out abdominally. The vagina is lifted by means of two sutures inserted into each side of the bladder and then attached to the iliopectoral ligament.

FISTULAE

Fistulae may occur between the vagina or uterus and the bladder, urethra or rectum (Figure 22.27). They can occur as a sequel to injury during labour and delivery, surgery, and disease processes, such as carcinoma, and radiation therapy.

When urinary fistulae develop, some urine leaks into the vagina or uterus. Rectal fistulae causes the escape of flatus and faeces into the vagina. In both instances, irritation to the tissues occurs. An offensive odour develops and causes much embarrassment for the patient. Since many fistulae spontaneously heal within a

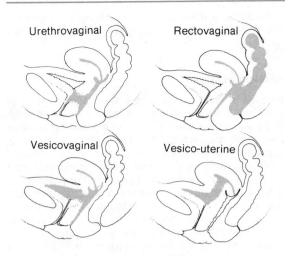

Urethrovaginal   Rectovaginal

Vesicovaginal   Vesico-uterine

Figure 22.27 Fistulae: urethrovaginal; rectovaginal; vesicovaginal; and vesico-uterine.

matter of several weeks, treatment may be postponed. During that period nursing care is very important to the patient. Frequent perineal care is required to keep the patient clean. Cleansing and deodorizing douches may be ordered. High enemas may be given to reduce the constant flow of faeces. Care should be taken to go above the fistula with the rectal tube. If the fistula does not heal spontaneously, surgery may be indicated. Following surgery involving the bladder, the patient may return from the operating room with a urethral as well as a suprapubic catheter. Drainage must be maintained so that pressure on the repaired area is kept at a minimum. Repair may also include implantation of the ureters elsewhere. Rectal fistulae may be repaired and a temporary colostomy established in order to provide time to heal. Ambulation may be postponed for a few days. The woman may be discharged home on restricted activity until the doctor advises that the repair is complete.

Benign and Malignant Disorders of the Reproductive Tract

IN THE MALE

SPERMATOCELE

A spermatocele is a cyst of the spermatic cord which contains sperm in a thin white fluid. It lies above the testis and is separate from it. The mass will transilluminate. Usually a spermatocele requires no treatment. Sometimes it may become large enough to be confused with hydrocele and to be aggravating to the patient. Then it may be excised. The aetiology is unclear.

VARICOCELE

Varicocele is the dilatation of the venous plexus about the testis. It occurs most frequently on the left side. Its appearance on the right side may indicate that a tumour is occluding the vein above the level of the scrotum. Some testicular atrophy may occur if the circulation is impeded for long periods of time. This may result in subfertility. On palpation behind and above the testis the doctor feels a mass of tortuous veins which empties when the patient lies down.

Treatment may consist of a scrotal support which relieves the dragging sensation. If fertility is an issue or the condition is severe, the internal spermatic vein may be ligated. The results are usually excellent. A scrotal support may be worn for 4–5 days following surgery, since scrotal oedema may be present.

HYDROCELE

A hydrocele is a collection of fluid in the tunica vaginalis. It may occur following local injury, infection or a neoplasm and may be unilateral or bilateral. More often it is chronic, and the cause is unknown. In newborn babies, the cause is usually a late closure of the processus vaginalis. This frequently closes spontaneously. In some young men a chronic type exists because the processus vaginalis never closes completely, and a connection remains between the peritoneal cavity and the tunica vaginalis.

Treatment is not required unless the testis cannot be palpated to rule out abnormality, circulation to the testis is impaired or the hydrocele becomes large, unsightly and uncomfortable. Then the hydrocele is aspirated, and a sclerosing drug may be injected. In chronic cases the tunica vaginalis is excised (hydrocelectomy). Postoperatively the scrotum is elevated on a pillow or bridge dressing, and a pressure dressing is applied. Depending on the operation, there may or may not be a drain present in the incision. The patient must be observed for haemorrhage which may be concealed in the hydrocele sac. When ambulatory the patient usually requires a fresh scrotal support daily. Immediately after the operation he may need a larger support than usual.

TORSION OF THE TESTIS

Torsion of the testis occurs when the testis rotates within the tunica vaginalis. Often this is due to spasm of the cremaster muscle which rotates the testis in what is usually an abnormally large vaginalis. The young man experiences a sudden severe pain in the area of the testis which is unrelieved by rest or support. Because the torsion reduces the blood supply to the testis, testicular atrophy follows rapidly. Sometimes under local anaesthesia the surgeon will attempt to reduce torsion. If this is unsuccessful, surgical reduction follows.

BENIGN HYPERPLASIA OF THE PROSTATE

The reason benign enlargement of the prostate gland occurs is unknown. However, it is estimated that over 50% of men over 60 show some signs of prostatic enlargement. Of these, about 25% will require treatment.

In the young adult male the prostate gland is encased

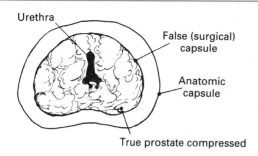

Figure 22.28 Transverse section of a hyperplastic prostate.

in a thin capsular membrane which is closely adherent to the underlying tissue. Gradually tissue begins to enlarge by new growth (hyperplasia) and the capsule of the prostate becomes thick and is loosely attached to the underlying tissue. This inner tissue can now be easily stripped away, leaving the thickened capsule intact (Figure 22.28). The enlarging prostate encroaches on the urethra and the base of the bladder, producing certain symptoms.

Effects on the patient

Gradually, the man may experience hesitancy in beginning the flow of urine. The stream of urine is reduced in force and size. Incomplete emptying of the bladder produces residual urine which reduces bladder capacity so that urgency and frequency result. Nocturia occurring three or more times in one night is a good indication of frequency. Often, cystitis occurs as well. In severe cases, the bladder becomes overdistended, and hypertrophy and small diverticula follow as weakened areas of bladder mucosa bulge out between the bands of muscle fibres. The back-up of urine causes hydroureter or even hydronephrosis. Over long periods of time renal function may be impaired.

Frequently, the patient does not seek medical attention until acute retention of urine occurs. Overdistension of the bladder is usually the precipitating factor. The patient is catheterized and urine is slowly released from the bladder. This prevents a sudden release of pressure in the abdomen which could cause shock and haemorrhage. Shock follows the rush of blood from vital centres to fill the newly released blood vessels. This sudden filling may cause small blood vessels in the bladder mucosa to rupture. The catheter remains in place for 2–3 days, after which normal voiding patterns usually return. The patient is cautioned to avoid an excessive intake of fluid in a short period of time, as this rapidly distends the bladder, precipitating retention. He should void frequently when he has the urge to do so in order to avoid overdistension of the bladder. If followed, these instructions should help the individual to avoid acute retention. However, one should remain alert for the patient with retention with overflow who voids frequent small amounts of urine. This may be seen in the chronic case with progressive upper urinary tract involvement.

Backache and sciatica may also bring the patient to the doctor, since the enlarged prostate exerts pressure on nerves.

Surgical treatment

Surgery is indicated to relieve the symptoms and to prevent infections of the urinary tract and renal damage. If the amount of residual urine in the bladder is above 75–100 ml, the surgeon may feel surgery is necessary even though the symptoms are not severe. Residual urine is estimated in several ways. Immediately after voiding, a catheter may be passed and any remaining urine is drawn off and measured. A radiopaque contrast medium can be injected into the bladder. The man is then asked to void and postvoiding films are made. Direct visualization of the bladder may be done by cystoscope, and any bladder changes will be noted. Intravenous urography will indicate the extent of ureter and kidney involvement. Renal function tests may be ordered as well.

A period of preoperative preparation may be necessary. Residual urine and hydroureter are treated by catheterization for a period of 1–2 weeks. The patient is prepared for surgery by explaining what may follow the operation so that the postoperative period is not so traumatic.

Several operations are commonly used to treat this condition. The choice of operation seems to depend on the size of the prostate, the condition of the patient and the preference of the surgeon. A prostate in excess of 50 g is considered by most surgeons to be too difficult to remove transurethrally. Therefore, an open route is chosen.

Transurethral prostatectomy
This procedure is the most frequently performed operation and is the closed method. Postoperative recovery is usually rapid; sexual potency is maintained and urinary results are good. The operation is performed with a resectoscope, an instrument similar to a cystoscope but equipped with cutting and cauterizing attachments. This slender instrument is inserted up the urethra to the prostatic urethra, and the enlarged prostate is chipped away. The capsule remains intact. During the operation, the bladder and urethra are continuously irrigated with a sterile, isotonic, non-conductive clear fluid. In this manner, debris and blood are washed away.

Immediately after the operation the catheter drainage is bloody. A closed irrigation system is usually initiated to prevent blockage of the catheter by any clots. The nurse must be alert for signs of haemorrhage by paying close attention to the blood pressure and pulse of the patient and the amount of drainage. The drainage is watery and blood-tinged for 24–48 hours postoperatively.

The fluid used to irrigate the bladder during the operation may be absorbed, causing haemodilution. The signs and symptoms of this may be those of sodium deficiency or excessive blood volume. Complaints of headache, nausea, vomiting or muscle weakness should not be ignored by the nurse but must be reported.

Hypertension, restlessness, apprehension, shortness of breath or blurred vision likewise should be reported. If the surgeon expects that the operation may be more than 2 hours long, fluid intake may be restricted for 12 hours before the operation. Following the operation, 200–300 ml of normal saline may be given intravenously over 2 hours. The nurse must observe the patient for signs of pulmonary oedema.

Complaints of spasmodic, intermittent pain by the patient in the suprapubic region or a constant desire to void are related to bladder spasms. In severe cases the patient will need medication to obtain relief. The nurse should explain bladder spasms and catheters to the patient and instruct him not to try to void. These instructions and explanations are best given preoperatively so that the patient is prepared for the postoperative period; they are then reinforced postoperatively.

Complaints of persistent pain in the suprapubic area may be due to an overdistended bladder from a catheter which is not draining properly or from haemorrhage into the bladder. Rarely the bladder may have been perforated during the operation and blood and urine seep into the abdominal cavity. First the nurse irrigates the catheter and patency is established. The pain should diminish proportionately; if not, other causes must be ruled out. Pain medication may be given to the patient to give some relief during this period but pain medication does not provide relief from an overdistended bladder.

Because haemorrhage remains a threat, even in the later postoperative period, care is taken to prevent its occurrence. The patient is cautioned against straining to pass stool, and a light diet is usually ordered. Enemas, rectal tubes and rectal thermometers are contraindicated during the first postoperative week.

Because of the danger of a urinary tract infection, a prophylactic antibiotic may be prescribed. The catheter is removed 3–7 days postoperatively and, for a short period following this, the patient is usually instructed to record and measure each voiding. If difficulty in voiding is still present, the catheter may be reinserted. The nurse should watch for signs of incontinence which may follow or signs of urinary retention which may indicate a urethral stricture. Before being discharged the patient should be told that an episode of bleeding may occur about the second to fourth week postoperatively. In that event, he should contact his doctor and come to the emergency department of the hospital. Also he is warned to avoid any straining, heavy lifting or vigorous exercise for about 1 month postoperatively.

Suprapubic prostatectomy

This operation may be chosen when the prostate is large and when some bladder surgery is indicated as well. Sexual potency is maintained following the operation.

A small abdominal incision is made above the pubis and directly over the bladder. The bladder is opened and, through another incision into the urethral mucosa, the prostate is excised. The prostatic capsule remains intact. Sometimes only a Penrose drain in the suprapubic incision is all that is judged necessary in the postoperative period. It is usually removed after 36 hours. If a cystostomy tube is present, it is removed 3–4 days postoperatively. The indwelling catheter usually stays until the incision is nearly healed. The suprapubic incision may take time to heal. Bladder spasm is a frequent difficulty for these patients.

Retropubic prostatectomy

This method is preferred by some surgeons. Urinary results are excellent and potency is maintained. An abdominal incision is made above the bladder. The bladder is not incised, but the surgeon dissects down between the pubis and the bladder to reach the prostate. The capsule is opened and the tissue is removed.

Perineal prostatectomy

In a perineal prostatectomy the surgeon excises the prostate through a semicircular incision in the perineal body. The prostatic capsule is opened and the gland is removed. Unfortunately, after this operation is performed the patient may be impotent, and some difficulty may be experienced in establishing urinary continence following surgery.

CARCINOMA OF THE PROSTATE

Carcinoma of the prostate gland is one of the most common tumours seen in men. Perhaps 16% of all malignancies in the adult male are due to prostatic lesions. The tumour most often arises in the posterior prostatic lobe and in 85% of cases is hormone related, depending upon androgens to retain its integrity. The tumour also causes an increase in the secretion of acid phosphatase which is normally high in prostatic secretions. This increased production is reflected in blood serum levels and may indicate a prostatic tumour. Cancer of the prostate is frequently seen in association with benign hyperplasia but does not result from it. In addition, surgery for benign hyperplasia is not prophylactic against cancer as the posterior prostatic lobe is retained.

Because of its frequency and the fact that early diagnosis can be made in most cases by a rectal examination, all men should be advised to have an annual check-up after the age of 40. Nurses are advised to include this advice whenever it is related in their health teaching in the community.

Effects on the patient

The symptoms are essentially those of benign enlargement of the prostate. On rectal examination, the examiner palpates a hard nodule. Since the nodule may resemble other conditions, a biopsy is often done. A transrectal ultrasound examination may help in locating and staging the malignancy. Needle biopsies can now be done by putting a needle gauge into the ultrasound probe. This has greatly increased the accuracy of biopsies. The patient receives a cleansing enema before the procedure. On discharge the patient is told that blood-stained urine is to be expected for a short time.

Classification

Carcinoma of the prostate is classified into four stages. These stages are based on the results of rectal examinations, serum acid phosphatase levels, X-rays of the skeleton, and metastases. Stage I, or carcinoma in situ, is often called latent, or focal. Usually there are no symptoms. In stage II the nodule may be palpated on rectal examination, and serum acid phosphatase levels are normal. When stage III is reached, the growth has spread to the seminal vesicles, the base of the bladder and outside the prostatic capsule, but no distant metastases are present. Seventy-five per cent of men will show elevated serum acid phosphatase levels. With stage IV carcinoma, excessive levels of serum acid phosphatase circulate in the bloodstream. Previously, the thick prostatic capsule has kept the lesion localized and prevented spread into the abdominal cavity. Now the blood and lymphatics have carried the disease to distant sites. The bones of the pelvis are most frequently affected, and elevated serum alkaline phosphatase levels reflect this spread. Also, because of bone and liver involvement, severe anaemia may occur, accompanied by the other symptoms of a terminal disease.

Treatment and nursing intervention

Stages I and II are treatable. Stages III and IV usually receive palliative therapy. Treatment is by radical prostatectomy by the retropubic or perineal routes. The entire gland and seminal vesicles are removed. The bladder neck is sutured to the urethral stump. A large Foley catheter is inserted which serves as a splint for the urethra as well as a drain for the bladder. Drains may be placed in the incision lines as well. Preoperative and postoperative care are similar to that of any prostatectomy.

Incontinence may follow temporarily or on a longer basis. The patient is usually relieved to be assured that this is likely to be temporary and that control can be regained by practising perineal floor tightening and relaxing a few times periodically throughout the day when permitted.

If the perineal route was used, care must be taken to avoid infection. The incision is cleansed two to three times daily and following bowel movements.

In Stages III and IV, therapy includes radiation therapy and the administration of oestrogens. Radiation therapy is used in stage III in higher doses to achieve a cure and in stage IV in lower doses to achieve palliation. The course of treatment extends over 5–6 weeks. Oestrogen suppresses the production of androgens upon which the tumour is dependent. The patient experiences relief, and life is prolonged. However, the side-effects may be severe, so that oestrogen is usually reserved for patients with metastases. Some doctors may give lower doses of oestrogens in the earlier stages to shrink the tumour before surgery. The side-effects include oedema of the ankles, tender gynaecomastia, some nausea and vomiting, impotence with loss of libido, and a significant increase in the incidence of death from thromboembolic disease. The patient on oestrogens is observed for these side-effects. Sodium intake is reduced in order to prevent oedema. Eventually the effect of the oestrogens is reduced, and an orchidectomy (removal of testes) may be done to reduce the amount of androgens in the body.

This combination of oestrogens and orchidectomy may produce good results for about 18 months. Then the adrenals seem to recover from the oestrogen-induced hormonal imbalance and begin producing androgens again. Cortisone may be given now in an attempt to depress this source of androgens. In extreme situations an adrenalectomy may be performed. Deep X-ray therapy reduces discomfort from bone metastases. Radioactive phosphate given orally or intravenously also lodges in the bone, bringing relief from pain. In the case of a bladder obstruction, a transurethral prostatectomy is done. Since the operation is merely palliative, no attempt is made to remove all of the growth.

The patient will require nursing care related to the special needs of the cancer patient and to the aforementioned prostatectomy therapies.

CARCINOMA OF THE TESTES AND PENIS

Most tumours of the testes are malignant. Only about 1% of all malignancies occur in this area. Men between the ages of 18 and 35 are at greatest risk and cancer of the testes is the most common cause of death from cancer in this age group. Because the organ is palpable and early detection is possible, all men should be taught how to examine the testes. This is especially important for men with a history of cryptorchism, whether surgically corrected or not, as they are at increased risk of the disease. Caucasians are at highest risk for the condition. Although the tumour is rare, and this should be stressed in teaching, each man should be alert to possible changes in his testes. Any painless lump felt in the testis should be examined by a doctor. The man should also be alert to a testis that feels enlarged, is firm, gives the impression of heaviness, and when squeezed, fails to elicit the deep visceral pain that is usually associated with testicular pressure.

Diagnosis and treatment

As in all cancers the type of neoplasm and stage of the disease will govern treatment. Treatment is bilateral orchidectomy and, for some types of tumours, the surgery is followed by radiation therapy to the lumbar lymph nodes. Other types will receive chemotherapy postsurgery.

Malignancies of the penis are essentially malignancies of the skin. The glans and prepuce are nearly always affected. The disease is less frequent among circumcised men. In populations with poor genital hygiene, frequent sex partners, low age at first intercourse and a high incidence of HPV infection, carcinoma of the penis also has a higher incidence. HPV is associated with or coexists in many cases. Treatment is by excision of the affected areas or by partial or total amputation of the penis.

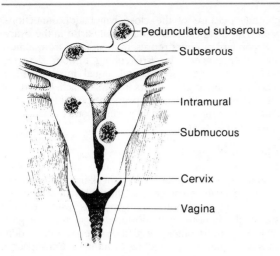

Pedunculated subserous

Subserous

Intramural

Submucous

Cervix

Vagina

Figure 22.29 Uterine myomas.

IN THE FEMALE

POLYPS

Polyps are common benign growths occurring mainly in the endometrium and cervix. The polyp has a characteristic smooth, shiny surface and is pink to deep red in colour. They are small in size, seldom exceeding more than 3 cm in length. The cause is unknown. No symptoms are usually present, but occasionally postcoital bleeding occurs. Treatment is by surgical excision of cervical polyps and may be followed by dilatation and curettage to remove endometrial polyps.

Myomas of the uterus

A myoma (fibromyoma, leiomyoma) is a benign tumour of the uterus composed of myometrium and fibrous tissue. Colloquially, myomas are known as 'fibroids'. At least 25% of women over 35 years of age show some evidence of myomas. The cause is unknown, but oestrogen stimulation is thought to play a part (Dewhurst, 1986; Llewellyn–Jones, 1986).

Myomas occur mainly in the uterine body. According to their position they are classified as subserous, submucous and intramural (Figure 22.29), and may become pedunculated. A pedunculated fibroid in the uterine cavity may be referred to as a fibroid polyp. This may be extruded through the cervix and may come to lie in the vagina. Myomas in the broad ligament or cervix are recorded, but these locations are rare. Several fibroids of varying sizes may be present in any one uterus. As the fibroids become larger, their blood supply may be reduced, causing some degeneration. The most common is a hyaline degeneration in the middle of the myoma. This causes a loss of cellular structure and, in extreme cases, a collection of gelatinous fluid lies at the centre. Sometimes the tumour shows signs of fatty changes and may even become calcified (womb-stone). A so-called red degeneration may occur, usually in association with pregnancy. The tumour looks like raw beef on the inside. The patient shows signs of malaise with fever, rapid pulse and pain over the fibroid. Following menopause all myomas atrophy and show slight shrinkage.

Effects on the patient

Symptoms vary with the size and location of the tumour. Frequently, with small tumours, there are no symptoms. Occasionally hypermenorrhoea occurs. Pain is rarely a symptom but most frequently is associated with torsion of a pedunculated myoma. Sometimes the myoma passing through the cervix causes cramps. Dysmenorrhoea may occur as a result of mechanical interference. Large myomas can cause frequency or retention of urine. Pressure on veins, lymphatics, and nerves of the pelvis may cause varicosities, unilateral or bilateral oedema of the lower extremities, or a radiating pain through the thighs. Occasionally, these tumours may be the cause of abortions or infertility. Some tumours become infected.

Treatment

Treatment depends on the age of the woman, her desire for more children and the size of the myoma. In the young woman who wishes children, a myomectomy is usually done. This is the enucleation of the myoma, but the uterus is retained. Blood loss during the operation may be extensive if the surgeon excises multiple myomas from a large uterus which may not contract efficiently. Persistent oozing of blood may occur postoperatively for the same reasons. The nurse should be alert to this possibility and monitor BP closely. In cases of very large myomas the treatment is hysterectomy.

In the young woman, myomas are not a contraindication to pregnancy and usually cause no difficulty. Rarely, they may obstruct labour or cause a postpartum haemorrhage.

TUMOURS OF THE OVARY

Tumours of the ovary are many and varied. The aetiology of most is unknown. For purposes of clarity they are roughly divided into non-neoplasms and neoplasms. Only a few are described in each group.

Non-neoplasms

Non-neoplasms are usually simple cysts or collections of fluid surrounded by a thin capsule. They do not grow but expand only as more fluid accumulates. These physiological cysts are seen mainly during the reproductive years. The follicular cyst is the most common of this group. Corpus luteum cysts may occur as well. Theca lutein cysts develop under the stimulation of high levels of chorionic gonadotrophins.

Occasionally, the Stein–Leventhal syndrome or polycystic disease of the ovary occurs. The syndrome appears in the late teens and early twenties with variable symptoms. These may include a history of sterility, secondary amenorrhoea, hirsutism and cysts bilaterally in the ovary. The ovary shows some enlargement and presents a glistening white appearance. Microscopically, many atretic follicular cysts are present. The syndrome is thought to follow an endocrine imbalance, probably arising in the ovary but affecting the hypothalamus. The ovaries produce an excessive amount of androgens which inhibit maturation of a follicle with subsequent disturbance of the ovarian-hypothalamic relationships. What triggers the imbalance is unknown. Medical treatment consists of a course of the drug clomiphene, with or without gonadotrophins, to produce an LH surge and ovulation.

Neoplasms

Pseudomucinous cystadenomas are the single most common neoplasms, occurring in about 40% of patients with a neoplastic ovarian growth. They may attain the largest size of any ovarian tumour. The tumour is characterized by multiple pockets filled with a thick fluid called pseudomucin. They may be bilateral and may become malignant.

Serous cystadenoma is the second most common of this group and appears to arise from germinal epithelium. The cyst contains a serous fluid. These cysts are frequently bilateral and often become malignant.

The dermoid cyst or teratoma may be cystic or solid. When it is soft, the cyst is filled with sebaceous material, hair and ordinary skin. The solid cyst frequently contains cartilage, bone, teeth, thyroid, and similar material. Rarely is the cyst malignant. It occurs most frequently in young women and may be bilateral.

Neoplasms of the ovary may also be divided into those which have some hormonal effect and those which do not. One tumour with no hormonal effect is a *dysgerminoma*. It arises from the primitive germ cells and is usually malignant. A *fibroma* is a benign solid neoplasm occurring most frequently in the postmenopausal patient. The fibroma arises from connective tissue in the ovary and may be associated with Meigs' syndrome, which is characterized by ascites and pleural effusion.

Those tumours which have hormonal effects may be further subdivided into feminizing and virilizing lesions. The most common of the rare feminizing tumours is the *granulosa cell tumour*. The tumour produces oestrogen and may induce precocious puberty or cause hypermenorrhoea or postmenopausal bleeding. It may be malignant or may be associated with carcinoma of the endometrium. The most common of the even rarer masculinizing tumours is *arrhenoblastoma*. By the production of androgens, presumably from the primitive male cell elements in the ovary, the woman is masculinized. In about 15–25% of cases it proves to be malignant.

Carcinoma of the ovary

Primary carcinoma of the ovary is usually the common adenocarcinoma. However, a review of ovarian growths is indicated, as almost any one of them has the potential to become malignant. The most common malignancy arises from the serous cystadenoma. Only one ovary may be affected but the other quickly follows, ap-

parently because of the close lymphatic connections. About 5% of all cancers in the female arise in the ovary.

Secondary tumours represent metastases from almost any other cancer. The Krukenberg tumour deserves mention. In this case bilateral, equal involvement is usually secondary to tumours in the stomach. Back-up of the lymphatic drainage appears responsible for this particular tumour, especially since other metastases usually occur later.

Effects on the patient
The ovarian tumour in its early stages is often symptomless. At regular yearly check-ups, palpation of the adnexa will reveal a mass. Often this may be the first discovery of the tumour. The symptoms result from the size of the tumour or its position. An increase in girth may be noticed but ignored. Pressure on the bladder causes frequency or a feeling of fullness. Constipation, oedema of the legs, anorexia and a full feeling in the abdomen may be present. Pain may be associated with stretching of the tissues as the tumour enlarges. Ascites may be present, accompanied by difficulty in breathing.

Treatment
Because of the danger of malignant growth, any ovarian mass is observed suspiciously. A rule of thumb says that any soft mass below 5 cm may be watched closely for 2–3 months. If no further growth occurs, then conservative treatment may be considered. Other tumours demand biopsy, and a laparotomy is indicated.

Ovarian tumours are staged as follows:

- Stage 1: Limited to ovaries
  - 1a: One ovary; no ascites
  - 1b: Both ovaries; no ascites
  - 1c: One or both ovaries with cytologically positive ascites
- Stage 2: Spread within the pelvis
  - 2a: Uterus and/or fallopian tubes; no ascites
  - 2b: Other pelvic tissues; no ascites
  - 2c: Other pelvic tissues with ascites
- Stage 3: Extension to small bowel, or intraperitoneal metastases
- Stage 4: Distant metastases

Following diagnosis, the surgeon strives to preserve as much ovarian function as is possible. In premenopausal women benign growths, if size permits, will be enucleated and ovarian function retained. Malignant growths are treated with total hysterectomy and bilateral salpingo-oophorectomy (removal of the fallopian tubes and ovaries). Surgery is followed by chemotherapy. Unfortunately, many malignancies have metastasized before discovery of the tumour. Prognosis is poor and surgery may be only palliative. Further treatment is directed toward relieving the symptoms of the terminally ill patient. Recurrent ascites may be a problem, and frequent paracentesis may be indicated.

Complications of ovarian tumours

Torsion or twisting of the growth on its stalk frequently occurs. Circulation is impeded, and necrosis may follow.

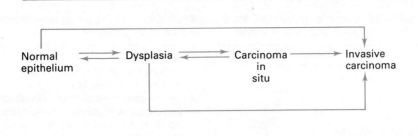

Figure 22.30 Patterns of development of cancer of the cervix.

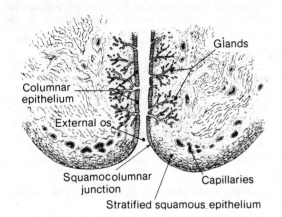

Figure 22.31 Squamocolumnar junction of the cervix.

The patient usually feels a sudden severe pain in the lower abdomen. Treatment is by excision of the tumour at an immediate laparotomy.

The cyst may rupture. Often the 'chocolate cyst' of endometriosis ruptures and drains fluid into the abdomen. Again the patient may present with an 'acute abdomen'.

Haemorrhage and infection occur in tumours as well. Usually, they are more common in the malignant tumour.

Postsurgical menopause is the result of a bilateral oophorectomy. The symptoms are similar to those of the regular menopause. Replacement therapy with oestrogens may begin before the patient leaves the hospital if it is not contradicted by malignancies which are aggravated by oestrogens.

CARCINOMA OF THE CERVIX

Carcinoma of the cervix is a common malignancy in women. The woman who has borne children or had an early sex life with several partners is more apt to develop the disease.

Cancer of the cervix is a complex disease which is preceded by several earlier cervical changes (Figure 22.30).

These changes usually occur at the squamocolumnar junction of the cervix (Figure 22.31), and initially are evident only on histological examination. They reflect a varied pattern of development. Some cases arise with no known precursor stage, while others appear to have gone through all the changes or any combination of them. The earlier changes may be reversible, and so do not always herald cancer. How many of these will reverse is unknown, but about 50% of women with carcinoma in situ are thought to develop invasive cancer; this development may take an average of 10 years. The cervical smear is the best method of early detection of these changes. Combined with treatment of these changes it is largely responsible for the declining mortality rates associated with cervical cancer.

Because 5-year survival rates are excellent in those cases which are discovered early, the Royal College of Nursing and the Royal College of Obstetricians and Gynaecologists both recommend that all women who are sexually active or over 25 should have cervical smear tests at least every three years. The nurse has a responsibility to disseminate this knowledge. The nurse emphasizes the hopeful aspects of cure following cases of early recognition. This may encourage more women to seek medical attention by reducing their anxiety. Fear of what she may discover often seems to prevent the patient from consulting her doctor. The nurse should do her utmost to persuade the woman confiding irregular bleeding to her to seek medical attention immediately.

Effects on the patient

A small lesion develops which, in the early stages, can be confused with other cervical conditions. The early stages may be asymptomatic, but eventually some bleeding from the vagina occurs. An unusual vaginal discharge may be present which may have an offensive odour. Pain is a late symptom and is followed by weight loss, anorexia and cachexia.

Carcinoma of the cervix is divided into stages. Stage 0 is carcinoma in situ. There is an intact basement membrane containing the malignant cells. Stage I is invasive cancer, which means that the basement membrane has been breeched and the cells are invading the surrounding tissue. Stages IA and IB refer to degrees of this invasion which is still within the confines of the

Table 22.8 Grading of smear test, cervical intra-epithelial neoplasia (CIN) grade and cancer stage.

Smear class	CIN grade	Cancer stage
I: normal cells	—	—
II: atypical cells	—	—
IIIA: mild dysplasia	I	—
III: moderate dysplasia	II	—
IV: severe, carcinoma in situ	III	0
V: invasive, below the basement membrane	—	IA,B
—	—	II
—	—	III
—	—	IV

Table 22.9 Cervical dysplasia: treatment and patient information guidelines.

Laser surgery:
- Uses carbon dioxide laser to vaporize cervical tissue and discrete vulvar lesions
- Can be done in the clinic with or without local anaesthesia
- Colposcope used during procedure allows for good visualization of the lesions and transformation zone. Precise aim and depth can be achieved
- Procedure takes an average of 20 minutes
- Post-treatment the patient can expect minimal vaginal bleeding and discharge, rapid healing
- Women's subjective experience: moderate cramps, pricking sensation
- Precautions: if bleeding is as heavy as menses, contact doctor; no vaginal insertion (tampons, intercourse, douches) for 3 weeks

Cryotherapy:
- Uses cryoprobe to freeze transformation zone
- Done in the clinic, usually without local anaesthesia
- Procedure takes less than 15 minutes on average
- No bleeding but profuse watery discharge can last up to 6 weeks
- Women's subjective experience: felt cold; mild-to-moderate cramps
- Precautions: as for laser surgery

Electrocautery:
- Uses electrically charged cautery tip to burn transformation zone
- Done in the clinic, usually without local anaesthesia
- Average procedure takes less than 5 minutes
- Usually no bleeding but vaginal discharge can last 2 weeks after treatment
- Women's subjective experience: heat; mild-to-moderate cramps
- Precautions: as for laser surgery

Extensive laser surgery:
- Indicated for extensive vaginal, vulvar, perianal lesions
- Done under general anaesthesia, usually as out-patient
- Post-treatment care: sitz baths 3–4 times a day with applications of topical analgesics such as xylocaine gel
- Women usually report improvement in vulvar pain/tenderness 5 days postoperatively
- Precautions: as above and if problems with voiding or passing stool occur

Modified from Toole & Vigilante (1990).

cervix. Unfortunately, about 20% of stage I will already have spread to the lymphatics. A small lesion similar to an erosion may be present on the cervix. In stage II the carcinoma has spread to close adjacent structures, and the upper third of the vagina may be involved. By stage III invasion has reached the pelvic walls and lower vagina. Stage IV is marked by extensive pelvic involvement, including the bladder or bowel, and distant metastases may be present (Table 22.8).

Treatment

Treatment is usually guided by the stage assigned to the situation by the gynaecologist. Since the main method of diagnosing Stage 0 carcinoma is the cervical smear test, the results of this test help to guide treatment. The smear results are organized into five classes. In classes I and II the cells are non-malignant. Class II may have atypical cells suggestive of viral changes. Both herpes and HPV are associated with atypical cervical cells. Other infections may contribute and the patient will be treated accordingly. Some of these altered cells will revert back to normal epithelium. Class III is suspicious and arouses concern. The patient is asked to have repeat smears done in 3 months or a biopsy is done. Classes IV and V are positive, indicating that definite changes are present which require biopsy.

Biopsy
A *punch biopsy* may be done with special punch biopsy forceps. Because of the paucity of nerve endings in the cervix, the biopsy may be done with relative comfort for the patient. She may feel something like a pinch when the biopsy is taken. A Schiller test can be done. Normally the cervix contains glycogen. This is depleted in areas of abnormal cell change. When Lugol's solution (iodine in potassium iodide) is swabbed on the cervix, the normal epithelium stains a dark brown. Glycogen-deficient areas are a pale colour by contrast, and these are the areas requiring biopsy.

Further treatment may be a *cone biopsy*. It is an operative procedure in which a cone-shaped segment of the central cervix is removed. The internal os remains intact (Figure 22.32). On examination the section may

contain all of the malignant area. In these cases the biopsy may be considered sufficient treatment. Pre-operative and postoperative care for the patient is similar to other vaginal surgery such as a D and C. The major difference is that these patients face the threat of a malignant disease and may be extremely anxious. Considerable skill in providing supportive nursing will be demanded of the nurse. Haemorrhage is a threat, and the patient should be warned of this. Bleeding from the biopsy site may occur up to a week after the biopsy

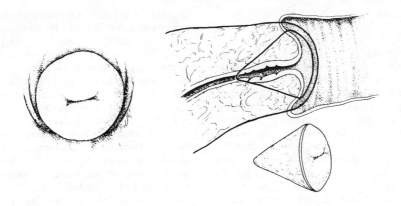

Figure 22.32 Cone biopsy of the cervix. The cone indicates the segment of cervix removed at biopsy.

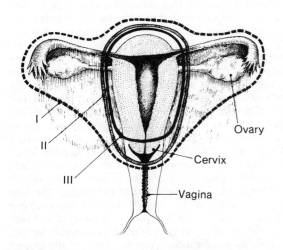

Figure 22.33 Types of hysterectomy. I, total hysterectomy with bilateral salpingo-oophorectomy; II, total hysterectomy; III, subtotal hysterectomy.

when the patient is at home. The nurse should inform the patient of this possibility before discharge so that she will notify her doctor and not be unduly alarmed. Sometimes the haemorrhage is severe enough to necessitate re-admission to hospital and a blood transfusion.

The biopsy results may indicate normal cells, dysplasia or invasive carcinoma. Carcinoma in situ may be treated with a cone biopsy. All carcinoma in situ must be treated to ensure prevention of invasive carcinoma. Invasive carcinoma of the cervix will be treated according to the stage in which it is classified.

Colposcopy is a method increasingly used to visualize the cervix and surrounding perineal tissues. The colposcope is an instrument that provides visualization of the cervix under a bright light and from 10–40 × magnification of the field.

In cervical intraepithelial neoplasia, therapy is directed at local eradication of the lesion. Table 22.9 outlines several treatment methods and guidelines for patient teaching.

Surgery and radiation therapy

Stages IA and IB and some early stage IIs are treated by radical surgery (modified Wertheim's hysterectomy), which attempts to eliminate the cancer, and radiation therapy. There is much debate over the optimum approach. Some prefer radiation alone; others prefer surgery with or without radiation. In major medical centres, with highly qualified surgeons and sophisticated radiation equipment and radiologists, higher cure rates have been recorded with a combination of surgery and radiation. In small centres lacking highly experienced surgeons some quote higher cure rates for radiation alone. Most seem to agree that stages III and IV are best treated by radiation and some palliative surgery. In cases where the surgeon feels that the tumour is surgically excisable a pelvic exenteration is done. Surgery is used in cases of a radioresistant tumour.

The patient who is having a total hysterectomy (Figure 22.33) for carcinoma in situ will have the uterus, cervix and upper third of the vagina removed. The ovaries are conserved in most cases of the premenopausal woman but may be removed in the older woman. The patient is prepared as for abdominal surgery. Postoperatively, any vaginal discharge must be observed. Some staining may occur from the vaginal cuff. A Foley catheter may be inserted and may remain in place for 1 or 2 days postoperatively. The nurse is alert to possible signs of hormonal imbalance following removal of the ovaries as well as signs of a urinary tract infection and thromboemboli.

In a Wertheim's hysterectomy, the uterus, ovaries, broad ligaments, surrounding tissue, upper half of the vagina and pelvic lymph nodes are removed. In a more extensive Wertheim's operation, the pelvic fascia and further lymph tissue will be removed. Preoperatively the patient has a cystostomy examination and her ureters are catheterized. This allows them to be easily identified during the extensive pelvic dissection. The patient's vagina and cervix are painted with an iodine solution to identify any glycogen-deficient areas which would indicate further vaginal resection.

Nursing intervention

When the patient returns to the ward she will require general postoperative care. Two Redivac drains may have been inserted, one in either lower quadrant, and attached to a drainage system. These are removed when there is no drainage. Drainage is usually more extensive if no radiation has been given before surgery, and less if radiation has been given. Occasionally two rubber drains, one on either side, may be draining into the vagina. They are shortened about the third postoperative day and removed about the fifth day if drainage has ceased. If oozing of blood was a problem during surgery, the pelvis may have been packed with a gauze pack, the tail of which is brought out through the vaginal cuff into the vagina. This is usually advanced in 48 hours and removed in 72 hours. The ureters and bladder have been handled during surgery and may be atonic. Care must be taken to see that the catheter is draining properly and that bladder distension does not occur. The catheter should drain clear urine. Observations are made for signs of thromboemboli postoperatively; the femoral areas as well as the calves are examined. Early ambulation is encouraged, but does not merely mean sitting in a chair by the bedside for extended periods of time. Better venous return is achieved by having a patient lie in bed with her legs elevated to about 15° than by sitting for long periods of time in a chair at the bedside. Ambulation refers to movement: getting up to sit in a chair for 10–15 minutes, back to bed with feet slightly elevated, getting up to walk to the bathroom, getting up to eat lunch and back to bed to rest. Leg exercises, coughing and deep breathing are important in promoting good circulation.

Fistula formation is a hazard and the risk is greater if radiation therapy has been given prior to surgery. Because these fistulae are a result of poor blood supply and the sloughing of tissue they are a later development, usually appearing in the second post-operative week. The most common are vesicovaginal and ureterovaginal. Thus, any unusual drainage of urine must be noted. In addition, any unexplained fever or lower quadrant or flank pain should alert the nurse. The fistula is usually not repaired immediately, but postponed until a more favourable time.

A pelvic exenteration includes all of the Wertheim's hysterectomy plus a total vaginectomy and removal of portions of the bladder or bowel, depending upon the spread of the disease. The patient may return postoperatively with an ileostomy, a colostomy or an ileal conduit. Nursing care for such conditions is elaborated in Chapter 16. In these operations preoperative bowel preparation is done. Postoperatively, drains may be left in areas of node dissection to prevent the pooling of blood and serum which may easily lead to infection. The drains may be draining freely or may be attached to suction. Usually they are advanced daily and removed by the fifth postoperative day.

The postoperative adjustment to life may be difficult. Preoperative discussions with the doctor and nurse should help to prepare the patient. In pelvic exentera-

tion sexual function of the vagina is lost; in a Wertheim's operation it may have to be modified. Menopause may occur as oestrogen therapy is frequently contraindicated. The care of the colostomy or ileostomy must be learned and accepted. The patient will require much understanding and support from the nursing staff while the nurses gently encourage her to retain as much independence as is compatible with her situation.

Frequently, external and internal radiation therapy is used in conjunction with, or instead of, surgery for these patients. Because a high oxygen concentration in the tissues and blood increases the radiosensitivity of the tumour, anaemia and low circulating blood volumes are corrected before radiation therapy by medication or blood transfusions. Radium in special containers is inserted into the cervical canal and into the lateral fornices of the vagina. The insertion of the radium is an operative procedure. During the procedure a urinary catheter is passed. This prevents a distended bladder from coming into contact with the radium, which would greatly increase the chance of a vesicovaginal fistula. After the radium is inserted, packing is placed in the vagina and may be sutured in place to maintain the position of the radium. Because the tight packing prevents voiding, the catheter drains the bladder. The patient's temperature is monitored, as radiation may stimulate a latent infection. The patient remains on bed rest with head and shoulders nearly flat. A slipper bedpan is used, and straining at stool is discouraged. The catheter is checked to see that it is draining. These measures help to ensure that the radium remains where it has been placed. Complaints of pain and any bloody discharge should be reported to the doctor. The time for removal should be carefully observed. Removal may be uncomfortable for the patient because of the tight packing, and the patient may need an analgesic for this. For further information on the care of the patient consult the section on care of the patient receiving radium inserts.

Clinical situation: Sally Barlow, a woman with cancer of the cervix

Sally Barlow is a 26-year-old with cancer of the cervix. Four years ago she was treated with two caesium insertions and a 6-week course of radiotherapy to her pelvic area. She has been undergoing investigations as an outpatient for a suspected recurrence involving her rectum and has today been admitted to the ward with a view to her having posterior pelvic exenteration. Sally was accompanied by Dave her boyfriend but he disappeared quickly saying that he would come back later in the day. Roper *et al.*'s Activities of Living were used as prompts during the assessment interview and information was documented in the order in which it was obtained.

Sally's problems are related to the forthcoming surgery and are prioritized to ensure she is physically

Table 22.10   Care plan for Sally Barlow: pelvic exenteration for cancer of the cervix.

Patient's problem	Goals	Nursing intervention
(1) Hazards of surgery (P).	No post-op complications.	Explain need for pre-op preparation. Follow standard procedures including bowel preparation.
(2) Breathing problems postanaesthetic (P).	Sally will stop smoking preoperatively.	Explain why smoking increases risks of complications. Help Sally set a time to stop. Suggest Sally set a time to stop. Suggest alternative stress-reducing strategies. Offer support and encouragement. Reinforce breathing and effective coughing techniques
(3) Discomfort associated with having bowels opened (A).	No discomfort.	Offer analgesia as prescribed.
(4) Anxiety and fear related to lack of knowledge about colostomy (A).	For Sally to be able to discuss the impact of a colostomy on her lifestyle without becoming tearful.	Refer to specialist stoma care nurse. Provide the opportunity for Sally to voice her specific fears. Provide verbal and written information for Sally. Arrange contact with ostomist of similar age if appropriate. Sally to try wearing bag filled with water. Mark suitable sites.
(5) Uncertainty about ability to have vaginal intercourse post-surgery (A).	For Sally to be able to state the potential outcome of surgery and identify some positive coping strategies.	Facilitate discussion with surgeons about this topic involving Dave according to Sally's wishes. Ensure privacy for this. Explain to Sally and Dave the resources that exist to give them support and advice with sexual difficulties post surgery.
(6) Fear of surgery and death (A).	Sally will verbally express confidence in her decision to proceed with surgery.	Allow Sally time to express all her fears. Ensure medical staff fully explain options and answer all her questions. Reinforce and help Sally interpret information given. Provide information about post-op care.
(7) Lack of sleep (A).	Sally will report 8 hrs sleep.	Offer night sedation. Teach relaxation techniques.

and mentally prepared for this. Problems (4), (5) and (6) are the most important. Problems (3) and (7) are related to the cancer and will be alleviated by the operation. Sally decided to proceed with surgery and problems (1) and (2) then became priorities.

Post-operatively Sally was nursed in a high-dependency unit. After 24 hours she was transferred back to the ward and a reassessment was undertaken. As a result of this a revised care plan was formulated for Sally's post-operative care.

Patient's problem	Goals	Nursing intervention
(1) Pain due to surgery (A).	Sally to rate pain less than 3 on a 10 point scale.	Administer analgesia via epidural infusion. Titrate prescribed dose against pain. Inform anaesthetist if not controlling pain. Substitute oral analgesia as pain diminishes. Encourage coping strategies —distraction, massage, etc.

Patient's problem	Goals	Nursing intervention
(2) Complications of immobility DVT chest infections, pressure sores, etc. (P).	No avoidable complication.	Assist Sally to change her position 2-hrly whilst in bed. Encourage 2-hrly deep breathing and coughing when awake. Refer to physiotherapist. Promote mobilization by use of effective analgesia.
(3) Dehydration (P).	Sally to have a fluid intake of 2–3 litres/24 hrs.	Monitor and care for IVI. Administer IV fluids as prescribed. Aspirate NG. tube. Maintain fluid balance record. Provide mouth care. Introduce oral fluids and diet as instructed by surgeon.
(4) Impaired healing due to infection (P) and previous radiotherapy (A).	Wound will be healed in 16 days.	Record vital signs 4-hrly. Administer antibiotics as prescribed. Abdominal wound—check dressing—leave intact for as long as possible. Perineal wound—repad and re-dress as necessary—shorten drain daily after 3rd day post-op. Leave all sutures for at least 14 days.
(5) Risk of urinary tract infection (P).	No UTI.	Observe, measure and record urine output. Ensure Sally remains in fluid balance and has an average urine output of > 35 ml/hr. Monitor temperature 4-hrly. Maintain closed drainage system. Meatal cleansing prn.
(6) Alteration in elimination habits.	For Sally to manage her colostomy independently in 14 days.	Check stoma for colour and evidence of retraction 4-hrly. Measure and chart drainage. Observe for passage of flatus and stool. Administer medication to solidify stool as prescribed. In conjunction with the stoma care nurse demonstrate change of appliance with full explanation. Encourage increasing level of participation. Encourage Sally to decide on an appliance system of her choice.
(7) Inability to perform own hygiene needs (A).	Sally to state she is satisfied with her appearance.	Give bed bath or assisted wash until Sally is independent. Encourage Sally to wear her own clothes.

By the ninth day post surgery Sally had made very good progress and resumed independence in all of the above activities of living with the exception of elimination. Two new problems were identified.

Patient's problem	Goals	Nursing intervention
(8) Reluctance to assume responsibility for her stoma (A).	Sally to touch and clean stoma within 24 hrs. Sally to complete a bag change in 2 days.	Support and reassure Sally. Encourage her to start participating right away in self care by removing bag, cleaning her stoma and preparing the new bag. To change bag with assistance tomorrow and with minimal supervision the day after. Discuss dietary changes that may help to reduce flatus and discuss products that can reduce odour. Discuss arrangements for coping with the stoma at home and follow up care.
(9) Anxiety about altered body image (A).	Sally to feel confident enough to sleep in the nude.	Encourage Sally to show Dave the stoma before discharge. Suggest interim coping strategies, e.g. wearing bag covers or a waist slip, etc.

Patient's problem	Goals	Nursing intervention
(10) Alteration in sexual behaviour (P).	Sally to report a satisfying sexual relationship (long term).	Get Sally's surgeon to explain what potential for vaginal intercourse exists. Identify potential problems with Dave and Sally and suggest alternative ways of love-making until healing is complete. Offer follow-up support and advice. Discuss reconstructive surgery if appropriate.

(A) = Actual; (P) = Potential.
Reproduced from Walsh M (1991) *Models in Clinical Nursing: The Way Forward.* London: Baillière Tindall.

CARCINOMA OF THE ENDOMETRIUM

This is a frequently occurring malignancy which appears to be increasing in incidence. Since it is a disease largely of older women, this may be due to a lengthened life span. Oestrogens aggravate the tumour and prolonged oestrogen therapy, especially in the premenopausal or postmenopausal woman, has been implicated as a contributing cause of endometrial cancer.

The first symptom is a painless, bloody vaginal discharge. Thirty to 40% of women with postmenopausal bleeding have cancer of the endometrium. Bleeding postmenopausally should therefore never be ignored but investigated immediately. A careful endometrial biopsy is usually done. The growth is usually in the fundus of the uterus, but may arise in or spread to the isthmus. The thick body of the uterus contains the growth and it metastasizes late in its growth.

Treatment is by intracavitary radiation followed by a careful total hysterectomy and bilateral salpingo-oophorectomy. Care is taken to pack the vagina or suture the cervix, and tie the fallopian tubes to prevent spread by seeding from the uterus. Surgery is often followed by radiation of the vagina as well in order to reduce the risk from stray malignant cells spread during surgery. Some surgeons may do the hysterectomy first and follow with radiation. More advanced cases are treated with combinations of external and internal radiation with surgery to relieve symptoms. Where radium is inserted, several containers attached to strings may be placed in the body of the uterus to irradiate the endometrium. Cure rates are excellent when the tumour has been discovered early.

Progesterone therapy retards the growth of the tumour and metastases. Treatment in the form of medroxyprogesterone acetate (Provera) may be started before surgery and continued for two years afterwards.

CARCINOMA OF THE VAGINA

In recent years there has been an increase in clear cell adenocarcinoma of the vagina in girls and young women. This is a result of in utero exposure to diethylstilboestrol (DES), a synthetic non-steroid oestrogen compound. DES was first synthesized in 1938; by 1940–1941 the drug was prescribed for women to help prevent or treat threatened spontaneous abortion, which was thought to be due to low progesterone levels. Unlike natural oestrogens, it stimulated the body to increase the production of progesterone. The drug was withdrawn from use for this purpose in 1971. Between

1940 and 1971 many thousands of women received treatment with DES. Prior to its withdrawal it had been shown to be a transplacental teratogen and carcinogen, producing a wide range of congenital anomalies of the genital tract in the offspring and a rare vaginal cancer in a few daughters of such pregnancies (Table 22.10). During organogenesis, exposure to DES affected müllerian duct tissue. This tissue remained inappropriately or, in many women, is in the wrong place.

Table 22.11 Effects on children of exposure to diethylstilboestrol (DES) in utero.

Women
1. Congenital anomalies:
   (a) Cervix—hooded, ridged, ringed by fibrous tissue
       —hypoplastic
   (b) Uterus—abnormally shaped, small, internal adhesions, constrictions
   (c) Vagina—transverse ridges
       —stenosis
   (d) Adenosis or ectopic tissue by vagina and cervix
       —this may disappear by age 30
       —not cancer precursor but usually present when cancer occurs
2. Cancer of the genital tract:
   Usually clear cell adenocarcinoma
   Most common between ages 14–20
   Rare, incidence 1–40 per 1000 at-risk women
3. Increased reproductive difficulties
   Secondary to abnormalities of cervix and uterus
   (a) Primary infertility
   (b) Spontaneous abortion
   (c) Ectopic pregnancy
   (d) Premature labour and delivery

Men
1. Congenital anomalies:
   (a) Testis—undescended
       —hypoplastic
   (b) Epididymis—benign cysts
   (c) Penis—microphallus
       —urethral stenosis
2. Fertility problems related to:
   Decreased sperm counts
   Alterations in density, motility and penetrating ability of sperm
3. Possible increased cancer risk:
   Testicular

Time of exposure was more important than amount of exposure. Disorders following DES exposure in utero include physical anomalies, adenosis and carcinoma of the vagina. Estimates vary but from 65–95% of at-risk women have cervical and uterine anomalies and about 90% have adenosis. By contrast the risk of developing cancer is small; perhaps 0.5% of women affected by DES exposure. There is less information concerning sons of women treated with DES but they appear to be at less risk of abnormalities. Perhaps 30% of 'DES sons' have testicular abnormalities. Although DES induces breast cancer in male mice, there is no evidence at present to indicate that it does so in either sex in humans.

Treatment and nursing intervention

The regular follow-up and screening visits of those who were exposed to DES begins with the first menstrual period or at age 14 years, whichever is first. Early monitoring of the girl to detect changes at the cellular level involves regular examinations every 6 months including cervical smears and a colposcopy examination. Cervical smears are only about 75% effective in detecting change in this condition and the cellular screening must be more rigorous and extensive. Women who have not been involved in this early screening programme present with bleeding or a suspicious lesion in the vagina.

Treatment is radical vaginal surgery followed by irradiation and possibly chemotherapy.

Nursing interventions are directed to case-finding by public education and by questioning of appropriate age groups during history taking. Once a case of DES exposure is suspected, teaching about the condition, attendant risks and necessary follow-up is done and the patient is referred to a doctor. The patient and the mother usually require support from professionals and from others in a similar situation.

Adenosis

The signs and symptoms of adenosis include complaints of a heavy clear mucoid discharge, dyspareunia and postcoital bleeding. On inspection, small bright red papillary or granular lesions may be seen on the smooth pink vaginal mucosa. Alternatively, large diffuse red patches may be seen. Numerous small cystic nodules beneath the epithelium are felt on the anterior and posterior vaginal walls. During palpation care must be taken to inspect and palpate the entire vagina as the blades of the speculum may obscure the adenosis. Most adenosis requires no treatment. Extensive adenosis may need cryotherapy or partial vaginectomy with skin grafting.

CARCINOMA OF THE VULVA

Carcinoma of the vulva is a less frequent malignancy, occurring mainly among women in their fifth and sixth decades of life. It is frequently preceded by vulvar changes.

Dystrophy of the vulva

Dystrophy of the vulva refers to changes in vulvar epithelium which are most often associated with ageing but may occur in the younger woman. Most are benign but some are premalignant. Because premalignancy must be assessed at the cellular level a biopsy is done on all lesions.

The patient complains of a shrinking of vulvar structures which progressively narrows the introitus. Dyspareunia, pruritus and soreness are frequent complaints. Smooth red or white patches of thick or thin epithelium may be evident. They may be only in the vestibule or scattered over the vulva and perineum. These patches crack easily, and fissures and excoriated areas develop. Pruritus is common and secondary infection of the scratched lesions occurs. Ulceration may develop.

Mild symptoms usually respond to improved perineal hygiene, control of pruritus and infection and topical appliction of oestrogen. Patients with more severe symptoms are admitted to the hospital. Nursing care will then involve keeping the vulva dry, cool and clean by daily baths. No pants or pyjamas are worn. The patient is nursed as much as possible with her legs apart and a bed cradle over the perineum to keep it dry and cool. A hair dryer may be used at intervals to blow cool dry air over the perineum. This helps relieve pruritus and promotes healing. It is wise to avoid powders and creams. Medication to reduce the pruritus may be needed as well. If the condition resists treatment or recurs, a simple vulvectomy may be done. These patients who show signs of cellular changes consistent with an increased risk of developing cancer will have periodical examinations and biopsies done or a simple vulvectomy.

In addition the nurse must observe the vulva and perineum in order to identify changes which would require further investigation and should encourage patients who confide symptoms to seek medical attention.

Treatment

Carcinoma of the vulva is treated by radical vulvectomy. Here the dissection is extensive for the clitoris, labia and all the perineal subcutaneous tissue; all the perineal glands and the femoral and inguinal lymphatics are removed.

Nursing intervention

Preoperative preparation includes all the measures common for perineal and abdominal surgery. The patient and nursing staff may react with repugnance at the thought of this surgery. It is frequently seen as mutilating. However, the results of the operation are quite favourable. Sexual function is retained, as the vagina is not removed. Young women have conceived following simple vulvectomy and have been delivered by caesarean section.

Postoperatively, the patient returns to the ward with an indwelling catheter. Much oedema is present and great care must be taken not to dislodge the catheter. It may be very difficult to replace. The operation may be done in two stages or all at once. In the former, the patient returns with an open area, requiring future skin grafting. Barrier isolation may be required for this patient both before and after skin grafting. A bed cradle over the pubic area will keep bed linen away. When the procedure is completed in one operation the patient may return with a bulky pressure dressing held in place by a T binding. In other cases there are bilateral stab wounds near the iliac fossa containing drains which are attached to suction; this arrangement may replace the pressure bandage. Thus, the fluid is drained away and the skin flap is kept in close approximation to the underlying tissue so that it becomes firmly attached to the tissue. Some necrosis along the incision lines may be expected, and occasionally skin grafting may be necessary to replace a necrotic area. The stitches are usually not removed for 2–3 weeks. Close observation is maintained for thromboemboli. Once ambulation is begun, the patient may need elastic stockings to avoid swelling of her legs. Standing for long periods of time should be avoided.

SUMMARY

Issues of patient care involving sex and reproduction are very sensitive and many patients, and also nurses, may feel very uncomfortable in dealing with such problems. The nurse therefore needs to be clear about his or her own sexuality and moral beliefs about sex and reproduction before addressing the needs of the patient. Empathy and sensitivity are essential for good nursing practice in this area together with a non-judgemental approach. The nurse has many opportunities to be a promoter of good health in the fields of sex and reproduction which should be seized upon at every opportunity. Male patients should be targetted for health education as well as females however as the responsibility for 'sexual health' falls on both partners in any relationship, be it heterosexual or gay.

LEARNING ACTIVITIES

1. Design a discharge pamphlet for a patient who has had a hysterectomy.
2. What teaching materials are available for:
   (a) A woman undergoing hysterectomy.
   (b) A young man concerned about testicular cancer.
3. How would you evaluate the effectiveness of a nursing intervention such as a discharge pamphlet?
4. What steps may a woman take to protect herself from AIDS? Discuss this with a colleague.
5. Consider these two statements:
   (a) Condoms should be freely available in prisons.
   (b) The presence of condoms in a woman's possession may be used as evidence in certain circumstances for a charge of soliciting for prostitution.
   What are the implications for health promotion of these statements?

REFERENCES AND FURTHER READING

Andrist L (1988) Taking a sexual history and educating clients about safe sex. *Nursing Clinics of North America* **23(4):** 959–973.

Annon JS (1978) The PLISSIT model: a proposed conceptual scheme for the behavioural treatment of sexual problems. *Journal of Sex Education and Therapy* **2:** 1–15.

Bartscher PWB (1983) Human sexuality and implication for nursing intervention: a teaching format. *Journal of Nursing Education* **22(3):** 123–127.

Bayles MD (1984) *Reproductive Ethics*, Prentice Hall Series in the Philosophy of Medicine.

Borg S & Lasker T (1982) *When Pregnancy Fails*. London: Routledge & Kegan Paul.

Brush M (1984) *Understanding Premenstrual Tension*. London: Pan.

Burgess A & Holmstrom L (1974) *Rape: Victims of Crisis*. Bowie, MD: Brady.

Clayton S, Lewis T & Puker G (1986) *Gynaecology by Ten Teachers* 14th edn. London: Edward Arnold.

Cowper A & Young C (1989) *Family Planning* 2nd edn. London: Chapman & Hall.

Cronin CJ & Mablebust J (1989) Case-managed care: capitalizing on the CNS. *Nursing Management* **20(3):** 38–47.

Dewhurst J (1984) *Female Puberty and its Abnormalities*. Edinburgh: Churchill Livingstone.

Dewhurst J (1986) *Dewhurst's Integrated Obstetrics and Gynaecology* 4th edn, chap. 47. London: Blackwell.

Dunn B & Rossler S (1985) *Nursing Care of Women*. London: Harper & Row.

Farrer H (1989) *Gynaecological Care* 2nd edn. Edinburgh: Churchill Livingstone.

Foucault M (1978) *The History of Sexuality*. Harmondsworth: Penguin.

Frater A & Wright C (1986) *Coping with Abortion*. London: Chambers.

Gillenwater J et al (1987) *Adult and Paediatric Urology*, vols 1 and 2. Chicago: Year Book Medical.

Glover J (1984) *Human Sexuality in Nursing Care*. London: Croom Helm.

Gould D (1990) *Nursing Care of women*. Englewood Cliffs, NJ: Prentice Hall.

Guillebaud J (1986) *Contraception: Your Questions Answered.* Edinburgh: Churchill Livingstone.

Houghton D & Houghton P (1984) *Coping with Childlessness.* London: Allen & Unwin.

Jones R (1988) With respect to lesbians. *Nursing Times* **84(20):** 48–49.

Katchadourian HA & Lunde DT (1987) *Fundamentals of Human Sexuality* 3rd edn. New York: Holt Rinehart & Winston.

Kuczynski J (1986) Liberal studies. *Nursing Times* **32(28):** 60–61.

Liu D & Lachelin G (1989) *Practical Gynaecology.* London: Butterworth.

Llewelyn SP & Pytches R (1988) An investigation of anxiety following termination of pregnancy. *Journal of Advanced Nursing* **13(4):** 468–471.

Llewellyn-Jones D (1986) *Fundamentals of Obstetrics and Gynaecology* 4th edn, vol. 2. London: Faber & Faber.

London Rape Crisis Centre (1984) *Sexual Violence: The Reality for Women.* London: Women's Press.

Loo R (1983) Nursing students: personality dimensions and attitudes towards women. *Psychological Reports* **52:** 504–506.

Mackenzie R (1985) *Menopause.* London: Sheldon.

Masters WH (1986) *Sex and Human Loving.* London: Macmillan.

Moldanado S (1985) Trends in public attitudes towards legal abortion, 1972–1978. *Nursing and Health* **8(3):** 219–225.

Neustatter A & Newson G (1986) *Mixed Feelings.* London: Pluto.

Oakley A (1972) *Sex, Gender and Society.* London: Temple Smith.

Roberts H (1981) *Women, Health and Reproduction.* London: Routledge & Kegan Paul.

Savage J (1987) *Nurses, Gender and Sexuality.* London: Heinemann.

Shields-Poë D (1981) Spontaneous abortion as an index of exposure to carcinogens. Master's thesis, University of Toronto.

Snitow A, Stansell C & Thompson S (1984) *Desire—the Politics of Sexuality.* London: Virago.

Toole K & Vigilante P (1990) Cervical dysplasia and condyloma as risks for carcinoma. *Maternal Child Nursing Journal* **15:** 170–175.

Webb C (1985) *Sexuality, Nursing and Health.* Chichester: John Wiley.

Webb C (1986) *Women's Health.* London: Hodder & Stoughton.

Webb C (1987) Sexual healing. *Nursing Times.* **83(32):** 29–30.

Wright B (1986) *Caring in Crisis.* Edinburgh: Churchill Livingstone.

Caring for the Patient with a Disorder of the Breast

23

OBJECTIVES

On completion of this chapter the reader will be able to:

- Describe the structure of the breast
- Describe the physiological development of the female breast through the adult life span
- Appreciate the role of the nurse in promoting breast awareness and regular screening for breast disorders
- Recognize the nurse's responsibility to include the woman's partner and family as active participants in the nursing plan of care for women with disorders of the breast
- Describe nursing strategies to alleviate the health problems common to women with breast cancer and their families

THE NORMAL BREAST

STRUCTURE AND DEVELOPMENT OF THE BREAST

The breasts, or mammary glands, lie on the anterior chest wall. The base of each rests on the fascia of the pectoralis major muscle, and supporting ligaments extend from the skin through the breast to the fascia. The breasts are undeveloped in both sexes until puberty. At this time, the female breasts enlarge and develop secreting cells and ducts in response to increased concentrations of ovarian and certain adeno-hypophyseal (anterior pituitary) hormones. The cylindrical projection on the skin surface forms the *nipple*, which is perforated by duct orifices. The pinkish area of skin around it is referred to as the *areola*; it becomes markedly pigmented during pregnancy and retains the darker colour following delivery. The male breasts remain rudimentary throughout life.

Following growth and maturation, the female breast is composed of 15–25 lobes, each with a duct that opens on to the surface of the nipple. Each lobe consists of clusters of secreting cells which form lobules (Figure 23.1). The main ducts (lactiferous ducts) are formed by the union of smaller ducts which drain the lobules. They are dilated just before entering the base of the nipple to form reservoirs, or ampullae, for the milk during active secretion. The lobes and ducts are separated and supported by areolar, fibrous and fatty tissues.

The blood supply to the breasts is abundant and is derived from the internal mammary arteries and branches of the thoracic and intercostal arteries. A large proportion of the lymph in the breasts is channelled through the axillary lymph nodes; the remainder drains through mediastinal nodes (Figure 23.2).

The female breasts change in size and shape in response to hormonal changes during the menstrual cycle, pregnancy and ageing. After menopause, the lobes and ducts undergo some atrophy and replacement with fibrous tissue.

PHYSIOLOGICAL FUNCTIONING

The breasts are subject to menstrual cyclical changes associated with alterations in the concentrations of various hormones. *Oestrogens* initiate growth of the duct system and promotes fat deposition in the breasts. They are responsible for the characteristic external appearance of the breasts at various stages of development and for the pigmentation of the areolas. *Luteotropic hormone* and *progesterone* are considered the chief stimulants for the development of the secreting cells in the lobules and alveoli. Progesterone causes the breast swelling and tenderness many women experience during the 10 days preceding menstruation. This is due to increased fluid in the subcutaneous tissue as well as to distention of the ducts and hyperaemia. All of these changes decrease during menstruation.

During pregnancy, the lobes and ducts enlarge in response to oestrogen stimulation in preparation for the secretion of milk. Progesterone acts on the oestrogen-primed ductal tissue and supports the secretory functions of the breast during lactation. Lactation is a function of the breasts that occurs in response to prolactin stimulation after the birth of a child.

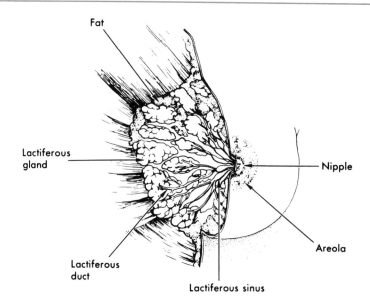

Figure 23.1 The female breast.

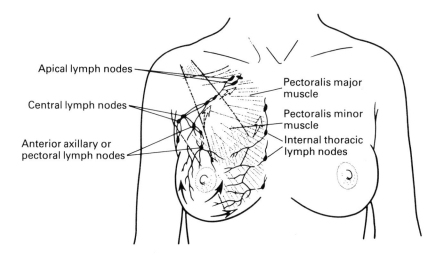

Figure 23.2 Lymphatic drainage of the breast.

DISORDERS OF THE BREAST

The breast evolves from puberty, through pregnancy, menopause and old age in response to hormonal changes. Breast disorders may occur and these vary during a woman's life cycle. Benign tumours are the most common disorder of the female breast. It is estimated that 1 in every 12 women will develop cancer of the breast at some time in her life. Cancer of the breast is the most common site of cancer in females and in the UK approximately 24 000 women annually are diagnosed as having this disease and around 15 000 women die from it each year. Although rare, breast cancer can occur in men; it is estimated that approximately 1% of breast cancer affects men.

The psychosocial implications which accompany breast disorders are varied and complex. The female breast carries significant yet different meaning for each woman, her partner and her family. The female breast is one symbol of a woman's sexuality; it is an integral component of her self-image. The importance of the breast has been reinforced throughout the ages by society, and today the media frequently idealize the perfect female breast.

CHARACTERISTICS

Symptoms of breast disorders may be insidious and may include: alterations in the size and/or shape of the breasts; palpable masses in the breast tissue and

Table 23.1 Interpretation of assessment findings related to breast disorders.

Presenting characteristics	Related assessment findings	Possible disorder
Thickened, nodular areas in breast (usually bilateral); may be slight; pain and tenderness possible, especially premenstrually	Female in childbearing years Exacerbated by caffeine intake Single or multiple breast masses; usually bilateral, mobile, well-defined, tender, in upper outer quadrant Cystic fluid (typically grey-green) from aspirated cysts	Fibrocystic disease (mammary dysplasia, cystic adenosis, chronic cystic disease, cystic mastitis, see p. 837)
Nipple discharge accompanied by nipple retraction; pain in affected areas; itching around nipple	Female in early-stage menopause Subareolar ducts that feel like rubbery lesions filled with a pastelike material Enlarged regional lymph nodes possible	Mammary duct ectasia (dilatation)
Nipple discharge, usually bloody; breast lump	Female, over age 35, with a family history of breast cancer, a personal history of long menstrual cycles, early menses, late menopause, or a first pregnancy after age 35 History of endometrial or ovarian cancer Enlarged, shrunken, or dimpled breast with no pain Nipple erosion, retraction, or discharge Non-tender, firm or hard lump that is irregularly shaped and fixed to skin or underlying tissues Enlarged surrounding lymph nodes	Breast cancer
Well-defined mass or masses in breast; no pain	Female in teens or early 20s Round, firm, discrete, movable mass 1–5 cm in diameter; usually solitary but may be multiple and bilateral	Fibroadenoma of breast (see p. 837)
Pain accompanied by tenderness in breast; hard, reddened breast	Female in third or fourth week postpartum History of cracked nipples Breast abscess Painful, enlarged, axillary lymph nodes Firm, tender, warm and reddened area in affected breast	Mastitis
Serous or serosanguineous discharge from one nipple duct unilaterally; moderate pain	Female aged 35 to 55 No palpable tumour or mass, or a soft mass that is difficult to distinguish from surrounding tissue	Interductal papilloma

From Morton PG (1989) with permission.

discharge from the nipples (Table 23.1). The size and shape of breasts vary among individual females and with age. Attitudes towards breast size are individual and may be influenced by social values, clothing styles and the person's self-image. Changes in the symmetry of the breasts may be caused by pathological processes. Palpable masses in the breasts may not be tender but frequently are discovered by women during self-examination of their breasts. Disorders of the breast in males are much less common than in females but alterations in size and shape do occur as a result of hormonal influences and abnormal tissue growth.

Anxiety and fear of cancer may accompany the discovery of a breast lesion. Both the woman and her partner experience stress and uncertainty about the potential loss of a very meaningful body part, the potential threat to life itself and the potential implications for any relationship. Research has demonstrated that patients frequently experience psychological prob-

lems following a diagnosis of breast cancer. A study by Maguire et al (1978) demonstrated that 27% of women undergoing mastectomy suffered from depression, and up to a third of patients developed sexual problems post mastectomy. Fallowfield et al (1986) also demonstrated that women undergoing conservative surgery for breast cancer suffered psychological morbidity.

RISK FACTORS

The identification of factors which contribute to the development of breast cancer has been the focus of many large and small studies of varying quality of design and control. All agree that the incidence of breast cancer increases with *age* and that it is predominately a *female* disorder. It rarely occurs under the age of 25. Women with a *family history* of breast cancer in a mother or sister, especially if it was premenopausal, are at greater than normal risk. *Early onset of menstruation* (before

12 years of age), a *late first pregnancy* and *late menopause* are additional risk factors. A personal health history of *benign fibrocystic breast disease* can predispose to the development of breast cancer.

Large international differences in the incidence of breast cancer suggest that *environment* and *diet* may be contributing factors. The incidence is five times greater in Western industrialized countries than in the less-developed countries of Asia, Africa and Latin America (London and Willett, 1988). Evidence, while not conclusive, supports a strong link between the amount of total dietary fat and the incidence and mortality rate of breast cancer.

Body size and *weight* have been extensively studied in relation to the risk of breast cancer. Obesity is believed to be a minor risk factor especially in postmenopausal women.

The use of hormonal replacement therapy and oral contraceptives has been questioned as possible risk factors, and the findings are ambiguous to date. There is no indication that oestrogen replacement therapy in menopausal women increases the risk for breast malignancy.

HEALTH EDUCATION

Although the public and health professionals are more aware of the need to prevent breast disorders, we still lack the knowledge for the primary prevention of breast cancer. Health education is directed largely toward secondary health promotion. There is strong evidence that early detection of breast cancer does reduce mortality (Tabar et al, 1985).

PRIMARY HEALTH PROMOTION

There are some measures women can take to prevent and alleviate minor breast problems:

- *Premenstrual breast swelling and tenderness* is common in many women and may be alleviated by reducing sodium intake during the immediate premenstrual period. A reduction in salt intake decreases water retention which contributes to the problem caused primarily by an increased progesterone production.
- *Breast support during exercise* can be improved with the use of newer sports brassières which are designed to eliminate irritation, decrease sagging and tension on the underlying muscles. These brassières have wide shoulder straps and do not have the usual metal hooks, fasteners and seams. Standard brassières can provide adequate support depending on the fit, amount of support provided and the intensity and duration of the exercise being undertaken.

SECONDARY HEALTH PROMOTION

The *goal* of secondary health promotion activities is to achieve a high rate of survival by diagnosing and treating breast cancer while it is still localized and confined to the breast (stage I).

Diagnosis and treatment of breast cancer at an early stage contributes to a 5-year survival rate of 87%. The early detection and treatment of breast cancer is therefore the best-known means of control. To date, early diagnosis is best achieved by identifying risk factors and the use and accessibility of mammographic screening.

BREAST AWARENESS

There is now a move away from the promotion of ritualistic breast self-examination towards encouraging breast awareness as part of general body awareness. The woman knowing her breasts might change at different times, and getting to know what is normal for her or abnormal and encouraging and supporting her to report without delay to her doctor anything she might feel is abnormal.

Champion (1987) demonstrated that combinations of attitudinal variables as perceived by women, susceptibility, seriousness, barriers to health action, motivation and control influenced the practice of breast self-examination. In view of the new emphasis on breast self awareness the nurse should consider how the above factors may influence a woman's approach to this new concept.

The role of the nurse

Nurses should include breast concerns as a component of their role in health education. Bathing and dressing activities alone provide the nurse with opportunities for for giving information. Clinical opportunities should also be used to educate.

The elderly in the community and in institutions rarely receive health education on this topic, yet we know that the incidence of breast cancer increases with age. Elderly women may also be less comfortable talking about their breasts and related concerns. Nurses have an obligation to this group and to all patients to assess their needs for breast examination and to carry out the procedure as indicated.

Teaching resources. A pamphlet outlining the concept of breast awareness has been produced for the National Health Service Breast Screening Programme for the guidance of women it outlines (Fig. 23.3):

1. What breast awareness is
2. The normal breast
3 Changes to look out for
4. What to do if a woman finds an abnormal change

Women should be aware that 90% of breast tumours are initially identified by women themselves. A high percentage of breast carcinomas are palpable and can be detected early at a size of about 1 cm. Being aware of any changes from what the woman perceives as normal increases the likelihood of early detection and thus improved prognosis, as the chance of metastasis is decreased in the early stages of the disease.

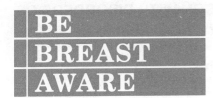

BE BREAST AWARE

WHAT IS BREAST AWARENESS

Breast Awareness is a part of general body awareness. It is a process of getting to know your own breasts and becoming familiar with their appearance. Learning how your breasts feel at different times will help you to know what is normal for you.

You can become familiar with your breast tissue by looking and feeling in any way that is best for you (eg. in the bath, shower, when dressing etc.).

Being **Breast Aware** and knowing what is normal for you will help you to be aware of any changes from normal, should these happen.

THE NORMAL BREAST

Before the menopause normal breasts feel different at different times of the month. The milk producing tissue in the breasts becomes active in the days before a period starts. In some women, the breasts at this time feel tender and lumpy, especially near the armpits.

After a hysterectomy the breasts usually show the same monthly differences until the time when your periods would have stopped.

After the menopause activity in the milk producing tissue stops. Normal breasts feel soft, less firm and not lumpy.

NHSBSP

Take care of your own well being

Know what is normal for you

CHANGES TO LOOK OUT FOR

Appearance. Any change in the outline or shape of the breast, especially those caused by arm movements, or by lifting the breasts. Any puckering or dimpling of the skin.

Feelings. Discomfort or pain in one breast that is different from normal, particularly if new and persistent.

Lumps. Any lumps, thickening or bumpy areas in one breast or armpit which seem to be different from the same part of the other breast and armpit. This is very important if new.

Nipple change. Nipple discharge, new for you and not milky. Bleeding or moist reddish areas which don't heal easily. Any change in nipple position - pulled in or pointing differently. A nipple rash on or around the nipple.

WHAT TO DO IF YOU FIND A CHANGE

There can be many reasons for changes in the breast. Most of them are harmless but all of them need to be checked as there is a small chance they could be the first sign of cancer.

If you are aware of any change in your breast from what is normal for you, **tell your doctor without delay**. Remember, you are not wasting anyone's time. If there is a cancer present, the sooner it is reported, the more simple treatment is likely to be. This offers greater prospects of benefit in terms of quality of life.

Breast cancer is very rare in women under the age of 40. The likelihood of developing breast cancer increases with age.

BREAST SCREENING

If you are aged 50 and over it is strongly recommended that you take advantage of the National Health Service Breast Screening Programme which offers 3 yearly mammography. This is an x-ray procedure which can detect breast changes at a very early stage. For more information about the breast screening programme ask your doctor.

Routine x-ray breast screening is not available for women under 50 as it has not been shown to be of benefit. If you have any cause for concern about your breasts tell your doctor.

Prepared for the
NHS Breast Screening Programme
by the

 Cancer
Research
Campaign

Oxford

Parts of this leaflet have been adapted from an original leaflet by Dr Barbara Thomas.

Know what to look and feel for

Report any changes without delay

Figure 23.3 'Be Breast Aware' Leaflet. Reproduced with permission of the NHS Breast Screening Programme.

MAMMOGRAPHIC SCREENING

Screening mammography is known to be of most benefit to women over the age of 50. Tabar et al (1985) demonstrate a 31% decrease in mortality from breast cancer in women over 50 years of age, and the Hospital Insurance Plan Study also reported similar findings (Seidman et al, 1987). High survival rates associated with this technique are attributed to the increased proportion of tumours detected in early stages. With the use of mammography it is possible to detect abnormalities too small to be palpable on clinical examination. It is estimated that mammography is capable of picking up 85–90% of all breast cancers in breasts examined.

The role of the nurse

The general public is becoming increasingly aware of the value and use of mammography with the introduction of the National Breast Screening Programme within the United Kingdom. Nurses can promote screening programmes by teaching about the importance of screening procedures and the availability of resources. Nurses can allay fears by assuring women that radiation exposure from a mammogram is minimal.

The United Kingdom breast screening programme

Research demonstrated that, with the introducing of a mammographic screening programme, mortality rates from breast cancer in women over the age of 50 years could be reduced by 31% (Tabar et al, 1985). A Government working party was therefore established to assess the evidence and consider the need for a National Breast Screening Programme within the United Kingdom. The report of the Working Party (Forrest, 1986) concluded that reductions in mortality rates could be achieved with the introduction of a mammographic screening programme and advised how such a programme might be implemented.

The Government established a mammographic screening programme for women of 50–64 years of age. Women are invited to partake in this programme and those who are identified as having screen-detected abnormalities are invited to an assessment centre for further diagnostic procedures. It is estimated that about 10% of those women who are screened will require further investigation but only a small minority will have breast cancer diagnosed and these women will be referred to treatment centres.

Nurses can contribute to this programme by offering women information and support whilst they are undergoing further diagnostic procedures within the assessment centres, and further support and care should a diagnosis of breast cancer be established.

THE PERSON WITH DISORDERS OF THE BREAST

ASSESSMENT

PHYSICAL EXAMINATION OF THE BREASTS

Breast examination is a very personal experience for the patient and requires understanding and consideration on the part of the health care team. Privacy should be ensured before the examination begins, and a warm environment provided.

Inspection. With the patient uncovered to the waist, the breasts are observed with the patient sitting upright, leaning forward and lying down. In each position the patient is asked to place the arms first at the sides and then to raise them above the head. The breasts are observed for: (1) nipple inversion, retraction and discharge; (2) retraction or dimpling of an area; (3) redness, excoriation, discoloration, oedema; and (4) changes in contour and symmetry.

Palpation. The breasts are palpated with the patient in the supine and then sitting position. Palpation begins with the patient's arms at the sides and is repeated with the arms raised over the head. The entire breast is examined in a systematic manner, beginning in one quadrant and moving around until the starting point is again reached. The palmar surface of the fingers is used, with the examiner's hands moving from the outer circumference toward the nipple or in concentric circles, from the nipple outward. With the patient in a sitting position, the breast is supported in one hand while being palpated with the other. The normal breast varies in consistency and may feel granular in older individuals. If any masses are discovered they are palpated for size, shape, consistency, mobility, discreteness of borders, location and tenderness. The intraclavicular, cervical and axillary areas are palpated for enlarged lymph nodes.

Following the breast examination, documentation of the size, shape and symmetry of the breasts and the size, shape, colour, mobility, consistency, tenderness and location of any palpable masses or abnormalities should be made.

DIAGNOSTIC TESTS

Mammography

Mammography is a radiological examination of the breast from several angles. Preparation is minimal. It is important to instruct the person to avoid using powder, perfume, deodorant or creams on the breasts or underarms prior to the procedure as they may cause misleading results. The women is told that she will be required to strip to the waist during the procedure.

The woman is placed in front of a mammographic X-ray machine and one breast at a time is placed between plates and compressed while a view is taken.

The procedure may cause some physical discomfort from compression of the tender breast tissue. During the procedure the woman is undressed and her breasts are exposed. This can be uncomfortable in a cold room and may be embarrassing. Care should be taken to ensure privacy and to support the woman through the procedure.

The films are examined for any areas of increased density and, if present, their characteristics (location, size, shape, regularity of borders). A lesion that is not palpable may be detected in a mammogram.

Biopsy. Biopsy provides a specimen of tissue for microscopic examination; the specimen may be obtained by aspiration, resection or excision. In the case of breast tumours, most surgeons prefer an excision biopsy, since it permits an examination of the complete tumour.

Bone scans. In patients with malignant tumours of the breast, bone scans may be carried out to identify bone metastases and to serve as a baseline for future bone scans.

DISORDERS OF THE NIPPLE

Causes

Drainage from the nipple in a non-lactating breast is usually a result of an intraductal papilloma, carcinoma, mammary dysplasia or ductal ectasia (distension).

Clinical characteristics

The discharge is usually serous or bloody but may be milky, brownish or purulent and may be unilateral or bilateral. It may be spontaneous or occur with manipulation. The breasts are assessed for a mass, and a history is taken to determine whether there is any relationship between the drainage and menstruation and if the patient is taking oral contraceptives or oestrogen therapy for postmenopausal symptoms.

An *intraductal papilloma* is a benign, wart-like growth usually involving a single collecting duct. It is located near the areola, is non-tender, may be soft or firm and bleeds or produces a yellow, pink or bloody drainage on pressure or with trauma. Treatment involves surgical excision of the papilloma and the involved duct.

Ductal ectasia is a form of fibrocystic mastitis characterized by dilation of multiple and usually bilateral ducts in the subareolar areas. Signs and symptoms include burning and itching, pain and swelling of the nipple and areolar area of the breast. Treatment may involve surgical excision of the involved ducts.

FIBROCYSTIC DISEASE AND BENIGN EPITHELIAL HYPERPLASIA

Causes

These are relatively common disorders of the female breast and are characterized predominantly by fibroplasia, epithelial hyperplasia and the formation of cysts. The lesions are influenced by a hormonal imbalance, are usually bilateral and occur most often in women 30–50 years of age, with a higher incidence in those approaching menopause.

Clinical characteristics

A painless mass is usually the first and only manifestation; occasionally there may be some tenderness. The woman may experience more severe soreness and pain of the breasts than is usual in the premenstrual period.

Treatment

The cysts may be aspirated with or without local anaesthesia. If a solid mass is encountered or the aspirated fluid contains blood, an incisional biopsy may be done to rule out carcinoma. Following the initial aspiration, the woman is re-examined periodically and aspiration of recurrent or newly formed cysts may be necessary. Fibrocystic disease is a recognized risk factor for breast cancer. The disease usually regresses with the onset of menopause.

FIBROADENOMA

Causes

Fibroadenoma is a benign tumour which develops most frequently in young women.

Clinical characteristics

It generally occurs singly, but may be multiple and bilateral. They do not change during the menstrual cycle. Although it is not usually encapsulated, it remains localized and is freely movable and usually painless. Medical authors indicate no increased tendency to subsequent carcinoma in patients who have had a fibroadenoma.

Treatment

The treatment consists of local excision of the tumour, which is submitted for cytological examination for confirmation of the diagnosis of non-malignancy.

NURSING MANAGEMENT

POTENTIAL HEALTH PROBLEMS OF THE WOMAN AND PARTNER/FAMILY

It must be realized that patients admitted for biopsy and

confirmatory diagnosis of a benign breast growth have very specific nursing needs related to their diagnosis:

- *Anxiety* related to the possible diagnosis of cancer, the significance of the breast and possible discomfort from the procedures.
- *Knowledge deficit* related to structure, development and hormonal influences of the breast; the diagnostic process; the potential for malignant breast disease; and measures to alleviate symptoms.
- *Coping*. Patients who are offered surgical removal of the growth are potentially at risk of developing many of the problems associated with surgery of malignant growths, especially those concerning self-image and the development of appropriate coping mechanisms.

GOALS

The person with a benign breast disorder and her spouse/family will be able to:

- Verbalize their emotional response to the experience.
- State the importance of being aware of any breast changes from normal.
- Describe measures to relieve physical symptoms of the breast disorder.

INTERVENTION

Nursing intervention for patients with *benign breast* disorders includes assessment of the person's emotional responses to the disorder and biopsy, instruction regarding being aware of abnormal breast changes and measures to reduce the physical symptoms.

Anxiety. The emotional response of individuals to the diagnosis of a benign breast tumour or scarring and possible disfigurement from a biopsy varies with the individual and the degree of the perceived threat to her self-image and femininity. The nurse assesses the woman's response and allows opportunity for the patient to express her feelings and concerns. A referral may be made to the general practitioner and a community nurse.

Knowledge deficit. Breast awareness is taught to all patients and the importance of this is stressed.

Measures which may help alleviate the physical symptoms of the disorder are explained if relevant to the individual. Such measures include: (1) wearing a brassiere 24 hours a day to provide firm support for the breast and to ease discomfort associated with movement; (2) use of heat or cold applications or mild analgesics to relieve discomfort.

Family coping. The person's partner and family will also be anxious about the possibility of malignant disease and the discomfort the person is experiencing during the diagnostic process. Their fears and anxieties should be identified and opportunity created to answer their questions and to teach them about the breasts, risk factors, common breast disorders and the importance of regular breast examination. The nurse should reinforce the positive behaviour of seeking health care and encourage communication and supportive activities among family members.

Evaluation

Evaluation of nursing intervention for the person with benign breast disease includes confirmation of the outcomes related to the spouse and family as well as the patient. The women should be able to demonstrate the techniques of breast self-examination. It is important that the woman and her family receive the results of the diagnostic procedures as soon as feasible to dispel their anxieties. The nurse should reinforce the need for regular, ongoing breast examination even though the disorder is benign.

Carcinoma

The breast is the most common site of cancer in the female. Approximately 20% of all female malignancies are breast cancers.

CONTRIBUTING FACTORS

Most breast cancers originate in the epithelial tissue of the ducts and account for approximately 70–75% of all breast cancers; the remainder arise from the secreting cells of the lobules. Approximately fifty per cent of breast carcinomas develop in the upper outer quadrant, 10% in the lower outer quadrant, 10% in the upper inner quadrant, 5% in the lower inner quadrant and 25% in the central portion of the breast (Robbins et al, 1981).

The cause of breast cancer is unknown. Three factors presently being considered are: (1) hormonal, (2) viral, and (3) genetic.

Many malignant tumours of the breast appear to be influenced by ovarian hormones, especially oestrogen. It has been demonstrated that some patients with cancer of the breast have a remission of their disease when the oestrogen concentration is reduced by endocrine therapy or by the administration of anti-oestrogenic agents.

Factors which might influence the risk of development of breast cancer are discussed above. Age, race, family history, early menarche, late menopause, late first pregnancy, fibrocystic breast disease and a high fat diet are the most significant of these factors.

The rate of growth of the cells of the neoplasm may depend on the immune response or resistance of the individual.

CLINICAL CHARACTERISTICS

The earliest symptom is generally a single, painless, non-tender mass which is poorly circumscribed and may have a nodular surface. It is usually discovered by the person when bathing or during a routine self-examination of the breasts. Other symptoms which may develop include change in the size or contour of the affected breast, retraction of the nipple or an area of the skin over the breast, bleeding or discharge from the nipple, a scaly rash around the nipple, enlargement of axillary or infra- or supraclavicular lymph nodes and subsequent oedema of the upper extremity or a bleeding, ulcerated area on the breast surface.

As the cancer grows, it spreads to adjacent tissues, such as the skin and underlying fascia and muscle. Retraction is due to involvement of the supporting fibrous tissue; there is a proliferation of fibroblasts and ensuing scar tissue within the breast and fascia of the chest muscles. The breast becomes firmer and cannot be moved as freely. Ulceration is associated with advanced disease which has spread to involve the skin.

METASTASES

Cancer of the breast may spread directly into adjacent structures or may metastasize to distant structures by emboli of tumour cells being transported through the lymphatics or the blood vessels. The axillary, supra-clavicular or mediastinal lymph nodes are usually the first site of secondary involvement. Other structures which frequently become the site of metastases are the bones, lungs, liver and brain.

TYPES OF BREAST CANCER

Cancers of the breast may be classified according to the primary breast tissue involvement or according to certain tissue changes. The most common type is *scirrhous carcinoma* characterized by marked fibrosing and hardness. The *medullary breast cancer* grows rapidly, forming a larger mass which is softer in consistency than the scirrhous type. There is less fixation of the breast. A third type which occurs rarely is the *inflammatory carcinoma*, which involves the skin and more superficial tissues as well as the lymphatics. *Lobular cancer* involves primarily glandular tissue and is less invasive than other types. This type of breast cancer accounts for approximately 15% of breast cancers. *Intraductal carcinoma*, which has a high incidence, originates in the epithelial tissue of one or more mammary ducts. *Papillary carcinoma* is charac-terized by small papillary growths within the duct system and usually causes bleeding from the nipple. *Paget's disease* is also an intraductal cancer that extends to involve the nipple and areola; a scaly rash and erosion of the nipple accompany this type.

The patient's disease may be classified by location (Figure 23.4) and whether it is infiltrating or non-infiltrating, or in stages (clinical staging) according to the characteristics of the primary breast *tumour*, regional lymph *node involvement* and *distant metas-tasis*. This classification is referred to as the TNM system (Table 23.2). Histological staging is carried out after examination of the removed axillary lymph nodes. It provides information on the proliferative activity of the tumour improving the prediction of five-year survival. Survival rates do not predict cure as the disease may recur as long as 20 years after initial surgery.

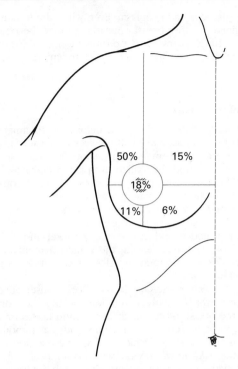

Figure 23.4 Incidence of breast cancer at various anatomical sites.

TREATMENT

The forms of treatment used in carcinoma of the breast are surgery, radiation, endocrine therapy which may be additive or ablative, chemotherapy and combinations of these treatments. There is no unanimous opinion as to the best method of treatment; the search continues for treatment that will provide more encouraging statistics than those currently recorded.

Currently, the choice of treatment is influenced by the stage of the disease, the age and general condition of the patient and the existing knowledge of the mechan-

Table 23.2 Clinical staging of breast carcinoma.

Stage I:	Tumour <2 cm in diameter
	Nodes, if present, not felt to contain metastases
	Without distant metastases
Stage II:	Tumour <5 cm in diameter
	Nodes, if palpable, not fixed
	Without distant metastases
Stage III:	Tumour >5 cm in diameter
	Tumour any size with invasion of skin or attached to chest wall
	Nodes in supraclavicular area
	Without distant metastases
Stage IV:	Tumour of any size
	Nodes either positive or negative
	With distant metastases

isms of spread of the neoplasm. Even when the tumour is confined to the breast, metastases may become apparent 10–20 years later. Consideration of the systemic nature of the disease influences treatment.

Surgical treatment

Radical mastectomy is the most deforming treatment and is not usually used today. It involves removal of the complete breast, the underlying pectoralis (major and minor) muscles and the axillary lymphatics and lymph nodes. This extensive operation leaves a long oblique scar and the chest wall may appear concave.

A *modified radical mastectomy* or Patey mastectomy involves the removal of the breast, axillary lymphatics and lymph nodes and leaves the pectoral muscles. Removal of the breast leaving the axillary lymphatics, lymph nodes and pectoral muscles intact comprises a *simple mastectomy*.

Primary tumour excision is the more conservative procedure which involves removal of the tumour, leaving the breast intact. The axillary lymph nodes may be sampled or removed en bloc with: a tumour resection (lumpectomy), which is a simple excision of the tumour; *wide local excision*, which is removal of the tumour with 1–2 cm of apparently normal adjacent breast tissue; or *quadrantectomy*, which is resection of the tumour and the involved breast quadrant and overlying skin.

Radiation therapy

External radiation therapy may be used as an adjunct to surgery, especially if the person had conservative surgery, or alone in cases in which the disease is advanced and inoperable, or in which there is a local recurrence after surgery. For the care of the patient receiving radiation therapy, see Chapter 10.

Chemotherapy

Chemotherapy may be offered to patients with early or metastatic disease as an adjunct to surgery. It may also be prescribed for persons with recurrence of the disease. Combinations of anticancer drugs are usually used. An example of a combination used in therapy is CMF, which is cyclophosphamide (Endoxana) (C), methotrexate (M) and fluorouracil (F). The schedule for administration may vary with patients. In the case of CMF, cyclophosphamide may be taken orally for 2 weeks and the other two drugs (methotrexate and fluorouracil) are given intravenously on days 1 and 8. This is followed by a treatment-free period of 2 weeks and then the 4-week cycle is repeated.

Adjuvant chemotherapy is prescribed for 6 to 8 months. The drugs are circulated in the blood throughout the body, reaching areas of metastatic disease. They are toxic to many normal cells in addition to cancerous cells, and have side-effects. See Chapter 10 for side-effects of these chemotherapeutic agents and the nursing responsibilities.

Endocrine therapy

Some patients with carcinoma of the breast experience a remission of their disease when the concentration of certain hormones (mainly oestrogen) is reduced. Their cancer is said to be hormone-dependent. Cells in some breast cancers have a high affinity for oestrogen; these cells are referred to as oestrogen-receptor cells. Moetzinger indicates that approximately 60% of breast cancers are oestrogen-receptor positive (Moetzinger and Dauber, 1982).

Oestrogen and progesterone receptor assays may be carried out on breast cancer tissue at the time of initial diagnosis. It is suggested that the presence of progesterone receptors, in addition to the oestrogen receptors, in breast cancer cells increases the response to endocrine therapy.

The patient may have an oophorectomy (removal of the ovaries), especially if she is premenopausal. This reduces the production of both oestrogen and progesterone. Non-steroidal anti-oestrogen drugs such as tamoxifen, which bind with oestrogen receptors, may be administered along with the standard chemotherapeutic agents and may be the treatment of choice in postmenopausal women. Tamoxifen is usually prescribed for a minimum of 2 years. Megestrol (Megace), an antioestrogenic drug, may be used when the patient has a recurrence of the disease following standard therapy with CMF or tamoxifen. Antioestrogen drugs may have side-effects but are usually well tolerated by patients.

TREATMENT OPTIONS

Nurses as patient advocates and educators and as participants in the clinical ethical decision-making process are likely to be asked about treatment options for the person with breast cancer. Today, the treatment options available are numerous but most are based on evidence obtained from large, multicentred, randomized control trials. It is extremely difficult for the patient and her partner and family to make such vital choices at a time of acute personal crisis. The nurse needs to be aware of the treatment options and the quality of the current scientific evidence supporting each choice. Nurses need to remain open and receptive to new developments in therapy while at the same time critically analysing the evidence on which the change was based. The final decision rests with the patient. Although the doctor is responsible for the medical plan of care, the nurse plays a major role in assisting the decision-making process and in supporting the choices of the patient and her family and in teaching them about the implications of their choices.

Current treatment options include:

- *Stage I breast cancer*. Treatment may involve limited excision of the tumour and lymph node sampling, or removal en bloc followed by radiation therapy to the remainder of the breast, or simple mastectomy usually with lymph node excision, or by modified radical mastectomy.
- *Stage II breast cancer* can also be treated and may be cured. Treatment options are similar to those for

stage I breast cancer. When cancer from the breast is present in the axillary lymph nodes, adjuvant chemotherapy or endocrine therapy may be used.

- *Stage III breast cancers* may be treated by mastectomy and/or radiation prior to surgery, and adjuvant chemotherapy or hormone therapy prior to or following surgery. Some stage III and most stage IV tumours are not operable. They may be controlled by radiation and chemotherapy and/or hormone therapy.
- *Metastatic breast cancer* can be treated but usually not cured. Treatment may depend on the hormone receptor levels of the tumour, the previous treatment and the time since initial treatment. Therapeutic interventions include combinations of surgery, radiation, chemotherapy and endocrine therapy.

Surgical procedures with or without radiation. Criteria for the selection of persons for conservative surgery plus radiation has been fairly well established based on the location and size of the tumour, and the woman's feelings about conservation of the breast. Tumours that involve the nipple area, those that are multifocal and large tumours are not usually suitable for conservative surgery. Conservative surgery plus radiation, has been shown to be equally as effective as partial mastectomy for selected patients with early or stage I or II lesions and has better cosmetic results (Fisher et al, 1989). If limited surgical excision is used without radiation, about one third of women will experience local recurrence in the involved breast.

Adjuvant chemotherapy. The use of single agent chemotherapy has not shown a significant reduction in mortality from breast cancer. Combination chemotherapy using the CMF regimen has been shown to have significant value in treating premenopausal women (Bonadonna et al, 1981).

Endocrine therapy. The use of tamoxifen has been found to be effective in women with breast cancer especially in postmenopausal women with hormone receptor positive tumours; tamoxifen (antioestrogen) therapy for at least 2 years has been shown to prolong the disease-free interval and to have a significant impact on survival (Bartlett et al, 1987; Baum et al, 1987; Early Breast Cancer Trialists' Collaborative Group, 1988). Much of the research on the use of tamoxifen has been carried out in the United Kingdom. An analysis of many clinical trials demonstrated that tamoxifen gave a survival benefit to women over 50 years of age (Peto, 1985). The role of endocrine therapy in the treatment of premenopausal women is less clear.

Reconstructive surgery. The option of reconstructive surgery should be discussed with the patient and her partner, if appropriate, prior to the initial surgery. Reconstructive surgery may be carried out at the time of the initial surgery or delayed. The patient should be aware that the surgery will not interfere with the diagnosis of recurrent disease. The patient's wishes should be considered but she does not have to make a final decision until later. Breast contour can be restored by either a silicone implant or by a flap of overlying skin

and muscle from the latissimus dorsi or rectus abdominis muscles. Implants are available in various sizes to accommodate breast size and shape. A nipple and areola can also be created by the surgeon from the skin overlying the area of reconstruction, from the other nipple or from a graft taken from the labia or upper inner thigh. Breast reconstruction may help a woman and her partner move toward restoration of self-image and previous life-style.

BREAST CANCER IN THE MALE

Carcinoma of the breast is relatively rare in the male, usually occurring in the older man. The course of the disease is similar to that in the female; it readily metastasizes to regional lymph nodes and other structures. It is often unrecognized and neglected in the early stage because of the low incidence in men; as a result, metastases have frequently developed when the patient is first seen. Treatment may involve a mastectomy or radiation therapy or chemotherapy. A bilateral orchidectomy (removal of the testes) and hormonal therapy may also be used.

The Person with Cancer of the Breast

The following clinical situation describes the experiences of a woman with breast cancer, her family and care-givers. The situation, which is divided into preoperative, surgical, postoperative, discharge and times when she was receiving chemotherapy after her operation, illustrates that life's problems rarely present as single events. The patient must be viewed within the context of her total situation.

The interdisciplinary as well as the multidisciplinary roles of the nurse are demonstrated. The primary care nurse, the associate nurses on the oncology unit and the clinical nurse specialist worked collaboratively and in partnership with the patient and her family to provide patient-centred, goal-directed nursing care. This situation is a composite from actual clinical practice. Although it illustrates a co-ordinated and comprehensive approach to nursing care, it also contains the realities of clinical practice and the unpredictable nature of life and people.

CLINICAL SITUATION

Rose Lewis is a 43-year-old Jamaican woman who emigrated in her youth. She was recently diagnosed as having carcinoma of the right breast and was admitted to hospital for surgical excision of the malignant breast tumour.

Jane Miles, her primary nurse, met Rose the afternoon prior to her scheduled surgery. Rose presented as a pleasant, reserved, almost retiring woman, with clear, dark complexion, and large brown eyes which expressed simultaneously anxiety and hope. She greeted Jane expectantly, and quietly admitted her anxiety. Jane explained that she would be primarily responsible for her care with the assistance of other nurses.

ASSESSMENT

Social History

Rose stated that she was married 7 years ago and lives with her husband and their 6-year-old daughter, of whom she is immensely proud. Conversation suggested her anxiety was more related to their well-being than her own. This is her second marriage. She was previously married at 19 years of age and has three older children: two sons, aged 21 and 23, and a daughter. Both sons are successfully employed and living independently but are geographically close and emotionally supportive. Her 19-year-old daughter lives at home and is working at two jobs, one full-time and one part-time, to save towards a long holiday. After her first husband left her, Rose brought up these three children essentially alone, while employed in a clothes factory.

Recently, with the assistance of a loan, Rose was able to realize a long-standing dream. She opened a small boutique selling women's clothing and accessories.

During this discussion with Rose, Jane mentally noted several social concerns which could be summarized as a *potential for alteration in family process* related to the crisis of illness and hospitalization of a primary care-giver and secondary wage earner. Rose had voiced the following concerns:

- Her husband, a shift-worker, was not always at home when their young daughter returns from school. Her husband, oldest daughter and a neighbour were sharing this responsibility.
- The youngster was already confused and saddened by her mother's absence. Her usual sunny disposition was being replaced by an unusual irritableness which was difficult for others to deal with effectively.
- The boutique was closed through the day because Rose could not afford to hire a replacement for herself. Although her youngest son opened the boutique in the evening after his day at his job, the store was losing valuable daytime business. Rose feared she would soon be unable to meet payments on the boutique rent and her loan.
- Rose was uncertain how her husband, who is 3 years younger than herself, would cope with: (1) her change in appearance postoperatively; (2) her temporary physical incapacity, loss of strength and well-being; (3) the added responsibility for their young daughter; and (4) their new financial concerns.
- Rose was understandably fearful that this diagnosis might (1) shorten the time she expected to have to raise her younger daughter and guide her growth to maturity; (2) diminish her immediate effectiveness as wife and mother due to continued illness.

In considering the above diagnosis, Jane also noted several *strengths* in the family system:

- Rose appeared to have strong emotional support from her immediate family and a few close friends.
- Her husband's salary was sufficient to support the small family at an adequate though basic standard of living.

- Her older children and some friends were willing to assist in a practical manner at this time.
- Rose was very open and was quickly establishing a relationship of trust.

The *goal* of care was that the family members would show a decrease in the existing stress level by addressing each of the above concerns constructively and supportively with a view to preventing family breakdown.

Planned nursing interventions were to:

- Facilitate the development of a feasible timetable for available care-givers and Rose's young daughter.
- Assure Rose that it is possible for her young daughter to visit her postoperatively and thus be reassured by her appearance and caring.
- Seek guidance from the social worker to discuss the future of her boutique and her loan payments. This information may help reduce Rose's anxiety.

Jane noted the following expected problems on Roses's care plan:

- *Knowledge deficit* related to essential pre- and postoperative care measures.
- *Anxiety* related to the threat of change in role function as wife, sexual partner, mother and business woman.
- *Fear* related to this life-threatening diagnosis with possible terminal outcome.

Physical History

Rose had a tendency to *obesity*. Her admission weight was 77.8 kg (height 162 cm). There was no familial history of breast cancer. Her mother was a diagnosed diabetic but had never had breast disease.

History of illness

In response to questions, Rose relayed the following sequence of events, alternately displaying frustration with the system, fear and tears, guilt, hopefulness, quiet resignation, and occasional brief smiles as she recounted a humorous incident.

- While showering, Rose felt what she perceived to be a large firm lump beginning near the nipple and extending to the upper outer quadrant of her right breast, 'about the size and shape of an egg'. She allowed Jane to examine it.
- Though she was initially fearful, she knew the lump might be a benign cyst, and with this hope decided to wait for her scheduled appointment, a decision which later generated some guilt. Her family doctor was very reassuring and dismissed her concerns, stating he was sure the lump was cystic.
- She was given an appointment for a mammogram.
- Her apprehension increased when informed that she must wait 3 more weeks for this appointment.
- The report, received 4 days later, recommended a biopsy of the lump be done to rule out malignancy definitely.

- Rose was referred to a surgeon and within the week had a needle biopsy of the tumour. The subsequent report confirmed a diagnosis of malignancy, though questions remained regarding the extent of the disease.
- Rose was admitted 2 days later. Though her worst fears seemed confirmed, she continued to hope that this experience was all a bad dream, and that nothing significant would be found. She completed all the preadmission laboratory and X-ray examinations.
- She was relieved to be in hospital but concerned that 2 months had elapsed since she discovered the lump and that she did not know how long it had previously existed.
- Blood tests showed that Rose had a highly elevated fasting blood sugar, which was further distressing information — a second new diagnosis. Further tests were completed and treatment for diabetes mellitus implemented that evening.

TREATMENT ALTERNATIVES

- The surgeon had explained to Rose that it was planned that she should have an excision biopsy and frozen section the following morning. The tissue would be examined and, if warranted, a modified radical mastectomy would follow while she was still 'under the anaesthetic'. She had signed the appropriate consent form for this procedure in case the surgical team deemed a mastectomy to be advisable following the biopsy report. Rose still had questions about the proposed procedure. She had desperately hoped that she would only have the lump removed, because she had seen a television programme which stated this procedure was just as successful. Women were urged to insist on discussion of alternatives but she hesitated to delay the surgeon for further explanations.
- Jane explained that a lumpectomy is satisfactory for smaller growths which do not invade the nipple. The surgeon's note indicated the operation of choice was complete removal of the breast based on the apparent size of the tumour and possible extension into the areola tissue. Jane requested that the house officer return for further discussion.
- The doctor corroborated Jane's information, stating the location of the tumour and its size made it unsafe to attempt to save the breast. Rose accepted these explanations and began the long process of adjustment.

Jane stated she would spend time with Rose and her family in the postoperative period to relay necessary information, advice and physical care. A second *goal*, to establish a therapeutic relationship based on trust, had been successfully initiated.

SURGICAL PERIOD

- In surgery, following the biopsy and a positive pathology report, a modified radical mastectomy and axillary node dissection were performed.
- Rose quickly regained consciousness in the recovery room. She was immediately aware of pain in her right thoracic region and a sore throat from the anaesthetic.
- Rose was returned to the ward with a heavy compression dressing in place over the wound and drainage tubes in situ. An intravenous infusion was running slowly. At the bedside, her husband and eldest daughter anxiously greeted her arrival and asked if they might speak with the surgeon.
- Jane completed her postoperative check of vital signs and wound area, recorded them and assured Rose the pain would be controlled with medication administered regularly. She supported Rose's affected arm comfortably on a pillow. Rose slept for long periods that evening and night.

POSTOPERATIVE PERIOD

- The next morning, Rose was still shocked and depressed that the tumour had proven to be malignant. Her denial and hope must now be replaced with truth. She had viewed her life more positively in the last few years that ever before. The situation seemed dreamlike and unreal. At intervals though, she was able to be quite realistic about the impact of this disease on her life expectancy.
- Rose was concerned now about her own response to the alteration in her appearance, apprehensive about viewing her incision, and doubtful if she would have the inner strength required to cope with this adjustment.
- Jane and the nursing team, although they could not alter the diagnosis and did not yet know the extent of disease or prognosis, believed that assisting Rose to develop a positive attitude and decrease internal stress would contribute to physical and emotional healing and general well-being.
- Following this evaluation of Rose's present emotional status, Jane continued her review of her status. Her further assessment revealed:
- Rose was not in pain, having received analgesia at 6 a.m.
- Her bedclothes and surgical dressing were dry externally.
- The drainage device suctioning blood and tissue fluid from the operative site had recently been emptied.
- Rose had not been out of bed postoperatively, but was turning slowly and carefully from her back to her unaffected side. She was moving the head and forearm of her affected side with hesitancy and great care.
- She was drinking satisfactorily and passing urine.
- She experienced no nausea that morning and agreed to try some light solid food for lunch.
- Her respiratory status was satisfactory.
- Her temperature was normal.
- The operative report indicated Rose had lost more than the expected amount of blood during the operation but did not require replacement therapy. Jane noted blood pressure and pulse rate were quite normal and stable since Rose's return from surgery and her intravenous infusion was running slowly.
- Rose was expecting her husband after lunch before his shift-work started at 3 p.m.

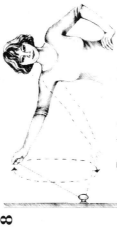

Hair-brushing exercise
(for hospital)

Rest elbow on bed-table. Keep head erect. Start by brushing one side only, then gradually increase to whole head. Don't overdo, but be persistent.

1

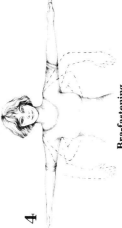

Squeezing and relaxing hand
(for hospital)

A rubber ball or similar object may be used.

2

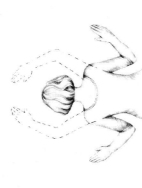

Arm-swinging

Place unaffected arm on back of chair and rest forehead on arm. Allow your other arm to hang loosely and swing from shoulder, forwards and backwards, then side to side and in small circles. As arm relaxes, increase length of swings and size of circles. Swing until arm is relaxed.

3

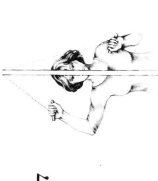

Bra-fastening

Extend arms, drop hands from elbows, then slowly reach behind back to bra level.

4

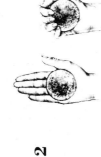

Wall-reaching

Feet apart for balance. Stand close to and facing wall. Start with hands at shoulder level and gradually work hands up the wall. Slide hands back to shoulder level before starting exercise again. Do slowly several times a day. Mark spot reached and aim higher each time.

5

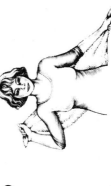

Bean-bag exercise
(A small purse or cosmetic bag will do just as well)

Drop bag from right hand over right shoulder into left hand at back. Repeat five times and do with opposite side.

6

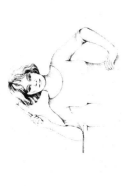

Rope-pulley exercise

Throw rope or dressing gown cord over top of open door. Sit with door between legs. Hold lower end in hand on the side of your surgery and gently pull other end. Raise arm as high as possible each time, until full elevation.

7

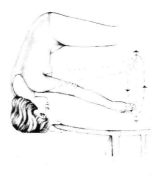

Rope/string exercise

Attach rope to doorknob or handle. Make small circles with rope moving entire arm from the shoulder. Do five times in one direction and five times in the other and gradually increase size of circle (by moving in closer) and number of circles.

8

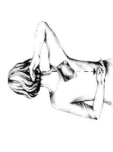

Back-drying exercise

With towel or similar item use a gentle back-drying motion. Reverse procedure.

9

Figure 23.5 Exercises for the postmastectomy patient. Reproduced with permission from the Breast Care and Mastectoomy Association of Great Britain.

Table 23.3 Nursing plan of care for Rose (postmastectomy).

Patient problem	Goals	Nursing intervention
1. Activity intolerance: impaired mobility	• Rose will increase activity tolerance daily	• Assist Rose to sit upright in bed with her legs over the side, supported as necessary • Assist Rose to stand and move to chair and sit down • Assist Rose to the toilet before returning to bed • Gradually encourage Rose to walk in hall with assistance and eventually to move about independently
2. Fluid volume deficit	• Rose will have a balance of fluid intake and output	• Empty drainage bottles as necessary and record volume of drainage • Observe dressing and bed linen periodically to assure there is no postoperative bleeding • Discuss with patient and surgeon the advisability of discontinuing infusion if no nausea or emesis occurs during morning • Regular check of all vital signs
3. Obesity	• Rose will lose weight gradually (0.5–1 kg/week)	• Determine likes and dislikes and discuss with dietitian • Refer to dietitian for diabetic meal planning • Reinforce teaching during remainder of hospitalization • Attempt to allay Rose's fears about diabetes with knowledge and support
4. Impaired breathing pattern and airway clearance	• Rose will have regular, rhythmic respirations	• Initiate deep breathing and coughing exercises immediately • Encourage Rose to continue this independently if no respiratory problem arises
5. Inability to carry out personal hygiene due to effects of surgery limiting movement	• Rose will demonstrate arm exercises, show increasing range of motion in right arm, and perform self-care activities	• Assist Rose to begin her bath. Complete bath for patient • Encourage increasing independent activity each day • Encourage Rose to begin range of motion exercises of fingers, hands, wrist and elbow of affected arm • Explain the necessity to avoid shoulder contractures on affected side (frozen shoulder) • Later, demonstrate simple exercises she can begin gradually in order to maintain normal function in all joints on affected side. Avoid pain. Give patient pamphlet with diagrams and explanations of postmastectomy exercises (Figure 23.5) • Work with the physiotherapist, who will guide patient in appropriate exercises

Table 23.3 Continued.

Patient problem	Goals	Nursing intervention
6. Pain	● Rose will verbalize absence of pain	● Explain the analgesic regimen. Offer analgesics 4-hourly initially as prescribed and ask Rose to request medication if uncomfortable ● Administer oral analgesics, as prescribed, when Rose tolerates fluids well
7. Altered body image	● Rose will select a temporary breast prosthesis, verbalize feelings of satisfaction with her appearance, socialize with family, patients and friends	● Refer Rose to clinical nurse specialist for ongoing support working towards developing a coping acceptance ● If Rose requires this refer to The Breast Care Mastectomy Association for support ● Assist Rose eventually to view the operative area and assume control of her care
8. Knowledge deficit related to postmastectomy care	● Rose will describe treatment plans and options available	● Refer patient to clinical nurse specialist for support and teaching about the availability of a permanent prosthesis and reconstructive surgery, and significance of pathology results when received ● Reinforce teaching received ● Practice techniques taught for postmastectomy exercises
9. Anxiety	● Rose will verbalize and share her feelings and concerns	● Initiate further discussion of Rose's feelings in order to determine her fears, apprehensions, hopes, needs and desires for the future. Improve her awareness of the help available to her in hospital and community (about cancer, mastectomy, diabetes) ● Foster the continuance of close and supportive family ties ● Encourage Rose's positive feelings and assist with resolution of problems, fears. Expect the normal grieving process, which includes anger ● Create a discharge plan for Rose and her family
10. Altered family coping	● Rose will utilize resources to communicate and resolve actual and potential family stresses, and re-establish a positive sexual relationship with her husband	● Be present to meet Rose's husband and other family members and offer information in conjunction with the clinical nurse specialist and assist them to adjust to this traumatic illness and temporary instability in the home

Table 23.3 Continued.

Patient problem	Goals	Nursing intervention
		• Arrange for youngest daughter to visit the following day to allay fears and to allow Rose to elicit her co-operation in 'helping' her father and sister at home. This might reverse the negative effect of mother's absence, reassure the youngster regarding mother's illness

Satisfied with this assessment of Rose's physical and emotional status, Jane now formulated her plan of care for the postoperative period (Table 23.3).

PREDISCHARGE PERIOD

Four days later, Rose was feeling considerably improved.

- She experienced very occasional operative discomfort which was controlled with analgesia.
- The drainage has ceased and the drains were removed that morning.
- The initial dressing had been changed but Rose has not yet viewed the incision.
- She was now independently completing such daily activities as bathing, eating, drinking, walking, reading, phoning the family and friends, and visiting other patients.
- Rose had many concerns about her diabetes but her fasting blood sugar level had dropped in response to the diabetic diet, decreased stress and an oral hypoglycaemic agent. The dietitian stated her knowledge was improving and planned to continue to counsel her as an out-patient.
- The social worker contacted a social worker in the community to begin working with Rose towards resolution of her financial concerns.
- The clinical nurse specialist had informed Rose about postsurgical care: the availability of volunteer help from the Breast Care Mastectomy Association. The staff had all encouraged the patient and family members to think positively about the future. This was most essential for Rose. In this domain, the clinical nurse specialist had assisted by providing patient education and support. She had introduced the topic of future reconstructive surgery. She had emphasized the importance of a healthy diet. Rose had been taught to decrease the fat content of her diet and to eat fruits and vegetables. Moderate exercise, preferably outdoors, was to be encouraged as an aid to improving muscle strength and creating a sense of well-being.

Chemotherapy

- The expected pathology report was received on the nursing unit on Rose's fifth postoperative day. The final diagnosis was 'infiltrating duct and intraductal carcinoma'. The report stated there was an extensive amount of residual tumour remaining following the excision biopsy but the mastectomy margins were free of tumour. Three of the ten excised regional lymph nodes were involved with metastatic disease, necessitating further therapy. The oestrogen and progesterone receptor assays were later reported as positive. Rose's bone scan, liver scan and chest X-ray showed no evidence of metastases.
- The surgeon immediately referred Rose to an oncologist who described the disease process as stage III. His decision was to proceed with adjuvant chemotherapy as soon as healing was sufficiently advanced. Rose was given an appointment in the chemotherapy clinic for 2 weeks later.
- The drugs of choice for Rose were CMF (cyclophosphamide, methotrexate and 5-fluorouracil).
- As she had promised, the clinical nurse specialist returned, at the request of the oncologist, to discuss this new development with Rose prior to her discharge. Rose had heard many horror stories from acquaintances at work about the side-effects of chemotherapy. She had discussed these concerns with Jane her primary nurse and the clinical nurse specialist in the earlier postoperative period and some of her fears had been dispelled. Although she would have preferred to avoid the necessity for further therapy, Rose accepted the fact that these adjuvant medications were required to prevent the development of metastatic disease in areas distant from the original tumour, commonly lungs, liver or bone. Although she had no evidence of disease in these structures at this time, the medication was intended to destroy possible microscopic disease and prevent widespread extension to other organs.
- Although each person responds differently to the same regimen, the nursing team were able to allay one of Rose's major concerns—hair loss. Because the cyclophosphamide would be taken orally over time, rather than intravenously, hair loss would be substantially decreased. Although her hair would

thin, and Rose would be aware of the loss, it would be less apparent to others. Few patients on this regimen actually need a wig. Although nausea can be an unpleasant experience, antiemetics are available to counteract this problem. Other common side-effects, such as myelosuppression, possible stomatitis, amenorrhoea, diarrhoea, nasal congestion, and lacrimation, were discussed and coping strategies suggested. Rose was given an explanatory pamphlet to read and an outline of the 28-day schedule which would be repeated from 6 to 12 times.

- Rose consented to the therapy.

Altered Body Image

- Rose was able to discuss with the primary nurse her concern about viewing her incision and caring for the area at home. She asked Rose what she expected the operative area to look like. The picture Rose imagined and tried to describe was much more drastic than the reality. Since Jane was preparing to remove alternate sutures and apply a lighter dressing, she and the clinical nurse specialist offered to assist Rose during this difficult moment, reassuring her that the neat, clean surgical wound, now healing well, would be less traumatic than the gaping, open area she had imagined. The more difficult adjustment would be accepting the change in her familiar body image. With their support, Rose was able to look at her operative area and quickly expressed relief that the area was already so well healed. She had not imagined such an ordinary surgical wound because a comparatively large structure had been removed.
- Although she could not touch her body at this time, she agreed with the help of Jane to participate in the wound-care the next morning. Rose was also encouraged to assist her husband to go through this same difficult experience in the privacy of their own home.
- Rose was looking forward to having a temporary prosthesis.

DISCHARGE

- Rose's discharge was arranged for her seventh postoperative day. After bathing that morning, with guidance from her nurse, she was able to remove her own dressing. She observed how the nurse gently washed her incision, removed the remaining sutures and covered the area with a light dressing. She had instructions to leave the incision uncovered as soon as the last evidence of the scab was removed by cleansing. As the wound was completely healed, she was given permission to shower as soon as she felt strong enough.
- When touching the surrounding area that morning, Rose noted the numbness around the incision in the axillary area and the inner aspect of the upper arm. She remembered Jane had warned her of this and that this feeling would take time to resolve and that there might be some permanent residual numbness. Rose wondered how long it would take to become accustomed to yet another new experience.

- She noted a puffiness and mild discomfort on the chest wall under her arm and asked the nurse if this signified a problem. She was told there was no sign of inflammation but the swelling might indicate a collection of some tissue fluid since the drains were removed. She was advised to mention this to the doctor at her appointment a few days later because it is occasionally necessary to aspirate this fluid.
- Rose experienced a sense of satisfaction that she had finally been able to participate in the care of her incision. As she dressed in preparation for going home, she realized that psychologically she was beginning to cope: 'It feels like part of me now.'

DISCHARGE PLAN

In Jane's absence the associate nurse reviewed the discharge plan that had been developed with Rose.

1. Wound

- When strong enough to shower (few days) wash scar area normally, gently.
- Leave dressing off when scab is gone.
- If signs of redness or tenderness occur, notify the doctor.
- Notify the doctor if puffiness is observed on chest wall (side, back) near incision.
- Numbness postoperatively over incision axilla and inner part of upper arm is normal. Exercise caution when shaving axilla; use electric razor if possible.

2. Exercise

- Check knowledge of postmastectomy exercises.
- Carry out each exercise at least once a day, preferably twice, avoiding extremes and pain.

3. Nutrition

- Review diabetic meal plan each evening and plan meals for the next day (later for a week at a time).
- Emphasize fruits and vegetables, especially those from the list containing large amounts of vitamins A and C.
- Decrease fat intake; red meat less often, fish and fowl in its place.
- Whole grain cereals and bread.
- Keep appointments with dietitian in 2 weeks and 1 month.
- Keep diary of food taken daily and review with dietitian.
- Keep appointment at hospital regarding diabetes management.

4. Chemotherapy

- Keep appointment at clinic for chemotherapy.
- When in clinic, ask to see clinical nurse specialist and social worker if necessary.
- Light breakfast the day of the clinic.

5. Self-care

- Gradually resume light household duties (e.g. dusting, washing/drying dishes, getting light meals).
- Assume responsibility for own care (bathing, dressing, shampooing, light laundry).
- Share in responsibility for your youngest daughter (clothing, school activities, play, friends, discipline, lunch, etc.).

6. Sexual Relations

- Assist husband to see, touch, adjust to new appearance of operative site.
- Share gentle physical contact.
- Resume sexual activity when appropriate.

7. Financial Concerns

- Make an appointment with social worker for help and advice about financial problems.
- Make a long-range plan to return to work once the body's response to chemotherapy was known.

8. Rest

- Rest as necessary, especially on the day chemotherapy is administered.

Before the nurse completed this review, Rose's eldest son arrived to transport her home because her husband was working. Although she knew the alteration in her appearance was not noticeable to others, she nevertheless felt apprehensive and 'different' as she left the safety of the hospital, and the compassion and empathy of so many staff members. She hoped some day she would feel an integral part of life again when this traumatic time was long past. There was no certainty about this, but there was hope and a positive attitude toward the future.

OUTPATIENT CLINIC

- Rose returned regularly to the clinic for her routine blood tests and chemotherapy. Her white blood cell count was low, as expected, but not unsafe. So far she has not missed any treatments. Her planned programme is not yet complete.
- The social worker has helped Rose. Rose is planning to return to the boutique if the loan payment can be refinanced. If not, she plans to find a position in a ladies' wear shop and get on with the arduous task of repaying the loan. She is looking forward to returning to the workplace and the social contact it provides.
- The social worker has also assisted Rose with grief counselling. She was most often cheerful and hopeful, but occasionally overwhelmed with distaste for her altered body image, the chemotherapy, the fear of recurrence of disease and death.
- The clinical nurse specialist reviewed Rose's clinical situation, her response to chemotherapy, advent of side-effects, her coping ability and need for assis-

tance. Rose did experience nausea for 24–36 hours after treatment but had only one episode of emesis. The oncologist prescribed an antiemetic for her to take at home.
- Although Rose wonders how worried her husband really is, she told the clinical nurse specialist that he remains outwardly controlled. They have been able to adjust to a quiet and gentle intimacy when she feels well.
- Rose has experienced some stomatitis and the clinical nurse specialist advised her on oral hygiene, to use a soft toothbrush, avoid extremes of temperature (hot, cold) in food and fluids and avoid highly spiced foods.
- Rose states she has carried out her postmastectomy exercises and has achieved close to a complete return to normal function.
- As a result of her diet, she has lost some weight but realizes she has a long way to go yet.
- Oestrogen/progesterone receptor assays were reported as positive.
- *Holidays*. Rose was anxious to return to Jamaica to visit her grandmother, her ailing mother and large extended family. She presumed her chemotherapy would not allow this. When she mentioned her wish, the clinical nurse specialist reviewed her protocol with her and indicated she had a 3-week period every 28 days during which she could be absent from the clinic. Rose was pleased and made the necessary arrangements. When she returned, she brought the sad news that her grandmother died suddenly a few days after she arrived. Her mother was at the funeral, but was not well. Within a week, she became very ill and died. These two losses were indeed a traumatic experience but she was happy to have seen both alive and grateful she went when she did. She is concerned because her mother's primary problem was diabetes and its complications.

EVALUATION

Rose, with her family and with the nursing staff, achieved many of the goals and outcomes, both preoperatively and postoperatively, which Jane and the nursing staff had outlined early in her hospital period.

1. Establishing a sense of trust with a great number of medical, nursing and allied health personnel who played vital individual roles on the team responsible for her care.
2. Adjusting to the hospital environment, and its established policies and procedures while maintaining her own individuality.
3. Responding favourably to general preoperative teaching about the operative and postoperative experience.
4. Monitoring herself to achieve various postoperative goals each day in her speedy return to independence and some normality in the activities of daily living.
5. Sharing some very intimate feelings, personal information, fears, hopes and problems with hospital personnel and allowing them the privilege of assisting her to cope.

6. Gradually gaining the strength to adjust to a new body image and begin to look positively at the future.
7. Learning basic facts about her particular chemo-therapy regimen and possible side-effects, and several coping strategies.
8. Assisting her husband, her three older children and her 6-year-old daughter to cope with this change in their family structure and with her period of hospitalization.
9. Coping with the additional diagnosis of diabetes, a fear she has had for many years because of her personal weight gain and her mother's history.
10. Co-operating with nursing staff and the physio-therapist in learning an exercise which has im-proved use of the affected right arm and shoulder.
11. Finding the inner strength and courage to over-come some of the dread and fear which normally accompany a life-threatening illness.
12. Allowing herself to set aside temporarily the concern about her business which was so worrying on her admission, recognizing that life and its immediate preservation is basic and essential to achieving any other goal.

SUMMARY

Breast cancer is the most frequent cause of cancer in women. Although much is known about risk factors for breast cancer, prevention is not yet possible. Breast screening is one of the few health promotion activities that is effective in reducing cancer mortality. Teaching women breast self-examination techniques is an area of nursing responsibility.

Partners and family are valued participants in the care of women with breast disorders. The nurse is respon-sible not only for the patient but also for identifying and alleviating the health needs of the partner and family, who are also affected by the patient's breast disorder. Scientific work has yet to identify definitive treatment(s) for breast cancer. The nurse plays an important role in helping the patient and family make choices regarding the best combination of therapies for her situation.

Although discussion in this chapter focuses on women with breast disorders, it is important to remember that men, although rarely, can also develop breast disorders and their experiences can be equally as disturbing to their lives and well-being.

LEARNING ACTIVITIES

Investigate the resources available in your community for:
(a) Breast cancer screening.
(b) Literature and learning resources for the prevention and/or management of breast disorders.
(c) Breast prostheses.
(d) Breast cancer patients and their partners.

REFERENCES AND FURTHER READING

Bartlett K, Eremin O, Hutcheon A et al (1987) Adjuvant tamoxifen in the management of operable breast cancer:-the Scottish trial. *Lancet* **ii**: 171–175.
Baum M, Brinkley DM, Dosset JA et al (1988) Controlled trial of tamoxifen as a single adjuvant agent in the management of early breast cancer: analysis at eight years by Novaldex Adjuvant Trial Organization. *British Journal of Cancer* **57(6)**: 608–611.
Bonadonna G et al (1981) Dose response effect of adjuvant chemotherapy in breast cancer. *New England Journal of Medicine* **304**: 10–15.
Champion VL (1987) The relationship of breast self-examina-tion to health belief model variables. *Research in Nursing and Health* **10(6)**: 375–382.
Clement-Jones V (1985) Cancer and beyond: the formation of BACUP (British Association of Cancer United Patients and Their Families and Friends). *British Medical Journal* **291**: 1021–1023.
Davita VT, Hellman S & Rosenburg SA (1985) *Cancer: Principles and Practice of Oncology* 2nd edn. Philadelphia: Lippincott.
Early Breast Cancer Trialists' Collaborative Group (1988) Effects of adjuvant tamoxifen and of cytotoxic therapy on mortality in early breast cancer: an overview of 61 randomized trials among 28,896 women. *New England Journal of Medicine* **319(26)**: 1681–1692.

Fallowfield LJ et al (1986) Effects of breast conservation on psychological morbidity associated with diagnosis and treat-ment of early breast cancer. *British Medical Journal* **293**: 1331–1334.
Fisher B, Redmond C, Poisson R et al (1989) Eight-year results of a randomized clinical trial comparing total mastectomy and lumpectomy with or without irradiation in the treatment of breast cancer. *New England Journal of Medicine* **320(13)**: 822–828.
Forrest APM (1986) *Breast Cancer Screening.* London: HMSO.
Ganong WF (1989) *Review of Medical Physiology* 14th edn, pp 370–387. Norwalk, CT: Appleton & Lange.
Gould D (1990) *Nursing Care of Women*, pp 355–381. New York: Prentice Hall.
Graham SK & Kalinowski BH (1981) Problems of the breast. In Fogel CI & Woods NF (eds) *Health Care of Women*, pp 334–360. St Louis: Mosby.
Graydon JE (1982) Physiological and psychosocial aspects of breast cancer. In Cahoon MC (ed.) *Cancer Nursing*, pp 39–53. Edinburgh: Churchill Livingstone.
Griffith-Kenney J (1986) *Contemporary Women's Health: A Nursing Advocacy Approach*, pp 546–587. Menlo Park, CA: Addison-Wesley.
Howard J (1987) Using mammography for cancer control: an

Kushner R (1984) *Alternatives*. Cambridge, MA: Kensington.

London SJ & Willet WC (1988) Diet, body size and breast cancer risk. *Reviews on Endocrine-Related Cancer* **31**: 19–25.

Lovejoy NC (1986) Family responses to cancer hospitalization. *Oncology Nursing Forum* **13(2)**: 33–37.

Maguire GP et al (1978) Psychiatric problems in the first year after mastectomy. *British Medical Journal* **1**: 963–965.

Mast D, Meyers J & Urbanski A (1987) Relaxation techniques: a self-learning module for nurses: unit 1. *Cancer Nursing* **10(3)**: 141–147.

Moetzinger CA & Dauber LG (1982) The management of the patient with breast cancer. *Cancer Nursing* **5(4)**: 287–291.

Morton PG (1989) *Health Assessment in Nursing*, p 349. Springhouse, PA: Springhouse.

Nielson BB & East D (1990) Advances in breast cancer: implications for nursing care. *Nursing Clinics of North America* **25(2)**: 365–375.

Northouse LL (1988) Social support in patient's and husband's adjustment to breast cancer. *Nursing Research* **37(2)**: 91–95.

Northouse LL & Swain MA (1987) Adjustment of patients and husbands to the initial impact of breast cancer. *Nursing Research* **36**: 221–225.

Peto R (1985) The breast cancer trials review meeting. Washington DC, September.

Pfeiffer CH & Mulliken JB (1984) *Caring for the Patient with Breast Cancer: An Interdisciplinary/Multidisciplinary Approach*. Reston, VA: Reston.

Robbins SL, Angell M & Kumar V (1981) *Basic Pathophysiology* 3rd edn, pp 585–594. Philadelphia: Saunders.

Seidman H, Gelb SK, Silverberg E, LaVerda N & Lubera JA (1987) Survival experience in the breast cancer detection demonstration project. *Ca-A Cancer Journal for Clinicians* **37(5)**: 258–290.

Tabar L et al (1985) Reduction in mortality from breast cancer after mass screening with mammography. Randomised trial from the Breast Screening Working Group of the Swedish National Board of Health and Welfare. *Lancet* **i**: 829–832.

Tschudin V (ed.) (1988) *Nursing the Patient with Cancer*. London: Prentice Hall.

Ward S, Heidrich S & Wolberg W (1989) Factors women take into account when deciding upon type of surgery for breast cancer. *Cancer Nursing* **12(6)**: 344–351.

Way LW (ed.) (1988) *Current Surgical Diagnosis and Treatment* 8th edn, pp 258–275. Norwalk, CT: Appleton & Lange.

White LN & Faulkenberry JE (1985) Screening by nurse clinicians in cancer prevention and detection. *Current Problems in Cancer* **IX(4)**: 17–23.

Caring for the Patient with Musculoskeletal Trauma

OBJECTIVES

At the end of this chapter the reader should be able to:

- Discuss the factors which affect healthy bone development
- Describe the functional classification of the major joints and explain the structural differences between them
- List the various types of fractures and describe the situations in which they are most likely to occur
- Describe the specific problems of a patient following trauma to bone including the factors that would indicate the presence of a fracture
- Assess patients following bone injury and use the information gained to plan care
- Implement and evaluate the care of a patient following:
  (i) the application of an external fixator
  (ii) the application of skin or skeletal traction
  (iii) internal fixation of a fracture
  (iv) application of a plaster cast
- Prepare a patient for discharge into the community using all the facilities available to enable them to be as independant as possible within the limitations of their reduced mobility

---

This chapter discusses the health care problems encountered by patients who have experienced skeletal and joint trauma and describes various approaches to their nursing care.

Alteration in mobility, either temporary or permanent, is the most common consequence of interruption in bone and joint function. The nurse needs to work with the patient, family and all members of the health care team in planning and implementing care, thus enabling the patient to return to the community with maximum independence.

STRUCTURE AND FUNCTION OF BONES

Bone Tissue

Bone is a rigid connective tissue consisting of bone cells, calcified collagenous intercellular substance and marrow. Each bone, except at joint surfaces, is covered by a tough, supportive membrane called the *periosteum*. It is firmly attached to the underlying bone by penetrating fibres, and its blood vessels give off many branches which enter the tissue to provide the essentials for growth, repair and maintenance. The inner layer of the periosteum gives rise to the osteoblasts, which function in the development and replacement of bone. The shaft of the long bones is hollow and is lined with a comparable membrane referred to as the *endosteum*. Although approximately two-thirds of bone tissue is inorganic mineral substance, which gives it the characteristic hardness and inert appearance, it is viable tissue undergoing constant metabolic processes, just as other tissues.

Bone tissue contains a network of minute anastomosing canals and spaces which contain blood vessels, lymphatics, lymph and bone cells. The rigid intercellular substance is formed in scale-like sheets or layers (lamellae) around the canals and spaces. It is composed of a tough collagenous network of fibres which becomes impregnated with mineral salts, principally tricalcium phosphate and calcium carbonate.

There are three types of bone cell: osteoblasts, osteocytes and osteoclasts. The *osteoblasts* are found beneath the periosteum on the surface of growing bones and in developmental or ossification areas within the bones. They are responsible for the formation of the collagenous fibres, the organic bone matrix and the deposition of the mineral salts. The *osteocytes* are matured osteoblasts which become imprisoned in small

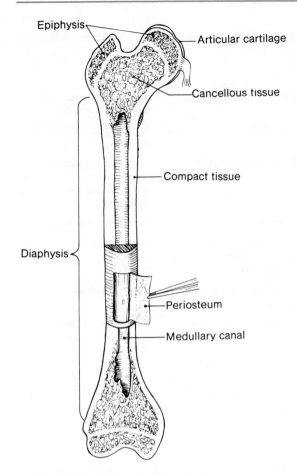

Figure 24.1 Diagram of a long bone.

TYPES OF BONE TISSUE

Each bone is composed of two types of tissue: compact and cancellous. Outer layers consist of dense, *compact* tissue (cortical bone), and the interior is of a spongy or porous nature (*cancellous*). The numerous larger spaces of cancellous tissue contain *red bone marrow*. The thickness of each type of tissue varies in different bones as well as in parts of the same bone.

In the long bones (e.g. humerus, tibia, femur), the extremities have a thin outer layer of compact tissue enclosing a larger mass of cancellous tissue (Figure 24.1). The shaft is formed mainly of two thick layers of compact bone separated by a small amount of porous tissue. The central hollow portion of the shaft forms the medullary canal, which is filled with fatty, *yellow marrow*. Flat bones (e.g. skull bones, scapula, ribs) have a thicker layer of cancellous tissue lying between two relatively thinner layers of compact tissue. Short and irregular bones such as those of the wrist and ankle have a thin shell of compact tissue enclosing a fair thickness of cancellous tissue.

FUNCTIONS OF BONES AND CONTAINED MARROW

The bones are bound together by ligaments and collectively form the skeleton, which provides a supporting framework for the body and protection for vital structures. They assist in body movement by providing attachment for muscles and leverage for their action. The bones also serve as the body's store of calcium. A constant level in the blood and tissue fluid is necessary for several physiological processes (e.g. blood clotting, normal muscular activity, normal heart action). If the blood calcium falls below the normal level, the deficit may be met by the withdrawal of calcium from the bones. Conversely, much of the excess in the blood is deposited in bone tissue.

The red bone marrow is a highly vascular haemopoietic tissue contained within the spaces of cancellous tissue. It produces erythrocytes, granulocytes and thrombocytes (blood platelets). During childhood, all cancellous tissue contains red marrow. In the adult, much of this is replaced by yellow marrow, and the cancellous tissue of the ribs, sternum, skull bones, vertebrae, pelvic bones and the proximal ends of the long bones play the major role in haemopoiesis. Yellow bone marrow consists mainly of fat cells and blood vessels; the largest amount is found in the medullary canals of long bones.

THE DEVELOPMENT AND GROWTH OF BONES

The development of the bones begins early in embryonic life and is not normally completed until the late teens or early twenties. They are composed of membranous connective tissue or cartilaginous tissue, which is gradually replaced by bone in the process of ossification.

The cranial bones and the mandible (lower jaw) develop by *intramembranous ossification*. There is a marked increase in the vascularity of the membranous tissue. This is followed by the appearance of localized

spaces by the calcification. It is believed these regulate bone metabolism. The *osteoclasts* are considered responsible for the breaking down and reabsorption of bone tissue. Normally, there is a constant turnover of the mineral deposits. This continuous breaking down, reabsorption and new bone formation is necessary, since old bone becomes weak and brittle. The bone cells respond by internal reconstruction according to the forces acting upon the tissue. The mineralization and strength of the bones are influenced by the amount of weight bearing and muscle pull to which the bones are subjected. Those of the active person and of an athlete are stronger and more resistant to stress than the bones of non-active persons. One of the complications of prolonged bed rest is the decalcification and weakening of the bones; the calcium is excreted by the kidneys and there is therefore a risk of the formation of renal calculi. In older persons the bones tend to become brittle and less resistant to stress, increasing the possibility of fractures. This is due to the general decline in cell reproduction which results in a slower rate of production of the collagenous matrix and mineralization as well as of reabsorption.

centres of ossification from which bone formation proceeds to the periphery. Radiating bundles of fibres and osteoblasts appear between the blood vessels, followed by the development of the collagenous fibrous matrix which becomes impregnated with calcium salts. The original membrane becomes the periosteum. As the conversion to bone proceeds outward, the edges of the membranous tissue continue to grow. When ossification overtakes the growth of the membranous tissue, the full size of the bone has been reached. The continued growth of the membranous tissue of the cranial bones accounts for the 'soft' areas or fontanelles in the skull in the infant.

The bones which are preformed of cartilage undergo *intracartilaginous (endochondral) ossification*, which involves destruction of the cartilage and its replacement by bone tissue. Osteoblasts develop at the surface of the cartilage and initiate the formation of surface layers of bone tissue by producing a collagenous fibrous matrix in which mineral salts are deposited. Then osteoblasts, osteoclasts and blood vessels invade internal areas of the cartilage, setting up ossification centres around which cartilage is progessively removed and replaced by bone tissue.

In long bones (Figure 24.1), an ossification centre appears within the shaft (*diaphysis*) and later at each end (*epiphysis*). As ossification proceeds, growth of the cartilage continues, resulting in a persisting thin strip of cartilaginous tissue between each epiphysis and the diaphysis, which is referred to as the *growth or epiphyseal plate*. The bones continue to grow as long as new cartilage develops to maintain this plate. Cessation of growth occurs when it becomes ossified, and the epiphyses are fused with the diaphysis. Bones grow in circumference by the formation of layers of bone beneath the periosteum.

Factors in bone development, growth and repair

Several factors influence the development, growth and maintenance of normal bone structure (Table 24.1). A diet which is adequate in calcium and phosphorus is essential for ossification and the constant formation of new bone to replace that which is reabsorbed. Vitamin D is necessary for the absorption and utilization of the minerals. Milk and milk products provide an abundant source of these minerals. Vitamin D may be formed by exposure of the skin to sunlight, which acts on sterol (7-dehydrocholesterol), a component of the skin. Adequate dietary amounts of protein and vitamin C are necessary for the formation of the collagenous, fibrous, intercellular matrix in which the minerals are deposited. Vitamin A, which is essential to all tissue growth, is also necessary.

Bone growth and ossification are also influenced by such hormones as the growth hormone produced by the anterior pituitary gland, thyroxine from the thyroid gland, and parathormone produced by the parathyroid glands. Bone metabolism is also affected by oestrogen, androgens and calcitonin.

In addition to these factors, the demand placed on the bones by weight bearing and muscle pull plays an important role in the shaping of bone. For example,

Table 24.1 Factors in bone development, growth and repair.

Factor	Action
Calcium and phosphorus	Ossification and constant formation of new bone
Vitamin D	Absorption and utilization of minerals
Protein and vitamin C	Formation of collagenous, fibrous, intercellular matrix in which minerals are deposited
Vitamin A	Essential to tissue growth
Somatotrophic and parathyroid hormones (see Chapter 19)	Bone growth and ossification
Oestrogen, androgens and calcitonin	Bone metabolism
Weight bearing and muscle stress	Maintenance of bone strength and shaping of bone

bony prominences, such as the greater and lesser trochanters of the femur, the tibial tuberosity and the deltoid tuberosity of the radius, develop as the result of specific muscle pull during growth.

STRUCTURE AND FUNCTION OF JOINTS

A joint or articulation is a point of contact between bones that permits flexibility in the skeletal system and allows for movement. Joints are classified according to their structure and the kind of movement that they allow. The *structural* classification of joints is based on the kind of tissue that connects the bones and on the presence or absence of a synovial (joint) cavity, while their *functional* classification takes into account the degree of movement they permit. The joints of the body will be described according to their functional classification, with reference made to their structure.

CLASSIFICATION OF JOINTS

There are three major functional classes of joints: immovable, slightly movable and freely movable.

* Structually immovable joints are classified as *fibrous*, with the bones united by fibrous connective tissue. The sutures between the bones of the skull are examples of such joints.
* Slightly movable joints are referred to as *cartilaginous* because the bones are held together by cartilage, a strong avascular material. The inferior tibiofibular joint and the symphisis pubis (in the pelvis) are examples of slightly movable joints.

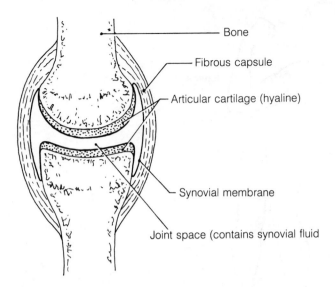

Figure 24.2 A synovial joint in frontal section.

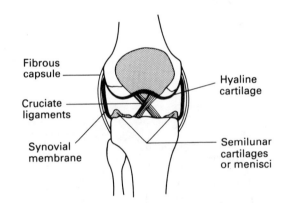

Figure 24.3 Knee joint, showing supporting ligaments and medial lateral menisci.

- Freely movable joints have a space between articulating bones called the synovial or joint cavity. These joints are classified structurally as *synovial* and include the hip, knee, shoulder and elbow (Figure 24.2). As most of the joints in the skeleton fall into this last category they will be described in detail.

SYNOVIAL JOINTS

Freely movable or synovial joints, consisting of articulating bones and the joint cavity, are enclosed in a tough fibrous capsule (the articular capsule) which is continuous with the periosteum of the bones. This arrangement serves to stabilize the joint and keep the bones in normal apposition. The joint may be further reinforced by ligaments extending from one bone to another.

The inner surface of the articular capsule is lined with synovial membrane that secretes synovial fluid. This fluid lubricates the joint, reduces friction and provides nourishment for the articular cartilage that covers the articulating surfaces of the bones of the joint. The amount of synovial fluid present in each joint varies, from only a thin film over the surfaces within some joints to about 3.5 ml of free fluid in a large joint such as the knee. Some freely movable joints also have flat, crescent-shaped pieces of cartilage interposed between the articulating surfaces to cushion and protect the bone surfaces. For example, in the knee joint, semilunar cartilages referred to as menisci are located between the condyles of the femur and tibia (Figure 24.3). Bursae are also situated between some body parts to further reduce the friction created by various movements of the body. These sac-like structures are lined with synovial membrane, with the walls of the sac separated by a film of synovial fluid. Bursae are located between tendons and bone, muscles and bone, and ligaments and bone.

Freely movable joints are also differentiated by the type of movement they permit. These movements are limited by several factors, including the shape of the articulating bones, the tension of the ligaments and the arrangement and tension of muscles. Generally, these joints permit one or more of the following movements: flexion, extension, abduction, adduction, rotation, circumduction, eversion, inversion, pronation and supination (Figure 24.4).

How movement occurs at joints

To enable movement to occur, each synovial joint has at least one pair of muscles surrounding it. These work together so that when one is contracting (the agonist) the other is relaxing (the antagonist). Each muscle is attached to bone by a tendon at either end. The proximal tendon is usually referred to as the tendon of origin, the distal tendon is referred to as the tendon of insertion. Thus, when the muscle on the inner aspect of the joint contracts, the distal (furthest) bone is brought

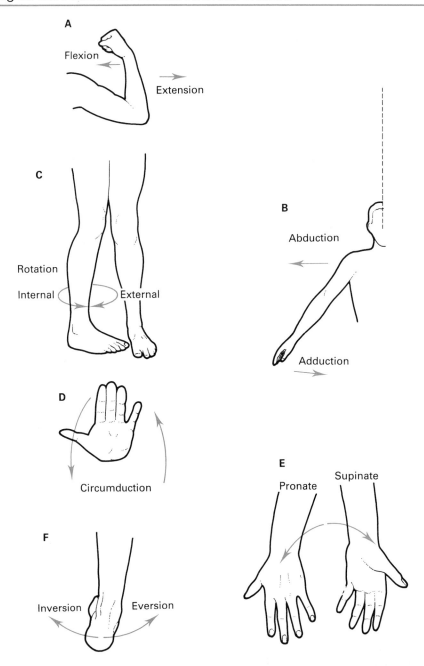

Figure 24.4 Joint movements.

nearer the body (flexion). To allow this movement the muscle on the outer aspect of the joint must relax. Similarly, when the muscle on the outer aspect of the joint contracts, the joint straightens (extension). Examples of this are the contraction of the hamstring muscle group behind the knee which produces flexion of the knee. This can only occur if the quadriceps muscle group relaxes sufficiently to allow flexion. This 'working in pairs' is essential for smooth joint movement.

Muscle Contraction
Skeletal muscle is composed of muscle fibres which, under a microscope, appear to be striated (striped). These stripes show the different proteins of which muscles are composed: actin found in the Z band or stripe and myosin found in the A band. The Z bands become closer together during a muscle contraction. The presence of calcium ions is necessary to activate the myosin and release the energy required for muscle contraction.

It would appear that during a muscle contraction 75% of the energy released is lost as heat (Green, 1978). In this respect the body would appear to be unusually inefficient.

ASSESSMENT OF THE PATIENT WITH TRAUMA TO THE MUSCULOSKELETAL SYSTEM

The patient who has been injured will have suffered an unpleasant experience which may well have been both frightening and painful. Whether a nurse encounters the patient in a first aid situation, an A & E Unit, or on the ward, these elements of psychological stress and pain should be carefully considered in assessing the patient.

In all acute trauma situations the priority is to assess the 'ABC of resuscitation' i.e. the patency of the person's *a*irway, their *b*reathing and *c*irculation (and *c*ervical spine). This should always precede the next stage of the assessment which should then focus on pain and psychological status alongside the actual injury itself. Assessment should then move on to consider the rest of the patient, checking for other less obvious injuries, unrelated but coexisting medical conditions (e.g. is the patient also diabetic?) as well as social factors.

It is important to obtain a history of the injury and the degree of force involved. Certain mechanisms of trauma produce characteristic patterns of injury, knowledge of how the accident happened will therefore focus the nurse's attention on certain possible injuries. For example a fall on an outstretched hand in an elderly person may produce a fracture of the lower extremity of the radius (colles fracture) but less obviously it may produce an impacted fracture of the upper humerus.

An injured limb should be assessed gently with the minimum amount of movement due to the pain this may cause and also the risk of making the injury worse.

Pain is obviously a key sign of trauma, however it is not necessarily always present or related in intensity to the severity of the injury. The cardinal sign of a fracture is localized bony tenderness, i.e. gentle pressure on the fracture site produces a painful response. In assessing a patient in a first aid or A & E situation this is a key observation for the nurse to make.

The cardiovascular status of the limb must also be assessed as trauma may occlude the arterial blood supply leading to ischaemia, nerve damage and in extreme cases loss of the limb itself. The nurse must locate and mark a peripheral pulse which should be monitored regularly. This is equally important on the ward after medical treatment such as manipulation of a displaced fracture and mobilization in a plaster cast as swelling and arterial compression within the limb can be sufficient to occlude the blood supply.

The limb should also be assessed for evidence of deformity or shortening. Dislocation of a joint will obviously lead to deformity as may a displaced fracture. Fractures of the femoral neck region characteristically produce shortening of the injured limb by approximately 2 cm and external relation of the limb.

In assessing the injured limb for localized bony tenderness, pain, cardiovascular compromise and deformity, the nurse must not lose sight of the whole person and their psychological status. They may be very tearful and obviously frightened, or stoically silent. Either way the person has recently had a very unpleasant and probably painful experience which may affect their life for months and even years ahead. Not surprisingly a wide range of thoughts and fears may be running through the injured person's head whether it be in A & E or the ward, and in order that the nurse may provide quality nursing care, these thoughts and fears must be explored (Walsh 1990).

An elderly woman living alone may have suffered a fractured wrist which can be treated usually on an outpatient basis once the fracture has been reduced and immobilized in a plaster cast, but how well can that patient manage at home with her arm in plaster? Can she manage to walk safely with her zimmer frame? What if the plaster becomes wet as a result of washing? Another common injury in elderly women is fracture of the femoral neck. The patient may be terrified of becoming a burden on relatives, she may feel her family will see this as too much of a burden and put her in a home or that she will have to sell the house she has lived in for the last 60 years because she cannot cope any more. These are just some of the fears and anxieties that may affect a patient and which the nurse needs to try and discover if help is to be offered.

Patient assessment therefore needs to be a continual process and incorporate far more than the injured limb.

MEDICAL INVESTIGATIONS

X-rays are always indicated following injuries to bones and joints. Since a film is a flat surface, at least two different views of each area of interest are taken, at different angles, to provide a three-dimensional guide to structure. This is particularly important when displacement is being identified.

In the acute stage of an injury care must be taken not to move the patient unnecessarily. Casts, immobilization devices or traction should not be removed while X-ray investigations are performed in order to prevent the risk of displacement of the fractured bone.

The following investigations may also be ordered for the patient following trauma to bone and/or joints.

Nuclear medicine studies differ from X-rays in that the radiation is introduced into the body circulation and carried by the blood to the target organ. In bone studies a radioactive isotope, usually technetium, is attached to a compound which will be preferentially taken up by bone when compared with other tissues. The radiation emitted by the technetium when it has become attached to bone can then be detected by special crystals that convert the energy to light to produce an image on film. There are two devices that do this, a scanner or a gamma camera. Most studies are now done with the camera.

Since the radioactive isotope is excreted by the kidneys, the patient's urine is slightly radioactive for a short time. This does not cause any particular hazard as the level of radiation is very small.

Computerized tomography (CT) provides cross-sectional images of the body by using a rotating beam of X-rays. The picture is produced through a computer on to a television screen. This provides a three-dimensional image.

Magnetic resonance imaging (MRI) is an imaging method that does not use hazardous radiation. The patient is placed within a tube that is a very powerful magnet, and is exposed to certain radiowaves that produce a signal which can be detected and manipulated by a computer. This provides sectional images of a body part that reveal considerable anatomical detail. It is used to study joints, bone tumours and bone marrow problems and to visualize the spinal cord.

Because of the powerful magnet there should be no magnetic materials close by. This includes metal stretchers, oxygen tanks, some monitoring equipment and metal objects such as scissors, badges, buckles, pins or watches; the smaller objects may become projectiles into the magnet.

Patients are warned that the procedure is somewhat noisy and ear plugs are often supplied. Some patients may become claustrophobic during the MRI scanning, precluding the completion of the examination. Because it is difficult to monitor patients in the scanner, very sick people are excluded from these examinations.

THE ROLE OF THE NURSE

The nurse manages the progress of patients through all stages of injury/illness. The nurse who knows the usual nursing care needs of patients with interruption in bone function and the activities that other health professionals undertake in the patients' care is able to formulate a critical path for each. This then allows a critical evaluation of the patient's responses to treatment and care. Accurate documentation and continuous communication among the health professionals caring for the patient ensures not only that the person's treatment plan is efficiently carried out but also that deviations from expected outcomes are identified and dealt with.

Fractures

A fracture is a break in the continuity of a bone, separating it into two or more parts, which are referred to as *fragments*. The soft tissues in the area surrounding the fracture are also injured.

CAUSES

The majority of fractures are due to violence incurred by falls, blows or rotational stresses. In each case the force is in excess of the bone's resistance and may have been applied directly or indirectly. In direct violence, the fracture occurs at or near the site of the applied force. When indirect violence is the cause, the force is applied at a point remote from the site of the fracture. For example, in a fall on the outstretched hand, the stress may be transmitted to the radius, ulna, humerus or clavicle. Occasionally a fracture may be due to a

Table 24.2 Types of fracture.

Type	Description
Traumatic or pathological	Traumatic: the result of violence; pathological is spontaneous or the result of disease
Incomplete	Break not all the way through bone; e.g. greenstick fracture in children
Complete	Bone is separated into two distinct parts
Closed (simple)	Overlying skin intact
Open (compound)	A wound exists over the fracture establishing communication between the fracture and the outside air
Complicated	Fracture includes injury to adjacent structures, e.g. blood vessels, nerves or organs
Comminuted	More than one line of fracture and more than two fragments
Transverse	Line of fracture is at right angles to the long axis of bone
Spiral	Curves in spiral fashion around bone
Impacted	One fragment is driven into another (cancellous bone usually involved)
Crush or compression	Fracture occurs in cancellous bone which is compressed beyond limits of tolerance
Avulsion	A ligament or tendon under excessive stress fractures or tears away its bony attachment
Depressed	A segment of cortical bone is depressed below the level of surrounding bone

sudden forceful contraction of attached muscles, this is known as an avulsion fracture.

A fracture can occur as the result of disease of the bone which has weakened its structure to the point that it can no longer withstand the normal stresses and strains of everyday life; this is known as a pathological fracture. Metastases, primary tumours (e.g. sarcoma, osteitis fibrosa cystica due to hyperparathyroidism), osteogenesis imperfecta (a congenital condition affect-

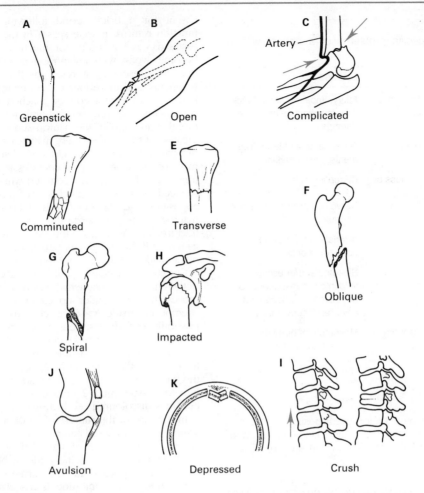

Figure 24.5 Types of fracture.

ing the formation of osteoblasts) and osteoporosis are examples of diseased conditions of bone that may lead to spontaneous fracture. Prolonged stress may also cause a fracture in certain bones. This is known as a stress fracture and may, for example, affect the fibula in professional sportsmen.

TYPES OF FRACTURE

The types of fracture are listed in Table 24.2 and illustrated in Figure 24.5. Injury and fracture of the spine and skull are discussed in Chapter 21 as there is often serious neurological involvement.

PHYSIOLOGICAL RESPONSES

Local

A fracture is always accompanied by some degree of damage to the surrounding soft tissues. Blood vessels within the bone, the periosteum and surrounding tissues are torn, resulting in haemorrhage and then the formation of a haematoma. The periosteum at the site may be stripped away from the underlying bone tissue, interrupting the blood supply into the area and thus contributing to the death of bone cells. There may also be haemorrhage into adjacent muscles and joints and damage to ligaments, tendons and nerves. Soon after a fracture occurs the muscles in the area go into spasm, causing severe pain and possible displacement of a fragment due to tendon pull.

Depending on the location of the fracture, visceral injuries may occur, which may threaten the patient's life. Examples of such injuries are rupture of the bladder by a fractured pelvis and rupture of the spleen or perforation of a lung by a fractured rib.

Systemic

The patient suffers some degree of shock which is influenced by the severity of the injury, the amount of soft tissue damage, associated disorders or multiple injuries, and the patient's age and general condition at the time of injury. A fracture of the femoral shaft results in a blood loss of approximately 1 litre and will probably lead to hypovolaemic shock, while a fracture of the tibia produces blood loss of approximately

Table 24.3 Specific problems of a patient with a fracture.

Patient problem	Causes
Sudden severe pain at site, (may or may not persist)	Injury, impaired nerve function, muscle spasm, tissue damage
Deformity or shortening of limb	Displacement of bone fragments, muscle spasm
Impaired mobility and loss of function	Disruption of bone
	Nerve compression by bone fragments
Loss of circulation	Arterial compression by bone fragments
Swelling	Bleeding and/or escape of fluid into tissues; after 2–5 days area may become discoloured (ecchymosis)
Crepitation (grating sound)	Movement of bone fragments at fracture end

500 ml. (See Chapter 12 for predisposing factors and manifestations of shock.) Usually a slight elevation of temperature and leucocytosis occur in the first 2 or 3 days.

CLINICAL CHARACTERISTICS OF FRACTURES AND PATIENT ASSESSMENT

A fracture may produce one or several well defined physical effects on the patient which are discussed below. The nurse is referred to the general discussion on patient assessment on p. 857 and this should be borne in mind in working through the next section. Throughout, it is important to be asking how the patient experiences the various clinical signs discussed below and what meanings the patient may place upon such signs, for it is out of those meanings that the patient constructs reality. In order to recognize patient problems, the nurse needs to share the patient's perceptions of reality i.e. try and see what the patient sees.

The following discussion is an important guide to assessment and care planning as it highlights potential and actual problems the patient may have.

The symptoms of a fracture vary with its location, type, the amount of displacement of the fragments and the degree of damage to soft tissue structures (see Table 24.3).

The patient or an observer usually relates a history of a fall, blow or sudden forcible movement, and the victim may actually say that he or she heard the bone break. Sudden severe pain at the site is experienced which may or may not persist. Frequently, because of injury, nerve function is impaired and pain may be absent for a brief period following the injury. As function returns, muscle spasm in the area, as well as tissue damage, accounts for much of the pain, which becomes worse with any movement. Obvious deformity may be present as a result of displacement of the fragments, and there may be shortening of the affected limb due to contraction of attached muscles; this is particularly apparent in femoral fractures. Impaired mobility and loss of mechanical support occur, and, in the case of long bones, there may be obvious movement in a part that is normally rigid. Complete loss of function may result from nerve compression by displaced fragments; this is usually restored when the fracture is reduced and the fragments are placed in normal apposition and alignment. The blood supply to a limb may be severely impaired if an artery is trapped in the fracture. In severe cases the limb may be lost due to gangrene if the blood supply is not quickly restored by manipulation of the fracture to restore normal anatomy.

Crepitation (a grating sound produced by movement of the ends of the fragments) may be noted if the patient moves the part. Under no circumstances should any attempt be made to elicit crepitus because of the possibility of further serious damage to soft tissues (e.g. blood vessels and nerves), unnecessary displacement of fragments and the possible production of an open fracture. Swelling may develop rapidly over the site of the fracture because of bleeding and the escape of fluid into the tissue. After 2 or 3 days this area frequently becomes discoloured (ecchymosis).

In the case of the rupture of an organ by a fragment, symptoms of impaired function of the damaged organ appear. With rupture of the bladder by a fractured pelvis, extravasation of urine gradually becomes evident, and blood appears in the urine. Although rare, perforation of the intestine is associated with pelvic fracture and causes severe shock and peritonitis; the abdomen becomes distended and board-like. A serious complication of a rib fracture may be puncture of a lung. The patient manifests severe shock, respiratory distress, coughing and haemoptysis.

Some fractures, especially those which are incomplete, or impacted, or of short bones, may produce few signs and symptoms. The fracture may be suspected only on the basis of the history of violence, tenderness on pressure over the site or the patient's complaint of pain upon use of the part or weight-bearing on it. Again, no attempt should be made to elicit symptoms by having the person move or stand. The patient is treated as having a fracture if there is any doubt.

Diagnosis of a fracture is based on the history of the accident, physical examination of the patient and X-rays of the affected part.

FRACTURE HEALING

Bone is different from many of the specialized tissues because of its ability to regenerate and hence restore the continuity which was disrupted by the fracture. Many tissues heal by laying down non-specialized fibrous scar tissue.

Immediately following a fracture, the space between the fragments and around the fracture line is filled with blood and inflammatory exudate. The haematoma and the exudate are invaded by fibroblasts and capillaries from adjacent connective tissue and blood vessels, forming granulation tissue. Simultaneously, osteoblasts proliferate, mainly from the inner surface of the periosteum (and endosteum in a long bone), and invade the granulation tissue. Calcium salts are deposited, forming a loosely woven, bone-like tissue referred to as a callus. It forms a 'collar' around the bone at the fracture site, giving it greater thickness than the original bone. The callus unites and helps to stabilize the fragments but is not strong enough to bear weight or withstand stress. If the blood supply is poor, or if it is disturbed by excessive mobility at the fracture site, cartilage may be formed instead of bone. As the osteoblasts increase, the callus is gradually restructured by ossification (production of a collagenous fibrous network which becomes impregnated with mineral salts) to form bone tissue. Remodelling is the final stage of fracture healing. The external bulbous bony area is remodelled by the action of osteoclasts.

In some instances, a fracture is complicated by malunion, delayed healing or non-union. *Malunion* implies healing of the fracture in an abnormal position. There may be angulation of the bone or overriding of the fragments which alters the shape and length of the limb. Function may be impaired. The cause is usually ineffective reduction and/or fixation during healing. *Delayed healing* simply implies that the fracture is not healing as rapidly as is normally expected. In *non-union*, the granulation tissue that formed between the fragments following the fracture is converted to dense fibrous tissue instead of normal callus and bone tissue. Causes of delayed union or non-union include too wide a gap between the fragments, the interposition of soft tissues or a foreign body between the fragments, poor blood supply to the site, loss of the initial haematoma by the escape of blood through an open wound or surgical intervention, infection of the bone, malnutrition and disease of bone, e.g. bone metastases.

The serum alkaline phosphatase level is a good indication of bone formation; it is secreted by osteoblasts which promote the deposition of calcium. The serum level of phosphatase rises with the increased osteoblastic activity during bone repair.

GENERAL PRINCIPLES AND METHODS OF TREATMENT OF FRACTURES

EMERGENCY CARE

Emergency treatment of a person with a fracture usually occurs at the site where the injury took place. The patient's general condition and the extent of injuries are quickly assessed and priorities are set. Respiratory insufficiency, haemorrhage or shock may be evident and take precedence over injured bones.

The first aid treatment is very important; movement of the patient or improper handling may cause serious tissue damage and increased pain; haemorrhage and shock. If a fracture is obvious or suspected, care at the site of the accident and during transportation to a hospital is directed toward reducing pain and preventing further tissue damage, including to underlying tissues and organs, and a closed fracture becoming open. The patient should receive a minimum of handling (unless there is danger of further injury) until the emergency services arrive. Before moving the patient, the fracture site and the joint above and below are immobilized; in order to reduce the risk of further damage and to relieve pain. A splint can be made from whatever is available (e.g. a board, two or three thicknesses of cardboard, a folded quilt or blanket, pillows). In the case of a board, the surface applied to the patient must be padded (towels or clothing may be used) to prevent pressure. If the limb is in an abnormal position, it is splinted in that deformed position; no attempt is made to reduce the fracture or restore the limb to a normal postion. The easiest splint is the patient's own body: an uninjured leg can act as a splint for an injured leg and the trunk can splint an injured arm. Thus a lower limb may be immobilized by placing a pillow or folded blanket between the legs and tying them together. In the case of an arm, it may be secured against the trunk by bandages and a sling. If it is an open fracture, the wound is covered with the cleanest material available in order to prevent further contamination and reduce infection risks. If the bone is protruding from the wound, no attempt is made to replace it or reduce the fracture. Nothing is given by mouth in case a general anaesthetic proves necessary.

When the patient arrives at the hospital a quick assessment is made of the general condition, and if there is respiratory insufficiency or shock, appropriate treatment is instituted before the fracture receives attention. When the general condition is satisfactory, X-rays are made of the fracture area.

The patient may be disorientated, frightened and agitated. An ongoing explanation of what is about to be done and what the patient can do to best assist in care often helps to keep the patient calm. This makes it possible to provide efficient on-the-scene care and prevent further injury.

TREATMENT

The treatment of a fracture usually involves reduction, fixation (immobilization) of the part, protection while the bone heals, and rehabilitation during and following the healing process to restore normal function. When possible, bone stress is utilized to increase the process of repair. The bone fragments are mechanically fixated to enable immediate use, creating stress at the fracture site which accelerates osteoblastic activity. Some fractures, such as those of distal phalanges of the fingers and toes, may heal without reduction and immobilization equipment. However, regular analgesia will be required to maintain mobility.

Reduction

This is the procedure by which fragments are brought into their preinjury position so that the normal shape and length of the bone are restored and union is promoted. Obviously, reduction is only necessary if

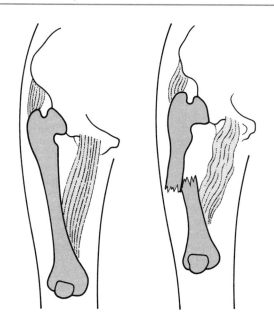

Figure 24.6 Fracture of the femoral shaft. The pull by the adductor muscles causes displacement of the fragments.

there is some displacement of the fragments (Figure 24.6). It is carried out as soon as possible. A delay makes it more difficult to obtain satisfactory alignment because of the rapid organization of the blood clot and the development of associated muscle spasm. Also, there is likely to be less tissue trauma with early reduction.

A fracture may be reduced by a number of methods, with the use of general or regional anaesthesia or an analgesic such as pethidine or papaveretum. Methods for reducing fractures include closed manipulative reduction, traction applied distal to the fracture, or open (internal) reduction. In *closed reduction*, the surgeon manipulates the fragments into position by manual traction, pressure, and/or rotation. In fractures in which one fragment is overriding the other and there is considerable muscle pull, continuous *traction* may be applied to the distal fragment to bring it into apposition and to maintain the alignment. This method of reduction is used most often in fractures of the femur because the pull of the strong thigh muscles tends to displace the fragments and cause overriding. The traction may be applied to the skin (skin traction) or directly to bone (skeletal traction). In some fractures, reduction can only be achieved through an *open surgical incision*.

Immobilization or fixation

Various methods are used to maintain reduction and fixate the fragments. They may be categorized as external fixation, external skeletal fixation, skin or skeletal traction or internal fixation. The method used depends upon the particular bone (e.g. location—short, long or flat), the type of fracture and the muscles involved.

External fixation
This is most commonly achieved by enclosing the part in a cast (Table 24.4). A *plaster cast* is most widely used and is made by the application and moulding of moist plaster of Paris bandages to the affected part. The bandages are strips of cotton material impregnated with gypsum (anhydrous calcium sulphate). They are immersed in warm water, 21–24°C (70–75°F), for a few seconds and then are lightly squeezed to remove excess water before application. The addition of water to the bandage causes the gypsum to crystallize. While wet it is possible to mould the soft moist bandage to the affected body part. As it is applied, each layer is rubbed with the palms of the hands into that below to prevent separation of the cast into layers. As the water evaporates from the bandages, the plaster hardens and the application becomes rigid. This takes over 24 hours to fully set; an alternative is to use fibreglass, synthetic casting materials which set fully in 30 minutes, however they are more expensive (see below).

Before the cast is applied, the skin is cleansed and examined for any contusions or abrasions. The part is then enclosed in circular stockinette for skin protection. Extra padding is used over bony prominences or to fill in spaces which might weaken the cast. It is also applied when swelling is anticipated.

When the application of the plaster bandages is completed, the stockinette which extends beyond the cast is turned back over the cast edges and is secured by incorporation into the cast or with adhesive tape. Newer cast materials are available that are lightweight, strong, do not soften in water and set faster. Such materials include: low temperature thermoplastics, which become pliable when heated and harden when cooled; fibreglass with photosensitive resin, which becomes rigid when exposed to ultraviolet light; fibreglass with polyurethane

Table 24.4 Types of cast.

Cast type	Description
Plaster	A cylinder which encases a fractured limb
Walking	A weight-bearing wooden heel and sole (rocker) is incorporated into the cast
Body (jacket)	Applied to the trunk
Spica (shoulder/hip)	Applied to the trunk and shoulder or hip
Bivalve	Moulded to trunk or limb and cut down each side when dry. Held in place with Velcro or bandages
Splint	Plaster of Paris, metal, fibreglass thermoplastic or polyurethane material moulded to support the affected limb

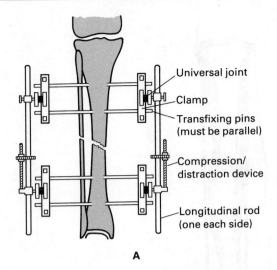

Universal joint

Clamp

Transfixing pins
(must be parallel)

Compression/
distraction device

Longitudinal rod
(one each side)

A

B

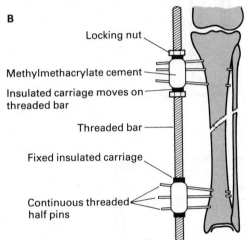

Locking nut

Methylmethacrylate cement

Insulated carriage moves on
threaded bar

Threaded bar

Fixed insulated carriage

Continuous threaded
half pins

C

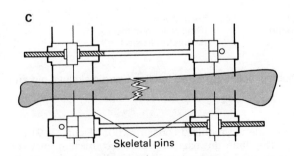

Skeletal pins

Figure 24.7 External skeletal fixation systems: (A)
universal day frame; (B) Portsmouth external fixation
bar (Denham external fixation compression); (C) the
Belfast fixator.

prepolymer which is activated by contact with water. A
walking cast may be applied with stable fractures of the
tibia and fibula. A 'rocker' or sole plate incorporated in
the base of the plaster enables the patient to be weight
bearing. A *bivalve cast* may be removed for brief
periods to allow skin or wound care or other treatment,

however this is rarely used for fracture prior to callus
formation due to the danger of loss of position. When
swelling of the limb is expected, for example in a recent
injury, a plaster back slab may be applied rather than a
cylindrical cast. This is made by the application of slabs
of plaster of Paris to the posterior of the limb; the slabs
are then secured in position with cotton bandages. The
rationale is that, if necessary, the cotton bandages can be
easily split to prevent circulatory and neurological
impairment.

External skeletal fixation
With this method of treatment the bone fragments are
held in alignment by skeletal pins. Two or more pins
are inserted into each fragment either side of the
fracture and the fracture is reduced. The pins are then
held in proper relation to one another by an external
support, usually a rigid mechanical system of clamps
and connecting rods is employed (Figure 24.7). External
skeletal fixation may be used in the treatment of
fractures associated with extensive damage to the soft
tissues where traction is not suitable and internal
fixation would carry a high risk of introduction of
foreign material into the wound. It may also be used in
the management of infected fractures, in multiple
fractures (to allow the treatment of other fractures by
traction) and in pelvic fractures with disruption of the
symphysis pubis. External skeletal fixation is designed to
hold the fracture without a plaster cast until union, and
allow access to any wounds. The disadvantages are the
risks of pin-track infections, the loosening of the pins,
and delayed union, as external callus formation may be
suppressed by tissue trauma and rigid immobilization of
the fracture.

Traction
Traction (which may also be employed to correct a
deformity, relieve pressure on a spinal nerve or prevent
a contracture deformity in cases in which there is
muscle spasm) is most commonly used to reduce and
maintain reduction in fractures of the limbs by
overcoming the effects of gravity and muscle pull. It
involves the application of a force along the long axis of
the bone distal to the fracture. For this force to be
effective, a force in the opposite direction is required
(countertraction). Countertraction is necessary and is
usually provided by elevating the foot of the bed in the
case of a lower limb; the weight of the body on the
incline supplies the required countertraction. An important use of traction is to overcome the deforming
muscle pull that is associated with many fractures. For
example, a fracture in the femur is accompanied by
marked displacement of the fragments due to the
contracture of the very strong muscles of the thigh and
hip. The adductor muscles produce a lateral bowing
(see Figure 24.6). The appliance used may produce
fixed traction or balanced (sliding) traction, with or
without suspension of the affected limb.

Fixed traction is traction between two fixed points,
for example a lower limb is supported in a Thomas
splint (a metal splint with a medial and lateral bar and a
leather-covered ring which surrounds the thigh at the
groin); traction is exerted by either skin extension tapes

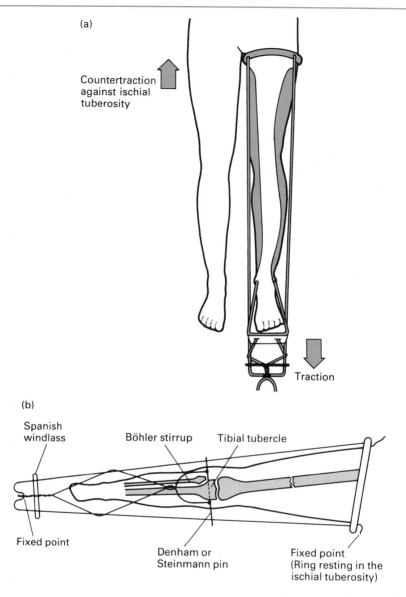

(a)

Countertraction
against ischial
tuberosity

Traction

(b)

Spanish
windlass

Böhler stirrup

Tibial tubercle

Fixed point

Denham or
Steinmann pin

Fixed point
(Ring resting in the
ischial tuberosity)

Figure 24.8 (a) Fixed traction using skin traction and a Thomas' splint. (b) Fixed traction using a skeletal pin and Thomas' splint.

tied to the distal end of the splint or by passing a pin through the tibia and pulling directly on the bone. Countertraction is obtained by the thrust of the ring against the ischial tuberosity (Figure 24.8).

In *balanced* or *sliding traction* there must also be two opposing forces (traction and countertraction). The forces are balanced and mobile, allowing the patient to move about the bed without disturbing the desired line of pull. Traction is applied by the use of a weight and pulley system. A cord passes over the pulley to the weights and is attached at the proximal end to skin extensions in skin traction, or to a skeletal pin which passes through the patient's bone in skeletal traction. Countertraction is obtained by elevation of the foot of the bed. Gravity together with the patient's body weight

provide the required countertraction (Figure 24.9).

The limb in fixed or balanced traction may be suspended off the bed surface, allowing the patient greater mobility in bed. Suspension of the lower limb is achieved by supporting the limb in a splint (e.g. Thomas' splint); this is suspended to an overhead frame by means of cords, weights and pulleys (Figure 24.10).

Skin traction is established by application of adhesive or non-adhesive tapes to the medial and lateral surfaces of the limb. These are secured by a firm encircling crêpe or elasticated bandage. The skin extension tapes extend beyond the foot and attach to a spreader, which must be wide enough to prevent the tapes from rubbing the malleoli and sufficient distance from the foot to allow for plantar flexion. A cord, connected to

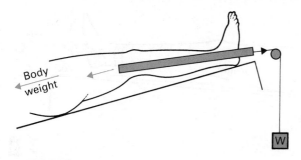

Figure 24.9 Balanced (sliding) traction. Note elevation of foot of bed uses patients own body weight as countertraction.

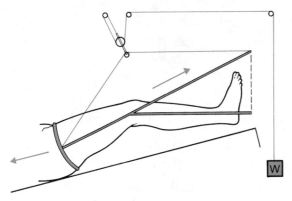

Figure 24.10 Suspension of a Thomas' splint.

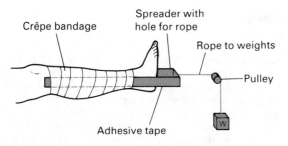

Figure 24.11 Skin traction of a lower limb.

the spreader, passes over a pulley on a cross-bar at the foot of the bed and suspends a prescribed weight (usually 2–4 kg for an adult) to exert the traction force (Figure 24.11). The disadvantage of skin traction is the limited traction weight that can be used without damaging the skin. The choice of the type of skin extension tapes to be applied is dependent on the condition of the patient's skin, hypersensitivity to adhesive strapping and the surgeon's preference. Non-adhesive skin traction kits with foam rubber or foambacked skin extensions are available but are of limited use in the treatment of fractures. If adhesive strapping is to be applied the surgeon may or may not want the leg shaved. An application of tincture of

benzoin will protect the skin and provide better adherence of the tapes. The adhesive is not applied over the malleoli or foot. The bandage must not be applied tightly around the limb as this may cause skin or vascular complications.

Skeletal traction is achieved by the insertion of a metal wire (Kirschner wire) or pin (e.g. Steinmann or Denham pin) through the bone distal to the fracture. By this means traction is applied directly to the skeleton. A special traction stirrup or U-loop is fastened to the protruding wire or pin (Figure 24.12); cord is attached to this which leads to a weight and pulley system. Countertraction is obtained by gravity and the patient's body weight on an inclined bed. The limb in traction is then usually suspended off the bed surface.

Various arrangements are used in applying traction to the lower limb. Those commonly employed are Buck's traction (or extension), Bryant's (Gallow's) traction, Hamilton Russell traction, Perkin's traction and balanced skeletal traction with a Thomas' splint and knee flexion piece.

Buck's traction involves simple skin traction (as previously described). The leg is supported on a soft pillow to keep the heel clear of the bed. Particular care is taken to avoid pressure from tight bandaging over the fibula head to prevent compression of the peroneal nerve which lies close to the surface. Damage, to the nerve could result in interference with normal ankle movement. Countertraction is obtained by elevating the foot of the bed. Buck's traction (Figure 24.13) is used for undisplaced fractures of the acetabulum, for the correction of minor fixed flexion deformities of the hip or knee, and following relocation of a dislocated hip or total hip replacement. Bilateral Buck's traction may be used for the treatment of a prolapsed intervertebral disc.

Bryant's or *Gallow's traction* is used in the treatment of a fracture of the femoral shaft of a young child (under 4 years). The traction may be fixed or balanced. Skin traction is applied to both legs which are then suspended at right angles to the body. For fixed traction the traction cords are tied to an overhead beam and the cord tightened sufficiently to raise the child's buttocks just clear of the mattress; countertraction is supplied by the weight of the pelvis and lower trunk. The traction may be balanced by means of weight and pulley system (Figure 24.14). Frequent observations on the state of the circulation in both limbs must be made, especially in the first 24–72 hours after the aplication of the traction, as vascular complications may occur in either limb. Any discoloration, fall in skin temperature, oedema, impaired loss of function or sensation of the feet must be reported immediately. All bandages and strapping are removed.

Hamilton Russell traction is used mainly in the preoperative treatment of a fracture of the neck of a femur. Vertical traction is applied at the knee; at the same time a horizontal force is exerted on the tibia and fibula. It is a straight Buck's traction with weights attached to the foot plate or spreader bar and a vertical pull from a sling under the patient's leg just above the knee. The traction simply reduces the amount of friction between the bone ends and reduces the patient's pain, thus facilitating the use of bedpans and pressure area

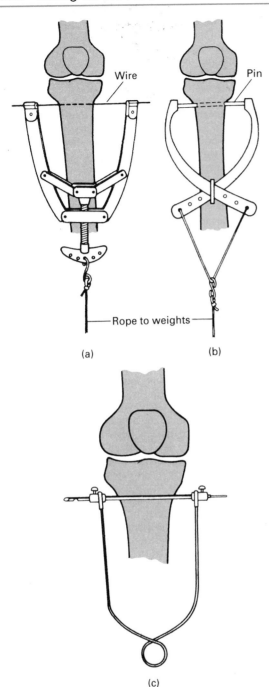

(a)

(b)

(c)

Figure 24.12 Skeletal traction may be applied by: (a) a Kirschner wire and traction stirrup; (b) A Steinmann pin and traction stirrup; or (c) a Steinmann pin and Böhler stirrup.

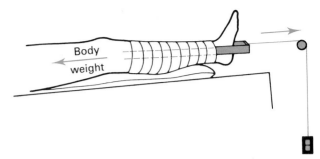

Figure 24.13 Buck's traction.

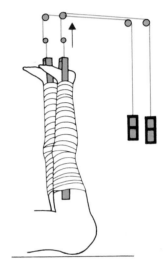

Figure 24.14 Bryant's traction.

care prior to going to the theatre.

An overhead bar is attached to the bed in line with the affected limb. A crossbar is provided at the foot of the bed to hold the necessary pulleys. One pulley is attached to the overhead bar in line with the tubercle of the tibia, two are secured to the bar at the foot of the

bed, one several inches above the other, and a fourth is attached to the spreader plate to which the traction tapes on the leg are attached. The cord attached to the sling leads vertically to the overhead pulley and then to the uppermost one on the crossbar. From there the traction cord passes over the pulley on the foot spreader and back to the lower pulley on the crossbar. It then attaches to weights which hang suspended well above the floor. The weight used with an adult patient is usually 2–3 kg. Pulleys are placed so that the patient's heel is kept clear of the bed.

The force exerted by the sling is that of the weight at the end of the rope. The horizontal pull on the leg is approximately twice that exerted on the knee by virtue of the pull of the two parallel traction cords at the foot. The vertical and horizontal tractions are exerted on the same point and together produce a resultant force in line with the femur. A thin pillow is usually placed lengthwise under the thigh; precautions are taken not to increase the slight flexion of the thigh. A second pillow is used under the leg, leaving the heel suspended and therefore free of pressure. The foot of the bed is elevated to provide countertraction. The popliteal area is padded to protect it from the pressure of the sling. A

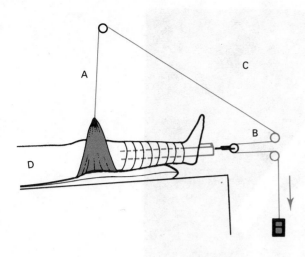

Figure 24.15 Hamilton Russell traction. Forces A + B = C, which is counterbalanced by the patient's bodyweight (D).

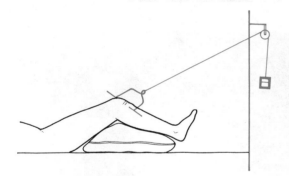

Figure 24.16 Perkin's traction.

monkey pole is attached to the overhead bar, enabling the patient to move.

Perkin's traction involves balanced skeletal traction without any form of external splintage. Active movements of the limb are commenced as soon as possible. Perkin's traction can be used in the management of fractures of the femur from the trochanteric region distally (Figure 24.16). A split bed in which the distal one third of the mattress and base of the bed can be removed is used when the patient has a fracture of the femur managed by Perkin's traction, as this will facilitate flexion of the knee.

Balanced skeletal traction with a half- or full-ring Thomas' splint with a Pearson's knee flexion piece is commonly used to obtain reduction of a fracture of a shaft of a femur and to maintain reduction until union occurs.

Firm cotton slings are secured to the upper part of the Thomas' splint to support the thigh and to the Pearson's knee flexion piece to support the leg. The

Thomas' splint extends from the groin to beyond the foot in line with the femur. The knee is in 10–20° of flexion to control rotation and prevent stretching of the posterior knee capsule and ligaments and subsequent joint instability. Some provision may be made to support the foot to prevent footdrop. The skeletal traction is usually applied to the proximal area of the tibia. The pull is exerted in line with the femur by means of a traction cord attached to the bow or stirrup that is fitted to the protruding ends of the pin that passes through the bone. The traction cord passes over a pulley and suspends a weight. The proximal and distal ends of the splint are suspended by separate cords, pulleys, and weights. Countertraction is obtained by elevating the foot of the bed. When the patient moves up or down in the bed the splint moves as well, and traction is maintained. The patient has greater freedom of movement and is usually more comfortable in this system of traction. It also has the advantage of allowing a certain amount of movement in adjacent joints.

Internal fixation

Some fractures require *internal surgical reduction and fixation*. Various types of internal fixation devices are used. These include stainless steel or vitallium wire, screws, plates, rods, and pins and bone grafts. They may be secured to the sides of the bone, placed through the fragments or passed through the intramedullary cavity of the bone. Internal fixation may be reinforced after the wound is closed by the application of a cast or splint. However, new devices of such strength and design are being made that external splintage is not always required, thus allowing immediate joint freedom, early weight bearing and short-term hospitalization. This system of fracture fixation has been developed by the Association for the Study of Internal Fixation (ASIF or AO).

Special internal fixation devices are used to immobilize the fragments in a hip fracture or fracture of the femoral neck. Three-flanged nails (Smith-Petersen pins or nails), Neufeld nail or a McLaughlin nail and plate or a compression hip screw may be used (Figures 24.17 and 24.18). In a few patients, especially the elderly with an intracapsular fracture through the neck of the femur, reduction may not be possible and there may be a risk of avascular necrosis of the femoral head (death of bone due to lack of blood supply); in these cases a hemiarthroplasty is performed by replacing the head of the femur with a metallic prosthesis. (A discussion of hip fracture occurs later in this chapter.)

Following any method of reduction and fixation a postoperative/reduction X-ray is vital to ensure that the position is maintained. X-rays are then made periodically to determine healing is occurring. In the case of traction, some adjustment in the amount of weight being used may be necessary. For instance, the X-ray may demonstrate too wide a separation of the fragments which would prevent healing and necessitate a reduction in the weight used. This is a particular problem following fractures of the shaft of femur, when heavy weights are required to overcome quadriceps spasm, especially in the first 48 hours after injury.

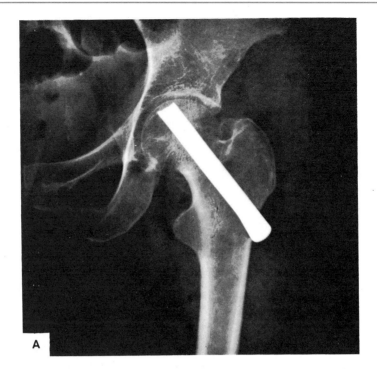

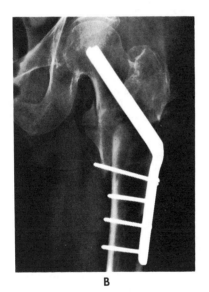

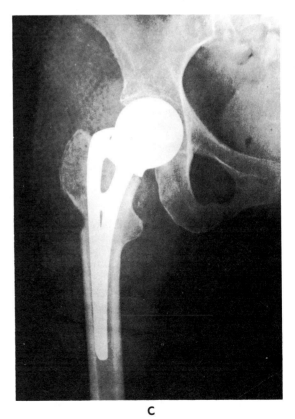

Figure 24.17 Radiographs showing: (A) Smith-Petersen nail; (B) McLaughlin nail and plate; (C) a femoral head prosthesis.

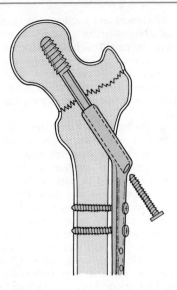

Figure 24.18 Compression (dynamic) hip screw for trochanteric fracture.

Open (compound) fractures

The patient with an open fracture requires special treatment as soon after the accident as possible. The site is potentially infected, and there is usually a greater amount of soft tissue damage and destruction. Infection and necrosis impede bone union and may result in serious disability. As soon as the patient's general condition permits, the wound is examined and cleaned. Gross contaminants and foreign material are removed, and the open wound is covered. The surrounding skin is then cleansed thoroughly with an antiseptic solution. The open wound may then be irrigated with sterile normal saline. The surgeon explores the wound and a debridement (the removal of foreign material and excision of dead tissue) is performed, if necessary. The repair of severed or torn tendons or nerves may be necessary. The fracture is reduced and then immobilized. If there has been gross contamination, the wound may be packed and left open until the danger of infection is past. Drains are inserted in the wound (e.g. Redivac drainage system). Antibiotic therapy may be prescribed.

Before the administration of the anaesthetic, it is determined if the patient has had previous immunization for tetanus. If so, a booster dose of tetanus toxoid may be ordered. If not, human tetanus immunoglobulin is given.

CARE OF THE PATIENT IN A CAST

The care of the patient following the application of a cast requires the following considerations.

Drying of the cast

Complete drying of a plaster cast following its application may take several hours or days, depending on the material used, its thickness and the temperature, humidity and circulation of the air. During this period, support of the cast and handling are very important, since the cast is vulnerable to pressure and cracking which could alter its shape, cause indentations that result in undue pressure on an area of the body or make it ineffective. When the part must be lifted, it is supported on the palms of the hands to avoid making indentations by the finger tips. In the case of a body or long leg cast, firm support along the line of the cast is ensured. Pillows with plastic or rubber undercovers are placed under the part encased in plaster so that the cast is not subjected to pressure by the firm mattress. Since it is moulded to the contours of the part to which is is applied, support by an extra pillow or folded flannelette sheet may be necessary under such regions as the lumbar or popliteal area.

Drying is promoted by exposure to dry, warm circulating air which evaporates the moisture from the cast. The bedding is arranged so that the cast is left uncovered. A fan may be placed approximately 45 cm (18 in) from the cast. Unless otherwise indicated, the patient is turned every 4–6 hours to facilitate drying of the complete cast. If it is a large or body cast, two or three persons act in unison and pillows are used to avoid strain on any part of the plaster. A moist cast has a dull grey appearance and produces a dull sound on percussion. When dry, it appears white and shiny and produces a resonant sound on percussion. Casts made of materials other than plaster of Paris usually dry more quickly. A study of the instructions that come with these materials will explain the drying time.

Weight bearing on a walking cast is begun when the cast is thoroughly dry, usually in 48 hours.

Unless the patient experiences complications or requires surgery, treatment is performed in the accident and emergency department. This greatly reduces the time the nurse has to assess the patient and/or family for their response to, or understanding of the injury and the care required. Rapid assessment and intervention is necessary.

PATIENT PROBLEMS

It is important to assess if there are any skin lesions (e.g. wounds, pre-existing skin conditions) as these will be enclosed in the cast, possibly for several weeks, leading to the risk of tissue necrosis, suppuration or infection. Swelling should be carefully assessed due to the risk of neurovascular compromise if the limb becomes compressed with the cast. It is important to check that any jewellery has been removed, a ring for example could act as a tourniquet around the finger if severe swelling develops.

Apart from such physical factors the nurse should assess the patient's level of comprehension of what is happening. After discharge from A & E the patient will be responsible for the self-care of the cast and fracture. This requires understanding of teaching about swelling and circulation, the condition of the cast, pain control etc. The nurse needs to assess the patient's grasp of language and intellectual functioning in order to ensure that teaching is delivered in an effective and appropriate way.

The social consequences of injury have already been raised and the nurse has a responsibility to assess whether the patient will have any significant social problems as a result of having a limb in a cast. This is particularly true of groups such as the elderly or single parents who may find coping alone very difficult in these circumstances.

The following is a summary of some of the principal health problems that assessment may reveal for the patient with a limb in a cast.

1. Potential problem of further injury related to pressure on soft tissue, nerves or arteries

Goals
The patient will:

* Understand the importance of the absence of pain and feeling of pressure, irritation or loss of sensation in the affected limb.
* Have normal temperature and colour in the fingers or toes.
* Demonstrate movement of the fingers or toes.
* Show no sign of skin breakdown.

2. Problem of immobilization due to limitation of movement by the cast

Goals
The patient will:

* Demonstrate a safe method of walking, and the use of aides such as crutches and walking sticks when these are being used.
* Demonstrate a safe method of transferring from bed to chair or chair to chair when walking is restricted.

3. Potential problem of a knowledge deficit due to changes in self-care

Goals
The patient and/or family will be able to:

* Describe the care of the cast.
* List risk factors related to potential for further injury or damage to the cast.
* Describe the action to undertake if the cast becomes loose.
* Describe the activities the person may engage in.
* Identify the out-patient clinic for follow-up treatment and where emergency care can be received.

Nursing management

Assessment and monitoring of the cast
Note. Examples of core care plans for patients following application of a plaster cast, an external fixator and skeletal traction have been designed for teaching purposes and are useful as guides when developing an individualized plan of care for a patient.

Assessment of an in-patient with a cast involves neurovascular evaluation of the affected limb every 30 minutes for the first 4 hours and then every 4 hours for several days. The affected extremity is compared with the uninjured one for alterations in colour, temperature, sensation, movement and swelling. Any blanching or the presence of a bluish colour indicates an interruption in circulation to the part. Touching the toes or fingers will identify temperature differences; pressure applied to these extremities will elicit from the patient any differences in sensation; patients should be asked to demonstrate movement of fingers/toes. Pain assessment is ongoing.

The nurse checks the cast with the palm of the hand for any warm or soft areas. Areas of discoloration or changes in discoloured areas are looked for. A musty smell will be present if infection has occurred, so any odour should be noted as part of the nurse's assessment. Since odour is a late sign infection may be suspected before a musty smell is detected due to localized pain, elevated temperature, etc. When an opening (window) has been made in a cast to allow for treatment of an incision or wound, the section is removed regularly to assess the status of the wound and surrounding skin. The skin next to the edges of the cast should also be inspected for signs of rubbing, soreness, etc., especially if a resin cast is used.

The mood of the patient should also be assessed, younger patients in particular may become bored and frustrated at their lack of activity.

Intervention
To alleviate and prevent further swelling, the affected limb is elevated above the level of the heart. This is achieved by the use of pillows, and elevating the foot of the bed when a leg is affected. To elevate the arm, it may be suspended by a Leslie sling to an intravenous stand. If such a sling is not available a draw sheet (or towel) may be used by folding the sheet in half and placing the flexed elbow on the fold with the fingers towards the sheet ends. Several large safety pins are carefully inserted on either side of the arm and the sheet ends are pinned over an intravenous stand. Ideally the hand should be well above the elbow and the elbow off the bed to promote drainage of tissue and reduce swelling. Once the oedema has gone, normal positioning may resume.

Swelling in the injured arm may be prevented by the use of a sling. When the lower limb is injured, it should always be elevated on a stool, to prevent swelling, when the patient is sitting down.

Care must be taken to avoid getting a plaster cast wet as it will disintegrate with resultant loss of immobilization and fracture position. The cast can be protected when bathing or in inclement weather by plastic bags or some other waterproof material which is sealed around the edges of the cast to prevent moisture from seeping under it. Casts of other materials may be allowed to become wet but saturation should be avoided.

To prevent skin irritation, exposed edges of a cast may be padded by folding the stockinette from under the cast over the top and bottom edges of the cast. If this cannot be done the cast can be 'petalled' by using 5 cm strips of adhesive tape. One end of the tape is pressed inside the cast edge and the other end is folded over the outside edge. The use of powder or lotion under a cast should be avoided as these tend to cake and cause more irritation. The patient should be cautioned against inserting objects such as knitting needles under the cast to try and relieve irritation as this may lead to serious skin breakdown and infection.

Patients with leg casts may be taught to use crutches. The nurse will walk with the patient initially to ensure safety. Walking casts should be protected with a boot or other covering.

The patient and/or family are taught to assess the cast and affected limb, the care of the cast and where to report any alterations in sensation, comfort or signs of drainage. Activities which may be undertaken should be discussed and reasons given for any restrictions. All patients discharged with a plaster cast should be given a leaflet reinforcing information given. The leaflet should also give details of who to contact if the condition of the limb or cast deteriorates.

Evaluation. Evaluation is achieved by discussion with and reassessment of the patient to see if the stated goals have been met.

REMOVAL OF THE CAST

When the cast is taken off, the rigid support to joints which have been immobilized for a considerable period of time is removed. The patient is likely to be discouraged by the stiffness, instability and weakness encountered and requires reassurance that with exercise and progressive use function will be restored.

The cast is removed by special cast cutters or a plaster saw. Since this may be frightening, the nurse describes the equipment and the process to the person before removal begins. The limb must be handled gently and with support under the joints. The skin is bathed gently, and an application of oil or lanolin is made to soften the accumulation of dry, scaly skin. Vigorous rubbing is discouraged to avoid skin irritation and abrasions.

REHABILITATION

A regimen of passive and active exercises and massage is established to restore joint and muscle function. Weight-bearing and activities are gradually resumed. When the cast is removed and the limb becomes dependent, oedema and swelling are likely to occur. The patient is advised to elevate the limb when sitting and lying, and elasticated tubular bandage (Tubigrip) may be applied when walking to control the oedema which gradually becomes less troublesome as muscle tone improves and there is increasing activity.

CARE OF THE PATIENT WITH EXTERNAL SKELETAL FIXATION

PREOPERATIVE PREPARATION

The length of time that elapses between the time of injury and surgery varies and is dependent on the patient's general state of health and associated injuries. Forms of treatment, such as traction, may be employed temporarily to immobilize the fracture prior to surgery. The care of the patient in the accident and emergency department and following admission to the ward includes observations of vital signs to detect signs of haemorrhage and shock, and observations of colour, temperature, sensation, movement of digits and pulse are made of the injured limb to detect impaired circulation or nerve damage; any abnormal signs are reported to the doctor immediately. Pain as a result of the injury and potential for infection as a result of an open wound are specific problems which will need to be addressed between arrival in the accident and emergency department and transfer to the operating theatre. Analgesics as ordered are administered to alleviate pain. Wounds and surrounding skin are cleansed according to the preference of the surgeon and covered with an antiseptic soak (e.g. Betadine and saline) and sterile dressings. This reduces the risk of infection and by keeping the tissue moist improves its viability, thereby promoting postoperative wound healing.

The operation is explained to the patient and the external skeletal fixation system is briefly described to alleviate some of the problems which could otherwise occur postoperatively, associated with altered body image. The nurse should make herself available to the patient and encourage free discussion of fears and anxieties concerning treatment and recovery.

POSTOPERATIVE CARE

The general principles of postoperative care are applicable (see Chapter 11). If the external skeletal fixation system has been applied to a fractured limb, the limb is elevated by means of suspension cords to a frame attached to overhead bars or the limb is elevated on a frame supported on the bed (Braun frame) in cases of fracture of the tibia. Elevation of the limb assists in the reduction of swelling.

In addition to the problems usually experienced postoperatively, the patient with external fixation has an added *potential problem of infection* at the pin sites. The nurse checks the external fixation system daily to ensure that the clamps and nuts are tight. This routine is explained to the patient so he or she understands that it is an expected procedure. The pin sites are observed for bleeding or leakage of exudate; they should be dry approximately 48 hours after surgery. Dressings to the pin sites are renewed when they become soiled or when the pin site requires close inspection. Strict asepsis is adhered to when dressing the pin sites and when dressing any skin wounds. Pain, tenderness, erythema, swelling and increased skin temperature at a pin site must lead the nurse to suspect pin site infection. Any of these clinical features must be reported to the doctor, and a wound swab should be taken and sent for microscopy, culture and sensitivity. Antibiotic therapy is prescribed and the pin may be removed by the surgeon. Any loosening of a pin must also be reported as this increases the risk of pin tract infection; the offending pin is usually removed. Any exposed pin tips must be covered by metal or plastic caps or corks to prevent damage by the sharp ended pin to the other limb or body or to the nursing staff.

The patient will usually require a strong analgesic at regular intervals during the first 48 hours following surgery. If severe or moderate pain persists after this time the surgeon must be informed as it may be an indication of infection. The patient is usually confined to bed until bone and skin healing is progressing satisfactorily. Exercises of all joints, including those of the affected limb, are commenced as soon as possible to maintain muscle tone, strength and mass and to maintain joint movements. The patient with a lower limb fracture is at high risk of the formation of deep vein thrombosis. Foot and leg exercises are commenced on the day after the application of the fixation device and observations are made to detect any signs of this complication.

Some patients may be upset on seeing their injured limb and the fixation system. The nurse needs to show patience and understanding and should encourage the patient to express any anxieties and fears. By encouraging the patient to take part in the planning of care and to take an interest in the care of the fixation system and the rehabilitation programme, the nurse may assist the patient in coming to terms with an altered body image.

The patient with a lower limb fracture is taught to mobilize with the aid of crutches; weight bearing on the affected limb is not permitted due to the risk of refracture and bone displacement until callus formation is detected by X-ray examination. Once callus has formed the patient may be taught to partial weight bear through the affected limb.

The external skeletal fixation device is removed once fracture union has occurred, as diagnosed by X-ray. After removal of the fixation system (from a lower limb) the patient is generally not permitted to fully weight bear for a further 2 weeks.

CARE OF THE PATIENT IN TRACTION

It is important that the nurse is familiar with the purpose of the traction and that the principles behind the use of the appliances are understood.

ASSESSMENT OF THE PATIENT IN TRACTION

The ongoing nature of assessment is well illustrated in the case of a patient on traction where several weeks may elapse before the traction is discontinued.

Of particular importance is the patient's skin condition due to the high risk of pressure sore development. Regular monitoring is therefore essential along with the pin sites to detect any early signs of tissue breakdown or infection. The use of a pressure sore risk calculator such as the Norton or Waterlow scale is strongly recommended.

The patient's normal bowel habits and diet should be assessed due to the risks of constipation associated with inactivity. Constipation should be detected early by frequent monitoring rather than at the late stage where the patient is impacted.

Micturition is difficult in traction, particularly for female patients. Any previous history of retention or incontinence needs to be noted and ongoing assessment of urinary output is essential to prevent the risk of retention developing.

The patient's hobbies and interests should be explored as inactivity and boredom can quickly become major problems. Worries about work, income, housing and family to name but a few social factors may develop and the nurse therefore needs to assess how the patient feels about these important areas.

PATIENT PROBLEMS

The nurse plans the care of the patient in traction to prevent the following potential problems

1. Potential problem of infection at the pin sites.

Goal
The patient will not develop an infection at the pin sites.

Intervention
See care of pin sites (p. 871).

Evaluation. While the pins are in place they should remain static and the patient pain free. On removal there should be no sign of infection and the pin sites should heal within a week.

2. Potential problem of general muscle wasting due to immobility

Goal
The patient will not suffer muscle wasting in the uninjured limb and it will be minimal in the injured limb.

Intervention and rationale

- Encourage the patient to be as self-caring as possible within the confines of the traction. This will promote the use of various muscle groups, particularly in the upper body, and may be more appealing to the patient than simply 'doing the exercises'.
- Teach the patient to lift himself or herself up the bed on to a bed pan using an overhead monkey pole. This will strengthen the muscles of the arms and chest, which will help the patient use crutches once mobilizing commences. It also helps prevent skin breakdown due to friction caused by dragging on the sheets.
- Commence a physiotherapy programme to ensure all muscle groups are put through a range of activity daily. The physiotherapist can identify muscles which are particularly at risk of atrophy and teach the patient the required specific exercises. The nurses and physiotherapist should work together with the patient to ensure the patient understands the exercises and the nurse can supervise them (if required) in the physiotherapist's absence.

Evaluation. When the traction is removed the patient's general musculature will be in good condition with minimal evidence of muscle wasting, enabling mobilization to commence.

3. Potential problem of skin breakdown due to traction and immobility

Goal
The patient will not suffer any break in skin due to traction or immobility.

Intervention and Rationale
- Four-hourly inspection of all vulnerable skin areas for the first 48 hours:
  (a) Under the ring of the Thomas' splint. When this is first applied the skin is at special risk as the thigh may continue to swell and the circulation in the skin become compromised. By gently moving the skin under the ring the nurse can see the skin and also relieve any pressure. It is essential that all the skin under the ring is inspected. It may require two nurses to lift the patient while one inspects the skin in the gluteal fold and the inside of the groin. The patient may find this uncomfortable and unnecessary and clear explanations are required beforehand. The use of padding under the ring is to be discouraged as it only creates pressure in other areas. If the ring appears to be getting tighter and the skin is in danger, the doctor should be informed and bolt cutters obtained in case the ring needs to be split and removed
  (b) In the popliteal area where slings may rub and the skin is quite vulnerable. When a Pearson knee flexion piece is used the knee will be partly flexed which increases the likelihood of rubbing. The skin should be protected from the rough sling by padding such as Gamgee.
  (c) Over the head of fibula where the skin and peroneal nerve are at risk of pressure from the side of the splint. This is a particular problem if the leg falls into external rotation and rolls outward, resting on the side arm of the Thomas' splint. Thus it is essential that the nurse ensures the patient's leg is positioned in the splint in such a way that it rests in the centre and any rotation is corrected by small pads of Gamgee strategically placed. The use of a foot piece may also correct this malalignment.
  (d) Over the Achilles tendon, which is superficial and frequently damaged by pressure from the edge of the last sling. If a foot piece is not used and the heel is left free to hang over the edge of the last sling (thus avoiding the heel rubbing), the area which is then at most risk is the skin over the Achilles tendon. If a sore develops the resultant injury to the Achilles tendon may mean further hospitalization and immobilization long after the original injury has healed.
  (e) The back of the heel of the injured leg. This should be free of the bed; if it is found to be lying on the bed the balance weight suspending the Thomas splint needs increasing, thus elevating the leg (helping to reduce swelling), making it easier for the patient to move, and lifting the heel free.
  (f) The back of the heel of the uninjured leg. This is subject to friction on the bedding, particularly while the patient is learning to lift himself or herself free of the bed. If counterpanes are traditionally used at the bottom of traction beds they should be removed because they are very rough. Occasionally the use of sheepskin bootees may be called for but these are only of any use if they are put on when the traction is first applied and if they are maintained in the correct position.
  (g) Buttocks and sacrum. These areas are at risk due to friction caused by the patient not being lifted properly or not lifting themselves properly. Shearing forces caused by the movement of muscle and bone under the skin may destroy the microcirculation to the skin and reduce the skin's viability. Unrelieved pressure is also a cause of skin breakdown in these areas. When patients are on traction it is very difficult to change their position so that their buttocks and sacrum are free from pressure. Simply asking the patient to lift themselves free of the bed for a short while and then replacing themselves in a slightly different position will help. Alternating pressure mattresses are another way of overcoming this problem. These include the Pegasus air bed and ripple mattresses, which can be effectively used with patients on traction. (For a more in depth discussion see Judd, 1989).
  (h) Elbows. Even in young patients elbows become quite sore from their use as 'body props'. To prevent this occurring, patients must be well supported by pillows in a position which is comfortable but allows them access to locker, books, etc. As elbows tend to be quite dry areas, cracking may be prevented by gently massaging hand cream into them.
- After 48 hours the skin will still need to be inspected in all these areas at least twice a day. However, there should be much more patient involvement, with the patient being told exactly what to look for in the early signs of skin breakdown. For some patients 48 hours is too early to even start to take on this responsibility, but many patients are ready and will take a much more active interest in their progress if given this responsibility in these early days.

Throughout the patient's time on traction the nurse should be aware of the danger of breaks in the skin, however small they may appear.

Evaluation. Even after several weeks on traction the patient should remain free of pressure sores. They are not inevitable in this situation but need to be actively prevented by assessment and reassessment of the patient, including the use of risk scales such as Norton or Waterlow (see Chapter 26).

4. Potential problem of constipation due to immobility
Goal
The patient will be able to defaecate naturally, in the usual pattern, without feeling discomfort or requiring artificial stimuli.

Intervention and Rationale

- The patient must be hydrated by the use of specific intake goals such as 2 litres of water per day plus other drinks. If the general condition does not allow for this, an intravenous infusion may be required. If the patient is dehydrated in the first 24–48 hours the faeces will become hard and painful to pass. This will make the patient reluctant to use a bedpan.
- The patient must be given some privacy, somewhere where nobody else will be aware of the noises and odours that may result in attempts to defaecate. In a ward area with only curtains around the bed this can be a problem. Sometimes a bathroom can be used, as long as there is a call bell to hand so that the patient can call for assistance. If a nurse has to keep going in every few minutes, privacy will be lost.
- Although hospital food is supposed to be high in fibre the patient might be encouraged to ask any friends or family who visit to bring in fruit, fruit juice or bran-based breakfast cereals, especially in the first few days when the problem of constipation appears to be at its worst.
- The nurse should ensure that being lifted on to a bedpan is not a painful experience. Ideally analgesia should be kept at an appropriate level from admission so that the patient will not equate being lifted with pain. If a patient is having difficulty opening the bowels, pain experienced due to being transferred to a bedpan will only make matters worse; the situation may be eased by the use of a slipper bedpan.

Evaluation. The patient will regularly pass a soft, well-formed stool, without discomfort, in accordance with his or her usual routine.

5. Potential problem of urinary retention

Goal
The patient will be able to empty the bladder in comfort when the need is felt.

Intervention and Rationale

- The patient must be hydrated and any evidence of hypovolaemia corrected. In both dehydration and hypovolaemia the level of diuresis falls dramatically.
- For female patients interventions are similar to those in problem 4. For male patients the problem is quite different as they find the position they have to adopt (lying on their back with the foot of the bed elevated) extremely difficult to come to terms with. The patient should be regularly offered a urinal and gently told about the need to pass urine. The nurse will need to give constant explanations about the importance of emptying the bladder, why he may be finding it more difficult than he expects and how it should not result in a wet bed. (Howver if it does, the patient will need to be reassured that the problem can be overcome). In exceptional circumstances the doctor may agree to lowering the foot of the bed to see if that helps the patient adopt a better position. However, as this may alter the fracture position it should not be under-

taken without written instructions. Occassionally the use of a sedative such as diazepam may be used to relax the patient, facilitating the passing of urine in these unnatural circumstances.
- Catheterization should be seen as the last resort and the catheter should be removed straight away. After a few days, passing urine usually becomes less and less of a problem but the patient needs to be reminded to continue drinking to prevent the renal complications of calculi and urinary tract infections.

Evaluation. The patient should have been able to empty his bladder in response to the natural urge and will not have developed a urinary tract infection.

6. Potential problem of boredom and depression due to enforced immobility

Goal
The patient will develop ways of coping with the inevitable boredom and will be able to express any feelings of depression that might occur.

Intervention

- Ensure the patient has sufficient diversions such as books, radio, television, etc. to hand. These might help the patient keep in touch with usual interests and activities.
- The nurse should spend time listening to the patient and concentrate on what the patient is trying to say. It sometimes takes time and practised skills by the nurse to produce a situation where the patient is ready to talk about what is really bothering him or her.
- The nurse must recognize that there are times when it is more appropriate to call in other professionals, e.g. social worker, counsellor, minister of religion. Simpson (1987) describes the 'traction intolerance syndrome' in which patients fiddle with their traction, become threatening or abusive and are subject to large mood swings. In this situation he suggests the need for referral to a psychiatrist to help the patient recognize the seriousness of his (it usually occurs in men) injury and the consequences of not following advice.

Evaluation. At the end of the stay in hospital the patient should feel able to return to home life feeling positive about the future.

CONVALESCENCE AND REHABILITATION

Patients may from time to time feel depressed and unhappy but progress may be aided by the free expression of needs and fears. When the traction is removed, the patient will probably be surprised and depressed by the weakness, joint stiffness and joint instability in the limb. Before being allowed up, the head of the bed is elevated so the patient may adjust to having the head and trunk in an upright position after being flat and in the countertraction position for so long. The elevation is gradual; otherwise faintness may be experienced.

Appropriate passive, active and resistive exercises of the affected limb are introduced. These may be planned and supervised by a physiotherapist, but the nurse must be familiar with the plan so that the necessary assistance is provided when the therapist is not at the bedside. In the case of a lower limb, arm and shoulder exercises are continued to strengthen the upper limbs in preparation for the use of a walking frame or crutches. When weight bearing is permitted, the person begins to relearn to walk using a walking frame, crutches or a walking stick. Firm, low-heeled walking shoes, preferably with a non-skid rubber heel, should be worn.

The patient may need prompting to maintain an erect posture (avoid bending forward) and to increase the degree of flexion of the thigh and leg when raising a foot off the floor to take a step in order to overcome the tendency to shuffle. Most patients require a good deal of encouragement and reassurance from the nurse. Physical assistance and support are gradually withdrawn, but the nurse remains with the patient when getting in and out of bed or a chair until it is evident that he or she can safely manage alone.

A home assessment may be carried out prior to discharge to determine what barriers to access and mobility may exist and whether there is someone who will be at home to assist the patient. If the patient experiences difficulties with self-care or mobilizing, a referral may be made to the primary health team so that assistance and supervision will be available. Resumption of the former occupation and activities will depend on progress in relation to mobility and independence.

That patient should know the date, time and place of appointments for follow-up examinations.

CARE OF THE PATIENT WITH INTERNAL (SURGICAL) FIXATION

PREOPERATIVE CARE

The preoperative preparation described in Chapter 11 is carried out. In addition, a person requiring internal fixation may need care for several complicating health problems. When the person has suffered injury there is a *potential problem of hypovolaemic shock* related to trauma. This should be treated in the accident and emergency department by the use of plasma expanding agents (e.g. Haemaccel) and blood transfusion. By the time the patient is transferred to theatre the condition should be stabilized and the patient pronounced fit for an anaesthetic.

How soon after injury the internal fixation occurs depends on factors such a the patient's general condition, the type of fracture, the position of the bone ends and the surgeon's preferences.

During the preoperative period, some temporary form of immobilization is applied to prevent the situation worsening. The injured limb should be handled as little as possible but the patient will need lifting on to a bedpan and for pressure area care so

some form of external splintage may be used, such as a vacuum splint, backslab or sandbags. In the case of an open fracture the wound should be kept moist and covered with a sterile pad soaked in a solution such as povidone-iodine (Betadine). This will promote tissue viability and reduce the risk of infection. In the specific situation of a fractured neck of femur, Hamilton Russell traction may be applied. Analgesia will need to be given and its effect monitored. When elderly patients are awaiting surgery the nurse must be aware of the psychological effects of the strange environment, the accident, pain, journey to hospital and perhaps several hours of lying in the accident and emergency department looking at the ceiling. The use of reality orientation should be employed to remind the patient exactly where he or she is, what has happened and what is going to happen in the near future in order to prevent anxiety and confusion. Prior to surgery most patients will have an intravenous infusion started to correct any evidence of dehydration and provide a drug route. A fluid balance chart should be started at the same time and all intake and output recorded. The patient's urine should be tested as soon as possible to detect any abnormalities such as bleeding into the urinary tract, particularly in patients who may have incurred even apparently minor pelvic injuries. Elderly patients may need an ECG if this was not done in the accident and emergency department in order to ensure their cardiovascular system is fit for a general anaesthetic and the stresses of surgery.

AIDS Precautions

With the suspected increase in the number of individuals carrying human immunodeficiency virus (HIV) being seen in accident and emergency departments it is vital that nurses working in this area ensure that they are familar with the local policy for such patients. There are sensible precautions the nurse can take with all patients to prevent the spread of infection both to other patients and among the staff. Ceccio (1988) suggests the use of gloves when blood or other body fluids are likely to be spilt, and cautious handling of syringes and needles. The latter should not be recapped and must be disposed of in the appropriate puncture-resistant container. Nurses must always wash their hands between patients and after removing gloves. These precautions should be used when caring for patients with open fractures when there is always the danger of spreading blood borne infections. All open fractures should be covered with a Betadine-soaked pad while a decision on treatment is made. All soiled pads should be disposed of in a sealed bag and incinerated.

POSTOPERATIVE CARE

Following internal fixation of fractures the general principles of postoperative care are applicable, with the following additions.

Where surgery is performed on a limb it should be elevated as soon as the patient is back in bed. If a plaster cast has been applied the patient's extremities should be examined for colour, sensation, warmth and movement

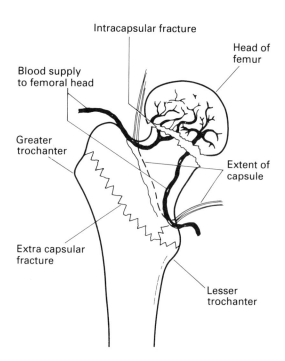

Figure 24.19 Intracapsular and extracapsular fractures of the neck of femur.

every 30 minutes to ensure there is no compromise of the circulation. The digits should be compared with those on the uninjured side and if any difference is observed the nurse in charge should be informed immediately. Sometimes the situation can be relieved by elevating the limb higher, thus reducing the swelling, but more often than not the plaster will need to be split to allow some 'give'. If a backslab has been applied the cotton bandages will need cutting down to skin, especially if there has been some haemorrhage as blood soaked bandages are notoriously harsh and do not 'give' and may act as a tourniquet (Morgan, 1989). Any blood staining on a plaster should be outlined after the first couple of hours so that continued bleeding can be monitored.

Where a plaster cast has not been applied, the circulation, to and sensation of, the limb distal to the surgery should be monitored to ensure no damage was incurred during the operation or preoperatively while the limb was splinted.

All wound drains should be inspected regularly and changed as required. The amount of drainage should be entered on the patient's fluid balance chart. Drains are removed when they have stopped draining, usually after 48 hours.

The patient should become self-caring after three or four days, within the limits of allowed mobility; assistance will be required then.

The patient may be allowed out of bed but, in the case of surgery on a lower extremity, is not usually permitted to bear any weight on it for several days or weeks. He or she may be allowed the use of a

wheelchair and is gradually introduced to the use of crutches. When sitting in either a stationary chair or a wheelchair, provision is made for elevation and support of the affected limb. Precautions against pressure sores and slumping posture are necessary when the patient is allowed up in a chair for long periods. Skin care is provided at regular intervals and patients are taught to shift the weight frequently so that no one area is subjected to continuous pressure. Adjustments may also be necessary to avoid prolonged pressure on the popliteal area of the unaffected, dependent leg and to prevent forward sagging of the shoulders.

Exercises of the affected part are started as soon as the surgeon permits. They may be limited to isometric contractions for a period, followed by the gradual introduction of passive and active movements and resistive exercises. In the case of a lower extremity, weight bearing is not introduced until X-rays indicate satisfactory healing. The overambitious patient is cautioned not to attempt standing or walking without the assistance of a physiotherapist or nurse. The patient should have a firm, non-skid pair of shoes and be assisted first to stand. The physiotherapist or nurse stands facing the patient and places the hands to the sides of the patient's lower chest. The patient is encouraged to stand erect, knees extended and head up. When sure of balancing in the upright position, the patient is then assisted with the next step, which may be the use of crutches, a walking frame or simply walking with only the assistance of one person. Support is given to the affected side.

Treatment and Nursing Care Required for Specific Injuries

In the final section of this chapter a brief summary of the more common injuries, their treatment and the nursing care required will be presented.

FRACTURES OF THE NECK OF FEMUR

Fracture of the neck of femur is one of the more common injuries to the musculoskeletal system. It occurs more often in elderly women, due in part to hormonal changes and the affect this has on bone reabsorption, leading to osteoporosis.

There are two categories of such fractures: *intracapsular* and *extracapsular* (Figure 24.19). Intracapsular fractures occur through the joint and capsule and include subcapital fractures, transcervical fractures and impacted fractures at the base of the neck of femur. An extracapsular fracture may pass through either the greater or lesser trochanter or the intertrochanteric area. These are called intertrochanteric fractures.

ASSESSMENT

The initial assessment in A&E should focus on how much pain the patient is experiencing and apart from gently examining the affected leg (which classically is shortened and externally rotated) the nurse should assess the rest of the patient for other injuries sustained at the same time. Such are the effects of ageing that the nurse should also be alert to other pathological processes which may exist at the same time. It is important therefore to screen for hypothermia (especially in winter), diabetes (possibly undiagnosed) or any signs of cardiovascular disorder (the patient may have suffered a stroke or serious cardiac arrhythmia).

Although these are ultimately medical responsibilities, before the patient is seen by a doctor in A&E, such information is essential for correct triage and nursing care.

Other important information concerns the patient's general condition and whether they look well cared for or neglected. Vital information about home circumstances is available from the ambulance crew in A&E that may not be available to the ward staff. The patient's orientation and understanding of their situation should also be assessed as confusion may speedily develop.

While the surgeon may carry out a technically correct repair to the fracture site, the patient's long term prognosis may depend far more on skilled nursing care preventing complications such as pressure sores, constipation, chest infections or confusion and on the resolution of social problems.

The principles outlined above, of assessing not only the obvious injury but also the rest of the patient, of checking for co-existing but unrelated health problems, assessing the patient's psychological status and exploring social factors apply equally to all types of injury.

Having seen the importance of this approach in discussing the care of an elderly patient with a fracture of the femoral neck region, the nurse should consider these factors while reading through the following summary of commonly seen types of injury, their treatment and the nursing care relevant to specific problems.

GENERAL PRINCIPLES OF TREATMENT

Surgical reduction and fixation of the joint is the treatment of choice. The limb may be temporarily placed in traction (e.g. Hamilton Russell) to hold it in alignment and alleviate muscle spasm while the person's condition is stabilized for surgery. A variety of metal nails, plates and screws may be used for surgical fixation (see Figures 24.17 and 24.18).

Intracapsular fractures are highly likely to damage the blood supply to the head of the femur if there is any displacement at the fracture site (Figure 24.19). If there is no displacement and it is thought the head will survive, two screws such as Garden screws are inserted in a relatively simple operation. However if there is any displacement the femoral head will need to be removed and replaced with a prosthesis such as Thompson's or an Austin Moore. In extracapsular fractures, head viability is not a problem and a fixation device such as a dynamic hip screw or nail and plate is used to hold the fragments.

After 48 hours, following a check X-ray and the removal of any wound drains (providing they have stopped draining), the patient should be able to mobilize. The amount of weight bearing allowed depends on the severity of the fracture, the precision

with which the bone fragments are held by the fixation and the ability of the patient to understand how much weight can be taken by the injured leg.

The nursing care for patients who have had a prosthesis inserted is much the same as that following a total hip replacement. The principles governing care is that the hip is in danger of dislocating if it is allowed to flex more than 45° or if it adducts and the injured leg crosses the good one. Patients are therefore nursed with their legs in abduction, with a frame or two pillows between them, and are not allowed to sit upright either in bed or in a chair.

FRACTURES OF THE SHAFT OF FEMUR

The causes of and the group of patients associated with this type of fracture differ considerably from those suffering a fractured neck of femur. It is caused by high energy trauma, frequently a road traffic accident, and involves men in the 16–35-year-old age group.

Anatomically these fractures range from the subtrochanteric region in the proximal third of the femur, through midshaft fractures, to supracondylar fractures in the distal third. The nurse will find these regional descriptive terms in frequent use and should be familiar with them. The fractures are often spiral, with at least three fragments, due to a twisting injury but direct trauma usually results in the more manageable transverse fracture.

COMPLICATIONS

The major complications which may result from fractures of the shaft of femur are:

- Hypovolaemic shock: even when there is no obvious sign of haemorrhage a litre of blood can be contained within the thigh from a fracture of the shaft of femur.
- Damage to the femoral artery, often a tear from a sharp bone fragment.
- Damage to the femoral nerve, again from a sharp fragment.
- Following an open comminuted fracture, loss of bone fragment at the scene of the accident. This will lead to a shortening of the limb. Occasionally the fragment may be found and used in the treatment.
- Fat emboli. There are two theories behind the explanation of the development of fat emboli following fracture of the shaft of femur: (i) that trauma causes disruption of the veins and fat cells in the bone allowing fat into the circulation, and (ii) catecholamine release due to the stress of trauma mobilizes lipids from adipose tissue which then become fat droplets. In the lung these droplets are converted to free fatty acids which are toxic to lung tissue and disrupt alveolar function (Mims, 1989). Small globules of fat may become enmeshed in the capillary network around the alveoli and prevent small amounts of gaseous exchange occurring; however, if large blood vessels in the pulmonary system are obstructed the result will be fatal. The presence and effect of fat emboli is monitored by the

concentration of oxygen in arterial blood; thus blood gas analysis may be performed every couple of hours in the first 24–48 hours of admission. Patients with bilateral fractures of the shaft of femur should be given high concentrations of oxygen immediately. Some orthopaedic surgeons would say this would be appropriate treatment for unilateral fractures as well. It is important that the nurse recognizes that oxygen therapy does not prevent fat emboli but helps the body cope with them by raising the oxygen content of the blood. As the oxygen content of arterial blood leaving the left side of the heart is usually assessed as $Po_2 = 13\,kPa$ (100 mmHg) and falls to $Po_2 = 5\,kPa$ (40 mmHg) by the time it enters the right side of the heart, any reduction in the oxygen content when it should be at its highest will have a 'knock-on effect' throughout the system. The effect on the patient will be similar to respiratory failure, i.e. cyanosis and cerebral hypoxia leading to confusion, coma and death. By artificially raising the Po_2, the reduction (which will still occur) will not have such a profound effect, especially on cerebral perfusion. Occasionally patients will need to be transferred to an intensive care unit for intubation and ventilation to ensure oxygen levels are maintained. Mims (1989) cites altered mental status as the most important clinical feature in the recognition of fat emboli.

TREATMENT

The treatment for fractured shaft of femur depends on the severity and position of the fracture and how well callus formation takes place. In most cases the patient is nursed in skeletal traction for the first 2–3 weeks until callus is seen on X-ray and the fracture is in an acceptable position. As most patients fall into a relatively young age group there is a need to obtain as good an anatomical result as possible, otherwise there may be considerable stress on the weight-bearing joints in the future. This could eventually lead to an early onset of secondary osteoarthritis. (For care of patient on skeletal traction see p. 872).

The alternative treatments following callus formation are:

1. Remain on traction until fracture has united.
2. Intramedullary nailing using a Küntscher or A.O. nail. An intramedullary nail acts as an internal splint and is inserted the length of the femur along the medullary canal. A piece of the nail is usually left protruding from the greater trochanter but under the skin to allow easy access for its removal 12–18 months later.

   The immediate care is outlined on p. 875. Once the wound drains have been removed and the check X-ray shows a satisfactory position the patient is usually allowed to commence mobilizing either partially or non-weight bearing using crutches. The patient will require a programme of exercises, particularly static exercising of the quadriceps, to ensure the retention or building up of the quadriceps muscles. The physiotherapist will also gradually introduce knee flexion, although this may be limited in the early stages of rehabilitation.

Once the patient is confident on crutches he or she may be discharged, although an appointment will be required for the removal of stitches and follow-up in the out-patient department. Prior to discharge the patient should be reminded that if the leg suddenly becomes painful or swollen or the wound becomes red and inflamed he or she should telephone the orthopaedic out-patient clinic (giving the name of the consultant concerned) or, if out of clinic hours, attend the casualty department. All internal fixation carries a risk of infection which should be treated aggressively at the first indication.
3. Femoral cast brace may be applied 2–6 weeks after fracture (Morgan, 1989). The main aims of such a brace are to encourage bone healing and prevent knee stiffness by early weight bearing and mobilization. The cast may be made of synthetic resins or plaster of Paris (resins are usually favoured as they are light and dry very quickly) and is applied in two sections, the thigh section and the lower leg section, by specially trained technicians. The two sections are joined by a pair of hinges. The position of the hinge is crucial to avoid undue stress on the patient's knee. (For a more detailed explanation of this technique see Morgan, 1989). The patient will require considerable help at the first attempts at weight bearing but should be able to be discharged within a few days of the application of the brace.

FRACTURES OF THE TIBIA

Tibial fractures are classified according to whether they are open or closed, their position and the degree of displacement at the fracture site. As the treatment and therefore the nursing care required depends on this classification, this section will start at the proximal tibia and finish with fractures of the malleoli. Fractures of the fibula will not be dealt with separately as the treatment is usually in association with that of the tibia. Isolated fractures of the fibula with no tibial involvement are relatively minor and are treated in the accident and emergency department.

TIBIAL PLATEAU FRACTURE

Although this frequently appears to be a minor fracture its position within the knee joint and its effect on future knee function mean that it is treated aggressively and every endeavour is made to retain and/or restore good anatomical position of the articular cartilage.

One of the overriding principles of treatment is the maintenance of knee movement. If the fracture is depressed the patient will require an elevation of the fragment under a general anaesthetic to restore the joint surface. Any displacement of the fracture will require internal fixation using a buttress plate, screws or bone graft in combination. Postoperatively the patient will be nursed on a continuous passive movement (CPM) machine. This machine (frequently used following total knee replacements) can be set to specific degrees of flexion and speed of movement. For the first few days the amount of flexion should be very small while the wound is healing and the swelling starts to subside. This may be gradually increased with time and within the patient's pain threshold. The nursing staff must be aware of the need to maintain a constant level of analgesia as the machine is moving the patient's knee 24 hours a day.

Patients with undisplaced tibial plateau fractures will be placed on the CPM machine after a period of Hamilton Russell traction. The nurse must know exactly why the machine is being used and be able to explain the need for 24-hour movement.

Because the patient's leg is held in the machine quite firmly it is crucial that the skin is examined every day for any sign of redness or breaks.

Once healing is beginning to take place and there is knee flexion of at least 45°, a femoral cast brace will be applied and the patient may be up weight bearing. Because the patient's weight is transferred through the upper component, the hinges and the lower leg piece of the brace there is no danger that the fragment will become depressed.

TIBIAL SHAFT FRACTURES

These fractures vary from the simple, undisplaced, closed fracture which is treated with an above-knee plaster of Paris cast in the accident and emergency department and the patient discharged, to the open, grossly contaminated, displaced comminuted fracture seen following a severe road traffic accident.

As tibial fractures, particularly in the middle to lower third, have a reputation for poor healing, if the fracture is open the problem of infection has to be considered very quickly. Harley et al (1986), in their paper on the comparison of plating and traction in the treatment of tibial shaft fractures, suggest that the problem of soft tissue swelling and fracture shape frequently make the use of plaster of Paris unacceptable. The alternatives in regular use are external fixators, which allow nursing access to any wounds while holding the fracture position, open reduction and internal fixation using a compression plate, and skeletal traction using a calcaneal pin or wire and a Braun frame. In their study of 115 patients, Harley and colleagues looked at the last two alternatives and found that the length of hospitalization was about the same (although the surgically treated group required two admissions), the surgical group healed 6 weeks sooner than the conservatively treated group but there was a 30% complication rate in the surgical group. The authors' conclusions were that, although new techniques for internal fixation have been introduced, the results are still not very good and that conservative treatment is a satisfactory method of care for patients with these fractures.

The *specific problems* patients with these fractures may develop include:

- Gross infection. The patient will require diligent observation of temperature, pulse and respiration 4-hourly until all the wounds are healed.
- Poor healing rate. A close observation of pedal pulses must be made to ensure adequate perfusion of the lower leg. Excessive soft tissue damage may produce swelling, leading to compartmental syndrome in

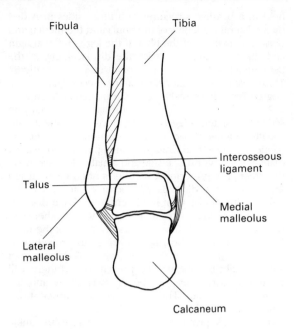

Figure 24.20 The anatomy of the ankle joint.

which the muscle fascia of the three compartments in the lower leg come under intense pressure, eventually compromising the major arteries. This situation requires prompt action; usually fasciotomies are performed in theatre to relieve the pressure and restore an adequate blood supply.

Every effort must be made to ensure the maintenance of the optimum position of the fracture. This entails the nurse checking the traction 4-hourly, ensuring the cords are over the pulleys and the patient's leg is in alignment, and that the bed remains elevated to maintain traction. Although the patient should be encouraged to be as self-caring as possible, moving around too much, especially in the first week, should be discouraged.

- Knee and ankle stiffness. The physiotherapist and the nurse will be responsible for ensuring that the patient's range of movements in these joints are kept at an optimum. Harley and colleagues cite ankle stiffness occuring in six patients out of 47 in the conservatively treated group and three out of 56 in the surgically treated group. Ankle stiffness will add considerably to the patient's mobilization problems when the fracture is united.
- Problems from the pin sites. These have been discussed earlier in the chapter and the reader is directed to the care plans for external fixation and skeletal traction.

FRACTURES OF THE MALLEOLI

These are usually the result of a twisting injury from stepping on to uneven ground. To understand the mechanism of the injury the nurse needs to know the anatomy of the ankle joint (Figure 24.20). The talus is held in a box-like structure, with three sides provided by the lateral malleolus of the fibula and the medial and posterior malleoli of the tibia. If the leg is held straight and the foot forced to twist, the displacement of the talus may break off one, two or three of the malleoli. These fractures are referred to a first-, second- and third-degree Pott's fractures, or bi- or trimalleolar fractures.

As the fracture is frequently displaced, especially in second- and third-degree Pott's fractures, patients are usually admitted for open reduction and internal fixation. The internal fixation is often performed using a plate and screws on one side and a malleoolar screw on the other. The posterior malleolus is often manipulated into place. If a diastasis has occurred in which the inferior tibiofibular joint has been displaced, a diastasis screw, which crosses from one bone to the other, will be used. It is crucial that the nurse is aware of the need for total non-weight bearing following this procedure as the normal movement at the inferior tibio-fibular joint when weight bearing will be prevented and there will be unnecessary stress on the diastasis screw and the surrounding bone. This can lead to further bone damage at the ankle.

The specific problems following surgery to the ankle are:
- Risk of infection. The nurse must be aware that the patient may have two wounds so the risk of infection is doubled. If the fracture was open the chances of infection are also increased. If it was initially a closed fracture it has now effectively been converted to an open fracture.
- Circulatory compromise due to swelling. On return to the ward the patient's leg should be elevated well above the level of the heart. Circulatory observations should be performed half-hourly for at least the first 12 hours; these should include pedal pulses if possible. Some surgeons use plaster of Paris following internal fixation, especially in severe fractures when it is felt that the fixation is less than perfect. Sometimes the patient will simply have wool and a crepe bandage around the wounds. If there is a plaster cast it should be split to allow for swelling.
- Wound drains, which require attention to ensure their patency is maintained. These should be changed as required until the wound(s) stop draining. Any drainage on the plaster should be outlined 4-hourly so that it can be monitored.

FRACTURES OF THE CALCANEUM

These fractures are the result of jumping or falling from a height and landing on the feet. The calcaneum is frequently crushed, with many fragments. Traditionally the treatment has been high elevation and ice packs to reduce the enormous swelling that can result. However more recently the use of internal fixation has been introduced.

SPECIFIC PATIENT PROBLEMS

- This injury is often seen following an unsuccessful

attempt to commit suicide. The result is that the patient has both the physical discomfort of often two very painful heels and the emotional trauma of still being alive and still facing the problems that prompted the suicide attempt, but also having to face the world in the knowledge of the failure of the attempt. The nurse on the trauma ward must be able to care for such patients with empathy, being non-judgemental and recognizing the need to bring in other professionals and take their advice on the best ways to care for such patients.
- Ankle stiffness. As soon as the swelling starts to subside the physiotherapist and the nurse must outline a programme to improve the patient's ankle movement. At first this might be mainly passive movement but will gradually progress to include more active exercises.

FRACTURES OF THE PELVIS

Pelvic fractures are second only to head injuries as the cause of death following road traffic accidents (Conolly and Hedberg, 1969). Fractures involving the posterior sacroiliac region have the highest morbidity and mortality, whereas those affecting the pubic rami appear to be painful but do not carry many dangers. Because of the difficulty in making exact diagnoses in some parts of the pelvis, the patient may require a CT scan to augment the X-rays. As the function of the pelvis is to protect key internal organs, when it is fractured there is a high risk of damage to the bowel, bladder and urethra. Also in danger are the abdominal aorta and internal iliac arteries and it is damage to these large vessels that is responsible for 60% of the deaths following this injury (Peter, 1987). Where there is some doubt if the patient is bleeding, peritoneal lavage will be performed in the accident and emergency department.

In displaced, open and complicated fractures the patient will usually require open reduction and application of an external fixation device. Some parts of the pelvis may also be fixed with a small plate and screws. This can only be performed once the general condition has been stabilized and any bleeding blood vessels repaired.

Undisplaced fractures, such as those sustained by the elderly when they fall and 'sit down' resulting in fractures of the pubic rami, are treated by bed rest and analgesia. This injury is extremely painful and the balance between helping and encouraging the patient to mobilize and ensuring they have sufficient analgesia to allow pain-free movement is important. Often there is little visible damage and the nurse may be dismissive of the pain; however, after 2–3 days the bruising starts to show and the whole of the perineum may turn purple.

Injuries resulting in diastasis at the symphisis pubis may be treated by nursing the patient on slings which cross over the front of the pelvis, pulling the pelvis into shape.

SPECIFIC PATIENT PROBLEMS

- Pin sites. The care required for these is slightly different as very often there are more than one inserted in adjacent bone. Instead of a puncture in the skin there may be a slash of 2–4 cm which will require regular dressings to prevent infection.

- Bladder and/or urethral involvement. All urine passed should be tested for haematuria for at least 24 hours or until it has been clear for 24 hours. A suprapubic catheter may be inserted to keep the bladder empty until it has healed and the risk of chemical peritonitis has subsided.
- Bowel involvement. Rupture of any part of the intestinal tract introduces the risk of peritonitis from spillage of the bowel contents into the peritoneum. Signs such as abdominal pain, pyrexia and shock indicate this complication may have occurred.
- Implications for child bearing in females. In females of child-bearing age, injuries to the pelvis carry with them the risk of creating the inability to carry a fetus to full term. Thus every effort must be made to restore the anatomical position of the pelvis. The situation must be discussed with the patient, who should be examined by an obstetrician. This would be an opportunity for all the problems to be aired and may provide the patient with some comfort.
- Neurological problems. These mainly affect the sacral plexus and the sciatic nerve. Such damage is recognized by absent plantar flexion and ankle jerk. However the damage is usually only temporary due to bruising and stretching of the nerves rather than to any more permanent damage.

Fractures of the *acetabulum* are usually caused by indirect violence and have their own problems. The head of the femur needs to be held out of the acetabulum by traction to allow healing to take place. A major worry is the development of secondary arthritis in the hip joint, especially in a young patient. Many of the patients requiring total hip replacements in their forties have a history of severe trauma to the hip in their twenties and thirties.

FRACTURES OF THE NECK OF HUMERUS

Most of the fractures of the neck of humerus occur at the surgical rather than the anatomical neck (McRae, 1989). They are caused by falling on an outstretched hand or on the side. Impacted fractures are treated symptomatically, using the support of a collar and cuff sling until the pain starts to subside, and then encouraging movement. For slightly displaced fractures the arm should be supported by a collar and cuff sling and the body bandaged for the first two weeks, after which the body bandage may be discarded. Movement should gradually be introduced; this is often limited and follow-up physiotherapy will usually be required.

Grossly displaced fractures of the neck of humerus will require open reduction and internal fixation using a Rush pin and/or AO plate and screws.

SPECIFIC PATIENT PROBLEMS

Patients with undisplaced or minimally displaced fractures will be treated in the accident and emergency department.

- Injury to the brachial plexus. As well as circulatory observations, sensation and motor function of the affected hand should be observed because stretching of the nerve plexus at the time of the accident or during surgery may occur. Usually this is only temporary; nevertheless it must be monitored in case it is of a more serious nature.
- Avascular necrosis of head of humerus. This is not common and tends to occur in fractures of the anatomical neck.
- Arterial obstruction. Occasionally a displaced bone fragment may cause occlusion of the axillary artery. This usually resolves following reduction of the fracture. Circulatory observations of the hand (including a radial pulse) must be performed half-hourly for at least the first 12 hours postoperatively.
- Maintenance of the position of the hand and arm postoperatively. The patient may have a collar and cuff sling, with or without a body bandage, after surgery. The nurse should ensure both are comfortable, not rubbing and are providing the support required.
- Joint stiffness. This is a particular problem with the elderly and, left untreated, quickly leads to loss of independence even when the fracture has united. The importance of performing exercises prescribed by the physiotherapist cannot be overemphasised.

FRACTURES OF THE SHAFT OF HUMERUS

Humoral fractures may be the result of indirect violence such as falling on an outstretched hand, or direct violence such as falling on the side. They may be open or closed fractures although open fractures are mainly found in those involving the middle third of the humerus (McRae, 1989). Conservative treatment of such fractures involves reduction of the fracture under sedation/general anaesthetic (if necessary) and the application of a hanging 'U' slab. The patient will require a broad arm sling under the clothes for support. If an above elbow plaster is applied with the elbow at right angles, a collar and cuff sling should be applied as the weight of the plaster is designed to act as traction on the fractured shaft. Occasionally internal fixation using an intramedullary nail or plate may be performed.

SPECIFIC PATIENT PROBLEMS

- Radial nerve palsy. This is recognized by a drop wrist and sensory loss on the back of the hand between the thumb and index finger.
- Non-union due to loss of position. To prevent this the nurse must be vigilant in ensuring that the correct sling is worn and that it is providing the correct support. This can be difficult if the patient is unable to get out of bed and unable to sit upright. Careful explanations of the rationale for care should be given to the patient and repeated as frequently as necessary.

FRACTURES OF THE WRIST

Colles' fractures are probably one of the most common

fractures the nurse is likely to encounter. Most are dealt with in the accident and emergency department. They are usually the result of falling on an outstretched hand, particularly in the elderly. The displacement of the radius leads to the 'dinner fork' deformity when the wrist is viewed laterally. Following reduction of the fracture, usually under intravenous regional anaesthesia (Bier's block), a below elbow backslab is applied. This will need to be completed when the medical staff are assured that the inevitable swelling is receding and that finger movement is good, usually up to a week later.

SPECIFIC PATIENT PROBLEMS FOLLOWING A COLLES' FRACTURE

- Stiffness and swelling of the fingers. All jewellery, including wedding rings, should be removed as soon after the accident as possible. Finger exercises should be taught, and a leaflet with a description of the exercises and information on who to contact if the fingers suddenly swell or movement becomes more difficult should be supplied.
- Carpal tunnel syndrome. This is caused by median nerve compression in the wrist and is recognized by paraesthesia over the anterior aspect of the thumb, index and second finger and half the ring finger. Surgical decompression is required.
- Loss of independence. As this fracture frequently occurs in the elderly, the nurse must ensure that the patient will be able to manage alone or has someone to help. For many old people, adapting to changes in circumstances takes a long time and 'young' hospital staff are in danger of dismissing the difficulty such patients encounter in coping with relatively minor fractures.

Smith's fractures are often described as reversed Colles' fractures. They are caused by falling on the flexed wrist; X-rays confirm the anterior displacement of the distal fragment. Unlike most Colles' fractures it is difficult to maintain a good position after reducing a Smith's fracture, therefore internal fixation using a buttress plate is usually required.

The foregoing is not an exhaustive list of fractures but highlights some of the more common fractures a nurse is likely to encounter. For a more detailed account of fracture care the reader should consult a specialist text.

Injuries to Joints

Injuries to joints may range from a mild sprain to complete dislocation with associated fractures. The overall aim of care is to allow the joint surface time to recover, in order to reduce the likelihood of secondary osteoarthritis, while keeping the patient as active as possible to overcome muscle wasting around the joint which may lead to permanent joint instability.

SHOULDER DISLOCATION

In this injury the shoulder is usually dislocated anteriorly. In the 18–35-year-old age group it is usually due to a sports or motor cycle accident in which the person is thrown and lands on an outstretched hand and the body rotates above the hand. It is also quite common in the elderly, usually following a more minor injury due to the lax musculature of the shoulder joint in this age group.

As soon as the injury has been confirmed by X-ray the shoulder should be reduced as the longer it is left the harder it is to relocate the humoral head. In some accident and emergency departments it is customary to give such patients intramuscular analgesia and lie them prone on a trolley with the affected arm hanging free over the side. Spontaneous reduction may occur due to gravitational traction and the muscle relaxant effect of the analgesia. However it must be recognized that some patients will find this position suffocating and very difficult to maintain. Reduction of the dislocation should take place in the accident and emergency department under intravenous diazepam and a narcotic analgesic. Occasionally a general anaesthetic will be required.

In younger patients the postreduction care includes the application of a body bandage (including the forearm) to prevent abduction and external rotation. Both these movements predispose to recurrence, which is about 50% in this age group (McRae, 1989). If recurrence becomes a problem the patient may eventually require a surgical repair.

In the elderly recurrence is not such a problem but there is a high risk of stiffness leading to loss of independence; thus mobilization of the shoulder may begin after a week.

SPECIFIC PATIENT PROBLEMS

- Axillary nerve palsy. This may be tested for in the accident and emergency department by a pin prick test over the outer aspect of the shoulder. The condition may be severe enough for the patient to lose deltoid function and although it is usually temporary, months of physiotherapy may be necessary for full recovery.
- Rotator cuff tear. The head of the humerus is held in place in the glenoid cavity of the scapula by the tendons of the shoulder joint muscles which fuse and form the rotator cuff. The cuff inserts at points around the greater and lesser tuberosities of the humerus. If it is torn the most common problem is in abducting the arm. The condition may be helped by physiotherapy but a repair of the tear may eventually be required.
- Loss of independence. Use of the shoulder is essential to perform many aspects of self-care. Ability to perform self-care must be assessed in all patients.

HIP DISLOCATION

This injury may range from incomplete dislocation (subluxation), when the head of the femur is partly out of the acetabulum, to complete dislocation, when the femoral head is lying behind the acetabulum (posterior dislocation). Once the hip has been reduced the joint should be rested, usually on skin traction and then 'free in bed' for several weeks, before weight bearing can take place.

The major problem for patients with this injury are as those for fractures of the acetabulum (see p. 881).

MENISCAL INJURIES IN THE KNEE

These injuries usually occur in young people who engage in sports and are the result of rotational stress on the flexed, weight bearing knee. The extent of the tear may vary from being small and undisplaced to one in which the whole of the meniscus is involved and displaced to such an extent there is complete loss of joint function. Arthroscopy may confirm diagnosis and a partial meniscectomy may be performed via the arthroscope. The aim of treatment is to leave as much of the meniscus intact as possible.

A major postoperative problem is instability of the knee joint following quadriceps wasting. The nurse should be aware of the patient's need to perform static quadriceps exercises to overcome muscle wasting in the thigh. The physiotherapist will need to be involved in organizing an exercise programme but as the patient is only likely to be in hospital for two or three days the nurse will need to be able to reinforce the necessity of practising the exercises and ensure they are being performed correctly for maximum benefit.

SOFT TISSUE INJURY OF THE ANKLE

These occur most commonly following inversion injuries, damaging the lateral ligament. The patient will complain of pain and swelling over the lateral malleolus although the X-rays will be normal. Following mild sprains the patient will require support of the ankle, such as double Tubigrip, and should be advised to rest at home with high elevation of the ankle to reduce the swelling. If weight bearing is painful a pair of crutches should be provided.

In more serious injuries where the lateral ligament is completely torn the patient will require complete immobilization in a below-knee weight-bearing plaster.

SPECIFIC PATIENT PROBLEMS

● Loss of independence. Some patients will need to be admitted overnight, even following relatively minor injuries, until they are safe to mobilize on crutches. This, of course, is particularly true of the elderly person who lives alone.
● Circulatory compromise due to swelling.
● In the long term, ankle instability may be the result of this injury and the patient will require surgery to reconstruct a stable joint.

Amputation of a Limb

The incidence of amputation of part of a limb increases sharply in the over-55 age group as a result of peripheral vascular disease (PVD). Amputation of a limb is a very mutilating procedure and an extremely devastating experience for the individual. However it frequently provides relief from severe intractable pain due to PVD or osteomyelitis and allows a significant improvement in mobility.

For those for whom an amputation is a necessity, the loss of the limb has become less obvious and less disabling nowadays as a result of improved prostheses and rehabilitation programmes.

REASONS FOR AMPUTATION

An amputation is performed to preserve the patient's life or may be undertaken to improve function and usefulness. The conditions which necessitate amputation include: (1) insufficient blood supply to the part (PVD) and resulting gangrene; (2) severe, uncontrollable infection such as gas gangrene (*Clostridium welchii* infection) or chronic osteomyelitis in which there is marked bone destruction; (3) malignant neoplasm (e.g. osteosarcoma); (4) an injury that has resulted in irreparable crushing of the limb or laceration of arteries and nerves; and (5) a handicapping deformity (e.g. flail limb).

LEVEL AND TYPES OF AMPUTATION

Occasionally an amputation is an emergency surgical procedure performed because of irreparable traumatic damage to a part. But, when possible, the level of the amputation is decided before operation so that the patient may be informed of the anticipated extent of the loss. The decision as to the level is based on achieving (1) complete removal of the diseased tissue, (2) viable tissue and an adequate blood supply to the remaining part of the limb, and (3) a stump that will allow for a satisfactory fitting and functional movement of a prosthesis. Adequate soft tissues (skin, subcutaneous tissue and muscle) are preserved so that the end of the bone is well padded and covered. If possible, the stump should be the optimum length for adequate leverage on the prosthesis. Too long a stump may interfere with the function of the prosthesis joint below. In amputation of the lower extremity the knee joint is maintained, if at all possible, since mobility and agility are more readily acquired. The prosthesis for the above knee amputation limits the person, especially if elderly, because of the high energy demands for locomotion.

Two types of operative procedures are used, the closed or flap type of amputation and the guillotine or open amputation.

In the *flap type* of procedure, fascia, probably muscle, and full-thickness skin flaps are brought over the end of the bone. In an above knee or through knee amputation, the anterior flap is usually longer in order to bring the suture line well to the posterior aspect. In a below knee or in a Syme's amputation, the posterior flap is usually longer, with the suture line situated on the anterior aspect of the stump. This arrangement prevents direct pressure on the scar by the prosthesis in weight-bearing.

A *guillotine or open amputation* is reserved for emergency cases in which the limb has been severely traumatized and contaminated or in which an infection such as gas gangrene has already developed. The skin and other soft tissues are severed at the same level as the bone. The wound is left open to promote adequate drainage and closed later when infection is brought under control. Traction may be applied to the skin while it remains open to prevent retraction of the soft tissues.

Traumatic amputation implies the loss of a whole or part of a limb in an accident. This is frequently a life-threatening situation because of the concomitant haemorrhage. A second problem incurred by such circumstances is contamination of the wound. Immediate emergency care is directed toward arrest of the bleeding and getting the person to where blood replacement may be instituted. Precautions are taken to handle and transport the amputated part with the patient carefully, since efforts may be made to reattach the separated unit.

Disarticulation is the term used when the amputation is at the level of a joint.

PREOPERATIVE NURSING INTERVENTION

Psychological preparation
When the amputation is an elective procedure, the surgeon, nurse and the rehabilitation team work together to inform the patient and family of the need for the operation and the level at which the limb will be removed and what functional restoration can be anticipated. When the patient is first advised of the loss of a part of the body, regardless of how functionally insignificant, the information is still likely to be a shock, causing considerable emotional disturbance. The patient's body image and independence are seriously threatened and encouragement is needed to talk freely about fears and anxieties. Good nurse–patient communication is essential both pre and post operatively to help the patient resolve these fears and adapt to a change in body image. Reactions vary among patients, depending on culture, personality, life situation and the impact loss of a limb is perceived as having on the individual's social circumstances.

The patient and family receive explanations of how the problems associated with the loss of a limb may be handled through a planned rehabilitation programme. The knowledge that the interest and assistance of specialists in this area are available may help the patient to develop a positive attitude toward overcoming the handicap. Opportunities are provided for questions and discussions about what is likely to take place before and after the operation. The patient may derive support from a visit by someone who has had a similar amputation and has been successfully rehabilitated.

Physical preparation
Normal preop preparation is required as for any major operation, but in addition exercises are introduced which will facilitate postoperative mobilization and rehabilitation. These include active exercises of the unaffected limbs to prevent loss of muscular strength. If the use of walking aids is anticipated, arm strengthening exercises using weight-lifting and push-ups may be introduced to strengthen the shoulder and arm muscles. Over-protection of an affected lower limb usually result in continuous flexion of the hip and knee joints, leading to contractures. This is discouraged by lying the patient in a prone position several times a day.

POSTOPERATIVE NURSING INTERVENTION

Assessment
The blood pressure, pulse and respirations are recorded, colour noted and the stump examined at frequent, regular intervals for the first 48 hours for early signs of shock and haemorrhage. The patient is observed for psychological distress following the amputation. Even though he/she was prepared for and consented to the operation, the actual loss of the body part may cause severe depression. The nurse is also alert for any indications of infection such as pyrexia, raised pulse, increased pain, erythema and wound discharge.

Potential patient problems following an amputation are listed in Table 24.5

1. Promotion of healing
The stump is usually enclosed in a thick soft dressing and elasticated bandages.

When a soft dressing is used, any blood staining is reported immediately. If serous drainage soaks through the dressing, it is promptly reinforced and pressure is applied until the bleeding is brought under control, if necessary, by the surgeon. Continuous closed wound suction drainage may be established to prevent haematoma formation. The wound dressing, providing it is comfortable, is generally left undisturbed until the wound drain is removed, thus reducing the risk of introduction of infection. The wound drain is removed 2–4 days following surgery and the sutures are left in place for 10–12 days for an above knee amputation and 3–4 weeks for a below knee wound, in order to ensure firm healing.

Unless the surgeon instructs otherwise, the patient should lie in a supine position with the stump resting flat on the bed. Following an amputation above the knee, the patient must be guarded against shortening of the hip flexors and abductors. In an amputation below the knee, the patient is encouraged to maintain extension of the knee to avoid contracture of the hamstrings (posterior thigh muscles).

The patient or a member of the family is taught the care of the stump and the correct application of the bandage. The stump is bathed as necessary with a mild soap and rinsed and dried thoroughly. Lanolin may be applied if the skin is dry and flaky. The patient is taught to inspect the stump twice daily, using a mirror, for redness, swelling, irritation and calluses. If any symp-

Table 24.5   Identification of patients' problems following amputation.

Problem	Causative factors	Goals
1 Failure of wound to heal	Infection Poor blood supply Haematoma formation	The wound will heal without any complications
2 Potential for injury	Surgical construction of a residual limb (stump) Altered balance Possible disorientation in the post-operative period Phantom limb phenomenom	1 To achieve a residual limb that will support activity with a prosthesis 2 Physical injury will not occur
3 Discomfort/pain	Surgical intervention Phantom pain phenomenon	1 Patient will be painfree 2 To understand and minimize the experience of phantom sensations
4 Disturbance in body image	Amputation of a body part	1 To express feelings about the loss of a body part 2 To attain an acceptable level of social and physical functioning
5 Nutritional intake lower than body requirements	Surgery and anaesthesia	To maintain nutritional and fluid balance
6 Impaired mobility	Surgery and loss of a body part	1 Complications of immobility will not occur 2 To increase physical activity and ambulation
7 Inadequate knowledge about the care of the residual limb and the prosthesis, application and use of the prosthesis and follow-up care	Lack of information, skill and resources	1 To develop self-care skills 2 To develop a plan for follow-up health management

toms develop, weight-bearing on the stump is avoided and the doctor or clinic consulted. Stump bandaging is resumed if the prosthesis is not worn during this time. Certain activities may be ordered which apply pressure to the stump in preparation for the use of a prosthesis and weight-bearing. Contact is first made with something quite soft and, as tolerance is developed, the firmness and resistance of the contact surface and pressure are progressively increased. If the patient complains of muscular spasms and discomfort, massage to the stump may provide relief. Fig. 24.21 illustrates points the patient is taught 'not to do' with the stump in order to prevent injury and promote healing.

2. Prevention of physical injury
The most common cause of falls is that the patient forgets momentarily that he has only one leg. He may experience the sensation that his limb is still present; this phenomenon is known as *phantom limb*. The majority of amputees experience this phenomenon, which is strongest immediately following surgery. Awareness that it is a common experience following amputation helps to decrease the patient's anxiety.

3. Control of pain
A narcotic analgesic is usually required by the patient at regular intervals during the first 48 hours after surgery.

Persistent pain 24–72 hours after surgery may indicate haematoma formation. This must be reported to the surgeon immediately, as breakdown of the wound could occur if the haematoma is not evacuated. If pain occurs later in the postoperative recovery period it may be due to wound infection or to the formation of a neuroma. If infection is suspected the wound is inspected, a wound swab is taken for microscopy, culture and sensitivity and the relevant antibiotic is prescribed. Some patients experience pain which is interpreted as originating in the portion of the limb which has been removed. This is referred to as phantom pain. It varies in severity and may be temporary, but if it persists, treatment in the form of local nerve blocks in the stump, transcutaneous nerve stimulation, ultra-sound, relaxation training or drug therapy including the use of anticonvulsant agents (e.g. carbamazepine) may prove effective. No single method of treatment has shown itself to be consistently successful. Research continues and other therapies are in use.

4. Adjustment to altered body image
Acknowledgement by the nurse of the patient's feelings of depression, anger and frustration and provision of opportunities for the patient and family members to discuss feelings help the patient to accept the situation. An understanding of the meaning of the loss is

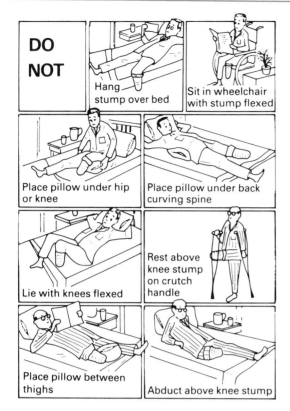

DO NOT

Hang stump over bed

Sit in wheelchair with stump flexed

Place pillow under hip or knee

Place pillow under back curving spine

Lie with knees flexed

Rest above knee stump on crutch handle

Place pillow between thighs

Abduct above knee stump

Figure 24.21 Positions to be avoided by lower extremity amputee during the immediate postoperative period.

necessary for the health professional to provide constructive support. The nurse and other health care workers may set expectations that the patient will increase mobilization, socialization and self-care activities. The patient may feel very differently however. Support and encouragement are therefore essential. Early mobilization and patient participation in decision-making promote the development of a more positive attitude. A temporary prosthesis is worn as soon as possible so the patient only briefly experiences an empty sleeve or empty trouser leg. The permanent prosthesis is fitted within a few weeks for most patients. As the patient's functional capacity increases, feelings of self-worth and tolerance of the change in body image may begin to emerge. Friends and relatives are encouraged to visit and opportunities for the patient to go home for an evening or weekend are created whenever possible.

Involvement of members of the rehabilitation team prior to surgery and during the postoperative period enables them to provide information about the expectations for functional restoration, develop plans for rehabilitation and establish a trusting relationship with the patient and family. Rehabilitation centres usually provide both individual and group sessions to allow patients to share experiences, gain support and learn new and effective coping strategies.

The patient is encouraged to discuss with the limb fitter how the artificial limb will look as well as function.

Help is provided in selecting shoes, trousers, skirts, shirts and blouses to promote a favourable and acceptable appearance.

Psychological and social adjustment is generally a longer process than is the relearning of physical functioning.

5. Maintenance of fluid and nutritional status
Intravenous fluid may be necessary during the first 24–48 hours to maintain an adequate intake. Oral fluids are given freely, and the patient progresses to a regular diet as soon as it is tolerated. An explanation is made, if necessary, of the importance of adequate nutrition in maintaining and promoting his muscular strength for the exercises that will assist in rehabilitation.

6. Promotion of mobility
An hourly routine of coughing and deep breathing and frequent change of position are necessary until the patient is allowed up and becomes sufficiently active to prevent limited ventilation and circulatory stasis.

As soon as the patient is well enough, a daily regimen of exercises is introduced to maintain and promote the muscular strength and joint mobility that are needed for rehabilitation. The tone of the trunk muscles, as well as that of the limb muscles, receives attention since adjustments and compensation are necessary for the amputee to maintain balance. If the leg has been amputated above the knee, the hip extensors and adductors play an important role in remobilization, as hip flexion and abduction deformity can occur. The patient should be taught active stump exercises to maintain and improve joint mobility and muscle strength. To prevent flexion contracture of a thigh stump, the patient lies in the prone position for a minimum of ½ hour two to three times a day (Fig. 25.22). If the leg has been amputated below the knee, particular attention is given to quadriceps exercises. Following the amputation of an arm, the shoulder muscles of that limb are exercised to prevent adduction and rounding of the shoulder.

The patient is allowed out of bed as soon as possible. Assistance must be available until he/she can maintain balance and is able to manoeuvre safely. In the case of a lower limb, the patient first learns to stand and gain balance, to transfer safely from bed to chair and from wheelchair to toilet. When fitted with a temporary prosthesis (pylon) the patient mobilizes using a walking aid such as a stick. A walking frame may be used by those unable to manage sticks, but it is generally not recommended as there is a risk of the patient falling backwards and also the frame limits the patient in various activities and pursuits because of its size and shape. Crutches should not be used as they hinder the patient in learning how to weight-bear. To ensure the patient is able to walk safely with walking sticks, he is first taught to walk between parallel bars, one hand holding a bar and the other a stick. The patient progresses to walking with the aid of two sticks, he is first taught to walk between parallel bars, one hand holding a bar and the other a stick. The patient progresses to walking with the aid of two sticks. If the patient has satisfactory gait and balance, he may walk with one stick, held in the opposite hand to the amputation, before his permanent prosthesis is fitted.

When the stump has sufficiently shrunk and is conditioned, measurements are taken, and a permanent prosthesis is made.

When learning to use a permanent lower limb prosthesis, the patient uses one or two walking sticks for support. When he achieves a satisfactory stable gait, he is encouraged to discontinue the use of a stick. All of this takes considerable time and perseverence; the amputee will require encouragement and support from his family and those working with him in rehabilitation. An elderly patient may feel more secure if he begins with a walking frame when he is instructed in wheelchair activities or the fitting of an appropriate prosthesis for weight-bearing is not possible.

7. Inadequate knowledge

Following an amputation, the patient and his family are taught to care for the stump and to inspect it several times daily for oedema, redness, drainage or breaks in the skin and to note any changes in sensation or tenderness. When the prosthesis is fitted, they are taught how to care for it, to assess for proper fit, what to do if the fit alters and when to return to the limb fitter for reassessment. The physiotherapist helps the patient develop a plan for continuing the exercise and activity programme at home. The nurse helps the patient and family plan how they may incorporate the recommended health care measures and activity programme into the daily routine of the patient. Referrals to a community nurse or resettlement officer are made as indicated. Arrangements are made for follow-up visits to the surgeon's clinic in the outpatient department.

EVALUATION

Expected outcomes

1 The skin over the stump is clean, dry and intact.
2 The patient indicates understanding of the phenomenon of phantom limb and phantom pain, if present.

3 The patient and family are able to express feelings regarding the loss of a body part and the change in body image.
4 The patient is able to apply the prosthesis and wear it with comfort.
5 The patient follows the planned exercise regimen to maintain and/or increase muscle tone and strength and joint function in all limbs.
6 The patient moves about safely.
7 Suitable body weight to aid mobilization is maintained or achieved.
8 The patient is able to assess the condition of the skin over the stump.
9 The patient knows how to contact the limb-fitting centre should problems occur.
10 The family takes part in the rehabilitation programme and is able to give assistance to the patient if required.

SUMMARY

Accidents can happen to anyone at anytime. For a fit young man a fractured little finger may be no more than a temporary inconvenience, whereas for an eighty year old grandmother a fractured neck of femur may lead to a major loss of independence.

Bone and joint injuries may be complicated by serious injuries to vital organs such as the brain, spinal cord and major blood vessels. Patients may have to endure many weeks of hospitalization in which a great deal of time is spent on bed rest. The nursing care, therefore, needs to reflect more than the patient's physical needs. It will need to encompass the patient's reaction to the stress of sudden immobility and accompanying dependence, in addition to possible major social problems.

Trauma nursing therefore demands a wide range of skills. Whatever the injury, all patients should be helped to maintain as much independence as possible while in hospital, to help prepare the person for as independent a life as possible in the community after discharge.

LEARNING ACTIVITIES

1. Measure a colleague with a tape measure for
   (a) Thomas Splint
   (b) Crutches
2. Teach a colleague how to use crutches in order that they might be ambulant but non weight bearing on their right leg.
3. Describe the psychological effects of sudden immobilization (of up to 4 months). What should be included in a care plan to meet the needs of such a patient?
4. Select a sample of 10 patients recently admitted after a fracture of the femoral neck region. What proportion were discharged to the same address that they were admitted from and what community arrangements were necessary? What was the age/gender distribution of these patients?

REFERENCES AND FURTHER READING

Ceccio C (1988) AIDS: scientific update, treatment and nursing care. *Orthopaedic Nursing* **7(5)**.

Ceccio C (1990) Understanding therapeutic beds. *Orthopaedic Nursing* **9(3)**: 57–70.

Clifford R, Lyons T & Webb J (1987) Complications of external fixation of open fractures of the tibia. *Injury* **18**: 174–176.

Furstenberg A (1986) Expectations about outcome following hip fracture among older people. *Social Work in Health Care* **11(4)**: 33–47.

Green JH (1978) *An Introduction to Human Physiology.* Oxford: Oxford University Press.

Harley JM, Campbell MJ & Jackson RK (1986) A comparison of plating and traction in the treatment of tibial shaft fractures. *Injury* **17**: 91–94.

Hoshowsky V (1988) Chronic lateral ligament instability of the ankle. *Orthopaedic Nursing* **7(3)**: 33–40.

Johnson L (1989) Operative management of unstable pelvic fractures. *Orthopaedic Nursing* **8(4)**: 21–25.

Jones-Walton P (1988) Effects of pin care on pin reactions in adults with extremity fracture treated with skeletal traction and external fixation. *Orthopaedic Nursing* **7(4)**: 29–33.

Judd M (1989) *Mobility: Patient Problems and Nursing Care.* London: Heinemann.

Katz K, Gonen N, Goldberg I, Mizrah J, Radwan M & Yosipovitch Z (1988) Injuries in attempted suicide by jumping from a height. *Injury* **19**: 371–374.

Lamb K, Mille J & Hernandez M (1987) Falls in the elderly: causes and prevention. *Orthopaedic Nursing* **6(2)**: 45–49.

McRae R (1989) *Practical Fracture Treatment.* Edinburgh: Churchill Livingstone.

Maheson M & Colton C (1988) Fractures of the tibial plateau in Nottingham. *Injury* **19**: 324–328.

Mims B (1989) Fat embolism syndrome: a variant of ARDS. *Orthopaedic Nursing* **8(3)**: 22–27.

Moore K & Thompson D (1989) Posttraumatic stress disorder in the orthopaedic patient. *Orthopaedic Nursing* **8(1)**: 11–18.

Morgan S (1989) *Plaster Casting: Patient Problems and Nursing Care.* London: Heinemann.

Peter N (1987) Care of patients with traumatic pelvic fractures. *Critical Care Nurse* **8(3)**: 62–77.

Schoen D (1986) *The Nursing Process in Orthopaedics.* New York: Appleton–Century–Crofts.

Simpson M (1987) Psychiatric problems on an orthopaedic ward and the traction intolerance syndrome. *Nursing RSA Verpleging* **2(8)**: 14–15.

Smith J (1990) Applying the continuous passive motion device. *Orthopaedic Nursing* **9(3)**: 54–55.

Unkle D & DeLong W (1989) Abdominal trauma associated with pelvic fractures. *Orthopaedic Nursing* **8(4)**: 27–30.

Caring for the Patient with Bone and Joint Disease

25

OBJECTIVES

By the end of this chapter the reader should be able to:

- Describe the common forms of bone and joint diseases and their effects on patients
- Assess patients with bone and joint disorders to discover actual and potential health problems
- Plan, implement and evaluate care for such patients
- Discuss the importance of social factors and the family in promoting recovery and maximum independence for the patient
- Appreciate the nurse's role in health education with regard to bone and joint disorders and its effect on patients

For the pathophysiology of bones and joints see Chapter 24. In this chapter the aim is to describe how the nurse can care for patients with diseases of the bones and joints by identifying problems, setting patient goals and giving a sound rationale of all nursing interventions.

INFLAMMATORY JOINT DISEASE

Rheumatoid arthritis

Rheumatoid arthritis is a chronic systemic disease of unknown aetiology, although current thinking suggests that there may be genetically susceptible individuals in whom a 'triggering factor' may lead to the disease.

The disease is a major health problem, being responsible for much of the existing chronic illness and crippling incapacity of adults. Women are affected about three times more often than men, although sex differences decrease with age as the prevalence of the disease increases; by the age of 69 years the sex distribution is equal (Dieppe et al, 1985). The onset is most frequent in the fourth and fifth decades of life.

In recent years, attention has been focused on an autoimmune reaction being the causative factor. Antibodies called rheumatoid factors are found in the blood of 70–80% of persons with rheumatoid arthritis. These antibodies interact with antigens in various connective tissues but the reaction is greatest in the synovium.

PATHOPHYSIOLOGY

There is some evidence that microvascular injury and mild proliferation of synovial lining cells are the initial events in rheumatoid arthritis. Leading contenders for the role of triggering factors include viruses and mycoplasms, although no confirmation exists of the role

Table 25.1 Criteria for diagnosis of rheumatoid arthritis

- Morning stiffness
- Pain and tenderness in one joint
- Swelling in one joint for 6 weeks
- Swelling in one other joint
- Symmetrical widespread joint involvement
- Nodules
- Radiological changes of rheumatoid arthritis
- Rheumatoid factor
- Characteristic synovial histology

    Seven of the above = classical rheumatoid arthritis
    Five of the above = definite rheumatoid arthritis
    Three of the above = probably rheumatoid arthritis

Major extraarticular features

• Anaemia	• Episcleritis
• Lymphadenopathy	• Keratoconjunctivitis
• Oedema	• Entrapment neuropathy
• Nodules	• Nailfold vasculitis
• Osteoporosis	• Peripheral sensory
• Muscle wasting	neuropathy

of any specific agent in the onset of the disease. The normal synovium becomes swollen and inflamed (synovitis) and eventually extends into the joint space. The process is reversible in the early stage, and the joint may be left undamaged and functional. As the inflammation continues the synovium proliferates and, with the fibrin of the inflammatory exudate, forms a thick spreading membrane of granulation tissue known as a *pannus*. It spreads over the joint surfaces, gradually eroding the cartilage, and may even destroy the denuded bone surfaces. An X-ray may show rarefaction of the ends of the involved bones. Instability and irritation of the joint may cause muscle contraction with a resulting flexion or extension deformity or subluxation of the joint. Fibrous

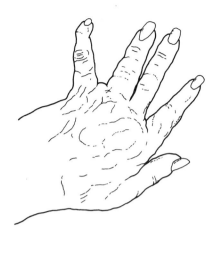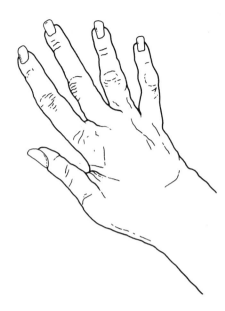

Figure 25.1 Metacarpophalangeal joint swelling with ulnar deviation.

scar tissue and adhesions develop between the opposing joint surfaces, leading to fibrous ankylosis of the joint. The exposed, roughened ends of bone tissue may eventually proliferate bone cells into the joint cavity, resulting in calcification and bony ankylosis.

The patient with rheumatoid arthritis may also have diffuse involvement of non-articular connective tissues. Degenerative lesions of the collagen component of the connective tissue may develop in muscles, tendons, blood vessels, pleura, heart or lungs.

CLINICAL CHARACTERISTICS

The onset is usually insidious; the person experiences a period of general fatigue, non-specific illness, and morning stiffness and tenderness in some joints. The small joints of the hands or feet or the wrists, elbows or knees are generally the first to be involved. The disease develops symmetrically and as it progresses, the affected joints become swollen, painful, red and increasingly difficult to move. Their range of motion is reduced. The overlying skin may take on a stretched, smooth, glossy appearance.

Muscle weakness and spasm are common in the early stages and are frequently followed by marked muscular atrophy. Unless early treatment is instituted, progressive joint tissue destruction and deformities develop, leading to permanent disability. Partial dislocation (subluxation) and flexion contractures occur. Deformities commonly seen include hyperextension of the distal phalanges, flexion contracture or ulnar deviation of the fingers due to metacarpal-phalangeal joint involvement and flexion contraction of the wrists, knees and hips (Figure 25.1). Subcutaneous nodules (*rheumatoid nodules*) appear principally on extensor surfaces or areas subjected to pressure. These are composed mainly of fibrinoid material (degenerative tissue cells) and granulation tissue.

General constitutional disturbances are manifested; the patient is pale and looks ill; anorexia, loss of weight, fatigue and depression may develop. Low-grade fever, tachycardia, anaemia and a mild leucocytosis may also be present. Later, leucopenia may develop. The erythrocyte sedimentation rate is usually elevated (normal: Westergren 3–5 mm in one hour for males and 4–10 mm in one hour for females) and, later in the disease, a blood examination may reveal the presence of the rheumatoid factor. When rheumatoid arthritis develops in children, it may be referred to as *Still's disease*. In addition to the symptoms mentioned for adults, children usually have some enlargement of the lymph nodes (lymphadenopathy).

The early stages of rheumatoid arthritis may be very similar to those of other conditions. A list of the characteristics of the disease has been formulated (Table 25.1) and these criteria, together with the extra-articular features also listed, should help the nurse to understand the widespread implications the diagnosis of 'rheumatoid arthritis' may have for a patient.

CLASSIFICATION

The disorder may be classified according to the pathological changes (clinical stages) and the loss of functional capacity (functional classification) (see Table 25.2).

Table 25.2 Classification of rheumatoid arthritis

Stage	By clinical stages Manifestations	Class	By functional classification Manifestations
1 (Early)	No evidence of joint destruction or osteoporosis	1	No loss of functional capacity
2 (Moderate)	Evidence of some destruction of cartilage and proabably of subchondral bone. No deformity but full range of motion may be limited. Adjacent muscle atrophy present	2	Able to carry out usual activities despite some discomfort and limited joint mobility
3 (Severe)	Cartilage and bone destruction quite evident. Muscle atrophy and joint deformities such as hyperextension, flexion contracture, ulnar deviation and subluxation present	3	Functional capacity impaired; occupational and self-care activities quite limited
4 (Terminal)	Criteria of stage 3 plus fibrous or bony ankylosis present	4	Confined to a wheelchair or bed; not able to carry out self-care. Dependent.

NURSING ASSESSMENT

Since rheumatoid arthritis is a systemic disease with a range of signs and symptoms that impact on all aspects of daily life, an extensive nursing *history* should be obtained that explores the following areas: (1) current local and systemic effects on the patient; (2) self-care abilities; (3) coping responses to the disease; and (4) knowledge of the disease and its management. Reliable and valid assessment tools such as the Arthritis Impact Measurement Scale (Table 25.3) may be useful as a guide to data collection.

Symptoms. The nurse should explore all symptoms the patient is experiencing to obtain some understanding of the extent of the disease. A plan of care can only be determined when the extent of the physical effects the disease has on the patient has been determined. The psychological impact will be discussed below. Determine which joints are involved and obtain a description of the severity, duration, precipitating, aggravating and relieving factors of the common problems: pain, swelling, stiffness and impaired movement. Explore the systemic symptoms of generalized weakness, fatigue, listlessness, anorexia and weight loss. Inquire about the presence of extra-articular symptoms including subcutaneous nodules, sensory loss in one or more of the extremities and dryness of the eyes.

Self-care abilities. Depending on the number and extent of symptoms present, the patient may be able to continue to perform self-care independently or may be completely dependent on others. The ability to walk and use the hands should be assessed along with general mobility. Determine from the patient what activities can be performed and how important each activity is to the patient. Continuing to perform personal hygiene is generally very important to the patient, while giving up houshold chores may be equally distressing as it represents a loss of independence.

Coping Responses. Coping with the pain, stiffness and decreased mobility of rheumatoid arthritis is often overwhelming. Equally distressing is the uncertaintly about when remissions and exacerbations may occur. The loss of self-care ability coupled with the physical effects of the disease described above can lead to the patient being depressed or very anxious and fearful for the future. The psychological effects of the illness need to be sensitively explored along with the possible social consequences if the nurse is to be able to plan care for all the patient's needs.

An assessment is made of factors influencing coping, as well as of the individual's present coping pattern. Wiener (1984) describes the arthritic patient as being caught between two imperatives: 'the inner or physiological world, monitored by pain and disability readings by day and sometimes the hour, and the outer world of activity of maintaining what is perceived as a normal existence'. Five coping strategies used by arthritic patients are cited by this same author. 'Covering up' is the principal strategy employed. Concealment of disability and pain are demonstrated by such responses as 'If anyone asks me how I am, I say fine'. The patient focuses on hiding the social significance of his handicap by making efforts to walk as normally as possible and to carry his weight in office or household tasks. This is termed 'keeping up'. 'Justifying inaction' results from use of the previous strategies and the fact that symptoms of arthritis are unpredictable. Some days the patient is successful in participating in daily activities, but is unable to do so the next day because energy has been drained by the previous efforts. The patient reacts by justifying inaction, leaving family and friends confused. 'Pacing' involves activities around periods of rest and accounting for the fact that it takes the patient longer to complete daily tasks. The ability to 'elicit help' from others varies with the individual and the person being asked for help. It may be relatively easy for a wife to ask her husband to open a jar but it may be very difficult for a single person to ask a neighbour to perform the same task. A husband may feel his role is threatened if he has to ask his wife or child to carry a heavy object.

Knowledge of the disease and its management. In order to maximize independence the patient must participate in ongoing care and this requires knowledge of the disease process and the treatment regimen. Determine the patient's knowledge base, interest level, ability to learn and degree of physical comfort. Teaching sessions in the hospital and reinforced in the community must be based on a thorough assessment (see Chapter 3).

Table 25.3 Arthritis impact measurement scales (AIMS)

Mobility

4 Are you in bed or in a chair for most or all of the day because of your health?
3 Are you able to use public transport?
2 When you travel around your community, does someone have to assist you because of your health?
1 Do you have to stay indoors most or all of the day because of your health?

Physical activity

4 Are you unable to walk unless you are assisted by another person or by a stick, crutches, artificial limbs/or braces?
3 Do you have any trouble either walking several blocks or climbing a few flights of stairs because of your health?
2 Do you have trouble bending, lifting or stooping because of your health?
1 Does your health limit the kinds of vigorous activities you can do, such as running, lifting heavy objects or participating in strenuous sports?

Dexterity

5 Can you easily write with a pen or pencil?
4 Can you easily turn a key in a lock?
3 Can you easily button articles of clothing?
2 Can you easily tie a pair of shoes?
1 Can you easily open a jar of food?

Social role

7 If you had to take medicine, could you take all your own medicine?
6 If you had a telephone, would you be able to use it?
5 Do you handle your own money?
4 If you had a kitchen, could you prepare your own meals?
3 If you had laundry facilities (washer, dryer), could you do your own laundry?
2 If you had the necessary transport, could you go shopping for food or clothes?
1 If you had household tools and appliances (e.g. vacuum, mops), could you do your own housework?

Social activity

5 About how often have you been on the telephone with close friends or relatives during the past month?
4 Has there been a change in the frequency or quality of your sexual relationships during the past month?
3 During the past month, about how often have you had friends or relatives to your home?
2 During the past month, about how often have you met socially with friends or relatives?
1 During the past month, how often have you visited friends or relatives at their homes?

Acitivities of daily living

4 How much help do you need to use the toilet?
3 How well are you able to move around?
2 How much help do you need in getting dressed?
1 When you bathe, by sponge bath, bath or shower, how much help do you need?

Pain

4 During the past month, how often have you had severe pain from your arthritis?
3 During the past month, how would you describe the arthritis pain you usually have?
2 During the past month, how long has your morning stiffness usually lasted from the time you wake up?
1 During the past month, how often have you had pain in two or more joints at the same time?

Depression

6 During the past month, how often have you felt that others would be better off if you were dead?
5 How often during the past month have you felt so down in the dumps that nothing could cheer you up?
4 How much of the time during the past month have you felt downhearted and depressed?
3 How often during the past month have you felt that nothing has turned out for you the way you wanted it to?
2 During the past month, how much of the time have you been in low or very low spirits?
1 During the past month, how much of the time have you enjoyed the things you do?

Anxiety

6 During the past month, how much of the time have you felt tense or 'strung up'?
5 How much have you been bothered by nervousness and your 'nerves' during the past month?
4 How often during the past month have you found yourself having difficulty trying to calm down?
3 How much of the time during the past month have you been able to relax without difficulty?
2 How much of the time during the past month have you felt calm and peaceful?
1 How much of the time during the past month have you felt relaxed and free of tension?

Higher scores reflect more limitations
From Meenan et al (1980).

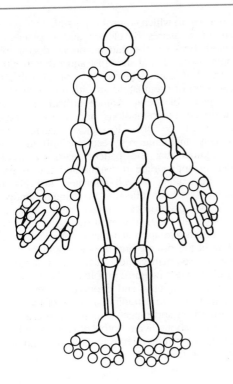

Figure 25.2 Illustration for use in joint assessment.

Lindroth et al (1989) describe a study in which patients with arthritis were involved in an education programme about osteoarthritis and rheumatoid arthritis. Previous papers (Vignos et al, 1976; Lorig et al, 1985) have suggested that informed patients would practise self-care more often and show reduced disability from these diseases. The intervention group of 100 patients was given six sessions by a health care professional covering all aspects of the diseases. They were given questionnaires at 1, 3 and 12 months after the programme. A control group of 95 patients was given questionnaires at the same time. The results confirmed previous findings that, following an educational programme, patients can demonstrate an increase in knowledge, enjoy better health and suffer less from the disabling effects of arthritis.

Individual joints or groups of joints and their surrounding tissues are observed, palpated and their range of motion determined. Joints are inspected for swelling, redness, physical deformity, discoloration, scars or discharge. The adjoining muscles are observed for signs of atrophy. Each joint is compared with the corresponding joint for symmetry and degree of change. Painful joints are supported by the examiner's hands and movements are performed gently and slowly. Joint function and muscle strength may be appraised also by using resistance. This involves the examiner applying pressure against which the patient actively performs a specific movement (for example, the examiner's hands are placed on the patient's lower arm, pressure is applied and the patient is asked to flex the forearm).

Illustrations of the human body may be used to record joint assessment and provide an overview of involved joints (Figure 25.2). A goniometer, which measures angles, may be used to measure degrees of movement of a joint. For example, the normal range of flexion of an elbow is 135–150°, and tension 0–5°; hip abduction varies from 45–50°, with hip adduction being approximately 20–30°. Some decrease in mobility of joints occurs with age.

DIAGNOSTIC PROCEDURES

Radiographs are made of the joint(s) and may include *arthrography*, in which a radiopaque contrast medium is injected into the joint cavity so that the soft tissue components may be visualized. This is generally done with investigation of a knee. The procedure takes 30–45 minutes. No special post-test precautions are necessary and the patient should be reassured that the contrast substance will be reabsorbed systemically and joint swelling will subside.

Aspiration of synovial fluid may be performed to obtain a specimen for laboratory examination for the presence of blood, pus, organisms, sodium urate crystals or malignant cells. A local anaesthetic is used and strict asepsis must be observed although use of sterile gloves and draping are not necessarily routine. A large-bore needle is inserted into the joint space to aspirate a fluid specimen. No special precautions are required after the procedure. The synovial fluid of a patient with rheumatoid arthritis may be cloudy or have a greenish hue and will have an elevated leucocyte level.

An *arthroscopy* may be done to provide endoscopic examination of a joint. It is used most often in knee disorders. The doctor is able to visualize and assess the synovium, articular surfaces, menisci and ligaments, and a biopsy of synovial tissue may also be done.

The examination is performed in the operating theatre under strict aseptic conditions.

A large-bore needle is introduced into the joint following anaesthesia and normal saline is introduced to 'fill out' the cavity. The arthroscope is then introduced. Following the examination the puncture area is sealed and a compression bandage applied. Activity is usually limited for approximately 3 days. Arthroscopic examination of the rheumatoid arthritis patient reveals cartilage destruction with fibrous scar formation. Synovial villi appear swollen, thick and pale.

The *electromyograph* (EMG) measures and records the electrical activity of skeletal muscles. Information is provided about the strength of the muscle's response. No physical preparation of the patient is necessary but the patient receives an explanation of the procedure beforehand.

Laboratory *blood and serum tests* that may be used in investigation of rheumatoid arthritis and other disorders include: (1) erythrocyte and leucocyte counts; (2) determination of haemoglobin, erythrocyte sedimentation rate (ESR), serum alkaline phosphatase, calcium and phosphorus concentrations and blood uric acid level; and (3) examination for rheumatoid (Rh) factors, antinuclear antibodies (ANA), lupus erythematosus cells (LE prep), anti-DNA and complement fixation.

The blood cell counts, haemoglobin and ESR are used to determine the presence of anaemia, infection or tissue destruction. The serum phosphatase level is elevated in malignant disease, as is the ESR. The phosphorus and calcium concentrations are significant in bone disease, and the blood uric acid level is increased in gout. The presence of rheumatoid factors and autoimmune antibodies in serum occurs in 85% of people with late stage rheumatoid arthritis. The *latex fixation test* is most commonly used to identify rheumatoid factor IgG. Antinuclear antibodies and lupus erythematosus cells are usually present in patients with acute, active systemic lupus erythematosus. The anti-DNA test detects antibodies which react with DNA and is considered a specific test for systemic lupus erythematosus.

PATIENT PROBLEMS

Assessment of the patient with rheumatoid arthritis will often reveal some or all of the following problems:

- *Reduced physical mobility* related to inflammation and deformity of joints, muscle weakness and atrophy, and limitation in range of motion of joints.
- *Activity intolerance* related to disease process and to prescribed treatments.
- *Alteration in comfort and pain*, related to the disease process and accentuated by movement.
- *Alteration in self-care activities* related to decrease in activity tolerance and to knowledge deficit.
- *Alteration in mood* related to pain and decreased mobility.
- *Alteration in nutrition* related to intake lower than body requirements.
- *Knowledge deficit* related to self-management of rheumatoid arthritis.

The nurse and patient should work together to determine patient centred goals.

The *goals* derive from the identified problems and generally include: maintain/increase mobility and activity tolerance; obtain relief of pain and discomfort; perform self-care in daily living; achieve an optimal nutritional intake and achieve/maintain a positive mood state. The overall goal is to achieve a maximum state of wellness within the limitations imposed by a chronic and potentially disabling health problem. Criteria for evaluation of goal attainment should be negotiated with the patient. The nurse uses assessment skills in determining the extent to which each goal is achieved. Criteria may include any of the following: (1) demonstrates stable or improved joint mobility; (2) demonstrates an optimal level of functional mobility; (3) performs therapeutic measures to minimize further impairment of joint function; (4) controls pain through appropriate use of treatment measures including medications; (5) maintains a satisfactory level of independence; (6) consumes a well-balanced diet; (7) demonstrates a satisfactory level of psychosocial health.

NURSING INTERVENTION

Rheumatoid arthritis is a disease for which there is no cure but one in which control is possible by the use of a variety of measures developed and implemented in teamwork between the patient, nurse, doctor, physiotherapist, occupational therapist and other health care workers. The patient plays the critical role in the management of rheumatoid arthritis and the attainment of the goals of therapy. Since arthritis is a disease characterized by remissions and exacerbations, the patient must be able to adjust management appropriately, including rest, exercise and medications. This requires that the patient learn to make and implement appropriate decisions and this is possible only if the patient is well informed. Arthritis patient education has been effective in changing knowledge, behaviours, psychosocial status and health status (Lindroth et al, 1989). The most successful programmes use an interactive approach that emphasizes an understanding of the disease and the development of a daily routine of self-management activities. Education that includes coping strategies, problem solving approaches to common problems, and endurance exercise should supplement the more traditional areas of focus such as joint protection and range of motion exercises.

Education about living with arthritis should include the family and can be offered in individual and/or group sessions (see Chapter 3).

Maintain/increase, mobility and activity tolerance. Maintenance of joint mobility and the promotion of optimal joint function and activity tolerance are achieved through a combination of planned rest and exercise, and by protecting the joints from unnecessary stress. Planning and implementation of care requires co-operation between the nurse, physiotherapist and occupational therapist, doctor, patient and family.

Rest. Rest is necessary for the patient with impaired joint mobility; it helps to control fatigue, inflammation and pain. The patient with limitation of joint function expends excessive energy in movement. Bed rest may be prescribed for a brief period during acute episodes of the disease when many joints are acutely inflamed and when systemic symptoms such as fever, anaemia and severe fatigue are present. Body positioning is important to prevent contractures and deformity during periods of bed rest and during sleep.

The patient should rest and sleep in a position as nearly anatomical as possible, that is with knees and elbows fully extended and with the neck and wrists in a near-neutral position. Pillows may be placed under the full length of the legs to maintain extension of the leg when the patient is supine, but never under a painful knee or elbow as this contributes to the development of contractures.

When an acute episode of the disease has passed, patients are encouraged to continue to have several rest periods throughout the day and to alternate periods of activity with periods of rest. Patients must be convinced that rest is as important a part of their treatment regimen as medications, exercise and splinting, and must be assisted to develop a balanced programme of rest and exercise. Relaxation techniques may also be

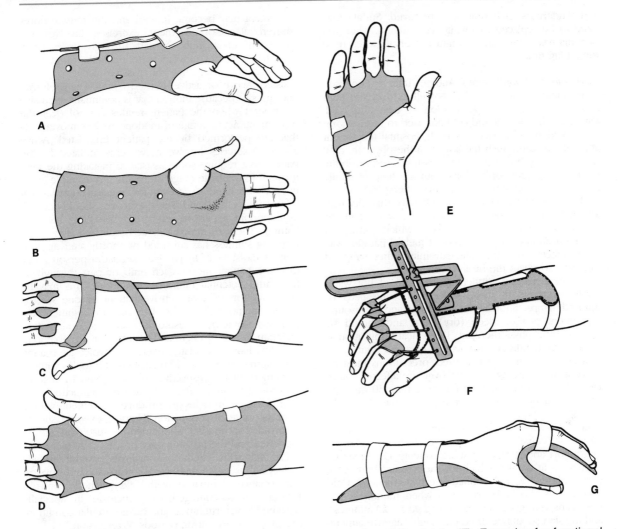

Figure 25.3 Different types of splint. (A)–(E), Resting splints to immobilize joints. (F), Example of a functional splint used to stabilize and support a joint during activity. (G), A corrective (dynamic) splint used to immobilize an involved joint, realign soft tissue or correct contractures or deformities.

used by the patient to promote body relaxation and decrease emotional stress.

Joint rest may involve the use of splints to support and protect involved joints. The type of splint which may be applied depends on the purpose to be achieved (Figure 25.3). Resting splints are used to immobilize inflamed and painful joints and are worn continuously during periods of acute inflammation. They are removed for short intervals for essential activities such as eating and cleansing of the skin. During chronic or inactive phases of joint disease, rest splints are worn only at night. Functional splints are designed to stabilize and support a joint during activity. Corrective or dynamic splints are used to immobilize an involved joint, realign soft tissues or correct contractures or deformities. Splints are usually made of a lightweight thermoplastic

material which is pliable when heated. They are moulded to the affected part and held in place with Velcro straps. The patient's skin is protected from the splint by a layer of cloth material. The protective layer is either placed on the patient (e.g. a tube stocking) or is incorporated into the splint. Splints may be used on the fingers, hands, wrists, knees or ankles. Cervical collars may be used to restrict movement of the head and neck and thus protect the extremely vulnerable joint between the first and second cervical vertebrae. Patients and family members should learn how to apply the splint and how to prevent any side-effects such as skin breakdown. A demonstration should be given to illustrate the pressure points that are created if the splint is not a proper fit or is not applied correctly. The patient is taught to inspect the skin under the splint for redness and tenderness each time it is removed. Splints may need to be replaced following acute illness, when the oedema has abated, and at regular intervals when used for a long time.

Heat and cold applications. Another intervention used to maintain/increase mobility as well as decrease pain and discomfort is the application of heat and cold. Various forms of heat and cold are used to reduce joint inflammation and muscle spasm. In hospital the patient generally receives such therapy from the physiotherapy department. At home the patient assumes responsibility for heat and cold applications, with the help of family and the community nurse and physiotherapist.

Moist heat is considered more effective than dry heat and may be applied in the form of a warm bath or shower, or paraffin wax immersion, which consists of the application of several layers of melted paraffin wax to the affected extremity. The extremity is then wrapped in plastic to retain the heat.

Dry heat may be applied in the form of hot water bottles wrapped in towels, electric heating pads or infrared lamps. Short-wave diathermy and ultrasound equipment provide deep (dry) heat and should be applied by a physiotherapist. Deep heat application is usually contraindicated for acutely inflamed joints.

Whatever form of heat is used, precautions must be used against burning the skin over the affected joints. Heat should not be applied for more than 30 minutes, and should not be used if the patient has decreased sensation or poor circulation.

Applications of cold in the form of ice packs may be more or equally as effective as heat in relieving discomfort and spasm for some patients. Cold may be applied as in ice water bath for the affected body part, or as a plastic bag pack applied directly to the joint. Cold applications should be removed when numbness has been achieved (generally not more than 15–20 minutes), and the skin should be dried thoroughly after treatment. Cold should not be used if the patient has impaired circulation. Selection of either heat or cold is usually based on patient preference and perceived effectiveness of the modality in relieving pain and spasm.

Exercise. General exercise and therapeutic exercises contribute to the maintenance and promotion of joint function. An individualized exercise programme is designed by the physiotherapist in consultation with the patient, nurse and medical staff. Patients are told the purpose and importance of exercise in the management of their disease. Although the exercise programme is supervised by a physiotherapist or nurse when it is first begun, it is eventually performed by the patient as independently as possible. Support, including family members, can provide encouragement and assistance to the patient as the exercise programme is incorporated into daily living. Patients are encouraged to report excessive fatigue or increased pain associated with the performance of their exercises so that the programme can be modified.

Any exercise programme includes a *range-of-motion* component. Normally, each joint is capable of a certain range of movement. In a joint disorder, that range of movement may become limited and the muscle fibres shorten. Range-of-movement exercises involves the movement of a limb or part through its maximal potential range of movement to maintain or increase joint function. They may be passive, active or active assisted. Active or active assisted exercise is preferred over passive because motion that is potentially excessive is avoided when the patient retains control over the movement. Active range of motion involves movements that are performed by the patient unassisted. Active assisted exercises involve movements initiated by the patient that require some assistance in taking the joint through its available range of motion. An example is the use of one hand to stretch the metacarpophalangeal joints of the other hand. These exercises should become as important a part of self-care as brushing teeth or bathing. They are most easily accomplished after initial morning stiffness has subsided or shortly after application of moist heat. In passive exercise a person other than the patient moves each limb or part through its maximum potential range of movement. This may be necessary for an apprehensive patient or one who is unable to move the limbs. The exercise regimen also includes isometric or isotonic exercises, designed to maintain muscle strength and maintain or promote joint mobility. Isometric (static) exercises involve alternating maximum contraction and relaxation of muscles without movement of the respective part and joint. In isotonic exercise (dynamic) there is active contraction and shortening of muscles to produce movement with a minimal force of contraction. Isotonic exercise should be avoided if the joint is inflamed because pain will be increased and the inflammatory process may increase.

Patients with rheumtoid arthritis exhibit greatly reduced muscle strength, aerobic capacity and physical performance compared with age-matched controls. Patients are encouraged to participate in specially designed long-term fitness and cardiovascular conditioning programmes during periods of remission.

Surgical procedures. Various surgical procedures may be used with arthritic patients to facilitate joint function and mobility, retard disease progress or correct a deformity. These procedures and the nursing care of the patient are described in the section on osteoarthritis (see p. 900).

Obtain relief of pain and discomfort. The pain associated with rheumatoid arthritis is variable in intensity and aggravated by movement. Although the amount of pain does not always correlate with the degree of inflammation present, it generally corresponds to the pattern of joint involvement. Pain is further caused by muscle spasm that develops adjacent to affected joints. Patients should be advised that the therapies for maintenance of joint function are also useful in the relief of pain. Rest, splinting, the use of heat and cold applications and the continuation of muscle strengthening exercises all help to prevent and relieve pain. The patient can be helped to identify those activities that aggravate and relieve pain and take action to improve pain control.

Drug therapy with one or more classes of phar-

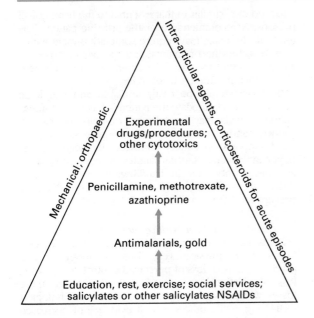

Figure 25.4 Treatment pyramid for rheumatoid arthritis.

macological agents has a vital role in the management of rheumatoid arthritis and the associated pain. The pyramid approach (Figure 25.4) provides a helpful guide to the addition of drugs to the non-pharmaceutical approach to treatment described above.

Drug therapy. Non-steroid anti-inflammatory agents (NSAID) provide the first line of therapy in rheumatoid arthritis. Their main purpose is to relieve joint pain and inflammation. The agent most commonly used is *acetylsalicylic acid* (aspirin). It is prescribed in relatively large doses and must be taken regularly at the intervals stated in order to maintain effective plasma salicylate levels. Salicylates have numerous side-effects that must be monitored by the patient and the nurse including gastrointestinal disturbance, tinnitus and loss of auditory acuity particularly in the elderly.

Other non-steroidal anti-inflammatory drugs are available should the salicylate compounds fail to control pain or be intolerable to the patient.

Ibuprofen (Brufen) is an anti-inflammatory, analgesic drug also used in the treatment of arthritis. The principal side-effects that develop with some patients are nausea, vomiting, diarrhoea and dizziness.

Indomethacin (Indocin) may be prescribed for its anti-inflammatory, analgesic and antipyretic effects. Some patients cannot tolerate it because of side-effects, which may be gastrointestinal irritation and ulceration, nausea, headache, depression, dizziness and a sense of detachment.

Other NSAIDs include: naproxen (Naprosyn), fenoprofen (Fenopron), piroxicam (Feldene) and sulindac (Clinoril). Salicylates are generally not used with other NSAIDs, nor is more than one NSAID used at one time because of the possibility of increased risk of side-effects.

If the pain and discomfort continue or if there is evidence of gastric erosions, second-line drugs including gold or antimalarials are added to the drug therapy. They have the capacity to alter the course of the disease but are used in conjunction with NSAIDs because they exert only minimal anti-inflammatory effects.

Gold compounds are preferred because of substantial evidence of their efficacy. When a preparation of *gold salts* such as sodium aurothiamalate (Myocrisin) is given, the patient is observed closely for signs of toxic reactions. The initial dose is small to test the patient for adverse reactions. Reactions that may be seen include stomatitis (inflammation of the oral mucous membrane), dermatitis, renal damage and bone marrow depression leading to severe anaemia, leucopenia (agranulocytosis) and thrombocytopenia. Gold therapy usually involves an intramuscular injection given each week for a period of 4–6 months. Most responses occur during the first 16 weeks of treatment. Once a response has been obtained, maintenance therapy should be continued. Urine analysis and blood cell counts are done weekly, and the patient is checked for possible signs or symptoms of adverse side-effects.

The *antimalarial drugs* such as chloroquine (Nivaquine) and hydroxychloroquine (Plaquenil) may be prescribed over a period of several months for some patients. Toxic effects that may develop include skin eruptions, headache, anorexia, nausea, vomiting and auditory or visual disturbances. Frequent blood cell counts are done because occasionally bone marrow depression occurs, and frequent eye examinations are required to check for keratopathy which is reversible or a serious irreversible retinopathy.

Adrenal corticosteroids are now usually reserved for patients whose rheumatoid arthritis is rapidly progressing, is very painful and has not responded to therapeutic courses of other antirheumatic drugs. Examples of oral preparations used are prednisone, prednisolone and hydrocortisone. The dosage is individualized and kept to a minimum because of the unfavourable side-effects which may develop. It is important that the patient understand that the drug will be given only for a limited period. The dosage is gradually reduced and then completely withdrawn. Adverse side-effects which are likely to develop with overdosage or prolonged therapy include reduced lymphocyte and antibody production, leading to increased susceptibility to infection, sodium and water retention, excessive potassium excretion, mood swings or euphoria, restlessness or overactivity, hyperglycaemia and glucosuria, fullness or rounding of the face (moon face) and growth of hair on the face in the case of a female. The patient who has experienced increased appetite, a marked sense of well-being and some remission of the disease while receiving a corticosteroid may feel quite depressed and let down when the drug is withdrawn, and will require considerble emotional support from the nurse.

Immunosuppressive drugs such as azathioprine (Imuran) and cyclophosphamide have been used in treating the patient with rheumatoid arthritis, using the rationale that the cause is an antigen-antibody reaction. These drugs are prescribed for patients who are unresponsive to any of the drugs mentioned previously in this section.

Table 25.4 Guidelines for joint protection.

- Maintain good posture and body alignment at all times
- Change position frequently
- Use the largest muscles and strongest joints available for any task
- Distribute weight of objects over several joints
- Perform activities slowly and smoothly
- Limit repetitive movements
- Minimize use of swollen, painful joints
- Stop activity when pain occurs
- Space activities to provide frequent rest periods
- Use assistive devices in the environment to eliminate unnecessary stress

The suppression of leucocyte and antibody formation makes the patient very susceptible to infection. The rheumatoid arthritic patient is frequently debilitated and already has a lowered resistance. Precautions are necessary to avoid exposure to infection; recognition of early symptoms is reported promptly so an antibiotic may be prescribed. The patient should be fully informed of the major side-effects which can occur with these drugs.

- *Carry out daily self-care.* Activities which previously seemed very simple and were taken for granted become difficult and time consuming for the patient with rheumatoid arthritis. Often there are some activities that are of particular importance to the patient, whether related to personal hygiene, housekeeping or social and recreational life. The nurse can help the patient identify key areas and encourage performance of self-care in these areas. The importance of alternating periods of rest with periods of activity should be reinforced. Self-help devices should be provided to maximize independence. The occupational therapist has an important role in providing such aids and the nurse reinforces their importance and usefulness.

Table 25.4 lists general guidelines which help a patient to protect a damaged, inflamed or painful joint from further injury. The patient learns new ways to perform activities to decrease stress on affected joints. Conditions and unnecessary movements which cause pain and discomfort are avoided and the person learns to perform tasks with the least effort and greatest efficiency to minimize joint stress.

Family members must be included in any discussion of self-care, since they must allow the patient to achieve maximum independence. This may be difficult for those who feel that 'doing for' the patient is helpful. Instead, they should encourage the patient to perform activities alone or with help as requested. They need to be aware of the additional time and patience required to allow the patient to achieve various activities that appear so simple.

- *Achieve an optimal nutritional intake.* Nutritional problems including anorexia, weight loss and anaemia frequently accompany rheumatoid arthritis. A well-balanced diet, similar to that essential to the health of all persons, is recommended for the arthritic patient. The total calorie intake may require some adjustment with a view to achieving or maintaining the person's normal weight. Obesity increases the strain on joints and may also reduce motivation to exercise.

Breakfast should be easily available and simple to prepare to accommodate the patient's morning stiffness. Eating utensils may be adapted to help the patient. Padded handles on cutlery make them easier to grip; hand supports on cutlery eliminate the need for fine finger movements; special handles on cups and glasses are easier and safer in handling; suction cups stop dishes from sliding; and high edges on dishware prevent food from spilling.

- *Achieve/maintain a positive mood state.* Rheumatoid arthritis may be accompanied by a number of significant losses, both physical (e.g. loss of mobility) and psychosocial (e.g. loss of perceived control, loss of role, loss of relationships). Some patients manage these losses without significant threat to their psychological well-being, while others exhibit evidence of decreased psychosocial health, including symptoms of anxiety, depression and a withdrawal from others. Psychosocial health in rheumatoid arthritis patients is influenced by many factors, including level of perceived support from others and a sense of helplessness toward the disease. Recent research suggests that severity of impairment and disability are not major factors in the mood state of rheumatoid arthritis patients. The nurse has an important role in assisting the patient to achieve and maintain a positive mood state, despite having rheumatoid arthritis. Since emotional and instrumental support from family and friends influences response to illness, the nurse needs to determine with the patient who makes up the patient's social network and who provides the most valuable support. If the patient receives limited support, the nurse can work with the patient to identify alternative sources of support such as self-help groups and home care agencies.

Helping the patient to learn management of the disease is essential. This decreases the feelings of helplessness and hopelessness that the patient may experience and influences the psychological health of the patient. The nurse and other health team members must continue to support the patient and family as they learn about the disease. Since this encouragement and support must continue in the community, referral to appropriate community agencies should be made.

Nursing intervention also involves helping the patient to identify feelings about the illness and what it means. By identifying how he or she copes in certain situations, the patient develops insight into his or her behaviour and looks at the consequences of that behaviour and the alternatives open. Is social interaction worth the cost of occasional embarrassment and/or excessive fatigue? Covering up and keeping up drain the patient's energy, and asking for help may reinforce fears of being dependent. Hope may be a positive factor that motivates the patient to comply with therapy and learn to control symptoms. It may also be a negative force, prompting the patient to self-treatment, use of home remedies and quackery. The patient and family need opportunities to discuss such ideas to help in making decisions about what is best for the patient. Family members and friends also need the opportunity to express their feelings and develop understanding of the patient's illness, limitations and potentials and how to respond to the daily or even hourly fluctuations in the patient's behaviour.

• *Preparation for discharge.* Specific actions are required to prepare the patient for discharge from hospital in addition to those actions taken throughout a patient's hospitalization. The quality of life of the patient with rheumatoid arthritis following discharge depends largely on the severity of the patient's disease and whether or not the pathological process in the joints is arrested. Obviously, if the disease is severe and more and more joints are progressively involved, the patient is less likely to be well enough to return to a former occupation and will require a more active and closely supervised care programme. Many patients are well enough to go to work and adjust their daily life to provide for extra rest as well as continuance of a daily physical exercise regimen. A period of vocational training or assessment by the Disablement Resettlement Officer (DRO) may be necessary before the arthritic patient can be re-employed.

If the patient is sufficiently handicapped to require physical care, a referral will be made to the community nurse. The community nurse and the occupational therapist can be of assistance in assessing the home situation and making recommendations for adjustments that will simplify the care of the patient and will increase mobility and independence.

The patient and family should be acquainted with the societies and organizations which are concerned with rheumatic disease and with publications that may be helpful. Transport is frequently a problem for the person with arthritis. If the patient is required to go regularly to physiotherapy as an out-patient or to a rehabilitation unit, hospital transport may need to be organized.

Evaluation

Evaluation of nursing action is an ongoing process that is directed by the goals negotiated with the patient. Nursing action is effective if it assists the patient to achieve optimal physical and psychosocial function.

DEGENERATIVE JOINT DISEASE

Osteoarthritis (osteoarthrosis)

Osteoarthritis, also known as osteoarthrosis or degenerative arthritis, is a common chronic joint disorder characterized by degenerative changes in articular cartilage and marginal bony overgrowth. The disorder affects both men and women, but has a higher incidence in women over the age of 55. The prevalence of the disease increases with age and is almost universal in individuals over the age of 75. The placement of stress on joints is implicated in the development of osteoarthritis regardless of age, so that previous trauma, athletics, obesity and strenous labour are all considered factors in the development of the disease. Genetic factors are important in certain presentations of the disease. Over 5 million people in the UK alone suffer significant pain and disability from osteoarthritis (Dieppe et al, 1985).

PATHOPHYSIOLOGY

The pathology of osteoarthritis is associated with biochemical and inflammatory changes that occur in response to ongoing stress on affected joints. The cartilage on the articular ends of the bones becomes thin and worn and gradually breaks down, leaving the denuded bone exposed. The reaction of the denuded bone is manifested in outgrowths of bone from the joint margins, resulting in thickening of the ends of the bones and protruding ridges and spurs (osteophytes) which impair joint movement. Spurs may break off and become loose in the joint, causing further impairment of movement and more pain.

The weight-bearing joints, such as the hip and knee, and the interphalangeal joints of the fingers are most frequently the site of degenerative joint disease. It may occur in a single joint or may involve several.

CLINICAL CHARACTERISTICS

The clinical manifestations of the disease include soreness and an aching, poorly-localized pain that occurs with use of the involved joint(s) and is relieved by rest. As the disease progresses, pain occurs even at rest. Joint stiffness is most pronounced in the morning and after periods of activity during the day, and usually lasts less than 30 minutes. The patient complains of stiffness, soreness and pain in the affected joint(s). Crepitation may be felt or heard on movement. The range of motion becomes increasingly limited because of pain, muscle spasm and the bony outgrowths. Joint enlargement and instability develop, and the joint feels hard and irregular. Bony outgrowths on the dorsal surface of affected interphalangeal joints give the knuckles a knobby or gnarled appearance; these knobby protrusions are referred to as *Heberden's nodes.* Affected joint protuberances occurring on the proximal interphalangeal joints of the fingers are called *Bouchard's nodes.* Systemic manifestations do not occur.

NURSING ASSESSMENT

Pain, stiffness and decreased mobility should be assessed. The nurse should ask the patient what makes the symptom better or worse, where the symptom is located, the onset, frequency and duration of each symptom and how the symptom rates on a scale of 0 to 5, with 5 being the worst. Assess how much each symptom interferes with the ability to perform self-care and work-related activities and what changes the patient has made in usual daily life. Equally important is an evaluation of the emotional response of the patient to the disease. Some patients feel helpless and hopeless because of the limitations imposed by the disease while others continue to enjoy life despite having osteoarthritis.

The patient's gait, movement and ability to walk are observed. All joints are assessed with particular attention to those most troublesome to the patient. Detail on the assessment of joints and surrounding structures is presented in the section on rheumatoid arthritis. It is important to gather data in this way not only to identify problem areas where nursing intervention is required, but also as a baseline against which to measure progress. A pain rating scale of 1 to 10 for example allows careful pain control while a progressively reducing stiffness rating allows both patient and nurse to see progress. This can act as a powerful reinforcer for the patient, encouraging maximum participation in a plan of therapy. Assessment should therefore be an ongoing activity rather than a one off activity performed on admission.

PATIENT PROBLEMS

Assessment of the patient with osteoarthritis will often identify one or all of the following health problems:

- *Alteration in comfort* related to the disease process and accentuated by activity.
- *Impaired physical mobility* related to limitations in the range of motion of joints.
- *Alteration in self-care activities* related to knowledge deficit and to decrease in activity tolerance.
- *Mood alteration* related to discomfort and reduced mobility.

The *goals* of patient care are formulated between the nurse and the patient and are directed to the identified health problems. Overall goals for patients with osteoarthritis include achieving optimal physical mobility, relief of pain and discomfort and attaining realistic levels of independence and hopefulness for the future. Medical and surgical interventions are important components of treatment as are physiotherapy and occupational therapy. Most patients are treated conservatively but if the pain becomes intractable and the disability severe, surgery is indicated. The nurse has a role in the total care of the patient, including the co-ordination of the various patient services. The nurse and patient work together to identify patient centred goals; these may include: (1) demonstrates optimal physical mobility; (2) demonstrates appropriate action to control pain; (3) maintains a satisfactory level of independence; and (4) demonstrates a satisfactory level of psychosocial health.

NURSING INTERVENTION

- *Achieving optimal physical mobility.* Appropriate exercises are prescribed to maintain muscle tone and movement and promote good alignment and joint stability. The patient is encouraged to be posture conscious and to review regular daily activities and posture. Work should be interspersed with short intervals of rest, and unnecessary walking, climbing

stairs, lifting and bending should be eliminated. A fitted corset may be helpful to immobilize and provide support in the case of degenerative changes in the spine. A firm mattress with a 'fracture' board between it and the bedsprings is recommended to promote good alignment and support for the affected joints.

- *Relief of pain.* Patients with osteoarthritis are encouraged to use the same measures for pain relief and joint protection as outlined for the patient with rheumatoid arthritis: application of heat and cold; splinting; use of assistive devices; rest alternating with activity and the maintenance of an exercise programme.

Medications used in treating the patient with osteoarthritis are prescribed primarily to control pain. They include analgesic agents and non-steroidal anti-inflammatory agents described in the section on rheumatoid arthritis. Since no medications are known that halt the disease process of osteoarthritis, medications such as gold compounds and hydroxychloroquine are generally not prescribed for osteoarthritis patients.

Local corticosteroids injected into the affected joint provide short-term relief. Joint surgery is indicated for pain and disability that is unrelieved by these measures.

- *Promoting maximum independence and hope for the future.* Achievement of both these goals is influenced by a programme of patient education and the input of family and other health professionals. The actions outlined for the patient with rheumatoid arthritis should also be implemented with osteoarthritis patients.

SURGICAL TREATMENT

When an arthritic or deformed joint causes intractable pain and severe disability, surgical intervention may be undertaken. The operative procedures used are osteotomy, arthrodesis or total replacement arthroplasty.

Osteotomy is the reshaping of the bone by cutting or curettement. This surgery is mainly used on young patients with osteoarthritis whose range of motion is still good but whose pain requires surgical relief.

Arthrodesis is the surgical fusion of a joint, which results in loss of joint movement. It is done to provide relief from pain or to correct joint instability. In this surgery, the articular cartilage is removed and bone grafts are implanted across the joint surface. Arthrodesis is rarely used now in the management of knee or hip osteoarthritis but is considered in the treatment of severe osteoarthritis of the cervical spine.

An *arthroplasty* is a reconstructive procedure that may entail replacement of part of the joint or of the whole joint with a prosthesis. It is done to relieve pain and permit patient mobility.

Total hip replacement

Total hip arthroplasty is being used frequently with

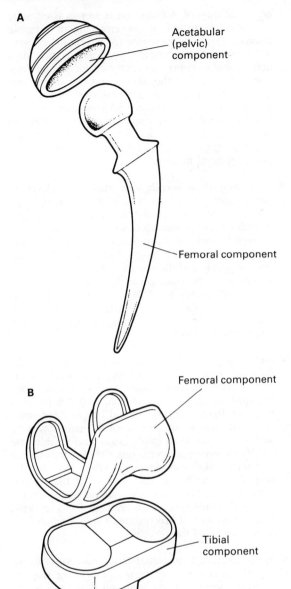

Acetabular
(pelvic)
component

Femoral component

Femoral component

Tibial
component

Figure 25.5 (A) Total hip arthroplasty prosthesis. (B) Knee replacement prosthesis.

patients with degenerative joint disease and involves surgical replacement of both articulating surfaces of the joint. The femoral head and neck are removed. The cartilage is removed from the acetabulum and a polyethylene cup is fitted into the socket. Surgical bone cement may be used to secure the plastic cup to the surface of the acetabulum or a porous, non-cemented prosthesis is used. The head and neck of the femur are then replaced by a metal prosthesis consisting of a spherical head and stem (Figure 25.5). The latter is implanted and cemented into the proximal portion of the femoral shaft. The ball part of the prosthesis is fitted into the acetabulum and tested for a range of motions to make sure it does not dislocate on movement. It is important that the nurse caring for the patient is familiar with the postsurgical position to be maintained and when movement may be resumed in order that the prosthesis does not accidentally dislocate. If surgical cement is not used, the period of immobility is longer. When the wound is closed, a closed drainage system is established to promote drainage of accumulating secretions and decrease the potential for infection, as blood is an excellent medium for the growth of microorganisms. Until adduction movements are judged safe by the surgeon the limb should be kept in abduction.

Nursing care of the patient experiencing total hip replacement includes thorough preoperative teaching, careful postoperative monitoring and preparation of the patient for discharge.

Preoperative care
Assessment should cover the usual physical parameters required for all patients who are to have surgery under general anaesthetic. In addition long term medication and possible side effects should be determined. The patient's psychological assessment should include examining how realistic the person is being about the benefits of surgery in order that unrealistic expectations may be dealt with appropriately. Family and social factors should also be explored. Prior to surgery, the patient should be given a simple but complete explanation of the surgical procedure, including information about the surgical incision required and the prosthesis to be used. Use of diagrams and written materials is helpful in conveying this information.

The patient must also be told what to expect postoperatively and how to help in the rehabilitation process. The importance of abduction of the hip is explained and techniques to maintain abduction demonstrated. These may include the use of abduction splints, wedge pillows or two or three pillows between the legs. The limits of hip flexion should be explained (45–60°). An overhead bed frame or pulley can be used to demonstrate how the patient can move about the bed after surgery.

The patient requires instruction in and practice of postoperative exercises. Emphasis should be placed on the purpose of each part of the exercise regimen. Deep breathing and coughing are important to facilitate venous return and to prevent hypostatic pneumonia. Exercises including quadriceps and gluteal contractions and plantar and dorsiflexion of the toes and ankles are essential to maintain function and aid circulation. A complete preoperative assessment is conducted by the surgical team and includes an electrocardiogram, chest X-ray and blood examination (e.g. blood cell counts and determination of haemoglobin, serum electrolyte levels and prothrombin time). The patient's blood is typed and cross-matched and blood is made available for blood replacement during the surgery, and postoperatively if necessary.

During the preoperative period, an anticoagulant and

antibiotic may be prescribed. The anticoagulant is administered to reduce the risk of thrombophlebitis and ensuing embolism, and to promote microcirculation in the operative site. Because infection is a very serious postoperative complication, the surgeon may commence antibiotic therapy before the surgery as a prophylactic measure. Local skin preparation will be indicated by the surgeon.

Postoperative Care

In the immediate postoperative assessment, the nurse monitors carefully for the complications and sequelae of any surgery, including the state of the wound, pain, shock and haemorrhage.

Patient centred goals include: (1) hip is maintained in correct anatomical position; (2) prescribed exercise plan is followed in hospital and plan for exercise post-discharge is described; (3) the patient is free of pain; (4) infection is prevented in the postoperative period and plan to prevent infection post-discharge is described; (5) satisfactory cardiovascular, neurovascular and respiratory function are maintained; (6) anxiety related to surgery is controlled; and (7) mobility is restored to the affected joint.

- *Preventing dislocation of the hip prosthesis.* Nursing actions to maintain the prosthesis in position include positioning of the patient in bed, assistance with early ambulation and instructions for physical mobility at home. The patient returns from surgery supine and will have abductor splints or pillows in place to keep the hip in abduction and maintain neutral rotation. Acute flexion of the hip must be avoided due to the risk of dislocation. Indications of dislocation, including severe hip pain, shortening of the affected extremity, a firm palpable mass in the operative area or internal or external hip rotation, and report possible dislocation immediately. Two nurses are generally required when turning the patient. One nurse supports the limb, maintaining the abducted position, while the second person turns the patient to the unaffected side. Pillows are placed anteriorly and posteriorly to provide support in the side-lying position.

A limited range of movement and slow flexion of the hip are introduced and gradually increased under the supervision of the nurse or physiotherapist. The patient is usually assisted from bed on the first postoperative day but this varies with the individual surgeon. Patients are instructed to avoid flexing the hip joint more than 90° when moving from bed to chair or wheelchair.

The patient is assessed for weight bearing and, if appropriate, crutches should be used for weight support. Walking is started using crutches or a walking frame. The patient usually remains in hospital for 5–10 days.

- *Preventing infection.* Infection is disastrous in arthroplasty as it results in destruction of bone and failure of the prosthesis to stabilize and fuse. A closed (Redivac) drainage system is established at the time of surgery and remains in place 1–2 days, depending on the amount of drainage. Strict asepsis is essential in wound care and in the emptying of portable drainage. The administration of a prophylactic antibiotic which was commenced one to two days before operation may be continued for several days. The appearance of the wound and the colour and amount of drainage should be assessed for any signs of infection so they can be detected and reported. Close observations for other signs of infection are also made, including elevation of temperature and pulse, complaints of pain and pressure in the affected hip, or general malaise.

- *Preventing thromboembolism.* Patients undergoing arthroplasty are at high risk for thromboembolism, due to a possible combination of advanced age, immobility and conditions conducive to venous stasis. Preventive measures are employed including encouragement of the prescribed exercises taught preoperatively and the use of antiembolic stockings. Prophylactic anticoagulants are administered as prescribed, usually for 7 days or until the patient is able to walk. Careful monitoring is conducted for indications of thromboembolism, such as calf oedema, tenderness or redness.

- *Reducing pain.* The patient normally experiences pain following arthroplasty, due to surgical trauma and to related muscle spasm. Assess the patient for the quantity and quality of pain and the patient's response to it. Analgesia should be provided regularly and consistently to control the pain, promote movement and early ambulation and enable the patient to receive adequate rest. Other pain relieving techniques like a change in position may also be helpful in maximizing the comfort of the patient. Extreme pain that does not respond to prescribed analgesia should be carefully evaluated and reported to the surgeon as it may indicate a complication such as dislocation of the prosthesis.

- *Reducing anxiety and maximizing function.* Patients experience anxiety over many aspects of the surgery. Concerns should be assessed and dealt with on an individual basis. Generally, all patients express concern over commencement of activity and ambulation. Having experienced so much pain and instability when walking before the operation, the patient is likely to require repeated reassurance that walking is now possible without discomfort or damage to the new joint. The patient needs much support, both physical and emotional, in the early phase of ambulation. The support is very gradually withdrawn when the patient has sufficient control to be safe and displays confidence.

Selman (1989), in her study of the impact of total hip replacement on quality of life, recognized the findings of other authors (Roush, 1985; Powell, 1986; Schoen, 1986) that patients awaiting total hip replacement appeared to be more motivated and looked forward to surgery more than patients awaiting other orthopaedic surgery. She investigated 46 mainly white, female patients post-total hip replacement, basing her questionnaire on Roy's model of nursing. This looked at the change in the patients' quality of life in four modes: physiological function, self-concept, role function and interdependence. The results of this small study showed a positive change in all four modes and an overall satisfaction in having had a total hip replacement.

Another area of potential anxiety concerns the return to sexual activity. Counselling should be offered to all patients, regardless of their age. The patient should refrain from intercourse for about 6 weeks postoperatively to avoid extreme hip flexion or adduction that could lead to dislocation of the prosthesis. Healing of the internal capsule takes about 6 weeks, after which sexual intercourse can be resumed.

- *Preparation for discharge*. To prepare for going home and becoming as independent as possible, the patient gradually takes over self-care and receives instructions for home care. It is most important not to flex the hip by more than 90° and to avoid extremes of other movements of the hip. The patient is advised to avoid lying on the affected side for at least 2 months. Legs should not be crossed and low, soft chairs should be avoided. Patients should choose a high, firm chair with arms and a raised toilet seat is recommended. The importance of continuing the exercises and walking is stressed, while excessive bending, heavy lifting and jogging is discouraged. Support stockings are helpful until no swelling remains in the legs or feet. This information should be reviewed verbally with the patient and written instructions given at discharge.

A referral to the community staff is appropriate to reinforce hospital teaching and to provide support to the patient and family as full activity is resumed. A home visit with the occupational therapist before discharge is helpful to assess the situation and for suggestions of any adaptations that would promote the patient's independence and safety.

Knee replacement

Total knee joint prostheses consist of two components: a tibial component and a complex femoral component with a channel in which the patella moves. These artificial joints allow for flexion and extension movement of the knee. The prostheses are secured by bone cement or by bony ingrowths through a porous base. Some devices combine the two methods to obtain firmer fixation to bone. A more recent development has been that of the unicompartmental or 'sledge' arthroplasty. In this operation either the medial or the lateral femoral condyle is replaced, together with the corresponding tibial articulating surface. The operation is performed in the relatively early stages of osteoarthritis of the knee and often offers the patient several years of pain-free mobility before a total knee replacement is performed.

Preoperatively the patient is taught and practises quadriceps, hamstring and gluteal setting exercises to maintain optimum strength. These exercises are per-

formed hourly postoperatively. The patient is also taught to transfer from bed to chair and may practise with a Zimmer frame or crutches prior to surgery.

Postoperatively, during the first 24–48 hours, a drain is left in place in the wound to promote drainage. The closed-drainage system is checked regularly to ensure it is draining and is not clogged. Postoperative leg exercises are started early.

Care of the patient following total knee replacement is similar to that following total hip replacement.

Evaluation

Nursing care of the patient with osteoarthritis is effective if the patient is able to achieve a maximum level of self-care while controlling pain and discomfort. For patients undergoing surgical intervention, the nursing care has been effective if complications of surgery are avoided (or detected and treated promptly) and the patient regains a satisfactory level of mobility and independence. Osteoarthritis can be controlled with ongoing collaboration of the patient, family and the health care team.

OTHER INFLAMMATORY JOINT DISEASES

Ankylosing Spondylitis

This is a chronic disorder characterized by inflammation and ensuing ankylosis of the sacroiliac joints and spinal articulations. The pathological process is similar to that seen in rheumatoid arthritis, but there is a greater tendency toward calcification. In most instances the disease remains confined to the joints cited above but occasionally does spread to peripheral joints.

The highest incidence was thought to be in young men, the onset occurring most often in the late teens or the twenties, however with increasing knowledge of the condition it appears that the incidence of ankylosing spondylitis in females accounts for about one-third of all diagnosed cases. It is also recognized that underdiagnosis in females is high, mainly due to the lack of knowledge about female incidence and reluctance to perform pelvic X-rays. The asymmetrical inflammatory arthritis of hips and knees, which is the early presenting problem of women years before the onset of any back problems, only adds to the difficulty of 'labelling the problem'. The cause is unknown, but heredity is suspected of having a role, since a large majority of those afflicted have a family history of some form of inflammatory arthritis.

CLINICAL CHARACTERISTICS

The onset of this disease is usually insidious; the patient first complains of stiffness in the back in the morning or following a period of inactivity. Progressively, this becomes more noticeable; limitation in the range of spinal flexion develops, chest expansion is reduced and there is low back pain radiating to the buttocks and thighs along the sciatic nerve pathways. General systemic symptoms are usually absent or are limited to unusual fatigue and probably some weight loss.

Laboratory examinations indicate an increase in the erythrocyte sedimentation rate, but in most cases the rheumatoid factor is absent. Recently it has been recognized that the histocompatibility antigen HLA-B27 is present in 90% of these patients; this has become a confirming diagnostic of ankylosing spondylitis. Leucocytosis and anaemia may be present and the protein concentration of the cerebrospinal fluid is frequently increased.

Remissions and exacerbations of the acute disease are common. In most advanced stages, some patients develop some peripheral rheumatoid arthritis. A few develop circulatory complications due to aortitis and aortic valvular insufficiency. Uveitis (inflammation of the iris, ciliary body and choroid of the eye) is also seen in about 25% of the patients.

Progressive involvement of spinal segments may continue over a period of years and eventually leave the patient with practically the whole spine firmly ankylosed, producing what may be referred to as a poker back or poker spine. Rarely, osteospondylitis has an abrupt, acute onset and spreads rapidly through the lumbar, thoracic and cervical segments, leaving the patient with a poker spine in a relatively short period.

NURSING ASSESSMENT

A patient with this condition may be admitted for two reasons, either for review and stabilization of the condition or as a result of an acute chest infection. The person's ability to fully expand the chest becomes progressively restricted as the disease advances leading to an increased risk of chest infection which may be so severe as to require in-patient treatment.

If the patient has been admitted for review and stabilization it is important the nurse assess mobility, pain levels and the possible side effects of long term drug therapy such as gastric disturbance. The patient's social circumstances should be assessed as these can have a profound effect upon mood and self concept. The condition may be seriously affecting the person's ability to work or may have led to loss of employment. The inability to be involved in favourite recreations or sports, or even to play with children, may contribute to a depressed mood state while self concept may be severely damaged.

During the in-patient period medical staff will be reviewing the patient's condition, drug regimen etc. and there will also be an intensive physiotherapy review. It is important that the nurse should be sensitive to the person's psychological and social problems in order to achieve the maximum benefit from the hospitalization and send the patient home with a positive, but realistic view of their future based upon an effective mix of physical therapy, psychological support and patient teaching.

If the patient has been admitted with a severe chest infection, assessment in the acute phase is focussed upon respiratory status, and other physical parameters such as pain and mobility. However, as the patient's condition resolves, assessment of the type of area discussed above becomes important. For example does the patient smoke? If he does this is an area for health education as not smoking will greatly reduce the risk of serious respiratory disorder.

NURSING CARE

In general terms goals for the patient with ankylosing spondylitis include the relief of pain, maintenance of good spinal alignment and preservation of maximum spinal function.

During acute phases, the patient usually receives a non-steroidal anti-inflammatory agent such as indomethacin (Indocid).

Rest and good posture at all times are extremely important so that ankylosis of the affected joints occurs while they are in the normal neutral position, thus preventing deformity and handicap. The patient is advised of the need for constant attention to good posture when up, with emphasis on contraction of the buttock and lower abdominal muscles and keeping the chest up, shoulders back and head erect. In some instances, the patient is fitted with a back brace to maintain optimum alignment of the affected joints. A fracture board and a firm mattress are placed on the bed, and it is suggested that the patient does not use a pillow or, if necessary, only a very small one. The patient is advised to sleep straight and flat on the back or in the prone position to discourage possible flexion of the spine.

A daily physical exercise programme is prescribed with the objective of strengthening the muscles which help to support the spine, maintain good alignment and promote the patient's functional capacity. Since ankylosis of the costovertebral joints may occur and reduce the ventilatory capacity, breathing exercises are also included in the suggested exercise regimen.

Heavy lifting and activities which place strain upon the back are restricted. The patient assists in determining the level of tolerance of physical activity; that which produces pain or exhaustion should be avoided; additional rest is important.

If hip and spinal deformities develop, surgical correction may be undertaken to facilitate the patient's mobility and rehabilitation. The most common deformity is fixed flexion of the spine (kyphosis).

METABOLIC JOINT DISEASE

Gout

Gout is a disorder of uric acid metabolism, characterized by recurring episodes of acute inflammation, pain and swelling in a joint. Any joint may be affected, but those of the foot are more susceptible; the condition usually develops first in the great toe. Gout occurs more commonly in men over 40 years of age and is rarely seen in females.

The disorder is caused by an excessive concentration of uric acid in the plasma (hyperuricaemia) which may be brought about by an overproduction or faulty disposal of the kidneys. Urate crystals may be precipitated and deposited within joint tissues, setting up irritation and a local inflammatory response. The small masses of crystals, which are called *tophi* may also form in cartilage, the kidneys or soft tissues in other areas of the body.

Secondary gout may develop in disorders such as blood dyscrasias in which there is a marked breakdown of cellular nucleic acid. When the urate crystals are deposited in joints and produce inflammation, the condition may be referred to as *gouty arthritis*.

CLINICAL CHARACTERISTICS

Acute episodes are characterized by the sudden onset of excruciating pain in the affected joint. It becomes very tender, red, hot and swollen. Veins in the area stand out because of congestion and distension. The patient may also experience anorexia, headache, fever and constipation. The blood uric acid concentration is elevated (normal: 0.18–0.42 mmol/l). Subcutaneous tophi are frequently apparent in the ears or over joints or knuckles. Precipitations of urates may occur in kidney tissue, leading to impaired renal function. In some patients, the excessive concentration of uric acid results in the formation of kidney stones.

The acute attack usually subsides in a few days, and in the early stages of the disease the joint returns to normal. Remissions may gradually become shorter, and the disease may become chronic. More joints become involved, and there are irreversible changes, leading to deformity and loss of function.

NURSING ASSESSMENT

Patients with gout are usually only admitted to hospital for a severe acute exacerbation. Assessment should include checking the principal vital signs, monitoring pain levels and mobility. As in the case of ankylosing spondylitis, it is important to find out how the condition is affecting the person's everyday life in terms of work, family relationships, recreation etc. Much unhappiness may result if these areas are adversely affected, which may in turn affect patient compliance with therapy. It may be very beneficial for the patient to use the time in hospital to talk freely and frankly about such worries and anxieties.

The nurse in the community may encounter a patient with gout if the urate crystal deposits lead to tissue breakdown and the formation of open lesions requiring dressing. Close monitoring of the size and appearance of such lesions is an essential part of assessment, in addition to the factors mentioned above.

NURSING CARE

During an attack of gout, the patient may be placed on bed rest and the affected part immobilized. Drug therapy is promptly instituted. The preparation most commonly used is colchicine. It may be administered orally or intravenously. If it is given intravenously, precautions are taken to avoid any of the drug being deposited in the subcutaneous or extravascular tissues because of its local irritating effect. Side-effects include nausea, vomiting, abdominal discomfort and diarrhoea. The drug generally relieves the pain fairly quickly but does not lower the hyperuricaemia. If the patient cannot tolerate or does not respond to colchicine a non-steroidal anti-inflammatory agent may be prescribed.

Hot or cold applications to the affected joint(s) may provide some relief, but frequently the patient cannot tolerate either. Discomfort is usually less when the part is protected as much as possible from any direct contact with applications and bedding.

A fluid intake of 2500–3000 ml is encouraged to promote dilution and renal elimination of the uric acid. This minimum daily intake should be continued during remissions.

Rigid dietary restrictions are usually not necessary. The patient is instructed to limit foods high in purines such as organ meats (liver, kidneys, heart, sweetbreads), shellfish, sardines and meat extracts and to limit also the intake of alcoholic beverages. Since it is more difficult for uric acid crystals to precipitate as urate crystals in alkaline urine, alkaline-producing foods are encouraged, such as milk, potatoes and citrus fruits.

Patients who are having frequent and severe attacks may receive a uricosuric drug routinely. This type of preparation promotes the urinary excretion of uric acid and lowers the serum uric acid level by inhibiting renal tubular reabsorption. Drugs that may be prescribed for the patient with chronic gout are allopurinol (Zyloric) or probenecid (Benemid).

CONNECTIVE TISSUE (COLLAGEN) DISEASE

Systemic Lupus Erythematosus (SLE) (Disseminated Lupus Erythematosus)

This disorder is a multisystem disease which is characterized by diffuse inflammation and biochemical and structural changes in the collagen fibres of connective tissues in organs and tissues throughout the body. Originally, lupus erythematosus, dermatomyositis and scleroderma comprised the collagen diseases. In recent years, some references include rheumatoid arthritis, rheumatic fever and polyarteritis nodosa in the classification of connective tissue disease.

Systemic lupus erythematosus is an autoimmune disorder characterized by antibodies which develop against cells' nuclear components. A sensitivity to the individual's own DNA develops and the antigen–antibody complexes damage the vasculature, structure and functions of tissues and organs. Several factors are suspected of having a role in precipitating the onset or an acute exacerbation of the disease; these include exposure to the sun's rays, emotional stress, infection and drugs (e.g. sulphonamide, penicillin, procainamide, isoniazid). The incidence is increasing and many patients are diagnosed with mild forms of lupus. The 15-year survival rate for patients with mild disease, is over 90%. Prognosis depends on the age of the patient (it is usually more severe in children; in the elderly it may be mild and respond well to treatment), severity of the disease, the organs affected, and the patient's response to treatment and ability to participate in the treatment plan.

CLINICAL CHARACTERISTICS

The disease may begin at any age in either sex, but is seen most often in young women between the ages of 20 and 30 years. It has a female:male incidence of 9:1. The signs and symptoms, especially at the onset, vary greatly from one person to another, depending upon the systems and organs involved. Those most commonly seen include fever, general malaise, excessive fatigue, weakness, anorexia, weight loss and joint pain. An erythematous rash may be evident on the face, neck and/or extremities. If the disorder is confined to the skin it is referred to as *discoid lupus erythematosus*. The lesions on the face typically spread over the nose and cheeks to form a butterfly pattern. Angioneurotic oedema with burning or itchy sensations, patchy vitiligo or areas of hyperpigmentation, mucosal ulceration and alopecia may develop. (*Angioneurotic oedema* is the temporary appearance of large oedematous areas in the skin or mucous membrane due to a disturbance in the innervation of the vasomotor system.)

In the systemic type of lupus erythematosus, generalized lymphadenopathy occurs. The patient may complain of impaired vision as a result of corneal involvement and retinopathy. Raynaud's phenomenon may be troublesome, especially if the patient is exposed to even slight cold. As the disease progresses, serious visceral involvement and ensuing dysfunction are likely to develop. Impaired pulmonary, cardiovascular and kidney function are common. Clinical renal involvement occurs in many patients with systemic lupus erythematosus. Central nervous system involvement is also common.

The erythrocyte sedimentation rate is elevated (normal: Westergren, 3–5 mm in one hour for males and 4–10 mm in one hour for females), and anaemia is a frequent development. The presence of the lupus erythematosus cell factor and other antinuclear antibodies in the serum facilitates diagnosis. The haematocrit falls and thrombocytopenia may be manifested in petechiae and purpura.

NURSING ASSESSMENT

The patient with SLE is likely to be encountered in hospital either as a result of an acute exacerbation or on admission for joint replacement surgery. However it should be remembered that the patient may have been admitted for other reasons not directly related to this condition, a consideration that applies to all the types of condition discussed in this chapter. Whether the patient has been admitted after a myocardial infarction or for surgery to the bowel, if he or she is affected by another disorder, then the assessment should reflect this.

If the patient has been admitted with an acute exacerbation of SLE the nursing assessment must be comprehensive yet tailored to individual needs, as the disorder can affect the patient in many different ways. Multi-system involvement is possible. The person who has been admitted for joint replacement surgery requires careful assessment to ensure they are fit enough for the anaesthetic and the stress of surgery, in addition to the normal assessment required for a patient undergoing joint replacement surgery.

NURSING CARE

The care of the patient is mainly supportive and symptomatic; at present, no therapy is considered curative. In remissions, the patient is advised against exposure to sunlight, infection and excessive fatigue which are thought to predispose or precipitate an exacerbation of the disease process. Lotions may be used to screen out the ultraviolet sun rays when the person has to be exposed. Cold should be avoided because of the vascular reaction (Raynaud's).

Medications which may be prescribed include aspirin to control fever and joint involvement, an antimalarial drug such as hydroxychloroquine (Plaquenil) for the patient with skin and joint involvement if the condition is unresponsive to salicylates, and an adrenocorticosteroid preparation. The latter is used for the more severe stage of systemic lupus erythematosus when there is renal, central nervous system, cardiovascular and haemopoietic involvement. The steroid drug is given in relatively large doses during an acute exacerbation, and then gradually reduced to a maintenance dose or withdrawn completely. If hydroxychloroquine is given, frequent ophthalmological examinations are necessary since the drug may precipitate retinopathy. Cyclophospamide (Endoxana) or azathioprine (Imuran) may be used when the patient with severe disease is unresponsive to the more conservative drugs.

Dialysis may be necessary when the disease attacks the kidneys. Infection is treated promptly with antibiotics. Emotional stress should be minimized and fatigue avoided.

New treatments, such as plasmapheresis, the use of monoclonal antibodies and pulse therapy which involves the intravenous administration of corticosteroids over a short period, are being used with some success.

Systemic lupus erythematosus is a serious chronic disease that is unpredictable in nature. The patient experiences remissions and exacerbations. Nursing intervention focuses on assisting the patient to manage the disease and adapt life-style to altered functional level. Emphasis is placed on the patient's strengths and the positive aspects of functional ability. The patient is helped to identify factors which precipitate flare-ups or exacerbation of symptoms and to create an environment free of stress. A daily routine is planned to provide adequate rest.

The following points are emphasized in teaching patients and their families about the disease and self-management:

1. Knowledge of the disease process, its management and signs and symptoms of disease activity.
2. Actions, dosage and possible side-effects of the prescribed drug(s) and adjustment of medication dosage in response to symptom changes.
3. The importance of carrying an identification card if the patient is receiving corticosteroid therapy.
4. Awareness of expected weight gains with corticosteroid therapy and measures to minimize and cope with the weight gain.
5. The necessity of regular medical supervision so that tissue changes can be detected early by laboratory tests and prompt adjustment made in drug therapy to help control tissue damage. (Regular medical supervision enables the doctor to keep medication dosages to a minimal level, preventing or decreasing harmful side-effects of drug therapy.)
6. The importance of prompt identification of infection and the action to take if infection develops.
7. The importance of regular rest, sleep and good nutrition.
8. Methods of decreasing physical and emotional stress.
9. Knowledge of community resources including self-help groups.
10. Avoidance of over-exposure to sunlight.

Dermatomyositis (Polymyositis)

In this form of connective tissue disease, the skin and voluntary muscles are the principal focal sites of the pathological inflammatory process. Contracture of the skin and muscles due to the fibrous scar tissue may lead to tightly drawn skin in the affected areas, muscle contracture and loss of function. Involvement of the respiratory muscles may cause respiratory insufficiency and frequently is the cause of death.

This collagen disease may be treated with an adrenocorticosteroid preparation, but the outlook is generally unfavourable.

Scleroderma (Progressive Systemic Sclerosis)

This is a chronic disorder in which the collagen component of the skin undergoes degenerative changes and becomes sclerotic. The dermal changes and contraction produce deformities and restricted movement. The pathological sclerosing process may spread to viscera, causing systemic disturbances and organ dysfunction similar to those that may occur in systemic lupus erythematosus. The rate of progress varies with patients; some survive many years, while the disease may prove fatal to others in a few months.

INFECTIVE BONE DISEASE

Osteomyelitis

When bone tissue becomes infected the condition is known as osteomyelitis. The pathogenic organisms may be introduced directly through an open fracture or from infected contiguous tissue but are more commonly carried by the blood to the bone from a distant primary focus such as boils (furuncles), an abscessed tooth or infected tonsils. When the infection is bloodborne, the condition is referred to as *haematogenous osteomyelitis*. The most common bacterial offender is *Staphylococcus aureus*, but the disease may also result from the invasion of streptococci, pneumococci or other strains of staphylococci.

Growing bone is more susceptible to haematogenous osteomyelitis and, as a result, the incidence is highest in children and adolescents. The infection usually develops in long bones at the diaphyseal side of the growth plate. In adults the pelvis and vertebrae are more often affected. The bone marrow is affected first. Unless it is checked at the onset, the inflammatory process forms a purulent exudate that collects in the minute canals and spaces of the bone tissue. The pressure of the exudate builds up because of the resistant, rigid bone and compresses the blood vessels, causing thrombosis and occlusion. The accumulation under pressure eventually breaks through the cortex of the bone into the subperiosteal space. The periosteum at that site becomes elevated and stripped from the bone, interrupting the blood vessels that lead into the bone. Interference with the blood supply results in an area of dead bone tissue, which is called a *sequestrum*. The periosteum may rupture, and the infection may then extend into the adjacent soft tissues, forming a sinus tract that discharges on to the skin surface. Small sequestra, separated from the living bone tissue, may escape with the exudate through the sinus. The infection may destroy the growth plate (epiphyseal plate), leading to reduced growth of the limb, or it may extend into the adjacent joint with ensuing permanent loss of joint function. The periosteum initiates the formation of new bone tissue around the affected area. The new tissue is called the *involucrum* (a covering or sheath, such as contains the sequestrum of a necrosed bone) and may enclose and trap sequestra and infecting organisms. These organisms continue to grow in the confined area and the osteomyelitis becomes chronic, characterized by recurring abscess formation and sequestration. Chronicity is more likely to occur in non-traumatic osteomyelitis.

The actual and potential *problems* of acute osteomyelitis include:

- Severe pain in the affected limb (caused by the pressure of accumulating exudate and bone destruction) aggravated by even slight movement.
- Protection of the limb by avoiding weight bearing, any movement and flexion of the adjoining joints.
- Tenderness and eventual redness and swelling of the affected part; a draining sinus may develop over the involved area.
- Restlessness and irritability.

- Nausea and vomiting.
- Increased leucocyte count and erythrocyte sedimentation rate may be present.
- X-rays show destructive bone changes and periosteal elevation after 1–2 weeks.

NURSING ASSESSMENT

The patient admitted with this condition after trauma has usually been affected over a lengthy period involving significant loss of mobility and function together with chronic pain. A careful assessment of the patient's social and psychological state is essential if nursing care is to address the patient's main problems, while pain assessment is also of prime importance. A patient who is self employed may, for example, face bankruptcy as a result of a prolonged period of inactivity and frequent hospitalizations, while the chronic nature of the pain and apparent lack of progress in resolving the condition may severely affect the person's morale. The patient may be aware that in some cases the only way of resolving the condition is by amputation.

If the condition is acute, it usually involves adolescents. The nurse needs to pay particular attention to vital signs as the patient may be very febrile and toxic in the initial stages; pain should also be carefully assessed. The developmental stage of the person should be considered as part of the assessment together with the family situation as this can have a significant bearing upon nursing care.

NURSING CARE

Antimicrobial drug therapy and rest in the early stage of osteomyelitis may bring the infection under control with minimal bone damage and before a sinus is formed. In more advanced cases, surgery may be necessary to provide drainage to relieve the pressure within the bone and periosteum and to remove dead bone tissue.

Efforts are made to identify the infecting organism by making cultures of the blood, nose and throat secretions and discharge from any skin lesions (e.g. boils). If a positive culture is obtained, sensitivity tests may then be made to determine the most effective antibiotic therapy.

Large doses of antibiotics are given, usually by parenteral channels. Antibiotic therapy is begun after culture and sensitivity tests are done. Effective oral antibiotic therapy has only recently been achieved. Ciprofloxacin has been shown to be effective in treating Gram-negative bacillary osteomyelitis when treatment extends from 4 to 6 weeks or longer. In some cases, when the acute phase of the illness is over, the patient may be discharged and continue therapy at home.

Large doses of antibiotics may be given parenterally over several weeks (usually a minimum of 4 weeks). If the response is favourable and the infective process controlled, antimicrobial therapy is generally continued for several weeks to ensure destruction of the organisms.

The patient is placed at rest, and the affected limb is handled very gently. It is positioned and supported to prevent contractures and deformities. A splint may be used to immobilize the adjacent joint or skin traction

may be applied if a lower limb is affected. Careful monitoring of pressure areas and rigorous pressure care are essential. A well balanced high calorie diet will be needed to help cope with the metabolic demands of what is a serious infective process.

If surgical drainage or a sequestrectomy is performed, the wound is packed and allowed to heal by granulation from within toward the surface. Antibiotic or sulphonamide preparations may be introduced locally into the wound. The dressing is changed often enough to keep the wound clean and to prevent the development of an offensive odour that may become very distressing to the patient and those in his environment. Precautions must be taken to observe aseptic technique when dressing or treating the wound to prevent the introduction of secondary infection and to prevent the transmission of the patient's infection to others.

When the patient is allowed up protection must be afforded against falls and injury to the limb. The loss of bone substance may weaken the bone structure, predisposing it to fracture when subjected to even slight injury or pressure. In the case of a lower extremity, weight bearing may be contraindicated for many weeks while new bone tissue is being formed. The patient may then have to be taught to use crutches and may be discharged from the hospital but is likely to require guidance and supervision for a considerable period of time.

OSTEOPOROSIS

Osteoporosis is a disease which results from an imbalance between calcium reabsorption and bone formation. This results in an overall loss of bone tissue and increases the risk of bone fracture, often with little trauma. Factors that influence the reabsorption, and the laying down of new bone are listed in Table 25.5.

NURSING ASSESSMENT

Osteoporosis is a condition which is likely to be present in many elderly patients, particularly women, although it is not usually the prime cause of admission. The nurse therefore needs to be aware of the likely existence of this condition in assessing elderly patients, whatever other health problems they may have.

Clinical Characteristics

Actual and potential *problems* may include the following:

- Fractures of any bone but most commonly of the vertebrae between T10 and L2, the femoral necks and the metacarpals. Fractures may be complete or compressed (see Table 24.2).
- Pain either localized or radiating.
- Tenderness.
- Muscle spasm.
- Loss of normal lumbar curve.
- Progressive development of kyphosis (curvature of the spine).

Table 25.5 Factors that influence bone formation and reabsorption.

Effect	Formation	Reabsorption
Increase	Exercise, stress on bone	Parathyroid hormone excess
	Growth hormone	Vitamin D hormone†
	Fluoride*	Vitamin A excess
	Vitamin C	Adrenocortical steroid excess
	Thyroid hormones	Calcium deficiency
	Insulin	Phosphorus deficiency
	Androgens	Anabolic steroid deficiency
	Vitamin D metabolites	Immobilization
	Parathyroid hormone	Acidosis
		Heparin
		Pregnancy and lactation
		Osteolytic neoplasms
		Prostaglandins
Decrease	Immobilization, disuse, bed rest	Calcium
	Growth hormone deficiency	Phosphorus
	Adrenocortical steroid excess	Parathyroid hormone deficiency
	Anticonvulsants	Calcitonin
		Magnesium deficiency
		Anabolic steroids
		Alkalosis
		Mithramycin
		Diphosphonates
		Colcichine

* Fluoride in excess causes deposition of uncalcified osteod and produces osteomalacia.
† Osteolytic effect of parathyroid hormone requires presence of vitamin D hormone.
Modified from Snyder (1985).

The presence of these problems leads to decreased mobility (which exacerbates the condition), and interferes with normal self-care.

RISK FACTORS

A number of factors are known to put people at risk for osteoporosis. Among these are:

- *Sex*. Women usually have less bone mass than men.
- *Race*. Europeans have less bone mass than Afro-Caribbean or Asian people.
- *Stature*. People who are underweight or who have small bones have less bone mass.
- *Activity*. Inactivity or immobility increases bone reabsorption. Women athletes experiencing secondary amenorrhoea may have an accelerated loss of bone.
- *Smoking/drinking*. Tobacco and alcohol decrease the body's ability to absorb and retain calcium.
- *Diet*. Inadequate calcium, vitamin D, protein and

vitamin C increase bone reabsorption.
- *Family history*. Osteoporosis tends to run in families.
- *Menopause*. With the gradual decline in oestrogen levels there is an accompanied increase in bone reabsorption.
- *Hypogonadism*. Men suffering from this condition experience bone loss.
- *Medical conditions*. Endocrine disturbances such as hyperthyroidism and Cushing's syndrome; persons receiving treatment with steroids may also experience a decrease in bone density.

NURSING CARE

Since treatment for osteoporosis cannot reverse the condition, it is directed at arresting or slowing the rate of calcium reabsorption, reducing discomfort and maintaining a satisfactory life-style. These goals are addressed through medication, diet, and exercise.

Medication. At this time, oestrogen replacement is the standard against which other treatments for osteoporosis are measured. Restoration of oestrogen to premenopausal levels slows bone loss and maintains bone levels in most women (Dieppe et al, 1985). Persons receiving oestrogen are thought to be at risk for biliary disease and cervical and endometrial cancer, although controversy exists about the influence of oestrogen in the development of breast cancer, although this may be minimized by using a low-dose (30 mg ethinyloestradiol) contraceptive pill. Women should be taught breast self-awareness (see Chapter 23).

Progesterone is known to prevent endometrial hyperplasia and prevent the increase in cancer incidence. It is therefore given to a woman receiving oestrogen therapy if she still has her uterus.

Calcitonin has been shown to be as effective as oestrogen in the reduction of bone reabsorption. Long-term effects are not yet known and, while side-effects are described as tolerable, it has the disadvantage of requiring parenteral administration. It may, however, be of short-term benefit.

Calcium preparations such as calcium gluconate (recommended dosage is 1200–1500 mg for women) and vitamin D may also be prescribed. Neither has been shown to reduce bone loss effectively but may slow the process.

Replacement of testosterone to normal levels stops bone loss and increases bone mass in men.

Recent studies (Watts, 1990) report that persons with osteoporosis treated with a non-steroid drug, etidronate, had 50% fewer fractures (spinal) than those persons treated with calcium. Further study on the action of this new drug is being recommended.

Diet. Diet therapy stresses the importance of the intake of foods high in calcium, supplementary vitamin D and protein, and of fluid intake, and the monitoring of the types of foods chosen to accomplish this. Emphasis is placed on the use of dairy products as a source of protein because excessive protein from meat sources is known to precipitate reabsorption of bone. Carbonated drinks are discouraged as they contain phosphorus which is also linked to bone reabsorption.

Exercise. Regular weight-bearing exercise is recommended to assist in the prevention of bone loss. Walking, jogging and stair climbing, while not proven to prevent bone loss, are influential in improving the general condition of individuals, which contributes to the prevention of falls and their sequelae.

Health promotion. Nurses should be aware that women are more likely to suffer from osteoporosis than men. Nurses have a responsibility to teach health habits related to a life-style believed to assist in the prevention of osteoporosis. The target group is premenopausal women, but all women may benefit from such teaching.

After assessing the patient for the risk factors listed above, a teaching plan should be developed with the patient; this should cover diet, exercise and any medication the person may be taking, and is directed towards the reduction of any risk factors identified.

The content of the teaching plan includes the importance of a recognized nutritional diet, high in calcium and low in animal fats. Vitamin D supplements may also be recommended. The fact that excessive intake of alcohol and caffeine can accelerate the onset of osteoporosis is stressed. It is important to know the patient's usual diet, and to use this as the core for any dietary planning.

While the long-term benefits of exercise programmes are as yet unknown, it is known that regular, weight-bearing exercise benefits a person's overall well-being and should therefore be included in the plan. If a regular exercise programme is already a part of the patient's life-style, encouragement to continue should be given.

OSTEOMALACIA

Osteomalacia is an adult disorder comparable to rickets in children, and, for this reason, it is occasionally referred to as adult rickets. It is characterized by an insufficient plasma concentration of calcium and inorganic phosphate for normal calcification of bone tissue.

Osteomalacia may be the result of an insufficient amount of calcium reaching the plasma or an excessive urinary excretion of the mineral. In the first instance, the deficiency of calcium may be due to a lack of calcium-containing foods in the diet, insufficient absorption of the mineral from the intestine (caused by steatorrhoea or prolonged diarrhoea), or a deficiency of vitamin D in the diet or as a result of renal failure, which is necessary for normal absorption of calcium and its deposition in bone tissue. Osteomalacia may also occur during pregnancy if the woman does not receive additional calcium to meet the increased demand incurred by the developing fetus.

The second major cause of the disease, an excessive urinary excretion of calcium, is usually the result of acidosis associated with renal failure or of renal tubular damage and malfunction.

Actual and potential *problems* may include:

- Softening and weakening of bone.
- Tenderness and aching.

- Deformity of the long bones.
- Loss of weight and muscular strength.
- Tetany.

The *treatment* consists mainly of the administration of calcium, phosphorus and vitamin D. If the serum calcium concentration is markedly low, calcium (e.g. calcium gluconate 10%) may be given intravenously.

PAGET'S DISEASE (OSTEITIS DEFORMANS)

Paget's disease is a chronic inflammation of the bone. The exact aetiology is not known.

The actual and potential *problems* may include:

- Softening, enlargement and production of imperfectly developed bones.
- Bone pain.
- Skeletal deformities.
- Changes in skin temperature.
- Pathological fractures.
- Symptoms of nerve compression.

It is most commonly found in persons over 50 years of age, but may affect younger persons as well. Men, in a ratio of 3:2, are more likely to contract this disease than women. However 10–20% of patients are asymptomatic.

NURSING CARE

When the disease is asymptomatic and weight-bearing bones are not involved, no treatment is necessary. Treatment and nursing intervention are supportive and directed toward alleviating presenting symptoms. The primary therapy is calcitonin. The objective of this treatment is to control the metabolic action of the disease, reduce the rate of bone turnover and ease pain. Diphosphonates may be given as an alternative drug for the same purpose. Patients are advised to eat a diet high in calcium and protein, with vitamin C and D supplements. An individualized exercise programme is taught and the person is encouraged to follow it unless symptoms recur.

BONE NEOPLASMS

Primary and secondary neoplasms may develop in bone tissue. Primary new growths may be benign or malignant; secondary bone neoplasms are metastases from malignant disease in another area of the body and have a much higher incidence than primary bony neoplasms. Primary sites that frequently cause bone metastases are the breast, prostate, lung, thyroid and kidney. The bones that are the most common sites of metastases are the vertebrae, pelvic bones, femora and humeri.

Most primary bone neoplasms develop in children and adults younger than 40 years. They may be classified by the type of cell from which they originate, whether they are benign or malignant, and whether the tissue

Table 25.6 Common primary bone neoplasms.

Cell of origin	Neoplasm	Benign/malignant	Comments
Osteocyte	Osteoid osteoma	Benign	Small, reactive lesion. Femur and tibia common sites. Especially painful at night. Treatment involves surgical removal
	Osteochondroma	Benign	Most common benign bone neoplasm; a hamartoma* consisting of bony outgrowth with a cartilage cap. Distal end of femur, proximal end of tibia and proximal end of humerus are common sites. Symptoms depend upon impingement on surrounding tissues
	Osteogenic sarcoma (osteosarcoma)	Malignant (rapid spread)	Destroys medullary and cortical bone tissue. Usually develops in end of long bone; almost 50% involve the knee joint. Severe pain and tenderness; area may be hot and swollen. Treatment consists of amputation and chemotherapy, or chemotherapy and endoprosthetic replacement
	Osteoclastoma	Benign—may become malignant	Develops most often in epiphyseal region of femur, tibia or humerus of young adults. Rarefaction of bone occurs. It causes pain, swelling and rarely pathological fracture. Treated by curettage or by resection of the bone and replacement with a bone graft. If malignant, the limb is amputated, or chemotherapy and endoprosthetic replacement
Chondrocyte	Endochondroma	Benign	Growth of tumour cells of the hyaline cartilage may cause a pathological fracture. Treatment is by curettage
	Chondroblastoma	Benign	Develops toward end of adolescence. Common sites are femur, tibia and humerus. Highest incidence in males. Causes pain and swelling in epiphyseal area. Treatment is curettage and bone grafts
	Chondrosarcoma	Malignant (slower spread than osteosarcoma)	Age group most often affected 30–60 years. Common sites are scapula, pelvis, humerus and femur. Treatment involves radical excision, amputation, or chemotherapy and endoprosthetic replacement
Fibrocyte	Non-osteogenic fibroma	Benign	Most common site is end of diaphysis of long bone. If asymptomatic, it may be left untreated. If painful, it is excised
	Fibrosarcoma	Malignant	Rare. Usually in adults. Treated by amputation if in a limb or chemotherapy plus endoprosthetic replacement
Uncertain; reticulocyte suggested	Ewing's tumour or sarcoma	Malignant	May involve ilia, ribs, vertebrae and shafts of long bones. Begins in marrow cavity and gradually erodes the bone tissue. Manifestations include severe pain, swelling, fever and leucocytosis. Treatment is combination of irradiation, chemotherapy and surgery, including endoprosthetic replacement

* A *hamartoma* is a benign tumour formed by an overgrowth of normal mature cells characteristic of the area.

response is osteolytic or reactive. The neoplasm may cause a breakdown of the bone structure, with loss of calcium from the tissue; this type of reaction is referred to as osteolytic. The response of bone tissue to some types of neoplastic cells is the formation of dense bone tissue around the lesion, which may be referred to as a nidus. This type of process is called reactive bone formation.

The more common primary bone neoplasms are listed in Table 25.6.

CLINICAL CHARACTERISTICS

Neoplasms of bones may be asymptomatic for a period of time and may only be discovered when the person has an X-ray for some other reason (e.g. sustained injury) or has a pathological fracture. Persistent pain, progressively increasing in severity, and limitation of activity of the affected part are common characteristics. Local tenderness, swelling and warmth may be present. If the neoplasm is malignant, systemic symptoms such as weight loss and anaemia develop.

Diagnosis is made by bone scan as this is more sensitive than radiography, although this may also be performed.

Benign bone neoplasms are treated by excision or curettage. The bone structure may have to be reinforced following the removal of the lesion by filling in the space with bone chips or small grafts. Treatment of primary malignant neoplasms involves a combination of surgery and chemotherapy. Radical excision is done if the lesion is accessible or, in the case of an extremity, the limb is amputated. Development has occurred in the preservation of mobility of many patients by the use of custom-made joint and bone replacement (endoprosthetic replacement, pioneered at the Department of Biomedical Engineering, Institute of Orthopaedics at Stanmore Royal National Orthopaedic Hospital). Suitable cases may be those where there is no diffuse spread of the tumour into surrounding secondary deposits. Extending prostheses have been developed in the last decade. They can be used in the tibia, femur and humerus of the growing child or adolescent.

The treatment of the patient with skeletal metastases depends principally on the origin of the primary malignant disease. Chemotherapy, hormones and/or irradiation may be used. Irradiation may be used to reduce the severity of the pain experienced by the patient. Analgesics are prescribed to keep the patient comfortable; a small dose is used at first, but usually has to be increased as the condition worsens and the patient develops a tolerance for the drug.

NURSING INTERVENTION

Nursing care is directed toward symptom management, psychosocial support and patient and family teaching.

The most common patient *problems* may include:

- *Pain* related to the disease process.
- *Potential problem of nausea and vomiting* related to treatment/disease.
- *Knowledge deficit* related to disease and treatment options.
- *Knowledge deficit* related to long-term management.
- *Potential problem of ineffective coping* related to diagnosis.

Pain. Specific points for assessment include the presence, location and degree of pain. It is important to determine the exact location of pain in order to learn if new areas of the skeleton are involved, particularly in metastatic bone cancer.

The *goal* is that the patient will be as free of pain as possible. Alleviation of pain may be best achieved through regular scheduling of optimum doses of narcotics with follow-up assessment of the effectiveness of each dose. Time-scheduled medication should prevent patients from experiencing pain. If this is not the result for any individual then the medication regimen should be reassessed with the patient and physician and the necessary changes made. Other approaches to pain control include frequent gentle change of position (at least every 2 hours); maintenance of good hygiene; and mental imaging.

Potential for nausea and vomiting. The *goal* is that the patient should be free of nausea and should not vomit. The patient should be closely assessed for nausea and vomiting as they have many causes and should not be quickly attributed to any particular one; radiation therapy, additive hormones, narcotics and hypercalcaemia may all contribute. Effective intervention to prevent nausea is only possible when the cause has been identified.

Knowledge deficit. Patient and family teaching includes issues related to treatment options and signs and symptoms of further advancing disease, including early indications of spinal cord compression and hypercalcaemia. Family members are taught basic care techniques in order to care for the patient at home. These include positioning, bathing, skin care, assisting the person in ambulation, and safety measures. The nurse also assists the patient and family to understand the need for a diet high in calories, fibre and fluids.

Potential for ineffective coping due to disease. The *goal* is that the patient may adapt to the disease in a positive way. The psychosocial needs of patients with bone neoplasms and their families are most severe when the neoplasm is malignant, particularly as a malignant neoplasm is usually metastatic. Supportive care in the form of guided questioning, attentive listening, use of touch, and information giving is provided. If this proves insufficient, referral for more intensive support should be made.

Evaluation

Evaluation of the effectiveness of nursing intervention is carried out by discussion with the patient and family concerning how effectively the goals have been met.

SUMMARY

Disease of bones and joints frequently result in the patient suffering years of chronic pain with occasional acute episodes. Hospital admission is often during the acute stages of the disease and the nurse must be aware of the way in which the patient usually copes with the disease if the patient is to be adequately cared for during the acute phase.

In caring for patients with orthopaedic conditions nurses may develop long term relationships with them. Individuals with a chronic condition will frequently return to the same ward or unit when they need hospitalization. There is a great scope in this situation for the patient's care to be discussed with the family and multidisciplinary team. For example, the work of the physiotherapist is closely linked to that of the occupational therapist and they both need the cooperation of the family at home for their ideas to be continued in the community. It is the patient's quality of life in the long term that must be of paramount importance and this may require specialist advice for chronic pain counselling, the involvement of social services and support groups for both the patient and/or the relatives in addition to a wide range of therapeutic interventions.

LEARNING ACTIVITIES

1. A restricted range of joint movement is a common patient problem. Progress may be monitored by use of a goniometer, an instrument which measures range of movement in degrees. Measure the range of movement of a colleague's knee and hip joints and compare this with that of 3 elderly patients.

2. Design a health education leaflet appropriate for general community distribution on osteoporosis.

3. For approximately the same cost it would be possible to perform hip replacement surgery on:
   i) A 35 years old female PE Teacher who has two young children or
   ii) Two elderly retired patients
   In this era of limited resources, how might a decision be made between these two alternatives? Discuss with your colleagues. Use Table 1.4 as a guide in your decision making.

REFERENCES AND FURTHER READING

Burton S (1989) Drugs to treat rheumatic disorders. *Nursing* Feb. 3(34).

Crosby LJ (1988) Stress factors, emotional stress and rheumatoid arthritis activity. *Journal of Advanced Nursing* July. 13(4).

Crossfield T (1990) Patients with scleroderma. *Nursing* May. 4(10).

Davis GC (1989) The clinical assessment of chronic pain in rheumatic disease: evaluating the use of two instruments. *Journal of Advanced Nursing* May. 14(5).

Dieppe P, Doherty M, Macfarlane DG & Maddison PJ (1985) *Rheumatological Medicine*. Edinburgh: Churchill Livingstone.

Donavon JL (1989) The patient is not a blank sheet: lay beliefs and their relevance to patient education. *British Journal of Rheumatology* Feb. 28(1).

Goodall C (1988) Living with pain. *Nursing Times* Aug. 10–16 84(32).

Green A (1989) What's happening to hips? *Nursing Times* Nov. **85(46):** 15–21.

Katzin L (1990) Chronic illness and sexuality. *American Journal of Nursing* Jan. 90(1).

Lindroth Y, Bourman A, Barnes C, McCredie M & Brooks PM (1989) A controlled evaluation of arthritis education. *British Journal of Rheumatology* **28**.

Lorig K, Lubuck D, Kraines RG, Seleznick M & Holman HR (1985) Outcomes on self help education for patients with arthritis. *Arthritis and Rheumatology* **28**.

Mate C et al (1987) Cervical myelopathy in rheumatoid arthritis. *Nursing Times* Oct. **83(40):** 7–13.

Meenan RF, Gertman PM & Mason JH (1980) Measuring health status in arthritis: the arthritis impact measurement scales. *Arthritis and Rheumatism* **23(2):** 146–152.

Perry GR (1988) Living with osteoporosis. *Geriatric Nurse* May–June 9(3).

Pinel C (1989) Metabolic bone disease. *Nursing* May, 3(37).

Powell M (1986) *Orthopaedic Nursing and Rehabilitation*. Edinburgh: Churchill Livingstone.

Pownell M (1987) Consensus on Osteoporosis. *Nursing Times* Dec. 83(45).

Redfern S (1989) Patients with Rheumatoid Arthritis. *Nursing* Feb. 3(34).

Roberts A (1988) Senior systems: locomotor system — bone. Osteoporosis, osteomalacia and Paget's disease. *Nursing Times* Dec. 84(50) Systems of Life no. 166.

Roush S (1985) Patient perceived functional outcomes associated with elective hip and knee arthroplasties. *Physical Therapy* 65(10).

Schoen D (1986) *The Nursing Process in Orthopaedics*. New York: Appleton-Century-Croft.

Selman S (1989) Impact of total hip replacement on quality of life. *Orthopaedic Nursing* **8(9)**.

Snyder M (1985) *Independent Nursing Interventions*, p. 466. Toronto: Wiley.

Thompson J (1989) A new lease of life. *Nursing Times* July 85(30).

Vignos PJ, Parker WT & Thompson HM (1976) Evaluation of a clinic education programme for patients with rheumatoid arthritis. *Journal of Rheumatology* **3**.

Watts NB et al (1990) Intermittent cyclical etidrorate treatment of postmenopausal osteoporosis. *The New England Journal of Medicine* **323(2):** 73–79.

Weiner CL (1984) The burden of rheumatoid arthritis. In Strauss AL et al (eds) *Chronic Illness and the Quality of Life* 2nd edn. St Louis: Mosby.

Caring for the Patient with a Disorder of the Skin

26

OBJECTIVES

On completion of this chapter the reader will be able to:

- Describe the structure and function of skin
- Describe the characteristics common to impairment of skin and tissue integrity
- Assess the individual for these characteristics
- Assess the individual for risk factors which contribute to impairment of skin and tissue integrity
- Identify, plan, implement and evaluate nursing interventions for the person with specific health problems related to skin integrity
- Develop strategies to assist the person with psychosocial problems resulting from skin impairment
- Assist individuals and families to acquire the knowledge and skill necessary to promote, maintain and restore skin integrity
- Provide comprehensive nursing care for persons at risk for or with pressure sores
- Provide comprehensive nursing care for persons during the emergent, acute and rehabilitative phases of recovery from burns

INTRODUCTION

The skin is the largest organ of the body and provides us with many invaluable functions. Examination of the integrity of the skin is a major component of the patient's assessment. Prolonged and intimate contact with patients puts the nurse in an ideal position to assess actual skin condition or the presence of risk factors which may influence skin integrity. The data collected during such an assessment form the basis of the plan for nursing intervention, teaching and evaluation of outcomes.

Health problems involving the skin vary from minor to catastrophic. Nurses require the skills necessary to provide not only the necessary physical care but also the much needed psychological support.

A preventive approach to the maintenance of skin integrity combined with specific education can be of greater benefit to a person than a delayed, reactive one. For example, the prevention of skin cancers by educating people about the hazards of overexposure to the sun is a far more desirable goal than successful treatment. Today's better-educated health care consumers expect to be involved in their own care. They are also more conscious of the need for information related to health promotion. For further information about health promotion and patient teaching refer to Chapters 2 and 3.

Structure and Functions of the Skin

The skin (integument) is composed of a thin, avascular

layer of epithelial cells called the epidermis, and a supporting layer of connective tissue (on which the epidermis rests) called the dermis or corium (Figure 26.1). Beneath the dermis is the hypodermis, or subcutaneous tissue, which contains the panniculus adiposus (fat), arrectoris pilorum (smooth muscle) and the tela subcutanea (areolar bed). Vital vascular, lymphatic and neural supplies are subjacent to and intertwined with these three layers.

The *epidermis*, the outermost, cornified layer of the skin, containing only 10% water, has five layers, and is composed of the stratum corneum and the stratum Malpighii. The stratum corneum (one layer thick) consists of dead, keratinized cells. The maintenance of fluid balance is an important feature of the corneum's overall barrier function.

Cells responsible for the regeneration of skin are produced in the basal (germinating) layer and then gradually move through the other layers to the surface. As they ascend, they progressively undergo degenerative changes. The nuclei disintegrate, the cell substance changes to a water-repellent, waxy, protein-like substance called *keratin*, and the cells become flat. They are continuously reproduced in the basal layer and cast off from the surface. It is thought that normally they reach the surface in approximately 27–30 days. The cells that are shed disintegrate, leaving their keratin on the surface; this keratin helps to protect the skin. The epidermis contains no blood vessels. The cells are nourished by intracellular fluid from the dermis, from which nutrients are diffused.

The thickness of the epidermis varies in different areas of the body from a minimum of 0.07 to 0.12 mm in

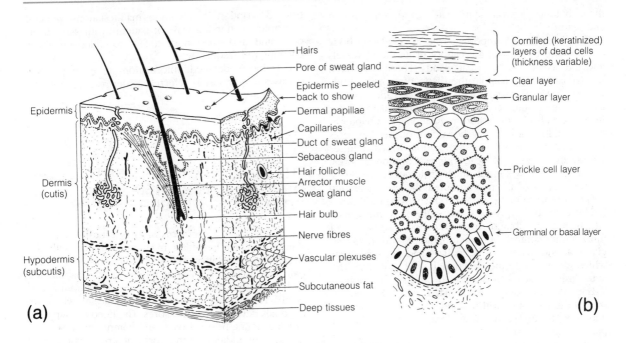

Figure 26.1 (a) Generalized structure of skin, showing epidermis, dermis and appendages. (b) Cell layers of the epidermis.

depth. It is thickest on the soles of the feet and palms of the hands and thinnest on the lips and eyelids. This provides maximum 'wear and tear' qualities for areas of maximum stress. Imparting physical strength to the skin and potential wounds remains, however, the role of the dermis.

The *dermis*, consisting of fibrous and elastic connective tissue, contains many blood and lymphatic vessels, nerves and their end-organs, sebaceous and sweat glands, ducts and hair follicles. The undersurface merges with the loose, *fatty subcutaneous tissue*, also known as hypodermis. The thickness of the dermis ranges from 1 to 2 mm with some variation, as with epidermal depth.

Lying between the epidermal germinating layer and the dermis are the melanocytes, which produce the pigment melanin and deliver it to the epidermal cells. The amount of pigment is mainly determined by the person's genetic inheritance. The activity of the pigment-producing cells may also be influenced by the melanocyte-stimulating hormone (MSH), which is released by the pituitary gland, and by exposure to sunlight and friction.

The *panniculus adiposus* or subcutaneous tissue contained in the hypodermis is composed primarily of fat cells and functions as a heat insulator, a cushion against mechanical pressure and a caloric energy store. The subcutaneous tissue is distributed in varying thicknesses over the entire body surface. Its thickness is influenced by sex and age.

The cutaneous sebaceous glands secrete an oily substance (sebum) which reaches the skin surface via the hair follicles. Glands are plentiful in the face and scalp, but are absent in the palmar and plantar aspects of the hands and feet. The secretion prevents drying of the hair and skin and helps to keep the skin soft and pliable. Blackheads are discoloured accumulations of sebum in hair follicles and frequently provide a medium for organisms, causing pimples or the condition acne. Sebaceous gland activity increases at puberty and decreases in later life due to the influence of gonadal hormones on the output of sebum. The growth of hair on certain areas of skin is also stimulated by gonadal hormones, principally the androgens.

The skin has many important functions, for example, protection, sensation, heat regulation, absorption and storage. By its continuity the skin protects the internal structures from injury, acts as a barrier to keep vital fluids and chemicals from leaking out, and prevents invasion of organisms. Its protective functions are enhanced by the water-repellent, waxy nature of the surface cells, desquamation (separation of the superficial cells) and an 'acid mantle', produced from keratinizing cells and cutaneous glands, resulting in an acid pH (4.5–6.5) between the cells and on the surface; it is hypothesized that this secretion has both antifungal and antibacterial properties.

The abundance of sensory receptors and afferent and efferent nerves in the skin function in the sensations of touch, pressure, pain and temperature. These sensations serve as an important protective mechanism for the body and also convey impulses that contribute information about the external environment. For example, through touch we can appreciate shape, composition and texture.

The skin plays an important role in regulating body temperature by varying the calibre of its blood vessels and the activity of the sweat glands. These controlled mechanisms may promote the dissipation of the body heat or conserve it according to the need indicated by the heat-regulating centre in the hypothalamus. For further details of temperature regulation, see Chapter 8.

The fluid sweat lying on the surface of the skin cools the body by the process of evaporation, which requires energy in the form of heat; thus evaporation of sweat results in heat loss, so reducing body temperature. Sweat contains traces of albumin and urea; therefore sweating helps to remove these waste products from the body.

There are two types of *sweat glands*; *eccrine* glands which are distributed over the body surface and function to control body temperature and *apocrine* glands found mainly in the axillary and perineal areas which do not become functional until puberty. The latter are stimulated by stress and produce an odour.

Hair is a cylinder of keratinized cells. Distribution over the body varies with human groups, and with age and sex within each group. Hair serves primarily psychological functions.

The absorptive function of the skin is mainly limited to the absorption of ultraviolet rays from the sun or special lamps; it then converts sterol substances in the skin to vitamin D. A few drugs which may be included in ointments or lotions may be absorbed in small amounts.

The dermis and subcutaneous tissue may act as a storage area for water and fat. For instance, when an excess of water is retained in the body, the accumulation in these tissues becomes evident as oedema. The subcutaneous tissue serves as one of the main fat depots and acts as a pad over muscle and bone, cushioning them from mechanical forces.

The sebaceous glands protect the skin from moisture and prevent desiccation. With advancing years, they become less active as a result of the decreased production of hormones, and the skin becomes dry.

Due to its high proportion of collagen bundles and elastin fibres, the dermis provides mechanical strength and serves to anchor the epidermis to the basal layer of the dermis. The epidermis and its various appendages receive nourishment and support from the dermis. With age, degenerative changes occur in the elastic tissue and collagenous component of fibrous tissue, and the skin becomes wrinkled. Frequently, areas of melanocytes produce more pigment, and 'brown spots' characteristic of ageing skin appear.

The Person with Impaired Skin Integrity

Impairment of skin integrity may be primary or may be secondary to a systemic disease or reaction. It is not the author's intention to present an all-inclusive discussion of many specific skin disorders but, rather, to offer a

brief description of common manifestations, general principles of nursing care of patients with skin disorders, and a discussion of a few conditions that are encountered frequently.

For more detailed information relating to skin diseases, the reader is referred to dermatology texts.

THE PERSON WITH POTENTIAL FOR OR ACTUAL IMPAIRED SKIN INTEGRITY: PRESSURE SORES

A pressure sore or *decubitus ulcer* is a localized area of skin breakdown resulting from interference with the circulation to the affected tissue(s). Pressure sores cause pain and discomfort, prolong illness, delay rehabilitation and discharge, and may contribute to disability and death. Health care costs rise dramatically when individuals develop pressure sores. The need for supplies, nursing hours, hospital days, and community resources increase, in addition to the personal stress experienced by the individual.

The nurse plays a major role in the prevention and management of pressure sores and in assisting individuals and families to acquire the necessary knowledge and skill to promote, maintain and restore skin integrity.

RISK FACTORS

The four major precipitating factors in pressure sore development are: pressure, shearing forces, trauma and moisture. The degree and duration of these extrinsic factors and the status of the underlying tissue determine the rate at which tissue damage occurs. Intrinsic factors which influence the status of the person's tissue and its ability to tolerate these external forces include: sensation, nutritional status, incontinence, infection and any debilitating concurrent illness (Versluysen, 1986), as well as cognitive/perceptual function and immobility (Judd, 1989). Certain individuals are especially prone to develop pressure sores. They include people who are comatose, anaemic, febrile, depressed, spastic and elderly. Diabetes mellitus, arteriosclerosis, loss of vasomotor control and incontinence also increase the person's susceptibility for tissue impairment. Healthy tissue is maintained when the extrinsic factors are minimized and the intrinsic factors are at an optimal level of functioning. When the intrinsic factor(s) are impaired, the tissue's ability to tolerate the external forces is decreased. An increase in the degree and duration of one or more of the extrinsic factors also contributes to the development of pressure sores.

Table 26.1 The Norton scale for identifying the patient at risk of developing pressure sores.

A General physical condition		B Mental state		C Activity		D Mobility		E Incontinence	
Good	4	Alert	4	Ambulant	4	Full	4	Not	4
Fair	3	Apathetic	3	Walk with help	3	Slightly limited	3	Occasionally	3
Poor	2	Confused	2	Chairbound	2	Very limited	2	Usually urinary	2
Very bad	1	Stuporous	1	Bed-fast	1	Immobile	1	Double	1

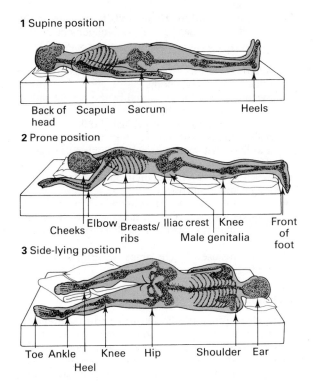

1 Supine position

Back of head   Scapula   Sacrum   Heels

2 Prone position

Cheeks   Elbow   Breasts/ribs   Iliac crest   Knee   Front of foot   Male genitalia

3 Side-lying position

Toe   Ankle   Heel   Knee   Hip   Shoulder   Ear

Figure 26.2 Risk areas for pressure sores.

The Person at Risk of Developing Pressure Sores

ASSESSMENT

Assessment of the person at risk for the development of pressure sores includes identification of the contributing factors. External factors are those which cause pressure, shearing and/or trauma to the skin as well as the presence of prolonged moisture. The individual's age, nutritional status, circulatory status, degree of mobility and dependence, ability to exercise, voluntary control (continence), sensory awareness, mental awareness and degree of alertness are assessed.

An assessment tool that assists in estimating the risk of skin breakdown has been developed: the Norton scale (Table 26.1). The maximum score used is 20; patients with high scores are least likely to develop a breakdown of their skin while those with lower scores are at greater risk. Although this scale is over 25 years old and has served as the standard for the development of subsequent scales, neither it nor other scales have been fully tested. Goldstone and Goldstone (1982) investigated the predictive ability of the Norton score. They concluded that it was a reliable guide to the incidence of pressure sores but that it tended to overpredict which persons would develop lesions. The physical and incontinence scores were found to be the most discriminatory. Other scales have been devised by Waterlow, Douglas and Knott. Barratt (1987) reviewed these scales alongside the Norton scale and stresses that while there is not sufficient research evidence to favour one against the other, the use of risk scales is to be encouraged as an objective measure of pressure sore risk. Further testing is needed to increase the usefulness of these scales in clinical practice for the identification of persons at risk and the prevention of pressure sore development. It should be remembered that Norton's scale was developed for use in the elderly; the validity of its application to younger patients is therefore open to challenge.

The skin is inspected at frequent intervals; areas subjected to weight bearing and friction should receive special attention. The vulnerable areas are the sacral region, buttocks, ischial tuberosity areas, spinal processes, scapular areas, occipital area, ears, elbows, knees and heels. The patient's body position is observed; the patient may favour one position, for example the dorsal recumbent or a lateral position, resulting in prolonged pressure on the respective vulnerable areas. In a lateral position, the area over the anterior iliac spine, greater trochanter, shoulder and malleoli become vulnerable. Figure 26.2 illustrates the areas receiving greater pressure in different body positions.

Body weight also influences the areas receiving greatest pressure. In the underweight individual, areas are more vulnerable in both the lying and sitting positions. In obese individuals pressure is distributed over larger areas. Casts, braces and underlying tubing are additional causes of pressure; the skin under these areas should be inspected regularly.

The skin over each pressure point should be carefully examined at frequent, regular intervals for redness, swelling, warmth, flaking and erosion.

The *goal* for the individual at risk for the develop-

Table 26.2 Nursing intervention to maintain skin integrity and prevent pressure sore development.

- Assess individual(s) for risk factors
- Ensure regular changes of position to relieve pressure on 'at risk' areas 2-hourly or more frequently if indicated by patient's condition
- Maintain cleanliness and hygiene
- Prevent mechanical, physical and chemical injury
- Ensure adequate nutrition and hydration
- Promote control of incontinence
- Ensure good body alignment and proper positioning
- Utilize devices to equalize pressure over pressure points
- Inspect the skin several times a day
- Promote mental alertness and orientation
- Educate the individual, family and care-givers in skin care measures

ment of pressure sores is to maintain the integrity of the skin.

NURSING INTERVENTION

Strategies and actions to promote skin integrity and to prevent the development of pressure sores are important aspects of the individual's health care that fall into the realm of nursing.

All individuals with suspected or known risk for pressure sores should be assessed for the degree of risk and identification of the specific factors. Assessments should be carried out on admission to hospital or nursing home, during community visits and whenever the person's health status changes. It should be remembered that it only takes a few hours for pressure sores to develop. For example, an elderly, immobile patient may develop a pressure sore while lying on a trolley in the accident and emergency department or during surgery.

Table 26.2 lists principles for nursing intervention directed at *maintaining skin integrity* and *preventing pressure sore development*. Nursing interventions include the following measures.

1. Promote ambulation and range-of-motion activities.
2. Have the patient change position frequently. If the patient is immobile, change body position every 2 hours throughout the day and night according to an established schedule. If redness is present, increase the frequency of the turning schedule.
3. Provide regular bathing and good perineal care twice daily and immediately following incontinence; keep skin dry but avoid friction and rubbing with towels.
4. Establish a programme to control or manage incontinence.
5. Encourage consistent intake of a nutritionally balanced diet with adequate fluid intake.
6. Use a mattress that distributes body weight over a large area and/or alternates pressure such as an alternating pressure mattress.

7. Keep sheets dry and free of wrinkles and crumbs. Flannelette sheets or pads provide protection from any underlying plastic or rubber covers.
8. Use devices to support specific pressure areas, such as foam pads, gel flotation pads, sheepskins and splints or pads over heels and elbows to relieve pressure on vulnerable areas and to decrease friction.
9. Use a footboard or cradle to prevent pressure on toes.
10. Provide space between the footboard and mattress for heels when the patient is lying supine, or the anterior part of the foot when lying in the prone position.
11. Use pillows and trochanter rolls in positioning the patient to maintain good body alignment and to relieve pressure on known risk areas (see Figure 26.2).
12. Keep connectors, tubes, pins and clamps from under the patient's body.
13. Avoid shearing forces caused by the patient sliding or slumping down the bed.
14. Those caring for the individual should keep their nails trimmed and remove rings, watches or other jewellery that might scratch or injure the patient during turning or care activities.
15. Teach people to inspect their skin regularly using a long-handled mirror.
16. Avoid the use of bedpans when possible for persons with sensory loss and paralysis. If the use of a bedpan is unavoidable, a slipper pan should be used.
17. Avoid the use of tight straps on urinary drainage leg-bags.

Evaluation

Strategies to promote skin integrity and to prevent the development of pressure sores are effective if the person's skin remains clean, dry and intact. If skin breakdown does occur, the nurse reassesses the total situation and determines if the original goal was realistic or if the person's status/situation has changed. Although the prevention of pressure sores is desirable, we must recognize that this is not always possible.

A quality assurance programme with defined standards for the care of persons at risk for skin breakdown provides a means for nurses to monitor the effectiveness of their practice. Information obtained from auditing health records is analysed by the nurses involved to identify areas of strength and weakness. The nurses define the standards they expect to achieve in preventing pressure sore development in their patients and develop and implement remedial actions to reinforce positive behaviours and to minimize negative behaviours.

The Person with a Pressure Sore

A pressure sore or decubitus ulcer is an area of inflamed and necrotic tissue. It develops as a result of sustained, localized pressure which compresses the blood vessels

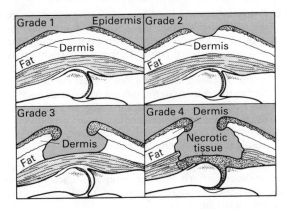

Figure 26.3 Classification of decubitus ulcers (pressure sores). *Grade 1*: Involvement of epidermis with some extension into the dermal layer, producing redness, induration, warmth and slight erosion of the epidermis. The reddened area blanches to the touch. *Grade 2*: Involvement of the epidermis and dermis with extension into the subcutaneous layer. The shallow ulceration shows induration, redness and heat and does not blanch to the touch. *Grade 3*: Involvement of epidermis and subcutaneous layers with extension down to and including muscle. The ulceration is deep, foul-smelling with a necrotic base and undermining of tissue. The borders are hyperpigmented. *Grade 4*: The ulcer involves all layers of the skin, the underlying muscles and communicates with bone or joint. The ulcer is deep; the tissue is necrotic and foul-smelling. Undermining is extensive. Borders are darkly pigmented.

in the area causing ischaemia of the skin and underlying tissues.

ASSESSMENT

The area may appear blanched and cool at first, followed by redness, warmth and a breakdown of the skin. As the necrotic tissue is sloughed off, an open, moist, inflamed excavation (ulcer) develops which is open to infection and is slow to heal by granulation.

The pressure sore area is examined closely to determine the extent and depth of tissue involvement and must be described accurately. The size of the lesion is measured in centimetres and is recorded at the onset and at frequent intervals until healing takes place. Figure 26.3 illustrates four different grades of decubitus ulcer according to the depth of the ulceration and involvement of underlying tissues. The pressure sore may be a reddened, slightly indurated area with only the epidermis sloughed off, forming a grade 1 decubitus ulcer. Grades 2, 3 and 4 indicate necrosis of progressively deeper tissues. The grading scale is useful for identifying the severity of tissue damage and changes that occur and in planning treatment. The lesion is examined for inflammation, bleeding, sloughing, infection and fibrous scar tissue formation. The area surrounding the lesion is inspected for discolouration, oedema and inflammation

which may signify extension of tissue damage.

Pressure sores may develop in underlying tissue as a result of internal pressure exerted by the bony prominences on the deep tissues adjacent to the bone. Such deep tissue necrosis may occur without any initial signs of damage to the overlying skin. Subsequently there is an area of swelling and tension and the skin becomes shiny and/or cyanosed. Erythema and a sinus develop at a later stage. If a sinus has formed, its depth and path may be determined by gently introducing a sterile probe; a sinogram may be ordered to define the length, size and exact location of the sinus and underlying tissue damage.

The person with a pressure sore is at risk of developing further lesions, therefore vulnerable areas are inspected every 2 hours or when the position is changed.

Nursing care for the individual is designed, whenever possible, to restore skin and tissue integrity and to prevent the development of further skin breakdown.

NURSING INTERVENTION

The number and variety of therapeutic measures and topical preparations used in the prevention and management of pressure sores indicate an urgent need for further controlled research studies. Multiple patient variables contribute to the complexity of the problem. Nursing intervention for a patient with a pressure sore has to be individualized, and is based on a detailed assessment of the patient as well as of the pressure sore; the general condition is important as well as the grade of the pressure sore. Consistency in carrying out the treatment plan is essential. The measures cited for the preventive care in the preceding pages are also applicable.

Further considerations include:

- Measures to correct existing health problems.
- The use of mechanical devices.
- Care of the lesion.
- Physical activity.
- The control of injurious factors in the environment.
- Surgical intervention.

Control of existing health problems

Optimal control of health problems is essential to promote healing as well as prevent a break in the skin. The reader is referred to the predisposing and causative factors cited on p. 916. Management of these problems requires the co-operative efforts of the patient, doctor, nurse and other individuals caring for the patient.

A high protein, high vitamin diet is important to combat the tendency toward a negative nitrogen balance associated with inactivity and to provide the essentials for healing and tissue resistance.

Mechanical devices

The mechanical devices used in the prevention and treatment of pressure sores may be divided into three categories:

1. Those designed to support specific pressure areas of

the body such as heels, sacrum, buttocks or elbows. These devices include gel flotation pads, sheepskins, splints and air-filled wheelchair cushions.

2. Those designed to aid in turning and moving a patient such as turning frames, rotating beds and hydraulic lifts.

3. Those designed to support the entire body surface by minimizing or equalizing pressure. Alternating pressure mattresses and beds, low air loss beds, which are individually pressurized according to the person's height and weight, and air fluidized beds in which air flows through ceramic-coated glass beads are examples of such devices.

A 5-month trial comparing the effectiveness of the commonly used, inexpensive, slab form of polyurethane foam cushions with the customized foam cushions found no significant differences in the preventive qualities of the cushions (Lim et al, 1988). More pressure sores occurred in the area of the ischial tuberosities in both groups of chronically ill, elderly persons. Since these sores were more severe in the subjects who used the slab cushions, the investigators supported the use of the more expensive customized cushions with this population only when an existing pressure sore in the ischial region has been a repeated problem.

Low air flow and air-fluidized flotation treatment strategies have been shown to be more effective than conventional therapy for hospitalized patients with large pressure sores (Allman et al, 1987). Turning and positioning of patients is often easier with these beds. Wounds can be kept moist or dryness can be promoted, depending upon the direction of air flow to the area. These devices supplement rather than replace the administration of excellent basic skin care and nutritional support.

Care of the pressure sore

Aseptic care of the lesion is necessary to reduce the infection potential of the open area. Gentleness is required when cleansing the area and when removing paste or ointment to avoid tissue damage. If there is a firm eschar on the surface of the ulcer, the scar must be scored with a scalpel to allow topical applications to penetrate. One must always assess the individual's pain before caring for the wounds. Appropriate pharmacological and non-pharmacological approaches for managing the level of discomfort can then be selected and reassessed on a consistent basis. Cultures are taken from the ulcer site after the surface slough has been cleared away to permit access to the underlying tissue.

A large variety of topical preparations are available for application in the prevention and treatment of decubitus ulcers (see Table 26.3). They are categorized according to their action and include: cleansing and antiseptic agents; protective preparations; debriding agents; and agents which promote granulation and epithelial tissue formation.

1. *Cleansing and antiseptic* agents are used to remove necrotic tissue, 'old' blood and exudate as well as inhibit the growth of organisms.

2. *Protective agents* provide a protective covering for the skin surrounding the lesion and may also be applied to the ulcerated area to protect granulation and new epithelial tissue. They are especially useful to protect surrounding skin when moist applications and a debriding agent are being used on the ulcer. Agents that adhere to the wound result in damage to the newly-formed granulation tissue and should be discontinued immediately.

3. *Debriding agents* may be enzymatic, keratolytic, autolytic or absorptive in action.

The enzymatic preparations used in debridement may be collagenic, fibrinolytic or proteolytic, according to the tissue component that reacts to the respective enzymatic agent.

A keratolytic agent promotes separation of the epidermal tissue and may also be antimicrobial and have a stimulating effect on granulation.

Autolytic preparations promote liquefaction of necrotic tissue by endogenous enzymes and keep the ulcer moist. A transparent adhesive dressing such as Opsite is applied to seal the wound or a hydroactive dressing (a transparent occlusive dressing with an underlying layer of gel) may be used (see Table 26.4 for a list of dressings for pressure sores).

A comprehensive review of the literature showed only four studies evaluating the effectiveness of moisture vapour permeable dressings in pressure ulcer care (Smietanka and Opit, 1981; Kurzuk et al, 1985; Oleske et al, 1986; Sebern et al, 1986). All studies demonstrated that the dressings promoted wound healing. Two studies showed increased pain relief (Smietanka and Opit, 1981; Sebern, 1986) and two demonstrated a saving in nursing time (Kurzuk et al, 1985; Sebern, 1986). These issues have been well discussed by Anthony (1987) who offers a useful review of valid pressure sore treatment.

Absorptive agents absorb the products of tissue breakdown. They are prepared in granular or bead-like forms and, sprinkled into the area, and can absorb copious amounts of exudate and debris.

Hypochlorite solutions (e.g. Eusol) have been shown to have serious harmful side-effects and their use should be discontinued immediately (Walsh and Ford, 1989).

Saline used as a soak, bath or compress is an effective and inexpensive cleansing agent. It softens and washes out necrotic and crusting tissues and exudate.

Physical activity. Pressure on the area is relieved as much as possible by having the patient change his position frequently. If unable to turn unaided, the patient is turned every 2 hours throughout the day and night. When turning or transferring a patient, precautions are observed to prevent further damage to the skin; the patient is gently lifted clear of the bed or chair to avoid dragging and a shearing force.

Patient activity is encouraged; it stimulates metabolism as well as circulation. A programme of regular exercises adapted to the person's ability to actively participate is established as soon as possible.

Control of environmental factors. A frequent assessment is made of the person's environment for possible sources of pressure and injury to skin. Again, the reader

Table 26.3 Topical agents used in the management of pressure sores.

Types of agents	Examples	Comments
Protective agents	Silicone cream Zinc oxide cream	• Should be avoided as they are of no demonstrated value
Cleansing and antiseptic agents	Soaps and detergents	• Should be avoided as they tend to dry and irritate tissue. If used, the skin should be rinsed well
	Antiseptics • Povidone-iodine • Chlorhexidine • Sodium hypochlorite solution	• Should be avoided as they are of no demonstrated benefit and some agents have been shown to be harmful. The spread of antiseptic-resistant strains may be encouraged by their use and allergic reactions are also possible
	Antibiotics (topical) • Neomycin • Gentamicin	• Should be avoided • Resistant strains of organism may develop • May cause allergic sensitization
Débriding agents	Enzyme preparation • Streptokinase-streptodornase • Deoxyribonuclease Dextranomer	• Before application, loose necrotic debris should be surgically removed and the wound cleansed with saline • Acts through capillary force • Cleans wound by drawing exudate, bacteria and other biological substances
Occlusive dressings	Opsite Duo Derm Comfeel Ulcus	• Occlusive dressings can remain on skin for several days • Keep wound surface moist to promote healing • Protect wound surface from mechanical injury or bacterial entry

is referred to the measures cited in the prevention of a pressure sore. The bedding, wheelchair, bedpan or commode, clothing and appliances such as a prosthesis and drainage tubes or bags are examples of factors in the patient's environment that could be a source of pressure or injury.

Surgical treatment. Surgical debridement of a pressure sore may be done on the ward. Overgranulation of an ulcer may require removal of some of the excess tissue with scissors or by the use of a silver nitrate stick. Grade III and IV ulcers may require surgical excision and repair by skin flaps. For care of the patient following surgery see Chapter 11.

Selection of the treatment and nursing care for the patient with a pressure sore should be a co-operative effort by all members caring for the patient and should take into consideration the patient's needs, overall status and resources. For example, if frequent dressing changes cause discomfort for the patient, consideration is given to a treatment method that requires dressing changes about every 5–7 days; an occlusive dressing (Opsite) has additional advantages of being easier for the person to manage at home, interfering less with daily activities and enabling the patient to have a bath without interfering with the dressing. A variety of interventions are usually required; selection is based on

evaluation of the effectiveness of care and assessment of the individual patient.

Patient/family education

The learning needs of the patient and family are assessed on an on-going basis. The individual and family are encouraged to participate in the care planning and in the management of the patient's pressure sores. They are taught to identify risk factors and to plan and carry out measures to prevent further skin breakdowns. If the patient is in the community or returning home before healing is complete, the patient, family and care-givers are taught the skills necessary to carry out the skin care regimen. They are also advised to make life-style changes to promote adequate nutrition, rest and activity.

Evaluation

The evaluation of nursing interventions designed to treat the individual's pressure sore(s) include documented evidence that healing is occurring. The size and depth of the lesions are decreased, exudate is absent and clean granulation tissue is present. When healing is complete, the area will be clean, dry and intact. Related outcomes include the absence of discomfort, and appropriate and realistic improvements in nutritional status, mobility and incontinence.

Table 26.4 Examples of dressings for pressure sores.

Classification	Examples	Comments	Frequency of change	Ulcer type
Foams	Silastic Synthaderm Lyofoam Coraderm	The surface that is applied directly to the wound is water-permeable while the back is non-absorbent Provide protection and a thermal effect Associated with a marked increase in exudate in the early stages Lyofoam is not very absorbent	2–10 days	Those that are not exudative with little slough and poor formation of granulation tissue
Polysaccharides	Debrisan	Can act as a cleaning or débriding agent Can stick to the wound if not enough moisture An additional dressing is needed on top	Daily preferred	Offensive and sloughy ulcer
Hydrogels and hydrolloids	Vigilon Geliperm Scherisorb Comfeel Ulcus Granuflex	Absorb exudate from the wound and reduce smell Do not adhere to wound Some need additional dressing on top Various formulations are available	Vigilon, Geliperm, Scherisorb — daily to every 3 days Comfeel Ulcus, Granuflex — up to every 7 days	Offensive and exudative wounds
Alginates	Sorbsan Kaltostat	Seaweed products which gel in contact with wound exudate	Daily to alternate days	Offensive and exudative wounds

If documentation indicates that the pressure sore is the same or that deterioration has occurred, the patient's status, the goals for care as well as the suitability of the strategies used are re-evaluated.

In conclusion, it should be noted that in their review of pressure sore treatment Walsh and Ford (1989) stated that much care is meaningless ritual that is of little value and may be of positive harm. The need is for rational, research-based pressure care, not ritual and tradition.

THE PERSON WITH IMPAIRED SKIN AND TISSUE INTEGRITY: BURN INJURIES

To sustain a burn injury is to be confronted by one of the most devastating and multifaceted trauma known to man. In addition to managing a multitude of physiological challenges for a prolonged period of time, the burn survivor has to contend with a complex array of psychosocial/quality-of-life sequelae. The family and significant others are also affected by the impact of the burn trauma. Nursing the person with a burn and the family can be one of the most complex, challenging and immensely rewarding opportunities in a nurse's career.

CAUSES

Causes of burn injuries include:

- *Dry heat*: direct contact with a flame or hot object.
- *Scalds*: moist heat such as boiling water, steam or hot liquid at more than 66°C.
- *Friction*: contact with a moving wheel, rope, wire or asphalt.
- *Radiation*: overexposure to sun and radiant heat sources, e.g. tanning lamps.
- *Chemical*: acids (sulphuric, nitric, hydrofluoric, hydrochloric) and alkalis (caustic soda, oven cleaners).
- *Electrical*: direct passage of current through the body, and lightning injuries.

RELATED FACTORS

A large proportion of burn injuries are due to carelessness, lack of knowledge and resources or personal feelings of invulnerability. Townsend et al (1982) showed that the incidence of burn injury was much more common in children of poorer families.

The age of the person is an important factor in the type and severity of the burn. Scalds are the most common cause of burn injury in the toddler for example, and the impact of any given burn injury is more severe in children and the elderly than in adults.

PREVENTION OF BURN INJURIES

Prevention of burn injuries is aimed at two levels: prevention of the occurrence of the injury and prevention of complications resulting from the burn injury. There are a number of well-organized burn and fire prevention programmes available through various fire departments and burn units/foundations. Health promotion activities planned for the population at greatest risk for sustaining a burn injury and joint collaboration with local fire brigades are excellent means for nurses to be seen disseminating health promotion messages to the public, while posters in waiting rooms of general practitioners' surgeries or accident and emergency departments are another useful means of getting the message across. Such messages can inform individuals about home safety tips, fire and burn prevention strategies and give important information on burn first aid. In-patient education focuses on different areas so as not to make the individual feel more responsible for the accident having occurred than may already be the case. Sensitive and well-timed discussions with patients can focus on prevention of a similar burn injury, first aid advice, and home safety tips. One must be alert to the person's readiness to learn about this sensitive topic. Experience with burn survivor support groups has indicated that, following their recovery, those people who have sustained a burn injury, regardless of the cause and circumstances, in most instances become avid fire and burn prevention advocates. Their support can and should be mobilized through prevention programmes.

We also have to battle with the common problem associated with most trauma prevention activities: the 'It will never happen to me' phenomenon. Increased interaction between the public and burn survivor organizations, together with straightforward, written material, help to decrease the sense of personal invulnerability, but at a painfully slow pace.

Education, however, is not the sole answer. National legislation and industrial awareness are necessary to make our world a safer place for adults and children. For example, legislation on childrens' and adults' flame-retardant sleepwear, banning cigarette smoking, smoke detector installation, use of short, flexi-cords for appliances, and hot water heater temperature regulation are all needed.

CHARACTERISTICS OF BURN INJURIES

Severity of a burn injury is determined by five factors:

1. Surface area of body burned
2. Depth of tissue damage
3. Age of patient
4. Past medical history
5. Part of body burned

Surface area. The most accurate estimation of the percentage of body surface burned may be based on the Lund and Browder chart (see Fig. 26.4). The chart assigns a certain percentage to various parts of the body and includes a table indicating the adjustments necessary for different ages, since the head and trunk

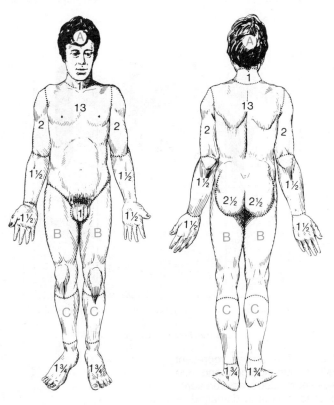

Figure 26.4 The Lund and Browder burn chart.

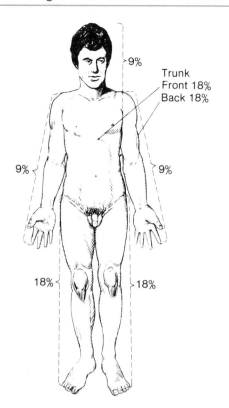

represent relatively larger proportions of body surface in children. The Berkow chart is a similar alternative to the Lund and Browder chart; it is accurate for all ages but is more time consuming to use. Copies of these charts should be kept available in the emergency department or intensive care unit so that the burned areas can be mapped out when the patient is examined and the percentage estimated.

If the Lund and Browder or Berkow charts are not available, a quick approximate estimate of the percentage of body surface burned may be made using the Rule of Nines (Figure 26.5). The Rule of Nines, unlike the Lund and Browder and the Berkow charts, is useful for adult patients only and should not be used for children under the age of 15 years. The body is divided into areas, each of which represents 9%. The apportionment is as follows: the whole of the upper limb is 9%, a thigh 9%, a leg (below the knee) 9%, the anterior chest 9%, the posterior chest 9%, the abdomen 9%, the lower half of the back (lumbar and sacral regions) 9%, the head and neck 9%, and the perineum 1%. If the burns are scattered, the palm of the patient's hand may be taken to represent 1% of his or her total body surface area.

If approximately *10% or more of the body surface of a child or 15% or more of that of an adult is burned, the injury is considered to be a major burn.* The patient requires hospitalization and fluid replacement to prevent shock.

Figure 26.5 Rule of Nines; used for estimating the percentage of body surface burned.

Depth. The depth of tissue damage is the result of two factors: the temperature of the burning agent and the duration of exposure. Burn depth is classified as

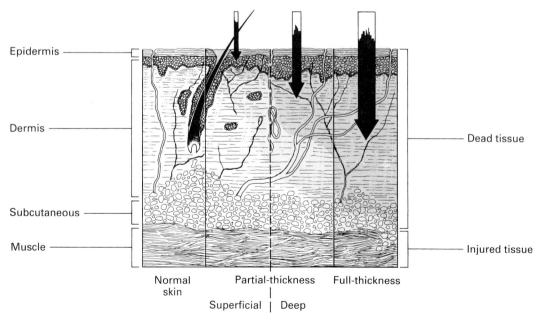

Figure 26.6 Depth of burn. The arrows represent degree of heat or intensity of burning agent and time of contact with skin. The darker shaded area represents dead tissue; the lighter shaded area is damaged or injured tissue which will heal with good care.

Table 26.5 Characteristics of partial-thickness and full-thickness burns.

Factor	Partial-thickness burn	Full-thickness burn
Sensation	Normal or increased sensitivity to pain	Anaesthetic to pain and temperature
Blisters	Large, thick-walled will usually increase in size	None or, if present, thin-walled and will not increase in size
Colour	Red, will blanch with pressure and refill	White, brown, black or red. If red, will not blanch with pressure
Texture	Normal or firm	Firm or leathery

From Feller and Archambeault-Jones (1973) with permission.

superficial partial-thickness, *deep partial-thickness* and *full-thickness* (Figure 26.6). Superficial burns, such as those produced by sunburn, are not taken into consideration when assessing extent and depth.

A superficial partial-thickness burn involves total destruction of the epidermis and very minor involvement of the dermal layers and appendages. Healing usually occurs within 7–10 days.

A deep partial-thickness burn involves total destruction of the epidermis and major involvement of upper dermal layers only. Lower dermal layers remain intact. Healing usually occurs within 14–21 days.

Table 26.5 illustrates the symptoms associated with partial and full-thickness burns. A full-thickness burn involves total damage to the epidermis and major damage to both upper and lower dermal layers. Subcutaneous tissue, muscle and bone may also be involved. Healing by the formation of normal epithelial tissue cannot occur, given the extensive damage to the body's skin reproducing cells; skin grafting therefore is required.

A *full-thickness* burn is characterized by the destruction of the full thickness of the skin and its appendages. Underlying tissues such as the subcutaneous fat, muscles, tendons and bone may also be burned. The skin's re-epithelializing cells are located throughout the dermis and along the dermal appendages, such as the shafts of the hair follicles and the sweat glands. Therefore, when the dermis is damaged, spontaneous regeneration and replacement of the skin is not possible. The area may be slowly filled in with granulation tissue and fibrous scar tissue, proliferated from marginal or underlying connective tissue. In order to avoid the contracture disability that occurs with the fibrous scar tissue, the area may be covered with a skin graft.

Age. Persons younger than 2 years and older than 50 have the highest incidence of morbidity and mortality. The severity of the burn increases with age. A person of 20 withstands a burn better than a 40-year-old, and the patient of 40 has a much better chance of survival than a 60-year-old, even though the percentage of body surface burned and the depth are the same. Infants and young children also tolerate burns less well than young adults.

PATHOPHYSIOLOGICAL EFFECTS OF BURNS

The person who suffers a major burn develops shock which, in some cases, may be irreversible. Immediately following the injury, the pain and fear which may be experienced by the injured person are considered to be responsible for widespread vasodilatation and subsequent hypotension and impaired circulation. This phase may be referred to as *neurogenic shock* or *nervous compensation*. The duration varies; it may be brief or may persist to become a part of the *hypovolaemic (oligaemic) shock* that develops rapidly as a result of the loss of fluid from the circulating blood volume. Increased permeability and dilatation of the capillaries in the burn area result in a shift of protein-rich fluid out of the vascular compartment into the interstitial spaces, causing the formation of blisters and oedema. Large volumes of the fluid, which is similar in composition to plasma, may seep into the tissues. Some is carried away via the lymphatics, but an amount in excess of what can be drained into the lymphatic system accumulates. The oedema is also promoted by the loss of blood proteins with the fluid and the ensuing reduction of the intravascular colloidal osmotic pressure. As a result oedema also occurs in non-burned tissue, resulting in generalized oedema. Oedema of the lungs from this cause can be life-threatening, even in the absence of any respiratory injury. In a full-thickness burn the fluid loss is extensive and, in areas of greater vascularization, such as the face, the oedema and swelling may be very severe.

In response to the massive inflammatory reaction post burn, there is an increased release of catecholamines. The intravascular volume is reduced, the blood pressure falls, the cardiac output may be decreased by as much as 30–50% (in burns greater than 40%, the decrease occurs within 15–30 minutes post burn), and the blood flow through the tissues is reduced. Other factors which contribute to decreased cardiac output include hypothermia (due to the release of a prostaglandin metabolite, which resets the hypothalamus), acidosis (due to increased lactic acid), decreased coronary artery perfusion, and the possible release of a myocardial depressant factor. *Hypovolaemic shock* develops unless there is adequate fluid replacement. The reduction in the intravascular volume produces a corresponding haemoconcentration, evidenced by an increase in the haematocrit and haemoglobin levels. (Normal haematocrit: males, 40–50%; females, 37–47%. Normal haemoglobin: males, 13–18 g/dl; females 12–15 g/dl.) The greater concentration of cellular elements in the blood increases the demand on the heart and predisposes to thrombosis and circulatory insufficiency.

An 8–10% decrease in the number of red blood cells occurs especially in deep burns, due to trapping and heat injury of those blood cells in the skin capillaries at the time of the injury. Often red cells, including transfused cells, may also be destroyed in the immediate post-burn period; blood transfusion may be delayed for at least 48 hours. Normal red blood cell production may also be reduced because of depression of the bone marrow.

Inhalation of smoke and chemical fumes can seriously impair ventilatory function; irritation of the mucosa may cause laryngeal oedema and airway obstruction or pulmonary oedema and severe respiratory insufficiency.

The urinary output is decreased as a result of the decreased intravascular volume and subsequent hypotension. If the blood supply is markedly reduced in the shock phase, renal tubular damage may also result. Providing intravenous fluid replacement is adequate, and shock is reversible, a fluid shift occurs in the opposite direction from the initial stage. Oedema decreases and blood volume increases, producing haemodilution and diuresis. Diuresis and increased sodium excretion occurring in 3–5 days are favourable signs. When there is massive red blood cell destruction, large quantities of haemoglobin are released. These blood pigments may block the renal tubules, causing renal shutdown. Another cause of renal failure in the burn injured patient is due to the breakdown of protein from damaged tissue, especially muscle, and the release of these products (e.g. myoglobin) into the renal tubules.

The appearance of brownish black urine indicates the presence of free haemoglobin and/or myoglobin; this is an ominous sign which requires urgent action to achieve diuresis.

In severe burns gastrointestinal peristalsis is depressed; nausea, vomiting and abdominal distension may occur. Haematemesis or melaena may develop, indicating the presence of stress ulcers. Gastric ulceration has been found to occur in 78% of those burns affecting more than 30% of the total body surface area.

Electrolyte imbalances develop because of the burn oedema, loss of fluid through the open wound, impaired renal function in the associated shock, and excessive release of potassium by the damaged tissue cells and erythrocytes. The disturbances are also influenced by the adrenocortical response (increased secretions) to the stress, which results in sodium retention and increased potassium excretion by the kidneys (if they are functioning satisfactorily). The adrenocortical hyperactivity also accelerates protein catabolism, resulting in a negative nitrogen balance. Immunologically, after a major burn, the patient is compromised, a condition which usually prevails until the patient dies or the wounds are resurfaced and there is a gradual increase in IgG, properdin, complement, factors I, V, VIII and fibronectin. All burn wounds are colonized with bacteria. Once the bacterial counts become high and infectious organisms enter the lymphatic system, the patient can develop septicaemia or is said to be septic. Sepsis accounts for 70% of the deaths post burn and the nurse plays a crucial role in identifying the subtle, soft signs of sepsis indicative of this change in status. Multisystem organ failure, often secondary to sepsis, is a serious and frequently fatal consequence of septicaemia.

The layer of burned tissues may form a dry, charred, coagulated surface, called an *eschar*, or a soft, moist non-coagulated area. Inflammation and oedema develop at the wound margins and below the layers of dead tissue. Many small blood vessels below the devitalized tissue may be thrombosed, promoting further cellular destruction. The decomposition of dead tissue and sloughing produce a favourable culture medium for organisms and the development of serious infection.

NURSING ASSESSMENT

Assessment of the person with a burn injury is a collaborative function between the nurse and physician.

Health history

Following the introduction to the patient, the nurse can begin to gather data about how the individual was burned, past medical history, existence of any known allergies, and medications the patient is currently taking. This information can be obtained from the patient, family, ambulance personnel, transferring health care personnel or colleagues accompanying the patient.

Physical examination

An assessment of the ABCs of trauma management should follow as soon as possible after admission. Although an assessment of the individual's airway, breathing patterns, circulation and cervical spine immobilization may have been performed at the accident scene, the nurse should conduct his or her own assessment in the hospital treatment area. The person should also be assessed for bleeding, shock and concomitant injuries.

The potential for ineffective airway clearance and ineffective breathing pattern is a primary concern. The airway should be checked for patency, the patient's vital signs and level of consciousness monitored and recorded, and the presence or absence of inhalation injury determined. If the patient is experiencing respiratory distress, the nurse can play an important role in calming the individual and providing support while interventions take place to restore an adequate airway.

Signs and symptoms of smoke inhalation include burns to the head and neck, singed nasal hairs, darkened oral and nasal membranes, carbonaceous sputum, stridor, history of being burned in an enclosed space and exposure to flame. Following an assessment of the status of the cervical spine, a laryngoscope and/or fibreoptic bronchoscope may be inserted in the airway to determine the extent of any inhalation injury and subsequent risk of impaired gas exchange. The nurse can provide much needed emotional support to the burned individual during these diagnostic tests.

Circulation to burned and unburned areas should also be assessed and noted on the health record. Altered tissue perfusion can occur with the oedema as a result of hypovolaemic shock and constriction of blood vessels in circumferential burns. If the nurse cannot feel the pulses with her fingertips, a Doppler may be used to determine their presence or absence.

The previously mentioned severity factors of extent and depth of burn and the part of the body burned are included in the physical assessment.

Following removal of all constricting items, such as jewellery and belts, and remaining clothing, the burn wounds can be inspected more closely. The extent of the burn can be determined by filling in one of a number of available burn estimation tools (see p. 923). This exercise should be performed by more than one person, e.g. doctor and a nurse, to ensure accuracy. The potential for fluid volume deficit exists if the extent of the burn is greater than 15% of the total body surface area. The resulting hypovolaemic shock makes fluid replacement a top priority.

The depth of the burn can be determined using criteria such as those described in Table 26.5. It may take several days of ongoing assessment before an exact determination of depth can be made. Burns can also convert (become deeper) if the burning process continues, if infection develops and/or if the wound is allowed to dry out.

The location of the individual's burns needs to be assessed and noted, e.g. the face, hands, feet and perineum. These particular areas pose specific functional and aesthetic challenges which should be identified early post burn.

The burned individual's renal and gastrointestinal function also need to be assessed. The nurse can pass a urinary catheter and assess the quantity and quality of the urine produced. Laboratory data such as a complete urinalysis and haemoglobinuria provide further objective information. Determining the presence or absence of bowel sounds, the insertion of a nasogastric tube and the assessment of gastric contents should also be performed by the nurse or the doctor.

The burned individual's comfort level should also be assessed and the request made for an analgesic and perhaps an anxiolytic to relieve pain and decrease anxiety.

Once the patient has been transferred or admitted to a burn treatment unit, physical parameters need to be monitored on a consistent basis to note changes in the patient's physical status.

Psychosocial concerns/developmental factors

These include an assessment of the individual's age, sex, ethnic origin, cultural background, usual coping mechanisms and responses to stress, responses to previous hospitalizations/illnesses and patient/family/significant other interactions. Other factors such as financial status, acceptance (adaptation to altered body image) and changes in roles and responsibilities need to be assessed at a later date.

Patient and family knowledge

The nurse can assist the patient and family in understanding the burn injury and treatment plan. It is important to assess the patient's and family's perception of the burned individual's health status, potential for rapid and fluctuating changes in that status, the educational level, readiness and willingness to learn, ability to comprehend what is being said and potential for non-compliance with treatment.

While the physical examination is taking place, someone from the health care team should be providing the family/significant others with information and emo-tional support. The burned individual should also be made aware of what is, and will be, taking place during the hospitalization and that loved ones are being kept fully informed.

Health Problems Common to the Person with Burn Injury

Impaired skin and tissue integrity is the major health problem experienced by the individual in relation to the burn injury. The restoration of skin and tissue integrity is a significant nursing concern. Much of what has been discussed in the previous sections of this chapter regarding this patient problem will apply to the individual with burns. Nursing care will be discussed in relation to the three phases of recovery: emergent, acute and rehabilitative. Associated health problems common to persons with burns will be discussed in relation to each phase.

EMERGENT PHASE

Care during the emergent phase is directed towards ensuring that the individual receives prompt, knowledge-able and appropriate first aid and initial medical and nursing care. The following key points require urgent attention:

- The patient should have a patent airway.
- The patient's wounds are protected.
- Further injury and contamination of wound(s) should not occur.
- The patient's pain is controlled.
- Prescribed treatment for hypovolaemic shock needs to be immediately implemented.
- The patient verbalizes concerns and feelings of anxiety.
- The patient and family verbalize awareness of the patient's status and care.

Care during the emergent period includes first aid at the site of the injury and the initial medical and nursing care. This initial care is directed toward establishing and maintaining an airway if necessary, reversing hypovolaemic shock and cleansing and assessing the severity of the burned areas. The emergent period may last for 2–7 days.

FIRST AID (SEE TABLE 26.6)

Nursing intervention

The overall *aim* of burn first aid is to stop the burning process. With flame burns, the words 'Stop — Drop — Roll — Cool' apply. Running fans the flames and increases the severity of the injury. Immediate cooling of the burn wound is the next priority. Water is usually accessible. The burned area must be held or immersed under cool, running water or cool moistened towels or compresses can be applied. Burn blisters should be left untouched in the first aid situation as they

Table 26.6 First aid: at the accident scene for the burned patient.

1. Stop the burning process
2. Maintain airway — resuscitation measures may be necessary
3. Assess for other injuries and check for any bleeding
4. Flush the burn with copious amounts of cold water
5. Protect wounds from further trauma
6. Provide emotional support — have someone remain with patient. Explain that assistance will be available
7. Transport the patient to where medical care can be obtained

Table 26.7 Dressing minor burn wounds.

Layer of dressing	Rationale
Flamazine cream (silver sulphadiazene)	Antibacterial cream prevents infection of wound
Non-adherent dressing pad (e.g. Melolin or Telfa) and paraffin gauze	Prevents damage to new tissue when dressing removed. Makes dressing changes less painful
Thick gauze pad	Absorbs wound exudate
Tubular bandage for limb (e.g. Tubigrip), elasticated net tubular bandage for trunk (e.g. Netelast); may be supplemented by traditional crêpe bandage	Holds dressing securely in place

help protect the wound from contamination. Cooling reduces pain and decreases the effect of heat transmission through the tissues. Ice is avoided because of the sudden vasoconstriction that it produces. Hypothermia is a potential complication that can be decreased through the use of sheets and then blankets over the patient and adjusting the temperature of the cooling agent.

Once the burning process has been stopped, the ABCs of burn trauma management become crucial.

Oils, ointments, lotions and other preparations *should not* be applied, and no attempt is made to remove clothing that is adherent. The burn area is covered with a moist, sterile or clean material to exclude air (which stimulates pain) and to reduce contamination. Cling film is an excellent first aid dressing. Non-burned areas are covered with warm, dry covers. While awaiting transportation, the patient is kept at rest. A minimal amount of movement and handling is important.

In the case of chemical burns, the area is washed with generous amounts of water for at least 20 minutes or until the pain is lessened. The patient's clothing and any contact lenses are removed, since they may possibly contain some of the chemical substance. Care-givers should also protect themselves from any residual chemical. Neutralizers are no longer indicated as they produce an undesirable thermal reaction with the acid or alkali.

The patient with severe burns is conscious unless other injuries interfere with awareness. Simple explanations of what is being done should be provided and repeated frequently. The presence of a nurse can be very supportive and helps reduce the considerable amount of anxiety and fear experienced by the patient.

Most superficial burns involving approximately *less than 10%* of body surface are treated at home or in the accident and emergency department. Systemic effects in such cases are minimal and are not considered sufficiently significant to require hospitalization.

Outpatient management

It is essential that nursing staff ensure the patient will be able to manage at home before discharge from the accident and emergency department is arranged. Attention should be paid to ensuring the wound is securely dressed and the patient has adequate analgesia. The patient should be encouraged to return to the department before their next appointment if they are worried about the state of their injury (Walsh, 1990).

Wound care. Before a dressing is applied, burned areas must be gently but thoroughly cleansed with normal saline solution. Burned tissue (eschar) must be removed (debrided) carefully, with sterile scissors and forceps, in order to reveal the presence of healthy tissue. A suggested dressing routine is shown in Table 26.7. The patient should return to the out-patient department or clinic to have the dressing(s) changed every 3–4 days, or more frequently if it is disrupted or if breakthrough drainage occurs. With facial burns, wound care should be performed twice daily, with ointment reapplied as needed to keep the area lubricated.

In selected circumstances non-debrided wounds may be managed on an out-patient basis.

An immediate *assessment* of the patient's general condition is made before attention is directed to the burn wound (Table 26.8). A history as to how the burn was sustained is obtained from the patient or the accompanying person; this may indicate the need to

Table 26.8 Treatment of the severely burned patient on admission.

1. Maintain an airway and administer oxygen if necessary
2. Assess severity of injuries and degree of shock
3. Initiate fluid replacement — establish an intravenous line
4. Insert an indwelling catheter
5. Insert a nasogastric tube
6. Control pain
7. Provide emotional support
8. Provide initial wound care
9. Initiate protective isolation measures
10. Administer tetanus prophylaxis

search for other injuries. The burn patient is usually sufficiently alert to provide information; if drowsy, confused or comatose, other disorders or injuries are suspected (e.g. hypoxia, head injury, cerebral aneurysm or stroke).

POTENTIAL FOR INEFFECTIVE AIRWAY CLEARANCE AND INEFFECTIVE BREATHING PATTERN

Damage to the respiratory tract and respiratory insufficiency demand prompt attention. Respiratory impairment is frequently associated with burns of the face or neck and may be the result of the inhalation of smoke, a gaseous chemical or flames. The presence of singed nasal hair or blackened oral or nasal mucosa are suggestive of inhalation burns. To assess ventilatory function, observe respiratory effects and listen for inspiratory wheezes, check odour of breath (a smoky or chemical odour may be detected which indicates inhalation of smoke or fumes), listen for hoarseness, and examine any sputum for blood and carbon particles. Humidified oxygen is administered, if necessary, and suctioning may be helpful to clear the airway of secretions. Intubation may be performed if respiratory embarrassment increases. If there is marked insufficiency, a mechanical ventilator may be used in conjunction with the endotracheal tube. Frequent estimations of the blood gases and expiratory or tidal volume may be done. See Chapter 15 for the care required in respiratory insufficiency and endotracheal intubation. In addition, a chest X-ray should be taken to establish baseline lung findings and ensure proper placement of invasive tubes and lines.

Respiratory insufficiency may develop later in circumferential or severe chest burns due to restricted respiratory excursion as a result of a firm unyielding coagulum or eschar. The doctor may have to make several incisions in the eschar to relieve the thoracic restriction. This is known as escharotomy and may also be performed on circumferential full-thickness limb burns to prevent neurovascular compromise from the tourniquet-like effect of the eschar. Following the initial assessment and treatment, the patient is required to breathe deeply and cough hourly to avoid the risk of chest infection.

When satisfactory ventilation is established, attention is directed toward fluid therapy and assessment of the extent and severity of the burn and any other injuries.

HYPOVOLAEMIC SHOCK

The control of shock resulting from the loss of intravascular volume in a severe burn is dependent upon prompt, adequate fluid replacement. The extent and depth of burn and the patient's age and health status determine the need for fluid therapy. Burns greater than 15% of the total body surface require intravenous therapy. A reliable intravenous route is established by the insertion of two large intravenous catheters, preferably through unburned tissue. The intravascular fluid shift commences immediately after burning but signs of shock may not appear for a few hours. The choice of a fluid

resuscitation formula depends upon the attending doctor's and the institution's burn care protocol. Solutions that may be administered include colloidal solutions (contain large, non diffusible particles of solutes that will not leak out of the capillaries) such as plasma, whole blood and a plasma expander (e.g. Haemaccel), or a solution of electrolytes (e.g. lactated Ringer's solution). The volume, composition and rate of flow of the intravenous fluids are based on the percentage body surface burned, the weight of the patient, the hourly urinary output, arterial blood pressure, haematocrit, and serum electrolyte concentrations, especially potassium and sodium. An adult may require as much as 500–1000 ml per hour intravenously to maintain a urinary output of 30–60 ml per hour. Close monitoring and frequent adjustment of the intravenous flow rate is essential. If oral fluids are permitted, the amounts ingested are recorded accurately.

Generally, after the first 24–36 hours, fluid extravasation into the tissues lessens and the intravascular volume tends to stabilize gradually. This physiological phenomenon of fluid remobilization signals the end of the emergent period of care. Nursing documentation of intake/output continues to be an essential part of the patient assessment. The intravenous fluid therapy is gradually reduced and may be discontinued when laboratory studies indicate satisfactory concentrations and the patient is able to take adequate amounts of fluid orally. Close observation is needed for signs of circulatory overload, since much of the fluid in the interstitial spaces is reabsorbed into the intravascular compartment as capillary integrity is re-established. Overloading of the circulatory system may be manifested by a urinary output greater than 100 ml per hour within the first 48 hours, pulmonary oedema, a central venous pressure in excess of 13 cm of water and a weak pulse. If renal function is satisfactory, the excessive amount is controlled by diuresis.

An indwelling (Foley) catheter is passed as soon as the patient requiring fluid resuscitation therapy is admitted so that the hourly urinary output may be noted. This serves as a guide in determining intravenous fluid requirement and also provides information about the patient's general circulatory status and renal function. The urinary output should be at least 25–30 ml per hour for an adult. A volume below the normal minimum is reported promptly and a bolus of fluid, an increased hourly intravenous rate or a diuretic may be ordered until an adequate urinary output is reported. Urine specimens are tested hourly for specific gravity and sugar, acetone and protein and blood. Dark urine, indicating the presence of haemoglobin and myoglobin, is brought to the doctor's attention promptly. A bolus of a diuretic with mannitol (100–200 ml i.v.) may be ordered in the emergent phase for electrical burns where there is a high incidence of haemoglobinuria and myoglobinuria.

The catheter is removed as soon as the patient's condition is stable and shock is reversed, since the indwelling catheter predisposes to bladder infection and loss of bladder tone.

Dialysis may be initiated if the urine output drops below 400 ml in 24 hours. Haemodialysis is usually the treatment of choice to remove toxic wastes and excessive body fluids.

The patient is observed closely during the early post-burn period for symptoms of shock. The blood pressure, pulse and level of consciousness are noted every 15–30 minutes and the urinary output per hour is recorded. A diminishing intravascular volume and subsequent circulatory failure may be reflected by a fall in blood pressure, weak pulse, abnormal drowsiness, disorientation and a urinary output of less than 30 ml per hour.

Frequent haemoglobin and haematocrit determinations are made; abnormal elevations indicate haemoconcentration due to loss of intravascular fluid into the tissues. After 6 or 7 days a deficiency of erythrocytes and haemoglobin may indicate the need for a blood transfusion. As a consequence of hypovolaemic shock, a nasogastric tube needs to be inserted to depress gastric dilatation and the patient is given nothing by mouth until bowel sounds return. H_2 blockers, antacids and enteral/parenteral feeds may also be indicated. Serum protein and electrolyte concentrations are also determined frequently; these help in selecting the type of intravenous solutions required. An accurate record of the fluid intake (oral and intravenous) and the output is of paramount importance. The patient is weighed daily. A gain is manifested at first because of the increased extracellular fluid and the intravascular infusion. Then a marked weight loss accompanies the diuresis that corresponds with the recovery from shock. Much of the fluid which escaped into the interstitial spaces is reabsorbed into the blood vessels. During this period, the patient is observed for any signs of overhydration. If the intravenous infusion is continued at the previous rate of administration at this time the vascular system may become overloaded, placing an excessive demand on the heart and causing pulmonary oedema. The reabsorption of the tissue fluid can usually be recognized by a marked increase in the urinary output.

After the emergent period the nurse is alert for an elevation of temperature, rapid pulse, odour and discharge from the burned area which may indicate infection.

The patient's position, especially that of the burned parts of the body, is checked frequently during the day and night for optimum alignment. Flexion contracture may develop very quickly and preclude restoration of function.

ALTERATION IN COMFORT: PAIN

Pain assessment is a highly individualized and subjective process. Analgesics are administered to decrease the physical pain and anxiolytics are used to decrease the emotional overtones of the trauma. Many burn units successfully use a pain control regimen based on continual narcotic infusion, delivered by one of the many regulating devices now available, which is supplemented for breakthrough pain. The intravenous route is used because the circulatory disturbances and oedema reduce absorption via alternative routes.

Pain assessment and intervention is an ongoing task, and varies from patient to patient, and from day to day in the same patient. The patient's subjective response is the best indicator of the efficacy of a chosen strategy. The nurse's role in pain assessment and management is even more crucial when the patient is ventilated and/or comatose/confused. For more information on pain management, see Chapter 9.

ANXIETY

Following a severe burn, the patient and family experience considerable emotional disturbance. As with any severe stress, the reactions and adaptive mechanisms may vary markedly from one person to another, depending mainly on the particular situation and past experiences of each person. Factors which generate fear and anxiety in both the patient and family include the actual threat to life, permanent incapacity and disfigurement, the prolonged period of treatment necessitating dependence as well as separation, and the uncertain future.

The nurse should encourage the patient and family to discuss their concerns and fears. It is important that they are kept informed of all activities and why certain procedures and actions are being carried out. Repetition of information is necessary as the patient and family are anxious and experiencing varied and rapidly changing phenomena over which they perceive minimal, if any, control. Questions such as 'Will I be scarred for life?' should be given the honest answer 'We do not know', and the patient should be encouraged to express fears and anxieties as the nurse explores the patient's self-concept.

ONGOING NURSING MANAGEMENT

Collaboration with the physiotherapist and occupational therapist is important since the nurse usually co-ordinates the patient's care and may assume some of the functional responsibilities in the 'off hours'. Splints, head rolls, hyperextension devices and exercise routines are implemented as soon as possible following admission to maintain functional alignment of affected body parts.

Evaluation of the person following the emergent phase

The care provided to the person with a severe burn injury during the emergent phase is multifaceted and demonstrates collaboration among first aid workers, nurses in accident and emergency departments and special burns units, doctors, physiotherapists and other health professionals.

The following criteria may be used to evaluate the effectiveness of nursing care: airway will be patent, the breathing pattern effective, the fluid balance maintained, initial wound assessment completed, initial wound care protocols initiated, and pain and discomfort controlled. The patient and family will be able to describe what has happened and what the patient's status and progress are. They acknowledge receiving emotional support relevant to the emergency situation.

ACUTE PHASE

Sepsis is the primary cause of death in 70% of patients who die from burn injuries. Pneumonia and cardiovascular, respiratory, gastrointestinal and renal system failures are the other main causes of death. Complications tend to be the rule rather than the exception for individuals with severe burns. Experience of patients with burn injuries indicates the need to take a proactive approach to their care to try and prevent complications.

There are two primary patient *goals* in the acute phase for individuals with burns: (1) healing and closure of the burn wound; and (2) coping with physical and psychosocial complications that cannot be avoided. Through effective management of the first goal, many of the complications can be avoided or kept to a minimum. By treating persons with moderate to large burns in specialized treatment units, patient outcomes are improving internationally.

The following criteria can be used to measure the success of care. The patient will demonstrate:

- Absence of further wound contamination.
- Negative wound and blood cultures.
- Verbalization of absence/alleviation of pain and discomfort.
- Body temperature within normal range.
- Weight loss of less than 10% of preburn weight.
- A clean wound; absence of drainage and odour.
- Evidence of wound closure by re-epithelialization or acceptance of the graft.
- Limited development of scar tissue and contractures.
- Together with family members, verbalization of concerns and feelings of psychological support.
- Together with family members, verbalization of alleviation of distress; verbalization of understanding of the wound management protocol and participation, as appropriate, in care.
- Awareness of a plan for ongoing rehabilitation.

INTERVENTION

Potential for and actual infection

Avoiding or minimizing infection involves appropriate use of topical antimicrobial agents, support for the patient's immune mechanisms, rapid elimination of reservoirs of infection, and prevention of the transfer of infection.

Fresh frozen plasma and cryoprecipitate may be administered to support the patient's weakened immune system. Strict, aseptic technique is used when inserting invasive lines and when applying sterile inner dressings. If the patient has dressings in place, universal barrier precautions are instituted for infection control. These focus on the safe handling of all body substances/fluids as potential sources of infection. In many burns units, isolation gowns, head covers, masks and gloves are used when changing burn dressings. Disposable, non-sterile gloves are suitable for removing soiled dressings and for assisting with many patient care activities. The more expensive sterile gloves can be reserved for the application of inner dressings and for procedures requiring strict aseptic technique.

Everything in the patient's room is considered a source of contamination to him or her. It is also acknowledged that hospital personnel serve as vectors in the transmission of organisms between patients. The nurse wears a protective, isolation gown when rendering physical care to the patient. Visitors may also be instructed to wear gowns. The importance of strict hand washing guidelines and strict adherence to them must be stressed.

Septicaemia can develop at any stage until complete wound coverage is achieved. It may have a sudden onset, with rigors and a rapid elevation of temperature, or it may develop gradually over 2–3 days. It is characterized by high fever which may fluctuate, rapid pulse, drowsiness and disorientation. Paralytic ileus is a common concomitant. Oozing from the burn wounds or the appearance of purulent exudate or petechiae require wound swabs for examination by microbiologists and infectious disease specialists. Blood cultures are necessary for a definitive diagnosis. *Staphylococcus aureus*, haemolytic streptococcus and *Pseudomonas aeruginosa* are common causes of septicaemia.

Nursing interventions for the patient whose wound(s) have shown organisms on culture and is at risk for or has become septic include: careful and continuous monitoring for the early signs of impending sepsis; the administration of antibiotics; assistance with the insertion of invasive lines for more sophisticated diagnostic monitoring; and scrupulous wound and skin care. If a patient does develop a resistant organism, strict isolation procedures are implemented and enforced at all times. Regardless of the type of isolation employed, however, the most definitive answer to the problem of infection and resultant complications due to burns lies with coverage of the burn wound.

Wound healing

Various forms of local treatment are used to prevent further wound contamination and tissue destruction, suppress the growth of bacteria in the area, and promote separation of the devitalized tissue and its replacement with skin. Initially, the burn is cleansed of dirt, foreign substances and detached epithelium, using gauze and a mild soapy solution, water or normal saline. The temperature of the burn bath solution is kept at 37–38°C to approximate body temperature. If a hydrotherapy bath is not available, the cleansing is done on the stretcher or in the patient's bed. The entire burned area is bathed during the admission procedure. Loose, sloughing skin and debris are removed with sterile forceps and the skin may be removed from blisters. The cleansing must be *very gentle* to avoid damage of exposed viable tissue and the area is rinsed with generous amounts of water or saline.

There are three methods used to treat burn wounds. In the *open method*, the wound remains exposed. A thin layer (2–4 mm) of topical antimicrobial ointment may be applied over the wound surface. The exposure results in drying and the formation of a protective coagulum of serum. A cradle is used over the patient to support a sterile sheet and blanket to reduce body heat

Table 26.9 Objectives for wound management.

Prevention of conversion to full-thickness burn due to infection or desiccation
Removal of devitalized tissue
Preparation of healthy granulation tissue
Minimization of systemic infection
Completion of the autograft process
Limitation of scarring and contracture

loss. Exposure is the preferred form of treatment for facial, neck, head and perineal burns. If infection develops under the coagulum, it is removed and baths and topical antimicrobials used.

With the *closed method*, a dressing may be left intact for 1–7 days. The burned areas may be covered with a topical antimicrobial preparation and gauze. The topical applications commonly used include silver sulphadiazine (Flamazine) or povidone-iodine (Betadine).

The most common approach is to make *multiple dressing changes*, from twice daily to every 4 hours, according to a fixed schedule determined by the wound's condition and the properties of the dressing being used. The choice of treatment method varies among institutions, and also according to the condition of the burn wound. Flexibility with the wound management approach is very important in burn care. All treatment approaches have certain common objectives (see Table 26.9).

If a patient has a circumferential burn on a limb, close observations are made for signs of interference with the circulation as a result of the constricting effect of the dry, shrinking eschar. In the case of a circumferential eschar of the trunk, the constriction may restrict chest excursion and embarrass respiratory function. If signs of constriction appear, in the emergent or acute periods of care, or both, an escharotomy is done immediately under aseptic conditions. If the wound is deep enough, fasciotomies may also be performed.

Infection may develop under the eschar as a result of organisms that were present deep in ducts or on adjacent areas which were not destroyed at the time of the burn. Topical antimicrobial coverage is selected according to the condition of the wound, desired results and properties of the topical agent. It is also important, whatever topical and dressing strategies are chosen, that basic aseptic wound management techniques are followed. It is imperative to prevent burned surfaces from touching each other. Burned fingers or toes should be wrapped individually, and web spaces should be maintained wherever possible.

Choice of dressings, determined by the doctor in collaboration with the nurse, should take into consideration those which best promote healing, alleviate pain, apply pressure, enhance debridement, permit immobilization or mobilization (as desired at the time), preserve function and provide the patient with the least amount of psychological stress.

In a partial-thickness burn, healing (i.e. re-epithelialization) occurs under the coagulum, which gradually

separates. When a full-thickness burn is sustained, the non-viable tissue changes in 3–5 days to a hard, tough black layer (eschar). The eschar eventually sloughs off, liquefies and detaches from the viable tissue. There may be considerable drainage before there is complete separation. The wound will not granulate until the eschar has been sloughed off, therefore treatment in wound care is directed towards the promotion of this process. Alternatively, the wound may be debrided surgically. As the eschar is removed (by slough or debridement) granulation tissue consisting of fibroblasts and capillaries is gradually formed. If the granulation tissue is allowed to mature to fibrous scar tissue, the natural shortening of the collagenous fibres results in contracture of the area and possible deformity or loss of function, depending upon the location. Some marginal growth of epithelium may take place but, unless the burn is very small, this is usually insignificant.

Those wounds which are full-thickness in nature do not have the capacity for self-healing. These patients have their wounds surgically excised and skin grafts placed to provide permanent coverage. The patient's general condition and the size of the burn area determine whether the grafting will require several stages. Priority is given to areas where scarring and contraction produce loss of movement and marked deformity. The grafts may be laid or sutured or stapled, depending on their thickness. They are dressed with a pressure dressing or may be left exposed. If the grafts are around or over a joint surface, a splint or plaster cast may be applied to immobilize the part.

Split-thickness grafts may also be applied to deep partial-thickness burns since they produce a much better scar with improved wear and tear tolerance. Further information is offered about skin grafts at the end of this discussion on the care of the burned patient.

The only graft which is permanent is the autograft. As the name implies, the skin is taken from an unburned part of the patient's body (the donor site) and placed over the debrided, granulation tissue. No tissue rejection is experienced but 100% graft take is not guaranteed with every procedure. If there are not enough donor sites available, a temporary skin covering may be used.

Temporary, biological dressings include homograft (cadaver skin) or heterograft (pigskin or amniotic membrane). Isografts are special in that they come from an identical twin and can be placed on the other twin's debrided area and not be rejected. This type of procedure is relatively rare, but very successful.

Temporary, synthetic dressings are also available when it is necessary to gain time for the patient awaiting further grafting. Such products include Tegaderm and Opsite. Normal saline and dressings can also be applied.

Recently, selected patients with major burns and with no available donor sites have been managed with autologous epidermal skin cultures or a bilayer 'artificial' skin covering with dermal components. Both strategies, whilst not widely available, hold promise for future burn survivors.

Donor sites are usually covered intraoperatively with a protective inner dressing. A normal saline and gauze dressing are placed on top of the inner dressing. After one to several days postoperatively, depending on the unit protocol, the outer dressings are removed and the wound redressed once daily. In 5 days or so, the inner dressing is removed and fresh paraffin gauze is placed on the wound. Great care must be taken with donor sites for they increase the open body surface area and put the patient at greater risk for infection. The donor sites can be reharvested in about 10 days, once they have healed, providing the patient with the opportunity to have several grafts taken from the same place. Donor sites can be very painful wounds.

Patient teaching related to skin grafts

The nurse who is involved in all stages of wound healing plays a very important role with respect to patient and family teaching and support around this crucial aspect of burn care. When the patient learns that skin grafts are needed, he or she can become apprehensive or have unrealistic expectations regarding graft 'take' and the 'finished product's' appearance. This support and teaching continue until the wound and scars have fully matured, a process which can take several years.

Positioning and exercises

The patient is turned every 2–3 hours to prevent respiratory congestion and circulatory stasis. If the back is burned or the involvement is circumferential, care is facilitated if the patient is nursed on an air-fluidized support system (Clinitron bed). Because of the oedema, burned extremities are elevated on pillows or another form of support during the initial phase. Frequent attention is paid to body alignment; flexion contractures, outward rotation of thighs and footdrop must be prevented.

Splints may be applied if the multiple-dressing change or closed wound care procedure is used. They may be used for immobilization to promote healing and to prevent contracture and deformity. The splint used must fit the contour of the part to which it is applied and be secured well enough to provide stability but not cause pressure or interfere with circulation.

Burned parts which involve joints are moved through their range of motion as soon as possible and as indicated by the doctor. Early skin grafting permits the patient to be mobile earlier and prevents contractures. The physiotherapist usually supervises the exercise programme. The patient in a bath is encouraged to exercise while soaking. As healing occurs, the activity programme is progressively increased to preserve normal range of motion and function.

Nutrition

In addition to fluid therapy, nutrition plays an important role in the recovery of the burned patient. In the initial shock period in severe burns the patient is sustained mainly by intravenous fluids. Oral food and fluids are usually restricted for 24–48 hours for patients with severe burns. The initial hypovolaemic shock produces depression of gastric motility. A nasogastric tube is inserted and connected to intermittent suction. The tube is removed in 2–3 days when bowel sounds have returned and a clear fluid diet initiated. Oral intake is carefully monitored in relation to the patient's fluid balance. The intake is progressively increased from fluids, through soft foods, to a full normal diet.

The patient develops a negative nitrogen balance as a result of tissue catabolism which increases susceptibility to infection and debilitation and delays healing. A high-calorie, high-protein and high-vitamin diet is recommended to provide the essentials for tissue repair and the production of antibodies and blood cells. Vitamin C is essential in the synthesis of corticosteroids and in tissue repair, and the vitamin B complex is needed in the many cellular enzyme systems essential to normal cellular responses.

Ingenuity and resourcefulness are necessary on the part of the nurse to have the patient take the essential food. The patient should be advised of the important role of nutrients in the diet, and small frequent feedings of high-calorie foods are offered. Supplements of protein concentrates may be added to fluids or given through a fine bore nasogastric tube. Likes and dislikes are determined and respected, and the family is encouraged to bring in favourite foods. Adequate assistance is provided so that taking meals does not require too great an effort. A close check is made of the patient's daily intake, and the weight is also recorded daily.

Evaluation of the acute phase

Following the acute period of care after a severe burn injury the following criteria may be used to evaluate progress.

The patient's wounds demonstrate healing and acceptance of skin grafts. The patient verbalizes absence or alleviation of pain and discomfort. Signs of infection are absent; the wound is clean and free from drainage and odour; body temperature is within normal range; body weight is within acceptable limits with a loss of not more than 10% of preburn weight; and wound and blood cultures are negative. Systemic complications are prevented or managed and rehabilitation is promoted. The patient and family understand the wound care protocol and are actively participating in the care as appropriate to the person's health status and the level of understanding and readiness of the individual and family. They are able to express their feelings and concerns and verbalize feelings of support from the burns team members.

During the acute period of care, the nurse assumes both independent and collaborative responsibilities for the assessment and management of the patient's wounds, for the identification of patient and family concerns and anxieties, and for teaching the patient and family about the wound and overall plan of care.

REHABILITATION PHASE

Rehabilitation of the burned patient is fostered throughout the acute stages by conscientious attention to good body alignment, the prevention of infection and contractures, and the maintenance of joint and limb mobility as much as possible. Following recovery from the burn, considerable reconstructive surgery and retraining may be required before the patient can resume independent and self-supportive functioning. Rehabilitation is a lengthy process for many, and they and their families may require social guidance and financial assistance as well as psychological support throughout. Retraining for a different occupation may be necessary. In some instances the patient finds it very difficult to resume social contacts and to take his or her place in society because of scarring and gross disfigurement.

The *goals* for the person are (1) to achieve maximum function and optimal reconstruction, and (2) to achieve an acceptable quality of life. The achievement of these goals may be shown by:

- Absence of infection.
- Intact skin.
- Range-of-movement exercises and functional movement in involved joints.
- A plan to continue the prescribed exercise programme.
- A diet plan to obtain adequate protein, vitamins, minerals and calories.
- Understanding of prescribed skin care routine.
- Independence in personal care.
- Return to social activities.
- Return to employment or plans for job retraining.
- Plans for continuing health care.

INTERVENTION

Skin and tissue integrity

Healed burns must be kept well moisturized since the sebaceous glands are unable to secrete sufficient lubricating oils. Frequent applications of mild, non-perfumed, water-based moisturizers are recommended; oil-based lotions can block pores and do not penetrate into the dermis. For 5 months, burn survivors must not exposure their healed burn or donor sites to direct or indirect sunlight. Sunblocks and clothing/hats must be worn to prevent sunburn and hyperpigmentation.

All wounds heal by the process of contraction. Burn patients must be made aware of the possibility that the splints and other corrective devices they may have been utilizing since the day of admission (in essence, day 1 is when rehabilitation begins) may not bring about a miraculous or 'good as new' result. Further corrective surgery may be needed to release the contracture and insert a skin graft.

Hypertrophic scarring is another result of healing from a burn injury. Some individuals have a greater propensity for scarring than others. The burns team may frequently be unable to give definite answers regarding the need or duration of use of pressure garments/devices for pressure therapy. Counselling should also include information on skin care and cosmetic camouflage. Future surgery may be necessary for these patients, but in the future, for it takes approximately 2 years for the pressure to exert its maximal effect and for the burn

scar to fully mature. It is important to stress that, when counselling these patients the nurse emphasizes that these time frames are estimations and that every patient responds to therapy in a unique manner. A good rule is to be cautiously optimistic, to repeat a number of times and to document what the patient and family have been told.

Compliance with positioning and exercises can be a difficult challenge for the burn survivor. Patient education and support from burns team members can be very helpful in meeting these challenges in a positive manner. In addition, the patient is encouraged to undertake more responsibility for self-care. The occupational therapist and nursing staff need to encourage the patient to perform self-care activities, such as personal hygiene, dressing and participating in recreational activities. It is the nurse who undertakes the activities that the physiotherapist, occupational therapist and the patient have worked hard on that day when the therapists are not here. In order not to lose valuable function, rehabilitation activities must be attended to with much energy by all concerned.

Alteration in individual and family coping

As the burned individual prepares to leave the protective environment of the burns unit, numerous feelings may be experienced. The nursing staff, who have formed a unique and trusting bond with patients and families, should be sensitive to and encourage the need for the patient to verbalize concerns and questions. The burned person may experience feelings of uncertainty, fear and anxiety about what lies ahead, decreased confidence due to weeks and perhaps months of dependence on hospital staff, concern about coping with treatment protocols and impaired physical mobility and learning to re-enter society, potentially with an altered body image and decreased sense of self-esteem. Nervousness about returning home after a prolonged absence and concerns about resumption of previous roles and responsibilities may also be experienced.

It is important to make the person aware that these concerns are very normal for the burn survivor at the same stage of recovery. Knowing that one is not alone can be very comforting. Introduction to previously discharged patients and members of a burns support group, if available, can be a helpful strategy and be part of an overall predischarge teaching programme aimed at assisting the burned individual and the family to gather information and receive support aimed at facilitating the smoothest transition as possible from hospital to home.

Family members generally experience anxiety since they are now assuming the caretaker role once held by burns team members. They may have many questions about their loved one's physical care and emotional readjustment. They may express concerns about how to support the burned individual emotionally as he or she adjusts to being home, re-enters society and begins to socialize with friends and be seen in the community by strangers, and contemplates what the future may bring. Family may have concerns about their own reactions to the burn survivor, and should receive support and advice in this regard. A common concern requiring attention revolves around setting limitations on what the family will and will not do for the burned person. If they have experienced or witnessed difficult behaviour by their loved one in hospital, they may be uncertain as to how to best handle such behaviour at home.

Both the burned person and family members will experience challenges upon the return home. Coping strategies must either be developed or previous positive strategies reinforced and applied to this particular situation.

A comprehensive discharge teaching programme should begin several days prior to the individual's discharge (or sooner, if possible). Attention should be paid to the individual's and family's readiness and willingness to learn. Important topics to discuss include skin care, emotional reactions to returning home, adjusting to alterations in appearance and mobility, coping with discomfort (itchiness and pain), nutrition, rehabilitation needs, family readjustment, and continuity of care, i.e. home care, burns clinic and rehabilitation department visits. The information conveyed and the opportunity to talk with nursing staff and other burns team members are both valuable means to support individual and family coping.

Both the burned individual and the family need to know that nursing staff are anxious to provide support, answer questions, assist in problem solving and conflict resolution, and offer a reassuring pat on the back for the courage and perseverance displayed during a very traumatic time. This supportive and informative presence can do much to assist in the individual's efforts at reaching the optimal level of physical and emotional recovery; in other words, establishing a 'new normal' pattern of living, incorporating the adaptations necessitated by the burn injury with positive activities from the past.

Clinical situation: Mr Brown, a man with burns

Mr Joshua Brown is a 56-year-old businessman who is recovering from a 40% flame burn sustained during a propane barbecue explosion. He received burns to both hands, arms, chest, neck and back. He is going to be discharged on home care in one week's time. He has a very supportive wife and two children, aged 25 and 29 years. The discharge teaching plan (Table 26.10) has been drawn up to assist in meeting the learning needs and emotional concerns of Mr Brown and his family.

Evaluation following the rehabilitation phase

The following criteria may be used to evaluate care following the rehabilitation phase after a severe burn injury.

- The patient has maximum function and optimal reconstruction, and has achieved an acceptable quality of life. The burn wounds remain healed and are well moisturized. The patient continues to participate in attempts at minimizing contractures and hypertrophic scarring.

- The patient and family members demonstrate an understanding of the individualized nature of rehabilitation results and of the difficulty in identifying when scar and contracture control measures are complete.
- The patient participates actively in care and performs activities of daily living as appropriate to the health status and level of understanding and acceptance. Support from family members/significant others is appropriate, i.e. emotionally supportive, but encouraging of the patient's attempts at self-care.

During the rehabilitative phase of care, the nurse provides much needed emotional support but has to continue to encourage self-care attempts by the patient. Use of a local burn survivor's support group or the unit's discharged patients/families group, appropriate for such a counselling role, can be invaluable sources of continuing support to the burned individual and the family.

The nurse should continue to answer the patient's and family's questions and to identify and allay their concerns and anxieties. The nurse can also continue to play an important teaching role concerning scar and contracture development, cosmetic camouflage, future surgeries and community re-entry concerns before discharge and following the return home.

GENERAL SKIN CONDITIONS

PROMOTION AND MAINTENANCE OF HEALTHY SKIN

The nurse plays a vital educational role by encouraging and instructing patients to take a health-orientated approach to skin care. As health care consumers, patients should be desirous of playing an active role in their own health care.

Issues which should be addressed concerning promotion and maintenance of healthy skin include:

- *Cleansing.* Essential to the health of one's skin is appropriate and thorough cleansing. There are a number of products available to care for the wide variety of skin types, i.e. dry, normal, oily, combination. Cleanliness is the first step in achieving and maintaining healthy skin.
- *Moisturizing.* The skin can become dry due to moisture loss through the use of inappropriate cleansing agents, illness, trauma, or exposure to sun, wind, pollution and hot water. Patients should be advised to use water-based moisturizers to replenish that which has been lost and for the maintenance of healthy, intact skin, which is the body's primary barrier against infection.
- *Noting changes in the skin's appearance.* Nurses should teach the individual to inspect the skin carefully for any changes in colour, texture or appearance and change in lesions, moles or other deviations. If changes are noted, the person should consult a health care professional immediately.

Table 26.10 Discharge teaching plan for the patient recovering from severe burn injury.

Patient/family problem	Goals	Nursing intervention
1. Anxiety (individual and family) related to limited understanding of injury, treatment plan and expected outcome	The individual and family will: • Verbalize feelings, concerns and questions • Participate in treatment plan • Achieve a degree of control over care • Verbalize realistic goals for the future • Cope effectively with the present situation and experience decreased anxiety • Demonstrate problem-solving skills and effective use of resources	• Provide frequent and repeated explanations and information about care procedures, after establishing individual and family's readiness and willingness to learn • Demonstrate willingness to listen and talk to individual/family at frequent intervals • Assess mental status to determine level of anxiety • Identify previous methods of coping with stressful situations • If individual is agreeable, arrange for meeting with discharged burn survivor who is coping well at home • Encourage and reinforce individual/family participation in care • Plan experiences for the individual/family to control and succeed in decreasing feelings of powerlessness (e.g. allow to make some decisions regarding scheduling and participation in care) • Arrange for social work and/or psychiatric consultation, if necessary
2. Knowledge deficit related to rehabilitation process, i.e. long-term rehabilitation and home care programme.	The individual will: • Identify realistic goals and plans for ongoing rehabilitation and home care • Verbalize understanding and demonstrate: (a) Wound and skin care (b) Use of therapeutic devices (c) Medications (d) Physical therapy	• Assess knowledge level regarding treatment measures and overall rehabilitation process • Discuss individual/family's role in successful physical and emotional rehabilitation • Encourage questions and discussion of anxieties regarding discharge routines • Explain and demonstrate procedures necessary following discharge • Have individual/family demonstrate/discuss procedures/care activities, i.e. daily bathing/skin care; wound care; participation in activities of daily living and range of motion exercises; application of therapeutic devices and pressure garments; gradual increase in activity; diet requirements, medications and side-effects; signs and symptoms to report to burn team members • Assist to plan for economic and social needs upon return to home environment • Assist to make follow-up appointments as necessary, i.e. burn clinic, rehabilitation department, and stress necessity of follow-up care • Set up home care referral when indicated

Table 26.10 *Continued*

Patient/family problem	Goals	Nursing intervention
		• Advise individual/family of potential for physical exhaustion, boredom, emotional lability, adjustment problems • Provide phone number for contact person at the burn unit • Identify community resources, i.e. burn survivor support group
3. Impaired physical mobility related to pain, dressings, wound contractures	The individual will: • Return to an optimal level of functioning, i.e. minimal disability, participation in maximum number of activities of daily living • Be as free from complications associated with immobility as possible	In consultation with rehabilitation therapists: • Maintain burned areas in position of physiological function • Assess burned areas prone to develop contractures for range of motion and strength • Explain rationale for activities and positioning • Assess, teach and observe demonstrations of active and passive range of motion exercises and application of splints and pressure garments • Instruct individual and family regarding appropriate application of dressings and tensor bandages • Encourage individual/family to participate in diversional activities, i.e. visits from friends/family, short walks for fresh air, exercise and change of scene • Ensure increased fluid and fibre intake to prevent constipation due to immobility and use of codeine-containing medications • Educate individual regarding use of pain mediation prior to sustained periods of activity
4. Potential disturbance in self-concept related to potential or actual change in body image, and potential or actual change in role responsibilities	The individual will: • Grieve in an adaptive, therapeutic manner • Verbalize feelings of loss and eventual acceptance of altered self-concept and change in role responsibilities • Develop effective coping mechanisms through this stage of recovery • Make social contacts with persons outside immediate family and close friends • Verbalize strategies to deal with problems as they might arise related to altered self-concept and role responsibilities • Express feelings to family/significant other • Develop realistic goals and plans for the future	• Assess meaning of loss/change with individual/family • Acknowledge and accept expression of frustration, dependency, anger, grief and hostility • Provide hope and maintain a positive attitude, within realistic limits • Communicate to the individual a sense of acceptance through verbal and non-verbal techniques • Offer to introduce the individual to another burn survivor with similar losses • Encourage family to express their feelings • Encourage family to demonstrate signs of acceptance to the individual; give them examples of helpful things to say and do, and to avoid non-constructive comments/actions

Table 26.10 *Continued*

Patient/family problem	Goals	Nursing intervention
	• Incorporate changes in self-concept and role responsibilities without losing positive sense of self-esteem	• If agreeable, introduce individual and family to burn support group members • Begin to discuss supportive alternatives such as cosmetic camouflage, when appropriate • Rehearse with the individual strategies to enhance self-esteem and assist with community re-entry
5. Alteration in comfort: pain and itchiness related to sensitive skin, wound care and wound healing process, rehabilitation routines	The individual will: • Verbalize relief or control of pain and itchiness • Increase participation in self-care • Require decreased amounts of analgesic/antipruritic medications	• Assess the individual's level of pain and itchiness using a verbal, subjective response • Assess the individual's response to pharmacological pain therapies and change as indicated • Assess the individual's response to pharmacological antipruritic therapies and change as indicated • Provide information to the individual regarding pharmacological therapies and outline the side-effects accordingly • Instruct the patient on the use of non-pharmacological therapies, i.e. relaxation techniques, distraction techniques, water-based lotions, loose, 100% cotton clothing • Consult other professionals, i.e. social work, psychology, psychiatry, regarding non-pharmacological strategies • Ask the individual what he or she has found useful in the past to relieve pain and itchiness, and try to incorporate such strategies into the plan of care • If necessary, suggest the individual takes medication prior to painful activities, i.e. dressing changes, rehabilitation activities, prolonged sitting, standing or walking

• *Avoiding exposure to ultraviolet radiation.* People are becoming increasingly aware of the dangers associated with exposing the skin to the sun and other sources of ultraviolet radiation, i.e. tanning lamps/beds. The increasing incidence of skin cancer is cause for alarm and individuals, health professionals and manufacturers alike are advocating education of consumers regarding the use of protective practices such as the use of sun screens/blocks, decreased time in the sun and the wearing of protective clothing, e.g. a wide-brimmed hat and a shirt.

During routine health examinations and wellness tests, the nurse is in an excellent position to teach the individual about the dangers and the appropriate proactive and reactive strategies to employ.

• *Diet.* Good nutrition is an essential component in the promotion and maintenance of healthy skin.

• *Annual physical examinations.* To encourage healthy patterns of skin care and to detect any changes which may have gone unnoticed by the individual, the nurse should advise each person to have an annual examination. This also provides an excellent opportunity for health teaching and for answering questions.

ASSESSMENT

Health history

Skin impairment cannot be examined 'in isolation'; information about the patient's total health can reveal very significant diagnostic factors and influence the therapeutic plan. The social and occupational history as well as the health history are significant.

In taking the patient's health history, particular attention is given to eliciting information about:

1. Any previous skin disorders, their nature, the patient's age, the season of the year at which they occurred and the treatment.
2. Any known allergy or drug reactions.
3. Drugs being taken, and for what reason.
4. Known food(s), fluid(s) or contact substances (e.g. soap, certain material) that worsen the condition.
5. Substances that are brought in contact with the skin throughout daily activities (e.g. cosmetics, chemicals at work).
6. Dietary habits.
7. Recreational customs or hobbies.
8. Family history, especially in relation to skin disorders, allergy and systemic disease.
9. Emotional stress resulting from job, interpersonal relations and other situations are identified. Stress and anxiety may influence the severity of skin disorders and the patient's responses to treatment.

In questioning the patient about the present skin condition, it is necessary to determine:

10. When it was first observed.
11. Whether the lesion(s) persist or come and go, or change in appearance.
12. The extent to which it has spread.
13. Whether it itches or hurts.
14. Whether the lesions are dry, moist or discharging.

Physical examination

The history-taking is followed by an examination of the skin. This involves touching, feeling and observing the person's skin. A good light and warm room are essential and the skin must be clean. Care is taken to prevent unnecessary exposure of the patient and to respect dignity by closing curtains or doors and protecting the patient with a gown or sheet.

A general survey of the skin is done, noting: *colour* (redness, pallor, cyanosis, yellowness or brownness); *vascularity* (any evidence of bruising or bleeding); *moisture* (dryness, sweating, oiliness); *temperature*; *texture* (roughness and smoothness); *thickness*; and *turgor* (the rate at which it returns into place when a section is pinched and lifted).

Lesions are inspected and the nature of the lesion (e.g. ulcer, etc.) is established and its characteristics recorded according to size, shape, colour and whether it has a dry or wet surface. It should be noted if an odour is associated with the affected areas. The entire skin surface of the body is examined to determine the general condition of the total skin in addition to the distribution and grouping of the affected areas. The latter is of assistance in diagnosis since certain disorders are known to develop more frequently in certain areas. For example, acne, impetigo, contact dermatitis, herpes simplex and discoid lupus erythematosus develop most commonly on the face. The oral mucosa is usually included in an examination of the entire skin. The fingernails and toenails are observed and palpated for colour, shape and the presence of lesions. The quantity, texture and distribution of hair is also noted.

Diagnostic tests

Many skin lesions can be diagnosed by physical examination and history. If the lesions are moist or discharging, a swab of the exudate may be obtained for culture. If the affected areas are dry or scaly, scrapings may be taken for cytological examination and/or culture. Other laboratory tests may be done, such as leucocyte and thrombocyte counts, examination for the lupus erythematosus (LE) cell, anti-D test for systemic lupus erythematosus (SLE) and erythrocyte sedimentation rate determination. A biopsy of a lesion may be done if malignancy is suspected or if the lesion is longstanding and obscure in nature. Toxic epidermal necrolysis syndrome (TENS) types I and II, a form of exfoliative dermatitis, are also definitively diagnosed by a skin biopsy. If the condition is dermatitis, patch, intracutaneous or scratch tests may be done during a remission to identify the allergen or substance to which the person is sensitive. The substances are administered intracutaneously or applied to the skin on the back and observed at intervals over 48 hours. If positive, the reaction is manifested by inflammation and papules or vesicles. Immunofluorescent tests may be done in certain skin diseases to identify antinuclear antibodies.

Although the skin lesions prompted the patient to seek medical assistance, the disorder may have internal or systemic components. This may necessitate other investigative procedures, such as urinalysis, X-rays, pulmonary function tests or further blood studies.

RISK FACTORS

Impairment of skin integrity is related to the presence of one or more risk factors (see Table 26.11).

- *Internal factors*: alterations in nutrition, metabolism, circulation, sensation, immune system, mental status, skin turgor, pigmentation, body fat and moisture, thickness and texture of the skin, the presence of infection, and actions of medications
- *External or environmental factors*: mechanical forces including pressure and shearing, chemical substances, radiation, temperature extremes, moisture and physical immobilization
- *Systemic disorders* such as:
  (a) Malnutrition (e.g. nutritional deficiency, obesity).
  (b) Metabolic disorder (e.g. diabetes mellitus, hypo- or hyperthyroidism).
  (c) Cardiovascular disease.
  (d) Neurological disorders that impair sensation and cause immobility (e.g. cerebral haemorrhage,

Table 26.11 Factors contributing to impairment of skin integrity.

External (environmental)
Hyperthermia or hypothermia
Chemical substance
Mechanical factors
   Shearing forces
   Pressure
   Restraint
Radiation
Physical immobilization
Humidity

Internal (somatic)
Medication
Altered nutritional state: obesity, emaciation
Altered metabolic state
Altered circulation
Altered sensation
Altered pigmentation
Skeletal prominence
Developmental factors
Immunological deficit
Alterations in turgor (change in elasticity)
Excretions/secretions
Psychogenic
Oedema

From NANDA (1989).

brain tumour, spinal cord injury, multiple sclerosis).
(e) Severe infection and fever.
(f) Debilitation (such as occurs in cancer and anaemia, for example).
- *Skin characteristics*:
(a) Thickness and texture of skin which vary in different areas of the body and are influenced by the person's genetic code and age.
(b) Turgor. Dehydration and oedema reduce the resistance of the skin.
- *Age.* The older person's skin is drier, less elastic and less turgid, predisposing it to breakdown when subjected to pressure or other mechanical forces or irritants.

CHARACTERISTICS OF IMPAIRED SKIN

Lesions

Various changes in areas of the skin may occur, and the exact nature of these is important in diagnosis and treatment.

Primary lesions. Characteristic primary lesions in which the skin is usually intact include the following:

- *Erythema* — an area in which the blood vessels become dilated, causing redness, warmth and increased firmness of the skin.
- *Macule* — a circumscribed, smooth, flat, discoloured area up to 1 cm in size.
- *Papule* — a small circumscribed elevated area which may or may not be discoloured and is not more than 1 cm in diameter.
- *Vesicle* — an elevated area which contains clear fluid.
- *Pustule* — a small elevation of the skin which contains pus.
- *Nodule* — a solid elevation larger than a papule, usually involving both the skin and subcutaneous layers.
- *Wheal* — a localized, elevated, oedematous area that is red at the margins with a blanched centre.
- *Bulla* — an elevation larger than 1 cm of superficial skin layers containing serous or purulent fluid.
- *Comedo (blackhead)* — a plug of sebum and keratin within a hair follicle.
- *Telangiectasia* — a lesion composed of a group of small blood vessels that are abnormally dilated.
- *Plaque* — a patch on the skin or mucous membrane.

Secondary lesions. These are those that develop as a result of a break in the skin and destruction of cells. They include:

- *Crust (scab)* — a rough, dry area formed by the coagulation and drying of plasma and exudate over a primary lesion.
- *Scales* — thin, flat, minute plates of dried epidermal cells which have not completely undergone the normal keratinization process before being separated. Desquamation is the term which refers to the separation of scales or patches of cells.
- *Fissure* — a split or crack in the surface, extending through the epidermal layers and possibly into the dermis. If it extends into the dermis, bleeding occurs. This type of lesion is most likely to occur in a natural skin or surface crease such as those located over knuckles, at the angles of the mouth, in the groin, between the buttocks and behind the ears.
- *Erosion (excoriation)* — loss of the epidermis producing a superficial, reddened, weeping lesion.
- *Ulcer* — a denuded area of irregular size and shape extending into the dermis or subcutaneous tissue due to necrosis of superficial tissue.
- *Lichenification* — the thickening and hardening of skin as a result of continued irritation.
- *Atrophy* — the skin is thin and wrinkled resembling tissue paper. Atrophy is seen with ageing.
- *Corn, callus (hyperkeratotic plaque)* — an excessive thickness of the epidermis caused by chronic pressure and/or friction. In the case of a corn, the hyperkeratosis is sharply circumscribed.
- *Leucoplakia* — a white plaque which is seen most commonly on the lips or mucous membranes of the oral cavity or tongue. About 10% of patients subsequently develop carcinoma in the lesions.
- *Scar (cicatrix)* — an area of fibrous tissue replacing tissue destroyed by trauma or disease.
- *Hypertrophic scars.* Normally a scar becomes paler and flatter as it matures. Hypertrophic scars become increasingly raised, red and itchy for several months after injury, due to excessive formation of fibrous

tissue within the scar. The scar is then classified as hypertrophic. Over the next few years these scars usually flatten and lose their vascularity, thus becoming paler. The hypertrophy is confined to the site of injury. If these scars are excised there is some tendency for the hypertrophy to recur. It may be very difficult to determine if a scar is hypertrophic or keloid (see below).

- *Keloids*. Histologically keloids are similar to hypertrophic scars, but keloids behave differently. Fibrous tissue formation is sometimes so excessive that the keloid has the appearance of a tumour, and the initial injury which produces the keloid may be so small as to appear insignificant, for example ear piercing, or an insect bite. Unlike hypertrophic scars, the keloid extends into surrounding uninjured skin and persists for many years. There is a high tendency to recur after excision. The incidence of keloid is highest in negroid skins.

It appears that tension within a scar encourages hypertrophy and keloid formation, therefore redistribution of the tension by use of elastic pressure garments usually produces some improvement in scar quality.

Pruritus

Generalized or localized itching is a common complaint in skin disorders. It may be associated with an internal disorder, such as diabetes mellitus or obstructive jaundice. Excessive dryness due to overbathing, a dry atmosphere and the ageing process can also cause pruritus. Emotional distress can play an important role in the development and control of this disturbing symptom. The sensory nerve endings or end-organs are irritated, giving rise to the desire to scratch. The patient is hard-pressed to refrain from scratching which further irritates the area and is frequently responsible for fissures, abrasions and subsequent secondary infection. Itching does not occur if the whole thickness of the skin has been removed as in a full-thickness burn.

Urticaria

Urticaria is a skin disorder characterized by itching wheals of varying size, which may develop rapidly and become widespread. The reaction consists of dilatation and increased permeability of the capillaries and arteriolar dilatation. The combination of these is referred to as the triple response.

A severe and possibly life-threatening form of the disorder is known as angioneurotic oedema on the skin and mucous membranes. The lesions frequently disappear in a few hours when the blood vessels return to normal. General malaise and fever may also develop if the urticaria is widespread. The most common cause of angioneurotic oedema is a severe allergic reaction to a drug, food or insect bite.

Pain

The pain associated with skin lesions may be described as prickly or burning. It may be caused by chemical, mechanical or pressure irritation of the cutaneous sensory nerves, actual cellular damage or exposure of the nerve endings due to tissue destruction and erosion.

Redness

Erythema or redness of the skin indicates vasodilatation and hyperaemia in the area. Erythematous lesions are initially macular but frequently become papular because of the oedema or developing exudate in the affected tissues.

Swelling

A puffy swollen area of the skin is usually due to localized oedema, resulting from increased permeability of the capillaries, or to localized inflammatory reaction.

Systemic disturbances

The skin reflects the individual's general physical and emotional status. Skin lesions are frequently manifestations of a systemic disorder (e.g. measles, systemic lupus erythematosus) or a systemic or emotional disturbance may be secondary to primary skin lesions. An elevated temperature is likely to be present if the skin disorder involves infection.

HEALTH PROBLEMS COMMON TO INDIVIDUALS WITH SKIN IMPAIRMENT

Regardless of the cause of impairment to an individual's skin, there are certain health problems which are common to all. Knowledge of what may be fairly typical for this group of patients helps the nurse in assessing each person and in planning care.

Each individual has to cope with varying physiological problems, depending upon the nature of the impairment. The nurse can explain the nature of the impairment to the patient and the rationale behind local skin/wound care, systemic therapy and nutritional support. The patient can then be encouraged to participate in as much of the care as is realistic. Emphasis on strategies to resolve the physiological problems associated with the patient problem of skin impairment will be addressed below in greater detail.

Along with the physiological sequelae, there are individual psychological responses. Emotional support and health teaching are important nursing functions in assisting the individual to understand and learn to cope with altered status in a positive manner. The nature of these nursing roles will be discussed in more detail.

GENERAL PRINCIPLES OF CARE FOR PERSONS WITH SKIN DISEASE

The nursing care varies greatly with these patients. The extent of the skin involvement as well as the nature of the condition determines whether or not the patient continues activities, is ambulatory and is treated at home. The patient's reaction to the disease also influences the plan of care and progress. The following are general considerations which will require adaptation and modification according to the individual.

PSYCHOLOGICAL SUPPORT

The person with skin lesions is likely to be quite sensitive about the condition. Many are self-conscious about their appearance, worry constantly and tend to withdraw, believing that a skin disease carries a stigma. The disease may be such that it persists over a long period, interfering with the individual's ability to work or go out socially. Many skin diseases are aggravated by emotional stress. The understanding nurse helps the patient identify any emotional factors which may contribute to the skin condition and carefully assesses her own responses to the person. Expression of revulsion at the patient's appearance adds to the distress. The nurse should make a conscious effort to touch the person's skin, thus reassuring him or her that the appearance and the texture of the skin are both accepted. The patient is advised whether or not the disorder is contagious, and there should be no hesitation on the part of the nurse to touch the affected parts when giving care. In accordance with institutional infection control guidelines and the introduction of universal and body substance precautions, gloves may be indicated. The rationale should be explained calmly and matter-of-factly to the patient so as not to add to the psychological distress. An effort is made to convey an appreciation of the patient's feelings, to make the patient aware that he or she is accepted and to provide the necessary support and care which will help to reduce anxiety.

LOCAL CARE

Cleansing. Cleansing of the skin or affected areas is determined for each patient. In some instances the application of soap and water may be contraindicated, and an alternative method of cleansing is necessary. For example, cleansing the skin with a vegetable oil may be necessary. If soap is permitted, it should be mildly alkaline and used very sparingly. A soft flannel is preferable, and the surface is washed lightly and gently to avoid injury and erythema. If there are open, discharging lesions, sterile gauze or a disposable absorbent cloth may be used. If the skin is dry, it may also be advisable to limit bathing to once or twice a week.

Special local or general therapeutic baths may be prescribed. These may be used to relieve itching, remove scales or crusts, or apply medications as well as for cleansing purposes. Caution is used against having the water or solution hot; a temperature higher than 35–38°C is likely to be too hot for the sensitive areas. Also, higher temperatures are likely to promote hyperaemia and itching. The patient is usually encouraged to remain in the bath for 10–20 minutes, and an attendant remains with the patient or close by, depending on condition and age. Measures are taken to prevent the patient from slipping whilst getting into and out of the bath. After bathing, excessive rubbing to dry the skin is avoided. The moisture is blotted gently with a towel.

Fingernails are kept short and clean, and the patient is advised to refrain from scratching due to the threat of skin damage and infection.

- *Moist compresses.* Wet dressings may be applied over lesions, especially if they are open and discharging. The compresses are generally left uncovered and dry out very quickly, necessitating frequent changing or resoaking. The prescribed solution is usually used at room temperature. Wet dressings are not usually applied to dry or scaly lesions; an ointment or creamy lotion is more appropriate.
- *Dressings.* In the TENS patient, care is given to scrupulous management of the exposed dermis. Multiple dressing changes with a protective 'greasy gauze' paraffin-type dressing such as Jelonet or the application of a biosynthetic skin substitute such as Biobrane may be most helpful. Both types of dressing encourage the re-epithelialization necessary for the resurfacing of open wounds.
- *Cold applications.* Application of cold dressings can cause vasoconstriction and decrease skin sensitivity and itching.
- *Clothing.* Woollens and other irritating clothing are avoided. Loose-fitting 100% cotton is best. The effectiveness of this strategy can be enhanced by maintaining a cool environment, when possible.

Topical applications. Many different drug preparations are used in treating skin diseases. Topical applications may be in powder, lotion, oil, cream, paste or ointment form. They may be classified according to their effect.

- *Antipruritic preparations* are applied to relieve itching. Examples are calamine lotion, corticosteroid cream or ointment and antihistamines.
- *Keratolytic agents* soften and remove scales and the horny layer. An example is salicylic acid ointment.
- *Antieczematous agents* are applied to relieve itching and remove the vesicular drainage. Examples are corticosteroid lotion or spray and coal tar solution.
- *Keratoplastic preparations* stimulate the epidermis, increasing its thickness. An example is a weak salicylic (1–2%) acid ointment.
- *Antimicrobial agents* destroy or inhibit the reproduction of bacteria and fungi. Examples are antibiotic ointments such as neomycin and gentamicin.
- Zinc undecylenate is a common *antifungal* agent.
- *Antiparasitic preparations* destroy or inhibit parasites. Examples are benzyl benzoate lotion and gamma benzene hexachloride.
- *Emollients* are used to soften the skin. Examples commonly used are lanolin, petroleum jelly and Alpha Keri bath oil. Agents which contain lanolin and/or mineral oil, in moderate to large quantities, do not offer moisturizing properties and should not be used as such.

Frequently topical preparations are a combination of two or more agents which have been selected for their specific effect.

Assessment. Following each cleansing and before each local therapeutic application, the lesions are examined carefully. Any increase or spread, or change in size, colour or appearance is noted. The nurse is constantly alert for factors in the individual's environment (e.g. contacts, diet, drugs) with which exacerbations of the condition may be associated. The person's responses to the skin disorder and treatment are documented in the health record and communicated to colleagues in order to promote continuity of care and enhance consistent communication regarding the patient's current and projected status.

The person with angioneurotic oedema may have intercutaneous patch or scratch sensitivity tests done to identify the offending substance. In the case of severe respiratory involvement, the patient experiences respiratory distress secondary to laryngeal obstruction. Total obstruction of the airway may ensue with alarming speed. If laryngeal stridor is present, the patient should be prepared immediately for emergency laryngostomy or tracheostomy. Prompt action is necessary. A corticosteroid preparation such as hydrocortisone is given intravenously; this usually reverses the reaction rapidly. However, as soon as one suspects that the airway is or will be compromised, the doctor should attempt to intubate the patient. When a patient is in respiratory distress, the nurse plays a very important role by calming and being with the patient throughout.

Physical agents. Ultraviolet rays may be prescribed in the treatment of psoriasis, acne and seborrhoeic dermatitis. Irradiation is used if the lesion is malignant. Electrosurgery or cautery may be employed in the removal of warts, leucoplakia and seborrhoeic or senile keratoses (areas of horny thickening of epidermis).

SYSTEMIC THERAPY

If the skin disorder is secondary to a systemic disease, treatment is directed principally toward the primary condition. Most TENS patients are best managed in a burn/plastic surgery unit due to the intense nature of the wound care and increased likelihood of infection.

Systemic drugs. The treatment of primary skin disorders may include the administration of systemic drugs. The drug will depend upon the nature of the disorder and the patient's general health and response to the condition. An oral corticosteroid (e.g. prednisone) is frequently prescribed in dermatitis, urticaria and pemphigus. If the skin lesions are infected, an antibiotic (e.g. tetracycline) may be ordered to be given orally. An antihistamine such as chlorpheniramine maleate (Piriton) may be used in urticaria. If the patient is very agitated and distressed, a sedative may be necessary. However, long-term use of antihistamines and sedatives is to be avoided. Through patient education, the nurse can emphasize the role of non-pharmacological approaches. Adrenaline 1:1000 may be ordered subcutaneously if the urticaria is widespread and causing considerable irritation. Vitamins may be given to improve the patient's appetite, general condition and resistance. In the case of the patient with TENS type II with a drug-induced reaction, discontinuation of the suspected allergy-producing drug is immediate, together with avoidance of drugs of a similar nature. Consultation with the pharmacy and infectious disease services is very helpful from a patient management perspective and for the discharge teaching these patients require.

Concern about the condition and fear of disfigurement and rejection as well as itching may result in a considerable loss of sleep for the patient. A sedative may be necessary to provide rest, which plays an important part in the patient's recovery. In the event of a significant degree of depression, psychiatric services may be appropriate for the patient.

NUTRITION

Attention is paid to the nutritional status and to whether the patient is taking sufficient food. Frequently severe anorexia is a problem with the dermatological patient because of the skin irritation experienced, as well as the emotional disturbance. Dressings, ointments, lotions or similar applications on the hands may make self-care in feeding difficult. A creative occupational therapist and nurse should be able to assist in choosing appropriate assistive devices if problems with feeding occur. Continuity of such practices in-hospital and following discharge are essential if such strategies are to bring about long-term gain.

PATIENT EDUCATION

In the clinic or during preparation for discharge from the hospital nurses have a key role in advising the patient and family members of the day-to-day care required and precautionary measures applicable to the prevention of an exacerbation of the skin disorder. Verbal and written directions are given about the local applications and taking of medicinal preparations. For example, adrenocorticosteroid preparations in the form of an ointment or cream are used topically to suppress inflammation and reduce sensitivity of the tissues. The patient must be cautioned to apply the corticoid preparation sparingly. If compresses or therapeutic baths are to be continued, specific details of the preparation, temperature and application are outlined and demonstrated if necessary.

DISCHARGE PLANNING

In the recovery phase, nurses can also help to boost the person's self-esteem and prepare for greater independence by assisting him or her to cope with an altered sense of self-esteem.

The need to consider changing employment should be discussed with the patient, and the occupational therapist and social worker may be consulted to discuss re-training facilities if appropriate.

DOCUMENTATION

Nursing documentation in the form of a 'wound documentation tool' might prove helpful in the assessment, planning, implementation and evaluation of care strategies. Sections for subjective and objective data, treatments given and an assessment of their effectiveness, together with the progress of the skin disorder are very helpful and appropriate in the nursing record.

THE PERSON WITH IMPAIRED SKIN INTEGRITY: COMMON CONDITIONS

PATIENT ASSESSMENT

In assessing patients suffering from skin diseases it is necessary to determine the history of the illness, paying attention to dietary or other possible causative factors such as allergic substances that the patient may have come in contact with. The extent of the skin disorder should be accurately recorded in order that progress can be monitored.

The patient's view of his or her condition should be determined, together with any coping mechanisms that are used. The patient's self-concept should be explored along with how the illness is affecting everyday life. Other psychosocial factors such as developmental status and family relationships should be explored.

Some common conditions and their causes will now be considered, together with patient goals and specific nursing care.

Acne Vulgaris

Risk factors

- Alterations in nutrition.
- Increased sex hormone levels.
- Increased stress levels.
- Sebaceous gland oversecretion of keratin, sebum and bacteria in the follicular duct.
- Age, i.e. greatest in adolescents after puberty.

Characteristics

- Initial formation of a comedo (blackhead) or mila (whitehead).
- Progressive formation of medones, papules, pustules or apts.
- Inflammation reaction results when comedonal material is released into surrounding skin by a ruptured follicle.
- Subsequent scarring in severe cases.

Patient goals

The patient will recover from the acne vulgaris condition with a minimum of residual scarring. The patient will maintain/achieve a positive body image and sense of self-esteem.

Nursing intervention

- Obtain wound swabs if deemed necessary to identify existing harmful bacteria.

- Explain the importance of cleansing procedures; encourage frequent washing of affected areas, hands and hair to prevent secondary bacterial infections.
- Instruct the patient not to scrub excessively and to dry the skin.
- Encourage and instruct the individual to participate in all aspects of care.
- Discuss the advantages of eating a well-balanced diet.
- Encourage ventilation of feelings.
- Provide for an atmosphere of positive acceptance of self in order to enhance self-esteem and a positive body image.
- If appropriate, discuss use of cosmetic camouflage and/or surgical dermabrasion to address problems of residual scarring.

Contact Dermatitis

This inflammatory disease of the skin is very common and, according to the cause, may be referred to as primary irritant dermatitis or allergic contact dermatitis. A less common form is referred to as exfoliative dermatitis. If mucosal involvement is present, it is referred to as toxic epidermal necrolysis syndrome (TENS), a form of erythema multiforme.

Risk factors

- Contact with an irritant substance such as strong soaps and some acids/alkalis.
- Contact of hypersensitive or allergic skin with an agent such as poison ivy, cosmetics, hair dye, soaps, clothing, material, dyes, plastic and insecticides.
- Exfoliation due to drugs such as antibiotics or anticonvulsants, and infectious agents (*Mycoplasma pneumoniae* and herpes simplex virus).

Characteristics

- Development of an erythematous area with small papular development and progression to vesicles.
- Vesicles may rupture and discharge contents, followed by crusting and scaling.
- Denuded areas may ooze a serous discharge and then be covered by regenerated epidermis.
- Itchiness and burning leading to scratching, which may result in infected lesions.
- With TENS, virtual universal erythema desquamation, peeling and itching of the skin and loss of hair; malaise, fever, headache and sore throat may precede lesions; extensive sloughing of epidermis (positive Nikolsky's sign); involvement of mucous membranes also evident.

Patient goals

The patient will recover from the contact dermatitis condition with a minimum of scarring and mucosal damage (TENS). The patient will maintain/achieve a positive body image and sense of self-esteem, and will demonstrate relaxation techniques to reduce emotional exacerbations.

Nursing intervention

- Local applications of cold, wet compresses, bland, unmedicated lotions or thinly applied steroid-based creams.
- If extensive, therapeutic baths may be helpful. Explain rationale to the patient.
- Antibiotic ointment may be applied if there is an infection. Advise the patient regarding use.
- Advise the patient to avoid scratching and keep nails short and clean. Mittens may be helpful with children.
- Advise the patient of correct use of corticosteroid (e.g. prednisone), for reduction of tissue response and inflammation, and antipruritic (e.g. diphenhydramine) for itchiness.
- Educate patient regarding stress reduction techniques.
- With TENS, early recognition, immediate débridement and coverage with biological and/or biosynthetic dressings are essential; excellent respiratory care, i.e. incentive spirometry, postural drainage, suctioning, chest physiotherapy and intubation/ventilation if necessary.
- Lubrication of ocular mucous membranes and use of glass rod to remove conjunctival discharge.
- Provide the patient and family with psychosocial support.
- Arrange for follow-up care.

Eczema

This superficial inflammatory process primarily involves the epidermis and can occur in adults, although it is also known as infantile dermatitis.

Risk factors

An allergic sensitivity to foods, dust, pollens, or similar inhalants; affects approximately 1–3% of the world's population.

Characteristics

- Red, minute papules and vesicles.
- Weeping, oozing, crusting and scaling present.
- Lichenification (thick hardened skin).
- Pigmentation and itchiness may be present.

Patient goals

The patient will recover from the eczema with a minimum of scarring; the patient will maintain/achieve a positive body image and sense of self-esteem.

Nursing intervention

- In collaboration with other team members, identify the allergen.
- Apply prescribed lotions and ointments aimed at symptom management, not cure.

- Teach the patient and family the use of prescribed lotions/ointments, the nature of the condition, and the goal of symptom management versus cure.
- Provide psychosocial support to the patient and family in relation to the chronic nature of the condition and the need to follow regimens closely.
- Teach the patient measures to prevent/decrease further occurrences of eczema.
- Arrange for follow-up care.

Psoriasis

Risk factors

- History of living in a temperate climate.
- Hereditary biochemical defect.
- Hormonal influences, i.e. decreased incidence during pregnancy.
- Onset common during adolescence.
- Association with rheumatoid arthritis, since elevated uric acid is present in some patients.
- May be precipitated by trauma, infections and psychological stress.

Characteristics

- Chronic inflammation of the skin, producing dry, scaly lesions; exacerbations and remissions.
- Dull, red, papular lesions form.
- Silvery white, waxy scales accumulate in layers, with epidermal replacement every 4 days (normal rate is every 28 days), therefore skin's normal protective layers are not able to form.
- Lesions may increase in size, coalesce and form large scaly plaques.
- Small, pinpoint bleeding areas are found when the plaque is removed.
- Nail involvement; pitting, discoloration and separation from thick, hard and dry underlying tissue.
- Onset may be gradual or sudden.
- Duration may be lengthy or short-lived.

Patient goals

The patient will recover from the psoriasis with a minimum of scarring; the patient will maintain/achieve a positive body image and sense of self-esteem.

Nursing intervention

- Teach the individual regarding the rationale and limitations of treatments, i.e. to reduce scaling and itchiness, not to cure the condition.
- Provide psychosocial support to individual and family, particularly about living with a chronic illness, and assist with the development of adaptive techniques as necessary.
- Apply and instruct the patient regarding various treatments, i.e. local applications, baths and exposure to ultraviolet rays.

- Topical applications may include pastes, ointments or creams, including salicylic acid, coal-tar derivatives or diethranol.
- Caution individual about the use of topical and systemic corticosteroids.
- Instruct the patient to soak in prescribed bath for 20–30 minutes and to gently scrub off scales. Daily shampooing may be necessary if the scalp is affected.
- If ultraviolet light therapy is used, teach the individual about the wearing of dark glasses during treatment and to begin at exposures of 1 minute duration, to be gradually increased under medical supervision.
- If dithranol paste is used, instruct the patient on the importance of protecting unaffected skin with petroleum jelly.
- Provide support to the patient as occlusive dressings, plastic bags, vinyl suits and shower caps may be necessary for these time-consuming and aesthetically unappealing treatments.
- Explain to the individual and family that topically-applied agents suppress epidermopoiesis, whereas tar therapies retard and inhibit rapid growth of psoriatic tissue.
- Reinforce the symptomatic management versus the cure nature of therapies.
- If appropriate, gently touch the patient's arm or hand in a gesture of acceptance, not revulsion or fear, of the sight of the skin lesions.
- Encourage the family to accept the individual's condition and not to be fearful that it is contagious or infectious.
- Encourage adequate rest, a balanced nutritional diet and prevention of skin irritations and infections.
- Arrange for follow-up care.

Parasitic Infestations

PEDICULOSIS (LICE)

Risk factors

- Poor hygiene.
- Intimate or casual contact with an infected person.

Characteristics

- Appearance of eggs (nits) or lice on body, head and/or pubic areas; may also be found on seams of clothing.
- Haemorrhagic points may be noted, along with hyperaemia, linear scratches and a slight degree of eczema.
- Thickened, dry, scaly darkly pigmented patches noted with long-term infestation.

Nursing assessment

1. *Health history*: present social situation, i.e. access to

bathing facilities; contact with an infected individual, clothing or bed linen
2. *Physical examination*: visually assess the involved areas in a well-lit room. Include the neck, thighs and trunk. Pubic lice and head lice can be found on hair shafts.
3. *Psychosocial concerns/developmental factors*: assess changes in patient/other interaction due to the contagious nature of the condition. Identify the patient's social situation, i.e. living conditions, health practices, non-compliance with health care treatments.
4. *Patient and family knowledge*: identify their perceptions of health status, disease condition and relationship to health practices/contacts with infected individuals, education level, readiness and willingness to learn.

Patient goals

The patient will have no evidence of pediculosis infestation and will learn preventive health care practices to avoid reinfestation and transmission to other people during the treatment period.

Nursing intervention

- Teach the patient/family regarding the cause, nature and prevention of pediculosis.
- Body lice — instruct individual/family to launder clothing to destroy lice and nits;
  — check family for infestation;
  — administer antipruritic, systemic antibiotic and topical corticosteroid applications as ordered;
  — teach patients to look for evidence of rickettsial disease (lice serve as vectors).
- Head lice — cleanse hair vigorously with gamma benzene hexachloride shampoos followed by a combing with a vinegar-soaked fine-toothed comb; repeat in 24 hours;
  — disinfect combs and brushes with shampoo;
  — instruct patient/family to wash all bed linen;
  — check family members for infestation and treat as necessary.
- Pubic lice — as above for head lice;
  — check sexual contacts for infestation and treat as necessary;
  — discuss the possibility of coexisting sexually transmitted disease.
- Establish a realistic plan of care including followup for the individual/others involved.

SCABIES

Risk factors

- Contact with parasite *Sarcoptes scabiei* (itch mite).

Characteristics

- Appearance of greyish-white, slightly elevated, zigzag lines on skin.
- Secondary lesions develop in form of vesicles or papules, pustules and encrustations.

Nursing assessment

1. *Health history*: contact with an infected person or scabies mite (via an alternate vector).
2. *Physical examination*: visual assessment of involved site in a well-lit room; common sites include flexor surfaces of the wrist, palms, between the fingers and toes, groin and areolae of the breasts; in addition to lines on skin and secondary lesions, individuals complain of severe itchiness.
3. *Psychosocial concerns/developmental factors*: identify changes in patient/other interaction due to infectious nature of the condition; social situation, i.e. living conditions, health practices.
4. *Patient and family knowledge*: perception of health status, disease condition and relationship to health practices/contacts with infected individuals; education level, readiness and willingness to learn.

Patient goals

The patient will have no evidence of scabies infestation and will learn preventive health care practices to avoid reinfestation and transmission to other people during the treatment period.

Nursing intervention

- Teach the patient/family about the cause, nature and prevention of scabies.
- Instruct the patient to take a hot bath and vigorously scrub open infested burrows.
- Apply a benzyl benzoate preparation (Ascabiol) or monosulfiram (Tetmosol) over entire skin surface.
- Instruct the individual to repeat bath and ointment application once again, usually the next morning.
- Instruct the individual/family to wash bed linen and clothing in boiling water or press with a very hot iron.
- Examine all close contacts of the individual for scabies and treat if necessary.
- Establish a realistic plan of care, including follow-up for the individual/others involved.

Skin Cancer

Risk factors

- Long periods of exposure to sunlight, radiation, chronic irritation (e.g. scars of poor quality which frequently break down), and long-standing contact with chemicals (e.g. oil, tar and paraffin).
- Ruddy or lighter skin complexion.

Health-seeking behaviours related to the prevention of skin cancer

Skin cancers can be prevented. Ninety-five percent of skin cancers are curable, if diagnosed and treated early. Health promotion programmes and the encouragement of health-seeking behaviours are therefore important for nurses to stress to the public.

Educational points to reinforce with individuals include:

- The avoidance of unnecessary sun exposure, especially between 1000 and 1400 hours when the ultraviolet rays are strongest.
- The application of sunscreens and/or sunblocks with high levels of para-aminobenzoic acid (PABA) whenever exposure to the sun is unavoidable. PABA-free lotions are available for people who are allergic to it.
- The wearing of protective clothing, i.e. long-sleeved shirts and broad-brimmed hats, but to recognize that sunscreens/blocks are still necessary.
- The treatment of moles if they are particularly prone to repeated friction and irritation.
- An awareness of indicators of potential malignancy, i.e. an increase in size, ulceration, bleeding or serous exudate from a mole or other skin lesion.

Characteristics

- Changes in moles or other skin lesions that may at first appear innocuous; changes include an increase in size, ulceration, bleeding, serous exudate, and brownish, scaly thickening of the dermis (Bowen's disease).
- Sores that do not heal and become enlarged; a small nodule which is waxy in appearance with a rolled, translucent border and grey or yellow plaque formation (basal cell carcinoma).
- Open sores, nodular lesions, long-standing scars which repeatedly break down (squamous cell carcinoma).
- Clearly pigmented lesions arising from an existing mole which has changed in size and/or colour (malignant melanoma).
- Kaposi's sarcoma (KS), a malignancy of lymphatic endothelial cell origin which presents as moderately infiltrated reddish-brown plaques located on the trunk of the body and face is a complication of HIV infection which particularly affects homosexuals. KS is also found amongst HIV-negative homosexuals in New York, indicating that perhaps an agent transmitted through sexual behaviour is at work. KS lesions have particular affinity for the tip of the nose, necessitating body image adjustments for the individual. Radiotherapy is useful in treating some KS lesions, being particularly useful for short-term cosmetic effect and pain management. When KS lesions are found systemically, either in the gastrointestinal tract or lungs, chemotherapy such as α-interferon or etoposide may be useful.

Individuals with HIV infection are also susceptible to attacks from viruses such as herpes simplex and varicella-zoster which may cause painful, deep and destructive ulcers in a variety of different locations

(Nily, 1988). Topical or intravenous acyclovir may be used if these conditions are diagnosed in early stages. Many people are also prone to seborrhoeic dermatitis, which may respond to cortisone preparations.

Nursing assessment

1. *Health history*: age; history of sun exposure; knowledge of changes in moles or skin lesions; occupation; recent changes in general health status (to rule out metastases); family history of cancer, in particular skin cancer.
2. *Physical examination*: visually assess the involved areas in a well-lit room. Exposed areas, especially of the upper extremities and of the face, lower lip, nose, ears and forehead are common sites.
3. *Psychosocial concerns*: anxiety, fear once the word 'cancer' is mentioned; patient and family interaction; coping abilities.
4. *Patient and family knowledge*: perception of health status and skin cancer; education level.

Patient goals

The patient will recover from the skin cancer, will have a minimum of scarring and will learn preventive health care practices to avoid/detect reoccurrences. If the cancer is malignant and/or has rapidly and extensively metastasized, the goals will include acceptance/adjustment to cancer treatment and/or palliative care measures.

Nursing intervention

- Provide the patient and family with psychosocial support once they hear the diagnosis of skin cancer.
- Teach the patient and family about the causes, treatments and outcomes of the particular type of skin cancer.
- Basal cell and squamous cell carcinoma: discuss with the patient, in collaboration with the attending physician what the treatment options are and what the individual wishes to do. Options may include surgery, radiation therapy or chemical destruction of the tumour.
- Malignant melanomas: prepare the individual educationally and psychologically for surgery to remove the tumour. Warn the patient that future surgery will be necessary to remove surrounding lymph nodes.
- Encourage the individual to engage in regular visual assessments for changes in moles or the appearance of lesions to the skin. If found, encourage him or her to seek medical help immediately.
- Reinforce the important role of prevention and the high cure rate with early detection.
- Capitalize on society's growing awareness of the alarming increase in skin cancer rates by encouraging the use of health promotion and disease prevention strategies.
- Arrange for follow-up care.

NURSING MANAGEMENT OF THE PATIENT WITH AIDS AND SKIN DISORDER

As there is a strong possibility of a patient with AIDS developing skin disorders the nurse should consider the following general principles which apply to the care of patients with AIDS.

Before providing care for the patient with HIV infection, the nurse must have confidence in the infection control measures that are being used. The nurse must also explore his or her feelings in caring for others who may have a sexual orientation that is different from his or her own or participates in behaviours such as intravenous drug abuse that the nurse may not approve of.

Care for people with HIV infection has historically focused on helping the individual cope with a terminal illness, and was primarily institutionally based because the patient was frequently compromised by opportunistic infections. As health care workers learn more about HIV disease and as patients become more skilled in self-care, the illness trajectory has greatly increased. It is more appropriate to talk about HIV infection and AIDS as a chronic illness. Care is now primarily based in the community with occasional short periods of stay in the hospital.

The type of care individuals require depends on the stage and severity of the illness. When the individual is newly diagnosed with HIV infection, particular consideration is given to helping the person adjust to the diagnosis and implications it has for quality of life. Nursing intervention focuses on learning self-care skills such as stress management techniques and assessing coping behaviours. Psychosocial concerns are heightened (see Chapter 6).

SUMMARY

This chapter discusses the important role that the skin plays in maintaining overall health and well-being. The skin fulfils a multitude of functions, many of which we are unaware of until something threatens to alter or impair its integrity. The consequences of an insult to the skin's integrity can be relatively minor or they can be devastating and life-threatening. The person with impairment of skin integrity must cope with changes in self-image as well as with minor or major disruptions to physiological functioning.

The nurse plays a key role in the prevention, assessment, planning, administration and evaluation of care strategies to manage potential and actual impairment of skin integrity. Patient and family teaching is a vital function of the nurse as a primary care-giver and one of those closest to the individual and family.

The care of persons with impaired skin integrity can be challenging and calls upon many facets of the nursing role. The nurse must be knowledgeable about the structure and function of the skin, measures to maintain skin integrity and to promote healing and tissue repair, and the impact of changes in body image on the individual and family.

LEARNING ACTIVITIES

1. Assess a patient's pressure sore risk score using the Norton scale, check your score with that of a colleague who should make the assessment independently of you. Repeat this on a sample of 5–10 patients and compare your results. What do these discrepancies suggest?

2. Repeat the above exercise with one of you using the Waterlow Scale while the other uses Norton on a further sample of 5–10 patients. How do your differences compare with those obtained above? What are the implications of these differences for care?

3. A patient who has been admitted to the A & E with 20% burns affecting the face, chest and arms turns to you and asks 'Will I be scarred for life?' Roll play with a colleague how you may respond.

4. Many burns occur as a result of domestic accidents. Identify the most likely causes of thermal and chemical burns in the home, the age groups most at risk and design a teaching package suitable for mothers attending a day nursery with young children.

REFERENCES AND FURTHER READING

Allman RM, Walker JM, Hart MK, Laprade CA, Noel LB & Smith CR (1987) Air-fluidized beds or conventional therapy for pressure sores. *Annals of Internal Medicine* **107(5)**: 641–648.

Anthony D (1987) Pointers to good care. *Nursing Times* **83(34)**: 27–30.

Barratt E (1987) Putting risk calculators in their place. *Nursing Times* **83(7)**: 65–68.

Bayley EW (1990) Wound healing in the patient with burns. *Nursing Clinics of North America* **25(1)**: 205–221.

Bernstein NR, Breslau AJ & Graham JA (eds) (1988) *Coping Strategies for Burn Survivors and Their Families*. New York: Praeger.

Caine RM & Bufalino PM (eds) (1987) *Nursing Care Planning Guides for Adults*, pp 99–104. Baltimore: Williams & Wilkins.

Clarke M & Kadhom HM (1988) The nursing prevention of pressure sores in hospital and community patients. *Journal of Advanced Nursing* **13(3)**: 365–373.

Dyer C & Roberts D (1990) Thermal trauma. *Nursing Clinics of North America* **25(1)**: 85–117.

Feller I & Archambeault-Jones C (1973) *Procedures for Nursing the Burn Patient*, p 41. Ann Arbor, MI: The National Institute for Burn Medicine.

Freeman JW (1984) Nursing care of the patient with a burn injury. *Critical Care Nursing* **4(6)**: 52–68.

Goldstone LA & Goldstone J (1982) The Norton score: an early warning of pressure sores? *Journal of Advanced Nursing* **7(4)**: 419–426.

Gonzales-McLaughlin E (ed.) (1990) *Critical Care of the Burn Patient: A Case Study Approach*. Rockville, MD: Aspen.

Harvey Kemble JV & Lamb BE (1987) *Practical Burns Management*. London: Hodder & Stoughton.

Holloway NM (1988) *Nursing the Critically Ill Adult* 3rd edn, pp 557–551. Menlo Park, CA: Addison-Wesley.

Judd M (1989) *Mobility*. Oxford: Heinemann.

Kurzuk-Howard G, Simpson L & Palmieri A (1985) Decubitus ulcer care: a comprehensive study. *Western Journal of Nursing Research* **25(2)**: 19–26.

Lim R, Sirett R, Conine TA & Daechsel D (1988) Clinical trial of foam cushions in the prevention of decubitus ulcers in elderly patients. *Journal of Rehabilitation Research and Development* **25(2)**: 19–26.

Martyn JAJ (ed.) (1990) *Acute Management of the Burned Patient*. Philadelphia: W.B. Saunders.

NANDA (1989) *Taxonomy 1: Revised 1989: With Official Diagnostic Categories*, p 47. St Louis: North American Nursing Diagnosis Association.

Oleske DM, Smith XP, White P, Pottage J & Donovan MI (1986) A randomized clinical trial of two dressing methods for the treatment of low-grade pressure ulcers. *Journal of Enterostomal Therapy* **13(3)**: 90–98.

Sebern MD (1986) Pressure ulcer management in home health care: efficacy and cost effectiveness of moisture vapor permeable dressing. *Archives of Physical Medicine and Rehabilitation* **67(10)**: 726–729.

Settle J (1986) *Burns — The First 5 Days*. Welwyn Garden City: Smith & Nephew.

Smietanka MA & Opit LJ (1981) A trial of transparent adhesive dressing ('Op-Site') in the treatment of decubitus ulcer. *Australian Nursing Journal* **10(8)**: 40–42.

Townsend P et al (1988) *Inequalities in Health*. London: Penguin.

Versluysen M (1986) Pressure sores: causes and prevention. *Nursing* **3(6)**: 216–218.

Walsh M (1990) *A & E Nursing: A New Approach*. Oxford: Heinemann.

Walsh M & Ford P (1989) *Nursing Rituals: Research and Rational Action*. Oxford: Heinemann.

Caring for the Patient with a Disorder of the Ear and Nose

27

On completion of this chapter the reader should be able to:

- Describe the anatomy of the ear and nose
- Understand how the sense of hearing functions
- Discuss the various tests used to measure hearing ability
- Discuss the principal disorders of the ear and nose together with the appropriate nursing care required for patients with such disorders

STRUCTURE AND FUNCTIONS OF THE EAR

The ear is concerned with the special sense of hearing as well as with the maintenance of equilibrium. It has three divisions: the external and middle ears for the collection and conduction of sound waves and the inner ear, which actually serves as the receptor. The eighth cranial (auditory or acoustic) nerve provides the afferent impulse pathway of the sensory unit. Part of its fibres carry impulses to the interpretive centres for sound in the temporal lobes, and the others transmit impulses to areas of the brain stem and cerebellum associated with control of body posture.

EAR STRUCTURE (FIGURE 27.1)

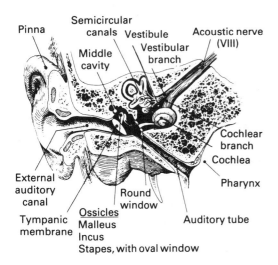

Figure 27.1 The parts of the ear.

External ear

The outer ear consists of the *auricle (pinna)* and the external auditory meatus. The auricle is an immobile cartilaginous framework covered with skin and may contribute slightly to the collection of sound waves. The external auditory meatus is an S-shaped tube approximately 2.5 cm (1 in) long. The tube ends at the tympanic membrane (eardrum), which separates the external and middle ears. The skin lining of the canal is covered with fine hairs near the opening and has special glands which produce a yellow waxy secretion called *cerumen* for protection against insects and dust particles. The *tympanic membrane* is a thin, semi-transparent membrane covered externally with skin and internally with mucous membrane which is continuous with that which lines the middle ear cavity. The middle layer is composed of thin elastic and fibrous tissue. A white streak is normally seen extending from the periphery towards the centre; this is the handle of the malleus in the middle ear (Figure 27.2).

Middle ear

This portion of the ear is contained within a small cavity in the temporal bone. The cavity communicates with the nasopharynx by means of the *auditory or Eustachian tube* and with the mastoid cells. The auditory tube permits the entrance of air into the middle ear; this equalizes the pressure on the internal surface of the eardrum with atmospheric pressure (that which is exerted on the external surface of the drum). The cavity is lined with mucous membrane which is continuous with that of the auditory tube and mastoid cells. The *mastoid cells* are small air spaces within the posterior portion of the temporal bone, just behind the middle ear. Obviously the continuity of the lining membrane provides a ready means for the spread of infection from

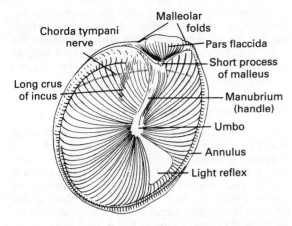

Figure 27.2 Diagram of a tympanic membrane.

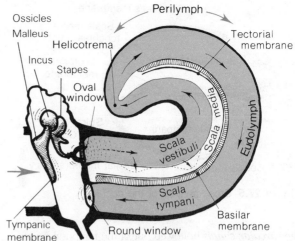

Figure 27.4 Schematic drawing of the cochlea.

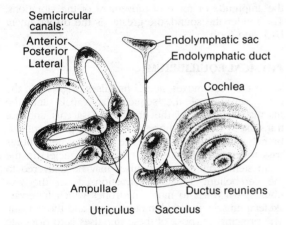

Figure 27.3 The membranous labyrinth of the ear.

the throat to the middle ear and from the middle ear to the mastoid.

The middle ear cavity contains three small bones called the auditory ossicles, which are movable for the purpose of transmitting sound vibrations. The first ossicle, the *malleus*, is attached to the eardrum and articulates with the second ossicle, the *incus*. The incus articulates with the third ossicle, the *stapes*, which is attached to the membranous oval window (fenestra ovalis) that leads into the inner ear. The middle ear also has two small muscles; one, the tensor tympani, is inserted on the malleus and the other, the stapedius, is inserted on the foot plate of the stapes. Contraction of these muscles reduces the amplitude of the sound waves entering the middle ear and cochlea.

Inner ear (labyrinth)

The inner ear consists of a system of irregularly shaped cavities which contain fluid and complex membranous structures which initiate nerve impulses as a result of sound waves or change of position. The *bony (osseous) labyrinth* is divided into a series of channels — the

cochlea, vestibule and semicircular canals. Within the bony labyrinth is a membranous labyrinth which conforms fairly closely to the shape of the bony-walled cavities (Figure 27.3). The fluid contained within the osseous cavities is called *perilymph*, and that within the membranous cavities is known as *endolymph*.

The complex snail-shaped structure, the *cochlea*, consists of three tubes wound two to three times around a central column called the modiolus. The channels formed by the tubes are called the scala vestibuli, scala media (cochlear duct) and scala tympani (Figure 27.4). The scala vestibuli is closed at one end by the membrane of the oval window. As a result, vibrations transmitted to the membrane by the stapes set up waves in the fluid within the scala vestibuli. The scala vestibuli communicates with the scala tympani at the apex of the cochlea so that when the fluid within the scala vestibuli is set in motion, the fluid in the scala tympani is similarly affected. The base of the scala tympani is closed off by the membrane covering an opening into the middle ear which is known as the *round window (fenestra rotunda)*.

The scala media is walled off from the scala vestibuli by Reissner's membrane and from the scala tympani by the basilar membrane. On the surface of the basilar membrane are special cells with hair-like projections which collectively are known as the organ of Corti. Contained within the organ of Corti are receptor cells which produce auditory nerve impulses when stimulated by vibrations of the basilar membrane (Figure 27.5).

The *vestibule* lies between the cochlea and the semicircular canals. The bony-walled cavity contains perilymph. The suspended membranous portion is divided into two sacs, called the utricle and the saccule, which contain endolymph. Within these cavities are hair-like projections and calcium carbonate concretions (otoliths) which respond to movements of the head by giving rise to neural impulses concerned with the maintenance of equilibrium.

The third division of the inner ear consists of three

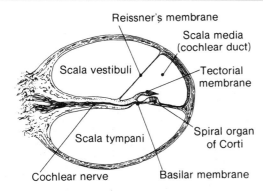

Figure 27.5 Cross-section of the cochlea.

semicircular canals hollowed out of the temporal bone at right angles to each other. They communicate with the osseous vestibule and contain perilymph. Three semicircular membranous ducts suspended within the osseous canals contain endolymph and communicate with the utricle. Each membranous semicircular canal has a dilated portion at one end, called the ampulla, which contains special sensory hair cells, forming the *crista acustica*, or crista ampullaris. The crista is sensitive to movement of the endolymph within the ampulla and initiates neural impulses that are transmitted by the vestibular portion of the acoustic (eighth cranial) nerve to the central nervous system.

AUDITORY PATHWAY

Sound waves passing into the external ear strike the tympanic membrane, causing it to vibrate with the same frequency as the sound waves. This in turn results in vibrations of the ossicles in the middle ear. The stapes, being attached to the oval window, causes its membrane to move in and out. The ossicles serve as amplifiers but, if the amplitude of the waves is excessive, producing excessive loudness, the vibrations may be modified by contraction of the tensor tympani and the stapedius. The tensor tympani decreases tympanic membrane contractions and the stapedius pulls the stapes away from the oval window, reducing the force of the vibrations which strike the oval window. The vibrations are transferred into the perilymph of the scala vestibuli of the inner ear and in turn through the Reissner's membrane and through the endolymph in the scala media to the basilar membrane. Movements of the endolymph and basilar membrane stimulate the receptor cells of the organ of Corti, initiating neural impulses which are transmitted via nerve fibres to a ganglion in the central core (the modiolus) of the cochlea. The axons of the ganglionic neurones form the cochlear branch of the acoustic (eighth cranial) nerve. The cochlear branch synapses with a group of neurones in the medulla (cochlear nucleus). The impulses are then transmitted to the inferior colliculi which are the centres for auditory startle reflexes, through the thalami and eventually reach a cortical area of the temporal lobe (auditory centre) where they are interpreted as sound. Each ear delivers impulses to both auditory centres.

The movements of the perilymph, initiated by the vibrations of the oval window, are transmitted through the helicotrema (communicating channel between the scalae at the apex of the cochlea) to the scala tympani and subsequently to the membrane of the fenestra rotunda (round window).

PITCH AND INTENSITY OF SOUND

The pitch of a sound depends upon the frequency of the vibrations (number per second). The number of vibrations or cycles per second (cps) are expressed as a unit of frequency referred to as a hertz (Hz) which is used in measuring the pitch of sound. The fibres of the basilar membrane vary in length. It is thought that different frequencies stimulate selective areas of fibres and cells of the membrane — that is, each place on the basilar membrane is sensitive to sound waves of a certain frequency.

The intensity, or loudness, of a sound depends upon the amplitude or force of movement of the vibrations. The louder the sound, the greater is the displacement back and forth.

PHYSICAL EQUILIBRIUM

When the head moves, neural impulses originate in the crista acustica of the semicircular canals and the maculae acusticae of the utricle and saccula and are transmitted by nerve fibres which form the vestibular branch of the acoustic nerve. The vestibular nerve fibres pass to groups of neurones (vestibular nuclei) in the brain stem from which impulses may be delivered to the cerebellum, reticular formation, down the vestibulospinal tracts to motor neurones which innervate skeletal muscle, the oculomotor centre and the thalami. The principal purpose of these impulses is to orientate the person in space, and to stimulate muscles in a reflex action so that he or she may assume an upright position or maintain the position that has been assumed against gravity.

THE PERSON WITH DISORDERS OF THE EAR

ASSESSMENT

HEALTH HISTORY

Previous illness. A nursing assessment of a patient with an ear disorder involves collecting information regarding previous ear disease or surgery that may have altered the normal architecture of the ear, history of ear infections, trauma and complications including perforation of the eardrum and aural discharge.

Any history of associated symptoms is recorded, i.e. upper respiratory tract infections, dizziness, (vertigo) tinnitus, hearing loss.

Medications. Information is obtained about exposure to ototoxic drugs that may produce hearing loss, dizziness or tinnitus. Common examples of such drugs are acetylsalicylic acid (aspirin) and aminoglycosides.

Family history of hearing loss and the type of hearing loss is obtained; congenital malformation of the auditory system or nerve damage may account for the loss of hearing.

Present disorder. The reason for seeking health care is identified. The manifestations being experienced and the duration and severity of the symptoms are determined. It is important to identify what the patient perceives as the problem and if someone else prompted him or her to seek care.

SOCIAL HISTORY AND BEHAVIOURAL CHANGES

Behavioural clues are often important indicators of hearing loss. Does the patient avoid social or work situations where several persons are talking at the same time? Have friends, relatives or the patient noticed evidence of inattentiveness, strained facial expressions, frequent requests to repeat instructions, increased volume of the radio or television, complaints about others mumbling, or postural change such as leaning forward or turning the head to one side to hear? Language development and school record are assessed if the patient is a child.

Use of hearing aids. It is important to document the use of a hearing aid and to communicate this to all health care personnel working with the patient.

PHYSICAL EXAMINATION

Physical examination of the ear may include inspection of the external ear, tests for Eustachian tube patency, evaluation of hearing, labyrinth tests, mastoid X-rays, blood tests and cultures. Obviously, the selection of investigational procedures depends upon the presenting signs and symptoms.

Inspection of the external ear

The ear is inspected inside and outside. The pinna (auricle) is examined for size, position, symmetry and lesions, and the mastoid process is palpated, especially if infection of the middle ear is suspected. The entrance of the ear canal is inspected for presence of debris or pus. The inside of the auditory canal is inspected with an auriscope (otoscope) which has a magnifying lens in addition to a light. The canal is inspected for lesions, foreign bodies and the amount and characteristics of the cerumen (wax). The tympanic membrane is viewed and the colour and tension noted (normal: light pearl-grey). It is examined for retraction or bulging, increased vascularity and perforation(s). During examination of the tympanic membrane, the patient is asked to take a breath and then to try to exhale forcibly through the nose with it tightly pinched and the lips closed. The normal Eustachian tube opens to admit air into the middle ear and the tympanic membrane may be seen to move outward. This latter procedure is referred to as Valsalva's manoeuvre (autoinflation) for testing the patency of the Eustachian tube.

Hearing evaluation

In hearing evaluation, the examiner assesses the degree of hearing loss and establishes whether it is due to conductive or nerve impairment. Conductive deafness results from failure of the conducting mechanism to transmit sound impulses from the external ear to the inner ear fluids. Neural deafness can be a result of disease of the sensor organ (the cochlea), auditory nerve or auditory cerebral centre.

Hearing screening. A quick evaluation of hearing acuity can be made using whispered and spoken voice tests and watch ticking. The patient occludes one ear while the examiner is positioned to the side with the lips 1 metre (3 feet) from the patient's unoccluded ear. The examiner exhales and softly whispers numbers which the patient is asked to repeat. A medium and then a loud whisper are used, and then, if necessary, a soft, medium and louder voice until the patient hears. (The normal ear can hear the spoken word at 7 m (23 feet) and the whisper at 5 m (16 feet).) The ability to hear high-frequency sounds is estimated by slowly moving a watch away from the patient's unoccluded ear and indicating when the ticking sound is no longer heard. The patient's hearing acuity is compared with that of the examiner, which is presumed to be within normal range.

Tuning fork tests. These are used to differentiate the type of deafness. The tuning fork may produce a frequency of 512 or 1024 cycles per second (cps). The tests should be made in a room free of noise.

- *Rinne test*. A tuning fork of 512 Hz is struck and held 2.5–5.0 cm (1–2 in) in front of the patient's external auditory canal. It is then placed firmly on the mastoid process and the patient is asked to state whether it is heard better by bone conduction (BC) or air conduction (AC).

  A more accurate method of performing the Rinne test is to hold the tuning fork 2.5–5.0 cm (1–2 in) in front of the external auditory meatus; the patient is asked to say when it can no longer be heard. It is then placed on the mastoid process and the patient states whether or not it can still be heard; if not, air conduction is better than bone conduction — a positive Rinne. Conversely if the tuning fork can be heard by bone conduction, then bone conduction is better than air conduction — a negative Rinne.

  In the normal ear air is a better conductor than bone (i.e. positive Rinne).
- *Weber's test*. This test is used to compare the degree of impaired hearing in the two ears. The tuning fork is set in vibration; the stem is held against the middle of the forehead or the vortex and the patient is asked if the sound is heard better in one ear than the other. Normally, the sound appears to be in the midline, being heard equally by both ears. If conductive

deafness is present the sound is greater in the affected ear. If the sound is heard equally well in both ears, the hearing loss is the same in both ears.

In sensorineural loss of hearing, the sound will be localized in the normal ear.

Thus, if the sound is louder in one ear there may be conductive loss of hearing in that ear or there may be a sensorineural deafness in the other ear.

- *Schwabach test.* This test compares the patient's bone conduction with that of the examiner, whose hearing is normal. The tuning fork is set in vibration and the stem is placed against the patient's mastoid process. The patient is instructed to indicate when the sound becomes inaudible. The stem of the tuning fork is then transferred to the mastoid bone of the examiner. If the sound is still audible to the latter, the patient has some sensorineural loss of hearing.

Audiometric tests. These tests provide information as to the degree of hearing loss. The unit used to express the intensity (or loudness) of sound is the *decibel* (*dB*). The audiometer is operated to produce sounds of known intensity and frequency (cps). Hearing is evaluated by recording the minimum intensity of sounds of various frequencies that are just audible to the patient. A normal adult ear is most sensitive to frequencies of 500–4000 Hz or cps. The normal ear in a child and young adult is sensitive to frequencies much lower and much higher. A soft whisper suggests about 20 dB; speech in normal conversation ranges from 55–60 dB.

Audiometric tests are conducted in a soundproof room and the patient wears earphones. The audiometric methods of assessing hearing that are commonly used are the pure-tone and speech tests.

- *Pure-tone audiometry.* The audiometer produces a range of pure tones of varying frequencies (cps or Hz). The intensity is adjusted in 5-decibel steps. The procedure is explained before the earphones are put on, and the patient is instructed as to when and how to signal. The test commences with a sound of high intensity which is gradually reduced to below the patient's threshold of hearing sound. The patient signals when the sound disappears. The intensity then is increased very slowly until the patient signals that the tone is just discernible. A range of frequencies is used, and the threshold intensity for each frequency is recorded on a chart called an audiogram. This indicates any hearing loss and the range of tones most affected. The test may be made of bone or air conduction. The greater the number of decibels recorded at which sound is perceived, the greater is the degree of defective hearing.
- *Speech audiometry.* In this test, a recording of lists of words representing normal vocabulary sound is played at varying volumes. The patient indicates the words heard. The percentage of words correctly heard for each intensity is recorded.

Tests for vestibular function

Tests used to assess the function of the vestibular system of the internal ear involve observing responses to certain stimuli. Strong stimulation normally produces vertigo or the falling to one side, nystagmus (involuntary, rhythmic eye movement) and nausea. Note that because the vestibular function tests may cause vertigo, nausea and vomiting, the nurse remains with the patient, prepared to provide the necessary support and assistance. Precautions are taken to prevent possible falls when the patient moves or attempts to walk.

Rotation test. The patient is seated in a chair that can be rotated, with the head tilted forward and the eyes closed. The chair is rotated quickly for ten full turns and stopped suddenly. The patient is asked to look at the doctor's finger which is held in front of the patient. Nystagmus is a normal response and its duration is timed. It should continue for about 25–40 seconds.

Caloric test. This test is also used in neurological investigation of the vestibular portion of the acoustic (VIII) nerve (see p. 711). The patient lies recumbent with the head raised at 30°. Water at 7°C above or below body temperature is injected into the external auditory canal and the patient observed for nystagmus. The nystagmus is timed, and past-pointing and testing for swaying to one side may be done. The test is carried out in each ear. The normal response to cold water is rotary nystagmus away from the ear being tested. If hot water is used, the normal movement of the eyes is toward the ear being irrigated. Pathological disturbances in the labyrinth may result in an absence of responses or excessive reaction.

Electronystagmography. This is an electroencephalographic recording of the eye movements in nystagmus. A study is made of the frequency, speed and amplitude of the eye movements. The recording is carried out in darkness or with the eyes closed to prevent fixation which suppresses nystagmus.

Radiological examination

Mastoid X-rays may be done to determine if mastoiditis has developed.

Blood examinations

Leucocyte and differential cell counts may be ordered if acute infection of the middle ear or labyrinthitis is suspected. In the case of acute infection and inflammation, the leucocyte count is usually above normal, the increase being principally in neutrophils.

Culture

Any discharge from the ear is usually cultured as soon as observed in order to identify the causative organism. Sensitivity tests to antibiotics may also be done.

CLINICAL CHARACTERISTICS

LOSS OF HEARING

The incidence of loss of hearing in varying degrees is very high and, in many instances, the person is unaware of it until it is well advanced. Hearing limitations interfere with the ability to communicate with others, which is extremely important. It may also result in the individual not being alerted to a threatening object or situation. Obviously, the effects and problems vary with the degree of loss and the age at which it developed. In the child, it retards development, affecting the learning of speech and normal adjustment within society. It creates physical, emotional and socioeconomic problems for both the person and family.

The degree of loss of hearing may be indicated by classifying those affected as 'hard of hearing' or 'deaf'. The hearing is defective in those who are hard of hearing but is not totally absent. They have sufficient hearing, either with or without the use of a hearing aid, to cope with ordinary activities. Persons who are described as deaf have a marked or total loss of hearing that makes it very difficult, if not impossible, to function normally.

Characteristics of impaired hearing

Indications of a hearing deficit may include failure to respond when addressed, frequent requests for repetition, and misinterpretation of what was said, especially of words that sound alike. A short attention span or lack of attention, lack of interest, a strained confused expression, turning of the head to direct the 'good' ear to the source of sound, irritability and fatigue because of the strain and withdrawal from the group may be manifested. The person who is hard-of-hearing may hesitate to acknowledge the handicap and may feign hearing when actually he or she does not hear. In some instances the person may talk continuously to avoid the situation of someone else speaking and being unable to hear what is said. Changes in speech, such as a lack of inflections, and a low or excessive volume, may also develop. A person with conductive deafness tends to speak softly; the person with nerve deafness usually speaks loudly.

In the case of a child, impaired hearing may be suspected if there is a failure in the development of speech, a lack of normal progress in school, no response to voice or sound, or no interest in noise-making toys. The severity of the speech defect depends on when the hearing deficit developed and the degree of loss. If the person is partially deaf with loss for high frequency (high pitched) sounds, he or she may hear vowels but not consonants. The deaf child responds more readily to movements than to sound and, when in need of comfort and reassurance, responds to cuddling or touch rather than to verbal expressions. The child may develop and persistently use gestures to indicate needs or wishes rather than producing vocal expressions.

Classification and causes of loss of hearing

A hearing deficit may be congenital or acquired and may be classified as conductive, sensorineural, central or combined.

In a *conductive hearing loss*, sound waves fail to reach the internal ear as a result of some disturbance in the external ear, middle ear or the oval window (fenestra ovalis).

The person with conductive deafness tends to speak softly as he or she can hear himself or herself.

In *sensorineural deafness*, which may also be called *nerve or perceptive deafness*, the disorder is located in the organ of Corti, cochlear division of the acoustic nerve, or auditory impulse pathway or centre within the brain.

The person with nerve deafness cannot hear anything, so tends to shout, hoping to hear.

Central hearing loss denotes a hearing deficit resulting from disturbances within the brain, principally the auditory centre in the temporal lobe.

Combined hearing loss occurs because of impairment within both the conductive and neural auditory mechanisms.

Congenital loss of hearing may be due to a prenatal malformation or lack of development of a part of the auditory apparatus. Heredity may play a role, or it may be the result of a viral infection in the mother during the first trimester of the pregnancy, the effect of a toxic drug taken by the mother during pregnancy, hypoxia or a birth injury.

Acquired impairment of hearing may be caused by obstruction of the external auditory canal by a foreign body or impacted cerumen, infection (e.g. otitis media, labyrinthitis, meningitis), a neoplasm (e.g. acoustic neuroma), an ototoxic drug (e.g. streptomycin, quinine), trauma associated with a skull fracture or excessively loud noise, obstruction of the Eustachian tube, or degenerative changes in the auditory pathway frequently associated with the ageing process (presbycusis).

TINNITUS

Tinnitus or ringing in the ears may be unilateral or bilateral and constant or intermittent. It may be of high or low pitch and vary in quality from a humming, buzzing, hissing, roaring, popping or pulsating sound. The sound sensation experienced by the patient is without a relevant external stimulus. It is usually heard only by the patient and rarely by others. Tinnitus is not a disease but a symptom. It may be a symptom of any abnormal condition of the ear, may be associated with deafness, or it may be drug related.

VERTIGO

Vertigo is a disturbance of equilibrium characterized by a sensation of movement or rotation of one's self or of one's surroundings. The patient experiences feelings of dizziness, light-headedness, falling or spinning. It may be accompanied by staggering or falling, clumsiness, nausea, vomiting or nystagmus which produces blurring of vision. It may occur suddenly, be transient in nature or recur as with Menière's syndrome. Disorders of the labyrinth are the most common cause. Disturbances in the pathways in the central nervous system may also produce vertigo.

OTALGIA (EARACHE)

Ear pain is usually severe and may be caused by infection, a neoplasm of the external or middle ear or may be referred pain from more distant disease processes. Inflammation of the middle ear produces pressure on the tympanic membrane and may lead to rupture. Obstruction of the Eustachian tube which is produced or aggravated by sudden changes in atmospheric pressure causes pain when the tympanic membrane is suddenly retracted.

OTORRHOEA

Otorrhoea is the term used for a discharge from an ear which may develop suddenly or gradually. It may be purulent, sanguineous, serous, waxy or mucoid in nature and may be associated with pain, vertigo, tinnitus and/or hearing loss. Causes include trauma and infection.

PATIENT PROBLEMS

The problem is a *sensory–perceptual alteration*; that is, an *auditory* deficit due to a disorder of one or both ears or the central nervous system.

The *goals* are that the patient will:

1. Preserve or maintain hearing.
2. Identify factors contributing to hearing loss.
3. Maintain or develop ability to communicate with others.

PRESERVATION OF HEARING

Nurses, especially those working with industrial workers and schoolchildren, have an important role in the prevention of hearing loss. The public requires education about the causes and early signs of impaired hearing and significant preventive measures.

Good prenatal care and the avoidance of contact with persons with measles or other viral infections are important in preventing congenital deafness. Immunization against measles should be promoted. Prompt treatment of respiratory infection and infectious diseases may allay the complication of otitis media. Prompt medical treatment and follow-up are urged for persons with an ear disorder.

The danger of introducing foreign objects into the external ear canal should be emphasized; for example, cleansing the ear with applicators, matches and hairpins is dangerous, as accidental perforation of the eardrum may occur. If the wax (cerumen) becomes dry and impacted or an insect or foreign body becomes lodged in the canal, a few drops of warm oil or sodium bicarbonate may be instilled and followed by a warm water or sodium bicarbonate irrigation in a few minutes. If this does not remove the foreign object or impacted wax, the person is advised to go to the doctor.

Routine tests of schoolchildren's hearing are important so that early recognition may be made of any impairment. Teachers and school nurses must be familiar with manifestations of a hearing deficit.

The nurse caring for a patient receiving a preparation of streptomycin, kanamycin or other ototoxic drugs and quinine must be alert for early signs of damage to the hearing.

The occupational health nurse, especially in an industry in which there is prolonged, intense noise in the work environment, must be cognizant of the possibility of noise-induced hearing loss. Frequently the employees tend to accept noise simply as a necessary part of the occupation and do not realize that hearing damage may be insidiously developing. Gradual loss of hearing usually involves, first, failure of response to high frequency sounds. Later, areas of the cochlea which respond to lower frequencies become damaged. In order to protect persons exposed to noise that endangers hearing, protective devices in the form of earmuffs, ear plugs or a special helmet should be provided. Employees should receive regular hearing tests and be exposed to an active educational programme.

High intensity music such as rock music is another source of noise pollution. Frequent exposure to the noise of firearms may also lead to hearing loss. Public education about the effects of noise pollution and the importance of the use of ear plugs or earmuffs to decrease the intensity of the noise is necessary and should be directed to high-risk groups.

SUGGESTIONS TO THOSE SPEAKING TO A PERSON WHO IS HARD OF HEARING

- Do not speak until you have the person's attention. The speaker's face should be in full view of the listener so that lip movement may be readily observed.
- Determine which is the better ear and go to that side if possible. Look directly at the listener.
- Speak slowly, enunciate clearly and avoid raising the pitch of voice. The volume is increased, but actual shouting is avoided. Guard against running words together. The natural form of conversation is used rather than broken statements and incomplete sentences.
- Exaggerated lip movement only confuses the listener.
- If repetition is necessary, rephrasing the communication may be helpful; remember that vowels are heard more readily than consonants.
- Patience, tact and understanding are needed. Avoid any irritation or annoyance; such reactions on the part of the speaker only discourage the listener.
- Do not prolong a conversation unnecessarily, since the listener tires under the strain.
- If a hearing aid is used, give the person time to adjust to it. Do not get within 4–5 feet of the aid and use natural volume and tone.
- A misinterpretation must not be ridiculed or treated as a joke.

- When a deaf person enters a room, an effort is made to draw him or her into the group. They should be advised of the topic of conversation and encouraged and given the opportunity to participate. Otherwise, they may tend to withdraw and become isolated.
- If it is not possible to communicate verbally, write the message.
- If a patient is totally deaf and does not lip-read, pictures or symbols that represent objects may be helpful to orientate the patient and for use during hospitalization.

SUGGESTIONS TO THOSE WHO ARE HARD OF HEARING

- Look directly at the speaker (preferably in a good light) since observation of lip movements proves helpful.
- Concentrate on the speaker.
- Observe the total situation, since this may give a lead to the topic of conversation.
- Acknowledge your hearing deficit; do not guess at things rather than ask for repetition.
- Indicate understanding of the speaker.

HEARING AIDS

Some persons with a hearing deficit may be helped by using a hearing aid, which is a small, battery-operated instrument which amplifies sounds. Aids are helpful to persons who have reduced conduction of sound waves into the inner ear. Few of those with sensorineural loss of hearing receive help from hearing aids; amplification of sound does not assist with the distortion and impaired discrimination resulting from impairment of the neural elements of the auditory apparatus. Before purchasing a hearing aid, the person with a hearing deficit should be examined by a doctor for evaluation of the residual hearing and identification of the type of hearing loss. The selection of the aid is based on the patient's particular type of hearing loss. If an aid is recommended, it should be worn for a trial period to determine if it does help.

AUDITORY AND SPEECH TRAINING

Auditory training is intended to help the individual utilize residual hearing effectively and improve communication skills. The process helps the patient develop good listening skills and increases his awareness of sounds and other clues.

Lip-reading or speech reading is the process of interpreting spoken words through the study of lip movements, facial expressions, body movements and gestures used in speech. Training helps the individual consciously and effectively use these cues.

Speech training is provided to maintain existing speech skills which deteriorate when the usual monitoring mechanism of hearing is lost. Hearing is necessary to assess loudness, clarity, tone and rate of speech. The congenitally deaf child requires a different type of programme to develop speech and language skills.

COMMUNITY RESOURCES

Those who are deaf or hard of hearing and their families should be familiar with the Royal National Institute for the Deaf and Hard Of Hearing. Assistance may be provided in the form of procuring medical examination and treatment, counselling as to the type of hearing aid that would be helpful, obtaining vocational training and employment, arranging for special classes (e.g. speech) and obtaining printed advice in pamphlets.

EVALUATION

The patient should demonstrate he/she can:

1. Understand the factors which contribute to hearing impairment.
2. Describe health practices to preserve hearing.
3. Understand how to obtain a hearing aid (if relevant).
4. Understand how to use and care for his or her hearing aid.
5. Understand the need for an auditory or speech training programme (if relevant).
6. Apply acquired skills in communicating with others, if so wished.
7. Be informed about the local branch of the Royal National Institute for the Deaf and Hard Of Hearing.

Common Disorders of the Ear

IMPACTED CERUMEN

The normal secretion of the external auditory canal (cerumen) may accumulate and become hard and dry. The retention may be due to abnormal narrowness of the canal, dryness of the skin or excess hair in the canal or misguided attempts to clean the ear with cotton-wool buds. It may also be associated with the person's occupation; it is a common problem for those working in a dusty or dry environment.

Symptoms develop with the obstruction of the canal; the person may experience a sense of fullness, noises, loss of hearing, irritation or, rarely, a cough. The latter is a reflex response to stimulation of the vagus nerve. Examination of the ear with an otoscope reveals a firm yellow or dark mass.

Removal of the mass may be by irrigation with warm water. It is important that any solution introduced into the ear be warmed to approximately 38°C; cold or hot solutions may stimulate the labyrinth and cause nystagmus, vertigo and nausea. It may be necessary to soften the wax prior to syringing. Instillation of sodium bicarbonate ear drops are recommended. If the mass cannot be removed by irrigation, the doctor may remove it with a Jobson–Horne probe.

OTITIS EXTERNA

This is a generalized inflammation of the external ear that may vary in severity from a mild dermatitis to cellulitis. The tympanic membrane may be affected. The cause is usually bacterial but, in some instances, may be a fungus (otomycosis). A predisposing factor is moisture in the ear. The incidence is higher in summer and may result from swimming in contaminated water (swimmer's ear). The infection is more likely to develop in a warm moist atmosphere or if the person swims frequently. It may be secondary to trauma inflicted by efforts to remove wax. External otitis may also be due to allergic dermatitis. Some people are prone to otitis externa because of a narrow external canal.

Characteristics

The patient may complain of pruritus if the disorder is dermatitis, and the skin may be dry and scaly at first. If the cause is infection, the ear is painful and examination may reveal redness, swelling, oedema of the walls of the auditory meatus and often the tympanic membrane and purulent lesions. An elevation of temperature and increased leucocyte count indicate a serious infection.

Treatment

Scrupulous aural cleansing is performed, and a swab obtained for culture; the topical application of an antibiotic preparation is prescribed in the case of infection of the canal. If allergic dermatitis is the cause a corticosteroid ointment or solution may be prescribed. Inflammation of the auricle (pinna) may be treated by warm compresses.

The patient with severe infectious otitis which has extended beyond the skin receives an oral or parenteral antimicrobial preparation as well as local treatment. An analgesic may also be necessary to provide relief from the pain. The patient should be advised to keep the ear dry and not to touch the ear. Antihistamines may be indicated to relieve irritation in dermatitis, especially at night.

ACUTE OTITIS MEDIA

This is an inflammation of the middle ear and is frequently a complication of an upper respiratory tract infection or an infectious disease, as in measles. Often the organisms gain access through the auditory tube and, less frequently, through a perforation in the tympanic membrane. The disorder is usually acute but may become chronic.

The initial inflammatory response causes congestion and swelling of the mucous membrane lining of the middle ear, and the cavity fills with exudate. The tympanic membrane bulges externally and, unless the infection is checked, the exudate generally becomes purulent. If the cavity is not surgically drained, the tympanic membrane may rupture spontaneously.

Characteristics

The patient with otitis media experiences a sensation of fullness in the ear and dullness of hearing at first, then severe pain, and increasing loss of hearing because of failure of the conduction of sound waves through the middle ear. The temperature and leucocyte count are elevated, and the patient feels generally ill. Examination of the eardrum by means of an auriscope reveals redness, hyperaemia and external bulging due to the pressure of the collection of exudate in the middle ear, or rupture and discharge in the advanced stage.

Treatment

The patient is given an antibiotic and a nasal vasoconstrictor may be administered to dilate the auditory tubes. A mild analgesic may be taken to alleviate pain. The eardrum may occasionally be surgically opened to permit drainage if the exudate is producing excessive pressure on the eardrum and there is danger of spontaneous rupture. The operative procedure is referred to as a *myringotomy*. Incision and drainage is preferable to leaving the condition until there is spontaneous rupture of the tympanic membrane. Delayed treatment of acute otitis media may predispose to mastoiditis, chronic otitis media and permanent hearing loss.

The patient having a myringotomy receives a local anaesthetic. Fluid is aspirated from the middle ear cavity through the incision, and a culture is taken. Absorbent cotton may be placed loosely in the outer ear to absorb the drainage. The patient is encouraged to lie on the affected side to promote drainage. A persistent elevation of temperature, pain and deep tenderness in the region of the mastoid, headache, drowsiness or disorientation is reported to the doctor. These may indicate the onset of a serious complication such as mastoiditis, meningitis or brain abscess.

SEROUS OTITIS MEDIA

Serous otitis media is characterized by an accumulation of fluid in the middle ear. The effusion is usually caused by obstruction of the Eustachian tube incurred by enlarged adenoids, severe nasopharyngitis or an allergic reaction. It may also develop following acute otitis media that has not been completely resolved. Rarely, the condition may be associated with a benign or malignant neoplasm of the nasopharynx or pharynx which blocks the Eustachian tube.

The fluid is a thin and watery transudate. Blockage of the Eustachian tube results in a negative pressure in the middle ear cavity which promotes movement of fluid out of the mucous membrane capillaries.

Characteristics

The patient experiences loss of hearing and discomfort in the affected ear. Examination of the eardrum reveals its immobility and an air–fluid level in the middle ear. The nasopharyngeal area is investigated for disease that is the likely primary cause.

Treatment

Any nasopharyngeal disorder is corrected; for example, if hypertrophied adenoids are found to be the cause, an adenoidectomy is performed. The allergic reaction is treated if it is found to be the problem. If nasopharyngitis due to infection is obstructing the auditory tube, the patient receives antibiotic therapy.

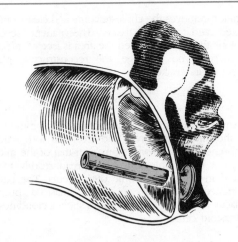

Figure 27.6 Grommet (tympanostomy tube).

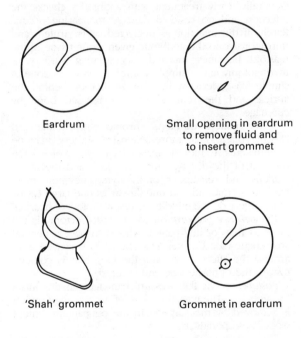

Eardrum

Small opening in eardrum
to remove fluid and
to insert grommet

'Shah' grommet

Grommet in eardrum

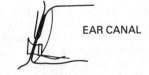

EAR CANAL

Grommet tube seen in cross section

Figure 27.7 The grommet tube.

A myringotomy is done and the fluid aspirated. This may be followed by repeated Valsalva manoeuvres to clear the Eustachian tube (see p. 953) and ventilate the middle ear. Following the myringotomy, a plastic indwelling tympanostomy tube (grommet) may have to be inserted via the external auditory canal. This permits continuous ventilation and drainage of the middle ear

(Figures 27.6 and 27.7). The tube is left in position until patency of the auditory tube is re-established; this may be a period of several weeks or months. The patient is closely supervised following the surgery and is usually seen in the out-patient department 6 weeks postoperatively, then every 3 months, when the tube and the patient's hearing are checked.

When the tube is inserted the nurse instructs the patient, and the parents if the patient is a child, about the care of the affected ear and the restrictions on activities. If the doctor prescribes the instillation of drops, an explanation and demonstration are given to the parents, and an opportunity provided for one of them to carry out the procedure under supervision. They are cautioned that if the medication causes pain following the instillation, the procedure is discontinued and the surgeon contacted promptly. The surgeon is also notified immediately of any increase or change in the fluid drainage, increasing deafness or pain. The patient must guard against getting water into the ear. During a bath or shower, a cotton ball coated with petroleum jelly is placed in the entrance to the ear canal. Swimming is allowed after the first 6 weeks and with the surgeon's consent. The ear should be prepared as for a bath or shower, and the patient is cautioned against diving.

CHRONIC OTITIS MEDIA

This chronic inflammatory disorder of the ear is associated with a permanent perforation of the tympanic membrane. It usually is a sequela of repeated episodes of acute otitis media that were not treated or were caused by virulent or antibiotic-resistant organisms. The perforation may also be the result of mechanical trauma or blast injury.

The location of the perforation is an important factor in the seriousness of the disease. If it is central or at least does not involve the margin of the eardrum, the perforation is less serious and can be treated more effectively. This type of perforation is categorized as *tubotympanic*. If the perforation involves the tympanic margin in the posterior-superior area, the disorder is a more serious problem. There are usually several perforations and, because of their location, may be referred to as *attic perforations*.

Characteristics

The otitis media associated with a central perforation is manifested by purulent discharge with an offensive odour. The discharge may be greatly increased during periods of acute upper respiratory infections or if water gets into the ear during bathing or swimming. Over a period of time, middle ear structures are damaged by the infection and necrosis. There is usually some impairment of hearing which worsens during exacerbations.

Treatment

The initial treatment of the patient with a *tubotympanic perforation* is directed towards eliminating any upper respiratory tract infection as well as that in the ear. An antibiotic is administered orally or parenterally. The ear is cleansed by suction and dry mopping, followed by the instillation of an antimicrobial solution. If the exudate is excessive, it may be removed by daily aspiration by the doctor. When the infection is cleared up, the perforated area very occasionally fills in with scar tissue. If the perforation persists, a tympanoplasty may be done to improve the patient's hearing and reduce the risk of reinfection by establishing a barrier between external and middle ears. The type of surgical procedure used depends upon whether there is damage to the middle ear structures or not and, if so, the extent of the involvement. Tympanoplastic surgery is only undertaken if infection is controlled.

Tympanoplasty type I indicates a myringoplasty in which a graft is used to repair the perforated eardrum when the middle ear structures are intact and functional. Epithelium from the ear canal, skin from the postauricular area, fascia stripped from the temporal muscle or a section of a vein may be used as a graft. Tympanoplasty types II, III, IV, and V operative procedures involve plastic correction of the perforated eardrum and repair of damaged middle ear structures. The operations progressively increase in complexity, involving more extensive surgery and structural replacement. The reparative and/or reconstructive procedures are directed toward re-establishing a conductive system from the eardrum through the ossicles and the oval window and providing sound protection for the round window. Re-establishing ossicular continuity may necessitate the replacement of ossicles by a graft or a prosthesis.

Postoperatively, the pressure dressing is left undisturbed for 48 hours. If necessary, the outer part may be reinforced. Dressings are changed and the packing is removed by the surgeon. Precautions are taken to avoid wetting the dressing during bathing. The patient is asked not to blow the nose and to avoid coughing and sneezing to prevent air being forced through the Eustachian tube into the middle ear. When first up, a nurse assists and remains with the patient for a while since dizziness and nausea may be experienced.

In *marginal (attic) perforations*, the disease involves the bony rim of the tympanic membrane and the mastoid cells as well as the middle ear structures. An invasive *cholesteatoma* may develop; this is a mass that forms in the middle ear as a result of the growth of epithelial tissue implanted in the middle ear from the collapsed and invaginated parts of the eardrum when it perforates. The inflammation causes hyperactivity of the basal layer of the epidermis. The epidermal tissue encloses sebum and desquamated epidermal cells; these serve as a good culture medium for organisms. The mass compresses middle ear structures and mastoid cells, causing necrosis and bone erosion. The presence of the cholesteatoma predisposes to the serious complications of labyrinthitis and brain abscess. Marginal perforation and the development of a cholesteatoma are treated by radical surgery. A mastoidectomy is done, the cholesteatoma and middle ear debris are removed and reconstruction undertaken to provide a conductive channel. The surgery is done in two stages; the first operation removes the cholesteatoma and clears out the infected and necrotic tissue. The patient receives antibiotic therapy and, when the area is free of infection and there is no drainage, the reconstructive plastic surgery is undertaken.

MASTOIDITIS

The small spaces (air cells) in the mastoid communicate with the middle ear cavity and are lined with mucous membrane which is continuous with that of the middle ear. As a result, infection may spread readily to the mastoid in acute or chronic otitis media. The patient experiences tenderness over the mastoid process, headache and fever. Mastoid X-rays show a cloudiness in the mastoid cells.

Treatment and nursing intervention

Generally, early treatment with antibiotics checks the infection and no residual damage to hearing occurs. Rarely, if the infection is neglected or is virulent and unresponsive to the antibiotic given, bone tissue of the mastoid becomes infected, necessitating surgery. A myringotomy and a simple mastoidectomy are done. A simple mastoidectomy involves an incision behind the auricle and the removal of the diseased bone by curettage.

If the patient develops chronic otitis media and chronic mastoiditis, more extensive surgery may be undertaken. A radical mastoidectomy involves the removal of the diseased mastoid tissue and the incus, malleus and remainder of the tympanic membrane, leaving the mastoid and middle ear as one large cavity. This surgery on the middle ear results in loss of hearing.

Preoperative preparation for a mastoidectomy is the same as that for any patient who is to have a general anaesthetic (see Chapter 11). The scalp is shaved 2 cm around the affected ear, and the long hair is combed toward the opposite side and secured.

Postoperatively, the pressure bandage remains intact for 48 hours. The meatal pack is left undisturbed until it is removed by the surgeon in the out-patient clinic 2 weeks postoperatively.

The patient is observed closely for nystagmus or any sign of facial paralysis. Facial paralysis is a threat in mastoidectomy because of the facial (seventh cranial) nerve's proximity to the operative site. Persisting headache, stiffness of the neck, elevation of temperature or disorientation is brought to the surgeon's attention, since it may indicate a complicating brain abscess or meningitis. Fluids are given freely and a regular diet is served as soon as it is tolerated.

The patient is generally allowed up on the evening of surgery or the following morning; someone remains at first in case of dizziness and nausea that may develop as a result of labyrinth disturbance, especially following a radical mastoidectomy.

If the patient suffers some hearing loss, he or she is reassured that assistance is available. The nurse advises the patient about trying to communicate with others and may also refer him or her to the Royal National Institute for the Deaf and Hard Of Hearing.

OTOSCLEROSIS

This is a chronic ear disease in which the stapes becomes immobilized because of progressive growth of bone tissue over the oval window and fixation of the stapes, interfering with the transmission of vibrations into the inner ear. Both ears are affected eventually.

The disease appears to be hereditary and has a higher incidence in females. The ability of the stapes to vibrate progressively decreases, and the loss of hearing usually becomes apparent in the teens or twenties, and during pregnancy. The person may complain of tinnitus as the deafness becomes more marked. The testing of hearing with a tuning fork reveals that the person has good bone conduction of sound but none by air.

Treatment

A hearing aid may be of some help for a period of time, but a stapedectomy has proved to be the treatment of choice at present. By means of a surgical microscope, the surgeon works through the external auditory canal and the middle ear. The stapes is removed, and a prosthesis introduced to transfer the vibrations of the incus through the oval window into the inner ear. Various forms of prostheses have been used and include a wire or teflon tube with a section of vein, a 'pad' of fat or Gelfoam. The teflon prosthesis is attached to the incus with its distal end in the oval window. The oval window niche is sealed using a free graft of fat or vein, and protected with Gelfoam. Only one ear is done at a time.

Postoperatively, dizziness and nausea may be troublesome because of the disturbance of the labyrinth. A specific directive is received from the surgeon about the position in which the head is to be maintained as practices vary in different hospitals. A close check is made for any sign of infection (elevation of temperature and leucocyte count, discharge and pain); if it is suspected, an antimicrobial drug is prescribed. The patient is instructed not to blow the nose to prevent air from being forced through the Eustachian tube to the middle ear. The patient is cautioned to move slowly and not to stoop over. If vertigo is experienced, ambulation may have to be delayed. The patient requires assurance that the dizziness is temporary. The patient should be observed closely for nystagmus or any sign of facial palsy.

Packing is placed in the ear upon completion of the surgery; this is removed by the surgeon in approximately 7–9 days. When the packing is removed, the patient may find the noise in the environment very confusing and disturbing. A nurse or family member should accompany him to provide support and reassurance.

MENIÈRE'S DISEASE OR SYNDROME

This is a disorder of the internal ear characterized by recurrent attacks of severe vertigo, nausea, vomiting, tinnitus and a progressive loss of hearing. The cause is not known but an excess of endolymph (endolymphatic hydrops) develops, resulting in increased pressure and dilatation of the canals. Vascular spasm and allergic reaction have been suggested as possible aetiological factors. The disorder usually makes its appearance between the ages of 40 and 60 years, and occurs more often in males.

The episodes have a sudden onset, and the patient is generally prostrated by the dizziness and nausea. The duration of an attack varies from hours to days.

During an attack the patient remains in bed in a quiet environment. Cot sides may be necessary for safety because of the vertigo. An antiemetic such as dimenhydrinate (Dramamine) and a sedative may provide some relief. Diphenhydramine hydrochloride (Benadryl) given intravenously may arrest an acute attack. In an effort to offset episodes, the patient is placed on a low-sodium diet and receives ammonium chloride; a diuretic such as hydrochlorothiazide (Esidrex) may also be prescribed to reduce the formation of endolymph. A vasodilator (e.g. nicotinic acid) to discourage vasospasm may be helpful. Recent usage of betahistine has provided good evidence that it is effective in Menière's disease, by increasing cochlear circulation. Although the acute attacks are episodic, the hearing loss tends to be permanent.

The condition can be very incapacitating and may necessitate surgery. The procedure entails the destruction of the membranous labyrinth. More recently, ultrasonic waves have been used. This form of treatment requires a mastoidectomy to permit the application of the probe. If the patient still has considerable hearing in the affected ear, ultrasonic treatment is used because it is thought to be less hazardous for the hearing.

STRUCTURE AND FUNCTIONS OF THE NOSE

The nose is concerned with the special sense of smell as well as being the first organ of the respiratory system. Air breathed in through the nose is warmed, filtered and moistened before entering the lower respiratory passages and the lungs.

NASAL STRUCTURE (FIGURE 27.8)

The two anterior nares (nostrils) form the openings into the nasal cavities, which are separated from each other by the nasal septum formed of cartilage and bone. Skin covers the external nose and lines the nostrils, and displays hair internally. The external skin separating the two nostrils is called the columella. The boundary of the external nose is the narrow opening into the nasal cavity. The roof of the nose is formed by the base of the skull. The floor is formed by the roof of the mouth and is composed of the maxillary bones, the palatine bones and the soft palate. The lateral walls of the nose are formed by bone of the maxilla, containing the maxillary sinuses, and the ethmoid bone, containing the ethmoid sinuses. Three bony ridges, the inferior, middle and superior conchae (or turbinates), project from the outer wall of each nasal cavity partially to divide it into three passages. At the back of the nose these passages lead to

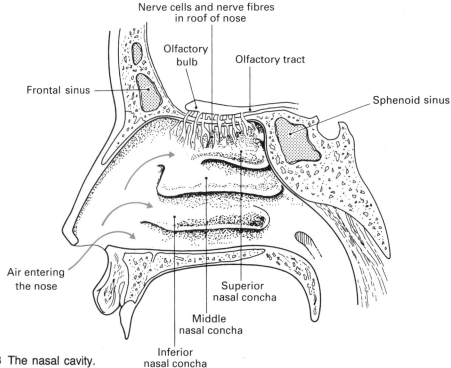

Nerve cells and nerve fibres
in roof of nose

Olfactory
bulb

Olfactory tract

Frontal sinus

Sphenoid sinus

Air entering
the nose

Superior
nasal concha

Middle
nasal concha

Inferior
nasal concha

Figure 27.8 The nasal cavity.

the pharynx. The interior of the nose is lined with mucous membrane. Most of this membrane is covered with minute hair-like projections called cilia. Moving in waves, these cilia filter the air passing through the nasal passages and sweep the debris out of the cavity, together with nasal mucous. The mucous membrane also acts to warm and moisten the inhaled air and is therefore a very vascular tissue.

The nasal cavities have connections with the middle ears by the pharyngotympanic (Eustachian) tubes, and with the eye region by the nasolacrimal ducts. The adenoids, two small areas of lymphatic tissue, can be found on the wall of the nasopharynx, behind the nose.

THE OLFACTORY REGION

The first cranial (olfactory) nerve provides the afferent sensory impulse pathway. The nerve endings, the olfactory receptors, are located in two pea-sized areas high in the interior of the nasal cavity.

All odorous materials give off particles of their substance and these chemical particles are carried into the nose with the inhaled air. They dissolve in the secretions of the mucous membrane and will only stimulate nerve cells when in solution. The air entering the nose is heated and convection currents carry the inspired air to the roof of the nose. Sniffing transmits the currents more rapidly so that delicate odours can be better appreciated. When an individual is continuously exposed to an odour, perception of the odour decreases and eventually ceases. This loss of perception only affects that specific odour. The sense of smell may be diminished or lost entirely as a result of nasal

obstruction or infection or trauma to the nasal tissue or the olfactory nerve. Mental illness or brain tumours can also affect the sense of smell. The complete absence of the sense of smell is called anosmia.

The two senses of smell and taste are inextricably linked. Taste registers only four qualities: salt, sour, bitter and sweet. Other qualities of taste depend on smell. The sense of smell may affect the appetite positively or adversely, depending on whether the smell is pleasant or unpleasant.

THE PARANASAL SINUSES

The paranasal sinuses are commonly referred to as nasal sinuses, or simply as 'the sinuses'. They are the eight cavities in the skull that are connected with the nasal cavity. They are arranged in four pairs, with members of each pair symmetrically placed on each side of the head. The pairs are:

- The *maxillary* sinuses in the maxillae.
- The *frontal* sinuses in the frontal bone.
- The *sphenoid* sinuses in the sphenoid bone behind the nasal cavity.
- The *ethmoid* sinuses in the ethmoid bone behind and below the frontal sinuses.

The function of the sinuses is not clearly understood but it is thought that they may help with the warming and moistening of inhaled air and provide a resonating chamber for the voice. Being air-filled chambers, they make the skull lighter than it would otherwise be.

The sinuses, all lined with mucous membrane, are each connected with the nasal cavity; their openings into the nasal cavity are called the ostia. One of the functions of the nose is to drain fluids discharged from the paranasal sinuses.

THE PERSON WITH DISORDERS OF THE NOSE OR NASAL SINUSES

ASSESSMENT

HEALTH HISTORY

Previous illness. A nursing assessment of a patient with a disorder of the nose or nasal sinuses involves collecting information about any previous trauma or surgery that may have affected the anatomy of the region. Any history of previous, associated symptoms should also be recorded.

Medications. Information is obtained about the drugs being taken for the current problem, which may include inhalations and decongestants, as well as other medications.

Present disorder. The reason for seeking health care is identified. The manifestations, the duration and severity of the symptoms are determined.

PHYSICAL EXAMINATION

The nose is examined both inside and out. The external nose is examined for asymmetry and lesions. The nostrils are examined for the presence of debris or discharge. The nurse may assist the patient while the doctor performs a full physical examination of the nose and sinuses. The inside of the nasal cavity can be examined (using nasal speculae and a light source) for lesions and foreign bodies, and to determine the amount and characteristics of the nasal mucous. Any oedema or congestion of the mucous membranes will be noted. Air entry via each nostril is assessed by occluding the other. The patient may be asked to sniff to aid this assessment. Examination of the posterior aspect of the nose may be performed via the oral cavity and nasopharynx using a dental mirror and light source.

Radiological examination

X-rays of the nasal bones will determine if fractures or displacement of the cartilage have taken place. X-rays of the maxillary or frontal sinuses will show sinusitis.

Common Disorders of the Nose and Nasal Sinuses

RHINITIS

Acute rhinitis is the medical term for the common cold.

Most adults experience, on average, 2–4 attacks of acute rhinitis per year. Children may have much more frequent attacks. The mucous membranes of the nose become swollen and there is a nasal discharge. Some types are accompanied by fever, muscle aches and general discomfort with sneezing and running eyes. Breathing through the nose may become difficult or impossible. Rhinitis is often accompanied by inflammation of the throat and sinuses.

Common rhinitis is caused by a virus but may be complicated by a bacterial infection. Hay fever is another common form of rhinitis and is caused by an allergen to a particular substance. It too may be complicated by a superimposed bacterial infection.

The best treatment for the common cold is rest, preferably in bed, a well-balanced diet and sufficient liquid intake. Mild analgesia may be taken to relieve headache or fevers. It must be remembered that the common cold is highly contagious, both by direct contact with the virus (on a handkerchief, for example) and by droplet inhalation (transmitted when coughing or sneezing).

Chronic rhinitis may result in permanent thickening of the nasal mucosa. Treatment involves treating the primary cause; nasal decongestants may be of some use.

EPISTAXIS (NOSEBLEED)

Epistaxis is usually due to the rupture of small blood vessels overlying the anterior part of the cartilaginous nasal septum. A minor nosebleed may be caused by a blow on the nose, irritation from foreign bodies (or fingers), or vigorous nose blowing. Treatment involves sitting the victim up with head tilted forward to prevent the swallowing of blood, which is a gastric irritant. Pressure should be applied to the soft portion of the nose by grasping it between the thumb and forefinger. Pressure may need to be applied for up to 15 minutes. Once the bleeding has been arrested, the victim should rest quietly for an hour or so, and avoid stooping or lifting for several hours. If bleeding persists, medical help should be sought as it may be necessary to pack the nose or to cauterize the bleeding vessel.

Sometimes nosebleeds have serious underlying causes such as arteriosclerosis, polyps or other growths in the nose, hypertension or vitamin deficiencies. Anyone who experiences frequent or profuse nosebleeds should therefore seek medical advice.

SURGERY TO THE NOSE

Nasal surgery is indicated in a variety of conditions ranging from removal of a foreign body (usually in children) to the correction of a deviation of the nasal septum (caused by irregular growth or injury). Polyps or other growths can be removed to restore normal nasal breathing. Adenoidectomy to restore normal nasal breathing is a common operation in children and is frequently performed routinely; grommets are inserted into the tympanic membranes (see p. 959). Cosmetic plastic surgery to correct disfiguring nasal anatomy is a common operation. Any surgery to the nose may result in swelling and bruising, which may last up to 6 weeks so the success of the surgery cannot be assessed immediately. The patient needs to be aware of this prior to the operation.

Postoperatively the most common complication is bleeding. Excessive bleeding is indicated if the patient becomes restless, swallows repeatedly or spits up blood. Nasal packing or a splint may be left in the nose to prevent the formation of a haematoma. These are usually removed by the surgeon or at the surgeon's direction. If severe swelling or bleeding are expected, ice compresses may be used to reduce these.

Most nasal surgery results in some mild discomfort. This is partly due to the swelling and bruising but also to the presence of crusts of dried blood and mucous in the nose. The patient must be discouraged from attempting to dislodge these by noseblowing or picking. Lubricants or humidification may be used to help soften crusts, but no swabs or other objects should be inserted into the nose. Mild analgesia may be given to reduce the discomfort.

SINUSITIS

Sinusitis is the inflammation of one or more of the paranasal sinuses. It tends to occur when an upper respiratory tract infection spreads from the nose to the sinuses but may be associated with allergies, air pollution, diving or swimming. Any alteration to normal nasal breathing, such as that caused by a deviated nasal septum or polyps, may lead to sinusitis. As the inflammation of the mucous membranes lining the sinuses increases, swelling occurs and partially or totally occludes the ostium (opening into the nasal cavity), preventing the exudate from draining. Mucous then accumulates and becomes infected, creating pressure within the sinus. Thus the symptoms of sinusitis are pain located in and around the affected sinus, headaches, nasal discharge, fever and general malaise.

Radiological confirmation of the diagnosis can be undertaken, and this helps to identify any underlying problem such as polyps or deviated septum. CT scanning may be used if more complex sinus disorders are suspected.

The treatment of acute sinusitis is with antibiotics and decongestants, with the inhalation of steam to help encourage drainage. Analgesia is given to relieve the discomfort and as an antipyretic.

Chronic sinusitis occurs when the mucous membranes become thickened and obstruct the ostium, even when infection is not present. This prevents normal drainage from the sinus so that build-up of mucous occurs and frequent infections exacerbate the condition.

Treatment involves the identification and treatment of any underlying pathology, such as polyps or a deviated nasal septum. Changing the quality and humidity of the air in the home or workplace by using air-conditioners or filters and humidifiers may reduce the number and severity of the attacks. Failing this, drainage of the sinus may be performed surgically. Chronic sinusitis may lead to complications due to the proximity of other structures, such as the bones of the middle ear, the mastoid process and the brain, and for this reason it needs to be treated aggressively.

SUMMARY

Although the nursing care of patients with specific disorders of the ear and nose tends to occur on specialized units, the nurse should be aware that impaired hearing can affect a patient in a multitude of settings. Throughout this text the importance of good communication and patient teaching have been emphasized. It is therefore appropriate to conclude this chapter by stressing the section within it which discusses communication with persons whose hearing is impaired. If the patient fails to hear the nurse, and understand what is being said, it is doubtful that effective nursing care can occur unless alternative avenues of communication are utilized.

LEARNING ACTIVITIES

1. Interview a colleague or friend to find out how a significant loss of hearing would affect that person's life. Reverse roles and repeat the interview.
2. Can you change the batteries in a hearing aid? If not find out how.
3. What are the principal sources of noise that disturb patients trying to sleep at night? Ask some patients and observe for yourself. What can nurses do to make wards quieter places at night?

REFERENCES AND FURTHER READING

Ballantyne J & Groves J (eds) (1979) *Scott Brown's Diseases of the Ear Nose and Throat. Vol. 2: The Ear* 4th edn. London: Butterworths.

Ballantyne J & Martin JAM (1984) *Deafness* 4th edn. Edinburgh: Churchill Livingstone.

Birrell JF (ed.) (1982) *Logan Turner's Diseases of the Nose Throat and Ear*, pp 286–443. Bristol: Wright.

Broder MI, Busis SN, Dewesse D, Friedman A & Lau FY (1981) Probing physical causes of dizziness. *Patient Care* **15(11)**: 41–44, 49–51, 55–57, 61, 62, 64, 66–71, 75–79, 82–84, 86, 89, 90, 91, 95, 99–102.

Browning GG (1982) *Updated ENT*, pp 1–68. London: Butterworth.

Burton RC, Frederic MW, Pulec JL & Rubin W (1981) Evaluating complaints of dizziness. *Patient Care* **15(10)**: 23–25, 28, 29, 33, 36, 43, 47, 54–56, 59–61.

Doyle J (ed.) (1981) *No Need to Shout*. London: ITV.

Fields WL & McGinn-Campbell KM (1983) *Introduction to Health Assessment*, chapt. 8. Reston, VA: Reston.

Ganong WF (1985) *Review of Medical Physiology* 11th edn, chapt. 9. Los Altos, CA: Lange.

Hanawalt A & Troutman K (1984) If your patient has a hearing aid. *American Journal of Nursing* **84(7)**: 900–901.

Hawke M et al (1984) *Clinical Otoscopy*. Edinburgh: Churchill Livingstone.

Hayes C (1981) Ergonomics: the body's reaction to noise. *Occupational Health* **33(1)**: 75–83.

Heller BR & Gaynor EB (1981) Hearing loss and aural rehabilitation of the elderly. *Topics in Clinical Nursing* **3(1)**: 21–29.

Holder L (1982) Hearing aids. *Nursing '82* **12(4)**: 64–67.

Innes A (1985) *Ear, Nose and Throat Surgery and Disorders*. London: Faber & Faber.

Krupp MA & Chatton MJ (1983) *Current Medical Diagnosis and Treatment*, pp 93–100. Los Altos, CA: Lange.

Ludman H (1988) *ABC of Ear, Nose and Throat*. London: British Medical Association.

Malkiewicz J (1982) How to assess the ears and test hearing acuity. *Registered Nurse* **45(3)**: 56–63.

Marshall KH & Attia EL (1983) *Disorders of the Ear*. Boston: Wright.

Miles EH (1980) *Lecture Notes on Diseases of the Ear Nose and Throat*, pp 1–85. Oxford: Blackwell.

Morgan RH (1983) Breaking through the sound barrier. *Nursing '83* **13(6)**: 112–114.

Nash & Nash (1981) *Deafness in Society*. Massachusetts: Lexington Books.

Nave CR & Nave BC (1985) *Physics for the Health Sciences* 3rd edn, chapt. 18. Philadelphia: Saunders.

Senra A, Bailey CM & Jackson P (1986) *Ear, Nose and Throat Nursing*. Oxford: Blackwell.

Smith LH & Thier SO (1985) *Pathophysiology* 2nd edn, pp 1113–1121. Philadelphia: Saunders.

Stafford N (1988) *Ear, Nose and Throat Colour Aids*. Edinburgh: Churchill Livingstone.

Caring for the Patient with a Disorder of the Eye

28

OBJECTIVES

On completion of this chapter the reader will be able to:

● Describe the structure and functioning of the eye.
● Discuss the assessment of vision.
● Demonstrate an understanding of the common causes of visual impairment.
● Discuss the care of a patient with impaired vision.

STRUCTURE AND FUNCTION OF THE EYES

Vision, like all other sensory mechanisms, requires receptors, an afferent pathway to carry the impulses into the central nervous system and an interpretive centre. The eyes serve as receptors which are sensitive to light rays, the pathway is formed by the optic nerves and tracts within the brain, and the interpretive centres are composed of groups of neurones localized in the cortex of the cerebral occipital lobes (visual centres). In addition, the visual apparatus includes intrinsic and extrinsic muscles which play an important role in vision. There are also several accessory structures which function to protect the eyes.

LOCATION OF THE EYE

Each eyeball rests in a cone-shaped cavity (the orbit) in the skull. The orbit is covered posteriorly by a fibrous sac lined with a smooth moist membrane which promotes smooth movement of the eye in its socket. The space between the intra-orbital structures contains fatty tissue which serves as a cushion for the eyeball.

The accessory structures include the eyelids, lacrimal system and extrinsic ocular muscles.

EYELIDS (PALPEBRAE)

The upper and lower eyelids are curtain-like structures lying in front of the eyeball. They serve as protective coverings by shutting out intense light, dust and foreign bodies. The space between them is referred to as the palpebral fissure; the angles or corners where the lids meet are known as the inner (medial) and outer (lateral) canthi. Each eyelid has an outer layer of skin, a layer of firm fibrous tissue (tarsal plate), sebaceous-like glands (meibomian glands) which secrete an oily substance on to the free margins of the lids, and a mucous membrane lining called the conjunctiva. The conjunctiva is reflected over the anterior portion of the eyeball forming the bulbar conjunctiva, and is continuous with the corneal epithelium. The secretion of

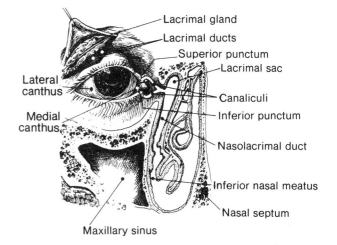

Figure 28.1 The lacrimal system.

the meibomian glands prevents adherence of the lids when the eyes are closed and also prevents the overflow of normal amounts of lacrimal secretion. The eyelashes emerge from the free borders of the eyelids to protect the eye from dust and perspiration.

LACRIMAL SYSTEM

The lacrimal apparatus protects the eye by continuously secreting a fluid that 'washes' over the anterior surface of the eyeball, keeping it moistened and cleansed. The system of each eye consists of a gland, ducts and a drainage system (Figure 28.1).

The lacrimal gland lies in a slight depression in the outer superior portion of the orbit. Several ducts carry the secretion of the gland onto the inner surface of the upper eyelid. The secreted fluid is distributed over the anterior surface of the eye and then drains through two small openings (puncta) in the medial canthus into two short canals (lacrimal canaliculi). The canals drain into a small sacular structure, the lacrimal sac, which narrows to form the nasolacrimal duct. The latter carries the secretion into the nasal cavity.

A volume of lacrimal secretion in excess of what the drainage system can handle results in fluid overflowing the eyelids and forming tears. Increased lacrimal secretion (lacrimation) occurs in response to irritation of the conjunctiva or to certain emotions. If there is excessive tear flow due to the blockage of the canaliculi or nasolacrimal duct, it may be referred to as *epiphora*.

EXTRINSIC OCULAR MUSCLES

Several external muscles have their origin in orbital structures and insert on the eyeball to provide movement of the eye within its socket. There are four straight muscles (*recti muscles*); each is named for the direction in which it moves the eye. The superior rectus turns the eye up, the inferior rectus turns it downward, the medial rectus turns it in, and the lateral moves it in the reverse direction. In addition to the recti muscles, two *oblique muscles* (a superior and an inferior) provide rotation and modification of straight movements. For most movements, more than one external ocular muscle generally operates; various combinations of recti and oblique muscle action are necessary (Figure 28.2).

The external ocular muscles include the levator palpebrae superioris muscle which inserts in the upper eyelid. It is responsible for raising the upper eyelid (opening the eye). The muscle responsible for closing the eye is the *orbicularis oculi*. This is a circular muscle situated in the eyelids.

EYEBALL

The eyeball is spherical with a slight anterior bulge. It is composed of three layers of tissue which enclose the iris and special transparent, refracting structures (Figure 28.3). The tough, outer coat forms the sclera and cornea. The *sclera*, which covers the posterior five-sixths of the eyeball, is white, opaque fibrous tissue. The *cornea* is a continuation of the sclera over the anterior portion of the eye. It consists of transparent, special connective tissue that is devoid of blood vessels. The corneoscleral junction is referred to as the *limbus*.

Underlying and attached to the sclera is a thin, heavily pigmented, vascular coat, the *choroid*, which extends forward to what is referred to as the ciliary body. The pigmentation prevents the reflection of the light rays.

The *ciliary body* consists mainly of muscle tissue which takes its origin at the corneoscleral junction and inserts in the suspensory ligaments that are attached to the lens, holding it suspended in position. The action of the ciliary muscle influences the curvature, and thus the refractive power, of the lens.

The second layer of the eyeball continues forward and inward beyond the ciliary muscle to form the iris. The *iris* is composed of circular and radial muscles and pigmented cells and is perforated centrally, creating the opening referred to as the *pupil*. Contraction of the circular muscle fibres (sphincter pupillae) constricts the pupil; dilatation is controlled by the radial fibres. The iris, ciliary body and choroid are known as the uvea or uveal tract.

The *retina* is the innermost and neural coat of the posterior two-thirds of the eyeball. It consists of several

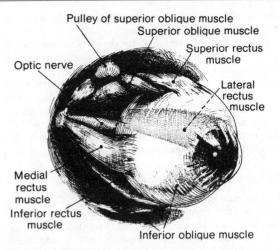

Figure 28.2 Extraocular muscles of the eye.

strata of cells through which light rays pass before reaching the outer layer of cells, which are light-sensitive receptors that convert luminous energy into nerve impulses. There are two types of receptor cells: the rods and cones. The rods have a lower response threshold, making them more sensitive to lower levels of illumination. The cones have a higher response threshold and, as a result, function in bright light and provide colour and detailed vision.

In the centre of the retina, a small area occurs in which the inner layers of cells are absent and only cones are concentrated. Light rays falling on this site strike the cones directly and produce the greatest visual acuity. This area is referred to as the *fovea centralis* and occurs as a slight depression in a small, elevated, yellowish area called the macula lutea, or yellow spot. Slightly medial to the macula there is a pale papillary area called the *optic disc*, or *fundus oculi*. It is at this point that the optic nerve and the central retinal vein and artery leave

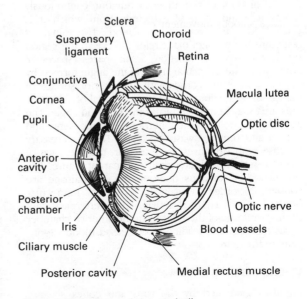

Figure 28.3 Parts of the eyeball.

and enter the eyeball. The disc is a blind spot, since the area is devoid of rods and cones.

The eyeball is 'filled out' by contents composed of fluids (aqueous humour), a biconvex disc (lens) and a jelly-like mass (vitreous humour).

The *lens* is elastic and crystal clear and is suspended just behind the iris by ligaments (suspensory ligaments or zonules) which attach to the ciliary body. Its shape varies with age; it is spherical' in infancy, gradually flattening to a disc shape with age. In the elderly, the lens tend to flatten and become less elastic.

Divisions of the interior of the eyeball

The interior of the eyeball is divided into the anterior and posterior cavities. The *anterior cavity* is the space between the cornea and lens and is subdivided into the *anterior and posterior chambers*, which are areas frequently referred to in clinical work. The anterior chamber lies posterior to the cornea and in front of the iris. The posterior chamber is situated posterior to the iris and anterior to the lens. The content of the two chambers is *aqueous humour*.

The posterior cavity lies posterior to the lens and is the remainder of the interior of the eyeball. It is filled with the *vitreous humour*, or *vitreous body*.

Fluid system of the eye and intraocular pressure

The interior of the eyeball is filled by the aqueous and vitreous humours and the crystalline lens. The vitreous humour is a clear, jelly-like mass enclosed in a hyaloid membrane. The vitreous humour fills out the larger and posterior portion of the eyeball that lies behind the lens.

The anterior and posterior chambers are filled with a clear fluid, the aqueous humour. There is a continuous flow into and out of the eye. The fluid originates from capillaries contained in processes of the ciliary body. After circulating around the posterior chamber, it flows through the pupil into the anterior chamber. From here, a small amount of the aqueous humour continuously drains into the canal of Schlemm, from which it is carried into the venous circulation. The canal of Schlemm is a channel that circles the eye in the region of the corneoscleral junction. Small spaces (spaces of Fontana) in the trabecular mesh at the angle formed by the junction of the cornea with the anterior surface of the iris allow the fluid to pass into the canal of Schlemm. This area may be referred to as the filtration angle. The aqueous humour carries nutrients to the lens and cornea and removes waste products. This is necessary because both structures are avascular; the presence of blood vessels would alter their transparent nature. The production of aqueous humour and its drainage are constant in order to maintain a normal intraocular pressure, which is 16–21 mmHg. Any interference with normal drainage of the fluid from the anterior chamber raises the pressure, leading to decreased blood supply, pain and impaired vision.

VISUAL IMPULSE PATHWAY

Impulses generated by the rods and cones synapse through several neurones to ganglionic cells whose

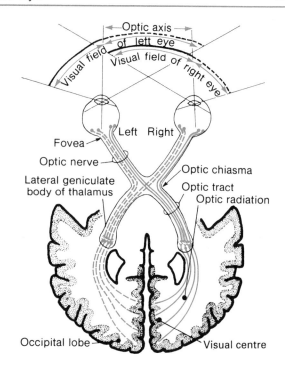

Figure 28.4 Left and right visual fields and the visual impulse pathway.

axons course toward the site of the optic disc where they unite to form the optic nerve. This nerve differs from most nerves in that it has no neurilemma; thus, it is even less capable of regeneration if damaged or destroyed. At the base of the brain, the nerve fibres from the medial half of the retina of each eye cross, going to the opposite sides of the brain. The fibres from the lateral halves of the retinae do not cross but continue on to the corresponding side of the brain. This arrangement forms the optic chiasma (Figure 28.4). Within the brain, the fibres from the lateral half of the right eye and those from the medial half of the left eye continue on as the right optic tract. The fibres of each tract synapse with the lateral geniculate in the thalamus on the corresponding side. From there, the impulses are transmitted along the postsynaptic fibres (optic radiations) to the visual centre in the occipital cerebral cortex of the same side, where they are interpreted as sensations of light, colour and form. Other cerebral areas are necessary for normal vision; correlation with information stored as memory in association areas has to occur in order to give meaning to what is seen. For example, a written word or an object may be seen but, unless the person has heard or experienced its meaning, he or she is unable to interpret it.

VISUAL FIELDS

The retinae of both eyes receive light rays at the same time from an object within the field of vision (binocular vision). Light rays from an object in the left outer visual field are received on the medial, or nasal, side of the left retina and on the lateral, or temporal, side of the right retina. The ensuing impulses are carried over fibres of the left and right optic nerves but, with the crossing of fibres in the chiasma, the impulses will travel along the right optic tract to the visual centre in the right occipital lobe for interpretation. Conversely, rays from objects in the outer right visual field will fall on the lateral area of the left retina and nasal area of the right retina, with the resulting impulses ending up in the visual centre of the left occipital lobe. There is some overlapping between the two halves of each retina and, as a result, the central half of each is represented in each hemisphere.

If the optic nerve of one eye is destroyed, blindness occurs in that eye, but destruction of fibres of the optic tract (i.e. beyond the optic chiasma) causes blindness to occur in half of each retina, limiting the field of vision. The term for this blindness is *hemianopia*.

EYE REFLEXES

The eye reflexes are used frequently in assessing the patient's condition. Some fibres of each optic tract terminate in a group of neurones referred to as the superior colliculus (superior colliculus quadrigeminae) in the midbrain. From here, efferent impulses originate, resulting in blinking of the eyelids, movement of the head, or dilatation or constriction of the pupil.

The conjunctival and corneal reflex of blinking is a protective response elicited by touching the conjunctival surface.

The pupils are normally round and of equal size. They adjust to light by constricting, and to darkness or dim light by dilating. A second reflex that may be noted is the accommodation reflex. The pupils are observed while the person shifts the gaze from a distant to a near

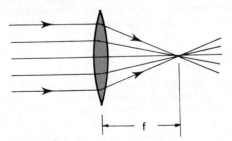

(a) A double convex lens focuses light

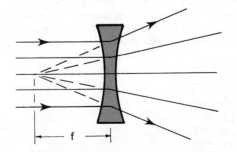

(b) A double concave lens causes light to diverge

Figure 28.5 Diagram showing refraction: (a) refraction of light rays by a double convex lens (convergence); (b) refraction of light rays by a double concave lens (divergence). f, Focal length of lens.

object. The normal response is constriction of the pupils. In some pathological conditions (e.g. syphilis), the response of the pupil to light may be absent while the accommodation reflex is present. This type of response is referred to as an Argyll Robertson pupil.

REFRACTION, ACCOMMODATION, PUPILLARY MODIFICATION AND CONVERGENCE

Several processes may be necessary to focus the light rays on the retina in order to form a clear image.

Refraction

When light rays pass obliquely from one medium to another of a different density their velocity is altered, and they are bent or deflected. The process is referred to as refraction (Figure 28.5). If the rays pass into a medium of greater density, they are deflected toward the perpendicular; conversely, in a medium of lesser density the rays are bent away from the perpendicular. Parallel rays striking a surface at right angles are not refracted. Parallel light rays striking the centre of the cornea and lens pass through unrefracted. At either side of the centre of the convex surfaces of the cornea and lens, light rays enter at an angle to the surface and are refracted toward the perpendicular. The greater the curvature or convexity of the surface, the greater is the degree of refraction.

The cornea and lens are the principal refractive media in the eye; the lens is particularly significant in that its curvature and degree of refraction can be varied by the ciliary body, according to the amount required to focus the light rays on the retina. The aqueous and vitreous humours also contribute to refraction but the degree, as with the cornea, remains the same. Without strain or modification, the normal eye will refract light rays from an object 6 or more metres away sufficiently to focus them on the retina. For objects that are near, refraction must be increased, and for distant objects, the eye must decrease its refraction. When greater refraction is necessary, the ciliary muscles contract and the suspensory ligaments, which are attached to the lens and the ciliary body, move forward, reducing their pull on the lens. As a result, the lens increases its convexity and thickness and, thus, its refractive power. When light rays reflected by distant objects enter the eye, the ciliary muscles relax, and the suspensory ligaments exert greater tension on the lens. This reduces convexity, thickness and refractive power of the lens, and focus of the light rays on the retina is achieved.

Various errors of refraction occur which interfere with the ability of the eye to focus light rays on the retina, resulting in impaired vision.

Emmetropia implies normal refraction.

Shortsightedness, called *myopia*, is the result of light rays from an object at 6 metres or more being focused at a point in front of the retina. Close objects can be seen, but distant objects are blurred. Correction may be made by use of a concave lens, since a concave lens produces divergence of light rays (Figure 28.6).

Long-sightedness (*hypermetropia*) is due to insufficient refraction and, as a result, light rays from an

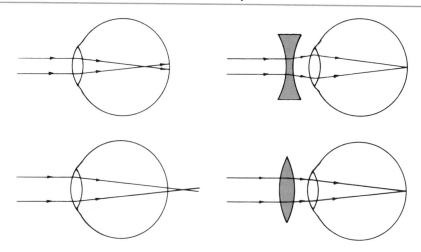

The use of lenses to correct common eye defects.

Figure 28.6 Diagram to show the use of lenses to correct common eye defects: (top) myopia and correction by concave lens; (bottom) hypermetropia and correction by convex lens.

object at 6 metres or less are focused at a point behind the retina. The person sees distant objects more clearly than close ones. Correction may be made by use of a convex lens, since a convex lens focuses light rays by convergence (Figure 28.6). In the later years of life, as part of the ageing process, the lens loses its elasticity and becomes thinner and flatter. This lessens the normal degree of refraction and the person becomes farsighted, a refractive error referred to as *presbyopia*.

In some persons, the horizontal and vertical curvatures of the cornea are uneven, producing differences in the degree of refraction. This results in different focal points; some light rays may be focused on the retina, but others may fall short or be carried to a point beyond the retina. This type of refractive error is known as *astigmatism*.

Accommodation

This is the process by which the degree of refraction by the lens is changed in order to focus rays from objects at various distances. This is made possible by the elastic nature of the lens and the action of the ciliary muscles on the suspensory ligaments, as explained under refraction (Figure 28.7).

Pupillary modification

The pupillary aperture is varied to control the amount of light entering the eye. For clear vision of near objects, the iris constricts the pupil of each eye to prevent divergent rays from entering. The opening is also reduced to restrict the entrance of excessively bright light, which may harm the retina. The iris constricts the pupil through parasympathetic innervation; sympathetic nervous stimulation produces dilatation of the pupil. In dim light and when focusing on a distant, wider visual field, the iris dilates the pupil to admit more light rays.

Convergence

Although light rays from the same object(s) fall on both retinae, only single vision is experienced. This is due to light rays from the object falling on corresponding points of the two retinae. This is brought about by convergence, which involves the extrinsic muscles (recti and oblique). The movements of the two eyes must be coordinated accurately. As an object is brought closer to the eyes, convergence of their axes occurs as they turn inward. For distant objects convergence is not necessary; the eyes remain parallel. *Strabismus* (squint) is a defect

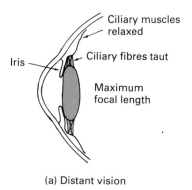

Iris

Ciliary muscles relaxed

Ciliary fibres taut

Maximum focal length

(a) Distant vision

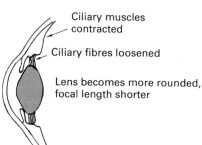

Ciliary muscles contracted

Ciliary fibres loosened

Lens becomes more rounded, focal length shorter

(b) Close vision

Figure 28.7 Diagram showing the ciliary body, suspensory ligaments and lens and the changes in accommodation: (a) distant vision and (b) close vision.

which interferes with co-ordination of the eye movements, and the light rays do not fall on corresponding points of the two retinae. It is usually due to an abnormal extrinsic muscle, or to an undiagnosed refractive error. Two images result and the person 'sees double'; this is termed *diplopia*.

LIGHT AND DARK ADAPTATION

Light adaptation. When exposed to intense light, adaptation takes place by constriction of the pupils and lowering the eyebrows, eyelids and head; the visual purple (rhodopsin) within the rods is bleached which reduces their sensitivity and responses.

Dark adaptation. When a person goes from a light to a dark area there is a period when nothing is seen, followed by the outlines of objects gradually becoming visible. This vision in dim light is due to an increased sensitivity of the rods as they produce a chemical pigment, visual purple or rhodopsin. Vitamin A is essential for the formation of the chemical; if it is deficient, the person experiences night blindness. At the same time that the rods increase their sensitivity, the pupils dilate to admit more light.

THE PERSON WITH HEALTH PROBLEMS RELATED TO VISION

ASSESSMENT

It is necessary, in most instances, that a thorough assessment is carried out before a diagnosis is made and, if appropriate, treatment prescribed. (*Immediate* action would be required if the patient's eye is damaged by accidental instillation of chemicals.) This includes a history of the patient's ocular disorder, general health, life-style, and an examination of the eyes. The latter involves inspection, palpation and the use of special equipment. The eye examination may require complex electrophysiological studies which are done by specialists in the field of ophthalmology.

HEALTH HISTORY

1. *Age.* The age of the person in relation to developmental changes and effects of ageing on the eyes is important.
2. *Occupation and life-style.* Information is obtained as to the demands for visual acuity, potential for eye injury and the use of protective devices. What are the patient's recreational activities? Is there participation in sports that have a potential for head or eye injury or exposure to bright sunlight? Are sunglasses worn?
3. *Family history.* Since many eye disorders are inherited, it is significant to learn of any family history of eye disorders, diabetes mellitus, cardiovascular disease and thyroid disease.
4. *Past health.* Any childhood and adult illnesses,

injuries and previous eye problems should be noted and the treatment and responses elicited. Ocular changes may be secondary to a disorder such as hypertension, diabetes mellitus, renal disease, hyperthyroidism and brain injury or tumour. Degenerative disease in the elderly is frequently the cause of their loss of vision.

It is determined whether corrective lenses are used, in what form and when the last eye examination was carried out.

CURRENT SYMPTOMS

What prompted the patient to seek health care? The following is a list of common symptoms:

● Changes in visual acuity
● Blurring of vision
● Halos
● Flashes of light
● Spots before the eyes (floaters)
● Excessive lacrimation or epiphora
● Double vision (diplopia)
● Light sensitivity (photophobia)
● Night blindness
● Recurring headache
● Discomfort, burning sensation or itching of the eyes.

What events led to or just preceded the symptom(s)? When did the symptoms begin and are there measures that provide relief?

EXAMINATION OF THE EYES

Macroscopic examination
Tests for ocular motility and measurement of visual acuity are usually performed before the examination of internal structures of the eye or tests which involve the touching of normally sensitive eye structures.

Initial observations of the eyes include noting: general appearance; symmetry of visual axes and physical features; any discharge and its characteristics; excessive or deficient lacrimal secretion; swelling or discoloration of extraocular structures or surrounding tissues; and the presence of a foreign body. The size and equality of the pupils are recorded. The medial canthi are examined for swelling and redness and *gently* palpated for tenderness.

The eyelids, lashes and brows are inspected for: redness or any discoloration; crusting; eversion or inversion of the lids; complete and equal opening and closing of the lids; swollen areas or oedema. The areas are very gently palpated for tenderness and nodules. The inner surface of the lower eyelid is examined by placing the index finger on the cheek and gently pulling down. The interior surface of the upper eyelid is examined by everting the lid over a cotton-tipped applicator; the lid is pulled gently downward by the eyelashes and then flipped upward over the applicator which is held against the outer surface of the lid, thus turning the eyelid 'inside out'. The colour of the conjunctiva of the lids is noted, as are any swollen or raised areas.

Assessment of extraocular muscle function
The patient sits facing the examiner, holding the head in a fixed position. The neuromuscular balance or straightness of the eyes is assessed by shining a light directly on the patient's eyes. The patient is asked to look at the light which should be reflected in corresponding positions in the pupillary corneas. If there is deviation of one eye, asymmetrical reflection occurs.

Movements of the eyes by the extraocular muscles are examined by having the patient in the position cited above; the examiner moves a light through several different positions while observing the eye movements. The patient is asked to look at the light and the movements of both eyes should be co-ordinated and symmetrical. Abnormal response may indicate paralysis of one or more extraocular muscles, muscular imbalance or injury.

Assessment of eye reflexes
Pupillary reflexes are observed in a dimly lit room by shining a light from the side on to the pupil of one eye at a time. Both pupils are observed; the normal response is constriction of both pupils when the light is shone in one. This is referred to as consensual pupil reaction.

The accommodation reflex is elicited by having the patient focus on a light held about 150 cm (20 in) from the nose. As the light is moved toward the patient, the eyes normally converge and the pupils constrict.

Measurement of visual acuity
Visual acuity implies the ability to distinguish details of objects and is measured as a means of evaluating ocular function. Each eye is tested separately; the eye not being examined is completely covered, but without any pressure being applied directly to the eye. A standard wall chart (Snellen chart) with rows of letters of gradually decreasing size is used and placed 6 metres from the patient and is well lit. The person is required to read the chart through to the line of smallest letters that can be seen. The distance from which the normal eye can read each line is known. The top line of the Snellen chart is perceived by the normal eye at 60 metres, the second line at 36 metres, the third at 24 metres, the fourth at 18 metres, the fifth at 12 metres, the sixth at 9 metres, the seventh at 6 metres, and the eighth line at 4 metres. Visual acuity is expressed as a fraction; the numerator represents the distance between the chart and the patient, and the denominator is the distance from which a person with normal vision could read the same line. Visual acuity recorded as 6/6 means normal vision. If the patient 6 metres from the chart can only read the line that the normal eye could read at 12 metres, the visual acuity is expressed at 6/12. The larger the denominator recorded, the poorer is the vision. In a person with severe impairment who can only see a hand moving in front of the face, the visual acuity may be recorded as HM (hand movements). If the person can only distinguish between light and dark, the recording is PL (perception of light) and if there is no light perception it is expressed as NPL (no perception of light). A recording of 3/60 or less in the better eye when wearing glasses or contact lenses indicates that the person is legally blind.

Near vision is assessed by also having the individual hold a card about 32 cm (13 in) from the eyes. The print on the card is sized proportionately to the 6 metres.

Refraction
The testing of the eyes' ability to focus the light rays on the retina is done by using a series of trial lenses as well as by assessing the person's visual acuity. In doing a refraction test in young children the doctor may require the instillation of a cycloplegic drug, such as atropine 0.5–2.0% which temporarily inhibits ciliary muscle action and dilates the pupil.

Visual field measurement (perimetry)
A special semicircular instrument, called a perimeter, which is marked in degrees, is used to determine if the patient's visual fields are normal or restricted. Defects in the visual fields are frequently associated with intracranial lesions or damage to an optic nerve.

Each eye is tested singly. Normal figures for perimetry evaluation are:

Lateral or temporal vision—90°
Looking up—50°
Looking down—70°
Medial—60°

Estimation of the visual field may also be made by the confrontation test. The patient faces the examiner (approximately 60–90 cm away) and has one eye covered. The examiner covers the opposite eye and holds an object which is moved slowly from beyond the patient's peripheral vision towards the central line of vision. The patient is asked to indicate when the object first comes into view and this is compared with when it was first seen by the examiner. The difference is recorded, taking for granted the examiner's vision is normal. The test is made using lateral, upper and lower fields.

Measurement of intraocular pressure
The detection of increased intraocular pressure is important; an excessive pressure may be very painful and progressively causes permanent damage within the eye, leading to loss of vision. The pressure is measured by an instrument called a tonometer. A few drops of a local anaesthetic (e.g. amethacaine 0.5–1%; oxybuprocaine 0.3%) are instilled in each eye. The tonometer is then placed on the corneal surface, causing indentation; the extent of the indentation reflects the intraocular pressure. If the pressure is high, the cornea resists indentation. The calibrated scale of the tonometer records the pressure in millimetres of mercury (mmHg). The normal intraocular pressure is approximately 16–21 mmHg.

A second instrument that is now generally employed to measure the ocular tension is the applanometer. This is an electronic device which is considered to provide a more accurate measurement of the intraocular pressure.

The patient with elevated intraocular pressure is at risk of serious impairment of vision due to ischaemic neuropathy.

Slit-lamp microscopy (biomicroscopy)

A more detailed examination of the internal structures of the eye can be made by the use of slit-lamp microscope. This instrument provides much clearer viewing and magnification of the tissues within the eye than obtained with the ophthalmoscope because of its intense light along with the increased magnification. It is helpful in locating foreign bodies in the eye and identifying ulcer erosion as well as degenerative and inflammatory conditions.

Fluorescein staining

A fluorescein strip, which is a sterile strip of paper that has been impregnated with a solution of sodium flurorescein, is moistened at one end and lightly applied to the lower conjunctival sac. A single-drop, disposable dispenser may be used as an alternative. The dye flows over the eye and abrasions and corneal ulcers readily stain a yellowish-green.

Following the examination, the eye is irrigated with a sterile saline solution to remove the dye.

Ophthalmoscopic examination

With an ophthalmoscope, the posterior, internal surface (fundus) of each eye is magnified and observed. The lens, vitreous body, blood vessels, retina, optic nerve and disc are viewed. In order to get a wider view, the pupil is dilated by the instillation of a mydriatic such as cyclopentolate hydrochloride (Mydrilate) 0.5–1% or tropicamide 0.5–1%. Ophthalmoscopy is valuable in the recognition of some systemic disorders, as well as in the assessment of ocular function. The optic blood vessels and disc may reflect a disorder such as hypertension, renal disease and increased intracranial pressure.

Fluorescein angiography

This test is done to assess vascular structures and blood circulation within the eye and the condition of the retina. Photographs are taken of the intraocular area and then a small dose (5 ml) of sodium fluorescein 10% is given intravenously and a series of photographs are taken at timed intervals.

The patient may experience a brief period of nausea and should be advised that the sclerae and possibly facial tissues will likely be a yellowish-green colour for a few hours as a result of the injection of the dye. The dye is eliminated in the urine which will be deeply coloured for approximately 24 hours.

Ultrasonography (echo-ophthalmography)

Ultrasound waves of very high frequency are directed into the eye and the echoes vary with the density of the tissues from which the sound waves are reflected. This test may be used to examine the fundus when the medium which transmits light rays becomes opaque (as in cataract), to detect retinal detachment or a tumour or to locate a foreign body.

Assessment of the retina

An electroretinogram may be done to record the extent of the electrical response made by the retina to light stimulation.

Gonioscopy

This involves the examination of the angle of the anterior chamber by means of an optical instrument (gonioscope).

CLINICAL CHARACTERISTICS

IMPAIRMENT OF VISION

The development of significant signs and symptoms of impaired visual function varies greatly. The onset of changes may be insidious in some cases, but in others, the onset may occur suddenly and be acute. One or both eyes may be involved. The manifestations may be principally subjective or may be objective only, with the abnormal structure or function being noted by an observer. In some instances manifestations may be recognized without tests or the aid of instruments.

The signs and symptoms of eye disorders include the following characteristics.

Subjective manifestations

1. Difficulty in reading and seeing objects clearly, blurred vision or headaches when reading or doing close work. These symptoms may be caused by simple refractive errors or by cataract, glaucoma, inflammation of the cornea (keratitis) and ulceration leading to scarring and opacity, degenerative changes, detachment of the retina or a systemic disease such as hypertension, diabetes mellitus and arteriosclerosis.
2. Photophobia (sensitivity to light) may be associated with inflammation of the conjunctiva, cornea or iris.
3. Excessive tear flow may indicate trauma, chemical irritation, allergy, inflammation of ocular tissue or obstruction of the tear duct.
4. Dryness of the conjunctival surface due to decreased lacrimal secretion which may be due to severe dehydration or cerebral trauma or disease (e.g. rheumatoid arthritis). It is frequently a problem in an abnormally dry environment and in the elderly. Some drugs may suppress lacrimal secretion.
5. Ocular pain may be due to irritation from a foreign body, infection, inflammation of eye tissues or accessory structures, or increased intraocular pressure (glaucoma).
6. Diplopia (double vision) is most frequently experienced by patients with a head injury or cerebral disorder (e.g. brain tumour) that incurs a paralysis or functional imbalance of the extraocular muscles.
7. Spots before or floaters in the eyes, single and occasional, are common and of no clinical significance. Frequent or sudden development of numerous spots or floaters may signify an intraocular haemorrhage or threatening of the retina. In the latter, the patient may experience flashing lights followed by a clouding across the eye.
8. Scotoma or blind spot develops as a result of damage to an area of the retina or optic nerve. It may be caused by an inflammatory disease process

within the eye or a degenerative disorder. If the scotoma occurs in the same area in each eye, the aetiology may be intracranial, affecting the fibres in the visual pathway.

9. Halos around lights are usually associated with increased intraocular pressure and glaucoma.

10. Extensive loss of visual acuity of 3/60 or less in the better eye with correction, or a restriction of the visual field to 20° or less indicates blindness according to the legal definition.

Objective manifestations

1. The person is observed holding reading material or an object nearer than 30 cm (12 in) to the face or beyond the distance of approximately 40 cm (16–18 in).

2. A strained expression or scowl may be noted when an effort to see is being made.

3. The younger person may fail to develop at a normal rate, make normal progress at school or relate normally to peers.

4. Errors are made because of misread information or directions.

5. Deviation of one eye (the visual axis of one eye differs from that of the other eye) indicates impaired extraocular muscle structure of function. The latter may be due to a disorder involving the oculomotor (third cranial) nerve.

6. Discoloration of the eyelid or surrounding tissue. Redness of the eyelids suggests infection, allergy or injury. Redness of the exposed area of the eye may be caused by conjunctival irritation by a foreign body, infection, or trauma or may be incurred by a subconjunctival haemorrhage associated with trauma, hypertension or inflammatory disease of intraocular structures.

   Yellow sclerae occur when the patient has an excessive concentration of bile pigment in the blood (jaundice) which may be due to liver or gallbladder disease or a blood dyscrasia, but many are idiopathic and resolve spontaneously.

   Discoloration of surrounding tissue may be the result of extravasation of blood related to an eye or facial injury.

7. Discharge (serous or purulent) or crusting may indicate infection, chemical irritation, allergy or trauma of the eyelid or eye.

8. Swelling or oedema may develop with local trauma, infection or cyst, or may be associated with renal or cardiac failure, a cerebral disorder or head injury.

9. Abnormal pupillary shape or reaction. Constriction, asymmetry, or failure of normal reaction to light is most often due to some cerebral disorder or iris collapse. A greyish white colour of the pupil suggests an opacity of the lens (cataract).

10. Exophthalmos or proptosis (prominence or bulging of the eyes) is usually caused by hyperthyroidism or brain tumour.

11. Ptosis or a lag in the closing of eyelid may indicate some oculomotor (third cranial) nerve involvement. The drooping of both eyelids is also characteristic of myasthenia gravis.

The Person with Visual Impairment

Humans are very dependent upon their sense of vision, since most of our knowledge of the environment is obtained through our eyes. The eyes are also used in expressing emotions. Any impairment or loss of vision is a serious threat. In many instances the ability to freely move about safely and the privilege of enjoying colour, form, depth, beauty and distance are lost. Loss of vision results in reduced sensory input and stimulation; this may lead to boredom and reduced responsiveness and disorientation to time and place on the part of the person unless stimuli by other channels (e.g. hearing and touch) are increased and the person's interest maintained.

The nurse should appreciate the incalculable value of sight and the natural anxiety and concern of the patient when it is threatened. Reduced vision affects the patient's whole way of life socially, physically, economically and emotionally. Effective nursing care can only be planned if the nurse has an understanding of the causes of visual impairment as this will allow the identification of appropriate goals for the individual.

CAUSE

Visual impairment may be due to a primary eye disorder or may be secondary to a neurological or systemic disorder. The causes include:

- Structural or functional defect in the eye or extraocular structures (e.g. malfunction of the extraocular muscles causing deviation of one or both eyes).
- Ageing (e.g. the lens becomes less spherical with age, may become opaque and the nucleus hardens).
- Infection.
- Trauma (chemical or mechanical).
- New growth.
- Impaired innervation of the eyes due to a neurological disorder (e.g. brain tumour or injury).
- Systemic disease (e.g. hypertension, diabetes mellitus, cardiovascular disease).
- Inadequate knowledge about the factors which contribute to the preservation of good vision (e.g. nutritonal requirements, protection of eyes in potentially hazardous situations).

Patient centred *goals* common to most patients with visual impairment are:

1. Vision will be preserved.
2. Factors contributing to visual impairment will be identified.
3. The patient will receive meaningful sensory input.
4. The patient will remain orientated.
5. Injury or complications will not occur.
6. If visual impairment is permanent, the patient will learn to be as self-caring as possible, retaining maximum independence.

Once the goals have been identified, appropriate nursing intervention can be planned and implemented. Goals relevant to other individual problems must also be identified in addition to the above common core of patient goals.

PRESERVATION OF VISION

The maintenance of vision and prevention of loss of sight includes consideration of the following:

Good general health
There is a tendency to consider vision as being independent of general health. It remains good in some serious bodily disorders, while others may have a serious effect on visual acuity. Occasionally, general body disease is discovered because of changes in the eyes and vision (e.g. hypertension, diabetes, brain tumour).

Optimum diet
A well-balanced diet contributes to good eye health as well as to good general health. Vitamins A, B complex and C are considered important; a deficiency of vitamin A may cause drying and changes of the cornea and conjunctiva and a decreased production of the retinal pigment, rhodopsin, leading to night blindness. A deficiency in the vitamin B complex may predispose to retinal changes. Vitamin C plays a role in resistance to infection.

Protection of infants' and children's eyes
Babies' eyes should be observed regularly after birth so that signs of infection (e.g. gonorrhoea) may be detected early. Failure to treat an infection could lead to corneal scarring and blindness. Congenital cataracts and blindness occur most often in infants whose mothers have a history of a viral infection, especially rubella, during the first trimester. Immunization for German measles is encouraged for women of child-bearing age. The nurse has an important role in preventing blindness in premature and underweight newborn infants by maintaining the prescribed level of oxygen. Administration of high concentrations of oxygen to these infants causes retrolental fibroplasia.

A child's eyes are not fully developed until at least 7 years of age. Toys and play-things should be selected to avoid broken, sharp and pointed parts that predispose to injury. Children are taught to keep dirty fingers and other objects away from their eyes and are also instructed in the necessary precautions when old enough to play with such things as fireworks.

It is sensible to ensure that for adults, when working, the light is adequate and that intensive detailed work is broken up by frequent rest periods. Close work should be avoided when fatigued.

Regular periodical eye examination
Some eye diseases and changes develop insidiously without markedly reducing vision or causing pain until they are well advanced. Regular eye examination may reveal early signs, and a serious disease may be checked before it progresses to loss of vision and blindness. If glasses are necessary, only those which have been properly prescribed should be used. Lenses are individually ground for each eye according to the testing

and examination findings (see Table 28.1 for a list of terms which relate to eye examinations and errors of refraction).

If glasses are worn, the importance of protecting the lens from scratches and maintaining good alignment is stressed. If glasses are not straight or if the distance between the eyes and lenses is not equal, the degree of refraction is altered. Lenses in spectacles are safer if made of impact-resistant material.

The correct care and application of contact lenses are extremely important in preventing eye disorders (e.g. infection and ulceration) and reduced vision. When the person receives prescribed fitted lenses, detailed instruction about the handling, wearing and cleaning of them is extremely important. The patient should be able to describe and demonstrate the necessary techniques and precautions to ensure correct and safe use.

Prevention of trauma
The loss of vision due to exposure to chemicals, dust, wind, glaring light or direct sun rays and eye injury by mechanical objects (e.g. flying pieces of metal or wood) is preventable in most instances by the use of standard safety measures and devices. The use of legislated safety helmets, shatter-proof goggles or shields in potentially hazardous situations should be observed. Sunglasses may be necessary to protect the eyes from bright sun rays. The use of adequate protective equipment as well as observance of established safety rules in sports where there is a potential for injury should be promoted.

Rubbing of the eyes should be avoided because of the possibility of trauma and the introduction of infection, especially if wearing contact lenses. Cautious use of sprays and caustic solutions and the wearing of protective goggles when exposed to caustic substances should be emphasized.

Prompt treatment
No 'eyedrops' or ointment should be instilled in the eyes unless prescribed by a doctor. In the event of a persisting foreign body which cannot be gently washed or wiped away, inflammation or any other disturbance in an eye, early treatment by a doctor or ophthalmologist should be secured.

If a chemical spray or irritating solution accidentally gets into the eye, immediate and extended irrigation with water or saline is recommended and prompt medical treatment sought to avoid potential ulceration and blindness.

PRINCIPLES TO BE OBSERVED IN GIVING EYE CARE PROCEDURES

1. The patient receives a full explanation of the procedure and is advised that it is important that the head is held steady.
2. Hands are washed thoroughly before and after doing any eye procedure.
3. Precautions are used to protect the unaffected eye from possible injury and cross-infection from one eye to another. Irrigation solution or eye drops being used in the affected eye must not be

Table 28.1 Terminology and abbreviations.

Term	Meaning
RE	Right eye
LE	Left eye
BE	Both eyes
Emmetropia	Normal vision (normal refraction)
Myopia (M)	Short-sightedness
Hypermetropia (hyperopia; H)	Long-sightedness
Presbyopia	Reduced accommodation associated with the ageing process
Astigmatism	Uneven curvature of the cornea; results in different focal points
Diplopia	Perception of two images of a single object (double vision)
Hemianopia	Loss of vision in one half of the visual field
Entropion	Turning in of the eyelid
Ectropion	Turning out of the eyelid
Ptosis	Drooping of the upper eyelid
Aphakia	Absence of the lens of an eye
Hyphaema	Haemorrhage into the anterior chamber of the eye
Hypopyon	White blood cells in the anterior chamber
Photophobia	Hypersensitivity to light
Ophthalmologist (oculist)	A doctor who specializes in the treatment of eye disorders
Optometrist	A person who examines the eyes to assess vision and prescribes corrective spectacles or lenses
Optician	A specialist who prepares spectacles or lenses according to prescription
Mydriasis	Dilatation of the pupil
Mydriatic	Drug that dilates the pupil
Miosis	Contraction of the pupil of the eye
Miotic	Drug that contracts the pupil
Proptosis (exophthalmos)	Bulging forward of the eyes
Epiphora	Excessive lacrimal secretion (tears)

permitted to enter the unaffected eye. Similarly, dressings from the affected eye should not touch the unaffected eye. Dressings and swabs are used only once.

4. Pressure on the eyeball is avoided.
5. When irrigating the eye, the solution is directed on to the nasal side of the eyeball. The eye is gently wiped from the inner canthus to the outer canthus.
6. Solutions and drugs should always be fresh; they are dated as to preparation and expiry.
7. Frequent, regular assessment of the eye and the patient's vision is made. The eye is examined before and after each procedure; alteration in comfort, change in colour, discharge, dryness, oedema or swelling is brought to the attention of the doctor.
8. If both eyes are involved, separate sterile equipment and solutions are used for each eye. In the case of infection, the eye manifesting less inflammation and discharge is treated before the other eye. These precautions are aimed at reducing the risk of cross-infection.
9. A separate sterile eye dropper is used for each drug used in the eye.
10. If the eyelid does not close, precautions are necessary when handling articles such as bed-linen, towels and clothing to avoid abrasions and injury of the conjunctiva and cornea. An exposed (open) eye may become dry and susceptible to ulceration; the

instillation of artificial tears may be prescribed as a prophylactic measure, as may ointment applied to the exposed conjunctiva.

11. It is important that the patient is warned of any effect the eye drops may have; for example cycloplegic agents will paralyse the muscles of accommodation, and cause blurring of vision.
12. Eye dressings are normally applied to protect, to absorb lacrimal secretions or exudate or to apply pressure. The skin around the eye should always be supported gently when the dressing is removed.
13. Drops are instilled at the *lateral* aspect of the inner lower lid, with the patient looking up, so that direct corneal contact is avoided and reflex squeezing of the eye prevented.
14. In order to keep the affected eye at rest, the unaffected eye may be covered. Adaptation to light is resumed gradually; the unaffected eye may first be exposed by wearing a shield with a small central opening. This minimizes eye movement. A similar shield may also be used later on the affected eye; however, it is more usual for the patient to wear dark glasses. Extreme gentleness is used when changing a dressing or doing any treatment; caution is used to avoid pressure on the eyeball.
15. Great care should be taken to prevent the eye opening under the dressing as this can cause corneal abrasion. The dressing should be secured firmly.

Care of the Visually Handicapped Patient

MAINTENANCE OF ORIENTATION AND REDUCTION OF ANXIETY

Impairment and threatened loss of vision arouse considerable fear, insecurity and emotional reactions. All the implications which impaired vision may have in the present and future 'crowd in' on the patient. Fears and worry may be greatly exaggerated, and the patient may become panicky and lose control. The patient's behavioural responses must be assessed frequently; with reduced or no vision, the patient (especially if elderly) may become disorientated, particularly if not in a familiar environment.

Individuals deprived of visual input become more dependent on other senses such as hearing and touch. The understanding of the nurse as to what the patient may be experiencing, the provision of emotional support and the use of communication techniques which promote the use of other senses contribute greatly to the care of this patient.

Factors which help to reduce the patient's anxiety include the following suggestions. The patient is carefully oriented to any new environment; if confined to bed, the orientation is by a verbal description. If allowed up, the verbal description is combined with helping the person explore the ward environment. An explanation is made of how the usual daily needs will be met.

The patient is given the opportunity and encouragement to express concerns and to ask questions. The person who cannot see is spoken to while being approached and is advised who is speaking. Any treatment or investigative procedure should be well described in advance. It means a great deal to the patient to always have the call-button within reach; it means that help is always at hand. The patient should not be left alone for long periods for although a lot of physical care may not be needed, support and contacts are still required. The nurse should take time to talk to the patient and, as required, indicate the time and describe the place and current situation and details of the environment. The patient may have visual memory from which it is possible to recall sufficiently to form a mental picture of what is being described. Some appropriate form of diversion, such as a radio and visitors to chat with or read to the patient, is encouraged to provide sensory input. Noisy, confusing situations are avoided; the visually handicapped patient is usually more sensitive to sounds and voice inflections. An effort is made to anticipate the patient's needs.

MAINTENANCE OF A SAFE ENVIRONMENT

Adequate orientation and frequent observations are important to prevent accidents when the patient's vision is seriously impaired. If the patient is disorientated, it may be necessary to have someone present to ensure the environment must be checked carefully for any hazards for the unseeing, ambulatory person. He or she should be escorted around the area until familiar with it and encouraged to move about alone. Stools, rugs or other such articles over which it is possible to trip should be removed. Furniture is not moved from its original position when possible, and doors are kept closed or wide open. The person is cautioned about nearby stairs and radiators. All members of the staff, medical, nursing, paramedical and ancillary, should be made aware of the individual's degree of visual handicap.

CONTINUOUS ASSESSMENT

Prompt recognition of change in the eye, visual acuity and orientation is very important, as failure to do so can lead to an increase in the amount of impairment. The nurse is required to be familiar with any specific observations that are important in certain eye disorders. Generally, significant factors that should be brought promptly to the doctor's attention include elevation of temperature, discharge, unrelieved pain, headache, any evidence of disturbance in the unaffected eye, and signs of bleeding, or infection/inflammation in the anterior segment.

POSITIONING AND ACTIVITY

The position which the patient with an acute eye disorder is to assume varies with different conditions and is usually indicated by the doctor. Prolonged restriction of activity is relatively rare; patients worry less and have fewer complications when allowed up as soon as possible. If the patient is required to remain in bed, lying flat with the head immobilized, the arms and lower limbs are moved through a range of motion, and active exercises of the legs are begun as soon as the doctor permits.

EATING AND DRINKING

The patient frequently experiences anorexia due to anxiety and because of the difficulty with taking food when vision is impaired. The necessary assistance is provided and, when feeding, the food is described; only small amounts are offered to avoid choking and coughing, since coughing raises the intraocular pressure. As soon as the patient is well enough, self-care and independence are major considerations; however, assistance is withdrawn gradually, not all at once.

The position of different foods on the plate may be described using the clock analogy. Aids such as plate guards and non-slide mats may also be useful.

Some visually handicapped patients are reluctant to socialize at meal times in case they cause embarrassment; the use of aids can help them overcome this. Drinks should be offered regularly and poured out if necessary; it is often difficult for the patient to do this, and they may just not drink. Aids are available to help with pouring drinks.

COMMUNICATION

Verbal communication should be clear and concise and may need frequent repetition. Touch and tone are very important, as they offer a form of non-verbal and verbal reinforcement of which the patient can be aware.

REHABILITATION OF THE BLIND

There are two official categories of visual handicap in the United Kingdom: (1) blindness, and (2) partial sight.

1. *Blindness*
   (a) 'So blind as to be unable to perform *any* work for which eyesight is essential'.
   (b) Visual acuity of below 3/60.
   (c) Visual acuity of 6/60 and below if there is considerable contraction of the visual field.
2. *Partial sight*. A visual acuity of 6/60 or less, the individual being substantially or permanently handicapped by defective vision. The category to which the person is assigned (according to the amount of visual impairment) dictates eligibility for help.

The patient with marked visual impairment or with total loss of vision needs a great deal of assistance in adjusting to the situation. The individual needs to realize that life still has meaning and potential. Emphasis is placed on what is possible given that the person still has visual memory of form, colour, and space and can learn that other senses can be put to greater use.

The development of independence is started as soon as possible, beginning with self-care (feeding, bathing, dressing and hair). Assistance is given with moving about the room and then from room to room, locating furniture and necessary articles by touch. The environment is organized to provide safety. Furniture is left in the same place unless the person is advised and oriented to its new position; rugs, foot-stools and other such hazardous objects are removed. Doors are kept wide open or closed.

Anyone walking with a blind person allows the individual to take an arm rather than grasping the person and pushing. Writing is practised, beginning with the person's signature. Differentiation by touch is also tested and practised. The person learns to tell the time by using a specially designed watch.

Various forms of diversion and recreation are introduced (records of books and music, radio games). The patient is referred to the Social Services and the Royal National Institute for the Blind, which provide vocational training, assistance in learning Braille and in finding a job, recreation, transportation, and financial assistance when necessary. The use of the white cane is introduced and the necessary guidance given on excursions beyond the house until the person is capable of safely getting around alone.

The patient and family are advised of the financial assistance available for the registered blind or registered partially sighted and are assisted in making application for it. The family may require help in accepting the blind patient and in organizing the home environment in the interest of safety and independence.

Common Eye Disorders

REFRACTIVE ERRORS

Various errors of refraction occur which interfere with the ability of the eye to focus light rays on the retina, normally resulting in impaired vision. (See p. 969 for a discussion of short-sightedness, long-sightedness, presbyopia and astigmatism.)

BLEPHARITIS

This is an inflammation of the eyelid; it is usually bilateral and affects the marginal area of the lids.

Characteristics

The patient may complain of itching or irritation. The margins of the lids are reddened and develop crusts or scales. It may be associated with seborrhoea (excessive sebaceous gland secretion) of the scalp and eyebrows.

Treatment

Therapeutic measures include gentle removal of the crusts once or twice daily with warm water, the application of the prescribed antibacterial ointment and if the cause is seborrhoea, a daily shampoo with an antiseborrhoeic shampoo is recommended.

CONJUNCTIVITIS

Inflammation of the conjunctiva may be caused by bacteria, viruses, chemicals or an allergic reaction and may be acute or chronic. Sources of eye infection include foreign bodies, dust, hands, infected neighbouring structures (nose, face, sinus) or contaminated equipment or solutions used in treatment. Viral infections are a very contagious form of conjunctivitis and prompt therapeutic measures are necessary to prevent its rapid spread to others. Infection may begin in the conjunctival lining of the eyelids and spread or remain confined to that area.

Characteristics

The inflammation is manifested by irritation, feeling of grittiness, pain, redness, encrustations and excessive lacrimation or serous or purulent discharge. The patient may complain of photophobia. When infection is present a culture may be made from a swab of the discharge for identification of the invading organism; this should be carried out before instilling an antimicrobial agent.

Treatment

Frequent gentle cleansing of the lid margins is necessary to prevent encrustations. Precautions must be observed to treat each eye separately so that infection is not transferred from one to the other. The patient is usually more comfortable in dim light or darkness and dark glasses ease the discomfort in the early stages. A specific antimicrobial ointment or solution may be prescribed for instillation. In an allergic reaction, an antihistamine preparation may be prescribed to relieve the irritation. The patient is advised to keep the hands away from the eyes and, if responsible for instilling medications, the patient must be cautioned to wash the hands thoroughly under running water before starting and after completing the medication procedure. The affected eye should be left uncovered.

If the conjunctivitis is due to allergy, efforts are made to identify the allergen so that it can be avoided if possible; it may be air-borne or transferred by the person's hands or by towels. A topical corticosteroid preparation may be prescribed to provide relief.

HORDEOLUM (STYE)

A hordeolum, or stye, is a small abscess that develops within a marginal sebaceous gland or hair follicle of an eyelash. A small, red, swollen tender area appears. Spontaneous drainage of pus may be hastened by a topical broad-spectrum antibiotic such as chloramphenicol, which should be instilled regularly. If necessary, the offending eyelash is removed.

CHALAZION

A chalazion is a cyst that forms in a meibomian (sebaceous) gland. It may remain as a small, firm, painless swelling in the lid for a long period. Eventually it may become infected and irritate the palpebral conjunctiva. Application of an antibiotic preparation is usually prescribed. Recurrence frequently necessitates a small incision for drainage and curettage.

GLAUCOMA

This disorder is characterized by an increase in the intraocular pressure above the normal, which causes damage to the optic disc and visual field loss. Normal pressure is generally maintained by a balance between the production of aqueous humour by the ciliary body and its drainage from the anterior chamber through the trabecular meshwork of the filtration angle into the canal of Schlemm. If an imbalance occurs between production and drainage, the pressure increases, compressing the retina and the blood vessels within the eye. Permanent optic nerve damage leading to blindness results unless there is early recognition and treatment of the disease.

Glaucoma is usually due to some interference with the outflow of aqueous humour from the anterior chamber into the canal of Schlemm. It may be classified as *primary*, *secondary*, or *congenital*. The primary acute form may be referred to as *acute angle-closure glaucoma*; the primary chronic type is called *open-angle* or simple chronic glaucoma.

Secondary glaucoma may be associated with infection, inflammation, trauma or a tumour within the eye.

OPEN-ANGLE (CHRONIC) GLAUCOMA

This chronic and more common type develops very gradually; the cause is not understood but the frequency of familial incidence points to hereditary aetiology that results in degenerative changes in the trabecular meshwork of the filtration angle. It is usually bilateral and has a high incidence in persons over the age of 35 or 40 years; this emphasizes the importance of regular eye examinations which include the measurement of intraocular pressure.

Characteristics

Because of the insidious onset of open-angle glaucoma, the central field of vision is not lost for some time. The disorder is frequently well advanced before the person seeks assistance. The visual field progressively diminishes, and the individual may become aware that something is wrong when discovering objects on either side that have been 'missed', or if halos are persistently seen around artificial lights. The condition may be discovered during a routine examination. As the condition progresses, the person may complain of some pain in the eye(s), especially in the morning on awakening. If chronic glaucoma is not recognized and treated in the early stage, the person eventually goes blind.

Treatment

In the early stages, treatment of open-angle glaucoma consists of instillation of a miotic 2–4 times a day which causes constriction of the pupil. Preparations are available now which have a more prolonged effect, requiring instillation only twice in 24 hours. An example of such a preparation is timolol maleate (Timoptol), a β-blocker which has the advantage of lowering the intraocular pressure, but does not constrict the pupil. Acetazolamide (a carbonic anhydrase inhibitor) is a diuretic which may be prescribed orally to lessen the formation of aqueous humour. Surgical treatment may become necessary. A trabeculectomy, creates an opening between the anterior chamber and subconjunctival space; aqueous fluid is absorbed into the conjunctival tissues. The procedure is used mostly for patients with advanced glaucoma which does not respond to previously cited methods of treatment.

Teaching the glaucoma patient

Because glaucoma accounts for such a large proportion of blindness, more effort has been directed toward informing the general public about the disease and the significance of early recognition.

Glaucoma cannot be cured, but blindness can be prevented by continuous use of a miotic as prescribed, by surgery and by medical supervision, if it is begun early in the disease.

An important nursing responsibility is to alert the patient to activities and situations that predispose to a rise in intraocular pressure. The condition is explained to the patient and family, and emphasis is placed upon the need for some precautions to prevent visual damage. Emotional and stressful situations are avoided as much as possible; the patient must learn to tolerate and live with what cannot be changed.

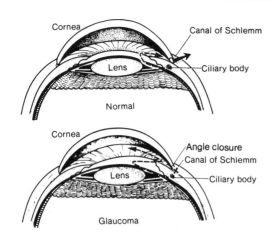

Figure 28.8 Diagram to show how a disturbance in the balance of fluid within the eyeball increases pressure in the eye and can result in glaucoma. ⟶, Normal direction of fluid movement; - - ➤, abnormal fluid movement in glaucoma.

The patient and family must appreciate the importance of regularly scheduled visits to the ophthalmologist for measurement of the intraocular pressure and visual field and acuity testing. They are taught the correct method of instilling the prescribed miotic, and cautioned against the use of any solution or medication that is not prescribed by the doctor. An identification card or Medic-Alert pendant indicating that the person suffers from glaucoma is recommended. Some job modification or change may be made by encouraging the patient to consult with the employer and occupational health department, but every effort should be made to continue employment. Patients with advanced glaucoma and loss of vision are referred to the Royal National Institute for the Blind or another appropriate agency.

ACUTE ANGLE-CLOSURE GLAUCOMA

This form of glaucoma is characterized by rapid marked increase in intraocular pressure as a result of a complete block in the outflow of the aqueous humour. The iris appears to have been pushed forward, narrowing the peripheral angle between it and the cornea (Figure 28.8), and, with dilatation of the pupil and the concomitant thickening of the iris, the openings in the filtration angle which led into the canal of Schlemm become occluded. The condition demands prompt emergency care because rapid compression of the retinal blood vessels develops, and destruction of the optic nerve cells and fibres occurs, with resultant loss of vision.

Characteristics

The patient with acute glaucoma experiences severe pain, nausea and vomiting, halos or rainbows around artificial lights and blurring of vision. On examination, the pupil is seen to be dilated and fixed, and there is evidence of congestion with a marked increase in

intraocular pressure. The cornea becomes oedematous losing its lustre and transparency.

Prompt treatment is necessary to prevent blindness. A miotic prepartion such as pilocarpine hydrochloride is instilled to constrict the pupil; this effects an increase in the peripheral angle by moving the iris away from the cornea. A drug such as acetazolamide (Diamox) may be administered orally or intravenously to reduce the formation of aqueous humour; or, an osmotic agent, such as intravenous urea or mannitol, or oral glycerol is given to reduce intraocular pressure. The latter can be unpalatable and sometimes an antiemetic is required.

A quiet environment is provided and the patient is helped to relax and is positioned with the head and shoulders elevated; analgesia is prescribed to relieve the pain.

If an immediate, satisfactory response to drug therapy does not occur, surgical intervention is undertaken. A small section of the iris is removed (iridectomy) to prevent it from being imposed on the drainage system. Newer techniques include the use of a laser beam to make a hole through the iris. *Laser irodotomy* may be done on an outpatient basis. Prophylactic surgery is always undertaken in the unaffected eye.

Postoperative management
An important nursing responsibility is the instillation of eye drops: a mydriatic and a corticosteroid are usually prescribed and the eye kept at rest. A topical antibiotic may also be prescribed. It is important that the cycloplegic effect of some mydriatics is explained to the patient *before* instillation, as they may cause a decrease in visual acuity which can be upsetting. Reassurance should be given that this alteration is temporary.

CATARACT

A cataract is a clouding of the crystalline lens, resulting in opacity. It may be classified as a *degenerative* or *developmental* (congenital or juvenile) cataract; the latter type of cataract occurs most often in infants whose mothers have a history of a viral infection (e.g. German measles) during the first trimester of pregnancy, or is associated with a genetic defect, which, for example, causes an inborn error of metabolism.

The degenerative cataract has a high incidence in persons over 50 years of age and may be referred to as a senile cataract. The cause is not known; metabolic changes in the lens substance are considered to be a major factor. It is also suggested that an inherited predisposition to develop the characteristic lens changes plays a role. Some deficiencies in nutrients, such as vitamins C and B, have also been suggested as possible aetiological factors. Degenerative cataract is frequently associated with diabetes mellitus. Opacity of the lens may also be secondary to eye trauma or to exposure to radiation or extreme heat. It may develop following uveitis or the prolonged use of the miotic echothiopate or a topical corticosteroid preparation.

Characteristics

The opacity develops very gradually, unless caused by

trauma and may be localized to the centre of the lens, incurring early impairment of vision, or it may start in the periphery. A cataract, even in its early stage, is readily recognized through the pupil, using an ophthalmoscope. As it matures, the examiner is not able to visualize the fundus or optic disc and the pupillary area appears grey or whitish because of the opaque lens behind it.

The loss of the normal refractive ability of the lens prevents light rays from being focused on the retina. Vision becomes blurred, objects may appear distorted and colour perception decreases. Visual loss is very gradual and is directly proportional to the degree of opacity of the lens. Cataract may be unilateral or bilateral; if bilateral the opacity does not usually develop at the same rate in both lenses.

Treatment

Cataract is irreversible but as loss of transparency of the lens develops, visual acuity and distant vision can usually be improved by increasing the correction of lens in the person's spectacles. Eventually, the opacity increases to the point that no light rays pass through the lens to reach the retina.

When the person's visual impairment becomes a handicap and interferes with usual life-style and activities, surgical treatment is undertaken. The operative procedure used may be classified as extracapsular or intracapsular cataract extraction.

In the *extracapsular extraction*, the anterior portion of the capsule and the lens content may be removed, or the procedure may involve phacoemulsification (a small incision is made in the anterior capsule and the lens content is aspirated). Phacoemulsification uses ultrasonic vibrations to fragment the lens content which prepares it for aspiration. The extracapsular extraction leaves the posterior part of the capsule intact and the vitreous body undisturbed. If the posterior capsule of the lens has lost its transparency, a small opening (a capsulotomy) may be made in it with a laser beam several weeks or months following the initial surgery.

In *intracapsular cataract extraction*, the lens is removed, complete with its capsule, usually by cryoextraction in which a probe-like instrument is introduced so that it lies against the lens and is cooled to $-30°C$ to $-35°C$. The lens and its capsule freeze to the probe, and are removed when the probe is withdrawn. To make the zonules (attaching fibres) more readily detachable, an enzymatic preparation of chymotrypsin (Zonulysin) may be instilled behind the iris a few minutes before the lens is removed, especially in younger patients.

Following either an extracapsular or intracapsular extraction, an *introacular lens implant* may be placed in the anterior or posterior chamber.

Usually cataract extraction is done in only one eye at a time; if both eyes are affected, they are treated (in most cases) in separate operations.

Management before an operation is necessary

During the period through which the lens is progres-sively losing its transparency, a nurse usually has contact with the patient only at the clinic, the surgery or on home visits that are for some other purpose. During such contacts, the nurse assesses the person in relation to the visual impairment.

Potential patient problems
1. Anxiety due to the visual impairment and fear of blindness and dependency.
2. Potential for injury.
3. Decreased mobility, usually due to a fear of moving about, especially outside the immediate familiar environment.
4. Alteration in self-image due to limitations.

Nursing intervention

1. Anxiety. The nurse explains what cataracts are to the patient and family and reassures them that it is a common problem. They should be advised that vision can be improved by corrective lenses in glasses for a period of time and that eventually the cataract can be treated by surgery. Details should then be given about what this will entail.

2. Potential for injury. Advice should be given to the patient and family about adjustments within the patient's environment that may be necessary to prevent accidents. Improved lighting may help and other aids, such as stair rails can be installed. Direct vision into sunlight and bright lights is avoided. Driving should be discussed with the patient and the advice of the ophthalmologist sought.

3. Decreased mobility. Because of the fear of falling, or making errors and being unable to read signs, price tags, etc., the patient becomes reluctant to venture beyond immediate familiar environments and activity may gradually decrease. Socialization decreases. The patient should be encouraged to go out with family members and friends, not to hesitate to ask for assistance when alone and to turn the head to the side when looking at something, since peripheral vision is usually decreased. The patient and family are informed that books in large print are available in public libraries. They are advised also of the services of the local branch of the Royal National Institute for the Blind. For example, when the patient is unable to read and watch television, recordings may be obtained. Registration as blind or partially sighted will make certain benefits and allowances available.

4. Alteration in self-image. The person with loss of vision may become depressed and lose self-esteem as activity and participation progressively become restricted and dependence upon others increases. The positive aspects of life should be emphasized and accessible forms of diversion discussed. Unless there is some existing complication that contraindicates surgery, the patient is reassured that this is a temporary problem that will be relieved by surgery.

Immediate preoperative care

Nursing intervention
The patient is alerted to any furniture or articles over which it is possible to trip or stumble. Contact lenses must be removed before leaving the ward. Spectacles and hearing aids can be removed in the anaesthetic room.

The nurse should check that the correct eye has been marked by the surgeon and that the consent form has been signed.

An example of a care plan for a patient about to undergo intraocular surgery is given in Table 28.2. This describes potential problems, full nursing intervention and expected outcomes.

Table 28.2 Preoperative care* of patients undergoing intraocular surgery.

Problem	Goal	Nursing intervention	Expected outcomes
1. Anxiety related to the unfamiliar environment and lack of knowledge about the surgical procedure and local anaesthetic; and fear of an undesirable outcome	• The patient will experience reduced anxiety levels • The patient will show an understanding of what will be done, what to expect and the patient's role	• Orientate the patient to environment and staff • Encourage the patient and family to express their fears and concerns • Identify specific fears, misconceptions and learning needs relevant to the disorder, surgery, postoperative care and the patient's future • Provide the necessary information; answer questions	• Anxiety is reduced, as evidenced by decreased restlessness and conversation that indicates understanding and acceptance of the situation and what may be expected
2. Inadequate knowledge about anticipated postoperative care	• The patient will show awareness of the activities and restrictions to be expected after surgery	• The anticipated restrictions in positioning and activities in the postoperative period and their significance are explained • The patient is informed about the following. If nauseated he or she should notify the nurse promptly so an antiemetic can be given to avoid vomiting. The eye should not be squeezed closed and sudden jerky movements, bending over, pushing, lifting and constipation are avoided • If both eyes are likely to be covered, explain the reason for this and assure the patient that assistance will be readily available as required	• The patient indicates understanding of anticipated procedures
3. Nausea and vomiting	• Nausea and vomiting will not occur	• Food and fluid may be withheld for 4–6 hours preceding surgery	• Nausea and vomiting are absent
4. Bowel elimination: potential for constipation	• Constipation and straining at stool postoperatively will not occur	• A high-fibre diet and adequate fluids are encouraged	• Bowel movements are soft, regular and are evacuated without strain

Table 28.2 *Continued*

Problem	Goal	Nursing intervention	Expected outcomes
5. Potential for injury related to infection and surgical intervention	• The eye will not become infected	• Inspect the eyes for irritation, redness, discharge and excessive lacrimation • A routine culture of the conjunctival sacs may be required • Specific directions are given by the surgeon; the eyelids and area around the eye are cleansed. If the eyelashes are to be cut, the blades of the scissors used are coated with chloramphenicol ointment to prevent lash remnants dropping into the eye • Some marking should be used to ensure identification of the eye to receive surgery • A prophylactic antibiotic may be instilled in the eye before surgery, as prescribed	• The patient is free of infection
6. Alteration in comfort: pain related to surgical procedure	• Pain and discomfort will be absent	• Instil drops prescribed by the surgeon (e.g. Mydrilate) prior to surgery and give any appropriate prescribed systemic premedication	• The patient's eye is at rest; the pupil is dilated or constricted as indicated • Patient is relaxed and free of pain and discomfort

* Therapeutic measures and care vary with the disorder, surgery to be performed and the surgeon. Specific requirements are cited with the discussion of the various disorders.

Postoperative care

Potential eye injury and complications are the major concern following cataract extraction. The period of bed rest and hospitalization varies considerably. The patient is usually allowed out of bed the day of or day after surgery and may be discharged home the first or second postoperative day. Day case cataract surgery is becoming very popular.

Identification of patients' problems and *nursing intervention* are discussed in Table 28.3.

Table 28.3 Postoperative care of patients following intraocular surgery.

Problem	Goal	Nursing intervention	Expected outcomes
1. Alteration in comfort: pain	• Pain and discomfort will be absent	• The patient may experience some burning or smarting sensation which may be relieved by a mild analgesic. Severe pain, particularly if it develops suddenly or if the patient expresses a 'feeling of pressure within the eye' is reported promptly to the surgeon	• The patient feels no pain or discomfort. However, if an episode of severe pain develops, it is identified promptly

Table 28.3 *Continued*

Problem	Goal	Nursing intervention	Expected outcomes
		• The patient is usually allowed to use the bathroom on the first postoperative day and walking is progressively increased, or may be discharged on the second postoperative day • If the patient is on bed rest for several days or longer, deep breathing at regular intervals is encouraged; secretions are less likely to be retained and cause infection and coughing • Lower limb and arm exercises are introduced for the bed patient to promote circulation but the patient is cautioned against moving the head while doing them	
2. Potential for injury related to surgical intervention	• The site of surgery will heal without complications • Intraocular haemorrhage, increased intraocular pressure and rupture of the incision line will be prevented	• The head is held steady and supported during transfer from operating theatre table to bed • If confined to bed, the patient is assisted to change position • After the initial dressing, prescribed drops or ointment are instilled 3 or 4 times daily. A pad may be reapplied or dark glasses worn, except at night when a dressing and protective shield should be worn • Restrictions in positioning and activity are indicated by the ophthalmologist and should be made familiar to staff and family members • The patient is sat up when the surgeon allows; the head is well supported and the patient is discouraged from lying on the affected side • The patient is reminded: to avoid straining at stool, to avoid any pressure on the eye, not to lean over the side of the bed or make sudden movements, to try to avoid coughing by taking	• The patient does not experience intraocular haemorrhage; increased intraocular pressure or rupture of incision line

Table 28.3 *Continued*

Problem	Goal	Nursing intervention	Expected outcomes
		a deep breath and if it cannot be avoided to cough with mouth open (lessens intracranial pressure), as these actions may increase intraocular pressure which may cause intraocular haemorrhage or prolapse of the iris, and to inform the nurse promptly of pain in the eye; severe pain should be brought to the surgeon's attention immediately, since it may indicate intraocular haemorrhage • Nausea and vomiting should also be controlled because of the associated strain; an antiemetic is prescribed if necessary • Monitor vital signs as necessary	
3. Potential for infection	• Infection of the eye will not occur	• The length of time a dressing is kept on depends on the surgery and the surgeon • The daily instillation of topical antibiotics may be prescribed; aseptic technique is observed • Each time the eye is uncovered or treated it is inspected for inflammation and discharge • If infection is suspected or present, prompt antibiotic therapy is prescribed (topical and systemic). A culture is usually made to identify the organism and determine its sensitivity • A topical corticosteroid preparation may be instilled in the eye to reduce the effects of the inflammation on intraocular structures	• The eye is free of infection
4. Potential for injury related to sensory deprivation or disorientation	• Injury will not occur • The patient will be orientated with regards to ward environment	• Reorientate the patient on return from the operating theatre (location, staff and time) and reassure as to assistance and care • The call-button is always ready within the patient's reach	• The patient is free from injury • The patient is orientated to time, place and person • The environment is free of physical hazards

Table 28.3 *Continued*

Problem	Goal	Nursing intervention	Expected outcomes
		• Do not leave the patient alone for long periods; frequent communication reduces sensory deprivation, especially if both eyes are covered or the room is darkened. On each visit, the person's orientation is assessed	
		• An effort is made to anticipate the patient's needs so avoiding premature activity. It may be helpful to have a family member or friend remain with the patient	
		• Articles that the patient is likely to want are replaced within reach and always in the same place	
		• The affected eye is protected by a shield; a plastic one is always used at night	
		• When ambulatory, the patient is assisted until familiarity with the environment is indicated. The environment is cleared of hazardous articles such as foot-stools, loose rugs; furniture should remain in its original position and doors kept wide open or closed	
		• If the patient becomes confused restraints on the arms may be necessary to prevent interference with the eye dressing. The use of body restraints are avoided because the resistance to them may increase intraocular pressure. Someone (e.g. a family member) may have to remain to ensure safety. Removal of dressings usually reduces the confusion	
		• Sedation may be prescribed	
5. Aleration in nutrition: less than body requirements	• Nutritional and fluid intake will be progressively increased to normal as tolerated	• The restoration of a balanced diet will aid healing. The patient should be given sips of water on return from theatre. Then a light	• The patient's usual body weight is maintained

Table 28.3 *Continued*

Problem	Goal	Nursing intervention	Expected outcomes
		easily digestible diet should gradually be introduced the following day. Fluid intake should be encouraged unless the patient complains of nausea in which case an antiemetic should be given. Fluid intake and output should be recorded until the patient is capable of taking control of eating and drinking. A high-fibre diet is encouraged in order to prevent straining at stool. Normal nutrition can be resumed immediately if a local anaesthetic has been given • It is important that the necessary assistance with eating is available for the person with severely impaired vision. Assistance is also necessary for the patient whose movement is restricted. The food is described and the patient fed slowly to avoid the possibility of aspiration and coughing. Sandwiches are useful in maintaining the patient's independence	
6. Inadequate knowledge about post-hospitalization care and rehabilitation	• The patient will show knowledge and skill essential to follow-up care	• The patient's home situation should be determined and the patient and a family member assisted to develop an appropriate plan of care. Instruction and/or demonstrations are given relevant to: —Restrictions to prevent intraocular haemorrhage and increased intraocular pressure (bending over, lifting, pushing, falls and bumps) —The prescribed therapeutic eye procedures (dressing, and how to clean away discharge and the instillation of drops or ointment) • Emphasis is placed on: —The need for the	The patient and family: • Indicate an awareness of the importance of compliance with the recommended restrictions • Demonstrate ability to perform the prescribed eye procedures safely • Express an awareness of the: need for an eye shield and dark glasses; symptoms that require prompt medical attention; and the correct care of corrective lenses • Describe plans for follow-up care and demonstrate awareness of community resources

Table 28.3 *Continued*

Problem	Goal	Nursing intervention	Expected outcomes
		washing of hands and careful handling of dressings	
		—securing the dressing so it does not abrade the eyes	
		—The wearing of dark glasses when the dressing is removed and the subsequent wearing of corrective spectacles or contact lenses (see text for details)	
		—The wearing of the eye shield at night for 2–3 weeks	
		—The avoidance of rubbing the eye	
		—The restriction on reading and driving for the period indicated by the ophthalmologist	
		—The care of corrective glasses or lenses. If an enucleation was done, the application, removal and care of the artificial eye	
		—The symptoms that indicate the need to promptly contact the ward (pain in the eye, increased redness and discharge, loss of vision)	
		—Subsequent appointments with the ophthalmologist or clinic	

Spectacles and contact lenses

When the dressing is removed, dark glasses are worn because the patient may experience discomfort in the eye with exposure to light; gradual adaptation is necessary. If an intraocular lens has not been implanted at the time of the surgery, the patient may be fitted with a contact lens some weeks after surgery. The lens may be of the type which has to be removed each night, or an extended-wear type which can be left in the eye for several weeks. With the latter, the patient returns to the clinic or ophthalmologist at regular intervals (approximately 90–120 days) to have the lens removed, cleansed and replaced.

When only one eye has had cataract extraction, spectacles are not useful since the thick biconvex lens that would be necessary magnifies considerably and would not produce binocular vision. When both eyes have had cataract surgery without intraocular lens implant, the patient is fitted for spectacles with thick biconvex lenses which are used for a few weeks or months before permanent glasses or contact lenses are provided. With spectacles, peripheral vision is restricted (Figure 28.9).

Implantation of an intraocular lens at the time of the cataract extraction or at a later date is becoming more common. The advantages are the provision of greater depth perception, full visual field, and binocular vision (less magnification than glasses).

Teaching patients in preparation for discharge

This includes the following considerations:

● The avoidance of lifting, bending over and straining at stool for about 3 weeks is stressed. The patient is cautioned against squeezing the eye closed or applying pressure on the eye. A shield is worn at

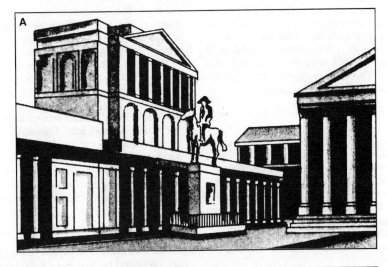

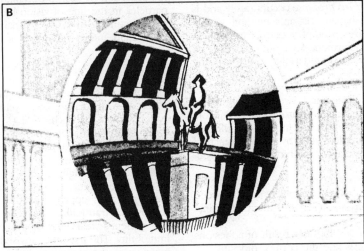

Figure 28.9 The Bank of England. (A) As seen normally. (B) Illustrates the loss of peripheral vision as seen through the eyes of a patient wearing cataract glasses. The central vision appears larger and nearer than it is. The side vision is bowed and outside this there is a ring area of no vision at all.

night for 2–3 weeks to avoid pressure and unconscious rubbing.

- A family member and the patient are instructed how to care for the eye following discharge (dressings and the instillation of drops and ointment).
- If redness, oedema or pain develops in the eye or vision deteriorates, the surgeon should be contacted promptly.
- If glasses are to be worn an explanation is made about the reduced peripheral vision. The patient is advised that in order to see, he or she must learn to look straight-on; this necessitates turning the head when making a side-on peripheral observation. Because of the magnification and difference in spatial judgement, the patient is advised of the necessary precautions when using stairs and handling objects.
- When the patient receives a contact lens, detailed instructions and demonstrations are necessary. A contact lens is a thin plastic disc shaped to fit the

anterior surface of the eye. The outer surface is ground to meet the patient's visual need. The patient is taught the daily procedure of putting in and removing the lens, the cleansing and care of it and the prevention of complications. Meticulous care is necessary to prevent complications, which are painful and could cause loss of vision. Washing the hands thoroughly with soap under running water before handling the lens is emphasized. If worn in both eyes, on removal each lens is stored separately in containers marked for right and left; the correction in one may be quite different to that of the other. Directions for cleansing are provided in writing. Before applying the lenses, they are rinsed free of any chemical that may have been used for cleansing and a wetting solution may be used. Solutions must be fresh and are not reused.

The patient is advised to use the lens for brief periods at first, progressively increasing the length of time until the eye is comfortable with it. Unless the lenses are of the extended-wear type, they are removed at the end of each day; they are *not* worn during sleep. If the eye is inflamed or painful or if there is excessive lacrimal secretion (tearing), the lens is not applied. The most common complications that develop are conjunctivitis, corneal abrasion and keratitis.

Complications

Complications that may occur following cataract extraction include the following:

Haemorrhage into the anterior chamber (hyphaema) is a serious complication that may occur in the early postoperative period. The patient experiences sharp pain in the eye and on examination, blood can be seen in the eye. The patient is placed at rest, the head is elevated and the ophthalmologist is notified immediately. A mydriatic preparation is usually ordered to dilate the pupil and rest the eye.

Wound rupture and iris prolapse occurs rarely and is manifested by a misshapen iris and bulging in the incision area. It requires prompt surgical treatment to avoid serious visual impairment. Mydriatics must not be instilled if a prolapse is suspected as this can worsen the condition.

Infection may develop; the eye becomes red, and painful. It is treated by topical and parenteral antibiotics.

A severe infection may manifest itself as a hypopyon: white cells in the anterior chamber. Intensive instillation of eye drops may be supplemented by a subconjunctival injection of a broad-spectrum antibiotic such as gentamicin or methicillin.

Retinal detachment occurs rarely as a result of the formation of adhesions within the eye, usually between the retina and the vitreous. (See treatment of retinal detachment, below.)

Glaucoma may also develop as a result of adhesions forming between the iris and the cornea, blocking the filtration angle, and secondary to a hyphaema.

Evaluation

The patient:
1. Does not experience discomfort in the affected eye.
2. Indicates understanding of the importance of avoiding activities which may cause increased intraocular pressure and, if pain or discomfort is experienced, the need for prompt contact with the ophthalmologist or clinic.
3. Is able to see because of the intraocular lens, contact lens or glasses.
4. The patient and/or a family member satisfactorily demonstrate the necessary procedures to care for the eyes and contact lenses.
5. The patient is free from post-cataract extraction complications.

DETACHMENT OF THE RETINA

Retinal detachment is separation of the pigmented epithelium of the retina from the layer of rods and cones; the pigmented layer remains attached to the choroid. The separation occurs as a result of tears or holes in the retina. These openings permit fluid from within the eye to leak through and accumulate in the retina, incurring the separation.

The cause may be degenerative retinal changes associated with the ageing process, aphakia (absence of the lens), trauma or tumour. The trauma may be directly to the eye (e.g. penetrating foreign body) or may be associated with a head injury. Retinal detachment may occur as a complication following cataract extraction or an inflammatory intraocular disorder. There is a higher incidence in those who have myopia and are over 50 years of age. The damaged areas are usually toward the periphery of the retina but may occur in the area of the macula, causing severe visual impairment.

Characteristics

Manifestations of a detached retina appear suddenly and are preceded by flashes of light, blurred vision, floating particles in the line of vision before the sensation of a curtain coming in front of a part of the eye, restricted visual field and eventual loss of vision occurs.

Treatment

The patient is placed at rest and both eyes may be covered. A mydriatic and cycloplegic drug such as cyclopentolate hydrochloride (Mydrilate) may be prescribed for instillation to dilate the pupils and arrest accommodation by depressing ciliary action. The ophthalmologist indicates the position the patient is to assume: left or right lateral or on the back (never prone). The position is such that the detached area of the retina will approximate the underlying layers. A sedative or tranquilliser may be prescribed to reduce the patient's fear and apprehension and promote immobility. The patient is advised of the importance of maintaining the recommended position and of avoiding sudden movements, bending over, coughing, sneezing and rubbing the eye. The patient should be informed that assistance is close at hand and how it may be summoned.

Surgical intervention is usually undertaken fairly early. Various procedures are used, but the underlying principle is scarring of the area. As the scar tissue forms, it fills in the retinal hole and provides attachment to the underlying sclera. The surgical procedures include electrodiathermy, encirclement plombage, cryosurgery (the application of extreme cold), photocoagulation which involves the application of heat by means of directing a very intense light into the eye (laser beam), and scleral buckling. In scleral buckling, the accumulated fluid is removed, the area is treated to produce scar tissue, and a fold is then made in the underlying sclera, which buckles the overlying choroid and retina bringing them in contact.

Victrectomy surgery is fast becoming a common method of treating complicated retinal detachments. The retina is reapposed to the underlying pigment epithelium by removing vitreous humour and replacing this with liquid gas or oil. This method requires strict positioning for 2–3 days postoperatively.

After the operation, a patch is placed over the eye for 24 hours. Dilating and antimicrobial eye drops may then be ordered. The patient is instructed to ask for assistance when ambulating and not to bend or strain. The light in the room is kept low to decrease light sensitivity when the patch is removed and dark glasses may be worn. Because of the amount of oedema within a confined space (the orbit) pain can be a problem and may be for 6–8 weeks postoperatively. A full explanation of the cause of pain and regular analgesia may be given. Analgesia to take home should also be prescribed.

Prior to discharge the patient is taught to instil the eye drops and is given written instructions about activity limitations. No heavy lifting or heavy work is undertaken for at least a period of 5–6 weeks. Appointments are made for follow-up care. The patient must be cautioned against bumping the head, rapid eye movements, reading and close work.

UVEITIS

Inflammation due to injury or infection may develop in the uveal tract, which includes the choroid, iris and ciliary body. It may also be associated with collagen disease (e.g. rheumatoid arthritis, sarcoidosis).

Characteristics of anterior uveitis

The eye is reddened and the patient complains of pain, photophobia, and impaired vision in the affected eye. The pupil usually remains constricted.

Treatment

Treatment may include rest of the eyes, the application of heat and the administration of an antimicrobial drug if infection is suspected as being the cause. A mydriatic (e.g. atropine, cyclopentolate, tropicamide) is instilled to dilate the pupil and prevent adhesions from developing between the iris and the lens. A corticoid preparation may be given systemically and also instilled in the eye(s) to arrest the inflammatory process and scar formation; scar formation is likely to cause loss of vision.

POSTERIOR UVEITIS OR CHOROIDITIS

Characteristics

Painless loss of parts of the visual field corresponding to the area of inflammation.

Treatment

Systemic corticosteroids are the treatment of choice. Monitoring and patient education is essential, as all forms of uveitis can have periods of exacerbation.

KERATITIS

This term is used for inflammation of the cornea, which is a serious condition. It may be due to infection or trauma and is likely to lead to ulceration and scarring.

The affected areas lose their transparency, diminishing the light rays entering the eye.

Debilitated persons and those with vitamin A deficiency and allergies develop corneal ulceration more readily with an eye infection or trauma. The inflammation may be superficial or deep and in some instances becomes chronic.

Characteristics

Keratitis is manifested by irritation, discharge if the cause is infection, redness of the eye due to injection of the peripheral areas of the cornea by blood vessels, photophobia and lacrimation. Ulcerated areas may be identified by the instillation of fluorescein which outlines the lesions.

Treatment

Prompt medical treatment is necessary to prevent perforation of the cornea and serious visual damage. Keratitis frequently may be prevented by early removal of foreign bodies as well as early treatment of injuries and infection.

Treatment includes rest, the use of antimicrobial drugs, the instillation of a mydriatic and the administration of a systemic analgesia to relieve pain. The eyes may be covered to protect them from light and to limit eye movement. If ulcers develop and are complicated by corneal perforation the aqueous humour escapes, the anterior chamber collapses and there may be intraocular bleeding. The patient is placed on complete bedrest, a mydriatic is instilled in the affected eye to dilate the pupil, and a pressure dressing is applied. Sometimes a soft contact lens called a protective membrane or bandage lens is applied.

If a cornea appears to be in danger of perforating, the lids may be closed over it, either by closure by tape or actually sutured shut, a tarsorrhaphy. In severe cases, surgery to the cornea (keratoplasty), may be required.

VITREOUS HAEMORRHAGE

The most common cause of vitreous opacity is bleeding from adjacent papillary, retinal or ciliary vessels. With minimal bleeding the patient may be conscious of floaters or 'small black dots'; more serious bleeding causes a sudden flood of floaters and subsequent loss of visual actuity so that the patient is only able to perceive light.

The haemorrhage may be associated with trauma, retinal tears and detachment, hypertension or diabetes mellitus. Many diabetics develop diabetic retinopathy, which is a common cause of blindness; increased vascular permeability, microaneurysms and atheroma (fatty plaques in the walls of the arteries) develop in the ocular blood vessels in diabetic retinopathy. Fragile vessels in the vitreous frequently bleed.

Loss of vitreous transparency may also be incurred by uveitis in which the inflammatory exudate and debris are carried into the vitreous and cause opacity.

Minor haemorrhages into the vitreous resolve fairly quickly. In more severe bleeding, which causes a serious visual impairment or where there is a loss of vitreous transparency due to other aetiological factors, a *vitrectomy* may be undertaken. This involves the removal of vitreous content and opacities with a special instrument to which there is a fibreoptic light attached. The vitreous is replaced with a liquid or gas.

KERATOCONUS

This is a rare degenerative disorder of the cornea that is seen in young persons, usually young men. There is a degenerative thinning and protrusion of the central cornea, usually of both eyes. Severe astigmatism develops, causing visual impairment.

An excessive amount of fluid collects posterior to the protruding cornea, and scar tissue develops as a result of the damage to tissue by stretching and rupture. The person experiences blurring of vision in the early stages but progressive changes may eventually led to complete loss of vision. The patient may be helped at first by the wearing of hard contact lenses but may finally require keratoplasty.

KERATOPLASTY (CORNEA TRANSPLANATION)

Loss of vision due to destruction of the cornea, keratoconus or loss of transparency may be corrected by a cornea transplanation. The central portion of the affected cornea is removed and replaced with a cornea obtained from a cadaver. The period between death and removal of the graft should not exceed 6–8 hours, and the transplant must be performed within 24–48 hours. Corneal tissue can now be preserved for up to 2 weeks as corneal buttons and still remain viable, which has reduced the need for the majority of patients to be sent for urgently, and this operation can now be planned for. During the interval following enucleation the donor eye is refrigerated at 4°C to minimize degenerative changes. Rejection is less of a problem with corneal transplanation than with other types of organ transplantation. It is suggested that this is due to the avascularity of the cornea. In the absence of blood vessels, donor tissue antigens do not get into the recipient's blood to initiate the formation of antibodies and sensitized lymphocytes.

Preoperative preparation

A detailed discussion of all that is involved in a keratoplasty occurs between the surgeon and the patient and family. The patient is informed that several weeks will elapse following the transplant before the results can be evaluated.

The immediate preoperative period is now a planned admission. Blood specimens are collected for the usual preoperative blood studies, and the surgeon usually prescribes the instillation of a miotic (e.g. pilocarpine 2–4%) in the affected eye to constrict the pupil so that the lens is protected during surgery. Acetazolamide (Diamox) or mannitol may be prescribed intravenously to reduce the intraocular fluid volume and tension (see Table 28.2).

Types of keratoplasty

The operative procedure may be a penetrating keratoplasty or a lamellar transplant. The penetrating transplant involves a full-thickness removal of the central portion of the affected cornea and replacement with an equivalent full-thickness section of the donor cornea. In a lamellar keratoplasty, a partial-thickness piece of the donor cornea replaces superficial layers of the recipient's cornea.

Postoperative management (see Table 28.3)

The patient experiences some pain and a mild analgesic may be prescribed. The main cause of discomfort is the presence of the sutures giving a continuous 'foreign body' sensation. The sutures stay in for 3–9 months, but the eyes usually become more comfortable, as the epithelium grows over the sutures.

The patient is allowed up as much as he or she wishes after recovery from the anaesthetic.

The eye is protected by a dressing. Sunglasses are worn during the day; at night a shield (usually of plastic) is applied.

Topical medications prescribed for instillation for a period of time may include, in addition to a mydriatic (e.g. Mydrilate), a corticosteroid preparation to suppress inflammation which would reduce the clearness and transparency of the cornea. A prophylactic topical antibiotic may also be used for a few days. When instilling ointments or drops, as always, precautions are observed to avoid any pressure on the eye and having the dropper or the tube applicator touch the eye.

During the weeks and months following the transplantation, the patient may have alternating periods of optimism and discouragement. It is important for the patient to be informed before leaving the hospital that healing will be slow because a transparent cornea does not have blood vessels.

A family member and the patient receive demonstrations and instructions in the care of the eye and the instilling of medications in preparation for leaving the hospital. If a family member or the patient is not able to undertake the care safely, a referral may be made to the district nurse. The patient is followed closely by frequent visits to the clinic or surgeon.

INJURY TO THE EYE

An eye may be traumatized by a foreign body, laceration or chemical agent. The patient may experience the discomfort associated with 'something in the eye', excessive lacrimation, pain, redness and sensitivity to light. Persisting pain, loss of vision and bleeding usually manifest a serious injury. With any type of injury, contact lenses should be removed promptly.

A *foreign body* may lodge on the conjunctiva or may be embedded in the conjunctival or corneal tissue, causing inflammation and possible ulceration. In some accidents, the injury may penetrate the lens or even the retina. If a foreign body is not easily and lightly wiped off or washed out, the patient is promptly referred to an ophthalmologist or accident and emergency department. Fluorescein dye may be used in the eye during the assessment to localize the foreign body. Deep metal foreign bodies may be removed by the use of a strong electromagnet. If the foreign body has caused an abrasion or was penetrating, an antibiotic ointment is instilled and a dressing may be applied.

Lacerations of the eyeball seriously threaten vision because of the formation of scar tissue in healing and by predisposing the eye to infection. Prompt treatment and strict asepsis are very important.

Various *chemicals*, acids and alkalis may cause serious irritation or burns of the conjunctiva and cornea. Emergency treatment consists of washing the eye with copious amounts of water or saline. The lids must be wide open and assistance may have to be provided in order to keep the eye open during the flushing. The person should be taken to an accident and emergency department as quickly as possible. A local anaesthetic may be instilled to provide relief and facilitate examination of the eye(s). Both eyes are covered to limit eye movement.

STRABISMUS (SQUINT)

Normally, both eyes perform an equal range of movement and assume corresponding lines of position when focusing on an object. Strabismus ('cross eyes') is characterized by the deviation of one eye from the position of the other. One eye (the normal or fixing eye) focuses directly on the object, but the other one (the deviating eye) appears to be focused on a different object or area.

The inequality in the movement of the eyes is due to an imbalance in the function of one or more extrinsic ocular muscles. The defect may result in the eye being turned medially, producing a convergent strabismus (*esotropia*). If the eye is turned laterally, the condition is referred to as divergent strabismus (*exotropia*). The result of the unequal movement and two points of focus is double vision (*diplopia*). Two images are formed on the retinae and the visual centres in the brain receive two sets of impulses, each producing a separate picture.

Strabismus may also be classified as being non-paralytic or paralytic and monocular or alternating. Non-paralytic strabismus (the more common) is the result of a congenital abnormality. The defect is in the central nervous system mechanism which co-ordinates the movements of the eyes in order to bring them into the positions that will focus the light rays from an object on corresponding areas of the two retinae. The person may be able to focus the right eye on an object of attention but the left deviates, presenting a second image. If the person has alternating strabismus it is possible to focus first with one eye on the object, then with the other. The eye that is in the correct position is referred to as the fixing eye; the other is called the deviating eye. If it is always the same eye, the strabismus is said to be monocular.

The person with strabismus develops single vision over a period of time, seeing only what the fixing or non-deviating eye perceives by involuntarily suppressing the confusing image presented by the deviating eye. Non-paralytic strabismus is generally recognized in early childhood.

Paralytic strabismus is due to the inability of the extraocular muscles to move the eye into the position corresponding to that of the other eye. As a result the person experiences diplopia. The cause of paralytic strabismus may be a defect in the muscle itself or a disturbance in the muscle innervation. The condition may be a manifestation of a disorder within the brain or orbit that interferes with the transmission of impulses by the third (oculomotor), fourth (trochlear) or sixth (abducens) cranial nerve.

Treatment

Strabismus requires medical treatment; unfortunately, in some instances parents think it will correct itself as the child becomes older. A delay may result in permanent damage; constant suppression of the image presented by the deviating eye may lead to loss of vision in that eye (amblyopia). The form of treatment will depend on the cause and severity of the strabismus. Obviously, if it is secondary to a lesion that is interrupting nerve impulses, the primary condition is surgically treated, if possible. Strabismus in the child may be corrected by the wearing of prescribed glasses. The unaffected eye may be covered for periods to enforce the use of the deviating (or so-called 'lazy') eye. Special eye exercises may be ordered (*orthoptics*).

If the condition does not respond to these conservative forms of treatment, surgical correction may then be undertaken. The procedure may involve shortening or lengthening of one or more extrinsic eye muscles. Following the surgery, exercise and the wearing of glasses may still be necessary for a period of time. The patient requires continual medical supervision.

NEOPLASMS OF THE EYE AND ACCESSORY STRUCTURES

Tumours that develop in the skin on other parts of the body may also occur on the skin of the eyelids. Neoplasms of the external structures are usually discovered in the early stages since they are visible.

Neoplasms of the eye may be benign or malignant and the latter may be primary or secondary. Secondary malignancies in the eye are rare. A biopsy is done if the neoplasm is accessible. Malignant melanoma is the most common intraocular tumour. It usually originates in the choroid, ciliary body or iris. Retinoblastoma which develops in both eyes is attributed to a genetic defect that is considered hereditary.

Early symptoms of an intraocular neoplasm depend on its location. As it enlarges and spreads, pain is experienced because of the increased intraocular pressure; retinal detachment, intraocular haemorrhage and loss of vision occur. Primary malignant tumours may be treated by radiotherapy, local excision or enucleation.

ENUCLEATION

Enucleation is the removal of an eyeball and may be necessary because of a malignant neoplasm, deep infection, severe trauma or persisting pain in a blind eye. Rarely, an enucleation is done to remove a disfiguring blind eye. When an eyeball is removed, the extrinsic muscles are severed close to their insertion, and the Tenon's capsule is retained. These may be arranged around a plastic ball to provide support and movement for an artificial eye. A plastic shell is inserted as soon as possible to maintain lid tone and prevent adhesions developing between the layers of conjunctiva which would make the fitting of a prosthesis difficult. The prosthesis is made as soon as the incision has healed and the oedema has subsided.

The patient should not be discharged until able to clean the socket and handle the shell proficiently. A district nurse may be asked to visit.

Occasionally, the operation performed is an evisceration in which the contents of the eyeball are removed, leaving the sclera. This is more usually performed when infection is present to prevent spread to the brain.

A more radical procedure may be necessary in malignancy or severe trauma. The operation performed is called exenteration and involves the removal of the eyeball and the surrounding structures. These operations can be psychologically very distressing as they alter the individual's body image. The patient should be given time to express feelings.

SYMPATHETIC OPHTHALMIA

Following an eye injury, especially a deep penetrating one, the patient may develop panophthalmitis (inflammation of the ciliary body, choroid and iris) in the uninjured eye. This response is not understood; it has been suggested that it may be an allergic reaction to the pigment released by the damaged eye. Any redness or tearing of the uninjured eye and any complaint of photophobia, pain or loss of vision must be reported promptly. The condition may develop soon after the injury or several months or years later. Unless the inflammatory reaction is checked promptly, loss of vision results. Corticoid preparations are used locally and systemically. Rarely, the injured eye is removed to prevent sympathetic ophthalmitis from developing.

SUMMARY

The importance of vision to normal human functioning and independence is apparent, therefore the psychological trauma of any threat to a person's eyesight must always be considered by the nurse in caring for such an individual. Although ophthalmic nursing is a specialized field, the student should remember that any person may ask advice about visual problems at any time and expect the nurse to be able to give an informed answer. Further, nurses in a wide range of clinical areas may care for patients with impaired vision, therefore it is essential to understand the principles of care for a person with visual defects if good quality nursing is to be practised.

LEARNING ACTIVITIES

1. Investigate what problems a visually impaired person may encounter in finding his or her way around your hospital.
2. What aids are available to help a patient with impaired vision cope with household jobs, employment and recreation?
3. If a person can have their blood pressure checked free of charge, why should they have to pay to have their eyes tested? Discuss.

REFERENCES AND FURTHER READING

Anonymous (1983) Cataract surgery: providing total patient care. *Nursing '83* **13(4):** 65–69.

Belmont O (1981) Some common visual symptoms: what they mean and what to do about them. *Occupational Health Nursing* **29(6):** 21–24.

Boyd-Monk (1981) Practical methods of how to examine the external eye. *Occupational Health Nursing* **29(6):** 10–14.

Bryant WM (1981) Common toxic effects of systemic drugs on the eye. *Occupational Health Nursing* **29(6):** 15–17.

Gardiner PA (1987) *ABC of Ophthalmology.* London: BMJ.

Gaston H & Elkington AE (1986) *Ophthalmology for Nurses.* London: Croom Helm.

Gillin SE (1981) Simple nursing procedures for the occupational health nurse. *Occupational Health Nursing* **29(6):** 18–20.

Glasspool M (1984) *Eyes—Their Problems and Treatment.* London: Martin Dunitz.

Hayes PL (1981) Treatment and nursing care of corneal disease. *Nursing Clinics of North America* **16(3):** 383–392.

Krupp MA & Chaton MJ (eds) *Current Medical Diagnosis and Treatment*, chap. 4. Los Altos, CA: Lange.

Lowe J (1983) Nursing management of eye injuries. *Nursing* **2(17):** 490–495.

Nave CR & Nave BC (1985) *Physics for the Health Sciences* 3rd edn, chap. 20. Philadelphia: Saunders.

Norman S (1982) The pupil check. *American Journal of Nursing* **82(4):** 588–591.

O'Cauaghan B & Wright M (1983) Structure and function of the eye. *Nursing* **2(17):** 485–512.

Pearce V (1981) Sensory changes in old age. *Nursing* **1(25):** 1111.

Perry J & Tullo A (1990) *Care of the Ophthalmic Patient: A Guide for Health Professionals.* London: Chapman & Hall.

Phillips CI (1984) *Basic Clinical Ophthalmology.* London: Pitman.

Rowley RS (1981) Chemical and thermal burns of the eye. *Occupational Health Nursing* **29(6):** 28–30.

Seewoodhary M (1983) Common presentations in accident and emergency. *Nursing* **2(17):** 498–501.

Shreeve C (1985) Understanding glaucoma. *Nursing Mirror* **160(17):** 18–19.

Stern EJ (1980) Helping the person with low vision. *American Journal of Nursing* **80(10):** 1788–1790.

Stoller R (1987) *Ophthalmic Nursing.* Oxford: Blackwell.

Walsh MH (1990) *A & E Nursing: A New Approach* 2nd edn. Oxford: Heinemann.

Watkinson S (1985) Dry eye syndrome. *Nursing Times* **80(43):** 32–35.

Useful Addresses and Telephone Numbers

Every effort has been made to ensure that the following addresses and telephone numbers are current and correct, but the Publishers will be most grateful for information regarding any recent changes, along with suggestions for new inclusions in future editions.

AAA (Action Against Allergy)
23–24 George Street
Richmond
Surrey
TW9 1JY

Accept Services UK (ACCEPT)
200 Seagrave Road
London SW6 1RQ
Tel: 071–381 3155

Action Health 2000/International
 Voluntary Health Association
The Bath House
Gwydr Street
Cambridge CB1 2LW
Tel: 0223 460853

Action for Research into Multiple
 Sclerosis (ARMS)
4a Chapel Hill
Stansted
Essex CM24 8AG
Tel: 0279 81553

Action on Smoking and Health (ASH)
5–11 Mortimer Street
London W1N 7RH
Tel: 071–637 9843/6

Active Birth Centre (ABC)
55 Dartmouth Park Road
London NW5 1SL
Tel: 071–267 3006

Age Concern England
60 Pitcairn Road
Mitcham
Surrey CR4 3LL
Tel: 081–679 8000

Age-Link
Suite 5
The Manor House
The Green
Southall
Middx UB2 4BR
Tel: 071–734 9083

Al-Anon Family Groups UK and Eire
 (AFG)
61 Great Dover Street
London SE1 4YF
Tel: 071–403 0888

Alcohol Concern
305 Gray's Inn Road

London WC1X 8QF
Tel: 071–833 3471

Alcoholics Anonymous (AA)
General Service Office
PO Box 1
Stonebow House
Stonebow
York YO1 2NJ
Tel: 0904 644026 (admin); 071–352 3001
 (helpline)

Alzheimer's Disease Society
158–160 Balham High Road
London SW12 9BN
Tel: 081–675 6557

Anorexia and Bulimia Nervosa
 Association
Tottenham Women's Health Centre
Annexe C, Tottenham Town Hall
Town Hall Approach
London N15 4RX
Tel: 081–885 3936

Anti-Racist Response and Action Group
 (ARRAG)
c/o 112a The Green
Southall
Middx UB2 4BQ
Tel: 081–574 6019

Arthritis Care
6 Grosvenor Crescent
London SW1X 7ER
Tel: 071–235 0902

Arthritis and Rheumatism Council
 (ARC)
41 Eagle Street
London WC1R 4AR
Tel: 071–405 8572

ASH
5–11 Mortimer Street
London W1N 7RH
Tel: 071–637 9843

ASPIRE (Association for Spinal Injury
 Research, Rehabilitation and
 Reintegration)
Royal National Orthopaedic Hospital
Brockley Hill
Stanmore
Middx HA7 4LP
Tel: 081–954 0701

Association for All Speech-Impaired
 Children (AFASIC)
347 Central Markets
Smithfield
London EC1A 9NH
Tel: 071–236 3632

Association for Improvements in the
 Maternity Services (AIMS)
40 Kingswood Avenue
London NW6 6LS
Tel: 081–960 5585

Association for Post-Natal Illness
7 Gowan Avenue
London SW6 6RH
Tel: 071–731 4867

Association for Prevention of Addiction
 (APA)
5–7 Tavistock Place
London WC1H 9SS
Tel: 071–383 5071

Association for Spina Bifida and
 Hydrocephalus
ASBAH House
42 Park Road
Peterborough PE1 2UQ
Tel: 0733 555988

Association of Breast Feeding Mothers
Order Department
Sydenham Green Health Centre
Holmshaw Close
London SE26 4TH
Tel: 081–774 4769

Association of British Paediatric Nurses
 (ABPN)
c/o Central Nursing Office
The Hospital for Sick Children
Great Ormond Street
London WC1
Tel: 071–405 9200

Association of Community Health
 Councils for England and Wales
22 Columbo Street
London SE1 8DP
Tel: 071–609 8405

Association of Continence Advisors
380–384 Harrow Road
London W9 2HO
Tel: 071–266 3704

Association of Medical Secretaries
Tavistock House South
Tavistock Square
London WC1
Tel: 071–387 6005

Association of Parents of Vaccine-
    Damaged Children
2 Church Street
Shipston-on-Stour
Warwickshire CV36 4AP
Tel: 0608 61595

Association of Professions for Mentally
    Handicapped People (APMH)
Greytree Lodge
Second Avenue
Ross-on-Wye
Herefordshire HR9 7HT
Tel: 0989 62630

Association of Radical Midwives (ARM)
62 Greetby Hill
Ormskirk
Lancs. L39 2DT
Tel: 0695 572776

Baby Life Support Systems (BLISS)
17–21 Emerald Street
London WC1N 3QL
Tel: 071–831 9393

Back Pain Association
31–33 Park Road
Teddington
Middx TW11 0AB
Tel: 081–977 5474

Breast Care and Masectomy Association
    of Great Britain (BCMA)
15–19 Britten Street
London SW3 3TZ
Tel: 071–351 7811

British Agencies for Adoption and
    Fostering
11 Southwark Street
London SE1 1RQ
Tel: 071–407 8800

British Association for Cancer United
    Patients (BACUP)
121 Charterhouse Street
London EC1
Tel: 071–608 1661

British Association for Counselling
37a Sheep Street
Rugby
Warwickshire CV21 3BX
Tel: 0788 78328/9

British Colostomy Association
13–15 Station Road
Reading
Berks RG1 1LG
Tel: 0734 391537

British Council of Organisations of
    Disabled People (BCODP)
St Mary's Church
Greenlaw Street
London SE18 5AR
Tel: 081–316 4184

British Deaf Association
38 Victoria Place
Carlisle CA1 1HU
Tel: 0228 48844

British Diabetic Association
10 Queen Anne Street
London W1M 0BD
Tel: 071–323 1531

British Epilepsy Association
Anstey House
40 Hanover Sq
Leeds LS3 1BE
Tel: 0532 439393

British Geriatrics Society (BGS)
1 St Andrew's Place
Regents Park
London NW1 4LB
Tel: 071–935 4004

British Heart Foundation
14 Fitzhardinge Street
London W1H 4DH
Tel: 071–935 0185

British Holistic Medical Association
179 Gloucester Place
London NW1 6DX
Tel: 071–262 5299

British Homeopathic Association (BHA)
27a Devonshire Street
London W1N 1RJ
Tel: 071–935 2163

British Kidney Patient Association
    (BKPA)
Bonden
Hampshire GU35 9JP
Tel: 0420 472021/2

British Medical Association (BMA)
BMA House
Tavistock Square
London WC1H 9JP
Tel: 071–383 6101

British Organ Donor Society (BODY)
Balsham
Cambridge CB1 6DL
Tel: 0223 893636

British Paediatric Association (BPA)
5 St Andrew's Place
Regents Park
London NW1 4LB
Tel: 071–486 6151

British Pregnancy Advisory Service (BPAS)
Austry Manor
Wootton Wawen

Solihull
West Midlands B95 6DA
Tel: 05642 3225

British Red Cross Society (BRCS)
9 Grosvenor Crescent
London SW1X 7EJ
Tel: 071–235 5454

British United Provident Association
    (BUPA)
24/27 Essex Street
London WC2
Tel: 081–466 6531

Brittle Bone Society
112 City Road
Dundee DD2 2PW
Tel: 0382 817771

Brook Advisory Centres
153a East Street
London SE17 2SD
Tel: 071–708 1390

Bureau for Overseas Medical Service
Africa Centre
38 King Street
London WC2E 8JT
Tel: 071–836 5833

Cancer Link
17 Britannia Street
London WC1X 9JN
Tel: 071–833 2451

Carers National Association
29 Chilworth Mews
London W2 3RG
Tel: 071–724 7776

Cancer Relief Macmillan Fund
Anchor House
15–19 Britten Street
London SW3 3TZ
Tel: 071–351 7811

Central Midwives Board for Scotland
24 Dublin Street
Edinburgh EH1 3PU

Centre for Policy on Ageing
25–31 Ironmonger Row
London ECN3 QPY
Tel: 071–253 1787

ChildLine
50 Studd Street
London N1 0QJ
Tel: 071–239 1000

Chest, Heart and Stroke Association
CHSA House
Whitecross Street
London EC1Y 8JJ
Tel: 071–490 7999

Christian Council on Ageing
The Old Court
Greens Norton
Nr Towcester
Northants NN12 8VS
Tel: 0327 50481

Cleft Lip and Palate Association (CLAPA)
1 Eastwood Gardens
Kenton
Newcastle-upon-Tyne
NE3 3DQ
Tel: 091–285 9396

Coeliac Society of the United Kingdom
PO Box 220
High Wycombe
Bucks HP11 2HY
Tel: 0494 437278

Commission for Racial Equality
Elliott House
10–12 Allington House
London SW1E 5EH
Tel: 071–828 7022

Confederation of Healing Organizations
(CHO)
113 High Street
Berkhamsted
Herts HP4 2DJ
Tel: 0442 870660

Committee Against Drug Abuse (CADA)
359 Old Kent Road
London SE1 5JH
Tel: 071–231 1528

Committee on Safety of Medicines
Market Towers
1 Nine Elms Lane
London SW8 5NQ
Tel: 071–720 2188

Compassionate Friends
6 Denmark Street
Bristol BS1 5DQ
Tel: 0272 292778

Coronary Prevention Group (CPG)
60 Great Ormond Street
London WC1N 3HR
Tel: 071–833 3687

Cruse (National Organization for the
Widowed and their Children)
Cruse House
126 Sheen Road
Richmond
Surrey TW9 1UR
Tel: 081–940 4818

Cystic Fibrosis Research Trust
Alexandra House
5 Blythe Road
Bromley
Kent BR1 3RS
Tel: 081–464 7211/2

Department of Health
Richmond House
79 Whitehall
London SW1A 2NS
Tel: 071–210 3000

Welsh Office
Crown Buildings, Cathays Park, Cardiff
CF1 3NQ
Tel: 0222 825111

Scottish Office
Dover House, Whitehall, London
SW1A 2AU
Tel: 071–270 3000

*Scottish Home and Health
Department*
St Andrew's House, Regent Road,
Edinburgh EH1 3DE
Tel: 031 556 8400

*Department of Health and Social
Services, Northern Ireland*
Dundonald House, Upper
Newtownards Road, Belfast
BT4 3SB
Tel: 0232 650111

Department of Social Security
Richmond House
79 Whitehall
London SW1A 2NS
Tel: 071–210 3000

Depressives Anonymous (fellowship of)
36 Chestnut Avenue
Beverley
North Humberside HU17 9QU
Tel: 0482 860619

Diabetes Foundation
177a Tennison Road
London SE25 5NF
Tel: 081–656 5467

Disabled Living Foundation
380–384 Harrow Road
London W9 2HU
Tel: 071–289 6111

Down's Syndrome Association
153–155 Mitcham Road
London SW17 9PG
Tel: 081–682 4001

Drugline Ltd
9a Brockley Cross
Brockley
London SE4 2AB
Tel: 081–692 4975

ENB Career's Advisory Office
PO Box 356
Sheffield S8 0SJ

English National Board for Nursing,
Midwifery and Health Visiting
(ENB)

Victory House
170 Tottenham Court Road
London W1P 0HA
Tel: 071–388 3131

Epilepsy Association of Scotland
48 Govan Road
Glasgow G51 1JL

Equal Opportunities Commission
Overseas House
Quay Street
Manchester M3 3HN
Tel: 061–833 9244

Families Anonymous (FA)
310 Finchley Road
London NW3 7AG
Tel: 071–731 8060

Family Planning Association (FPA)
Margaret Pyke House
27–35 Mortimer Street
London W1N 7RJ
Tel: 071–636 7866

Family Welfare Association
501–505 Kingsland Road
London E8 4AU
Tel: 071–254 6251

Florence Nightingale House
173 Cromwell Road
London SW5 0SE
Tel: 071–235 2369

Foresight Charity for Preconceptual
Care
The Old Vicarage
Church Lane
Witley
Godalming
Surrey GG8 5PN
Tel: 0428 684500

The Foundation for the Study of Infant
Deaths (Cot Death Research and
Support)
35 Belgrave Square
London SW1X 8BQ
Tel: 071–235 1721

Gamblers Anonymous and Gam-Anon
PO Box 88
London SW10 0CU
Tel: 071–352 3060

Gay Bereavement Project
Unitarian Rooms
Hoop Lane
London NW11 8BS
Tel: 081–445 8894

Gay Men's Disabled Group
PO Box 153
Manchester M60 1LP

Gemma (Lesbians with/without
disabilities)

BM Box 5700
London WC1N 3XX

General Medical Council (GMC)
44 Hallam Street
London W1N 6AE
Tel: 071–580 7642

Gingerbread
35 Wellington Street
London WC2E 7BN
Tel: 071–240 0953

Guillain Barre Syndrome Support
    Group
Foxley
Holdingham
Sleaford
Lincs NG34 8NR
Tel: 0529 304615

Haemophilia Society
123 Westminster Bridge Road
London SE1 7HR
Tel: 071–928 2020

Health and Safety Executive
Baynards House
1–13 Chepstow Place
Westbourne Grove
London W2 4TF
Tel: 071–229 3456

Health Education Authority
Hamilton House
Mabledon Place
London WC1H 9TX
Tel: 071–631 0930

Health Rights Ltd
Unit 110
BonMarché Building
444 Brixton Road
London SW9 8EJ
Tel: 071–274 4000 ext. 442

Health Service Commissioner
Church House
Great Smith Street
London SW1P 3BW
Tel: 071–276 3000

Health Services Superannuation
    Division
Hesketh House
220 Broadway
Fleetwood
Lancs FL7 8LG
Tel: 0253 856123

Health Unlimited
3 Stamford Street
London SE1 9NT
Tel: 071–928 8105

Health Visitors' Association (HVA)
50 Southwark Street
London SE1 1UN
Tel: 071–378 7255

Help the Aged
16–18 St James's Walk
London EC1R 0BE
Tel: 071–253 0253

Her Majesty's Prisons and Borstal
    Institutions Nursing Service
Her Majesty's Prison
Holloway
London N5 1PL
Tel: 071–607 6747

Herpes Association
41 North Road
London N7 9DP
Tel: 071–609 9061

Hodgkin's Disease Association (HDA)
PO Box 275
Haddenham
Aylesbury
Bucks HP17 8JJ
Tel: 0844 291500 (8.30–10 pm)

Hospice Information Service
St Christopher's Hospice
51–59 Lawrie Park Road
Sydenham
London SE26 6DZ
Tel: 081–778 9252

Hospital Saving Association
Hambledon House
Andover
Hants SP10 1LQ
Tel: 0264 53211

Huntingdon's Disease Association
108 Battersea High Street
London SW11 3HP
Tel: 071–223 7000

Hysterectomy Support Group (HSG)
The Venture
Green Lane
Upton
Huntingdon
Cambs PE17 5YE
Tel: 081–690 5987

Identity Counselling Service
Beauchamp Lodge
2 Warwick Crescent
London W2 6NE
Tel: 071–289 6175

Imperial Cancer Research Fund (ICRF)
PO Box 123
Lincoln's Inn Fields
London WC2A 3PX
Tel: 071–242 0200

Institute for Complementary Medicine
21 Portland Place
London W1N 3AF
Tel: 071–636 9543

Institute for the Study of Drug
    Dependence
1 Hatton Place
Hatton Garden
London EC1N 8ND
Tel: 071–430 1991

Institution of Environmental Health
    Officers (IEHO)
Chadwick House
Rushworth Street
London SE1 0QT
Tel: 071–928 6006

International Confederation of Midwives
10 Barley Mow Passage
London W4 4PH
Tel: 081–994 6477

International Council for Nurses
3 Place Jean-Marteau
1201 Geneva
Switzerland
Tel: 010 41(22)7312960
For addresses of the ICN Member
    Associations see the list at the end
    of this section

International Voluntary Service (IVS)
(British Branch of Service Civil
    International)
162 Upper New Walk
Leicester LE1 7QA
Tel: 0533 549430

Invalid Children's Aid Nationwide
    (ICAN)
198 City Road
London EC1V 2PH

Invalids at Home
17 Lapstone Gardens
Kenton
Harrow
Middlesex HA3 0EB
Tel: 081–907 1706

Jewish Bereavement Counselling Service
1 Cyprus Gardens
London N3 1SP
Tel: 071–387 4300 ext 227

Jewish Care
Stuart Young House
221 Golders Green Road
London NW11 9DQ
Tel: 081–458 3282

Jewish Social Services
221 Golders Green Road
London NW11 9DW
Tel: 081–458 3282

Kerland Foundation
The Kerland Clinic
Marsh Lane
Huntworth Gate
Bridgewater

Somerset TA6 6LQ
Tel: 0278 429089

Kidscape Campaign for Childen's Safety
World Trade Centre
Europe House
London E1 9AA
Tel: 071–488 4200

King Edward's Hospital Fund for
London (The King's Fund)
148 Palace Court
London W2 4HT
Tel: 071–727 0581

King's Fund Centre (KFC)
126 Albert Street
London NW1 7NF
Tel: 071–267 6111

Lady Hoare Trust for Physically Disabled
Children (Associated with Arthritis
Care)
37 Oakwood
Bepton Road
Midhurst

Lepra (British Leprosy Relief
Association)
Fairfax House
Causton Road
Colchester
Essex CO1 1PO
Tel: 0206 562286

Lesbian and Gay Employment Rights
(LAGER)
St Margaret's House
21 Old Ford Street
London E2 4PL
Tel: 081–983 0694

Leukaemia Research Fund
43 Great Ormond Street
London WC1N 3JT
Tel: 071–405 0101

Leukaemia Care Society
PO Box 82
Exeter
Devon EX2 5DP
Tel: 0392 64848

Listeria Support Group
2 Wessex Close
Faringdon
Oxon SN7 7YY

London Lesbian and Gay Switchboard
BM Switchboard
London WC1N 3XX
Tel: 071–837 7324

London Lighthouse
111–117 Lancaster Road

London W11 1QT
Tel: 071–792 1200

Malcolm Sargent Cancer Fund for
Children
14 Abingdon Road
London W8 6AF
Tel: 071–937 4538

Margaret Pyke Centre
15 Bateman's Building
Soho Square
London W1V 5TW
Tel: 071–734 9351

Marie Curie Cancer Care
(Marie Curie Memorial Foundation)
28 Belgrave Square
London SW1X QG
Tel: 071–235 3325

Marie Stopes Clinic
Well Woman Centre
108 Whitfield Street
London W1P 6BE
Tel: 071–388 0662

Maternity Alliance
15 Brittania Street
London WC1X 9JP
Tel: 071–837 1265

Medic-Alert Foundation
17 Bridge Wharf
156 Caledonian Road
London N1 9UU
Tel: 071–833 3034

Medical Council on Alcoholism (MCA)
1 St Andrew's Place
London NW1 4LB
Tel: 071–487 4445

Medical Research Council (MRC)
20 Park Crescent
London W1N 4AL
Tel: 071–636 5422

Mental After Care Association
Bainbridge House
Bainbridge Street
London WC1A 1HP
Tel: 071–436 6194

Midwives Information and Resource
Service (MIDIRS)
Institute of Child Health
Royal Hospital for Sick Children
St. Michael's Hill
Bristol BS2 8BJ
Tel: 0272 251791

Migraine Trust, The
45 Great Ormond Street
London WC1N 3HD
Tel: 071–278 2676

MIND (National Association for Mental
Health)

22 Harley Street
London W1N 2ED
Tel: 071–637 0741

Minority Rights Group
379 Brixton Road
London SW9 7DE
Tel: 071–978 9498

Miscarriage Association
PO Box 24
Ossett
West Yorkshire WF5 9KG
Tel: 0924 830515

Motor Neurone Disease Association
PO Box 246
Northampton NN1 2PR
Tel: 0604 250505

Motor Neurone Disease Society
36 Portland Place
London W1N 3DG

Multiple Births Foundation (MBFI)
Queen Charlotte's and Chelsea Hospital
Goldhawk Road
London W6 0XG
Tel: 081–748 4666

Multiple Sclerosis Society of Great
Britain and Northern Ireland
25 Effie Road
Fulham
London SW6 1EE
Tel: 071–736 6267

Muscular Dystrophy Group
Nattras House
35 Macaulay Road
London SW4 0QP
Tel: 071–720 8055

Myasthenia Gravis Association
Keynes House
77 Nottingham Road
Derby DE1 3QS
Tel: 0332 290219

Narcotics Anonymous
PO Box 417
London SW10 0DP
Tel: 071–351 6794

National Association for Colitis and
Crohn's Disease (NACC)
98a London Road
St Albans
Herts AL1 1NX
Tel: 0227 763133

National Association for Gifted Children
Park Campus
Boughton Green Road
Northampton

Northants NN2 7AL
Tel: 0604 792300

National Association for Premenstrual
    Syndrome (NAPS)
PO Box 72
Sevenoaks
Kent TN13 1QX
Tel: 0732 459378; 0227 763133
    (Helpline)

National Association for the Relief of
    Paget's Disease
Teaching Unit 4
Withington Hospital
Nell Lane
Manchester M20 8LR

National Association for the Welfare of
    Children in Hospital (NAWCH)
Argyle House
29–31 Euston Road
London NW1 2SD
Tel: 071–833 2041

National Association of Bereavement
    Services (NABS)
122 Whitechapel High Street
London E1 7PT
Tel: 071–247 1080 (24-hour
    answerphone for referral requests);
    071–247 0617 (admin.)

National Association of Citizens' Advice
    Bureaux
115–123 Pentonville Road
London N1 9LZ
Tel: 071–833 2181

National Association of Laryngectomy
    Clubs (NALC)
4th Floor
39 Eccleston Square
London SW1V 1PB
Tel: 071–834 2557

National Association of Widows
54–57 Ellison Street
Digbeth
Birmingham B5 5TH
Tel: 021–643 8348

National Asthma Campaign
300 Upper Street
London N1 2XX
Tel: 071–226 2260

National Board for Nursing, Midwifery
    and Health Visiting for Northern
    Ireland
RAC House
79 Chichester Street
Belfast BT1 4JE
Tel: 0232 238152

National Board for Nursing, Midwifery
    and Health Visiting for Scotland

22 Queen Street
Edinburgh EH2 1JX
Tel: 031–226 7371

National Council for Civil Liberties
21 Tabard Street
London SE1 4LA
Tel: 071–403 3888

National Directorate of the National
    Blood Transfusion Service
Gateway House
Picadilly South
Manchester M60 7LP
Tel: 061–237 2087

National Ethnic Minority Advisory
    Council (NEMAC)
2nd and 3rd Floors
13 Macclesfield Street
London W1V 7HL

National Federation of Kidney Patients'
    Associations
6 Stanley Street
Worksop
Notts SS1 7HX
Tel: 0909 487795

National Health Service Retirement
    Fellowship
Botleys Park Hospital
Chertsey
Surrey KT16 0QA
Tel: 0932 874032

National Marriage Guidance Council
Herbert Gray College
Little Church Street
Rugby
Warwickshire CV21 3AP

Natural Medicines Society (NMS)
Edith Lewis House
Back Lane
Ilkeston
Derby DE7 8EJ
Tel: 0602 329454

National Osteoporosis Society
PO Box 10
Barton Mead House
Radstalk
Bath
Avon BA3 3YB
Tel: 0761 32472

National Rubella Council
Bray Business Centre
Weir Bank
Monkey Island Lane
Bray-on-Thames
Berks SL6 2EP
Tel: 0628 770011

National Schizophrenia Fellowship
28 Castle Street

Kingston-upon-Thames KT1 1SS
Tel: 081–547 3937

National Society for Epilepsy
Chalfont Centre for Epilepsy
Chalfont St Peter
Gerrards Cross
Bucks SL9 0RJ
Tel: 02407 3991

National Society for Mentally
    Handicapped People in Residential
    Care (RESCARE)
Rayner House
23 Higher Hillgate
Stockport
Cheshire SK1 3ER
Tel: 061–474 7323

National Society for Phenylketonuria
    and Allied Disorders
Worth Cottage
Lower Scholes
Pickels Hill
Keighley
W. Yorks BD22 0RR
Tel: 0535 44865

National Society for the Prevention of
    Cruelty to Children (NSPCC)
67 Saffron Hill
London EC1N 8RS
Tel: 071–242 1626

Nuffield Nursing Homes Trust
Nuffield House
1–4 The Crescent
Surbiton
Surrey KT6 4BN
Tel: 081–390 1200

Nurses' Fund for Nurses
1A Winders Road
London SW11 3HE
Tel: 071–738 0004

Order of St John
St John's Gate
London EC1M 4DA
Tel: 071–253 6644

PARENTLINE–OPUS
Rayfa House
57 Hart Road
Thundersley
Essex SS7 3PD
Tel: 0268 757077

Parkinson's Disease Society
36 Portland Place
London W1N 3DG
Tel: 071–255 2432

Partially Sighted Society
Queen's Road
Doncaster
South Yorks DN1 2NX
Tel: 0302 323132

Phobic Action
Greater London House
547–551 High Road
London E11 4PR
Tel: 081–558 6012

Phobics Society
4 Cheltenham Road
Chorlton-cum-Hardy
Manchester M21 1QN
Tel: 061–881 1937

PlayMatters (National Toy Libraries
Association)
68 Churchway
London NW1 1LT
Tel: 071–387 9592

Poisons Unit
New Cross Hospital
Avonley Road
London SE14
Tel: 071–955 5095

Primary Nursing Network
Barbara Vaughan
Nursing Developments
King's Fund Centre
126 Albert Street
London NW1 7NF

Pregnancy Advisory Service
13 Charlotte Street
London W1P 1HD
Tel: 071–637 8962

Princess Mary's Royal Air Force Nursing
Service (PMRAFNS)
Ministry of Defence
First Avenue House
High Holborn
London WC1V 6HD
Tel: 071–430 5555

Psoriasis Association
7 Milton Street
Northampton
NN2 7JG
Tel: 0604 711129

Queen Alexandra's Royal Army Nursing
Corps (QARANC)
Ministry of Defence
First Avenue House
High Holborn
London WC1V 6HD
Tel: 071–430 5555

Queen Alexandra's Royal Naval Nursing
Service (QARNNS)
Ministry of Defence
First Avenue House
High Holborn
London WC1V 6HD
Tel: 071–430 5555

Queen's Nursing Institute
3 Albermarter Way

London EC1V 4JB
Tel: 071–490 4227

Release
169 Commercial Street
London E1 6BW
Tel: 071–377 5905

Renal Society
41 Mutton Place
London NW1 8DF

Restricted Growth Association
103 St Thames Avenue
Hayling Island
Herts PO11 0EU
Tel: 0705 461813

Royal Association in Aid of Deaf People
27 Old Oak Road
London W3 7HN
Tel: 081–743 6187

Royal British Nurses' Association Club
94 Upper Tollington Park
London N4 4NB
Tel: 071–272 6821

Royal College of General Practitioners
14 Princes Gate
Hyde Park
London SW7 1PU
Tel: 071–581 3232

Royal College of Midwives (RCM)
15 Mansfield Street
London W1M 0BE
Tel: 071–580 6523

Royal College of Nursing of the United
Kingdom (RCN)
20 Cavendish Square
London W1M 0AB
Tel: 071–409 3333

Royal College of Nursing and Council of
Nurses of the United Kingdom
(RCN) Scotland
44 Heriot Row
Edinburgh EH3 6EY

Royal College of Nursing and National
Council of Nurses of the United
Kingdom (RCN) Welsh Board
Tŷ Maeth
King George V Drive
East Cardiff CF4 4XZ

Royal College of Obstetricians and
Gynaecologists (RCOG)
27 Sussex Place
Regent's Park
London NW1 4RG
Tel: 071–262 5425

Royal College of Physicians
11 St Andrew's Place

London NW1 4LE
Tel: 071–487 5218

Royal College of Psychiatrists
17 Belgrave Square
London SW1X 8PG
Tel: 071–235 2351

Royal College of Surgeons of England
35–43 Lincoln's Inn Fields
London WC2A 3PN
Tel: 071–405 3474

Royal College of Radiologists
38 Portland Place
London W1N 3DG
Tel: 071–636 4432

Royal Institute of Public Health and
Hygiene
28 Portland Place
London W1N 4DE
Tel: 071–580 2731

Royal National Institute for the Blind
(RNIB)
224 Great Portland Street
London WIN 6AA
Tel: 071–388 1266

Royal National Institute for the Deaf
(RNID)
105 Gower Street
London WC1E 6AH
Tel: 071–387 8033

Royal National Pension Fund for Nurses
Burdett House
15 Buckingham Street
Strand
London WC2N 6ED
Tel: 071–839 6785

Royal Society of Health
38a St George's Drive
London SW1V 4BH
Tel: 071–630 0121

Royal Society of Medicine (RSM)
1 Wimpole Street
London W1M 8AE
Tel: 071–408 2119

Royal Society for the Prevention of
Accidents (ROSPA)
Cannon House
The Priory
Queensway
Birmingham B4 6BS
Tel: 021–200 2461

Samaritans
17 Uxbridge Road
Slough
Berkshire SL1 1SN
Tel: 0753 32713

SANE (Schizophrenia – a National
Emergency)
5th Floor
120 Regent Street
London W1A 5FE
Tel: 071–494 4840

Schizophrenia Association of Great
Britain (SAGB)
Bryn Hyfryd, The Crescent
Bangor
Gwynedd LL57 2AG
Tel: 0248 354048

Scoliosis Association (UK)
380–384 Harrow Road
London W9 2HU
Tel: 071–289 5652

Scottish Council for Single Parents
13 Gayfield Square
Edinburgh EH1 3NX
Tel: 031–556 3899

Scottish Council on Alcohol, The
137–145 Sauchiehall Street
Glasgow G2 3EW
Tel: 041–333 9677

Scottish Society for the Mentally
Handicapped
13 Elmbank Street
Glasgow G2 4QA
Tel: 041–226 4541

Sickle Cell Society (SCS)
54 Station Road
Harlesden
London NW10 4BO
Tel: 081–961 7795

Sikh Cultural Society of Great Britain
88 Mollison Way
Edgeware
Middlesex HA8 5QW

Society for Advancement of Research
into Anorexia (SARA)
Stanthorpe
New Pound
Wisborough Green
West Sussex RH14 0EJ
Tel: 0403 700210

Spastics Society
840 Brighton Road
Purley
Surrey CR8 2BH
Tel: 081–660 8552

Spinal Injuries Association
Newpoint House
76 St James Lane
Muswell Hill
London N10 3DF
Tel: 081–444 2121

SPOD (Association to Aid the Sexual and
Personal Relationships of People
with a Disability)
286 Camden Road
London N7 0BJ
Tel: 071–607 8851

St John Ambulance Association (StJAA)
1 Grosvenor Crescent
London SW1X 7EF
Tel: 071–235 5231

Standing Committee on Sexually-Abused
Children (SCOSAC)
73 St Charles Square
London W10 6EJ
Tel: 081–960 6376

Standing Conference of Ethnic Minority
Senior Citizens
Ethnic Minority Resource Centre
5–5a Westminster Bridge Road
London SE1 7XW
Tel: 071–928 0095

Standing Conference on Drug Abuse
(SCODA)
1–4 Hatton Place
Hatton Garden
London EC1N 8ND
Tel: 071–430 2341

Student Nurses' Association
Royal College of Nursing
20 Cavendish Square
London W1M 0AB
Tel: 071–409 3333

Stress Syndrome Foundation
Cedar House
Yalding
Kent ME18 6JD

Sue Ryder Foundation
Cavendish
Sudbury
Suffolk CO10 8AY
Tel: 0787 280252

Tavistock Institute of Human Relations
Tavistock Centre
Belsize Lane
London NW3 5BA
Tel: 071–435 7111 ext 2383

Tay-Sachs and Allied Diseases
Association
17 Sydney Road
Barkingside
Ilford
Essex IG6 2ED
Tel: 081–550 8989

Tenovus-Cancer Information Centre
142 Whitchurch Road
Cardiff CF4 3NA
Tel: 0222 619846

Terence Higgins Trust
52–54 Gray's Inn Road
London WC1X 8JU
Tel: 071–242 1010

Toy Libraries Association
Seabrooke House/Wyllyots Manor
Darkes Lane
Potters Bar
Herfordshire EN6 5HC

Travellers' Community Social Workers
Haringey Area 6 Office
Willoughby Road
London N8
Tel: 081–341 1100

Travellers' Rights Organization
S. Crawley
4 Toneborough Estate
Abbey Road
London NW6

Tuberous Sclerosis Association of Great
Britain
Little Barnsley Farm
Catshill
Bromsgrove
Worcs B61 0NQ
Tel: 0527 71898

Turkish Cypriot Cultural Association
(TCCA)
14 Graham Road
London E8 1BZ
Tel: 071–249 7410

Twins and Multiple Births Association
(TAMBA)
51 Thicknall Drive
Pedmore
Stourbridge
W. Midlands DY9 0YH
Tel: 0384 373642

Union of Muslim Organizations of UK
and Eire (UMO)
109 Campden Hill Road
London W8 7TL
Tel: 071–229 0538

United Kingdom Central Council for
Nursing, Midwifery and Health
Visiting (UKCC)
23 Portland Place
London W1N 3AF
Tel: 071–637 7181

United Kingdom Thalassaemia Society
107 Nightingale Lane
London N8 7QY
Tel: 081–348 0437

United Nursing Services Club
40 South Street
London W1Y 5PF
Tel: 071–499 1564

Urostomy Association
'Buckland'
Beaumont Park
Danbury
Essex CM3 4DE
Tel: 024–541 4294

Vegan Society
7 Battle Road
St Leonards-on-Sea
East Sussex TN37 7AA
Tel: 0424 427393

Vegetarian Society of the UK Ltd
Parkdale
Dunham Road
Altrincham

Cheshire WA14 4QE
Tel: 061–928 0793

Welsh National Board for Nursing,
    Midwifery and Health Visiting
13th Floor, Pearl Assurance House
Greyfriars Road
Cardiff CF1 3AG
Tel: 0222 395535

Women's Health Concern
PO Box 1629
London W8 6AU
Tel: 071–938 3932

Women's Natural Health Centre
1 Hillside

Highgate Road
London NW5 1QT
Tel: 071–482 3293 (9.30 am–1 pm)

Women's Therapy Centre
6–9 Manor Gardens
London N7 6LA
Tel: 071–263 6200

Women's Royal Voluntary Service
    (WRVS)
234–244 Stockwell Road
London SW9 9SP
Tel: 071–733 3388

World Health Organization (WHO)
Geneva
Switzerland

International Council of Nurses'

HEADQUARTERS: 3 place Jean-Marteau, 1201 Geneva, Switzerland. Phone: 01041 (22) 731 29 60

ICN MEMBER ASSOCIATIONS

Argentina

Federación Argentina de Enfermería
Rivadavia 3518
1204 Buenos Aires
Tel: (541) 87 06 02

Aruba

Aruba Nurses' Association
PO Box 499
Oranjestad
Tel: (2978) 34283

Australia

Australian Nursing Federation
373–375 St Georges Road
North Fitzroy
Victoria 3068
Tel: (613) 482 27 22

Austria

Osterreichischer Krankenpflegeverband
Mollgasse 3a
A – 1180 Wien
Tel: (431) 346397

Bahamas

The Nurses' Association of the
    Commonwealth of the Bahamas
Longley House
PO Box N – 1691
Nassau
Tel: (1809) 32 22461

Bangladesh

Bangladesh Nurses' Association
c/o Registrar

Bangladesh Nursing Council
86 Bijoy Nagar
Dhaka 2
Tel: (8802) 418116 or 259668

Barbados

Barbados Registered Nurses' Association
"Gibson House"
PO Box 120 C
Bridgetown 5
Tel: (1809) 4275627

Belgium

Fédération Nationale Neutre des
    Infirmier(ière)s de Belgique
18 rue de la Source
B – 1060 Bruxelles
Tel: (322) 535 4488; 535 4481

Bermuda

Bermuda Nurses' Association
PO Box HM 1466
Hamilton HM FX

Bolivia

Colegio de Enfermeras de Bolivia
Casilla No. 9346
La Paz
Tel: (5912) 322713

Botswana

The Nurses' Association of Botswana
PO Box 126
Gaborone
Tel: (267) 2044

Brazil

Associaçao Brasileira de Enfermagem
    (ABEn)

Av. L–2 Norte, Módulo B. Quadra 603
CEP 70.830 Brasilia
Tel: (5561) 226 0653; (5561) 225 4473

British Virgin Islands

BVI Nurses' Association
PO Box 3055
Road Town
Tortola
Tel: (1809) 4943497

Brunei

Brunei Darussalam Nurses' Association
PO Box 557 Seri Complexs
Bandar Seri Begawan
Negara Brunei Darussalam

Burkina Faso

Association Professionnelle des
    Infirmiers/ières du Burkina (APIIB)
BP 2066
Ouagadougou

Canada

Canadian Nurses' Association
50 The Driveway
Ottawa K2P 1E2
Ontario
Tel: (1613) 237 2133

Chile

Colegio de Enfermeras de Chile
Miraflores 563
Casilla No 9752-Correo Plata de Armas
Santiago
Tel: (562) 398556; 393718

China

Chinese Nursing Association
42 Dolg Si Xi Da Jie
Beijing

Colombia

Asociación Nacional de Enfermeras de
    Colombia
Carrera 27 No. 46 21
Apartado Aéreo No. 059871
Bogotá D.E.
Tel: (571) 2692095

Costa Rica

Colegio de Enfermeras de Costa Rica
Avenida 8 calle 14 y 16
Apartado No. 5085 1000
San José
Tel: (506) 33 6963

Cuba

Sociedad Cubana de Enfermería
Calle 15 No. 9 Apto. 6B, 6to Piso
Entre N y O, Vedado
Ciudad Habana
Tel: (537) 32 3614

Cyprus

Cyprus Nursing Association
PO Box 4015
Nicosia
Cables: CYNURSA NICOSIA

Czechoslovakia

Czechoslovak Society of Nurses'
Mickiewiczova 18/1
813 22 Bratislava CSFR
Tel: (427) 571 88; 503 54

Denmark

The Danish Nurses' Organization
Vimmelskaftet 38
PO Box 1084
DK – 1008 Copenhagen K
Tel: (45) 33151555

Dominican Republic

Asociación Dominicana de Enfermeras
    Graduadas
San Bosco No. 50
Santo Domingo

Ecuador

Federación Ecuatariana de Enfermeras/
    os
Apartado 3523
Quito

Egypt

Egyptian Nurses' Syndicate
5 Sarai Street
Manial
Cairo

Ethiopia

Ethiopian Health‑Professionals' Union
Ethiopian Nurses' Association
PO Box 467
Addis Ababa

Fiji

Fiji Nursing Association
PO Box 1364
Suva
Tel: (679) 312841

Finland

The Finnish Federation of Nurses'
Asemamiehenkatu 4
00520 Helsinki
Tel: (3580) 1551

France

Association Nationale Française des
    Infirmier(ère)s Diplômés et Elèves
    (ANFIIDE)
BP 133
73001 Chambéry
Tel: (33) 79690909

Gambia (The)

The Gambia Nurses' Association
PO Box 2341
Serre-Kunda
Kombo St. Mary's Division
Tel: Banjul (220) 27673

Germany

DBfK – Bundesverband
Hauptstrasse 392
6236 Eschborn
Tel: (4969) 740566

Ghana

Ghana Registered Nurses' Association
PO Box 2994
Accra
Tel: (23321) 665401 ext 6578

Greece

Hellenic National Graduate Nurses'
    Association
Athens' Tower (C. Building)
115 27 Athens
Tel: (301) 7702861

Guatemala

Asociación Guatemalteca de Enfermeras
    Profesionales
14 Calle # 1–15 Zona 3, Apto. 6
Guatemala
Tel: (5022) 517265

Guyana

Guyana Nurses' Association
178 Alexander and Charlotte Streets
PO Box 10462
Lacytown, Georgetown
Tel: (59) 202 72188

Haiti

Association Nationale des Infirmières
    Licenciées d'Haïti
Boîte postale 410
Port-au-Prince

Honduras

Colegio de Profesionales de Enfermería
    de Honduras
Apartado 1144
Tegucigalpa, DC
Tel: (504) 32 8579

Hong Kong

The Hong Kong Nurses' Association &
    Hong Kong College of Nursing
12th Floor, Hyde Centre
221–226 Gloucester Road
Wanchai
Hong Kong
Tel: (852) 5729255, 5729256

Hungary

Hungarian Nursing Association
Budapest PF: 200–H–1518
Tel: (361) 868807

Iceland

Icelandic Nurses' Association
Sudurlandsbraut 22
Reykjavik 108
Tel: (3541) 687575

India

Trained Nurses' Association of India
L–17 Green Park
New Delhi 110016
Tel: (9111) 666665

Iran

The Nurses' Association Tohid Square
Nossrat Ave
Next to Nursing School of Teheran
    University
Teheran

Ireland

Irish Nurses' Organization and National
    Council of Nurses'
11 Fitzwilliam Place
Dublin 2
Tel: (3531) 760137; 760138

Israel

The National Association of Nurses' in
    Israel
The Histadrut
93 Arlosoroff Street
Tel-Aviv
Tel: (97236) 431111

Italy

Consociazione Nazionale delle
    Associazioni Infermiere-Infermieri
    ed altri Operatori Sanitario-Sociali
Via Arno 62
I – 00198 Roma
Tel: (396) 8840654

Jamaica

The Nurses' Association of Jamaica
4 Trevennion Park Road
PO Box 277
Kingston 5
Tel: (1809) 92–95213; 92–66585

Japan

Japanese Nursing Association
8–2, 5-chome
Jingumae, Shibuya-ku
Tokyo
Tel: (81) 33400 8331

Jordan

Jordan Nurses' and Midwives' Council
PO Box 10076
Amman

Kenya

National Nurses' Association of Kenya
PO Box 49422
Nairobi
Tel: (254) 29083

Korea (Republic of Korea)

Korean Nurses' Association
88–7 Sang Lim Dong
Choong Ku
Seoul
Tel: (82) 279 3618/19

Lebanon

Federation of Nursing Associations in
    Lebanon
c/o Syndicat des Hôpitaux du Liban
Place du Musée
Immeuble Georges Salamé –
    B.P. 165–662
Beyrouth
Tel: (9611) 447678

Lesotho

Lesotho Nursing Association
PO Box 473
Maseru 100

Liberia

Liberia Nurses' Association
PO Box 1608
Monrovia

Luxembourg

Association Nationale des Infirmier(e)s
    Luxembourgeois(es)
Boîte postale 1184
Luxembourg
Tel: (00352)

Malawi

The National Association of Nurses' of
    Malawi
PO Box 30128
Capital City
Lilongwe 3

Malaysia

Malaysian Nurses' Association
PO Box 11737
General Post Office
50756 Kuala Lumpur
Tel: (603) 2543846

Malta

Malta Nurses' Association
140 Manoel Street
Gzira
Tel: (356) 337984

Mauritius

Nursing Association of Mauritius
SSRN Hospital Pamplemousses
Mauritius
Tel: (2222) 03 1661

Mexico

Colegio Nacional de Enfermeras, AC
Czda Obrero Mundial 229
Apartado Postal 12–986
06300 México D.F.
Tel: (525) 5436637

Monaco (Principauté de)

Association des Infirmières et Assistantes
    Sociales de la Croix-Rouge
    Monégasque
27, boulevard de la Suisse
Monte-Carlo 98000
Tel: (33) 93506701

Myanmar (Union of)

Myanmar Nurses' Association
80/84 Shwebontha Road
Yangon

Nepal

Trained Nurses' Association of Nepal
Mahabouddha Bhotahity Galli

Post Box No 4780
Kathmandu

Netherlands

National Nurses' Association
"Nederlandse Maatschappij voor
    Verpleegkunde"
PO Box 6001
3503 PA Utrecht
Tel: (3130) 964144

Netherlands Antilles

O.D.E.A.N.
PO Box 645
Curaçao
Antilles néerlandaises
Tel: (5999) 623736

New Zealand

New Zealand Nurses' Association
Executive Director
CPO Box 2128
Wellington
Tel: (644) 850–847

Nicaragua

Asociación de Enfermeras/os
    Nicaragüenses
Apartado No 3289
Managua
Tel: (5052) 44 749

Nigeria

The National Association of Nigeria
    Nurses' and Midwives
PO Box 3857
Ikeja Post Office
Lagos

Norway

Norwegian Nurses' Association
PO Box 2633, St Hanshaugen
0131 Oslo 1
Norway
Tel: (472) 382000

Pakistan

Pakistan Nurses' Federation
Director General Nursing
146–A–1, Township
Lahore
Tel: (9242) 841403

Panama

Asociación Nacional de Enfermeras de
    Panamá
Apartado 5272, Zona 5
Panamá
Tel: (507) 25 4717

Paraguay

Asociación Paraguaya de Enfermeras
    (A.P.E.)

Departamento de Enfermería
Hospital de Clinicas
Casilla de Correo 3306
Asunción

Peru

Federación de Enfermeros del Peru
Jirón Washington No. 1651 – Oficina No.
201
Lima

Philippines

Philippine Nurses' Association
1663, F.T. Benitez Street
Malate
Manila – 1004
Tel: (632) 583092; 501545

Poland

Polskie Towarzystwo Pielegniarskie
Koszykowa 8
00–564 Warszawa
Tel: (4822) 21 50 66

Portugal

Associaçâo Portuguesa de Enfermeiros
Rua Duque de Palmela No. 27–4o D
Lisboa – 1200
Tel: (3511) 535543

Puerto Rico

Colegio de Profesionales de la
Enfermeria de Puerto Rico
GPO Box 3647
San Juan, Puerto Rico 00936
Tel: (1809) 7537192

St Lucia

St Lucia Nurses' Association
PO Box 819
Castries

Salvador (El)

Asociación Nacional de Enfermeras
Salvadoreñas
Calles: Gabriel Rosales y Matias Alvarado
No. 157
Reparto Los Heroes
San Salvador
Tel: (503) 731850

Senegal

Association Nationale des Infirmiers et
Infirmières Diplômés d'Etat du
Sénégal (ANIDES)
Hôpital A. Le Dantec
B.P. 353
Dakar RP
Tel: (221) 230085

Seychelles

Nurses' Association of the Republic of
Seychelles

Secretary
PO Box 52
Victoria
Tel: (248) 24 400 ext 3076

Sierra Leone

Sierra Leone Nurses' Association
PO Box 971
Freetown
Tel: (23222) 24326

Singapore

The Singapore Nurses' Association
151 Chin Swee Road
Manhattan House # 09–13
Singapore 0316
Tel: (65) 7333985

Spain

Consejo General de Colegios de
Diplomados en Enfermería de
España
Buen Suceso, 6–2do.
28008 Madrid
Tel: (341) 5416073

Sri Lanka

Sri Lanka Nurses' Association
Room 123, Nurses' Home
93 Regent Street
Colombo 10
Tel: (941) 01 91111

South Africa

South African Nursing Association
PO Box 1280
0001 Pretoria

Sudan

Sudan Professional Nurses' Association
Khartoum North Teaching Hospital
Khartoum
Att. Sister Amna Shobbo
Tel: (24911) 224426

Swaziland

Swaziland Nursing Association
PO Box 1771
Mbabane

Sweden

Swedish Association of Health Officers
PO Box 3260
S – 103 65 Stockholm
Tel: (468) 147700

Switzerland

Association Suisse des Infirmières et
Infirmiers
Secrétariat Central
Case Postale
CH – 3001 Bern
Tel: (4131) 256427

Taiwan

The Nurses' Association of the Republic
of China
Fl 12, No. 315
Hsin I Rd, Section 4
Taipei 10666
Tel: (8862) 7552291; 7552292

Tanzania

Tanzania Registered Nurses' Association
Secretary General
PO Box 4357
Dar-es-Salaam
Tel: (25551) 26211 Ext 220

Thailand

The Nurses' Association of Thailand
12/21 Rang Nam Road
Bangkok 10400
Tel: (662) 2474463; 2474464; 2450148

Togo

Association nationale des infirmiers et
infirmières du Togo
Synpersanto
BP 163
Lomé
Togo

Tonga

Tonga Nurses' Association
PO Box 150
Nuku'alofa
Tel: (676) 22870 or 22610

Trinidad and Tobago

Trinidad and Tobago Registered Nurses'
Association
No. 4 Fitz Blackman Drive and
Wrightson Road, Extension
Port-of-Spain
Tel: (1809) 6231567

Turkey

Turkish Nurses' Association
Yüksel Caddesi No. 35/2 Yenisehir
Ankara 06420
Tel: (904) 1318099; (904) 1350689

Uganda

Uganda National Association of
Registered Nurses' and Midwives
PO Box 8322
Kampala

United Kingdom

The Royal College of Nursing of the
United Kingdom
General Secretary: Ms Christine
Hancock
20 Cavendish Square
London W1M 0AB

United States of America

American Nurses' Association, Inc
Suite 500
2420 Pershing Road
Kansas City, Missouri 64108
Tel: (1913) 474 5720

Uruguay

Asociación de Nurses' del Uruguay
Colonia 1854, Piso 6, Esc. 607
Montevideo
Tel: (5982) 490900

Venezuela

Colegio de Profesionales de Enfermería
de Venezuela
Av. Luís Roche, entre 8va. y 9na.
Transveral

Qta. Acuarela. Altamira
Dtto. Sucre. Zona Postal 1062
Caracas
Tel: (582) 2613444

Western Samoa

Western Samoa Registered Nurses'
Association, Inc.
PO Box 3491
Apia
Tel: (685) 24439

Yugoslavia

Nurses Association of Yugoslavia
Klinika za kirurgiju "REBRO" KBC
Kispaticeva 12
41000 Zagreb
Tel: (3841) 233233

Zaire

Association des Infirmiers(ères) du
Zaïre (A.I.Za)
BP 12–156
Kinshasa I
Tel: (24312) 61591

Zambia

Zambia Nurses' Association
PO Box 50375
Lusaka
Tel: (2601) 252457

Zimbabwe

Zimbabwe Nurses' Association
PO Box 2610
Harare
Tel: (2634) ZINA 790 597

Index